■■■ VITAL SIGNS

Blood Pressures: Girls and Boys, Ages 1–17 Years*, for 95th Percentile in Height†

Age	Height Percentile	GIRLS: Systolic			GIRLS: Diastolic			BOYS: Systolic			BOYS: Diastolic		
		5%	50%	95%	5%	50%	95%	5%	50%	95%	5%	50%	95%
1	95th	100	104	107	56	58	60	98	103	106	54	56	58
2	95th	102	105	109	61	63	65	101	106	110	59	61	63
3	95th	104	107	110	65	67	69	104	109	113	63	65	67
4	95th	105	108	112	68	70	72	106	111	115	66	69	71
5	95th	107	110	113	70	72	74	108	112	116	69	72	74
6	95th	108	111	115	72	74	76	109	114	117	72	74	76
7	95th	110	113	116	73	75	77	110	115	119	74	76	78
8	95th	112	115	118	75	76	78	111	116	120	75	78	80
9	95th	114	117	120	76	77	79	113	118	121	76	79	81
10	95th	116	119	122	77	78	80	115	119	123	77	80	82
11	95th	118	121	124	78	79	81	117	121	125	78	80	82
12	95th	119	123	126	79	80	82	119	123	127	78	81	83
13	95th	121	124	128	80	81	83	121	126	130	79	81	83
14	95th	123	126	129	81	82	84	124	128	132	80	82	84
15	95th	124	127	131	82	83	85	126	131	135	81	83	85
16	95th	125	128	132	82	84	86	129	134	137	82	84	87
17	95th	125	129	132	82	84	86	131	136	140	84	87	89

*Blood pressure percentile determined by a single measurement.
†Height percentile determined by standard growth curves.
Complete tables found in Cardiovascular chapter of this text.
From National High Blood Pressure Education Program Working Group on High Blood Pressure in Children and Adolescents: The Fourth Report on the Diagnosis, Evaluation, and Treatment of High Blood Pressure in Children and Adolescents, *Pediatrics* (114):555-576, 2004. Available at *www.nhlbi.gov*

Respirations: Normal Respiratory Rates In Children

Age (years)	Respiratory rate (breaths/minute)
0-1	24-38
1-3	22-30
4-6	20-24
7-9	18-24
10-14	16-22
15-18	14-20

Slightly higher respiratory rates in the neonatal period (i.e., 40-50 breaths/min) may be normal in the absence of other signs and symptoms.

Pulse

Normal Heart Rates (Beats per Minute) in Infants and Children

Age	Resting (Awake)	Resting (Asleep)	Exercise/Fever
Newborn	100-180	80-160	Up to 220
1 week-3 months	100-220	80-200	Up to 220
3 months-2 years	80-150	70-120	Up to 220
2-10 years	70-100	60-90	195-215
10-20 years	55-90	50-90	195-215

■■■ NUTRITION
Caloric Needs of Infants and Toddlers

Daily Estimated Energy Requirements (EER) for Infants and Toddlers in Kilocalories

Age	Calculation of Daily Kilocalorie Needs	Estimate Based on 50th Percentile of Weight
0-3 months	EER = (89 × weight of infant [kg] − 100) + 175 (kcal for energy deposition)	100 kilocalories/kg/day
4-6 months	EER = (89 × weight of infant [kg] − 100) + 56 (kcal for energy deposition)	85 kilocalories/kg/day
7-12 months	EER = (89 × weight of infant [kg] − 100) + 22 (kcal for energy deposition)	80 kilocalories/kg/day
13-35 months	EER = (89 × weight of child [kg] − 100) + 20 (kcal for energy deposition)	83 kilocalories/kg/day

Robertson J, Shilkofski N: *The Harriet Lane handbook: a manual for pediatric house officers,* ed 17, Philadelphia, PA, 2005, Elsevier/Mosby

Calories Per Day Based On Level Of Activity For Children Ages 2–18 years

Gender	Age in years	Sedentary	Moderately Active	Active
Males	2-3	1000	1000-1400	1000-1400
	4-8	1400	1400-1600	1600-2000
	9-13	1800	1800-2200	2000-2600
	14-18	2200	2400-2800	2800-3200
Females	2-3	1000	1000-1400	1000-1400
	4-8	1200	1400-1600	1400-1800
	9-13	1600	1600-2000	1800-2200
	14-18	1800	2000	2400

From US Department of Health and Human Services and US Department of Agriculture: *Dietary guidelines for Americans, 2005,* ed 6, Washington, DC, 2005, US Government Printing Office.

FLUID REPLACEMENT CALCULATIONS FOR DEHYDRATION

Mild	Oral rehydration solution	40-50 mL/kg over 4 hours
Moderate	Oral rehydration solution	60-100 mL/kg over 4-6 hours
Severe	IV fluids	See Chapter 33 for protocol

Number of Servings and Serving Sizes for Age and Calorie Intake

Food Groups	1-3 Years Old* Servings	4-6 Years Old* Servings	6-21 Years Old 1600	2000	2600	3100	Serving Size 1600–3100 Calorie Diets
Grains	6: ¼-½ slice bread; 4 tbsp cooked cereal, rice, pasta; ¼ cup dry cereal; 1 or 2 crackers	6	6	7-8	10-11	12-13	1 slice bread; 1 cup of ready to eat cereal; ½ cup rice, pasta, or cereal
Vegetables	2-3: 1 tbsp/year age cooked vegetable	3-5	3-4	4-5	5-6	6	1 cup raw leafy, ½ cup cooked or raw other vegetables, ¾ cup vegetable juice
Fruits	2-3: ½ piece fresh fruit, ¼ cup fruit canned/cooked, ¼-½ cup juice	2	4	4-5	5-6	6	¾ cup fruit juice; 1 medium fruit; ¼ cup dried fruit; ½ cup fresh, frozen, canned fruit
Low-fat or fat-free dairy foods	2: 1-2 year olds should have whole milk, 500 mg calcium/day	2: 800 mg calcium/d	3: 1200-1500 mg calcium/d 9-18 years of age	3	3	3-4	1 cup milk, 1 cup yogurt, 1½ oz cheese
Meat, poultry, fish, egg	2	2	2	2	2	2-3	2-3 oz cooked meats, poultry, fish; 1 egg
Nuts, seeds, legumes	2: (a) 2 tbsp cooked beans or peas (b) Only creamy peanut butter spread thinly on a cracker/bread (c) Omit seeds and nuts	2	3-4/week	4-5/week	1	1	1 tbsp peanut butter, ⅓ cup nuts, 2 tbsp seeds, ½ cup cooked dry beans or peas
Fat, oils	Moderate use until 2 years of age (about 30% of total calories)	sparingly	2	2-3	3	4	1 tsp soft margarine; 1 tbsp low-fat mayonnaise, salad dressing, vegetable oil

*Because of the inconsistency in recommendations for calorie intake in young children among expert sources, the table focuses on the areas of agreement in terms of serving sizes and number of servings.

REFERENCES

American Academy of Pediatrics: *Pediatric nutrition handbook*, ed 5, Elk Grove Village, IL, 2004, American Academy of Pediatrics.

Dietz WH, Stern L, editors: *Guide to your child's nutrition*, New York, 1999, Villard.

US Department of Health and Human Services and US Department of Agriculture: *Dietary guidelines for Americans, 2005,* ed 6, Washington, DC, 2005, US Government Printing Office.

PEDIATRIC
Primary Care

FOURTH EDITION

PEDIATRIC
Primary Care

Catherine E. Burns, PhD, RN, CPNP, FAAN
Professor Emeritus
Primary Health Care Nurse Practitioner
 Specialty
School of Nursing
Oregon Health & Science University
Portland, Oregon

Margaret A. Brady, PhD, RN, CPNP
Professor
Department of Nursing
California State University Long Beach
Long Beach, California;
Co-director
PNP Program
School of Nursing
Azusa Pacific University
Azusa, California

Ardys M. Dunn, PhD, RN, PNP
Associate Professor Emeritus
School of Nursing University of Portland
Portland, Oregon;
Professor, retired
School of Nursing Samuel Merritt College
Oakland, California

Nancy Barber Starr, MS, RN, CPNP
Pediatric Nurse Practitioner
Advanced Pediatric Associates
Aurora, Colorado

Catherine G. Blosser, MPA:HA, RN, APRN, BC (PNP)
Pediatric Nurse Practitioner
Multnomah County Health Department
Portland, Oregon

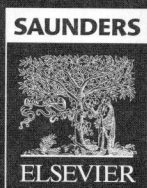

SAUNDERS

ELSEVIER

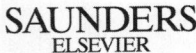

11830 Westline Industrial Drive
St. Louis, Missouri 63146

Pediatric Primary Care   **ISBN 978-1-4160-4087-3**

Notice

Knowledge and best practice in this field are constantly changing. As new research and experience broaden our knowledge, changes in practice, treatment and drug therapy may become necessary or appropriate. Readers are advised to check the most current information provided (i) on procedures featured or (ii) by the manufacturer of each product to be administered, to verify the recommended dose or formula, the method and duration of administration, and contraindications. It is the responsibility of the practitioner, relying on their own experience and knowledge of the patient, to make diagnoses, to determine dosages and the best treatment for each individual patient, and to take all appropriate safety precautions. To the fullest extent of the law, neither the Publisher nor the Editors/Authors assumes any liability for any injury and/or damage to persons or property arising out of or related to any use of the material contained in this book.

Previous editions copyrighted 2004, 2000, 1996

ISBN: 978-1-4160-4087-3

Senior Acquisitions Editor: Sandra Clark
Publishing Services Manager: John Rogers
Senior Project Manager: Helen Hudlin, Doug Turner
Designer: Andrea Lutes

Printed in the United States of America

Last digit is the print number: 9 8 7 6 5 4 3 2 1

The Child's Name is Today

We are guilty of many errors and faults,
but our worst crime is abandoning the children,
neglecting the fountain of life.
Many of the things we need can wait.
The child cannot.
Right now is the time his bones are being formed,
his blood is being made,
and his senses are being developed.
To him we cannot answer, "Tomorrow."
His name is "Today."

Gabriela Mistral (1889-1957) 1945
Nobel Laureate in Literature, Chile

...

This book is dedicated to the infants, children, and adolescents
and their families about whom this book was written, wishing them health,
loving support, and happiness, the real goals of this book.

...

Contributors

Michele E. Acker, MN, ARNP
Pediatric Nurse Practitioner
Senior Lecturer and Graduate Faculty
Director, Pediatric Nurse Practitioner Program
School of Nursing
University of Washington
Seattle, Washington
Chapter 33: Dental and Oral Disorders (with Peter Milgrom,
    Ohnmar K. Tut, Donald L. Chi, and Mary Ann Draye)

Jan Bazner-Chandler, RN, MSN, CNS, CPNP
Assistant Professor
Azusa Pacific University
Azusa, California
Chapter 37: Musculoskeletal Disorders
    (with Margaret A. Brady)

Anita Berry, MSN, CNP/APN
Director
Healthy Steps for Young Children Program
Project Director
Enhancing Developmentally Oriented
    Primary Care (EDOPC)
Advocate Health Care
Park Ridge, Illinois
*Chapter 4: Developmental Management in Pediatric
    Primary Care* (with Barbara Jones Deloian)
Chapter 5: Developmental Management of Infants
    (with Barbara Jones Deloian)
*Chapter 6: Developmental Management of Toddlers
    and Preschoolers* (with Mary A. Murphy)

**Catherine G. Blosser, MPA:HA, RN, APRN, BC
(PNP)**
Pediatric Nurse Practitioner
Multnomah County Health Department
Portland, Oregon
*Chapter 14: Activities and Sports for Children and
    Adolescents*
Chapter 19: Sexuality (with Teral Gerlt and Ardys M. Dunn)
Chapter 23: Infectious Diseases and Immunizations
    (with Margaret A. Brady and William J. Muller)
Chapter 27: Neurologic Disorders (with Melissa
    Reider-Demer)
Chapter 28: Eye Disorders
Chapter 30: Cardiovascular Disorders (with Julie Martchenke)
Chapter 42: Complementary Medicine
Appendix A: Medications in Pediatric Practice

Margaret A. Brady, PhD, RN, CPNP
Professor
Department of Nursing
California State University Long Beach
Long Beach, California;
Co-director
PNP Program
School of Nursing
Azusa Pacific University
Azusa, California
Chapter 18: Role Relationships (with Ardys M. Dunn)
Chapter 22: Introduction to Diseases and Pain Management
Chapter 23: Infectious Diseases and Immunizations
    (with Catherine G. Blosser and William J. Muller)
Chapter 24: Atopic and Rheumatic Disorders
    (with Catherine J. Goodhue)
Chapter 31: Respiratory Disorders
Chapter 36: Dermatologic Diseases (with Peggy Vernon and
    Nancy Barber Starr)
Chapter 37: Musculoskeletal Disorders
    (with Jan Bazner-Chandler)

Constance B. Brehm, PhD, MS, MPh, RNP, RN
Associate Professor
Azusa Pacific University
Azusa, California
Chapter 39: Common Injuries

Melissa L. R. Burchett, RN, MSN, CPNP
Pediatric Nurse Practitioner
Legacy Emanuel Children's Hospital
Portland, Oregon
Chapter 25: Endocrine and Metabolic Diseases
    (with Cheryl E. Hanna and Robert D. Steiner)

Catherine E. Burns, PhD, RN, CPNP, FAAN
Professor Emeritus
Primary Health Care Nurse Practitioner Specialty
School of Nursing
Oregon Health & Science University
Portland, Oregon
Chapter 2: Child and Family Health Assessment
    (with Sheila M. Kodadek)
Chapter 9: Introduction to Health Promotion
Chapter 15: Sleep and Rest
Chapter 40: Genetic Disorders (with Janet K. Williams)
Chapter 41: Environmental Health Issues (with Ardys M. Dunn)
Appendix B: Growth Charts
Appendix C: Normal Laboratory Values (with Steven Goodstein)

Donald L. Chi, DDS
Resident
Department of Pediatric Dentistry and
    Preventative and Community Dentistry
College of Dentistry
University of Iowa
Iowa City, Iowa
Chapter 33: Dental and Oral Disorders (with Peter
    Milgrom, Ohnmar K. Tut, Mary Ann Draye,
    and Michele E. Acker)

Barbara Jones Deloian, PhD, RN, CPNP
Pediatric Nurse Practitioner
Director, Health Services for Children with Special Needs
Colorado Department of Public Health and Environment
Denver, Colorado
*Chapter 4: Developmental Management in Pediatric
    Primary Care* (with Anita Berry)
Chapter 5: Developmental Management of Infants
    (with Anita Berry)

Mary Ann Draye, MPh, ARNP
Assistant Professor
Director, Family Nurse Practitioner Program
School of Nursing
University of Washington
Seattle, Washington
Chapter 33: Dental and Oral Disorders (with Peter Milgrom,
    Ohnmar K. Tut, Donald L. Chi, and Michele E. Acker)

Karen G. Duderstadt, PhD, RN, CPNP
Associate Clinical Professor
School of Nursing
University of California at San Francisco
San Francisco, California
Chapter 1: Child Health Status in America

Ardys M. Dunn, PhD, RN, PNP
Associate Professor Emeritus
School of Nursing
University of Portland
Portland, Oregon;
Professor
School of Nursing
Samuel Merritt College
Oakland, California
Chapter 3: Cultural Perspectives for Pediatric Primary Care
Chapter 8: Developmental Management of Adolescents
*Chapter 10: Health Perception and Health Management
    Patterns*
Chapter 11: Nutrition
Chapter 13: Elimination Patterns
Chapter 18: Role Relationships (with Margaret A. Brady)
Chapter 19: Sexuality (with Teral Gerlt and Catherine G. Blosser)
Chapter 21: Values and Beliefs
Chapter 41: Environmental Health Issues
    (with Catherine E. Burns)

Bonnie Gance-Cleveland, RNC, PNP, PhD
Director, Center for Improving Health Outcomes in
    Children, Teens, and Families
Arizona State University
Phoenix, Arizona
*Chapter 7: Developmental Management of
    School-Age Children* (with Yvonne Yousey)

Dawn Lee Garzon PhD, APRN, BC, CPNP
Assistant Professor, Pediatrics
University of Missouri - St. Louis
St. Louis, Missouri
Chapter Discussion Forums (with Rita Marie John)

Nan M. Gaylord, PhD, RN, CPNP
Associate Professor
College of Nursing
University of Tennessee
Knoxville, Tennessee
Chapter 34: Genitourinary Disorders
    (with Nancy Barber Starr)
Chapter 38: Perinatal Conditions (with Robert J. Yetman)

Teral Gerlt, MS, RNC, WHCNP, PNP
Instructor
Oregon Health & Science University School of Nursing
Portland, Oregon
Chapter 19: Sexuality (with Catherine G. Blosser
    and Ardys M. Dunn)
Chapter 35: Gynecologic Conditions (with Nancy Barber Starr)

Catherine J. Goodhue, MN, RN, CPNP
Research Nurse Coordinator
Children's Hospital of Los Angeles
Los Angeles, California;
Adjunct Faculty
Azusa Pacific University
Azusa, California
Chapter 24: Atopic and Rheumatic Disorders
    (with Margaret A. Brady)

Steven Goodstein, MS, MT (ASCP)
Assistant Professor
Department of Pathology
Oregon Health & Science University
Portland, Oregon
Appendix C: Normal Laboratory Values (with Catherine E. Burns)

Mary Margaret Gottesman, PhD, RN, CPNP, FAAN
Associate Professor, Clinical
Pediatric Nurse Practitioner Special Program Director
College of Nursing
The Ohio State University
Columbus, Ohio
*Chapter 20: Coping and Stress Tolerance: Mental Health
    Problems* (with Gail M. Houck)

Denise A. Hall, BS, ACMPE (Nominee)
Administrator
Advanced Pediatric Associates
Centennial, Colorado
Chapter 43: Practice Management Strategies for a
    Health Care Practice

Cheryl E. Hanna, MD
Associate Professor of Pediatrics
School of Medicine
Oregon Health & Science University
Portland, Oregon
Chapter 25: Endocrine and Metabolic Diseases
    (with Melissa L. R. Burchett and Robert D. Steiner)

Pamela J. Hellings, RN, PhD, CPNP-R
Professor Emerita
Oregon Health & Science University
Portland, Oregon
Chapter 12: Breastfeeding

Gail M. Houck, RN, PhD, PMHNP
Professor and Program Director
Academic Graduate and Interdisciplinary Programs
School of Nursing
Oregon Health & Science University
Portland, Oregon
Chapter 20: Coping and Stress Tolerance: Mental Health
    Problems (with Mary Margaret Gottesman)

Rita Marie John, CPNP, DrNP
PNP/NNP Program Director
Assistant Professor of Clinical Nursing
Columbia University
New York, New York
Chapter Discussion Forums (with Dawn Lee Garzon)

Sheila M. Kodadek, RN, PhD
Professor, Child and Family Nursing
School of Nursing
Oregon Health & Science University
Portland, Oregon
Chapter 2: Child and Family Health Assessment
    (with Catherine E. Burns)

Julie Martchenke, RN, MSN, PNP
Nurse Practitioner
Pediatric Cardiology
Doernbecher Children's Hospital;
Instructor
School of Nursing
Oregon Health & Science University
Portland, Oregon
Chapter 30: Cardiovascular Disorders (with Catherine G. Blosser)

Shirley Becton McKenzie, MS, APRN, BC, PNP
Pediatric Nurse Practitioner
Emergency Department
The Children's Hospital
Denver, Colorado;
Colorado Kids Pediatrics
Centennial, Colorado
Chapter 29: Ear Disorders (with Ann M. Petersen-Smith)
Chapter 32: Gastrointestinal Disorders
    (with Ann M. Petersen-Smith)

Peter Milgrom, DDS
Professor of Dental Public Health Services
Director, Northwest/Alaska Center to Reduce Oral Health
    Disparities
Adjunct Professor of Pediatric Dentistry
University of Washington
Seattle, Washington
Chapter 33: Dental and Oral Disorders (with Ohnmar K. Tut,
    Donald L. Chi, Mary Ann Draye, and Michele E. Acker)

William J. Muller, MD, PhD
Assistant Professor, Pediatric Infectious Diseases
Children's Memorial Hospital
Chicago, Illinois
Chapter 23: Infectious Diseases and Immunizations
    (with Catherine G. Blosser and Margaret A. Brady)

Mary A. Murphy, CPNP, PhD
Developmental Consultant
The Children's Hospital
University of Colorado at Denver and Health Sciences Center
Denver, Colorado
Chapter 6: Developmental Management of Toddlers
    and Preschoolers (with Anita Berry)

Bridget O'Boyle-Jordan, PNP, MSN
Assistant Professor
School of Nursing
Oregon Health & Science University
Child Development and Rehabilitation Center
Child Development Clinics
Portland, Oregon
Chapter 16: Cognitive-Perceptual Problems:
    Attention-Deficit/Hyperactivity Disorder, Blindness,
    Deafness, and Autism (with Kathleen C. Shelton)

Ann M. Petersen-Smith, PhD, RN, AC-CPNP
Pediatric Nurse Practitioner
Emergency Department
The Children's Hospital;
Associate Professor
University of Colorado at Denver and Health Sciences Center
Denver, Colorado
Chapter 29: Ear Disorders (with Shirley Becton McKenzie)
Chapter 32: Gastrointestinal Disorders
    (with Shirley Becton McKenzie)

Melissa Reider-Demer, MSN, CPNP
Neurology Pediatric Nurse Practitioner
Childrens Hospital of Los Angeles
Los Angeles, California
Chapter 27: Neurologic Disorders
    (with Catherine G. Blosser)

Kathleen C. Shelton, PNP, PhD
Training Director, LEND Project
Child Development and Rehabilitation Center
Oregon Health & Science University
Portland, Oregon
Chapter 16: Cognitive-Perceptual Problems:
    Attention-Deficit/Hyperactivity Disorder, Blindness,
    Deafness, and Autism (with Bridget O'Boyle-Jordan)

Nancy Barber Starr, MS, RN, CPNP
Neurology Pediatric Nurse Practitioner
Aurora Pediatric Associates
Aurora, Colorado
Chapter 17: Self-Perception Issues
Chapter 34: Genitourinary Disorders (with Nan M. Gaylord)
Chapter 35: Gynecologic Conditions (with Teral Gerlt)
Chapter 36: Dermatologic Diseases
    (with Peggy Vernon and Margaret A. Brady)

Robert D. Steiner, MD
Professor, Pediatrics and Molecular and Medical Genetics
School of Medicine
Oregon Health & Science University
Portland, Oregon
Chapter 25: Endocrine and Metabolic Problems
    (with Melissa L. R. Burchett and Cheryl E. Hanna)

Martha K. Swartz, PhD, RN, CPNP
Professor and Associate Dean
Office of Clinical and Community Affairs
School of Nursing
Yale University
New Haven, Connecticut
Chapter 26: Hematologic Disorders

Ohnmar K. Tut, BDS
Preventive Services Dentist
Ministry of Health
Majuro, Republic of Marshall Islands;
Department of Dental Public Health Sciences
University of Washington
Seattle, Washington
Chapter 33: Dental and Oral Disorders (with Peter Milgrom,
    Donald L. Chi, Mary Ann Draye, and Michele E. Acker)

Peggy Vernon, RN, MA, C-PNP
Dermatology Nurse Practitioner
Sorkin Dermatology
Grenwood Village, Colorado
Chapter 36: Dermatologic Diseases
    (with Margaret A. Brady and Nancy Barber Starr)

Janet K. Williams, PhD, RN, PNP, FAAN
Kelting Professor of Nursing
College of Nursing
University of Iowa
Iowa City, Iowa
Chapter 40: Genetic Disorders (with Catherine E. Burns)

Robert J. Yetman, MD
Professor of Pediatrics
Director, Division of Community and General Pediatrics
University of Texas-Houston Medical School
Houston, Texas
Chapter 38: Perinatal Conditions (with Nan M. Gaylord)

Yvonne Yousey, RN, CPNP, PhD
Senior Instructor
Department of Pediatrics
School of Medicine
University of Colorado at Denver and
    Health Sciences Center
Denver, Colorado
Chapter 7: Developmental Management of School-Age
    Children (with Bonnie Gance-Cleveland)

Preface

We are delighted to introduce the fourth edition of *Pediatric Primary Care*. This book was first designed for advanced practice nurses serving the primary health care needs of infants, children, and adolescents. Pediatric nurse practitioners (PNPs) and family nurse practitioners (FNPs) were, and still are, our primary audience. However, our audience has grown so that physician assistants, pediatricians, family physicians, pediatric clinical nurse specialists, community health nurses, pediatric ambulatory care nurses, school nurses, and other primary care providers also find the book to be a valuable resource. Our goal has been to provide a textbook for health care students, as well as a resource for clinicians. Feedback from our readers over the past several years indicates that we achieved our goal: both students and experienced clinicians find *Pediatric Primary Care* to be a key resource for their work and study. The first edition won an award from *Nurse Practitioner* journal, and the third edition received an AJN Book of the Year Award for primary care, an indicator of the quality of our work.

Each of the authors brings a special perspective to the subject of pediatric primary health care: nurse practitioner educators, practicing PNPs, and a PNP with long experience working in and teaching community health. Each author has unique areas of expertise—development, nursing theory, cultural competence, and extensive experience with a variety of health care problems. Additionally, we have drawn on contributors from a variety of specialties to address specific content of the book. These include physicians in a variety of specialties, a dentist, a health care administrator, a laboratory specialist, and nurse practitioners in other specialties.

▌▌ ORGANIZATION OF THE BOOK

After three introductory chapters that discuss child health issues and assessment of children in the context of their families and cultures, the book is organized into three major sections—Management of Development, Approaches to Health Management in Pediatric Primary Care, and Approaches to Disease Management. Some features of the fourth edition that we are excited about include the following:

- A Discussion Forum at the end of each chapter written by nurse practitioner educators to assist students to think about the implications for practice of the material they have just read
- Color figures of some important ear, skin, and dental pathologies to help with diagnosis
- A chapter on practice management, an area of increasing concern and interest for clinicians
- An especially updated chapter on environmental health of children that addresses more key toxicants with resources for diagnosis and management
- More in-depth discussion of management of childhood obesity
- More in-depth discussion of management of mental health problems, including those of infants
- An extensive table of current medications used in pediatric primary care
- More tables to facilitate differential diagnosis of related conditions or conditions that have some common elements
- More tables to summarize management strategies for common conditions
- Resource boxes that are at the end of chapters and include websites to access organizations and printed materials that may be useful for clinicians and their clients
- Improved formatting of the text to make it even easier to read

Every chapter has been updated to bring the most current information available to the reader.

We have maintained key features that have made the first three editions so successful:

- An assessment chapter that emphasizes a holistic approach, including identification of both medical and nursing problems within the context of the family
- Attention to cultural factors
- Emphasis on prevention and management of problems from the primary care provider's point of view and scope of practice
- Explicit reference to *Healthy People 2010* guidelines (U.S. Department of Health and Human Services, 2000), *Bright Futures,* (Hagan et al, 2007), *Guidelines for Adolescent Preventive Services (GAPS)* (Elster & Kuznets, 1994), nurse practitioner competencies, and practice guidelines from the U.S. Preventive Services Task Force, the American Academy of Pediatrics, and others
- Introduction of key concepts and foundations for care in a narrative format followed by identification and management of diagnoses discussed using an outline format
- Organization of information into tables and appendices for quick access and efficient use by working primary care providers and nurses
- Selection of an expanded list of common medical and nursing diagnoses that are managed by primary care providers in practice
- Emphasis on best practice guidelines for asthma, otitis media, obesity, and elevated bilirubin in the newborn

The authors assume that the reader has a baccalaureate degree in nursing or a related field and advanced course work in physiology, child development, health assessment, pharmacology, and family systems. Thus, this book guides clinical application of concepts important to primary health care of children and their families.

INTRODUCTORY SECTION

Chapter 1 begins with a review of the major morbidity and mortality statistics highlighting the health problems of children in the United States. The chapter then identifies the important goals for health care of children and describes several sets of current guidelines and standards designed to safeguard primary care of the nation's children. Working with managed care organizations is discussed. Chapter 2 presents the health assessment of the child and family, including both history and physical examination data. The chapter uses a model that supports identification and management of development, functional health patterns, and disease problems. Chapter 3 highlights important cultural components of care to be incorporated into the assessment and management plans for all clients.

DEVELOPMENT SECTION

The development section includes five chapters—an introduction to development for primary care and chapters on infants, toddlers and preschoolers, school-age children, and adolescents. Each chapter begins with a review of the major developmental theories used to understand children in a particular age group. The assessment of developmental needs of children in primary care is then reviewed. Topics for discussion with parents are outlined, including parenting and discipline. Several important developmental issues for each age group are discussed from a problem-oriented perspective. Application of principles of child development to primary care is the key feature for these chapters. Red flags are described to alert the clinician about key developmental problem indicators.

APPROACHES TO HEALTH MANAGEMENT IN PRIMARY CARE SECTION

Functional health patterns (Gordon, 1987) serve as the organizational framework of this section. Eleven patterns are common to people of all cultures and ages. The first seven chapters provide a platform for discussing health promotion through the various components of healthy living—health maintenance, nutrition, breastfeeding, elimination, sleep, and activity and sports participation. The remaining functional health pattern chapters are more psychosocial in nature—self-perception; role relationships where issues of child abuse are addressed; coping and stress tolerance to explore mental health problems of children; cognitive/perceptual patterns to discuss attention-deficit/hyperactivity disorder and problems of blindness, deafness, and autism; sexuality; and values and beliefs. In all of these chapters, foundations of psychology and the basic sciences are first introduced and then applied to common problems of children. NANDA International nursing

diagnoses related to the respective health pattern are identified in boxes near the end of each chapter. Normative behaviors are discussed, and the assessment process is reviewed. Current guidelines, standards for care, and management strategies with which the clinician should be familiar are identified. Common problems of each pattern are presented with the aid of a problem-oriented framework.

DISEASE MANAGEMENT SECTION

The section of the book related to diseases is organized with a chapter for each of the main components of the *International Classification of Diseases*, 22 chapters in all. This section begins with an introductory chapter that outlines approaches to diseases and their management. The infectious diseases chapter then reviews key communicable diseases and includes a comprehensive subsection on immunizations. A major set of chapters focuses on principal body systems, with additional chapters devoted to neonatology, genetics, and uncomplicated trauma. An environmental health chapter discusses these important emerging issues. A chapter on complementary therapies promotes the primary care provider's knowledge about many of the less traditional health care strategies that families may be using.

Each chapter follows the same format throughout, standards and guidelines for care are highlighted, the physiologic and assessment parameters are discussed, management strategies are identified, and management of common problems is presented in a problem-oriented format. Each disease or condition is explained as follows:

- Description
- Epidemiology
- Clinical findings (history, physical examination, laboratory and other studies)
- Differential diagnosis
- Management
- Complications
- Preventive and patient education measures

Tables highlight and summarize differential diagnoses, management, and other pertinent information. The scope of practice of the primary care provider is always kept in mind with appropriate referral and consultation points identified. At the end of many chapters, useful resources are listed, such as national organizations for various disorders.

PRACTICE MANAGEMENT SECTION

In the current health care marketplace, it is increasingly important that the clinician be aware of issues of productivity, compliance with state and federal laws, quality-of-care indicators, and successful business practices that will ensure viability. The chapter on practice management provides information for developing practices.

APPENDICES

The appendices include sections on common drugs used in pediatric primary care settings, growth parameters, laboratory data, and the most current guidelines for management of asthma in children. The appendices are designed for easy access to reference data.

SUMMARY

This book is written by and for nurse practitioners and other clinicians interested in the primary health care of children. It provides a comprehensive resource for students and serves as a reference for practicing clinicians. The book is conceptually organized around domains of interest to pediatric primary care providers—development; functional health patterns related to health maintenance and psychosocial well-being of children and their families; and diseases of children that require intervention, monitoring, and/or referral. The book uses a problem-oriented focus consistent with the education of nurse practitioners and other health care providers and has been written using the latest standards and guidelines available. Content is consistent with the major recommendations for primary care of children in the United States. We are delighted to bring forward a fourth edition of this much-needed resource.

Catherine E. Burns, PhD, RN, CPNP, FAAN
Ardys M. Dunn, PhD, RN, PNP
Margaret A. Brady, PhD, RN, CPNP
Nancy Barber Starr, MS, RN, CPNP
Catherine G. Blosser, MPA:HA, RN, APRN, BC (PNP)

REFERENCES

Elster A, Kuznets N: *AMA Guidelines for Adolescent Preventive Services (GAPS)*, Baltimore, 1994, Williams & Wilkins.

Gordon M: *Nursing diagnosis: process and application*, New York, 1987, McGraw-Hill.

Hagan J et al: *Bright futures: guidelines for health supervision of infants, children, and adolescents*, ed 2, Elk Grove, IL, 2007, American Academy of Pediatrics.

US Department of Health and Human Services: *Healthy People 2010: understanding and improving health*, ed 2, Washington, DC, 2000, US Government Printing Office.

■■ ACKNOWLEDGMENTS

A book of this size and complexity could never have been completed without considerable help—the work of the contributors who researched, wrote, and revised content; the consultation and review of experts in various specialties who critiqued drafts and provided important perspectives and guidance; and the essential technical support from those who managed the production of the manuscript and the final product. We want to especially thank Drs. Ritamarie John and Dawn Garzon for their excellent contributions of discussion questions for each chapter. Another kind of help came from family and friends who offered unending support and encouragement for the duration of the project. We are indebted to so many people and want to say thanks to them all. The following are some of the many people we want to acknowledge.

CONTRIBUTORS TO THE THIRD EDITION

These people were instrumental in helping us develop the third edition of the book. Although they are not authors in this edition, their ideas and work have contributed greatly to our work, and we are deeply indebted to them:

Jeanette Broering, NP
Kevin Hale, DDS
Janie Huff-Slankard, MN, CPNP
Margaret A. MacDonald, CPNP, PMHNP
Jan Freitas-Nichols, MSN, RN, CPNP
Deborah Parks, DSN, PNP
Charles Poland III, DDS
Jean Betschart Roermer, MSN, CPNP
Teri Moser Woo, MSN, CPNP
Linda M Kollar, MSN

OUR THANKS TO FAMILY AND FRIENDS

Jerry Burns; Jennifer, Dusty, and Jessica Lee; Jill, Cory, Alyssa, and Kyla Nordstrom and other family and friends.
Catherine E. Burns

Marvin and Malcolm Dunn; Philip Dunn and Liz Flynn, and Miles Christopher; and other family and friends.
Ardys M. Dunn

Martha, Larry, Greg, and Katie, and other family and friends and in memory of Grandma Mary.
Margaret A. Brady

Jon and Jonah and AnnaMei Starr, my APA colleagues, and in memory of Janet Barber.
Nancy Barber Starr

Terry Dolan, family, and special acknowledgement of my sister, Cris.
Catherine G. Blosser

Contents

UNIT ONE

Pediatric Primary Care Foundations

Real Little Kids
Wear Black
Sox

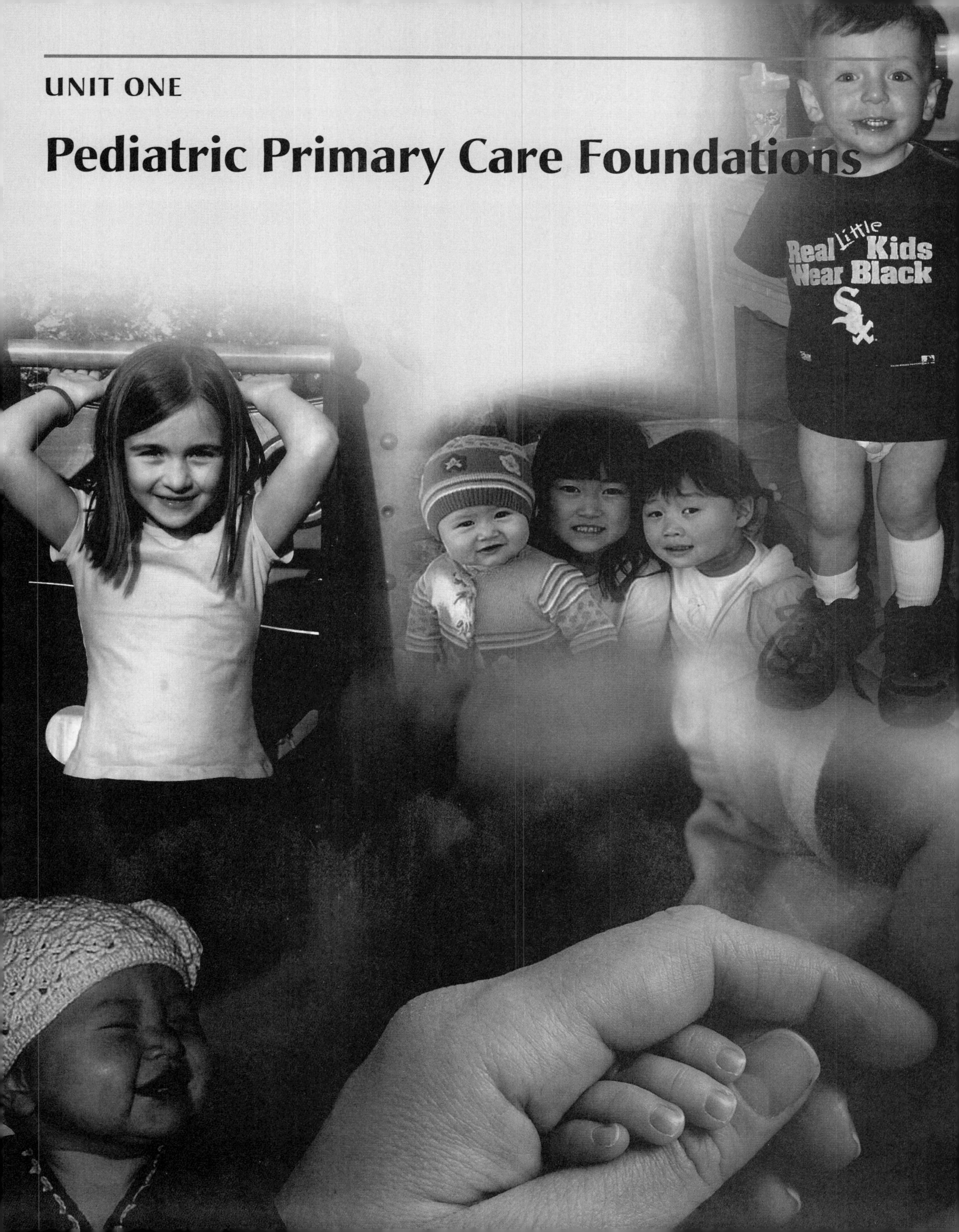

CHAPTER 1

Child Health Status in America

Karen G. Duderstadt

The worth of a society is often measured by the health and well-being of its children. Recent reports from the U.S. Department of Health and Human Services (USDHHS) (2001) and other federal agencies indicate that the health of America's children is in an uneasy balance. Gains have been made in many areas including reduction in teen birth rates and exposure to second-hand smoke, reduction of unintentional injuries, and improved immunization rates. At the same time, rates of infant mortality remain significantly higher than other industrialized nations; the rate of low- (less than 2500 g) and very low- (less than 1500 g) birth-weight infants continues to rise, the proportion of children and teens with emotional and behavioral difficulties is increasing, and far too many children are raised in families that lack adequate resources with the number of children living in poverty increasing from 17% in 2001 to 19% in 2005 (Annie E. Casey Foundation, 2007). Increased vigilance is required in the U.S. to improve the health outcomes of children and ensure that children are well cared for, well served by public institutions, safe, and protected as our most vital resource—the next generation.

This chapter presents an overview of the state of children's health in the U.S. and reviews current pediatric morbidity and mortality statistics. The chapter reviews the leading health indicators for children, including access to care and barriers to use of health care services, and the impact of health disparities on the overall health of children. The health priorities from *Healthy People 2010* are presented along with updated health supervision guidelines for pediatric care. Finally, the important role that pediatric primary health care providers play in improving child health status through health promotion and continuity of care for all children is defined and discussed as an integral part of improving the health of all children.

◼ INDICATORS OF CHILD HEALTH STATUS

In 2004, children under 18 years old constituted 25% of the U.S. population. By 2020, the number of children is expected to increase by 80 million and represent 24% of the U.S. population. Multiple indicators are used to measure the health of children: rates of low-birth-weight infants, infant mortality, child deaths, teen deaths, and births to teen mothers. Immunization rates; limitations in physical activity; rates of homicide, suicide, and unintentional injuries; violent crime arrest rates;

the percentage of teens who are high school dropouts; and the percentage of children who live below the federal poverty threshold are also indicators of child health status. These measures inform pediatric health care providers and other professionals who work with children and teens, guide practice, and provide evidence on the health of children. The health of children is an important indicator of the future health of the nation because many lifelong health problems begin in childhood.

CHILD AND YOUTH MORBIDITY AND MORTALITY
Infants: Birth Rates, Birth Weight, Births to Teenage Mothers

The U.S. continues to rank poorly in international comparisons of infant mortality. The five leading causes of death in infants birth to 12 months old remain congenital malformations (20%), complications of low birth weight (17%), sudden infant death syndrome (8%), newborns with complications of pregnancy (6%), and newborns with birth complications (4%). Whereas infant mortality in the U.S. remained high from 2000 to 2004 compared with other industrialized nations, the birth rate decreased. In 2004, there were 14 births per 1000 population in the U.S., down 1% from the rate for 2003. This represents the second lowest birth rate recorded in the U.S. since national data have been available. In 2004, 23% of all births in the U.S. were to Hispanic women 15 to 44 years old as compared with 15% in 1990 (Hoyert et al, 2006).

Birth by cesarean section has continued to increase. The rate of cesarean delivery rose to 29.1% in 2004, up 6% from 2003 and 41% since 1996. Recent increases in multiple births, increased use of infertility therapies, and older ages of mothers when bearing children place infants at risk for low birth weight, very low birth weight, and subsequent infant mortality (CDC, 2006).

The adolescent birth rate has continued to decline. The teen birth rate in 2004 was the lowest rate ever recorded (22 births per 1000 females 15 to 17 years old). Although birth rates among racial and ethnic groups vary, the decline has been particularly dramatic among African-American teens. The rate among African-American females 15 to 17 years old dropped from 86 births per 1000 in 1991 to 37 per 1000 in 2004. The birth rate among Hispanic females 15 to 17 years old decreased slightly in 2004, but remained high at 50 births per 1000 females (America's Children, 2006). These figures represent the race of the mother and not the child. Beginning in 2003, several states began multiracial reporting, a trend that has continued and more accurately reflects the increasing numbers of children born to parents of different races.

The proportion of infants with low and very low birth weight has increased. In 2004, the rate was 9.3% of births nationally (CDC, 2006), up from 6.8% in 1980. Racial and ethnic disparities persist for this health status indicator, with the rate of low birth weight and very low birth weight consistently higher among African-American women.

The proportion of infants born to unmarried mothers continues to rise. In 2004, 36% of all births were to unmarried women. Births to unmarried women 20 years old and older were higher in 2003 than rates recorded in 1994. In low-income communities, the proportion of infants born to unmarried women was 70% to 80%. More favorable health outcomes are associated with children living in two-parent families, and parents in two-parent families are healthier, have higher sustained incomes, and have fewer emotional problems (AAP, 2003).

Children

For children 1 to 4 years old, the death rate has steadily declined over the past two decades. In 2004, the death rate was 31 deaths per 100,000, down from 33 deaths per 100,000 in 2001. The decline primarily reflects a drop in motor vehicle deaths because of increased use of safety seats and other child restraints. With improved installation of safety seats and compliance with new child restraint laws, this death rate could be reduced even further in the coming decade.

Adolescents

Risk-taking behaviors often have severe long-term consequences for teens and for society. Tobacco, alcohol, and illicit drug use cause significant morbidities; engaging in violent crime and other risk-taking behaviors contribute to deaths of many youth each year. Intentional injuries (e.g., homicide and suicide) and unintentional injuries were responsible for 3 of every 4 deaths among adolescents 15 to 19 years old in 2004. Firearm injury and motor vehicle crashes were the two leading causes of deaths among adolescents. On the positive side, the rate of firearm injuries declined by more than half since 1994. In 2003, the rate of firearm injury death was 12 per 100,000 adolescents compared with 28 per 100,000 in 1994 (America's Children, 2006). The death rate from motor vehicle crashes among 15- to 19-year-olds also decreased slightly to a rate of 25 deaths per 100,000 adolescents.

IMMUNIZATIONS

Over the past decade, immunization rates have significantly improved among U.S. children and adolescents, surpassing the 80% level set by the *Healthy People 2010* objectives. In 2004, 83% of children 19 to 35 months old received the recommended combined series of childhood vaccines compared with 76% in 1996. Coverage rates for varicella and pneumococcal vaccines increased as well, reaching 88% and 73% respectively in 2004 (America's Children, 2006). This represents a significant accomplishment on the part of pediatric health care providers and parents who have recognized the benefits and values of immunizations.

Despite these advances, immunization coverage rates still vary significantly among states. In 2004, the coverage for the recommended initial immunization series was 92% in Massachusetts, 91% in Rhode Island, and 90% in Florida. In contrast, immunization coverage in Nevada was 71% and 75% in Texas, Oklahoma, and Utah. More needs to be done in individual states where coverage is lagging behind the national average and where there is persistent disparity of immunization coverage rates among racially and ethnically diverse groups.

Teenagers also fall short in immunization coverage rates. About 25% of teens in the U.S. lack at least one of the currently recommended immunizations: hepatitis B; measles, mumps and rubella (MMR); varicella; meningococcal; or tetanus, diphtheria, and acellular pertussis vaccines.

The nation cannot afford to be complacent. Recent outbreaks of vaccine-preventable diseases illustrate the importance of full immunization. The largest U.S. measles outbreak in a decade occurred in 2005 (Mulholland, 2006). Thirty-four people in Indiana were infected by a 17-year-old girl who had traveled to Romania without receiving recommended immunizations. Only 2 of the 33 individuals had been vaccinated against measles. The majority were children whose parents had chosen not to vaccinate them because of perceived safety concerns regarding vaccines. Three individuals were hospitalized, though no deaths occurred. A mumps epidemic also occurred in the Midwest in 2005 (CDC, 2006), and the recent upsurge in pertussis infections (CDC, 2005) among adolescents has impacted unimmunized and underimmunized infants, children, and adults. Increased vigilance is required to achieve herd immunity and lower the human and health care costs of vaccine-preventable diseases.

EXPOSURE TO TOBACCO

The percentage of children exposed to environmental tobacco smoke, measured with blood cotinine levels, decreased from 88% in 1994 to 59% in 2004 (America's Children, 2006). Teen smoking rates have also declined since 1997 when data were first reported. Daily cigarette smoking declined from 10% to 4% in eighth graders, 18% to 8% in tenth graders, and 25% to 14% in twelfth graders (America's Children, 2006). One reason for these decreases may be the decline over the last decade in the number of youth ever initiating smoking, which, in turn, may be due to the national public health campaign to prevent cigarette smoking among adolescents.

CHILDREN LIVING IN POVERTY

Seventeen percent of America's children live in families with annual incomes at or below the federal poverty threshold. In 2004, this was $15,067 for a family of three and $19,307 for a family of four. This proportion has remained steady since 2003. Over the past 15 years, the rate of children living in poverty reached a high of 22% in 1993 and a low of 16% in 2000.

Economic security is a major factor affecting the health and well-being of children and families. The lack of adequate economic resources affects the physical and emotional growth and development of children. Likewise, poverty is a predictor of poorer academic success, especially at the higher education levels (Haveman & Smeeding, 2006). Family structure greatly affects household income, and children living in single-parent families experience higher poverty rates than children living in two-parent families. In 2005, 33% of children living in single-parent households were below the poverty line, whereas only 7% of children living in two-parent households were living at or below the federal poverty threshold (Annie E. Casey Foundation, 2006).

Children from ethnically and racially diverse populations have far less economic security as measured by poverty levels than do children from white populations in America. The rate of African-American children living at or below the federal poverty threshold was 36% in 2005 as compared with 29% of Hispanic children and 11% of non-Hispanic white children (Annie E. Casey Foundation, 2006). Economic insecurity corresponds to poorer levels of health.

CHILD WELL-BEING

In 2006, the Foundation for Child Development published an update on trends for the well-being or quality of life of children and youth from birth to 17 years old in the U.S. The analysis reviews a 30-year period from 1975 to 2005 and reports on seven summary indices including family economic well-being, safety and behavioral concerns, educational attainment, community connectedness, social relationships, emotional and spiritual well-being, and health. Fig. 1-1 presents the Child and Youth Well-Being Index for 2005 (Foundation for Child Development, 2006). Children and youth have experienced substantial improvements in two domains according to this report: safety and behavioral concerns and family economic well-being. There was also improvement in the domain of emotional and spiritual well-being from a low in 1990. Two domains remain below baseline levels: health and social relationships. The health domain is almost 30% below the baseline measured in 1975. Health is measured by the rate of infant mortality, low birth weight, child mortality (children 1 to 19 years old), children in very good or excellent health by parental report, children with activity limitations by parental report, and the rate of childhood overweight for 6 to 19 years old. Despite overall improvements in infant and child mortality rates, the other health indicators continue to decline as a result of increasing levels of childhood overweight and obesity.

OVERWEIGHT: THE NEW MORBIDITY

The most concerning indicator of child health status in the U.S. is the number of children who are overweight and at risk for becoming overweight. This new morbidity presents a substantial challenge to health care providers seeking to prevent cardiovascular complications, diabetes, and pulmonary compromise in future generations. It will also lead to excess expenditure of health care dollars on preventable morbidities. Overweight is the primary challenge confronting pediatric health care providers today and will be discussed more fully in Chapter 11.

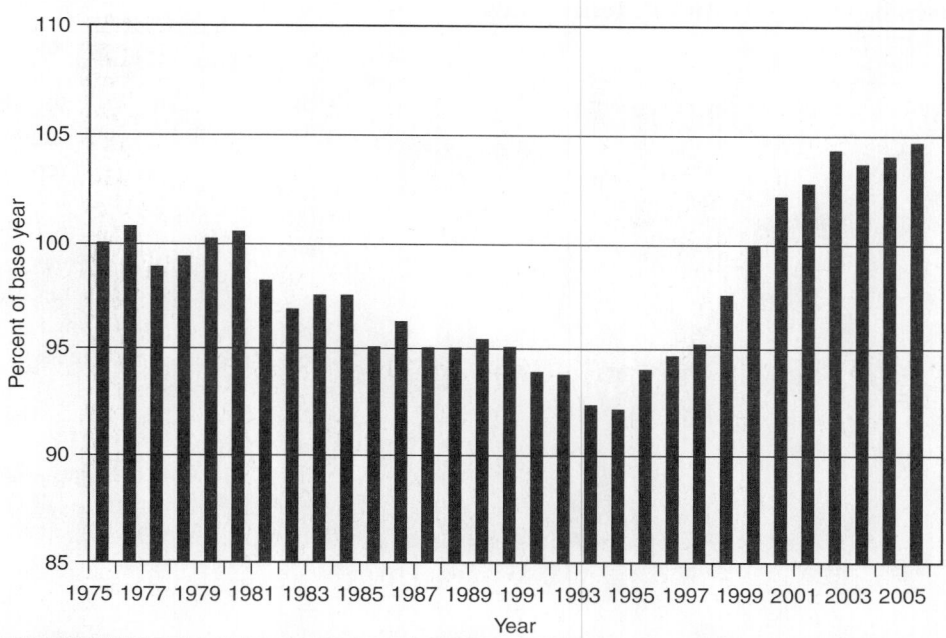

FIG. 1-1 The FCD Child and Youth Well–Being Index (CWI) is a national measure of how American children have fared since 1975. It assesses specific aspects of children's lives and gives both an overall measure of changes in child well-being over time and a detailed examination of key indicators of well-being. (From Foundation for Child Development: *The Foundation for Child Development Child and Youth Well-Being Index [CWI], 1975-2004, with projections for 2005*, Durham, NC, 2006, Duke University. Available at *www.fcd-us.org* [accessed June 30, 2007].)

■ HEALTH DISPARITIES AND CHILDREN'S HEALTH

RACIAL AND ETHNIC DISPARITIES

Despite improvements in health among immigrants and racially and ethnically diverse populations, disparities persist among Hispanic and African-American children compared with other groups. Race and ethnicity have an independent effect on having a usual source of primary care and on a child's health status in the U.S. Racially and ethnically diverse children with the same socio-demographics and insurance status as white children are less likely to have a usual source of care and more likely to have fair or poor health status. These children are also more likely to be uninsured, to have poorer health status, and to experience inadequate access to health care (Guendelman & Pearl, 2004; Hughes & Ng, 2003; Newacheck et al, 2000; Newacheck et al, 2004; Weinick & Krauss, 2000).

Nonwhite and Hispanic racial and ethnic groups, in aggregate, will become the majority population in the U.S. in the next few decades (Hernandez, 2004). Currently, 1 in 5 children live in immigrant families in the U.S., most of whom are U.S. citizens (Shields & Behrman, 2004). Children born to immigrant mothers are healthier than those born to U.S.-born mothers, on average, and more likely to be living in two-parent families. They are also more likely to be living in poverty and be uninsured (Shields & Behrman, 2004).

Eliminating racial and ethnic disparities in health has become a national priority to reduce health care costs. The USDHHS (2003) implemented a policy to better understand the nature of persistent disparities and to identify potential solutions. Research has shown that no single factor accounts for racial disparities in health and health care among children, and the causes are dynamic and vary across individuals and groups (Shone et al, 2003). A recent report, *Closing the Gap: Solutions to Race-Based Health Disparities*, published by the Northwest Federation of Community Organizations, presents a summary of institutional causes of health disparities and potential policy responses to the inequalities (Table 1-1) (NWFCO, 2005). Understanding the health care needs of racially and ethnically diverse children, designing programs to meet those needs, providing culturally and linguistically appropriate services, and monitoring health outcomes by race and ethnicity are activities that can assist in reducing or eliminating disparities in children's health and health care.

ACCESS TO HEALTH CARE: HEALTH INSURANCE DISPARITIES

Children with health insurance have better access to care, greater use of health care services, and better overall health outcomes than uninsured children (Shone et al, 2003). In 2004, 11% of children lacked health insurance nationally, with a wide disparity in the proportion of uninsured children reported by state. In that year, 20% of children under 17 years old in Texas lacked health insurance whereas only 4% of children in Vermont were uninsured (Annie E. Casey Foundation, 2006). This disparity by state reflects the level of economic resources available for families and sources for health insurance. The proportion of children living in families with private

---

TABLE 1-1 **Causes of Disparity and Potential Responses**

Root Cause of Disparity	Potential Policy Response
Inaccessible health care for people of color as a result of financial and geographic barriers	• Universal health care • Expand employer contributions and responsibility for health care • Expand Medicaid, SCHIP, Medicare coverage
Lower quality or culturally inappropriate care for communities of color	• Increased funding for understaffed hospitals and clinics • Access to specialized or urgent care • Resource support and incentives for building relationships • Recruitment and on-the-job training programs for people of color
Lack of comprehensive interpretation and translation services within hospitals and clinics	• Provide access to highly trained medical interpreters • Translate written materials and signage into multiple languages • Implement federal CLAS standards
Lack of understanding or integration of alternative and traditional medicine	• Insurance coverage for appropriate alternative health care • Training of physicians to understand alternative treatments

SCHIP, State Children's Health Insurance Programs. *CLAS,* Culturally and Linguistically Appropriate Services.
From Northwest Federation of Community Organizations: *Closing the gap: solutions to race-based health disparities* (p 10), Seattle, 2005, Northwest Federation of Community Organizations.

health insurance has continued to decline from 70% in 1999 to 66% in 2004. The proportion of children with publicly funded health insurance continues to increase and reached 26.7% of the pediatric population in 2005 (AAP, 2006).

Uninsured children are more likely to lack a usual source of care, have unmet health needs, delay seeking health care, have lower immunization rates, and use fewer well child care services than insured children (Newacheck et al, 2000). Although health insurance alone does not eliminate health disparities or guarantee access to health care services, reducing disparities requires access to care, links to a health care home for children, increased surveillance of the use of health care services, and reduced nonfinancial barriers to care for children living in low-income families. Public health insurance has the potential to play a critical role in reducing and eliminating racial and ethnic disparities in health care for all children.

■ THE NEW MORBIDITY: CHILDHOOD OVERWEIGHT

Childhood overweight represents an example of a significant childhood health problem with important policy, economic, and public health implications. It also illustrates the health care disparities evident in the U.S.

EPIDEMIOLOGY AND RISKS

Overweight has increased globally among children and adolescents and is now recognized by the World Health Organization (WHO) as one of the most important public health issues. The problem is most prominent among developed countries, and the U.S. has the highest prevalence of overweight children and adolescents in the world. Overweight is defined using the body mass index (BMI), which is calculated as weight in kilograms divided by the square of height in meters. Children who have BMIs in the 85th to 95th percentiles are children "at risk" for overweight, and those children with BMIs greater than the 95th percentile are defined as overweight. The proportion of children 6 to 17 years old who are overweight continued to rise from 15% in 2000 to 18% in 2004. Rates of overweight in children 10 to 17 years old are reported as 31% (America's Children, 2006).

Most concerning in the current epidemic of overweight is the overrepresentation of children living in low-income families, particularly among racially and ethnically diverse children (Graham, 2005). The rate for non-Hispanic black children 2 to 19 years old who are overweight is 20%, while another 35.1% are at risk for overweight (Ogden et al, 2006). The rates for overweight and at risk for overweight in Mexican-American children (2 to 19 years old) are 19.2% and 37%, respectively (Story et al, 2003). Prevalence rates for overweight Native-American children, although varying greatly among tribes, have been estimated at as high as 40% (Story et al, 2003).

Childhood overweight is associated with significant comorbidities and both immediate and long-term health risks. Children who are overweight are predisposed to type 2 diabetes, hypertension, dyslipidemia, and mental health problems (Barlow & Dietz, 2002). In addition to health risks, there are considerable economic costs. The estimated annual cost of obesity and over-

weight in children and adults in the U.S. in 2002 was $117 billion, accounting for an estimated 31% of the total direct costs of 15 comorbid conditions (Finkelstein et al, 2003).

Most concerning of comorbidities reported is the link between suicide ideation and overweight. Adolescents who perceive themselves as slightly overweight (85th to 94th percentile) or very overweight (95th percentile or greater) were significantly more likely to experience depression than those who thought their weight was appropriate (Eaton et al, 2005). Teens who were overweight were also 2.5 times more likely to have suicide ideation than those teens who perceived their weight as normal (adjusted odds ratio for adolescents at 95th percentile or greater). How adolescents perceive their body weight may be more important than their actual weight in terms of increased likelihood of suicidal behavior. Regardless of body mass index, extreme perceptions of weight appear to be a significant risk factor for suicidal behavior (Eisenberg et al, 2003; Eaton et al, 2005).

OBESITY AND OVERWEIGHT PREVENTION: PROGRAMS AND POLICIES

The prevention of obesity has now risen to the top of the list of public health priorities (USDHHS, 2001; America's Childern, 2006). The burden of obesity in the population, particularly high-risk and ethnically diverse populations, will exceed the capacity of the current health care delivery system to deliver treatment for obesity or for the associated conditions (Kumanika & Obarzanek, 2003). Further the treatment of obesity cannot necessarily reverse the long-term health effects of overweight, particularly when it begins in childhood. This represents a significant challenge to health professionals and health care organizations to design strategies to identify children at risk for overweight and to implement programs for children and adolescents with sedentary lifestyles. Prevention focuses on good nutrition and physical fitness for all children as opposed to treatment of obesity and its associated morbidities.

Establishing programs with good nutrition and physical activity for children is an important first step, and integrated programs are built around sound health policy. Health policies reflect governmental choices, influence the health of individuals, and change the health outcomes of a society (DePalma, 2002). Building sound health policy requires a clear recognition of the causes of the problem and good science. The development and implementation of health policy is *ideally* shaped by a process similar to evidence-based health care. Evidence-based policy design incorporates a firm foundation of the best data, individual expertise, and a policy maker willing to partner and facilitate the process (DePalma, 2002). Often, however, policy efforts are influenced by an inadequate research base or by fragmented bills offering a variety of incremental changes, not a comprehensive model for system-wide change.

Pediatric health care providers, including nurse practitioners, and others working with children have expressed their strong concern with the growing numbers of overweight and severely overweight children seen in their practices every day, especially among children and adolescents from ethnically diverse backgrounds. The National Association of Pediatric

Nurse Practitioners (NAPNAP), as the leading nursing organization representing the health of children in the community, has used its member expertise to establish clinical practice guidelines for the prevention of childhood weight problems. With current indicators attributing the increase in overweight to changes in environmental factors influencing energy intake and physical activity levels, the Healthy Eating and Activity Together (HEAT) guidelines have effectively included physical activity guidelines and mandates for advocacy in the community along with dietary recommendations to assist children and families in promoting healthy lifestyles. NAPNAP's emphasis on prevention begins the movement of evaluating point-of-care intervention (Gottesman, 2003). The HEAT guidelines and management strategies for this clinical condition are presented in Chapter 11 of this book.

IMPROVING THE HEALTH OF CHILDREN: HEALTH PROMOTION FOR ALL

DEFINING CHILDREN'S HEALTH

The Institute of Medicine (IOM) defines child health as the extent to which an individual child or groups of children are able or enabled to develop and realize their potential; satisfy their needs; and interact successfully with their biological,

physical, and social environments (IOM, 2004). This definition acknowledges the context of health and the myriad of influences that contribute to the health of the pediatric population. The IOM further defines three distinct domains that can be used to measure children's health: (1) *functioning* (the manifestations of health in a child's daily life), (2) *health conditions* (disorders or illnesses of bodily systems), and (3) *health potential* (captures the developmental potential and positive assets of health). Factors that influence these domains include the child's physical and social environment, the receipt of available health care services, and local and national health policies. Fig. 1-2 represents the IOM's conceptual framework for children's health and its influences (IOM, 2004). It correlates well with the conceptual framework for this book, which includes three domains for analyzing and managing child health status: development, functional health problems, and diseases.

This text also promotes the position that pediatric health care providers must focus on prevention and health education to ensure children's health and well-being. The IOM's broad definition of child health will assist pediatric providers to shift from a disease-focused health care system to one with primary prevention at its very core. Providers need to work with members of the health care team, third party payers, health maintenance organizations, policy analysts, and legislators to move toward a prevention-based health care system.

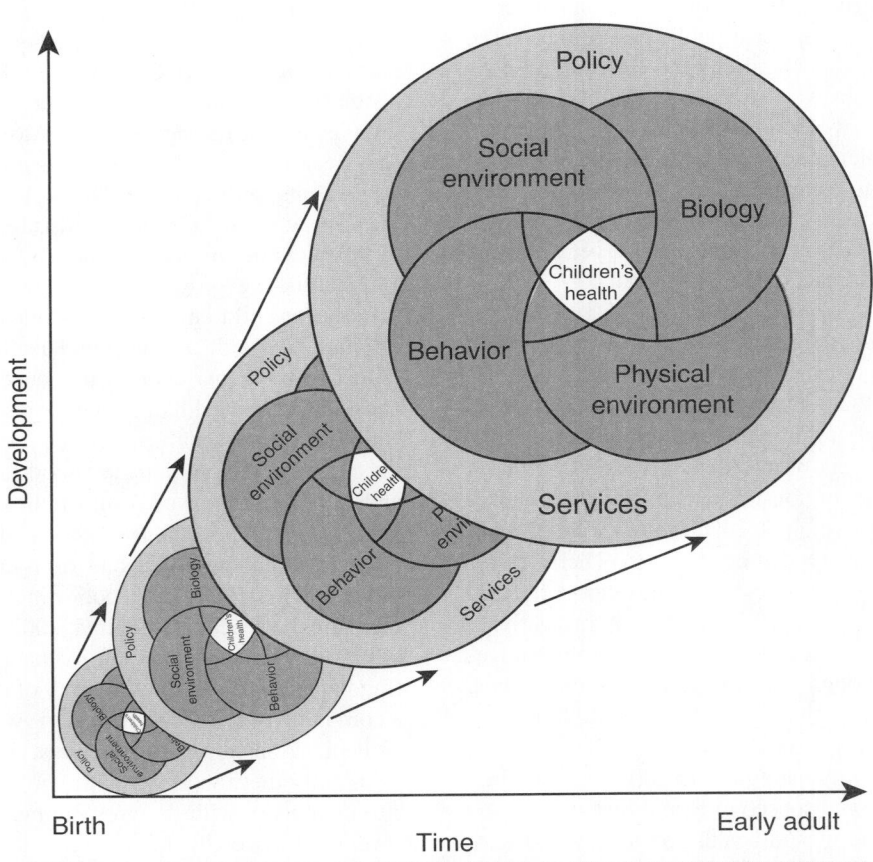

FIG. 1-2 Model of children's health and its influences. (From Institute of Medicine: *Children's health, the nation's wealth: assessing and improving child health*, Washington DC, 2004, Institute of Medicine.)

PRIMARY CARE AND CHILD HEALTH STATUS

Defining Primary Care

The most widely quoted definition of primary health care remains the work of the IOM. "Primary care is the provision of integrated, accessible health care services by clinicians who are accountable for addressing a large majority of personal health care needs, developing a sustained partnership with patients, and practicing in the context of family and community" (IOM, 1996). To achieve a goal of primary care for all of America's children will require continuous innovation and improvement in the health care system. The Institute laid out a road map to do just that. The objectives based on this definition of primary health care include:

- Organizational arrangements for health care that are built on a foundation of strong primary care and that facilitate the coordination of the full array of services essential for maintaining and improving the individual's health status
- Improved information systems and quality assurance programs for primary care
- Ways to make primary care available to all Americans, regardless of economic status, geographic location, language, or cultural background
- Financing mechanisms that encourage quality primary care rather than episodic interventions late in the disease process
- An enhanced knowledge base for primary care, drawn from clinical and health services research
- Program evaluation, dissemination of innovations, and continued education of both clinicians and patients to continually improve the primary care system in an era of rapid change
- A primary care workforce sufficient in numbers to meet the needs for primary care, equipped with appropriate skills and competencies, and prepared to work in teams that include primary care physicians, nurse practitioners, physician assistants, community health workers, and other health professionals

Achieving Primary Care Goals

This road map could lead to a primary care system of services for all. Nurse practitioners play a key role in the delivery of primary health care to all segments of the population and are a key element in the primary care workforce required to achieve the vision laid out by the IOM (2004). The competencies and guidelines for nurse practitioner education developed by the National Organization of Nurse Practitioner Faculties (NONPF) and the American Association of Colleges of Nursing under contract with the USDHHS ensure that nurse practitioners are prepared to provide culturally appropriate, quality health care services to diverse populations (USDHHS, 2002).

Improving and strengthening primary care will require a strong evidence-based foundation. To develop this evidence base, funding and infrastructure to support primary care research must be increased. Currently, most clinical research efforts focus on expanding the knowledge of diseases (often single disease entities) and treatment options. Much of the basis for primary care is not yet evidence-based. This is particularly true in relation to well child care. This deficit provides an area of research open to nurse practitioners and other pediatric primary health care providers. Increased evidence in the primary health care domain could help to move the public dialogue toward a greater emphasis on prevention and away from a disease-focused health care system.

The U.S. health care system spends far more on the "technology" of care than on achieving equity in the delivery of health care. Within the health care arena, the national dialogue has focused on cuts to critical health care programs, such as Medicaid coverage for children rather than eliminating inequalities in access and quality of care (Woolf et al, 2004). The racial disparities in health constitute a national crisis as health care costs continue to rise. From 1991 to 2000, medical advances eliminated 176,633 deaths, but equalizing the mortality rates of African Americans with whites would have averted 886,202 deaths. Ultimately, achieving quality in health care delivery may do more to decrease health care costs than further protecting the technology of care (Woolf et al, 2004).

Immunizations

Pediatric primary care providers need evidence on the manufacture and safety of newer vaccines to combat the widespread misinformation about vaccine safety, assure parents of safeguards in the vaccine supply, and provide support services for parents and answers to their questions about particular vaccines. These measures can be used to help achieve full vaccine coverage for children.

HEALTH SUPERVISION GUIDELINES

Healthy People 2010

The objectives of the *Healthy People 2010* initiative continue to challenge local, state, and national agencies and insurers, in addition to pediatric health care providers. The objective of achieving optimal health for individuals to contribute to a healthier, happier, and more productive society is laudable. Box 1-1 presents the ten leading indicators for *Healthy People 2010*.

BOX 1-1   ***Healthy People 2010* Major Health Indicators**

- Physical activity
- Overweight or obesity
- Tobacco use
- Substance abuse
- Responsible sexual behavior
- Mental health
- Injury and violence
- Environmental quality
- Immunizations
- Access to health care

From US Department of Health and Human Services: *Healthy People 2010: understanding and improving health,* ed 2, Washington, DC, 2000, US Government Printing Office.

In some areas of child health, the U.S. is meeting the objectives. Of the ten leading indicators, three areas have shown significant progress toward meeting the 2010 goals: tobacco use, immunizations, and injury prevention. Yet progress in other areas has been slow or has even reversed. In the areas of physical activity and overweight, the trend has been reversed since 2000. Model programs exist to curb this trend, but it will take sustained commitment on the part of pediatric health care providers; local, state, and federal agencies; leading health organizations; and child health advocates to change the current trajectory.

Bright Futures

Bright Futures is a national health promotion initiative of the Maternal and Child Health Bureau and the American Academy of Pediatrics (AAP) dedicated to the principle that "every child deserves to be healthy and that optimal health involves a trusting relationship between the health professional, the child, the family, and the community as partners in health practice" (Green & Palfrey, 2002). The *Bright Futures* Children's Health Charter was developed by advocates for children's health. Box 1-2 presents the principles that are the foundation for the initiatives. The complete guide to *Bright Futures* is available to health care providers and to parents at *www.brightfutures.org*.

Recent additions to the *Bright Futures* website include four developmental tools based on the *Bright Futures in Practice: Mental Health* publication. The tools offer a framework for discussing the social and emotional development of children in infancy, early childhood, middle childhood, and adolescence. The *Bright Futures* website features a companion referral tool for providers and families to connect with community resources.

QUALITY OF CHILDREN'S HEALTH CARE SERVICES

The quality of preventive care services for children varies greatly, and many children are not receiving the recommended preventive and developmental services that meet a basic threshold. Quality standards for well child care have not been specified (Belamarich et al, 2006), and many services are not meeting the needs of children and families, particularly families with children with special health care needs. There are many barriers to effective well child care including time constraints, low level of reimbursement for preventive care services and developmental screening services, limited training of health care providers in emotional and behavioral problems impacting children and families, and lack of community referral sources to assist children, teens, and families.

■ SUMMARY

Nurtured, healthy children will be productive citizens and leaders for coming generations. Far too many children, however, are growing up without the benefits of families with adequate resources. Millions of children grow up hungry, neglected, and abused, living in unsafe environments, and receiving inadequate education. The nation's commitment to children should involve providing for them directly and ensuring opportunities for families to be successful in their child-rearing efforts. Primary health care providers have unique opportunities to be involved with families and children as they work to solve the problems of living to achieve and maintain hopeful, fulfilled lives.

BOX 1-2 *Bright Futures* **Children's Health Charter**

Every child deserves:
- To be born well, to be physically fit, and to achieve self-responsibility for good health habits.

Every child and adolescent deserves:
- Ready access to coordinated and comprehensive preventive, health-promoting, therapeutic, and rehabilitative medical, mental health, and dental care. Such care is best provided through a continuing relationship with a primary care professional or team and ready access to secondary and tertiary levels of care.
- A nurturing family and supportive relationships with other significant persons who provide security, positive role models, warmth, love, and unconditional acceptance. A child's health begins with the health of his parents.
- To grow and develop in a physically and psychologically safe home and school environment free of undue risk of injury, abuse, violence, or exposure to environmental toxins.
- Satisfactory housing, good nutrition, a quality education, an adequate family income, a supportive social network, and access to community resources.
- Quality child care when her parents are working outside the home.
- The opportunity to develop ways to cope with stressful life experiences.
- The opportunity to be prepared for parenthood.
- The opportunity to develop positive values and become a responsible citizen in his community.
- To experience joy, have high self-esteem, have friends, acquire a sense of efficacy, and believe that she can succeed in life. She should help the next generation develop the motivation and habits necessary for similar achievement.

From *Bright Futures,* National Center for Education and Maternal and Child Health and Georgetown University. Available at *www.brightfutures.org/charter.html* (accessed June 30, 2007). Used with permission of the National Center for Education in Maternal and Child Health.

☑DISCUSSION FORUM

1. Forty percent of children are not being raised by two parents who live in the same household. How can you improve the quality of care that you deliver to nontraditional families?

2. Childhood overweight is very prevalent in the community in which you work. What can you do as a primary care provider on a community level to address this issue? Please do not consider your clinical care of individual overweight children as a strategy for this question.

3. The AAP writes that children will grow and thrive best when cared for by "two mutually committed adults who respect one another, who have adequate social and financial resources, and who both are actively engaged in their upbringing" (AAP, 2003). Explore the various aspects of this definition:
   - Who would qualify in the definition of "two committed adults who respect one another"?
   - What constitutes "adequate social and financial resources"?
   - What does "actively engaged in their upbringing" mean? When is a person "actively engaged?"

4. The *Bright Futures* Charter (Box 1-2) sets high ideals for the well-being of children.
   - Take any one of the charter points and discuss the ways in which that right is met for children in a community you designate. In what ways and for which children is that right not met currently? What needs to be done to improve the status of children in the community you have identified?

REFERENCES

American Academy of Pediatrics (AAP) Task Force on the Family: Family pediatrics, *Pediatrics* 111:1549-1587, 2003.

American Academy of Pediatrics (AAP): *Children's health insurance status and Medicaid/SCHIP eligibility and enrollment,* 2005, American Academy of Pediatrics, September 2006. Available at *www.aap.org/research/cps.pdf* (accessed Feb 12, 2007).

America's Children: *America's children in brief: key national indicators of well-being,* Forum on Child and Family Statistics, 2006. Available at *www.childstats.gov/americaschildren* (accessed Feb 12, 2007).

Annie E. Casey Foundation: *KIDS COUNT data book.* Available at *www.kidscount.org/sld/databook.jsp* (accessed Feb 11, 2007).

Barlow SE, Dietz WH: Management of child and adolescent obesity: summary of recommendations based on reports from pediatricians, pediatric nurse practitioners, and registered dieticians, *Pediatrics* 111:236-238, 2002.

Belamarich P et al: Drowning in a sea of advice: pediatricians and American Academy of Pediatrics policy statements, *Pediatrics* 118(4):e964-e978, 2006.

Centers for Disease Control and Prevention (CDC): Assisted reproductive technology surveillance–United States, 2003, *MMWR Surveillance Summaries* May 26, 2006/55(S S04):1-22, 2006.

Centers for Disease Control and Prevention (CDC): *Pediatric and pregnancy nutrition surveillance system data–12/2006 report.* Available at *www.cdc.gov/pednss/pednss_tables* (accessed Feb 11, 2007).

Centers for Disease Control and Prevention (CDC): Update: multistate outbreak of mumps–United States, Jan 1-May 2, 2006, *MMWR Dispatch* 55(Dispatch):1-5, 2006.

Centers for Disease Control and Prevention (CDC): Pertussis–United States, 2001-2003, *MMWR* 54:1283-1286, 2005.

DePalma J: Proposing an evidence-based policy process, *Nurs Adm Q* 26(4):55-61, 2002.

Eaton DK et al: Associations of body mass index and perceived weight with suicide ideation and suicide attempts among U.S. high school students, *Arch Pediatr Adolesc Med* 159(6):513-519, 2005.

Eisenberg M, Neumark-Sztainer D, Story M: Associations of weight-based teasing and emotional well-being among adolescents, *Arch Pediatr Adolesc Med*:157:733-738, 2003.

Finkelstein EA, Fiebelkorn IC, Wang G: National medical spending attributable to overweight and obesity: how much, and who's paying? *Health Aff* [serial online] 22:219-226, 2003. Available at *http://content.healthaffairs.org/cgi/content/full/hlthaff.w3.219v1/DC1* (accessed June 30, 2007).

Foundation for Child Development: *The Foundation for Child Development Child and Youth Well-Being Index (CWI), 1975-2004, with projections for 2005,* Durham, NC, 2006, Duke University.

Gottesman MM: Healthy eating and activity together (HEAT): weapons against obesity, *J Pediatr Health Care* 17(4):210-215, 2003.

Graham EA: Economic, racial, and cultural influences on the growth and maturation of children, *Pediatr Rev* 26(8):290-294, 2005.

Green M, Palfrey JS: *Bright Futures: guidelines for health supervision of infants, children, and adolescents,* ed 2, Arlington, VA, 2002, National Center for Education in Maternal and Child Health.

Guendelman S, Pearl M: Children's ability to access and use health care, *Health Aff* 23(2):235-244, 2004.

Haveman R, Smeeding T: The role of higher education in social mobility, *The Future Child* 16(2):125-150, 2006.

Hernandez DJ: Demographic change and the life circumstances of immigrant families, *The Future Child* 14(2):17-47, 2004.

Hoyert DL et al: Annual summary of vital statistics: 2004, *Pediatrics* 117: 168-183, 2006.

Hughes DC, Ng S: Reducing health disparities among children, *The Future Child* 13(1):153-167, 2003.

The Institute of Medicine (IOM): *Primary care: America's health in a new era,* Washington DC, 1996, National Academies Press.

The Institute of Medicine (IOM): *Children's health, the nation's wealth: assessing and improving child health,* Washington DC, 2004, Institute of Medicine.

Kumanika SK, Obarzanek E: Pathways to obesity prevention: report of National Institute of Health workshops, *Obes Res* 11(10):1263-1274, 2003.

Muholland EK: Measles in the United States, 2006, *N Engl J Med* 355: 440-443, 2006.

Newacheck PW et al: The unmet health needs of America's children, *Pediatrics* 105(4):989-997, 2000.

Newacheck PW et al: Trends in private and public health insurance for adolescents, *JAMA* 291(10):1231-1237, 2004.

Northwest Federation of Community Organizations (NWFCO): *Closing the gap: solutions to race-based health disparities,* Seattle, 2005, Applied Research Center.

Ogden CL et al: Prevalence of overweight and obesity in the United States, 1999-2004, *JAMA* 295:1549-1555, 2006.

Shields MK, Behrman RE: Children of immigrant families: analysis and recommendations, *The Future Child* 14(2):4-15, 2004.

Shone LP et al: The role of race and ethnicity in the State Children's Health Insurance Program (SCHIP) in four states: are there baseline disparities, and what do they mean for SCHIP? *Pediatrics* 112(6):e521-532, 2003.

Story M et al: Obesity in American-Indian children: prevalence, consequences, and prevention, *Prev Med* 37:S3-S12, 2003.

USDHHS: *The Surgeon General's call to action to prevent and decrease overweight and obesity,* Rockville, MD, 2001, Office of the Surgeon General.

USDHHS: *Nurse practitioner primary care competencies in specialty areas: adult, family, gerontological, pediatric, and women's health,* April 2002, NONPF. Available at *www.nonpf.com/finalaug2002.pdf* (accessed Feb 15, 2007).

USDHHS: *Initiative to eliminate racial disparities in health,* 2003. Available at *www.raceandhealth.hhs.gov* (accessed June 1, 2003).

Weinick RM, Krauss NA: Racial/ethnic differences in children's access to care, *Am J Public Health* 90(11):1771-1774, 2000.

Woolf SH et al: The health impact of resolving racial disparities: an analysis of U.S. mortality data, *Am J Public Health* 94(12):2078-2081, 2004.

Child and Family Health Assessment

Catherine E. Burns and Sheila M. Kodadek

Family-centered, community-based primary care for children is recognized as the best possible practice model for providing health care services to children and their families. The family is the most influential factor in a child's life (American Academy of Pediatrics [AAP] 2003) and its functioning is totally intertwined with the child's health and well-being.

Nurse practitioners (NPs) perhaps understand this point better than any other group of primary care providers, but they, like their colleagues, face significant challenges in implementing family-centered care. At minimum, family-centered care is perceived as time consuming. In addition, families are still too often viewed from a pathology-based model borrowed from psychiatry and psychology, and primary care providers often report feeling inadequate to the task of working with the complex and often stressed families they meet in their practices. Assessment of family psychosocial risks among U.S. clinicians has been rated low according to data from the National Survey on Early Childhood Health (Bethell et al, 2004).

Delivery of family-centered care for children requires the provider to shift focus from child-as-the-unit-of-analysis to family-as-the-unit-of-analysis depending upon the problem at hand. Although the child's welfare is ultimately the goal, the family is so integral to a child's well-being that unless the family is healthy, the child cannot achieve true physical, developmental, and psychological health. Moving from child to family and back again during the assessment process is a complex task, but an essential one for providing excellent care.

This chapter presents a child assessment model that integrates some family issues and a family assessment model that is useful when greater focus on the family is needed.

The outline for assessment of children in this chapter is consistent with the organization of the entire text. Development, functional health problems, and diseases are the three domains for pediatric practice and are the major units of this book. Each chapter provides comprehensive coverage of topics that are categorized within one of those domains. Throughout the book, family is considered integral to the child's life and his or her care.

![] PEDIATRIC NURSE PRACTITIONER (PNP) ASSESSMENT COMPETENCIES

In 2002 the U.S. Department of Health and Human Services (USDHHS), Division of Nursing, published a document of NP primary care competencies (USDHHS, 2002). Representatives of all major NP organizations worked to develop competencies

for all NPs and for specialty NPs, such as pediatric nurse practitioners. These competencies serve as standards for practice, which can be used to develop curricula, test graduates for board certification, and educate the public and health care industry about the care that an NP is expected to provide. Competencies related only to assessment, decision-making, and family-centered care for NPs in general and for PNPs in particular are found in Box 2-1.

![] FOUNDATIONS FOR CHILD AND FAMILY ASSESSMENT
CHILD HEALTH ASSESSMENT

A careful, complete, and thoughtful assessment of the child's health status is absolutely essential to providing excellent primary health care. This assessment is based on knowledge of child development, family structure and functions, culture, anatomy and physiology, pathophysiology, pharmacology, health care delivery systems, communities, and standards of primary health care for children. The assessment must also be viewed through the lens of the provider's experience to allow the provider to modify perceptions and validate data on the basis of previous work. When providers analyze patient care situations, they are engaged in critical thinking. This chapter cannot teach critical thinking nor does it teach physical assessment. Rather, it provides frameworks for gathering data to facilitate expert decision-making. It is assumed that the reader knows how to do a complete physical examination and has some experience working with children and families in health care settings. It is also assumed that clinicians have the requisite knowledge in the foundation areas listed above.

When analyzing patient problems, most NPs and other providers are comfortable with classification of diseases using categories found in the *International Classification of Diseases, edition 9 revised, Clinical Modification (ICD-9-CM)* (USDHHS, 2003), including infectious, endocrine, nutritional, metabolic, immunologic, respiratory, and cardiovascular. Providers consistently record the disease diagnoses they make for problems in these body systems. One reason that providers use this classification system so easily is that the classic health history format drives decision-making into these categories. Box 2-2 on p. 15 shows this classic health history format.

The classic medical history is written to expand on the chief complaint, which is generally a physical problem. Issues such as nutrition, development, and activities of daily living are included, primarily as they relate to various diseases.

BOX 2-1   Assessment and Management Competencies for Nurse Practitioners

Items selected for this box reflect the content of this chapter—collection of the health history, completion of the physical examination, diagnostic reasoning, communication via charting and verbal reports, and communication with the patient and family to promote the caregiving role of the NP. Many other competencies that relate to other aspects of the NP's work are found in the original competencies document (USDHHS, 2002).

COMPENTENCIES: ALL NURSE PRACTITIONERS
Domain 1: Management of Patient Health and Illness Status

1. Demonstrates critical thinking and diagnostic reasoning skills in clinical decision-making.
2. Obtains a comprehensive and problem-focused health history from the patient.
3. Performs a comprehensive and problem-focused physical examination.
4. Analyzes the data collected to determine health status.
5. Formulates a problem list.
6. Assesses, diagnoses, monitors, coordinates, and manages the health and illness status of patients over time and supports the patient through the dying process.
7. Demonstrates knowledge of pathophysiology of acute and chronic diseases or conditions commonly seen in practice.
8. Communicates the patient's health status using appropriate terminology, format, and technology.
9. Applies principles of epidemiology and demography in clinical practice by recognizing populations at risk, patterns of disease, and effectiveness of prevention and intervention.
10. Uses community and public health assessment information in evaluating patient needs, initiating referrals, coordinating care, and program planning.
11. Applies theories to guide practice.
12. Applies and conducts research studies pertinent to areas of practice.
[...]
19. Orders, may perform, and interprets common screening and diagnostic tests.
20. Evaluates results of interventions using accepted outcome criteria, revises the plan accordingly, and consults and refers when needed.
21. Schedules follow-up visits to appropriately monitor patients and evaluate health and illness care.

Domain 2: The Nurse Practitioner–Patient Relationship

1. Creates a climate of mutual trust and establishes partnerships with patients.
2. Validates and verifies findings with patients.
3. Creates a relationship with patients that acknowledges their strengths and assists patients in addressing their needs.
4. Communicates a sense of "being present" with the patient and provides comfort and emotional support.
5. Evaluates the impact of life transitions on the health and illness status of patients and the impact of health and illness on patients (individuals, families, and communities).
6. Applies principles of self-efficacy and empowerment in promoting behavior change.
7. Preserves the patient's control over decision-making; assesses the patient's commitment to the jointly deter-

mined, mutually acceptable plan of care; and fosters the patient's personal responsibility for health.
8. Maintains confidentiality while communicating data, plans, and results in a manner that preserves the dignity and privacy of the patient and provides a legal record of care.
[...]
12. Evaluates patient's and caregiver's support systems.

PEDIATRIC NURSE PRACTITIONER COMPETENCIES
I. Health Promotion, Health Protection, Disease Prevention, and Treatment
A. Assessment of Health Status

1. Obtains and documents a relevant health history for children.
2. Performs age-appropriate screening for developmental and behavioral concerns, such as speech and language development, learning disabilities, and behavioral and mental health concerns.
3. Assesses the child's developmental status based on developmental theories recognizing the individual differences in temperament, reactions to selected developmental tasks and situational crises, and coping styles and strategies.
4. Identifies and analyzes factors that affect the child's growth and development, such as the following:
   Genetic background, prenatal factors, temperament, family and cultural influences, parenting style, environmental milieu (e.g., day care, school, neighborhood, community), health status, significant life events (trauma, loss, violence, etc.).
5. Adapts and performs the history and screening procedures according to the child's developmental age, behavior, and reason for contact.
6. Performs and records a complete, accurate, and systematic pediatric physical assessment.
7. Recognizes variations of normal including genetic, ethnic, physiologic, and anatomic differences.
8. Assesses for evidence of child abuse and neglect and the effects of violence on the child.
9. Analyzes the family system to identify factors that influence the health of the child and adolescent, including, but not limited to, the following:
   Parental occupation, education and developmental level, family support system, family dynamics, family values and beliefs, family management style, family stresses, social morbidities including poverty and illiteracy, management of and coping with chronic illness.
10. Assesses patient's health risks, including, but not limited to, the following:
   Developmental level, genetic and family history, immunization status, nutritional status, risk-taking behavior, environmental factors, family issues, social support.
11. Assesses patient's and family's knowledge and behavior regarding leading health indicators, including, but not limited to, the following:
   Physical activity, eating disorders, tobacco use, substance abuse, responsible sexual behavior, mental health, injury and violence, environmental quality, immunizations, access to health care.

Continued

BOX 2-1   Assessment and Management Competencies for Nurse Practitioners—Cont'd

B. Diagnosis of Health Status

The pediatric nurse practitioner (PNP) is engaged in the diagnosis of health status. This diagnostic process includes critical thinking, differential diagnosis, and the integration and interpretation of various forms of data. These competencies describe this role of the PNP.

1. Differentiates between normal and abnormal development in relation to anatomic findings, physiologic findings, motor findings, cognitive findings, psychological findings, and social behavior of the child.
2. Identifies cause, natural history, developmental considerations, pathogenesis, and clinical manifestations of common disease processes in children.
3. Identifies nutritional conditions and behavioral feeding issues.
4. Orders and interprets age- and situation-appropriate screening, laboratory tests, and other diagnostic tests, including, but not limited to, hematocrit, lead level, tuberculosis testing, ova and parasites.
5. Collaborates in the diagnosis of children with special health needs and disabilities.

C. Plan of Care and Implementation of Treatment

The objectives of planning and implementing therapeutic interventions are to return the patient to a stable state and to optimize the patient's health. These competencies describe the PNP's role in stabilizing the patient, minimizing physical and psychological complications, and maximizing the patient's health potential.

1. Promotes healthy nutritional practices, including promotion and management of breastfeeding, national nutritional programs, and nutritional intake considering food preferences and avoidance of food sensitivities.
2. Provides interventions to modify behavior associated with health risks, such as tobacco and substance use, lack of physical activity, nutritional patterns, sexual activity, and violence.
3. Refers children with developmental disabilities and chronic illnesses to appropriate community agencies and for family support and specialty care as needed.

4. Incorporates health objectives into individual educational plans (IEPs) for children with special needs.
5. Assists the parent and/or child in coping with developmental behaviors and in facilitating the child's developmental potential.
6. Manages common pediatric illnesses and conditions and behavioral problems of children.
7. Performs common primary care procedures, including, but not limited to, suturing, splinting, Papanicolaou (Pap) tests, and microscopy.
8. Develops, implements, and evaluates health maintenance and health promotion services for the child and/or family by including teaching, counseling, advising, and anticipatory guidance.
9. Activates child protective services and other resources on behalf of children at risk.
10. Prescribes drugs and other therapies, recognizing the pharmacodynamic and pharmacokinetic processes and the effects of drug selection and dosing regimens on children.
11. Collaborates in planning for transition to adult health care.
12. Applies child-centered research that contributes to positive change in the health of or the health care delivered to children.

II. Pediatric Nurse Practitioner–Patient Relationship

Competencies in this area demonstrate the personal, collegial, and collaborative approach, which enhances the PNP's effectiveness in patient care. The competencies speak to the critical importance of interpersonal transactions as they relate to therapeutic patient outcomes.

1. Adapts the PNP-patient relationship to the changing nature of the child's cognitive and psychosocial environment.
2. Communicates effectively with children of all developmental levels.
3. Communicates effectively with family members, including multigenerational family members.

Note: Competencies continue within the teaching-coaching, professional role, managing and negotiating health care delivery systems, monitoring and ensuring the quality of health care practice, and cultural competence domains.
From US Department of Health and Human Services: *Nurse practitioner competencies in specialty areas: adult, family, gerontological, pediatric, and women's health,* Rockville, MD, 2002, USDHHS.

This classification system works well and has generally been taught to physicians, NPs, and other providers. The system fails, however, to provide a framework for integrating nursing aspects of NP work into the problem list and management plan. Without that framework, NPs may fail to clearly identify and document the unique contributions they make as nurses providing primary health care. Without that identification, the special aspects of their work with patients remain invisible.

An alternate model is offered in this chapter that integrates the nursing and medical aspects of NP work conceptually and clinically (see Box 2-4 discussed later). This assessment model (Burns, 1991a, 1992a, 1992b) is based on the assumption that patient problems can be grouped into three distinct domains: developmental problems, functional health problems, and diseases (Box 2-3). Although it was originally developed for NPs, the framework is useful to all pediatric health care providers.

The pediatric health history has several unique aspects. First, the participants in the conversation include more than just the patient and provider. Second, the topics emphasized vary significantly depending on the child's developmental stage. Third, the process of communication with the child and the extent to which he or she is involved with health care decisions varies with his or her age.

BOX 2-2	The Classic Health History

I. Patient identifying information: name, birth date, sex, address, record number, and name of historian, along with relationship to the patient stated
II. Chief complaint (CC)
III. History of present illness (HPI)
IV. Past medical history (PMH)
  A. Prenatal, natal, postnatal
  B. Past illnesses
  C. Allergies
  D. Accidents
  E. Hospitalizations
  F. Immunization history
  G. Nutrition history
  H. Growth
  I. Development
V. Review of systems (ROS): as found in disease domain database described previously with the following added:
  A. Psychological—colic, breath-holding, thumb sucking, head banging, fears, tics, behavior disorders, temper tantrums, nail biting, hair pulling, masturbation. Adjustment to home, school, neighborhood. Temperament—activity level, predictability, moods, intensity of reactions, adaptability, initial responses, distractibility. Sleep—amount, habits, problems
VI. Family history (FH)
VII. Socioeconomic (SE)
  A. Occupations of father and mother
  B. Time spent with child by parents, activities together
  C. Finances—adequacy
  D. Persons in the home
  E. House or apartment living arrangements
  F. General relationship of family members
  G. Community support systems—friends, church, agencies involved with family

Developmental Problems

This domain includes the long-term issues of development and maturation over the life span. In pediatrics, developmental issues are prominent. Failing to identify a developmental problem or to plan for its management is as serious as missing diabetes mellitus or a dislocated hip. Both physical and developmental problems can affect the child's entire future if not remedied or managed to minimize their effects. Clinicians assess for developmental problems in the areas of gross motor, fine motor, speech and language, cognitive, and social and adaptive behaviors. Developmental surveillance is considered integral to every pediatrics visit (AAP, 2006). A recent study, however, found that developmental assessments were completed for only 57% of children 10 to 35 months old (Halfon et al, 2004).

Functional Health Problems

Functional health problems are derived from Gordon's functional health patterns (Gordon, 1987) and are used by the nursing diagnosis association, NANDA International,

in their taxonomy of nursing diagnoses (NANDA, 2007). These patterns provide a way of thinking about the problems that nurses have always managed independently. They represent the universal health behavior patterns of all humans, regardless of culture, sex, age, or economic status. Gordon's 11 patterns include health beliefs and behavior, nutrition, elimination, activity, sleep, role relationships, coping, self-perception, cognition and perception, sexuality, and values and beliefs. Nursing's primary mission is management of problems related to these patterns to maximize a person's health. In hospital settings, nurses help patients eat or receive nutrition, facilitate sleep, promote coping with illness, and maximize activity (even if only rolling a comatose patient from side to side). In primary care, NPs are also concerned with these issues, although their management strategies differ with the nature and complexity of the problem. All functional health problems involve the family since the family really is the primary caregiver for infants and children. NPs and other providers become involved when the family's knowledge and experience are insufficient to meet the needs of the child or when the family directly contributes to the child's problems as with the role-relationship problem of child abuse.

Labels for the problems in the functional health domain are derived primarily from the NANDA taxonomy terms (NANDA, 2007). The NANDA taxonomy is expanded and updated every 2 years. It was first developed in the 1980s and thus represents a taxonomy of phenomena in its early stages which is important to nursing as compared, for instance, with the taxonomy for disease diagnoses which is more than 100 years old. Diagnoses can be statements of health, health risks, or health problems.

Diseases

Diseases are conditions assessed and managed at the tissue or organ level of analysis. The diagnoses found in the disease domain generally come from the ICD-9-CM and from some NANDA physiologic diagnoses. Otitis media, streptococcal pharyngitis, and appendicitis are examples of disease diagnoses. It is not expected that NPs use nursing diagnosis language for traditional disease diagnoses. For example, "seborrheic dermatitis" would not be called "alteration in skin integrity."

The *International Classification of Diseases* is designed to represent the phenomena of concern to physicians. It is broad and mature in scope. It represents physiologic problems of patients extremely well, but includes few labels, or rubrics, for the behavioral, social, and developmental problems that NPs also manage. The ICD-9-CM listings are recognized by many insurance carriers for billing purposes and, as such, have become the "currency" for much health care delivery in the U.S., whereas the NANDA nursing diagnoses have not yet achieved that recognition. Fortunately, a variety of diagnoses similar to those in the NANDA classification can be found among the medical listings, thus facilitating reimbursement for nursing aspects of NP work.

BOX 2-3   Integrated Classification System of Diagnoses for Use by Nurse Practitioners

Domain I: Development Diagnoses
Cognitive development
  Cognitive delay
  Learning disorder
Language development
  Language delay
  Speech delay
Motor development
  Gross motor delay
  Fine motor delay
Social development
  Social development delay
  Attachment failure

Domain II: Functional Health Diagnoses
Health perception and health management pattern
  Adjustment impaired
  Decisional conflict
  Health maintenance alteration
  Health-seeking behavior
  Home-care resources inadequate
  Home-maintenance management impaired
  Knowledge deficits
  Noncompliance
  Risk of injury–suffocation, poisoning, trauma, aspiration
  Self-care deficits, dressing, toileting, hygiene
  Skill deficit
  Therapeutic regimen management ineffective–individual
    or family
Nutritional-metabolic pattern
  Anorexia
  Anorexia nervosa
  Breastfeeding ineffective or interrupted or effective
  Bulimia
  Colic
  Infant-feeding pattern ineffective
  Nausea
  Nutrition alterations < > body requirements
  Swallowing impaired
Elimination pattern
  Constipation
  Encopresis
  Enuresis
  Incontinence, bowel or urinary
Activity and exercise pattern
  Activity intolerance
  Diversional activities deficit
  Fatigue
  Physical mobility impaired
Sleep pattern
  Sleep pattern disturbance
Cognitive and perceptual pattern
  Attention-deficit disorder
  Disorganized infant behavior
  Memory impaired
  Potential for enhanced organized infant behavior
  Sensory-perceptual alteration
    Blind
    Deaf

Self-perception and self-concept pattern
  Body image disturbance
  Depression
  Personal identity disturbance
  Self-esteem disturbance, chronic or situational
Role relationships pattern
  Abuse
  Caregiver role strain
  Communication impaired–verbal
  Family coping ineffective, disabling, compromised, potential
    for growth
  Family process alteration
  Family process alteration: alcoholism
  Loneliness, risk for
  Parenting alteration
  Parental role conflict
  Risk of alteration in parent-infant-child attachment
  Role performance alteration
  Social interaction impaired
  Social isolation
Sexuality pattern
  Pregnancy
  Sexual dysfunction
  Sexual pattern alteration
Coping and stress tolerance pattern
  Anxiety
  Comfort alteration
  Coping, individual, ineffective, defensive
  Fear
  Grieving, anticipatory, dysfunctional
  Hopelessness
  Ineffective denial
  Pain, chronic pain
  Posttrauma response
  Powerlessness
  Rape-trauma response
  Self-mutilation risk
  Substance misuse
  Violence potential, self or others
Values and beliefs pattern
  Potential for enhanced spiritual well-being
  Spiritual distress

**Domain III: Pediatric Disease Diagnoses (Diagnoses
included are examples, not an exhaustive list.)**
Infectious diseases
  Candidiasis
  Chickenpox
  Chlamydia
  Diarrheal infection
  Giardiasis
  Gonorrhea
  Herpes simplex
  Haemophilus influenza
  Infection, potential for
  Influenza
  Measles
  Mumps
  Parasites

BOX 2-3   Integrated Classification System of Diagnoses for Use by Nurse Practitioners—Cont'd

Roseola
Scabies
Staphylococcus
Streptococcus
Tuberculosis
Viral hepatitis
Warts
Endocrine, nutritional, metabolic, and immune diseases
　Diabetes mellitus
　Fluid volume excess
　Fluid volume deficit
　Food allergy
　Immune deficiency disease
　Thyroid disorders
Diseases of blood and blood-forming organs
　Anemias and red blood cell disorders
　Jaundice
　Leukemia and white blood cell disorders
　Platelet disorders
Neurologic and sense organ diseases
　Central nervous system–epilepsy or seizures, cerebral palsy
　Ear–otitis externa, otitis media, serous otitis
　Eye–amblyopia, conjunctivitis, dacryocystitis, myopia, strabismus
Circulatory system diseases
　Cardiac output decreased
　Congenital heart disease
Respiratory system diseases
　Acute nasopharyngitis
　Airway clearance ineffective
　Allergic rhinitis
　Asthma
　Bronchiolitis
　Croup
　Pharyngitis
　Pneumonia
　Tonsillitis
Digestive system diseases
　Acute abdomen
　Constipation (not encopresis)
　Diarrhea
　Gastroesophageal reflux disease
　Hernia
　Swallowing impaired
　Vomiting
Dental disorders
　Caries
　Dentition impairment

Malocclusion
Oral mucous membrane alteration
Genitourinary system disorders
　Adhesions
　Cryptorchidism
　Hydrocele
　Hypospadias
　Incontinence
　Urinary tract infection
　Urinary elimination alteration
　Urinary retention
Gynecologic disorders
　Menstrual disorder
　Vaginitis
Skin diseases
　Acne
　Atopic dermatitis
　Cellulitis
　Congenital lesion
　Contact dermatitis
　Folliculitis
　Impetigo
　Nevus
　Seborrhea
　Urticaria
Musculoskeletal diseases
　Developmental dislocated hip
　Genu varum or valgum
　Internal tibial torsion
　Lordosis
　Metatarsus adductus
　Osgood-Schlatter disease
　Scoliosis
　Strain or sprain
Symptoms, signs, ill-defined conditions
　Hypotonia
　Jaundice
　Lack of physiologic maturity
　Temperature alteration–hypothermia, hyperthermia
Injury and poisoning
　Abrasion
　Bee sting
　Burn
　Contusion
　Corneal abrasion
　Fracture
　Insect bite
　Sprain or strain
　Injury, high risk for

Data from Burns C: Development and content validity testing of a comprehensive classification of diagnoses for use by pediatric nurse practitioners, *Nurs Diagn* 2:93-104, 1991; and Burns C: *Development and content validity testing of a comprehensive classification of diagnoses for use by pediatric nurse practitioners,* unpublished doctoral dissertation, University of Oregon, Eugene, OR, 1989.

Problem Interactions

The concept of interactions of problems across domains is important to understand. For instance, iron deficiency anemia can be considered a disease if looked at from the effects of lack of iron on heme production, red blood cells, oxygen transport, and cellular metabolism. The clinician can diagnose this disease and prescribe an iron supplement to manage the problem at this physiologic level. However, if the problem is found to be related to a lack of iron in the diet, the NP can choose to intervene at the functional health-nutrition level, call the problem "nutrition: less than body requirements for iron," and teach the family how to increase the selection of iron-rich foods for the table. Iron deficiency has also been shown to cause developmental delays (Glader, 2004). If a goal for the visit is to provide additional support in the school setting, a developmental problem would be diagnosed.

A particular domain can also serve as the context for the problem in another area. For instance, Down syndrome, a chromosomal disorder, can be the cause or context for a cognitive development problem. If the intervention is for cognition, a developmental problem of cognitive delay is listed. Content issues for which the clinician is planning interventions are the diagnoses. The contextual issues are not the diagnoses.

The most important point to remember is that interventions must be based on or derived from diagnoses. A situation should never arise in which the provider intervenes without explicit reasons for doing so. The reasons are stated as diagnoses, either actual or potential, and enumerated in the problem list. The preventive work (i.e., to avoid potential problems) done by clinicians also needs to be identified. Diagnoses, in addition to interventions, must be recorded.

FAMILY ASSESSMENT

The Family's Role in Health Care of Children

However daunting the perceived barriers to family-centered care, investing in family assessment and management is essential in contemporary pediatric primary care practice. Duffy (1988) wrote that understanding family health promotion begins with understanding family dynamics. Research has repeatedly demonstrated that a mother's level of education, her beliefs and attitudes about health, and her own health practices have a significant influence on the health status of her children. Mothers' depression also affects children's receipt of health care, among other things (Minkovitz et al, 2005). As fathers become increasingly involved in their children's health care, questions about relationships between characteristics of fathers and family health behavior are being raised. Fathers, too, need to be involved with the health care of their children (Garfield & Isacco, 2006). It is not surprising that parents who believe that they can improve their health status by practicing health promotion behavior tend to raise children who share similar beliefs.

Research has provided definitive evidence that children, from birth through adolescence, need nurturing and attention from the significant adults in their lives. These significant adults most often are the child's birth or adoptive parents, but they may also be grandparents, extended family members, or foster parents. Evidence is strong that when children are raised without this consistent, affectionate attention and without sensitive interactions with a caring adult, the results can be devastating for both the child and society (Belsky et al, 2001). In contrast, when a parent or another significant adult responds consistently and sensitively to a child's needs, such as a need to play, to eat, to sleep, to be comforted, or to be left alone, the child is likely to grow up competent to initiate and build strong, nurturing relationships.

Although inadequate or poor parenting is linked in the literature to factors such as poverty, substance abuse, and minimal education, research suggests that a poor "fit" between a child and a significant adult can occur in any family, including those in which the adults are well educated, socially competent, and economically successful (Perry & Pollard, 1998). For example, parents who value competition and athletic success may be a good parenting fit with a daughter who is star of her soccer team. However, they may not be able to connect with their younger son who prefers reading to sports and avoids competition in all forms.

Family assessment begins with the assumption that families are central to and inseparable from the health of children. It is based on a family health promotion framework that assumes that the vast majority of family members are competent, want to do what is best for their children, and desire to be active participants in their children's health care. Family assessment in primary care practice with children requires attention to family structure, family life cycle stage, family functioning, and social network. In other words, a basic family assessment addresses characteristics of the family, transitions that the family is experiencing, how family members interact and get things done, what they believe and value, and how they interact with the community.

It is important to recognize that providers' own definitions of family and healthy family functioning are culturally and temporally bound, determine who is and who is not family, and can profoundly affect assessment, treatment, and outcomes. Providers might find it useful to periodically examine their own assumptions and beliefs regarding families and use the knowledge gained to foster increased sensitivity and openness to the rich diversity that their clients present.

Legal definitions of *family* usually address bonds of blood, marriage, and adoption. A significant number of contemporary families do not fit such restrictive definitions. To address this reality, Whall (1986) defined *family* as "a self-identified group of two or more individuals whose association is characterized by special terms, who may or may not be related by bloodlines or law, but who function in such a way that they consider themselves to be a family." Wherever practitioners' personal definitions might fall on a continuum of inclusiveness, it is imperative that they know and understand the implications of that definition in practice.

Family Structure and Roles

Assessment of a family's structure and roles includes the composition of the family or household, demographic data, intergenerational data, and information about family roles. Implicit in the data is the way the family defines itself and how the family gets its work done.

Families come in many forms today, including two-parent families, single-parent families, families headed by grandparents or other family members, blended families or stepfamilies, foster families, and others. Specific issues are addressed for these and other forms in the section on targeted assessments later in this chapter and in Chapter 18.

Family Life Cycle

Family life cycle assessment includes data on the present family life cycle stage (such as a family with young children), family life cycle transitions or developmental crises (such as serious illness of a frail, elderly grandparent), and family life cycle events that are untimely or "out of sync" (such as the terminal illness of a young wife and mother).

Family Functioning

Healthy family functioning should result in what Terkelsen, in his classic paper, called the "good-enough family" (Terkelsen, 1980). Families have both strengths and limitations, but the majority of families are able to meet most of their members' needs most of the time. This is a hopeful stance, one that allows for the less than perfect family to feel successful and empowered.

Characteristics of healthy family functioning have been identified by a number of researchers, and lists of characteristics differ. For example, deChesnay (1986) used an extensive research literature review to identify healthy families as those characterized by open communication, mutual respect and support, differentiation, shared problem-solving, shared decision-making, flexibility, and enhancement of personal growth of members. Additions to that list might include a sense of play and humor and a shared value of service to others (Curran, 1983). The American Academy of Pediatrics (AAP) states that the child will thrive best when cared for by two mutually committed parents who respect and support one another, who have adequate social and financial resources, and who both are actively engaged in the child's upbringing. Characteristics of the successful family are described by the AAP as being cohesive, enduring, and mutually appreciative. Such families communicate effectively and often, adapt to changing circumstances, spend time together, are committed to the family, and embrace a common religious or spiritual orientation (AAP, 2003).

Family Social Network

The family's social network includes those persons, activities, agencies, and institutions that have the potential to support, harm, or drain energy from the family. Assessing the family's relationships with extended family, friends, and the community provides information on which to base recommendations and further assessment.

THE ENVIRONMENT FOR DATA COLLECTION

Health care is a family event in pediatrics, and pediatric primary health care is delivered in many settings, not just examination rooms in outpatient clinics. Wherever the patient and the family are to be cared for, privacy must be ensured. People should have places to sit down, and the room in which the examination is conducted should be well lighted and allow the patient to lie down comfortably. The examiner must be able to work comfortably, too. The environment must be safe, given the developmental ages of the children to be cared for, and should present an atmosphere of warmth and welcome. All those in the room need to be addressed by name at one time or another.

The health care provider should sit down during the history to make data collection a conversation, to equalize the status of clients and examiner, and to help clients feel that they have time to talk. Sitting also helps the provider conserve energy for a busy day.

For young children, the conversation time gives them the opportunity to become familiar with the examiner and setting, which is essential for cooperation when needed. Remember that young children are learning the "script" for health care visits. The visit should help them learn a script that is understandable and not too stressful. When the script is to be varied (e.g., no immunizations this visit), alert them to the change with cues and explanations for the new experiences of this visit and the likelihood that the new script will be repeated at future visits.

The provider is also observing parent-child interactions during the visit. For example, are the parents responding to their baby? Do the parents contribute to the school-age child's self-esteem? Cues to mental health problems in any family member or the child should be addressed.

For adolescents, the history can be started with the parents and teen together; however, they then need to separate, with the provider getting information from the parents and the teen independently. Interviewing teens requires patience as they are learning to take responsibility for their own health care. Interactions will change as teens mature developmentally or as the situation is modified (Cottrell et al, 2006).

Data can be collected verbally, through record review, via written forms completed by the family, or through a combination of these methods. It might not be practical for data to be fully collected on the first visit; rather the collection can be staged according to the visit priorities. When time with patients is limited, it is common to ask new families to come early for their first appointment to complete a written history before meeting the clinician. Notation of any missing data should be made so that further baseline data can be collected at the next visit.

Since more than 9.7 million children speak a language other than English in the home (Annie E. Casey Foundation, 2006), interpreter services must be available if the clinician and family are not fluent in each other's languages. These services are mandated by law. Use of family members as interpreters is not recommended. Family members may try to protect the patient by hiding important information. Legally the provider may be at risk if information was not transmitted correctly or completely either to or from the clinician (Lehna, 2005).

■■■ THE DATABASE
THE CHILD HEALTH HISTORY

It is said that 80% of diagnoses are made on the basis of the history. The physical examination only provides a partial view of the situation as it is at the moment. It is often a cloudy picture because the body frequently responds similarly to different assaults. It is the history of the problem—its onset, duration, progress, associated symptoms, meaning, and effects on daily living—that brings the health care provider to an understanding in sufficient depth to choose appropriate management. Functional health and developmental problems present the same issues for the provider. A thorough, thoughtful history is essential.

The database described in this chapter summarizes the child health history and physical examination and the family assessment. The model presented uses a basic problem-oriented format that begins with subjective data (the history), moves to objective data (the physical examination, laboratory, and test data), then lists the problems by domain (identified through the subjective and objective data), and finally, plans care, problem by problem (Box 2-4). The items listed under each topic are suggestions; they are not required data to obtain from every patient. As children age, the emphasis will change (e.g., less time spent on birth and infancy histories). The history needs to be individualized, considering family, culture, health status, and environment. The complete format should be mastered so that it becomes core to the provider's approach to all patient situations. If data are omitted, the omissions should be by choice, not by an error committed through haste, distraction, ignorance, or habit.

The adolescent history needs special modification because adolescents' health care needs, risks, and developmental characteristics are so different from those of infants and young children and because they are interviewed directly. See Box 2-5 for a modification of the initial health history for adolescents.

BOX 2-4 **Problem–Oriented Health Record With Consideration of Disease, Functional Health, and Development Domains**

I. Preliminary Information
 Date:
 Name:
 Birth date:
 Record no.:
 Corrected age for preterm infant younger than 2 yr:
 Caregiver's name:
 Address:
 Phone:
 Informant, relationship to patient, reliability as historian:
 Referral source:

II. Database: Subjective Information–Child and Family
 A. Chief complaints (CC) child or family
  1. Concern #1:
   History of present illness (HPI):
  2. Concern #2:
   HPI:
 B. Disease history database–child
  1. Past medical history
   a. Prenatal:
   b. Perinatal—birth weight, length, head circumference, delivery, and postpartum course
   c. Past disease profile:
   d. Current health problems (put in table below):

Diagnosis	Date	Provider	Current status
1.			
2.			
3.			

   e. Operations and hospitalizations:
   f. Injuries:
   g. Allergies–food, environmental, medications:
   h. Growth:
   i. Immunizations:
   j. Medications:
  2. Review of systems
   General:
   Skin:
   Head:
   EENT:
   Respiratory:
   Cardiovascular:

   GU:
   GI:
   Musculoskeletal:
   Neurologic:
   Endocrine:
   Hematologic:
   Dental:
  3. Family history of diseases
   Mother, father (age, health):
   Mother's pregnancy history:
   Familial diseases:
   Pedigree for single disease genetics history, if appropriate to explain genetic transmission in family or health of various family members:
  4. Environmental history
   Air quality, tobacco smoke
   Water quality
   Exposures to soils with toxins, pesticides, or heavy metals
   Food-borne exposures
   Noise exposure
 C. Functional health problems database–child
  1. Health maintenance and health perceptions
   Primary care provider: Last visit:
   Dentist: Last visit:
   Knowledge and skills for caregiving and self-care:
   Safety measures:
    Car:
    Smoke alarms:
    Occupational and pesticides and poisons:
    Guns locked:
   Sports equipment:
   Home and health management and resource issues:
  2. Nutrition
   Diet—breakfast, lunch, dinner:
   Supplements:
   Feeding strategies and patterns:
   Restrictions–calories, other:
  3. Activities
   Amount and type of activities:
   Play:
   Limitations and equipment:

BOX 2-4 **Problem-Oriented Health Record With Consideration of Disease, Functional Health, and Development Domains—Cont'd**

4. Sleep
   Number of hours–night, naps:
   Disturbances:
5. Elimination
   Urinary:
   Bowel:
6. Role relationships
   Family patterns:
   Parenting patterns:
   Peers and social support:
   Communication–verbal, nonverbal:
7. Coping and temperament and discipline
   Substance use and abuse–alcohol, drugs, tobacco:
      Indicators of depression, anxiety, mental health disorders:
8. Cognitive and perceptual problems
   Cognitive disturbances and school performance:
   Hearing deficit:
   Vision deficit:
   Kinesthetic disturbance:
   Attention deficits and hyperactivity:
9. Self-perception and self-concept
   Role identity:
   Self-concept and self-esteem, body image:
10. Sexual and menstrual patterns
11. Values, beliefs, and religious patterns

D. Developmental issues database–past milestones and current skills of child
1. Motor development:
   Gross motor development:
   Fine motor development:
2. Language development:
3. Cognitive development:
4. Social development:
5. Development test scores:

E. Family contextual information:
1. Family structure and roles
   People living in the home:
   Type of family–two-parent, single-parent, divorced, family, etc:
2. Family functioning: primary caregiver
   Family care issues (time, energy, needs of other family members, emotional stresses):
3. Family social network: agencies involved with family, support systems
4. Family environment and resources:
   Home environment description, day care
   School and employment

III. Database: Objective Information
   A. Physical examination
Age: Sex: Height: Weight:
HC: BP: TPR: BMI:

1. General appearance:
2. Skin:
3. Head:
4. Eyes:
5. Ears:
6. Nose:
7. Mouth:
8. Neck:
9. Chest and breasts:
10. Lungs:
11. Heart:
12. Abdomen:
13. Genitalia:
14. Anus and rectum:
15. Musculoskeletal:
16. Neurologic
    Motor—tone, strength:
    Reflexes:
    Primitive reflexes:
    Cranial nerves:
    Responsiveness:
    Extraneous movements:
    Gait and position:
    Cerebellar, including coordination, balance, nystagmus:
    Sensory function:

B. Screening and laboratory data
1. Hct and Hgb:
2. Hearing:
3. Vision:
4. TB:
5. Metabolic and newborn screens:
6. Other:

C. Data from other disciplines
Physical therapy, occupational therapy, speech therapy, audiology, social work, psychology, medical specialties, home health, education:

IV. Problem List (Use classification of diagnoses list.)
Include all CCs and problems identified during the assessment. Categorize diagnoses by the following:
1. Diseases:
2. Functional health problems:
3. Developmental problems:
4. Family problems

V. Plan
For each problem, describe plans, including diagnostic, therapeutic, and educational activities:
A. Disease problems:
B. Functional health problems:
C. Developmental problems:
D. Family problems:

VI. Disposition and Return Appointments and Purpose:

BP, Blood pressure; *EENT,* eyes, ears, nose, throat; *GI,* gastrointestinal; *GU,* genitourinary; *HC,* head circumference; *Hct,* hematocrit; *Hgb,* hemoglobin; *TB,* tuberculosis; *TPR,* temperature, pulse, respirations; *BMI,* body mass index.
Adapted from Burns C: A new assessment model and tool for nurse practitioners, *Pediatr Health Care* 6:76-79, 1992a.

BOX 2-5   **Problem-Oriented History for Adolescents**

I. Database–subjective information

A. Contextual and family information
1. With whom do you live?
2. In the past year, have there been any changes in your immediate family, such as:
   Marriage, separation, divorce
   Serious illness or injury
   Loss of job
   Move or change of address
   Change of school
   Births, deaths
   Other (explain):
3. What languages are spoken in your home?

B. Chief complaint

C. Past medical history
1. In the past year, have you had any injury or illness that made you miss school or cut down on activities, or that required medical care?
2. Have you been hospitalized in the past year?
3. Do you have any illnesses or medical conditions?
4. Are you taking any medications?
5. Have you been exposed to tuberculosis in the past year?
6. Have you stayed overnight in a homeless shelter, jail, or detention center in the past year?
7. Girls only: Have you had a period? Date of last one. Do you do breast self-examinations?
   Boys only: Have you had wet dreams? Do you do testicular self-examinations?

D. Review of systems
1. Do you have any questions or concerns about any of the following?
   Height or weight
   Blood pressure
   Headaches and migraines
   Eyes or vision
   Hearing, ears or earaches
   Nose
   Frequent colds
   Mouth and teeth (frequency of tooth brushing, flossing)
   Neck and back
   Chest pain
   Coughing and wheezing
   Breasts
   Heart
   Stomach
   Nausea and vomiting
   Diarrhea and constipation
   Skin (rash, acne, sore, use of sunscreen)
   Muscle or joint pain
   Frequent or painful urination
   Sexual organs or genitals
   Menstruation or periods
   Sexual activity
   Future plans or job
   Physical or sexual abuse
   Masturbation
   Cancer or dying
   Other (explain):

II. Functional health database

A. Health maintenance and health perception
1. Do you usually wear a helmet for rollerblade, bicycle, skateboard, motorcycle, or all-terrain vehicle use?
2. Do you usually wear a seat belt when riding in a car, truck, or van?
3. In the past year, have you been in a car when the driver has been drinking or using drugs?
4. Do you use electric tools or heavy equipment at work or home?
5. Do you have questions or concerns about preventing accidents or injuries?

B. Nutrition
1. Do you eat from the four food groups almost every day?
2. Do you have any diet, food, or appetite concerns?
3. Are you eating in secret?
4. Are you satisfied with your eating patterns?
5. Do you prefer a change in your current weight?
6. Have you tried to lose weight or control weight by vomiting, taking diet pills or laxatives, or starving yourself?
7. Do you have concerns about your weight?

C. Activities
1. Do you watch television or play video games more than 2 hours per day?
2. Are you involved with exercises that make you sweat and breathe hard at least 3 times per week?
3. What do you do after school?
4. Do you have physical problems that limit your exercise?
5. Do you have questions or concerns about exercise or physical activity?

D. Sleep
1. Do you have trouble sleeping?
2. Do you have trouble with tiredness?

E. Elimination habits
1. Do you sometimes wet the bed?

F. Role relationships
1. Do you have at least one friend you really like and feel you can talk to?
2. Do parents or guardian usually listen to you and take your feelings seriously?
3. Do you and your parents or guardian do things together on a regular basis, such as eating meals, attending religious activities, performing chores or errands, playing sports, or watching television?
4. Is there a lot of tension or conflict in your home?
5. Do you have questions or concerns about family or friends?

G. Coping and temperament and discipline
1. Alcohol
   In the past year, did you or friends get drunk or very high on alcoholic beverages?
   Have you ever consumed alcohol and then done any of the following: driven a vehicle, gone swimming or boating, gotten in a fight, used tools or equipment, done something you later regretted?
   Have you been criticized or gotten in trouble because of drinking?
   Do you have any questions or concerns about alcohol?

BOX 2-5   **Problem-Oriented History for Adolescents—Cont'd**

2. Drugs

Do you or your friends ever use marijuana or street drugs?

Some drugs can be bought at a store without a physician's prescription. Do you ever use nonprescription drugs to get to sleep, stay awake, calm down, get high, or enhance your sports performance?

Have you ever used steroids without a physician telling you to do so?

Do you have any questions or concerns about drugs or drug use?

3. Tobacco

Do you or your friends ever smoke cigarettes or use smokeless tobacco?

Does anyone you live with smoke cigarettes or use smokeless tobacco?

Do you have any questions or concerns about cigarettes or other tobacco products?

4. Emotions

Have you had fun during the past 2 weeks?

In general are you happy with the way things are going for you these days?

During the past few weeks, have you often felt sad or down with nothing to look forward to?

Have you ever seriously thought about killing yourself, made a plan to kill yourself, or actually tried to kill yourself?

Do you think counseling would help you or someone in your family?

Do you have any questions or concerns about physical, sexual, or emotional abuse?

5. Weapons and violence

Do you or does anyone you live with have a gun, rifle, shotgun, or other firearm in your home?

In the past year, have you ever carried a gun, knife, razor blade, club, or other weapon?

Have you been in a physical fight during the past 3 months?

Are guns or violence a problem in your neighborhood?

Have you ever witnessed a violent act?

When you are angry, do you ever get violent?

Do you have any questions or concerns about violence or your safety?

H. Cognitive and perceptual problems

1. In general do you like school? Why?
2. Are your grades this year better on worse than the year before? What are your usual grades?
3. Have you ever had to repeat a grade in school?
4. Do you cut classes or skip school?
5. How many days of school have you missed this year?
6. Have you ever been suspended or dropped out of school?
7. Do you have any questions or concerns about school or your learning?

I. Self-perception and self-concept

1. Do you have any concerns about the size or shape of your body or your physical appearance?
2. What do you like about yourself?

3. What do you do best?
4. If you could, what would you change about your life or yourself?

J. Sexual and menstrual

1. Do you date?
2. Do you or your friends have sexual intercourse or oral or anal sex?
3. Do you think you might be gay, lesbian, or bisexual?
4. Have you ever been told that you have a sexually transmitted disease, such as gonorrhea, genital herpes, chlamydia, trichomonas, syphilis, hepatitis, genital warts, AIDS, or HIV infection?
5. Do you have any questions or concerns about sex or relationships?
6. Are you worried about getting pregnant (girls) or do you worry about getting someone pregnant (boys)?
7. Have you ever been forced to do something sexual that you did not want to do?
8. Do you practice abstinence?
9. Do you use a birth control method? If so, which one(s)?
10. Do you want information or supplies to prevent pregnancy or sexually transmitted diseases, including HIV?

K. Values and beliefs and religious

1. Are you involved with any religious groups or activities on a regular basis?
2. Do you have any strong ethical, moral, or religious beliefs?

III. Development database

Throughout the history, listen for data that allow you to assess the following areas (see Chapter 8):

A. Motor development

1. All teens should be active and skilled in a variety of physical activities and sports.
2. Fine motor development should also be mature. Special arts or crafts or occupational activities may be learned.

B. Cognitive development

1. Early adolescents are still concrete and generally present rather than future oriented. Questions can be answered quite literally.
2. Middle adolescents can use and understand if-then statements. They are able to understand long-term consequences and think of the future. They might challenge many ideas and rules with their newfound skills in logic and reasoning.
3. Late adolescents are able to consider options before making decisions, engage in sophisticated moral reasoning, and use principles to guide their decisions.

C. Social development

1. Early adolescents are egocentric in thinking. They can vacillate between childish and mature behavior, especially around their parents. Their peers are usually of the same sex. Group activities are the norm.

Continued

BOX 2-5   **Problem-Oriented History for Adolescents—Cont'd**

2. Middle adolescents are concerned with their identity within society and less concerned with their sexual identity unless they are struggling with recognizing their homosexuality. They tend to distance themselves from parents, spend less time at home, and increasingly challenge parental control. Cliques or friends prevail, with only a few close friends. Physical intimacy can occur during this stage, and romantic partners are common.
3. Late adolescents have distanced themselves from parents and then reestablished relationships with family on a new basis of independence. Romantic, emotional intimacy appears.

D. School and vocational development
1. Early adolescents are usually adjusting to the expectations of middle school. Setting priorities and completing homework independently can be a challenge. Future goals are often unrealistic and change frequently.
2. Middle adolescents are entering high school and beginning to develop an awareness that their performance in school will affect their future options for work or college. They do not usually have specific ideas about future vocations in mind.
3. Late adolescents are making decisions about vocations, college, working, or entering the military.

Adapted from American Medical Association, Department of Adolescent Health: *Guidelines for adolescent preventive services (GAPS) user's manual,* Chicago, 1994, American Medical Association.

The Initial (Complete) Health History

Patient Identifying Information.   Data here are standard to medical records: date, name, medical record number, birth date, sex, address, phone number, and names of other family members. Information about the informant is designed to give the reader a sense of the probability that the history is accurate, complete, and from a knowledgeable source.

The Database-Subjective Information
Chief Complaint and History of Present Problem

- *Concerns:* The health care visit should begin with open-ended questions to allow child and family to voice their concerns. What brings the child to the clinic today? The chief complaint is a brief statement of the problem and its duration. Remember that new concerns can arise at any point during the visit. Agendas can be hidden or unconscious. The chief complaint or complaints can involve disease, the functional health pattern, or development, and the problem may lie primarily with either the child or family.
- *Present problem history:* For each concern, a chronologic description should be made that includes a symptom analysis (i.e., onset, duration, characteristics or symptoms, exposure to illnesses or other causative factors, similar problems in other family members or neighbors, previous episodes of similar illnesses or symptoms, previous diagnostic measures, pertinent negative data, things that have been tried in attempts to manage the concern and their success, and the meaning of the concern for the family and child).

Disease Domain Database
1. **Past medical history:**
   - *Prenatal:* Planned pregnancy? When did prenatal care begin? What was the mother's health during pregnancy? Drug, alcohol, and tobacco use? Illnesses and medications? Weight gain? Accidents? (With age and history of a healthy baby, these sections may become less significant.)
   - *Perinatal:* Where was the baby born and who delivered the infant? Duration and process of labor? Vaginal or cesarean delivery and process? Infant response to labor and

delivery (breathing, crying)? Resuscitation needed? Apgar scores? Birth weight, length, and head circumference? Gestational age? Neonatal course: Infections or other health problems, physiologic stabilization, feeding, responsiveness? Jaundice? Weight at discharge? Hospital duration? Neonatal follow-up over the first few weeks? (Again, with age and health, this section is given less attention.)

- *Past disease profile:* What health problems has the child experienced, and what have the outcomes been? Who has provided care? Infectious diseases?
- *Other current health problems (not related to the chief complaint):* What problems does the child have now? What was the date of onset? Who is the principal health care provider for each problem, and what is the current status (e.g., medications, awaiting surgery, problem in remission)?
- *Operations, hospitalizations, emergency department visits:* Has the child been hospitalized for any reason? Why, when, where, outcomes? Response to hospitalization? Problems resolved? Emergency department visits? Why, when, and outcomes?
- *Injuries:* What significant injuries has the child experienced? What care was needed, was care sought at emergency department(s), and does the child currently have any sequelae?
- *Allergies:* Allergies to foods, medications, or environmental factors? How are the allergies manifested? What care is given?
- *Growth:* What has the child's growth pattern for height, weight, and head circumference been? (Always plot growth data and body mass index [BMI] on a growth grid to assess progress.) Is the child similar in size to peers? Are clothing sizes changing? Has growth been a worry for the child or family?
- *Immunizations and laboratory tests:* Obtain a record with dates for all immunizations received in the past. Reactions? Blood tests and screening tests?
- *Medications:* Is the child taking any medications (prescription drugs, over-the-counter agents, or folk remedies)? What? Why? How much? Responses to the medication?

2. **Review of systems:** Remember that this section documents the history of body systems, not the physical assessment findings. The goal is to seek information about all the body systems that may be related to the present problem or the patient's general health status.
   - *General*: Is the child considered to be well, happy, and developing normally?
   - *Skin:* History of birthmarks, lesions, or skin conditions including hair and nails?
   - *Head:* Head trauma? Head growth–microcephaly, macrocephaly? Headaches?
   - *Eyes, ears, nose, throat:* Vision and eye problems? Hearing and ear problems? Nose–discharge or bleeding episodes, breathing interference? Throat problems or infections?
   - *Respiratory:* Breathing problems? Respiratory infections? Blue spells? Cough? Snoring at night or obstructive sleep apnea?
   - *Cardiovascular:* Heart murmur history? Cyanosis? Blood pressure problems? Activity intolerance? Syncope?
   - *Gastrointestinal:* Infections, diarrhea, constipation, vomiting, or reflux? Structural problems? Anal itching or fissures? Stomachaches? Weight loss?
   - *Genitourinary:* Infections, discharges? Structural problems? Stream appearance? Frequency or burning?
   - *Gynecologic:* Menarche and menstrual history including length of menses, frequency of cycle, cramps, and clots? Vaginal discharge or bleeding? Itching?
   - *Musculoskeletal:* Movement or structural problems? Broken bones or joint sprains? Joint inflammation?
   - *Neurologic:* Seizures? Movement disorders? Tremors? Tics? Loss-of-consciousness episodes? Headaches?
   - *Endocrine:* Problems with growth or pubescence?
   - *Hematologic:* Anemia history or symptoms? Blood transfusions? Bleeding disorders?
   - *Dentition:* Number of teeth and eruption pattern? Dental trauma? Dental care? Use of fluoride? Teeth brushing? Toothaches? Use of appliances?

3. **Family history of diseases:** Classically the three-generation pedigree is used to map out risks for genetic diseases in families, but can be used more broadly to detect conditions with modifiable risk factors. In a broader form, the pedigree is also a genogram (Beery & Shooner, 2004; Wattendorf & Hadley, 2005). The genogram is described in more detail later in this chapter. Families can use checklists to note conditions or construct a pedigree online (*www.hhs.gov/familyhistory*).
   - *Mother and father:* Ages and health history.
   - *Mother's pregnancy history:* Number of pregnancies, births, status of offspring.
   - *Familial diseases:* Age, sex, and health status of each family member. Familial and communicable diseases, such as diabetes, epilepsy, tuberculosis, hypertension or heart disease, cancer, sickle cell anemia, birth defects, known genetic disorders?
   - *Genogram or pedigree:* Draw out a genogram of the family members, including sex, age, and health status of each member. (See Chapter 40 for pedigree notations.)

4. **Environmental history:** This section is used to consider toxic exposures. What foods does the child eat and how are they prepared? What is the quality of the child's living environment(s)—water and air quality? Pesticides used? Chemicals or heavy metals near or in the home? Tobacco smoke and lead exposure? Noise levels?

Functional Health Domain Database. The questions in this section are organized by functional health patterns and relate to the nursing diagnoses for each pattern. This text devotes an entire chapter to each of the 11 patterns, including assessment and management of identified problems.

1. **Health maintenance and health perceptions:** All people take steps to influence and protect their health. These choices include selection of health care providers, use of safety devices, learning how to take care of oneself, and daily care of the body. Nursing diagnoses can include health-seeking behavior, altered health maintenance, or noncompliance with a preventive or adaptive health care regimen. Usual data include the following:
   - Usual primary care provider–last visit?
   - Dentist–last visit?
   - Child's self-care or caregiver needs for more knowledge of caregiving?
   - Health care recommendations that the family chooses not to or is unable to follow?
   - Safety measures used: Car seats or seat belts? Smoke and carbon monoxide alarms? Window screens? Home safety measures? Pools? Firearms in the home? Helmet use?
   - Routine health promotion regimens?
   - Home and health management resource issues for the chronically ill or handicapped child? Home nursing? Equipment needs? Transportation needs?

2. **Nutrition:** Quality and quantity of the daily diet and the processes of feeding and swallowing, in addition to data to support diagnoses, such as nutrition, less than or greater than body requirements; anorexia; bulimia; impaired swallowing; and breastfeeding issues would be found in this section.
   - Daily diet–breakfast, lunch, snacks, and dinner? Aversions and preferences?
   - Cultural patterns related to diet and eating?
   - Supplements and vitamins?
   - Feeding patterns–meal times and snack times? Feeding strategies? Self-feeding skills? Breastfeeding and bottle-feeding issues?
   - Nutritional restrictions or special needs–calories, other?
   - Satisfaction with weight?
   - Difficulties chewing or swallowing? Reflux?

3. **Activities:** Physical mobility and the diversional and occupational activities of daily life should be described here.
   - Amount, timing, and types of physical activities? Other play opportunities and activities?
   - Television and computer or electronic games time?
   - Reading time?
   - Sports, organized activities, and hobbies of older children and adolescents?

- Activity limitations caused by health problems?
- Special equipment used or needed to support mobility?

4. **Sleep:** Sleep and rest patterns are described here. Hours? Disturbances for the child or family? Sleep aids? Sleep position for infants? Signs of sleepiness?

5. **Elimination:** Problems of elimination can be analyzed at the physiologic level of the genitourinary or gastrointestinal systems or in terms of daily living patterns. Enuresis and encopresis are daily living problems (bowel and bladder habits) that fall in this area. Physiologically, the child is well, but the elimination habits are problematic.
   - Urinary patterns: Bed-wetting? Toilet training? Voiding schedule?
   - Bowel patterns: Constipation or soiling? Stooling patterns? Toilet training?

6. **Role relationships:** Role relationships include family relationships and relationships with peers and friends in the community. Both family and individual diagnoses need to be considered here. Family coping, family process alteration, parenting alteration, abuse, and social interaction or isolation can be addressed. This section assesses family functioning in greater depth than the introductory family functioning section of the history.
   - Family interactions: Between parents? Parents and children? With other family members?
   - Parenting style and activities?
   - Peers and social supports for the child and family? Special adults in the child's life?
   - Communication with and by the child: Verbal? Nonverbal?
   - School performance for school-age children and teens.
   - Concerns that anyone has abused the child.

7. **Coping and temperament, mental health, and discipline issues:** People select and use a variety of coping strategies in their daily lives. Temperament is also important to understand child behavior and likely responses to the environment. Discipline strategies used in families are important to identify. Anxiety, fear, hopelessness, grief, powerlessness, substance abuse, pain, and potential for violence might be identified nursing diagnoses.
   - Stressors for the child and family? Losses?
   - Coping strategies of the child and caregivers?
   - Use of alcohol or drugs?
   - Temperament characteristics of the child and the "fit" with other family members?
   - Problem behavior, discipline strategies used and their outcomes?
   - Indications of depression, suicide, violent behavior, anxiety?

8. **Cognitive and perceptual:** Cognitive or perceptual problems are identified here. Attention deficit disorder is an example.
   - Hearing or vision problems?
   - Learning disorders or attention problems?
   - Adaptations made at home and school to assist the child, especially for problems of comprehension.

9. **Self-perception or self-concept:** Personal role identity, body image, and self-esteem are issues identified in this functional health domain.
   - Satisfaction with self?
   - Feelings of depression?

10. **Sexuality:** All people have sexuality issues that affect their lives. Within their sexual preferences and habits, problems are identified when these patterns are interrupted or viewed as problematic by the client or family. Pregnancy, viewed from the psychosocial perspective, is also a sexual issue that should be explored.
    - Sexual habits?
    - Sexual relationships?
    - Development of sexual identity?

11. **Values and beliefs:** This last section explores spiritual patterns and personal values and beliefs that affect the child's health.
    - Involvement with church?
    - Religious rituals?
    - Sense of alienation?
    - Sense of spiritual meaning in one's life
    - Values the family wants to impart to their children?

Development Domain Database. The levels of different aspects of development are assessed and documented in this area. Both past milestones and current functioning are important. Developmental surveillance is expected at all visits, and screening tests should be administered periodically to infants and young children (AAP, 2006).

- *Motor landmarks*–gross and fine motor: sitting, standing, walking, use of hands and arms, and so on
- *Language landmarks*–words, sentences, intelligibility, comprehension
- *Personal and social*–play, attachment, self-care, peer and family relationships
- *Scholastic grade and progress*

The Interval History

The complete history usually needs to be completed only once for new patients. After that for routine scheduled health maintenance visits, the history is updated only from the last contact to the present. The format remains the same as for the complete history; however, questions are modified to verify that the situations are as they were in the past or to add new information. All areas of the history should be assessed.

The Episodic History

Many times patients come for help with specific problems. The history includes the chief complaint and history of present illness sections of the complete history. The framework for dealing with these problems is as follows, with each symptom analyzed in chronologic sequence.

Symptom Analysis

1. Onset–initial and episodic; date and time, sudden or gradual, setting
2. Location of pain–local, radiation, generalized, superficial, or deep
3. Duration–how long, has it eased, gotten worse?
4. Characteristics and course:
   - Symptom quality: Nature of symptoms
   - Symptom quantity: Severity, frequency, volume, number, size or extent, degree of functional impairment
   - Course: Continuous or intermittent, pattern of variation
5. Activating (precipitating) and aggravating factors

6. Relieving factors
7. Tests and treatment, including complementary therapies: What, when, where, who, and results, including complications and sequelae
8. The meaning of the symptoms to patient and family and patient's reactions to symptoms

Even though the patient comes in for a specific problem, always ask some screening questions that tap into the other domains of the history–disease, functional health, and developmental. At visits for minor illnesses, health promotion and disease prevention issues should be considered in addition to the problem at hand. An immunization history, if appropriate, should be completed at every visit.

The Psychosocial Problem History

Psychosocial or behavioral problems also must be assessed (Green et al, 2002). Some considerations are summarized in Box 2-6. Much of the data related to psychosocial concerns will be collected in the functional health pattern domain database. Additional suggested material is included in the Family Database section to be discussed later in this chapter.

For adolescents, the HEADSS method is often recommended as a psychosocial review of systems, (i.e., *h*ome environment; *e*ducation, *e*ating, and *e*mployment; peer-related *a*ctivities; *d*rugs; *s*exuality, suicide and depression; and *s*afety from injury and violence (Goldenring & Rosen, 2004).

FAMILY DATABASE

The intent of this section is to identify basic family, day care, school, work, or community agency factors that form the context of the child's life and need to be considered in planning care. The provider also needs to shift to the family-as-unit-of-care here to identify family problems–another level of issues. Family problems might include impaired communication among family members, social isolation, family violence, impaired parents, alterations in parenting, caregiver role strain, and others. This section of the history could be obtained using a genogram and/or ecomap format, both of which are discussed in greater detail later or, at least, provide preliminary data if those assessment strategies are used. In general families appreciate concerns and inquiries related to the health of their family though, in one study, mothers preferred to answer domestic violence questions away from the children (Zink et al, 2006). Providers should not hesitate to ask questions about the family.

Family Structure and Roles
- People living in the home
- Type of family–two-parent, single-parent, divorced, foster, etc.
- Meaning of the family structure to the child

Family Life Cycle
- Family life cycle issues; "out of sync" issues, such as seriously ill parent, young teen parent

Family Functioning
- Primary caregiver? Who helps? Stresses of caregiver. Is the caregiver well both physically and emotionally?

- Does anyone require more attention from the primary caregiver than the patient?
- How much time do parents and child spend in the home together?
- How are family decisions made? How are arguments worked out?
- How would you describe your relationship with your partner?
- Do you feel safe in your current relationship?

Family Social Network
- What community resources and family support systems are used?
- What agencies work with this child and family?

Family Environment and Resources
- Home environment description: apartment, home, or farm? Fenced yard or perceived unsafe neighborhood?
- Family financial resources–health insurance? Money for necessities. What are the sources of money for the family–jobs or government assistance?
- Family stresses over resources and home environment?
- Where does the child go for day care, school, work (teens), and what is the quality of each setting?

Genograms and Ecomaps
Many family assessment models and tools can be used in primary care practice (see Box 2-7 on p. 36). The following provides

---

| BOX 2-6 | Suggestions for the Psychosocial Complaint History |

1. Use good communication skills–listen. Nonjudgmental approach. Seek a balanced give and take of information.
2. Interview the child or adolescent alone and with parents. Time alone with the preschooler may be used for play or drawing.
3. Have questionnaires or checklists from parents, teachers, child care workers available. Use the information in the interview.
4. Be alert to emotional tone and interactions among family members.
5. Review the context for the concern:
   - Information about parents and family members: illnesses, mental health problems, poverty, employment, violence, social isolation
   - Information about the child: school, peer relationships, temperament, neglect or abuse history, foster home placements, losses
   - Information about child-parent relationships: attachment disorder, unrealistic expectations, poor family communication, lack of knowledge of child development and appropriate parenting
6. The history of present illness becomes an amalgam of information from the multiple sources—child, parents, others. Do not assume that both parents have the same views of the issues.
7. Remember that the interview itself may be therapeutic.

From Green M, Sullivan P, Eichberg C: Avoid a "Swiss cheese" history when psychosocial complaints are on the menu, *Contemp Pediatr* 19:115, 2002.

a baseline assessment model that provides clinicians with essential data on which to build a management plan. It is tailored for a relatively busy practice, can be done in stages across visits, and invites additional data entries to update the family database over time.

The construction of genograms and ecomaps, two approaches to developing a family database, is described in the following sections. Neither requires the purchase of standardized assessment tools, and both can be updated over time, a characteristic making them valuable to pediatric providers in understanding patterns in children and families. Together, the genogram and ecomap assist clinicians in assessing family structure and roles, life cycle transitions, family functioning, and social networks in a relatively quick and efficient manner. Both have the advantage of providing a means for interacting with children and their family members in a focused, nonthreatening way around potentially complex and difficult issues. Both also are inherently appealing to families. They help families see themselves in new ways and provide ways for families to be partners in their own diagnosis and management. Even if not explicitly constructed during a visit, conceptually, they assist the provider to organize family data for analysis and identification of problems (Olsen et al, 2004). Thus, every pediatric provider should be familiar with these two models. Studies have shown that assessment of family issues and resources does not always occur in primary care, but families generally welcome the opportunity to discuss the family-as-the-unit-of-care with clinicians (Kogan et al, 2004).

Providers who use genograms and ecomaps in their practice frequently come to the conclusion that the tools are as useful for intervention as they are for assessment. In addition, those working with children find that including the children in the construction and updating of genograms and ecomaps helps children be active in their own care and provides data on family interactions (Visscher & Clore, 1992).

Genogram Construction.   Genograms are sociometric, paper-and-pencil tools used to depict a family's composition and history across generations (Fig. 2-1). Although not essential, computer programs to facilitate genogram data management have become available in recent years and can be easily included in computerized patient records. These programs have made updating genogram data easy and efficient. Genograms are appealing to providers because they provide graphic representations of complex family data; they allow the providers to map the family structure clearly and to update the picture as it emerges. Further, genograms are an efficient clinical summary making it easier for providers to keep in mind family members, patterns, and events that may have recurring significance in a family's ongoing care. Genograms also help providers think systematically about how events and relationships in their clients' lives are related to patterns of health and illness, and they are a subjective, interpretive tool to help generate tentative hypotheses for further systematic evaluation.

Priorities for organizing genogram data for clinical use rely less on formal blood and legal links and more on repetitive symptoms and relationships or functioning patterns seen across the family or over generations. They are most effective when constructed during an initial visit with children and their families and then revised as new information becomes available.

The provider begins by drawing a basic family tree, with the present family members guiding identification of family members. It is clinically useful to identify members of the current household in which children live. In fact, it can be more informative and useful to learn who is living in a household than who is related by blood or birth. This objective can be met by drawing a circle around the members of the genogram who currently live together (e.g., the circle may include parents and 3 children, or it may include 1 of 2 parents, 2 of 3 children, and a grandparent). It is also useful to include at least 3 generations of the family. Standardized symbols can be found at *www.genopro.com/genogram_components/default.htm*.

Health history information, including serious medical, behavioral, and emotional problems, can be noted on the genogram (e.g., drug or alcohol problems, serious problems with the law, and causes of death). Likewise, family information that is significant to the health of the child can be included, such as ethnic background, language spoken in the home, education of parents, occupations, religious affiliation, major family moves, and current location of family members. Significant others who live with or are important to the family should be included, for example family friends, foster children, and baby sitters. In some cases, the significant other is a family pet.

Practical pointers include using pencil instead of pen, unless there are legal or institutional requirements to use a pen; leaving space at the bottom of the page for notes; and including a key to notations or unusual symbols. It also is useful to provide child patients with their own paper and pencils or crayons to use while conducting the interview; they might even draw a picture of their family for you.

The genogram interview can begin with an open question, such as "Tell me about your family." It can be addressed to children, to parents, or to both. As the genogram is being constructed, questions can be used to elicit information about family functioning. McGoldrick and Gerson (2007) suggest the following order of questions; specific suggested questions are found in Table 2-1. They are examples only and should not be viewed as exhaustive. Therapeutic interviewing questions relate to all the issues of the genogram discussed below.

Family Composition and Structure.   The provider needs to know who makes up the family as the family defines it.

Current Family Situation.   An understanding of the current family situation is helpful, especially if a significant time period has elapsed since the child and family were last seen. Understanding changes that the family is facing and where they are in the family life cycle is also important.

Extended Family Context.   Data about the extended family may not seem relevant to parents or children, but patterns that can have an impact on children's health often do not become evident until this kind of intergenerational mapping is done. This more extensive mapping of a family may be used when the clinical picture includes conflicting information or when the effectiveness of a prevention activity is a concern. For example, knowing that both the mother and grandmother of

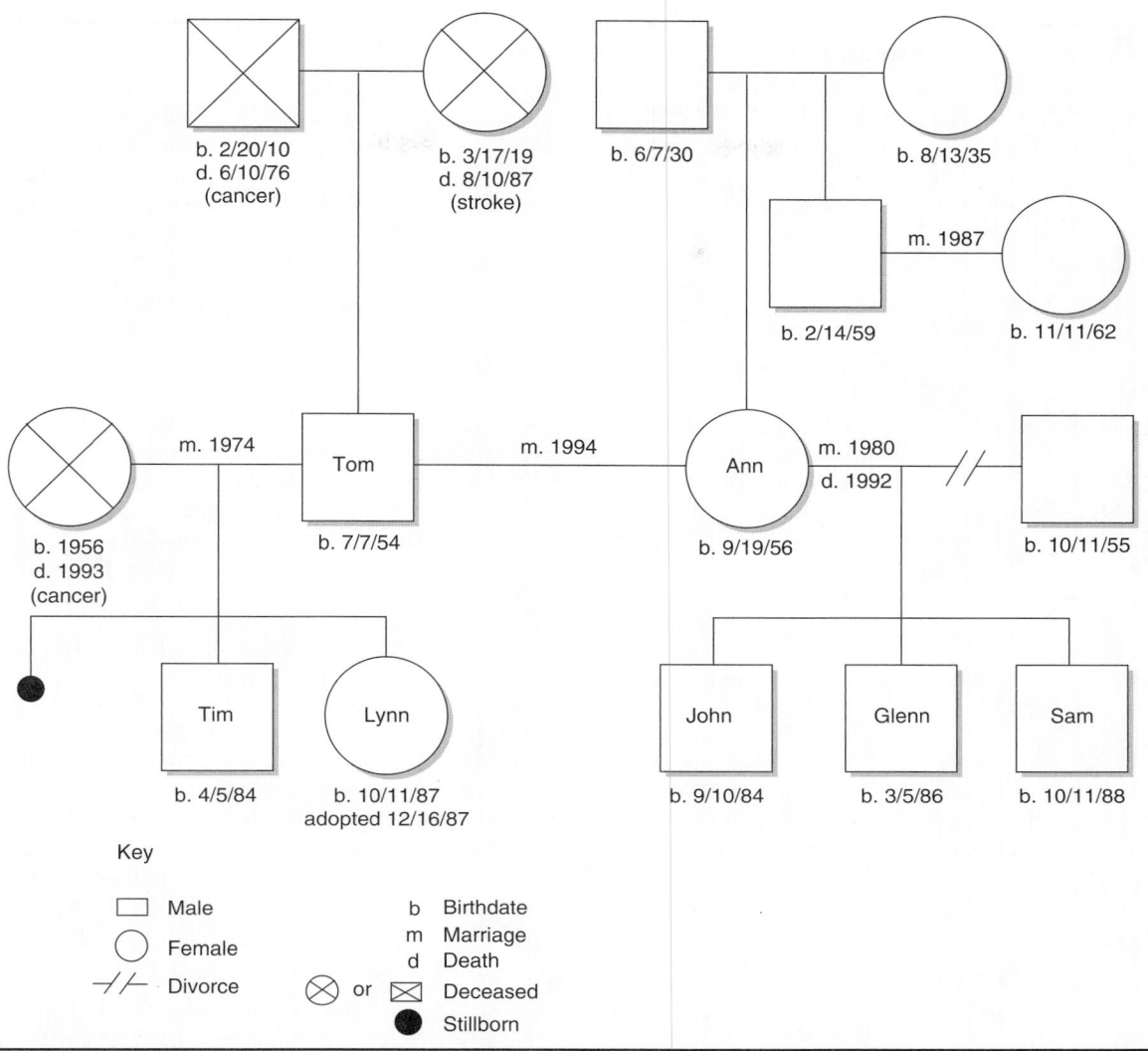

Key

☐ Male	b Birthdate
○ Female	m Marriage
⧸⧸⧸ Divorce	d Death
⊗ or ⊠ Deceased	
⬤ Stillborn	

FIG. 2-1   A 3-generational genogram of a blended family.

the young adolescent in your office became pregnant at 14 and dropped out of high school may be helpful in deciding how to best use a brief visit.

"It would help me to help your child if I knew more about your child's grandparents, aunts, uncles, and other relatives. Let's begin with your mother's family...."

Demographic Data.   Demographic data include dates of birth, death, adoption, marriage, separation, divorce, significant illness, and major family events; culture and ethnicity; religion; education; and occupations. The provider can probe for more information about specific data as they appear to be significant in a given situation. For example, faith and strength of adherence to a specific religion may have an unexpected impact on care decisions for a child. Disagreement about adherence within a family may result in mixed messages and uneven follow-through with a treatment plan.

Historical Perspective.   Knowledge of the timing and repetition of significant family events or behavior may be helpful. For example, adolescent pregnancy, alcohol abuse, dropping out of high school, and suicide may be patterns of behavior in a family's intergenerational history.

If gaps in data become evident, they need to be explored. It is also helpful to keep in mind events external to the family that may have influenced family choices. For example, the years of conflict in Vietnam and Iraq have interrupted many life plans. Immigration, voluntary or forced, can have an impact on family health status. Natural disasters, such as floods, hurricanes, and droughts, have changed family histories and the health status of family members.

Family Relationships and Roles.   In developing the database, providers can begin to probe for family relationships and roles. For example, understanding how parents make decisions and solve problems can be useful in helping parents improve health promotion practices or to recognize the positive actions they take with their families.

Ecomaps.   Ecomaps are similar to genograms in their inherent and deceptive simplicity (Fig. 2-2). Ecomaps depict, in a clear and dynamic way "the major systems that are a part of the family's life and the nature of the family's relationship with the various systems" (Hartman, 1995). A lack of family social support is related to feelings of isolation, hopelessness, depression, and other negative feelings, which will

TABLE 2-1   **Family Assessment Questions for Genogram**

Family History Topic	Suggested Questions

Family composition and structure	• Who is in your family?
	• Who currently lives with you and your child?
	• If the relationships are not clear: How are you related to the members of your household?
	• If divorce or separation is involved: Where does the child's other parent live? What are the custody and visitation agreements? How often does the child see or hear from the other parent?
	• Who in your family was involved in the decision to come here today?
	• If a health-related problem is involved:
	  ○ How do other members of your family see this problem?
	  ○ With whom will you discuss today's visit when you go home?

Current family situation	• Have there been any changes in your family since your last visit? • What, if any, changes do you anticipate in the near future?
Extended family situation	• When was your mother born? Where? Who were her parents? • Who was in her family while she was growing up? • Is she living? (If yes) Where does she live now? How often do you have contact with her? (If no) When did she die? What was the cause of death? • How did she meet your father? When were they married (if applicable)? (And so on.)
Family relationships and roles	• How would you describe your parenting style? How does it compare with your partner's? • Who in your family is responsible for monitoring your children's health? • What does your family enjoy most about this child? • What are some of the things you do together as a family? How often? • How do you generally make important decisions in your family? • To whom does your child tend to tell problems and concerns? • How do family members show their support for one another? • How well do you think your family adapts to change? • How does your family nurture the interests and talents of each individual family member? • To whom do you go for advice about being a good parent? Why do you go to that person? • How do you deal with unwanted advice from family members about raising your child(ren)?
Two-parent families	• How do you decide who does what at home? • Who has primary responsibility for daily child care? How is that working? • Who has primary responsibility for health care and appointments? How is that working?
Working parents and child care	• How many hours do you work outside the home in a typical week? How does that affect your family life? • What tensions do you anticipate (or are you experiencing) to be associated with balancing work and home? • What child care arrangements have you made? How satisfactory are they? What would you change if you could? • How do you manage care for a child who is ill on a workday?
Multiple births	• Have things gone as you expected with the babies? • When you have questions about their care, whom do you ask? • Have you had help from your partner? Family members? Friends? • How are your babies similar? How do they differ from one another? • How have you managed those times that happen to all new parents when you feel overwhelmed? • How have the babies' sibling(s) responded to them?
Families with a child with a chronic illness	• How are things going on a day-to-day basis with your child's care? • How is the management affecting your child's relationships with other children? • How is school going? • How is the management affecting family life? • What are your hopes for the future? Your concerns? • What do you need most right now to better care for your whole family?
Blended families	• Have things gone as you expected they would in your new family? • How is each child coping with the new family? • How do their responses vary with their ages and developmental levels? • How has their child care or school situation changed, and how have they responded?

TABLE 2-1	Family Assessment Questions for Genogram—Cont'd
Family History Topic	**Suggested Questions**
	• What do the parents identify as the most significant loss for each child in the blended family? The most significant benefit?
	• How are the relationships between parents (including stepparent) and children?
	• How are the relationships among the stepsiblings?
Single-parent families	• How are the parents handling discipline issues?
	• What is the best thing about being your child's only parent?
	• What is most challenging for you about being a single parent?
	• How do you get the support you need as a parent?
	• What would most help you raise your child at this point in time?

secondarily affect the child's well-being. Mapping of family relationships within and outside family boundaries highlights the nature of those relationships, their potential for support, conflicts in the relationships, and areas of current or potential strain and stress. The ecomap uses a genogram as a foundation, so the genogram should be constructed first (McGuiness et al, 2005).

As with genograms, all that is needed is a piece of paper and a pencil. A large circle representing the family boundary is drawn in the center of the paper; smaller circles representing different parts of the environment (individuals, organizations and institutions, hobbies, work, and so on) are drawn around the large circle. Inside the large circle, a genogram depiction of the family members in the household is drawn. Family members are then asked to label the smaller circles with those people, places, and activities, whether enjoyable, stressful, or both, that make up their world. Examples of labels include extended family members, friends, work, school, band practice, church or synagogue, camping, exercise, and health care. Connections between individual family members or the family as a whole and the smaller circles are then drawn. Coded lines and brief descriptions are used to indicate the strength and quality of the relationships. Common codes for the lines are found in the key in Fig. 2-2.

Direction of the flow of energy, resources, or interest can be indicated by drawing arrows along the connecting lines. An example is a family with 3 children, one of whom loves school and does well (3 solid lines with arrows pointing from school to the child); one of whom is an indifferent student, but likes the social aspect of school (a dotted line with no arrows); and one who has serious academic problems and dreads going to school each morning (a solid line with hatch marks and arrows pointing from the child to school) (see Fig. 2-2).

Sometimes the whole family is connected to an activity, and the energy flow is similar for all members. For example, a family might identify a particular family friend as supportive. In other cases, the experience differs across family members. For example, family vacations may be positive for all members of the family except adolescents, who would prefer to stay home near their friends. A scarcity of connections outside the household suggests isolation and may be a problem if the family needs significant support during a crisis. A sheet full of circles may indicate a family overcommitted and overwhelmed by activities and responsibilities.

In summary ecomaps provide both additional data about a family's social network and potential for social support. They also provide a way of validating information from the genogram interview, especially around family relationships and roles (Ray & Street, 2005).

Targeted Family Assessments

Families come with a variety of issues, some related to the composition and structure of the family, others related to variables, such as socioeconomic and health status. Family-related issues have the potential to influence the health and well-being of children and adolescents in significant ways. Although much about family assessment remains constant across families, it is useful to pay attention to some of the unique potential family variations. Again, Table 2-1 provides some examples of questions for the family options identified later.

Two-Parent Families.   Two-parent families include married couples with children, unmarried couples with children, remarried couples with blended families (or stepfamilies), and gay or lesbian couples. Two-parent families experience the same stressors as do single-parent families, but children in two-parent families tend to have social, economic, and health advantages. Parent educational levels, economic status, and health status are generally higher in two-parent families than in single-parent families (Annie E. Casey Foundation, 2006). There is also the fact, seldom researched but often cited by parents, that even when the division of labor is uneven, it is still a relief to have another adult with whom to share the work of raising children. Several studies, however, show that children's well-being depends upon composition of the household and not just the number of adults present. For example, mother-stepfather families have no better child outcomes than single-parent families (Whitehead & Popenoe, 2004).

Working Parents and Child Care.   When a single parent works outside the home or both parents in a two-parent family work outside the home, specific considerations involve all members of the family. Carter (1999) identified three "unresolved problems" related to work and families that

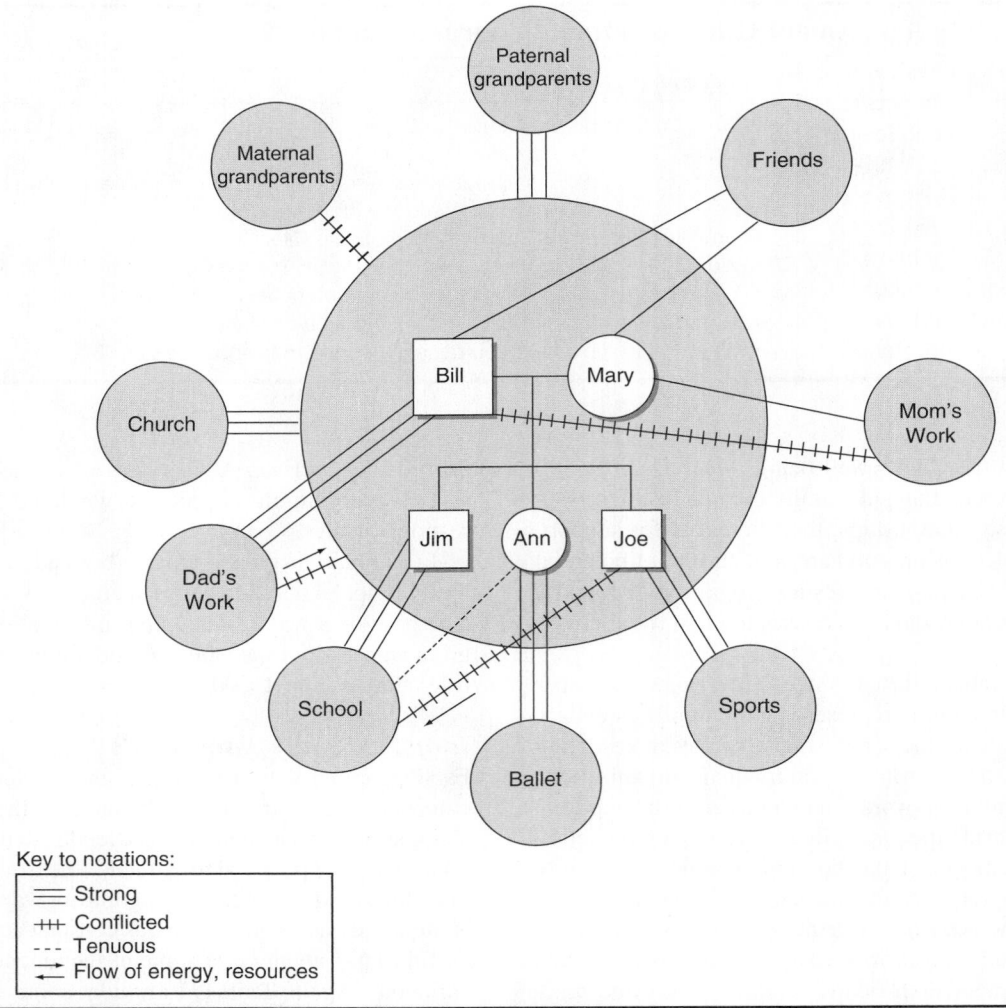

Key to notations:

═══	Strong
+++	Conflicted
- - -	Tenuous
⇄	Flow of energy, resources

FIG. 2-2 Ecomap of family with 3 children. Ecomaps can provide additional data about the major systems in a family's life and the nature of the family's relationships with those systems.

can affect parenting: men's unequal contributions to housework, workplace inflexibility, and the increasing number of hours both men and women are spending outside the home. Many studies have explored the impact of maternal employment on children's maternal attachment, with mixed results. Whereas some researchers have found weakened attachment bonds, others have found no effect. Researchers have identified protective factors that are in the socioeconomic realm, including educated parents, financial security, and parents' psychological well-being (Kneipp, 2002). Studies have found decreased school readiness scores at 36 months for children whose mothers were employed by 9 months, even when controlled for child care quality, home environment quality, and maternal sensitivity. This is a real issue for child health (Brooks-Gunn et al, 2002). It has also been shown that children's temperaments and behavior problems have negative effects on mother's work outcomes (Hyde et al, 2004).

Multiple Births. A family faced with caring for newborn twins, triplets, or more, even while delighted, can be quickly overwhelmed by the responsibility and amount of

work involved. Assessing parents' level of fatigue, ability to seek and accept support, and plans for ongoing care is useful to both the provider and the parents.

Families with a Premature Infant. Low-birth-weight and premature infants present special issues for new parents. There may be an extended time between the birth of the child and being able to bring the child home. Concerns about the child's physiologic vulnerability may arise. Almost certainly, costs and time commitments around the care of the infant will be increased. Parents may have the same concerns as parents of a full term newborn, but their fears and anxieties about being responsible for a seemingly fragile newborn may be close to overwhelming. Similar to the situation of a multiple birth, exploring who is caring for the child and who is helping the parents is a priority.

Families Raising a Child with a Chronic Illness. Parents caring for a child with a significant medical or developmental challenge, whether it is a chronic illness, a disabling condition, or a developmental disability, are responsible for their child's daily medical care, monitoring, and management. The care can be minimal or consume hours of every day and night.

The monitoring can be casual or meticulous; the management, routine or complex. Survival may be a realistic concern.

The health, both physical and psychological, of the caregiver is essential to that person's ability to care for the child and family. Raina and colleagues (2005) found that the best predictors of caregiver well-being for 468 families with a child with cerebral palsy were (1) child behavior, (2) caregiving demands, and (3) family functioning. A study of 36 families caring for technology- dependent children found that time demands around the clock, a lack of trained respite care providers, and limits on school, employment, and social life were significant problems (Heaton et al, 2005). Families "live worried," and they are often overwhelmed but feel the need to stay in the struggle on behalf of their child. They also worry about how to survive as a family (Coffey, 2006).

The impact of a chronic illness or disabling condition on a family, including the child, parents, siblings, and extended family, is influenced not only by the diagnosis and its sequelae, but also by the meaning it has for the family and individual members. Time may or may not help (e.g., the overall stress of living with the aftermath of a diagnosis may not lessen, but specific concerns may). Families of children with a developmental disability rated primary care physicians low on understanding the impact of the child's condition on the family (Liptak et al, 2006).

Whereas all developmental levels present challenges and opportunities for these families, the interface between families and schools around developmental and health issues can be particularly difficult. Parents generally want their child to be placed in a situation in which he or she has the maximal opportunity to be successful. Parents also want their child to be as "normal" as possible. Both of these goals may require a great deal of planning and negotiation with school teachers and staff. Sydnor-Greenberg and Dokken (2000) identified five recommendations to help parents and children cope with schools, camps, and other settings:

- Communicate details about the child's needs.
- Recognize that education and knowledge about chronic illness vary widely among individuals.
- Be flexible around rules surrounding treatment.
- Advocate for parents' needs.
- Promote self-care and self-advocacy for the children themselves.

The process of normalization in such families is important to their health. Parents acknowledge the condition and potential impact, redefine (or adapt) their definition of normal to fit their family, engage in behaviors that fit the definition of normal, develop a treatment regimen that also fits, and interact with others based on the view that the child and family are normal (Knafl et al, 2001). Promoting normalization can be a powerful nursing intervention.

Often parents become both medical experts in their child's diagnosis and management and experts in their child's idiosyncratic responses. They expect to be treated seriously and with respect, and they set high standards for their child's health care providers.

Health care providers can find it a challenge to work with parents raising a child with a significant health problem. Providers can feel tested and challenged; they may be taken by surprise by angry responses from parents, responses that do not appear to be justified. In a classic paper, Thorne and Robinson (1988) described three phases of this relationship between health care providers and health care recipients or family caregivers. Naïve trusting was the first stage, a time when the family assumed that its perspective was shared by the professionals who cared for their family members and that the family members' involvement as caregivers would be respected and acknowledged. Family members also assumed that all professionals would be highly knowledgeable and skilled and would be honest and direct in communications. As ongoing interactions with health care professionals taught families that these assumptions were not valid, a second phase, characterized by disenchantment, occurred. Anger was often the primary expression of this disenchantment, reflecting the loss of trust in health care providers, and family members moved toward trying to protect their family member. Finally, but not inevitably, family members moved to a phase called *guarded alliance*. The no longer naïve family members were able to reconstruct trust on a more sophisticated level. Trust was now shared with individual professionals, and it had to be earned.

Blended Families.   A blended family is one in which two adults create a reorganized family by joining together with their children from previous relationships. Although this term usually refers to families created by remarriage after divorce, it is also used to describe families created by remarriage after the death of spouses. Assessing how the children are coping with the significant changes in their lives can help both the provider and the parents direct their attention.

Single-Parent Families.   The number of children living in single-parent households rose from 12.8 million in 1990 to 16.8 million in 2000 (Annie E. Casey Foundation, 2006). Although the vast majority of single parents are women, increasingly fathers are raising their children in single-parent homes. Today, single parents may be adolescents enrolled in welfare programs or company executives with live-in nannies. Clearly, understanding the family context is fundamental to assessing these families.

Single-parent households may be headed by a divorced parent or by a parent who has never been married. In general, children living with a divorced parent have an advantage; divorced parents tend to be older, with more years of schooling completed, and with higher levels of income than do parents who have never been married. Children in single-parent families benefit when both parents are involved in their lives, regardless of marital or living arrangements.

Single parents across socioeconomic parameters all experience the demands and burdens of raising a child alone. Even with help, the weight of responsibility is felt and exacerbated by lack of time and role strain (Kneipp, 2002; Lipman et al, 2002; Lutenbacher, 2002). Single parents sometimes have difficulty accessing health care. Research suggests that affordability is a more significant issue than time pressures or workplace demands (Kneipp, 2002). The relatively large proportion of single parents who are classified as "working poor" puts them above the income level for subsidized care and below the level where they could realistically afford health insurance. Black children are more likely (58.1%) to live in a single-parent household than a two-parent one unlike children from all other racial groups (Annie E. Casey Foundation, 2006). In a study of 93 black single mothers, financial strain was related to increased depressive symptoms, which, in turn, affected parenting quality (Jackson et al, 2000).

Cohabitation of a parent and a nonparent is considered to be more detrimental to children than a single parent living alone. Rates of divorce are higher among those who later marry, and breakups occur during the cohabitation period. More children may experience child abuse, and poverty rates tend to be higher than with married families (AAP, 2003).

Adolescent Parents. Adolescents who become parents generally face the problems inherent when a major role is assumed before the adolescent is developmentally ready. Adolescent parents have developmental needs of their own, and not infrequently, their needs are in conflict with those of their children. In addition, children of adolescent mothers are more likely than children of older mothers to have a low birth weight, to have ongoing health problems during childhood, to grow up in homes without fathers, and to be raised in poverty or near poverty. Questions that can help formulate an idea about the environment in which a child will be raised include exploring the adolescent parent's own support system, attitudes toward parenting, and source of parenting advice. In addition, it is helpful to understand the adolescent's school status, child care arrangements, financial situation, and plans for the future (Stiles, 2005).

Gay and Lesbian Parent Families. Gay and lesbian parents face the same problems as all parents do, with an added concern about societal attitudes and behavior that add stress to their lives and the lives of their children. These parents generally need support in raising their children to deal with beliefs and attitudes that may include isolation and teasing. Assessing the ability of these families to find and use community support is important, as is exploring their ideas about how they will prepare their children to handle curiosity, possible negative responses, and the experience of "being different."

Adoptive Parent Families. Adoptive parents come in every variety–married couples, single parents, gay and lesbian parents, grandparents, or other extended family members. Assessment of these families includes asking about the legal status of the adoption, the timing of the adoption in the child's life, arrangements regarding involvement of the birth parents or other family members, decisions about how and when to tell the child about being adopted, and potential health concerns related to the birth parents or family, if known.

Grandparents Raising Grandchildren. According to the 2000 U.S. census, 6.3% of U.S. children under 18 years old live in grandparent-headed households, a 29.7% increase since the 1990 census; these percentages include all socioeconomic and ethnic groups. About 5.7 million grandparents

lived with their grandchildren, and 2.4 million individuals were raising their grandchildren (U.S. Census Bureau, 2003). The reasons why grandparents assume parenting responsibility for their grandchildren vary, but they rarely do so unless the parent is unable or unwilling to parent. In the U.S., substance abuse, parental illness, and parental immaturity are primary reasons (Monsen, 2001). Death of a parent, child abuse and neglect, and incarceration also are reasons for placement with grandparents.

Grandparents face significant legal issues around custody, adoption, guardianship, and foster care. Trying to enroll a grandchild in school can lead to a minefield of legal issues. In addition, although some states provide financial assistance to grandparents, others do not. Grandparents may have difficulty accessing and paying for health care. For example, some insurance carriers do not allow grandchildren as dependents. More than 90% of grandparents do not receive social security, and 85% do not receive public assistance. Only a few have foster family status, which would provide some help with child care, remuneration, developmental assessments, and tutoring (Dellman-Jenkins et al, 2002). Grandparents may be in their thirties or their eighties, and may have boundless or flagging energy. They may be still active in a job they love, or they may have looked forward to enjoying their retirement and new challenges. They may be thrilled to be parenting again, or they may be clinically depressed. There is no "one size fits all" template.

The incidence of diabetes, hypertension, depression, and coronary heart disease is greater among caregiving grandparents than it is for noncaregiving ones (Hayslip & Kaminski, 2005). Compounding the practical economic and health issues are the psychological and emotional responses of all involved. Grief, anger, confusion, resentment, and depression all can describe reactions of both grandparents and their grandchildren. At the same time, relief that the grandchildren are safe, loved, and nurtured can be present. Sensitivity and openness to grandparents can allow them to express their ambivalence and concerns. Expressed respect and appreciation can help form a working partnership.

Knowledge of resources can be especially helpful (Monsen, 2001). The American Association of Retired Persons (AARP) has a website for grandparents, which lists excellent resources, including information for grandparents parenting grandchildren. The site includes information about financial assistance, including the Temporary Assistance to Needy Families (TANF) program, online and community-based support groups, books and other literature, and a wide range of other resources (see Resource Box: Grandparents Raising Grandchildren). Support groups have been shown to be helpful in reducing the stress of raising grandchildren (Hayslip & Kaminski, 2005; Gerard et al, 2006).

Foster Parent Families. Children are placed in foster care for a variety of reasons. Substance abuse by biologic family members is the leading cause; the effects of family substance abuse on children are many and profound (Barton, 1999). Children may be placed in foster care because they need specialized medical, psychiatric or mental health, and developmental assistance beyond the ability of their biologic parents to provide. The children may need to be removed from a chaotic and unsafe family environment. They may have been abandoned or orphaned. These children, first and foremost, are at risk for deep-seated feelings of insecurity, loss, and anger. Assessment of these families includes exploration of the child's history that resulted in foster family placement, identification of health issues that precipitated or resulted from separation from the birth parents, and evaluation of the foster parent.

Foster parents have a difficult role in society. They want to be treated with respect and to have their care and knowledge of the foster child acknowledged. They want to have the assistance they need to provide the best care possible to the children in their care. However, they report that their concerns and needs often are not recognized by health care professionals (Pasztor et al, 2006). Exploring concerns the foster parent has with his or her parenting, with attention not only to the child's needs, but also to the foster family's needs, may help establish a working relationship that can work for the benefit of all (Gottesman, 2001; Pasztor et al, 2006). Again, providing resources can be helpful. The Child Welfare League of America's website has excellent information and resources about and for family foster care providers. In addition, the National Foster Parent Association provides support and caregiving information for foster families (see Resource Box: Foster Families at the end of the chapter).

Displaced or Homeless Families.   The number of homeless children in the U.S. is growing, with substance abuse and poverty as prime reasons for this increase. Homeless children and their families have difficulty with the most basic needs of food, shelter, and clothing. Accessing education and health care may be difficult to impossible. The health care visit may be in response to a crisis that could not be denied, but assessment should include well child care, including immunizations, on the operating principle that every child should receive the maximum care possible.

Poverty and Families.   Families are facing poverty in increasing numbers, and children are the most at risk. Two-parent families, with both working, may be struggling to meet basic needs. For example, in some states welfare reform has resulted in the working poor, who make too much to qualify for subsidized health care, having to choose between keeping a job that helps feed their family or meeting their children's health needs. Forty percent of children living with their single-parent mother are classified as living in poverty (Annie E. Casey Foundation, 2006). Further, data from the National Longitudinal Survey of Youth show that single mothers who were previously on welfare with health limitations for themselves or their children are at higher risk for losing their jobs. They are also less likely to have paid sick time or flexible hours, despite the fact that they are more likely to have children with chronic illnesses (Earle & Heymann, 2002; Heymann & Earle, 1999).

Selected Family Assessment Tools

The process of constructing a genogram and ecomap results in a fairly complete picture of the family's composition, social network, and family functioning. However, at times additional information is needed. The following assessment models and tools offer providers other resources that are clinically relevant and reasonably efficient. In addition, the tools have research evidence of reliability and validity supporting their use in practice (Box 2-7).

THE PHYSICAL EXAMINATION AND LABORATORY AND OTHER STUDIES

The Physical Examination

The physical examination is conducted following the history, although younger children might do better with developmental testing preceding the physical examination. Height, weight, head circumference, BMI, and vital signs are recorded. Principal findings that the provider is expected to identify are presented in the following list. Screening tests for hearing and vision, in addition to laboratory data and data from other disciplines, are included as other types of objective information. More experienced providers collect some of the history while conducting the physical examination. Content of the examination will vary depending upon the child's age and the various problems under consideration. Further discussion of physical examination techniques and findings are found in Specific Disease chapters.

1. *General appearance:* Ill or well, distressed, alert, cooperative, body build. Reaction to parents. Characteristic position, movements, nutrition, developmental appearance as contrasted with the stated age.
2. *Skin:* Color–pigmentation, cyanosis, jaundice, carotenemia, erythema, pallor. Vascular–visible veins, arteries. Eruptions, petechiae, ecchymosis, hives, rashes. Lesions. Texture, scaling, striae, scars. Sweat, edema, turgor. Subcutaneous tissue. Distribution and color of hair. Nail appearance.
3. *Lymph nodes:* Occipital, postauricular, preauricular, cervical, parotid, submaxillary, sublingual, axillary, epitrochlear, inguinal. Size, mobility, tenderness, heat.
4. *Head:* Position, shape, sutures, fontanelles. Size–circumference, microcephaly, macrocephaly, hydrocephaly. Facial paralysis, twitching.
5. *Eyes:* Vision, visual fields, cover test. Blinking. Position: exophthalmos, enophthalmos, hypertelorism, hypotelorism. Movements: strabismus, extraocular movements, nystagmus. Ptosis, eyelids, sclera, conjunctivae. Lesions–styes, chalazion. Corneas, corneal reflex. Discharge. Pupils, accommodation, iris. Retina, red reflex, fundus.
6. *Ears:* Anomalies. Position. Discharge. Tenderness. Canals. Tympanic membranes: redness, light reflex, landmarks, bulging or retraction, perforation, mobility. Mastoid. Hearing. Vestibular function.
7. *Nose:* Shape. Alae nasi, flaring. Mucosa, secretions, bleeding, airway. Septum. Polyps, tumors.
8. *Mouth:* Odor. Teeth–number, edges, occlusion, caries, formation, color. Gums–discoloration, bleeding. Buccal

---

BOX 2-7   Family Assessment Tools

Comprehensive Family Assessment Models
These models provide ways to organize family assessment material. They can provide a database characterized by both breadth and depth.
- Calgary Family Assessment Model (CFAM) (Wright & Leahey, 1994)
- Family Health Assessment Form (Friedman, 1986)

Family Assessment Screening Tool
This screening tool is quick to administer (5 minutes) and provides an overview assessment of family functioning.
- Family Apgar (Smilkstein, 1978)

Family Functioning Tools
These tools vary in length and complexity, but all are easy to score and provide in-depth data about family functioning.
- Family Adaptability and Cohesion Evaluation Scale (FACES IV) (Olson et al, 2004).
- Family Environment Scale (FES) (Moos & Moos, 1994)
- Feetham Family Functioning Survey (FFFS) (Feetham & Humerick, 1982)

Family Stress and Coping Tools (McCubbin et al, 1996)
These tools provide clinicians with information about how families define and manage stress. They can be used to help families self-diagnose their strengths and identify areas needing modification.
- Assessing adolescent stress: Adolescent-Family Inventory of Life Events and Changes (A-FILE)
- Family Inventory of Life Events (FILE)
- Family Coping Strategies (F-COPES)

---

mucosa, tongue–coating, protrusion, color, tremor, lesions. Palate–cleft, arch. Tonsils–size, color, exudate. Pharynx–appearance, color, lesions.

9. *Neck:* Size. Anomalies–webbing, edema, nodes, masses. Sternocleidomastoids. Trachea. Thyroid. Vessels. Motion–head drop, tilting, nodding, range of motion.

10. *Chest:* Shape–circumference, symmetry, Harrison groove. Movement–flaring, expansion, abdominal or thoracic breathing, intercostal retractions.

11. *Breasts:* Tanner stage of development, symmetry, redness, heat, tenderness, lumps. Gynecomastia.

12. *Lungs:* Respiration–type, rate, dyspnea. Exercise tolerance. Cough, hemoptysis, sputum. Palpation–masses, tenderness, fremitus. Percussion–dullness, hyperresonance, diaphragm location. Auscultation–breath sounds, crackles (rales), rubs, rhonchi, wheezes, vocal resonance.

13. *Cardiovascular and heart:* Blood pressure and pulse rate. Inspection–Vascularity, bulging, impulse. Distress, cyanosis, edema, clubbing, pulsations, venous distention. Palpation–Femoral pulses, point of maximal impulse, thrill. Auscultation–First and second heart sounds, rhythm, split, third heart sound, gallop, friction rub, venous hum, murmurs.

14. *Abdomen:*
    Inspection–Shape, distention, transillumination. Umbilicus, diastasis rectus, veins. Peristaltic, gastric waves.
    Auscultation–Bowel sounds, bruits.

Palpation–Superficial or deep tenderness, rebound. Spleen, liver, masses, kidneys, bladder, uterus.
Percussion–Masses, fluid, flatus.

15. *Genitalia:* Discharge, foreign body. Tags. Labia, adhesions, vagina, clitoris. Penis–hypospadias, epispadias, phimosis. Meatus, scrotum, testes, hydrocele, hernia. Cremasteric reflex. Tanner staging. Vaginal, bimanual examination for teenage girls. (Pelvic examination observations are discussed further in Chapter 35.)

16. *Anus and rectum:* Buttocks, fistula, fissure, prolapse, polyps, hemorrhoids, rashes. Rectal–rectum, fistula, megacolon, masses, prostate, tenderness. Sensation.

17. *Musculoskeletal:* Anomalies, length, clubbing, pain, tenderness, temperature, swelling, shape, symmetry.
    Gait–Stance, balance, limp. Foot position.
    Spine–Tufts of hair, dimples, masses, spina bifida, tenderness, mobility, scoliosis.
    Posture–Lordosis, kyphosis.
    Joints–Heat, tenderness, mobility, swelling, effusion.
    Muscles–Development, pain, tone, spasm, paralysis, rigidity, contractures, atrophy.

18. *Nervous system:*
    General impression, abilities, responsiveness, position, spontaneous movements, play activity.
    Development–consistent with age or current level.
    State of consciousness, irritability, seizure activity.
    Gait, stance, limp, ataxia.

Coordination, Romberg sign.

Tremors, twitching, choreiform movements, athetosis, spasticity, paralysis, flaccidity.

Reflexes: Superficial, deep tendon, clonus, Chvostek sign.

Primitive reflexes for infants and children with neurologic impairments: Moro, tonic neck, Babinski, grasp, suck. Thumb position.

Sensation: Hyperesthesia, paresthesia, temperature, touch. Stereognosis.

Cranial nerves I to XII.

Hearing and vision.

Other Data

Laboratory and Radiographic Data. Record hearing, vision, hematocrit or other blood tests, lead, urinalysis, newborn screening tests, tuberculosis screening.

Developmental and Psychological Test Scores. Scores need to be recorded and considered when problems are being identified.

Data from Other Disciplines. Summarize social work, nutrition, physical therapy, occupational therapy, medical specialist, speech pathology, education, and other reports.

▆▆ CREATING THE PROBLEM LIST

The problem list is derived from analysis of the subjective and objective data collected. Differential diagnosis is the clinical decision-making process used to derive the problems listed (Fig. 2-3). To use this process, the provider considers all the possible diagnoses for the problems presented by the patient. Then the factors that support or rule out each of the various options considered are analyzed. Identification of the best fit of the patient's subjective and objective data with the possible diagnoses is the goal. If further data are needed to confirm a diagnosis, collection of these data is incorporated into the plan. For example, the differential diagnoses for coryza (a runny nose) include, among others, allergic rhinitis, upper respiratory infection, and a foreign body in the nose. The clinician uses data about related symptoms (e.g., itchy eyes, a sore throat, systemic symptoms, or bilateral or unilateral drainage from the nostrils) to choose which diagnosis best fits the child's picture. That analysis for fit is the diagnostic reasoning process.

Functional health problems and developmental problems are also subject to the notion of differential diagnosis. For example, a child who is not sleeping well might be fearful, a trained night feeder, or experiencing episodes of obstructive sleep apnea. The interventions for each problem are different. Thus the provider must use the differential diagnosis process to identify the problem or problems at hand. A problem should never be included on the problem list that is not supported by subjective and objective data found and recorded in the database. "Rule out" should not be listed as a diagnosis. (It may be considered part of a plan). The diagnosis would be the unexplained symptom (e.g., "dysuria").

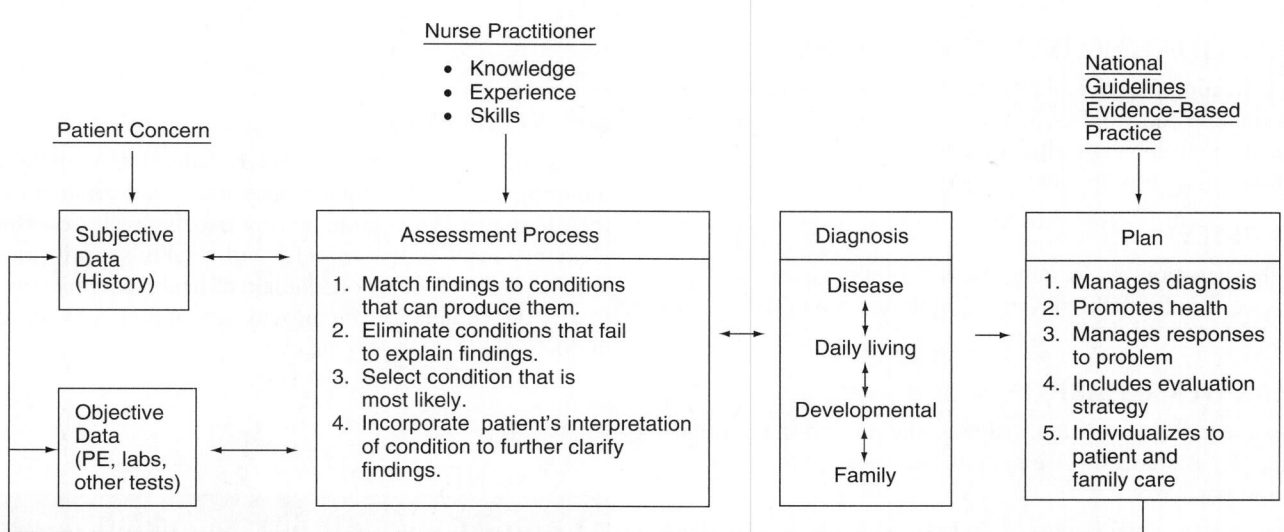

FIG. 2-3   Model for clinical decision-making. The provider takes the patient's concern and clarifies it with subjective and objective data, using past experience and skills to facilitate the assessment process. The process, which happens both during and after data collection, involves decision-making to find the best match between standardized diagnoses and the patient's findings. Once the diagnosis is made, a plan is developed, using national evidence-based guidelines where appropriate, to achieve the five goals listed. Sometimes the development of the plan requires further data collection. (Data from Burns C: Development and content validity testing of a comprehensive classification of diagnoses for use by pediatric nurse practitioners, *Nurs Diagn* 2:93-104, 1991).

CREATING THE MANAGEMENT PLAN

A plan must be developed for every identified problem. It is helpful to consider diagnostic, therapeutic, and educational interventions for every problem listed. Of course, not every problem requires work in all three areas, but they should be considered. The management activities are listed in the record. The plan should always include a recommendation for the next visit and what is to be done at that visit in an attempt to move the patient into a health maintenance pattern rather than being seen only episodically. Just as the problem list must be consistent with the data at hand, plans must address diagnoses that are included in the problem list. In other words, the plan is internally consistent with the data and diagnoses.

COMMUNICATING ASSESSMENT DATA

An important corollary to health assessment is the skill to communicate information obtained in both oral and written forms. A record of the care given must always be written to communicate the provider's logical thinking based on data obtained. This record is important because it provides information for later care, serves as a communication link with other providers, documents the quality of care provided, may be used for research purposes, and serves as a legal and billing document. Verbal communication of health care information is also essential. The words must paint a picture of the child and family for the reader (e.g., a consultant). Knowledge of the classic format used by other health care providers is important. Using that same format or one that is closely related facilitates efficient communication about patient problems.

VALIDATING DATA COLLECTION

Data collection for clinical practice, just as for research, must be as reliable and valid as possible. To assist with reliability, consider the following techniques (Burns, 1991b): test-retest, interrater reliability, and internal consistency.

TEST-RETEST

Ask the question again later. Take a blood pressure reading twice. Look for the physical finding a second time a bit later.

INTERRATER RELIABILITY

Ask someone else to listen, palpate, and so on for the same finding. Does someone else get the same answer to the same question you asked?

INTERNAL CONSISTENCY

Look for a logical consistency to the findings obtained. If something is "out of sync," question it. For example, do the height points on the graph line up, or is one significantly off the trajectory? If there is significant variation, consider a measuring error before looking for a health problem that has altered growth. Does the history support the physical findings? Does the story keep changing?

Algorithms, protocols, and flow sheets can improve the consistency and reliability of the data collected, especially when several staff members are involved with the data for a given patient.

To assess the validity, or meaning, of data collected, the provider should consider sources of error:

- Do the cumulative data fit and support a given diagnosis? If not, perhaps the diagnosis was inadequate or an error in data collection, sequencing, or interpretation occurred.
- Was the diagnosis made on the basis of one isolated finding or a cluster? For instance, diagnosing pneumonia after hearing a cough and diagnosing failure to thrive with one growth measurement are mono-operation bias errors.
- Sometimes two problems occur with overlapping findings. One problem might be missed, whereas the other is pursued.
- The patient might change the data provided because of stress or worry about the outcomes of the assessment visit. Both findings and their meaning to patients need to be explored with the patient and family.
- Provider expectations can also threaten accurate diagnosing.
- Were cues missed or questions unasked?
- Data are often compared with specific criteria (e.g., heights and weights for age are known, developmental milestones are established, laboratory norms are set for children of different ages). Which test has been used? What is its specificity and sensitivity? Is the right criterion being used?
- Providers constantly need to attend to age, sex, race, culture, and other issues when they consider data. Is it likely for a white child to have sickle cell disease? What diagnoses should one consider when a teenage girl has abdominal pain, as opposed to the diagnoses possible for a boy of the same age (Burns, 1991b)?

SUMMARY

Assessment of children and their families is complex. An inquiring mind, time, efficiency, accuracy, and communication that demonstrates genuine caring and interest are essential elements. Further, the provider will need to set priorities yet not lose sight of the whole domain of health care information that is the foundation for providing optimal care for every child.

$\mathcal{R}$ESOURCE BOX

Grandparents Raising Grandchildren

American Association of Retired Persons (AARP)
Grandparenting Information Center
www.aarp.org/families/grandparents

Grandparents **Magazine**
www.grandparentsmagazine.net

RESOURCE BOX

Foster Families

Casey Family Programs National Center for Resource Family Support
www.fostercaremonth.org

Child Welfare League of America, Family Foster Care
www.cwla.org/programs/fostercare

Children's Bureau Express
www.cbexpress.acf.hhs.gov

Connect for Kids
www.connectforkids.org

Rowell Foster Children's Positive Plan
www.rowellfosterchildren.org

The National Foster Parent Association
www.nfpainc.org

☑ DISCUSSION FORUM

1. How do the health impacts of otitis media differ depending on whether the person uses the functional health, developmental, or disease problem orientation? Would there be a difference between a toddler and an adolescent? If so, discuss which frameworks would differ and provide examples of the differences.

2. How might a provider's own personal definition of family and family roles impact the ability to assess a child and their family? List at least three strategies than can be used to overcome family-related beliefs and biases.

3. Compare and contrast history assessment techniques for a child from a blended family, a foster family, a single-parent family, and a grandparent-led family. How are these families similar? What unique issues are inherent in each of these family types?

4. Conduct a complete health history and physical examination on a child. Make sure you do a problem-oriented and a functional health history. What information is the same? What information is different?

REFERENCES

American Academy of Pediatrics (AAP), Council On Children With Disabilities, Section On Developmental Behavioral Pediatrics, *Bright Futures* Steering Committee, and Medical Home Initiatives For Children With Special Needs Project Advisory Committee: Identifying infants and young children with developmental disorders in the medical home: an algorithm for developmental surveillance and screening, *Pediatrics* 118(1):405, 420, 2006.

American Academy of Pediatrics (AAP): Family pediatrics: report of the task force on the family, *Pediatrics* 111:1541-1571, 2003.

Annie E. Casey Foundation: *Kids count state-level data online.* Available at *kidscount.org/sld/databook.jsp* (accessed Sept 26, 2006).

Barton SJ: Family matters: promoting family-centered care with foster families, *Pediatr Nurs* 25(1):57-59, 1999.

Beery T, Shooner K: Family history: the first genetic screen, *Nurs Pract* 29:14-25, 2004.

Belsky J et al: Child-rearing antecedents of intergenerational relations in young adulthood: a prospective study, *Dev Psychol* 37(6):801-813, 2001.

Bethell C et al: Measuring the quality of preventive and developmental services for young children: national estimates and patterns of clinicians' performance, *Pediatrics* 113(6 suppl):1973-1983, 2004.

Brooks-Gunn J, Han WJ, Waldfogel J: Maternal employment and child cognitive outcomes in the first three years of life: the NICHD study of early child care, *Child Dev* 73(4):1052-72, 2002.

Burns C: Development and content validity testing of a comprehensive classification of diagnoses for use by pediatric nurse practitioners, *Nurs Diagn* 2:93-104, 1991a.

Burns C: Parallels between research and diagnosis: the reliability and validity issues of clinical practice, *Nurs Pract* 16:42-50, 1991b.

Burns C: A new assessment model and tool for nurse practitioners, *J Pediatr Health Care* 6:73-81, 1992a.

Burns C: Using a comprehensive taxonomy of diagnoses to describe the practice of pediatric nurse practitioners: findings of a field study, *J Pediatr Health Care* 7:115-121, 1992b.

Carter B: Becoming parents: the family with young children. In Carter C, McGoldrick M, editors: *The expanded family life cycle: individual, family, and social perspectives,* ed 3, Boston, 1999, Allyson & Bacon.

Coffey J: Parenting a child with a chronic illness: a metasynthesis, *Pediatr Nurs* 32(1):51-59, 2006.

Cottrell LA, Nield LS, Perkins KC: Effective interviewing and counseling of the adolescent patient, *Pediatr Ann* 35(3):164-6, 169-72, 2006.

Curran D: *Traits of a healthy family,* New York, 1983, Ballantine.

deChesnay M: Promoting healthy family functioning in acute care units, *J Pediatr Nurs* 1:96-101, 1986.

Dellman-Jenkins M, Blankemeyer M, Olesh M: Adults in expanded grandparent roles: considerations for practice, policy, and research, *Educ Gerontol* 28:219-235, 2002.

Duffy ME: Health promotion in the family: current findings and directives for nursing research, *J Adv Nurs* 13:109-117, 1988.

Earle A, Heymann S: What causes job loss among former welfare recipients: the role of family health problems, *J Am Womens Assoc* 57:5-10, 2002.

Feetham SL, Humerick SS: The Feetham Family Functioning Survey. In Humerick SS, editor: *Analysis of current assessment strategies in the health care of young children and childbearing families,* East Norwalk, CT, 1982, Appleton-Century-Crofts.

Friedman MM: *Family nursing: theory and assessment,* ed 2, East Norwalk, CT, 1986, Appleton-Century-Crofts.

Garfield C, Isacco A: Fathers and the well-child visit, *Pediatrics* 117(4):e637-e645, 2006.

Gerard J, Landry-Meyer L, Roe J: Grandparents raising grandchildren: the role of social support in coping with caregiving challenges, *Int J Aging Hum Dev* 62(4):359-383, 2006.

Glader B: Iron deficiency anemia. In Behrman R, Kliegman R, Jenson H, editors: *Nelson textbook of pediatrics,* ed 17, Philadelphia, 2004, WB Saunders.

Goldenring J, Rosen D: Getting into adolescent heads: an essential update, *Contemp Pediatr* 21:64-90, 2004.

Gordon M: *Nursing diagnosis: process and application,* New York, 1987, McGraw-Hill.

Gottesman MM: Children in foster care: a nursing perspective on research, policy, and child health issues, *J Soc Pediatr Nurses* 6(2):55-64, 2001.

Green M, Sullivan P, Eichberg C: Avoid a "Swiss cheese" history when psychosocial complaints are on the menu, *Contemp Pediatr* 19:115-125, 2002.

Halfon N, Regalado M, Sareen H: Assessing development in the pediatric office, *Pediatrics* 113(6):1926-1933, 2004.

Hartman A: Diagrammatic assessment of family relationships, *Fam Soc* 76(2):11-122, 1995.

Hayslip B, Kaminski P: Grandparents raising their grandchildren: a review of the literature and suggestions for practice, *The Gerontologist* 45:262-269, 2005.

Heaton J et al: Families' experiences of caring for technology-dependent children: a temporal perspective, *Health Soc Care Community* 13(5):441-50, 2005.

Heymann SJ, Earle A: The impact of welfare reform on parents' ability to care for their children's health, *Am J Public Health* 89(4):502-505, 1999.

Hyde J et al: Children's temperament and behavior problems predict their employed mothers' work functioning, *Child Dev* 75(2):580-94, 2004.

Jackson AP et al: Single mothers in low-wage jobs: financial strain, parenting, and preschoolers' outcomes, *Child Dev* 71(5):1409-23, 2000.

Knafl KA, Deatrick JA, Kirby A: Normalization promotion. In Craft-Rosenberg M, Denehy J, editors: *Nursing interventions for infants, children, and families,* Thousand Oaks, CA, 2001, Sage.

Kneipp SM: The relationships among employment, paid sick leave, and difficulty obtaining health care for single mothers with young children, *Policy Polit Nurs Pract* 3(1):20-30, 2002.

Kogan MD et al: Routine assessment of family and community health risks: parent views and what they receive, *Pediatrics* 113(6 suppl):1934-43, 2004.

Lehna C: Interpreter services in pediatric nursing, *Pediatr Nurs* 31:292-296, 2005.

Lipman EL et al: Child well-being in single-mother families, *J Am Acad Child Adolesc Psychiatry* 41(1):75-82, 2002.

Liptak G et al: Satisfaction with primary health care by families of children with developmental disabilities, *J Pediatr Health Care* 20(4):245-252, 2006.

Lutenbacher M: Relationships between psychosocial factors and abusive parenting attitudes in low-income single mothers, *Nurs Res* 51(3):158-167, 2002.

McCubbin HI, Thompson AI, McCubbin MA: *Family assessment: resiliency, coping, and adaptation: inventories for research and practice,* Madison, 1996, University of Wisconsin Publishers.

McGoldrick M: History, genograms, and the family life cycle. In Carter C, McGoldrick M, editors: *The expanded family life cycle: individual, family, and social perspectives,* ed 3, Boston, 1999, Allyn & Bacon.

McGoldrick M, Gerson R, Shellenberger S: *Genograms: assessment and intervention.* New York, 2007, Norton.

McGuiness T, Noonan P, Dyer J: Family history as a tool for psychiatric nurses, *Arch Psychiatr Nurs* 19(3):116-124, 2005.

Minkovitz C et al: Maternal depressive symptoms and children's receipt of health care in the first 3 years of life, *Pediatrics* 115(2):306-314, 2005.

Monsen RB: Raising kids, grandparents bear a burden, *J Pediatr Nurs* 16(2):130-131, 2001.

Moos R, Moss B: *Family environmental scales manual,* ed 3, Palo Alto, CA, 1994, Consulting Psychologists Press.

NANDA International: *NANDA-I nursing diagnoses: definitions & classification 2007-2008,* Philadelphia, 2007, NANDA International.

Olsen S, Dudley-Brown S, McMullen P: Case for blending pedigrees, genograms, and ecomaps: nursing's contribution to the 'big picture,' *Nurs Health Sci* 6:295-308, 2004.

Olson DH, Bell R, Portner J: *Family inventories,* St Paul, 1982, University of Minnesota.

Olson DH, Gorall D: *FACES IV,* Roseville, MN, 2006, Life Innovations.

Pasztor E et al: Health & mental health services for children in foster care: the central role of foster parents, *Child Welfare* 85(1):33-57, 2006.

Perry BD, Pollard R: Homeostasis, stress, trauma, and adaptation: a neurodevelopmental view of childhood trauma, *Child Adolesc Psychiatr Clin North Am* 7:33-51, 1998.

Raina P et al: The health and well-being of caregivers of children with cerebral palsy, *Pediatrics* 115(6):e626-e636, 2004.

Ray R, Street A: Ecomapping: an innovative research tool for nurses, *J Advanc Nurs* 50:545, 2005.

Smilkstein G: The family APGAR: a proposal for a family function test and its use by physicians, *J Fam Pract* 6:1231-1239, 1978.

Stiles A: Parenting needs, goals, and strategies of adolescent mothers, *Am J Maternal Nurs* 30(5):327-333, 2005.

Sydnor-Greenberg N, Dokken D: Helping parents and children cope with chronic conditions in school, *J Child Fam Nurs* 3(6):447-451, 2000.

Terkelsen KG: Toward a theory of the family life cycle. In Carter EA, McGoldrick M, editors: *The family life cycle: a framework for family theory,* New York, 1980, Gardner.

Thorne SE, Robinson CA: Health care relationships: the chronic illness perspective, *Res Nurs Health* 11:293-300, 1988.

US Census Bureau: *QT-02. Profile of selected social characteristics, 2000.* Available at *http://factfinder.census.gov/servlet/QTTable?ds_name= D&geo_id=D&qr_name=ACS_C2SS_EST_G00_QT02&_lang=en* (accessed Feb 23, 2007).

US Department of Health and Human Services (USDHHS), Centers for Disease Control and Prevention: *International classification of diseases, ninth revision, clinical modification,* ed 6, Hyattsville, Md, 2003, Centers for Medicare and Medicaid Services.

US Department of Health and Human Services (USDHHS): *Nurse practitioner primary care competencies in specialty areas: adult, family, gerontological, pediatric, and women's health,* Washington, DC, 2002, USDHHS.

Visscher EM, Clore ER: The genogram: a strategy for assessment, *J Pediatr Health Care* 6:361-367, 1992.

Wattendorf D, Hadley D: Family history: the three-generation pedigree, *Am Fam Physician* 72:441-48, 2005.

Whall AL: The family as the unit of care in nursing: a historical review, *Public Health Nurs* 3:240-249, 1986.

Whitehead B, Popenoe D: *The state of our unions: the social health of marriage in America 2004.* Available at *http://marriage.rutgers.edu/ Publications/SOOU/TEXTSOOU2004.htm* (accessed Sept 15, 2007).

Wright LM, Leahey M: *Nurses and families: a guide to family assessment and intervention,* ed 4, Philadelphia, 2005, FA Davis.

Zink T et al: Mothers' comfort with screening questions about sensitive issues, including domestic violence, *J Am Board Fam Med* 19(4):358-67, 2006.

CHAPTER 3

Cultural Perspectives for Pediatric Primary Care

Ardys M. Dunn

Primary health care providers in the U.S. increasingly work with culturally diverse clients, families, colleagues, and communities. According to U.S. census data, approximately 35.7 million individuals or 12.4% of the U.S. population are immigrants, a number larger than the population of California (US Census, 2006). Approximately 53.3% were born in Latin America, 25% in Asia, 13.7% in Europe, 3% in Africa, and the remainder in other countries (Larsen, 2004; Wilson, 2003). A recent study by the Pew Hispanic Center found that 7.2 million undocumented workers hold jobs in the U.S., making up 4.9% of the overall labor force; some 24% of farm workers and 14% of construction workers are undocumented (Passel & Suro, 2005). Many immigrants arrive in the U.S. without documents, and many come as refugees from war-torn countries, both stressful circumstances that put them at high risk for physical and psychological health problems. Health care providers must consider these circumstances when assessing and managing care for immigrant clients.

In addition, there are significant health disparities among minority cultural groups in the U.S. For example, infant mortality for non-Hispanic blacks is 13.61 per 1000 live births, in contrast to an overall rate of 6.84 per 1000 live births and 5.7 for non-Hispanic whites (Mathews & MacDorman, 2006). These disparities have been attributed in part to a lack of communication between providers and patients that may be related to cultural differences (Fadiman, 1997).

In response to these demographic changes and in an effort to mitigate health disparities, many health education institutions have created curricula with courses to develop culturally competent providers (Kripalani et al, 2006). Evaluation of these curricula is just beginning, and data vary on the difference they make in provider attitudes and health outcomes (Shapiro et al, 2006; Thom et al, 2006; Crosson et al, 2004). Some theorists contend that the focus on a traditional "cultural competence" approach is misguided (Gray & Thomas, 2006), and some educators are calling for a move "beyond cultural competence into transnational competence" (Koehn & Swick, 2006). Educational programs must prepare clinicians to deal effectively with the complex interrelationship of variables that influence health behaviors, decisions, and outcomes, only one of which is culture per se (Airhihenbuwa & Liburd, 2006; Underwood et al, 2005). Having this skill gives clinicians the ability to provide high-quality health care to all populations.

This chapter outlines some of the basic principles of cultural dynamics, emphasizing that environmental, economic, and social factors are integrally woven into the fabric of every client-provider encounter and that clinicians must consider the reality of individual history, experience, and meaning in every interaction.

■ CULTURE

Culture is defined as a set of "patterns, explicit and implicit, of and for behavior." It is "acquired and transmitted by symbols" and is based on "traditional (i.e., historically derived and selected) ideas and … their attached values; culture systems may, on the one hand, be considered as products of action, on the other as conditioning elements of further action" (Kroeber, 1952). In an anthropologic and sociologic sense, culture is a social construction of the relationships within and among groups of human beings, specifically created through the ongoing interactions of individuals with others and with their environment (Berger & Luckmann, 1966). It is based on ethnicity, race, religion, class, and geography. The term *ethnicity* is used to identify groups of people within society, each of which shares distinctive traits and customs. *Race,* in contrast, classifies humans according to specific physical characteristics (e.g., pigmentation, facial features). Humans also differ by religion, social class, and the physical place or environment in which they experience life. All of these qualities contribute to shaping the culture of the social group.

UNIVERSAL CHARACTERISTICS OF CULTURE

Although a cultural group may possess unique qualities, all cultures have certain common characteristics. These universal characteristics of culture represent the framework within which cultures exist (Table 3-1). As health care providers, it is helpful to approach all individuals using this framework, since no one quality is definitive of a culture, and within cultural groups, individuals show great variation in behavior and beliefs.

Culture Is Dynamic and Shared

As both a product and function of human interaction, culture is constantly evolving; there is no absolute, reified quality that can be attributed to human groups. In most societies,

TABLE 3-1   Universal Characteristics of Culture

Characteristic	Significance
Culture is dynamic.	Beliefs and practices of groups are created through interactions among people and between people and their physical and social environments.
	Beliefs, customs, and values change over time as new interactions occur and to meet the needs of the social group.
	Although cultures evolve, there is a tendency for stability and cultural continuity.
Culture is shared.	Members of a cultural group share group ways of thinking, doing, and interacting.
Culture is learned.	Cultural groups teach members the "rules" or expectations of that culture.
Culture is based on symbols.	Language is the primary mechanism for transmitting and interpreting culture.
	Humans use artifacts (e.g., clothing, food, music, religious icons) and rituals to communicate within and among cultures.
Culture is integrated.	Cultural norms, beliefs, customs, and values span all areas of social life (e.g., the lessons learned in the family extend into the school setting), providing coherence to the social group.
	There may be significant variation from one arena of social life to another (e.g., language used in the home may differ from that used in school or workplace).

a dominant group is clearly evident. The culture of this group largely shapes the lifestyle and collective consciousness of the community, functions as the guardian and sustainer of the controlling value system, and is the prime allocator of rewards. Generally, individuals in a society learn to identify with the dominant cultural framework and incorporate its traditions and customs into their daily life and decision-making. The extent to which this adaptation of culture occurs is termed *cultural embeddedness.* Many factors influence the degree of cultural embeddedness, including level of education, socioeconomic status, social class, country of origin of individuals or their ancestors, exposure to other cultures, lifestyle, length of stay in the host country, and the exact region of the host country in which individuals grow up, reside, or both.

Individuals may also identify with a minority group (i.e., a group that shares racial or ethnic characteristics that differ from those of the majority group) or may have a number of subcultural affiliations based on gender, social class, religion, occupation, or socioeconomic status. In diverse societies, especially where minority groups are large or their members are vocal proponents of retaining their cultural integrity, assimilation into the dominant culture may not be easy or automatic, and cultural confusion or conflict may occur. Characteristics (e.g., skin color, religion) that set a minority group apart from the dominant group may result in collective discrimination within the society. Ethnocentrism and racism create and perpetuate the distinctions of dominant and minority groups. *Ethnocentrism* is the belief that one's own ethnic culture or subculture is superior to all others. *Racism* is the assumption of inherent racial superiority or inferiority with consequent discrimination.

An individual or group that straddles two or more cultures and embraces more than one set of values is termed *bicultural,* but efforts to achieve this status can be a source of considerable stress. Tremendous intraethnic diversity may exist in life perspective, values, problem-solving strategies, and customs among individual members of dominant and minority groups.

Thus, one can expect to see variations within and between cultures. In diverse societies, all cultural groups will change as a result of their interactions.

Culture Is Learned

The elements of culture are transmitted from one generation to another through a complicated process of social interaction. This socialization process shapes a child's reality; through it children learn how to perceive the world, the values, ideologies, and rules that motivate and define behavior. This learning is facilitated by the long period of dependency that humans have before reaching physical and social maturity and depends on the child's temperament (Carey & McDevitt, 1995) and biologic capabilities.

A number of social institutions influence and support cultural socialization, including the family, school, peer groups, and the media.

Family.   The family is the first socializing force on individual encounters. A powerful primary group, the family exposes the child to a set of values in the context of intensely personal relationships, in addition to material and psychological support. It is here that children first learn patterns of socially appropriate (or inappropriate) behavior. Each culture possesses its own values, attitudes, and practices with regard to families and child rearing, providing care and guidance in culturally prescribed ways. Family dynamics can facilitate conformity to the prevailing standards and codes of behavior. As active family members, children develop their personalities and a sense of self; they are given the opportunity to identify feelings and emotions, express ideas and thoughts, and practice interactional skills that they will use throughout their lives.

School.   The school functions to expand the child's socialization beyond the boundaries of the family. Schools serve as models for much of the adult social world, providing the groundwork for developing methods of negotiating one's way within the institutions of adult society (e.g., workplace, politics, or organized recreation). For many children, schools may provide stability, opportunities for creative expression, and learning. A sense of collective identity and responsibility to the group may grow as children engage in school activities. For others, school experiences can have a negative impact on the child's sense of self, leading to a feeling of rejection and isolation from the group.

Peer Group.   Peer groups also play a powerful role in socializing children to their culture. Peer groups can place children in a position of social equality unlike the socially inferior position that they may experience at home or in their school role. Through peer interactions, children explore their identities, give and receive validation of appropriate behavior, and further consolidate a sense of self.

Media.   Television, radio, magazines, newspapers, films, and electronic media (e.g., Internet, chat rooms) have an enormous influence on the cultural socialization of children, especially in contemporary America. As an audience, Americans are conditioned to receive mass culture passively via these vehicles. Through the media, the child is exposed to a wide array of values, many of which conflict with those of the family or the school.

Culture Is Symbolic

Communication takes place between humans using cultural symbols such as language (verbal and nonverbal), dress, food, music, dance, sports, and other activities. The extent to which individuals understand and master these cultural symbols will shape their self-concept, how others perceive them, and their ability to function within and contribute to their culture.

Culture Is Integrated

Culture is reflected in and influences every aspect of an individual's life. The cultural values, beliefs, and behaviors taught are embedded in the fabric of one's life and can be generalized from one social arena to another. Ideas about the appropriate behavior of children may extend from the family to the school to the community (e.g., "children should be respectful to adults"). On the other hand, a cultural group may have different expectations in different roles; for example, language used among peers in the street may be very different from that used in the school or at home. Attitudes and behaviors regarding health, wellness, disease, and disability are an intricate part of this cultural framework.

▰ PROVIDING CULTURALLY COMPETENT CARE

As national economies become more global and as transportation and communication systems become more sophisticated, interdependence among countries and their peoples will continue to increase. Health care providers in the U.S. will see more clients from cultures different than their own, and they will need to become more culturally competent in the care they provide. This effort to develop cultural competency to provide high-quality care is an excellent example of the dynamic nature of culture–U.S. health care providers are members of a particular personal and professional cultural group, and health care in America will change because of the intercultural exchange among clients and providers.

DEVELOPING CULTURAL COMPETENCE

Cultural competence is the ability to communicate among cultures and demonstrate cultural skill outside one's culture of origin (Dunn, 2002). It is based on empathy, respect, and knowledge (Campinha-Bacote, 2002) and requires a fundamental recognition and valuing of culture as a distinctive way of life. The culturally competent provider's focus is not on how to interact with clients so that they will comply with a medical regimen. Instead culturally competent providers work with clients to increase mutual understanding, share information and knowledge, strengthen clients' control of their health, and construct more healthful decisions.

To achieve cultural competence, providers must work to:
- Understand and, if necessary, change their *worldview*
- Become familiar with *core cultural issues*
- Increase their knowledge about *core cultural issues related to health and illness*
- Become knowledgeable about the *cultural groups with whom they work,* in general, and in terms of health and illness
- Develop skills that provide a basis for *effective communication and negotiation* between client and provider

Worldview

A worldview is a conceptual framework that allows members of a social group or culture to answer fundamental questions such as "How does the world function?" "Why does it operate that way?" "Where is it going?" "What does it mean? What values, ethics, and moral standards is it working from?" "How should we act?" and "What is true or false? What is knowledge?" In the U.S., the dominant worldview tends to reflect an activist, rational-mastery, future-oriented approach to life. It is based on a sense of independence and autonomy, and it values acquisition and power. Diversity of ideas, race, ethnicity, and lifestyle may be given little value unless they are useful to those in power. Incidents of discrimination based on race, gender, age, or sexual orientation can be outcomes of this perception.

Various aspects of worldviews have been identified and are often presented as dichotomies for purposes of comparison: for example, individualism versus collectivism; masculinity versus femininity; linear thinking versus global thinking. An example related to health care would be the U.S. culture of "individualism," in which clients make their own decisions about treatment, as opposed to a Southeast Asian culture (e.g., Hmong), in which the family is actively involved in deciding what treatment will be done. The dualistic thinking reflected in these taxonomies has come under criticism as being too simplistic, however, because it does not help explain the subtle nuances of cultures or the complexities of behaviors of members of social groups (Turiel, 2004). Critics assert that to understand human behavior, one must look at interaction within the larger socio-ecological context. Not all Hmong clients rely on family members to help them make decisions about health treatments, for example; nor do all Americans make their decisions independently. Though culture is a vital element in why people make the choices they do, those choices depend on many other factors as well.

For health care providers working with clients from a cultural group other than their own, this means two things: first, they need to examine their own worldview, look at what social and cultural dynamics affect their thinking and behavior, and determine how this influences their practice and interaction with clients. A relevant example might be clinicians who work with adolescents. Clinicians are part of an "adult culture." To effectively work with adolescents, they need to reflect on what their "adult" perceptions are regarding teenagers and how those perceptions structure their approach to the client. There are additional dynamics to consider: Providers have experienced their own adolescence and have had their worldview shaped by that experience. They bring those perceptions to the interaction with their adolescent client (some providers have said, "Two people walk into the exam room when I see an adolescent—me as an adult caregiver, and me when I was 16 years old"). How do health care providers' worldviews affect their thinking about this client? How do those worldviews influence the way they interact with clients? Additionally the current life situation of the provider may be important to consider; perhaps he or she is struggling with a rebellious teenager at home. This personal concern could change their ability to provide high-quality care to adolescents.

Second, health care providers must be open to understanding the worldview of their clients and be willing to adapt their own in order to find the most effective way of providing health care. For example, problem-solving approaches vary among cultures. Not everyone solves problems in the linear, cause-and-effect way often attributed to the dominant culture in the U.S. If clinicians present a health problem and its solution in a linear fashion and insist that their patients and families use the same perspective, they should not be surprised if the patient is sometimes "noncompliant." An example might be a child who has a fever. Based on their worldview, clinicians begin a diagnostic process of examination and laboratory testing to rule out causes, with some idea of an infectious agent in the back of their mind that may need to be treated with an antibiotic. The family, however, may have a more reflective, circuitous problem-solving style, part of which is a wait-and-see attitude, letting the child's body do what it will in response to the fever; and part of which means providing support in traditional cultural ways that involve preparation and time (e.g., sweats, prayer, chicken soup).

Core Cultural Issues

Core cultural issues are those qualities that are "universal (i.e., every culture has them) but specific (i.e., every culture expresses them differently)" (Dunn, 2002, p. 107). One cannot know all there is to know about all cultural groups, but knowledge will be enhanced if core cultural issues are used to learn about and understand different cultural groups. Table 3-2 outlines these issues and provides several examples of each. Clinicians can work with their clients from specific cultural groups to identify how that culture expresses these core issues.

Core Cultural Issues Related to Health and Illness

In addition to examining general cultural characteristics of clients, one needs to look at how culture influences clients' understanding and management of health and illness. Categories in which beliefs and values may influence health behavior include the following:

- Definition or meaning of illness
- Causes of illness or disease
- Appropriate ways in which, when ill, an individual should behave
- Best treatments and appropriate individuals to seek out for treatment and healing

---

TABLE 3-2 Core Cultural Issues

Cultural Characteristics	Example
Physical and biologic characteristics	Bone structure, hair, skin.
Self-orientation and worldview	Individualistic (centered on self and one's needs) vs collectivistic (person is part of larger whole, functions within context of community and history).
Concepts of time, space, and physical distance	What is the comfortable distance between individuals during conversation; when and how is it appropriate to touch a client?
Style and pattern of communication	Who speaks for the family, and when do they do so, what language is used; are introductory comments or questions expected; is language formal?
Physical and social activities expected of group members	Muslim women are expected to cover their faces when in public; young Latino women may be expected to have a male family member escort when they go out.
Relationships with others, often based on gender, age, or social class	Father in family may make decisions for other family members; grandmother may be first person consulted for health problems.
Systems of social organization	Older children in Southeast Asian family may live at home with parents, contribute to family income; attendance at religious services and participation in church activities may be focus of social life.
Relationships with nature	Belief in animism (inanimate natural objects [e.g., wind, earth, rocks] have spiritual quality); sense of responsibility and stewardship toward environment; view that environment is unsafe (e.g., "cleanliness is next to godliness").

Assessment questions that allow clients and families to explain what they think the illness means, what they believe about the causes of their illness, and what they think might be a way to treat it can give providers significant insight into how to best work with clients (Kleinman et al, 1978) (Box 3-1).

When developing the plan of care, incorporate culture-related practices whenever possible and appropriate. Delivering care in an accepting, "nonjudgmental" manner that is congruent with the individual's cultural beliefs and practices does not mean that providers must lower their standards. Rather they should think in terms of the context within which those standards exist. It is helpful to ask the following questions: Is the culture-related practice efficacious? Is it safe? If it is beneficial, the clinician should encourage it. A home remedy may be safe, but have no therapeutic benefit; the client, however, may believe in it, and this belief can have a powerful placebo effect that should be encouraged. If the treatment is not safe, further negotiation must ensue with an explanation as to why the practice is harmful and what options would be better. An example might be treatments for gastrointestinal distress in children used by some Mexican families: One treatment involves rubbing the child's abdomen and body with an uncooked egg in the shell, a technique that is not likely to affect the biologic cause of the gastritis. The egg treatment is not harmful, however, and may comfort both parent (being able to do something) and child (because of the massage and attention). If the family wishes to use it, it should be encouraged. Another treatment for gastritis, however, is *greta,* a lead-based powder that is mixed with water and given to the child orally. *Greta* does not treat the cause of the gastritis and is a serious health risk to the child; it is the providers' responsibility to explain why it should not be given and explore with the family what alternatives are possible. Most families will not persist in treating their children with clearly harmful remedies.

Specific Cultural Groups

Becoming knowledgeable about specific cultural groups is essential to provide sensitive, relevant care. Interaction with and study about specific cultural groups, languages, and worldviews can greatly increase one's knowledge base. When doing cultural assessments, however, cultural characteristics must be viewed as being on a continuum, recognizing that not all individuals from the same social group have the same characteristics. Intraethnic variations must be anticipated and incorporated into the plan of care for a truly individualized approach. Attempting to fit a family or individual into any preconceived cultural framework is not cultural sensitivity—it is stereotyping. Stereotyping and cross-cultural comparisons are to be avoided because they interfere with the development of basic trust and threaten the success of the therapeutic relationship and the plan of care.

Communication and Negotiation Strategies

Communication strategies used in interactions with clients can facilitate trust and convey the message that the clients' beliefs and approaches to health and illness are recognized and respected. This allows both clinicians and clients to actively negotiate for mutually acceptable interventions of care. A basic communication course discusses these strategies; successfully using them in the clinical setting requires ongoing practice, evaluation of their effectiveness, and reflection on ways to change them to strengthen communication.

In the health care setting, effective communication requires listening in a way that allows clients to explain their meaning of the situation (see Box 3-1). Providers must clearly explain their perspective and understanding of the situation, explore a common ground of understanding with clients, and discuss and adapt possible solutions to meet the client's needs (Box 3-2) (Berlin & Fowkes, 1983). As mentioned above, generating a solution based on the client's cultural context does not mean that providers compromise quality of care; indeed care should be enhanced since it is tailored to the unique needs of the client.

Although the style of each provider will vary and the characteristics and needs of clients will create a multitude of variations in each client-provider interaction, there are several considerations that should be kept in mind when communicating with clients in a pediatric health care setting:

Respect. All communication should be respectful. Though this seems obvious, providers do not always convey a clear message of respect. Initially addressing parents, grandparents, and other adults by their formal name and shaking hands can be a good beginning. Acknowledging all individuals in the room is important. Taking notes should be deferred if it interferes with conversation and engagement with the child and family. Actively listening and speaking clearly, calmly, and responsively encourages the child and family members to express their ideas and concerns. Include the child in conversation as is age-appropriate, encourage

---

BOX 3-1 **Identifying Cultural Meaning of Illness for Families**

- What is the problem or illness called?
- What does the family believe is happening?
- What do you think caused the problem or illness?
- Why do you think it started when it did?
- How has this illness affected you and the family?
- What are the chief problems this sickness has caused?
- How severe is the sickness?
- Will it have a short or long course?
- What kind of treatment should the patient receive?
- What are the most important results you hope to have happen from this treatment?
- What treatments have you already tried?
- What helped in the past?
- What do you fear most about this illness?
- Are you afraid to tell your relatives or friends? What are you fearful might happen?

Adapted from Kleinman A, Eisenberg L, Good B: Culture, illness and care: clinical lessons from anthropologic and cross-cultural research, *Ann Intern Med* 88:251-258, 1978.

BOX 3-2 **Steps in Culturally Competent Client-Provider Interaction**

- Listen to client's explanation of situation.
- Explain provider's understanding of problem.
- Acknowledge differences and similarities of understandings.
- Explore possible treatment options—from both provider and client perspective.
- Negotiate a mutually agreeable treatment plan.
- Validate roles of client and provider in carrying out plan.
- Review, evaluate, and change plan as appropriate, using steps above.

Data from Berlin EA, Fowkes WC Jr: A teaching framework for cross-cultural health care: application in family practice, *West J Med* 139:934-938, 1983.

---

questions and check frequently for understanding. Be alert to the style of interaction of the family: a direct approach can be threatening to some; in these situations, using indirect questioning, hypothetical situations, and open-ended questioning can be more helpful.

Context. In some cultural groups, the context in which a message is presented may have more significance than what is actually said. In such a culture, for example, if elders are held in high esteem, a grandmother's comment can represent a definitive statement and should be listened to carefully. Individuals from high-context cultures tend to be less direct in their verbal statements and extremely sensitive to nonverbal and situational cues, such as body language. Communication is facilitated by use of nonverbal methods rather than direct verbal directions.

In low-context cultures, the emphasis is on the content of the verbal message. Verbal communication is direct and explicit, and nonverbal and situational cues are not as significant as in high-context cultures. The provider should be very clear in verbal communication with clients from low-context cultures, recognizing that they may not pick up on situational and nonverbal cues.

Time and Space as Forms of Nonverbal Communication

Time. Some cultures view time as steady, predictable, and mobile. It is always moving forward, and the impressions of past, present, and future are distinct–it is "monochronic," one thing at a time. For others the reality of time exists only in relation to events occurring. "Polychronic" time is characterized by "the simultaneous occurrence of many things and by a great involvement with people" (Hall, 1990, p. 14). From this perspective, there is no such thing as early or late. The future is less important than the present, and problems of daily survival take priority over far-reaching goals. An understanding of these differences can aid providers in looking at their clients' actions, especially failed treatment plans, from a different and more accepting perspective.

Space. Human beings seek to maintain a certain spatial distance from others. An expression of boundaries, this desire for control over a certain amount of personal space is known as *territoriality,* and although it varies from one individual to another, based on gender, age, and situation, there is a correlation between personal space requirements and culture (Watson, 1980). Three dimensions or zones of spatial distancing are recognized: The *intimate zone* allows close proximity and is reserved for family members and those in the roles of caregiver, comforter, and protector; the *personal zone* provides more spatial distance between individuals and is reserved for friends and close acquaintances; and the *public zone* is the spatial distance expected between co-workers and individuals in business encounters. This sense of personal space can be perceived not only visually, as with the establishment of a comfortable distance or with direct or indirect eye contact, but through sound, smell, and touch.

Most people are not consciously aware of their personal space requirements and unconsciously may give nonverbal cues, such as turning to avoid direct face-to-face contact or stepping back, to indicate that they need more personal space. A tendency to move closer, lean forward, and maintain direct eye contact for sustained periods indicates the need for less spatial distance.

Failure to recognize and respect an individual's personal space needs may be interpreted as a threatening invasion of personal space or a lack of caring and compassion, depending on the situation. An awareness of boundaries, territoriality, and appropriate responses to cues received with regard to the spatial needs of an individual client or family enhance the development of a satisfactory client-provider relationship.

Language and Use of Interpreters. Providers are encouraged to become "linguistically appropriate." As a part of this effort, federal standards relating to linguistic competence have been developed—Culturally and Linguistically Appropriate Services (CLAS). These guidelines encourage providers to recognize that there are linguistic variations within cultural groups and that individuals who speak the same language may not share the same cultural background. Also there may be a wide range of literacy levels in all language groups (USDHHS Office of Minority Health, 2001).

It is helpful to speak the client's language, but that ability alone is not sufficient and may not always be possible or necessary to be linguistically appropriate. Interpreters can be used very effectively. Federally funded managed care networks and community health centers are required, as part of the federal grant, to have interpreters accessible for all non-English speaking clients. The importance of using a qualified interpreter cannot be overemphasized. Interpreters who are familiar with the culture and the language are especially helpful because they are likely to be more sensitive to the nonverbal cues inherent in a patient's presentation of the complaint. The term *cultural broker* is used to describe an individual who bridges two or more cultures and can translate both linguistic and cultural meaning.

In some immigrant communities, especially those that are small, there may be few qualified interpreters. Also, as members of a small, closely knit community, both interpreter and client may find it awkward to discuss sensitive personal information in a clinical setting and then return to their culturally prescribed social roles in the community. In larger immigrant communities, several languages or dialects may be spoken; language barriers may arise even among people who speak the same language because communication patterns differ among classes, subcultures, and regions of the country of origin. Contracting with a commercial telephone interpreter service may be a possibility in cases such as these.

Qualified interpreters must be well-trained professionals who are able to communicate to the client that they can be trusted to keep information confidential. When family members or unqualified persons are relied on to translate, patient confidentiality, in addition to provider and family understanding, can be jeopardized.

The qualified interpreter stands or sits behind the provider so as not to interfere with eye contact between the patient, the parent, and the provider. In some instances, the interpreter can even stand or sit behind a screen if privacy is an issue. If topics related to sexuality are to be discussed, interpreters should be of the same sex as the patient.

The interpreter should make an effort to translate the dialogue as closely and accurately as possible for both parties. When a provider's yes-or-no question results in a lengthy response, the interpreter must ensure that the provider is apprised of the whole statement, including any seemingly unrelated data. It is especially difficult to convey emotion through verbal translation, and this component of communication may be lost or diminished when interpreters are used. This should not be perceived as lack of concern on the part of the client or family, and the clinician should be alert for nonverbal cues. Nonverbal cues may have their own cultural connotative meaning, however, so clarification may be necessary (e.g., "You seem very upset; I noticed your face changed when we talked about _____. Are you worried about _____?"). Regarding instructions for home management, it may be helpful if the interpreter can write instructions for the family in the family's language and review them again before the family leaves.

Interpreters should work toward the following goals:
- Make the clients' description and understanding of the problem clear to the provider.
- Communicate accurately the provider's interpretation and explanation of a health problem (e.g., pathophysiology) to the client.
- Facilitate the discussion to develop a management plan.
- Assess patient and parents' level of knowledge and understanding of what is being said.

Culturally Sensitive Patient Education.   It is incorrect to assume that all clients and their families value and benefit from patient education material. Although members of low-context cultures may seek and appreciate written educational material, it may be overwhelming for members of high-context cultures who are trying to interpret a myriad of nonverbal and situational cues as well as the verbal message associated with the visit. The best approach is to make clients aware of the written educational material that is available, and let them know they may take it if they wish.

Any instructions for home management should be written in simple terms in the client's native language or in the language in which parents or caregivers are literate (this may not be the same as the native language), and educational efforts should be directed toward adult family members present, fathers and mothers. Abbreviations should be avoided, and all written material should be reviewed with the patient, parent, or both, with the help of an interpreter when necessary. Do not assume that all parents can read English or their own native language. However, assessing literacy must be done with sensitivity because illiteracy is a source of shame among some peoples.

RECOGNIZING CULTURE SHOCK

The process of emigrating—leaving one's homeland to settle in a different country—presents the individual and the family with many challenges. Changes in diet, exposure to unfamiliar environmental hazards, and lack of appropriate immunity may threaten physical health. Familiar resources are absent, and unfamiliar behaviors, expectations, symbols, and language are barriers to meeting basic daily needs. Considerable energy is required to interpret and respond to this new environment. The feelings of helplessness and exhaustion that may ensue are part of the phenomenon known as *culture shock,* first identified by anthropologists in the 1950s (Oberg, 1960).

Culture shock affects the physical, emotional, and psychological well-being of every member of the family and may take many months to overcome. Generally, individuals progress through stages of culture shock. Initially, they may be fascinated with the novelty of the new culture, then become hostile or highly critical, before moving on to adjustment and acceptance. The degree of culture shock that is experienced depends on many variables, including social status, personality characteristics, age, occupation, available support systems, familiarity with the dominant language, general state of health, and the extent of cultural differences between the home and host countries. For immigrants from areas of the world where they have experienced displacement, violence, trauma, abuse, and fear, culture shock is complicated by difficulty coping with stress.

In the presence of health care providers, clients and family members may appear inappropriately complacent or overreactive. Rather than being noncompliant or uncooperative, they may, in reality, be experiencing culture shock. Successful management of culture shock can be facilitated by clearly and patiently explaining what is happening with the client; providing clear, relevant information about how the health system works; acknowledging the client's sense of confusion as normal; and giving positive feedback for the client's efforts.

TABLE 3-3   Health Issues Found in Cultural Groups

Cultural Group	Health Issue
African American	High infant mortality rate
	Sickle cell trait and disease
	Hypertension
	Obesity
	Type 2 diabetes mellitus
	Type 1 diabetes mellitus with beta-cell destruction
	Slipped capital femoral epiphysis
	Blount disease
	Lead poisoning caused by environmental exposure in urban areas
	Violence
Asian American	Lactose intolerance
	Tuberculosis, dental caries, malnutrition among some recent immigrants
	Cleft lip and palate
Caucasian	Rett syndrome (girls)
	Tay-Sachs disease (Ashkenazi Jewish; French Canadian)
	Tyrosinemia (French Canadian; Scandinavian)
	Celiac disease
	Cystic fibrosis
	Phenylketonuria (Northern European)
	Pyloric stenosis (Northern European)
	Blount disease (Northern European)
	Lactose intolerance
	Type 1 diabetes mellitus
	Glutaric aciduria type 1 (Amish and Hutterites; Canadian)
	Lice
Latino	Dental caries
	Obesity
	Type 2 diabetes mellitus
	Blount disease
	Asthma
Native American (American Indian)	Otitis media
	Poor prenatal care, low–birth-weight babies, high infant mortality rate
	Alcoholism
	Unintentional injury
Samoan or Polynesian	Dermatologic conditions
	Obesity
	Slipped capital femoral epiphysis
Russian American	Obesity
	Alcoholism

Health care providers working with clients and families from culturally diverse backgrounds frequently experience culture shock, too. Lack of knowledge of differences in diseases, cultural practices, beliefs, and values can result in feelings of helplessness, frustration, and inadequacy for everyone involved in the helping relationship. Clinicians can reduce their own culture shock and that of their clients by learning about the different cultural groups they work with and recognizing the signs of culture shock in their clients and themselves.

■ CULTURES IN AMERICAN SOCIETY

The population of the U.S. consists of numerous ethnic groups, races, and subcultures and is becoming increasingly diverse. It is often broken down into the dominant white middle class and a number of minority groups, including African Americans, Hispanic Americans, Asian Americans, Native Americans, Russian Americans, and Arab Americans. Within each of these categories, there are many subgroups. For example, most providers would include families from Iran, Syria, and Iraq in the category of "Arab Americans," yet the cultural differences between each are immeasurable, and, though they may share some common characteristics, each is unique and constantly changing.

To present descriptions of each cultural group is beyond the scope of this text. Instead Table 3-3 lists some of the more common health issues found in some cultural groups, and the Resource Box lists a number of resources that providers can use to access information that best suits their particular practice. It must be remembered that these health issues are not exclusive to a particular culture; they may be, however, overrepresented in some groups (e.g., lead poisoning in African-American children) because of environmental, social, economic, and class factors, not intrinsic cultural characteristics. Thus, though cultural competence on the part of providers is essential, institutional, political, and social change will also have to occur before full equity in health care is realized. That, too, is a discussion beyond the scope of this text.

Providing culturally competent care is increasingly required of health care providers. It is a challenge that requires personal reflection as well as significant change in beliefs, attitudes, and practices. By working sensitively with clients of diversity, sharing ideas and information, learning from and about each other, and celebrating differences and similarities, both clients and clinicians can become full participants in creating a new cultural context for the health and illness experience.

*R*ESOURCE BOX

Cultural Perspectives

Center for Medicaid and Medicare Services/American Indian Alaska Native
www.cms.hhs.gov/aian

Child Family Health International
www.cfhi.org
Opportunity for U.S. pediatric health care providers and students to work in an international setting

Diversity, Healing, and Health Care
www.gasi-ves.org/diversity.htm
Sponsored by the Stanford Geriatric Education Center and On Lok Senior Health; cultural and religious information relevant to health care providers

DiversityRX
www.diversityrx.org
Sponsored by the National Conference of State Legislatures (NCSL); Resources for Cross Cultural Health Care (RCCHC); and the Henry J. Kaiser Family Foundation of Menlo Park, CA
   Educational opportunities for professionals; legislative, policy, and advocacy information about cultural groups

EthnoMed
www.ethnomed.org
Detailed information regarding cultural characteristics of diverse populations

Health Resources and Services Administration (HRSA) and Office of Minority Health Resource Center
www.hrsa.gov/culturalcompetence
www.omhrc.gov
www.omhrc.gov/clas
A wide range of resources for health care workers, including assessment tools, technical assistance, training programs and curricula, and information about diseases, research, standards of care, etc.
   Guidelines for medical practices to develop and implement culturally and linguistically appropriate services

National Center for Cultural Competence
www.georgetown.edu/research/gucchd/nccc
Training opportunities; links to national resources for health care to diverse populations

National Network of Libraries of Medicine: Cultural Competency Resources
www.nnlm.gov/mcr/resources/community/competency.html
Resources and tools for providers; independent learning modules; extensive links to other sites

Northwest Translators and Interpreters Society (NOTIS),
Chapter of American Translators Association (www.atanet.org)
NOTIS Medical Interpreters SIG (www.notisnet.org/notis/org/SIGS/medsig.html)
   Inherited objectives of the Society of Medical Interpreters (SOMI); provides educational offerings, networking, list of medical interpreters for a wide range of languages

State University of New York Institute of Technology
www.culturedmed.sunyit.edu/bib/medica/
Extensive bibliographies, information, and links on a wide range of cultural groups, refugees and immigrants, standards, interpreters, dictionaries, etc

The Cross Cultural Health Care Program
www.xculture.org
Cultural competence training, interpreter training, research, and educational materials; links to community profiles for range of diverse populations

University of Buffalo, Health Sciences Library: Cultural Competency Resources
http://ublib.buffalo.edu/libraries/units/hsl/resources/guides/culturalcompetence.html
Highlights resources that assist with independent learning. Focused on nursing faculty and other interested professionals hoping to incorporate cultural competence skills into nursing curricula and practice

University of California, San Francisco, The Network for Multicultural Health, The Center for Health Professions
www.futurehealth.ucsf.edu/TheNetwork

☑ DISCUSSION FORUM

1. How do your cultural beliefs affect your ability to provide culturally competent care? List at least three strategies to overcome conflicts between your and your patient's cultural beliefs.
2. You see a child whose family believes in natural therapy for illnesses (e.g., diet therapy, massage, avoiding traditional medical treatments). How can you incorporate the family's beliefs if the child has an upper respiratory infection? What if the child has a more serious condition, such as leukemia?
3. Compare and contrast how the two main cultural groups in your community view family, gender roles, child rearing, and health.

REFERENCES

Airhihenbuwa CO, Liburd L: Eliminating health disparities in the African American population: the interface of culture, gender, and power, *Health Educ Behav* 33(4):488-501, 2006.
Berger P, Luckmann T: *The social construction of reality,* New York, 1966, Doubleday.
Berlin EA, Fowkes WC Jr: A teaching framework for cross-cultural health care: application in family practice, *West J Med* 139:934-938, 1983.
Campinha-Bacote J: The process of cultural competence in the delivery of health care services: a model of care, *J Transcult Nurs* 13:181-184, 2002.
Carey WB, McDevitt SC: *Coping with children's temperament: a guide for professionals,* New York, 1995, Basic Books.
Crosson JC et al: Evaluating the effect of cultural competency training on medical student attitudes, *Fam Med* 36(3):199-203, 2004.

Dunn AM: Culture competence and the primary care provider, *J Pediatr Health Care* 16:105-111, 2002.

Fadiman A: *The spirit catches you and you fall down,* NY, 1997, Farrar, Straus and Giroux.

Gray P, Thomas DJ: Critical reflections on culture in nursing, *J Cult Divers* 13(2):76-82, 2006.

Hall ET: *Understanding cultural differences,* Yarmouth, ME, 1990, Intercultural Press.

Kleinman A, Eisenberg L, Good B: Culture, illness and care: clinical lessons from anthropologic and cross-cultural research, *Ann Intern Med* 88:251-258, 1978.

Koehn PH, Swick HM: Medical education for a changing world: moving beyond cultural competence into transnational competence, *Acad Med* 81(6):548-556, 2006.

Kripalani S et al: A prescription for cultural competence in medical education, *J Gen Intern Med* 21(10):1116-1120, 2006.

Kroeber AL: *The nature of culture,* Chicago, 1952, University of Chicago Press.

Larsen LJ: The foreign-born population in the United States: 2003, *Curr Popul Rep* P20-551, Washington, DC, 2004, US Census Bureau.

Mathews TJ, MacDorman MF: Infant mortality statistics from the 2003 period linked birth/infant death data set, *Natl Vital Statistics Rep* 54(15), Atlanta, 2006, Centers for Disease Prevention and Control.

Oberg K: Culture shock: adjustment to new cultural environment, *Practical Anthropol* 7:177-182, 1960.

Passel JS, Suro R: *Rise, peak, and decline: trends in U.S. immigration 1992-2004*, Washington, DC, 2005, Pew Hispanic Center.

Shapiro J et al: "That never would have occurred to me": a qualitative study of medical students' views of a cultural competence curriculum, *BMC Med Educ* 6:31, 2006.

Thom DH et al: Development and evaluation of a cultural competency training curriculum, *BMC Med Educ* 6(1):38, 2006.

Turiel E: Beyond individualism and collectivism: a problem, or progress? *New Dir Child Adolesc Dev* (104):91-100, 2004.

Underwood SM et al: Nursing contributions to the elimination of health disparities among African-Americans: review and critique of a decade of research, *J Natl Black Nurses Assoc* 16(1):31-47, 2005.

US Census Bureau News: *Census Bureau data show key population changes across nation. American Community Survey provides first data for many cities since 2000,* Press release, Washington DC, Aug 15, 2006, US Department of Commerce.

US Department of Health and Human Services (USDHHS) Office of Minority Health: *National Standards for Culturally and Linguistically Appropriate Services in Health Care: final report,* Rockville, MD, 2001, USDHHS.

Watson OM: *Proxemic behavior: a cross-cultural study*, The Hague, Netherlands, 1980, Mouton.

Wilson JH: *African immigrants in metropolitan Washington: a demographic overview, presentation to the African Immigrants and Refugees Foundation*, Washington DC, Nov 18, 2003, The Brookings Institution.

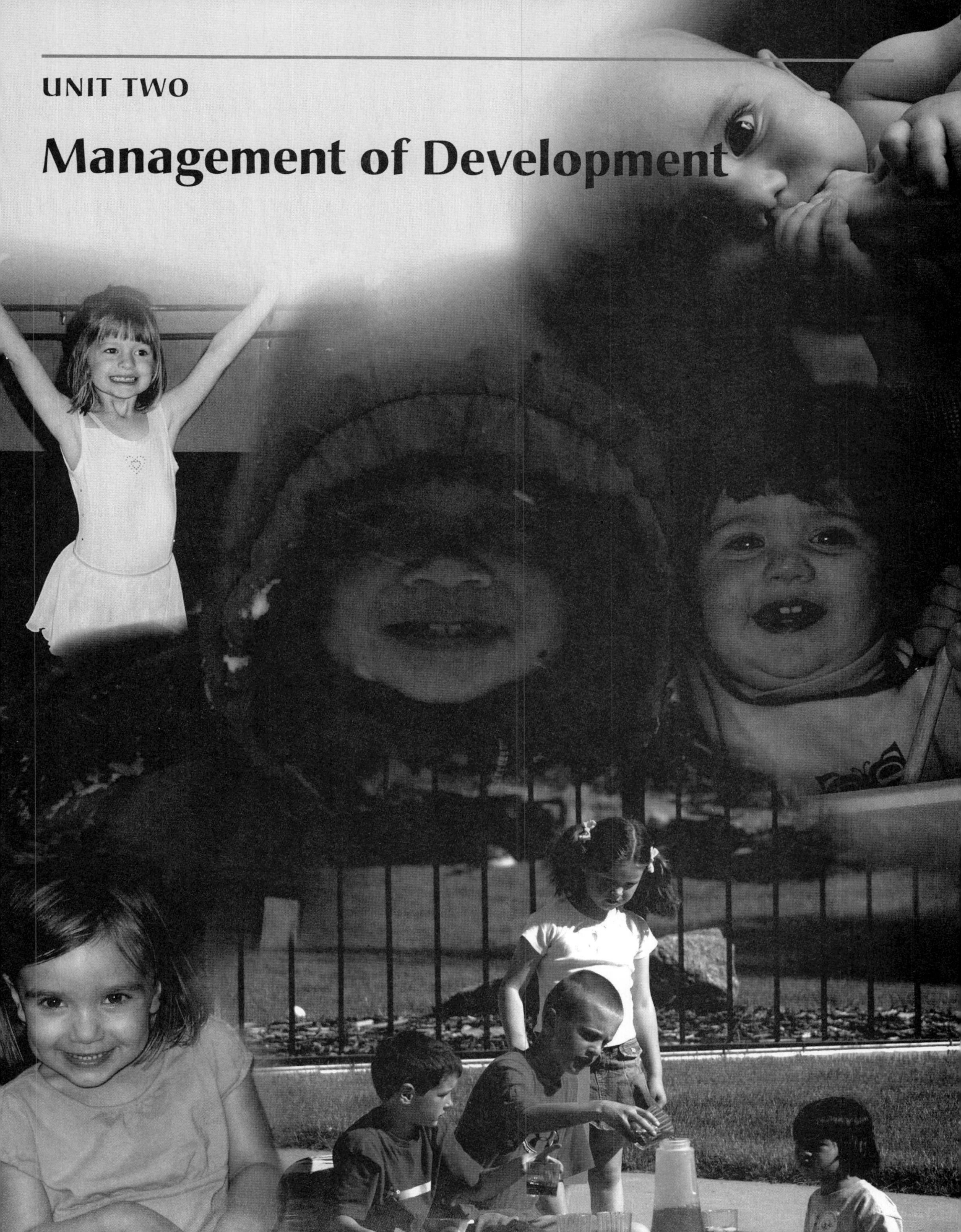

UNIT TWO
Management of Development

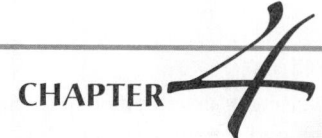

Developmental Management in Pediatric Primary Care

Barbara Jones Deloian and Anita Berry

Modern approaches to managing children's well-being differ dramatically from those that prevailed at the turn of the last century, when health supervision often consisted of a brief examination to detect communicable or contagious diseases. In the twenty-first century, significant social, economic, and demographic changes continue to influence the American family and affect children's health. Children's health supervision must take a broader approach than would be necessary only for detection of disease. Pediatric primary care providers have a responsibility to monitor children's overall physical, cognitive, and psychosocial development and to provide anticipatory guidance to families as children grow. This requires a strong background in child development, knowledge of strategies that help parents understand and adjust to their child's development, and an ability to establish effective relationships with children and their parents.

The Classification of Child and Adolescent Mental Health Diagnoses in Primary Care: Diagnostic and Statistical Manual for Primary Care (DSM-PC), Child and Adolescent Version (Wolraich et al, 1996) presents a comprehensive description of the physical and psychosocial developmental concerns of childhood and adolescence. An estimated 17% of American children have developmental or behavioral disorders (Bhasin et al, 2006). Thus, the pediatric primary care provider must have a sound knowledge of developmental and behavioral norms and variations (Dixon & Stein, 2006).

Pediatric providers offer parents support and can suggest diverse approaches to child rearing. They help parents to understand the challenges that new accomplishments create and how parents may best handle these challenges. Providers who develop a close relationship with parents and their children share in the parents' pride as their child grows.

Not all health care providers satisfy the parents' needs for guidance, however. A national survey of early childhood health (Blumberg et al, 2004) gathered data on parents' perceptions of the anticipatory guidance received from their child's primary health care provider. Parent reports indicated there were unmet needs, particularly for discussion related to discipline strategies and toilet training (expressed by 36% of parents with children 4 to 9 months old and 56% of parents with children 10 to 35 months old). Other areas in which

parents wanted more information included reading, vocabulary development, social development, child care, and burn prevention (Olson et al, 2004). To meet the needs of parents and children, it is imperative for primary care providers to have a sound foundation regarding all aspects of evaluating, assessing, and managing child development.

This chapter presents an introduction to principles of development, developmental theories, methods of developmental assessment, and identification and management of developmental problems. Chapters 5 through 8 review developmental theories, describe normal patterns of development, identify "red flags" related to development, and recommend anticipatory guidance for families of infants, toddlers and preschoolers, school-age children, and adolescents.

DEVELOPMENTAL PRINCIPLES

Development is a lifelong, dynamic process. Achievement of changes in one phase sets the stage for the next phase. Development is also a dynamic and reciprocal process that occurs between the child's internal and external environment. Key principles are often used to understand concepts of development. Exactly how these principles are manifested in a particular child depends on the child's genetic background, personality, and intrauterine and extrauterine environmental factors.

Principle 1. Growth and development are orderly and sequential. Although children differ in rates and timing of developmental changes, they generally follow certain predictable stages or phases. Specific examples include the rapid growth during the first year of life, progress toward independence throughout childhood, and the unfolding of secondary sex characteristics during adolescence.

Principle 2. The pace of growth and development is specific for each child. Developmental changes vary considerably for each child. Some children demonstrate early skill in motor coordination, others in language acquisition. These changes represent the uniqueness of each child.

Principle 3. Development occurs in a cephalocaudal and proximodistal direction. An example of this principle is seen as infants develop increasing motor coordination, gaining head control before sitting and walking. Similarly, developmental progress is seen in controlled movements that occur near the midline of the body first, such as rolling over. Eventually, distal coordination of the hands, such as mastery of the pincer grasp, occurs.

The authors would like to thank Mary A. Murphy for her contributions that remain unchanged from the third edition.

Principle 4. Growth and development become increasingly integrated. Behavior that is often taken for granted, such as self-feeding, occurs as a result of numerous small changes and skills acquired by the child. Simple skills and behaviors are integrated into more complex behaviors as the child grows and develops.

Principle 5. Developmental abilities become increasingly organized and differentiated. As a result of increasing maturation and experience, children's behaviors and responses to internal and external cues become more regulated, organized, and differentiated. The infant's crying and body movements in response to hunger cues are different from the toddler's walking to the refrigerator in response to the same cues.

Principle 6. Growth and development are affected by the child's internal and external environment. Opportunities for play, societal norms, cultural values, family traditions, and family beliefs all influence the development of children. Similarly, children influence their environment to achieve desired experiences and opportunities.

Principle 7. Certain periods are critical during growth and development. Critical periods are defined as points of time when developmental advances occur more readily than they do at other times. The occurrence of congenital anomalies when the fetus is exposed to certain viruses during fetal growth is one example.

Principle 8. Growth and development is a dynamic process influenced by many factors. Development is a continual process, often without smooth transitions. Phases of development are marked by periods of change, growth, and plateaus of stability. Efforts to predict and control the developmental process often emphasize the individual nature of development and the numerous individual factors that influence developmental outcomes (Cech & Martin, 2002).

▓ DEVELOPMENTAL THEORIES

The study of developmental theories reveals a fascinating array of ideas about how children progress from infancy through adolescence, providing many perspectives on children's growth and development. Health care providers need to stay abreast of changing ideas of child development and appreciate new developmental theories relating to children. Developmental theories are based on various cultures, personalities, environmental issues, philosophic beliefs, and investigative methods. Thus when using a developmental perspective in practice, the provider should understand how the theory was developed and how it may relate to a particular family and child. Developmental theories provide guidelines for understanding the unfolding of the child's behavior, personality, and physical abilities, and it is usually necessary to combine several theories to understand the child as a whole person.

Criticism has been expressed that early theorists' work lacked experimental support, especially related to different cultural and socioeconomic settings and that many theories were too linear in their thinking, missing the subtleties of the interaction of "nature" and "nurture." More research is being conducted to validate and test developmental theories, to incorporate new concepts, and to gain a better understanding of children's learning mechanisms, especially children who have special needs.

ETHOLOGY: ANIMAL STUDIES

The study of animal behavior, looking at the concepts of bonding, altruism, social intelligence, and dominant and submissive behavior, has led to some theoretic assumptions that assist in the study of child development. Bowlby (1969) first generalized theories developed about animal behavior to bonding for humans, articulating the concept of attachment theory. Ainsworth and colleagues (1971) continued to examine the elements of early attachment and separation in child development and personality. This was followed by Klaus and Kennel's work (1976), which emphasized the importance of early mother-infant contact that later became the basis for changes in hospital rooming-in care.

MATURATIONAL THEORIES: DEVELOPMENTAL MILESTONES

Early theories about human behavior set the stage for studies in child development. Rousseau's descriptions in 1762 of the natural, innately good growth of the child, if not misled by a "corrupt social environment," provided the foundation for maturational theories. Gesell (1940) is credited with the term *maturation* in reference to the orderly, sequential developmental changes that occur over time. He also described cycles of behavior that correspond to certain chronologic ages. His work resulted in the chronologic growth and development norms for motor, affective, linguistic, and social domains that are now used to assess developmental progress.

Lewin (1936) identified growth principles and the currently acknowledged stages of infancy, early childhood, and adolescence. He also provided an understanding of the play and decision-making phases through which children progress.

Havighurst's work (1953), a summation of ideas from many theorists, popularized the concept of developmental tasks as "successful achievement which leads to... happiness and to success with later tasks, while failure leads to unhappiness in the individual, disapproval by society, and difficulty with later tasks."

COGNITIVE-STRUCTURAL THEORIES: LANGUAGE AND THOUGHT

Cognitive-structural theories examine the ways in which children think, reason, and use language. They are based on assumptions of maturation of the central nervous system and children's interactions with their environment. Individual differences are ascribed to genetic endowment and environmental influences.

Jean Piaget's observations, many of which were of his own children, provide an understanding of children's cognitive development and their perception and use of the world around them. Piaget (1969) described how children actively use their life experiences, incorporating them into their own mental and physical being over time. He emphasized how children modify themselves depending on their environmental experiences and their stage-related level of competencies. Piaget described four stages of cognitive development (Table 4-1).

Sensorimotor Stage (Birth to 2 Years)

At this stage, children learn about the world through their actions and sensory and motor movements. Key concepts during this period include object permanence, spatial relationships, causality, use of instruments, and combination of objects. The child's framework for learning is the self, and there is little cognitive connection to objects outside the self.

Preoperational Stage (2 to 7 Years)

Children next attempt to make sense of the world and reality. However, this is based on an egocentric perspective and is accomplished through certain mental operations that are linked to concrete objects. Children at this stage are not able to understand cause and effect. Therefore their reasoning is often flawed. Children begin to use semiotic functioning, or the use of one thing to represent another. Intuitive reasoning emerges toward the end of this stage, but reasoning continues to be connected to the concrete reality of the here and now.

Concrete Operational Stage (7 to 12 Years)

Children use symbols to represent concrete objects (here and now) and perform mental operations in their head. This requires cognitive skills to organize experiences and classify increasingly complex information. Most schoolwork requires functioning at this level with flexibility of thought, declining egocentrism, logical reasoning, and greater social cognition.

Formal Operational Stage (13 Years Through Adulthood)

At this stage, children begin to think abstractly and to imagine different solutions to problems and different outcomes. Adolescents begin to develop increased awareness of degrees of illness and personal control of one's health. Renewed egocentrism may be noted early in this stage as a result of lack of differentiation between what others are thinking and one's own thoughts. This egocentric thinking eventually gives way to an appreciation of the differences in judgment between the adolescent and other individuals, societies, and cultures. It becomes the basis of an adolescent's ability to think about politics, law, and society in terms of abstract principles and benefits rather than focusing only on the punitive aspects of societal laws.

Piaget's work was expanded by theorists such as Flavell (1977) and Siegler and colleagues (1973), who looked at specific intellectual capabilities via the information processing model. This model included concepts of attention, perception, memory, and inferencing and provided an initial understanding of how mental activity leads progressively to more sophisticated ways of handling information.

Kohlberg (1969) focused on theories of moral development and socialization, emphasizing the process by which children learn the expectations and norms of their society and culture (see Table 4-1). Kohlberg's work primarily involved male participants. Gilligan (1982) suggested that female thoughts and actions involve significantly different objectives and goals; specifically that girls tend to think more in terms of caring and relationships, basing their moral judgments on complexities they perceive in human interactions.

Fowler's theory (1981) described the spiritual dimension of human life, or the development of faith. This theory addressed the process by which humans develop meaning for daily life. Faith is described as the structure that people use to build their lives. Fowler emphasized that achieving the stages is not due to intelligence but rather occurs through valuing, thinking, and interacting with others.

PSYCHOANALYTIC THEORIES

Personality and Emotions

Psychodynamic theorists have studied factors that influence the emotional and psychological behavior of individuals. Personality includes the characteristics of temperament and motivation, in addition to concepts related to self-esteem and self-concept. Sigmund Freud (1938) was one of the most influential theorists in this area. Freud sought to find links between the conscious mind and the body through the unconscious mind (see Table 4-1). Some of his most significant contributions were his descriptions of the interactions of id, ego, and superego (Thomas, 1985).

Anna Freud continued the work of her father, focusing particularly on children. It was through her studies that the implications of psychoanalysis for raising normal children were developed. She believed that psychoanalytic theory could help parents gain "insight into the potential harm done to young children during the critical years of their development by the manner in which their needs, drives, wishes, and emotional dependencies are met" (Freud, 1974).

Erikson (1964) also expanded Freud's theories, describing the stages of the individual through the life span (see Table 4-1). Each stage presents problems that the individual seeks to master. Erikson believed that if problems were not resolved, they would be revisited again at future stages.

Sullivan (1964) emphasized the importance of self-concept and the environmental influences that modulate it. He defined the most crucial cultural environment as the home and the parent. Sullivan posited that progression toward mature relationships is based on communication skills and the integration of social experiences inhibited or enhanced by the parents' relationship between themselves.

Mahler and colleagues (1975) analyzed the development of an infant's evolving independence through study of the mother-infant dyad. Three phases of development were proposed: autism, symbiosis, and separation-individuation. They posited that these phases account for the gradually increasing awareness of the infant's sense of self and others. In the autistic phase (3 to 5 weeks old), the infant has no concept of self, but is working, physiologically, to achieve homeostasis in the extrauterine world. The second phase, symbiosis, refers to a period of undifferentiation or fusion with the mother in which infant and mother form a dual unity. Separation-individuation (from about 4 to 5 months old onward) is characterized by a steady increase in awareness of the separateness of the self and the other.

TABLE 4-1 Comparison of Early Developmental Theorists

Age	Freud	Kohlberg — Stages	Piaget — Stages/Substages	Piaget — Characteristics	Erikson — Psychological Crisis	Erikson — Themes
0-12mo	Oral stage	"Amoral" pre-conventional level 1: Punishment and obedience	Sensorimotor stage 1. Reflexive stage: 0-1mo 2. Primary circular stage: 1-4mo 3. Secondary circular stage: 4-8mo 4. Coordination of secondary circular stage: 8-12mo	Innate infant reflexes Repetitive responses Outward-directed behaviors Object permanence and goal-directed behaviors	Trust vs. mistrust	To get; to give in return
12-18mo			5. Tertiary circular reactions stage: 2-18mo 6. Mental combinations stage 18-24mo	Causality and object permanence through several steps Memory used for problem-solving	Autonomy vs. shame	To hold on; to let go
18-36mo	Anal stage	Stages 1-2 conventional level 2: Instrumental realistic orientation				
3-6yr	Oedipal stage	Stages 1-3 3: Interpersonal acceptance of "nice" girl and "good" boy social concept	Preoperational stage: 1. Preconceptual stage: 2-4yr 2. Intuitive stage: 4-7yr	Increased use of symbols, especially language; representational thought, egocentrism, assimilation, and symbolic play Increased symbolic functioning, language, decreasing egocentricity, imitation of reality	Initiative vs. guilt	To make things; to play

Age				Concrete/Formal operational stage		Erikson	
6-11 yr	Latency stage	Stages 2-5	4: The "law and order" orientation 5: Social contract and utilitarian orientation	Concrete operational stage	Flexible thought: understands rules of reversibility and deconcentration, conservation, and identity Declining egocentrism: ability to understand another's perspective Local reasoning: understands concepts of relation, ordering, conservation; able to classify objects Social cognition: improved sense of equality and justice	Industry vs. inferiority	To make things; to complete
12-17 yr	Adolescence (Oedipus complex)	Stages 4-6	6: Universal ethical principle orientation	Formal operational stage	Development of logical thinking, able to work with abstract ideas; able to synthesize and integrate concepts into larger schemes	Identity vs. role confusion	To be oneself; to share being oneself or not being oneself
17-30 yr	Young adult	Stages 4-6		Formal operational stage		Intimacy vs. isolation	To lose and find oneself in another

Infant attachment within the context of separation and connectedness has been explored by Stern (1985), Emde and Buchsbaum (1990), and Rogoff (1990). They propose that the quality and consistency of infant-caregiver relationships help the infant develop an affective, or emotional, sense of self. The early beginnings of the sense of self are based on three biologic principles: self-regulation, social fittedness, and affective monitoring (Emde, 1988). Infants with attachment security and a sense of connectedness are more likely to explore and be autonomous; they also have what is called an *internal working model* to guide them in later attachments.

The concept of *intersubjectivity,* or mutual understanding of meaning and mutual engagement in social interactions, underlies attachment theory. Observing that even very young infants demonstrate an ability to interact beyond an instinctive or reflexive manner with a sympathetic individual, Trevarthen and Aitken conducted an extensive review of the literature on the topic of infant intersubjectivity (2001). They concluded that the infant's capacity for self-regulation may be based in the operation of an intrinsic motive formation (IMF) developed in the parietotemporal region of the prenatal brain. Studies of the brain and infant behavior suggest that this IMF guides the newborn's ability to integrate sensory-motor coordination, orient to preferred stimuli (e.g., mother's voice), sustain mutual attention with an affectionate other, and anticipate what to expect in the environment. Successful development of the infant's "purposive consciousness" and ability to cooperate with and learn from another depends on the neurologic functioning and the presence of a supportive environment. The parent guides the infant in connecting with others and experiencing mutuality. Social interactions and engagement of infants with their parents and objects in their world are major developmental influences.

These theories help the provider assist parents to understand why, for example, 9-month-old infants (who now understand object permanence) will look over the side of the highchair for food or a toy that has fallen to the floor and smile and laugh when they spot it–they knew it would be there. These same infants may call a parent to their room in the middle of the night; they now have "person permanence." They can picture their parent in their mind and, perhaps experiencing normal separation anxiety, they want the parent to come to them. The provider can use the concepts of attachment theory and intersubjectivity to explain that this behavior is that of a normal developing infant trying to have his or her needs met. The behavior reflects an infant who is attached and who uses the parent as a secure base from which to explore the world; it is not a problem nor is the child being "bad."

BEHAVIORAL THEORIES: HUMAN

Actions and Interactions

Behaviorism, the study of the general laws of human behavior, focuses on the present and ways that the environment influences human behavior. Skinner's view of child development examined learning that was controlled through classic operant conditioning (1953). Behavior modification therapy is largely based on Skinner's work. Bandura's social learning theory looked at imitation and modeling as a means of learning, emphasizing the social variables involved (Mott, 1990; Thomas, 1985). Bijou and Baer (1965) responded to critics of behaviorism's view of the child as a passive object, arguing that children's responses to environmental stimuli are dependent on their genetic structure and personal history (Thomas, 1985).

HUMANISTIC THEORIES

Innermost Self

Maslow (1971), Buhler and Allen (1972), and Mahrer (1978) are among the most well-known humanistic theorists, examining development throughout the life span. Maslow's hierarchy of needs included physiologic, safety, belongingness and love, esteem, and self-actualization needs. He differentiated deficiency needs from growth or self-actualization needs. Rather than proposing stages through which children or adults mature, the humanists believe that individuals and those around them are responsible for any movement they make from one plateau of needs to another; intrinsic forces do not move them along.

ECOLOGIC THEORIES

The key concepts of human ecology theory (Bronfenbrenner, 1979) emphasize the interdependence between environmental settings (roles, interpersonal relations, and activities) and the developing child. Development is described as the growing capacity to discover, sustain, or alter the self or the environment. Children are viewed as dynamic entities who are increasingly able to restructure the settings in which they live. Environments are seen as influencing children, leading to mutual accommodation and reciprocity. Children's perceptions of the environment influence their behavior and development more than the objective reality does.

Children are influenced by the home and family, child care settings, schools, entertainment and recreational activities, their parents' work, and broad economic opportunities in society. Recognition is given to ecologic transitions or changes in an individual's role or setting, such as the birth of a sibling or changes in family structure. Routine and ritual within the family system can be powerful mediators of children's development (Fiese, 2002; Kubicek, 2002). The parent-child interaction also may be inhibited or enhanced by the parents' relationships. When parents experience positive mutual feelings, the parent-child relationship can be strengthened. Alternatively, when parents experience mutual antagonism or interference, the parent-child relationship may be impaired (Kelly & Barnard, 2000). These theories are especially useful to better understand the impact of domestic violence on a child's development and future.

TEMPERAMENT

The work of Chess and Thomas (1995) seeks to explain the role that temperament plays in children's behavior. They identified characteristics or qualities of temperament and introduced the concept of "goodness of fit" to describe the degree to which the child's environment and parents' characteristics, including the parents' temperament, are

TABLE 4-2	Characteristics of Temperament

Temperament Characteristic	Description
Activity	What is the child's activity level? Is the child moving all the time he or she is awake, some of the time, or rarely?
Rhythmicity	How predictable is the child's sleep/wake pattern, feeding schedule, and elimination pattern?
Approach or withdrawal	What is the child's response when presented with something new such as a new toy, a new experience, or a new person? Does he or she immediately approach or turn away?
Adaptability	How quickly does the child get used to new things? Quickly or not at all?
Threshold of response	How much stimulation does the child require for calming? A quiet voice and touch or more intense, loud voice or firm grasp?
Intensity of reaction	Are the child's responses (crying or laughing) very subtle or extremely intense?
Quality of mood	Is the child's mood usually outgoing, happy, joyful, pleasant or unfriendly, withdrawn, or quiet?
Distractibility	How easily is the child distracted by outside disturbance such as a phone ringing, TV, siblings?
Attention span and persistence	How long will the child continue to play with a particular toy or engage in a certain activity? Does this continue even when there are distractions?

congruous with the child's natural temperamental characteristics. During a child's infancy, the health care provider can explore with parents the variations in the temperament of their child and help parents understand how temperament may affect the child's behavior (Carey, 1998). The provider can discuss with parents how they view their child's temperament, how it "fits" with the parent's temperament or that of other family members, and what parent-child strategies can be used if there is a mismatch of temperament. The intent is to alleviate guilt and frustration and to assist parents in developing skills that enhance positive behaviors rather than exaggerate difficult temperamental characteristics. Scales that can be used to assess an individual child's temperament are listed in the Resource Box at the end of Chapter 5. Table 4-2 further defines characteristics of temperamental differences.

SELF-REGULATION

Self-regulation involves a transition from mutual regulation between mother and newborn and emphasizes the importance of both "nature and nurture" in a child's development (Shonkoff & Phillips, 2000; Trevarthen & Aitken, 2001). Self-regulation is reflected in early infant sleep patterns and ability to self-sooth, the toddler's ability to manage emerging emotions, the preschooler's ability to transition from home to school, the school-age child's ability to focus attention on important tasks, and the adolescent's sense of confidence and competence. Learning to regulate the self is related to differences in temperament, genetics, abilities of the child, and characteristics of the child's environment (Kochanska et al, 2001). The ways in which the social environment interacts with the individuality of the child, and the types of interventions that will contribute to successful self-regulation continue to be explored. One important variable influencing the child's development appears to be a need for a predictable and consistent environment and a caring, emotionally available caregiver (Bronson, 2000).

CULTURAL FACTORS INFLUENCING DEVELOPMENT

Cultural and ethnic traditions are important considerations in the development of infants, children, adolescents, parents, and families. Differences have been identified in achievement of childhood developmental milestones for some cultural groups. Group differences, however, may be irrelevant when providing individualized care for a particular child and family. More accurate assessments of families and children come from understanding the specific culture of a family and community. To gain this knowledge about a family, additional assessment is needed beyond the traditional health history and physical examination.

Tools, such as the genogram, ecomap, and family functioning model (Minuchin, 1974), can be particularly helpful in identifying family structure, strengths, and resources, in addition to individual family health responses, beliefs, and practices. The childhood health assessment questionnaire (CHAQ) and child health questionnaire (CHQ) have also been adapted to a number of cultural groups (Ruperto et al, 2001). The interview process is valuable for clarifying families' unique qualities and resources and serving as an avenue for communicating interest in, and understanding of, individual families and their ethnic or cultural values, differences, and commonalities (see Chapters 2 and 3).

Nugent (1994) discusses three invaluable outcomes that can be achieved through cross-cultural studies of child development. First, these studies add an understanding of the diversity of parenting styles and belief systems, and, as such, they allow providers to move beyond their own worldview. Second, cross-cultural research provides a better understanding of the dynamic aspects of child-environment relationships and development. Third, providers become aware that conventional programs and assessment tools may not be appropriate for all populations.

Providers need to be aware of their own cultural biases and how their culture and ethnic traditions affect approaches to certain aspects of the well child visit. By gaining this awareness and understanding, they will be more effective in their work with others, especially those who are very different from themselves (see Chapter 3).

■ DEVELOPMENTAL ASSESSMENT

SIGNIFICANCE FOR THE HEALTH CARE PROVIDER

Monitoring children's developmental progress brings the pleasure of watching them master expected developmental milestones. With time, many providers develop an intuitive sense about the general ages at which particular milestones should occur. Experience also brings an appreciation of individual differences in infants, families, and ethnic groups.

Many variables can make it difficult to appreciate intuitively all the various developmental skills of any particular child, however. For example, a premature infant at or below the 5th percentile for height and weight may physically appear much younger. The discrepancy between size and age can result in an inaccurate estimate of the child's abilities. Consider an infant who is 15 months chronologically, 12 months adjusted age, but physically and developmentally at the 9-month level. If the provider evaluated this infant developmentally based on physical size, the development level might appear appropriate (size and development at 9 months). Adjusting for age because of the infant's prematurity (adjustment to 12 months), the infant might still appear normal, and the need for intervention and referral might be missed. When a valid and reliable standardized developmental screening tool is used, it is more readily apparent that the infant requires referral and intervention services. It is important to note that even the developmental assessment tools with the highest standards may not be predictive for extremely low-birth-weight infants (Hack et al, 2005).

As a result of the understandable inconsistency in a practitioner's intuitive knowledge of child development and the importance of early identification of developmental concerns, the American Academy of Pediatrics (AAP) Committee on Children with Disabilities recommends that developmental surveillance be incorporated into each well-child preventive visit (AAP, 2001a). Further, a standardized screening test is recommended for children at 9 months, 18 months, and 24 to 30 months (AAP, 2006). There are now many developmental screening tools that have psychometric qualities including sensitivity, specificity, validity, and reliability and have been standardized on diverse populations.

DEVELOPMENTAL SURVEILLANCE

The concept of developmental surveillance as described by Dworkin (1989; 1993) provides the framework for this discussion. Surveillance encompasses all primary care activities related to the monitoring of the development of children, including the following:
- Eliciting and attending to parental concerns
- Obtaining a relevant developmental history

- Making accurate and informative observations of children
- Sharing opinions and concerns with other relevant professionals

Developmental surveillance involves more than simply asking developmental questions, completing a developmental screening checklist, asking how a child is doing in school, or completing a school physical examination. Emphasis is placed on monitoring development over time within the context of the child's overall well-being rather than viewing development during an isolated testing session.

Several assumptions underlie developmental surveillance. These include the following:
- Development is a self-fueling, ongoing process that requires physical and emotional energy.
- Development occurs in stages and is dynamic and interactional.
- Development is influenced by the child and his or her environment.
- Development occurs in "spurts and lulls." Periods of disorganization, disharmony, and turbulence are usually followed by periods of harmony, balance, and organization as new skills are integrated.
- All areas of development are interrelated.

Providing supportive care for children through developmental surveillance also is based on certain assumptions. These include the following:
- Children are generally healthy and have adaptive capabilities. Therefore the goal of the provider is to maximize health and development and a child's overall potential, rather than solely to resolve problems.
- Individual differences among children are reflected in developmental variations that reflect the unique characteristics of families, cultures, and social circumstances. Individual developmental variations and positive adaptations should be appreciated and facilitated.
- Children and families have the capacity to learn from and grow beyond their limitations when interventions are based on their abilities.
- Preventive health care for children includes developmentally supportive mental health care.

One focus of developmental surveillance is to build parental competence and confidence, which, in turn, enhances the child's overall well-being. When providers teach parents about the child's unique development strengths and skills, parents increase their knowledge of development and create their own parenting style. When parents feel success in their current parenting role, they do a better job meeting their child's future needs. Developmental surveillance is further supported by developmental screening and assessment as discussed below (Rydz et al, 2005).

DEFINITIONS

Developmental Screening

Screening is considered a first-level contact with an individual to identify potential and actual developmental concerns. Developmental screening is a brief, inexpensive method to identify children who may need a more comprehensive assessment and diagnostic evaluation. It allows the practitioner to document a child's progress over time and objectively identify and reinforce a child's developmental strengths. It may also serve as a tool to stimulate parent questions about development and facilitate parent education (Perrin & Stancin, 2002).

Developmental screening strategies are appropriate for all children, although culture and life experiences may affect some outcomes and need to be taken into consideration. Screening is conducted with the assumption that some children's developmental skills will fall outside the normal limits identified by the screening tool, thus requiring a referral for a more in-depth developmental evaluation. In addition, parent education to facilitate the "next steps" of development for the child may also be needed.

Developmental Assessment

A developmental assessment, more in-depth than a developmental screening, is conducted when a definitive diagnosis and a more individualized approach to guide the plan of care and management of the child's concerns is required. Assessment is considered to be at a second level of analysis, focusing on a more narrow, often complicated problem. Generally, assessments will confirm a developmental problem; identify the type of problem; describe the level of functioning in one or more developmental domains; and provide parents with anticipatory guidance and referrals to appropriate therapy, early intervention services, or community resources.

AREAS OF DEVELOPMENTAL SCREENING AND ASSESSMENT

Typical areas of developmental screening and assessment include language, motor, social-emotional, and cognitive skills. Screening and assessment should also examine the regulatory and sensory systems as a part of the child's overall development and functioning. Regulation refers to infants' daily patterns of sleep/wake cycles that include sleeping, eating, moving, responding, and reacting to their internal and external environment. Examination of sensory systems includes evaluation of the child's ability to receive, process, and respond to both internal and external stimuli. Finally, although it is conceptually a part of the child's social skill set, review of parent-child interactions and the family and environmental context in which the child is living is important. A comprehensive approach to developmental screening and assessment that includes the areas of regulation and adaptive skills in daily routines will be presented for each age group in the following chapters. Table 4-3 provides examples of information to gather within each of these areas.

STRATEGIES FOR DEVELOPMENTAL SCREENING AND ASSESSMENT

Several key strategies are involved in both screening and assessment:
- Parent interview
- Child interview
- Observation of child's behavior
- Observation of child-parent interaction
- Parent questionnaire

TABLE 4-3 Areas of Child Development	
Developmental Area	**Definition**
Physical development	Physical stability, growth, sexuality
Regulatory skills	State control and modulation, ability to manage sensory (e.g., light, noise, touch, movement) input from the external and internal environment; self-regulation and control
Adaptive skills and fine motor skills	Self-care skills that are involved in daily routines (e.g., feeding, bathing, dressing, brushing teeth)
Motor skills	Skills that facilitate overall movement and locomotion
Communication and language	Verbal and nonverbal communication skills including behaviors, gestures, signs
Social-emotional development and parent-child interaction	Ability to interact with others and the environment and overall affect; the reciprocal relationship between the child and his or her caregivers
Cognitive and intellectual development	Cognitive and intellectual skills, including problem-solving, decision-making, and goal setting

Success using these strategies begins when the health care provider builds rapport and a trusting relationship with both parent and child. Gaining the parent's and child's trust and engagement in the interview process is critical to obtaining accurate and reliable information. The parent interview is one in which the provider supports parents to share sensitive information, ask questions, and express concerns about their child's development. The interview of the child requires an understanding of child development and ages. The provider must be skilled in the use of age-appropriate strategies to engage the child and sensitive to the unique needs of each child. Providers need to have the ability to relate to the child verbally and physically. One example would be to sit at the same level as the child in order to establish eye contact. Targeted questions around daily routines often provide insight into a child's daily activities and parents' areas of concern. Examples of these questions are provided in Box 4-1.

A trusting relationship also enhances the health care provider's ability to accurately observe the child's behaviors. Observation of the child and the child's attention, activities, verbalization, connection with the parent, processing of information, quality of movements, cooperation, and ability to follow requests are all components of developmental screening and assessment. Box 4-2 lists specific observations that may be made during an infant feeding in a clinic or home visit, and Box 4-3 lists observations that can be made during a play or teaching activity with the parent.

BOX 4-1 Interview Guide for Daily Routines

- Tell me about your child's typical day.
- What aspects of your child's day are easy? What aspects are more challenging?
- How does your child communicate what he or she wants?
- Does your child show an ability to understand the feelings of others?
- How does your child act around others?
- To what extent has your child developed independence in eating, dressing, and toileting? Responsibilities at home, school, and community?
- How does your child get from one place to another (e.g., running, walking, transportation)?
- What do you like best about your child?
- What nicknames does your child have?

BOX 4-2 Observations During a Feeding

- Positioning of the infant or child and the caregiver
  - Eye contact
  - Infant holding
  - Environmental distractions
- Suck, swallow, breathing coordination, and physiologic stability
- Infant or child comfort with eating
- Oral motor functioning
- Lip closure, tongue, jaw movements, swallowing
- Endurance for feeding
- Sustained attention to feeding
- Stability of head and trunk control
- Ability to reach, grasp, hold, transfer objects
- Self-feeding skills and utensil use
- Coordination and quality of movements during feeding
- Infant's or child's anticipation of feeding
- Clarity of behavioral cues and use of vocalizations
- Responsiveness to caregivers' actions and verbalizations

BOX 4-3 Observations During Spontaneous Play or a Teaching Activity

- Positioning of the infant or child and the caregiver
  - Eye contact
  - Placement of toys within reach
  - Environmental distractions
- Success of gaining child's attention and sustained attention to play or teaching activity
- Tracking or following both visually or with verbal instructions and modeling
- Initiation of play activity
- Anticipation of songs or games
- Ability to reach, grasp, hold, transfer objects
- Coordination and quality of movements
- Clarity of behavioral cues and use of vocalizations
- Responsiveness to caregivers' actions and verbalizations
- Use of a toy in the manner it was meant to be used
- Ability to use representational play

Many standardized screening tools are now available and recommended for developmental screening (Rydz et al, 2005). Many of these tools have been developed to meet the demands of a busy, efficient office practice. Each of the following chapters will provide suggested developmental screening or assessment tools that are age-appropriate.

Strategies Specific to Developmental Screening

Aspects of the screening should be incorporated into the physical exam. By doing this, the provider not only sees the child "in action," but also has an opportunity to demonstrate to parents the infant or child's current or emerging skills. After completion of developmental screening, the provider should review the findings with parents. A parent-report screening tool can be completed by the parent in the waiting room or exam room, scored by a nurse or medical assistant, and then reviewed by the provider with the parent. This discussion helps families

focus on concerns they may have, provides opportunities to answer specific parent questions, addresses parenting issues, and is conducive to providing anticipatory guidance.

When developmental screening is omitted or delegated to medical assistants or volunteers and not reviewed by the primary provider, the significance of subtle variations of normal behavior or behavior that is very near the abnormal range may be overlooked. Nurse practitioners should be leaders in the use of standardized developmental screening tools in their practices to enhance both the efficiency and quality of the practice. Such tools provide a consistent, reliable, and efficient method of documentation of care provided and set standards for referral. Use of developmental screening tools involves engaging other providers and office staff with some minimal training and imparting knowledge of community resources. Implementing this standard of practice increases parent satisfaction and engagement as experts on their child and recognizes the provider-parent partnership in the care of the child (Earls & Hay, 2006).

Strategies Specific to Developmental Assessment

Developmental assessment tools are significantly different from screening tools and are appropriate when concerns require more in-depth developmental or diagnostic evaluation. Assessment tools for developmental and behavioral diagnosis, home assessment, family assessment, parent-child interaction assessment, parent stress, and parental competency are most frequently used in research, but may also be of value in the clinical setting. These tools can be used for a thorough assessment of the child within the family context, to look at the parent-child interaction, and to develop a substantiated diagnosis for the child. The information also improves the practitioner's ability to structure individualized interventions for both the child and the parents, and it can be used to evaluate the effectiveness of recommended interventions. Tools used for overall development include the Bayley Scales of Infant Development

(Bayley, 1993) and the Mullen Scales of Early Learning (Mullen, 1989). Tools used to evaluate specific behaviors or characteristics include the Autism Diagnostic Observation Scale—Generic (ADOS—G) (Lord et al, 1998), Childhood Autism Rating Scale (CARS) (Schopler et al, 1986), and the Nursing Child Assessment Satellite Training (NCAST) Feeding and Teaching Scales (Barnard, 1976; 1979).

Because of the complexity of issues that might need evaluation, developmental assessment tools require more knowledge, practice, and skill to perform reliably, interpret the findings, and plan appropriate interventions. These tools generally require special training or credentials to administer accurately.

▉ MANAGEMENT STRATEGIES IN CHILD DEVELOPMENT

PROMOTING PARENT DEVELOPMENT AND PARENT-CHILD INTERACTION: ANTICIPATORY GUIDANCE

Parental role development is described by authors using the ecologic model (Barnard, 1999; Bronfenbrenner, 1979; Sameroff & Chandler, 1975). This model stresses the fluid nature of early parent-child relationships and the importance of understanding the interactive and reciprocal relationships among parent, infant, and environment. Based on this model, the parental role develops in concert with the child's development, within the context of a unique environment. Barnard (1979) described two major nursing interventions that can be used to promote parental role development:

- Provide information and anticipatory guidance to parents and caregivers to assist them to facilitate the child's growth.
- Support parents so that they are able to center their energy and motivation on caring for their child.

The goal of anticipatory guidance is to help parents plan for and cope with anticipated changes and to increase parenting skills, confidence, and competence in problem-solving. The guidance is intended to assist parents to adapt parenting styles and strategies to their child's temperament, growth, and development. The following should be included:

- Assess the child's developmental status.
- Determine the parents' knowledge of child development.
- Determine the parents' knowledge of and experience with the parent role.
- Assess the parents' problem-solving and coping skills.
- Instruct parents about normal child development and variations of that development as indicated. Provide educational information and materials as appropriate. Written materials that are age- and development-appropriate are valued by most parents.
- Assist parents to develop realistic expectations of their child's development.
- Instruct parents about parenting strategies and concepts.
- Guide parents to appropriate community resources and support networks.
- Reassess and obtain feedback; reinforce healthy parental role development.

The responsibility to promote parent development through anticipatory guidance has often been more of a challenge than providing physical care, especially in primary care practices where time is limited. The standard of care in pediatric practices should include opportunities for providers to address parenting issues or concerns. Quick, pat answers to complex parenting issues do not facilitate parental growth. Creative strategies can be used to structure prenatal visits, hospital discharge rounds, early discharge newborn follow-up, breastfeeding consultations, well-child visits, and referrals to achieve this standard. An organized parent support program in practice settings, for example, can help providers listen, hear, and act on parent concerns. Without an organized plan that connects the child's developmental needs, parents' concerns and educational needs, providers' abilities and resources, and community resources, it is easy to overlook, delay, or deny important parenting issues.

The interview and counseling conducted during anticipatory guidance should be based on a consistent framework. Programs such as *Touchpoints* (Brazelton, 1992), *Bright Futures* (Green & Palfrey, 2000), *Healthy Steps* (Minkovitz et al, 2001), and *The Incredible Years* (Webster-Stratton, 2005) (Fig. 4-1) can be used. Specific questions are suggested to elicit responses from parents and guide the visit, in addition to providing anticipatory guidance and counseling. Stein (1998) emphasized the need for such an organized framework when approaching developmental and behavioral issues. He suggested focusing on four basic areas: developmental themes, temperament, family support, and resiliency (the ability to withstand stressors). He also emphasized the use of the teachable moment and role modeling during the office visit.

There is a wealth of popular literature available for parents to guide them as they raise their children. The primary pediatric health care provider can be an invaluable resource for parents in three major ways: by accurately assessing and competently caring for the child's needs; by supporting positive parent behaviors or actions; and by providing the information, suggestions, strategies, and guidance they need to be good parents. Providing parents with positive feedback, being open to teaching, and listening to parent concerns builds parent confidence, creates a trusting relationship, and establishes comfort for bringing forth more difficult concerns if such discussion is necessary. The provider-family relationship can be a powerful tool to guide family members' management of their child's temperament, behavior, and development. The benefit of establishing a long-term, continuous relationship with a child and family cannot be overestimated (see Chapter 17 for a more in-depth discussion of parenting strategies).

Certain "red flags" related to parent-child interactions indicate that assessment of the home environment, parent-child interaction, and child's development is indicated. Box 4-4 identifies some of these parental red flags.

DISCIPLINE

Children do not always behave the way their parents want them to. The question of how parents should deal with children's misbehavior has led to a wealth of parenting books, books on

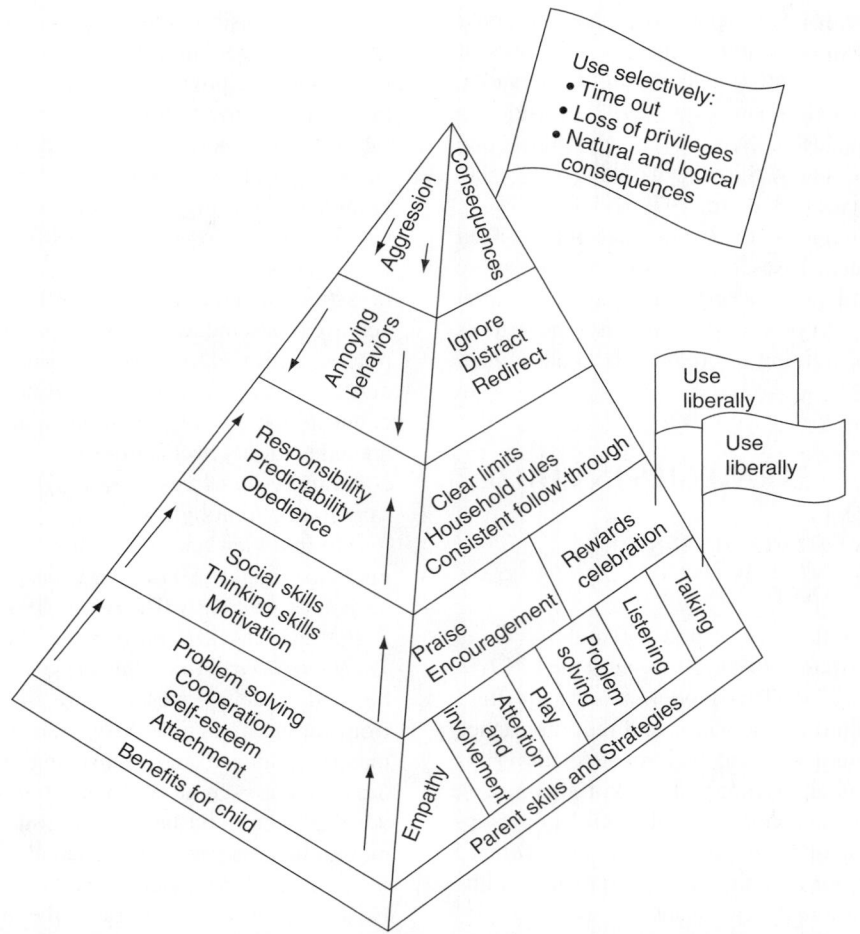

FIG. 4-1 Parenting pyramid. (From Webster-Stratton C: *The incredible years: a trouble shooting guide for parents of children aged 2-8,* Seattle, WA, 2005, Incredible Years Press).

BOX 4-4 **Parenting Red Flags**

Moderate Concern

Disinclination to separate from child or prematurely hastening separation

Signs of despondency, apathy, or hostility

Fearful, dependent, apprehensive

Disinterested in or rejecting of infant or child

Overly critical, mocking, and censuring of child; tendency to undermine child's confidence

Inconsistent in discipline or control; erratic in behavior

Highly restrictive and overly moralistic environment

Turning away from eye-to-eye contact

Extreme Concern

Extreme depression and withdrawal; rejection of child

Intense hostility; aggression toward child

Uncontrollable fears, anxieties, guilt

Complete inability to function in family role

Severe moralistic prohibition of child's independent strivings

Domestic abuse or violence in the home

Self-destructive behaviors: alcohol or drug abuse

Untreated mental health issues (e.g., parent with diagnosis of bipolar, schizophrenia, delusional)

---

discipline, strategies for child development, and many frustrated parents. Parents tend to use a combination of strategies–spanking, yelling, timeout, taking away a favorite toy, or reasoning with the child (Regalado et al, 2004), and each family brings differing temperaments, styles, and beliefs to the process. There are, however, some basic principles and guidelines about discipline that providers can discuss with parents to help them handle discipline. The AAP, in their 1998 policy statement (reaffirmed in 2004), stated that "effective discipline requires three essential components: (1) a positive, supportive, loving relationship between the parent(s) and child; (2) use of positive reinforcement strategies to increase desired behaviors; and (3) removing reinforcement or applying punishment to reduce or eliminate undesired behaviors" (AAP, 1998, p. 723). All three of these components guide the principles discussed below:

• Parents should talk with each other to come to agreement on how they will handle discipline and their child's misbehavior.

• A distinction must be made between discipline and punishment.

  ○ Discipline is training or education that molds the behavior, mental capacities, or moral character of an individual. Discipline is used by the parent to teach the child appropriate behavior and to keep the child safe.

○ Punishment, on the other hand, is loss, pain, or suffering that is administered in response to behavior; it is a form of retribution.

- Parents should focus their interactions with children on discipline, rather than punishment. As with the food pyramid in which wholesome grains, proteins, fruits, and vegetables form the base for good nutrition, a "parenting pyramid" has been constructed in which teaching, play, guidance, role modeling, and thoughtful correction of a child's behavior form the broad base for parent-child interactions (see Fig. 4-1; Webster-Stratton, 2005). Like nutrient-empty foods, punishment should be used as little as possible.
- Misbehavior can often be prevented. When a child appears willful, bored, or out-of-sorts, distraction and active engagement with the parent (e.g., giving the child something to do; talking to, playing with, dancing with the child) can be used to stop misbehavior before it starts.
- Parents need to be alert to when children are reaching their limits (i.e., are nearing "meltdown" because they are tired, hungry, or overstimulated) and intervene to prevent problems from occurring.
- Children who are at a "meltdown" stage are not able to relate rationally to a parent's reasoned explanation or request; the underlying problem—hunger, lack of sleep, etc.—must be dealt with first. Conversely, parents are not always at their best and may need to take a "timeout" from the child to cool down and regain self-control. Parents should have a plan for help when they need respite.
- All children need rules, limits, and expectations. These rules, limits, and expectations should be reasonable and appropriate to the age and developmental capabilities of the child. A 3-month-old, for example, cannot be expected to stop crying when her parents tell her to. As children grow, they should negotiate with their parents to help set the rules. This parent-child interaction helps children learn how to be active, valued family members and builds their social skills.
- Parents should be sure that the rules are clear and specific and should strive for consistency in adhering to them. Even young children benefit when the parent explains what the rules are and why they are necessary.
- Be flexible when responding to a child's behavior. Parents should agree about what issues are important to stand firm on. A wise mother said she had learned to "not sweat the small stuff," and chose to ignore very minor infractions while rewarding positive behaviors.
- Parents should role model expected behaviors.
- Adhering to rules should be rewarded. Parents should be encouraged to catch their children "being good" and give praise or rewards. Praise is a powerful reinforcement for good behavior. Some parents find a 4:1 ratio to be a good rule of thumb: four positive reinforcements for every negative.
- Praise and rewards for following the rules are different from "bribes" for being good (e.g., "If you stop crying, I'll get you an ice cream cone"), which should be discouraged.
- Children should be treated with respect and empathy, even when being reprimanded for misbehavior.
- Breaking rules should lead to natural consequences.

- Consequences should be given immediately, be fair, and should relate to the rule broken.
- Consequences should be appropriate to the age and developmental capabilities of the child. Timeout, being sent to the child's room, restricting a favorite activity, turning off the television or video games are all examples of consequences that have been successfully used. For example, if a 6-year-old child begins to play with his food, he can be sent to his room for "alone time," without his dinner. If a 4-year-old pushes or punches her sibling, she can be given "timeout" or not be allowed to play with a friend. If a 10-year-old breaks the neighbor's window with her baseball, she can be expected to apologize, help clean up the mess, and work to pay for the new window. As children grow, they should help determine the consequences for misbehavior.
- Parents should follow through on limits set. Frequent threats ("If you do that one more time, I'll send you to your room!") without follow-through teach the child that they can continue their misbehavior without consequence. Learning early that they are accountable for their behavior is an invaluable lesson for children.
- Punishment should never be a withdrawal of the parent's love or affection.
- Corporal punishment is unnecessary and has the potential to cause physical and/or psychic damage.

No parent is perfect, and parents bring their own upbringing to the role, Parental behavior may reflect efforts to "be like my parents were" or, as seems more often the case, "not do things wrong, like my parents did with me." Providers should acknowledge that parents are trying to do the best they can and encourage them to relax and discover how they and their child can best interact.

■ CONCERNS ABOUT DELAYED DEVELOPMENT

DEVELOPMENTAL RED FLAGS

Development among children is exceptionally varied. A 2-year-old girl may use full complex sentences, whereas her 3-year-old neighbor relies on three-word directives (e.g., "want milk, peeze") to get what he desires. Both can be normal, but the differences may be striking, and parents may express concern that their child is "delayed." Health care providers should keep in mind certain red flags related to normal child development when seeing infants and children for well child care or minor acute illnesses. These red flags are highlighted in each of the following chapters in this unit.

If a concern is noted during a routine visit, a standardized developmental screening is the next step, followed by a developmental assessment as appropriate. Subsequently, a decision must be made as to whether the child is progressing appropriately or whether intervention is indicated. Information from the history, physical examination, developmental screening and assessment, hearing and vision screening, and other tests that are indicated is essential in making this decision. It is also important to consider the cause of developmental delays when making a judgment to intervene directly or refer (Box 4-5).

BOX 4-5 Etiologies of Developmental Delays

- Central nervous system dysfunction
- Mental health problem
- Chronic disease affecting either functional abilities or activity tolerance (e.g., cardiovascular, visual, auditory)
- Child abuse and neglect
- Maternal or paternal stress
- Developmentally inappropriate animate or inanimate environment, or both
- Lack of parental knowledge of development
- Genetic syndromes
- Depression
- Attention-deficit hyperactivity disorder
- Autism spectrum
- Regulatory or sensory dysfunctions
- Unknown causes

Children with screening findings that are very near normal may be mildly delayed, but not eligible for early intervention services (criteria for early intervention vary from state to state, and a child may need to be between 25% and 35% delayed to be eligible in some states). Children with a mild delay and/or those who are at risk may benefit from activities such as encouraging "tummy time" when awake (for an infant who is not yet rolling over). Providers can use a manual such as *The Hawaii Early Learning Program (HELP) at Home Manual* to assist them with suggestions to parents for mild delays in various domains. These suggestions can also allow parents to begin working on an area while waiting for early intervention services to begin.

Understanding the possible cause helps the provider plan appropriate developmental care, including parent counseling, educational programs, and referral choices (e.g., Which developmental specialist is most appropriate to further assess the child? Which treatment modality, such as speech or physical therapy, would be most effective?). The discussion in Chapter 27 of the management of cerebral palsy illustrates the decision-making process used in cases of developmental delay. One should not assume that waiting will remedy a problem when parents express a concern or developmental delays are noted; even though developmental progress may occur, the rate and quality can be abnormal. In addition, parental stress and anxiety about their child may cause further problems. Neither can one assume that all developmental problems can be fixed with home remedies (e.g., changing parenting or environmental factors). Sometimes developmental problems are indicators of serious systemic, particularly neurologic, dysfunctions.

Vulnerability and resilience are two characteristics under current discussion in the child health literature. *Vulnerability* refers to a person's sensitivity and inclination to decompensate in the face of life stressors. *Resilience* (sometimes called *hardiness*), in contrast, is a person's capacity to survive intact, both psychologically and physically, despite adversity. In children these characteristics affect outcomes as stressors come and go in the child's life experiences. Many children demonstrate remarkable resilience despite significant risks. Any child who fails to move ahead as expected, however, or, worse yet, begins to deteriorate developmentally requires an immediate developmental assessment and diagnostic evaluation.

TALKING WITH PARENTS ABOUT DEVELOPMENTAL DELAYS

Talking with parents on a routine, ongoing basis about their child's development will usually make it easier should a specific developmental problem appear. It can be a challenging process. Typically, parents notice differences in the child first and seek reassurance or confirmation of problems from their health care provider. Should a problem be found, a "strength-based" approach can help sooth the experience of receiving "bad news." Each infant and child has areas in which development is progressing, even if the progress is not consistent with usual development. Discussing these areas, in addition to the parents' concerns, is important. Discussing these areas *first* provides parents with a framework for understanding their child's unique strengths along with any particular developmental challenges.

Parents may be overwhelmed with the news that their child has a developmental problem. To determine whether parents have understood what they have been told, the provider can ask the parent how they are going to explain what has been discussed to others at home. To increase parents' follow-through, providers need to be very familiar with referral resources; they should walk the parent through the next steps in the process; and then, after allotting time for the family to complete the referral visit, follow up with a phone call or office or home visit with the family.

Above all, it is important to be honest, positive, and realistic. Most often, the long-term prognosis for developmental delays is unknown because of continuing brain development. Parents want to know what they can do and, specifically, how they can assist their child. They also need support and time to cope with their own feelings. Different families have different expectations for their children, so a child with mild delay may be more devastating to one family than a child with severe developmental delays may be to another. Parents may report that they have expressed their concerns to their health care provider only to be reassured. Later on, as problems become more obvious and a referral is finally made, they are frustrated that they were not listened to initially and that services to their child have been delayed.

Implementing Individualized Interventions

Early Intervention Programs. Children with developmental delays should receive appropriate referral or more frequent visits, or both, particularly during the first year of life (see Chapter 22 for a discussion of issues related to children with chronic illnesses) (Batshaw, 2002). Many later learning problems, difficulties with parent-child interaction, behavioral problems, and attachment problems can be managed effectively during the first year of life simply by offering parental counseling or referral to appropriate community services. The longer the problem lasts, the more difficult it is to resolve. Most communities have early infant education programs for infants and young children (birth to 3 years old) provided for under Public Law 108-466, Individuals With Disabilities Education Improvement Act of 2004, which was a reauthorization of P.L. 99-457, enacted at the federal level in 1986. This legislation requires developmental screening and early intervention programs for infants and young children at risk for developmental delay. The individualized family service plan (IFSP) is a process that includes the family in planning services for children. Primary care providers may be asked to participate in the meetings in which the IFSP is developed with the family. These programs can be established through school systems, health departments, or developmental programs and vary significantly in quality and comprehensiveness from one community to another. The importance of structured programs that stimulate growth of all children cannot be overestimated (Emde et al, 2001). Providers need to be familiar with such community resources and educate community leaders and legislators about the developmental and health needs of children and families.

Children with developmental delays may require special attention in many areas, including assessment of medical and dental needs, feeding, sleep, elimination, activity, temperament, and behavior. Nursing interventions, such as education regarding medications, modifications of therapies as a result of the child's health status, referrals to parent groups, and assistance regarding organization of the child's health records, are greatly appreciated by the family.

School Intervention Resources.   Public Law 94-142, enacted in 1975, addresses the needs of children older than 3 years old. Under this legislation, schools are mandated to provide appropriate education to all children with developmental delays, including opportunities for mainstreaming children with developmental delays or handicaps into regular classrooms. Special education services assist in this process through the development of an individualized education plan (IEP).

Planning sessions for IFSPs or IEPs determine the school services that will be offered during a designated period of time for a particular child, usually each school year. If a child's or family's needs are not identified, services are not made available. Often, health care needs are not considered in these planning sessions. Primary health care providers should be available as advocates for families and children. In this role, they can help clarify children's health needs and ensure that parental concerns, health care services, and educational services are appropriately coordinated (Jackson Allen & Vessey, 2004).

Family-Centered Care.   The National Association of Pediatric Nurse Practitioners (NAPNAP) pediatric health care home position statement (NAPNAP, 2002), Public Law 99-457, and the AAP (AAP, 2001b) all emphasize the importance of the family within the child's life. The need to develop a partnership with the family is crucial so that families are comfortable and engaged in creating the plan of care for their own child. Each family's cultural values, learning styles, and health beliefs and practices must be respected. The shift from child-centered to family-centered care is represented in Table 4-4.

Care Coordination.   The Maternal and Child Health Bureau (MCHB) and the AAP define children with special needs as "children with special health care needs beyond those who have or are at increased risk for chronic physical, developmental, behavioral, or emotional conditions and

---

TABLE 4-4   **Comparison of Child-Centered and Family-Centered Care**

Child-Centered Care	Family-Centered Care
Goal: To take care of the child for the short term.	*Goal:* Parental empowerment and child advocacy for life of child.
• Child's needs are primary focus.	• Family needs to assist the child are the focus.
• Professionals decide on the plan of care.	• Family and professionals decide on the plan of care.
• Parents' opinions are not consistently requested.	• Parents' ideas are requested and valued.
• Families are considered part of a particular group.	• Families are all considered to be unique.
• Parents participate as observers.	• Parents are considered to be equal members of the team at whatever level they are comfortable.
• Parental differences are judged as not being in the best interest of the child.	• Family culture, language, ethnicity, and structure are respected.
• Test results of the child are the most important factor used to plan care.	• Focus is on addressing parental concerns, issues, questions, and their need for assistance in problem-solving.
• One-way communication, professional to parent.	• Two-way communication, with parents encouraged to have input into the child's care plan.

RESOURCE BOX

Pediatric Primary Care Developmental Management

American Academy of Pediatrics, Section on Developmental and Behavioral Pediatrics (SODBP)
www.dbpeds.org
Provides up-to-date information on developments in pediatrics related to development

***Bright Futures* in practice**
www.*brightfutures*.org
Guidelines for assessment, anticipatory guidance, and health promotion for infants, children, and adolescents

Facts for families
www.aacap.org
American Academy of Child and Adolescent Psychiatry facts for families and other resources

Growth charts
www.cdc.gov/nchs/about/major/nhanes/growthcharts/charts.htm
New National Center for Health Statistics growth charts

Growth charts for Down syndrome
www.growthcharts.com

Hawaii Early Learning Program (HELP) at Home Manual
www.vort.com
Curriculum-based assessment of cognitive, language, gross motor, fine motor, social, and self-help skills for working with children from birth to 6 years old and their families

Healthy Steps
www.healthysteps.org

Interactive multimedia training and resource kit integrate developmental screening and anticipatory guidance into primary care practices for children birth to 3 years old

Parents as Teachers
www.parentsasteachers.org
Born to learn model implemented through existing programs for parents of children up to kindergarten entry

NCAST
www.ncast.org
NCAST programs for nursing child assessment

The Commonwealth Fund
www.thecommonwealthfund.org
Provides web casts and information on the integration of developmental screening into pediatric offices

Touchpoints
www.touchpoints.org
Training based on the work of Dr. T. Berry Brazelton; incorporates relationship building and child development into professionals' practice

Zero to Three
www.zerotothree.org
Multidisciplinary focus on care, research, and education for the first years of life

who require health and related services of a type or amount beyond that required by children generally" (McPherson et al, 1998). The need to coordinate services is identified as one of the key elements for children with special needs, and the primary care provider is often seen as the one providing this coordination (AAP, 1999; Antonelli & Antonelli, 2004). Nurse practitioners (NPs) have the unique skills to function in this role as a result of their nursing background and appreciation for the complex needs of families and children with special health care needs. NPs may help families understand the importance of accessing parent and community resources to sustain their long-term care of the child. It is important for the NP to become "community wise" through professional networks, parent groups, and educational connections. It is essential to develop a system within the office of up-to-date referral agencies and contact information. Through public health agencies, these resources may also be easily identifiable and invaluable in assisting parents. However, it is not enough simply to give a family a name and phone number of a referral source. All too often, parents' calls lead to busy signals, disconnected numbers, or the wrong agency for their needs. These deterrents can discourage even the most willing

family from pursuing needed resources for their child. Parents can also hesitate to seek resources because of apprehension about the outcome of the referral, costs, time constraints, or lack of understanding about the need for timely follow-up. When the provider intervenes to guide families through the referral process and coordinate services, parents have greater confidence in the new health care or educational resource and are more likely to achieve appropriate follow-up for their child.

NURSING DIAGNOSES
Related to Development

Risk for disproportionate growth
Delayed growth and development
Risk for delayed development

From NANDA International: *NANDA-I nursing diagnoses: definitions & classification 2007–2008,* Philadelphia, 2007, Author.

✓ DISCUSSION FORUM

1. List strategies that might be used by a pediatric primary care provider to incorporate developmental anticipatory guidance into the following sick visits: (1) an 18-month-old with an acute upper respiratory infection, (2) 4-year-old with stool withholding and constipation, (3) a 9-year-old with chronic headaches, (4) a 15-year-old with dysmenorrhea.
2. Using the developmental theorists (where appropriate) listed in Table 4-1, explain the following child behaviors: A 3-year-old child has nighttime fears of the dark; an 8-year-old girl wants to be involved in a scouting group and is an avid collector of snow globes; a 13-year-old male wants to go to a camp sponsored by his religious denomination with a group of friends from school.
3. Conduct a developmental assessment on a child of your choice. Be sure to look at physical, developmental, social, and emotional growth. What changes to the assessment would you anticipate in 1 year? In 3 years?
4. You receive a phone call from a parent of a 4-year-old who fits the following temperament: high activity, high rhythmicity, low adaptability, low threshold of response, high intensity of reaction, outgoing and friendly mood, and high distractibility. His parent reports that the child is acting out against his younger sibling by kicking, hitting, and yelling. What anticipatory guidance related to discipline and parenting are appropriate for you to give the parents of this particular child and why?

REFERENCES

Ainsworth M, Bell S, Stayton D: Individual differences in strange-situation behavior of one year olds. In Schaffer HR, editor: *The origins of human social relations*, London, 1971, Academic Press.

American Academy of Pediatrics (AAP), Committee on Children With Disabilities: Care coordination: integrating health and related systems of care for children with special health care needs, *Pediatrics* 104:978-981, 1999.

American Academy of Pediatrics (AAP), Committee on Children With Disabilities: Developmental surveillance and screening of infants and young children, *Pediatrics* 108:192-196, 2001a.

American Academy of Pediatrics (AAP), Committee on Children With Disabilities: Identifying infants and young children with developmental disorders in the medical home: an algorithm for developmental surveillance and screening, *Pediatrics* 118:405-420, 2006.

American Academy of Pediatrics (AAP), Committee on Children With Disabilities: Role of the pediatrician in family-centered early intervention services, *Pediatrics* 107:1155-1157, 2001b.

American Academy of Pediatrics (AAP), Committee on Psychosocial Aspects of Child and Family Health: Guidance for effective discipline, *Pediatrics* 101(4):723-728, 1998.

Antonelli RC, Antonelli DM: Providing a medical home: the cost of care coordination services in a community-based, general pediatric practice, *Pediatrics* 113:1522-1528, 2004.

Barnard K: *NCAST II learners' resource manual*, Seattle, 1976, NCAST Publications, University of Washington.

Barnard K: *NCAST instructors' manual*, Seattle, 1979, NCAST Publications, University of Washington.

Barnard K: *Beginning rhythms: the emerging process of sleep wake behavior and self-regulation*, Seattle, 1999, NCAST Publications, University of Washington.

Batshaw ML: *Children with disabilities*, ed 5, Washington, DC, 2002, Paul H Brookes Publishing.

Bayley N: *Manual for the Bayley Scales of Infant Development*, ed 2, San Antonio, TX, 1993, The Psychological Corp.

Bhasin TK et al: Prevalence of four developmental disabilities among children aged 8 years–metropolitan Atlanta developmental disabilities surveillance program, 1996 and 2000, *MMWR Surveill Summ* 55(1):1-9, 2006.

Bijou S, Baer D: *Child development II: universal stages of infancy*, New York, 1965, Appleton-Century-Crofts.

Blumberg SJ, Halfon N, Olson LM: The national survey of early childhood health, *Pediatrics* 113(6 Suppl):1899-1906, 2004.

Bowlby J: *Attachment and loss, vol 1, attachment*, New York, 1969, Basic Books.

Brazelton B: *Touchpoints: your child's emotional and behavioral development*, New York, 1992, Addison-Wesley.

Bronfenbrenner U: *The ecology of human development: experiments by nature and design*, Cambridge, MA, 1979, Harvard University Press.

Bronson MB: *Self-regulation in early childhood—nature and nurture*, New York, 2000, The Guilford Press.

Buhler C, Allen M: *Introduction to humanistic psychology*, Monterey, CA, 1972, Brooks/Cole.

Carey WB: Let's give temperament its due, *Contemp Pediatr* 15:91-113, 1998.

Cech DJ, Martin S: *Functional movement development across the life span*, Philadelphia, 2002, WB Saunders.

Chess T, Thomas A: *Temperament in clinical practice*, New York, 1995, Guilford Press.

Dixon S, Stein M: *Encounters with children: pediatric behavior and development*, St Louis, 2006, Mosby.

Dworkin PH: British and American recommendations for developmental monitoring: the role of surveillance, *Pediatrics* 83:619-622, 1989.

Dworkin PH: Detection of behavioral, developmental, and psychosocial problems in pediatric primary care practice, *Curr Opinions Pediatr* 5:531-536, 1993.

Earls MF, Hay SS: Setting the stage for success: implementation of developmental and behavioral screening and surveillance in primary care practice: the North Carolina Assuring Better Child Health and Development (ABCD) project, *Pediatrics* 118:183-188, 2006.

Emde R: Development terminable and interminable. I. Innate and motivational factors from infancy, *Int J Psychoanal* 69:23-42, 1988.

Emde R, Buchsbaum H: "Didn't you hear my mommy?" Autonomy with connectedness in moral self emergence. In Cicchetti D, Beeghly M, editors: *The self in transition: infancy to childhood*, Chicago, 1990, University of Chicago Press.

Emde RN, Mann TL, Bertacchi J: Organizational environments that support mental health, *Zero to Three* 22:67-69, 2001.

Erikson E: *Insight and responsibility*, New York, 1964, Norton.

Fiese BH: Routines of daily living and rituals in family life: a glimpse at stability and change during the early child-raising years, *Zero to Three* 22:10-13, 2002.

Flavell J: *Cognitive development*, Englewood Cliffs, NJ, 1977, Prentice-Hall.

Fowler J: *Stages of faith: the psychology of human development and the quest for meaning*, New York, 1981, Harper & Row.

Freud A: *The writings of Anna Freud*, vol V, New York, 1974, International Universities Press.

Freud S: *An outline of psychoanalysis*, London, 1938, Hogarth.

Gesell A: *The first five years of life*, New York, 1940, Harper.

Gilligan C: *In a different voice: psychological theory and women's development*, Cambridge, MA, 1982, Harvard University Press.

Green M, Palfrey J: *Bright futures: guidelines for health supervision of infants, children, and adolescents*, ed 2, Arlington, VA, 2000, National Center for Education in Maternal and Child Health.

Hack M et al: Poor predictive validity of the Bayley Scales of Infant Development for cognitive function of extremely low birth weight children at school age, *Pediatrics* 116:333-341, 2005.

Havighurst R: *Human development and education*, New York, 1953, Longmans, Green.

Jackson Allen P, Vessey J: *Primary care of the child with a chronic condition*, ed 4, St Louis, 2004, Mosby.

Kelly JL, Barnard KE: Assessment of parent-child interaction: implications for early intervention. In Shonkoff JP, Meisels SJ, editors: *Handbook of early childhood education*, New York, 2000, Cambridge University Press.

Klaus M, Kennel J: *Maternal-infant bonding*, St Louis, 1976, Mosby.

Kochanska G, Coy KC, Murray KT: The development of self-regulation in the first four years of life, *Child Devel* 72(4):1091-1111, 2001.

Kohlberg L: Stage and sequence: the cognitive-development approach to socialization. In Gastin D, editor: *Handbook of socialization: theory and research,* New York, 1969, Rand McNally.

Kubicek L: Fresh perspectives on young children and family routines, *Zero to Three* 22:4-9, 2002.

Lewin K: *Principles of topological psychology,* New York, 1936, McGraw-Hill.

Lord C, Rutter M, Le Couteur A: Autism Diagnostic Observation Interview—Revised: a revised version of a diagnostic interview for caregivers of individuals with possible pervasive developmental disorders, *J Autism Dev Disord* 24:659-685, 1998.

Mahler M, Pine F, Bergman A: *The psychological birth of the human infant,* New York, 1975, Basic Books.

Mahrer A: *Experiencing: a humanistic theory of psychology and psychiatry,* New York, 1978, Brunner/Mazel.

Maslow A: *The farther reaches of human nature,* New York, 1971, Viking.

McPherson M et al: A new definition of children with special health care needs, *Pediatrics* 102:137-140, 1998.

Minkovitz C et al: Early effects of the Healthy Steps for Young Children program, *Arch Pediatr Adolesc Med* 155:470-479, 2001.

Minuchin S: *Families and family therapy,* Cambridge, MA, 1974, Harvard University Press.

Mott S: Developmental theories: how the child grows. In Mott S, James SR, Sperhac A, editors: *Nursing care of children and families,* New York, 1990, Addison-Wesley.

Mullen E: *Mullen Scales of Early Learning,* Cranston, RI, 1989, T.O.T.O.L. Child.

National Association of Pediatric Nurse Practitioners (NAPNAP): *Position statement: the pediatric health care home,* 2002. Available at *www.napnap. org* (accessed Aug 27, 2006).

Nugent JK: Cross-cultural studies of child development: implications for clinicians, *Zero to Three* 15:1-8, 1994.

Olson LM et al: Overview of the content of health supervision for young children: reports from parents and pediatricians, *Pediatrics* 113(6 Suppl):1907-16, 2004.

Perrin E, Stancin T: A continuing dilemma: whether and how to screen for concerns about children's behavior, *Pediatr Rev* 23:264-275, 2002.

Piaget J: *The theory of stages in cognitive development,* New York, 1969, McGraw-Hill.

Regalado M et al: Parents' discipline of young children: results from the National Survey of Early Childhood Health, *Pediatrics* 113(6 Suppl):1952-8, 2004.

Rogoff B: *Apprenticeship in thinking: cognitive development in social context,* New York, 1990, Oxford University Press.

Ruperto N et al: Cross-cultural adaptation and psychometric evaluation of the Childhood Health Assessment Questionnaire (CHAQ) and the Child Health Questionnaire (CHQ) in 32 countries. Review of the general methodology, *Clin Exp Rheumatol* 19(4 suppl 23):S1-S9, 2001.

Rydz D et al: Developmental screening, *J Child Neuro* 20(1):4-21, 2005.

Sameroff A, Chandler M: Reproductive risks and the continuum of caretaking casualty. In Horowitz FD, editor: *Review of child development research,* Chicago, 1975, University of Chicago Press.

Schopler E, Reichler RJ, Renner BR: *The Childhood Autism Rating Scale,* Los Angeles, 1986, Western Psychological Services.

Shonkoff JP, Phillips DA: *From neurons to neighborhoods: the science of early childhood development,* Washington, DC, 2000, National Academy Press.

Siegler R, Liebert D, Liebert R: Inhelder and Piaget's pendulum problem, *Dev Psychol* 9:97-101, 1973.

Skinner BF: *Science and human behavior,* New York, 1953, The Macmillan Free Press.

Stein M: Preparing families for the toddler and preschool years, *Contemp Pediatr* 15:88-110, 1998.

Stern D: *The interpersonal world of the infant: a view from psychoanalysis and developmental psychology,* New York, 1985, Basic Books.

Sullivan H: *The fusion of psychiatry and social sciences,* New York, 1964, Norton.

Thomas RM: *Comparing theories of child development,* Belmont, CA, 1985, Wadsworth.

Trevarthen C, Aitken KJ: Infant intersubjectivity: research, theory, and clinical applications, *J Child Psychol Psychiat* 42(1):3-48, 2001.

Webster-Stratton C: *The incredible years: a trouble shooting guide for parents of children aged 2-8,* Seattle, WA, 2005, Incredible Years Press.

Wolraich ML, Felice ME, Drotar D, editors: *The classification of child and adolescent mental health diagnoses in primary care: diagnostic and statistical manual for primary care (DSM-PC), child and adolescent version,* Elk Grove Village, IL, 1996, American Academy of Pediatrics.

CHAPTER 5

Developmental Management of Infants

Barbara Jones Deloian and Anita Berry

Infancy is an exciting time for everyone involved—the infant, his or her immediate family, extended family members, and others in the infant's community. Pediatric health care providers are privileged to be able to work with families during this period of rapid, predictable (yet unique), and challenging change. When providing care to infants and their families, practitioners have a responsibility to assess and monitor growth and development; educate parents about child development; offer guidance about ways to foster healthy growth and development; identify and manage health problems; guide, counsel, and support parents when dealing with their infant's health or illness; and collaborate with other providers as necessary.

Research on brain development has validated the notion that the child's experiences during the first years of life are critical to healthy physical, emotional, and intellectual development (Shonkoff & Phillips, 2000). During pregnancy and early life, the infant is affected by both internal physiologic and neurologic factors and external factors. such as light, sound, touch, positioning, taste, and movement. An infant's ability to develop consistent and predictable responses to these internal and external stimuli during the first year of life is influenced by physical growth, brain development, the surrounding environment, and, particularly, the actions of the infant's caregivers (Trevarthen & Aitken, 2001). The infant's mastery of self-regulating behaviors depends on healthy biorhythms and sensitive, consistent caregivers (Anders et al, 1998; Barnard, 1999). Nurturing relationships between infants and their adult caregivers strengthen all aspects of an infant's development (Dixon & Stein, 2006). Providers can give parents the information, support, and encouragement they need to be successful in their new role and ensure that their infant achieves optimal growth and development.

BIRTHRATES AND INFANT MORTALITY

As noted in Chapter 1, birthrates in the U.S. decreased slightly from 2001 to 2004 (14.7 to 14.2 births per 1000 population, respectively). The teen (15- to 19-year-olds) birthrate continued to decrease from 61.8 births per 1000 population in 1991 to 41.2 in 2002. The number of twin deliveries increased to 31.5 per 1000 births in 2002 and 2003 compared with 29.3 per 1000 live births in 2000. Triplet births increased from 180.5 per 100,000 births in 2000 to 187.4 per 100,000 live

births in 2002 and 2003 (CDC, 2004). The infant mortality rate increased from 6.8 deaths per 1000 births in 2000 to 7 deaths per 1000 births in 2002, with increased deaths found primarily among infants with low birth weight. The leading causes of infant mortality continue to be congenital malformations and chromosomal abnormalities, short gestation, or low birth weight, and sudden infant death syndrome (SIDS). SIDS continues the decline that began in 1988, reflecting the success of the back-to-sleep campaign. The U.S. still ranks poorly in comparison with international infant mortality rates, being 28th overall. The disparity of infant mortality rates between black, non-Hispanic and white American infants is also of grave concern. In 2004, black, non-Hispanics had a rate of 13.65 infant deaths per 1000 compared with 5.65 per 1000 births for white Americans. Unintentional injuries also remain high, and almost 25% of infants and toddlers in the U.S. live in poverty.

DEVELOPMENT DURING THE FIRST YEAR

BIRTH TO 1 MONTH

Physical Development

The assessment of the neonate must begin with a determination of gestational age using the Dubowitz or similar gestational age scale (see Chapter 38). It is important to be aware of significant prematurity, intrauterine growth retardation (IUGR), and size for gestational age (i.e., either large for gestational age [LGA] or small for gestational age [SGA]). The reported gestational age, birth weight and length, and head circumference data are compared with the infant's gestational age as assessed by observation.

The infant may initially lose up to 5% to 8% of birth weight, but should regain birth weight within 10 to 14 days. Weight loss of 10% or more requires close monitoring and may require further evaluation. Weight gain after the initial loss will average 0.5 to 1 oz per day, or about 2 lb per month. Nutritional needs to promote growth are about 110 kcal/kg per day (see Chapter 11).

The stability of the infant's autonomic nervous system can be evaluated through heart rate, respiratory rate, temperature control, and color changes. The infant should demonstrate some degree of regulation of state and ease of transitions from deep sleep through quiet alert to active alert and crying. A variety of techniques can be used to arouse the newborn for feedings. The newborn infant sleeps about 16 out of 24 hours and, if encouraged to breastfeed every 2 to 3 hours, may have one longer stretch of 4 hours at night. Assessment for a normally pitched cry is important because problems such as hypothyroidism and genetic disorders (e.g., cri du chat syndrome) can cause voice alterations.

Motor Skills Development
The newborn's flexed posture provides the infant with the ability to self-console when positioned so that the hands reach the face and mouth. Primary reflexes, such as sucking, rooting, asymmetric tonic neck, Moro, and grasp, should be present and symmetric. Passive muscle tone is evaluated within gestational age scales through observation of shoulder (scarf sign) and knee flexibility (popliteal angle). Arm and leg recoil provide information about the infant's active movements, particularly symmetry and coordination. Jerkiness and tremors may be noted. The neonatal period begins a remarkable series of fine and gross motor skill milestones for the infant (Table 5-1).

Communication and Language Development
The newborn infant is able to give clear signals of distress, such as crying, arching, or gagging. These help the caregiver respond to the infant's needs. The newborn also should be able to habituate to sound and light. Newborns use self-consoling or self-calming behaviors, such as sucking, moving hand to mouth, or grasping clothing, to keep organized or maintain their state.

Articulation, or the way that the structures of the nose and mouth mold the sounds emitted by the larynx, begins at birth with the infant's first cry. In the first few weeks of life, infants will make sounds of comfort and discomfort.

Social and Emotional Development
Social skills are evident as the newborn quiets readily, turns to the parent's voice, and demonstrates a brief smile. Using a soft voice, touching, and picking up the baby are ways the caregiver can console the newborn.

Social emotional development is closely linked to the mother's emotional state. Sixty to 80% of mothers will experience "baby blues," 10% to 15% will have postpartum depression, and 1% to 2% will manifest a postpartum psychosis during the first year of the infant's life. The health care provider is one of the few professionals who sees mothers with any regularity in the first year of life. Infants' well child visits should be used as opportunities to screen mothers and families for factors such as depression and domestic violence that can affect the infant's growth and development. A screening tool such as the 10-question Edinburgh Postnatal Depression Scale can be used to identify mothers needing further evaluation, referral, and close follow-up (Cox et al, 1987; Wisner et al, 2002) (see Chapter 38 for a copy of this scales).

Cognitive/Sensory Development
Vision is limited, but the newborn does have the ability to focus briefly on a face or bright object when it is brought into visual range (about 8 to 12 inches from the infant's face). The infant is also able to visually track an object to midline. Of all the senses, the sense of smell is most acute in newborns. Hearing is also fairly well developed.

1 THROUGH 3 MONTHS
Physical Development
During months 1 through 3, the infant experiences many physical and developmental changes. Length increases about 3.5 cm per month and head circumference about 2 cm per month, with more rapid growth for the younger infant. The infant will continue to gain 0.5 to 1 oz per day with 8 to 10 feedings in 24 hours, each lasting 30 to 40 minutes. Feedings lasting longer than 40 minutes should be evaluated further. At about 6 to 8 weeks, the infant may experience a growth spurt and fuss to eat more frequently. Mothers who are breastfeeding need extra encouragement during this time because they may believe that they do not have enough milk for their baby. Providers should instruct mothers to follow their infant's cues for feeding, pointing out that the extra suckling will increase the milk supply sufficiently to meet their growing infant's needs. Elimination patterns become more regular, with several stools a day for formula-fed infants; breastfed infants may stool less frequently. Wet diapers can be expected after each feeding.

Sleep cycles become more regular, about 15 to 16 hours per day, with defined sleep/wake patterns. The infant may need more organized play periods as sleep periods become consolidated with consistent naps. Many infants have fussy periods in the late evening that may last 1 to 3 hours. This age tends to be the height of infant crying but, fortunately, this fussiness usually lasts for a short period. Regular nap or nighttime routines can help keep infants calmer. The provider should have a discussion with parents about how they plan to cope with crying before this time is upon them. This would also be a time to explain "shaken baby syndrome" to parents and encourage them and others who care for the infant to have a repertoire of coping skills.

Motor Skills Development
Fine motor skills begin to emerge as primitive reflexes become integrated. Infants attempt to grasp rattles, fingers, and clothing. They also are able to demonstrate visible head control, lifting the head off the bed about 45 degrees when in the prone position and showing little head droop when held in suspension. All their body movements should be symmetric (see Table 5-1).

Communication and Language Development
Parents should be encouraged to notice how their infant looks at them when they are talking and how intently the infant looks at faces, especially during the quiet alert state, the time when the infant is most interactive. Infants are able to "connect" with parents, even if only for a few moments. By talking to their infant during caregiving activities, parents encourage early language development. Infants will start to

TABLE 5-1 Fine Motor and Gross Motor Development Milestones for Infants and Preschoolers

Age	Fine Motor Movement	Oral Movement	Gross Motor Movement
Birth	Flexion	Suckling tongue movements, extension-retraction of tongue, up-and-down jaw movements, low approximation of lips	Momentary head control when held sitting
1 mo	Extension, non-directed swipes	Rooting	Turns head when prone
4 mo	Directed swipes, corralling, reaching		Sits with support, rolls over, head steady in sitting
4-5 mo	Ulnar-palmar grasp		"Swims" in prone position, no head lag
6-7 mo	Radial-palmar grasp, raking	Sucking with negative oral cavity pressure, rhythmic jaw movements, firm approximation of lips	Sits independently, rocks on hands and knees, free head lift in supine
7-8 mo	Radial-digital grasp	Phasic bite reflex, rhythmic bite and release pattern	Supports weight standing, bounces when held
7-9 mo	Scissors grasp	Munching, early chewing	Sits alone well, may crawl
9-10 mo	Voluntary release		Cruises, pivots while seated, pulls to stand
12 mo	Picks up pellet with pincer grasp	Chewing with spreading and rolling tongue movements, tongue lateralization, rotary jaw movements, controlled sustained bite	Walks with one hand held, stands alone momentarily
18 mo	Makes tower of 4 cubes, imitates scribbling, dumps pellet, puts blocks in large holes, drinks from cup with little spilling, can take off socks		Directed throwing, walks well independently, climbs into adult chair
24 mo	Makes tower of 7 cubes, does circular scribbling, folds paper once imitatively, turns doorknobs, turns pages one at a time, unbuttons or unzips large fasteners, puts on coat with assistance		Throws overhand, runs well, kicks ball, up and down stairs placing both feet on each step
30 mo	Makes tower of 9 cubes, makes vertical and horizontal strokes, imitates circle, buttons large button, uses fork in fist, twists jar lids		Jumps off ground with both feet
36 mo	Makes tower of 10 cubes, imitates bridge of 3 cubes, copies circle, snips with scissors, can brush teeth but not well, puts shoes on feet		Broad jumps, walks up stairs alternating feet, may pedal tricycle, balance one foot 2-3 sec
48 mo	Copies bridge from model, copies cross and square, cuts curved line with scissors, dresses self, strings small beads		Pedals tricycle, runs smoothly, hops on one foot, catches large ball
60 mo	Some can print name; copies triangle, opens lock with key, bathes self, cuts out simple shapes, pours from small pitcher		Walks downstairs alternating feet, catches bounced ball, skips, stands on one foot 7-8 sec

make cooing and babbling sounds, much to the delight of their parents (Table 5-2). However, body movements (e.g., snuggling, turning the head, arching the body) continue to be the primary form of communication, and providers can help parents identify and become more skilled at interpreting their infant's cues.

Social and Emotional Development

The infant begins to become highly social, imitating the parent's expressions and visually following the parent. Infants are more responsive to sounds in their environment, attending to sounds by quieting body movements or demonstrating visual responses. By

3 months, infants demonstrate a social smile and will most often smile in response to their parent's voice. As infants become more active, alert, and responsive, parents may mistakenly assume that they can handle more activity and irregular stimulation than they are truly capable of. Developing sensitivity to infant cues for the need to rest or to have decreased stimulation is important.

Cognitive Development

By 4 to 8 weeks, infants readily begin to take in more of their environment, and, when a face or toy is brought into visual range, the infant begins to visually track past midline, vertically,

---

TABLE 5-2   Speech and Language Milestones: Areas for Assessment

Age	Receptive Language	Expressive Language
0-3 mo	Attends to voice, turns head or eyes Startles to loud sounds Quiets in response to voice Smiles, coos, gurgles to voice	Undifferentiated but strong cry Coos and gurgles Single-syllable repetition /G/, /K/, /H/, and /NG/ appear
3-6 mo	Actively seeks sound source May look in response to name Responses may vary to angry or happy voice	Increased babbling, vocal play Laughs Increased repetitive babbling (gaga) Vocalizes to toys Spontaneous smile to verbal play Increased intensity and nasal tone Vocalizes to removal of toy Experiments with own voice
6-9 mo	May look at family member when named Inhibits to "no" Begins interest in pictures when named Individual words begin to take on meaning	Babbles tunefully Increased sound combinations Uses /M/, /N/, /B/, /D/, /T/ Initiates sounds such as click or kiss Uses nonspecific "mama" and "dada"
9-12 mo	Will give toy on request Understands simple commands Turns head to own name Understands "hot," "where's …?" Responds with gestures to "bye-bye"	Increased imitating efforts Has one word with specific reference Accompanies vocalizations with gestures Jargon increases Imitates animal sounds

12-18 mo	Follows simple one-step commands
	Understands new words weekly
	Increased interest in named pictures
	Differentiates environmental sounds
	Points to familiar objects and body
	  parts when named
	Understands simple questions
	Begins to distinguish "you" from "me"
		All vowels, many consonants present
		Increased use of true words
		Jargon is sentence-like
		Shows "no" behavior
		Names a few pictures, 10 words
		Can imitate nonspeech sounds
		  (cough, tongue click)
		Names some body parts

18-24 mo	Follows two-step commands Vocabulary increases rapidly Enjoys simple stories Recognizes pronouns	Imitates two-word combinations Dramatic increase in vocabulary Speech combines jargon and words Names self Answers some questions Begins to combine words
24-30 mo	Understands prepositions *in* and *on* Seems to understand most of what is said	Jargon reduced 2- to 3-word sentences Repeats 2 digits

TABLE 5-2	Speech and Language Milestones: Areas for Assessment—Cont'd	
Age	**Receptive Language**	**Expressive Language**
	Understands more reasoning ("when you are done, then …") Identifies object when given function (wear on feet, cook on)	Increased use of pronouns Asks simple questions Joins in songs and nursery rhymes Can repeat simple phrases and sentences
30-36 mo	Listens to adult conversations Understands preposition *under* Can categorize items by function Begins to recognize colors Begins to take turns Understands "big" and "little," "boy" and "girl"	Answers questions (wear on feet, to bed) Repeats 3 digits Uses regular plurals Can help tell simple story
36-42 mo	Understands *fast* Understands prepositions *behind* and *in front* Responds to simple 3-part commands Increasing understanding of adjectives and plurals Understands "just one"	Understands and answers (cold, tired, hungry) Mostly 3- to 4-word sentences Gives full name Begins rote counting Begins to relate events Lots of questions, some beginning prepositions (on, in)
42-48 mo	Recognizes coins Begins to understand future and past tenses Understands number concepts— more than one	Uses prepositions Tells stories Can give function of objects Repeats larger than 6-word sentences Repeats 4 digits Gives age Good intelligibility
48-60 mo	Responds to 3-action commands	Asks "how" questions Answers verbally to questions such as "How are you?" Uses past and future tenses Can use conjunctions to string words and phrases together

and horizontally. Even very young infants may demonstrate various facial expressions, respond to sounds, and attempt to imitate mouthing movements. By 3 months, infants begin to enjoy toys and may wave their arms when a toy is brought into sight.

4 THROUGH 5 MONTHS

Physical Development

Infants 4 through 5 months old usually begin to settle into regular patterns of eating, sleeping, and playing. Babies sleep 12 to 15 hours a day with 5 feedings during the day and one during the night; by this age, the infant may sleep through the night without feeding. Somewhere between 4 and 6 months, infants will double their birth weight, gaining about 5 oz a week during this time. Their length increases about 2 cm per month, and head circumference increases about 1 cm per month. Growth may appear in spurts, rather than along an even curve. Weight gain can also be influenced by the amount of play activity and the sleep schedule. Although the infant's primary source of nutrition comes from breast milk or formula,

parents may ask about when to begin feeding the infant solid foods. Many parents introduce some infant cereals by 4 months, but nutritionally, full term babies need nothing other than breast milk or iron-fortified formula until 6 months old (see Chapter 11). As other food is added, changes in stool consistency will be noted.

Motor Skills Development

Fine motor skills are demonstrated as infants play with their hands and begin to reach for and pull at clothing or other objects that are close. Eventually, they grasp toys and begin to grab at other objects, such as the parents' hair, earrings, or eyeglasses. They also start to place their hands on the breast or the bottle in an attempt to hold or pat it.

Motor skills progress (see Table 5-1) as the Moro and asymmetric tonic neck reflexes are integrated, and there is no longer the obligation of arm extension with head turning. The Landau reflex emerges. Infants begin to roll, first from front to back and then from back to front, and can roll from one place to another. Head control becomes stronger and more sustained, and there should be no head lag when the baby is pulled to sit. When in the prone position, infants hold the head up at 45 degrees, gradually progressing to 90 degrees for sustained periods of time. The infant learns to sit, first in the tripod stance, then unassisted with the head held erect. When lying supine, infants are able to lift their legs and bring their feet to their mouth. They bear full weight when standing and enjoy bouncing up and down in their parent's lap. All their body movements should be symmetric.

Communication and Language Development

Infants' social skills are increasing and verbal skills are becoming more evident (see Table 5-2). They begin babbling, using vowel sounds, cooing, and laughing quietly. They experiment with variations in tone and pitch, such as low-pitched chuckles and deeper laughs. Eventually, they begin to laugh out loud, much to the enjoyment of those around them. Their responses to sounds gradually become more localized, and they search for the sound of a bell or rattle.

Oral-motor development is a prerequisite for speech. Throughout infancy, oral development progresses from sucking and rooting to rhythmic biting and chewing. Beginning at about 6 months and continuing through 2 years, the child learns to chew by moving the jaw up and down while flattening and spreading the tongue and to control biting by using rotary jaw movements with lateralization of tongue placement. These motor skills, essential for the production of speech, are among the most complex movements that the young child must master.

Social and Emotional Development

During this time, infants' social skills become more evident. Smiling spontaneously at parents and others while visually following the caregiver around the environment and turning the head a full 180 degrees is usual behavior. Babies at this age should promptly look at an object when it is placed in front of them; they notice things. The infant's increasing awareness of the environment facilitates more complex social interactions. Infants begin to recognize that their parents are responding to their needs. The infant will notice, for example, as the parent prepares to offer the breast or get a bottle ready for feeding. Because infants notice other things as well, parents can often distract them from demanding immediate gratification by talking, playing, or using other social interactions such as reciprocal vocalizations and eye contact. As a result, infants learn that their hunger needs will be met, but that there are other satisfying interactions they can have with their parents. Infants at this age begin to more actively reciprocate their parents' attention and enjoy playing with their parents. Crying may reflect tiredness or a need for social interaction, not just hunger. Parents are able to acknowledge their child's unique personality, and this reciprocal recognition is an important aspect of infant-parent attachment.

Cognitive Development

Visual exploration increases during this age, as infants seek out objects in the environment to look at such as mobiles, mirrors, their hands, and the toys that they are holding. Their preference, however, is looking at their parents' or another person's face. Chewing and mouthing are other means of exploration that infants use to differentiate textures, tastes, and shapes. As their muscle control improves, they are able to bring a toy to their mouth first when lying on the back and then when sitting.

6 THROUGH 8 MONTHS

Physical Development

As infants reduce their breast milk or formula intake and add solids to their diet, growth curves can change. Weight gain slows to 3 to 4 oz a week, or about 1 lb a month; length gains are about 1.2 to 1.5 cm per month; and head circumference increases about 0.5 cm per month. If concerns about a large head circumference exist, note each parent's hat size and continue to monitor the infant carefully. Teething for central incisors can begin at about 6 months, and lateral incisors appear at about 8 months. The first childhood illness might occur at this time, if it has not already done so, and either of these events can disrupt the infant's previous sleep routine.

Motor Skills Development

Motor skills at this age need little encouragement for development because of infants' desire to explore the environment. Infants sit erect for longer periods of time and may scoot while in a sitting position. Crawling begins with the infant pushing up to hands and knees and rocking in place, then eventually mastering the rhythm of hands and knees working together. Infants may stand, fully supporting their weight, when their hands are held at shoulder height.

Fine motor skills continue to be refined, and babies are more adept at using their palm and all of their fingers to pick up objects. Initially, they rake at small objects and are able to hold a small cube, lifting it off the table. Gradually, they use fingers and thumb to pick up objects. They reach for and grasp toys, can hold a toy in each hand at the same time, and can transfer objects from one hand to another.

Communication and Language Development

Vocalizations continue to show increasing variety in pitch and tone, and imitation of specific speech sounds begins. Infants articulate single-sound units that may be vowels, consonants, or blends such as "ah," "ba," "da," "ga," "ch," and "bl." Gradually, they progress to double-consonant sounds (e.g., "dada") and occasionally will vocalize using three or more different syllables. They use "mama" and "dada," but not specifically for their parents. Infants can delight their parents as they respond to verbal cues and play at making sounds and noises when alone. They enjoy imitating oral sounds such as raspberries and coughing.

Although infants' expressive language skills are limited, their receptive language can clearly be seen as they listen and respond to their parents' talking. Infants are able to distinguish facial expressions and gestures, may stop or quiet when their parent uses "no" or a different tone of voice, and will turn toward their parents' voices and other sounds, localizing directly to the sound.

The provider should encourage parents to begin reading to their child daily at a very young age, at least by 6 months. This can be introduced as part of the bedtime routine. Watching TV or videos should be discouraged since it is a passive medium, and infants learn language best when they interact with another person, by listening to parents' voices and looking at a face that responds to them.

Social and Emotional Development

Infants now greatly enjoy social play, and their individual personality and temperament continue to be expressed. At times infants' increased ability to do things for themselves puts them at odds with their parents; even if parents have learned to understand their infant's cues and allow reciprocity between themselves and the infant, control issues can arise. Infants use gestures such as pointing, reaching with outstretched arms, tugging, and throwing things to get their parent's attention and communicate their needs. As infants' abilities and desires become more complex and they expand their repertoire of communication cues, parents need to learn new parenting skills (e.g., how to handle a determined child) to meet their infant's social development needs.

Stranger anxiety may appear at this time, depending on the variety of caregivers infants have had and their individual temperament.

Cognitive Development

From 6 through 8 months, infant cognitive development demonstrates significant growth. The infant is able to see cause-and-effect relationships in activities such as ringing a bell; pulling on a string to retrieve a ring, train, or phone; and dropping a toy from the crib or highchair. They can follow a toy if it falls and remains within their visual field. For some older infants, beginning object permanence is evident because they will look for partially hidden objects and play peek-a-boo. The infant is increasingly aware of surroundings and begins to express individual preferences more clearly. This is often a time when resistance to bedtime, feeding, and parental separation occurs.

9 THROUGH 12 MONTHS

Physical Development

At 9 to 10 months, the infant's growth may have begun to follow a different growth curve than the one established early in infancy. Growth spurts become more apparent to parents as the infant seems to outgrow clothes "overnight." At the same time, illnesses, decreased solid food intake caused by teething, and the infant's increased activity level can slow the rate of growth. It becomes important to estimate the infant's total caloric intake if there is a significant decrease in the infant's growth or if feeding problems are present. Early intervention in feeding problems at this time can result in a much easier resolution (see Chapter 11).

Infants begin to show regular patterns in bowel and bladder elimination. Some parents interpret their ability to predict their infant's bowel movements as toilet training (see Chapter 13).

Sleep problems, if managed with consistency, begin to resolve. Otherwise there might still be struggles with bedtime.

Between 11 and 12 months, infants gain about 1 lb per month. Growth in length continues to occur in spurts. Eleven- to 12-month-olds usually eat solids well, want to feed themselves, and are able to recognize their own hunger or satiation needs. They usually do not eat the same amount at each meal and often demonstrate specific food preferences. Because infants do not have full dentition, food choices should be limited to soft or puréed foods or foods that turn soft when chewed (e.g., breadsticks). Feedings begin to follow a routine of breakfast, lunch, and dinner, with midmorning, afternoon, and bedtime snacks.

Motor Skills Development

Fine motor development allows older infants to entertain themselves for extended times. They are able to hold objects of different sizes and pick up small objects using the sides of the fingers and eventually a fine pincer grasp, most often transferring the object directly to their mouth. Infants at this age enjoy putting objects into containers and taking them out again and, by 11 or 12 months, can stack blocks one on top of the other. They often begin to hold a cup with two hands, but may still have difficulty sealing their lips around the edge of the cup to take sips.

At 9 to 10 months, most infants sit for long periods and crawl on hands and knees. They begin to "cruise," walking around furniture holding on with both hands, and are able to pull themselves off the floor to a standing position. They may begin to let themselves down from furniture with fairly good control. They also take steps if someone holds two hands and then one hand. Eventually, they take a few steps from one object or person to another. They may momentarily stand alone, and some infants walk independently.

Communication and Language Development

Receptive language skills improve, and infants participate in games such as pat-a-cake and peek-a-boo. Babies at this age momentarily stop activity when they hear "no," but they do not truly understand what "no" means. They are still very focused on observing activities in their environment and, when given names of things, attend well to the new information. They enjoy songs and rhymes and may participate by "singing" along.

By 12 months, infants' expressive language has expanded to a total of 3 or 4 words. Words such as "dada," "mama," or "ba-ba" (for bottle) can be recognized. They are able to name a picture in a book, visually look for an object when named, and follow simple one-step requests.

Social and Emotional Development

Infants at this age demonstrate stranger wariness, and some demonstrate fear of new situations or experiences. As a result, they will look to their parent for reassurance and attempt to engage the parent in eye contact while watching their parent's expression. Emotions such as affection, anger, jealousy, and anxiety become more evident in late infancy. However, once familiar with new people, particularly if introduced by their parents, babies enjoy initiating interactive games and social interchanges. Overall, 11- to 12-month-olds appear to be in love with the world, love to explore, and have little understanding of those things that can cause them harm. They assist in dressing by extending an arm or leg and are able to retrieve the bottle if it is dropped. They take great pride in mastering new skills or overcoming their fears, and they look to others around them to take notice as well.

Cognitive Development

Cognitively, older infants are completing more complicated tasks, such as stacking and container play. They master object permanence and easily locate a toy placed out of sight or under a cloth. This skill allows them to take a more active role in playing hide-and-seek or peek-a-boo. They hold a crayon or pencil with their whole hand and will make dots on a piece of paper imitating a drawn line.

Infants' curiosity blossoms as they begin to explore not only visually and with mouthing and chewing, but also by grasping, poking, shaking, pushing, pulling, and stacking. They often develop their own games or explore different ways of playing with familiar toys or objects. Play and other activities become more spontaneous and self-directed, and the parent begins to follow the lead of the child in play, imitating the child's interest and modeling newer activities related to the same toy or game (e.g., playing pat-a-cake and then adding a song).

■ DEVELOPMENTAL ASSESSMENT OF INFANTS

Monitoring the overall growth and development of the infant is critical because of the rapid changes during this time. If a delay or concern is detected early, treatment can be started, and outcomes are likely to be more positive. It is also very important to discuss the infant's development with parents so that they can anticipate changes and plan ways to support their infant's emerging developmental skills. Good assessment is facilitated through consistent visits with the same provider. Seeing the same provider on a regular basis strengthens the parent-child-provider relationship and makes it easier to pursue follow-up questions and concerns, validate the efforts of parents, and reinforce their successes.

SCREENING STRATEGIES FOR INFANTS

As noted in Chapter 4, there is a distinction between screening and assessment for diagnosis. Providers use both strategies when working with infants. One of the most informative questions that can be asked of the parent is, "Tell me about your infant's day." This will elicit information about daily routines of feeding, bathing, naps and sleep, elimination, and play activities. It will also gather data about what areas may be most difficult for the parents and areas where suggestions may be most helpful. Listening carefully to parents' responses to this question from visit to visit helps providers truly understand the life of the infant and how best to assist an individual family.

Every well child visit should include developmental surveillance in which the provider assesses parents' concerns, obtains a relevant developmental history, and completes a thorough and accurate examination, looking particularly at the child's development over time. Screening, using a standardized, valid, and reliable screening tool, should be conducted at the 9-month well child visit or whenever there is a parent or provider concern (AAP, 2001).

The Ages & Stages Questionnaire or the Parents' Evaluation of Developmental Status (PEDS) are recommended for infants and can be completed by parents before the visit (e.g., could be mailed with a reminder of the upcoming visit) or while waiting to see the provider. Other tools may be used for specific areas of concern, such as speech and language, social and emotional behavior: Ages & Stages Questionnaire: Social Emotional (ASQ: SE), the Infant-Toddler and Family Instrument (ITFI), the Temperament and Atypical Behavior Scale (TABS), and the Receptive-Expressive Emergent Language Scale (REEL). Simply completing a checklist of developmental milestones or asking about specific milestones does not adequately screen an infant for developmental status, especially an infant who was born prematurely.

DIAGNOSTIC DEVELOPMENTAL ASSESSMENT STRATEGIES FOR INFANTS

Developmental assessment tools include the Brazelton Neonatal Behavioral Assessment Scale, the HOME Scale, the Bayley Scales of Infant Development, and the Nursing Child Assessment Satellite Training (NCAST) Scales (feeding scale, teaching scale, sleep activity record, and personal environment assessments). These tools require special training to use and take longer to administer than screening tools. Use of developmental assessment tools can ensure more timely, appropriate referrals and help establish individualized intervention strategies for clients.

It is beyond the scope of this chapter to provide a complete review of the screening and assessment tools available in the areas of infant development, parent-child interaction, and family assessment. The Resource Box at the end of this chapter lists additional information about commonly used screening and assessment tools.

■ ANTICIPATORY GUIDANCE FOR INFANTS

Many of the issues of infancy can be addressed through education and anticipatory guidance of parents. New parents can be bombarded with more information and opinions than they can manage—from their own parents, neighbors, friends, the popular media, and others. Health care providers can help parents sort through the information, understand what it means, and decide what is best for their family. Acknowledging specific positive aspects of the parents' skills, before offering anticipatory guidance, will help ensure that parents are more receptive to new ideas. It can help to ask parents what they have tried that has worked, reinforce success, and suggest other options as necessary and in the best interest of the child.

Developmentally supportive care engages infants in activities that are tailored to their unique developmental capabilities. These "developmentally appropriate" activities are integrated into all aspects of the infant's daily routines. Parent education can be used to help parents learn about infant development, what activities will promote healthy development, and what the parent can do to provide secure, safe relationships in an environment that supports their child's development.

Steward and Steward (1973) first introduced the concept of a teaching loop, in which teaching interactions between the parent and child consist of four specific teaching behaviors (Table 5-3). These behaviors provide the infant with verbal instruction, modeling, and positive feedback. Providers can instruct parents about the teaching loop and encourage them to use it with their children in all areas of development. In fact, parents are often observed using the teaching loop as infants learn to walk but are unaware they are using a formal teaching strategy.

Providers can also use this teaching-loop model as they teach parents: verbal instruction, modeling, and positive feedback. When offering anticipatory guidance, providers must be sensitive to parents' interest in and tolerance of the information presented. Too much information, or information that the parent feels is irrelevant, can be overwhelming. If parents express a concern, listening carefully to their perception of the problem is important. Information can then be structured to more directly address specific concerns.

Frequently, time limitations in a clinic or office setting lead to use of a "laundry list" of topics for anticipatory guidance rather than information individualized to the infant and family being seen. Alternative approaches (e.g., parent groups or classes that focus on commonly shared parenting issues) can be used for effective parent education.

In addition to giving verbal instruction, providers can model developmentally appropriate activities during the well-child examination, showing parents ways to interact with their infant that stimulate, comfort, or soothe the baby. During these demonstrations, parents can be asked to give examples of things they have done at home as they care for their infant. If a problem was discussed at a previous well child care visit and a plan made to try certain activities (e.g., creating a nighttime ritual to manage a 10-month-old who refuses to go to sleep in her own bed), the outcome should be reviewed with the parent, and positive feedback and encouragement for the efforts made and successful results should be given. Providers should also be alert for developmentally appropriate parent-child interactions in the office and reinforce the parents' behavior with positive feedback. Observing the child's development in the office visit offers opportunities for "teachable moments," which can be a beginning point for a shared discussion around an issue of concern.

The goal of parent education in the early years is to provide tools that parents can use in the many challenging years to come. It also intends to give parents the skills to become their child's advocates, capable and knowledgeable about their child's individual needs. By understanding the infants' capabilities, such as hearing, vision, states and state transition, and self-calming and self-consoling techniques, parents are better able to read infant cues and provide timely and appropriate care. In turn, the infant's responsive behaviors assist in building the parents' confidence and aid in their receptiveness to future anticipatory guidance. The following are specific topic areas in which practitioners' anticipatory guidance can help parents through the remarkable, fast-moving first year of their child's life.

THE PRENATAL VISIT

Meeting with parents prenatally provides an opportunity to assess parents' knowledge and receptiveness to anticipatory guidance. The prenatal visit should include a discussion of the partnership between the primary care provider and the parent on instruction about newborn care, and the management of possible sibling rivalry or toddler jealousy situations. The prenatal visit can also be a time to look for risk factors for perinatal depression (e.g., previous history of depression or previous postpartum depression; lack of social support). These meetings provide a foundation for later visits and establish the pediatric provider as a resource for the parents.

THE NEONATAL VISIT

The hospital visit is the least opportune time to discuss infant care because of the short stay and the mother's physiological

TABLE 5-3	**The Teaching Loop**
Behavior	**Description of Behavior**
Alerting	The parent gets the infant's attention and makes sure that the child is paying attention. This may occur by calling the infant's name, making a noise, or directing the child to the toy.
Instruction	The parent gives a specific instruction to the infant or child about the toy or task and what is to be done. This instruction should be short and may be either verbal or a demonstration, or both.
Performance	The parent then gives the infant or child time to explore the material, to attempt to practice the task or play with the toy as shown, or just to explore the toy, depending on the child's age. Many parents have trouble allowing the child the time just to explore the task; others may offer excessive time without offering any assistance.
Feedback	The parent makes some comment that may be positive or negative, such as "Good job," "Good try," or "No, that's not quite right; try it this way."

Data from Steward D, Steward M: The observation of Anglo-Mexican and Chinese-American mothers teaching their young sons, *Child Dev* 44:329-337, 1973.

state, which reduces her ability to absorb new information. A 48- to 72-hour newborn home or office visit should be arranged to assess evidence of jaundice, breastfeeding needs, weight change from birth, status of newborn screenings, maternal well being, and needed infant care teaching. A postpartum visit at 1 week is also needed to assess the infant's weight gain, elimination pattern, sleep/wake cycle, continuation of breastfeeding, parent-infant interaction, and family support needs. This visit is a good time to discuss how parents and siblings are adjusting and to look for mothers who are having difficulty with "baby blues." Postpartum psychosis generally presents during the first 3 weeks after delivery; identifying it early and making timely referral is critical. Mothers should be given information on perinatal depression. The 1-week visit is also important to determine and document the results of newborn hearing tests that have been done and complete necessary metabolic screening tests.

BIRTH TO 1 MONTH

Regulation and Sleep-Wake Patterns

- Infants need assistance to develop day-night cycles because most infant's days and nights are mixed up. Using a consistent daily routine will help the infant establish a good sleep-wake cycle.
- Placing the infant in a bassinet or crib for naps during the day will allow an easier transition from the parent to bed at night.
- Infants need a variety of movement, voice, or touch to move them from sleep to wake states. Rhythmicity of voice, movement, or touch will calm an infant or lower their state, and a parent's slow, easy movements in caregiving will decrease the affect of the infant's startle or Moro reflex.
- Some infants benefit from external stimuli such as music, voice, or movement to help calm them down and support their own self-regulation. Gentle massage or swaddling can help some infants adjust to state changes.

Strength and Motor Coordination

Infants' gradual increase in strength makes it possible for them to lift their heads. Parents should be instructed to place their infants in the supine position for sleep, but to give their babies "tummy time" when awake and alert, placing them in a prone position once the umbilical cord has fallen off. Parents can be encouraged to interact with their infants during these "prone-to-play" periods, at least once or twice every day.

Feeding and Self-Care

- A primary developmental activity of the newborn is organizing feeding responses. Bringing the infant slowly to an awake state for feeding is the first step. If the infant becomes overstimulated or disorganized, it might be necessary to reduce external stimuli (e.g., lights and noise), increase the infant's flexion of arms and legs, or bundle the infant to assist with central nervous system control and improve feeding responses.
- Infants need to develop a regular suck-swallow and breathing rhythm for feeding. If milk flows through the breast or bottle too rapidly or too slowly, adjustments may be needed to help the baby manage the feeding. Feedings that are lon-

ger than 40 minutes or shorter than 20 minutes should be evaluated further.
- The face-to-face feeding position is important because it encourages eye contact and parent-child communication and interaction.
- The infant's reach for breast or bottle represents beginning exploratory learning and should be encouraged. Parents also can encourage the grasp reflex while the baby is feeding through finger play or finger holding.
- Infants generally are very good at regulating how much they need to eat. It may not always be consistent from one meal to the next. Understanding and respecting an infant's hunger and satiation cues helps protect against later feeding and nutritional concerns. Burping may also be different for each infant and is an important time for a rest during feeding, in addition to social interaction.
- Urinary output is one indicator of adequate intake, but not the only one. Weight gain, feeding type (breast milk or formula), frequency and duration, frequency of spit ups, and activity level of the infant must be evaluated to ensure the infant's adequate nutrition.
- Some infants need more opportunities for sucking. Nipple confusion may be an issue for some infants; avoid giving a bottle or pacifier to breastfed infants until breastfeeding is well established, usually by 3 to 4 weeks (see Chapter 12).
- Support and guidance for breastfeeding mothers may require additional counseling, observation of feedings, and referral to a lactation consultant, in addition to guidance on strategies for returning to work while breastfeeding (see Chapter 12).

Communication and Language

- Newborn's communication skills are seen during state changes, periods of alertness, feeding, and sleep routines. Parents must be alert to nonverbal infant communication (e.g., fussiness, turning the head away) to understand their infant's needs.
- Attending promptly to infant crying helps the infant to develop a sense of trust.
- Imitating infant sounds encourages an infant to vocalize and experiment with different types of sounds.

Social and Emotional Growth

- Newborns are able to tolerate brief periods of social interaction when they are in an alert state. Orienting to visual stimuli (e.g., a parent's smiling face) helps the infant keep a stable alert state. It is helpful to demonstrate for parents how the infant achieves this alert state and how a newborn can easily be overstimulated by the environment.
- Being gently touched and held are very important for the newborn. Encourage parents to hold their infant and assure them that holding does not spoil a baby, but meets their need for emotional support and tactile contact.
- Facilitating overall family development and emotional growth is important, especially for siblings. Based on the age of the sibling, parents may need ideas of what would be appropriate involvement for them with the newborn.

- Pointing out concrete ways that parents are meeting the needs of their infant (more than just "You are doing a good job") will help reinforce parents' confidence and promote their development as parents. Parents' concerns should be followed up closely with support, guidance, and reassurance when appropriate. Early success while caring for the new infant is essential for parents to enjoy their new role.

Cognitive and Environmental Stimulation

Encourage opportunities for the infant to look at things in the environment. Placing mobiles at the side of their bassinet or crib will help prevent overstimulation. As infants develop, a variety of objects will encourage them to visually explore their surroundings and move their heads from side to side. It is also helpful to place infants at different ends of the bed periodically. Including infants in family activities during their awake times exposes them to many sounds and visual images.

1 THROUGH 3 MONTHS

Regulation and Sleep-Wake Patterns

- Structuring an infant's day will help meet the infant's ongoing need for external routines and facilitate state organization.
- The use of repetitive stimulation (e.g., rocking or a soothing voice) for quieting and a variety of stimulation (e.g., undressing, stroking, or voice intonations) for awakening will continue to be an important parenting strategy.
- Parents need to understand their infant's need for swaddling and sensitive movements because of the immature nervous system (e.g., continuation of Moro or asymmetric tonic neck reflex).
- Sleep location, safety, position (back to sleep), and the establishment of a nap time and nighttime ritual all influence later sleep habits for the infant. Helping the infant learn to go to sleep on their own begins with the infant becoming drowsy in their parent's arms and then being placed in the bassinet or crib while still awake.

Strength and Motor Coordination

- Placing the infant in different positions for playtime, especially the prone position, encourages upper body strength, neck, arm, and head control. Other family members may be especially good at encouraging this as the infant lies prone on their chest and looks up into their face.
- A supine position stimulates movement of the fingers, hands, feet, and legs, and makes it easier to hold toys.

Feeding and Self-Care

- Feedings become more consistent and the infant continues to have a strong need for sucking, especially for non-nutritive sucking, such as sucking on fingers and toys. For a short period of time, a pacifier may be helpful.
- Feedings continue to be important to meet both nutritional and developmental needs. This is a time for close, affectionate communication between parent and baby.
- Each infant will demonstrate unique cues for readiness to eat and satiation. As the parent gets ready for the feeding, they will recognize that their infant begins to anticipate that they will be fed.

- Positive reinforcement for continued breastfeeding is still needed and problem-solving strategies for the mother who is returning to work are beneficial (see Chapter 12).

Communication and Language

- Talking and singing to infants during routine daily activities should be encouraged. The value of hearing the parent's voice is great, even if the infant does not understand the words.
- Helping parents understand and respond to their infant's cues and sleep-wake states supports communication between parent and infant.
- Reading as part of daily or evening routine should be stressed.

Social and Emotional Growth

- Parents' observations and intuitions about their infant need to be reinforced as they become "watchful wonders" of their infant. Recommendations associated with the parents' own observations are the most supportive and educational; parental competence will grow as their increasing skills are validated.
- Infant's hands are often described as an infant's "first toy." In addition, their hands are used for self-consoling and hand-to-mouth exploration.
- Continuing to respond to infants' cries as soon as possible reassures them that their needs will be met and decreases the chances of crying later on.
- The infant's emerging temperament and the parents' perceptions of the infant's behaviors will need to be resolved if there are conflicts (Carey, 1998).
- Infants have an increasing social need and desire to play with the caregiver. Often fussing or crying is misinterpreted for hunger. Parents may need assistance to set up "play stations" (different play activities) so the infant can be moved easily from one activity to another. As a result of the infant's short attention span, approximately 10 to 15 minutes at each "station" over an hour's time will usually lead to a tired, happy baby.
- Parents need to develop strategies to have time together as a couple. Providers can help them identify criteria for child care resources and locate those resources.

Cognitive and Environmental Stimulation

- The infant's visual awareness is increasing and more visual diversity will be needed, such as changes in position and location and changes in stimulating objects, such as a mobile or mirror.
- Toy selection and equipment should include criteria for safety and developmental appropriateness for the infant. Toys should be semirigid, unpainted, and have varying textures. Toys that rattle and make sounds are appropriate. These encourage waving arms and kicking legs.

4 THROUGH 5 MONTHS

Regulation and Sleep-Wake Patterns

- Infants need to resume sleep independently when they awaken at night. Help parents prepare for future changes in the infant's sleep-wake pattern by putting the infant to sleep in the crib while drowsy but not yet asleep. If they awaken at night, they are more likely to resume sleep without comforting from the parent.

- Nighttime rituals continue to be an important aspect of helping the infant anticipate what is going to happen next, which builds a sense of security.
- Parents' perception of their infant's temperament will play an important role in how they respond to their infant. They may describe their infant as easy, average, or challenging, and they may compare their infant with other babies. Parents may need encouragement to understand their infant's uniqueness and can be shown how individualizing their activities to their baby's style makes parenting much easier.
- Varied parenting approaches to infants of different temperaments, including patterns of eating and sleeping, can be discussed.
- Consistent, prompt responses to infant crying continue to be an important aspect of caregiving.

Strength and Motor Coordination
- As the infant becomes more mobile, safety measures become more critical; parental supervision is essential for child safety.
- Childproofing the home, relatives' homes, and child care or day-care settings (e.g., locks on cabinets and gates for stairs) is essential for safety.
- Floor-time play encourages motor strength and coordination. Playpens can be limiting, but some families may need to put a child in one briefly as a safety measure. Movable walkers have been found to be unsafe and should be discouraged (Shields & Smith, 2006). If parents choose to use a walker, it should not have wheels and should only be used for brief periods (e.g., 10 to 15 minutes) as a safe place to set a child.

Feeding and Self-Care
- Drooling is less about teething and more about salivary gland maturation. The infant gradually develops the ability to swallow excessive saliva.
- Responding appropriately to the infant's hunger cues and satiation cues continues to be important.
- An infant is ready for solids as the gastrointestinal tract matures. Listen closely to parents' questions and beliefs and the influence of others on the introduction of solids. Although the AAP recommends exclusive breastfeeding until 6 months old, they also note that it is appropriate to start solid foods between 4 and 6 months; not every infant is ready to start solids at the same age (American Heart Association et al, 2006).
- When solids are introduced, a spoon should be used instead of placing cereal in the bottle. This helps the infant develop new oral-motor skills. Skills needed to suck and swallow milk from a bottle or breast differ from those needed to take cereal from a spoon.
- Interacting with the infant during feeding fosters the parent-child relationship and makes feeding time fun rather than just a routine.

- Allowing infants to pat the breast or bottle and place their hands on the bottle promotes self-feeding later as they learn to hold their bottle or cup. Bottle propping can cause an infant to aspirate and is discouraged.

Communication and Language
- Parents' use of reciprocal or "back-and-forth talking" with their infant, especially using changes in voice inflection and intonation, is important in developing communication skills.
- Parents talking to their infant during caregiving activities holds the infant's attention, especially when the infant is fussy. Talking to the infant makes it easier to change diapers, prepare meals, and attend to the infant's needs in other ways. It also stimulates the infant's language skills.
- Reading to an infant and looking at picture books, describing the pictures, colors, and actions, is beneficial even at this early age. The importance of developing habits of quiet time, reading time, and parent-child together time can also be stressed. Providers may want to participate in the national early literacy program for children 6 months through 5 years old, Reach Out and Read (ROAR). See the Resource Box at the end of this chapter.

Social and Emotional Growth
- The infant continues to need nonnutritive sucking as a means of self-regulation. Sucking on fingers or toys requires different oral-motor movements from those needed to suck on a pacifier.
- Discipline can be discussed and differentiated from punishment. The important role of "parents as teachers" may be a new concept to some parents. Helping parents understand the importance of modeling desired behaviors and redirecting behavior should be discussed before it is needed. (see Chapters 4 and 17).
- Information about age level child development and strategies to deal with difficult behaviors is important. Referral to parenting classes that provide information on developmental milestones and anticipated changes may be helpful. Although parents may have books on development, a one-page handout addressing a particular subject of immediate concern, given to the parent by the provider, is likely to be more useful. Such handouts are available through Healthy Steps and Bright Futures (see Resource Box).
- Both parents need to be involved in ongoing communication about their roles, responsibilities, and expectations. Fathers may be more comfortable handling the infant at this age, as the infant becomes responsive. Differences between parent's expectations need to be discussed (e.g., to allow an infant to cry at bedtime or not).
- Helping mothers find time for themselves, manage life stresses, or return to work may be needed. Mothers' feelings are often reflected in infants' behaviors.
- The parents' emotional well-being and availability is an important aspect of the infant's overall care. Helping parents value their time together may need to be reinforced.
- Counseling about how to select safe and appropriate child care should be included in visits.

Cognitive and Environmental Stimulation

- With the infant's increasing activity and awake time, parents will need strategies to provide more attention and play activities. The infant will make every effort to obtain their parents attention by smiling, making sounds, or crying. Using a variety of types of activities and toys such as soft stuffed toys, rattles, a crib gym or busy box, and toys of different sizes, weights, shapes, materials, and colors can be suggested. Home objects that infants see every day can be used as "toys" for stacking, shaking, and rolling.
- Infants may also enjoy looking at themselves in a mirror and placing a mirror next to the changing table is a good diversion.
- Activities such as walks to the park, visiting neighbors, or trips to the grocery store are all part of an infant's learning experiences.

6 THROUGH 8 MONTHS

Regulation and Sleep-Wake Patterns

- Infants may have settled into a good sleep routine through the night, only to have it interrupted with teething or illness. They may need assistance to resume their regular sleep-wake patterns. Parents may need to go to the child to assure them they are safe, but should not feed infants for comfort or to help them return to sleep.
- An increased need for consistency of nighttime rituals to help the infant transition from playtime to sleep time (e.g., bath time and a story) may be evident.
- Teaching infants to sleep in their own crib can be a struggle for some parents. Begin by putting them to bed while they are drowsy but still awake. If the infant wakes in the night, parents can help them return to sleep with the least amount of intrusion (e.g., use face, voice, touch, and then holding).
- Infants are now more capable of waiting for gratification and thus parents can use talking and tone of voice to distract, calm, and reassure the infant that their needs will be met.

Strength and Motor Coordination

- Floor time is essential for the infant to learn to crawl and walk. Providing for infant safety, however, remains a major responsibility for parents. Movable walkers are unsafe and may actually hinder walking.
- Childproofing the home becomes increasingly important. Putting gates on stairs, padding sharp corners, covering electrical outlets, and keeping the cord on an iron safely out of the way needs to be stressed. Make sure that parents and other caregivers have the telephone number for a poison control center handy.

Feeding and Self-Care

- Solids should be introduced at 6 months. Breastfed infants need iron-fortified foods. Parents often need specific information about types of foods to start with, quantity, and feeding positions (see Chapter 11). Use an infant seat or a highchair (properly seated high enough that the infant's back and sides are supported and arms are at the level of the tray).
- Having structured mealtimes is important to help the family maintain regular routines for the infant.

- Allowing the child to hold a spoon or cup will encourage self-feeding and begin to prepare the infant for later weaning from bottle or breast.
- Often parents are uncomfortable with the messiness of infant feeding. Discuss ways they can minimize the mess (e.g., sheet or plastic table cloth on the floor, small-sized portions of food) and still allow the infant to explore, look at, touch, smell, and taste the new foods. Assure the parents that there will always be some mess.
- Introducing solid foods and infant teething often occur simultaneously. Cleansing the teeth (use a soft cloth or soft tooth brush) and providing fluoride supplements, if the water supply is not fluoridated, is important at this time (see Chapter 33).

Communication and Language

- Using the names of objects, encouraging gestures, continuing to talk about everyday activities, and responding to the infant's increasing vocalizations is important.
- Showing the infant picture books and magazines and talking about the pictures are early lessons in "reading" to an infant.
- Naming body parts while changing diapers and during bath time becomes a new and enjoyable activity for parents. To demonstrate the infant's responsiveness, the provider can model this behavior during the physical examination.

Social and Emotional Growth

- Identifying and encouraging the child to have a "transitional object" (e.g., a favorite toy or blanket) can ease the coming developmental phase of separation anxiety.
- Continuing to discuss parents' feelings regarding limit setting, consistency of care, and parental consensus about discipline is important.
- Positive parental responsiveness and attention continues to support both social and emotional growth of the infant.

Cognitive and Environmental Stimulation

- Toys that involve cause-and-effect reactions, stacking, and container play can be demonstrated and encouraged. Most often common favorite toys will be common household objects such as wooden spoons, plastic bowls, pull toys, or a telephone. Especially popular will be any object that the parents use.
- Interactive games continue to be important, and infants should be encouraged to initiate actions and guide play.

9 THROUGH 12 MONTHS

Regulation and Sleep-Wake Patterns

- The "transitional object" can ease transitions in new situations and provide a sense of comfort or familiarity.
- Predictability in the daily schedule allows the infant to gain mastery over new situations. Efforts to establish and maintain regular mealtimes, a nighttime routine, and consistent caregivers increase the infant's sense of security during the transitions.
- The infant's temperament becomes more evident in activity level, level of curiosity, and ease of adjusting to new situations. The infant's temperament, however, may not always be compatible with that of other family members. This discrepancy

can become an area of conflict and turmoil. Inquiring about such, and discussing positive parenting strategies, can generate creative solutions.

Strength and Motor Coordination

- The parents' natural tendency to "cheer" their infants on as they refine old and achieve new motor skills can be used as an example of positive reinforcement for the child in other areas of development.
- "Childproofing" the environment continues to be a major issue as the infant is increasingly mobile and curious. Parents need help to anticipate their infant's next major developmental achievement and prepare for the child's natural curiosity. Babies at this age are often able to get into trouble but not get themselves out (e.g., falling in a slippery bathtub).
- Safe storage of medicines, cleaning agents, matches, and firearms (in locked cabinets, not just out of reach) are essential precautions for mobile older infants with increased fine motor skills and unbounded curiosity.
- Bath-water temperature must be checked, and infants should never be left alone even for a few seconds in the tub.
- As fine motor skills improve, oral exploration is still one of an infant's primary learning methods, so most everything ends up in the mouth. Having the 24-hour poison control telephone number available and posted for caregivers is critical.
- Outings for both parents and child help relieve stress and provide wonderful learning opportunities for the infant. Because of the infant's increasing mobility, close supervision is required.

Feeding and Self-Care

- The division of responsibility in feeding becomes more obvious during this time. Parents are responsible for providing healthful foods in an environment that is pleasant and conducive to eating. Children are responsible for determining how much they will eat. Nine- to 12-month-old infants are beginning to self-feed and demonstrate clear preferences and dislikes. Discussing the division of responsibilities and the control issues that may arise at this time can help families establish healthy eating patterns for a lifetime (see Chapter 11).
- Dental hygiene and caries prevention includes use of a soft cloth or soft toothbrush to cleanse teeth and gums. Fluoride supplements should be given if water supply is not fluoridated (see Chapter 33).
- Transitioning from purées to blended foods, finger foods, and soft solids involves major changes for infant and parent. Remind parents that it can take 10 to 20 exposures for infants to accept a new food into their diet.
- Practicing with spoons and cups in play and at mealtime helps develop the infant's skills at using them and promotes eventual self-feeding.
- Establishing consistent mealtimes and snack times and avoiding the habit of "grazing" (i.e., having food constantly available) will encourage appropriate intake of foods. Because hunger is inconsistent for infants, 3 meals and 2 to 3 snacks will ensure adequate nutrition. Having the infant sit in a highchair to eat sets a pattern and expectation for eating at the table, rather than "grazing."
- Eating together as a family is important for infants at least once a day. As they observe the foods others are eating, the likelihood that they will try the new foods increases. Eating with others also keeps the infant focused on meals. Distracters, such as toys and television, should be avoided. Using verbal reinforcement and talking about the meal are important.

Communication and Language

- Reinforcing the infant's effort to communicate through gestures, pointing, and ambiguous vocalizations should be encouraged. This "practice" with language provides the groundwork for future speech skills. Parents should not try to anticipate exactly what the child needs.
- Naming utensils and the color, smell, taste, and texture of foods can build language skills and keep the infant engaged during mealtime.
- Naming body parts and pointing to them also provides distraction during diaper changes and bath time.
- Reading becomes much more interactive as the infant is able to point to pictures in a book, imitate animal sounds, and assist in turning pages. Encourage parents to read to their infant often (see the Resource Box for reading program information).

Social and Emotional Growth

- As infants reach 12 months, their emerging will, desire for autonomy, need for control, and sense of initiative become more evident. They begin to distinguish themselves from their parent.
- The concept of the teaching loop (see Table 5-3) can be used to explain the parents' "teaching role" as the child develops.
- Helping parents understand the role of discipline as a process of guidance to teach positive behaviors (as compared with punishment where constraints are applied to negative behaviors) is important.
- Distraction continues to be very effective in guiding an infant's curiosity by redirecting their behavior to desirable activities.
- The infant's stranger anxiety may be difficult for parents to handle. They may need help establishing a separation ritual by which the child understands the parent is leaving but will return. Parents may also need to express their feelings of concern or even disappointment when their infant enjoys the time away from the parent.
- Parents may have difficulty finding the energy needed to deal with busy, mobile infants and will appreciate suggestions on how to cope when exhaustion occurs.
- In two-parent families, parents may need an opportunity to discuss how to delegate and share parental role and responsibilities.
- Parents need positive reinforcement for their continually developing skills, just as their children do.

Cognitive and Environmental Stimulation

- Playing with the child is a creative way to strengthen the parent-child bond and stimulate the infant's cognitive development.
- Allowing the child to take the lead in play activities is important, but parents can also use play to model new activities and skills.
- Interactive games such as peek-a-boo, pat-a-cake, and rolling a ball back and forth encourage reciprocal social play. Interaction with the caregiver is still the most important activity for the infant.
- Books, music, blocks, stacking toys, container toys, and pull toys all allow self-initiated activities.
- Many 12-month-old children have a box of toys that they enjoy dumping out for play. Having parents put some toys away and then bring them out at a later date can sustain an infant's curiosity and interest.
- Bath time and sandboxes often provide a safe opportunity to engage in messy play that most infants enjoy. Infants need this type of tactile stimulation.
- Providing parents with factual information regarding the physiologic and cognitive development that is necessary for toilet training can prevent unrealistic expectations later on.

▰ COMMON DEVELOPMENTAL ISSUES FOR INFANTS

Parents' concerns during the infant's first year of life are often related to inexperience or lack of knowledge about what to expect as infants grow and develop. A minority of infants has a true developmental delay. The fact that their baby is "normal," however, does not make the parents' concern any less compelling, and the health care provider has a responsibility to answer parents' questions; provide essential information about development; make accurate assessments to rule out problems; treat or refer problems appropriately; and provide follow-up care and support. Some of the more common developmental issues that trouble parents are discussed in this section. When parents understand the complexity of infant growth and development, they are better able to make healthy decisions for their infants and family.

SLEEP

Should babies sleep in the same bed with their parents? How much sleep does an infant need? How can an 8-month-old be encouraged to sleep through the night? These are just a few of the questions parents may have about their infant's sleep. The answers to these and other questions will differ for each family and infant. A fuller discussion of children's sleep and rest patterns is found in Chapter 15. There are some general principles that can help guide parents, including the following:

- The first month of life is one of transition from the warm, dark uterine environment in which the fetus lived with the rhythm of the mother's body, heartbeat, and respirations. Being in a similar environment, close to those rhythms, helps many infants relax and sleep.

- Parents must ensure a safe environment for their infant's sleep: a supine sleep position on a firm surface in a crib or bassinet, from which the infant cannot fall is recommended. No blanket, or only a thin blanket that comes up to the chest and can be tucked into the bottom of the bed, should be used. Pillows, bumper pads, and numerous soft toys can be sources of suffocation and are not recommended. The space between crib slats should be no more than $2\frac{3}{8}$ inches, and the space between the mattress and slats, no more than the width of two adult fingers.
- Cosleeping is no longer recommended, especially if parents are obese, exposed to alcohol, drugs, or medications that would cause either parent to sleep more soundly than usual.
- Infants often need assistance transitioning from an awake state into sleep. Helping parents understand the natural consolidation of sleep states in the first year of life will help them appreciate this challenge.
- Feeding facilitates transition to sleep, especially for young infants.
- Self-regulation of state is an important skill for infants to learn; learning to put themselves to sleep and to sleep as long as they need is an important developmental task.
- As the infant matures neurologically, ease of state transition increases and self-regulation skills develop.
- A consistent and predictable sleep routine, in a consistent and predictable location (for both naps and nighttime sleep), provides the infant with a foundation to establish self-regulation.

FEEDING

Exclusive breastfeeding for the first 6 months of life and breast milk with solids from 6 to 12 months are current recommendations (see Chapters 11 and 12). Feeding concerns or problems in infancy (particularly a less than expected weight gain or decrease in weight) should be assessed through an observation of a feeding in the clinic (or at home, if resources allow). A detailed feeding history, a minimum of a 3-day diet history, and calorie analysis may be needed for a full assessment. The infant's oral motor skills and general development should also be assessed since early feeding concerns may indicate other subtle developmental delays that can benefit from early intervention. A standardized feeding assessment using a tool such as the NCAST Feeding Scale, provides information about the parent-child relationship and assists in the development of individualized recommendations for the parents (see Chapters 11 and 12).

CRYING

Infant crying and irritability can cause parents to worry that something is wrong. It also can become a great disruption to the family and create a strained parent-child relationship. Labeling the crying as "colic" when it occurs more than 3 hours a day, 3 times a week, and between 3 weeks and 3 months may or may not console stressed parents. It is advisable to evaluate the crying duration and intensity, what factors contribute to it, and what factors offer relief. Assessment of the infant's sleep-wake activity and amount of direct holding also provides insight into how to assist the family. Parents can use a tool such as the NCAST sleep activity record to evaluate the infant's daily feeding, sleep routine, and fussiness.

Teaching parents to understand their infant's behavioral cues and communication is an important first step in resolving frequent crying. Most often, infant irritability is reduced as the infant establishes a consistent sleep-wake cycle, especially daily naps. The sleep-deprived infant is likely to become irritable and demonstrate poor feeding routines. Parents can be instructed to be alert to the infant's cues of tiredness and assist their infant to transition more easily from the wake to sleep state.

SPITTING UP

Differentiating between normal infant "spit up," regurgitation, reflux, and vomiting is critical to provide appropriate care. In addition to describing the differences to parents, it can be valuable to have them complete a 3-day diary with the frequency and events surrounding these episodes. Spitting up may be influenced by the infant's daily routine and schedule, including feedings, lack of sleep-routines, and burping pattern. Incomplete feedings resulting in grazing or overfeeding may be precursors. Reflux, crying and arching while feeding, and vomiting require more in-depth assessment and management and are discussed in Chapters 11 and 32.

DISCIPLINE AND BEHAVIORAL GUIDANCE

Parents may express concern that their infant does "not mind," misbehaves, or is "spoiled." The first year of life is one in which the infant needs to establish a sense of trust and attachment; infants need to feel secure and safe, able to rely on the parents or caregiver to meet their needs. From this base, the infant learns self-regulation and the ability to reciprocate in affectionate, mutually satisfying interactions with others. If parents are struggling with behavioral or discipline concerns in the first year of life, early intervention should be initiated. Provider's time is well spent helping parents understand the needs of infants and develop an appropriate parenting style. Establishing a regular routine, especially for sleep and feeding, facilitates the infant's social and emotional growth. At times there is a mismatch in temperament between the parent and child. The child's challenging behaviors or external demands on the parent can leave the parent little energy to provide the assistance the child needs. Efforts spent early in a child's life are important in setting the stage for later emotional and behavioral patterns (AAP, 1998; Bronson, 2000).

■ CLASSIFICATION OF DEVELOPMENTAL DISORDERS IN INFANTS

When evaluating for possible developmental delay in an infant, it is important to distinguish disorders that manifest as motor problems (e.g., cerebral palsy), communication problems (e.g., receptive or expressive communication and behavior), or cognitive problems (e.g., problem solving, mental retardation, specific deficits in processing information). Processing disorders include peripheral problems such as deafness and blindness; central processing that results in motor, language, and perceptual dysfunction; and behavioral problems.

Although there are some limits to the history, it usually provides the best clues to the diagnosis of developmental delay. Some problems, such as fetal alcohol syndrome or uterine drug exposure, autism, and fragile X syndrome, may not have clear symptoms in infancy. Early behaviors of autism, for example, are just beginning to be explored. In some cases, parents may not be able to recall exactly when their child achieved a particular milestone or how long the infant has been demonstrating a particular behavior.

It is important to determine whether the problems are the result of neurodegeneration as opposed to a static encephalopathy. Developmental delays that appear during infancy are usually connected to dysfunctions of major organs, physiologic abnormalities, and physiologic imbalances. Thus early indications may be associated with alterations in feedings, sleep, or interactions. Later presentations may include motor coordination problems, hearing and vision problems, or more severe interaction problems. Gross motor deficits are most often identified after 9 months, although parents may report concerns earlier. The Diagnostic Classification Task Force (1995) has developed a systematic approach for organizing, describing, and managing developmental and mental health issues. The *Bright Futures* program also provides practical tools for clinicians (Green & Palfrey, 2002; Jellinek et al, 2002a, 2002b).

■ RED FLAGS FOR INFANTS

Developmental problems may be difficult to identify in infants, but the provider must be alert to "red flags" that place the infant at risk or indicate a particular problem. These need closer developmental surveillance and more frequent developmental and social-emotional screening, often requiring referral to developmental centers for more in-depth assessments. As the well child history is taken, specific risk factors that contribute to development delays can be identified, including the following:

- Prenatal exposure to street drugs or alcohol
- Prematurity
- Low birth weight, SGA, intrauterine growth retardation
- Anoxia or birth trauma
- Neonatal intensive care and long-term hospitalization
- Cardiovascular illnesses
- Endocrine and metabolic problems
- Genetic syndromes
- Failure to thrive
- Cerebral palsy
- Sensory problems
- Parental or environmental deficit in meeting the infant's needs (e.g., alcohol or drug abuse by parent; parental depression)

Table 5-4 outlines developmental findings that are indications for referral to a child development center, a state's early child development identification program, or a child

TABLE 5-4   Developmental Red Flags: Newborns and Infants

Age	Physical Development (Autonomic Stability, Regulation, Sleep, Temperament)	Gross Motor (Strength, Coordination)	Fine Motor (Feeding, Self-Care)	Language and Hearing	Psychosocial and Emotional Skills	Cognitive and Visual Abilities
Newborn–1 mo	Lack of return to birth weight by 2 wk examination Poor coordination of suck-swallow Tachypnea or bradycardia with feedings Poor habituation to external stimuli	Asymmetric movements Hypertonia or hypotonia Asymmetric primitive reflexes	Hands held fisted Absent or asymmetric palmar grasp	No startle to sound or sudden noises No quieting to voice High-pitched cry	Diffuse nonverbal cues Poor state transitions Irritable	Doll's eyes No red light reflex Poor alert state
3 mo	Poor weight gain; less than 1 lb weight gain in 1 mo Head circumference increasing greater than 2 standard deviations on growth curve or showing no increase in size Continuing problems with poor suck-swallow Difficulty with regulation of sleep-wake cycle Fussy baby	Asymmetric movements Hypertonia or hypotonia No attempt to raise head on stomach	Hands fisted with oppositional thumb No hand-to-mouth activity Feedings taking longer than 45 min Consistently awakening hourly for feeding	Does not turn to voice, rattle, or bell No sounds, coos, squeals	Lack of social smile Withdrawn or depressed Lack of consistent, safe child care	No visual tracking Not able to fix on face or object
6 mo	Less than double birth weight Head circumference shows no increase Continuation of poor feeding or sleep regulation Difficulty with self-calming	Persistent primitive reflexes Does not attempt to sit with support Head lag with pull to sit Scissoring	Does not reach for objects, hold rattle, hold hands together Does not grasp at clothes	No babbling Does not respond to voice, bell, rattle, or loud noises even with startle	No smiles No response to play Solemn appearance	Not visually alert Does not reach for objects Does not look at caregiver

Continued

TABLE 5-4   Developmental Red Flags: Newborns and Infants—Cont'd

Age	Physical Development (Autonomic Stability, Regulation, Sleep, Temperament)	Gross Motor (Strength, Coordination)	Fine Motor (Feeding, Self-Care)	Language and Hearing	Psychosocial and Emotional Skills	Cognitive and Visual Abilities
9 mo	Parent control issues with feeding or sleep Night awakening that persists Offered bottle in bed for sleep Difficulty with self-calming, self-regulation	Does not sit even in tripod position No lateral prop reflex Asymmetric crawl, handedness, or other movements	No self-feeding No high chair sitting No solids Does not pick up toy with one hand	Lack of single- or double-consonant sounds Lack of response to name or voice Does not respond to any words Lack of reciprocal vocalizations	Intense stranger anxiety or absent stranger anxiety Does not seek comfort from caregiver with stress	Lack of visual awareness Lack of reaching out for toys Lack of toy exploration visually or orally
12 mo	Less than triple birth weight Losing more than 2 standard deviations on growth curve for weight, length, or head circumference Poor sleep-wake cycle Extreme inability to separate from parent	Not pulling self to stand Not moving around the environment to explore	Persistent mouthing Not attempting to feed self or hold cup Not able to hold toy in each hand or transfer objects	Inability to localize to sound Not imitating speech sounds Not using 2–3 words Does not point, or uses only gestures or pointing	No response to game playing No response to reading or interactive activities Withdrawn or solemn	Not visually following activities in the environment

mo, month(s); *wk*, week(s); *min*, minute(s).

development specialist. When clear indicators are present, referral should be made rather than waiting some months to validate observations.

Some primary care practices have providers with expertise in minor developmental problems; in consultation with a specialist, this provider may take an initial "wait-and-see" approach. Providers with more in-depth expertise in developmental, sleep, feeding, behavioral assessments, and par-

enting issues can be a valuable resource in the primary care practice. They can conduct ongoing assessments as the infant grows and can help parents implement interventions to foster healthy development. If the infant is to be referred, primary health care providers work with the parents to connect them to community resources, advocate for necessary services, and continue to provide the infant with long-term primary care.

RESOURCE BOX

Developmental Management of Infants

SCREENING TOOLS

Ages & Stages Questionnaire (ASQ) and Ages & Stages Questionnaire: Social Emotional (ASQ:SE)
www.brookespublishing.com
Birth through 5 years

Batelle Developmental Inventory Screening Test
www.riversidepublishing.com

Child Development Inventories
www.dbpeds.org/screening/index.cfm
3 months through 6 years

Communication and Symbolic Behavior Scales Developmental Profile (CSBS DP)
www.brookespublishing.com

Denver Screening Scales (Denver II)
www.denverii.com

Early start online library
www.edgateway.net
Resource library of developmental and educational materials for assessment and teaching

Infant-Toddler and Family Instrument (ITFI)
www.brookespublishing.com
Age 6 through 36 months

Milani-Comparetti Motor Development
www.unmc.edu/mmi

Parents' Evaluation of Developmental Status (PEDS)
www.pedstest.com
Birth through 8 years

Prescreening Developmental Questionnaire, Inc (PDQ-II)
www.denverii.com

Receptive-Expressive Emergent Language Scale, second edition
www.proedinc.com

Temperament and Atypical Behavior Scale (TABS)
www.brookespublishing.com

DIAGNOSTIC DEVELOPMENTAL ASSESSMENT TOOLS
The following tools generally require training for use:

Bayley Scales of Infant Development, second edition
www.parinc.com
Age 1 through 42 months

Gesell Developmental Screening Inventory (Revised)
Birth through school age
Order from Lorraine Coulson (e-mail: lrcoulson@ualr.edu)

Home Observation for Measurement of the Environment (HOME) Scale
www.ualr.edu/crtldept/home4.htm
Order from Lorraine Coulson (e-mail: lrcoulson@ualr.edu)

Nursing Child Assessment Satellite Training (NCAST) Scales
www.ncast.org
Feeding and teaching scales (birth through 3 years)
Personal environmental assessments (manual only needed)
Sleep activity record (manual only needed)

Neonatal Behavioral Assessment Scale
www.brazelton-institute.com

PARENT AND PROVIDER EDUCATIONAL RESOURCES
Brazelton TB, Sparrow JD: *Touchpoints three to six: your child's emotional and behavioral development*, Cambridge, MA, 2001, Perseus Publishing Services.

Bright Futures
www.*brightfutures*.org
Project of National Center for Education in Maternal and Child Health

Goldberg S: *Baby and toddler learning fun*, Cambridge, MA, 2001, Perseus Publishing Services.

Healthy Steps for Young Children
www.healthy steps
A National Initiative to Foster Healthy Growth and Development

Holland K: *Johnson's your baby from birth to 6 months*, New York, 2002, DK Publishing.

Continued

RESOURCE BOX

Developmental Management of Infants—Cont'd

Mackonochie A: *Your baby's first year: month by month,* New York, 2001, Lorenz Books.

Masi W, Leiderman RC: *Gymboree baby play,* San Francisco, 2001, Creative Publishing International.

Reach Out and Read National Center
www.reachoutandread.org

Satter E: *How to get your kid to eat...but not too much,* Palo Alto, CA, 1987, Bull Publishing Company.

Schmitt B: *Your child's health: the parent's guide to symptoms, emergencies, common illnesses, behavior, and school problems,* New York, 1991, Bantam Books.

Shelov S, Hannemann R: *Caring for your baby and young child: birth to age 5,* Elk Grove Village, IL, 1999, American Academy of Pediatrics.

Weissbluth M: *Healthy sleep habits, happy child,* New York, 1999, Fawcett Books, Ballantine Publishing Group.

Zero to Three
www.zerotothree.org

✓ DISCUSSION FORUM

1. Many providers are required to see 25 to 30 patients per day in their primary care practice. Discuss ways providers can assess parents' sleep needs, expectations regarding crying, and maternal depression while providing education about infant sleep/awake states, feeding patterns, and emotional development during a 20- to 25-minute newborn exam.
2. Identify developmental behaviors of an infant that would require in-depth assessment as referral for developmental evaluation.

REFERENCES

American Academy of Pediatrics (AAP), Committee on Children with Disabilities: Identifying infants and young children with developmental disorders in the medical home: an algorithm for developmental surveillance and screening, *Pediatrics* 118:405-420, 2001.

American Academy of Pediatrics (AAP), Committee on Psychosocial Aspects of Child and Family Health: Guidance for effective discipline, *Pediatrics* 101(4):723-728, 1998.

American Heart Association et al: Dietary recommendations for children and adolescents: a guide for practitioners, *Pediatrics* 117(2):544-559, 2006.

Anders TF, Goodlin-Jones BL, Zelenko M: Infant regulation and sleep-wake state development, *Zero to Three* 19:5-8, 1998.

Barnard K: *Beginning rhythms: the emerging process of sleep wake behaviors and self regulation,* Seattle, 1999, NCAST, University of Washington.

Bronson MB: *Self-regulation in early childhood-nature and nurture,* New York, 2000, The Guilford Press.

Carey WB: Let's give temperament its due, *Contemp Pediatr* 15:91-113, 1998.

Centers for Disease Control and Prevention, National Center for Health Statistics: *National vital statistics reports* 53(9), Nov 23, 2004. Available at *www.cdc.gov/nchs/data/hestat/prelimbirth04_tables.pdf* (accessed Sept 9, 2006).

Cox JL, Holden JM, Sagovsky R: Detection of postnatal depression: development of the 10-item Edinburgh Postnatal Depression Scale, *Br J Psychiatry* 150:782-786, 1987.

Diagnostic Classification Task Force: *Diagnostic classification 0-3: diagnostic classification of mental health and developmental disorders of infancy and early childhood,* Arlington, VA, 1995, Zero to Three/National Center for Clinical Infant Programs.

Dixon SD, Stein M, editors: *Encounters with children: pediatric behavior and development,* St Louis, 2006, Mosby.

Green M, Palfrey J, editors: *Bright Futures: guidelines for health supervision of infants, children, and adolescents,* ed 2, Arlington, VA, 2002, National Center for Education in Maternal and Child Health.

Jellinek M, Patel BP, Froehle MC, editors: *Bright Futures in practice: mental health—volume I. Practice guide,* Arlington, VA, 2002a, National Center for Education in Maternal and Child Health.

Jellinek M, Patel BP, Froehle MC, editors: *Bright Futures in practice: mental health—volume II. Tool kit,* Arlington, VA, 2002b, National Center for Education in Maternal and Child Health.

Shields BH, Smith GA: Success in the prevention of infant walker-related injuries: an analysis of national data, 1990-2001, *Pediatrics* 117(3):452-9, 2006.

Shonkoff JP, Phillips DA, editors: Committee on Integrating the Science of Early Childhood Development, Board on Children, Youth, and Families: *From neurons to neighborhoods: the science of early childhood development,* Washington, DC, 2000, National Academies Press.

Steward D, Steward M: The observation of Anglo-Mexican and Chinese-American mothers teaching their young sons, *Child Dev* 44:329-337, 1973.

Trevarthen C, Aitken KJ: Infant intersubjectivity: research, theory, and clinical applications, *J Child Psychol Psychiat* 42(1):3-48, 2001.

Wisner KL, Parry BL, Pointek CM: Postpartum depression, *N Engl J Med* 347(3):194-199, 2002.

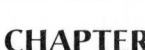

CHAPTER 6

Developmental Management of Toddlers and Preschoolers

Mary A. Murphy and Anita Berry

Developmental changes in the second through fifth years of life are subtler than those seen in the first year, yet they are highly significant. Children enter toddlerhood as babies, dependent on parents and caregivers for their very survival and leave as accomplished children with elaborate and sophisticated skills. Ready to enter the social world of school and community, 5-year-olds have a sense of self that will shape the quality of their character as older children, adolescents, and adults. Children begin this process of change by refining abilities acquired in the first year, learning, for example, to walk smoothly with control and speed, to run and climb, and to combine words into phrases and sentences. They add to their repertoire of skills, growing stronger, bigger, and more socially, emotionally, and intellectually capable. This chapter reviews some of the many changes that occur for toddlers (usually defined as a child 12 to 24 months old) and preschoolers (a child 2 to 5 years old), in addition to the primary health care provider's role when working with these children and their families.

DEVELOPMENT OF TODDLERS AND PRESCHOOLERS

PHYSICAL DEVELOPMENT

Physical and physiologic changes in toddlers and preschoolers continue at a much slower pace than in the first year of life (see Table 11-6 for a review of yearly gains in weight, height, and head circumference). Statistically, children are gaining weight faster and earlier, as one study of infant safety seats suggests (Trifiletti et al, 2006); however, growth charts continue to show the average 2-year-old weighs 26 to 28 lb (12.5 to 13.5 kg), with boys being slightly heavier than girls, and is 34 to 35 inches (85 to 90 cm) tall. Head circumference in the average 2-year-old is 19 to 19.5 inches (48 to 50 cm). Most toddlers have no palpable fontanelles by 12 months; for all children, the anterior fontanelle should be completely closed by 18 to 19 months. During the fourth and fifth years, skeletal growth continues as additional ossification centers appear in the wrist and ankle and additional epiphyses develop in some of the long bones. For the 4- to 5-year-old, the legs grow faster than the head, trunk, or upper extremities. Changes related to body systems are highlighted in Table 6-1. More detailed discussion of development, systems, and disease processes can be found in Units 3 and 4 of this text.

MOTOR DEVELOPMENT

Motor development is divided into 2 components—gross and fine. Gross motor refers to the development and use of the large muscles. Fine motor includes hand and finger development and oral-motor development. See Table 5-1 for a review of gross and fine motor milestones by age.

Use of the dominant hand may appear as early as 8 to 12 months but generally emerges between 2 and 4 years. The 4-year-old can thread small beads on a chain; grasp a pencil appropriately to copy some letters (v, h, t, o); draw a person with head and features, legs, trunk, and arms; use scissors to cut on a line; fasten buttons; and eat with a fork. By 5 years, these movements expand to copying a square and additional letters (x, l, a, c, u, y), writing some letters spontaneously, producing identifiable pictures, counting fingers on one hand, and using all eating utensils appropriately.

Two-year-olds may still be "toddling," using their arms for balance and frequently falling as they try to run or move quickly. They begin to master climbing and by 3 to 4 years are walking smoothly. The following are gross motor behaviors that an average 5-year-old could demonstrate:
- Walks with control
- Steps easily over a balance beam
- Climbs stairs with alternate feet both up and down to any height, up ladders
- Runs around corners, stops voluntarily, lightly on toes
- Rides a tricycle using the pedals to move from place to place
- Shows more control in throwing, catching, bouncing, and kicking a ball
- Skips using alternate feet
- Walks a narrow line easily
- Moves rhythmically to music

COMMUNICATION AND LANGUAGE DEVELOPMENT

Language uses symbols for thoughts; thus it emerges with Piaget's preoperational stage of development. Beginning around 2 years old, toddlers use words to convey their thoughts and feelings. Once the process begins, it develops rapidly. Cognitive development is a basic requirement for language development because the child must decipher the rules of language independently, problem solve to understand the communication of others, and create symbols that reflect his or

91

TABLE 6-1	Physical Development of Toddlers and Preschool-Age Children
Body System	**Developmental Changes**
Dental	By 12 mo, the child usually has 6 to 8 primary teeth. By 2 yr, the child has a complete set of 20 primary teeth. By 3 yr, the second molars usually erupt. During the second year, calcification begins for the first and second permanent bicuspids and second molars. Most growth and calcification of the permanent teeth occur within the gums; it is not visible.
Neurologic	Continued myelinization and cortical development occurs. Fine motor movements are more detailed and sustained: • 2-year-olds can easily manipulate fingers to stack 2 blocks. • 3-year-olds can create a tower of 8 or more blocks. • 4-year-olds can easily build a 12-block step design. • 5-year-olds can grasp a pencil appropriately to copy simple geometric designs accurately and write their name in block letters. Gross motor skills are smoother and more coordinated. Sensory function is more mature. Visual acuity is 20/70 for 2-year-olds; 20/30 for 5- to 6-year-olds.
Cardiovascular	Little change occurs in the second and third year. By the fifth year, the heart has quadrupled in size since birth. By 5 yr, the heart rate is typically 70 to 110 bpm. Normal sinus arrhythmia may continue, and innocent murmurs are common. The hematologic system should produce only adult hemoglobin by the fifth year. The hemoglobin level stabilizes at 12 to 15 g/dL.
Pulmonary	Abdominal respiratory movements continue until the end of the fifth or sixth year. Respiratory rate steadies and slows to about 30 breaths per minute.
Gastrointestinal	By 2 yr, the salivary glands reach adult size. The stomach becomes more bowed and increases its capacity to about 500 mL. Many children still require a nutritious snack between meals because of small stomach size. During the second year, the liver matures and becomes more efficient in vitamin storage, glycogenesis, amino acid changes, and ketone body formation. The lower edge of the liver may still be palpable. By 4 to 5 yr, the gastrointestinal system is mature enough for the child to eat a full range of foods. Stools are more like those of adults.
Renal	Kidneys begin descending deeper into the pelvic area and grow in size. Ureters remain short and relatively straight. A 2-year-old may excrete as much as 500 to 600 mL of urine a day. A 4- to 5-year-old excretes between 600 and 750 mL daily.
Endocrine	Quiescent time for sexual growth, with few physical or hormonal changes. Growth hormone stimulates body growth.

bpm, Beats per minute; *mo,* month(s); *yr,* year(s).

her ideas and emotions and can be understood by others. The development of language requires mastery of the following:

- Oral-motor ability to articulate sounds
- Auditory perception to distinguish words and sentences
- Cognitive ability to understand syntax, semantics, and pragmatics
- Psychosocial-cultural environment to motivate the child to engage in language use

Language milestones are evident in two general categories—receptive and expressive language. These are presented for infants and children younger than 5 years old in Table 5-2.

Articulation

Articulation skills are practiced daily, and by 24 months, speech sounds are 25% intelligible to a stranger. The intelligibility rate jumps to about 66% between 24 and 36 months, with 90% intelligibility by 3 years old. By 4 years, speech should be completely intelligible with the exception of particularly difficult consonants; by 5 years the tongue-contact sounds of n, t, d, k, g, y, and ng are more intelligible. Some sounds, such as the zh sound, are not added until the child is 6 to 8 years old. Fig. 6-1 identifies sounds articulated by children at specific ages.

During the second year, the child practices playful changes in pitch and loudness. Three- and 4-year-olds can show normal hesitance in speech or stuttering. These dysfluencies should pass if ignored and are no longer expected in 5-year-olds.

Children usually progress through a regular sequence of mispronunciations as they learn new articulation skills. At first they simply omit the new sound, and then they try to substitute a more familiar sound for the new one (e.g., the "w" for "r" substitution, as in "wabbit" for "rabbit"). Distortion is

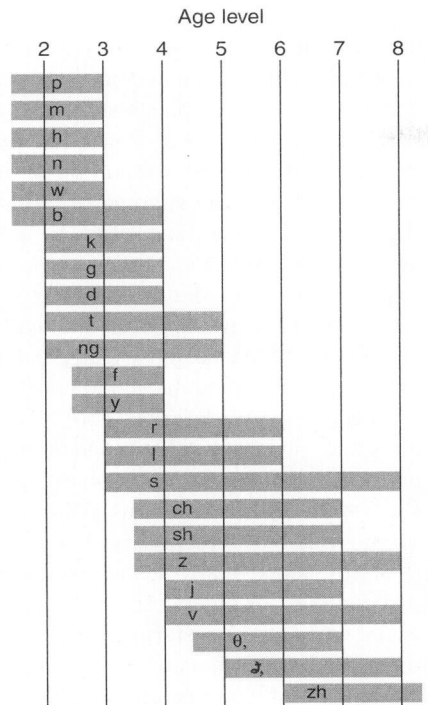

FIG. 6-1   Norms for development of speech sounds. *θ, th* as in *thin; ᴣ, th* as in *this.* (From Van Riper C, Erickson RL: *Speech correction: an introduction to speech pathology and audiology,* ed 9, Needham Heights, MA, 1996, Allyn & Bacon, p 98. Reprinted by permission.)

followed by "addition" as the child adds an extra sound (e.g., "gulad" for "glad"). Knowing each of these steps allows the examiner to assure the parent that the child is developing normally or needs monitoring.

Lexicon

Lexicon refers to vocabulary. Size of vocabulary is influenced by many factors, including environment, stimulation, intelligence, bilingualism, culture, and personality. Children usually understand more words than they are able to express, and addition of words to their expressive vocabulary comes with continued practice. Girls typically say their first word between 8 and 11 months, boys about 14 months. Most 2-year-olds have more than 200 words in their vocabulary, and most 4- to 5-year-olds add approximately 50 words a month to their vocabulary. Five-year-olds should be able to define some words with other words (e.g., "cup" is "you drink with it," or "chair" is "to sit on").

Syntax

Syntax, or grammar, refers to the structure of words in sentences or phrases. The ability to construct sentences that convey meaning is a complex skill, proceeding through several stages in children: receptive, holophrastic, and telegraphic speech. Much of this skill is developed between 8 months and 3.5 years. By 8 months, children are developing receptive language (i.e., they understand others who use a new word

or structure before they are able to use it themselves). When asked "Where is the ball?" an 8-month-old searches for the ball. Between 12 and 18 months, children begin to use holophrases or single words to express whole ideas. The child says "milk," perhaps to mean the whole sentence, "Give me a glass of milk." A complex idea is expressed in one succinct word. Holophrastic sentences are denominative (labeling) or imperative (commanding).

Around 18 months, children begin using telegraphic speech, phrases that have many words omitted and sound like a telegram, to convey their message (e.g., "get milk" "go bye-bye"). McNeill (1970) reviews research to support the idea that a child's linguistic structures in this phase are made up of two classes: pivot and open. The pivot class consists of a few frequently used words, and the open class contains newly learned words. Thus, the child may use the pivot word "daddy" with open-class words for "daddy eat," "daddy all gone," or "daddy sleep." During this stage, which typically lasts 2 to 3 months, the child begins to use articles (the, an, a), demonstrative pronouns (this, that, these, those), and adjectives and possessives. Sentence structure becomes more complex as children move from active sentences, to questions, to passive and negative construction, and then add plurals (at 3 years old) and past tenses (at 4 years old) to their grammar. Three- to four-word sentences should be evident by 3 years, and by 5 years old, the child's syntax is close to adult style, including use of future tense and complete sentences of five to six words in length.

Semantics

Semantic development, the understanding that words have specific meaning and the child's use of words to convey specific meaning, is an ongoing process extending into adulthood. This development occurs in stages from global to more specific and requires interaction through conversation, listening, and reading. Words used in any language have both denotative (the specific, concrete referent of the word) and connotative (a broader range of feelings aroused by the word) meanings. Even though children may be quite adept at using words correctly, they may have only a vague, diffuse connotative understanding of these words. For example, the 3-year-old who drops a toy and uses an expletive she heard when her father dropped a dish does not understand the connotative meaning of what she has said. As language progresses from simple to more complex, meaning and cognitive understanding evolve.

Bilingualism

Although some parents may choose to raise their children bilingually or monolingually, many families do not have that choice and struggle with the new language they are forced to learn. Bilingualism can help preserve the family culture and heritage, and studies suggest that fluent bilingual children have greater mental flexibility and enhanced employment and lifestyle opportunities. Normal toddlers in bilingual homes show mild delays in initial spoken words and can mix the words and phrases within the two languages. Children who associate a clear environmental context for each language (e.g., home is Spanish, and school is English) may progress faster in acquiring both languages

(Feldman, 2005). Maintaining bilingualism should be encouraged, but it requires time and effort as the child learns to read and write and maintain fluency in both. For families anxious to integrate culturally in a society with a different language, emphasizing skill in the language of the new community may be viewed by the family as a first priority.

Simultaneous bilingualism occurs when children hear and learn two languages from infancy. These bilingual children should be equally competent in both languages by 3 years old. Sequential bilingualism occurs when the child, usually 3 years or older, learns one language and then is immersed in another. Children learning sequentially may have more apparent differences in their skills from language to language until they have developed proficiency in both.

Bilingual preschoolers experience no delays in development of their vocabulary and are proficient in sorting one language from the other, although they may "code switch" to the other language for clarity as they talk. They switch languages depending on the person with whom they are speaking and the circumstances. Some even translate for others, seeming to understand that not everyone speaks or understands both languages. Ultimately, whether a second, third, or even more languages are learned simultaneously or sequentially, most children have one dominant language.

SOCIAL AND EMOTIONAL DEVELOPMENT

Psychosocial changes in toddlers and preschoolers are remarkable. Emotions and cognition are interconnected so that assessment of any one area of development is somewhat arbitrary. Toddlers spend most of their time up, running about, verbalizing, and demanding to join in family activities. These are years of intense learning about and managing feelings such as love, happiness, anger, frustration, aggression, and jealousy, and social skills such as sharing, giving, and receiving affection. They learn the words that go with their feelings and, with guidance, the appropriate behaviors. A major developmental milestone for this age is the achievement of a sense of independence and autonomy. The road from depending on parents for everything to doing some things for themselves, however, can be rocky and uneven.

The toddler and preschooler's ability to achieve independence is influenced, in part, by the strengths in their social environment. In particular, maternal depression (chronic and postpartum) has a significantly negative effect on the development of normal infant engagement behaviors that can persist into the toddler and preschool years. Based on the child's emerging sense of identity, maternal depression can lead to social, emotional, and language concerns (Cornish et al, 2005; Pascoe et al, 2006).

Toddlers need a great deal of love, warmth, and comfort, primarily from their parents and caregivers. Toddlers learn to give love and find satisfaction in pleasing their parents. They learn to respond to kisses, hugs, and cuddles they have received by giving kisses, hugs, and cuddles in return. Toddlers who make these early attempts at giving love and are rejected or ignored soon stop trying and begin to find pleasure elsewhere. Toddlers with sensory issues learn to avoid some gestures unless they are in control and decide they can handle the tactile or sensory feelings. Some toddlers find that thumb sucking, rhythmic body movements, and body manipulation are more pleasurable and reliable than person-to-person contacts.

Preschoolers develop more sophisticated ideas about feeling, giving, and sharing. The 4- to 5-year-old moves away from the extremely self-centered attitude of earlier toddlerhood. Parents are viewed as the epitome of wisdom, power, integrity, and goodness. If early stages of the love relationship have not been satisfied, preschoolers can show more fears, inhibitions, explosive behavior, and demands for attention.

Toddlers and preschool-age children gradually increase their ability to follow commands consistently as they work to gain and maintain approval of adults and to behave as "good" children are expected to do. By preschool years, children begin to show some interest in table manners, being polite, saying "Thank you" without a reminder, sharing, saying (and meaning) "I'm sorry," and taking turns. These social skills are learned through daily interactions at home, school, and church, from parents, peers, relatives, and neighbors. Children learn to read social cues of others' behavior (e.g., the voice tone, slight facial expression, posture) and correct their own behavior. Some children, frequently boys, find these cues vague and difficult to learn, and parents can help by explaining and discussing them.

Children at this age vacillate between being a big boy or big girl and mommy's baby. They take great pride in doing as many things as possible for themselves, yet they need to feel totally secure in their parents' care. On some days, toddlers cling to mother's skirt, not letting her out of sight; on other days, the child can play for short periods in the next room, trotting back every so often to see, touch, and hear the mother and be reassured by her presence. Gradually the periods of separation lengthen, and the child needs only to hear the mother's voice or to check occasionally for security. Separation anxiety is frequent during these years and can be traumatic for both parents and child.

Preschool children are much less dependent on their parents and frequently can tolerate physical separation for several hours. As this sense of separateness increases, children are more aware that they are different from their surroundings, their families, and their friends. They begin to realize that other persons also have feelings, fears, and doubts. Peer dependence and learning about how to have and be friends begins to be important.

Toddlers like to have a choice in matters and quickly learn the power of the word "no." They can become extremely negative, practicing the power of "no" every day for months. As toddlers practice making choices, they are clumsy, awkward, and frequently wrong. This can be very frustrating for them, and their outraged responses can be equally annoying for their parents. Toddlers discover the delights of control over others and themselves. This increases their sense of power but can also lead to misunderstandings and hurt feelings if their parents do not read their moods properly. With time, they become more skilled, make better choices, have more successes, and feel more powerful. They no longer have to work so hard to show others their power, and the negative stage passes.

Preschool-age children respond more verbally than toddlers and are able to perform many more self-care tasks (e.g., feed themselves using appropriate utensils, blow their own noses, and go to the bathroom unassisted). Interactions become easier and more enjoyable as the child learns to verbally express needs and feelings.

Sibling Interaction

Interaction patterns between siblings vary and are affected by factors such as opposite gender, temperament, insecure attachment, family discord, corporal punishment, and perceptions of unequal treatment. Many toddlers or preschoolers regress when a new baby arrives, whereas older children may experience excitement, love, and enhanced self-esteem with a new sibling. Parents need to promptly limit any aggression expressed by the older child, provide love and attention, and talk about feelings. When older children fight, parents need to describe the situation and provide even-handed control. Blaming a child, except in a clear-cut instance of misbehavior, is usually unproductive. Promoting support, loyalty, and friendship are important goals for sibling interactions (see Chapter 18).

Morality

Morality, or the ability to know right from wrong, is based on external control during the toddler years, stemming from children's love of their parents and a desire to please them. Parent teaching generally focuses more on helping the child to make safe decisions rather than moral ones. Toddlers cannot be expected to make correct choices if left alone in potentially dangerous situations because their internal sense of conscience is rudimentary and judgment is absent. Any room with electrical sockets, knobs for technical equipment, open windows, or hot food represents a risk. As toddlers gain language skills, they begin to echo the parent's firm "no," but they do not understand the full meaning of the term. By 24 months, many toddlers show beginning internalization by saying "no" to themselves and stopping the act; they may continue with the act as they talk to themselves, still saying "no."

For the 4- to 5-year-old, morality becomes more internally controlled. Instead of basing all decisions on the knowledge of the consequences of the act (e.g., "If I take a cookie, I will be sent to my room"), older children show an elementary understanding of what is right and wrong, fair or unfair. They begin to think ahead and are able to plan and control their urges, thus avoiding punishment. Four-year-olds can internalize some demands from their parents, and feelings of guilt can be elicited after some transgressions.

Peer Relationships

Toddlers may be fascinated by children their own age and can demonstrate curiosity by examining the other child closely, poking and probing. However, they generally do not engage with their peers in an interactive way. Parallel play is the norm. Preschoolers learn to interact with peers as their social world grows. Play becomes more interactive, cooperative, and shared, with use of more symbolic language. Imaginary play leads to "let's pretend," role-playing, and creation of imaginary friends. Fantasy and make-believe are very important during these years. Children need both structured and free play. Burdette and Whitaker (2005) reported a drop in free playtime by 25% between the years of 1981 and 1997 and suggested that free play should be resurrected by creating and maintaining playgrounds that allow children unstructured time to experience the fun of movement, creativity, and friendship.

Shared or cooperative play makes simple games of hide-and-seek and tag possible. Games with complicated rules can be frustrating to the preschooler, who prefers simple games with the option of making up the rules as the game proceeds. Cheating is common because the boundaries of acceptable play are not yet clear, and the earliest stages of moral behavior are only beginning to emerge.

Body Image

Toddlers are often highly concerned about body image. They realize that they are separate persons and begin to take notice of their own bodies. They may become fascinated with the different parts of the body and how they work. Bodily injury becomes a concern, and cuts and bruises elicit much discussion. Toward the end of the second year, children may notice the inner feelings of their bodies (e.g., the urge and tension to move the bowels, the release and relaxation resulting from going to the bathroom, the discomfort of hunger, and the pleasure of eating). These are abstract feelings that toddlers cannot put into words but can show with actions.

Preschoolers are equally curious about their bodies but are more capable of understanding and expressing themselves. They reexamine themselves frequently, and worries over a lost tooth or a skinned knee are common. Curiosity about their bodies and those of others generates a wealth of innocent questions that generally require only a simple answer. They learn that genital manipulation brings pleasure, and masturbation peaks around 3 to 4 years.

COGNITIVE DEVELOPMENT

Cognitively, toddler thinking is highly concrete. According to Piaget (see Table 4-1), 18- to 24-month-old children begin to use mental imagery and infer a cause when they can see only the effect. By the end of the second year, children enter the preoperational stage with preconceptual and intuitive thinking. Primitive conceptualization processes begin with the development of symbolic thinking. A block becomes a car; words become symbols for ideas. The 3-year-old continues to develop symbolic thinking, such as drawing and acting out elaborate play scenarios. However, children at this age generally are unable to take another's perspective but continue to view the world egocentrically. Attending to one characteristic at a time is another feature of preschool thinking. For example, the child will try to fit a jigsaw puzzle piece using either color or shape but not both.

Parents have difficulty understanding the thoughts of preschool children. On the surface, preoperational thinking has many characteristics that resemble adult thinking, and parents are often deceived into believing that children are able

TABLE 6-2 **Examples of Preschool Children's Thinking Using Piaget's Preoperational Stage**

Characteristic	Example
Egocentricism	"It's snowing, so I can go play in it."
Unable see another's viewpoint	If John is holding a doll with its face toward Ann, Ann thinks John can also see the doll's face.
Mental symbolization of the environment	"The wind is crying." "The (flushing) toilet is an angry animal."
Incomplete understanding of sequence of time	Knows names of time components: today, tomorrow, yesterday, minutes, days, weeks, etc., but uses them inconsistently: "I'm not going to take a nap yesterday." Yesterday means any time before now; tomorrow means any time in the future. Historical events are conceptualized in terms of the present: "Mommy, do you know George Washington?"
Developing sense of space: from experiencing space as a part of their activity to moving through it to understanding space in terms of detail and direction	Frequently used words: in, on, up, down, at, under.
Evolving ability to categorize or order objects and phenomena	Early preschooler: no understanding of concept of class or groups; undisturbed to see new Santa Claus on every corner. Cluster phenomena: when asked to sort a series of blocks, the child may cluster a small, medium, and large block as a "baby," "mommy," and "daddy" block. By 4-5years, child is able to consistently use 1 or 2 categories to arrange objects in some order (color, number, form, or size).
Developing ability to establish causality (realism, animism, artificialism)	*Realism:* Intellectual (dreams are actually real) and nominal (a horse can only be called a horse, not, for example, a stallion or filly). *Animism:* 2- to 3-year-olds think objects possess innate personlike qualities that cause results: "The chair made me fall down." *Artificialism:* 3- to 4-year-olds think things are caused by some controlling force that controls the world.
Transductive reasoning: from particular to particular	If the child does not like one particular vegetable, he or she will not like another particular fruit: "I can't eat my banana because my potatoes are burned."
Developing sense of conservation of quantity, weight, mass	Preschooler is usually unable to conceptualize that change in shape does not affect quantity, weight, or mass of an object. Generally, 50% of 5-year-olds have mastered conservation of quantity, and 50% of 6-year-olds have mastered conservation of weight or mass.
Rigidity	Generally, children in the preoperational stage are very rigid in their thinking.

to think as adults do. Preschool children, for example, are developing the use of language and the ability to symbolize concepts mentally. Some of their verbalizations appear quite precocious, as evidenced by the 3-year-old who stares out the window and then states, "Look, mommy, the trees are saying yes and no." Preschool children continue to be concrete and egocentric in their thinking, and their logic is the source of many communication problems between parents and children. Table 6-2 identifies major characteristic of the thinking of preschool children and gives examples of each.

Language development through the toddler and preschool years remains one of the most sensitive indicators of cognitive development, and assessment tools plot language ability as a way of measuring cognitive levels. Social development and adaptive skills are a major factor during this development. Differentiation of the self from others, with increasing sensitivity not only to the rules and norms for social interaction but also to the perception of the perspectives and feelings of others, requires ever increasing cognitive capability. Finally, quality of play can be used as an indicator of cognitive development. Through play children manipulate and learn to control their environment in safe yet stimulating ways.

DEVELOPMENTAL ASSESSMENT OF TODDLERS AND PRESCHOOLERS

Developmental assessment is an essential part of each health maintenance visit and can include both screening and diagnostic testing. Its goal is to monitor the growth and development of the child and determine at an early stage if problems exist. The process begins by building rapport with the parents, encouraging them to share developmental concerns, and listening to their comments with care and attention. Data are collected through parent interviews, use of screening tools, observation of the interactions between child and parents, physical examination, and laboratory or other diagnostic measures. If there are questions about the child's development, diagnostic assessments are needed for a more individualized approach to decide if a developmental problem exists and how to manage it.

SCREENING STRATEGIES FOR TODDLERS AND PRESCHOOLERS

Toddlers and preschoolers should be screened for physical and motor skills, communication and language, and social, emotional, and cognitive development. This screening can be done at well child visits and at visits for episodic illnesses. Validated screening tools provide a quick, inexpensive method of identifying potential problems. These tools are generally appropriate for all children, although culture and experience can affect outcomes and must be taken into consideration. In each area of screening, providers ask questions directly of the parent, make sure they have understood the parents' responses, and follow up with more probing questions as appropriate to clarify any concerns. Table 6-3 lists a variety of developmental screening tools, and the Resource Box in Chapter 5 provides information on how to obtain these tools. Tables 6-4, 6-5, 6-6, and 6-7 list questions that can be used to assess behavior and include the purpose or rationale for these questions.

Physical Development

Toddlers and preschool children should be screened for anthropomorphic measures and, after 3 years old, blood pressure. Vision, hearing, dentition, tuberculosis, lead, and cholesterol screening are recommended at certain ages or for those

---

TABLE 6-3   Screening Tools for Toddler and Preschoolers

Screening Tool	Appropriate Age; Screening Time	Characteristics
ASQ: Ages & Stages Questionnaire: a parent completed child-monitoring system	4-60 mo; 10-20 min	32 individual questions FM, GM, adaptive social and personal
ASQ: Ages & Stages Questionnaire: Social Emotional (ASQ:SE)	4-60 mo; 10-20 min	32 individual questions social and emotional
BDI: Battelle Developmental Inventory Screening test (BDI-2)	0-8 yr; 10-30 min; complete test 1-2 hr	100 standardized items, personal and social, adaptive, motor communication, cognitive
CDI: Child Development Inventory	15 mo-6 yr; 10-20 min	Questions: social, self-help, GM, FM, expressive language, language comprehension, letters, and numbers
DASE: Denver Articulation Screening Examination	2.5-7 yr; 5 min	30 repeated words
DENVER II: Denver Developmental Screening test	Birth-6 yr; 20-30 min	Standardized items in FM, GM, language, social
ESI-R: Early Screening Inventory Revised	3-6 yr; 15-20 min	Standardized items motor, language, and cognition; parent interview about self-help skills, social-emotional
HSQ: Home Screening Questionnaire	0-3 and 3-6 yr; 15-20 min	Parent questionnaire, 80 questions on environment
MAP: Miller Assessment for Preschoolers	2.9-5.8 yr; 20-30 min	Screens for preschool readiness for kindergarten: motor, language, sequencing, memory, visual-spatial perception
PEDS: Parent's Evaluation of Developmental Status	Birth-8 yr; 2 min	Parent interview with open-ended questions
PDQ-II: Prescreening Developmental Questionnaire	0-9 mo, 9-24 mo, 2-4 yr, 4-6 yr; 5-10 min	Parent questionnaire, FM, GM, social, language
TABS: Temperament and Atypical Behavior Scale	Birth-6 yr; 15-20 min	Parent interview, 55 questions on detached, hypersensitive and hyperactive, underreactive, dysregulated behaviors
SSP: Short Sensory Profile	Birth-adult; 15-20 min	Parental questions in 7 areas: tactile sensitive, taste-smell sensitivity, movement, underresponsive, auditory filtering, low energy and weakness, visual and auditory

FM, Fine motor; *GM,* gross motor; *min,* minute(s); *mo,* month(s); *yr,* year(s).

TABLE 6-4	Assessment of Physical Development and Motor Skills: Questions and Rationales

Question	Rationale for Question
How does your child usually feel?	Invites discussion of somatic issues and complaints.
Does your child appear to be developing in a way similar to other children of the same age?	Assesses parent perceptions of physical development; developmental milestones.
Describe your child's elimination patterns.	Provides parents' framework for systematically assessing child; can be especially helpful for children with a chronic illness.
Has any illness interfered with daily activities?	Assesses possible chronic medical problem and effects on development.
Tell me about your child's daily habits: toilet training, sleeping, eating.	Assesses parent understanding of readiness, child's cues, changing behaviors and current status.
How does your child get from place to place?	Assesses gross motor skills (e.g., walks, climbs, runs, pedals tricycle).
How does your child feed him or herself? (e.g., cup, bottle, utensils)	Assesses fine motor skills.
Tell me about your child's play activities.	Assesses gross and fine motor skills.

TABLE 6-5	Assessment of Communication and Speech Development: Questions and Rationales

Question	Rationale for Question
How does your child communicate needs and desires?	Assesses verbal and nonverbal communication strategies, vocabulary, and expressive language.
What do you think your child understands?	Evaluates cognitive level and receptive language.
How does your child respond to simple commands? To 2- or 3-step commands?	Evaluates receptive language; evaluates short-term memory and auditory sequencing.
Does your child use plurals, pronouns, phrases, and sentences?	Indicates increased understanding of more complex structures.
How well can you understand your child's speech? How well can others?	Indicates increased articulation ability.

children at risk (see Appendix D for American Academy of Pediatrics [AAP] recommendations for health supervision visits).

Motor Skills Development

Toddlers and preschoolers continue to develop and refine their motor skills, driven by curiosity, desire for independence, and endless energy. Gross and fine motor skills are best assessed using standardized screening tools, such as the Ages & Stages Questionnaire or parents' evaluation of developmental status.

Fine motor development is evaluated by assessing finger, hand, and oral movements. Gross motor skills are evaluated by assessing the child's ability to crawl, sit, walk, run, hop, skip, and climb. The quality of the child's movements during these activities is important to note as well.

Communication and Language Development

Communication is a vital part of being a happy, functioning human being, and assessment of language is important during early childhood. Much of the essential information can be obtained from a careful history of the child's abilities and pattern of learning (e.g., when did they first articulate words?). A physical examination is important to determine if physical structures necessary for speech are intact (e.g., a cleft uvula may indicate an occult cleft palate that could interfere with the child's ability to shape words). Finally, diagnostic testing, using tools such as the Early Language Milestones (ELM) test or the Denver Articulation Screening Exam (DASE) may be necessary to refine the assessment (Table 6-8). Listening to children and talking with their parents is essential, but the provider should also remember that parents may not be fully sensitive to speech problems because they are accustomed to hearing the child's current speech.

Language screening is divided into expressive and receptive language skills (see Table 5-2). Because language and cognitive skills are intricately interwoven, most intelligence tests have language sections that can be useful in assessing the total child. Expressive language screening places emphasis on articulation and vocabulary. Receptive language looks at comprehension, repetition, and follow-up of language heard (e.g., child's ability to follow directions).

Social and Emotional Development

Assessment of psychosocial and emotional development addresses children's roles in the family, success in making friends and working with peers, self-esteem, and feelings of contentment and security. The social emotional questionnaire section of the Ages & Stages Questionnaire can be used to assess these behaviors.

Cognitive Development

After 2 years old, as thinking moves into the preconceptual stages, cognitive development is increasingly expressed through symbol systems and language. Toddlers begin to enjoy make-believe; preschoolers love stories and can become masters at games of pretend and fantasy.

TABLE 6-6   **Assessment of Psychosocial and Emotional Development: Questions and Rationales**

Question	Rationale for Question
How able is your child to feed, dress, and take care of his or her own toileting?	Assesses adaptive skills, comfort with own abilities.
How does your child behave within the family and with other family members?	Assesses child's development of roles with the family system; attachment should be evident.
How do you guide or discipline your child without always saying "no?"	Evaluates adaptability, creativity, repertoire of parent's skills in response to child's behaviors.
How does your child respond when you set limits?	Assesses child's understanding of limits of appropriate behavior, social rules, and self-control.
How does your child react to strangers or new situations?	Evaluates child's ability to deal with increasingly complex social situations.
Tell me about any tantrums your child has had. What causes them? How does he or she behave?	Evaluates responses to stress, development of independence, and social control.
What does your child do for play?	Indicates social and emotional well-being.
How does your child behave around other children?	Considers social development with peers and development of appropriate play.
What is your child's best friend's name? Does he or she have shared activities with peers?	Indicates child is developing social circle and increasing opportunities for practicing new social skills.
Does your child seem to understand the feelings of others?	Assesses empathy.
Is your child afraid of anything in particular? How do you handle that fear?	Evaluates parents' responses to child's emotional stresses and understanding of child's view and feelings.
Does your child have imaginary friends? Does she or he have a fantasy play time?	Allows child to explore emotions and developing roles in a safe way.

TABLE 6-7   **Assessment of Cognitive Development: Questions and Rationales**

Questions Asked of 1- to 3-Year-Olds	Rationale for Questions
Tell me about a typical day. What sorts of things does your child do? Who does she or he play with? (ask of parent)	Assesses complexity of manipulation of objects, parallel and cooperative play, role-playing.
What is your name? Are you a boy or girl? How old are you? (ask of child)	Three-year-olds should know beginning facts.
Can your child follow simple instructions? (ask of parent)	Assesses ability to retain and process instructions and respond to input.
Does your child speak clearly? Can he or she understand what you say to them?	Assesses progress in decoding, encoding, and using a language system effectively.
How does your child behave in the family and with other children?	Indicates understanding of social systems and norms.

Questions Asked of 4- to 5-Year-Olds	Rationale for Questions
Ask child general information questions (e.g., colors, numbering, objects).	Assesses general fund of knowledge.
Ask child what makes the sun come up.	Illustrates child's belief about causality.
Ask child about concepts of time.	Assesses understanding of a relatively sophisticated concept.
Ask child about spontaneous play (e.g., with puppets or dolls), imaginative use of play materials (e.g., clay, crayons, other toys).	Assesses imagination and magical thinking.
Ask child to draw a person.	50% of 4-year-olds draw a 3-part person; by 5 years old, child can draw an 8-part person.
How does the child behave in preschool? (ask of parent)	Assesses language, social, and play development in relation to peers in a setting where expectations differ from those at home.

TABLE 6-8 **Speech and Language Evaluation Tools**

Evaluation Tool	Age Assessed and Test Characteristics	Source
The Capute Scales: Cognitive Adaptive test and Clinical Linguistic and Auditory Milestone test (CAT/CLAMS)	0-36 mo Interview and some observation Tests language and problem-solving skills to help clearly identify between the two	Paul H Brookes Publishing *www.pbrookes.com*
Clinical Evaluation of Language Fundamentals–Preschool (CELF-P)	3-6 yr Assesses receptive and expressive language	Harcourt Assessment The Psychological Corporation (Publisher) *www.psychcorp.com*
Clinical Evaluation of Language Fundamentals–School Age (CELF-3)	6-21 yr Assesses receptive and expressive language	Harcourt Assessment The Psychological Corporation (Publisher) *www.psychcorp.com*
Denver Articulation Screening Examination (DASE)	2.5-7 yr Screens articulation only (not a complete assessment)	Denver Developmental Materials *www.denverii.com/DASE.html*
Fluharty Preschool Speech and Language Screening test	3-6.11 yr Direct testing Vocabulary, articulation, comprehension, repetition (expressive)	Pearson Assessments *www.ags.pearsonassessments.com*
Early Language Milestone Scale (ELM Scale-2)	0-36 mo Tests visual and auditory receptive, auditory expressive History, testing, observation 3-5 min	Pro-Ed *www.proedinc.com*
Goldman-Fristoe Test of Articulation	2-22 yr Assesses articulation skills	Pearson Assessments *www.ags.pearsonassessments.com*
Peabody Picture Vocabulary test	2.5-40 yr Screens for receptive vocabulary	Pearson Assessments *www.ags.pearsonassessments.com*
REEL: Receptive and Expressive Emergent Language	0-36 mo Interview or direct observation of expressive and receptive language	Pearson Assessments *www.ags.pearsonassessments.com*

mo, Month(s); *yr*, year(s).

DIAGNOSTIC ASSESSMENT STRATEGIES FOR TODDLERS AND PRESCHOOLERS

Once a child has been identified through screening as having a possible problem, more definitive diagnostic testing or referral to an appropriate specialist is necessary. Some diagnostic assessment tools commonly used in this age group are listed in the Resource Box in Chapter 5.

■ ANTICIPATORY GUIDANCE FOR TODDLERS AND PRESCHOOLERS

Anticipatory guidance for toddlers and preschoolers is directed at helping parents and children transition from a highly dependent relationship to one in which the child has established a sense of autonomy with an evolving understanding of the self as a separate, creative, and powerful being. In the process, parents learn new skills of communicating and interacting with their children. Although the toddler and preschool years can be frustrating at times, the ultimate outcome of good communication and relationships that support the potential of both

child and parent is worth the effort. Providers should offer anticipatory guidance in all of the following areas of growth and development.

REGULATION AND SLEEP-WAKE PATTERNS

- Discuss the need to assist toddlers and preschoolers to transition from one state to another. Consistent sleep and naptime schedules are essential. Use of a comfort object (e.g., teddy bear) and bedtime rituals can help.
- Explain that children's ability to process information and control themselves at this age can be overwhelmed if they have too much stimulation.
- Explain that some children may have sensory integration problems that require even more structuring and modulation of their environment.
- Discuss how to help children identify and name their feelings. This ability will help them to more successfully organize and integrate the sensations they are experiencing and respond appropriately (Brazelton & Sparrow, 2001).

- Encourage parents to provide opportunities for children to have some control and choice in daily activities (e.g., can select the story to be read at bedtime), while maintaining important rituals.
- Discuss sleep problems that may appear at this time, including sleep resistance, bruxism, nightmares, and somnambulism (see Chapter 15).
- Encourage parents to offer naps and opportunities for rest but not to force them on children. It is the parents' job to make sure the child has ample time to rest.

STRENGTH AND MOTOR COORDINATION

- Discuss the importance of play as a way for toddlers and preschoolers to practice their developing physical, social, and emotional skills and to maintain a healthy lifestyle and weight.
- Encourage parents to provide their children with a variety of play activities that use both fine and gross motor skills, such as the following:
  - Take children to a park to run, throw balls, play on the swing set, and roll on the grass.
  - Provide children with pencils, crayons, paper, paints, utensils, blocks, and age-appropriate building toys.
- Explain how parents can incorporate practice with motor skills as part of daily routines (e.g., have child help pour the milk, hold the cup, or squeeze the toothpaste; encourage child to do own buttons, snaps, and zippers).
- Emphasize the need for constant adult supervision of children's activities.
- Discuss how parents can make the environment safer for their child: securing doors and windows; removing toxic substances and dangerous objects; providing toys that are developmentally appropriate and safely constructed.
- Reinforce teaching about car seat use and explain the need for larger car seats and booster seats as the child grows.

FEEDING AND SELF-CARE

- Provide parents with information about healthy foods and nutritional needs of their child (see Chapter 11). Three meals and two nutritious snacks per day are encouraged, if possible.
- Discuss the parents' responsibility to provide children with healthy foods and to allow children to make choices from healthy food options. Young children may go on "food jags," refusing some foods or requesting the same food day after day. Parents need to make sure the food eaten is nutritious.
- Explain how changes in toddlers' eating habits are caused by developmental changes (e.g., child has a decrease in appetite, is easily distracted, demonstrates more curiosity about what is going on around him or her than in eating, is more interested in using gross motor skills than in sitting still).
- Explain nonnutritive value of food and eating (e.g., finger foods stimulate fine motor and cognitive development, in addition to child's sense of control and independence; eating together as a family can strengthen relationships and develop social skills).

- Encourage self-feeding to help child gain new skills.
- Encourage parents to structure family meal times that are pleasant and interactive; this may mean offering the toddler foods that can be eaten in short periods of sitting. Avoid making meals a power struggle.
- Discuss weaning (if not already done by 12 months).
- Explain the importance of the child gaining mastery of self-care (e.g., toileting, bathing, dressing, eating) and the valuable role the parent plays as teacher in the process. Assist parents to cope with the frustration or tensions generated by toddlers and preschoolers wanting to "do it myself."

COMMUNICATION AND LANGUAGE

Children learn and refine communication and language skills best through their interactions with others. When parents and caregivers listen to them, talk interactively with them, and read to them, the child's language blossoms (Roberts et al, 2005). Encourage parents to stimulate their child's language skills by doing the following:

- Reading to children daily, using short, simple stories or picture books (see information on Reach Out and Read [ROAR] program in Resource Box, Chapter 5)
- Modeling appropriate language
- Talking to their child, explaining in clear, simple language what is happening around the child; this helps increase vocabulary and the child's understanding of the world
- Listening with care and responding actively to the child's verbalizations
- Providing the child with opportunities to interact verbally with other children and adults

Providers can also suggest the following strategies to parents to enhance their child's language development:

- No television viewing for children under 2 years old and limit television viewing and videos to 1 to 2 hours or less of appropriate programs per day for older children. Remove televisions from children's bedrooms (AAP, 2001; Gentile et al, 2004; NAPNAP, 2006).
- Explain that children need constant reinforcement of their speech and language efforts, but that nonverbal language, especially touch, continues to be crucial.
- Give parents an opportunity to explain their expectations for their child; discourage parental pressure on child to perform (e.g., use of flash cards, requirement that child articulate sounds correctly) but point out that daily activities provide a wealth of opportunities to practice language skills.
- Reassure parents that language errors of young children usually disappear as the child grows.
- Instruct parents that children learn receptive language first, then expressive, and that children may not fully understand the meaning, especially connotative meaning, of what they are hearing or saying (e.g., a 4-year-old may innocently ask a stranger about their private body parts). Parents should explain clearly, simply, and unemotionally which words are appropriate and in which settings.

SOCIAL AND EMOTIONAL GROWTH

The emotional development of toddlers is an area in which parents may need a great deal of anticipatory guidance and support. The balance between dependence and independence is constantly in flux for toddlers and their parents, and conflict can develop as a result of inconsistent or extreme behavior. Toddlers and preschoolers need to master multiple social tasks during these years. They need to learn how to identify, control, and manage their feelings and emotions around anger, joy, love, and frustration. They learn about making and keeping friends, sharing, cooperative play, and living socially within a family. They learn to handle separation from parents, home, and neighborhood (Green & Palfrey, 2002). In helping families with this process, providers should do the following:

- Reemphasize the role of parents in guiding their child's social and emotional growth. Parents must actively engage with their children, showing interest in their activities and giving them instruction on appropriate behavior (see Table 5-3).
- Encourage parents to give their children opportunities to expand social skills and form important attachments outside the immediate family by doing the following:
  ○ Provide toys that children can use creatively.
  ○ Allow children to explore, guiding them to activities that are fun.
  ○ Allow children to make choices when possible; do not give children a "choice" when there really is none (e.g., "Do you want to go to bed?").
  ○ Discuss differences among people openly and positively.
  ○ Help children identify, name, and express feelings, both positive and negative.
  ○ Teach children to manage anger and resolve conflicts without violence.
  ○ Discuss television programs and movies to help children distinguish fantasy from reality.
  ○ Take children on trips to places of interest in the community.
  ○ Arrange play times with other children; encourage cooperative play (e.g., tag, hide-and-seek).
  ○ Reinforce positive child behavior ("catch the child being good").
  ○ Make the limits of what is expected of children clear and achievable; try for consistency.
- Differentiate discipline and teaching from punishment.
- Discuss parenting and discipline (see Chapters 4 and 17).
- Clarify each parent's expectations of child's behavior.
- Discuss how parents plan to resolve differences in expectations.
- Provide information to parents related to child development and what parents can expect their child to be able to do.
- Recommend parenting classes that provide information on developmental milestones, anticipated changes, and management strategies as children grow.
- Encourage parents to show affection in the family.
- Explain to parents that myths or fables can be important ways of teaching children abstract concepts, such as love, sharing, and giving.
- Instruct parents on the need to provide a feeling of safety and security for children. Parents can do the following:
  ○ Support use of comfort or transitional objects to allay fears (e.g., blanket).
  ○ Consider use of a night light.
  ○ Provide reassurance if nightmares or fears occur and respond to child's fears.
  ○ Explain about "good" and "bad" touches to private parts.
  ○ Reinforce that the child can always come to the parent for comfort.

COGNITIVE AND ENVIRONMENTAL STIMULATION

- Explain to parents that toddlers and preschoolers are concrete and preoperational in their thinking. As a result, parents need to be ready to explain things over and over patiently, without expecting the child to understand the adult's interpretation clearly. Also, children may use words to convey thoughts and feelings, but many responses are repetitive, and trial-and-error problem solving is usually crude. They frequently attend to only one aspect of a problem, giving partial answers.
- Emphasize that parents should avoid putting their own meaning on the child's behavior or statements. For example, the child's statement, "What if you just bought a new house, and I was allergic to something in the house? I guess you'd have to get rid of me," should not be interpreted to mean the parents have somehow failed to show the child how much they love him or her. Rather the child can be exploring the concepts of place, ownership, belonging, size, or importance. In the child's mind, a house is much bigger than he or she is and may be more important. An appropriate response from the parent might be, "No, we'd probably have to get a new house or take out whatever you are allergic to. Even if we just bought it, you are more important than any house, and we wouldn't want to lose you."
- Reassure parents that "Why?" will not continue to be the child's most frequent question. Toddlers and preschoolers are actively exploring meaning in their world and have learned that asking "Why?" brings them more information—and attention. As parents answer them, children begin to show threads of symbolic and more abstract thought.

▩ COMMON DEVELOPMENTAL ISSUES FOR TODDLERS AND PRESCHOOLERS

FEARS

As the 2- to 3-year-old's world expands and the ability to fantasize develops, fears can appear about things that might happen. "Magical thinking," characteristic of preschoolers, can accentuate these fears. Early fears include fear of separation, strangers, water, loud noises, crowds, the dark, and animals. Four- to 5-year-olds add wild animals, masks, and aggressive actions to the list. Fears may be expressed in a variety of ways: flight, requests for help, sudden shyness, irritability, hyperactivity, frustration, or aggressive actions (Dixon & Stein, 2006). By 4 years old, children can identify nightmares as "not real," although they may still be afraid. Adults should not dismiss the fears as trivial but offer reassurance with words and their presence; this helps children work through the anxiety and tension they feel. Preschool children may still express fear of the dark or of harm to their bodies, but if the fears do not decrease with time, the child and family need referral for counseling.

TEMPER TANTRUMS

Temper tantrums are episodes in which the child is frustrated and angry and loses control of his or her feelings. The tantrum may be as mild as whining and pouting, or it may be a full-blown display of crying, yelling, flinging oneself on the floor, kicking, and screaming. Some children can hold their breath until they turn cyanotic and/or pass out (Dixon & Stein, 2006).

Temper tantrums are common, with as many as 50% to 80% of children experiencing them; they usually peak at about 18 to 28 months. Tantrums stem from the child's striving for power and control and the sudden loss of both. There are so many activities that toddlers want and struggle to do but are not developmentally ready to perform. Being tired or hungry exacerbates the frustration children can feel when their wishes are thwarted.

Ultimately, children will learn how to regulate the self, to identify a feeling and manage the actions appropriate to that feeling, and will thus "outgrow" the temper tantrums of toddlers. Management involves helping children master self-regulation and learn that there are better ways to handle frustration; this is a process that requires parents to engage in many of the interactions discussed earlier in this chapter (see Anticipatory Guidance for Toddlers and Preschoolers). Management also requires that parents deal with the immediate event of the tantrum itself. Some parents are aghast that their child would show such a violent display of emotions; others may express being frightened. Parents' responses usually depend on their comfort level. Some parents go to the child and hold, comfort, and distract him or her; some remove the child from the stimulation of the moment, putting him or her in "timeout"; and some physically restrain the child in a "bear hug" until the crying and thrashing-about behavior subsides. Generally, the most effective measures are thought to be the following:

- Ignore the child's behavior (give no physical or eye contact).
- Ensure that the child is safe and will not be injured.

Health care providers can prepare parents for the possibility of temper tantrums by discussing them at the 12-month visit. The provider should describe the developmental stages the child will be progressing through (autonomy, independence, and preoperational thinking) and explain how those stages can contribute to high levels of frustration for the child. When parents understand the dynamics of tantrums, they can minimize the likelihood that they will occur. Parents can do this by not putting children in positions that they cannot easily handle, providing support for the child or redirecting the child early in the emotional cycle if frustration appears to be building, and making sure that external factors (e.g., hunger,

sleepiness) are managed well. Providers should also give parents an opportunity to discuss how they would like to handle the tantrum should it come. Parents should be counseled to avoid hitting or spanking the child because it only teaches the child that hitting is permitted if you are an adult, and, when emotions are high, hitting can quickly escalate to abuse.

DISCIPLINE

Limit setting and discipline are methods of helping a child learn rules, regulations, guidelines, and goals that make the world a more predictable place and are best taught by someone who loves the child (see Chapter 4). Discipline should encompass love, self-esteem, guilt, praise, and discomfort. Parents teach the child how to live within their family, what activities are expected, limits, and consequences. The child is helped to learn respect for authority, even if they disagree. Discipline protects and keeps the child safe from environmental dangers.

Discipline as guidance begins at birth when babies begin learning what brings smiles, warmth, and food. By toddlerhood the parents must control the child's environment while offering limited challenges (e.g., a verbal "no" and physical removal). Reasonable consistency helps. Parents need to understand their limits and tolerances in how they guide their toddler. Methods can include verbal "no," physical removal, isolation, withdrawal of privileges, and natural consequences. Modeling good behavior, praising, and rewarding can reinforce "correct" behavior. Cause and effect need to be short and timely since toddlers may not remember what they did after minutes or hours.

CHILD CARE AND PRESCHOOLS

Many parents return to work during the first year of their child's life and must make arrangements for child care. In 2002 about 72% of mothers with children 1 year old and older were in the work force; 55% of mothers of infants were working outside the home (Downs, 2003). By 2002, approximately 63% of children under 5 years old were in some kind of regular child care arrangement (Overturf Johnson, 2005). Parents need to be able to evaluate child care options for their children and feel secure that their children are in safe, appropriate situations. Table 18-9 outlines important criteria for parents to consider when making choices about day-care placement.

Entering a setting outside the home that has a teacher, curriculum, and learning expectations can be a stressful experience. Suddenly, parents find their child compared with 20 other children. A child with developmental delays (e.g., speech, motor, physical) may be singled out as different, not fitting in, or a behavior problem. Preschool and kindergarten were originally intended to help the child learn separation, sharing, listening, paying attention, and some simple social skills. Curriculum planning has changed over the years. Kindergarten children are often expected to show preacademic skills such as writing, counting, and letter and word recognition in addition to the preschool social skills of paying attention and sitting still.

School readiness criteria are outlined in Table 7-6. Parents can make more appropriate decisions about their child's ability to handle the demands of a structured preschool setting by considering school readiness factors, in addition to the following characteristics of their child:

- Social skills (e.g., ability to separate from parent for several hours)
- Language skills, both expressive and receptive
- Physical size of the child
- Energy level of child (e.g., able to participate actively)
- Neurologic maturation required for fine and gross motor activities (e.g., writing, cutting, coloring, climbing, running, walking)
- Neurologic maturation of sensory and cognitive function (e.g., visuospatial perception, tactile maturation, auditory processing, attending skills, memory)

TOILETING

Toileting skills and training are a major milestone for a child and the parents. It is a complex developmental skill that many children master effortlessly, but some children and families need guidance and support along the way (see Chapter 13).

SAFETY

As children grow and develop, their world expands and exposes them to ever-increasing dangers. Safety should be a topic of every well-child visit, and the discussion should focus on the developmental age of the child. Toddlers are not to be trusted, even for a moment, but it is easier to monitor their environment because it is generally restricted to the house, the yard, or the parent's side. For preschoolers the world is bigger and more dangerous and includes the house, the yard, the neighborhood, the preschool, and traveling (e.g., car, bike, scooters). See Chapter 10 for a discussion of causes and management of unintentional injuries.

◼ RED FLAGS FOR TODDLERS AND PRESCHOOLERS

Although a wide range of normal development may be seen when assessing children, the provider needs to be alert to developmental red flags, signs of delayed or abnormal development. In addition to obvious abnormalities, minor problems that are left untreated can develop into major concerns; minor signs and symptoms that persist can indicate a more serious underlying problem, or a major problem can occur as a one-time event (e.g., child who sets a fire). Some children and families are at high risk and need careful monitoring and guidance to detect problems at an early stage or to prevent their occurrence (e.g., very early premature infants, families with history of violence, families with chronic medical or mental health problems, some single-parent families). The warning signs, or red flags, can be found in Table 6-9. Children who demonstrate these behaviors should be referred. Immediate referral is required for children who stop eating, demonstrate cruelty to animals or other people, are self-harmful, start fires, or talk of harming themselves, their peers, or others.

PHYSICAL DISORDERS

Children should be monitored for missing or delayed physical growth milestones. Most growth or milestone charts give a range that is normal. When the child falls outside that limit, there should be investigation, screening, and referral, if appropriate. When children are following a normal progression for weight and begin to level off or fall below that range, this should not be ignored. If a child begins to have symptoms—stops eating, complains of tiredness, is not as active as usual, or the parents state that the child has regressed—it is time to investigate.

COGNITIVE DISORDERS

Mental and cognitive delays are more difficult to recognize and categorize without the help of a screening tool or more in-depth assessment. These tools rank children on the basis of a standardized score or against standardized criteria (e.g., word definition). Children with scores below 85 on intelligence scales, for example, predictably have more difficulty in school. Significant discrepancies between test scores taken over time also suggest problems. The causes of delay must be carefully assessed as well because some children may have a neurologic limitation, whereas others may be delayed as a result of material or environmental deprivation. Identifying the causes is necessary to plan effective interventions. In any case, when delays are suspected, prompt referral to development centers for more detailed assessment is essential.

LANGUAGE DISORDERS

Language delays or disorders are problems in learning the systems of communication and, when present, can affect other areas of development, especially cognitive, social, and emotional development. Because language development is the best indicator of cognitive development, language delays can lead to serious issues needing developmental and educational intervention.

Children with language delays can experience problems in receptive or expressive language, or both. They can start saying words late, talk very little as toddlers, and have prolonged stages of normal stuttering, distortion, and substitution.

Language delays are caused by cognitive, familial, environmental, or cultural factors. Language delays or disorders may occur if the child does not hear, is not immersed in a language-rich environment, or has a psychological disorder, such as severe deprivation or autism. Speech disorders (problems producing sounds) are often associated with physical problems (e.g., cleft lip, cleft palate, cerebral palsy, hearing impairments), or they can be idiopathic.

Language evaluation must involve assessment of the total child, including physical, cognitive, social, emotional, and perceptual characteristics. Both expressive and receptive language must be evaluated.

TABLE 6-9   Red Flags of Development: Toddlers and Preschoolers

Age	Growth, Rhythmicity, Sleep, and Temperament	Psychosocial and Emotional Skills	Cognitive and Visual Abilities	Gross Motor, Language and Hearing	Fine Motor, Feeding, and Self-Care	Strength, and Coordination
15mo	No nighttime ritual Difficulty with transitions Parents express concern about temperament or control issues	Problems with attachment to caregiver	Lack of object permanence	Lack of consonant production Does not imitate words No gestures or pointing	No self-feeding	No attempts at walking
18mo	Poor sleep schedule Problems with control and behavior	Does not pull person to show something	Primary play: mouthing of toys No finger exploration of objects Lack of imitation	Unable to follow simple directions (e.g., "no," "jump")	Does not try to scribble spontaneously Unable to use spoon	Not yet walking or frequently falls when walking
24mo (2yr)	Less than 4 times birth weight or falling off growth curve Poor sleep schedule Awakens at night; unable to put self back to sleep	Absent symbolic play No evidence of parallel play Displays destructive behaviors Always clings to mother		Use of noncommunicative speech (echolalia, rote phrases) Unable to identify 5 pictures Unable to name body parts No jargon History of greater than 10 episodes of otitis media	Unable to stack 4 to 5 blocks Still eating puréed foods Unable to imitate scribbles on paper Unable to dump pellet from bottle	Unable to walk downstairs holding a rail Persistent waddle walk Persistent toe walking
30mo	Resistance to regular bedtime Beginning behavior issues	Problems with biting, hitting playmates, parents	Does not try to get toy with stick	No two-word sentences Unable to name some body parts	Unable to feed self Unable to build a tower of 6 blocks Unable to imitate circle shape Unable to imitate vertical stroke	Unable to jump in place Unable to kick ball on request
36mo (3yr)	Problems with toilet training Unable to calm self	Not able to dress self Does not understand taking turns		Unable to give full name Unable to match two colors Does not use plurals Does not know 2 to 3 prepositions Unable to tell a story Unclear consonants Unintelligible speech Unable to construct a sentence	Unable to build a tower of 10 blocks Holds crayon with fist Unable to draw circle	Unable to balance on one foot for 1 sec Toeing in causes tripping with running

Continued

TABLE 6-9 Red Flags of Development: Toddlers and Preschoolers—Cont'd

Age	Growth, Rhythmicity, Sleep, and Temperament	Psychosocial and Emotional Skills	Cognitive and Visual Abilities	Language and Hearing	Fine Motor, Feeding, and Self-Care	Gross Motor, Strength, and Coordination
48 mo (4 yr)	Lack of bedtime ritual Behavior concerns: withdrawn or acting out Stool holding Problems with toilet training	Unable to play games, follow rules Unable to follow limits or rules at home (e.g., put toys away) Cruelty to animals, friends Interest in fires, fire starting Persistent fears or severe shyness Inability to separate from mother	Unable to count 3 objects Unable to recall 4 numbers Unable to identify what to do in danger, fire, with a stranger Consistently poor judgment	Difficulty understanding language Problems understanding prepositions Limited vocabulary Unclear speech	Lack of self-care skills—dressing, feeding, Unable to button clothes Unable to copy square	Unable to balance on one foot for 4 sec Unable to alternate steps when climbing stairs
60 mo (5 yr)	Continued sleep problems Concerns with night terrors Hair pulling— scalp or eyelashes	Difficulty making and keeping friends; no friends Difficulty understanding sharing, school rules, organization of daily activities Cruelty to animals, friends Interest in fires, fire starting Bullying or being bullied Prolonged fighting, hitting, hurting Withdrawal, sadness, extreme rituals	Unable to count to 10 Unable to identify colors Difficulty following 3-step command	Speech pattern not 100% understandable Cannot identify a penny, nickel, or dime Abnormal rate or rhythm of speech	Unable to copy triangle Unable to draw a person with a body	Difficulty hopping, jumping

mo, Month(s); *yr,* year(s); *sec,* second(s).

The inability to use the symbols of language may be characterized by the following:
- Improper use of words and their meanings
- Inappropriate grammatical patterns
- Improper use of speech sounds

Speech disorders involve problems producing correct speech sounds and may be characterized by difficulty in the following:
- Producing speech sounds (articulation)
- Maintaining speech rhythm (fluent speech)
- Controlling vocal production (voice)

Management of children with language disorders requires a clear understanding of the nature of the problem. Referral to a specialist (e.g., pediatric speech pathologist) to make that determination is often the first step. Deficits identified in Table 6-9 are cause for referral for additional testing. Other criteria that warrant referral include the following:
- There is excessive, indiscriminate, irrelevant verbalizing after 18 months old.
- The child is not talking by 2 years old.
- There is consistent and frequent omission of initial consonants, which are generally mastered by early in the second year; the child uses mostly vowel sounds after 1 year.
- Sentence structure is consistently faulty after 5 years old.
- There are many substitutions of easy sounds for difficult ones after 5 years old.
- Word endings are consistently dropped after 5 years old.
- There are unusual confusions, reversals, or telescoping in connected speech.
- There is a loss of previously acquired language skills.
- The child stops talking.
- The child reacts to his or her own speech with embarrassment or withdrawal.
- The child's voice is monotone, extremely loud, largely inaudible, or of poor quality.
- Pitch is not appropriate to the child's age and gender.
- Hypernasality or lack of nasal resonance occurs.

▇ SUMMARY

During the toddler and preschool years, children learn the social skills of living with others. With healthy development, they become able to express temperament, demonstrate behavioral control, manage stress, seek support, articulate feelings, and foster family relationships. This growth begins with the self-centered, self-preoccupied toddler and evolves to the more mature, albeit still self-centered, preschool child. The preschooler is more aware of the responsibilities of being part of the family and group and is able to share and contribute. Preschoolers know right from wrong and are beginning to control emotional states, delay gratification, demonstrate patience, manage frustration, separations, fears, anxieties, and anger. The "terrible twos" are followed by the "terrific threes," and the "fierce fours" are followed by the "fantastic fives." By the end of the preschool years conflict and worries decrease, and family life is relatively calm. The process is facilitated by responsive parents who provide guidance, give their children a wide

variety of experiences, set limits, and ensure safety. Deviations, delays, and voids need to be assessed, monitored, and managed. Participating in the process of his or her child's growth and development can be one of a parent's many treasures. Having the support of a caring provider can make it easier and smoother.

☑ DISCUSSION FORUM

1. A parent expresses concern that her 3-year-old is stuttering. Further questioning reveals the child repeats entire words, not syllables, and word repetitions are more common at the start of a sentence or thought. The physical examination is normal, and you detect no speech deficits. What management will you provide?
2. Create a plan for anticipatory guidance related to diet and discipline for a 15-month-old, a 24-month-old, a 3-year-old, and a 4-year-old. What developmental influences have the greatest effect on these areas during these ages?
3. A mother of an 18-month-old child tells you that she is very concerned about her son's lack of interest in playing with others. She says he plays side by side with other children without any problems, but becomes quite upset if other children use the toys he is playing with. The mother says she encourages him to share, but he does not always respond to her encouragement. Physical examination reveals a healthy child with no developmental deficits in fine motor, gross motor, or language. What techniques might be used to evaluate peer relationships for a child this age? How will you respond to the parent?
4. Compare and contrast the developmental assessment of a 13-month-old, a 30-month-old, a 3-year-old, and a 4-year-old. Which issues are unique to each of these ages?
5. Develop a management and educational plan for the management of toddler temper tantrums. How might these strategies differ for an older preschooler?
6. Identify resources in your community that can be used for the evaluation and management of toddlers and preschoolers with the developmental red flags identified in this chapter.

REFERENCES

American Academy of Pediatrics (AAP), Committee on Public Education: Children, adolescents, and television, *Pediatrics* 107(2):423-426, 2001.

Brazelton TB, Sparrow JD: *Touchpoints three to six, your child's emotional and behavioral development,* Cambridge, MA, 2001, Perseus Publishing.

Burdette HL, Whitaker RC: Resurrecting free play in young children: looking beyond fitness and fatness to attention, affiliation and affect, *Arch Pediatr Adolesc Med* 159:46-50, 2005.

Cornish AM et al: Postnatal depression and infant cognitive and motor development in the second postnatal year: the impact of depression chronicity and infant gender, *Infant Behav Dev* 28:407-417, 2005.

Dixon S, Stein M: *Encounters with children: pediatric behavior and development,* ed 4, St Louis, 2006, Mosby.

Downs B: *Fertility of American women: June 2002, current population characteristics,* Washington DC, 2003, US Census Bureau.

Feldman HM: Evaluation and management of language and speech disorder in preschool children, *Pediatr Rev* 26:131-140, 2005.

Gentile DA et al: Well-child visits in the video age: pediatricians and the American Academy of Pediatrics' guidelines for children's media use, *Pediatrics* 114(5):1235-1241, 2004.

Green M, Palfrey JS, editors: *Bright Futures: guidelines for health supervision of infants, children and adolescents,* ed 2, Rockville, MD, 2002, National Center for Education in Maternal and Child Health.

McNeill, D: The development of language. In Mussen PH, editor: *Carmichael's manual of child psychology,* ed 3, New York, 1970, John Wiley & Sons.

National Association of Pediatric Nurse Practitioners (NAPNAP): *Identifying and preventing overweight in childhood: clinical practice guideline,* Cherry Hill, NJ, 2006, NAPNAP.

Overturf Johnson J: *Who's minding the kids? Child care arrangements, Winter 2002, current population reports,* Washington DC, 2005, US Census Bureau.

Pascoe JM, Stolfi A, Ormond MB: Correlates of mothers' persistent depressive symptoms: a national study, *J Pediatr Health Care* 20:261-269, 2006.

Roberts J, Jurgens, J, Burchinal M: The role of home literacy practices in preschool children's language and emergent literacy skills, *J Speech Lang Hear Res* 48(2):345-359, 2005.

Trifiletti LB et al: Tipping the scales: obese children and child safety seats, *Pediatrics* 117:1197-1202, 2006.

Developmental Management of School-Age Children

Bonnie Gance-Cleveland and Yvonne Yousey

School-age children are busy, active, curious, and creative. With guidance and encouragement, they eagerly apply the skills they learned as toddlers and preschoolers as they move into more structured school environments, home schooling, or community settings. Their physical abilities advance, and they may join organized sports activities and engage in casual play with friends or siblings. Cognitively and emotionally, school-age children face daunting challenges. They must master the intellectual skills of reading, writing, mathematics, science, and other academic work. They are also expected to become skilled socially, separating from home and family, establishing friendships, negotiating with siblings and other family members, and working on developing a sound sense of who they are as unique members of the community.

School-age children pass through several phases on their way from preschool innocence to the complexity of adolescence. The school-age years can be divided into early childhood (5 to 7 years), middle childhood (8 to 10 years), and late childhood (11 to 12 years) (Dixon & Stein, 2006). Children in each of these phases demonstrate different developmental goals and achievements. Each school-age child is unique, and patterns of "normal" development have broad parameters. The goals of school-age children's development include laying the groundwork for achievement, creating a sense of self-worth, developing the ability to contribute to the group, and, ultimately, gaining satisfaction with life.

Primary health care providers must be familiar with theoretic models of psychosocial development in this age group, in addition to the physical parameters of growth. Parents often turn to their health care provider for understanding and guidance. Some authors have characterized the school-age period as one of quiescence, but a remarkable amount of growth takes place, and the route is not always smooth. Providers can support children and their families to successfully achieve during these important years.

◼ DEVELOPMENT OF SCHOOL-AGE CHILDREN

PHYSICAL DEVELOPMENT

School-age children gain strength and coordination and become more physically capable, setting the stage for participation in sports, dance, gymnastics, and other activities. Social status among children is often based on physical competence; therefore the child's feelings about physical development can be as important as the physical growth itself.

The rate of growth of school-age children increases significantly from that of the toddler and preschooler and occurs in "spurts." The child can literally "grow out of his or her clothes" in a matter of weeks (see Table 11-6). The best way to evaluate an individual child's growth is to monitor his or her progress for height, weight, and body mass index (BMI) on a growth chart. Head circumference increases slowly. By middle childhood, the brain is about 90% of its adult size. Full adult size is reached by about 12 years old. Myelination of the brain, which is necessary for information processing, is not complete until early adulthood. The cerebral cortex (responsible for intelligence) and the frontal lobe (responsible for problem-solving and decision-making) are the last to fully develop. The increasing maturation of the brain allows children to complete increasingly complex skills and have greater control over their bodies (Shonkoff & Phillips, 2000) (see Chapter 27). Organ development is complete. Most school-age children sleep about 10 hours per night (range 8 to 14 hours) without naps, particularly during the school year. Night terrors or sleepwalking may emerge (see Chapter 15).

Traditionally, school-age children had decreased fat; however, recent national data indicate a steady increase in overweight school-age children. National health and nutrition examination survey data indicate that in 2003 to 2004, 37.2% of children 6 to 11 years old were overweight or at risk for overweight, up from 29.8% in 1999 to 2000; 17.1% of all children and adolescents were overweight. The number of overweight girls, 2 to 19 year old, increased from 13.8% in 1999 to 2000 to 16% in 2003 to 2004. For boys the increase was from 14% overweight in 1999 to 2000 to 18.2% in 2003 to 2004. Although these data represent a significant increase, even more alarming is that fact that in 1980, only 5% to 6% of children were overweight (Ogden et al, 2006). In less than 25 years, the number of overweight children in the U.S. has more than tripled, and the trend continues.

A comprehensive discussion of the physical growth of school-age children can be found in general pediatric texts. Table 7-1 looks briefly at significant changes in body systems; discussion of the health issues and disease processes related to these systems can be found in Units Three and Four of this text.

MOTOR SKILLS DEVELOPMENT

In middle childhood, gross motor skills continue to be refined, allowing children to run, jump, climb, hop, skip, tandem walk,

The authors would like to thank Barbara Jones Deloian for her contributions that remain unchanged from the third edition.

TABLE 7-1   Physical Development of School-Age Children

Body System	Developmental Change
Skin and lymph	• At about 6 yr, tonsils and adenoids are largest size. • Prepubescence is characterized by more active sebaceous glands and vasomotor instability that can lead to uncontrolled blushing.
Head, eyes, ears, nose, and mouth	• By early childhood, head size becomes smaller in proportion to body size. • Undeveloped sinus cavities contribute to increased susceptibility to upper respiratory infections, sinus irritation, and sinus headaches. • By 6–7 yr, retina is fully developed, and visual acuity is 20/20. • By middle childhood, eustachian tube grows longer, narrower, and more slanted. • By 5–6 yr, first primary teeth are shed, and first permanent teeth erupt, usually the central incisors. • Each year after 6 yr, approximately 4 teeth are replaced, one set in the upper jaw, one set in the lower jaw.
Pulmonary	• Through childhood, lungs gradually descend into the thoracic cavity. • By 8 yr, alveolar development is complete. • During middle childhood, tidal volume increases; normal adult respiratory rate is achieved, 18–30 breaths per minute. • Increased maturation of macrophagocytic activity of mucus and ciliary function in lungs make child more resistant to respiratory infections.
Cardiovascular	• By 5 yr, heart is 4 times larger than at birth. • By 7 yr, left ventricle thickens; is 2–3 times greater in size than right; blood pressure increases to 90–108/60; cardiac volume increases; heart rate declines to 60–100 bpm. • Atherosclerosis begins in childhood: In one study, approximately 50% of 2 to 15-year-olds had fatty streaks in their coronary arteries (Berenson et al, 1998). In another study, 1 of 6 adolescents had coronary atherosclerosis, although they were asymptomatic (Tuzcu et al, 2001).
Gastrointestinal	• By middle childhood, the GI system is of adult size and function.
Genitourinary	• By 6 yr, elimination patterns are established; greater than 90% of children are toilet trained. • Bladder capacity continues to expand. • Between 10 and 14 yr, puberty begins but can be normal in any child after 8 yr. • Delayed puberty is diagnosed as no secondary sex changes (e.g., breast budding; penis or testicle growth) at 13 yr in girls and 14 yr in boys.
Musculoskeletal	• Long bones grow, leading to taller, thinner school-age child. • Spine becomes straighter; legs become straighter. • Facial bones are actively changing, as nasal accessory sinuses grow.
Immune system	• Rapid maturation of immune system during middle childhood. • Allergic conditions may appear.

bpm, Beats per minute; *yr*, year(s).

alternate their foot patterns, and use an overhand motion. Activities that require balance and coordination such as riding a bicycle, swimming, and roller skating demonstrate children's expanding skills. In late childhood, gross motor skills become more controlled and purposeful. Skills are perfected with much practice. A sense of competition is high as children try to outlast or outperform one another.

Mastery of fine motor skills includes finer dexterity and better control of scissors and writing tools such as crayons and pencils. In early childhood, children become adept at dressing themselves, including being able to tie knots and manage buttons and zippers. Their drawings become more recognizable, showing details of eyes, ears, and other body parts. Self-care skills (e.g., combing hair, brushing teeth) are improved. In late childhood, hand-eye coordination improves, and the child is able to use each hand independently with speed and smoothness. During this time, skill in playing musical instruments emerges.

COMMUNICATION AND LANGUAGE DEVELOPMENT

The child's language patterns provide insight into the status of the neurologic system because the maturing brain is capable of increasingly complex language skills. Both receptive and expressive language skills improve. Six-year-olds have a well-developed vocabulary and are able to retrieve words quickly. They have simple syntactic abilities and can follow simple directions. The language demands of school can be challenging for 6-year-olds. First, they may not be accustomed to attending to total auditory stimuli as in the classroom environment. Second, they are still mastering connotative and semantic skills such as understanding the concepts "before" and "after," relative clauses (e.g., "the cat was chased by the dog"), and the structures of sentences. These factors can make it difficult for them to follow complicated directions or cope with the increased demand to recall information within a specific time frame. Narrative skills can be poor, and reading may be difficult. The expressive language of 6-year-olds should be fully intelligible. Stuttering has usually resolved by school age, but may be seen if young children are overly eager to express themselves. Stuttering should be ignored at this age.

Seven-year-olds' receptive language is strong; they generally have language decoding mastered and are working on encoding information. They can organize previous knowledge and express it verbally or in writing. They are able to solve word problems. Mastery of articulation may not be achieved until 7 or 8 years old with the sounds of "l" and "th."

Eight- to 9-year-old children demonstrate significant syntactic growth with better use of pronouns, allowing them to understand convoluted sentences. Comparatives are learned, and the child is able to distinguish qualities such as more or less, near or far, and heavy or light. By 8 years old, children can follow complex directions. They are beginning to tell jokes because they understand different meanings of words. In their expressive language, children have better narrative abilities and significantly improved storytelling and summarization skills needed for such activities as explaining a task to other children. Vocabulary grows, and there are gradual improvements in grammar (e.g., noted by the use of past and future tenses and plural forms of nouns, particularly irregular nouns and verbs).

At 10 years, children are able to discuss ideas and understand inflections and metaphors. Their ability to understand these ambiguities of sentence structure, word meaning, and language contributes to their increasing ability to enjoy jokes and riddles. Using concrete operational thinking, they can also analyze and interpret language and become more aware of the inconsistency in spoken languages. Children in late childhood understand that the literal meaning of words may not be the only meaning. By 12 years old, children should be able to answer questions involving sophisticated concepts. Expressively, their sentences should be grammatically correct, and they have more detail in their verbal skills. The ability to express emotions also develops. Language has become a means of socializing, and fewer gestures are used. Language can become a game as children make up words and participate in storytelling using proper sequence and pronouns.

SOCIAL AND EMOTIONAL DEVELOPMENT

The psychosocial development of school-age children puts to rest the notion that childhood is a "quiescent" period. Challenges that school-age children face are especially difficult because the child's skill and ultimate success are dependent on abilities that are only just evolving. Gaining social acceptance from one's peers, for example, depends on skills, such as being socially responsive, understanding the group "rules," using the group jargon, being appropriately assertive, and being empathetic (Coleman & Lindsay, 1998). Children who do not yet have those skills can experience a sense of failure when they are compared with their peers who do. Erikson posited that school-age children are eager to learn

and internally motivated to achieve mastery and recognition. They need to be given experiences in an environment that recognizes, adjusts for, and supports their maturing set of skills, where they can explore creatively, learn actively, and be recognized for their successes.

It is believed that the stages through which children progress as they become more socially and emotionally mature are sequential and have been built on since birth, with each being a prerequisite for the next (Table 7-2) (see Table 4-1 and discussion in Chapter 4 on theoretic models of development). In particular, school-age children must develop social interactional skills including how to:

- Understand meaning in social situations and interpret the social cues of others
- Initiate interactions
- Terminate interactions positively
- Gain impulse control and manage emotions
- Resolve conflicts
  Mastering these skills enables children to:
- Refine their role within the family system
- Separate self from family
- Develop and maintain peer friendships
- Develop positive relationships with adults outside the family
- Achieve social acceptance
- Strengthen a sense of self

The earliest school-age milestone in the psychosocial area occurs when children learn to separate easily from family, allowing them to go to school. As they move into the community, children maintain their role and feelings of belonging to a family, but also develop secondary attachments with other adults outside the home. Having good relationships with adults outside the home is especially important when the family is not wholly functional—not responsive and supportive—to the child (Schor, 1998).

Peer Relationships

A major task of school-age children is to develop competence in social relationships. "Friendships promote resilience, enhance self-image, fill emotional needs, and help compensate for stresses in other areas of life" (Coleman & Lindsay, 1998). Studies have shown that attraction to gang involvement may occur during late childhood for youth without a positive social support group (Taylor et al, 2002). Social acceptance is especially important at this age. Friends are generally chosen because of shared skills, interests, personality, and loyalty. Children come to see themselves in the eyes of their friends. As early as 7 years old, some children are more concerned about a friend's opinion than about adults' opinions. They develop "best friends" and dress and talk like their peers. A special-friend phase should occur at around 10 years old. This is an intense attachment to a same-sex child. With that friend, the child expands the self, learns altruism, shares feelings, and learns how others manage problems. Talking on the telephone and sleepovers become more common. These early friendships are the basis for later relationships. Family conflicts can arise when peer activities and expectations conflict with family rules and values.

TABLE 7-2 Developmental Characteristics of the School-Age Child

Approximate Stages and Ages	Psychosexual Development	Social and Emotional Development	Cognitive and Problem-Solving Development	Moral Development
Early childhood (5-7 yr) (carried over from the toddler and preschool years to about 6yr)	*Phallic stage (Freud):* Attachment to the parent of the opposite sex. Usually sexual identity occurs at the end of this phase, and sexual urges are submerged.	*Initiative vs. guilt (Erikson):* Moving into a larger social environment and thus able to initiate activities on their own. Begin to learn to modulate their own behaviors through development of a consciousness as to what is appropriate for parents and society.	*Preoperational period (Piaget):* Representative language and early reasoning. Problem-solving intuitive rather than logical. Thought process involves magical thinking, egocentrism, centration, syncretism, juxtaposition, animism, artificialism, participation, and irreversibility.	*Preconventional stage (Kohlberg):* Stage 1: Reasoning based on rewards and punishment or the consequences of behavior. Stage 2: Begins to base behaviors on own needs and at times the needs of others. Reciprocity is concrete. Other's feelings are secondary.
Middle childhood (7-10yr)	*Latency stage (Freud):* The superego or conscious is internalized. Energy is put into acquiring cultural and social skills. Guidelines established by the family are followed.	*Industry vs. inferiority (Erikson):* Begins to appreciate individual interests and skills and seeks to become a successful member of a group. Internal motivation to achieve, compete, and obtain recognition. If unsuccessful, learning motivation is lost.	*Early concrete operational (Piaget):* Begins to use logic and become more objective using an external point of view. Thinking becomes dynamic, decentralized, using conservation, transitivity, seriation, classification, and reversibility. The ability to understand size, shape when the physical properties can be manipulated.	*Conventional stage (Kohlberg):* Stage 3: Begins to act to please others. Stage 4: Begins to conform to rules.
Late childhood (10-12 yr) (carried into adolescence)	*Genital stage (Freud):* Reemergence of sexual impulses.	*Industry vs. inferiority (Erikson):* Continuation of socialization with other children and groups. Development of hobbies and interests outside of school allows recognition of individual worth.	*Late concrete operational (Piaget):* Able to conceptualize size, shape, quantity, space, and thus able to problem-solve using abstract thought. Able to classify items into a hierarchical system. *Formal operational (Piaget):* Distinguished by the ability to use abstract thinking, complex reasoning, flexibility, and hypothesis formation. Become more aware of contradictions, falsehoods, and shortcomings in previous beliefs. Become aware of how others think of them.	*Postconventional stage (Kohlberg):* Stage 5: Begins to appreciate that their behaviors benefit society. Stage 6: Begins to form principles from conscience, even if they differ from what is generally acceptable in society. Look for rationale in rules. Respect for authority and maintaining social order.

yr, Year(s).

Children's temperaments affect the way they interact with peers, teachers, family, and others in their environment. Emotional problems during these years often follow frustrations, losses, and situations in which the child's self-esteem is threatened or the child is faced with adversity.

Morality

Although there is variability in moral development, moral reasoning in early childhood is usually determined by the consequences of behavior: to avoid punishment, receive rewards, or meet one's needs. There is some consideration of the feelings of others, but only as it serves one's needs. By 7 years old, most children can name a site for their conscience (heart or brain), and, consistent with concrete thinking, school-age children tend to be rather rigid in their views of right and wrong. They can understand the relationships between responsibility and privileges and realize that choices between right and wrong behaviors are within their control. Some children at this age act appropriately to get a direct reward, whereas others do their duty, viewing moral behavior as following the rules of higher authority (see Table 21-2). In late childhood, children begin to move into Kohlberg's postconventional stage (Kohlberg, 1981) where respect for authority and social norms develop.

The ability to reason through difficult situations with a variety of factors operating is heavily dependent on cognitive development, however, and school-age children do not have the cognitive maturity to cope with all situations. The school environment, where rules and values differ from those of the immediate family, must be confronted and negotiated daily. This presents a challenge to the child's concepts of right and wrong. Social pressures also may make it difficult to choose actions that the child believes are right. The pressures of gangs, drugs, and peers push many children to make decisions about their activities and behaviors before they are developmentally ready. Furthermore the values of the family are challenged as the child learns that other families make decisions and have beliefs that differ from their own.

Body Image

School-age children can appear to be totally unaware of their bodies (e.g., the 9-year-old who does not change his shirt for 3 days) perhaps because they are so busy with their daily lives. In fact, children at this age are extremely curious about changes happening to them as they grow, and they are sensitive to others around them. Highly literal in their thinking, they can be very frank with questions to people they trust (e.g., "Grandma, why are you growing a moustache?"). At the same time, they are learning the importance of social politeness—what is appropriate in certain situations and how to behave themselves—so they may be uncomfortable or shy about new or unusual situations. Modesty is characteristic of school-age children.

Sexual exploration, including masturbation, is common. Children in early childhood, 5 to 7 years old, often play "doctor," and in middle childhood, children will compare their bodies with friends of the same sex.

Physical growth and neurologic maturation give children the ability to master many new skills in which they use their bodies. Young swimmers, runners, skateboard enthusiasts, and soccer players all emerge at this time. Their achievements—and failures—help them define who they are and are the basis for their evolving self-image. The images they have about their bodies come from the experiences they have and from the feedback from family, peers, teachers, and others in the community. This feedback can help clarify their understandings and allow the child to gain in self-confidence and feelings of worth (see Chapter 17).

Coping Skills

As a part of the process of developing relationships with others, school-age children refine their ability to identify, label, and manage their feelings. However, their experiences are limited and their cognitive abilities still expanding; they continue to need help labeling complex emotions such as sadness, depression, worry, and envy. They also need help in consciously managing those and other feelings in acceptable ways.

An important coping skill learned by school-age children is impulse control. Without impulse control, random behavior occurs; on the other hand, overly controlled children appear hostile, uncreative, or both. By 7 years old, children should have developed sufficiently to function in a variety of settings (e.g., home, school, playground) with increasing competence.

School-age children face a variety of stressors in society today, including violence, parental divorce, substance abuse in the family, early responsibilities, and lack of support in school. Violence is a constant problem for many, not only in neighborhoods where they live and play but also within their families and in the schools where they go to learn.

Based upon the Substance Abuse and Mental Health Services Administration's (SAMHSA) national survey on drug use and health in 2002, 7.2 million parents of children under 18 years old reported drug abuse in the past year. More than 11% of all parents (10.7% of mothers, and 12.2% of fathers) stated they abused drugs. Five million parents also met the criteria for alcohol dependence, and 10% of children under 5 years, 8% of children 6 to 11 years, and 9% of children 12 to 17 years were living with an alcohol-dependent parent (USDHHS, 2005). Substance abuse by parents has led to many children being placed in foster care. In some states, 60% to 70% of all foster care placements are drug related, many directly connected to methamphetamine use (Carta, 2006).

Some children are given heavy responsibility at a young age. When parents work, many children must care for themselves after school. Latchkey children remain alone, housebound, and unsupervised, until adults return at the end of the day. Some also have responsibility for caring for younger siblings.

Many schools lack resources to maintain small class sizes or offer special programs for children with learning difficulties. As a result, children are passed on from grade to grade without remediation of their fundamental learning problems and with the stigma of failure.

Children with chronic illnesses or disabilities may have trouble adapting to their disorders during the school-age years and may need special help to foster independence and a sense of self-esteem. Latchkey children with chronic illnesses are especially vulnerable because they may need to make decisions about their health care without adult advice, such as whether to take more medication or complete a treatment. Such children need to understand their illness, medications, where to go for emergency care, how to write down instructions or messages, and how to follow important rules. Children mature at different rates in their ability to manage their self-care throughout the school-age years. A child's capacity for self-care of chronic illnesses depends on the illness, its stability, and the child's age and cognitive skills (Jackson Allen & Vessey, 2004).

COGNITIVE DEVELOPMENT

In early childhood, children transition from a preoperational mode of thinking that uses intuitive problem-solving to early concrete operational thinking. At this stage, they are capable of logical thought processes described in Box 7-1. When they make this transition, children are more likely to be ready for school. Magical thinking and egocentric logic fade, and concepts of conservation, transformation, reversibility, decentration, seriation, and classification emerge. Children's ability to mentally manipulate the world, relationships, and viewpoints of others is facilitated when they have the opportunity to physically manipulate concrete materials (e.g., using paints, paper, and glue; building things; making dams and forts of mud, snow, or rocks).

By middle childhood, children need to be able to understand relationships of mass and length and multiple variables relating to objects. School-age children should be able to classify or group materials in relation to other information they have. By late childhood, children should have well-developed concrete operational thinking. They should be able to focus on more than one aspect of a problem and use logical thinking. For effective cognitive work, young people must be able to process information, recognize salient cues in the environment, organize their thoughts, consider relationships with other information, use short- and long-term memory retrieval and storage skills, make decisions based on the analysis of information, take action, and use feedback to further their learning.

These concrete operational abilities allow children to read, write, and communicate thoughts effectively. Learning about the world, its people, and the views and values of others becomes possible. With the ability to understand the viewpoints of others and the decline of egocentricity, logical thinking and new social skills appear. Empathy, or the ability to share and understand another's feelings, emerges and with it the capacity for making deep friendships.

School-age children should be developing a sense of personal competence as they experience success in school.

██ DEVELOPMENTAL ASSESSMENT OF SCHOOL-AGE CHILDREN

Some authorities have questioned the value of screening tests and the physical examination because few physical problems are identified in school-age children (4%), and parents may experience some overconfidence when a child "passes" the physical examination (Hoekelman, 2001). The real value of preventive health visits may be in the monitoring, screening, and anticipatory guidance related to developmental, behavioral, and emotional issues. It is by reviewing the child's progress, offering suggestions, and validating parent's efforts that providers can best assist families as they move through the school-age years. Table 7-3 summarizes some key points to discuss with children and their families.

Developmental surveillance (see Chapter 4) is an essential aspect of each contact with the school-age child because visits are less frequent during the school years. Most visits are for minor acute illnesses rather than health maintenance. Data must be collected on the child's physical, nutritional, neurodevelopmental, psychosocial, behavioral, and emotional status during these visits. As with all children, assessment of the family system is crucial; for the school-age child, it is particularly important to evaluate how well the family is nurturing the child while supporting the child's efforts to separate, become more independent, and create a unique self in the community.

The assessment process begins by building rapport with the parents and the child. Direct questions are asked first to the child, encouraging him or her to share aspects of daily routines, family experiences, school activities, and sensitive developmental concerns. Parents can then be invited to expand on data collected, providing information not only about the child's abilities but also about interactions between child and parents.

BOX 7-1 **Piaget's Concrete Operational Stage: Characteristics of Thought Process**

Decentration—can focus on more than one aspect of a situation at a time (e.g., keeping track of both color and shape when working on a jigsaw puzzle)

Conservation—can understand that some aspects of things, such as weight and mass, remain the same despite changes in appearance (e.g., one cookie, though broken into 2 pieces is still one cookie)

Transitivity—can deduce new relationships from sets of earlier ones (e.g., if a first-grade rule is to sit still when the teacher talks, and if all grades have the same rules, then children in the second grade should sit still when the teacher talks)

Seriation—can sequence in order (e.g., ordering triangle shapes from smallest to largest)

Classification—can group objects on the basis of common features (e.g., separating out all the triangles from circles, squares, and stars)

Reversibility—can mentally reverse a process or action (e.g., ice can melt to water and then refreeze)

TABLE 7-3	Topics for Preventive Health Visit	
5-7 Years	**8-10 Years**	**11-12 Years**
Adaptation to school	Progress at school	Progress in school
After-school activities	After-school activities	After-school activities
Development of peer relationships	Peer relationships: friendships, bullying, or victimization	Peer relationships
Family relationships	Family relationships	Family relationships
Activities that support positive self-esteem	Activities that support positive self-esteem	Activities that support positive self-esteem
Problem-solving away from home, without parents immediately available	Sexual education	Community safety; membership in gangs
Nutrition and physical activity at each visit	Community safety; joining gangs	Problem-solving away from home—avoiding drugs, alcohol, and smoking
	Problem-solving away from home	Handling emotions—sadness, anger, worries
	Handling emotions— sadness, anger, worries	Completion of basic education in sexuality and reproductive health
	Nutrition and physical activity	Nutrition and physical activity

SCREENING STRATEGIES FOR SCHOOL-AGE CHILDREN

Formal developmental screening tools and/or questionnaires should be used with all children (Pinto-Martin et al, 2005). These tools allow the child, parent, and teachers to provide specific information about a child's development, behaviors, and emotional status. They also document a baseline status, highlight potential need for referrals, and evaluate the effectiveness of intervention strategies. Differing parental, school, and child perceptions about specific issues may be noted. Parental reports of skills and concerns about language, fine motor, cognitive, and emotional-behavioral development have been shown to be highly predictive of true problems. The information can give the provider insights into areas needing further investigation and those that may require counseling, therapy, or other intervention strategies. The Resource Box at the end of this chapter provides a list of different developmental and behavioral screening tools (also see Chapter 5 Resource Box; some tools used in infant years are appropriate for school-age children).

In addition, the American Academy of Pediatrics (AAP) recommends six routine health visits for children during the school years at 5, 6, 8, 10, 11, and 12 years (AAP, 2000) (see Appendix D for specific recommendations; the AAP is currently reviewing and may revise this recommended schedule of well-child supervision visits [Kuo et al, 2006]).

Physical Development

A traditional history should be obtained and physical examination conducted and findings documented (Table 7-4). Growth measurements (weight, height, BMI) and blood pressure should be evaluated and compared with age-appropriate norms at each visit. Hearing and vision should be screened at routine health visits. Hemoglobin or hematocrit is done during early childhood (between 15 months and 5 years) and

again during late childhood (about 13 years); girls should be screened again after beginning menstruation. Perform fasting glucose, insulin, and lipid levels; total cholesterol; and liver function tests to assess for diabetes mellitus, hyperlipidemia, and metabolic syndrome in children 4 years or older with a BMI equal to or greater than 95%. Immunization status is an important aspect of these preventive health visits. Tanner staging should be a part of the physical examination because school-age children can begin pubertal changes as early as 8 years old, and some endocrine problems may emerge in the school years. Also evaluation for specific conditions listed in Box 7-2 can provide direction for the provider in the physical examination.

Motor Skills Development

Strength and coordination can be evaluated using a systematic musculoskeletal and neurologic examination as identified in Table 7-5. Concerns about balance, coordination, strength, and mobility should be followed up depending on attention, school performance, and overall developmental function. Problems in this area may account for school performance or learning problems.

Communication and Language Development

Assessment of communication and language development is ongoing during the health care visit as the provider talks directly with the child, probing for the child's level of understanding (e.g., can child follow directions? does the child understand explanations given by the provider?); listening to the child's articulation, vocabulary, sentence structure, and grammar; and noting the child's ability to interact socially with the examiner, the parent, and others in the setting. The child can be asked to write something on a sheet of paper to screen writing skills. Assessment is also based on reports from the parent and/or teachers.

TABLE 7-4   Guidelines for the History and Physical Examination of the School-Age Child

Assessment Area	Findings
Chief Complaint	Common concern (e.g., school performance: inattention, fidgeting, difficulty completing tasks, stays on tasks forever, forgetful, angry, frustrated, poor academic performance, moody, irritable, talks excessively)

Subjective Data and History

Assessment Area	Findings
Birth history	Early development, including feeding, sleep-wake cycles, colicky or fussy baby, poor suck; Apgar scores; length of hospitalization; oxygen or phototherapy
Past medical history	Illnesses that may explain the child's problems (e.g., otitis media, chronic illness, vision problems, dental problems, food allergies, reflux, voiding and stooling issues, or undiagnosed pain); chronic conditions such as asthma, congenital cardiac conditions, accidents, injuries, hospitalizations, or surgeries
Allergies	Type of allergies and reactions
Past development	Early developmental progress, especially in language and social skills (e.g., toilet training)
Interim history	Onset of problems; description of when it occurs; note child's use of alcohol, drugs, and cigarettes; systems review related to any chief complaint; any medications taken for acute or chronic conditions
Daily activities	Daily sleep-wake pattern, routines and schedule, amount of passive activities (TV and computer) vs. active play and recreational activities; note family routines, family activities, family expectations of the child, and child's ability to complete chores or jobs around the house
Temperament and personality	Identify difficulty with change and transitions, establishing routines, or finishing tasks; difficulty with mood, new situations, making or keeping friends
School history	School progress, subjects liked and disliked, peer relationships, match with teacher and school philosophy
Family history	Family and home routines and environment, family support systems, activities, involvement in social and school activities, parent's knowledge of child's friends and involvement with child's friends; family history of medical problems or congenital anomalies
Family review of systems	Family history of ADHD, learning problems, mental retardation, autism, emotional or psychiatric problems, sleep problems, drug or alcohol abuse, diabetes, obesity, asthma or allergies, domestic violence, criminal activities

Objective Data and Physical Examination

Assessment Area	Findings
Measurements and vital signs	Child's growth percentiles, especially if below the 5th percentile or above the 85th percentile; note head circumference for all children (even adolescents); note BMI and blood pressure and compare with norms for age of child; hematocrit
General	Child's overall appearance, cooperation, parent-child interaction, parent's responsiveness to the child, and the child's responsiveness to the parent
Skin and lymph	Rashes, lesions, edema, and shape of the nails, hemangiomas, hirsutism, fat tissue, and skin folds; note enlarged lymph nodes, or mottling of the skin
Head, eyes, ears, nose, mouth	*Head:* Unusual skull shape, hair swirls and unruly hair, and hairline; identify any problems with the temporomandibular joint *Face:* Flat midface, short mandible, asymmetric facial movements, and unusual facies, fetal alcohol syndrome facies *Eyes:* Eye position (hypertelorism/hypotelorism), asymmetries, small epicanthal folds or palpebral fissures; lid: ptosis; conjunctiva: clarity; pupils: PERRLA and cover test, especially for strabismus; EOM: visual fields, nystagmus; fundus: light reflex, vessels, disc, and macula *Nose:* Size, shape, bridge, and anteverted nostrils *Mouth, lips, fulcrum, tongue:* Thin upper lip, micrognathia or retrognathia, long or flat philtrum, prognathism or malocclusion; tongue: fasciculations, symmetry, suck, swallow, and strength *Teeth:* Enamel, shape, dentition, and signs of bruxism *Palate:* Pharynx, palate shape, size of tonsils, movement of uvula, gag reflex *Neck:* Asymmetric strength of movement, swallow, trachea, lymph; thyroid: position, asymmetry, movement
Chest	Shape, pectus excavatum, and short xiphoid
Breasts	Tanner stage; asymmetry or supernumerary nipples
Lungs	Inspiratory and expiratory wheezing or absence of breath sounds; peak flow if history of asthma
Cardiac	PMI, heart sounds, murmurs, and thrills; pulses: equality, symmetry, and strength
Abdomen	Bowel sounds, abdominal shape and movements, umbilicus position, tenderness, masses, organ size, bladder distention or bowel distention

TABLE 7-4	Guidelines for the History and Physical Examination of the School-Age Child—Cont'd	

Assessment Area	Findings
Musculoskeletal	Note size of muscles, symmetry, hypertonia or hypotonia, range of motion, posture, joints, dactyly
	Back: Evaluate spine for scoliosis, cysts, dimples, hair tufts, and CVA tenderness
	Upper and lower extremities: Evaluate active and passive strength (tone), symmetry, hyperextension of fingers and joints, and presence of tremors; movement: observe body while sitting, standing, running, walking, jumping, skipping, hopping, and kicking; note hip dysplasia, foot position, palmar creases, short fifth finger, incurved fifth finger, tapered phalanges, nail hypoplasia, flexion of elbow
Genitourinary, gynecologic	Evaluate anatomy and Tanner stage
	Male: Note testes size, placement; note if circumcised or not; evaluate for hydrocele, hernia, or hypospadias
	Female: Note hypoplastic labia; evaluate for hernia

BMI, Body mass index; *PERRLA,* pupils equal, round, reactive to light and accommodation; *EOM,* extraocular movements; *PMI,* point of maximal impulse; *CVA,* costovertebral angle.

BOX 7-2	**Physical Conditions to be Identified in the School-Age Child**

- Cataracts
- Congenital heart disease
- Congenital hip dysplasia
- Cryptorchidism
- Encopresis
- Enuresis
- Genetic syndromes
- Glaucoma
- Lymphadenopathy
- Obesity
- Scoliosis
- Tumors (benign and malignant)

Social and Emotional Development

Assessment of social and emotional development is an important aspect of the well child examination since 20% to 25% of children in the U.S. are affected by mental health, psychosocial problems, and risk-taking behaviors. Parent and teen surveys indicate children's top five worries are how to cope with stress in their lives, anxiety, depression, self-esteem, and parent-child relationships (Melnyk & Moldenhauser, 2005). These five concerns should be assessed. It is also important to observe the interaction between parents and child during the examination and to examine children's roles in the family, discuss their success in making friends and working with peers, and explore their feelings of contentment and security (see the Resource Box at end of this chapter for recent mental health screening guidelines; also see Ecomap, Chapter 2).

Cognitive Development

Assessment of cognitive development is difficult in school-age children. Generally, standardized paper-and-pencil tests are more accurate than clinical judgments. Knowledge about the child's performance compared with that of peers in the classroom, the child's grades, and information from conferences with teachers provide some data. Often a psychologist is asked to test children cognitively if more definitive information is needed.

DIAGNOSTIC ASSESSMENT STRATEGIES FOR SCHOOL-AGE CHILDREN

If problems are suspected, additional testing can be performed (e.g., bone age can be determined by using x-rays of the wrist to determine epiphyseal fusion; intelligence testing can establish cognitive abilities). Further endocrine, nutrition, genetic, or other assessments may be necessary if the child does not meet the norms for physical growth.

ANTICIPATORY GUIDANCE FOR SCHOOL-AGE CHILDREN

Anticipatory guidance should be an individualized discussion with parents that helps them understand, respond to, and guide their child's behavior and development. Some discussion points are identified in this section. Because children will assume more responsibility for self-care as they grow, these topics should be discussed with them as well, as is age-appropriate. The lists are not intended to be used exhaustively at visits, but to illustrate how developmental concepts can be applied in everyday living. If problems emerge from discussions in these areas, the provider is referred to the appropriate chapter for ideas for assessment and management (e.g., sleep problems are discussed in Chapter 15).

PARENT DEVELOPMENT

The role of parents is central in preparing and supporting their child's transition during the school-age years. Often families are constrained by social and economic conditions as they raise their children, and parents need help to fulfill their responsibilities (McAllister et al, 2005). They will welcome

TABLE 7-5   Guidelines for Neurodevelopmental Assessment of the School-Age Child

Assessment Area	Findings
Overall impression	Behavior, attentional skills and distractibility, motor activity level, impulsivity, degree of cooperativeness, strategies for and persistence in task completion, problem-solving, organizational skills, ability to follow directions and ask for assistance.
Cerebral	State control, attention, behavior, orientation, cooperation, participation, and separation from parents. Are judgment, orientation, memory (short- and long-term ability to remember eight familiar objects in "memory box"), affect, and calculation age appropriate or immature?
Cranial nerves	Note any asymmetries or oral-motor dyspraxia.
Cerebellar functioning	*Fine motor movements:* Evaluate for dysfunctions, including problems with balance, fine motor control (rapid alternating movements), and pincer or pencil grasp. *Coordination:* Evaluate coordination, including balance (Romberg, balance on one foot), tandem walk (heel-toe walk), duck walk, and coordination while throwing and catching a ball (use a small ball with older children).
Sensory functioning	Evaluate problems recognizing body parts or body position, sensitivity to touch, asymmetric or poor graphesthesia (letters or numbers) or stereognosis (objects).
Gross motor function	Evaluate overall gait, coordination for age while skipping, running, walking on balance beam. Appropriateness for age. Note posture, ability to sit in chair straight vs. leaning on desk. Ability to stand for periods of time without leaning on something.
Extraneous movement, tremors	Evaluate for synkinesis (motor overflow), dyskinesis (incomplete or fragmented movements), mild dyspraxic movements, dysdiadochokinesia (inability to perform rapid movements), motor impersistence.
Auditory perceptual abilities	Evaluate discrimination, processing, integration, memory, and comprehension of auditory information. Evaluate ability to follow 2-fold and 5-fold directions. Note directionality and consistent or inconsistent use of right or left eye, hand, foot. Note ability to remember series of spoken words and numbers forwards and backwards and ability to understand or comprehend a written paragraph. Note expressive language ability (word retrieval, formulation, and articulation). Evaluate conversation spoken spontaneously through story or history. Evaluate ability to define words appropriate for age.
Visual perceptual abilities	Identify memory recall (short- and long-term), visual discrimination, visuospatial perception, visual memory for objects, visual discrimination of subtle differences in words (e.g., ten and tin), object assembly, and decoding.
Organization	Observe problem-solving of math problems.
Visual motor integration and coordination	Note ability to copy a design (+, 0, square, or triangle) and handwriting. Evaluate picture of a person drawn by the child for age appropriateness.
Learning style	Evaluate concrete and abstract thinking, sequential or stimulus processing, thought integration, perseveration, ritual and routine; control; adaptation to changes; modulation of behaviors; exaggeration (overdo or underdo) activities.

the support, suggestions, and connection to resources that providers can give them.

A child's entry into school can be emotionally stressful for parents because they must adjust to a new social situation, routine, and a changing relationship with their child. Some parents feel that they have "lost" their child, watching him or her move from dependence on the family to participation in a new world of which the parent is not a part. Other parents anticipate the new opportunities facing the child and family and are ready to help their child cope with challenges that emerge in the school environment. Parents are expected to support the school's standards, and research indicates that parents' education expectations for their children help determine the child's school success (Davis-Kean, 2005). Parents also have

a responsibility to provide an environment that reinforces their children's educational efforts; research indicates that frequent television viewing, little parental control of media content, and viewing of R-rated movies damages children's school performance (Sharif & Sargent, 2006). As children move through the years from 6 to 12, parents will continue to extend freedoms along with adding new responsibilities. They need to provide opportunities that allow children to experience and master new challenges and adjust family patterns of nutrition, sleep, activities, health maintenance, safety, and communication to fit with the child's needs and emerging skills. Parents need to be available to children to ensure the child has both the social and emotional skills essential to move into and succeed in school environments.

REGULATION AND SLEEP-WAKE PATTERNS

Family routines provide a support to the daily life of the child and help the child self-regulate. If children have routines that they can rely on, they are more comfortable exploring in new areas and trying new skills. Family routines strengthen the relationship between parent and child, provide family stability and continuity, and serve as a buffer during times of change and transition (Kubicek, 2002). Stronger family relationships also serve as protection against risk factors such as divorce, alcoholism, substance abuse, or violence. Suggestions the provider can make to parents include the following:

- Encourage the family to establish and recognize traditions or family activities that are special (e.g., birthday celebrations, Sunday afternoon walks, videos and popcorn on Saturday night).
- Help parents explore ways to adapt the child's new schedule in an effort to maintain previous routines or readjust routines to meet the new schedule (e.g., if the child must meet a school bus at an early hour, making a school lunch the night before can become part of a new evening routine).

School-age children who do not receive adequate sleep often demonstrate irritability, fatigue, poor attention, and poor learning. Bedtime is still difficult, and delay tactics are not uncommon. Parents can be encouraged to do the following:

- Continue a regular nighttime routine to transition from active daytime play to evening quiet play.
- Set a regular time for morning awakening, giving the child extra time to come fully awake without being rushed.
- Minimize stimulation (e.g., no scary television programs) before bedtime.

STRENGTH AND MOTOR COORDINATION

Because of the maturity of the central nervous system and cognitive advances, most children are physically capable. Most enjoy playing hard so that they can develop physical skills, strength, and coordination. Parents can support this growth if they do the following:

- Encourage children's participation in daily exercise.
- Provide for activities that are fun, involve family or peers, and require cognitive or social skills, including rules, strategies, and skills.
- Include children's friends in family activities (e.g., hiking, skiing, swimming).
- Support children's interest in preferred physical activities that are healthful; personal achievement in an activity can be crucial to children's self-image.
- Encourage hobbies and activities that foster fitness and increased motor skills.
- Encourage activities that require training, commitment, and effort, especially for older children.
- Help children prevent the stress of overscheduling.
- Limit activities that include TV, video games, or computer time.

- Let the children "own" the activity (e.g., Little League baseball games should be fun for the children, not a contest among parents over whose child is the best).
- Explore ways children with physical limitations can participate in preferred activities and with their peers (see Chapter 14 regarding Special Olympic sports activities for families and children with physical challenges).

NUTRITION, SELF-CARE, AND SAFETY

Nutrition

School-age children have good appetites. Diets can be deficient in iron or vitamin C, however, and high-fat snack foods can become a habit, with resulting obesity. Choosing nutritious foods while away from home and learning to eat new foods are areas for learning. Because food is not readily available all day at school, eating well at breakfast and dinner becomes especially important. High-calorie snacks and other high-calorie foods have contributed to obesity in school-age children; nearly 18% of school-age children are overweight (Ogden et al, 2006), and monitoring and weight control programs are needed at earlier ages (see Chapter 11). Parents should be advised to do the following:

- Ensure that the child has three nutritious meals and two nutritious snacks daily.
- Know that food jags are common.
- Establish an eating routine, with at least one daily meal together as a family. Maintain family meals as much as possible to preserve family time and share interests and experiences from the day's activities.
- Monitor food choices and opportunities to determine best foods.
- Teach children to understand the importance of eating healthy foods.
- Encourage participation in meal planning, food shopping and selection, and meal preparation.
- Discuss making nutritious choices at fast-food restaurants.

Self-Care

For school-age children, learning to take responsibility for their own health begins with simple goals and moves to more complex decision-making strategies. For example, children may begin by deciding to have a fruit or vegetable at each meal and then progress to helping plan some meals and participate in their preparation. Other areas in which children take increasing responsibility are dental health, hygiene and grooming, snacking, and exercise. Children at this age see health in positive terms and equate it with being able to participate in desired activities (Story et al, 2002). Parents can do the following things to assist the child's achievement in self-care:

- Explain the relationship between good health and self-care.

- Supervise personal hygiene such as brushing teeth, combing hair, and doing nail care; for older school children, supervision is minimal, with an occasional reminder.
- Set clear limits on expectations for cleanliness, healthy exercise, hours of sleep, and other health promotion behaviors.
- Recognize that children may be "noncompliant" as a means of exerting independence; a discussion about decision-making and healthy choices may be needed to resolve the issue.
- Be flexible.
- Provide children with opportunities to experiment with appropriate healthy behaviors that allow them to develop self-expression (e.g., school-age children can enjoy new hair styles or having their hair dyed).
- Encourage shared decision-making and self-care during illnesses and for chronic disease management.
- Give children an opportunity to ask questions about sexuality, drugs, alcohol, and tobacco; encourage discussion about these topics as a family; teach about puberty changes.
- Model healthy behaviors.

Safety

Unintentional injuries are common among school-age children. Often their growing bodies allow them to get themselves into situations that they cannot get out of without help. They need guidance and direction to be safe and make safe choices. Although parents do not provide the constant supervision they did for toddlers and preschoolers, it is important that they work with their school-age child to ensure safety. The health care provider can give guidance to parents and encourage them to do the following:

- Help children learn "survival skills" (e.g., name, telephone number, address, use of 911, how to ask adults for help, what to do if lost).
- Require use of protective gear when riding bicycles, skateboards, or scooters.
- Wear seatbelts.
- Encourage use of sunscreen (sun protection factor 15 or higher) before going outside to play.
- Teach children to swim; supervise their activities near water.
- Educate children about hazards, both physical and social (e.g., pedestrian traffic on busy streets; facts about pregnancy, intercourse, and sexually transmitted diseases; what to do if they find a weapon or syringe).
- Monitor children's use of website chat rooms; limit access with use of parental filters. Control children's access to television programming with use of V-chip.
- Get rid of firearms or ensure that they are unloaded and locked, with ammunition in a different location.
- Help children to think about safety aspects of activities; talk about safety.

COMMUNICATION AND LANGUAGE

Mastering the ability to read, comprehend, and write is essential for the school-age child's academic success. Parents can help children learn these skills by doing the following:

- Provide structured time and space for children to complete school writing and reading assignments.
- Read stories to children; even older children enjoy listening to stories that are exciting or relevant to them.
- Listen to the child read aloud.
- Role model by reading and writing often.
- Encourage the child to make notes, keep a journal, and write letters to friends and family members. Skill with writing supports reading and vice versa (Altemeier et al, 2006).
- Play word games with the child (e.g., finding all the things that "start with B" while on a road trip can entertain a 6-year-old; Junior Scrabble or Boggle is fun for older children). Let the child lead the play; the parent should not be "out to win," and the child should not be made to feel inadequate for not knowing everything.
- Talk with the child and actively listen as the child talks.
- Enroll the child in structured, voluntary after school programs that offer an opportunity to engage in active conversation with other children and adults (Vandell et al, 2005).
- Never punish a child by removing books or writing materials.
- Limit television and video games to 1 to 2 hours per day.

SOCIAL AND EMOTIONAL GROWTH

Finding support in his or her family system and peer group while establishing individuality and independence is the hallmark of successful social and emotional growth for the school-age child. Providers can help foster that growth by encouraging parents to do the following:

- Enhance goal setting with charts, calendars, and tally sheets. Care should be taken not to reward children too much because this can decrease motivation. Let children set goals while parents monitor activities and point out options.
- Appreciate the products of the child's work at home and at school; encourage successful activities.
- Provide positive expressions of love, concern, and pride to promote a sense of belonging to the family.
- Share family history and visits with relatives to help children be proud of their heritage.
- Help children feel that the home base is secure to increase their confidence as they move into other domains.
- Make home rules and expectations clear and use consistency in applying them.
- Discuss family values and rules and explain the differences that the child may face when away from home.
- Play and work together as a family to teach children how to work together with their classmates and to function as a team; children should maintain their responsibilities to the family (e.g., jobs or chores around the house).
- Provide opportunities for children to make and develop friendships with a variety of children, teaching them how to initiate, sustain, and terminate relationships with friends.
- Include the child's friends in some activities and outings.
- Teach children how to read social cues.

- Provide social skills training and supervise experiences in which child can practice new skills successfully.
- Help children learn to communicate well with other adults.
- Teach respect for authority and rules away from home.
- Help children identify and appropriately express their emotions.
- Provide fantasy play opportunities to allow children to deal safely with their emotions and concerns and to develop their creativity.
- Provide guidance about how to appropriately express feelings of aggression and emerging sexuality; discuss sexual values.
- Help children with decision-making and accepting consequences of actions.
- Model positive conflict resolution and good communication.
- Teach anger-management and conflict-resolution skills.
- Help children learn delayed gratification and increase their frustration tolerance, while still remaining sympathetic.
- Provide children with opportunities for appropriate behavior when values are challenged (e.g., "You can say, 'No, my mom won't let me do that,' and then walk away").
- Recognize that parents are role models and that children internalize parental values as they begin to form a conscience.
- Recognize that children may identify with a special person, such as a movie star or athlete.
- Recognize that having a strong sense of self-esteem helps "inoculate" children against some of the negative peer pressures children may experience.

COGNITIVE AND ENVIRONMENTAL STIMULATION

The school is a major source of intellectual stimulation and an arena in which the child experiences cognitive growth. Expectations for performance increase over the school years with examinations, graded papers, and homework assignments. Reading becomes a tool to attain and master knowledge rather than being an end in itself. Thus poor readers begin to experience broader academic failure and can become increasingly frustrated. Unless these children are provided with social and remedial support, they may see school as an unpleasant burden, develop feelings of failure, and look for validation through nonacademic experiences. Social supports can help children cope with this stress, and interacting with healthy, interested, and caring adults is the strongest support children can have.

The family also provides the child with stimulation for cognitive growth. Parents can be counseled to do the following:

- Read to the child and have the child read to the parent.
- Stimulate the younger child's thinking about comparisons and differences (e.g., changes in shape, volume, directions to and from school) to facilitate cognition at the concrete operations level.
- Discuss variables in objects or situations as experienced, seen on television, or read about to help move the child's thinking away from the earlier egocentric style.

- Provide opportunities to gain knowledge through books, outings, classes, and family discussions.
- Engage children in experiences with other languages, music, and cultural groups.
- Explore and explain the environment and community to the child to promote broader understanding of the world.
- Establish a regular homework time and place to help the child maximize time for cognitive practice.
- Establish an environment that encourages children to focus and complete tasks with limits clearly defined.
- Provide help early if children experience school problems to lessen secondary problems with emotions and conflict.
- Volunteer at the child's school or participate in school activities for parents.
- Recognize academic achievement because success motivates further work.
- Stay involved with school assignments and evaluate progress to support the child's work.
- Encourage problem-solving efforts.
- Provide more complex opportunities to plan and complete projects that use skills learned at school, such as planning and cooking meals, planning family outings, and managing money and a budget.

◼◼◼ COMMON DEVELOPMENTAL ISSUES FOR SCHOOL-AGE CHILDREN

SCHOOL READINESS

Description

In 1992, the national education goals panel declared that school readiness was dependent upon "children who are ready for school, schools that are ready for children, and communities and parents that support the child's developmental processes" (Zuckerman & Halfon, 2003). School entrance is currently based on chronologic rather than developmental age. What children bring with them from other life experiences to school years either enhances or inhibits their capacity to learn (McAllister et al, 2005). School entry is stressful for all children, but immature children have increased stress because the expectations for performance are beyond their abilities, and they may not have adequate coping resources. Children who lack necessary skills to meet school demands and expectations may be unsuccessful, and early school failure can result in significant negative consequences. Health care providers have a responsibility to work with parents and their communities to promote optimal development and school readiness for children.

School participation requires skills to perform self-care, interact with a variety of new people, act with a sense of responsibility, and emotionally separate from the family and home base. Children need to meet school standards, which may be different from those at home. There is a social expectation to gain an awareness of "the group"—an ability to go along with the group while meeting some personal needs through the group's achievements.

Studies conducted in the early 1990s indicated that teachers believed up to 35% of children were not ready for school as a result of deficiencies in language, emotional maturity, general knowledge, social confidence, and physical maturity (Boyer, 1993). More recent studies indicate that many parents have ambivalent attitudes toward the schools that their children attend and do not feel that the schools have the capacity to meet children's educational needs (McAllister et al, 2005). Socially and economically disadvantaged children are at greatest risk for difficulties. Attention to social and emotional factors and to nurturing relationships in the life of a child will facilitate healthy development in preparation for success in school (Currie, 2005).

CLINICAL FINDINGS

History

- *Child experiences:* Evaluate opportunities for participating in activities away from home, following directions, playing with other children, habits, and interest in school.
- *Parents and family:* Assess the parents' feelings about their child entering school. What do they think their child will experience at school (e.g., racism, bullying, teachers who do not recognize or appreciate their child's unique strengths)? What do they think the school will expect of their child (e.g., to be appropriately sociable, to sit still, to learn quickly)? Do they think their child will be able to handle the demands of school? Do they think that the chosen school can meet the child's needs? Reluctance on the parents' part may be communicated to their child. Ask what parents have done to prepare their child for school. Ask about family activities, sibling school experiences, traumatic events, or separation on the part of the child or parents.
- *Home environment:* Inquire about daily routines, family activities together, parent- versus child-initiated activities for learning.
- *Developmental progress:* Ask about the child's developmental opportunities and skills in communicating needs, fine motor and gross motor activities, behaviors, fears, separation from parents, play with other children.
- *Other issues:* Ask about other concerns (e.g., chronic illness, economic issues, homelessness) that might compromise regular school attendance or school success.

Physical Examination

The child should have a complete physical examination with special focus on the following:
- Neurologic development, including sensory, cognitive, and language
- Height, weight, BMI, blood pressure
- Dental health
- Immunization status

Diagnostic Tests

- Hearing
- Vision
- Urine
- Hematocrit

TABLE 7-6	Basic First-Grade School Readiness Skills
Language skills	Counts 10 or more objects
	Uses complete sentences of at least 5 words
	Uses future tense
	Gives first and last name
	Recognizes 4 colors
	Defines 5 to 7 words
	Communicates needs
	Recalls parts of a story
	Follows 3-part commands
	Understands number concepts
Personal and social skills	Separates easily from parent
	Dresses without supervision
	Plays interactively with other children
	Has toilet skills
	Follows instructions
	Feels support from other adults
Fine motor and adaptive skills	Copies geometric shapes (circle, square, triangle)
	Draws a person (6 parts with distinct body)
	Prints some letters
	Classifies similar objects
Gross motor skills	Hops on one foot
	Catches bounced ball
	Walks backward heel to toe
	Balances on each foot 6 sec

Other Testing or Evaluations

Developmental Evaluation. Normative skills are included in Table 7-6.

Ancillary Studies. Screening tests to evaluate school readiness have established norms and are generally reliable in predicting developmental outcomes. They should be used to consider all areas of readiness (social, behavioral, cognitive) and to provide an explanation of readiness for parents. Test results should be evaluated in conjunction with history, observation, family situation, and previous experiences.

Management

Preventive strategies for high-risk children begin before the school-age years and include enrollment in preschool, interactive reading with the child from an early age to promote language mastery, increased time for young children to play with peers and engage in creative play activities, and interaction with caring adults (Byrd, 2005).

Ensuring school readiness involves sharing data with school counselors and teachers, parents, and primary care providers, and offering anticipatory guidance in the following areas:

- Teach and encourage parents to assist their child with skills that will be needed for school (e.g., knowing colors and numbers, behavioral expectations).
- Encourage parents to visit the school, meet the teacher, and discuss their child's characteristics with the teacher.
- Instruct parents to rehearse school activities with their child before school begins (e.g., getting to school, finding class, eating meals, going to the bathroom, asking for help, getting home, and following the rules).
- Help parents deal with their own stress of separation. Review their expectations of the child and identify what will be new and different.
- Provide parents with available community and school resources they may need to access to meet the developmental needs of their child.
- Encourage children to start school with their developmental-appropriate group. Children who are not ready often need extra support at school, and they would benefit by spending another year at home.
- Be an advocate for parents and children with identified deficits to ensure that the school adequately assesses both strengths and weaknesses of children and develops a program of study (e.g., an individual education plan [IEP]) that maximizes children's strengths.
- Counsel parents that deficits in a child's readiness may occur even with the best of parenting.
- Develop a "catch-up" or "tutorial plan" with parents to address deficits in a comprehensive way while preserving the child's self-esteem.
- Monitor the child's progress through the year, advocating as necessary.

LEARNING PROBLEMS

Description

Learning problems can be a hidden handicap that appears during the school-age years. Ability to manage school learning expectations requires growth in four areas: basic processing of information, memorization, increased attention span and recall of important events, and beginning problem-solving skills.

Knowledge (the sum of what children know) rapidly expands as a result of schoolwork, experiences at home, and activities with friends. The organization of knowledge improves as school-age children grow older and integrate knowledge into existing concepts. Self-awareness, reflected by children's ability to predict performance, develops slowly and in areas in which children have the most knowledge (Table 7-7).

Although children with learning problems generally have difficulties with basic thinking skills, they may have specific problems in linguistic skills, attention, and organizational skills; higher cognitive functions, such as memory and sensory function; motor capacities; visuospatial analysis and neuro-motor function; and social awareness and behavior (Tanner, 1995).

Clinical Findings

History. A complete, in-depth history is needed to examine underlying or related issues because learning difficulties are attributed to many different causes. The history will often provide the most information about how a child's learning affects aspects of the child's life. It should also identify areas of strength on which the child and family can build strategies for managing the learning difficulties. The history includes the following:

- *Medical history:* Prenatal history (including exposure to drugs and alcohol), neonatal history, recurrent or chronic medical conditions, allergies, medications (including in utero exposure), hospitalizations, syndromes; congenital, neurologic, metabolic, or endocrine conditions; current illnesses; vision and hearing problems, fetal alcohol

---

TABLE 7-7 **Developmental Changes in Thinking Skills**

Component	Developmental Changes	Examples
Basic skills	Improvements in the speed and efficiency of memory, attention, language processing, motor implementation	Longer digit span Ability to work for longer stretches of time The use of adultlike logical principles The development of reading skills
Strategies	Use of active, complex strategies to improve basic skills	Greater spontaneous use of strategies Wider repertoire of strategies Greater likelihood of generalization to new areas
Knowledge	Expansion of what is known and greater organization of knowledge	Development of hobbies and special areas of interest More complex network of concepts
Metacognitive awareness	Development of explicit self-conscious knowledge about how to think	Ability to predict success or failure Ability to plan and to modify strategies

From Feldman H: Development of thinking skills in school-aged children, *Pediatr Ann* 18:358, 1989.

syndrome and fetal alcohol effects (the leading cause of preventable mental retardation in the U.S. [USDHHS, 2006]); history of accidents, concussions, or other brain injury

- *Developmental history:* Achievement or regression of developmental milestones, especially in language; experiences for achieving developmental skills at home or in preschool, daily routines and preferred play activities; temperament and behavioral concerns of the parents; ability of the child to handle transitions and change; child's initiation of activities versus parent-guided activities; repetitive behaviors
- *Family medical history:* Family history of difficulties in school or school dropout, learning difficulties, attention-deficit/hyperactivity disorder (ADHD) or attention-deficit disorder (ADD), mental retardation, genetic disorders, and overall family members' functioning, substance abuse
- *Family social history:* Problem-solving and decision-making skills, use of community resources, financial resources, family stressors, substance abuse, homelessness, violence, criminal behavior

Physical examination. A complete physical examination, with special attention to the neurodevelopmental assessment (see Table 7-5) should be performed.

Diagnostic Testing or Evaluations

- *School records:* Information needs to be obtained from the school system to evaluate the child's school performance and to review any educational testing that has been done. Testing provides a picture of the child's strengths and weaknesses, revealing the cognitive styles that teachers and parents will be most successful in tapping. The Pediatric Examination of Educational Readiness at Middle Childhood (PEERAMID), a neurodevelopmental examination for 9- to 14-year-olds, may be administered (Levine et al, 1988).
- *Psychologic testing:* The school may or may not have the capacity for psychological evaluations. Often parents must ask for this, and they may need to seek outside evaluations. Schools are required, under Public Law 94–142, to provide appropriate education to all children identified with developmental delays.
- *Cognitive testing:* The school's ability to provide cognitive and learning evaluations may be limited, and some school districts do not recognize dyslexia as a legitimate problem, requiring the parents to seek outside testing. An evaluation for a learning disorder is not complete without this information (see Resource Box, International Dyslexia Association).
- *Developmental assessment:* A multidisciplinary developmental evaluation through a developmental program may be needed to provide the most appropriate plan of care for an individual child. Additional testing may be recommended such as genetic testing with chromosome studies, brain scans, and endocrine and metabolic testing.

Differential Diagnosis
The following diagnoses need to be considered in children with learning problems:
- Vision problems
- Hearing problems
- Mental retardation—genetic syndrome, neurologic insult, or malformation
- Cognitive developmental delay
- Speech or language delay
- Depression
- ADHD
- Autism spectrum disorder
- Toxin-related delay (e.g., lead, fetal alcohol syndrome and fetal alcohol effects, other intrauterine substance exposure)
- Medication-related delay (e.g., anticonvulsant, antihistamine)
- Substance abuse
- Neurologic problems
- Traumatic brain injury
- Dyslexia

Management
Providers can encourage parents to obtain an early diagnosis and identify and access appropriate school programs. Some children qualify for special educational support through IEPs. Parents need to review educational plans, provide an environment rich with experiences for children, and set realistic goals. They also need to act as advocates for their children during every school year because classrooms and teachers change. Parents should work to correct secondary problems, such as poor self-esteem, hopelessness, or depression. Finally, parents need to be encouraged to avoid the use of the many unsubstantiated cures for learning disabilities (see Chapter 16 for further discussion of ADHD and other cognitive-perceptual problems).

SCHOOL REFUSAL (PHOBIA)
Description
School refusal is a term that was introduced in the 1970s to describe the heterogeneity of its causes. The prevalence ranges from 0.4% to 18% of all school-age children. The disorder includes, but is not limited to, separation anxiety disorder, simple and social phobias, and depression. The criteria for a diagnosis include the following: (1) severe difficulty attending school or refusal to attend school; (2) severe emotional upset when attempting to go to school; (3) absence of significant antisocial disorders; and (4) staying at home with the parent's knowledge (Marino, 2001). Children may request to stay home from school with a variety of physical complaints, including stomachaches, headaches, dizziness, fatigue, or a combination of these. The symptoms gradually improve as the day progresses and often disappear on weekends. Unexcused school absences peak with the beginning of school attendance and again at 11 to 12 years old.

Clinical Findings

History. Because child, parent, family, and school environmental factors may all play into the causes of school refusal, an in-depth history exploring these areas is needed. Specific areas include the following:

- Frequent somatic complaints or sleep difficulties
- Parents' ambivalent feelings about children's attendance at school, evidence of overindulgence or overprotection
- Difficult home situation (e.g., children may try to stay at home to care for a chronically ill parent or may have a substance abusing parent who is not attending to the child's academic needs)
- Recent or anticipated loss or separation
- School environment and evidence of bullying, violence, humiliation, lack of privacy (in bathroom especially), mismatch with teacher

Physical Examination. A complete physical examination and any indicated laboratory testing should be done to rule out specific indications of organic disease.

Diagnostic Testing and Evaluations. Laboratory testing that is symptom specific, noninvasive, and cost effective to rule out organic disease is appropriate to assure child and parents that the problem is taken seriously. Both parent and child may then be more willing to accept the lack of organic disease and work toward addressing the underlying psychological issues and cooperating in the development of a treatment plan.

- Depression and anxiety questionnaires (see Chapter 20)
- ADHD evaluation tools (see Chapter 16)

Differential Diagnosis (Marino, 2001)

- Anxiety disorder. This is the most common reason for school refusal, usually manifesting as an inability to cope with anxiety, especially anxiety stemming from separation.
- Somatic illness or overresponse to minor illness. Avoid provider overresponse with excessive diagnostic testing.
- Depression: Isolation from peers, withdrawal from activities, sleep disturbances, erratic moods, poor self-esteem, and decreased activity level.
- ADHD and conduct disorder. Children who are unsuccessful in school, either academically or socially, may try to withdraw from the school environment.
- Sexual or physical abuse. Children who are being abused or who experience violence either at home or at school can feel intimidated to the point that they refuse to attend school.
- Chronic physical illness with poor adaptation.
- Learning disability with poor adaptation.
- Substance abuse in the family.
- Parental criminal activity.
- Pregnancy.
- Family dysfunction.
- Truancy.

Management

Intervention is generally successful when behavioral measures are combined with supportive counseling of parents. The physical complaints must be reasonably evaluated to rule out organic disease without excessive medical attention or diagnostic testing. Once the possibility of organic disease is set aside (or a plan is established to evaluate somatic problems), children must go to school. Generally, once they are at school, symptoms resolve.

- Support parents in getting children to school and insist on full attendance.
- Notify school personnel and encourage them to support and expect children's attendance and intervene to improve any situation related to children's anxiety.
- Assess home situation and identify issues that must be handled. Provide referrals as needed for family and parent problems for counseling, social service, or other resources. Notify child protection services in the case of threat of harm from parental inability to provide for adequate supervision and needs.
- Refer for psychiatric care if no improvement occurs within 2 weeks.
- Criteria for mental health referral include the following (Munro, 2001):
  - Unresponsive to pediatric management
  - Out of school for 2 months
  - Psychosis
  - Depression
  - Panic reactions
  - Parental inability to cooperate with plan

RECURRENT PHYSICAL SYMPTOMS

Description

Complaints of recurrent symptoms such as headaches, abdominal pain, and limb pain are frequent in school-age children. There is no good medical explanation for these symptoms, but the frequency of complaints in school-age children suggests a correlation with developmental factors. Children with recurrent symptoms may have parents with increased psychosocial problems and preoccupation with somatic complaints, but many times the cause is not clear. Often children receive a great deal of attention for these symptoms (see Chapter 32 for evaluation and management of recurrent abdominal pain).

Clinical Findings

History

- Vague and intermittent complaints of abdominal pain, headaches, nausea, or malaise, but absence of significant findings on physical examination
- Normal function between episodes
- No symptoms of vomiting, diarrhea, or constipation
- Possible family member with similar symptoms
- Stress in school or home environment (e.g., new social situation, new sibling, school, teacher, examination, peer group conflict, moving, family illness or loss, parental or self-initiated pressure for achievement or perfection)

Physical Examination. No evidence of organic disease.

Differential Diagnosis

- Chronic, recurrent abdominal pain (see Chapter 32): consider irritable bowel syndrome, lactose intolerance, acid peptic disease, inflammatory bowel disease, sickle cell anemia, porphyria, hereditary angioedema, systemic lupus erythematosus, and dysmenorrhea in adolescent females (see Chapter 35)
- Neurologic conditions (see Chapter 27 for discussion of headaches)
- School refusal

Management

The following are keys to management of recurrent symptoms:

- Try not to "medicalize" the problem with a barrage of tests if the initial history and physical examination do not indicate systemic symptoms.
- Encourage the child to keep a food or pain diary.
- Reassure the child and expect normal participation in activities.
- Refer for mental health counseling if symptoms persist.
- Discuss coping strategies to deal with stressors.
- Discuss family strategies that are supportive but that do not reinforce the illness behavior.

■■■ RED FLAGS FOR SCHOOL-AGE CHILD

Children have unique personalities and characteristics and are strongly influenced by the environments in which they live. Therefore, "red flags" during school years must be identified and addressed within the context of the child's family and their expanding world. Identification of problems in school-age children involves consideration of both developmental processes and risk-taking behaviors of the child in the family and school environment. Since many chronic illnesses that impact development have already been identified, the emphasis shifts to addressing issues that may arise from these illnesses.

The identification of risk behaviors in school-age children is the basis for health teaching and prevention. Both the child's interest in engaging in risk-taking behaviors and the specific behaviors need to be considered. It is unclear if risk-taking behaviors in school-age children are indicators of risky behavior in adolescence. As children progress through elementary school, they have more knowledge of health behaviors, but do not necessarily practice those behaviors. Research shows that the temperament of school-age children plays a role in risk-taking behaviors, and boys have been found to engage in risk behaviors more than girls (Cartland & Ruch-Ross, 2006). The family maintains an influential role, but increasingly, peers and influences outside the family during school years impact children's decisions related to risk-taking behaviors.

In addition to identifying high-risk behaviors, the health care provider must be alert to "red flags" that jeopardize children's school success and be ready to intervene with families and school professionals to obtain necessary evaluations and resources to address these problems. Learning problems may not surface until the child is in school, and early identification is important to ensure that children are able to access resources that result in a positive school experience.

The wide variation in the growth and development of school-age children necessitates looking at problems based on age and developmental tasks of each age. The status of the family significantly impacts the child's ability to move through developmental stages during school years. The well child history, focusing on specific accomplishments by age, provides the foundation for identifying developmental issues and behavioral risk factors. For school-age children, it includes the following:

- Presence of chronic illness
- Accidents and injuries (number and severity)
- Vision and hearing problems
- Progress, interest, and success in school
- Identification of learning problems with appropriate school plans and placement based on needs and abilities
- Sudden changes in school performance
- Changes in vocabulary and receptive language
- Cognitive processes: logical reasoning and ability to problem-solve
- Socialization: friends, involvement with peer group, community
- Antisocial behavior and/or destructive acts
- Participation in group sports
- Development of self-concept and self-identity
- Socialization away from family to peer or community groups
- Family circumstances such as death of a family member, divorce, changes in parents' health

Table 7-8 outlines red flags in five areas: psychosocial and emotional, cognitive and verbal abilities, language and hearing, fine motor, and gross motor for children 6 to 12 years old. Primary care providers have skills to address risk factors with families to prevent further problems. In situations where the child has been referred, the primary care provider has a crucial role in working with other professionals to ensure that children and families receive appropriate services.

TABLE 7-8   Developmental Red Flags: School-Age Child

Age	Psychosocial and Emotional Skill	Cognitive and Visual Abilities	Language and Hearing	Fine Motor	Gross Motor
6 years	Problems with peer relationships Latchkey: stays home alone Unable to state special quality about self Flat affect, depression, withdrawn Cruelty to animals, friends Interest in fires or fire setting	School problems with grades, behavior, interest in school Unable to sit still in class Unable to give age Watching television more than 2 hours per day Unable to name interests	Language partially unintelligible	Unable to copy "+" Picture of self includes less than 8 parts	Unable to catch a ball
8 years	Lack of hobbies Lack of best friend Cruelty to animals, friends Interest in fires or fire setting Flat affect, depression, withdrawn Defiant attitude	Unable to state days of the week Unable to add and subtract Unable to identify right and left	Unable to read simple phrases Unable to relate simple story	Unable to copy a diamond and square Unable to print name Unable to tie shoes Picture of self includes less than 12–16 parts	Unable to walk a straight line Poor coordination, endurance, strength
10 years	Lack of team sports or extracurricular activities at school Lacks understanding of rules Poor peer influence, interest in gangs Cruelty to animals, friends Interest in fires or fire setting Flat affect, depression, withdrawn	Lack of operational thinking: cause and effect, relationships of whole and parts, nonegocentric thinking	Problems with reading and math	Difficulty holding pencil with penmanship or cursive writing	Problems throwing or catching
12 years	Risk-taking behaviors: smoking, alcohol, sex Inappropriate for age sexual behavior Cruelty to animals, friends Interest in fires or fire setting Flat affect, depression, withdrawn Defiant, rebellious attitude	Difficulty with school work Lack of organizational skills for homework	Problems understanding, following through with verbal instructions Problems with reading comprehension	Problems getting written homework done because of difficulties holding pencil or doing paper-and-pencil tasks	Unable to list strengths and physical things he or she likes to do

$\mathcal{R}$ESOURCE BOX

Screening and Assessment

Screening Tests to Evaluate School Readiness

Test	Source	Content
Beery Visual-Motor Integration, Fifth Edition (VMI-5)	Pro-Ed Inc. www.proedinc.com	Test of visual motor integration
Denver Developmental Screening Test II	Denver Developmental Materials, Inc. www.denverii.com	Divided into four areas: Gross motor Language Fine motor Personal and social
Pediatric Examination of Educational Readiness (PEER) and Pediatric Examination of Educational Readiness at Middle Childhood (PEERAMID)	Educators Publishing Service, Inc. www.epsbooks.com	Combined neurodevelopmental, behavioral, and health assessment

Screening and Assessment Tools for the School-Age Child

Tools	Ages	Reference	Reporter	Item no.	Strengths	Weaknesses
Pediatric Symptoms Checklist (PSC)	6-12 yr	Jellinek et al, 1988; Jellinek et al, 1999	Parent report for 6-16 yr. List of behaviors followed by never, sometimes, often.	35	Measures psychosocial dysfunction. Normative data, reliable, valid. Specificity of 68% and sensitivity of 95%. Used extensively in pediatric populations.	Not for older adolescents. No depression-specific subscore, measures global dysfunction.
Child Behavior Checklist (CBCL)	6-18 yr	Jensen et al, 1996	Parent report for 4-18 yr. Checklist.	138	Multidimensional. Widely accepted and used; provides normative data for age and gender. Reliable and valid. Studied in many languages and countries. Often used to validate other screens.	Requires 20-25 min. Not easily scored. Computer scoring recommended. May not be feasible for mass screening. Subscales may have lower sensitivity than total scores.
Child Depression Inventory (CDI)	7-16 yr (used up to 18 yr)	Brooks & Kutcher, 2001; Myers & Winters, 2002	Child selects 1 of 3 statements.	27	Well studied, reliable, and internally consistent.	CDI scores vary with age and sample, making cutoff scores difficult for mass screening. Some studies failed to distinguish between depressed and nondepressed children. Does not ask if suicide was attempted.

*R*ESOURCE BOX

Screening and Assessment—Cont'd

Tools	Ages	Reference	Reporter	Item no.	Strengths	Weaknesses
Child Depression Inventory— Parent (CDI-P)	6-16 yr	Wierzbicki, 1987	Parent selects 1 choice from 3 statements.	27	Ability to ask a second informant. Studied in a nonclinical population.	Noted to be an experimental screen in 1987. Validity of the CDI-P based on the validity of the instruments from which it was derived (CDI and BDI).
Psychosocial Screening (PSC—youth)	9-14 yr	Gall et al, 2000	Self-report. List of behaviors followed by never, sometimes, often.	35	Addresses psychosocial impairment. Used in nonclinical populations.	Fewer validation studies than the parent version.
Children's Depression Rating Scale (CDRS)— revised	6-12 yr	Brooks & Kutcher, 2001	Interviewer based; 14 items for parents, 3 items based on child observation.	17	Reliable. Valid. Combines multiple informants. Interviewer does not need to be qualified clinician. All depressive symptoms.	Takes more than 30 min to complete. Recommended method is for trained interviewer to speak separately with parent, child, and another adult, such as the teacher. Involves training.

min, Minute(s); *yr,* year(s); *BDI,* Beck Depression Inventory.

*R*ESOURCE BOX

Websites

American Academy of Pediatrics
www.aap.org

Bright Futures
www.brightfutures.org
Guidelines for health supervision of infants, children, and adolescents (Green & Palfrey, 2002)
Bright Futures in practice: mental health, Volume I, *Practice Guide* (Jellinek, Patel, & Froehle, 2002a)
Bright Futures in practice: mental health, Volume II, *Tool Kit* (Jellinek, Patel, & Froehle, 2002b)

Child Development Institute
www.childdevelopmentinfo.com

Institute for Multisensory Education
www.orton-gillingham.com

International Dyslexia Association
www.interdys.org

NAPNAP
www.napnap.org
Keep Your Child/Yourself Safe and Secure (KySS) Guide to Mental Health Screening, Intervention and Health Promotion (Melnyk & Moldenhauser, 2005)

National Association for Child Development
www.nacd.org

Search Institute
www.search-institute.org

☑ DISCUSSION FORUM

1. A mother says she is concerned that her 7-year-old daughter "has no friends at school," seems "unhappy and very shy," and often "complains of a stomachache" before school begins. What assessment will you conduct to determine if there is a potential problem? What information can you share about development of children at this age? What guidance or suggestions will you give this mother?

2. While conducting an annual physical exam on a 12-year-old boy, you note that he is in the 85th percentile for weight, 50th percentile for height, has gynecomastia, and is at Tanner stage 1. What health issues are of greatest concern for you, and what will be your plan(s) for intervention?

3. The school nurse refers a 6-year-old boy for assessment of ADHD. What might the long-term management plan for this child be? Consider assessment, anticipatory guidance for the child and family, consultation with the school nurse, arrangements for an IEP, and treatments.

4. A 10-year-old girl's mother is killed in a motor vehicle accident; the family was very close, and the child is severely affected. Discuss the developmental characteristics and changes that guide the way this child might respond to her loss and examine how you will be able to help her most effectively.

REFERENCES

Altemeier L et al: Executive functions in becoming writing readers and reading writers: note taking and report writing in third and fifth graders, *Dev Neuropsychol* 29(1):161-173, 2006.

American Academy of Pediatrics (AAP), Committee on Practice and Ambulatory Medicine: Recommendations for preventive pediatric health care, *Pediatrics* 105:645, 2000.

Berenson GS et al: Association between multiple cardiovascular risk factors and atherosclerosis in children and young adults, *N Engl J Med* 338(23):1650-1656, 1998.

Boyer E: Ready to learn: a mandate for the nation, *Young Child* 48:54-57, 1993.

Brooks SJ, Kutcher S: Diagnosis and measurement of adolescent depression: a review of the commonly utilized instruments, *J Child Adolesc Psychopharmacol* 11:341-376, 2001.

Byrd RS: School failure: assessment, intervention, and prevention in primary pediatric care, *Pediatr Rev* 26(7):233-243, 2005.

Carta K: *The impact of meth on foster care, children, and families: field report of panel discussion,* Washington DC, 2006, Generations United. Available at *www.connectforkids.org/node/4292* (accessed Jan 30, 2007).

Cartland J, Ruch-Ross HS: Health behaviors of school-age children: evidence from one large city, *J Sch Health* 76:175-180, 2006.

Coleman W, Lindsay R: Making friends: helping children develop interpersonal skills, *Contemp Pediatr* 15:111-129, 1998.

Currie J: Health disparities and gaps in school readiness, *Future Child* 15(1):117-138, 2005.

Davis-Kean PE: The influence of parent education and family income on child achievement: the indirect role of parental expectations and the home environment, *J Fam Psychol* 19(2):294-304, 2005.

Dixon S, Stein MT: *Encounters with children: pediatric behavior and development,* ed 4, St Louis, 2006, Mosby.

Feldman H: Development of thinking skills in school-aged children, *Pediatr Ann* 18:358, 1989.

Gall G et al: Utility of psychosocial screening at a school-based health center, *J Sch Health* 70:292-298, 2000.

Green M, Palfrey JS: *Bright Futures: guidelines for health supervision of infants, children, and adolescents,* Arlington, VA, 2002, National Center for Education in Maternal and Child Health.

Hoekelman RA, editor: *Primary pediatric care,* ed 4, St Louis, 2001, Mosby.

Jackson Allen P, Vessey JA: School and the child with a chronic condition. In Jackson Allen P, Vessey JA, editors: *Primary care of the child with a chronic condition,* ed 4, St Louis, 2004, Mosby.

Jellinek MS et al: Use of the pediatric symptom checklist to screen for psychosocial problems in pediatric primary care, *Arch Pediatr Adolesc Med* 153:254-260, 1999.

Jellinek MS et al: Pediatric symptom checklist: screening school-age children for psychosocial dysfunction, *J Pediatr* 112:201-209, 1988.

Jellinek MS, Patel BP, Froehle MC, editors: *Bright Futures in practice: mental health, vol I, practice guide,* Arlington, VA, 2002a, National Center for Education in Maternal and Child Health.

Jellinek MS, Patel BP, Froehle MC, editors: *Bright Futures in practice: mental health, vol II, tool kit,* Arlington, VA, 2002b, National Center for Education in Maternal and Child Health.

Jensen PS et al: Scales, diagnoses, and child psychopathology: II. Comparing the CBCL and the DISC against external validators, *J Abnorm Child Psychol* 24:151-168, 1996.

Kohlberg L: *The philosophy of moral development,* San Francisco, 1981, Harper & Row.

Kubicek LF: Fresh perspectives on young children and family routines, *Zero to Three* 22:4-20, 2002.

Kuo AA et al: Rethinking well-child care in the United States: an international comparison, *Pediatrics* 118(4):1692-1702, 2006.

Levine M et al: Neurodevelopmental readiness for adolescence: studies of an assessment instrument for 9- to 14-year-old children, *Dev Behavior Pediatr* 9:181-188, 1988.

Marino RV: School absenteeism and school refusal. In Hoekelman RA, editor: *Primary pediatric care,* St Louis, 2001, Mosby.

McAllister CL et al: "Come and talk a walk:" listening to Early Head Start parents on school-readiness as a matter of child, family, and community health, *Am J Public Health* 95(4):617-625, 2005.

Melnyk BM, Moldenhauser Z: *KySS Guide to child and adolescent mental health screening, early intervention and health promotion,* Cherry Hill, NJ, 2005, National Association of Pediatric Nurse Practitioners.

Munro R: Mental health: recovery is a state of mind, *Nurs Times* 97:12, 2001.

Myers K, Winters NC: Ten-year review of rating scales. II. Scales for internalizing disorders, *J Am Acad Child Adolesc Psychiatry* 41:634-659, 2002.

Ogden CL et al: Prevalence and trends in overweight among US children and adolescents, 1999-2004, *JAMA* 295(13):1549-1555, 2006.

Pinto-Martin JA et al: Developmental stages of developmental screening: steps to implementation of a successful program, *Am J Public Health* 95(11):1928-1932, 2005.

Schor E: Guiding the family of the school-aged child, *Contemp Pediatr* 15:75-93, 1998.

Sharif I, Sargent JD: Association between television, movie, and video game exposure and school performance, *Pediatrics* 118(4):e1061-70, 2006.

Shonkoff JP, Phillips DA, editors, Committee on Integrating the Science of Early Childhood Development, Board on Children, Youth, and Families: *From neurons to neighborhoods: the science of early childhood development,* Washington, DC, 2000, National Academies Press.

Story M, Holt K, Sofka D, editors: *Bright Futures in practice: nutrition,* ed 2, Arlington, VA, 2002, National Center for Education in Maternal and Child Health.

Tanner J: Neurodevelopmental variation in school-aged children, *Compr Ther* 21:499-506, 1995.

Taylor CS et al: Individual and ecological assets and positive developmental trajectories among gang and community-based organization youth, *New Dir Youth Dev* 95:57-72, 2002.

Tuzcu EM et al: High prevalence of coronary atherosclerosis in asymptomatic teenagers and young adults, *Circulation* 103:2705-2710, 2001.

United States Department of Health and Human Services (USDHHS), Substance Abuse and Mental Health and Human Services. Substance Abuse and Mental Health Services Administration: Office of Applied Studies: *Results from the 2004 National Survey on Drug Use and Health: national findings,* Rockville, MD, 2005, SAMHSA.

United States Department of Health and Human Services (USDHHS), Substance Abuse and Mental Health and Human Services. Substance Abuse and Mental Health Services Administration: *Fetal alcohol spectrum disorders: the basics,* Rockville, MD, 2006, SAMHSA.

Vandell DL, Pierce KM, Dadisman K: Out-of-school settings as a developmental context for children and youth, *Adv Child Dev Behav* 33:43-77, 2005.

Wierzbicki M: A parent form of the children's depression inventory: reliability and validity in nonclinical populations, *J Clin Psychol* 43:390-397, 1987.

Zuckerman B, Halfon N: School readiness: an idea whose time has arrived, *Pediatrics* 111:1433-1436, 2003.

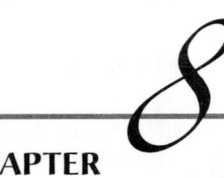

Developmental Management of Adolescents

Ardys M. Dunn

The changes a young person experiences during the transition from childhood to young adulthood are dramatic. The extent of physiologic growth and maturation rivals that occurring during infancy. Social and psychological changes are also extreme and can create a tenuous sense of balance during this phase of development. The common question on the minds of most adolescents is "Am I normal?" Anticipatory guidance and reassurance during well child care are perhaps the most valuable services a health care provider can offer the adolescent. This chapter focuses on the normal physical and psychosocial growth and development of adolescents and provides practitioners with a framework for structuring care of the adolescent client.

■ DEVELOPMENT OF ADOLESCENTS

Puberty is the term for the biologic process that ultimately leads to fertility. The hormonal regulatory systems in the hypothalamus, pituitary, gonads, and adrenal glands undergo major changes between the prepubertal and adult states. Accompanying these changes are rapid growth in height and weight, development of secondary sex characteristics, and onset of fertility (Fig. 8-1) see Chapters 25 and 35. Limits of normal can be difficult to define and are, at best, approximations rather than precise parameters. However, even though the timing (tempo) of adolescent development is variable, the sequence of events is orderly (Fig. 8-2).

Adolescence refers to the psychosocial and emotional transition from childhood to adulthood. The physical changes of puberty are accompanied by significant cognitive and psychosocial development that affects how adolescents view themselves and how the world views adolescents. Successful development in adolescence culminates in achievement of goals that can provide the basis for a healthy and productive adult life (Table 8-1).

PHYSICAL DEVELOPMENT

Tanner Stages

Pubertal growth and maturation can be divided into five stages ranging from prepubertal (sexual maturity rating [SMR] 1) to adult (SMR 5). These divisions are termed

The authors would like to acknowledge Judith W. Fisher for her contributions that remain unchanged from the third edition.

Tanner stages (Tanner, 1962) (Figs. 8-3 and 8-4). Pubertal changes occur on a continuum, with individual differences in timing or tempo.

Female Stages. Females enter puberty earlier than males do, and their puberty usually progresses sequentially in the following pattern:

- Ovaries increase in size; no visible body changes occur.
- Breast budding (thelarche) occurs, on average, at 11 years old, with 95% of normal girls having initial breast development between 9 and 13 years old. Most girls (85%) experience the development of breast buds approximately 6 months before the appearance of pubic hair. However, some females have pubic hair before the development of breast buds. The timing of onset of breast development in females has no relationship to breast size at the completion of puberty.
- Rapid linear growth usually begins shortly after the onset of breast budding and reaches its peak about a year later. Most girls experience peak height velocity (PHV) at about SMR 3, generally between 11 and 12 years old, and PHV is completed by about 13 years old. Early developers may experience a height spurt between 9 and 10 years old, whereas late developers may not experience a height spurt until between 13 and 14 years old. Final height is determined by the amount of bone growth at the epiphyses of the long bones. Growth stops when hormonal factors shut down the epiphyseal plates.
- Appearance of pubic hair (adrenarche or pubarche) commences at about 11.5 years old and is related to adrenal rather than gonadal development, not to thelarche; therefore it is less valid than other secondary sex characteristics in assessing sexual maturation.
- First menstrual period (menarche) occurs, on average, at 12.5 years old. More than 95% of girls experience menarche between 10.5 and 14.5 years old. The mean age of menarche is highly dependent on ethnic, socioeconomic, and nutritional factors. Menarche generally occurs 1.5 to 2.5 years after thelarche. It may be 18 to 24 months after menarche before females establish regular ovulatory cycles. To some degree, menstrual cycles can be affected by the athletic activity of the female (Theodoropoulou et al, 2005; Fujii & Demura, 2005).

Changes in the body composition of females occur during puberty, and adolescent girls will benefit from the primary health care provider's reassurance that these changes

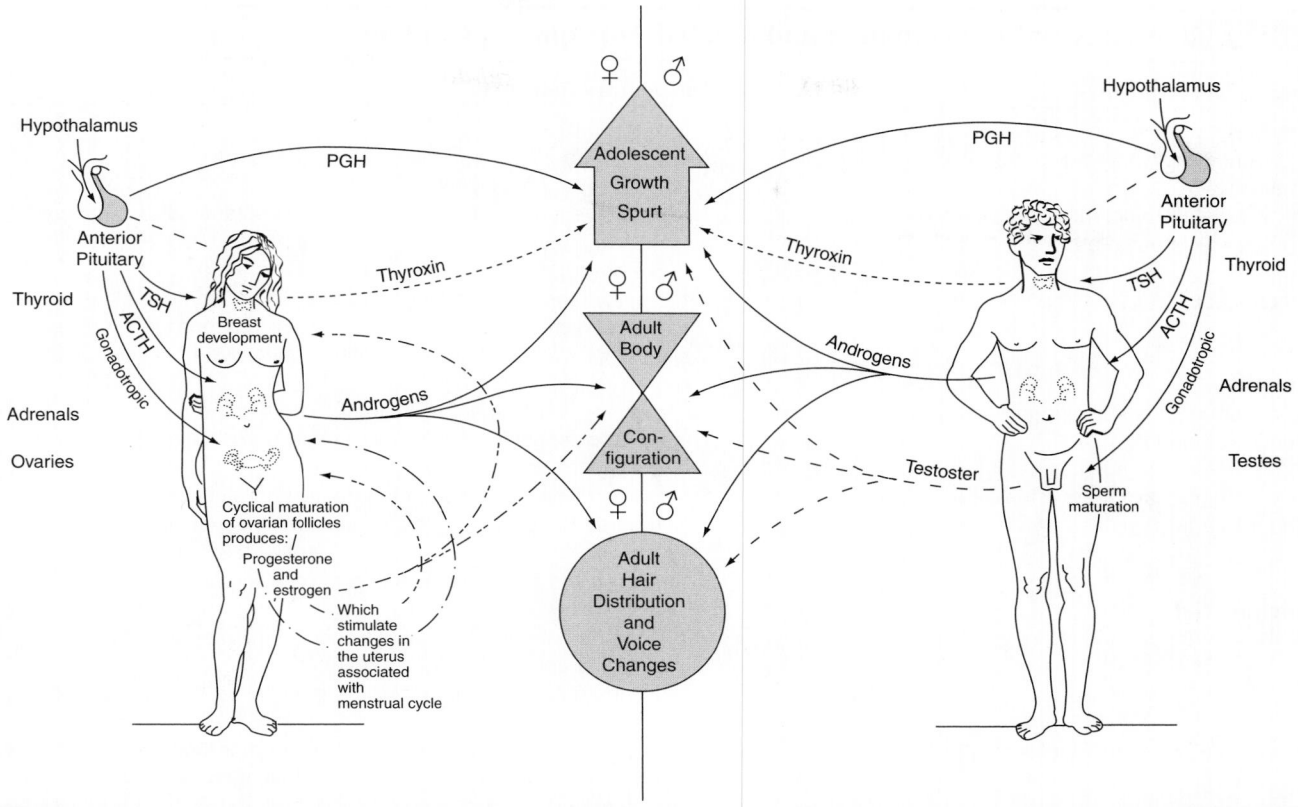

FIG. 8-1   The endocrine system at puberty. *ACTH,* Adrenocorticotropic hormone; *PGH,* pituitary growth hormone; *TSH,* thyroid–stimulating hormone. (From Valadian I, Porter D: *Physical growth and development from conception to maturity,* Boston, 1977, Little, Brown.)

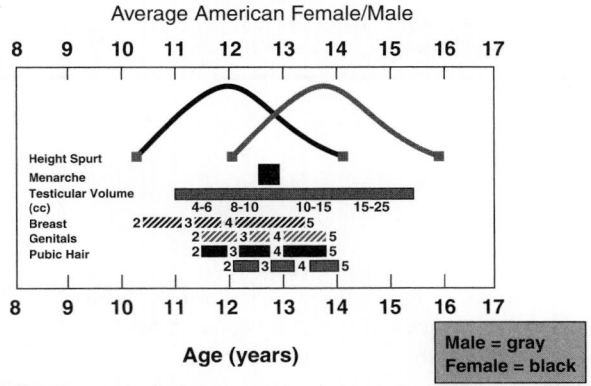

FIG. 8-2   Sequence of pubertal events. Breast, genital, and pubic hair development indicate Tanner stages 2 to 5. (Adapted from Division of Adolescent Medicine, Children's Hospital Medical Center, Cincinnati, OH, 1995.)

are normal. Girls often have asymmetric breasts and need assurance that breasts become more or less the same size within a few years after the onset of breast budding. The female body shape changes as girls progress through puberty, with broadening of the shoulders, hips, and thighs. Girls experience a continuous increase in proportion of fat to total body mass during puberty. They enter puberty with approximately 80% lean body weight and 20% body fat. By the time puberty ends, lean body mass drops to

about 75%. Body fat is an important mediator for the onset of menstruation and regular ovulatory cycles. An average of 17% of body fat is needed for menarche, and about 22% is needed to initiate and maintain regular ovulatory cycles.

Male Stages.   Physical body changes of puberty generally occur sequentially in males as follows:

- Growth of the testes occurs approximately 6 months before the development of pubic hair in most males. If testicular enlargement does not precede other changes, the provider should consider whether the youngster is taking exogenous anabolic steroids. Once puberty begins, the left testis generally hangs lower than the right.
- Pubic hair development follows a pattern similar to that of girls (see Fig. 8-4).
- First release of spermatozoa (spermarche) generally occurs in midpuberty at a mean age of 13.5 to 14.5 years. However, it can occur at any stage of development from SMR 2 to 5.
- Elongation and widening of the penis usually begins in SMR 3 and continues through SMR 5 (see Fig. 8-4).
- Rapid growth in height occurs. The PHV for males tends to occur late in middle puberty to early in late puberty. Boys generally lag about 2 years behind girls, but the height spurt can begin as early as 10.5 years or as late as 16 years. One fifth of normal adolescent males do not reach their PHV until SMR 5, and there is some evidence that late

TABLE 8-1   Adolescent Development and Related Anticipatory Guidance

Area of Development	Anticipatory Guidance
Physical	
Experience growth from prepubescence to sexual maturity.	Teach child about body functions (e.g., menstruation, nocturnal emissions) of both sexes.
Reach adult parameters of height and physical growth by late adolescence.	Provide prevention counseling regarding substance abuse, safety, and unintentional injuries (e.g., bicycle helmet use, seat belts, gun storage).
Become comfortable with one's body.	Offer reassurance that physical findings are normal; explain what to expect; listen to adolescents' concerns; encourage exercise, sports participation and body fitness; encourage healthy nutrition.
Cognitive	
Move from concrete thinking to ability to reason abstractly.	Emphasize value of successful completion of school.
	Engage adolescent in conversation, explain procedures, and answer questions; listen.
Develop personal value system and moral integrity.	Encourage discussion of what the adolescent believes is important and what the adolescent finds of value.
	Help the adolescent develop skills in conflict resolution and prevention.
	Discuss respect for rights, needs, and opinions of others.
Psychosocial	
Establish independence from parents.	Explain to parents an adolescent's need for privacy and that not joining in all family activities is not a sign of rejection.
	Discuss the notion that increased independence also requires increased responsibility.
Develop sense of self-identity.	Encourage adolescents to take responsibility for their own health care.
	Encourage adolescent to take on new challenges; discuss plans for the future (e.g., school, work, family).
Create new relationships with peers and other adults.	Discuss importance of activities with peers; identify healthy ways to be part of a group.
	Encourage the adolescent to participate in community activities.
	Provide information and opportunity to discuss questions regarding sexuality, how to differentiate between "love" and "infatuation," how to be sexually responsible, and how to protect against pregnancy and sexually transmitted diseases.

maturers may achieve greater PHV (Sherar et al, 2005). Males can continue to grow, although minimally, well beyond their teenage years.

• Change in the male voice occurs; this coincides with the PHV.

• Development of axillary, facial, and body hair occurs. Axillary hair generally does not appear before SMR 4 pubic hair. Facial hair appears only after SMR 4 pubic hair and does so in an ordered sequence. It starts at the outer corners of the upper lip and moves inward, then appears on the upper parts of the cheeks and middle of the lower lip, and finally grows along the sides and lower border of the chin. The extent of body hair is determined to a large extent by genetic factors. Body hair develops gradually after facial hair. The hair changes should not, however, be used to assess pubertal maturation related to changes in the endocrine system.

As with girls, the body composition of adolescent boys changes, sometimes causing great concern for the adolescent. The provider can be an invaluable source of information and reassurance. In contrast to females, males generally increase muscle mass and lose body fat during puberty.

Some changes associated with puberty may be unwelcome. For males, approximately half the population experiences *gynecomastia,* a transient enlargement of breast tissue. Gynecomastia generally lasts 12 to 18 months and resolves completely in nearly all cases by late puberty. In a small percentage of males, however, some palpable breast tissue may persist. Acne starts in early puberty, and by midpuberty many males have moderate to severe acne, which becomes somewhat worse by the end of puberty. In cases of persistent gynecomastia or severe acne, the provider should ask questions about the use of alcohol, marijuana, and anabolic steroids, all of which can exacerbate these conditions.

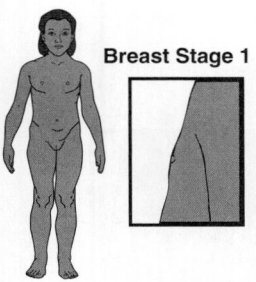

Breast Stage 1

Prepubertal; no noticeable change is seen in the size of the brest.

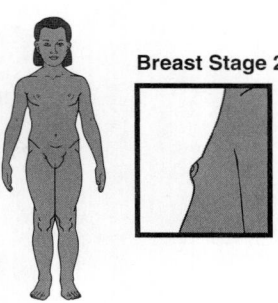

Breast Stage 2

Breast bud stage (thelarche); a small mound is formed by elevation of the breast and papilla, and the areolar diameter enlarges.

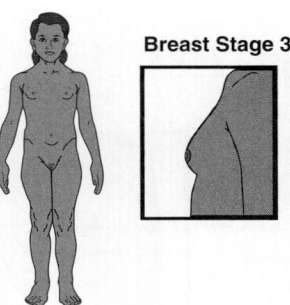

Breast Stage 3

Further enlargement of the breast and areola with no separation of their contours.

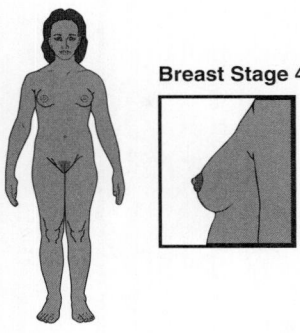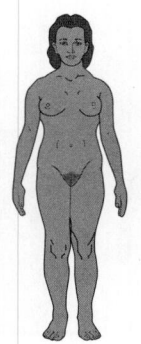

Breast Stage 4

Distinctive projection of the areola, with the papilla forming a secondary mound above the level of the breast. It is important to view the breast both anteriorly and laterally to appreciate this secondary mound.

Breast Stage 5

Adult-like; the areola has recessed to the general contour of the breast, and the overall size of the breast is increased. Not all women complete SMR 5.

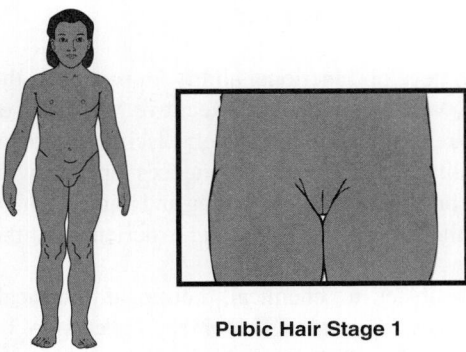

Pubic Hair Stage 1

Prepubertal or child-like; no pubic hair is present.

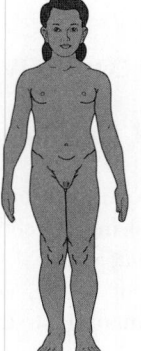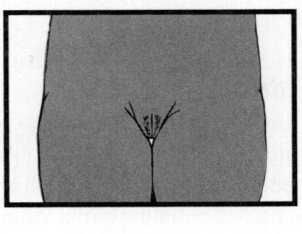

Pubic Hair Stage 2

First appearance of sexual hair (adrenarche or puarche); pubic hair is sparse, long, slightly pigmented, downy, straight or only slightly curled, and primarily located along the labia.

FIG. 8-3   Tanner stages: female. (Adapted from Division of Adolescent Medicine, Children's Hospital Medical Center, Cincinnati, 1995.)

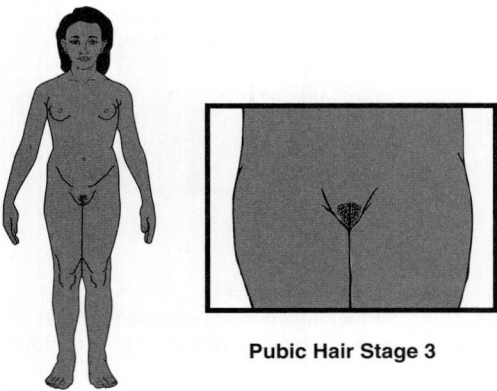

Pubic Hair Stage 3

Pubic hair is coarser, darker, and more curled; spreads over the middle of the pubic bone.

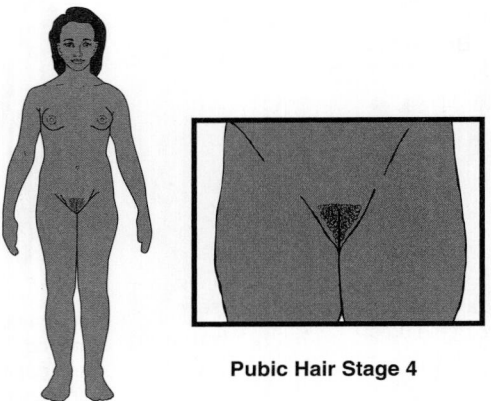

Pubic Hair Stage 4

Pubic hair is adult-like in appearance but not in distribution; does not extend onto the thighs.

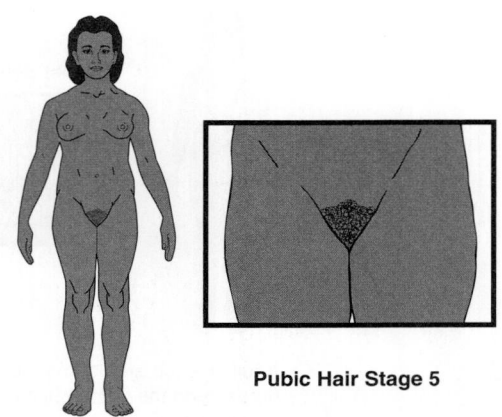

Pubic Hair Stage 5

Pubic hair is adult-like in appearance and extends onto the thighs; may extend in the midline in the shape of a broad-based triangle. Generally, females reach pubic hair stage 5 before reaching breast stage 5.

FIG. 8-3 Cont'd.

PSYCHOSOCIAL, EMOTIONAL, AND COGNITIVE DEVELOPMENT

Principles of Adolescent Psychosocial, Emotional, and Cognitive Development

As they transition from childhood to adulthood, all adolescents should achieve specific cognitive, emotional, and psychosocial developmental milestones. They should be able to:

- Feel a sense of belonging in a valued group
- Acquire skills and master tasks that are important to the valued group
- Develop a sense of self-worth
- Develop at least one reliable relationship with another individual
- Demonstrate cognitive potential

The adolescent's ability to achieve these goals depends in part on brain functioning. Although full sized, the adolescent brain continues to develop functional ability. In particular the prefrontal cortex, which coordinates executive functions of abstract thinking, reasoning, judgment, self-discipline, ethical behavior, personality, and emotions, experiences rapid growth. As with the infant brain, a process of pruning and reinforcement occurs, based on the stimuli, activities, and experiences of the teenager.

The brain is subject to chemical, hormonal, physical, and biologic changes. The adolescent brain appears to be particularly vulnerable to schizophrenia and to addiction. Schizophrenia most often appears in the second decade of life, during late adolescence or early adulthood, and is characterized by disturbances in memory and concentration, a decreased sense of connectedness, and changes in emotional responses. The individual often experiences hallucinations or hears voices. Though its cause is unknown, schizophrenia may

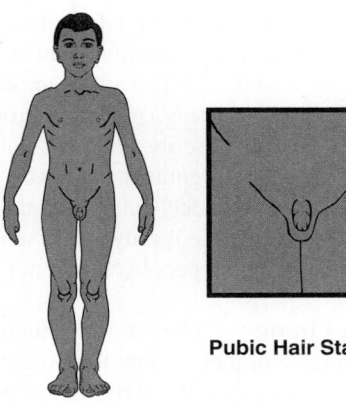

Pubic Hair Stage 1

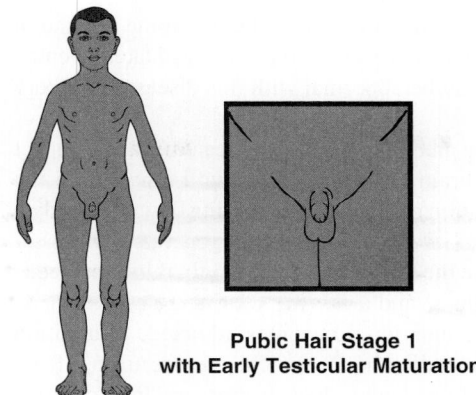

**Pubic Hair Stage 1
with Early Testicular Maturation**

Prepubertal; no pubic hair is present; penis, testes, and scrotum are child-like in size. The prepubertal testis is generally less than 4 mL in volume and less than 2.5 cm in greatest diameter.

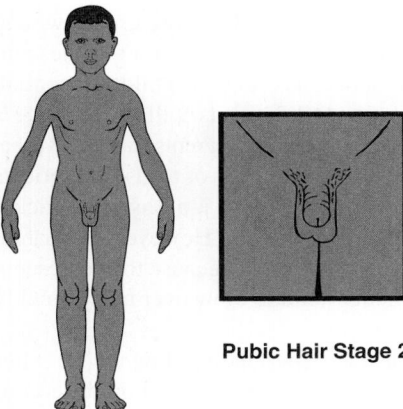

Pubic Hair Stage 2

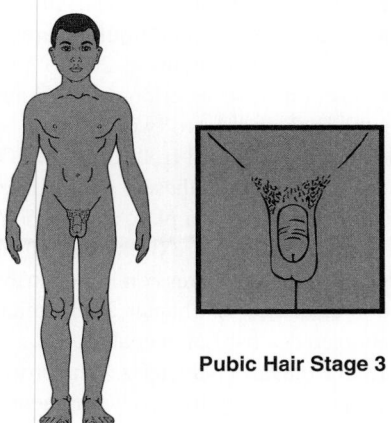

Pubic Hair Stage 3

First appearance of sexual hair (adrenarche or pubarche); sparse growth of fine, downy hair along the base of the penis. Enlargement of the scrotum and testes begins, but the penis usually does not enlarge. The scrotal skin reddens.

Pubic hair is darker, coarser, and curlier and extends over the middle of the pubic bone. Further growth of the testes and scrotum occurs, with enlargement of the penis, mostly in length.

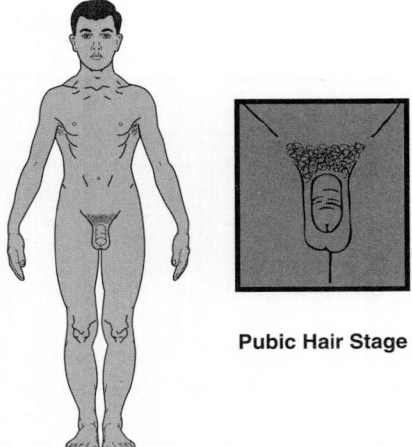

Pubic Hair Stage 4

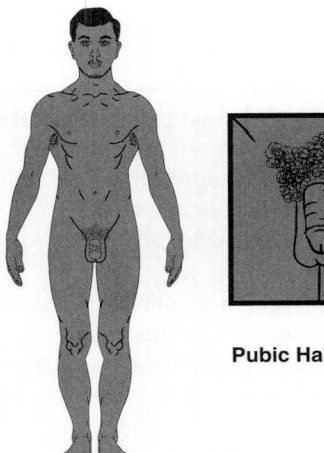

Pubic Hair Stage 5

Pubic hair is adult-like in appearance but not in distribution; does not extend onto the thighs. Growth of the testes (10 to 15 ml) and scrotum continues. The penis increases in size, especially in width, because of growth of the corpora cavernosa in response to testosterone.

Pubic hair is adult-like in appearance and extends onto the thighs; may extend toward the umbilicus. Gentials are adult-like in size. Growth of the penis is generally complete before full development of the testes or pubic hair.

FIG. 8-4   Tanner stages: male. (Adapted from Division of Adolescent Medicine, Children's Hospital Medical Center, Cincinnati, OH, 1995.)

be due to previous brain damage, and there is some indication that neurodevelopmental processes (e.g., enlarged lateral ventricles in the brain) may be abnormal with this disease (Pagsberg et al, 2007).

Drugs, including alcohol, have a significant negative impact on the adolescent brain, damaging the neural circuitry in the "reward" or motivation pathways and shutting down the body's ability to respond to stimuli that normally generate feelings of pleasure. In essence the drug becomes the only thing that leads to pleasurable feelings, and a craving for the drug is "etched" into the brain—the individual becomes addicted. In addition to contributing to addiction, brain changes resulting from exposure to alcohol can lead to loss of memory and cognitive function (Zeigler et al, 2005; Sher, 2006). Genetic structures of individuals vary, however, and not all brains respond to drugs in this way, but the adolescent brain is highly vulnerable.

Suicide and homicide are also risks for adolescents. Although motor vehicle accidents and unintentional injuries are the major causes of adolescent mortality, as many as 20% of teens in grades 9 to 12 across the country have seriously considered suicide, and 11% of deaths in the ninth- to twelfth-grade age group are due to suicide. In data collected from October 2004 to January 2006, an average of 16% of these teens had seriously considered suicide; 13% had made a plan, and 8.4% had attempted suicide. Particularly vulnerable are younger (ninth and tenth grade) white and Hispanic girls. Depression is a contributing factor to suicide and is discussed in Chapter 20. Homicide represents 15% of all teen-aged deaths (Eaton et al, 2006).

A wide variety of normal behavior characterizes the process of psychosocial, emotional, and cognitive development in adolescents. Three general principles may be used to understand the changes seen:

- Transition is continuous and generally smooth.
- Disruptive family conflict is not the norm.
- The quality of thinking changes from concrete to formal operational thinking.

Smooth Transition. The first principle of adolescent psychosocial development is that the transition from adolescence to adulthood is continuous and generally smooth. A commonly held myth is that adolescence is a period of "storm and stress." This view was originally described by G. Stanley Hall in 1904 (Hall, 1904). Although his argument was not based on research, this myth continues to be widely believed today. It is important to remember that adolescence is only one of many transitional phases in life and, for many people, it may not be particularly difficult.

Family Relationships Change. The second principle of adolescent psychosocial development is that the biologic, cognitive, and emotional changes experienced by adolescents prompt a reworking of family relationships. Some degree of adolescent-parent conflict is to be expected because of this reworking of relationships, but disruptive family conflict is not the norm. Mundane, everyday issues such as which clothes to wear, hairstyles, household chores, curfew, and friends continue to be the usual sources of parent-adolescent conflict, and negotiation between parent and child is essential. Inexperienced in negotiation, adolescents will often argue a point to excess. It may help to remind parents that this verbal debate, or "arguing," is a normal behavior of teens that reflects their use of more abstract thinking skills. It is a way of practicing abstract thinking and engaging parents. However, the parent should not become too deeply engaged because the adolescent rarely is, and the "arguments" tend to blow over fairly quickly (Box 8-1).

Families should not be experiencing one crisis after another. If family crises are the norm, one should be concerned. When true turmoil exists, it usually represents psychopathology and will not be simply "outgrown." Careful assessment and treatment are required. Behavior that results in negative consequences is cause for concern (e.g., red hair dye grows out, but being expelled from school has long-term consequences).

BOX 8-1 **Tips for Parents: Adolescent Survival Guide**

- Start with clear rules and expectations before children are teenagers. Work on developing good communication with children early and continue through adolescence. State expectations and future consequences before trouble has occurred (e.g., before the dance, not when the teen comes home late).
- Be firm and follow through.
- Try to be flexible and allow teenagers to negotiate. Discussing principles and negotiating solutions are valuable life skills for the future. Do not negotiate rules that are nonnegotiable.
- Fighting and arguing are typical, often employed by teens as they practice their developing reasoning skills. Often teens are engaged more recreationally than emotionally. Therefore, when the parent is tired, disengage and walk away. Try not to take what they say personally.
- Teenagers want parents to be involved, concerned, and asking questions. They just may not know it or know how to express their desire.
- Know who their friends are and call those parents from time to time. Compare household rules if possible.
- Be involved at their school if possible. Try to meet their teachers and stay in contact with them.
- Continue to involve teenagers in family activities, even when they no longer want to. Bringing friends along will help.
- Keep promises made to teens. This builds trust and respect and makes you a role model.

Cognitive Changes.   The third principle of adolescent psychosocial development is about change in cognitive abilities. Adolescents develop what Piaget referred to as *formal operational thinking,* characterized by the use of propositional thinking and abstract reasoning. The principal difference between concrete and formal operational thinking is the ability to reason using verbal manipulation rather than in terms of concrete objects. In early adolescence, thinking tends to be very concrete. The classic example is an adolescent who when asked, "Are you sexually active?" responds, "No, I just lie there" or when asked, "What brought you here to see me today?" answers, "The bus." Around 14 years and throughout adolescence, most teenagers acquire increasing sophistication in abstract thought. They learn to conceptualize about past and future events and to relate actions to consequences. During this process, adolescents begin to:

- Consider values. The ones they challenge most are those with which they are most familiar (e.g., in the past they always attended church on Sundays or always went to their grandmother's for Sunday dinner, but now they do not want to).
- Understand concepts of good and evil and understand human nature (e.g., not all authority figures are good people).
- Be aware of contradictions between what is said and what is done (e.g., adolescents are acutely aware when parents tell their children not to smoke or drink even though they do or when they tell them to wear their seat belts although the parent does not).
- Understand the significance of the concept of time (past, present, future) and begin thinking about what they will be doing in the future (e.g., college, technical school, job, marriage, and family).

Although most teenagers develop the ability to translate experiences into abstract ideas and think about the consequences of actions, approximately one third do not achieve more fully sophisticated thinking abilities, even as adults. Children who have demonstrated intellectual skill continue to be more successful in academic or intelligence testing as adolescents and adults (Shaw et al, 2006). Neurologic changes underlying development of executive function, memory, social inhibition, intelligence, and cognition in adolescence are being investigated; additional research is needed to clarify relationships among environment (e.g., drugs, alcohol, noise, etc.), innate traits, and cognitive ability (Blakemore & Choudhury, 2006; Paus, 2005; Steinberg, 2005; Dahl, 2004).

Emotional Changes of Adolescence

Hormones present during puberty cause emotional and physical changes. As with physical growth and development, emotional changes appear differently in males than in females. Some males may experience an association between an increase in testosterone and sad or anxious feelings, acting out, aggressive behavior, or sexual activity.

Some emotional changes that occur are not directly associated with hormonal changes. Research has shown that boys with adultlike physiques are given more leadership roles, are more proficient in sports, are perceived as more attractive and smarter than their peers, and are more popular than others in their age group. In general, they also demonstrate higher self-esteem in early adolescence. Late-maturing boys who are short and childlike in appearance until 15 years or older tend to show more personal and social maladjustment over the entire course of adolescence. They can be insecure, suggestible, vulnerable to peer pressure, and subjects of bullying or seen as weak, immature, and less competent than average. Males, as they progress through puberty, typically develop a more positive self-image and mood, whereas females may feel a diminished sense of attractiveness as their bodies mature. Boys tend to be more satisfied with their body image and, depending on their current size, may want to either gain or lose weight, whereas girls are more likely to express a desire to lose weight (Kostanski et al, 2004; Muris et al, 2005). This dissatisfaction with body image can appear before adolescence (in one study of third graders, 17% of boys and 24% of girls had dieted or were dieting to lose weight [Robinson et al, 2001]), may be related to weight changes in early childhood (Angle et al, 2005), and can continue into the teen years (McCabe & Ricciardelli, 2001).

The emotional affect and behavior of pubescent females differ in other ways from those of boys. Both early-maturing boys and girls demonstrate more risky behaviors than do adolescents who are late maturing, but girls are at greater risk as a result of romantic liaisons. Often these early bloomers get "bumped up" to an older group of peers and become the objects of sexual attention from older males. The developing body of early-maturing females may not match their chronologic age or emotional maturity. This difference can influence their behavior and place them at risk for early sexual involvement, smoking, and drinking (Halpern et al, 2007).

Egocentrism of Adolescents

Changes in the quality of adolescent thinking coupled with physical and emotional changes give rise to a form of egocentrism. This change may result in a rather self-centered, but not necessarily selfish, view of the world. Although there are recommendations that this prototype requires more research for validation (Vartanian, 2000) and evidence that adolescent egocentrism continues into adulthood (Frankenberger, 2000), four major types of egocentrism in the adolescent are generally recognized (Elkind, 1984):

- *Imaginary audience:* Everyone is thinking about them.
- *Personal fable:* They are special.
- *Overthinking:* They make things more complicated than they are.
- *Apparent hypocrisy:* Rules apply differently to them than to others.

Imaginary Audience.   Abstract thinking allows teenagers to wonder what others are thinking about. At the same time, adolescents are obsessed by the physical changes brought about by puberty. These changes and their new thinking abilities create the notion that everyone is thinking about the same thing that they are (i.e., them). Teenagers may believe that one can read minds and know what others are thinking. For example, a boy who goes to the drugstore to purchase a condom may feel that he is "on stage," the object of everyone's scrutiny. An adolescent wearing orthopedic braces may think that everyone is staring at him. A young girl who has a pimple on her nose may feel that it is the first thing others see when they look at her.

Personal Fable. The second type of egocentrism is the personal fable. If everyone is watching you and thinking about you (thanks to the imaginary audience), you must be someone special. The personal fable is the concept that the laws of nature do not apply to oneself and that one's thoughts and feelings are totally unique. The personal fable has a very positive aspect in that it provides adolescents with a sense of importance, purpose, and hope; it helps them to imagine possibilities and opportunities in their lives and futures. Personal fable can also have a negative impact (e.g., when adolescents believe that they will never grow old, cannot get pregnant [especially the first time], cannot get a sexually transmitted infection despite engaging in unprotected intercourse, or will not suffer long-term consequences from substance use).

Overthinking. Overthinking involves making things more complicated than they need to be. An example might be an adolescent who attributes complicated motives to simple oversights (e.g., an adolescent boy who thinks that his parents would not have divorced if only he had helped more with the chores around the house or an adolescent girl who breaks up with her boyfriend because she assumes that he does not like her because he did not compliment her on her new red dress).

Apparent Hypocrisy. Apparent hypocrisy is the notion that rules apply differently to adolescents than they do to others. For example, an adolescent girl may believe that she should have free access to her parent's clothes and electronic equipment (such as the stereo or home computer), whereas her parents entering her room to borrow a tape constitutes an invasion of privacy.

■ DEVELOPMENTAL SCREENING AND ASSESSMENT

APPROACHES TO ASSESSMENT OF ADOLESCENTS

Throughout infancy and the preschool and school years, the focus of the health care visit is the parent or caregiver and the child as a unit. This dyad changes with adolescence. Teenagers must be evaluated independently of their parents, and developmental issues must be discussed privately with the adolescents themselves. Nonetheless, parents remain concerned, and it is ideal that they be involved in their child's health care. Adolescents continue to be part of the family system, and providers should work with adolescents to maximize communication with parents around health issues. Some providers may believe that involving parents or other significant adults in the adolescent's care is essential. However, that decision is not always the provider's to make,

and it may not always be in the best interest of the adolescent. Recently for example, some counties and states have passed laws requiring parental notification before providing contraceptives to minors. Rather than having the intended consequence of encouraging adolescents to talk with their parents and decrease sexual activity, the birth rate in the areas where the laws were passed increased significantly (Zavodny, 2004). Adolescents must be actively included in decisions about sharing information with others. For many sensitive health issues, providers will need to help the teenager understand and evaluate the risks and benefits of involving family members. They must also provide guidance and support on how to best inform the family, if that is the final choice. This approach can help protect a teen from the parent who may be abusive or unsafe. It also can reduce the problem of parents who are upset if they feel they are denied information about the child they love and for whom they feel responsible.

Effective interviews with adolescent clients are based on the use of good general interviewing techniques: demonstrating respect for the client; establishing parameters of what can be accomplished during the visit; using appropriate body language, active listening, and communication techniques; and working with the client to develop a realistic, individualized treatment plan. The provider gives the message that the teenager and his or her concerns are important, that no judgments will be made, and that the provider and teenager are a team, working together to achieve the healthiest outcome possible.

Preserving confidentiality with the teenager is essential. Adolescents should be reassured that the provider will not share information with the child's parent or caregiver (general confidentiality) unless the adolescent agrees, or unless the health of the child or others may be compromised (e.g., threat of potential suicide, violence, evidence of an eating disorder). Providers must inform the teenager that there are limits to confidentiality (limited confidentiality). As "mandatory reporters," primary health care providers are required by law to report information that puts the child or others in danger (e.g., physical or sexual abuse; some states require reporting teen sexual activity, even if consensual, if an age difference of 3 or more years exists between the couple). If adolescents perceive that their provider will maintain confidentiality, they are more likely to disclose more sensitive, relevant information (Thrall et al, 2000); and it has been found that even when providers tell adolescents there are limits to their confidentiality, teens continue to disclose (Ford et al, 1997).

The American Medical Association (AMA) has developed a thorough interview format for teens in their published *AMA Guidelines for Adolescent Preventive Services (GAPS)* program (Elster & Kuznets, 1994), and basic health assessment of adolescents is discussed in Chapter 2. The HEADSS technique can be used to assess risk behaviors of adolescents (see discussion later in this chapter).

For teenagers who are hesitant to discuss sensitive issues, a questionnaire or checklist may be an effective way to collect information. Questionnaires used to identify adolescent strengths have also been created by the Search Institute and have been used by communities to enhance adolescent self-concept (see Chapter 17).

PHYSICAL DEVELOPMENT

Adolescents should have height, weight, body mass index (BMI), and blood pressure measured at each health maintenance visit. The growth trajectory should be evaluated, using growth grids to identify norms. The Tanner stage should be recorded at each visit to evaluate progression of pubertal changes initiated by the endocrine system. Testicular growth can be directly assessed by palpation of the testes in the scrotum and comparison of their size with a standardized orchidometer. Self-assessment is generally reliable, and adolescent males can be asked to evaluate their own level of development if provided with standards against which to compare themselves. Varicocele, or enlarged veins palpable in the scrotum, may develop at sexual maturity and are not cause for alarm unless a discrepancy in testicular size is noted on examination. Gynecomastia in boys should be noted. Scoliosis may develop rapidly at this age, and assessment should be done annually. The thyroid gland should be palpated because goiter may appear in this age group. Additionally, the teen should be questioned about attitudes regarding physical growth and development. Dissatisfaction with body appearance might warrant further probing to elicit unhealthy behavior (e.g., bingeing and purging, steroid use).

COGNITIVE DEVELOPMENT

Assessment should include questions about school attendance, school performance, and educational or career goals. Children who are behind a grade have a 20% to 30% greater chance of dropping out of school, and school failure could be viewed as "failure to thrive in adolescence" (Reiff, 1998). Chronic absenteeism, class skipping, and other types of school avoidance indicate a problem that may be related to cognitive ability and should be assessed in depth. Objective assessment of cognitive development, as with school-age children, requires formal psychological testing, which is best done through schools.

SOCIAL AND EMOTIONAL DEVELOPMENT

Key areas to assess in relation to social and emotional development include adolescents' emerging independence from family, relationships with peers, and goals for the future (an area that older teenagers should address more specifically than younger adolescents).

Adolescents should be interviewed about school, family, and peer relationships; safety (e.g., use of seat belts); exposure to violence, abuse, or weapons in their home or community; mental health issues such as mood, depression, anger problems, or suicidal ideation; sexuality, sexual activity, and sexual orientation; and involvement in risk behavior such as tobacco, alcohol, and prescription or street drug use and eating disorders.

PARENT ASSESSMENT

As at other developmental stages of childhood, parents are also changing in response to the adolescent's pressure on the family. Parents, too, need advice, support, and encouragement.

GAPS (Elster & Kuznets, 1994) also offers recommendations for health guidance for parents. The parent interview should occur on three occasions during adolescence: early, middle, and late. The interview should consist of parents' concerns about adolescents relating to:

- Health problems
- Physical development
- Social and emotional development
- Parenting issues
- Changing family structures

If problems exist in the parent's view or a discrepancy and potential conflict emerge in the interviews, the provider should bring the teen and parent together to clarify the concern and offer counseling.

■ ANTICIPATORY GUIDANCE DURING ADOLESCENCE

One simple way to understand adolescence is to divide it into three psychosocial developmental phases: early, 11 to 14 years old or junior high school; middle, 15 to 17 years old or high school; and late, 18 to 21 years old or college, work, or vocational-technical school.

Each phase is characterized by certain behavior. Understanding such behavior can assist in identifying behavior of concern to the adolescent or family. Within each developmental phase, adolescents deal with issues of autonomy, body image, peer group involvement, and identity development.

EARLY ADOLESCENCE (11 TO 14 YEARS)
Parameters of Normal Development
Early adolescence is the most difficult adjustment period for young people (Larson et al, 2002). Rapid changes are occurring simultaneously in all parts of the adolescent's life; cognitive skills may not be able to keep pace with physical changes; emotional reactions may overwhelm the child's ability to understand and cope. Early adolescents are often confused, even frightened, by the changes they are experiencing. They can be difficult people to be around, and the responses their behavior elicits from parents and other adults may be exactly the opposite of the support, caring, and understanding they desperately need.

Young adolescents begin to renegotiate relationships with parents and other significant adults and develop more intimate contacts with their peers. At the same time, lacking experience and social skills, they may not yet be a part of an adolescent subculture and can be very lonely. At this stage, teenagers can appear to be antiadult, preferring to spend more time with friends than with family, and suddenly finding their parents to be an embarrassment. This behavior is a normal and healthy step toward maturity and a first step toward independence. One way of demonstrating independence is to challenge parental authority. The adolescent may become more argumentative and disobedient, refuse to do chores, and want to renegotiate rules (e.g., curfews, allowance, household responsibilities).

Wide mood swings—from euphoria to sadness—can occur within a matter of minutes. Normative fluctuations of mood are linked to adolescent developmental processes and are characterized by their transient nature, commonly measured in hours or days. These emotional fluctuations can and should be distinguished from the unremitting, long-standing mood and behavior changes of serious depressive disorders.

During this period, adolescents become extremely conscious of their bodies as they adjust to the physical changes they are experiencing. They begin to spend more time in front of the mirror combing their hair, checking their skin, and putting on makeup. Clothes and appearance become more important for all teenagers, including those with a developmental delay or chronic handicap.

The most important question for an early adolescent is "Am I normal?" Health care providers for adolescents must never lose sight of this concern. Early adolescents often use their friends as the measure by which they determine standards of normal appearance. They become overly sensitive and critical of their own appearance, certain they are too tall, too short, too fat, too thin, too developed, or not developed enough. Health care providers should allay anxiety during an adolescent's examination by actively affirming normalcy.

As their thinking abilities develop, teenagers daydream frequently. Parents and teachers need to be reminded that daydreaming is cognitive work for adolescents and that they need time to participate in this activity. At the same time, adolescents should be given the opportunity to use their growing reasoning skills to actively solve problems, explore values, and examine principles on which they make decisions.

Early adolescents set idealistic goals that change frequently. One day they want to be an engineer and the next day a pilot or a parent who stays home to raise children. Typically, these adolescents experience a drop in academic performance in junior high school, which is related to motivation rather than ability. Much of adolescents' time is used in the development of new friendships as a greater number of opportunities become possible.

Adolescents have a desire for greater privacy. They often spend more time in their room alone listening to music or talking on the phone. They magnify their problems and believe that no one could possibly understand what they are feeling.

Early adolescents begin to develop their own value system. They may try value systems other than the one that they have learned from their family, often leaving family members befuddled or even threatened. However, once adolescence is complete, young adults often have a modified value system very similar to the one with which they grew up.

The onset of secondary sex characteristics increases anxieties about menstruation, wet dreams, masturbation, and size of the breasts or penis. This is an opportune time to dispel myths (e.g., masturbation causes blindness and acne) and to provide anticipatory guidance (e.g., a premenarchal girl often

has vaginal leukorrhea, which is generally a clear, mucoid discharge). Same-sex friendships occur, usually with one best friend. These strong friendships may lead to fleeting same-sex experimentation and the further development of a sexual identity. Contact with the opposite sex is usually in groups (e.g., middle school dances with boys on one side of the gym and girls on the opposite side). The peer group serves the purpose of aiding continued identity development.

Sexual feelings emerge, and behavior includes masturbating, telling dirty jokes, making lewd remarks to others, demonstrating interest in watching explicit sexual scenes in the media, or looking at magazines of nude individuals. The type of sexual experimentation may vary greatly, depending on the adolescent's subculture. For example, by this age, some teenagers have already experienced sexual intercourse or pregnancy, whereas others have not even held hands.

Developmental Anticipatory Guidance

Anticipatory guidance should be an individualized discussion with teenagers that helps them understand, respond to, and take responsibility for their own behavior and development. Separate discussions need to be conducted with parents to help them understand and support their child' maturation and need for independence. In these discussions, the provider should clarify what values and expectations parents have for their child and how the teenager perceives those expectations. Some discussion points are outlined here. These topics are not all-inclusive, and they should not be covered exhaustively at each visit. They can be used to apply developmental concepts to the adolescent's daily experiences. Ideas for assessment and management of any problems that emerge from these discussions can be found in the following chapters (e.g., sexuality issues are discussed in Chapter 19).

Physical and Sexual Development

- *Rapid physical growth:* Knowing what to expect and understanding the implications of growth (e.g., for injury) help adolescents become more comfortable with their bodies.
- *Physical activity:* Finding ways to enjoy physical activity (e.g., team, club, or individual sports) is an important part of adolescence and sets the stage for lifelong health.
- *Sexuality:* Discussion should include the following:
  - Menstruation and its management
  - Masturbation and nocturnal emissions
  - Pubertal development of the opposite sex
  - Anticipated sexual changes
  - Abstinence counseling
  - Protection against sexually transmitted diseases and pregnancy

Cognitive Development

- Discuss with the adolescent how meeting academic responsibilities is a priority activity that needs to be integrated with other activities.
- Discuss with the adolescent how changes in cognitive abilities may contribute to "overthinking" or a sense of confusion; encourage him or her to do "reality checks" with a trusted adult.

Social and Emotional Development

- *Family interaction:* Parents should not interpret their child's refusal to join in all family activities as rejection of the family.
- *Feelings:* Discuss how learning to identify feelings is the first step in understanding how "feelings" influence body processes.
- *Peers:* Peer interaction is important for all teenagers.
- *Dating relationships:* Healthy relationships are based on mutual respect.
- *Diversity:* Maturation involves understanding and appreciating multicultural differences.
- *Independence and responsibility:* Developing increased independence and accepting responsibilities at home and school and in the community are essential to maturation.
- *Privacy:* Some privacy within the home should be expected.

Self-Care

- *Accident prevention:* Correct and consistent use of helmets, seat belts, and proper sports equipment should be taught and encouraged.
- *Weapons:* Access to guns and other weapons should be restricted, with emphasis on safety and responsibility.
- *Abusive behavior:* Counseling should be provided on the following:
  - Avoiding gang involvement
  - Preventing the use of drugs, cigarettes, and alcohol
  - Stopping substance use for those who are using
  - Preventing date rape or other abusive relationships
- *Health care:* Immunization for human papillomavirus (HPV), diphtheria and tetanus toxoids and acellular pertussis vaccine (DTaP), and meningococcal meningitis are recommended.

MIDDLE ADOLESCENCE (15 TO 17 YEARS)

Parameters of Normal Development

Parental conflict peaks as middle adolescents continue to argue and renegotiate issues such as curfew, allowance, going to parties or movies, and dating. Rules and expectations must be clear by this stage. Physical development is nearing completion. Middle adolescents have less concern about body changes, but increased interest in making themselves more attractive. As body attractiveness increases in importance, teenagers spend more time with hairstyles, clothes, and, for some, dieting or activities to build muscle mass. Teenagers with apparent handicaps are equally concerned about their body image and participate in the same activities to improve their appearance. Middle adolescents defy the limits of their bodies, and many have periods of excessive physical activity followed by periods of lethargy.

Middle adolescence is the essence of adolescence and its subculture. Picture in your mind's eye what typical adolescents look like and how they behave (e.g., jocks, nerds, skaters, druggies, Goths). What are they wearing? How do they act? What language are they using to communicate to adults and to one another? The picture that probably comes to mind is that of a middle adolescent. Middle adolescents stand out for their unique appearance. Peer group involvement is intense and includes the establishment of a dress code, communication style, and code of conduct. They tend to be more nonadult than antiadult, a characteristic of early adolescents. By this time, more than twice as much of adolescents' time is spent with peers as with adults. The need for peer contact is equally important for teenagers with developmental disabilities, chronic handicaps, or both. However, peer involvement may be more limited for this group for any number of reasons (e.g., ostracism by the peer group, parental overprotectiveness, lack of social skills).

Sexual drive emerges, and middle adolescents begin to explore their ability to attract a partner. Dating activity and sexual experimentation and intercourse are beginning at younger ages. Frequently, physical urges precede emotional maturity, and societal pressure to experiment with sex is great. Adolescents of today are much more sexually tolerant than their predecessors. They are more sexually active than their parents were at the same age and may be more sexually active than adolescents of any earlier time, including their older siblings. Ambivalence about desire for pregnancy is not uncommon, especially among adolescents lacking clear future goals.

Intellectual sophistication and creativity increase in middle adolescents. Practicing these skills of reasoning, logic, and decision-making strengthens the adolescent's ability to establish healthy patterns as an adult. They demonstrate increased concern with neighborhood issues and certain societal issues, such as war or peace and the environment.

Because of the developing egocentrism and the concept of personal fable, with feelings of omnipotence, invulnerability, and immortality, risk-taking and behavioral experimentation intensify. This stage may include smoking, use of alcohol, sexual activity, or drinking and driving.

Developmental Anticipatory Guidance
Physical and Sexual Development

- *Physical growth:* Rapid growth and increasing skill allow adolescents to engage in a wider variety of activities.
  - Recommend fitness and sports activities; discuss the dangers of performance-enhancing drugs.
  - Recommend involvement in other activities (e.g., clubs, hobbies, sports).
  - Discuss nutrition and the relationship between good nutrition and health and a positive body image.
- *Sexuality:* Provide discussion and counseling about the following:
  - Responsible sexual behaviors
  - Implications of sexual intercourse
  - Postponement of coitus or the choice of abstinence
  - Prevention of sexually transmitted diseases
  - Birth control, including emergency methods
  - Breast or testicular self-examination

Cognitive Development

- Discuss the importance of completing schooling and making plans for the future.
- Acknowledge and validate more abstract reasoning.

Social and Emotional Development

- Family interactions:
  - Families should set reasonable limits for adolescents' behavior.

- Families need to show interest in teenagers' work, interests, and activities.
- Peers:
  - Adolescents should establish relationships with peers based on mutual respect, not promiscuous behavior.
- *Independence and responsibility:* Discuss how the adolescent is:
  - Learning to constructively resolve conflicts and manage feelings of anger
  - Learning to identify symptoms of stress and use of stress-reducing techniques

Self-Care

- *Accident prevention:* Encourage correct and consistent use of helmets, seat belts, and proper sports equipment.
- *Weapons:* Access to guns and other weapons should be restricted, with emphasis on safety and responsibility.
- *Abusive behavior:* Counseling should be provided on the following:
  - Avoiding gang involvement
  - Preventing the use of drugs, cigarettes, and alcohol
  - Stopping substance use for those who are using
  - Preventing date rape and other abusive peer relationships
  - Avoiding self-harm (e.g., cutting, bingeing and purging)

LATE ADOLESCENCE (18 TO 21 YEARS)

Parameters of Normal Development

Many late adolescents are preparing for high school graduation or entry to college. They are working, entering the military, marrying, or participating in a vocational or technical training program. These are all examples of normal behavioral autonomy. This period of late adolescence is a time when decisions are made about how to contribute to society as a responsible adult.

By now, adolescents usually relate to the family as adults. Relationships with parents and family are gradually renegotiated to a more adult-adult basis. The role of the parent during late adolescence should be one of support. By the end of late adolescence, this status has optimally progressed to autonomy for adolescents in the context of continuing strong ties of affection to the family.

Late adolescents have attained an adult level of reasoning skills. They are generally capable of understanding the consequences of their actions and behavior and can make complex and sophisticated judgments about human relationships. They no longer base their judgments about people on overt behavior, but have a good understanding of inner motivations, including multiple determinants of an action. Of course, neither teenagers nor adults consistently use this mature level of thinking, and some never reach this level of cognitive maturity.

A substantial number of late adolescents have established their sexuality and entered into an intimate, committed partner relationship. Selection of a partner is based more on individual preferences and less on the peer group's values.

Much of the final shaping of identity centers on adolescents' perceptions of their future options as adults. Among contemporary late adolescents, roughly half attend college, and the other half enter the adult world of work, though increasing cost of higher education is making it more difficult for many young people to afford college. In many significant ways, the

years in college offer a "moratorium," a time to engage in further consolidation of identity. College life offers both maximal autonomy and a structured, supportive environment in which to complete developmental tasks. In some ways, it could be considered a prolonged adolescence. Those adolescents who enter the workforce and leave home immediately out of high school have quite different tasks and experiences. Their identity may be consolidated earlier because they do not have the added time and supportive structures of the college experience. They cannot delay facing the issues of earning a living, forming a family, and accepting other adult responsibilities. Some late adolescents opt to join the military and, especially in times of war, face demands that force them to take on adult responsibilities, for which they may not be psychologically or emotionally prepared. For adolescents who are unsuccessful in the educational system or the workplace (underemployed or unemployed), identity may be established by joining peers in gangs or by becoming socially isolated. Individuals in the military can experience years of posttraumatic stress that jeopardize their sense of self. All of these have negative implications for achieving healthy adult roles.

Developmental Anticipatory Guidance

Physical and Sexual Development

- *Physical growth:* Exercise, nutrition, and rest are important to optimal physical growth; encourage adolescent to incorporate them into lifestyle.
- *Sexuality:* Discussion and counseling should be provided about the following:
  - Responsible sexual behaviors
  - Implications of sexual activity—sexual feelings for the same or opposite sex should be discussed with a trusted adult or health professional
  - Postponement of coitus or the choice of abstinence
  - Prevention of sexually transmitted diseases
  - Birth control, including emergency methods
  - Breast or testicular self-examination

Cognitive Development

- Discuss the importance of completing academic work.
- Validate choices made to achieve positive future goals and plan for the future—college, vocational training, military, and job or career.

Social and Emotional Development

- *Family interactions:*
  - Closer relationships with and an interest in the family should be reemerging.
  - Families need to be supportive of independence efforts.
- *Peers:*
  - Intimate relationships are established.
  - Respect for the rights, needs, and views of others is a measure of maturity.
- *Independence and responsibility:* Adolescents should be encouraged to do the following:
  - Take on new challenges that increase self-confidence.
  - Identify talents and interests to be pursued.
  - Continue to clarify values and beliefs. Ethical and behavioral role modeling behavior is valued.

- Develop skills in conflict prevention; resolution reflects cognitive growth and maturity.
- Learn to manage stress.
- Find a balance between job and school or vocational training.

Self-Care

- *Accident prevention:* Encourage correct and consistent use of helmets, seat belts, and proper sports equipment.
- *Weapons:* Access to guns and other weapons should be restricted, with an emphasis on safety and responsibility.
- *Abusive behavior:* Counseling should be provided on:
  - Avoiding gang involvement
  - Preventing the use and selling of drugs, cigarettes, and alcohol
  - Stopping substance use for those who are using
  - Preventing date rape and other abusive relationships
- *Health care:* Assist the adolescent to learn about health insurance, how to enter and use the health care system, and to take responsibility for self-care.

■ COMMON DEVELOPMENTAL ISSUES FOR ADOLESCENTS

RISK BEHAVIOR

Description

Risk behavior consists of actions that jeopardize adolescents' physical, psychological, or emotional health. Although health-risk behaviors among adolescents have decreased in the past few years, they continue to be the major cause of morbidity and mortality for adolescents (Eaton et al, 2006). It is a paradox of adolescence that developmental tasks (i.e., gaining independence, developing one's own values, becoming comfortable with one's body, and establishing meaningful relationships) may be achieved (albeit in negative ways) through risk-taking behavior (Alsaker, 1996). Adolescents needing peer affiliation and striving for increased autonomy are likely to explore, experiment, and otherwise push the limits of their personal experience—often in ways that put them at risk for health-compromising outcomes. However, many adolescents engage in risk behaviors without apparent negative outcomes. Is an adolescent who is sexually active but uses condoms on a regular basis engaged in risk behavior? Is an adolescent who goes to a party on the weekend and has a beer or smokes marijuana at risk? On the other hand, some teenagers who seem at high risk do not engage in risk behavior. What factors keep them from doing so?

Epidemiology

Although it is normal for behavioral experimentation to occur during this time, adolescents vary tremendously in their ability to think abstractly about the consequences of risky behavior. Their thinking is often characterized by the notion that "it can't happen to me" (personal fable). Although adolescents have an increase in abstract cognitive skills, thinking related to emotionally charged topics (e.g., substance use, sex, school performance, peer pressure) is often less sophisticated. An adolescent who is drinking may be doing so in part to be accepted by friends or to feel a sense of independence and maturity. Because

the behavior meets important developmental needs, it may be difficult for the adolescent to look at it objectively and give it up. In addition, the impact of alcohol on brain function further limits the adolescent's reasoning ability.

Environmental factors, both social and physical, can influence adolescents' decisions to take risks. Factors that contribute to the adolescent engaging in risk behaviors include, but are not limited to, the following:

- Poor academic performance or low intellectual function
- Impulsivity or attention-deficit/hyperactivity disorder
- Role models for deviant behavior (e.g., parents who abuse drugs or engage in criminal behavior)
- Lack of constructive support or encouragement from others in social environment
- Low self-esteem
- Sense of hopelessness or helplessness
- Child abuse or other types of early emotional trauma
- Depression or other mental-emotional disorders
- Illiteracy or lack of job skills
- Poverty

Protective Factors

Protective forces may help counter the effects of risk factors and help adolescents make healthier lifestyle choices. Parent monitoring and direction in the child's life has a particularly strong protective influence (Dalton et al, 2006; Ancheta et al, 2005), and community support of positive adolescent behavior appears to minimize risk-taking (see Chapter 17). Examples of possible protective factors are:

- High self-esteem
- Sense of future
- Academic success
- Parental direction
- Involvement in the family
- An interested adult
- Community involvement

Adolescents with multiple risk factors and few protective factors are more likely to engage in risk behavior, with potential health- and life-threatening results. These adolescents need prompt attention and assessment to determine the likelihood of negative outcomes. Conversely, resilient adolescents who are doing well, despite multiple risk factors, should be acknowledged and applauded.

Assessment

All adolescents should be assessed for their level of risk-taking behavior. The provider's approach to a discussion of sensitive issues should include ensuring confidentiality, providing privacy, using constructive communication strategies, and establishing rapport.

The HEADSS technique is a method of assessing risk behavior. Areas for assessment include **H**ome, **E**ducation and employment, **A**ctivities, **D**rugs, **S**exuality, and **S**uicide and depression (Ehrman & Matson, 1998). Providers should also be alert for red flags at each developmental stage because delays in development may contribute to negative behavior (Table 8-2).

TABLE 8-2   Developmental Red Flags: Adolescent

Age	Physical and Sexual Development	Psychosocial Development	Cognitive Development

Early adolescence (11-14 years)	Difficulty reading close or distant
	Female kyphosis or scoliosis
	Less than Tanner stage 2
	Female short stature or lack of height spurt
	Poor nutrition, poor oral health, caries, malocclusion
	Loss of appetite
	Chronic disease, such as heart disease, diabetes, or a family member with a chronic or lifelong illness
	No physical activity; overweight
	Sleep disturbance
	Sexual experimentation
		Social habits:
		  Early experimentation with drugs or alcohol (including tobacco)
		Relationships:
		  Permissive or authoritarian parental style
		  No participation in home chores
		  History of family violence
		  School fights
		  No close or "best" friend
		  Friends or siblings in gangs
		  Cruelty to animals
		Sexuality:
		  Sexual orientation worries
		Mood:
		  Pervasive sad mood, feelings of hopelessness, suicidal thoughts or gestures, history of previous suicide attempt
		  Flattened affect without expressions of joy, sorrow, or excitement
		  Excessive worrying or rumination
		Self-concept:
		  Believes self to be "ugly" or "fat"; is dieting despite normal body size and shape
		  Negative feelings of self-worth
		  Does not fantasize or dream about adult career
			Low IQ
			Behind in grade or failing classes
			Chronic absenteeism or class skipping
			Attention problems
			Lack of organizational skills for homework
			Disruptive behavior
			Unable to identify feelings
			Unable to control own behavior (e.g., anger, impulsivity)

Middle adolescence (15-17 years)	Difficulty reading close or distant
	Male kyphosis or scoliosis
	Less than Tanner stage 4
	Male short stature or lack of height spurt
	Male muscular growth without testicular maturation
	Male persistent gynecomastia and acne
	Female primary or secondary amenorrhea
	Poor nutrition, poor oral health, caries, malocclusion
	Loss of appetite
	Chronic disease such as heart disease, diabetes, or a family member with a chronic or lifelong illness
	No physical activity; overweight
	Sleep disturbance
	Unprotected sexual intercourse
	Multiple sexual partners
		Social habits:
		  Recurrent experimentation or frequent use of drugs or alcohol; blackouts
		  Drinking and driving
		Relationships:
		  Excessively oppositional, defiant of all authority
		  Abusive dating relationships
		  School fights
		  No identified peer group
		  Gang association or involvement
		Sexuality:
		  Sexual orientation worries
		Mood:
		  Pervasive sad mood, feelings of hopelessness, suicidal thoughts or gestures, history of previous suicide attempt
		  Flattened affect without expressions of joy, sorrow, or excitement
		  Excessive worrying or rumination
		Self-concept:
		  Believes self to be "ugly" or "fat"; is dieting despite normal body size and shape
		  Negative feelings of self-worth
			Low IQ
			Behind in grade or failing classes
			Chronic absenteeism or class skipping
			Attention problems
			Disruptive behavior
			Unable to differentiate emotional states from physical states
			Unable to control own behavior (e.g., anger, impulsivity)
			Poor judgment

	TABLE 8-2 **Developmental Red Flags: Adolescent—Cont'd**		
Age	**Physical and Sexual Development**	**Psychosocial Development**	**Cognitive Development**

Late adolescence (18-21 years)	Difficulty reading close or distant
	Less than Tanner stage 4 or 5
	Poor nutrition, poor oral health, caries, malocclusion
	Loss of appetite
	Chronic disease such as heart disease, diabetes, or a family member with a chronic or lifelong illness
	No physical activity; overweight
	Sleep disturbance
	Unprotected sexual intercourse
	Multiple sexual partners
		No life goals
		Does not fantasize or dream about adult career
		Social habits:
		  Substance abuse
		  Drinking and driving
		Relationships:
		  Lacks intimate relationships
		  Abusive dating relationships
		  Unable to separate from peer groups
		  Unable to separate from parents
		  Gang association or involvement
		  Unable to keep a job
		Sexuality:
		  Sexual orientation worries
		Mood:
		  Pervasive sad mood, feelings of hopelessness, suicidal thoughts or gestures, history of previous suicide attempt
		  Flattened affect without expressions of joy, sorrow, or excitement
		  Excessive worrying or rumination
		Self-concept:
		  Believes self to be "ugly" or "fat"; is dieting despite normal body size and shape
		  Negative feelings of self-worth
			Low IQ
			Behind in grade or failing classes
			Dropout
			Attention problems
			Disruptive behavior
			Persistent egocentrism
			Unable to control own behavior (e.g., anger, impulsivity)
			Unable to reason or plan based on future and abstract concepts
			Poor judgment
			Chronic health care seeking for psychosomatic complaints

Clinical Findings

The following are considered examples of risk behavior:

- Substance use or abuse
- Poor academic performance
- Unprotected sexual intercourse
- Drinking and driving
- Delinquency or involvement with gangs
- Violence-related behavior, such as carrying weapons

The consequences of such behavior can be addiction, school failure, pregnancy and sexually transmitted diseases, accidents, convictions for driving under the influence, incarceration, or death. Engaging in chronic risk-taking behavior often arrests developmental progression toward adult emotional maturity.

Management

Interventions should be considered when the adolescent's behavior threatens the accomplishment of developmental tasks or the adolescent's health, safety, and well-being. Generally, when adolescents' behavior supports the achievement of developmental tasks, such behavior should be encouraged. Adolescents who pierce their noses, shave half of their heads, and spend evenings with friends, for example, may be irritating to parents, but their behavior can help them establish their autonomy, identity, and ability to relate to others. On the other hand, such behavior may be an indicator of more serious problems. Tattoos and body piercings, especially among younger adolescents, have been shown to have a strong correlation with high-risk behaviors (Carroll et al, 2002). It is important to understand the meaning of the behavior for the adolescent before making decisions about intervention.

The approach used when providing care to teenagers differs from that used with younger children. Earlier, parents were central to the success of interventions. Although parents are still critical to successful intervention, health care providers must recognize that the teenager makes the decisions, and mediation between parent and teen may be necessary at times. The provider's role is to give the adolescent information and guidance to make the best decisions possible. Such information can have a big impact. For example, two 10- to 15-minute counseling sessions during clinic visits ("brief interventions"), followed by two nurse-made phone calls reinforcing the advice given by the provider, significantly reduced drinking and decreased ER visits and motor vehicle crashes among a group of Wisconsin teenagers (Grossberg et al, 2004).

Generally, high-risk teenagers require numerous services. Health care providers need to know their state laws regarding adolescent health issues, how to access community resources, and how to use other professionals collaboratively. The following list identifies basic services that at-risk teenagers may need:

- Food resources for teenage parents and their offspring
- Temporary shelters for teenagers
- Counseling and mental health services for teenagers and their families
- Foster care services for teenage parents and their offspring
- Local medical and social work services
- Local juvenile justice system and protective services
- Drug rehabilitation programs for teenagers
- Alternative school and vocational education programs
- Sports, fitness, and community activities for teenagers; after school programs may be a particularly successful means of preventing risky behavior (Cabral, 2006)
- Support programs for teenagers, such as Big Brothers or Big Sisters

Advocating for children and adolescents at risk; involving their families, communities, and schools; and helping young persons identify an individual who cares for them and trusts them are important actions all health care providers can take.

■ SUMMARY

As adolescents struggle with issues of autonomy, body image, peer relationships, and, ultimately, identity, parents and health care providers must be aware of and sensitive to the phase of development and the range of normal behavior. Both risk and protective factors must be assessed accurately. Intervention requires weighing the balance of risk versus protective factors, the actual behavior, and the potential threat to health and well-being. At-risk situations cannot always be avoided; therefore adolescents and their families need anticipatory guidance and strategies for managing risk. The desired outcome is for the teen to emerge into adulthood with a healthy mind, body, and identity.

ℛESOURCE BOX

Adolescents

RESOURCES FOR PROFESSIONALS
Alliance of Professional Tattooists, Inc. (APT)
www.safe-tattoos.com
Organization for education of health professionals and the public

American Academy of Family Physicians
www.aafp.org

American Academy of Pediatrics
www.aap.org

Centers for Disease Control and Prevention (CDC)
www.cdc.gov

Kids Counsel: Center for Children's Advocacy
www.kidscounsel.org
Legal resources, information, and advocacy for children and adolescents. Project of Center for Children's Advocacy, University of Connecticut, School of Law

Search Institute
www.search-institute.org
Nonprofit group to promote healthy children, youth, and communities. Support service for parents: Mvparents.com

Society for Adolescent Medicine
www.adolescenthealth.org
Health professional group focused on adolescents

RESOURCES FOR PARENTS
Wolfe AE: *Get out of my life, but first could you drive me & Cheryl to the mall: a parent's guide to the new teenager*, NY, 2002, Farrar, Straus, and Giroux.

Riera M: *Staying connected to your teenager: how to keep them talking and how to hear what they're really saying*, Cambridge, MA, 2003, Perseus Books Group.

Riera M: *Uncommon sense for parents with teenagers*, Berkeley, CA, 2004, Celestial Arts.

Parenting Teens
www.parentingteens.com

MVParenting
www.Mvparenting.com
Project of Search Institute that provides parents with information and resources

RESOURCES FOR TEENS
Adolescent Health Transition Project
http://depts.washington.edu/healthtr
Resource for adolescents with special health care needs, chronic illnesses, physical or developmental disabilities

National Runaway Switchboard
www.1800runaway.org
1-800-621-4000
1-800-RUNAWAY (786-2929)

National Sexual Assault Hotline
RAINN
(www.rainn.org)
1-800-HOPE (4673)

Sex, etc.
www.sexetc.org

☑ DISCUSSION FORUM

1. A mother asks you whether her daughter (13 years old) should get the "new sex shot" (HPV vaccine). How do you solicit her concerns about the vaccine? What information and guidance do you give this mother? What other immunizations should this child receive?

2. During a routine sports physical exam on a 16-year-old girl, she tells you "a friend" has been "cutting herself" and asks for your advice. What counsel do you give her? What other issues may be confronting this child (e.g., abuse, depression, suicidal ideation)? What will be your plan for long-term care?

3. Discuss the best approach to interviewing adolescent clients. What issues and challenges do adolescents present to the primary care provider being able to gain their trust and confidence? How can you relate to adolescents to develop a healthy, interactive, and constructive patient-provider relationship?

REFERENCES

Alsaker FD: Annotation: the impact of puberty, *J Child Psychol Psychiatry* 37:249-258, 1996.

Ancheta R, Hynes C, Shrier LA: Reproductive health education and sexual risk among high-risk female adolescents and young adults, *J Pediatr Adolesc Gynecol* 18(2):105-111, 2005.

Angle S et al: Weight gain since infancy and prepubertal body dissatisfaction, *Arch Pediatr Adolesc Med* 159(6):567-571, 2005.

Blakemore SJ, Choudhury S: Development of the adolescent brain: implications for executive function and social cognition, *J Child Psychol Psychiatry* 47(3-4):296-312, 2006.

Cabral L: Twenty-first century skills for students: hands-on learning after school builds school and life success, *New Dir Youth Dev* (110):155-161, 2006.

Carroll ST et al: Tattoos and body piercings as indicators of adolescent risk-taking behaviors, *Pediatrics* 109:1021-1027, 2002.

Dahl RE: Adolescent brain development: a period of vulnerabilities and opportunities, *Ann NY Aca Sci* 1021:1-22, 2004.

Dalton MA et al: Parental rules and monitoring of children's movie viewing associated with children's risk for smoking and drinking, *Pediatrics* 118(5):1932-42, 2006.

Eaton DK et al: Youth risk behavior surveillance—United States, 2005, *MMWR Surveill Summ* 55(SS5):1-108, 2006.

Ehrman WG, Matson SC: Approach to assessing adolescents on serious or sensitive issues, *Pediatr Clin North Am* 45:189-204, 1998.

Elkind D: *All grown up and no place to go: teenagers in crisis,* Reading, MA, 1984, Addison-Wesley.

Elster A, Kuznets N: *AMA guidelines for adolescent preventive services (GAPS),* Baltimore, 1994, Williams & Wilkins.

Ford CA et al: Influence of physician confidentiality assurances on adolescents' willingness to disclose information and seek future health care: a randomized controlled trial, *JAMA* 278:1029-1034, 1997.

Frankenberger KD: Adolescent egocentrism: a comparison among adolescents and adults, *J Adolesc* 23(3):343-354, 2000.

Fujii K, Demura S: An approach to verifying delayed menarche in Japanese female athletes: analysis by wavelet interpolation method, *J Sports Med Phys Fitness* 45(4):580-593, 2005.

Grossberg PM, Brown DD, Fleming MF: Brief physician advice for high-risk drinking among young adults, *Ann Fam Med* 2(5):474-480, 2004.

Hall G: *Adolescence: its psychology and its relations to physiology, anthropology, sociology, sex, crime, religion and education,* Englewood Cliffs, NJ, 1904, Prentice-Hall.

Halpern CT, Kaestle CE, Hallfors DD: Perceived physical maturity, age of romantic partner, and adolescent risk behavior, *Prev Sci,* 8(1):1-10, 2007.

Kostanski M, Fisher A, Gullone E: Current conceptualisation of body image dissatisfaction: have we got it wrong? *J Child Psychol Psychiatry* 45(7):1317-1325, 2004.

Larson RW et al: Continuity, stability, and change in daily emotional experience across adolescence, *Child, Dev* 73:1151-1165, 2002.

McCabe MP, Ricciardelli LA: Parent, peer, and media influences on body image and strategies to both increase and decrease body size among adolescent boys and girls, *Adolescence* 36:225-240, 2001.

Muris P et al: Biological, psychological, and sociocultural correlates of body change strategies and eating problems in adolescent boys and girls, *Eat Behav* 6(1):1-22, 2005.

Pagsberg AK et al: Structural brain abnormalities in early onset first-episode psychosis, *J Neural Transm* 114(4):489-498, 2007.

Paus T: Mapping brain maturation and cognitive development during adolescence, *Trends Cogn Sci* 9(2):60-68, 2005.

Reiff MI: Adolescent school failure: failure to thrive in adolescence, *Pediatr Rev* 19:199-207, 1998.

Robinson TN et al: Overweight concerns and body dissatisfaction among third-grade children: the impacts of ethnicity and socioeconomic status, *J Pediatrics* 138:158-160, 2001.

Shaw et al: Intellectual ability and cortical development in children and adolescents, *Nature* 440(7084):676-679, 2006.

Sher L: Functional magnetic resonance imaging in studies of neurocognitive effects of alcohol use on adolescents and young adults, *Int J Adolesc Med Health* 18(1):3-7, 2006.

Sherar LB et al: Prediction of adult height using maturity-based cumulative height velocity curves, *J Pediatr* 147(4):508-514, 2005.

Steinberg L: Cognitive and affective development in adolescence, *Trends Cogn Sci* 9(2):69-74, 2005.

Tanner J: *Growth at adolescence,* Oxford, 1962, Blackwell.

Theodoropoulou A et al: Delayed but normally progressed puberty is more pronounced in artistic compared with rhythmic elite gymnasts due to the intensity of training, *J Clin Endocrinol Metab* 90(11):6022-6027, 2005.

Thrall JS et al: Confidentiality and adolescents' use of providers for health information and for pelvic examinations, *Arch Pediatr Adolesc Med* 154(9):885-892, 2000.

Vartanian LR: Revisiting the imaginary audience and personal fable constructs of adolescent egocentrism: a conceptual review, *Adolescence* 35:639-661, 2000.

Zavodny M: Fertility and parental consent for minors to receive contraceptives, *Am J Public Health* 94(8):1347-1351, 2004.

Zeigler DW et al: The neurocognitive effects of alcohol on adolescents and college students, *Prev Med* 40(1):23-32, 2005.

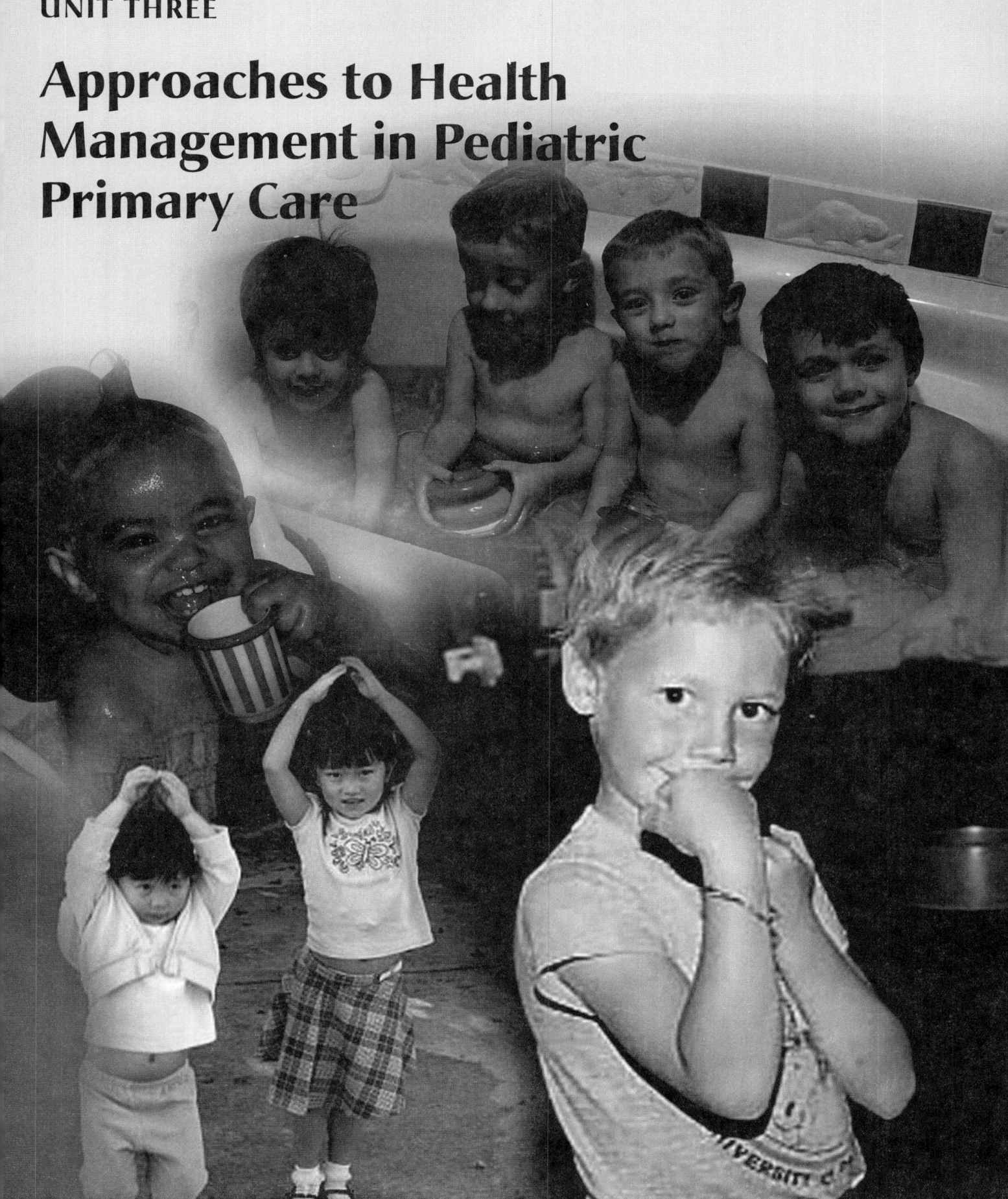

UNIT THREE

Approaches to Health Management in Pediatric Primary Care

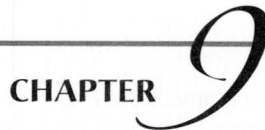
Introduction to Health Promotion

Catherine E. Burns

Health care is considered by many to be a birthright, and health is highly valued by all cultures in the world. Although valued, health is often compromised by behaviors of daily living. The landmark paper by McGinnis and Foege (1993) linked 50% of the mortality in the U.S. to lifestyle-related behaviors, such as tobacco use, poor dietary habits and inactivity, alcohol misuse, illicit drug use, and risky sexual practices. The majority of life-threatening and debilitating conditions of children are preventable. The goals of *Healthy People 2010 (HP 2010),* the health promotion and disease prevention objectives for 2010 (USDHHS, 2000), focus on essential lifestyle and behavioral factors related to health with benchmarks related to the above health-related behaviors. If the *HP 2010* goals are to be met, proactive, comprehensive health promotion and disease prevention strategies directed at individuals, families, and communities are absolutely essential.

Because meeting the *HP 2010* goals is a complex endeavor, the clinical prevention and population health curriculum framework was developed by an interdisciplinary team to assist students in all health professions to learn to meet *Healthy People 2010* goals (Allan et al, 2005). The framework presents four components—evidence base for practice, clinical preventive services, health systems and health policy, and community aspects of practice. The skilled clinician must take a broad view of practice and outcomes—it is not just the work of the clinician with individual patients that will make the difference, but working in an interdisciplinary way at the individual, family, community and health care systems, and policy levels (IOM, 2001). A broad array of professionals and citizens must be involved. Nurses, teachers, health educators, city planners, legislators, the industrial community, volunteers, and others from all levels of society need to guide development of an infrastructure that supports health care for all. Although this section of the book focuses on management of individual children within families, a broader perspective on community intervention and support for health also needs to be maintained. When opportunities to work with communities on their primary health care issues arise, the provider is strongly encouraged to become involved.

The nurse practitioner (NP) is in an excellent position to influence the health care outcomes of the nation through work in the health promotion arena. Teaching and modeling healthy behaviors help children learn to promote their own health, and because many health problems of children are carried into adulthood,

working with children has long-term health effects on the whole population. The broad perspective used by NPs serves as a framework to encompass all the factors that have an impact on health. The use of functional health patterns, a construct unique to nursing, focuses one's practice directly on lifestyle and health behaviors. Consistent and vigorous attention to issues of nutrition, activity, coping and stress tolerance, tobacco and drug use, accident prevention, and other factors of lifestyle has as much or more impact on achievement of national goals as time spent managing minor illnesses that occur in daily practice.

This chapter introduces the functional health patterns unit of the book. In this chapter, models that predict health behavior, factors that influence health promotion behaviors, functional health patterns used to describe the lifestyle domains that health promotion strategies must address, and specific management strategies for use with children and families are presented and discussed. Subsequent chapters in this unit examine each functional health pattern and its relationship to health.

MODELS TO PREDICT HEALTH BEHAVIOR

Four models are often used to predict health behaviors: the health belief model, the self-efficacy model, the health promotion model (Pender, 1996), and the transtheoretical (stages of change) model of behavior change (Prochaska, 1995; Prochaska et al, 1992; Prochaska et al, 1994). These models address issues of motivation, the first step toward action. They provide guidance for assessment of the motivation of the client, in addition to cues to plan efforts that will encourage the client to take positive action.

HEALTH BELIEFS AND SELF-EFFICACY MODELS

The health beliefs model explains behavior that seeks to prevent disease rather than behavior that attempts to promote health. According to this model, people engage in preventive behaviors if they have a reason or motive to do so and if they hold certain beliefs. They must meet the following criteria:
- Feel vulnerable or susceptible to the disease or health problem
- Believe that the disease will have negative consequences for them if they get it
- Be convinced that taking some action will reduce the risk
- Accept that the benefits of action outweigh the costs

The health beliefs model can be illustrated by assessing the motivation for tooth brushing behavior: the client must believe that caries are possible; that tooth loss, pain, or disfigurement would be unfortunate consequences of caries; that brushing teeth can prevent caries; and that the benefits of brushing outweigh the inconvenience, time, and costs of maintaining a supply of toothbrushes and toothpaste over time. This is a simple example. Getting a teenager to change the content in his or her diet after considering the consequences of obesity and perhaps heart disease in later life is not so easy.

Bandura's (1977) concept of self-efficacy augments the health belief model. Self-efficacy is the belief that the self is capable of acting effectively. "Expectations of personal efficacy determine whether coping behavior will be initiated, how much effort will be expended, and how long it will be sustained in the face of obstacles and aversive experiences." Bandura thought that two kinds of expectations were important. First, one estimates one's capacity to do what is required to achieve the goal. This expectation is based on performance accomplishments in the past, vicarious modeling experiences (watching the consequences of someone else's efforts), and verbal persuasion (someone saying, "You can do it"), with emotional arousal providing additional energy for action. Second, the person needs to believe that if he or she performs as well as expected, the outcome will be influenced favorably.

HEALTH PROMOTION MODEL

Pender (1996) developed a much more comprehensive model with a focus on health promotion rather than on disease prevention. The model consists of two main domains—cognitive-perceptual factors and modifying factors—that explain participation in health promotion behaviors (Fig. 9-1). The cognitive-perceptual factors include all the concepts in the health belief and self-efficacy models, locus of control notions, and individuals' definitions of health and their own health status estimates. Modifying factors in the model include demographic, biologic, behavioral, and situational factors, in addition to interpersonal influences. Together the two groups of factors are important in helping a person decide whether to engage in health promotion behaviors. This model was developed by a nurse and used most often by nurses.

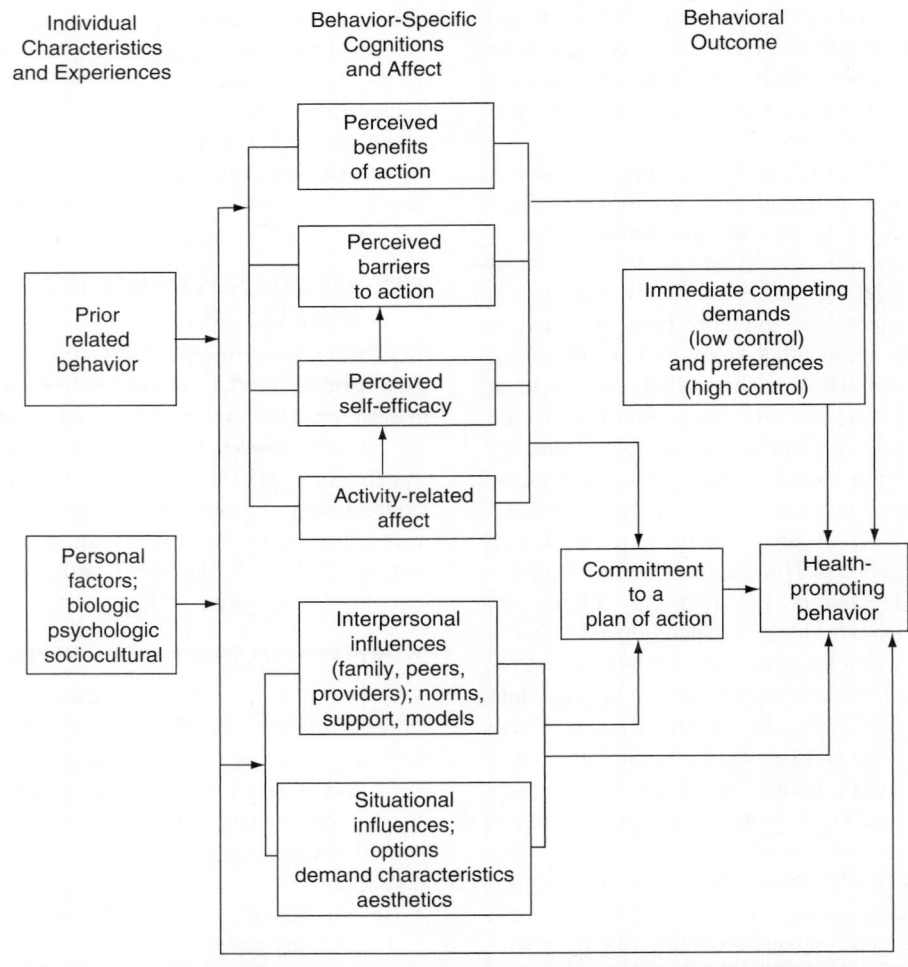

FIG. 9-1   Health promotion model. (From Pender N: *Health promotion in nursing practice,* ed 3, Norwalk, CT, 1996, Appleton & Lange.)

TRANSTHEORETICAL MODEL

The transtheoretical model is currently the most broadly used of the four models. It incorporates elements from health belief and self-efficacy theories to develop a model that can be used to describe the stages of change that individuals go through as they initiate behaviors that promote health. The model describes five stages of change, ten processes that facilitate movement from one stage to another, and four patterns that individuals use to progress through the various stages (Fig. 9-2) (Prochaska et al, 1992).

Stages of Change

The stages are precontemplation, contemplation, preparation, action, and maintenance. Shifts in attitudes and behaviors occur at each stage. The time required in each stage depends on the individual and the task to be attempted.

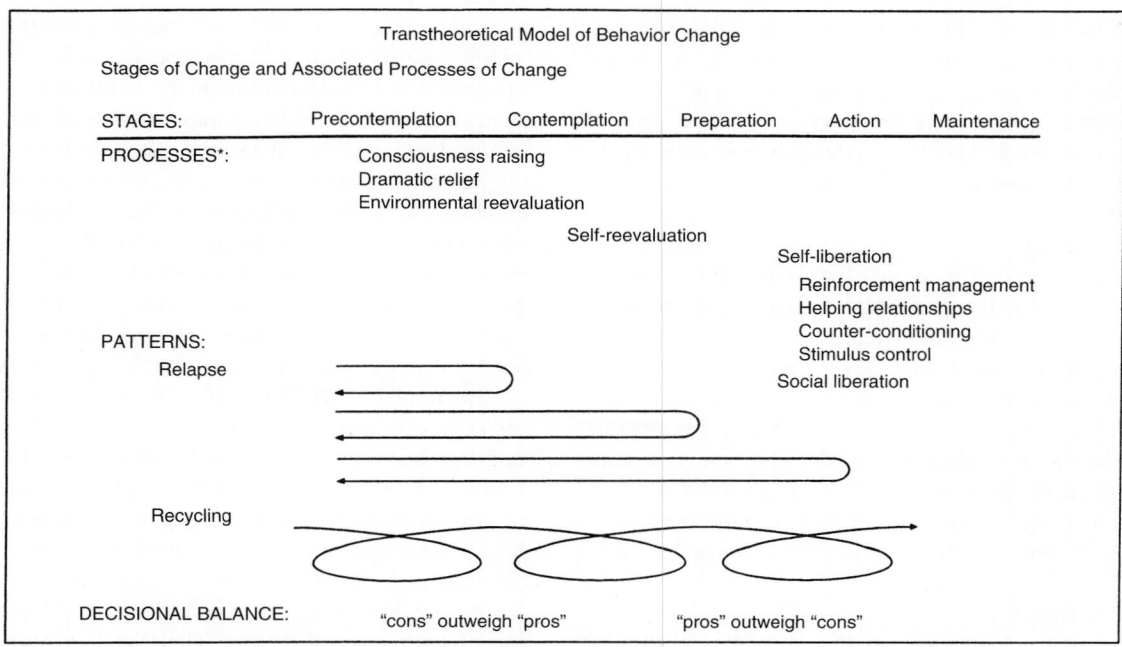

Explanations of Processes of Change | Associated Interventions

Consciousness raising: gathering information about self and problem[†] — Observation of others, confrontations; Classes, bibliotherapy, interpretations

Dramatic relief: feeling and expressing feelings related to problem — Role play, psychodrama, grief work

Environmental reevaluation: assessing one's behavior on environment — Documentary information, empathy, training

Self-reevaluation: exploring one's feelings about self and the problem — Value clarification, imagery; Corrective emotional experience

Self-liberation: choosing to act, changing belief in ability to change[‡] — Decision-making training; Making resolutions, commitment-enhancing techniques

Social liberation: increasing alternatives and support for health behaviors — Empowerment and advocacy activities, policy interventions

Reinforcement management: establishing a reward system — Overt and covert reinforcement, contingency contracts

Helping relationships: trusting and sharing problem with a caring person[*] — Therapeutic alliance, buddy system, self-help/support groups

Counter-conditioning: substituting alternatives for problem behavior — Relaxation, desensitization, assertive skills, self-affirmations

Stimulus control: avoiding triggers of problem behavior — Restructuring environment, avoidance techniques, cue identification

[*]Most frequently used. Used more frequently for psychologically distressing problems.
[†]Second most frequently used.
[‡]Third most frequently used. Used more frequently for weight control.

Adapted from Prochaska, DiClemente, and Norcross, 1992.

FIG. 9-2   Transtheoretical (stages of change) model. (Adapted from Prochaska J, DiClemente C, Norcross J: In search of how people change: applications to addictive behaviors, *Am Psychol* 47:1102–1114, 1992.)

Precontemplation. At this stage, the individual does not acknowledge that a serious problem exists, although a wish to change may be expressed. Resistance to change is the hallmark of this stage, and the reasons not to change are most clear to the individual.

Contemplation. Awareness of the problem exists, and the individual struggles with the costs and energy required for change. Many individuals remain stuck in this phase.

Preparation. Planning begins in this stage. Small behavior changes may occur in preparation for commitment to the actual plan.

Action. Behaviors to eliminate the problem occur in this stage. These may include initiating new behaviors, accessing resources, modifying the environment, and mitigating barriers.

Maintenance. Plans occur here to prevent relapse, consolidate gains, and establish new behaviors as long-term changes. Maintenance occurs after at least 6 months in the action stage.

Patterns of Change

Most people are not able to proceed through all five stages in a linear way. Rather there are relapses back to the precontemplation stage. Environmental barriers, external pressures to change beyond the individual's own desires, or problems with maintenance of steps not mastered at earlier stages can contribute to relapses. *Recycling* is defined as regression to the contemplation or preparation stages. The person spirals through small increments of change, recycling and moving forward again. Success with the change is increased with effort, action, and mastery of the tasks of each stage.

Decisional Balance

Another component of the model is the cognitive exercise of weighing the pros and cons of change. In the precontemplative stage, the pros of no change are dominant over the pros of change (e.g., "If I stop smoking, I'll gain weight"). To sustain behavior in the action stage and move to the maintenance stage, the pros of change must outweigh the cons of returning to old ways (e.g., "No smoking is cheaper than when I smoked"). Because most people at risk for health problems are in a precontemplative stage, programs need to be designed to move them to the contemplative stage. Also programs designed to maintain changes made are important. Many dieting, smoking cessation, and drug rehabilitation programs fail to initiate and sustain changes because assessment of readiness and readiness training to assist individuals to move through stages successively is not included in the initial plans. Motivational interviewing is a strategy based on the stages of change that appears to have excellent success rates for many health-related behaviors (Rubak et al, 2005). It will be discussed later in greater depth.

How the various factors that influence health behaviors develop in children and how and at what ages effects will occur is not well understood. These same factors also influence parents, so adult models are important to understand. Health care providers may also be affected by motivational factors—do they feel that they have the requisite teaching and knowledge skills, limited barriers, and the like to influence their clients' health-related behaviors, such as smoking or lack of physical activity?

CHILDREN'S CONCEPTS OF HEALTH AND ILLNESS

Children's health promotion behaviors are influenced by their own understanding of health and illness, the views and behaviors of their family, and community variables. The latter include direct effects of standards and practices in child care, school, and other community settings, in addition to indirect effects, such as cultural and community values related to health.

Children's concepts of health and illness must be considered within a developmental framework. Cognitive development is often used as a framework to analyze children's understanding of health and illness. More current models consider children to be developing their own theories of how things work, including health and illness processes. Many studies offer evidence of children's views, but the knowledge base is relatively weak, with more research needed in the area. Providers need to understand the health beliefs of their young patients and their goals, hopes, priorities, health interests and concerns, perceptions about seriousness of problems, feelings of vulnerability to health problems, and perceptions of benefits and barriers to taking action.

One model for understanding children's cognitive processing of health information, used more in the 1970s and 1980s, is Piaget's theory of cognitive development. Following this framework, preschoolers are in Piaget's preoperational stage of cognitive development. They have an egocentric view of health. Children at 3 to 5 years old are just learning about the differences between being sick versus being well for themselves and their family members. They have little understanding of their internal bodies. Their lack of understanding of time and transformations means that the process of healing, for example, is not clearly understood. School-age children are in the concrete operations cognitive development stage. They can list specific acts and rules used to maintain health and generally need overt signs of illness or health to recognize the health status of a person. Adolescents, who are in the formal operations stage, are able to understand the difficulties of defining health (e.g., a person who looks well, but has a cancerous tumor inside versus a person whose mobility is limited, but is actually healthy). Teenagers understand the difference between the sick role and actual pathologic conditions, are sensitive to feeling states, and differentiate mental health from physical health. Nevertheless, the provider should not consider adolescents ready for explanations at an adult level because they vary in their use of formal operations thinking with age and issue. Miller and Armstrong (2006) found that the Piagetian framework helps explain some developmental concepts of nicotine addiction. Understanding the model helps in designing effective smoking prevention and cessation interventions that are appropriate to children at different ages.

Many developmental theorists have become disappointed in the Piagetian framework, which they believe underestimates children's cognitive abilities. Further they argue that Piaget's theory describes children's logic and capabilities, not their understandings of specific concepts.

Recent research investigates children's understanding of illness and health in light of their concepts of biologic processes. Accordingly, with more experience and knowledge, children can incorporate more elaborate concepts into theories of how the body works, contagion, differences between physical and mental well-being, and the like. An excellent study by Myant and Williams (2005) explores the understanding of four different conditions, injuries (bruises and broken leg), chickenpox, colds, and asthma by children at 4 to 5, 7 to 8, 9 to 10, and 11 to 12 years old. The children were asked to describe the condition, its cause(s), prevention, time course to onset of symptoms, recovery process, and time for recovery. Children had the best understanding at earlier ages for injuries and colds, conditions they had experienced in some form. Their understanding became more sophisticated with age. They had the least understanding of asthma, which was neither visible nor commonly experienced. Similarly, adults may be cognitively sophisticated, but demonstrate very elementary understanding of specific conditions based on lack of experience and knowledge rather than inability to process information. Providers should provide information based on the child's current base of knowledge and experience. If providers assume, on the basis of a child's age, that he or she has a certain level of knowledge, experience, or cognitive abilities, they may fail to provide the most useful information to the child.

A significant health factor for adolescents is their risk-taking behavior. Questions the health care provider must consider when caring for teenagers include the following: What is the adolescent's perception of risk? When do teenagers identify behaviors as risky, but choose to engage in them anyway for the perceived social value?

OTHER DETERMINANTS OF HEALTH BEHAVIOR OF CHILDREN

A variety of studies have considered the determinants of health behavior of school-age children and adolescents, not just their cognitive understanding of health or illness.

Family Involvement With Health of Children

The family is the basic unit of health care management. The family influences lifestyles and the health status of its members. Providers need to understand family dynamics, especially the influence of the mother; decision-making patterns; and parenting styles, including autonomy and rewards for children and reasoning used to teach children. The psychological characteristics of the family, belief that members can make a difference, and the role of the family as a natural support system are all important in planning effective health promotion strategies. Knowledge of the family's composition, health, lifestyle, nutrition, economic resources, and recent changes is helpful. Exercise, diet, hygiene, and rest patterns are family routines affecting the health of individual members.

Peers

LaGreca and colleagues (2002) identify a variety of studies that support the proposition that peers offer support, influence adherence to treatment regimens, and affect both health promotion and health risk behaviors. For example, in adolescents with diabetes, friends provide more support for certain aspects of treatment, such as exercise and emotions. On the negative side, peer smoking is the best predictor of adolescent smoking.

Community Involvement With Health of Children

The community influences health promotion behaviors of families with children. The community provides options for health care, an economic base for family survival and prosperity, social norms, and regulation of the environment and behaviors of citizens. The community also provides many direct services, including schools, day care centers, social services, community organizations, and health care centers, that support or impede family efforts to maintain the health of the members.

Use of community resources benefits families positively if recommendations for access and use are appropriate and timely. Adoption of community standards and health values by individual families can effectively influence their health behaviors. According to Rogers' (1983) diffusion theory, innovators are the first to adopt new ideas in a community. They are followed by early adopters, then the early majority, the late majority, and finally late adopters. When between 10% and 25% of the population adopt an idea, it diffuses through the rest of the population. Thus, for example, when the use of bicycle helmets reaches a critical mass of 10% to 25%, use should become common enough so that the remaining families are persuaded to buy helmets and expect their children to use them.

Health care delivery systems are also beginning to use community services more effectively. Within a 20- to 30-minute preventive health care visit, health care providers cannot deliver all the information about health to families, nor can families absorb the information. Newer models of health care delivery are exploring opportunities to integrate services among different professions and agencies. The Healthy Steps for young children program is one example. It was designed to support young families using a new type of provider, the healthy steps specialist (HSS), working alongside traditional providers but doing many of the developmental screening, anticipatory guidance, and follow-up services of the agency. Among the other role activities, the HSS assists families to use appropriate community services. Studies of the model have noted positive outcomes in terms of parental knowledge, practice, well-being, and satisfaction (Minkovitz et al, 2003; Zuckerman et al, 2004).

Another example of a new model is the prescription for health: promoting healthy behaviors in primary care research networks initiative sponsored by the Robert Wood Johnson Foundation. Projects using this model were implemented in 120 primary care practices across the country. The project focuses on four leading health risk behaviors—smoking, risky drinking, unhealthy diet, and physical inactivity. Projects have increased use of community resources, reorganized their services to reduce barriers to health care counseling, focused on self-management and decision supports for patients and families making health behavior changes, and set up clinical information systems to monitor patients more systematically and effectively. The data are emerging about improvements to practices, which should translate to improved outcomes for patients (Cifuentes et al, 2005; Cohen et al, 2005). Margolis and colleagues (2001) provide a third example in which a community-wide intervention was implemented in Durham, North Carolina. Interventions were designed at the community, practice, and family levels for low-income women and children to improve health outcomes.

In summary many factors influence the health behaviors of children and their families. Pediatric providers helping families change lifestyle and behaviors to promote health need broad understanding of the health perspectives of their clients, in addition to an awareness of age, sex, education, and peer and community influences. Fig. 9-3 provides a model for use of these many factors to design behavior-change strategies in primary care. It incorporates the community, the practice in a broad sense, and then the examination and direct interventions with the individual client. The model is designed to demonstrate strategies for increasing physical activity of adults, but could easily be adapted for use with children and adolescents.

FUNCTIONAL HEALTH PATTERNS—THE BEHAVIORS OF HEALTH

The functional health patterns that Gordon (1987) used to describe the domain of nursing practice serve as the framework for the chapters in this unit. The patterns describe the health-related behaviors in which people engage. These functional health patterns are universal, applying to all humans regardless of age, sex, culture, health status, or other factors. All people need to eat, sleep, and eliminate, for example. Each pattern is described as follows:

Health perception-health management pattern: Describes client's perceptions of personal health and health care behaviors, prevention, and compliance with prescriptions for management of health and illness problems.

Nutrition-metabolic pattern: Describes patterns of food and fluid intake. Includes choice of foods and food supplements, eating habits, and schedules.

Elimination pattern: Describes patterns of bowel and bladder excretion. Includes schedule and habit patterns and use of laxatives or other methods to facilitate excretory functions.

Activity-exercise pattern: Describes patterns of activity and exercise, including type of activity, schedule of participation, vigor, effect on leisure, physical state, and meaning of activity to the client.

Sleep-rest pattern: Describes patterns of sleep and rest, including schedule, habits, aids to sleep, and perceived feelings of renewal, fatigue, or exhaustion.

Cognitive-perceptual pattern: Describes sensory-perceptual and cognitive patterns, including adaptations to hearing, vision, or other perceptual losses; includes the process of finding meaning from environmental stimuli and the effectiveness of efforts to compensate for deficits. Pain perception is a component.

Self-perception–self-concept pattern: Describes patterns of perception and valuing of the self, in addition to evaluation of strengths and weaknesses and sense of self-worth.

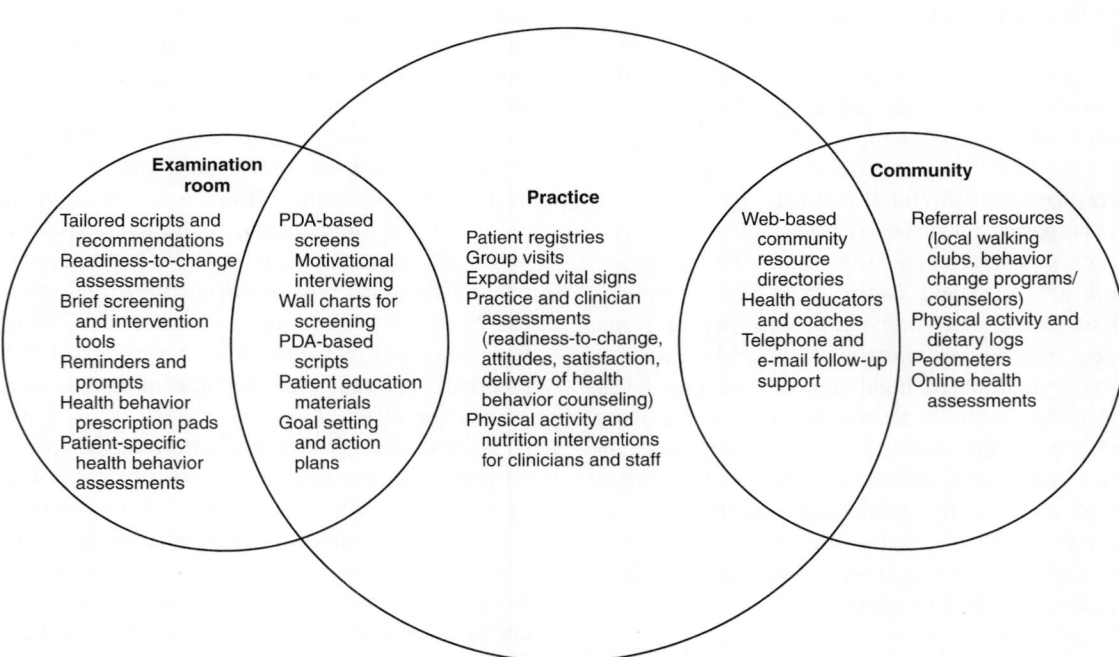

PDA = Personal digital assistant (i.e., handheld computer).

FIG. 9-3   Integration of health behavior change strategies in primary care. (From Cifuentes M et al: Prescription for health: changing the health care practice to foster healthy behaviors, *Ann Fam Med* 3:S8, 2005.)

Role-relationships pattern: Describes pattern of roles and responsibilities of the client and patterns of relationships with family and others.

Sexuality-reproductive pattern: Describes patterns of satisfaction or dissatisfaction with sexuality and sexual relationships. Involves perception and development of sexual identity, in addition to reproductive expectations, behaviors, and outcomes.

Coping-stress tolerance pattern: Describes patterns of coping with the range of stresses experienced. Includes strategies used, effectiveness, support systems, and perceived ability to control and manage difficult situations.

Values-beliefs pattern: Describes patterns of values and beliefs that influence daily living activities, guide decision making, and provide meaning to life. Involves religious and spiritual activities and personal values and beliefs.

SCREENING AND ASSESSMENT OF FUNCTIONAL HEALTH PATTERN DISORDERS

The same diagnostic reasoning methods are used by the provider to manage both health and illness issues. One must look at risk factors, comorbidities, cause, epidemiology, differential diagnosis, and options for management that are safe, efficient, effective, and acceptable to the client.

Screening for the presence of lifestyle and health behavior problems is a first step. In pediatric practice, the majority of screening is done in the clinical interview. Questions are asked about sleep, nutrition, elimination, play, discipline, use of primary care services, and others. Questionnaires can be used to ask about diet, smoking, exercise, use of seat belts, and feelings of satisfaction with self and health status. The clinical interview is more than taking a history of medical problems. It involves learning about concerns and worries, in addition to goals, lifestyle, family life, and cultural background. It produces information to put the child and family into a context necessary to plan for care. For instance, if a family has little money, decisions about care need to factor in the inability to pay for services, medications, or equipment.

If information generated by the clinical interview is appropriate, given the child's age and other factors, no further probing of the area is done. On the other hand, if an answer to a screening question is atypical, the provider begins the assessment mode to identify the nature, severity, duration, and effects of the problem to plan appropriate interventions. For example, if a mother notes that she has not been very happy lately, the Beck Depression Scale or a postpartum depression scale might be administered to assess whether she is depressed or not. Assessment might involve use of daily diaries of food intake, activity, or sleep-wake patterns. Screening methods are used for all children of a given age in the practice, whereas assessment is individualized and should yield information about the extent of the problem and comorbidities for a given client. The goal of assessment is diagnosis and development of a plan of care to manage the problem effectively and efficiently.

Health supervision using a clinical preventive services model involves regular visits timed to offer periodic screening opportunities. The visits need to be scheduled infrequently enough to be economic, but frequently enough to identify changes in the patterns of growth and development or early physiologic, psychological, or social problems that might be detrimental to the child's health. Health supervision includes the clinical interview, developmental and educational surveillance, observation of parent-child interaction, physical examination, and screening procedures, such as measuring height, weight, head circumference, body mass index (BMI), vision, hearing, blood pressure, and hemoglobin or hematocrit. The purpose of the health supervision visit is to assess strengths and weaknesses in health and to intervene to promote the best health possible. This will involve behavioral counseling and immunizations and other activities. The content of health supervision visits throughout infancy, childhood, and adolescence is addressed in Chapters 2 and 10. The details of screening, assessment and management of functional health problems identified are found in the remaining chapters of this unit. The American Academy of Pediatrics Recommendations for scheduling preventive health visits is found in Appendix D.

NURSING DIAGNOSES—A WAY TO LABEL FUNCTIONAL HEALTH PATTERN PROBLEMS

Nursing diagnoses developed by the North American Nursing Diagnosis Association, now called NANDA International (NANDA), provide a way to label, describe, and categorize the problems that NPs manage in the nursing part of their role. One advantage to the use of nursing diagnoses lies in systematically identifying the health problems that NPs manage with labels that allow data retrieval for evaluation of practice outcomes and research purposes.

Nevertheless, nursing diagnoses are not used systematically by all NPs. The first problem is that some NANDA diagnoses are not stated specifically enough for clinical application, although they identify an area of patient difficulty. For example, "sleep pattern disturbance" does not tell the NP whether the issue involves getting to sleep, staying asleep, or waking early. Each problem would be managed differently. Second, many senior NPs (those who are more likely to teach students) were educated as NPs before the development of nursing diagnoses. Thus, individuals might not have had role models using the system. Third, nursing diagnoses are not reimbursed, although some ICD-9-CM (*International Classification of Diseases, 9th revision, Clinical Modification*) diagnoses (see inside back cover) can be substituted. Fourth, there is a misconception on the part of some NPs that they should use nursing labels for medical diagnoses. NPs should use medical diagnoses for the pathophysiologic problems and nursing diagnoses for the problems of lifestyle and health behaviors not covered by medical diagnosis labels. The use of both sets of labels makes the scope of practice of the NP explicit. Therefore, for example, "impetigo" is best for describing the skin infection, but "alteration in parenting" alerts other professionals to look at parenting behaviors.

Though perhaps not reimbursable, using the labels in charting ensures that the range of services that providers render is made explicit. Without labeling the problems of sleep, nutrition, coping, and so forth, no one knows what the NP does while in the room with the patient and family aside from managing medical problems. The services provided become invisible, and the perception is left that NPs are slower in managing diseases than other primary care providers. To be valued, the NP's total work must be recognized. The use of nursing diagnosis labels can make the work in the health promotion domain of functional health patterns more visible.

In the functional health patterns chapters (Chapters 10 to 21) nursing diagnoses that might be appropriate to label problems in a particular pattern are identified for those who wish to use them. However, the content of each chapter is organized conceptually around the nature of the pattern and not the nursing diagnosis framework.

◼ MANAGEMENT STRATEGIES FOR HEALTH PROMOTION

This section discusses some management strategies for promoting health and working with functional health pattern problems. To provide excellent health promotion care, the provider must:

- Give consistent, credible health messages
- Merit trust and confidence
- Understand clinical preventive service recommendations and provide preventive services consistent with those recommendations
- Have working relationships with other provider colleagues, social services, and educational professionals in the community
- Ensure that the clinic setting creates an environment consistent with good health and is developmentally appropriate
- Use motivational, patient education, and behavioral strategies effectively

In *Nursing Interventions Classification* (NIC), Dochterman and Bulechek (2004) classify nursing interventions into six domains: (1) physiologic: basic, (2) physiologic: complex, (3) behavioral, (4) safety, (5) family, and (6) health system (Box 9-1). For the problems of functional health patterns and health maintenance and promotion, interventions in domains 1, 3, 4, 5, and 6 are most appropriate. The interventions of domain 2 (physiologic: complex) are most appropriate for the disease and pathophysiologic problems NPs manage. This text does not formally use the NIC. However, it is a useful tool when developing management strategies relevant to specific problems. For example, the interventions most specifically designed to result in behavioral changes desired for health promotion and disease prevention include those in NIC domain 3 (behavior therapy, cognitive therapy, communication enhancement, coping assistance, patient education, and psychological comfort).

Pediatric primary care providers face the difficult task of transmitting an enormous amount of information to their patients to promote health goals, but, more importantly, providers are expected to facilitate health behavior changes in patient's lives. Knowledge does not automatically result in behavior change.

Moyer and Butler (2004) have studied gaps in well-child care. They found that 42 preventive service interventions were recommended by two or more of the major authorities, such as the American Academy of Pediatrics, *Bright Futures* (Green & Palfrey, 2002), the American Academy of Family Practice, and *Guidelines for Adolescent Preventive Services* in the behavioral counseling, screening, and prophylaxis domains. *Bright Futures,* for example, suggests between 80 and 100 discrete counseling interventions. Although in 2001 greater than 30% of visits to physicians were for well-child care, clinicians were not able to complete all the recommended actions within 20- to 30-minute visits using current patterns of practice.

Moyer and Butler (2004) studied evidence to support the recommended health promotion interventions through clinical trials rather than expert opinion. They hypothesized that if it were clear which interventions were most effective, then time and costs could be used more effectively without sacrificing quality through omission of needed guidance or insufficient time and effort directed toward the most effective activities. Much work needs to be done in this area, and providers need to be alert to research that supports or refutes some of the standard interventions typically recommended in well-child care.

Health care providers need to use evidence-based practice wherever possible, set priorities, and focus precious time upon the most risky behaviors using the most effective interventions possible. Practice barriers, such as time, symptom-driven care, inadequate reimbursement, inadequate clinician training, and lack of self-confidence need to be addressed also (Whitlock et al, 2004).

BEHAVIORAL COUNSELING INTERVENTIONS

Whitlock and colleagues (2004) evaluated behavioral counseling interventions used in primary care. Rates of behavioral counseling interventions are far below national targets, though brief interventions integrated into primary care visits have been shown to be effective for many behaviors including smoking cessation and problem drinking. Behavioral counseling is usually directed at more complex behaviors; the term "counseling" implies a cooperative mode of interaction between client and provider rather than a more directive teacher-learner model. The goal is self-management of the problem behavior by the client to change and sustain healthy patterns of living.

The Whitlock group (2004) found many studies supporting behavioral counseling. Most of the behavioral counseling interventions are based upon the health beliefs, self-efficacy, and transtheoretical models that were discussed earlier. From their analysis of the studies, they developed several constructs that are useful for practicing providers. First, certain attributes of clients predispose them to successful behavior change:

- There is a desire to change for clear, personal reasons.
- Few obstacles to behavior change are perceived.
- The client has the needed skills and self-confidence for the needed changes.
- The client feels there will be benefits to the change.
- The changes are viewed as congruent with the client's self-image and norms of his or her social group.

BOX 9-1 **Nursing Interventions Classification: Domains and Classes of Interventions**

1. *Physiologic, basic:* care that supports physical functioning
   A. Activity and exercise management
   B. Elimination management
   C. Immobility management
   D. Nutrition support
   E. Physical comfort promotion
   F. Self-care facilitation
2. *Physiologic, complex:* care that supports homeostatic regulation
   A. Electrolyte and acid-base management
   B. Drug management
   C. Neurologic management
   D. Perioperative care
   E. Respiratory management
   F. Skin and/or wound management
   G. Thermoregulation
   H. Tissue perfusion management
3. *Behavioral:* care that supports psychological functioning and facilitates lifestyle changes
   A. Behavior therapy
   B. Cognitive therapy
   C. Communication enhancement
   D. Coping assistance
   E. Patient education
   F. Psychological comfort promotion
4. *Safety:* care that supports protection against harm
   A. Crisis management
   B. Risk management
5. *Family:* care that supports the family unit
   A. Childbearing care
   B. Child-rearing care
   C. Life-span care
6. *Health system:* care that supports effective use of the health care delivery system
   A. Health system mediation
   B. Health system management
   C. Information management
7. *Community:* care that supports the health of the community
   A. Community health promotion
   B. Community risk management

From Dochterman J, Bulechek G, editors: *Nursing interventions classification,* ed 4, St Louis, 2004, Mosby.

- Reminders, encouragement, and social support at key times and from persons and the community whom the client values will support the behavior changes.

They also found that the quality of the client-provider relationship is important. The provider must be viewed as an empathetic partner who interprets information and provides advice with exploration of options rather than "prescribing" needed change. Coercive techniques create resistance in clients, not change.

Another construct that Whitlock and her colleagues named "the five As" was found helpful in looking at common elements of various behavioral counseling strategies. They are as follows:

- *Assess:* Ask about behavioral health risks and factors affecting behavioral choices, goals, and methods used. For example, the Healthy Teen Project (Olson et al, 2005) used one innovative method to assess for behavioral risks of adoles-

cents. Teens were given a personal digital assistant (PDA) with 90 items while in the waiting room. The teen could use the PDA to respond to the items privately—even if a parent was nearby. The answers were forwarded electronically to the provider before the visit began so that time could be best spent by focusing on identified strengths and risks of the teen's health behaviors.

- *Advise:* Give clear, specific information including both harms and benefits of various behavioral options. In many ways, this step comprises models of patient education, assuming that with information, patients will choose to change.
- *Agree:* Find a collaborative plan that both provider and client can agree on that is based upon the client's goals, interest, and willingness to change.
- *Assist:* Using behavior change techniques, aid the patient to achieve the skills, confidence, and social supports necessary.

• *Arrange:* Schedule follow-up contacts with the client to provide further guidance, support, and encouragement to continue with the plan or make adjustments as needed. This step might also involve referral to special sources of help.

MOTIVATIONAL INTERVIEWING AS A STRATEGY

Motivational interviewing (MI) is a specific behavioral counseling method to help patients recognize and change risky behaviors. The method was developed by Miller and Rollnick (1991) as they worked with clients with problem drinking behaviors. It fits well with the notions of Whitlock et al (2004) previously discussed. Miller and Rollnick discovered that motivational interviewing was particularly helpful with clients who were reluctant to change or ambivalent about the need to change. In their experience, persuasion rather than coercion, and support rather than argument proved more effective. Using the client's intrinsic motivation was most powerful. MI has since been used effectively to support change in a variety of behaviors including smoking, drug addiction, inactivity, obesity, diabetic care, and asthma. It works with adolescents particularly well since developmentally they are trying to make their own decisions. In a meta-analysis of studies comparing motivational interviewing with other strategies, Rubak and colleagues (2005) found that MI outperformed traditional advice in approximately 80% of studies. No studies reported it to be harmful. Rubak et al (2005) also found that it can be effective in brief encounters of only 15 minutes, though more than one encounter will increase the likelihood of effects.

Sindelar and colleagues (2004) completed an extensive review of MI in pediatric practice and found it to be an effective strategy for decreasing adolescent substance abuse, decreasing health risk behaviors, and increasing adherence to regimens for treatment of various conditions. It also works with parents.

The strategy used the transtheoretical model. One first identifies the patient's readiness for change stage. The session then begins with discussion of pros and cons for change based upon that readiness. The discussion needs to match the patient's stage of change, or problems will result. For example, if the therapist tries to enter a discussion of pros and cons of various change goals (preparation stage) when the patient is still considering whether behavior change is needed or desired at all (precontemplation stage), resistance by the patient will result. The patient must be moved through the stages at his or her own pace. The discussions focus upon the ambivalence that one feels at each stage and helps the client come to a decision that motivates action. Some actions that Sindelar and colleagues (2004) recommend for pediatric providers are as follows:

1. Develop rapport with the patient. Studies support the ideas of active listening, forming a working alliance, and clarifying the patient's views with reflective comments.
2. Set an agenda. "What would you like to discuss today?"
3. Once the agenda is set, ask scaling questions to assess the patient's confidence in making a behavior change and then discovering the barriers to improvement in confidence. "Why do you feel you are at 4 out of 10 in terms of confidence

in yourself to be able to quit smoking? What would help raise your score? Why isn't it lower?" (Sindelar et al, 2004).

Skilled motivational interviewing can best be learned through short training sessions (a couple of hours) for providers. Students and clinicians are encouraged to seek out the support and knowledge to use the techniques. Use of open-ended questions, reflective listening, double-sided reflections (recognizing both pros and cons) are essential techniques. In the early stages of change, one elicits advantages and disadvantages of poor adherence from the patient and all the possible details regarding the advantages of nonadherence, affirming acceptance of the patient's views and summarizing to be sure the patient has been understood correctly. As the patient moves into a preparation stage, the focus shifts to the equally weighted advantages and disadvantages of adherence; in the action stage, the therapist focuses on the advantages of adherence (Lask, 2003). See Box 9-2 for some essential features of motivational interviewing. Encounters may last 15 or 20 minutes, but the time spent will be more effective than simply providing quick information or persuading or coercing change, which generally results in resistance to change rather than compliance.

PATIENT EDUCATION STRATEGIES

Patient education is the most commonly used strategy for guiding patients to increase health promotion behaviors and manage lifestyle problems. This strategy involves providing clients with information about ways to prevent contracting preventable diseases, ways to change lifestyle to reduce risks, and methods to maintain a healthy environment. Within the more current perspectives on helping clients make positive health behavior changes, it could be considered the *assess*

BOX 9-2   **Essential Features of Motivational Interviewing**

• Motivation to change comes from within the patient and is not externally imposed by the therapist or others.
• Ambivalence must be articulated and resolved by the patient, not the therapist. The therapist can help facilitate the patient's expressions of both sides of the issue and guide the patient toward a resolution that triggers a desire for change.
• Direct persuasion by the therapist will not resolve ambivalence.
• An intervention style that is quiet and eliciting works best.
• Readiness for change is not a patient trait, but a changing product of interpersonal interaction.
• The therapist-patient relationship must develop as a partnership rather than an expert-novice or teacher-student relationship.

Adapted from Sindelar et al: Motivational interviewing in pediatric practice, *Curr Problems Pediatr Adolesc Health Care* 34(9):322-339, 2004.

and *advise* step of "the five As" model (the other three As are *agree*, *assist*, and *arrange*). Patient education is an essential feature to help patients who need to change health behaviors, but is not sufficient in itself unless the patient and family are already quite motivated and self-sufficient. Patient education is also effective with groups, assuming that providers can also work with individuals to help them implement changes suggested in the group session. In pediatrics the learner may be the parent, caregiver, or a child or teen who is able to manage some of his or her own health behaviors.

The core methodology for patient education for individuals and groups is reviewed here and summarized in Box 9-3.

1. *Set the climate for learning.* Patients, families, or groups need to be in an environment that is comfortable, free of distractions, and provides cues that learning activities will occur. Introductions and a mutually agreed-on time limit are helpful. For example, mothers who are worried about being home when the school bus drops off their children attend poorly to teaching, no matter how skilled the provider.

2. *Assess.* Establish a structure of mutual planning. Identify learner and provider goals. If learning is to be successful, the client must recognize a need for new knowledge. It becomes the provider's responsibility to identify client (child, parent, class) needs. Getting the client to express questions is the most direct way to identify client needs. The provider can also ask about the client's health goals. Sometimes it is necessary to provide information that alerts clients to potential or emerging problems if lifestyle or behavior changes do not occur. In other words, the client does not always come to the provider with preestablished goals or needs; however, the client must agree with the provider that change is necessary for the mutual planning requirement of patient teaching to be met.

3. *Assess the learner.* Assessment includes readiness, attitudes and feelings, style of learning, level of knowledge and competency, and physical and developmental capabilities. Use of one of the health belief models identified earlier can provide the necessary information about the readiness, attitudes, and feelings factors. Questions in the following areas may be useful:

Readiness
- Does the client ask questions?
- Does the client have multiple stresses in his or her life that would inhibit concentration on learning?
- Is the client coping with survival issues, such as chronic poverty, debilitating chronic illness, unemployment, or rehabilitation from substance abuse, that inhibit learning?
- When is the best time to meet with the client, given other daily expectations?

Attitudes and Feelings
- Have there been past attempts at learning with successful outcomes?
- Does the client have a sense of control over his or her future, as demonstrated by an ability to set and achieve goals, a positive feeling about life, and an ability to care for himself or herself adequately?
- Does the client have worries, depression, or a life situation that would decrease learning?
- Does the client feel vulnerable?
- Does the client feel that actions could make a difference?
- Does the client feel that the benefits of taking action outweigh perceived costs?
- Does the client feel capable of taking the necessary actions?

Style of Learning
- What are the preferred modalities of learning for the client? (e.g., "Do you learn best by reading or listening?" "Does watching a videotape help you learn?")
- What does the client already know about the subject?
- Judging from the developmental level of the client, how concrete or abstract can the teaching be?

4. *Plan.* The plan is formulated using objectives that specify the behaviors that will demonstrate learning. Objectives need to be realistic, achievable, and relevant to the goals of the client. Both short-term and long-term objectives are written if the goals will not be achieved in one teaching session. The use of both types of objectives helps the client and provider set priorities and stage education in achievable steps. Generally, in routine pediatric visits, objectives are verbally stated, not written, but both client and provider should agree on what is to be achieved. Various aids facilitate

---

BOX 9-3 **The Patient Education Process**

1. Set the climate for learning—make introductions, provide comfortable environment.
2. Establish a structure of mutual planning—identify learner and provider goals.
3. Assess the learner's style of learning, level of knowledge and competency, readiness, physical and developmental capabilities, attitudes, and feelings.
4. Plan—provide knowledge, role modeling, practice, discussion. Various aids facilitate teaching—books, pamphlets, diagrams, videos, and models. The plan is formulated with objectives specifying the behaviors that the learner should exhibit to demonstrate learning.
5. Manage the learning intervention—use methods and resources for instruction with the patient or family (or both) to implement the plan.
6. Evaluate the outcomes—judge achievement of objectives and then reformulate the plan to move the learner to the next level.

learning—books, pamphlets, diagrams, videos, and models. Modalities for learning that are most appropriate for the client should be used. Methods for teaching include formal classes, role-playing, demonstration and return demonstration, lecture and discussion, reading, viewing videos, or other activities. The plan should facilitate clear presentation of material to the client, provide for frequent reinforcement and feedback, and include some kind of active involvement of the client. Passive listening does not ensure learning.

5. *Advise*. Manage the learning intervention. During implementation of the teaching plan, the process is carefully orchestrated to actively engage the client in successful learning. Progress is constantly evaluated, new information added, success reinforced, the pace of feedback assessed, the pace adjusted, and outcomes and achievement of objectives evaluated.

6. *Evaluate the outcomes*. Judge achievement of objectives and then reformulate the plan to move the client to the next level. Learning is evaluated using a variety of methods, such as asking questions that require use of new knowledge to answer, watching for new behaviors, and looking for feelings of achievement and expressions of new understanding.

PATIENT EDUCATION WITH CHILDREN AND ADOLESCENTS

Teaching children includes all the aforementioned steps and careful assessment of the child's developmental level because the concepts the child can learn vary with cognitive abilities. Children's attention spans are often short; therefore information needs to be presented in small bites, with frequent reinforcement and opportunities for doing rather than just listening. Reading skills may not be developed, so verbal and demonstration strategies are more effective for younger children. Terminology might need to be adjusted to use simpler words and concepts. Verbal and nonverbal reinforcement and feedback need to be appropriate for the child. The use of star charts is a good way to reinforce behaviors visually and concretely. Such strategies are consistent with school-age children in Piaget's concrete operations cognitive stage.

For adolescents assessment of developmental level is also important. The young adolescent (13 to 14 years old) understands and engages in learning differently from the 18-year-old. Motivators for teenagers do not include knowledge of long-term effects. The use of several modalities, such as discussions with peers, reading, reviewing, and viewing audiovisual media, is helpful. Advice needs to be practical. Teenagers do best when they are viewed as decision makers who need information to make good choices. Identification of strengths and weaknesses is always important. The use of peer groups can be extremely effective.

PATIENT EDUCATION WITH PARENTS

When working with parents, the provider must keep in mind that parents are experts for their child and home environment, whereas the health care provider has more knowledge about children as an aggregate. Thus collaboration between parents and providers produces the best outcomes for the child at hand. Adult education has some unique aspects. First, adults usually want knowledge to help them make decisions for change, not just to gain knowledge per se. Furthermore, they usually have expectations or goals and ideas about activities that will help them. Finally, adults may have to unlearn previous knowledge that is outdated or irrelevant to the situation at hand.

Roberts (1981), a nurse, developed a model of levels of parent education that is useful to providers (Table 9-1). The model identifies four levels of parental needs with related levels of responses by nurses. When parents have no obvious needs (level I), they may gain from anticipatory guidance. The nurse's role is one of providing prospective advice and information for future use. When parents feel uneasy about some aspect of child rearing (level II), the nurse begins to serve as a resource to help with the specific issue. At level III, problems overtly affect children in particular areas. The nurse, at this point, moves into a collaborative mode, taking more direct action to support the family rather than merely offering advice for the parents to use. For example, the nurse might begin to make telephone calls to arrange consultation appointments for the family or arrange transportation as needed. Finally, at level IV, the parents' resources are inadequate to meet the child's needs, so the nurse moves into a protective mode on behalf of the child.

Parent teaching is most effective at levels I and II. At level III, the parent generally needs more than teaching. At level IV, the activities of the nurse are designed to support the child first.

Anticipatory Guidance

Anticipatory guidance has been considered the principle intervention for well-child care in the U.S. for many years. It is a particular form of patient teaching. It is used when the provider wants to be sure that the patient and family have

TABLE 9-1	Levels of Parent Education
Parent Need Level	**Nursing Intervention**
I. No obvious needs	"Prospective mode"—provide anticipatory guidance
II. Parents uneasy or engaging in some child care practices that may cause difficulties in the future	"Resource mode"—respond to specific issues of parenting
III. Parents have obvious needs because children display difficulties	"Collaborative mode"—take more direct actions to support family
IV. Parents' resources inadequate to meet the needs of their children	"Protective mode"—protect the children and sometimes the parents

Adapted from Roberts E: A model for parent education, *Image J Nurs Scholarship* 13:89, 1981.

BOX 9-4   Anticipatory Guidance Steps

1. Scan. Discover the problem.
2. Formulate. Explore the issue, specify, and name it.
3. Appraise. Patient decides whether the issue is worth working on—readiness and willingness.
4. Negotiate. Develop willingness on part of both parties.
5. Plan. Divide labor, plan action, and follow-up.
6. Implement.
   Orient—develop or change feelings about the issue.
   Guide—identify actions to occur.
   Develop decision-making rules and problem-solving strategies.
   Practice.
7. Evaluate.

---

information for decision making about issues predicted to arise at some time in the future, usually between the current and the next scheduled visit. With the rapid growth and developmental changes occurring in childhood, anticipatory guidance is essential if competent child-rearing practices are to be maintained and developed. Skilled anticipatory guidance involves a process outlined in Box 9-4. The process involves a finely tuned cooperative discussion with the client about issues of client concern. Following the principles of patient education, it should not be a rote recitation of information automatically provided at a specified visit. Skilled anticipatory guidance is individualized teaching, with outcomes mutually agreed on by provider and client. Part of the skill of the provider relates to making issues of anticipated change in the child relevant to the parent so that those issues can become topics for guidance.

Problems with anticipatory guidance have developed over time. Principally, so many national guidelines exist and so many topics are deemed important to raising a child that there is too much information to be provided within the time limits of a well-child visit. Olson and colleagues (2004) used data from the National Survey of Early Childhood Health to describe the content of anticipatory guidance provided to parents of infants and toddlers and to identify unmet needs as reported by parents and pediatricians. Immunizations, feeding issues, and sleep patterns were most frequently discussed. Developmental needs and family issues were less commonly addressed. Topics that parents felt would be helpful but were rarely discussed included discipline strategies, toilet training, burn prevention, child care, reading, vocabulary development, and social development. The mean length of well-child visits was about 18 minutes. Greater unmet anticipatory guidance needs were noted among parents with lower income, lower maternal education, and those receiving public assistance or lacking insurance. Race and ethnicity were also factors, with black and Hispanic parents more likely to report unmet needs.

Providing Data

Often providing data about a child's status to the parents or adolescent is a powerful yet easy intervention. The height and weight grid and developmental screening or laboratory test scores with interpretation are often significant motivators or reinforcers for the work that parents have been doing. The key is interpretation of information so that the parents know how their child compares with appropriate norms. Data provided should include both normal outcomes and areas of concern.

Role Modeling

Social learning theory suggests that modeling is an effective way for people to learn. Modeling appropriate parenting techniques can be most effective, especially when the parent then rehearses the desired behaviors with positive reinforcement. The provider must be careful to create a situation in which parents are left feeling competent—that they are doing a fine job rather than that someone else could do it better. Parents need to feel new confidence as a result of working with the provider and trying out new behaviors. Parenting classes and support groups often provide more time for role modeling and practice of new behaviors than can occur during a primary care visit. Several visits are often needed to help parents learn new responses to children's behavior. Part of the developmental process requires that parents make decisions about when to use the new responses they are learning.

Contracting

Establishing a contract with a client or family is an effective intervention that is interactive and collaborative in style. It requires shared responsibility and control on the part of patient and provider. Contracting can involve either contingencies (rewards) for completion of the client's actions to meet the contract or noncontingencies with the implied reward of better health consequences for progress made. It is important to make the contract with all the parties involved.

The contracting process involves three major phases. Phase one includes mutual identification of needs and problems and mutual agreement on goals, resources, and a plan of action. In phase two, the provider and client divide up the labor and responsibilities, establish a time frame, and then implement the plan. Mutual evaluation and renegotiation occur along the way. In phase three, the contract is terminated. A key factor is to keep the goals achievable.

Bibliotherapy

Promoting use of reading materials can be an excellent intervention in primary care. Books or pamphlets provide information that is well organized and presented in a manner that facilitates its retention. Furthermore, written materials allow patients or families to pace their learning at their own rate, and they serve as a familiar source of reference when needs arise at unexpected times. Redman (1993) refers to printed teaching material as a "frozen language that is selective in its description of reality (which is both a strength and a weakness). It encourages limited feedback, but is constantly available." The good reader uses reading materials efficiently, scanning for important words, stopping to summarize the material learned, and using illustrations to enhance the meanings derived from the text. On the other hand, the unskilled reader either spends an inordinate amount of time trying to master the material at hand or sets aside the task, usually without letting the provider know of the difficulties encountered. Thus, the reading levels of the client and the materials must be considered.

Reading also provides vicarious role models for both children and parents, acts as a support by acknowledging the feelings and problems encountered by others with similar problems, and expands perspectives on various health-related issues. Stories can help children, especially adolescents, explore new ideas, clarify their own feelings and perceptions, and serve as an impetus for change.

Of course the Internet also provides information on many subjects, but readers must be cognizant of the source to sort out reliable information from biased sources. Video libraries also provide helpful information with role modeling played out in many cases.

Reframing

Reframing is a counseling strategy in which one changes the context of an experience to give it a new meaning. The goal is to create a frame of reference that focuses upon a desired outcome rather than a current problem. It redirects interpretation. Patients who can find meaning in their illness may become more invested in self-care. Optimizing one's condition in comparison with others is an example. "I thought I was bad off with condition Y until I talked with a person with condition X. He was much worse off than I am." Support groups are often useful in helping people reframe their current condition; clarifying life values and committing to family or self are all improvements to life. All behaviors are appropriate in some contexts; yelling at a ballgame is OK, but not at home or work; pain is a sign of illness, but may be an indicator that braces on a teen's teeth are beginning to work and move the teeth into a new alignment. Surgery is a risk, but it is also an opportunity for healing. A child can be viewed as stubborn, but persistence may be a trait that will be helpful during life (Shea, 2006). One needs to be careful, however, not to use reframing to discount, deny, or ignore real problems faced by families. For example, the child who is setting fires should not be described as "demonstrating scientific curiosity."

HEALTH SYSTEM INTERVENTIONS: THE ARRANGE STEP OF "THE FIVE As" MODEL

Families with children have many complex needs, which are often met by different organizations such as governmental agencies; health care resources, including clinics, screening programs, health promotion programs, and hospitals; and volunteer programs.

Referrals should be considered whenever there is need for expertise, a more accessible resource, more time for intervention than is available in the current setting, or special types of intervention, such as a support group, class, or practice opportunities. Managed care settings, in some cases, seem to discourage use of referrals outside the system. However, solving problems efficiently and effectively, even if that means using another resource, is generally a cost-effective intervention.

Identifying and using various community resources requires knowledge and skills that some families do not have. Locating

services and helping families learn to use them might be necessary. Transportation, financial resources, the process for entering the system, and the services that can be anticipated are all factors to be discussed with families.

■ SUMMARY

Health promotion management is as important to the health of children as is illness management. The process of diagnosis and treatment is the same for both domains of providers practice. Interventions for both health promotion and disease management include preventive and therapeutic strategies, with patient education essential to ambulatory management. The clients include children and their parents, in addition to other family members or foster parents. For adolescents, the client increasingly becomes the adolescent as the independent decision maker.

Because children change so rapidly, their functional health patterns are stable for only short periods of time. The patterns need continual reassessment in light of developmental progress. Parents also need continuing information and new skills, such as teaching behaviors, to manage their children's evolving health care needs adequately. In addition, a multitude of factors, such as family practices and attitudes, peer influences, and community effects, shape the health behaviors of children. In many ways, health promotion care for children is more difficult than is management of their physical status. Developing skill as a manager of health promotion for clients is no easy task, but it is worth the effort. It is in the area of functional health pattern management that the unique contributions of providers to the health care of their pediatric clients are confirmed.

☑ DISCUSSION FORUM

1. How could you integrate the use of the models to predict health behavior into your daily counseling?
2. The Olson study cited in the chapter reported parents had unmet anticipatory guidance needs that were related to lower income, lower maternal education, public assistance, race, and ethnicity. What are some of the ways that providers could make use of technology and informatics to improve education of these families? What are some concepts that need to be considered in the development of these programs?
3. What strategies can busy practices use to help parents manage their children's growth and development needs until the next well-child visit?
4. What are some similarities and differences between anticipatory guidance and motivational interviewing? When should a provider switch from an anticipatory guidance mode to a motivational interviewing mode?
5. What community, state, and Internet resources are available to help families in smoking cessation, weight control management, and mental health issues?

REFERENCES

Allan J et al: Clinical prevention and population curriculum framework: the nursing perspective, *J Profes Nurs* 212:259-267, 2005.

Bandura A: Self-efficacy: toward a unifying theory of behavioral change, *Psychol Rev* 84:191-215, 1977.

Cifuentes M et al: Prescription for health: changing the health care practice to foster healthy behaviors, *Ann Fam Med* 3(suppl):S4-S12, 2005.

Cohen D et al: Implementing health behavior change in primary care: lessons from prescription for health, *Ann Fam Med* 3(suppl 2):512-519, 2005.

Dochterman J, Bulechek G, editor: *Nursing interventions classification,* ed 4, St Louis, 2004, Mosby.

Gordon M: *Nursing diagnosis: process and application,* New York, 1987, McGraw-Hill.

Green M. Palfrey J: *Bright Futures: guidelines for health supervision of infants, children, and adolescents,* ed 4, rev, Arlington VA, 2002, National Center for Education in Maternal and Child Health.

Institute of Medicine (IOM): *Crossing the quality chasm: a new health system for the 21st century,* Washington DC, 2001, National Academies Press.

LaGreca A, Bearman K, Moore H: Peer relations of youth with pediatric conditions and health risks: promoting social support and healthy lifestyles, *J Dev Behav Pediatr* 23:271-280, 2002.

Lask B: Motivating children and adolescents to improve adherence, *J Pediatr* 143:430-433, 2003.

Margolis P et al: From concept to application: the impact of a community-wide intervention to improve the delivery of preventive services to children, *Pediatrics* 108(3):e42, Sept 2001.

McGinnis M, Foege W: Actual causes of death in the United States, *JAMA* 270:2207-2212, 1993.

Miller K, Armstrong M: Developmental concepts of nicotine addiction, *J Pediatr Nurs* 21:108-114, 2006.

Miller WR, Rollnick S: *Motivational interviewing: preparing people to change addictive behavior,* New York, 1991, The Guilford Press.

Minkovitz C et al: A practice-based intervention to enhance quality of care in the first 3 years of life: the Healthy Steps for Young Children Program, *JAMA* 290(23):3081-3091, 2003.

Moyer V, Butler M: Gaps in the evidence for well-child care: a challenge for our profession, *Pediatrics* 114(6):1511-1521, 2004.

Myant KA, Williams JM: Children's concepts of health and illness: understanding of contagious illnesses, non-contagious illnesses and injuries, *J Health Psychol* 10(6):805-819, 2005.

Olson A et al: The Healthy Teen Project: tools to enhance adolescent health counseling, *Ann Fam Med* 3(suppl 2):563-565, 2005.

Olson L et al: Overview of the content of health supervision for young children: reports from parents and pediatricians, *Pediatrics* 113(6):1907-1916, 2004.

Pender N: *Health promotion in nursing practice,* ed 3, Norwalk, CT, 1996, Appleton & Lange.

Prochaska J: Disease management needs new paradigms, *J Gen Intern Med* 10:472-473, 1995.

Prochaska J, DiClemente C, Norcross J: In search of how people change: applications to addictive behaviors, *Am Psychol* 47:1102-1114, 1992.

Prochaska J et al: Stages of change and decisional balance for 12 problem behaviors, *Health Psychol* 13:39-46, 1994.

Redman B: *Patient education,* ed 7, St Louis, 1993, Mosby.

Roberts F: A model for parent education, *Image* 13:86-89, 1981.

Rogers EM: *Diffusion of innovations,* New York, 1983, Free Press.

Rubak S et al: Motivational interviewing: a systematic review and meta-analysis, *Br J Gen Pract* 55:305-312, 2005.

Shea K: Reframing: a fresh outlook helps patients envision positive outcomes. In *2006 Pathways Professional Development,* Gannett Healthcare Group, Falls Church, VA, pp 56-60.

Sindelar H et al: Motivational interviewing in pediatric practice, *Curr Problems Pediatr Adolesc Health Care* 34(9):322-339, 2004.

US Department of Health and Human Services (USDHHS): *Healthy people 2010: understanding and improving health,* ed 2, Washington, DC, 2000, US Government Printing Office.

Whitlock E et al: Evaluating primary care behavioral counseling interventions: an evidence based approach, *Am J Prev Med* 22(4):267-284, 2004.

Zuckerman B et al: Healthy Steps: a case study of innovation in pediatric practice, *Pediatrics* 114(3):820-826, 2004.

Health Perception and Health Management Patterns

Ardys M. Dunn

Children's health depends on a multitude of factors, including appropriate nutrition, stimulation, exercise, rest, and emotional and social nurturance. In addition to healthy lifestyle behaviors, prevention and management of illness and injury is essential to children's growth and development. This chapter discusses ways health care providers can work with parents, children, and families to ensure that decisions made and actions taken regarding health management are best suited to growing children's needs. This chapter explores factors that influence the health behavior of children and their families and summarizes the health maintenance needs of infants, toddlers, preschoolers, school-age children, and adolescents.

■ HEALTH PERCEPTION AND HEALTH MANAGEMENT PATTERN

DEFINITION

The health perception and health management functional health pattern offers a framework to assess children's health status and the behaviors that contribute to health. Relevant health perception and management questions include the following: How is health perceived? What characteristics of children contribute to their health status (e.g., is there an underlying chronic illness or genetic disorder)? What decisions have families made and what actions have been taken to bring children to their current level of health? What resources to support good health are available to families? How can providers intervene to support healthy behaviors or to help change those that are unhealthy?

SIGNIFICANCE FOR PRIMARY HEALTH CARE PRACTICE

Effective health management requires a commitment to good health, prevention of illness and injury, knowledge of ways to achieve optimal health, and access to and use of necessary health care resources. This functional health pattern is most concerned with the primary level of prevention (i.e., actions taken to promote health or protect against specific factors that threaten health, or both).

Use of this functional health pattern gives providers a better understanding of why certain decisions about health care are made. For example, in some communities, fewer than 50% of children under 2 years old are fully immunized. Parents do not bring their children for regular well child examinations or for scheduled immunizations. These behaviors could be attributed to many factors, such as the parents' belief that immunizations are unnecessary or even dangerous or a lack of knowledge about community health resources that provide immunizations. Transportation, child care problems, and lack of financial resources can contribute to a parent's failure to bring children for regular well child visits. By identifying factors that influence the decisions families make, providers can intervene more effectively so that parents and children will actively engage in positive health management.

■ NORMAL PATTERNS OF HEALTH PERCEPTION AND HEALTH MANAGEMENT

Health perceptions are the ways that a person thinks about and defines health-related experiences. Health management is the action taken to deal with these experiences. Health management is based on health perceptions and reflects the judgments of individuals and families, the ways they solve problems, and the decisions or choices they make. Positive health management assumes that wise decisions are made and that resources are available for families to implement these decisions. These concepts are also discussed in Chapter 9.

COMPONENTS OF HEALTH PERCEPTION

By exploring a family's health perceptions, providers can begin to see reasons behind the health decisions a family makes. Components of health perception include (1) how individuals perceive and feel about their general state of health, past, present, and future and (2) the belief that there is a relationship between health status and health practices.

Perception of Health

How parents, caregivers, and children themselves perceive and feel about children's health status is shaped by several interrelated variables, including:

- Perception of one's susceptibility to the condition
- Severity of the condition
- Extent to which the condition has an impact on one's ability to function
- Knowledge about the condition
- Knowledge about how children's developmental stages affect their response to illness
- Developmental stage of the child
- Cultural or social cues about the condition

Belief That Health Practices Can Affect Health Status

The degree to which parents and children believe that they can influence their health status varies. In general, individuals and families with an internal locus of control believe that their behavior affects their health status. They are motivated to take action, seek information, and set goals, believing that such behaviors will make a difference in the outcome. Even when confronted with the stress and uncertainty of illness, they are active problem-solvers, engaged in the process of decision-making. Families with an internal locus of control often are able to more effectively cope with their child's illness (Dunn et al, 2001). In contrast, many individuals and families with an external locus of control tend to believe that factors outside their control determine illness outcomes. These families can be passive and dependent, lack motivation to engage in self-care, or fail to follow through with recommended treatments. Rather than actively seeking to change the condition, they let things happen to them.

A variety of factors affect the extent of belief in one's ability to control health outcomes (Steptoe & Wardle, 2001). Age and gender are two factors noted in children, with older children and girls having a more internal locus of control. Also, families who are usually self-directed can experience excessive stress related to their child's illness or other life circumstances and may temporarily feel inadequate to cope. Providing parents with specific strategies about how to manage their child's health can give them a sense of competence, decrease stress, and contribute to healthier family dynamics (Raina et al, 2005).

COMPONENTS OF HEALTH MANAGEMENT

Health management is the process of making decisions, taking action, and using resources to maintain and promote health. Health management reflects the underlying beliefs and perceptions that families, parents, and children have about health (Table 10-1).

Decision-Making

Although the ways in which people make decisions vary greatly, decision-making styles may fall into the following categories:

- The decision-maker examines and reexamines all options and selects one, but may alter the choice if new information or variables arise.
- The person making the decision looks at options, but is comfortable making a quick decision without excessive reflection.
- The person making the decision is overly concerned, shifts back and forth from one option to another, and never focuses on one as viable.
- The person elects not to make a decision, procrastinating or avoiding the situation entirely. Not taking action is a decision too.

Many factors help shape the health-related decisions a family makes, including:
- Social support structures
- Perception of current health status
- Emotional competence of family members, which may be situational (e.g., the family is confronted with a condition that severely disrupts their emotional or psychological health, such as severe, unexpected trauma to a child)

TABLE 10-1 **Relationship Between Health Perception and Health Behaviors**

Variable Affecting Health Perception	Related Health Behaviors
Perception of susceptibility	Increased sense of susceptibility contributes to taking precautions (e.g., immunizations) and seeking early treatment.
Severity of condition	Severity of condition usually, but not always, results in health-seeking behaviors; if signs and symptoms are subtle or appear minor, care may be delayed.
	Minor conditions with alarming signs (e.g., urticaria) may be responded to aggressively.
Impact on ability to function	Decreased function motivates health-seeking behaviors (e.g., child with minor illness may not be brought for care unless the condition disrupts sleep or eating patterns).
Knowledge about condition	Increased understanding of condition usually increases family's ability to manage, either by seeking appropriate health care or providing self-care.
	Increased education has not always contributed to health promotion activities.
Knowledge regarding child development	Knowledge of child development gives parents ability to anticipate behavior and recognize variations of normal.
	Parents who lack knowledge of child development may interpret normal behavior as problematic or may not perceive atypical behavior as a problem.
Developmental stage of child	Children's conceptualization and response to illness vary by developmental stage.
Cultural or social cues	Cultural beliefs shape health perceptions (see Chapter 3).
	Messages or cues may be mixed (e.g., children are encouraged not to smoke, yet movie stars are increasingly shown lighting up cigarettes) and can lead to positive and negative health behaviors.

- Past experience
- Education and knowledge level
- Cognitive abilities of family members
- Values and cultural perspectives
- Economic conditions
- Environment
- Information and advice from the health care provider

Health Behaviors

The decisions that a family makes lead directly to their health practices and behaviors. Within this functional health pattern, several behaviors are expected that promote health and prevent problems. Specifically, healthy families will:

- Establish an ongoing relationship with a primary health care provider
- Use health and community resources to promote health
- Demonstrate lifestyles that promote health and prevent illness and injury

Primary Caregiver Relationship. It is expected that the family will establish an ongoing relationship with a primary health care provider, ensuring that the child receives regular physical and developmental evaluations; health maintenance care, such as immunizations; early intervention for minor acute health problems; and information and guidance related to growth and development issues of the child and the family. Having a regular provider also offers the family a stable contact and access to health care resources in case the child requires hospitalization, surgery, or long-term care.

Health and Community Resources to Promote Health. Families with a positive health management pattern identify, access, and use appropriate social, community, family, and health-related resources effectively and efficiently.

The way parents use health care services will be based on past experiences that reinforce their beliefs about what causes illness, what is the most appropriate treatment, and how effectively the parents can care for their child. For example, if parents of an ill child have once managed a fever successfully, they are more likely to feel confident coping with a fever in the child's current condition. If they believe that their child remains free of illness as a result of their care and nurturing, they are more likely to continue health promotion activities. In contrast, if the child is healthy or ill despite what the parents do, they can be more inclined to depend on the provider for advice or care or not to seek care at all.

Effective use of health resources includes the ability to know when it is necessary to have a child seen by the primary care provider and how to interact appropriately with providers by telephone, via e-mail, or during the health visit.

Health management of children with special needs is challenging. Children with chronic illness receive expert illness care from a number of specialists, but their primary care needs may often be neglected. Primary care providers can serve to coordinate health maintenance care with ongoing specialty illness management. Communication and collaboration with the child's specialty physician are essential, as is clear communication with the parents about the role of each provider in the child's care. Providers also need to adapt normal intervention techniques when providing primary care to children with chronic illness. The regular immunization schedule may need to be adjusted, for example, or special techniques for obtaining height and weight or vital signs might be necessary. Parents and children should be assisted to develop ways to meet daily living needs consonant with the child's ability. Children with physical handicaps, for example, require special intervention to meet activity and exercise needs for growth and development.

Many community resources are available to families (e.g., school nurses or school-based clinics provide case management or primary care in the school setting). Providers can inform parents about these resources, explain their purpose, and encourage parents to communicate with school personnel about children's health needs. School-based health services are especially important for children with chronic illnesses.

Social supports offer a buffer against the stress of daily living, allowing the individual and family to respond more positively to both usual and unexpected events. Families isolated from a social network find it much more difficult to structure health maintenance into their lives or to cope with a child's illness. Connection to a network of community resources (e.g., schools, day care, recreational facilities) also provides structure to support families in daily living activities.

Families need economic and material resources for optimal health management. The high cost of health care services or lack of health care insurance coverage are barriers to access that contribute to delay or neglect in seeking essential treatment. There must also be a sufficient number of providers and health care services in the community. For many children, economic barriers prevent access to health care, but for others, adequate resources are simply not available in their communities.

Healthy Lifestyles. Healthy families demonstrate lifestyles that enhance health and prevent illness and injury. Although some factors causing disease, illness, and injury are beyond the control of individuals and families, in many cases, lifestyle choices directly affect health status. There are specific categories of behavior in which lifestyle change has an impact on health status (Box 10-1). In addition to changing their own behavior, individuals can act to significantly change their external environment, thus influencing forces that affect their health and the health of family members.

Environment

Environmental conditions relate to health management on two levels: first, the nature of the environment affects health status (see Chapter 41), and, second, as noted earlier, resources to support health may or may not be present in the physical environment. Many children experience environmental factors, such as urban crowding, air and noise pollution, streets with heavy traffic, inadequate housing, poor nutrition, lack of appropriate stimulation (e.g., no playgrounds or recreational facilities), violence, and physical and emotional stress. In addition, families with few economic resources have limited

Lifestyle Choices That Affect Health Status

- Nutrition
- Exercise
- Social-interactional patterns (family and community relations)
- Coping and stress management skills
- Motor vehicle use
- Sexual behavior
- Smoking
- Alcohol use
- Drug use

access to health care services. Frequent moves from one neighborhood, area, or state to another prevent families from establishing ongoing connections with a health care provider, and continuity of care is lost.

Rural environments often lack health-related resources, with few providers, clinics, or hospital services easily available. To compound this problem, children living in rural settings are at high risk for injury because of exposure to animals, farm machinery, pesticides, herbicides, unsafe transportation, and other physical hazards (AAP Committee on Injury and Poison Prevention and Committee on Community Health Services, 2001; Kmet & Macarthur, 2006).

ASSESSMENT OF HEALTH PERCEPTION AND HEALTH MANAGEMENT PATTERN

Assessment of this functional health pattern focuses on health perception, health management, and decision-making.

HISTORY

Components of Health Perception

Perception of Health. Health perception is assessed by examining the family's health belief structure and level of knowledge. Perceptions can be strongly shaped by the family's cultural background (see Chapter 3). During the initial intake history, the focus is on the family's general perception of health. At subsequent visits, questions look at the particular condition (e.g., "Tell me what this illness means to you"). General assessment questions include the following:

- How would you describe your child's health right now?
- Compared with other children, how healthy would you say your child is?
- What does it mean for you to say that your child is "healthy"?
- How do you describe good health in your family?
- Do you have any questions or concerns about your child's health, growth, or development?
- How important is it to you to have a regular health care provider?

- What makes you decide to call your health care provider or take your child in for an examination (e.g., as a way to stay well, for a serious problem such as a high fever, an accident, or a problem you have never seen before or one that will not go away)?
- What do you know about this current condition?
- Has your child had a problem like this before?
- How do you expect your child to respond when sick? To this particular sickness?
- What things can you do to help your child cope with being sick?

Belief That Health Practices Affect Health Status. General intake questions can yield important information about whether the family and child believe that their health practices affect outcomes. These include the following:

- Has your child ever had this type of problem before?
- What have you done for it in the past?
- What do you do or have you done that you believe makes a difference in how your child responds to illness?
- What kind of personality would you say your child has? How would you describe your child's temperament?
- When confronted with sudden changes in plans or a disruption of normal routine, feelings often change. What kinds of feelings do you have when this happens? How do you deal with those feelings?
- Describe the feelings you have when your child gets ill. How do you deal with those feelings?
- How do you think those feelings affect the way you handle your child's health and illness?

Locus of control can also be assessed using classic rating scales, such as Rotter's (1966) internal-external scale, the health locus of control scale (Wallston et al, 1976), the perceived health competence scale (Smith et al, 1995), or the multidimensional health locus of control scale (Wallston et al, 1978). Measures of the effect of locus of control on a particular health condition, such as weight and injury treatment, have been explored (Holt et al, 2001; Reicks et al, 2004).

Components of Health Management

Decision-Making. The family's decision-making is assessed by examining how active the family is in making decisions about the child's health care, the process used, and the factors that influence those decisions. Questions in this area include the following:

- What do you do when your child has health problems?
- Who makes decisions about health care in your family?
- How do you make those decisions? Do you talk things over? Do you get advice from others?
- Why do you think that you make decisions in that way?
- What are the most important things that you consider when making a decision about health care for your child?
- What is most difficult for you when you have to make decisions related to your child's health?

Health Behaviors and Use of Resources. The following questions refer to actions taken and resources used to promote health and healing:

- Do you have a regular health care provider for your child?
- What health care resources are available to you? Is there a primary care provider you can get to conveniently? Clinics? Pharmacies?
- When was the last time your child visited a regular health care provider or dentist?
- What makes it hard for you to follow the advice of your health care provider?
- What immunizations has your child received?
- What have you done to protect your child from injuries? What are your patterns of seat belt use?
- Does your child have any special health problems? How do you manage them?
- There has been much focus on healthy lifestyles lately, such as eating right and exercising. What does your family do regularly to stay healthy?
- Does anyone in your family (adolescents, you yourself) smoke, drink, or use drugs? How often? What kind? Are there other things that your family does that you think are bad for your children's health?
- How does your family fit into your neighborhood? Do you feel like part of the community? Do you have relatives or neighbors on whom you can call if you need help or advice?
- Who cares for your child when you are not at home and the child is not in school?
- For this illness:
  - How are you managing household, work, school, and other child care responsibilities? What is most difficult for you?
  - Having sick children can create a financial strain on families. Is this a problem for your family? What is the most difficult part?
  - How comfortable do you feel managing this illness? Have you had experience in the past that helps you manage?

Environment. Environmental conditions are difficult to assess during a clinic visit, even if the parent is open, cooperative, and willing to share information. If there is a question about a child's health because of possible environmental problems, it may be appropriate to arrange for a community health nurse to visit the family at home to gain a thorough understanding of the family environment. See Chapter 41 for a more full discussion of children's health as it is related to the environment. Some questions that can be asked in the clinic include the following:

- Do you use booster seats, seat belts, or child restraints when riding in a car?
- Where does your child play? Do you believe it is safe? Why?
- Is your home childproof? If you have firearms, are they unloaded and locked; is ammunition locked separately? Are pools fenced and gated?
- How do you heat or cool your home? Is it comfortable?
- Is there any danger of falls? Is he or she dressed warmly for cold weather? Do you have a working smoke alarm?

- What would you do if your child had a health emergency? Do you have a car, or is there a friend, family member, or neighbor close by who could help you?
- What other conditions in your child's environment do you think could be a health risk?

Children With Special Needs. Assessment of the health perception and management pattern for children with special needs encompasses all questions in the categories just discussed such as the following:

- What does it mean for you to say that your child is "healthy"?
- How did you feel when your child's problem was diagnosed? What did you do? What coping strategies do you currently use as you care for your child?
- How has managing a chronic illness changed your family functioning? How does your family function?
- Who is providing specialty care to your child? Do you believe this is adequate? What other special needs do you believe your child has that require care?
- How comfortable are you in providing home care? What would you need to be more comfortable?
- How are your child's regular health needs met (i.e., those not directly related to the chronic illness, such as immunizations)?
- What resources do you know about that can help you understand and manage your child's illness?
- What special physical arrangements have you made to accommodate your child's illness? At home? In the car? At school or day care?

MANAGEMENT STRATEGIES FOR POSITIVE HEALTH PERCEPTION AND HEALTH MANAGEMENT

Parents and providers work together to manage children's health. This section discusses areas of intervention relevant to health perception and health management.

PROVIDING HEALTH MAINTENANCE FOR CHILDREN BY DEVELOPMENTAL AGE

Health supervision visits for children are more than simple physical checkups. Visits with the provider also allow assessment of home, family, and social life, teaching about growth and development, and problem-solving related to issues that affect children's health status. The visits can be used to enhance children's sense of independence and positive self-concept and to encourage children to make healthy lifestyle decisions. As children mature, they should be actively involved in the visit, with the provider asking them questions directly and providing appropriate feedback to their responses. In addition to screening interventions recommended by the AAP Committee on Practice and Ambulatory Medicine (2000) (see Appendix D), the health supervision visit examines the child's daily living and functional health patterns as identified in Table 10-2.

TABLE 10-2 **Health Supervision Visits: Daily Living and Functional Health Patterns**

	Infant	Toddler	Preschool Child	School-Age Child	Adolescent
Parent-child interaction	Degree of mutual and reciprocal response between infant and parents Emotional status of parents Appropriateness of parental response to infant's cues	Parental confidence in role Emotional status of parents Appropriateness of parental response to toddler's cues Degree of affection demonstrated between toddler and parents Parental encouragement of independence, yet active involvement with child	Consistency in parents' behavior Emotional status of parents Appropriateness of parental response to child's cues Degree to which parents provide affection, praise, and emotional support and encourage child to express feelings Parental encouragement of independence, yet active engagement with child	Clear, consistent, but flexible expectations expressed by parents Appropriate limits set by parents Degree to which parents provide attention, affection, praise, approval, and emotional support and encourage child to express feelings Degree to which parents support independence, yet participate with child in activities Degree to which child demonstrates self-confidence, industriousness, cooperation, and consideration	Parental confidence and pleasure in role Open communication with mutual respect for privacy Parental encouragement of independence and activities with peers Reasonable and consistent limits Active parental interest in adolescent's activities, friends, school performance Parental pride and pleasure in adolescent's achievements
Developmental assessment to determine extent to which child has achieved milestones and received emotional nurturing	See Chapters 5 and 17	See Chapters 6 and 17	See Chapters 6 and 17; look for child who is friendly, secure, cooperative, proud, and happy Conduct speech evaluation	See Chapters 7 and 17; conduct speech evaluation	See Chapters 8 and 17
Nutrition and metabolic	Choice of feeding, breastfeeding versus bottle feeding (see Chapter 12) When to introduce solids; management of feeding problems or special nutritional needs (see Chapter 11) Fluoride beginning at	Management of self-feeding, feeding problems, or special nutritional needs (see Chapter 11) Pattern of dentition, need for good oral hygiene (see Chapter 33) Fluoride as indicated Skin care: apply sunscreen whenever child is exposed to sun	Need for well-balanced diet Parents' responsibility to provide nutritious foods, pleasant atmosphere for meals, and healthy role models for child; child's responsibility to select appropriate foods from those provided (see Chapter 11)	Healthy food selections with child making more independent choices (see Chapter 11) Daily dental hygiene (see Chapter 33) Fluoride as indicated Skin care: apply sunscreen whenever child is exposed to sun	Nutritional needs, dietary patterns with adolescent making choices (see Chapter 11) Body image and self-perception as they relate to eating habits Good oral hygiene, regular dental care (see Chapter 33), orthodontia

Continued

TABLE 10-2 Health Supervision Visits: Daily Living and Functional Health Patterns—Cont'd

	Infant	Toddler	Preschool Child	School-Age Child	Adolescent
	6mo as indicated according to fluoride level in water source Skin care: apply sunscreen whenever child is exposed to sun		Pattern of dentition, need for dental assessment (see Chapter 33) Fluoride as indicated Skin care: apply sunscreen whenever child is exposed to sun		Fluoride until 16yr, as indicated Skin care: apply sunscreen whenever child is exposed to sun Acne management as appropriate
Sleep and rest: sleep needs, patterns, and changes as child grows (see Chapter 15)	Importance of bedtime ritual, infant cues for sleep and wake states Position infant on back for sleep	Importance of bedtime ritual	Typical night fears, night terrors	Sleepwalking and night terrors	Sleep needs during rapid growth of adolescence
Activity and exercise (see Chapter 14); injury prevention (see Tables 10-4 through 10-7)	Physical developmental needs and skills of infant	Set limits and provide safe environment for expression of physical needs and developing skills	Set limits and provide safe environment for expression of physical needs and skills Active, pretend and fantasy play; discourage passive activities such as watching television Child's tendency to become overtired, often needing parent's help to calm down	Encourage regular physical activity Bicycle, skateboard, pedestrian, swimming safety Balance of nutrition with exercise to achieve appropriate weight gain Scoliosis in child 10-12yr	Regular physical activity, participation in fitness and organized sports activities Scoliosis evaluation Sports fitness and safety
Elimination (see Chapter 13)	Diapering, infant patterns of stooling and urination	Toilet training	Management of occasional "accidents" in toilet-trained child Good hygiene, hand washing	Good hygiene, hand washing Explain relationship between nutrition, exercise, and elimination	Good hygiene, hand washing Explain relationship between nutrition, exercise, and elimination
Sexuality (see Chapter 19)	Infant's sense of physical comfort and pleasure related to stimulation of genitalia Parents to express their perceptions of sexuality in infant and child Testes and inguinal canal for abnormalities	Toddler's sense of physical comfort and pleasure related to genital stimulation, masturbation Parents to express their perceptions of sexuality; ways parents communicate with toddler about sexuality	Child's natural curiosity related to sexuality Parents to answer questions at age-appropriate level Concept of "good" and "bad" touch; private body parts	Children's natural curiosity and exploration related to sexuality Parents to answer questions at age-appropriate level, set appropriate limits for sexual activity in child Sexual maturation (SM) stage (Tanner)	Developing sense of sexual identity, masturbation, degree of intimacy with others Sexual responsibility to self and others, how to say "no" and how to deal with potential sexual abuse or "date rape"

Pattern	Infant	Toddler	Preschool/School	School Age	Adolescent
					Prevention of sexually transmitted diseases and pregnancy; birth control options Sexual maturation stages, gynecomastia in boy Pelvic examination in sexually active girl, girl with menstrual problems, or those with history of mother taking diethylstilbestrol (DES) Breast and testicular self-examination Folic acid 400 mcg/day for girl
Role relationships (see Chapters 4 and 18)	Infant's interaction with siblings and other family members; impact child has on family system, place of child in family	Discipline strategies Interaction of toddler with siblings, other family members; impact child has on family system, place of child in family Day care needs and plans	Discipline strategies Interaction of child with siblings, other family members; impact child has on family system, place of child in family Day care needs and plans School readiness for older preschool-age child	Increasing child's participation in family activities, taking more responsibility for tasks in household Nature of child's interaction in school and with peer group Parents encourage and participate in hobbies, reading, other activities with child and peer group	Increasing independence in adolescents; responsibilities at home, school, or workplace Need to keep communication open among adolescent, peers, and parents
Self-concept and self-perception (see Chapter 17)	Infant's developing an awareness of self as separate from parents and others	Importance of giving child positive feedback on achievements Parents to relate to child in warm, loving manner; avoid harsh words, punitive and inconsistent parental behavior	Parents to give children choices, allowing children to express selves and participate in family tasks Children's sense of absolutes at this age; discourage teasing and threats Parents to participate in child's activities (e.g., school field trips)	Parents to give child attention and positive reinforcement of choices, allowing child to express self and expecting participation in family tasks	Opportunities to discuss changes in self and to openly ask questions about development Parents to give adolescent positive attention, reinforcement for healthy choices and appropriate activities, allowing adolescent privacy and expecting reasonable participation in family activities

Continued

TABLE 10-2 Health Supervision Visits: Daily Living and Functional Health Patterns—Cont'd

	Infant	Toddler	Preschool Child	School-Age Child	Adolescent
Coping and stress tolerance; for all ages, examine the following: Family support network Knowledge of community resources Knowledge of child development Level of parenting skills (see Chapter 20)	Parents' health habits (e.g., smoking, exercise, diet) may affect child	Discipline styles and options Parent to guide and instruct child's positive social behavior (e.g., sharing, not hitting or biting)	Discipline styles and options; need to set limits Parents to help child name and identify feelings and ways the child can manage feelings	Discipline styles and options; need to set limits Parents to praise child's efforts at self-control, management of feelings Depression assessment	Discipline styles and options Parents to provide appropriate limits while fostering independence Adolescent's emotional states related to rapid growth and changes of puberty Depression assessment
Values and beliefs (see Chapter 21)	Parents' expectations of self and child as family grows	Parents to identify their value and belief framework; how they demonstrate their beliefs to their child	Parents to provide opportunities for child to express ideas, feelings, and emotions Child included in family spiritual activities	Parents to provide opportunity for child to explore understanding of emotions, values, and beliefs in more formal settings (e.g., religious institutions, spiritual activities)	Adolescent, as part of normal process of developing self-identity, may appear to reject family values Encourage adolescent to discuss values and beliefs

FACILITATING COMMUNICATION BETWEEN FAMILIES AND HEALTH CARE PROVIDERS

Effective communication between families and health care providers requires sensitivity and skill. Families must be given the message that their values and beliefs are important, that providers recognize they are making their best effort to do the right thing, and that those efforts are to be applauded. If families are listened to, they are more likely to participate in health care decision-making and be more invested in the process and outcome. Communication is facilitated by two strategies in particular, one focused on content, one on process.

First, providers, parents, and children must develop a mutual understanding of the perspectives that each brings to the encounter (Kleinman et al, 1978). To do this, family members must be encouraged to explain their understanding of the child's illness, in addition to their expectations for its outcome and the role each player has in working toward that outcome. Providers must explain their perspective, usually biomedical, focusing on similar areas of concern: cause, symptoms, pathophysiology, nature and course of the illness, and treatment. Kleinman and his associates (1978) outlined a set of questions to elicit information about a family's health beliefs. These questions can be adapted and used with parents when asking about their child's illness (see Box 3-1). With this information in hand, providers, parents, and children can compare similarities and differences between their perspectives and create a mutually agreed-on plan of care.

A second strategy that strengthens communication and contributes to families having a greater sense of control in the situation relates to the process of the client-provider interaction. Marshall (1988) asserted that to arrive at the appropriate interpretation of what the clinical situation means, clients and providers must engage in a process of interpretation at the conversational level. This "conversational cooperation" is enhanced when family members and the provider do the following:

- Use cooperative turn-taking in the conversation.
- Use similar patterns of conversation, such as open-ended questions or narrative discussion. Communication is at risk, for example, if parents are using a narrative form of discussion and the provider is using closed-ended questions.
- Listen for the images clients use in speech patterns and try to respond in kind. Parents may use visual, auditory, or kinesthetic imagery when they talk and may better understand providers who respond with similar imagery. For example, the parent may state, "I don't see any change …"; the provider responds, "You're looking for …." Or the parent states, "I want to do something …" and the provider answers, "One action we could take…" (Howard, 1998).
- Confirm assumptions.
- Develop a clear understanding of differences in perspectives or meaning of the illness.
- Remain open to alternative explanations and solutions, not limited to following an isolated path of clinical reasoning.
- Explain or provide the context of pronouns used (e.g., if the provider says, "I'll check on that for you," be sure the parent understands what "that" means).

HELPING FAMILIES DEVELOP SOUND DECISION-MAKING SKILLS

Providers serve a vital role in helping families and children develop sound decision-making skills by providing information and health education and by giving families an opportunity to explore options for action. The way in which information is given may be as important as the information itself. Parents are more likely to accept information or suggestions from providers with whom they have established a high level of rapport and trust. These are providers who have worked to establish effective communication; generate mutual understanding of problems; and listen actively to parents' feelings, perceptions, fears, and anxieties. Providers can also structure the time and place for parents to discuss feelings, clarify points of confusion, and receive validation for their choices in this decision-making process. The process of making health care decisions includes the following steps:

- Identify the problem being confronted. Review the facts and feelings one has about the problem.
- Generate alternative solutions to the problem.
- Evaluate the alternatives. Which are feasible? Which are cost effective? What are the consequences of each? Which best fits the family's belief system?
- Select a solution.
- Develop and implement a plan of action based on that solution.
- Review the outcomes of the decision and the action taken.

For this process to function well, families must be able—or be assisted—to communicate effectively, understand abstract concepts, and mobilize resources. Children should be encouraged to participate in the process consistent with their developmental abilities. Adolescents, especially, are at a stage at which they can make many decisions independently of their parents.

HELPING FAMILIES GAIN ACCESS TO HEALTH CARE RESOURCES

Strategies to increase parents' ability to access resources occur on two levels: (1) giving parents the information to more easily and appropriately gain access and (2) removing barriers to access.

Giving Parents Information to Gain Access
Teaching Telephone Triage and E-Mail Communication

The nature of the telephone interaction between parent and provider can be a critical factor in accurately interpreting a child's condition, deciding on appropriate measures of care, and establishing confidence and trust. See Chapter 22 for a discussion of how pediatric care providers can work with parents to use the telephone in the management of illnesses. Increasingly, health care practices use e-mail communication to assess and give advice or treatment to patients. This trend is just beginning, and many questions remain about safety and appropriate use (Masters, 2006; Griffiths et al, 2006). As with any form of communication, providers who use e-mail should clearly establish with the parent how the technology is to be used (e.g., which types of questions, how quickly can a response be expected).

Identifying Resources. Providers serve as advocates by helping families locate local, regional, or national health care resources to meet their health needs. It is important that providers develop and maintain a resource list relevant to their practice. Using a resource list facilitates referrals and recommendations to parents; it gives the clear message that the family is not alone with their concern, that help is available, and that the primary care provider is a knowledgeable ally in the family's effort to maintain good health.

Assisting in Contact of Support Networks. As advocates, providers make every effort to encourage independent action and decision-making by families, but if the family's coping abilities are compromised, it is not enough simply to give the name of a resource or contact to the family. In these situations, providers may need to contact the resource themselves or assist the family to make the contact. For some families in crisis, it is appropriate to refer them to a community or mental health nurse for help to establish and maintain contact with a supportive network.

Removing Barriers to Access

Among the primary barriers to health care access are cost, geography, and lack of essential infrastructure services such as transportation and child care. The high cost of care is a major factor that prevents children from receiving regular well child care. Lack of primary care resources in rural and isolated areas also prevents families from obtaining regular care. If a family does not have adequate transportation or child care services, the cost of seeking well child care or treating minor acute problems that worsen without medical intervention often outweighs the perceived benefits.

Providers can work with parents and social workers to identify resources in the community that help overcome some of these barriers. For example, transportation may be available through some managed care plans or local volunteer organizations (e.g., churches), or a relative may have time to care for other children while the parent takes one child to the clinic. For other barriers, however, the solution lies in making changes in the way health care services are organized and financed. This task goes far beyond the primary care setting, but it is nonetheless the responsibility of all pediatric primary care providers to be aware of and to participate in the process of restructuring and reorganizing the health care system within their community.

■ ALTERED PATTERNS OF HEALTH PERCEPTION AND HEALTH MANAGEMENT

INEFFECTIVE USE OF HEALTH CARE SYSTEM

Description

Ineffective use of the health care system includes seeking care primarily when children are ill or when there is an external mandate (e.g., when immunizations are required to attend school), using emergency departments for routine care needs, or using outpatient services for emergency care, not establishing an ongoing relationship with a primary care provider, underusing health care resources, or failing to comply or follow-up with prescribed regimens. For behavior to be labeled "noncompliant," the child or caregivers must actively choose not to adhere to health recommendations despite knowledge of the benefits and risks.

Epidemiology

Ineffective use of the health care system can be caused by long-standing patterns of misuse, knowledge deficit about how to gain access to and use the system, and knowledge deficit about health and illness, such as the seriousness of illness in children. Access to care can be limited by social, physical, or economic barriers. Health care in the U.S. is largely connected to employment, but can be purchased independently. Some employees receive no health insurance coverage benefits and, for others, insurance coverage is inadequate. In addition, the unemployed or those with low incomes may not be able to afford insurance. As a result, the number of uninsured individuals in the U.S. has increased to 15.9% of the population or approximately 47 million in the past 5 years (DeNavas-Walt et al, 2006). The Medicaid program reimburses providers for primary health care services for families whose income is low enough to qualify for welfare, but reimbursement is often less than the cost of the services provided; some providers lose income and refuse care to Medicaid clients.

Cultural perceptions of care and the perception that health care providers do not understand or value the family or their cultural beliefs can discourage use of health care services. Values, beliefs, and perceptions of risk and benefits contribute to the choices made. For example, a client may refuse chemotherapy for leukemia, believing that there is greater risk associated with the treatment than with the disease itself. Finally a lack of health care resources can contribute to incomplete care. Rural and poor urban communities often lack health facilities, or the facilities there are understaffed, leaving residents with inadequate care.

Clinical Findings

The following are found with ineffective use of the health care system:

- No regular provider for child
- History of lack of continuity or fragmented care
- Use of emergency department for nonemergent conditions
- Lack of follow-up care for child seen in emergency department
- Failure to adhere to prescribed medical treatment or standards for well child health supervision after having adequate information for decision-making
- Child at risk for delayed or ineffective treatment or both
- Poor health status of children as a result of untreated illness or other health problem
- Underimmunization
- Parents' dissatisfaction with health care providers

Differential Diagnosis

- Dysfunctional family systems related to cognitive, emotional, or psychological variables

Management

Interventions vary depending on the reasons families ineffectively use the system.

LACK OF AN IDENTIFIED PRIMARY CARE PROVIDER

- Assist the family to establish a permanent relationship with a provider.
- Encourage and reinforce positive, ongoing communication with the primary care provider.
- Establish a positive, accepting environment of trust and mutual respect, encouraging the family and child to take an active role in health care.
- Assist the child and family to develop an understanding of the importance of regular care.

BARRIERS TO HEALTH CARE SERVICES

- Inform families of health care resources available in the community.
- Teach the family how to access and use health care services most effectively.
- Assist families to identify strengths and resources within their social and family network.
- Refer to social services or other resources to deal with financial concerns.
- Work with community, local, state, and federal leaders to change the way health care services are organized and financed.

KNOWLEDGE DEFICIT ABOUT CHILDREN

- Assess knowledge level of families related to development and health care needs of children.
- Educate parents about normal growth and development of children.
- Provide anticipatory guidance about variations of normal and health care needs of children at different ages.

KNOWLEDGE DEFICIT RELATED TO ILLNESS

- Explain what can be expected during minor illnesses or with conditions that change the child's health status.
- Strengthen the family's ability to make appropriate decisions regarding care of ill children in the home. Provide information needed to care for children in the home. Discuss family's plan for care of ill children at home.
- Establish a plan with the family about when and who to call for help. Although minor conditions can often be managed and more serious conditions prevented by actions taken in the home, many problems require professional intervention or advice. Families should be encouraged to initiate contact with the provider when they have questions and doubts about their child's condition. Parents should be given clear instructions on when to use the telephone, when to bring the child back to the office, or when to use the emergency department (see Tables 22-4 and 22-5).

NONCOMPLIANCE WITH HEALTH REQUIREMENTS

- Develop a partnership with the family around health care decision-making.
- Ensure that clients are active participants, invested in the decisions made.
- Assist the family to identify the bases of their decision-making.
- Identify differences between the families' and provider's approaches to health care.
- Clearly state when and why the provider disagrees with the client's decisions. In some cases, clients and providers can "agree to disagree" on one issue, finding others on which they can work together. In other cases, providers can feel so strongly about an issue that they need to refer clients to another clinician or intervene as an advocate for the child.
- Provide positive reinforcement for healthy decisions.

RISK-TAKING BEHAVIORS

Description

Risk-taking behaviors include activities that threaten the health and well-being of the child or adolescent. Although these include behaviors such as substance abuse, unprotected sexual activity, abuse, and violence, this section focuses on smoking in adolescents. Smoking appears within a cluster of risk-taking behaviors, and adolescent smokers are more likely than their nonsmoking peers to use marijuana and hard drugs, sell drugs, have multiple drug problems, drop out of school, and experience early pregnancy and parenthood. These adolescents are also at higher risk for low academic achievement and behavioral problems at school, stealing and other delinquent behaviors, and use of predatory and relational violence (Ellickson et al, 2001). More in-depth discussions of abuse and sexuality are found in Chapters 18 and 19.

Epidemiology

During the 1990s, cigarette smoking among non-Hispanic black, non-Hispanic white, and Hispanic high school students increased significantly in three assessed areas: "lifetime smoking (defined as having ever smoked cigarettes, even one or two puffs), current smoking (defined as smoking on more than one of the 30 days preceding the survey), and current frequent smoking (defined as smoking on more than 20 of the 30 days preceding the survey)" (Centers for Disease Control and Prevention [CDC], 2002). From 1997 to 2005, however, there has been a significant decline in smoking among U.S. youth 12 to 17 years old. In 1997, 36.4% of high school students were current smokers and 16.7% were frequent smokers. In 2005, approximately 2.4% of 12- to 13-year-olds, 9.2% of 14- to 15-year-olds, and 20.6% of 16- to 17-year-olds stated they were current smokers. Data from 2004 to 2006 show that of all high school students, 28.4% use some tobacco product (Eaton et al, 2006). Despite this decline, youth smoking continues to be a serious public health problem, with girls and boys smoking at about the same rates, and increased smoking among youth internationally (Mochizuki-Kobayashi et al, 2006) (see Chapter 41 for a discussion of environmental tobacco smoke [ETS]).

Smoking is positively related to the tobacco industry advertising cigarettes. Tobacco industry advertising that is focused on tobacco prevention does not appear to decrease smoking among adolescents (Wakefield et al, 2006). Portrayal of smoking in films (Sargent, 2006), parent smoking (Kalesan et al, 2006), access to cigarettes in the home, close peer or sibling smoking (Johnson et al, 2004), and stress and lower social status (Finkelstein et al, 2006) are all related to increased smoking.

Clinical Findings

In the clinical setting, adolescents' smoking patterns are best assessed through direct questioning. At every visit, children should be asked whether they or their friends smoke or use other forms of tobacco. Biochemical tests to measure tobacco by-products (e.g., carbon monoxide in serum or expired alveolar air; urine cotinine, a primary metabolite of nicotine; and thiocyanate, a detoxification product of hydrogen cyanide in tobacco smoke) are used primarily in the research setting and are not appropriate as a diagnostic tool in primary care.

Increased incidence of respiratory disease in children, including asthma, is a clinical finding in smokers or in families in which parents smoke (see Chapter 41).

Management

Management of adolescent tobacco use takes place on two levels: (1) primary, with a goal of preventing the child from starting to use and (2) secondary, with a goal of cessation (Table 10-3). Many adolescents experiment with tobacco use, but may stop after a short period before becoming addicted to nicotine. High recent cigarette consumption, slow nicotine metabolism, and higher depressive symptoms have been found to be related to tobacco dependence in adolescents (Karp et al, 2006; Mei-Chen et al, 2006). Tobacco dependence varies from one individual to another, however, and can appear at any time after initiating tobacco use, so prevention and early intervention is essential.

Educating young people about the actual use of tobacco in their age group may be a means of preventing them from initiating tobacco use. This approach is based on the social norms theory, which states that the perceptions an individual has of group norms of behavior will influence one's own behavior. The social norms approach has effectively reduced alcohol misuse on college campuses and appears to reduce violence against women (Perkins et al, 2006; Fabiano et al, 2003). Applying the social norms approach to tobacco prevention, if young people believe that "everyone is smoking," or even a majority of youth are smoking, they are more likely to begin smoking as well. Informing the child that nearly 98% of very young adolescents and 80% of older adolescents do not smoke can support a personal decision to not smoke.

Prevention may also be facilitated by increasing costs of tobacco products (Ding, 2005), implementing school-based programs (Unger et al, 2004; Valente et al, 2006), using antitobacco industry messages aimed at adolescents (Thrasher et al, 2006), and supporting positive parenting styles (O'Byrne et al, 2002). Intervention by dental providers can also prevent initiation or support smoking cessation (Ellison et al, 2006).

Many children are exposed to nicotine in utero or to secondhand smoke of parents or other caregivers. This not only puts them at risk for cognitive deficits, low test scores, and poorer school performance (Yolton et al, 2005), but children who live in a family with smokers are more likely to become smokers themselves. Although pediatric providers are not the parents' primary caregivers, they can intervene with parents in several ways. Parents can be encouraged to talk to their children about the dangers of smoking; there is evidence that when parents teach their children that smoking is bad, children are less likely to begin, even if the parent continues to smoke (Jackson & Dickinson, 2006). Parents should also be encouraged to stop smoking (see Chapter 41 for "the five As" smoking cessation guidelines for providers from the U.S. Agency for Health Care Policy and Research [USAHCPR]).

In addition, medical practices could implement population-based interventions to help their clients stop tobacco use. These include tracking and monitoring smokers, providing insurance coverage for tobacco-cessation services, educating employees not to use tobacco, and lobbying for public antismoking campaigns and increased taxes on tobacco products.

TABLE 10-3 **Primary and Secondary Prevention and Tobacco Use Cessation Strategies for Adolescents**

Primary Prevention	Secondary Prevention
Provide multimedia, multisite health information, not limited to schools	Ask at every visit whether adolescent or friends use tobacco
Emphasize skills to avoid peer pressure	Inform adolescent of health risks of tobacco use and process by which one becomes addicted to nicotine; emphasize that it is easier to stop early
Focus on adolescents' developmental need to belong to a social group	Develop mutual understanding of problem
	Determine realistic stop-use date
	Help adolescent identify barriers to stopping and ways to overcome those barriers
	Provide information about self-help and support groups; encourage adolescent to try to stop smoking with a friend
	Provide nicotine patches protocol if adolescent feels this will help
	Schedule follow-up visits to monitor progress; reinforce positive efforts
	Assess parents' tobacco use patterns; provide information and support to stop use

UNINTENTIONAL INJURIES

Description

Unintentional injuries are traumatic events that are unanticipated and accidentally caused (see Chapter 39 for a more complete discussion of injuries in children).

Epidemiology

Unintentional injury in children results from many factors, including the presence of hazards in the environment, unsafe or risky behaviors, and inadequate adult supervision. Injuries are one of the most serious health problems faced by the pediatric population, and morbidity secondary to injury is significantly more common than mortality. The nature and severity of childhood injuries vary by age, gender, race, and socioeconomic status (Behrman et al, 2004). Motor vehicle trauma is the major cause of pediatric mortality in the U.S. in children 3 to 14 years old. Mortality and morbidity related to falls, poisoning, drowning, near drowning, fires and burns, and trauma secondary to weapons are significant in children. Male children are more likely to experience injury than female children. Native-American children have the highest rate of injuries, followed in order by black, Hispanic, white, and Asian children. Children from lower socioeconomic groups experience more injuries than those from higher income groups. Injury rates are also high for many sports (see Chapter 14).

Clinical Findings

Clinical presentation of injuries varies, depending on the nature and extent of the trauma experienced. A thorough history of the child with an injury is essential, and the following information should be gathered to construct a clinical picture:

- Description of environment in which injury took place
- Condition of child before injury
- Actions of child and others immediately before injury
- Mechanism of injury
- Extent of supervision by adults
- First-aid management at scene of injury

Differential Diagnosis

The differential diagnoses for unintentional injuries include the following:

- Child abuse and neglect
- Suicide attempt
- Disease condition that makes the child more susceptible to injuries (e.g., osteogenesis imperfecta or hemophilia)

Management

Prevention is the key treatment. A discussion of safety issues needs to be incorporated into the providers' anticipatory guidance at every well child and adolescent visit, clarifying how the potential for injury and the type of injury varies by the child's age and developmental level. Effective management of unintentional injuries requires that parents understand how, at each age, developmental characteristics influence children's behavior and put them at risk for injury. Once aware of how children may be at risk, parents can more clearly see how they can intervene to prevent an injury from occurring. Tables 10-4 through 10-7 outline major injuries, developmental characteristics of children, the risks for injury these present, and strategies for intervention that parents can use to decrease the potential for injury (National Center for Injury Prevention and Control, 2003).

Efforts to prevent injury include the following:

- Restructure the environment to make it safer.
  - Place devices in the environment to protect children (e.g., automobile restraint systems, electrical outlet covers, fenced swimming pools).
  - Remove hazards from the environment (e.g., childproof the home).
  - Adjust environmental conditions (e.g., lower the water heater temperature).
- Mandate and enforce behavior or use of devices that protect the child (e.g., bicycle helmets, seat belts).
- Implement school policies and procedures to ensure that playground equipment and activities are well maintained and suited for children's developmental abilities.
- Teach children age-appropriate safe behavior to decrease risks of motor vehicle accidents, burns, drowning, poisoning, weapons, and falls.
- Advocate for school curricula that teach safety at every grade level.
- Provide health education regarding safety and protection, including first aid and safety and cardiopulmonary resuscitation techniques for both children and adults.
- Teach importance of adult supervision of children's activities.
- Encourage and instruct about proper training for sports in children and adolescents.
- Provide parents with poison control center telephone numbers.

Management of Motor Vehicle Trauma

Motor vehicle trauma continues to be the leading cause of death among children in the U.S., with significant mortality and morbidity rates in all age groups. In 2004, 1638 children birth to 14 years old died in motor vehicle crashes, and approximately 214,000 were injured. Alcohol was a contributing factor in 21% of pediatric motor vehicle fatalities. More than half of children killed were passengers in a car of a drinking driver; 96 children were passengers in a car hit by a drinking driver; and 48 children were pedestrians or cyclists hit by an alcohol-impaired driver (National Center for Statistics and Analysis [NCSA], 2006).

Positioning young children in rear seats and correctly using child restraint systems (CRSs) can prevent fatalities from motor vehicle trauma and can reduce the number and severity of injuries to children (Elliot et al, 2006; Brown et al, 2006). Nonetheless, many children ride unrestrained or incorrectly restrained. Half of the children who died in motor vehicle accidents in 2004 were unrestrained (NCSA, 2006), and 97.7% of the 263 children injured by airbags between 1998 and 2002 were improperly restrained (Quinones-Hinojosa et al, 2005). In states with primary seat belt enforcement laws (i.e., drivers can be stopped and cited

TABLE 10-4   Primary Injury Prevention Related to Developmental Characteristics of Infants

An estimated 1403 infants died of external causes in the United States in 2004. Unintentional injuries account for 70% of all deaths; 62% of these were caused by asphyxiation, ~15.5% by motor vehicle trauma and ~5.3% by drowning. Of grave concern, 299 children or about 20% of all injury deaths were due to homicide (Miniño et al, 2006). In 2004, more than 125,000 infants were seen in emergency departments for falls, the leading cause of nonfatal injuries among infants in the United States (National Center for Injury Prevention and Control, 2004).

Age and Developmental Characteristics	Potential Injuries	Strategies for Prevention
All infants		
	Burns	Do not hold infant in lap when drinking hot beverage or smoking Set water heater thermostat below 120° F Install smoke detectors in home and check batteries routinely
	Sunburn	Use coverup (e.g., hat) whenever child is exposed to sun; prevent exposure
	Motor vehicle trauma	Correctly use approved child safety restraint units in cars
	Fire	Install smoke detectors in home and check batteries routinely Install carbon monoxide detectors in home
Birth to 6 months		
Poor head control at younger ages	Injury to neck	Handle child with care when picking up or moving Support neck of young infant Supervise other children when they are playing with infant Never shake infant
Reflex behavior; especially strong suck reflex in early months	Aspiration of foreign objects	Keep occlusive materials, especially plastic, out of child's bed Check toys, mobiles for sharp, detachable parts, strings, or cords
Skin thin and sensitive	Suffocation Friction burns	Handle child with care when picking up or moving Dress infant appropriately
Poor body temperature control	Hypothermia Hyperthermia	Never leave child alone in car
Rolls, turns, and scoots	Falls	Do not leave infant alone on bed, changing table, or other area from which infant may fall Use playpen as safe area
	May slide between mattress and crib slats	Make sure mattress fits tightly against bed railings; railings are no more than 2⅜ inches apart
	Slips in bath	Place washcloth under infant in bath; always stay with infant during bathing
Age 6 to 12 months		
Grasps and mouths objects	Aspiration of foreign objects	Keep small, sharp objects off floor and play area, out of reach
	Suffocation	Check toys for detachable parts Keep balloons, plastic wrappers, and plastic bags out of reach
	Poisoning	Use childproof caps on medications Keep medications out of reach in locked cabinet Keep household, garden, and car products out of reach; decrease use of chemicals around child as much as possible Supervise children's activity Keep poison control numbers near telephone and alert older siblings and baby sitters about them Wash fruits and vegetables well; provide foods grown without pesticides or other chemicals
Sits, rolls, scoots, crawls, may stand while holding support, cruises, may walk	Falls	Do not use walkers Supervise children's activities Survey home for all accident hazards, sharp objects, table edges, stairs, loose rugs; remove those possible, provide protection of infant for others; use gates

TABLE 10-4	**Primary Injury Prevention Related to Developmental Characteristics of Infants—Cont'd**	
Age and Developmental Characteristics	**Potential Injuries**	**Strategies for Prevention**
	Drowning	Keep pool or water ponds behind closed and locked gates Never leave children alone in bath Use playpen as a safe area
Pulls and reaches	May pull objects down onto self	Remove tablecloths, dangling cords, appliances that may be in infant's reach
Developing fine pincer grasp	Electrocution	Insert plastic plugs in electrical outlets
	Swallowing, aspiration, or insertion of foreign body in body orifices	Keep small objects out of reach

TABLE 10-5	**Primary Injury Prevention Related to Developmental Characteristics of Toddlers and Preschoolers**	

Injuries cause more death and disability than all contagious diseases combined in children 1 to 4 years old. In 2004, more than 200,000 U.S. toddlers and preschoolers were seen in emergency departments for the 10 leading causes of nonfatal injuries; falls rank as the leading cause of injury morbidity (~50% of the top 10 causes) (National Center for Injury Prevention and Control, 2004). According to 2002 data, 77% of all injury-related deaths in children 1 to 4 years old were unintentional; about 25% were due to motor vehicle trauma, followed closely by drowning (~23%) (Miniño et al, 2006).

Developmental Characteristics	**Potential Injuries**	**Strategies for Prevention**
Increased gross motor skills and control: Able to walk, run, climb, throw objects, ride tricycle	Falls	Confine play to fenced area Always supervise play, especially in areas where climbing occurs Use gates or screens to block off stair; lock windows and doors
Engages in more active play outdoors, with peers	Contusions and bites	Supervise interactive play of children Teach children how to share, control temper; use adult interaction or distraction to stop harmful behavior or tantrum trauma
Increased fine motor skills:	Poisoning	Use childproof caps on medications; keep medicines locked in cabinet out of reach
Can open doors, gates, drawers, bottles, boxes		Keep household, garden, and car products locked or out of reach
Increased curiosity		Decrease use of chemicals around child as much as possible Place Mr. YUK stickers on toxic materials Have telephone number of poison control center readily available
	Sunburn	Use sunscreen whenever children are exposed to sun
	Motor vehicle trauma	Use approved child safety restraints Provide tricycle or bicycle helmet Teach children sidewalk, street, and highway safety Never let children cross street alone or play unsupervised on sidewalks near streets
Increased curiosity; reaches, stretches, and pulls	Burns, scalding	Turn handles of cooking utensils away from outer edge of stove Use caution in kitchen with children about Adjust hot water thermostat to 120° F Keep matches out of reach

Continued

TABLE 10-5 Primary Injury Prevention Related to Developmental Characteristics of Toddlers and Preschoolers—Cont'd

Developmental Characteristics	Potential Injuries	Strategies for Prevention
Increased curiosity, desire to explore Easily distracted, lacks judgment, unaware of danger of heights, water, fire, toxic materials, electricity, weapons, animals, or strangers	Drowning Other injuries	Fence swimming pools Supervise use of swimming and wading pools Never leave children unattended in a car or alone at home Do not allow children to play near running machinery, mowers, cars, or tools Provide plastic covers for electrical outlets; teach children safety with electrical appliances and cords Do not allow children to use pointed objects in play Do not allow children to run or walk with sticks, lollipops, or other such objects Remove weapons from the house, or keep in locked cabinet, with guns unloaded; store ammunition in separate, locked area Teach children to avoid strange animals, especially ones that are eating
	Abuse	Teach stranger safety
Easily distracted, not always attentive	Choking, aspiration	Do not give foods that can be easily aspirated, such as nuts, gum, popcorn, hot dogs, grapes Supervise mealtimes and snacks

TABLE 10-6 Primary Injury Prevention Related to Developmental Characteristics of School-Age Children

Motor vehicle and pedestrian accidents, burns, drowning, and choking are the most common fatal injuries among 5–14-year-olds in the U.S. (National Center for Injury Prevention and Control, 2003). About 79% of injury-related deaths are unintentional (Miniño et al, 2006), and as many as 4 million children in this age group are seen in emergency departments for one of the top 10 nonfatal injuries each year; falls predominate with nearly 1.5 million cases (National Center for Injury Prevention and Control, 2004).

Developmental Characteristics	Potential Injuries	Strategies for Prevention
Motor skills improve; becomes more physically agile and coordinated	Motor vehicle trauma as passenger, pedestrian, or cyclist	Use approved safety restraints in car Provide bicycle helmet and insist on its use Teach importance of seat belt and helmet use Teach bicycle safety Do not allow children to ride tricycles or bicycles with training wheels in the street Prohibit use of all-terrain vehicles Teach pedestrian safety
Engages in sports and strenuous exercise Enjoys physical activity Works hard to improve skills Can strain self with excessive activity	Sprains and strains, fractures, and other bodily injuries	Use kneepads, elbow pads, wrist support, and helmets when skateboarding Encourage child to be active and stay conditioned; if engaged in organized sports, provide supervised strength training Ensure use of properly fitted equipment and safe playing area for each sport
Is adventurous and more independent, looks for new challenges; may accept dares Engages in group activities, subject to peer approval	Drowning	Teach to swim; teach rules of water safety: swim in a supervised area with a buddy, check depth before diving, use life preservers in boats

TABLE 10-6 **Primary Injury Prevention Related to Developmental Characteristics of School-Age Children—Cont'd**

Developmental Characteristics	Potential Injuries	Strategies for Prevention
Is curious and exploring	Falls	
	Burns	Teach children dangers of flammable and toxic materials; how to handle them safely
		Supervise use of matches
		Develop a family plan for fires
	Poisoning	Keep hazardous materials out of reach, in locked location; supervise their use
Easily distracted by environment	Choking	Teach first aid, what to do in case of burns, choking, or poisoning
		Keep poison control center telephone number readily available
	Sunburn	Use sunscreen whenever children will be exposed to sun
Accepts explanations and is responsive to reasoning	Abuse	Teach child to memorize telephone number and address, use of 911
		Warn child never to go with or accept things from strangers

TABLE 10-7 **Primary Injury Prevention Related to Developmental Characteristics of Adolescents**

In 2002, 5522 adolescents 15 to 19 years old died as a result of motor vehicle trauma in the U.S., nearly 78% of all unintentional injury deaths among teenagers. Homicides were the second leading cause of injury death (approximately 18%). More than 914,000 teens were seen in emergency departments for motor vehicle injury, but sports injuries were the most common nonfatal injury (greater than 980,000 treated in ED) (Miniño et al, 2006; National Center for Injury Prevention and Control, 2004).

Developmental Characteristics	Potential Injuries	Strategies for Prevention
Able to legally drive motor vehicles	Motor vehicle trauma as passenger, pedestrian, or cyclist	Use approved safety restraints
		Take driver's education classes
		Use bicycle and cycling helmet
		Encourage to learn how to maintain bicycle
		Teach proper use of all-terrain vehicles
		Reinforce pedestrian safety
		Emphasize danger of driving, drinking, and drug use; support peer group efforts to control inappropriate behavior
Increased physical strength and ability	Falls	Use kneepads, elbow pads, wrist support, and helmet when skateboarding
More participation in structured sports activities	Sprains, strains, fractures, and other bodily injuries	Encourage adolescent to stay active and conditioned, engage in supervised strength training
Use of complex equipment, tools, weapons	Bodily injury	Teach gun safety; ask if families of child's friends have weapons in their homes
Perception of invulnerability; may take risks	Burns	Teach first aid and cardiopulmonary resuscitation: what to do in the event of injuries, burns, choking, or poisonings
	Choking	Teach to swim
	Drowning	Reinforce rules of water safety: swim in a supervised area with a buddy, check depth before diving or jumping, use life preservers in boats and when water skiing
Strong peer influence	Poisoning (drug and alcohol abuse)	Teach dangers of drug and alcohol use
Need for independence and peer approval		Provide an opportunity to discuss values, perceptions, fears, and needs related to high-risk behaviors and self-harming actions (e.g., cutting or suicide ideation); discuss how adolescent deals with anger and violence and how to prevent trauma related to violence; encourage healthy options
Able to problem-solve, reason, and think abstractly		

by law enforcement for failure to wear a seat belt) versus those with secondary enforcement laws (i.e., drivers can be cited if they are stopped for another traffic violation and are not wearing a seat belt), seat belt usage is significantly higher. Among adolescents, usage is twice as high if primary seat belt enforcement laws are in effect (Durbin et al, 2007; Houston & Richardson, 2006).

In addition to not using restraints, a number of common errors have been found in the way CRSs are used (Box 10-2). The National Highway Traffic Safety Administration (NHTSA) examined CRS use in six states between September 2002 and January 2003 and found 72.6% (of 3442 observed CRSs) had one or more critical errors in use of the child restraints. Most common were loose vehicle safety straps attached to the CRS and loose harness straps that secured the child to the CRS. More than 80% of infant seats were not correctly used (NHTSA, 2004). Providers should assess the parents' use of CRSs and correct errors. This may mean accompanying parents to the parking lot to observe how children are placed in the restraint. Use of CRSs should be reviewed at each well-child visit, and children should be involved in the discussion from a very early age. Both parents and children should receive positive reinforcement for proper use of CRSs. Current information from the NHTSA on which restraint system is appropriate for the size, age, and condition of the child should be shared with parents (Table 10-8).

In 2002 the NHTSA promulgated rules requiring most new vehicles and child safety seats to have hardware that makes installation of safety seats easier and more likely to be done correctly. These rules led to creation of the lower anchors and tether for children (LATCH) system that secures safety seats without using a seat belt. When the child safety seat is correctly attached to lower anchors and an upper tether built into the vehicle itself, it is less likely to move in a collision, and the child is less likely to be injured. Not all vehicles have the lower anchor bars (found in the bight of the seat), however, and those that do may not have them in the middle of the rear seat, which is the safest place for a child to ride. Many parents may not be familiar with the LATCH system or know if their vehicle is equipped with it.

Airbags were developed to prevent serious injury in the event of a motor vehicle accident. Designed to protect a 165-pound, 5-foot, 9-inch-tall man who is not wearing a seat belt in a 30-mph frontal crash, airbags have caused serious injuries and fatalities in infants and children (Quinones-Hinojosa et al 2005) and can be equally hazardous for small adults. Based on the nature of these injuries, children should always be restrained, and children younger than 12 years old should not ride in the front passenger seat if an airbag can be deployed. The optimal position for children is in the center back seat, with infants weighing less than 20 pounds placed in a rear-facing child seat (see Table 10-8).

Pedestrian injuries or injuries involving bicycles, skateboards, and automobiles are common among children. Providers should discuss this issue with parents at each well child visit, ask children about their pedestrian safety habits during the well child visit, and support educational efforts to instruct children on pedestrian safety and age-appropriate safe use of cycles or boards. Children of all ages need adult supervision related to motor vehicles. Adult supervision is especially important for younger children who are unaware of the dangers.

Adolescents, especially new drivers, are often involved in motor vehicle accidents because of their inexperience, immature judgment, or a tendency to take risks. Legislation has been passed in some states, Victoria, Australia, some Canadian provinces, and New Zealand to restrict adolescent driving. "Graduated licensing" legislation requires teenagers to complete driver education classes, restricts their driving to certain times of day, or prevents them from driving with other teenagers in the car. As adolescents gain experience and age, restrictions on driving decline. Implementation of this law has led to a significant decrease in fatal crashes among teenagers, with an approximately 20% reduction in fatalities among 16-year-old drivers in one review (Chen et al, 2006). Successful implementation of the law depends on parents acting as advocates for safety and supporting their adolescents' compliance with the regulations. Providers also can reinforce the message to teenagers that driving is a privilege that requires skill and maturity.

Management of Firearms Safety

Unintentional deaths caused by firearms among children under 14 years old declined 80% from 1987 to 2002 (Safe Kids Worldwide, 2006). In 2002, 1567 children 15 to 19 years old in the U.S. died as a result of an assault with a gun (a slight increase from 2000); 742 committed suicide using a firearm (a 17% decrease from 2000), and accidental gun fatalities ranged from 0.7% among 1- to 4-year-olds to 2.2%

| **BOX 10-2** | **Common Errors in the Use of Child Restraint Systems** |

- Seat belt is not tight enough.
- Rear-facing seat is not positioned at a 45-degree angle.
- Harness straps are not snug (infant may be wrapped in a "cocoon" of blankets).
- Harness straps in infant, rear-facing seat are not at or below shoulders of infant.
- Harness straps in child, forward-facing seat are not at or above shoulders of child.
- Retainer clip in child, forward-facing seat is not at armpit level.
- Seat belt is not in locked mode.
- Infant less than 1 year old is placed in forward-facing position.

| TABLE 10-8 | Vehicle Child Restraint Systems: Recommendations for Use | | |

Age of Child	Weight of Child	Type of Restraint	Seat Position
Birth-1 yr	Up to at least 20 lb	Infant only or rear-facing convertible Harness straps at or below shoulder level	Rear-facing seat only In rear seat
Under 1 year	20-35 lb	Rear-facing convertible seat (select one recommended for heavier infant) Seats should be secured to vehicle with safety belts or by LATCH system	
1-4 yr (toddler-preschooler)	20-40 lb	Convertible, forward-facing seat Harness straps at or above shoulder level; snug on child. Harness clip at armpit level Seats should be secured to vehicle with safety belts or by LATCH system	Forward-facing seat In rear seat
Ages 4-8	More than 40 lb; height less than 4 ft 9 in	Belt positioning booster seat, no back or high back Used with adult lap and shoulder belt NEVER use with lap-only belt NEVER place shoulder belt under arm or behind back	Forward-facing seat In rear seat
Older children	Height greater than 4 ft 9 in	Belt positioning without booster seat Shoulder belt snug across chest NEVER place shoulder belt under arm or behind back	Forward-facing seat In rear seat until 12 yr
Children with Special Needs (see variety of options at www.aap.org/family/specialcarseatschart.doc)			
Very small infants	Less than 5-7 lb	Infant only; maximum distance from crotch strap to back of seat is 5.5 in; height of harness straps should be less than 10 in If too small for infant seat, use side-lying car bed with restraints	Rear-facing seat or side-lying car bed In rear seat
Children with physical disabilities	Birth to adolescent (systems available for children up to 130 lb)	Spelcast (Snug Seat) is designed for children in spica cast; Snug Seat Car Bed (Snug Seat) for infants up to 21 lb who cannot ride seated semiupright; a number of systems are designed for older, heavier children (see NHTSA, Resource Box)	

ft, Foot/feet; *in*, inch(es); *lb*, pound(s); *yr*, year(s).

among 10- to 14-year-olds of all unintentional injury deaths (Miniño et al, 2006). Gun locks and load indicators could prevent more than 30% of these deaths; and safe-storage laws passed by states in an effort to prevent easy access to guns are estimated to reduce unintentional firearm deaths in children under 14 years old by 23% (Safe Kids Worldwide, 2006). Nonetheless, gun-related injuries still represent a serious public health problem requiring community-based solutions. Providers should work with families and community agencies to decrease gun-related injuries by doing the following:

- Include questions about children's access to guns in primary care assessment data.
- Educate parents and children about gun safety.
- Support parents' efforts to reduce children's exposure to guns (e.g., encourage parents to ask other parents if they have guns in their households and not allow their children to play in households with guns).
- Advocate for laws that mandate responsible sale, storage, and use of guns.
- Advocate to reduce violence in media.

NURSING DIAGNOSES

Related to Health Perception and Health Management: Functional Health Pattern

Diagnoses relate to concepts of therapeutic regimen management, health-seeking behaviors, health maintenance, and home maintenance:

- Decisional conflict
  - Readiness for enhanced decision making
- Deficient knowledge (specify)
  - Readiness for enhanced knowledge
- Effective therapeutic regimen management
  - Readiness for enhanced therapeutic regimen management
- Ineffective therapeutic regimen management
  - Ineffective family therapeutic regimen management
  - Ineffective community therapeutic regimen management

- Ineffective health maintenance
- Impaired home maintenance management
- Health-seeking behaviors (specify area of concern)
- Impaired adjustment
- Noncompliance
- Readiness for enhanced immunization status
- Risk for injury
- Self-care deficits—bathing, dressing/grooming, feeding, toileting
  - Readiness for enhanced self-care

From NANDA International: *NANDA-I nursing diagnoses: definitions & classification 2007–2008*, Philadelphia, 2007, Author.

RESOURCE BOX

Health Perception and Health Management

Bright Futures
www.brightfutures.org
Materials for health professionals on healthy child assessment and health promotion

Health Perception and Management in Nursing Care to Children
www.accd.edu/sac/nursing/r2201/plinks1.html
Links to several parent-child focused resources

Kids Health (Nemours Foundation)
http://kidshealth.org
Patient and parent educational information

GENERAL SAFETY RESOURCES
Children's Safety Network (funded by U.S. Maternal and Child Health Bureau)
www.childrenssafetynetwork.org

National Program for Playground Safety
www.uni.edu/playground

National SAFE KIDS Campaign
www.safekids.org

U.S. Consumer Products Safety Commission
www.cpsc.gov

WATER SAFETY
American Red Cross
www.redcross.org/services/hss/tips/healthtips/safetywater.html

United States Lifesaving Association (USLA)
www.usla.org

FIREARMS
American Academy of Pediatrics: Firearm Injury Prevention Project
www.aap.org
For AAP members, firearm prevention kit and presentation

Center to Prevent Handgun Violence
www.cphv.org
Lobbying and educating to establish gun regulations

Common Sense About Kids and Guns
www.kidsandguns.org

Join Together Online
www.jointogether.org
Educational materials, funding advice; alcohol and drug information

Violence Policy Center
www.vpc.org
Legislation and litigation activities

MOTOR VEHICLE SAFETY
Car Seats for Larger Children with Special Needs
www.adaptivemall.com
Produced by Columbia, Sammons Preston, and Snug Seat

Child Restraint Systems
www.aap.org/family/specialcarseatschart.doc
List of a variety of car seat options for children with special needs

National Highway Traffic Safety Administration
www.nhtsa.dot.gov
Statistics on injuries; guidelines for use of restraint systems: proper child safety seat use chart
Comprehensive child passenger safety information

Snug Seat
www.snugseat.com
Side-facing car bed for infants who cannot sit upright; restraint for child in spica cast, both rear and forward facing; car seats for larger children with special needs

☑DISCUSSION FORUM

1. You see a 2-year-old child who has not received any immunizations because the parents have concerns about the "link between autism and shots" and an expressed concern that stimulating a child's "immature immune system may have long-term damaging effects." Both parents are well-read and pay special attention to their child's diet and environment because they "believe in a focus on health not illness." Create a plan of care to validate this family's positive health behaviors and address their health behavior deficits.

2. Given the information in Table 10-2, create a plan of care to maximize the health perception and health behaviors of the family with a 7-year-old.

3. List health care resources in your community that can be used by families for health care services and education. Make special note of the agencies that can assist families with children with special health care needs.

4. Unintentional injuries are a leading cause of pediatric morbidity and mortality. List at least 5 strategies that can be used to incorporate injury prevention into preventative health care. At least 1 strategy should address health perceptions and 1 should address barriers to adopting injury prevention strategies.

5. You are asked by the parents of a 9-year-old for ways to help keep their son tobacco-free. How will you respond?

REFERENCES

American Academy of Pediatrics Committee on Injury and Poison Prevention and Committee on Community Health Services: Prevention of agricultural injuries among children and adolescents, *Pediatrics* 108:1016-1019, 2001.

American Academy of Pediatrics Committee on Practice and Ambulatory Medicine: Recommendations for preventive pediatric health care, *Pediatrics* 105:645-646, 2000.

Behrman RE, Kliegman RM, Jenson HB, editors: *Nelson textbook of pediatrics*, ed 17, Philadelphia, 2004, WB Saunders.

Brown JK et al: Patterns of severe injury in pediatric car crash victims: crash injury research engineering network database, *J Pediatr Surg* 41(2):362-367, 2006.

Centers for Disease Control and Prevention, Office on Smoking and Health and Division of Adolescent and School Health, National Center for Chronic Disease Prevention and Health Promotion: Trends in cigarette smoking among high school students United States, 1991-2001, *MMWR* 51:409-412, 2002.

Chen LH, Baker SP, Li G: Graduated driver licensing programs and fatal crashes of 16-year-old drivers: a national evaluation, *Pediatrics* 118(1):56-62, 2006.

DeNavas-Walt C, Proctor BD, Lee CH: *Income, poverty, and health insurance coverage in the United States: 2005,* Washington DC, 2006, US Census Bureau.

Ding A: Curbing adolescent smoking: a review of the effectiveness of various policies, *Yale J Bio Med* 78(1):37-44, 2005.

Dunn ME et al: Moderators of stress in parents of children with autism, *Comm Ment Health J* 37:39-52, 2001.

Durbin DR et al: Seat belt use among 13-15 year olds in primary and secondary enforcement law states, *Accid Anal Prev* 39(3):524-529, 2007.

Eaton DK et al: Youth risk behavior surveillance—United States, 2005, *MMWR Surveill Summ* 55(SS5):1-108, 2006.

Ellickson PL, Tucker JS, Klein DJ: High-risk behaviors associated with early smoking: results from a 5-year follow-up, *J Adolesc Health* 28:465-473, 2001.

Elliot MR et al: Effectiveness of child safety seats vs. seat belts in reducing risk of death in children in passenger vehicle crashes, *Arch Pediatr Adolesc Med* 160(6):617-621, 2006.

Ellison J et al: Characteristics of adolescent smoking in high school students in California, *J Dent Hyg* 80(2):8, 2006.

Fabiano PM et al: Engaging men as social justice allies in ending violence against women: evidence for a social norms approach, *J Am Coll Health* 52(3):105-112, 2003.

Finkelstein DM, Kubzansky LD, Goodman E: Social status, stress, and adolescent smoking, *J Adolesc Health* 39(5):678-685, 2006.

Griffiths F et al: Why are health care interventions delivered over the internet? A systematic review of the published literature, *J Med Internet Res* 8(2):e10, 2006.

Holt CL, Clark EM, Kreuter MW: Weight locus of control and weight-related attitudes and behaviors in an overweight population, *Addict Behav* 26:329-340, 2001.

Houston DJ, Richardson LE: Safety belt use and the switch to primary enforcement, 1991-2003, *Am J Public Health* 96(11):1949-1954, 2006.

Howard BJ: *Working with difficult families.* Paper presented at the 1998 Pediatric Update, Portland, OR, Nov 1998.

Jackson C, Dickinson D: Enabling parents who smoke to prevent their children from initiating smoking: results from a 3-year intervention evaluation, *Arch Pediatr Adolesc Med* 160(1):56-62, 2006.

Johnson CC et al: Profiles of the adolescent smoker: models of tobacco use among 9th grade high school students: Acadiana Coalition of Teens Against Tobacco (ACTT), *Prev Med* 39(3):551-558, 2004.

Kalesan B, Stine J, Alberg AJ: The joint influence of parental modeling and positive parental concern on cigarette smoking in middle and high school students, *J Sch Health* 76(8):402-407, 2006.

Karp I et al: Risk factors for tobacco dependence in adolescent smokers, *Tobacco Control* 15:199-204, 2006.

Kleinman A, Eisenberg L, Good B: Culture, illness and care: clinical lessons from anthropologic and cross-cultural research, *Ann Intern Med* 88:251-258, 1978.

Kmet L, Macarthur C: Urban-rural differences in motor vehicle crash fatality and hospitalization rates among children and youth, *Accid Anal Prev* 38(1):122-127, 2006.

Marshall RS: Interpretation in doctor-patient interviews: a sociolinguistic analysis, *Cult Med Psychiatry* 12:201-218, 1988.

Masters K: For what purpose and reasons do doctors use the Internet: a systematic review, *Int J Med Inform* epub ahead of print, Nov 28, 2006.

Mei-Chen H, Davies M, Kandel DB: Epidemiology and correlates of daily smoking and nicotine dependence among young adults in the United States, *Am J Public Health* 96(2):299-308, 2006.

Miniño AM et al: Deaths: injuries, 2002, *Natl Vital Stat Rep* 54(10):1-125, 2006.

Miniño AM, Heron MP, Smith BL: Deaths: preliminary data for 2004, *Natl Vital Stat Rep* 54(19):1-50, 2006.

Mochizuki-Kobayashi Y et al: Use of cigarettes and other tobacco products among students aged 13-15 years—worldwide, 1999-2005, *MMWR* 55(20):553-555, 2006.

National Center for Injury Prevention and Control: *National estimates of the 10 leading causes of nonfatal injuries treated in hospital emergency departments, United States, 2004,* Centers for Disease Control and Prevention. Available at *www.cdc.gov/ncipc/osp/charts.htm* (accessed Feb 1, 2007).

National Center for Injury Prevention and Control: *Ten leading causes of injury death by age group: highlighting unintentional injury deaths, United States-2003,* Centers for Disease Control and Prevention. Available at *www.cdc.gov/ncipc/osp/charts.htm* (accessed Feb 1, 2007).

National Center for Statistics and Analysis [NCSA]: *Traffic safety facts: 2005 data.* Available at *www.nhtsa.dot.gov* (accessed Nov 8, 2006).

National Highway Traffic Safety Administration: *Misuse of child restraints,* DOT HS 809 671, Mar 2004.

O'Byrne KK, Haddock CK, Poston WS: Parenting style and adolescent smoking, *J Adolesc Health* 30:418-425, 2002.

Perkins HW, Haines MP, Rice R: Misperceiving the college drinking norm and related problems: a nationwide study of exposure to prevention information, perceived norms and student alcohol misuse, *J Stud Alcohol* 67(3):482-483, 2006.

Quinones-Hinojosa A et al: Airbag deployment and improperly restrained children: a lethal combination, *J Trauma* 59(3):729-733, 2005.

Raina P et al: The health and well-being of caregivers of children with cerebral palsy, *Pediatrics* 115(6):626-636, 2005.

Reicks M, Mills J, Henry H: Qualitative study of spirituality in a weight loss program: contribution to self-efficacy and locus of control, *J Nutr Educ Behav* 36(1):13-15, 2004.

Rotter JB: Generalized expectancies for internal versus external control of reinforcement, *Psychol Monogr* 80:1-25, 1966.

Safe Kids Worldwide: *Facts about unintentional firearm injuries to children.* Available at *www.usa.safekids.org/tier 2_nl.ofm? folder id-510* (accessed Nov 17, 2006).

Sargent JD: Smoking in film and impact on adolescent smoking: with special reference to European adolescents, *Minerva Pediatr* 58(1):27-45, 2006.

Smith MS, Wallston KA, Smith CA: The development and validation of the perceived health competence scale, *Health Educ Res* 10:51-64, 1995.

Steptoe A, Wardle J: Locus of control and health behaviour revisited: a multivariate analysis of young adults from 18 countries, *Br J Psychol* 92 (pt 4):659-672, 2001.

Thrasher JF et al: Using anti-tobacco industry messages to prevent smoking among high-risk adolescents, *Health Educ Res* 21(3):325-327, 2006.

Unger JB et al: Project FLAVOR: 1-year outcomes of a multicultural, school-based smoking prevention curriculum for adolescents, *Am J Public Health* 94(2):263-265, 2004.

Valente TW et al: The interaction of curriculum type and implementation on 1-year smoking outcomes in a school-based prevention program, *Health Educ Res* 21(3):315-324, 2006.

Wakefield M et al: Effect of televised, tobacco company-funded smoking prevention advertising on youth smoking-related beliefs, intentions, and behavior, *Am J Public Health* 96(12):2154-2160, 2006.

Wallston BS et al: Development and validation of the health locus of control (HLC) scale, *J Consult Clin Psych* 44:580-585, 1976.

Wallston KA, Wallston BS, DeVellis R: Development of multidimensional health locus of control (MHLC) scales, *Health Education Monogr* 6:160-170, 1978.

Yolton K et al: Exposure to environmental tobacco smoke and cognitive abilities among U.S. children and adolescents, *Environ Health Perspect* 113(1):98-103, 2005.

CHAPTER 11

Nutrition

Ardys M. Dunn

■ INTRODUCTION TO NUTRITION

DEFINITION

Nutrition is a complex science that examines the processes by which organisms ingest, digest, absorb, transport, use, and excrete food substances and how food, nutrients, and other substances found in foods interact with the body to foster growth and health or contribute to disease. Adequate nutrition is essential for normal growth and development of children and plays a critical role in maintenance and restoration of good health. Nutrition affects children's ability to interact with their environment. The effect of nourishment on children's behavior can be immediate and dramatic, as with the hungry, irritable infant who eagerly nurses and falls asleep; or nutrition can have long-range implications, as in the relationship between childhood cholesterol levels and adult coronary heart disease. Nutritional knowledge also requires an understanding of social, economic, cultural, and psychological implications of food and eating. Patterns of eating have social implications and are not related to nutrients alone.

ROLE OF THE NURSE PRACTITIONER

Pediatric primary health care providers must assess accurately the nutritional status of children, determine parents' and children's knowledge related to nutrition and eating behaviors, identify ways in which food is managed and used, and work to ensure that children are adequately nourished. Interventions aimed at helping children and families meet nutritional requirements and preventing problems related to poor nutrition are based on certain assumptions, including the following:
- Children's nutritional needs vary as they grow.
- Children's nutritional needs are influenced by their state of health.
- A wide range of food choices and feeding behaviors are used to meet nutritional needs.
- Recommended dietary allowances are guidelines only.
- Parents and other caregivers are responsible for providing food choices that are nutritionally adequate and for establishing healthy eating patterns; to do so, they must be well informed.
- The primary care provider is a source of information regarding nutrition, feeding patterns, and health.
- The primary care provider works with a network of specialists (e.g., registered dietitians) to manage children's nutrition status.

STANDARDS FOR PREVENTIVE CARE

A number of recommendations have been developed related to nutrition. The American Academy of Pediatrics recommends exclusive breastfeeding until 4 to 6 months old, and continued breastfeeding, supplemented with appropriate foods for infants, until at least 12 months old (AAP, 2005). The American Medical Association (AMA) also supports breastfeeding as the best nutrition for infants. It recommends that providers calculate body mass index (BMI) measures in routine physical examinations of children "recognizing ethnic sensitivities and its relation to stature" and states that the AMA school health advocacy agenda includes attention to healthy eating and exercise in schools and for school-age children (AMA, 2005). *Bright Futures in Practice: Nutrition* (Story et al, 2002) provides an overview of nutritional guidelines, discussion of issues and concerns related to pediatric nutrition, and tools for providers to assess and manage nutrition in children. Although it recognizes that the number of overweight and obese children and adolescents has increased drastically since the 1970s and that these children are at increased risk for health problems, the U.S. Preventive Services Task Force (USPSTF) has concluded that the evidence is insufficient to recommend for or against routine screening for overweight in children and adolescents (USPSTF, 2005). Nutrition recommendations for children emphasize that:
- Breast milk is the best food for infants.
- Children's diets should include a wide variety of foods.
- Iron-rich foods are essential, especially for infants and adolescents.
- Fat intake, particularly saturated fats and cholesterol, should be limited.
- Calories and carbohydrates should be appropriate to metabolic needs.
- Sugar intake should be limited.
- Extra calcium, iron, and folic acid are important nutrients in adolescent girls' diets.
- Children's diets should include adequate fiber and sodium.

■ NORMAL PATTERNS OF NUTRITION

GENERAL CONSIDERATIONS

Energy

Energy intake, measured in kilocalories, should meet the basic needs of body metabolism, growth, and activity. Resting energy expenditure (REE), a concept used interchangeably with basal metabolic rate (BMR), is the largest source of energy consumption in the body. Growth, a second source of energy consumption, is greatest in infancy and again during adolescence. Finally, activity, exercise, and other metabolic demands, including illness, increase the level of calories needed to sustain good health. The body meets these energy demands, or estimated energy requirements (EER), by using stored energy sources or nutrients and calories consumed on a daily basis. EER for healthy children can vary significantly by age, health status, and activity level (Table 11-1).

Macronutrients (protein, carbohydrates, and fats) and alcohol provide calories necessary to meet the body's energy needs. There is wide latitude on how much of each macronutrient is necessary for optimal nutrition; the body will use whichever is present for its energy needs. Of critical importance is that basic energy needs are met and that other essential nutrients (e.g., vitamins, minerals) are consumed. Table 11-2 presents recommended macronutrient intake based on age for children who are of average height, weight, and physical activity level. Macronutrient intake is expressed in recommended grams per day and in the form of "acceptable macronutrient distribution range" (AMDR). AMDR is the percent of the total daily energy intake recommended for that macronutrient and is considered to be a range that provides adequate overall nutrition while minimizing risks for chronic disease associated with an excess or deficit of the macronutrient (Food and Nutrition Board, Institute of Medicine [IOM], 2005). Healthy individuals maintain a balance between the body's energy demands and caloric intake. Currently, many children have limited physical activity and are at risk for excess weight gain. These children should engage in regular physical exercise to balance energy use and caloric intake.

Water and Electrolytes

Water.   Water is the primary component of body tissue, and maintaining fluid balance is essential to good health. Because of the wide variation of healthful intake and output, there is no specific recommended daily requirement for water (Manz et al, 2002). Infants present special concerns: they have a large skin surface per unit of body weight, their renal systems are not fully mature to process solutes, they have a high daily water turnover (up to 15% of body weight), and they are unable to express thirst. All these factors make infants uniquely susceptible to rapid variations in water balance.

Water loss is influenced by illness, activity level, altitude, and temperature and dryness of ambient air. If a child is vomiting and has diarrhea, water loss can be significant, leading to dehydration and other complications. Children who exercise strenuously, especially in a warm, dry environment, require additional water intake. When more than 10% of body weight is lost without replacement, dehydration can become life threatening. After strenuous or prolonged exercise, high water intake without electrolyte replacement can lead to water intoxication.

Sodium.   Sodium functions primarily to regulate extracellular fluid volume. It also regulates osmolarity, acid-base balance, and the membrane potential of cells and is involved in the cell membrane transport pump, exchanging with potassium in intracellular fluid. Sodium loss occurs with vomiting, diarrhea, and perspiration.

TABLE 11-1   Daily Estimated Energy Requirements (EER) of Infants, Children, and Adolescents: Calculations (EER = Total Energy Expenditure [TEE] + Energy Deposition)

Age	Formula
0-3 mo	EER = (89 × weight of infant [kg] − 100) + 175 (kcal for energy deposition)
4-6 mo	EER = (89 × weight of infant [kg] − 100) + 56 (kcal for energy deposition)
7-12 mo	EER = (89 × weight of infant [kg] − 100) + 22 (kcal for energy deposition)
13-35 mo	EER = (89 × weight of child [kg] − 100) + 20 (kcal for energy deposition)
Boys 3-8 yr	EER = 88.5 − (61.9 × age [yr]) + (PA × [26.7 × weight (kg) + 903 × height (m)]) + 20 (kcal for energy deposition)
Girls 3-8 yr	EER = 135.3 − (30.8 × age [yr]) + (PA × [10 × weight (kg) + 934 × height (m)]) + 20 (kcal for energy deposition)
Boys 9-18 yr	EER = 88.5 − (61.9 × age [yr]) + (PA × [26.7 × weight (kg) + 903 × height (m)]) + 25 (kcal for energy deposition)
Girls 9-18 yr	EER = 135.3 − (30.8 × age [yr]) + (PA × [10 × weight (kg) + 934 × height (m)]) + 25 (kcal for energy deposition)

Physical activity coefficient (PA) varies by gender, age, and body weight as follows:

Physical Activity Level Category (see below)	Physical Activity Coefficient Boys, 3-19 yr	Physical Activity Coefficient Girls, 3-19 yr
Sedentary	1	1
Low active	1.13	1.16
Active	1.26	1.31
Very active	1.42	1.56

| Physical Activity Level (PAL) Category | Walking Equivalence (mile/day* at 2-4 mph) for | | |
	Heavy Weight (120 kg)	Middle Weight (70 kg)	Light Weight (44 kg)
Sedentary	—	—	—
Low active	1.5	2.2	2.9
Active	3-5.3	4.4-7.3	5.8-9.9
Very active	7.5-17	10.3-23	14-31

*The low, middle, and high miles/day values apply for relatively heavy-weight (120 kg), middle-weight (70 kg), and light-weight (44 kg) individuals, respectively.
mo, Month(s); *yr,* year(s); *m,* meter(s); *mph,* miles per hour.

TABLE 11-2 Recommended Daily Allowance or Adequate Intake*of Nutrient by Age for Children of Average Height, Weight, and Physical Activity Level

Nutrient	Age								
	0-6 mo	7-12 mo	1-3 yr	4-8 yr	Boys 9-13 yr	Boys 14-18 yr	Girls 9-13 yr	Girls 14-18 yr	Pregnant <18 yr
Protein, g	9.1*	11	13	19	34	52	34	46	71
Protein (AMDR)	ND	ND	5-20	10-30	10-30	10-30	10-30	10-30	10-35
Carbohydrates, g	60*	95*	130	130	130	130	130	130	175
Carbohydrates (AMDR)	ND	ND	45-65	45-65	45-65	45-65	45-65	45-65	45-65
Fats, total, g	31*	30*	—	—	—	—	—	—	—
Fats, polyunsaturated fatty acids (linoleic acid), g	4.4*	4.6*	7*	10*	12*	16*	10*	11*	13*
Fats, total (AMDR)			30-40	25-35	25-35	25-35	25-35	25-35	20-35
Vitamin A (RAE) mcg	400*	500*	300	400	600	900	600	700	750
Thiamin (B_1), mg	0.2*	0.3*	0.5	0.6	0.9	1.2	0.9	1	1.4
Riboflavin (B_2), mg	0.3*	0.4*	0.5	0.6	0.9	1.3	0.9	1	1.4
Niacin (NE), mg	2*	4*	6	8	12	16	12	14	18
Pyridoxine (B_6), mg	0.1*	0.3*	0.5	0.6	1	1.3	1	1.2	1.9
Folate, mcg	65*	80*	150	200	300	400	300	400	600
Vitamin B_{12}, mcg	0.4*	0.5*	0.9	1.2	1.8	2.4	1.8	2.4	2.6
Vitamin C, mg	40*	50*	15	25	45	75	45	65	80
Vitamin D, mcg	5*	5*	5*	5*	5*	5*	5*	5*	5*
Vitamin E, mg	4*	5*	6	7	11	15	11	15	15
Vitamin K, mcg	2*	2.5*	30*	55*	60*	75*	60*	75*	75*
Calcium, mg	210*	270*	500*	800*	1300*	1300*	1300*	1300*	1300*
Fluoride, mg†	0.01*	0.5*	0.7*	1*	2*	3*	2*	3*	3*
Iron, mg	0.27*	11	7	10	8	11	8	15	27
Zinc, mg	2*	3	3	5	8	11	8	9	12

*Adequate intake.
†Fluoride supplement is not necessary if the water supply contains ≥0.6 parts per million fluoridation.
AMDR, Acceptable macronutrient distribution range; *ND*, not determinable; *RAE*, retinol activity equivalents. To calculate RAE from RE (retinol equivalent) of provitamin A carotenoids in foods, divide the RE by 2. For preformed vitamin A in foods or supplements or for provitamin A carotenoids in supplements, 1 RE = 1 RAE.
mo, Month(s); *yr*, year(s).
Adapted from Food and Nutrition Board, Institute of Medicine (IOM): *Dietary reference intakes for energy, carbohydrate, fiber, fat, fatty acids, cholesterol, protein, and amino acids, Washington*, DC, 2005, The National Academies Press.

Sodium requirements vary with the rate of extracellular fluid expansion, which is most rapid in infants and very young children. With the older child, it is not necessary to add sodium to the diet, even for children who exercise and perspire heavily. In fact, the typical North American diet far exceeds minimum requirements for sodium intake, with most sodium coming from salt added during processing and manufacturing of foods.

Potassium. Potassium serves to maintain intracellular homeostasis and contributes to muscle contractility and transmission of nerve impulses. Severe potassium deficit (hypokalemia) can lead to cardiac arrhythmias and death. Excessive potassium (hyperkalemia) can cause cardiac arrest. The urinary and gastrointestinal systems function to regulate potassium levels, and extreme imbalances are almost always due to disease processes or medication rather than to dietary factors. Potassium requirements are related to increases in lean body mass and are proportionally higher during the rapid growth of infancy and adolescence than during middle childhood. Fruits, vegetables, and fresh meat have high potassium content.

Chloride. Chloride functions in conjunction with sodium to maintain fluid and electrolyte balance. Loss of chloride occurs through the same routes as sodium loss: vomiting, diarrhea, and perspiration. The major source of chloride is salt (NaCl or KCl) added to foods during processing. There is no recommended daily allowance for chloride, but adequate amounts are ingested with a normal diet.

Protein

Protein is a fundamental component of all body cells. Dietary protein is broken down into amino acids, which are necessary for the synthesis of body cell protein and nitrogen-containing compounds. The body requires sufficient caloric intake to break down dietary protein so it can be used for protein synthesis. Amino acids are also required in some enzyme and hormone activity, cell transport, and tissue growth and development. Ten amino acids, called "indispensable" or essential amino acids, are not synthesized by the body and must be provided for in the diet (phenylalanine, leucine, methionine, lysine, isoleucine, valine, threonine, tryptophan, histidine, and arginine [arginine is required in diet for infants but not adults]). Depending on their age, children should receive approximately 5% to 30% of daily calories from proteins (see Table 11-2).

Protein and amino acid deficiencies rarely appear alone but follow other dietary deficits. Extreme stress and disease can deplete nitrogen, a process that contributes to tissue wasting and creates an increased demand for protein. Growth needs of the premature infant require higher levels of protein intake than those of infants born at term. The demand for protein is not generally increased with normal activity except as needed to build additional muscle tissue during body conditioning or during some illnesses.

Carbohydrates

Carbohydrates are the body's major dietary source of energy. More than half (45% to 65%) of children's body energy requirements should be supplied by carbohydrates (Food and Nutrition Board, IOM, 2005). In addition to providing energy, adequate carbohydrate intake is essential to facilitate protein synthesis. Carbohydrates are either simple sugars (the monosaccharides and disaccharides of sucrose, fructose, and lactose found in fruits, vegetables, milk, and prepared sweets) or complex carbohydrates (starches found in cereal grains, potatoes, legumes, and other vegetables). Most dietary carbohydrates should be in the complex form. Refined food products (e.g., products made with white flour, white sugar, white rice, and corn syrup) should be limited.

If dietary carbohydrates are extremely limited or absent (e.g., with a ketogenic diet used to manage intractable seizures of epilepsy; see Chapter 27), the body lipolyses stored triglycerides, oxidizes fatty acids, and breaks down dietary and tissue protein. This process contributes to accumulation of ketone bodies.

Fats

Lipids, fats, and fatty acids are used by the body to provide energy, to facilitate absorption of the fat-soluble vitamins (A, D, E, and K), and to maintain integrity of cell membranes and myelin. There are two essential fatty acids (not produced by the body) that must be included in the diet. Linoleic acid (LA) and alpha-linolenic acid (ALA) are precursors of omega-6 and omega-3 fatty acids, respectively. LA is found in soy oil; corn oil; and sunflower, safflower, pumpkin, and sesame seeds. ALA is found in large quantities in flax seed and flax seed oil and in lesser quantities in walnuts, canola oil, and wheat germ. Adequate amounts of omega-3 and omega-6 fatty acids are produced in the body if there is adequate intake of these two essential fatty acids and the vitamins and minerals necessary to facilitate their conversion.

It is recommended that there be no restrictions on fat intake for children less than 2 years old; that children more than 2 years old gradually adopt a diet of 30% (maximum) and 20% (minimum) of total calories from fats, with less than 10% of total calories in the form of saturated fat; and that daily diets have no more than 300 mg of cholesterol (Joint Working Group of the Canadian Paediatric Society [CPS] &

Health Canada, 2001). The Food and Nutrition Board of the IOM recommends that children 2 to 3 years old receive 30% to 35% of total calories from fats; children more than 3 years old should have a diet in which 25% to 35% of total calories come from fats. Saturated fats, trans-fatty acids, and cholesterol in the diet are unnecessary, and their intake should be minimized, with zero intake of trans-fatty acids (Food and Nutrition Board, IOM, 2005). Studies indicate that lower-fat diets (approximately 28% fat as a source of energy) in children 8 to 10 years old and in children between 7 and 36 months old who also have high vitamin and nutrient intake reduce cholesterol levels without affecting normal growth and development (Van Horn et al, 2003; Niinikoski et al, 1997). Providers should strive for balance when counseling parents about fat in their children's diets. A diet with about 30% of calories from fat easily provides for energy and growth needs; below 20% total fat, the child can be at nutritional risk. A well-balanced diet, with an emphasis on limited saturated fats and cholesterol and no trans fats, is associated with healthier "nutritional and plasma lipid profiles" (Royo-Bordonada et al, 2006). Children should be encouraged to eat a variety of foods, including many complex carbohydrates, and to engage in regular, vigorous physical activity.

Vitamins

A number of fat-soluble and water-soluble vitamins are essential for good health. Table 11-2 lists recommendations for daily vitamin intake. Table 11-3 identifies specific metabolic functions, dietary sources, and signs of deficiency or excessive intake of these vitamins.

Fat-Soluble Vitamins. Several characteristics of the fat-soluble vitamins (A, D, E, and K) have implications for dietary assessment and management:

- They can be stored for long periods of time in body tissues. As a result, temporary dietary deficiencies may not affect the body's growth and development. If stores are depleted and nutritional intake is inadequate, signs of vitamin deficiency appear. If intake is excessive, as can occur with supplementation, toxic effects can appear.
- They are absorbed in the intestines along with fats and lipids in foods. Low-fat diets and increased intestinal motility or malabsorption syndromes may put individuals at risk for vitamin deficiency.
- They are fairly stable when heated, as in cooking. Food preparation does not destroy fat-soluble vitamins as readily as water-soluble vitamins.
- They require bile for absorption. Conditions that compromise the hepatobiliary system put the individual at risk for decreased vitamin absorption.
- They do not contain nitrogen and do not act as coenzymes in cellular metabolism of nutrients.

Water-Soluble Vitamins. Unlike fat-soluble vitamins, water-soluble vitamins (C and B complexes) are stored in very small amounts in the body. If water-soluble–vitamin intake is above that needed by the body, absorption (primarily in the jejunum) decreases, and excess vitamins are excreted. As a result, daily intake of water-soluble vitamins is necessary, and

TABLE 11-3 Vitamins: Function, Dietary Sources, Interactions, Deficiency, and Excess

Vitamin	Function	Dietary Sources	Interactions Affecting Absorption or Utilization	Signs of Deficit	Signs of Excess
Fat-Soluble Vitamins					
Vitamin A	Vision, cellular differentiation and growth, reproductive and immune system function	Liver, fish liver oils, fortified milk, eggs, carrots, dark-green leafy vegetables	Absorption and utilization are facilitated by dietary fat, protein, and vitamin E Absorption of vitamin A is hindered by lack of protein, iron, or zinc	Anorexia, dry skin, keratinization of epithelial cells of respiratory tract, night blindness, corneal lesions, increased susceptibility to infections	Headache, vomiting, double vision, hair loss, dry mucous membrane, peeling skin, liver damage Toxic at 10 times the RDA No toxicity with excessive intake of carotenoids (e.g., carrots)
Vitamin D	Bone growth and development; regulates intestinal absorption of calcium and phosphorus	Sunlight, artificial ultraviolet light, fortified food products, especially milk	Utilization compromised in patients with renal failure Increased exposure to sunlight increases intake Darker skin and aging skin inhibit synthesis	Inadequate bone mineralization, rickets or skeletal malformations, delayed dentition	Anorexia, nausea, vomiting, diarrhea, weakness, hypercalcemia, hypercalciuria, calcium deposits in soft tissue, permanent renal or cardiovascular damage
Vitamin E	Antioxidant, traps free radicals, prevents oxidation of polyunsaturated fats	Vegetable oils, margarine, nuts, wheat germ, green leafy vegetables	Low serum levels have been associated with prematurity and congenital defects of the hepatobiliary system (e.g., cystic fibrosis, biliary atresia)	Macrocytic anemia and dermatitis in infants; neurologic defects in severe malabsorption	Unknown, if any
Vitamin K	Forms proteins that regulate blood clotting	Green leafy vegetables, milk, dairy products, liver	Inhibited by long-term antibiotic use, hyperalimentation, chronic biliary obstruction, or lipid malabsorption syndromes	Defective coagulation of blood, hemorrhages, liver injury	Vitamin K-responsive hemorrhagic condition, especially if patient is being treated with anticoagulants
Water-Soluble Vitamins					
Vitamin C	Essential for collagen formation and function; promotes growth and tissue repair; enhances iron absorption; improves wound healing	Vegetables and fruits, especially citrus fruits, broccoli, collard greens, spinach, tomatoes, potatoes, strawberries, peppers	Vitamin C is easily lost in food storage and preparation owing to exposure to heat, oxygen, and water Exposure to cigarette smoke increases vitamin C requirement	Scurvy, cracked lips, bleeding gums, slow wound healing, easy bruising	Unknown; excessive vitamin is excreted in urine

Continued

TABLE 11-3 Vitamins: Function, Dietary Sources, Interactions, Deficiency, and Excess—Cont'd

Vitamin	Function	Dietary Sources	Interactions Affecting Absorption or Utilization	Signs of Deficit	Signs of Excess
Thiamine (vitamin B₁)	Necessary for carbohydrate metabolism; promotes normal appetite and digestion	Whole grains, brewer's yeast, legumes, seeds and nuts, organ meats, lean cuts of pork	Availability inhibited by presence of thiaminase (found in raw fish); alcohol contributes to thiamine deficiency	Beriberi: muscle weakness, ataxia, confusion, anorexia, tachycardia, heart failure in infants	None by oral intake; excess excreted in urine
Riboflavin (vitamin B₂)	Necessary for oxidation-reduction reactions, essential for function of vitamin B₆ and niacin; helps maintain integrity of skin, tongue, and lips	Dairy products, meat, poultry, fish; enriched or fortified grains, cereals, and breads; green vegetables, such as broccoli, spinach, asparagus, turnip greens	Positive nitrogen balance contributes to function of riboflavin	Oral-buccal cavity lesions, generalized seborrheic dermatitis, scrotal and vulval skin changes, normocytic anemia, dimness of vision	None known
Niacin (vitamin B₃)	Essential for energy metabolism, glycolysis, fatty acids; maintains nervous system, integrity of skin, mouth, tongue	Meats, fortified grains, legumes Milk, eggs, and meats contain tryptophan	Requires riboflavin for absorption and utilization Grains treated with lime have more biologically available niacin Dietary tryptophan converts to niacin	Pellagra: dermatitis, diarrhea, inflammation of mucous membranes, indigestion	No known toxicity with dietary doses; heat rush flushing with excessive doses
Vitamin B₆ (pyridoxine)	Essential for metabolism of amino acids, lipids, nucleic acids, and glycogen	Chicken, fish, kidney, liver, pork, red meat, eggs, unrefined rice, soybeans, oats, whole wheat, peanuts, walnuts	Riboflavin enhances function Increased protein intake increases requirements for vitamin B₆ Processing of foods destroys vitamin B₆	Seen in combination with other B-complex vitamin deficiencies; dermatitis, anemia, convulsions, neurologic symptoms, and abdominal distress in infants	Ataxia, sensory neuropathy when taken in gram quantities for months or years
Folate (folacin)	Essential for amino acid metabolism and nucleic acid synthesis; red blood cell formation	Liver, yeast, dark-green leafy vegetables, legumes, fruits, oranges, brewer's yeast, milk	Only about 25% of folate in foods is directly bioavailable for absorption in intestine; more efficiently absorbed if serum levels are low Boiling milk destroys about 50% of folate present	Poor growth, megaloblastic anemia in severe cases; macrocytic anemia, glossitis, gastrointestinal disturbances; increased risk of neural tube defects in infants of folate-deficient mothers	None known in dietary doses; excessive folic acid supplementation may inhibit uptake of phenytoin and contribute to seizures in epileptic cases controlled by phenytoin
Vitamin B₁₂	Essential for metabolism, adequate red blood cell formation	Animal products: meat, eggs, and milk; shellfish	Absorbed in ileum; intrinsic factor mediated In strict vegetarians, the vitamin excreted in the bile is reabsorbed	Megaloblastic anemia, neurologic symptoms, sore tongue, weakness	None known

RDA, Recommended dietary allowance.

there is little risk of toxicity from large doses. The B vitamins also contain nitrogen and serve as essential coenzymes in the body's metabolism of nutrients. Niacin (vitamin B_3) plays a significant role in increasing high-density lipoproteins (HDLs).

Minerals and Elements

Major minerals are defined as those present in the body in amounts greater than 5 grams. Calcium, magnesium, and phosphorus are considered major minerals. Dietary reference intakes (DRI) have been set for boron, calcium, chromium, copper, fluoride, iodine, iron, magnesium, manganese, molybdenum, nickel, phosphorus, selenium, silicon, vanadium, and zinc (Food and Nutrition Board, IOM, 2005). Table 11-2 identifies recommended allowances for calcium, fluoride, iron, and zinc.

Peak bone density is directly related to calcium intake during the years of bone mineralization. Most mineralization takes place by the time an individual is 20 years old, but calcification can continue for several years more. To ensure maximum peak bone density, dietary calcium needs remain high until about 25 years old. Breastfed infants or those who are fed an approved infant formula receive sufficient calcium and should not be given a supplement.

Minerals and essential trace elements, their functions, dietary sources, and signs of deficiency or excess are presented in Table 11-4. Foods rich in iron are listed in Table 11-5.

Use of Vitamin and Mineral Supplements

National surveys reveal that many U.S. children have suboptimal nutrient intakes, especially a deficit of fruits and vegetables that contain many vitamins and minerals. The National Health and Nutrition Examination Survey (NHANES) data from 1999 to 2000, for example, show that only 0.7% of boys 14 to 18 years old met the daily recommended intake (DRI) of vegetables (Guenther et al, 2006). School-age children, especially girls, are at high risk for vitamin and mineral deficits (Suitor & Gleason, 2002).

DRIs for most foods should be evaluated over a 3-day period (i.e., children do not need to achieve a DRI for all foods every day to be healthy). Vitamin and mineral supplements are not necessary for children who consume a varied, healthy diet, and caution should be used to prevent oversupplementation, especially since safe upper limits have not been identified for some elements. Children at risk for nutritional deficit, however, may benefit by supplementation with multivitamins, and pregnant teenagers should receive prenatal vitamins. Risk factors for vitamin and mineral deficiency may include economically deprived families, neglect or abuse, anorexia, poor and capricious appetites, fad diets, dietary restrictions to manage obesity, and vegetarian diets. Preterm or low-birth-weight babies and children with chronic illness also may need supplementation.

Developing Eating Habits

Good nutrition for children is not just a matter of meeting dietary nutritional requirements. Healthy eating habits are also essential. The role that food plays in the family, the meaning it has for family members, and the way it is incorporated into family dynamics (e.g., parents often use sweets to reward children for good behavior) must be considered as providers counsel families about nutrition.

The development of healthy eating habits begins during gestation and continues through the life span. A healthy pregnancy most often leads to a healthy term newborn, ready to learn and master the skills of eating. The toddler and preschool years are critical to establishing lifelong patterns of eating. Many eating problems, including obesity, are in part due to poor eating habits learned in infancy and early childhood that are reinforced through the school-age and adolescent years.

As children develop their eating habits, it is the parents' responsibility to provide healthful food, adequate to meet the child's nutritional needs, in an environment that makes eating enjoyable; it is the child's responsibility to decide what and how much of these healthful foods to eat. Critical to this interaction is a parent who is knowledgeable about which foods are healthy and which are not, and who is aware of and responsive to the cues being given by the child. Also essential is the parents' ability to provide healthful foods; this can be extremely difficult for some low-income families. Federal programs (e.g., Food Stamps; Women, Infant, and Children [WIC]) have been created to increase parents' options, and providers may need to refer families to public health nurses for assistance in finding adequate food sources.

Special considerations related to developing healthy eating habits are presented for each of the age-specific sections that follow.

AGE-SPECIFIC CONSIDERATIONS

Newborns and Infants

Energy.   Rapid growth in infancy requires high caloric intake. Table 11-1 can be used to calculate the energy needs of infants to meet demands of metabolism and growth. Adequate intake of breast milk or infant formula meets all energy needs for infants until 4 to 6 months old.

Fat.   For proper myelinization to occur, infants must have adequate fat intake. Children younger than 2 years old can require more than 30% dietary fat for neural development. The lipid content of breast milk and formulas meets infants' dietary requirements. During the second year of life, cow's milk can be included in children's diets. Because the majority of fat in the diet is derived from milk and milk products, skim milk is not recommended for infants. The American Academy of Pediatrics recommends whole milk for children between 12 and 24 months old, although 2% milk, as part of a varied diet, can contribute to adequate fat intake and has no negative effect on growth or body composition (Wosje et al, 2002).

Vitamins.   Vitamin and mineral supplements, except iron, are usually not necessary for healthy term infants who are breastfed or formula fed and who receive mixed feedings of cereal, fruits, vegetables, and proteins after 4 to 6 months old. Breastfed infants and infants who receive a formula not fortified with vitamin D (which is rare) need supplementation. Infants also should have an adequate source of vitamin C, especially after 4 to 6 months old. A multivitamin supplement is recommended for infants at nutritional risk.

TABLE 11-4 Minerals and Trace Elements: Function, Dietary Sources, Interactions, Deficiency, and Excess

Minerals	Function	Dietary Sources	Interactions Affecting Absorption or Utilization	Signs of Deficit	Signs of Excess
Calcium	Development of bone tissue; vital role in nerve conduction, membrane permeability, blood clotting, and muscle contraction	Milk and milk products, green leafy vegetables, broccoli, kale, and collards, soft bones of fish, foods processed or fortified with calcium	Absorption enhanced in the presence of vitamin D, adequate protein intake, during periods of rapid growth, and if dietary intake of calcium is low	Decreased bone strength, increased risk for fractures	Constipation, increased risk for urinary stone formation; risk for decreased renal function
Phosphorus	Essential for bone integrity and general metabolism; provides essential energy during the metabolic process	Almost all foods, especially meat, poultry, fish, milk, cereal grains; food additives in processed foods	Aluminum hydroxide in antacids prevents absorption	Bone loss, weakness, malaise, anorexia, and pain	None known
Magnesium	Activates enzymes, facilitates cell metabolism, maintains electrical potential of cell membranes, enhances transmission of nerve impulses, assists to maintain adequate serum levels of calcium and potassium	Nuts, legumes, whole (unmilled) grains, green vegetables; bananas provide some magnesium	High-fiber diet may reduce absorption slightly	Nausea, muscle weakness, irritability	None in healthy individual; with impaired renal function, excess may contribute to nausea, vomiting, hypotension, bradycardia, central nervous system depression
Iron	Formation of the heme molecule; used in oxygen transport	Meat, eggs, vegetables, cereals, foods fortified with iron additives; Table 11-5 identifies a number of iron-rich foods	Absorption is enhanced if iron stores or daily intakes are low; presence of ascorbic acid increases absorption Heme iron in meats is more bioavailable than nonheme iron from grains, fruits, and vegetables Absorption inhibited if the iron-rich food is ingested with milk or caffeine or in presence of phytic acid, oxalic acid, and tannic acid	Anemia Children are particularly susceptible to iron deficiency during periods of rapid growth combined with low dietary iron intake: from about 6 mo to 4 yr old and during early adolescence; adolescent girls are at risk owing to menstruation	Iron poisoning can be fatal; for a 2-yr-old, a fatal dose is approximately 3 g; for adolescents and adults, 200–250 mg/kg may be fatal
Zinc	Cellular metabolism, growth, and repair	Meats, animal products, seafood (especially oysters), eggs	Absorption may be decreased if taken with high-fiber diet	Anorexia, growth retardation, skin changes, immuno-logic abnormalities	Gastrointestinal disturbances, vomiting, acute toxicity, impaired immune response

Mineral	Function	Sources	Special considerations	Deficiency	Toxicity/Excess
Iodine	Production of thyroid hormones	Water, seafood, airborne water from ocean mist, iodized salt, food processing related to milk and bread	None known	Thyroid dysfunction ranging from simple goiter to cretinism and mental retardation	Thyrotoxicosis; goiter, rare and not seen in children with intake up to 1mg/day; toxic levels not known
Trace elements					
Selenium	Unknown	Seafood and organ meats; may be in grains grown in soil containing selenium	Intake linked to vitamin E intake; if vitamin E is adequate, selenium is likely to be also; may need to supplement in lactating women. Total parenteral nutrition (TPN) feedings contribute to deficiency	May be related to muscle weakness and pain, cardiomyopathy (Keshan disease) in young children	Nausea, abdominal pain, diarrhea, fatigue, nail and hair changes or loss; toxic levels not known
Copper	Normal growth	Organ meats, seafood, nuts, seeds; infants store copper in liver during gestation	TPN feedings contribute to deficiency; high vitamin C, molybdenum, or zinc intake may reduce retention or bioavailability	Bone loss, anemia, neutropenia, growth impairment	Liver disease, gastrointestinal symptoms, diarrhea, vomiting
Manganese	Unknown, may be related to reproductive health, normal growth	Whole grains and cereals	Increased absorption during third trimester of pregnancy	Unknown, may be related to growth retardation	Unknown, may be related to learning disabilities, anemia
Fluoride	Prevents dental caries, enhances bone health	Fluoridated water, tea, meat and bones of marine fish, potatoes, wheat germ	Processing foods in fluoridated water or cooking with Teflon increases content; cooking foods in aluminum reduces fluoride	Dental caries, may be related to poor bone health	Mottling of teeth, kidney disease, bone disease, may affect muscle and nerve function
Chromium	Assists in glucose metabolism	Brewer's yeast, calves' liver, American cheese, wheat germ	TPN feedings can contribute to deficiency	May be related to impairment of glucose tolerance	Unknown, requires further study
Molybdenum	Enzyme function	Milk, beans, breads, cereals	TPN feedings can contribute to deficiency	Unknown	Related to loss of copper, may lead to goutlike symptoms

*Nearly all trace minerals are toxic in large quantities because many are metals.

TABLE 11-5   Iron-Rich Foods

Food	High Levels (5 mg/Serving)	Moderate Levels (2-4 mg/Serving)	Low Levels (<2 mg/Serving)
Breads, grains, cereals, seeds*	Almonds (1 cup, whole, oil roasted)	Bagel (1, egg or plain)	Biscuits (1 each)
	Cashews (1 cup, dry roasted)	Bread, Indian fry (1 piece)	Bread (1 slice, whole wheat)
	Pumpkin seed kernels (¼ cup, roasted)	Breadstick (10, plain, without salt)	Egg noodles (1 cup, cooked)
	Fortified cereals	Filberts (1 cup, dried)	English muffin (1 each)
	Mixed nuts (1 cup, dry roasted with peanuts)	Gingerbread (1 piece)	Pancakes (1 each)
		Muffin (1 wheat)	Peanut butter (2 tbsp)
	Brown glutinous rice (1 cup, cooked)	Peanuts (1 cup, dried)	Oatmeal (1 cup, cooked)
	Sunflower seeds (1 cup, dry roasted)	White rice (1 cup, enriched, regular, cooked)	
	Watermelon kernels (1 cup, dried)	Waffles (2 each)	
	Wheat germ (1 cup, toasted)	Walnuts (1 cup, dried)	
Fruits*	Apricot (1 cup, dried halves)	Avocado (1 whole)	Apple (1 medium, unpeeled)
		Currants (1 cup, dried Zante)	Apple juice (1 cup)
		Fig (10 each, dried)	Banana (1 medium)
		Pear (10 each, dried halves)	Dried mixed fruit (2 oz)
		Prune juice (1 cup)	Orange (1 medium)
		Raisins (½ cup)	Orange juice (1 cup)
Vegetables*	Kidney beans (1 cup, cooked, fresh)	Black beans (1 cup, cooked)	Kidney beans (1 cup, canned)
	Lentils (1 cup, cooked)	Garbanzo beans (1 cup, cooked)	Green beans (1 cup, raw or cooked)
	Soybeans (1 cup, cooked)	Refried beans (1 cup, canned)	Broccoli (1 cup)
	White beans (1 cup, cooked)	Beet greens (1 cup, cooked)	Carrots (1 cup)
	Spinach (1 cup, cooked)	Potatoes (1 medium, with skin, baked)	Corn (½ cup)
	Tofu (½ cup)	Peas (1 cup, fresh, cooked)	Lettuce (1 cup)
		Snow peas with pods (1 cup, raw or cooked)	Potato (½ cup, baked, with skin)
			Spinach (1 cup, raw)
		Molasses (2 tbsp, blackstrap)	Sweet potatoes (1 cup, fresh, boiled, mashed)
		Spinach (1 cup, frozen, cooked)	Tomatoes (1 cup fresh)
			Tomato juice (1 cup, canned)
			Turnip greens (1 cup, cooked)
Meats, poultry, fish, other protein sources†	Clams (3.5 oz, 5 each, or 1 cup) = 22 mg Fe	Ground beef (3 oz, cooked lean)	Roast beef (3 oz, lean)
	Oysters (3.5 oz)	Catfish (1 piece, floured, fried)	Chicken (1 cup, dark or light meat)
	Beef heart meat (3.5 oz, cooked)	Tuna (1 cup, canned, water packed)	
	Beef liver (3.5 oz, simmered)	Lamb (3.5 oz, cooked)	Egg (1, whole)
	Veal liver (3 oz, simmered)		Halibut (1 piece, baked or broiled)
	Chicken liver (3.5 oz, cooked)		Ham (1 cup, roasted)
	Turkey liver (3.5 oz, cooked)		Bacon (3 pieces, cooked)
			Pork (3 oz, lean shoulder roast)

*Iron in plant foods is better absorbed when eaten with vitamin C or meat products.
†Iron in meat, poultry, and fish is more bioavailable than iron in other food sources.
Fe, iron.
Adapted from Hands ES: *Food finder: food sources of vitamins and minerals*, ed 3, Salem, OR, 1995, ESHA Research and Hands ES: *Nutrients in food*, Philadelphia, 2000, Lippincott Williams & Wilkins.

Iron.   Iron deficiency is the leading cause of anemia in children, and iron supplementation is appropriate in some cases. Term infants who are breastfed usually have adequate iron supplies until 4 to 6 months old. Premature or low-birth-weight infants, infants who are exclusively breastfed beyond 4 to 6 months old, and infants who are fed cow's milk before they are 12 months old are at high risk for iron deficiency anemia. Iron-fortified cereals and iron-fortified formulas are excellent sources of dietary iron supplements for infants 6 to 12 months old. Earlier supplementation may be necessary for breastfed premature infants.

Fluoride.   The American Dental Association recommends fluoride treatment starting at 6 months old (American Dental Association, 2002). See Chapter 33 for recommended fluoride dosages. The fluoride level of the water used to mix formula should be measured to ensure that infants do not receive excess fluoride. If the water supply is fluoridated, formula-fed infants can be given ready-to-feed formula, or nonfluoridated bottled water can be used to prepare fluoride-supplemented formula.

Infant Formulas. Breast milk is the ideal food for newborns and infants and should be promoted unless it is medically harmful to the infant. Most iron-fortified infant formulas provide adequate nutrition and, for some families, may be an appropriate alternative. Box 11-1 outlines various types of commercial formulas available.

Occasionally, infants demonstrate intolerance to formula, showing irritability, weight loss or slow gain, emesis, diarrhea, constipation, other gastrointestinal problems, or atopic dermatitis. The provider must work closely with parents to identify a formula tolerated by the infant, being careful to allow sufficient time for the baby to respond to a new formula as it is introduced. This can be a time- and energy-consuming process in which parents need support, reassurance, and encouragement. Referral to a registered dietitian can be helpful. See the discussion on food intolerances (Altered Patterns of Nutrition) later in this chapter for management of infants who are lactose- or protein-intolerant.

Introduction of Solids. A number of variables converge at about 6 months that make this an appropriate time to introduce solids into infants' diets:

- Infants' sucking patterns have changed sufficiently to allow mastery of chewing and swallowing.
- Infants can sit with some support, and they are able to purposefully move their heads.
- Infants are able to grasp, pick up, and bring objects to their mouths.
- Iron stores present at birth are being depleted.
- Growth demands require nutrients other than those provided in milk alone.
- Developmental needs (cognitive, sensory, and motor) are stimulated by new foods, textures, smells, tastes, and use of utensils.

The specific foods that parents provide for their children vary by cultural and family customs, and there are no set recommendations as to a sequence by which to introduce solids. Commercial baby foods provide adequate nutrition, but labels should be examined to determine their content, especially looking at calories, fats, additives, salt, and sugar. Commercial baby foods are not essential, since home-prepared foods, such as rice, mashed bananas, applesauce, puréed squash, cooked vegetables, and blenderized meats, can provide adequate nutrition if the diet is well balanced. Box 11-2 lists some principles to keep in mind when beginning solids.

Eating Habits. While infants are being exclusively breastfed or formula fed, the parents need to be alert to cues of satiety. Feeding on demand in early infancy is important, and neonates should not be allowed to sleep for long periods

---

BOX 11-1 **Categories of Infant Formulas Available***

- Premature formulas (hospital and transitional)
  - Higher caloric content more nutrient dense than regular cow's milk–based formulas
  - Protein source: human milk, nonfat cow's milk, whey
- Cow's milk–based formulas
  - Standard formula for healthy term infants
- Nutrient-dense cow's milk–based formulas
  - Similar to premature formula, but with less phosphorus and calcium; some preparations have up to 27 kcal/oz (vs. 20 kcal/oz in regular formula and 24 kcal/oz in premature formula)
- Hypoallergenic formulas
  - Partially hydrolyzed whey-based formulas
  - Soy-based formulas (protein source: soy protein isolate with L-methionine)
  - Casein hydrolysate formulas
  - Amino acid–based formulas (elemental)
- Formulas with long-chain polyunsaturated fatty acids
  - More closely approximates human milk with content of docosahexaenoic acid (DHA, an omega-3 fatty acid) and arachidonic acid (ARA, an omega-6 fatty acid)
  - May enhance visual and mental development, especially in preterm infants (Fleith & Clandinin, 2005)
- Formulas for feeding beyond 4-6 months of age, supplemented with solids
- Nutrient-dense formulas for older child
  - Caloric content up to 30 kcal/oz; other nutrients increased over regular infant formula
- Specialized formulas
  - Higher caloric content (24-30 kcal/oz); nutrient dense; free amino acid and peptide-based formulas
- Protein supplements
- Nitrogen-free calorie supplements
- Oral electrolyte solutions

*For names of formulas and detailed description of formula content, see *Infant formulas: approximate composition of pediatric formulas.* Available at *http://depts.washington.edu/growing/Nourish/Ftable.htm* (accessed Mar 23, 2007).

of time without feeding. But feeding primarily to comfort a child should be discouraged; every time a child cries, he or she is not necessarily hungry. Bottle-fed infants, whether formula or breast milk is used in the bottle, can easily be overfed (e.g., the caregiver often urging the infant to take that extra half-ounce just to empty the bottle). As a result, infants can learn to ignore feelings of satiety. Self-regulation of intake is evident in young infants, but even by the early toddler years, children can be influenced by other social cues around feeding and eat more than they need to (Fox et al, 2006). Recent research indicates that normal weight term infants who rapidly gain weight in the first 5 months of life are at higher risk for obesity as toddlers and preschoolers (Dennison et al, 2006).

When solids are introduced, parents should be counseled to respond early and promptly to a child's feeding cues and to allow the child to initiate and guide the feeding interaction. A selection of varied, healthful foods can give the older infant a chance to explore textures, smells, colors, and taste. Feeding is also a time when older infants and toddlers learn physical skills of fine motor control, cognitive skills of relationships between action and consequence (the dog will eat whatever is dropped on the floor), and interactional skills of social exchange among family members.

Toddlers and Preschoolers

Energy and Protein. The growth rate of toddlers and preschoolers is slower than that of infants, resulting in decreased energy needs per unit of body weight. But because of increased size and activity, these children require an increased number of total calories. Addition of muscle mass also demands a continued high protein intake.

Eating Habits. Toddlers become more skilled in managing eating, using utensils, joining the family for regular mealtimes, and demonstrating more distinctive likes and dislikes of food. They learn how and what to eat by observing adults around them and by responding to what adults provide for them to eat. Older infants and toddlers may show an initial aversion to new foods. Parents should be advised that, rather than forcing the child to try the new food or giving in to the child's feeding demands, the food should be removed without comment then offered again at another meal. Children may reject a food up to 15 times before they become accustomed to it and enjoy eating it. Parents should continue to be responsive to the child's cues for hunger and satiety, providing age-appropriate portions and not insisting on the "clean-plate" approach to nutrition.

Use of Vitamin and Mineral Supplements. Vitamin supplements are usually not necessary for young children since many foods are fortified. Findings from the Feeding Infants and Toddlers Study (FITS) show that most children who do not use supplements receive adequate amounts of vitamins, and adding a multivitamin supplement can actually place children at risk of excessive vitamin intake; 97% of children who received supplements had above the tolerable upper intake level for vitamin A, 66% for zinc, and 20% for folate (Fox et al, 2006; Briefel et al, 2006). Evaluate a child's intake over the course of a week. If children persist with *extremely* limited food choices or picky eating behavior, they might benefit from a children's multivitamin plus mineral supplement.

School-Age Children

Energy and Protein. Energy and protein needs of school-age children vary greatly, depending on body size, growth patterns, and activity and exercise levels. Protein needs increase in older children as they acquire more muscle mass. Boys older than 10 years generally need between 2500 and 3000 calories a day, whereas girls require about 2200 calories daily (see Table 11-1).

Eating Habits. Food likes and dislikes carry over from the preschool years. There is great variation in appetite and intake as a result of uneven growth and activity levels. School-age children have a tendency to skip meals and are more likely to snack as they become engrossed in activities. This tendency is exacerbated in families with hectic schedules, unstructured mealtimes, and reliance on fast foods. Parents and children can identify healthful "fast" foods (e.g., homemade burritos, stir-fry chicken, peanut butter sandwiches, an apple, carrot sticks,

---

BOX 11-2 **Principles for the Introduction of Solids into the Infant's Diet**

Introduce one food at a time, waiting 3 to 5 days before offering another to assess for adverse reaction.
Offer rice cereal, the least allergenic of cereal grains, as the first food.
Introduce fruits, vegetables, and other cereals in any sequence desired.
Feed only iron-fortified cereals.
Avoid allergenic foods (e.g., wheat, nuts [especially peanuts], shellfish, egg whites, citrus) before children are 12 months old.
Prepare food appropriate to child's developmental abilities (e.g., strained, mashed, or finger foods).
Use home-prepared or commercially-prepared foods.
Provide a variety of foods.
Help child develop healthy patterns of eating:
• Be alert and responsive to child's cues when eating.
• Use a spoon to feed solids.
• Offer about 1 tbsp per year of age as a serving for infants; for older children, about one-fourth to one-half an adult serving.
• Never force a child to eat.
• Include the child in family meal times.

string cheese and a bagel on the way to soccer practice) that fit a busy school-age child's schedule. High-fat, high-calorie, low-nutrient snacks, such as chips, soda, and pizza, should be a very small part of the child's diet.

Use of Vitamin and Mineral Supplements. Poor eating habits place school-age children at risk for deficiencies in iron, thiamine, vitamin A, and calcium. Teaching children about specific nutrient sources and encouraging healthy eating habits can prevent many problems; supplementation with a daily multivitamin is usually not necessary.

Adolescents

Energy and Protein. The growth rate of adolescents is remarkable (Table 11-6), and the description by some parents that their children never seem to stop eating is apt. High levels of energy are needed to support adolescents' rapid growth, and if children participate in sports or other exercise programs, additional caloric intake can be needed. Adequate protein intake is essential to produce muscle mass. The average intake of protein in the U.S. diet is significantly above the DRI, so additional supplementation is usually not necessary.

Eating Habits. Eating habits of adolescents are influenced by their increasing independence and social activity, perceptions of body image, and physical growth patterns. Adolescents often have erratic eating patterns; skip meals; eat high-fat, high-calorie, low-nutrient snack foods; and consume calories late in the day. Teens who participate in sports and adolescents who eat a mainly vegetarian diet tend to have healthier eating habits than their nonsports-involved or meat-eating counterparts (Croll et al, 2006; Dunham & Kollar, 2006).

Use of Vitamin and Mineral Supplements

Thiamine, riboflavin, niacin, folate, iron, zinc, and calcium needs increase during adolescence (see Table 11-2). Most adolescents who eat a well-balanced diet need no supplements, but their irregular eating habits put them at risk for deficits. Adolescent girls are at risk for iron deficit when menstruation begins, and children who eat a vegan diet will need vitamin B_{12} supplements.

Pregnancy in Adolescence. Pregnancy presents an added complication to the normal adolescent's nutrient intake. Nutrition needs are high for the pregnant teenager, particularly if she is younger than 15 years old, in the midst of her pubertal growth spurt. During this period, teenagers' bodies are still growing and compete with their fetuses for nutrients. Infants born to teenage mothers are at higher risk for prematurity, low birth weight, chronic illness, disabilities, and death. Proper nutrition and early prenatal care can increase the chance of a successful pregnancy.

The nutrition needs of pregnant teenagers also are the highest at a time when it is most difficult to meet them. Irregular eating patterns typical of adolescents contribute to poor nutritional status. Calcium; iron; zinc; vitamins A, D, and B_6; riboflavin; folic acid; and total calories—all of which are essential to fetal growth—are often found to be inadequate in the diets of female adolescents (Lytle et al, 2002).

When managing the pregnant teenager, providers should carefully assess dietary intake and counsel the adolescent to eat a varied and healthful diet. A prenatal multivitamin and mineral supplement, including iron and folic acid, is advised, and calcium supplements can be indicated. The pregnant teenager should strive for a total of 1300 to 1500 mg

---

TABLE 11-6 Average Weight, Height, and Head Circumference Gains in Infancy Through Adolescence

Age	Weight	Height	Head circumference	Comments
Infant (mo)	Average weekly gain:	Average monthly gain:	Average monthly gain:	
0-3	210 g (8 oz)	3.5 cm	2 cm	Regain or exceed birth weight by 2 wk
3-6	140 g (5 oz)	2 cm	1 cm	Birth weight doubles by 4-6 mo
6-12	85-105 g (3-4 oz)	1.2-1.5 cm	0.5 cm	
Toddler	Average yearly gain:	Average yearly gain:	Average yearly gain:	
1-3 yr	2-3 kg (4.4-6.6 lb)	12 cm	3 cm	Height at 2 yrs approximately half of adult height
Preschool-age child				
3-6 yr	2 kg (4.5 lb)	3-7 cm	1 cm	
School-age child				
6-12 yr	3-3.5 kg (7 lb)	6 cm	2-3 cm during entire period	Growth is discontinuous, in spurts lasting about 8 wk, occurring 3-6 times a year
Preadolescent and adolescent	Average total gain:	Average yearly gain:		Weight gain follows linear growth, with several months delay; adolescents first grow taller, then fill out
Girl, 10-14 yr	17.7 kg (39 lb)	6-8.3 cm		95% linear growth achieved by onset of menarche
Boy, 12-16 yr	22.2 kg (50 lb)	6-9.5 cm		95% linear growth achieved by 15 yr

Adapted from Needlman RD: Growth and development. In Behrman RE, Kliegman RM, Jenson HB, editors: *Nelson textbook of pediatrics*, ed 17, Philadelphia, 2004, WB Saunders.

of calcium through diet and supplements each day (Chan et al, 2006). Daily folic acid intake of 0.4 mg is recommended for all girls capable of becoming pregnant, increased to 0.6 mg during pregnancy (Food and Nutrition Board, IOM, 2005).

Weight gain in pregnant teens should be carefully monitored. Healthy teens who are still growing themselves (i.e., less than 4 years after menarche) should gain the amount they would normally gain in 9 months if they were not pregnant plus a normal pregnancy weight gain. For adolescents who are 4 years past menarche, pregnancy weight gain should be similar to that of adult women. In one study of pregnant African-American teenagers, extra weight gain for normal-weight girls was not shown to be beneficial (Nielsen et al, 2006). Adolescents who begin pregnancy when overweight are at high risk for neonatal and perinatal morbidity (Sukalich et al, 2006). All adolescents would benefit from comprehensive prenatal nutrition programs (Nielsen et al, 2006). For those adolescents who meet income guidelines, the federal supplemental food program WIC is a valuable resource. In addition to providing nutritious foods, the program offers nutrition education and counseling.

■ ASSESSMENT OF NUTRITIONAL STATUS

The goals of nutritional status assessment are to determine dietary adequacy and to identify deviation from normal growth and development. Data collected include a history of food and fluid intake, physical findings, and laboratory and diagnostic indicators.

HISTORY

Questions to elicit a history of nutritional status can be grouped into several categories:
- Food and fluid intake:
  - Nutritional status of mother during pregnancy.
  - Type of feeding method used during infancy. If not breast-fed, formula name and preparation. Any problems? When weaned? When solids started? Any allergies or intolerances noted?
  - Current nutritional intake of child (if child is still an infant, ask more specifically about frequency and amounts of feedings in 24-hour period).
  - Type of foods and fluids.
  - Amounts eaten (may use 24-hour recall, 3-day diet history, or length of time and frequency that child is at breast).
  - Additional intake (e.g., vitamin, fluoride, or iron supplements).
- Eating patterns:
  - Frequency of eating (nursings, meals, snacks).
  - Feeding patterns or behaviors for both child and family.
  - Bottle feeding: Is bottle propped? Does child take bottle to bed at night or at nap time? Who feeds child?
  - Breastfeeding: On demand or scheduled? How flexible is mother to demands of infant? Is mother working? Is breast milk frozen and fed by someone other than the mother?

- Describe mealtimes: Does family sit down together? Are meals prepared at home? Does child eat at school? How often are "fast foods" eaten? What amount of time is spent eating? How long does it take to feed child?
  - Does family eat out frequently? How many times per week?
- Reactions to and attitudes about foods:
  - Any reaction to particular foods (e.g., vomiting, diarrhea, rash)?
  - Food preferences or dislikes.
  - Cultural factors: What beliefs or attitudes does family have about how and what child should eat or how family should eat?
  - What is child's attitude about foods and eating?
  - Feeding abilities of child. For example, does child choke, gag, vomit, have suck or swallow difficulties, or refuse certain foods, perhaps because of texture or smell?
- Management of foods in the family:
  - Who plans, purchases, and prepares food and meals for family?
  - Economic and environmental factors that influence how food is managed. For example, are finances adequate to supply nutritious foods? Is there a refrigerator? Does family have a car to carry larger amounts of food from store? Is there a full-service grocery store in the neighborhood? What is the socioeconomic status of family? Is food shopping budgeted? Are food stamps or other supplemental programs used?
- Health status affected by nutrition:
  - Special considerations for children or family related to food. For example, does child have a chronic illness that requires a special diet or formula? Are any medications being taken?
  - Elimination patterns.
  - Dental status and care of teeth.
  - Patterns of wound healing, infections, colds, and mild illnesses.
  - Any change in hair, nails, skin, or mucous membranes?
  - Tolerance for hot or cold weather?
  - Growth, activity, and exercise pattern. For example, has child been growing as parent expects? Has there been a history of unusual weight gain or loss? Does child have energy to play?
  - Family history: hypertension, diabetes, hyperlipidemia, obesity, heart disease, allergies, eating disorders.

PHYSICAL EXAMINATION

The physical examination should include the following:
- Body temperature
- Height, weight, and head circumference measurements (see growth charts, Appendix B; also see Table 11-6 for average weight and height gains expected during childhood); arm circumference and triceps and subscapular skinfold caliper measurements for children at risk for obesity or malnutrition
- BMI (see growth charts, Appendix B)
- Skin condition (clear, smooth, firm, with good turgor)
- Muscle tone, posture, skeletal development (body erect, tone good)

- Hair (smooth, full, shiny; no dryness, broken ends, bare patches, or discoloration)
- Mucous membranes, eyes (moist, shiny, no dark circles, conjunctiva pink)
- Teeth (eruption appropriate to age, gums healthy, no bleeding)
- Neck (thyroid, parotid glands of normal size)
- Abdomen (flat, soft)
- Cardiovascular (no pathologic murmur; normal heart size; skin warm, pink, less than 3-second capillary refill; peripheral pulses equal, strong)
- Neurologic and behavior (alert, active, reflexes present, no complaints of headache, neuritis)

DIAGNOSTIC TESTS

- Laboratory and diagnostic tests are performed as indicated:
- Hemoglobin or hematocrit
- Iron and/or ferritin levels (see Chapter 26)
- Serum levels for various elements: albumin, nitrogen balance, minerals, lipids
- Bone radiographs for suspected iodine, vitamins C and D, or copper deficiency or to compare bone age with height age (age at which 50% of children reach the patient's height)

■ MANAGEMENT STRATEGIES FOR OPTIMAL NUTRITION

Pediatric health care providers can work to ensure that dietary intake adequately supports optimal growth and development through nutritional education, counseling, and anticipatory guidance. Parents should be given information and guidance about children's age and developmental abilities and characteristics, nutritional requirements, foods that meet children's nutritional needs, and strategies to facilitate the development of healthy eating behaviors. The relationship between disease and dietary intake should be discussed. Cultural issues related to food should also be considered.

NUTRITIONAL EDUCATION

Developmental and age variations of children related to nutrition and children's nutritional requirements have been discussed previously.

MyPyramid

MyPyramid is a recent adaptation of the well-known food guide pyramid and is a useful tool for educating families and children of all ages about a healthful diet. MyPyramid allows individuals to calculate their personal nutrient needs based on age, gender, and activity level. It illustrates the proportions of a healthy diet, emphasizing a foundation of grains, fruits, vegetables, beans, peas, and lean meats, fish, and poultry. The Oregon Dairy Council (2006) has adapted MyPyramid to identify a range of foods that are nutrient rich and to specify serving sizes. Called "Pyramid Plus," this adaptation encourages selection of nutrient-rich (N-Rich) foods, limitation of "other" and "sometimes" foods, and participation in regular exercise (Table 11-7).

Cultural Variations

N-Rich foods are found in all cultures and ethnic groups, although not all cultures officially categorize foods in the

TABLE 11-7 **MyPyramid Plus: Nutrient-Rich (N-Rich) Foods**

Grains	Vegetables	Fruits	Milk	Meat and Beans
Make half your grains whole	Vary your veggies	Focus on fruits	Get your calcium-rich foods	Go lean
Fiber, B vitamins, folic acid, iron, magnesium	Fiber, potassium, vitamins A, C, and E	Fiber, potassium, vitamin C, folic acid	Calcium, potassium, vitamin D, protein, magnesium	Protein, B vitamins, iron, magnesium, zinc, vitamin E
Whole grains: 100% whole grain cereals, oatmeal, 100% whole grain breads, bagels, tortillas, crackers, popcorn (lite), wild rice, barley, whole wheat pasta, brown rice	(Fresh, frozen, canned): Spinach, bok choy, mustard greens, asparagus, leaf lettuce, broccoli, celery, cauliflower, zucchini, iceberg lettuce, bell peppers, mushrooms, green beans, cabbage, tomatoes, winter squash, sweet potatoes, artichokes, cucumbers, salsa, beets, eggplant	(Fresh, frozen, canned in juice): Cantaloupe, papaya, grapefruit, blackberries, oranges, strawberries, apricots, kiwi, raspberries, pineapple, tangerines, mango, honeydew, watermelon, avocado, peaches, plums, blueberries, grapes, cherries, bananas, apples, pears	Fat-free and low-fat dairy: Milk, flavored milk, plain yogurt, flavored yogurt, cottage cheese, part-skim ricotta, 2% milk, reduced-fat cheese, part-skim mozzarella	Lean meats, fish, poultry: Shellfish, fish, beef (flank, top round, lean ground), pork (loin, lean ham), eggs, poultry (skinless light meat, lean ground) Beans and peas, vegetarian burger, lentils, soy beans (edamame), tofu, beans (black, kidney, garbanzo, pinto), peas (black-eyed, split) Seeds and nuts: seeds (flax, pumpkin, sunflower), nuts (almonds, hazelnuts, peanuts, walnuts), peanut butter

From Oregon Dairy Council: *Pyramid Plus*, 2006, Nutrition Education Services. Available at *www.oregondairycouncil.org* (accessed Mar 25, 2007).

same way (e.g., the Philippines has no milk category; some cultures place potatoes in the vegetable category, others list it as a protein; some categorize nuts as a protein, others as a fat or oil [Painter et al, 2002]). Pollan has suggested that poor nutrition, obesity, and subsequent health problems among Americans may have a cultural base and could be solved if individuals were to "Eat food. Not too much. Mostly plants." with meat as a source of "flavor" rather than protein (Pollan, 2007). This suggestion can form the basis for all healthy diets, incorporating a wide variety of foods from numerous ethnic and cultural groups.

STRATEGIES TO DEVELOP HEALTHY EATING BEHAVIORS

As noted above, basic eating patterns are established in the infant, toddler, and preschool years; these patterns tend to continue through the child's life. Children learn eating behaviors by observation and instruction, and parents are the primary teachers in this process. Often that teaching is done without conscious reflection or planning on the part of parents. Studies indicate that children tend to eat what their parents do and that parents who exert overt pressure on their children to eat less fat or more fruits and vegetables—without changing their own habits—actually contribute to poor eating patterns (Spruijt-Metz et al, 2006). The responsibility of parents to provide healthful foods cannot be overemphasized. Parents may rationalize giving their child "empty" calories rather than food that contains essential nutrients by stating, "That's all my child will eat, and I know she needs the energy," or "But he cries and carries on if I don't give it to him; I'm just doing it to make him happy." Providers need to remind parents that the parent decides if an 18-month-old's "treat" is French fries or blueberries, not the child. Parents have a choice and a serious responsibility to their children's long-term health. If children learn early that healthy, nutrient-filled foods are readily available and that mom and dad enjoy them, they will enjoy them as well. High-fat, high-sugar, and high-salt foods provide taste and calories, but little in the way of nutrition. They should make up a very small part of the diet; but overly restricting them, especially in children, can contribute to unhealthy attitudes toward food. If these foods are occasionally available, children learn to make better choices about how to fit them into a healthful diet. Providers can have parents do a "pantry evaluation" to see what types of snack foods are available for their children. If "empty-calorie" foods are not available in the home, children will not eat them.

Often parents will try to decide exactly what and how much their child should eat (e.g., they may make a child sit at the table to finish his vegetables). Appetite fluctuations and preferences are typical of children, and parents should be aware that children may appear to eat less than the parent thinks is sufficient or too much of one particular food to the neglect of others. If parents punish a child for not eating or force a child to eat, they have taken away the child's responsibility to choose. In response, the child may develop an aversion to certain foods, overeat, or act out in other ways. Mealtimes can become contests of will between parents and children, creating feelings and

patterns of interacting that extend far beyond the dinner table. Parents need to find out what healthy foods their children enjoy (it is perfectly alright to eat only carrots and broccoli for several weeks in a row!) and make those available. If provided a nutritious variety of foods they like, children tend to select those necessary for their healthy growth, in terms of both amount of calories and other nutrients. A general principle to keep in mind when considering portions is to serve 1 tablespoon of food per year of age. Thus for children younger than 5 years old, 1 serving is about one-fourth to one-third of an adult serving; for older children, one-fourth to one-half of an adult serving. Children's appetites vary, however, and parents should be alert to cues that the child wants more or less of any particular food.

Providers can help parents make the process more positive by having them examine their own values and patterns related to eating, identify and reinforce those they would like to foster in their children, and eliminate those they see as negative. Providers can inform parents about age differences and offer suggestions for effectively managing the eating experience. Parents should be encouraged to provide the following:

- Positive examples of healthy intake; parents are the child's role model
- An adequate supply of a wide variety of age-appropriate, nutritious foods and snacks
- Limits, but not prohibitions, on consumption of nonnutritious sugars and "sometimes" foods
- Food prepared in a form that stimulates children's appetites
- Regular, structured mealtimes where the family sits down to eat together; this may occur only once a day
- A pleasant, relaxed environment for mealtimes
- Clear, developmentally-appropriate expectations for children's behavior at mealtimes
- Developmentally-appropriate access to and instruction in the use of utensils
- Appropriate supervision during mealtimes
- Developmentally-appropriate opportunities to participate in preparing and serving meals
- Adequate exercise, sleep, and rest to stimulate appetites

The introduction of new foods can create tension between parents and children, with children refusing to try or rejecting new tastes or textures. Parents should be informed that this is a normal reaction for many children. Strategies that can be used to increase the chances of children accepting a new food include the following:

- Offer the food when children are hungry.
- Allow children to taste a little of the food rather than eating a full portion.
- Expose children to the food by preparing and serving the food without expecting them to eat it.
- Provide an example of parents eating and enjoying the food.
- Prepare the food the way children prefer: few spices, lukewarm, recognizable.
- Associate food with pleasant experiences.
- Never force food on children.

Finally, remind parents that individuals do not need to eat all foods. The parent may not eat some foods because of a personal dislike (e.g., anchovies, sushi, or cilantro); children should be afforded the same courtesy if they have been offered the food numerous times and repeatedly demonstrate dislike (some children may refuse a food 15 to 20 times before accepting it). There are many food options for attaining the same nutrients. As children become older, parents can help them master the social skill of politely trying new foods in new situations (e.g., visiting friends or dining in public places).

PHYSICAL ACTIVITY

Physical activity is integrally related to healthy nutrition. It is recommended that children and adolescents engage in 60 minutes of exercise that makes them breathe hard (moderate intensity) most days of the week and preferably daily (USDHHS & USDA, 2005). Increased activity creates a demand for more calories and nutrients; more sedentary behavior means the body needs fewer calories. Low physical activity among children has made a significant contribution to the epidemic of obesity among children in the U.S. (see discussion later in this

chapter). Fig. 11-1 presents an integration of the food guide pyramid with a physical activity pyramid and can be used by providers to proactively counsel children about the importance of being active (Reinhardt & Brevard, 2002).

VEGETARIAN DIETS

An increasing number of individuals are adopting a meat-free lifestyle. Vegetarian diets are nearly as varied as the children who eat them and may be initiated based on religious, ecologic, or health beliefs; economic necessity; or other reasons.

Description

In contrast to omnivores (individuals who eat all forms of food), vegetarians fall into one of the following categories:
- Vegans, or strict vegetarians, eat only foods of plant origin, including fruits, vegetables, grains, nuts, seeds, and legumes (e.g., beans, peas, lentils, tofu, and peanuts).
- Lactovegetarians include milk and dairy products in their diet, in addition to all plant-based foods.

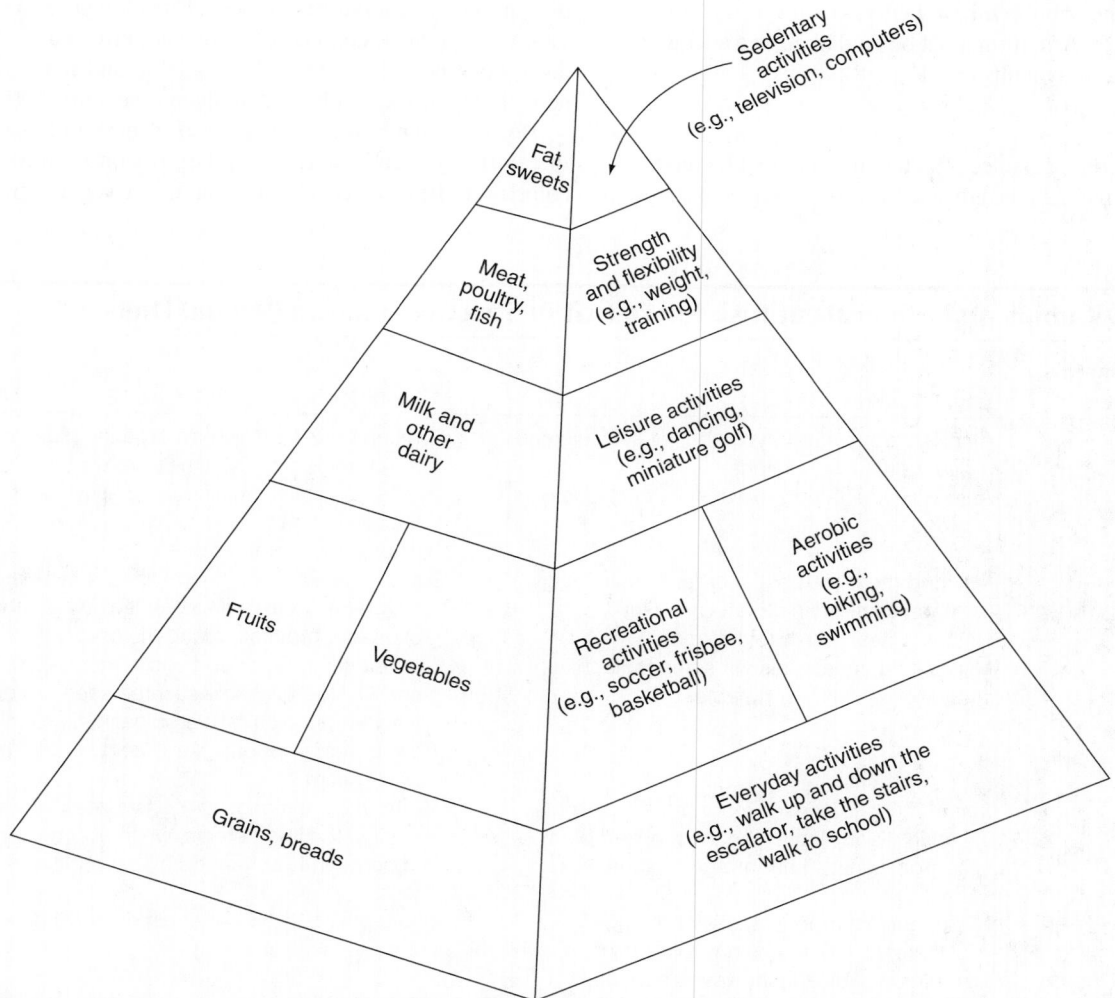

FIG. 11-1   Physical Activity Pyramid. (Data from Reinhardt WC, Brevard PB: Integrating the Food Guide Pyramid and Physical Activity Pyramid for positive dietary and physical activity behaviors in adolescents, *J Am Diet Assoc* 102:596-599, 2002.)

- Lacto-ovovegetarians consume eggs, dairy products, and all plant-based foods in their diet.
- "Sometimes" vegetarians have a diet that consists mostly of plant-based foods, but they occasionally eat fish, chicken, or some seafood.

Vegetarian and vegan diets can meet the nutritional needs of children (American Dietetic Association & Dietitians of Canada, 2003; Mesina et al, 2003). For children who are lacto- or lacto-ovo-vegetarians, or who from time to time eat nonred meat, it is not difficult to achieve adequate nutrients needed for proper growth and development. In fact, the diet of these children is often healthier and more likely to meet the *Healthy People 2010* goals than that of their red meat-eating peers (Perry et al, 2002; American Dietetic Association & Dietitians of Canada, 2003). Both vegetarian and nonvegetarian adolescents who place a high value on personal health tend to have better dietary intake (Greene-Finestone et al, 2005). If they continue to follow a plant-based diet into adulthood, vegetarian children can expect to have a lower incidence of obesity, high blood pressure, heart disease, diabetes, and perhaps cancer. On the other hand, strict vegan diets may be deficient in some nutrients: specifically, protein, Vitamin B_{12}, iron, calcium, zinc, riboflavin, and (if exposure to the sun is limited) Vitamin D. Attention must be paid to ensure adequate intake of essential fatty acids (Table 11-8).

Management

Families and children who select vegetarian diets should be counseled about potential deficits, educated about alternative sources of nutrients that may be lacking in the diet, and assessed regularly to ensure adequate growth and development is occurring. They should also be supported for their healthy dietary decisions.

Nutrition assessment of the child with a vegetarian diet should include regular growth measurements, diet recall and analysis, and laboratory assessment of vitamin B_{12}, zinc, and iron status.

Parents should be counseled that plant sources of protein are considered "incomplete" because they lack the full array of amino acids needed to synthesize new tissue. To ensure adequate intake of essential amino acids, these children need to consume plant-based proteins that "complement" each other and that together provide a complete protein. The daily diet needs to include these complementary proteins, but not necessarily in the same meal. Examples of foods that provide complete proteins include combinations of legumes and grains, nuts, or seeds (e.g., peanut butter on wheat bread, beans and rice, lentils and rice, lentils and sunflower seeds, peas and rye or wheat, or tofu and almonds).

Vitamin B_{12}, in the form of a supplement or in a fortified food (such as fortified soy milk or nutritional yeast), is required for the child who is a vegan because bioavailable vitamin B_{12} is present only in animal-based foods. Use of algae as a source of vitamin B_{12} may be counterproductive because vitamin B_{12} from algae does not appear to be bioavailable and may, in excess, actually block vitamin B_{12} metabolism (Dagnelie, 1997).

Because plant-based diets tend to be high in fiber and low in calories, the child may fill up before consuming sufficient calories and nutrients. Children eating a vegetarian diet are

TABLE 11-8 Vitamins and Minerals at Risk for Deficit in Strict Vegetarian (Vegan) Diets

Vitamin and Minerals at Risk for Deficit	Usual Sources	Alternative Sources in Vegan Diet
Vitamin D	Animal products: egg yolk, butter, liver, salmon, sardines, tuna; sunlight	Fortified cereals, milk, or margarine; sunlight (20-30 mins/day, 2-3 times per week)
Vitamin B_{12}	Animal products only: meat, fish, eggs, dairy products	Fortified soy milk, fortified soy-based meat substitutes, nutritional yeast, fortified cereals, vitamin supplements
Riboflavin	Milk and meat are best sources; also in eggs, dried yeast, grains, dark-green leafy vegetables, avocado, broccoli	Brewer's yeast, wheat germ, beans, almonds, soybeans, tofu, dark-green leafy vegetables, avocado, broccoli, orange juice
Calcium	Milk is best source; also in some fruits, nuts, dark-green leafy vegetables	Fortified soy milk, dried fruits, almonds, sunflower seeds, filberts, whole sesame seeds, green leafy vegetables (avoid spinach, Swiss chard, beet greens, whose oxalic acid hinders calcium absorption)
Iron	Iron in meat sources is more bioavailable than iron in plants; lentils, beans (cooked black, soy, garbanzo, lima) are good sources	All legumes, almonds, pecans, dates, prunes, raisins, fortified cereals, white or brown rice; absorption is enhanced by ascorbic acid–rich foods
Zinc	Meats, animal products, seafood (especially oysters), eggs; found in whole grains, brown rice, nuts, spinach; however, best plant sources also contain phytic acid, which inhibits zinc absorption	Whole grains, brown rice, almonds, wheat germ, tofu, pecans, spinach

advised to eat frequent meals and snacks, concentrating on nutrient-dense foods to achieve adequate energy and nutrient intake.

It is important that providers offer advice and counseling within the context of the child's and family's belief system. But in extreme cases, such as a highly restrictive macrobiotic diet resulting in growth failure or if the child is using vegetarianism as a form of eating disorder, intervention on behalf of the child is necessary, with referral to appropriate health professionals and agencies.

Complications

A high incidence of vitamin B_{12} deficiency and suboptimal zinc status has been noted in children who eat a strict vegan diet, and children are at risk for developmental retardation without these nutrients. If girls who are vegetarian become pregnant, the fetus is also at risk for vitamin B_{12} deficiency, with potentially permanent and severe neurologic damage. A study of more than 3000 Midwestern children also found that adolescents, especially adolescent boys, who were on a vegetarian diet were at risk for eating disorders (Perry et al, 2001).

◼ ALTERED PATTERNS OF NUTRITION

Many children have chronic illnesses, developmental disabilities, developmental special needs, or handicapping conditions that affect their nutritional status. As many as 79% to 90% of developmentally delayed children birth to 3 years old in early intervention programs have been identified as having nutritional risk indicators (American Dietetic Association, 2004b; Ekvall & Ekvall, 2001).

The numbers of children identified with chronic conditions requiring specialized nutrition care are increasing as a result of expanded screening programs, increased survival rates in children with certain chronic disorders, and improved prognosis for the very small (less than 1500 g), underdeveloped neonate. Increased rates of pediatric human immunodeficiency virus (HIV) infection and prenatal exposure to drugs and alcohol also contribute to the population of children with special health care needs. The nutritional management of children with special health care needs requires input from a multidisciplinary team and includes interventions directed at specifically diagnosed feeding problems. Physical, occupational, and speech therapists, particularly speech pathologists, can assess head and trunk control, positioning, body mechanics, and oral-motor skills as they relate to feeding. Depending on the child's symptoms and diagnosis, gastroenterologists, allergists, endocrinologists, and other specialists may need to participate in the child's care; surgical and medical intervention may be necessary. For children who are socially or economically deprived, or both, social workers and psychologists are central to appropriate assessment, counseling, and referral to outside services and agencies. The family should be included as an integral component of the team.

In addition to coordinating the medical management of children with special health care needs, primary care providers must carefully assess the nutritional status of this population and make appropriate referrals. Children who meet the criteria outlined in Box 11-3 should be referred to a registered dietitian for comprehensive nutrition assessment and further referral or treatment.

DISORDERS REQUIRING INCREASED CALORIC INTAKE

Description

A common nutrition problem in children with special health care needs is inadequate weight gain and delayed growth. Inadequate caloric intake should be suspected in any child with a weight-to-age ratio below the 10th percentile on standardized growth and BMI charts. For children who are genetically small or have a disabling condition that limits growth, a weight-to-length ratio or weight-to-height ratio below the 10th percentile indicates suboptimal nutrition.

Epidemiology

The actual incidence of children requiring an increased caloric intake is not known, but it occurs commonly.

BOX 11-3 **Suggested Criteria for Nutrition Referral**

- Markedly overweight or underweight (height or length for weight below the 5th or above the 95th percentile)
- Mechanical feeding difficulties or neuromotor dysfunction
- Feeding skills below those anticipated for developmental level or mental age
- Unusual food habits (e.g., pica or food faddism)
- Inadequate or imbalanced dietary intake, according to dietary history or 24-hour recall
- Nutrition treatment central to medical management (e.g., inborn errors of metabolism, diabetes, malabsorption syndromes, allergy)
- Overt physical signs of nutritional deficiency (e.g., extreme underweight, anemia)
- Emotional disturbances and associated feeding and nutrition problems (e.g., anorexia nervosa, autism)
- At high risk for compromised nutritional status (e.g., takes stimulant or anticonvulsive drugs, family below poverty level, inadequate housing, pregnant adolescent)

Data from Ekvall SW, Ekvall VK, Frazier T: Dealing with nutrition problems of children with developmental disorders, *Topics Clin Nutr* 8(4):51-57, 1993.

Caloric needs of children are influenced by multiple factors, and a number of conditions put children at risk for insufficient caloric intake, including the following:

- Conditions in which activity level is increased, either by purposeful or by involuntary muscle work, such as athetoid cerebral palsy, attention-deficit/hyperactivity disorder, or chronic lung conditions
- A hypermetabolic state (sometimes complicated by secondary malabsorption), which may be present in the child who has acquired immunodeficiency syndrome (AIDS), cancer, burns, fever, or frequent infections, or who has recently had surgery
- Chronic renal insufficiency
- Psychosocial factors, such as inadequate resources, poor feeding relationship with caregiver, and improper dilution of formula, which can lead to delayed growth and require increased calories for the child's catch-up growth
- Oral-motor impairment or chronic conditions, such as congenital heart disease, which can contribute to fatigue and poor feeding
- Low-birth-weight or premature infants
- Medical treatment (e.g., a child receiving corticosteroid treatment for Crohn's disease)
- Conditions in which malabsorption occurs (e.g., cystic fibrosis)

Clinical Assessment and Findings

History.   A thorough history should be taken, assessing for the following:

- Type and amount of foods and liquids consumed (e.g., nutrient content and consistency)
- Amount of food that falls from utensils, cups, or bottles during feeding and is not ingested
- Physical effort and time required for meal
- Any impaired oral functions (e.g., poor suck and swallow, tongue thrust, drooling, difficulty chewing, choking, or aspiration)
- Position of child during feeding
- Family's pattern of feeding child (e.g., time, place, utensils used)
- Child's apparent food likes and dislikes

Physical Examination.   Anthropometric measures are reliable indicators of a child's growth and development, especially if accurately measured and compared over time. Appendix B provides standard growth and BMI charts, in addition to growth charts for premature infants. These charts can be used to determine whether the child is following a consistent growth curve. Growth charts specific to children with Down syndrome, myelomeningocele, Prader-Willi syndrome, sickle cell anemia, and Turner syndrome have also been developed (see Resource Box). Anthropometric measures taken at each visit include the following:

- Height
- Weight
- Weight-to-height ratio
- BMI
- Head circumference
- Arm circumference
- Triceps skinfold measurements

A feeding evaluation can be included in the physical examination, particularly for the child with oral-motor or behavioral problems associated with eating. In this type of assessment, parents or caregivers are asked to replicate the home experience, using the same types of foods, utensils, and positioning. If possible the parents should videotape the child eating at home, and providers should review the video with them. By observing the interaction between the child and the caregiver during feeding, the health care team can more accurately assess feeding success and problems, along with emotional or psychological issues related to feeding.

Diagnostic Tests.   Laboratory studies are done as indicated:

- Hematocrit or hemoglobin
- Serum ferritin and transferrin levels
- Metabolic screening (chemistry screen)

Initial basic work-up for failure to thrive (FTT) (see Chapter 32) includes the following:

- Complete blood count (CBC) with reticulocytes
- Thyroid studies
- Chemistry screen
- Urinalysis, with culture and sensitivity
- Stool for ova and parasites
- Stool culture for enteric pathogens (e.g., *E. coli*)
- Bone age

Clinical Findings.   When a child is malnourished, regardless of cause, the nutritional insult follows a predictable course. In the early stages, the child maintains or begins losing weight. If poor intake continues, the child's linear growth slows or ceases. Finally, head circumference, indicating compromised brain development, levels off.

Other signs of inadequate nutrition include the following:

- Anemia
- Pallor
- Fatigue
- Vulnerability to infections
- Delayed healing
- Behavior problems
- Inactivity
- Irritability
- Poor academic performance, poor vocabulary
- Perceptual difficulties

Management

The management of the child with delayed growth or poor weight gain varies with the underlying cause of the problem and can require the intervention of specialists. Although the primary provider can coordinate the plan of care, a team approach to management is needed.

A child with an increased activity level, a metabolic condition that increases energy requirements, or a condition that decreases the body's ability to absorb nutrients needs to receive caloric- and nutrient-dense meals and snacks frequently, at 2- to 4-hour intervals.

A child with a chronic disease that decreases the appetite (e.g., AIDS, cancer) needs creative approaches that consider food preferences, optimal times of day for snacks and meals, and family dynamics that encourage eating.

A child with a condition that affects oral-motor control will need special equipment, specific feeding techniques, proper positioning, and use of foods and liquids with appropriate consistency to improve oral intake.

A child who is not receiving enough food because of neglect, inadequate financial resources, or other psychosocial factors requires referral to appropriate health care professionals and social services. The community health nurse can be an invaluable resource for these children.

Although feeding by the oral route is preferable from a developmental perspective, tube feedings or parenteral feedings may be indicated. Frequently, a medical crisis precipitates the use of supplemental feedings.

Premature or low-birth-weight infants (particularly those with a poor suck) frequently require supplemental feedings. Breastfeeding is both possible and desirable for these infants and ensuring that they receive higher-fat hindmilk is important; pumping may be necessary (see Chapter 12). Human milk fortifiers or premature formulas that increase the caloric density from 20 kcal/oz to 24 kcal/oz can be used. Regular infant formulas can be mixed to increase the kcal/oz ratio from 20 kcal/oz to 24 kcal/oz or 27 kcal/oz, and nutrient-dense formulas for older infants and children are available (see Box 11-1). Care must be taken that infants do not receive too much protein in concentrated infant formulas because the breakdown and excretion of excess protein by the kidneys may place an excessive demand on the renal system.

Practical suggestions for increasing calories, protein, and nutrients needed for weight gain and growth are outlined in Box 11-4. A "complete" multivitamin and mineral supplement is also recommended because it contains the entire spectrum of these nutrients and can usually be chewed or crushed and mixed into soft foods. For children who are underweight or growth retarded, it is not sufficient to simply increase intake of calories, protein, and nutrients to age-specific norms. These children require an excess of calories and protein for "catch-up" growth until growth is normalized. A method for calculating calories and protein required for catch-up growth is presented in Box 11-5. Calculations for catch-up growth in children with chronic diseases that contribute to poor weight gain (e.g., cystic fibrosis) can be found in more detailed nutrition texts. Additionally, some chronic conditions may require more complex treatment, such as growth hormone therapy. Frequent monitoring of the child with inadequate caloric intake is necessary. Infants should be weighed at least weekly, and length and head circumference measured once a month. Children older than 2 years should be measured for height and weight at least once a month.

Complications

Children with a chronic medical condition that requires increased caloric intake are at risk for frequent illness, medical complications, and impaired development, including growth retardation. In some cases, restoring nutritional status does not ultimately resolve growth deficits. In the case of environmental deprivation, the success of catch-up growth depends on the timing, length, and severity of the nutritional insult.

| BOX 11-4 | **Suggestions for Increasing Energy Intake** |

- Use readily available, economic foods that are familiar to the child.
- Fortify milk by adding 1 cup of nonfat dry milk powder to 1 quart of whole milk. Drink or use to prepare cooked cereals, creamed soups, pancakes, pudding, milkshakes (do not use with children younger than 24 months).
- Add additional margarine or cheese to potatoes, vegetables, casseroles, rice, pasta, cooked cereals, etc.
- Encourage high-calorie snacks, such as fruit juice, dried fruits, nuts, bananas, cheese cubes, pudding or custard, cereal with whole milk, fruit yogurt (alone or as a dip for fruit), cheese or peanut butter on crackers, olives, sliced or mashed avocado (as a dip for vegetables or crackers).
- Add instant breakfast mixes to whole milk.
- Use commercially prepared formula with high caloric content.
- Use commercial liquid supplements, such as PediaSure or PediaSure with fiber (Ross Laboratories) for children with lactose intolerance.
- Establish regular times for meals and snacks, 2 to 4 hours apart. Do not allow the child to nibble continually on small amounts of food.
- Keep mealtimes relaxed and pleasant. Avoid scolding, nagging, or force feeding.
- Allow the infant or child to provide cues regarding hunger and satiety.

Complications of treatment must also be considered for children with caloric deficits. Providers must be alert to negative effects on body systems caused by a sudden change to a high-calorie, high-protein diet. The child on a high-protein diet should be counseled to drink adequate fluids, for example; diarrhea can result from an abrupt increase in carbohydrate intake. Gradually changing the child's diet can decrease these negative effects.

DISORDERS REQUIRING DECREASED CALORIC INTAKE

Description

Health conditions that contribute to decreased metabolic activity in children can require a decrease in caloric intake. If children's caloric intake exceeds their metabolic needs, excessive weight gain, even obesity, can occur, placing the child at risk for additional health problems. The assessment and management of obesity is discussed later in this chapter as an eating disorder. This section looks specifically at medical conditions that contribute to excessive weight gain.

Epidemiology

Any disorder or disability that reduces energy output places the child at risk for overweight. Obesity is common, for example, in children with Prader-Willi syndrome, myelomeningocele,

---

BOX 11-5   **Estimating Catch-Up Growth Requirements**[*]

$$\text{Catch-up growth requirement (kcal/kg/day)} = \frac{\text{Calories required for weight age (kcal/kg/day)} \times \text{Ideal weight for age (kg)}}{\text{Actual weight (kg)}}$$

1. Plot the child's height and weight on the CDC growth charts.
2. Determine at what age the present weight would be at the 50th percentile (weight age).
3. Determine recommended calories for weight age (see Table 11-1).
4. Determine the ideal weight (50th percentile) for the child's present age.
5. Multiply the value obtained in step 3 by the value obtained in step 4.
6. Divide the value obtained in step 5 by actual weight.

Estimated protein requirements during catch-up growth can be calculated similarly (see Table 11-2):

$$\text{Protein requirement} = \frac{\text{Protein required for weight age (g)} \times \text{Ideal weight for age (kg)}}{\text{Actual weight (kg)}}$$

[*]Guidelines are used to estimate catch-up growth requirements. Precise individual needs vary and are mediated by medical status and diagnosis.
Adapted from Rathbun JM, Peterson KE: Nutrition in failure to thrive. In Grand RJ, Sutphen JL, Dietz WH, editors: *Pediatric nutrition*, Boston, 1987, Butterworth.

---

or Down syndrome. Overweight occurs in 50% of children with spina bifida.

The child with Prader-Willi syndrome is hypotonic and may demonstrate dysphagia and FTT as an infant. By 3 to 4 years old, the child becomes hyperphagic, lacking the internal regulation responsible for satiety. In addition to abnormally high food intake, children with Prader-Willi syndrome are short in stature.

Most children with Down syndrome have short stature, and, before they are 3 years old, children with Down syndrome may have a low weight-to-height ratio. The Down syndrome growth chart should be used to evaluate height and weight. As a result of a lower resting metabolic rate or hypothyroidism, the child with Down syndrome requires fewer calories than children without the syndrome, and overweight is common, but not inevitable; its incidence can be decreased with healthy eating and exercise habits begun in early childhood.

Clinical Assessment and Findings

History.   The history should assess the following:
- Level of physical activity in which child engages (see Table 11-1)
- Diet recall (3 days)
- Mealtime patterns
- Concerns and attitudes of parents and child regarding weight gain
- Previous interventions or attempts to control weight
- Risk for overweight and its complications (e.g., diabetes mellitus, limited mobility, family history of obesity)

Physical Examination.   Key components of the physical examination include the following:
- Weight-to-height or weight-to-length ratio. Ratio greater than 75th percentile on growth chart indicates at risk for overweight greater than 95th percentile indicates overweight.
- Triceps skinfold measurement (greater than 85% of norm indicates overweight).

- Midarm circumference.
- Body frame type; central adiposity and waist circumference (used more in adults).
- Muscle mass.
- BMI 85th to 95th percentile indicates at risk for overweight; 95th percentile is overweight. (See discussion of Overweight later in chapter).

A child's growth pattern is evaluated over time. A child who is consistently in the 85% weight-to-height ratio may be genetically programmed to be big, whereas a child who suddenly zooms from the 60% to the 90% weight-to-height ratio can be developing a weight problem.

Diagnostic Tests.   Laboratory studies include those to rule out metabolic conditions that may cause overweight (e.g., thyroxine and TSH to rule out hypothyroidism). Because of complications of obesity (e.g., hyperlipidemia, hypercholesterolemia), children more than 4 years old should be monitored annually for risk factors, and laboratory tests should be done as appropriate, including the following (see Chapter 25):
- Hypertension
- Blood sugar
- Complete lipid profile
- Liver function

Management

The goal of nutritional management of children with medical conditions that reduce energy expenditure is to ensure that the child receives adequate nutrients without excessive caloric intake. Families should be referred to a registered dietitian to establish an appropriate caloric level and eating plan individualized to each child's growth needs. A complete multivitamin with mineral supplement is recommended because a restrictive diet can result in nutrient deficiencies. Whenever possible, these children should be encouraged to increase their energy expenditure through physical activity. Though they may not be able to meet the recommended 60 minutes of moderate to vigorous activity each day, the goal is to both increase calories used and increase the child's level of fitness. A team approach, involving a physical or recreational therapist or both, is advised when developing exercise strategies.

In some cases, access to food needs to be rigidly enforced (e.g., in children with brain dysfunction affecting hypothalamic control or Prader-Willi syndrome). The family, school, and other care environments need to provide limited access to food, which may include locks on refrigerators, cupboards, and garbage cans.

Frequent monitoring is necessary to assess compliance and devise alternate strategies as indicated; weekly weight and monthly height measurements are recommended.

Support for families and children is essential. Despite the best efforts, many children gain excess weight. Primary care providers can model and encourage a positive, accepting attitude toward the child, independent of weight gain or loss (National Association of Pediatric Nurse Practitioners [NAPNAP], 2006).

DISORDERS REQUIRING RESTRICTED OR SUPPLEMENTAL DIETS

Description

The body's ability to absorb and metabolize nutrients is compromised when hormone, enzyme, or cofactor activity necessary for metabolism is either excessive or deficient or when physiologic conditions limit absorption of nutrients. Under these conditions, nutritional intake must be adjusted to maximize the body's ability to use foods. Diet restrictions or supplemental nutrients, or both, can be essential for optimal growth and development.

Table 11-9 lists several metabolic conditions seen in the primary care setting that affect children's nutritional status. A number of defects of absorption or transport affect nutritional status in children. Most are rare, but primary care providers may be part of the team managing the care of a child with inflammatory bowel disease (Crohn's disease or ulcerative colitis), short bowel syndrome, celiac disease, or other conditions falling into this category.

Epidemiology

Most metabolic disorders are rare, although in the U.S., type 1 diabetes mellitus affects about 1.9 in 1000 school-age children, and cystic fibrosis is seen in 1 in 3500 white infants and 1 in 17,000 black infants. Approximately 1 in 14,000 to 20,000 children are born with phenylketonuria (PKU) (Rezvani, 2004).

Metabolic disorders have a number of causes including inborn errors of metabolism, genetic conditions other than inborn errors of metabolism, and autoimmune diseases. Surgical intervention, drugs and medications, tumors, and infectious disease also contribute to metabolic dysfunction and problems of absorption or transport. For some individuals, a genetic

TABLE 11-9 **Metabolic Conditions Affecting Nutrition in Children**

Organ Affected	Excessive Hormone/ Enzyme Production	Deficient Hormone/ Enzyme Production
Pancreas	Reactive hypoglycemia Organic or fasting hypoglycemia	Diabetes mellitus Cystic fibrosis
Thyroid	Hyperthyroidism Graves' disease	Hypothyroidism
Parathyroid	Hyperparathyroidism	Hypoparathyroidism
Adrenal	Cushing syndrome	Addison disease
Cortex	Corticosteroid therapy	Congenital adrenal hyperplasia
Inborn Errors of Metabolism		PKU (deficiency of phenylalanine hydroxylase) Maple syrup urine disease Tyrosinemia Galactosemia

predisposition to the disorder can be triggered by environmental factors, and the disorder appears later in life.

Clinical Assessment and Findings

Clinical findings related to specific disorders are discussed in Unit IV. If nutrition is inadequate in children with these chronic conditions, clinical signs and symptoms worsen, pathophysiologic processes of the disorder accelerate, and growth is compromised.

Management

Disorders of absorption and metabolism are usually managed with specialized diagnostic tests and treatments and require the efforts of a coordinated health care team. Although not a cure for disease, nutrition is an essential component of treatment plans and can make a critical difference in the child's outcome. The goals of nutritional intervention include the following:

- Provide adequate nutrients for normal growth and development.
- Maintain optimal level of health.
- Prevent or delay development of complications associated with disease progression (e.g., diarrhea, fistulas).
- Prevent or delay need for more aggressive intervention (e.g., surgical bowel resection).

Nutritional intervention in chronic disorders can be extremely complex. Referral to a registered dietitian is necessary, and primary providers should consult frequently with the dietitian when providing care to the child.

In some conditions, dietary restrictions are lifelong requirements, and success of dietary intervention depends on the child's and family's willingness to adhere to the plan of care. Cooperation is enhanced if the child and family are actively included in decision-making and if meal plans are developed that minimize disruption to the family's lifestyle and maximize flexibility and normalcy for the child. Families and children must be given ample opportunity to express their concerns and frustrations regarding the child's condition. Support, empathy, and encouragement from providers can be vital elements in determining how well a family copes with the child's chronic condition.

Certain principles of nutrition related to disorders of absorption and metabolism guide the dietitian, primary care provider, and family as they create diet plans. Boxes 11-6 through 11-9 outline these principles for several specific conditions.

Complications

See Unit IV for complications of specific disorders. Additionally, fetuses of women with higher than normal phenylalanine levels are at risk of microcephaly, congenital heart defects, and other birth defects. Approximately 1 in 30,000 women in the general population has a phenylalanine level high enough to damage her fetus or contribute to a spontaneous abortion, but not necessarily high enough to hurt her. All pregnant women should be questioned about a history of PKU or special diets during childhood, and maternal PKU should be considered in any woman who has delivered an infant with microcephaly or has experienced spontaneous abortion.

DISORDERS REQUIRING PHYSICAL ALTERATIONS IN DIET MANAGEMENT

Description

Physical conditions, such as cleft lip or palate, esophageal atresia, cerebral palsy, gastroesophageal reflux, and pyloric stenosis, can create difficulty sucking, chewing, swallowing, or retaining food and liquids in the gastrointestinal tract.

BOX 11-6   Principles for Dietary Management of Diabetes Mellitus

- Individualize diet. There are many types of meal planning systems for diabetics; identify one that works best for child and family. Many current programs rely most upon a liberal diet plan with close insulin coverage.
- Space food intake to account for type of insulin used.
- Structure diet to include foods that everyone else eats; do not be overrestrictive; use insulin coverage to allow child to eat as typical a diet as possible.
- Vary specific nutrient intakes depending on child's age, size, and activity level.

General guidelines for nutrients include the following:

Energy
- Intake is essentially same as for child without diabetes; energy demands vary with growth spurts, exercise.
- Maintain plasma glucose as near normal physiologic range as possible.

Carbohydrates
- Obtain 55% to 60% of total calories from carbohydrates. Complex carbohydrates are recommended; limit simple sugars; small amounts can be acceptable as part of a mixed meal.
- Emphasize consistent intake of carbohydrates from day to day.
- Include 25 to 40 g/1000 kcal/day of fiber; increase fiber as complex carbohydrates are increased.
- Increase carbohydrates 10 to 30 g/hr (depending on level of exertion) for intensive exercise; best effect if intake is several hours preceding exercise.

Protein
- Same as for child without diabetes.

Fat
- Same as for child without diabetes.

Vitamins and Minerals
- Same as for child without diabetes; if diabetes is poorly controlled, supplements are recommended.

Sweeteners
- Noncaloric sweeteners such as aspartame and saccharine are acceptable but not encouraged; no long-term adverse effects of artificial sweeteners have been noted.
- Caloric sweeteners, such as fructose, sucrose, glucose, sorbitol, and mannitol, can be used (with caution) as a substitute for carbohydrate calories.
- Excess sorbitol intake can contribute to diarrhea.

BOX 11-7   Principles for Dietary Management of Cystic Fibrosis

- Nutrients needed (high protein, high fat, high energy) may cause physical distress; work with family to help them understand the balance between comfort and adequate nutrition sought.
- Small, frequent meals, eaten slowly are better tolerated.
- Consume nutrient-dense foods; avoid "empty calories."
- Increase fluid intake to prevent dehydration and help liquefy secretions.
- Assess intake on a 3- to 5-day diet record rather than daily.

General guidelines for nutrients include the following:

Energy
- Energy needs are increased as a result of malabsorption of nutrients, extra effort needed for respirations and frequent pulmonary infections. At least 120% of RDA caloric intake is recommended.
- Vary caloric intake for each child, depending on condition, activity, and growth.

Carbohydrates
- Obtain 40% to 50% of total calories from carbohydrates. Simple sugars may be better tolerated than complex carbohydrates.
- Include extra fiber; increase fiber as complex carbohydrates are increased.

Protein
- Higher need than for children without cystic fibrosis; 15% to 20% of caloric intake should be in proteins.
- Breastfed children may need supplements (e.g., casein hydrolysates).

Fat
- Increase to level of tolerance, minimum of 35% and as much as 40% to 50% of total caloric intake.
- Use medium-chain triglyceride oils to enhance absorption and decrease steatorrhea.
- Use corn or soy oil and include absorbable linoleic acid in diet to ensure essential fatty acid intake.

Vitamins and Minerals
- Daily multivitamin supplement and water-soluble preparation of vitamins A, D, and E are advised; 50 to 100 mcg/day of vitamin K is recommended.
- Daily calcium supplements are necessary.
- Normal diet is usually adequate to replace sodium lost through excessive sweat; can use salt tablets (intake is more easily monitored than adding salt to diet) if exercise or fever leads to profuse sweating.

Supplements
- Pancreatic enzymes are indicated.
- Other supplements include casein hydrolysates and powdered or liquid nutrient-dense preparations.

Epidemiology

Most of these conditions are congenital in nature, and a combination of environmental, hereditary, and behavioral factors appears to influence their development. Stenoses, atresias, or fistulas can also be secondary to environmental trauma, such as a chemical burn. Incidence varies by condition, with approximately 1 in 750 white children born with cleft lip and 1 in 2500 with cleft palate in the U.S. each year. Boys are more likely to have a cleft lip with or without a cleft palate, and Asian children are most likely and black children least likely to have clefts. Pyloric stenosis, occurring in about 3 in 1000 births, is four times more common in boys, especially firstborns; it is more frequent in children with Down syndrome and white children of Northern European heritage. It is rare in Asian children. Esophageal atresia occurs in 1 in about 4000 live births. In more than 90% of cases, it is accompanied by a tracheoesophageal fistula (Orenstein et al, 2004).

Gastroesophageal reflux (GER) is common in normal individuals following a meal and can be exacerbated by increased intraabdominal pressure (as with crying, coughing, defecation, or external pressure from movement or position). GER in infants can occur during, immediately after, or several hours after a feeding. Children with insufficient lower esophageal sphincter tone are especially susceptible to GER. Reflux becomes symptomatic early in life, peaks at about 4 months old, and spontaneously resolves for most children by 12 to 24 months old (Orenstein et al, 2004).

Children with cerebral palsy or other neurodevelopmental problems can have difficulty chewing or maintaining coordinated suck-swallow skills. GER is also a common problem in children with cerebral palsy, and, if the cause for food refusal cannot be determined, GER may be a likely explanation.

BOX 11-8 **Principles for Dietary Management of Phenylketonuria**

- Intervene promptly. Infants who begin treatment before 3 weeks old do not suffer mental retardation secondary to PKU.
- All children require phenylalanine in their diet.
- The goal of PKU dietary therapy is to prevent excess phenylalanine accumulation in the body.
- Recommended daily intake of phenylalanine decreases with age. Dietary restrictions continue for life.
- Most foods contain phenylalanine (approximately 5% of all protein is phenylalanine).
- Involve older children in preparation of nutritional supplements.
- Supplements may be more palatable if served as frozen drinks or flavored with juices or fruits.

General guidelines for nutrients include the following:

Energy, Carbohydrate, Fat, Vitamin, and Mineral
- Requirements are same as for child without PKU. Restrictions on high-phenylalanine carbohydrates.
- Daily multivitamin is recommended.
- Nutrient requirements not met by commercial formulas must be supplemented by a phenylalanine-deficient food.

Protein
- Same protein requirements as for child without PKU.
- Phenylalanine intake is restricted. Dietary intake to maintain serum phenylalanine levels between 2 and 10 mg/dL in children. Plasma phenylalanine levels greater than 6 mg/dL should be controlled with dietary therapy.
- Low or minimal phenylalanine medical foods are necessary to meet protein requirements.

BOX 11-9 **Principles for Dietary Management of Inflammatory Bowel Disease**

- Restrict irritating and poorly absorbed foods (e.g., carbonated beverages, fried foods).
- Decrease intake of foods that stimulate peristalsis (e.g., high-fiber foods) during inflammatory periods. High-fiber foods, especially those that retain water, can be introduced as clinical signs and symptoms decrease.
- Small, frequent meals are better tolerated.
- Vary specific nutrient intakes depending on child's age, size, activity level, and severity of disease. Mild disease can still require supplemental formulas; severe disease can require enteral elemental nutrition via tube feeding, or total parenteral nutrition.
- Condition can be complicated by lactose or gluten intolerance.

General guidelines for nutrients include the following:

Energy
- Teens need 40 to 50 kcal/kg of ideal body weight per day; younger children need up to 120 kcal/kg of ideal body weight per day.

Protein
- Greater than 1.5 g/kg of ideal body weight per day.

Fat
- Low fat (40 g/day) intake is necessary.
- Emulsified fats or medium-chain triglycerides (commercial preparation) are better tolerated.

Vitamins and Minerals
- Take a 100% to 150% daily multivitamin with minerals supplement.
- May need additional vitamin and mineral supplements (e.g., water-soluble vitamins, vitamin B_{12} intramuscularly), folic acid, iron, zinc, copper, calcium, potassium, and magnesium.

Clinical Assessment and Findings

History. A thorough history of the infant's feeding patterns, incidence of gagging or vomiting, arching and crying during feeding, timing of emesis in relation to feeding, character and quantity of emesis, and associated symptoms is essential.

Parents also should be asked about treatments they have tried and whether they have been successful.

Physical Examination. Clinical signs can be present at birth, and a diagnosis of the underlying condition, such as cleft lip or palate, can be made in the delivery room.

Roentgenography and endoscopy are diagnostic techniques used to confirm atresias or fistulas. Some conditions, such as pyloric stenosis, occur later in the neonatal period (see Chapter 32).

Management

The treatment goals related to conditions that require biomechanical or physical intervention include the following:

- Provide adequate nutrients for normal growth and development.
- Provide increased calories to add more weight if needed before surgical procedures.
- Strengthen infant's resistance to infection.
- Prepare infant to tolerate stress of surgical procedures.
- Facilitate healing processes postoperatively.
- Ensure correct development and use of oral-facial and oropharyngeal muscles and structures.
- Minimize disruption of family processes.
- Prevent development of feeding problems.

Some conditions require surgical correction of the underlying condition. In many cases (e.g., a simple cleft lip), initial surgical intervention is sufficient, and the child progresses normally. In others, especially for the child with serious or multiple anomalies, long-term treatment is required. However, the treatment itself can lead to problems that require further management. For example, correction of esophageal atresia, tracheoesophageal fistulas, or presence of a tracheostomy can result in scarring and strictures, which, in turn, put the child at risk for impaired swallowing, choking, and aspiration. See Table 11-10 for strategies related to feeding in children with cleft lip or palate.

GER usually can be managed in the outpatient setting. All babies "spit up," especially when burped or placed in certain positions directly after a feeding. A small regurgitation of undigested formula or breast milk is usually not of concern, but GER puts the infant at risk for esophagitis, pulmonary infection, and FTT. See Table 11-11 for specific suggestions related to managing GER.

Providers must also support parents emotionally and psychologically as they care for their children. Parents of a child with birth anomalies can suffer shock, loss, guilt, anger, or disappointment and may find it difficult to accept their child. Difficult feeding or uncertainty about the child's long-term prognosis adds additional pressure to parents who are already facing an extremely stressful situation. Creating a positive feeding experience can facilitate a healthy parent-infant bond. Providers can intervene in the following ways:

- Encourage parents to express their feelings.
- Listen without judging, acknowledging those feelings.
- Demonstrate techniques that increase feeding success.
- Explain the child's condition, treatments, and prognoses, both short and long term.
- Emphasize how the parent can be involved in the child's progress.
- Encourage parents to make decisions related to their child's care; provide suggestions and guidance as the child grows, as treatment is carried out, and as needs change.

TABLE 11-10 Strategies for Feeding in Children with Cleft Lip or Palate

Age	Problem Presented	Management Strategies
Infants	Poor suction when nursing	Individualize position used to feed infant; semiupright (60–90 degrees) position is often most effective.
	Nasal regurgitation	Breastfeed if possible; experiment with nipple position: position nipple toward side of mouth, do not put nipple into cleft.
		Use of longer, soft, or cross-cut nipples and squeezable bottles assists in infants with weak suck.
		Use of prosthetic device may be helpful.
		Wean child by 12 months old.
		Tube or gavage feedings may be necessary in severe cleft.
	Swallows air	Burp frequently.
	Fatigue	Allow sufficient time for feeding; work toward providing adequate nutrients in 30 minutes.
Toddlers	Risk of aspiration	Encourage use of cup, spoon, finger foods as developmentally appropriate.
	Nasal regurgitation	Avoid small, hard, sticky foods that can lodge in palate opening; supervise feeding.
School-age children and adolescents	Malocclusion	Dental referral and treatment are essential.
	Difficulty coordinating chewing, swallowing, and breathing	Teach child how to chew, swallow, and breathe, not to talk and chew at the same time.
	Aspiration	Cut food into small pieces; child can take sips of water while eating.
		Inform parents that child will chew with mouth open.
	Anorexia secondary to decreased sense of taste and smell	Plan diets that stimulate appetite; provide child's favorite foods.

TABLE 11-11 Strategies for Feeding in Children With Gastroesophageal Reflux

Condition	Management Strategies
Mild	Keep child in slightly upright position (10-15 degrees) after feeding; do not elevate head too much because it will cause scrunched over or slouched position that puts pressure on abdomen. Burp frequently during feeding. Thicken formula with rice cereal if bottle feeding to decrease episodes of vomiting.
Moderate to severe	Position infant on left side or supine after feeding; use folded and rolled blankets to keep child in position. Prone position should be used only if complications of gastroesophageal reflux outweigh risk of sudden infant death syndrome (SIDS) (Rudolph et al, 2001). Consult with pediatric gastroenterologist. Medication may be indicated (see Chapter 32). Surgical referral may be necessary in cases that do not respond to medical management.

Complications

Aspiration with damage to lung tissue, FTT, poor parent-child bond, esophagitis, and esophageal strictures are complications of difficulty in feeding.

EATING DISORDERS

An eating disorder is defined as "a situation where the time spent eating (or not eating) in response to an external stimulus is greater than the time spent eating in response to internal hunger cues" (Hahn, 1998). Anorexia nervosa and bulimia are two eating disorders seen in the pediatric population. The DSM-IV also lists binge eating as a disorder (APA, 1994). Obesity is listed as a general medical condition in the DSM-IV, but is included in the eating disorder discussion here since many people who are obese focus on food and its external cues rather than their body's messages about hunger and satiety, and many factors related to obesity are similar to those of eating disorders. Eating disorders may present in very subtle ways (e.g., persistent, low-level dieting) or be very severe (e.g., adolescent with cachexia). They are associated with serious medical conditions; place children at higher risk of suicide, hospitalization, and mortality; and are related to long-term health problems, such as physical illness (e.g., cardiac complications, osteoporosis, disorders of metabolism), depression, anxiety disorders, and substance abuse.

Anorexia Nervosa and Bulimia

Description. Individuals with *anorexia nervosa* often claim to feel fat even when underweight or emaciated, have an intense fear of becoming obese (the fear does not decrease as weight loss progresses), and actively seek to reduce their weight further. Anorexia nervosa is also characterized by weight loss to a body weight that is 15% less than ideal body weight for age with no known physical illness that would account for such loss and, in girls, absence of at least three consecutive menstrual cycles when they are expected to occur (Litt, 2004).

Bulimia is defined as a pattern of binge eating, followed by attempts to lose weight through excessive exercise, self-induced vomiting, severely restricted diets, fasting, and use of laxatives or diuretics. Bulimia may be present in underweight children, children of normal weight, and children who are overweight or obese.

Epidemiology. Anorexia nervosa occurs most often in adolescent girls (about 1 in 100), although approximately 10% of anorexics are males; a bimodal distribution of the condition is present, with peaks at 14.5 and 18 years old. Initially found only in middle- and upper-class girls in the U.S., anorexia has been diagnosed in all social classes and in other countries. Bulimia peaks in later adolescence, at about 18 to 19 years old, with binge eating occurring approximately 2 years before purging begins (Stice et al, 1998).

A specific cause for these eating disorders is unknown, though a number of etiologic theories are suggested, including psychodynamic, biologic, behavioral, sociocultural, and family systems theories. A relationship between eating disorders and child sexual abuse before puberty is evident, and, though the specific mediating effects are controversial, dissatisfaction with the body following abuse may be a major factor (Carter et al, 2006; Preti et al, 2006). Poor attachment, insecurity, and fear of abandonment have been identified as contributing to eating disorders in some young women (Ramacciotti et al, 2001). Bulimia appears to have a significant element of learned behavior, acquired through modeling among peers (Stice et al, 1998), and negative affect may lead to purging (Tyrka et al, 2002). Eating disorders may stem from dieting to control overweight (Haines et al, 2006; Neumark-Sztainer et al, 2006).

Clinical Assessment and Findings. Diagnosing anorexia or bulimia can be difficult. Some clinical findings characteristic of these eating disorders are also seen in the healthy adolescent. For example, it is not uncommon for a 14-year-old girl who is neither anorexic nor bulimic to express concern about her body appearance, stating that she is too fat or ugly. Additionally, adolescents with anorexia or bulimia and their families commonly work hard to hide their condition and actions, deny problems, or present a mature, self-sufficient, and successful facade. Early in the disease process, the family system may appear to be coherent, making it difficult to collect accurate data about family relations and behavior patterns that contribute to eating disorders.

Assessment using the Eating Disorder Screen for Primary Care (ESP) or the SCOFF questionnaire has been found to be highly reliable in the primary care clinical setting (Box 11-10). The Eating Disorder Diagnostic Scale (EDDS), a 22-item self-report questionnaire based on DSM-IV criteria, is also a reliable means to identify anorexia, bulimia, and binge eating (Stice et al, 2000; Stice et al, 2004).

Clinical Assessment and Findings—Anorexia Nervosa

History. The history should assess for the following:
- FTT as a child
- Amenorrhea
- Dizziness, syncope
- Expresses pleasure with weight loss
- Denies hunger
- States, "I feel fat," even though not overweight
- Preoccupied with food; often fixes elaborate meals but does not eat; has rituals associated with food
- Attempts to lose weight through diets, exercise, or self-induced vomiting
- Hides eating habits, lies about intake
- Engages in self-harmful thoughts and behaviors (e.g., cutting) that are not related to suicide ideation
- Displays social isolation and mood changes: irritable, sullen, hostile, introverted, unhappy, intolerant of others, can have suicidal ideation
- Has fixed, highly structured schedule, inflexible to change

Physical Examination. The physical examination may reveal the following:
- Growth parameters: decreased height-to-weight ratio; weight 25% below ideal for age and height
- Abdomen: pain and distention, decreased bowel sounds
- Skin: dry, rough, cracked, yellowish or grayish color; mucous membranes dry, dull; edema
- Hair: thin, brittle, dull, can have alopecia, bristle hairs on scalp, lanugo on body
- Muscles: weak, decreased definition and mass
- Sensory: lack of concentration, drowsy, confused, irritable, apathetic
- Vital signs: decreased temperature, pulse, respirations, blood pressure for age and weight

Diagnostic Tests. Laboratory studies are done as indicated:
- Hematocrit, hemoglobin, transferrin (decreased amounts)
- Serum glucose, albumin, electrolytes (decreased); may have hypernatremia
- Liver enzymes (elevated liver function)
- Thyroid function (low thyroxine)
- Creatine phosphokinase (elevated)
- Electrocardiogram (ECG) (abnormalities)

Clinical Assessment and Findings—Bulimia

History. The history may include:
- Excessive concern about weight
- Weight fluctuation
- Pattern of strict dieting followed by eating binges
- Plans for binge eating
- Frequent overeating, often used as a coping mechanism to manage stress
- Guilt expressed about eating
- Self-induced vomiting after bingeing; hematemesis
- Excessive exercise after bingeing
- Pattern of hiding information about bingeing and purging

BOX 11-10 Screening Questions for Eating Disorders

SCOFF questions*
[†]Do you make yourself **Sick** because you feel uncomfortably full?
[†]Do you worry you have lost **Control** over how much you eat?
Have you recently lost more than **One** stone (14 lb or 7.7 kg) in a 3-month period?
Do you believe yourself to be **Fat** when others say you are too thin?
Would you say that **Food** dominates your life?

Eating Disorder Screen for Primary Care (ESP) questions
[‡]Are you satisfied with your eating patterns? (No = abnormal answer)
[†]Do you ever eat in secret? (Yes = abnormal answer)
[‡]Does your weight affect the way you feel about yourself?
[§]Have any members of your family suffered with an eating disorder?
[†]Do you currently suffer with or have you ever suffered in the past with an eating disorder?

*One point for every "yes"; a score of 2 indicates a likely case of anorexia nervosa or bulimia.
[†]Best questions for ruling in an eating disorder. Cotton and colleagues (2003) recommend using these four questions as a basic screening tool; needs to be tested further on large-scale population for validation.
[‡]Best questions for ruling out an eating disorder.
[§]Question was not helpful in distinguishing eating disorders; recommend deleting from screening tool.
SCOFF questions from Luck AJ et al: The SCOFF questionnaire and clinical interview for eating disorders in general practice: comparative study, *BMJ* 325:755-756, 2002. ESP questions from Cotton MA, Ball C, Robinson P: Four simple questions can help screen for eating disorders, *J Gen Intern Med* 18:53-56, 2003.

- Complaints of frequent diarrhea or constipation
- Gregarious behavior but evidence of mood swings, especially depression
- High anxiety
- Isolation
- "Black and white" thinking
- Other destructive behaviors: shoplifting, substance abuse, self-harm
- Family history of chaos, abuse, sexual abuse

Physical Examination. The physical examination may indicate:
- Usually normal weight, can range from obese to severely underweight
- Tooth decay, lost enamel, especially on the lingual surfaces
- Enlarged parotid glands
- Skin: dry, rough, cracked, sores on mucous membranes of mouth and around fingernails, broken blood vessels in face; edema
- Weakness, fatigue
- Cardiac arrhythmias
- Decreased blood pressure for age or weight

Diagnostic Tests. Laboratory studies are done as for anorexia nervosa.

Differential Diagnosis (Anorexia and Bulimia). The differential diagnoses for anorexia and bulimia include:
- Diabetes
- Hyperthyroidism
- Inflammatory bowel disease
- Malignancy, central nervous system neoplasm
- AIDS
- Pregnancy
- Systemic lupus erythematosus
- Depression
- Substance abuse

Management. Management of children and adolescents with anorexia nervosa or bulimia is difficult, in part because the child, family, and even the health care provider often deny the significance of the problem. Even though early detection and treatment is helpful in reducing physical complications, diagnosis can be delayed and treatment may be inadequate. Because the issue is not food, but rather sociopsychological dynamics of control in the child's life, effective treatment is complex and long term (American Dietetic Association, 2006). Treatment must include both psychological and physiologic interventions, and referral to psychiatric therapists and medical specialists is essential. The multidisciplinary team approach is most effective (Joy et al, 2003). It is important to remember that eating disorders are a psychological problem that results in physical complications, not the other way around. Patients do not choose to suffer with this disorder and should not be subject to blame. Supportive, engaging relationships in which the provider gives the message that the child is unconditionally accepted will help the child respond to treatments with less resistance. Establishing trust and understanding is key to successful treatment.

Specific treatment modalities vary, depending on the age of the child, the severity of the condition, and causal factors and can include the following:

- Hospitalization to stabilize fluids, electrolytes, and nutrient intake
- Medications and supplementation
- Antidepressants and anxiolytics (e.g., fluoxetine)
- Estrogen and progesterone
- Minerals (potassium, calcium, phosphate, zinc, magnesium, iron)
- Folate
- Individual psychotherapy
- Group psychotherapy
- Family therapy (essential component)
- Nutritional counseling
- Assertiveness training
- Body work: relaxation, biofeedback, movement therapy

Prevention of eating disorders may be possible. An experimental 8-week, Internet-based cognitive behavioral intervention (Student Bodies) for college-aged women significantly prevented eating disorders among women who began the study with higher BMIs (Taylor et al, 2006).

Complications. The complications of anorexia nervosa or bulimia include:
- Death, usually secondary to cardiac arrhythmia, hypokalemia, congestive heart failure, or suicide
- Altered metabolism (chronic)
- Alcohol and drug addictions
- Osteoporosis
- Gastrointestinal disturbance: ulcers, motility disorders
- Fertility problems
- Gynecologic problems related to prolonged amenorrhea
- Growth retardation
- Dehydration

Overweight

Description. Excessive adipose tissue is the hallmark of obesity, often referred to as *overweight* in children, and may be due to an increase either in the size of fat cells (hypertrophy) or in the number of fat cells (hyperplasia). Childhood-onset overweight that is hyperplastic in nature is especially difficult to control because fat cells can be reduced in size but not in number. Ideal body weight-to-height ratio and BMI are used to define parameters of overweight. Ideal body weight is calculated based on the Centers for Disease Control and Prevention (CDC) growth charts (Table 11-12).

In adults, normal BMI ranges from 18.5 to 24.9, and an individual is defined as obese if BMI is 30 or greater. In children the definition of obesity and overweight varies. The CDC states that for children older than 2 years, those with a BMI at or higher than the 95th percentile for age and gender are considered overweight; if the BMI is at the 85th percentile, the child is at risk for overweight (CDC, 2007). The Expert Committee on the Assessment, Prevention, and Treatment of Child and Adolescent Overweight and Obesity (2007) recommends that children 2 to 18 years old with a BMI at above the 95th percentile for age and sex, or those with a BMI at or above 30 (whichever is smaller) be considered obese. Children with a BMI between the 85th and 95th percentile for age and sex are overweight. BMI measurements must be used cautiously to

TABLE 11-12 **Calculation of Ideal Body Weight from Centers for Disease Control and Prevention Growth Charts***

% Ideal Body Weight for Healthy Children	Interpretation
>120%	Overweight
90%-110%	Normal
80%-90%	Mildly underweight
70%-79%	Moderately underweight
<70%	Severely underweight

*% Ideal body weight = Current weight divided by weight at 50th percentile for current stature multiplied by 100.
From Centers for Disease Control and Prevention: *Growth charts*. Available at *www.cdc.gov/growthcharts* (accessed Mar 25, 2007).

assess individual children (see Appendix B). Some children are genetically large boned and have a body weight or BMI in excess of the norm for their age, gender, and height without having excess fat; athletic adolescents may have a higher BMI as a result of heavier muscle mass with little body fat.

Epidemiology. Studies indicate a decline in dietary fat intake since 1990, but rates of childhood overweight have increased dramatically, and overweight and obesity are becoming more common in infants and toddlers. Although findings vary from study to study, as many as 20% to 30% of U.S. children are overweight. Seventeen percent to 19% of children and adolescents between 6 and 19 years old were overweight in 2003 to 2004 (National Center for Health Statistics, 2006). NHANES data indicate that 24% of a sample of preschool children were overweight or at risk for overweight, and 10.7% were overweight (O'Connor et al, 2006). Chapter 1 discusses overweight in children as the "new morbidity" and presents additional statistics to illustrate the scope of this problem.

The cause of overweight among children is a topic of much controversy. It is safe to say that obesity results from a complex relationship of genetics, environment (e.g., exercise, caloric intake, dietary patterns), and the body's response to environmental factors (e.g., neurohormonal regulation). A number of factors clearly put children at risk for being overweight, including having obese parents, maternal smoking during pregnancy, bottle feeding, maternal control of feeding (either restricting or urging intake), middle and low socioeconomic status, binge eating in response to overvaluation of body image, social pressure to be thin, depression, use of food as a mechanism to cope with stress, and low self-esteem (Dubois & Girard, 2006; Bergmann et al, 2003; Stice et al, 2002; Farrow & Blissett, 2006; Spruijt-Metz et al, 2006).

Overweight in late childhood and early adolescence is related to overweight in young children and infants. Rapid weight gain in infants from birth to 5 or 6 months old appears to be a strong predictor of overweight in preschoolers (Dennison et al, 2006). Analysis of longitudinal data from more than 1000 U.S. children found that toddlers and preschoolers with BMIs more than 50% were more likely to be overweight at 12 years old; those with BMIs greater than 85% were five times as likely to be overweight at 12 years old; and a child who was ever overweight during early childhood was at higher risk for continued overweight

or obesity into adolescence (Nader et al, 2006). Based on this evidence, prevention of overweight from birth or early intervention for children at risk for overweight is essential.

Biologic factors may affect one's susceptibility to obesity. Resistance to insulin and to leptin, two hormones that normally serve to control satiety, may contribute to the body's failure to register satiety and to subsequent overeating in children (Sinha et al, 2002; Caro et al, 1996). Lustig (2006) posits that the biologic factors occurring in obesity may actually be "a pathological process of excess energy storage," and that "obesity is the same process in the CNS as starvation." His thinking, based on an extensive review of research literature, is thus:

- In the nonobese, healthy individual the following process normally takes place:
  - Leptin is produced by adipose tissue; when there are adequate stores of energy (i.e., fat tissue), leptin production is high. and the message to increase energy expenditure is sent to the ventromedial hypothalamus (VMH).
  - The VMH signals the sympathetic nervous system (SNS) to increase energy expenditure.
  - The SNS responds by reducing appetite (mediated through innervation of the hypothalamus and appetite centers in the medulla); increasing TSH secretion; innervating skeletal muscles (more ATP is produced, which leads to increased muscle contractility, and protein activity in the mitochondria increases heat loss from cells); and innervating receptors in white adipose tissue to increase lipolysis (use energy stores).
  - The VMH also signals the vagal nerve to reduce activity; as a result of decreased vagal activity, heart rate increases, peristalsis and absorption of energy substrates in the intestine decreases, insulin secretion decreases, and insulin sensitivity in adipose tissue decreases. As a result, energy expenditure increases and fat stores decrease or remain steady.
  - Therefore if the body is leptin replete and caloric intake is not excessive, an energy-storage balance is achieved.
  - With leptin depletion, as occurs when fat stores decrease (i.e., starvation), the body seeks to conserve energy by decreasing SNS activity and using calories more efficiently. Physical activity decreases, the individual becomes more lethargic, and energy consumption per kilogram of fat-free mass decreases.

- In obesity, the individual has become resistant to leptin, so the normal processes of stimulating the SNS and vagal nerve do not occur, even though there is a high level of leptin in the blood. Instead the body believes itself to be in a perpetual state of starvation, spontaneous activity decreases, and calories are used more sparingly. The result is further storage of energy in the form of adipose tissue, so the obese individual will become fatter, even if an effort is made to reduce caloric intake.
- Chronic hyperinsulinemia may be the source of this leptin resistance. Insulin and leptin share the same "signaling cascade" in the VMH; therefore if insulin levels are high, leptin is prevented from signaling its message that the body has adequate energy stores.
- Hyperinsulinemia in children has three sources: genetics, epigenetics (small- and large-for-gestational-age infants experience hyperinsulinemia and insulin resistance), and environment.
- Environmental dynamics contributing to hyperinsulinemia are threefold:
  ○ Increased stress leads to increased cortisol production, which can lead to insulin resistance.
  ○ Decreased physical activity contributes to insulin resistance.
  ○ Diet, especially high levels of fructose and decreased fiber, leads to excess insulin secretion.

Therefore, Lustig asserts, "hyperinsulinemia turns the leptin negative feedback system into a 'vicious cycle' of obesity...Externally, this appears as 'gluttony and sloth,' but it is biochemically driven" (Lustig, 2006, p. 906). Restoring the body's leptin feedback system to its normal function is key to increasing energy expenditure and reducing weight. This can be done through forced weight loss (Rosenbaum et al, 2002) and by decreasing insulin production (through diet change and increased exercise).

Unfortunately, American children are participating less in physical activity and more in sedentary behavior. A National Institute of Child Health and Human Development study found that one group of third-grade children participated in less than 25 minutes per week of moderate physical activity during physical education classes (Nader, 2003). The Youth Risk Behavior Surveillance for the U.S. in 2005 found that only 35.8% of high school students participated in the recommended amount of exercise (60 minutes of exercise that made them breathe hard for at least 5 of the last 7 days). More than 68% reported that they had participated in vigorous physical activity for at least 20 minutes on more than 3 of the previous 7 days and/or moderate activity for at least 30 minutes on 5 of the previous 7 days. Nearly 10% of adolescents stated they did no physical activity at all in the 7 days before the study (CDC, 2006). Children with chronic conditions that limit physical activity are especially susceptible to excessive weight gain.

Watching television, playing computer games, and talking on the telephone are all examples of sedentary behaviors in which children engage. Despite the fact that the American Academy of Pediatrics recommends no television for children under 2 years old, a recent study indicates about 63% of 0-to-2-year-olds, 82% of 3- to 4-year-olds, and 78% of 5- to 6-year-olds watch television each day (Vandewater et al, 2007). Older children watch even more television and are more likely to be overweight and eat fewer fruits and vegetables than recommended (Sanchez et al, 2007). Besides replacing active play, watching television exposes children to snack-food advertising and increases the likelihood that children will eat more low-nutrient-dense foods and clearly predicts overweight in children (Gable et al, 2007). This pattern of overweight and poor nutritional intake related to watching television is international in scope (Vereecken et al, 2006).

The contribution that genetics versus environment makes in the overweight or obese child is not entirely clear, and further research is recommended in this area (Kral & Faith, 2007). Just as parents pass on genetic traits, they also influence lifestyle habits and set patterns associated with eating and activity. Some racial and ethnic groups are at risk for excess insulin production and insulin resistance and are predisposed to obesity (Preeyasombat et al, 2005), and recent research in mice suggests that prenatal exposure to endocrine disruptors, such as bisphenol-A, may predispose to overweight and obesity (Sakurai et al, 2004).

Psychosocial factors also contribute to the increased incidence of obesity, particularly in regard to family dysfunction. Children who suffer neglect or abuse or have an overcontrolling parent may turn to food for comfort and solace, with overeating as a result.

Clinical Assessment and Findings

History. Assessment must consider underlying factors and comorbid conditions, such as hypothyroidism, polycystic ovary disease, depression, diabetes, and cardiovascular disorders, in addition to examining patterns of eating and exercise for both the child and the family system. The history should include the following:

- Dietary intake
- Total caloric intake
- Fat intake as percentage of total calories
- Carbohydrate intake as percentage of total calories
- Nutrient adequacy of diet
- Eating patterns, including breakfast, eating outside home, portion sizes, frequency and quality of meals
- Exercise pattern
- Parental obesity
- Time of onset of excessive weight gain
- Family history of diabetes and cardiovascular disease (hypertension, congenital heart disease [CHD])
- Family or child history of hypothyroidism or other medical conditions that could contribute to overweight
- Episodes of sleep apnea
- Social adjustment, peer group, friends
- Family and child readiness to participate in a weight management treatment program based on healthy eating and activity
- Barriers to exercise and healthy eating

Physical Examination. A complete physical examination is necessary to determine the child's level of fitness and anthropomorphic status, looking especially at the following:

- Blood pressure (measured with cuff that covers 80% of arm [Expert Committee, 2007])
- Vital signs
- Height and weight (height-to-weight ratio is a better indicator than BMI of overweight in infants and children under 2 years old)
- Ideal body weight (see Table 11-12)
- BMI
- Triceps skinfold (not recommended in routine assessment by Expert Committee [2007])
- Midarm circumference
- Skin (for acanthosis nigricans)

Diagnostic Tests
- Fasting lipid screen
- Fasting glucose tolerance test
- Thyroid screen, thyroid-stimulating hormone, T_4
- Metabolic panel

Differential Diagnosis. The differential diagnosis includes medical conditions such as hypothyroidism, polycystic ovary disease, Down syndrome and Prader-Willi syndrome that are related to obesity in children.

Management. The primary goal of weight management for most children is to normalize, not necessarily reduce weight. Because children are growing and developing, recommendations for treating risk for overweight focus on slowing the rate of weight gain, thereby allowing children to grow into their weight. Restricting fat intake for infants is not recommended because of the rapid neurologic development occurring at this age. If the child is beyond a weight into which he or she will reasonably "grow," weight reduction is the treatment goal.

If a child's body is able to signal to the brain that it has reached satiety before the child overeats, and if the child responds to the body's cues of satiety, caloric intake will decrease. Recent research indicates that young infants are highly sensitive to satiety and stop eating when full; but it appears that this natural regulator can be overridden by overfeeding the infant or providing high-caloric foods that are quickly absorbed as glucose (e.g., juice or juice drinks) (Lustig, 2006). In essence, the child no longer knows when he or she is full—when the body has received enough calories. As mentioned previously, infants who experience rapid weight gain in the first 5 months of life are at higher risk for overweight and obesity as toddlers and preschoolers and ultimately for their entire life. Breastfed infants tend to gain weight more slowly than formula-fed infants, and breastfeeding should be encouraged as a way to prevent possible overweight.

Children must be monitored for height and weight on a regular basis, but progress should be measured by other parameters as well. Improved dietary habits; increased physical activity, fitness, and strength; and enhanced self-esteem are significant end points that should be acknowledged and praised by the family and health care team alike.

Motivational interviewing as described in Chapter 9 may be a helpful strategy when working with adolescents and parents of overweight children. Guidelines developed as part of the National Association of Pediatric Nurse Practitioner (NAPNAP) Healthy Eating and Activity Together (HEAT) Initiative (2006) are consistent with recommendations for developing healthy eating habits (see previous discussion in this chapter) and include:

- Educate parents about:
  - Children's growth patterns and nutritional needs
  - Ways children communicate hunger and satiety
  - Strategies for developing healthy eating habits
  - Strategies to encourage physical activity in children
  - Risk factors for overweight
  - Early indicators of overweight
- Implement behavioral change interventions including:
  - Early intervention (in infancy if necessary)
  - Family-centered treatment, with counseling regarding communication and eating habits
  - Increased activity
  - Decreased intake of high-fat and high-calorie foods
  - Appropriate portion sizes
- Provide ongoing support to families

In addition, depending on the child's age, baseline BMI, presence of medical complications, and weight status of parents, treatment can include either weight-loss or weight-maintenance strategies that focus on the following:

- Modify diet to increase fruits and vegetables to five or more per day and eliminate sugared drinks
- Decrease "screen time" to less than 2 hours per day with no television in child's bedroom
- Exercise 1 hour or more per day
- Eat a daily breakfast
- Decrease meals eaten outside home
- Have a family meal at least five to six times a week
- Allow child to self-regulate meals; avoid being overly restrictive

The Expert Committee on the Assessment, Prevention, and Treatment of Child and Adolescent Overweight and Obesity (2007) recommends these strategies in a staged management approach with active monitoring by the primary care provider and involvement of the entire family. If initial efforts are unsuccessful, more rigorous management that may include behavior modification, highly structured monitoring and control, multidisciplinary interventions, medication, or surgery is recommended.

Overeating, overweight, and obesity are complex phenomena involving social cues and expectations and physiologic dynamics, and their management requires that both the child and family change lifestyle patterns. When the entire family changes to a more healthful diet and engages in regular physical activity, the overweight child has a much greater chance to normalize weight. Box 11-11 provides useful approaches and suggestions to use when counseling obese children and their families.

Several medications are used to control weight in adults and adolescents, including sibutramine (increases sensitivity to insulin), orlistat (decreases fat absorption), and phentermine (a stimulant that suppresses appetite). Other appetite suppressants include rimonabant and metformin; the latter does not have FDA approval for use in treatment of obesity, but has

---

BOX 11-11 **Guidelines for Managing Childhood Weight Problems**

- Do not put child on a diet. Instead gradually modify the entire family's eating habits. For example, serve fruit as a substitute for dessert, switch to nonfat or 1% milk, experiment with low-fat recipes and methods of food preparation, and use reduced-fat margarine, salad dressings, and other low-fat condiments. Serve nutritionally dense foods that reflect recommendations of MyPyramid, including whole grains, fruits, vegetables, lean protein foods, and low-fat dairy products.
- Do not force children to clean their plates. They should eat only until they are full.
- Schedule and enforce regular times for meals and snacks. Do not skip meals. Do not allow children to nibble throughout the day.
- Have low-calorie, nutritious snacks readily available, such as air-popped popcorn, pretzels, low-fat yogurt, frozen fruit juice bars, skim milk, low-sugar cereals, fresh fruit, and raw vegetables.
- Do not have high-calorie snacks readily available (e.g., potato chips, cookies, cakes, pies, ice cream, candy, soda pop, and doughnuts).
- Promote physical activity. Start slowly, with low-weight–bearing exercise. Set reasonable goals and celebrate achieving them. Make daily exercise a priority. Encourage family participation, individual exercise, and team sports and structured activities with peers as appropriate.
- Limit television viewing. Children who watch 4 or more hours of television per day are twice as likely as other children to become obese. Children are more sedentary when they watch television, and frequent food advertising has been linked to increased snacking.
- Scale back television watching slowly, replacing time with activities, hobbies, or chores.
- Praise and reward children for the progress they make in reaching nutrition, activity, physical fitness, self-esteem, or weight goals.
- Emphasize the uniqueness of each child, pointing out special talents, abilities, and positive qualities.
- Do not overly restrict children's diets or demand children eat when they are not hungry. This approach actually leads to overeating and subsequent overweight.

---

been used off label (Kay et al, 2001). All these medications have potential side effects and should be considered only when other treatments, especially lifestyle changes, have been ineffective (Padwal & Majumdar, 2007). The use of bariatric surgery for morbidly obese adolescents is increasing, and some believe that having surgery during adolescence (rather than waiting until adulthood) may be more beneficial for individuals with childhood-onset obesity (Inge et al, 2007).

Complications. Children who are overweight are at much higher risk for related conditions, including hypertension, impaired glucose tolerance, sleep apnea, orthopedic problems (e.g., slipped capital femoral epiphysis), social rejection, lowered self-esteem, depression, and suicide. In the child with a physical disability, overweight can further impair mobility and reduce energy expenditure.

ADVERSE FOOD REACTIONS

Description

A distinction is made between *food allergy*, a hypersensitivity to a food or food additive with either an immediate or a delayed immune system response (e.g., anaphylactic reaction to ingestion of nuts), and *food intolerance*, a nonimmunologic inability to process or tolerate the food product (e.g., enzyme deficiencies [lactase] or PKU secondary to the body's inability to metabolize phenylalanine) (Fig. 11-2). Food can also be toxic (e.g., food poisoning or toxins from bacteria growing in the food) or create pharmacologic effects (e.g., headaches after eating ice cream). All are considered adverse reactions to food; this section discusses food allergy and intolerance.

Epidemiology

Many individuals believe they have a food allergy or intolerance, with up to 20% changing their diets because of this belief.

Actually, far fewer people have true food allergies. Research reported in 1998 indicated that only 1% to 2% of individuals met the criteria of having "either a positive double-blind, placebo-controlled food challenge or an unequivocal report of a reaction with the typical features of an immunoglobulin E (IgE)-mediated severe allergic or anaphylactic reaction" (Hourihane, 1998). Current research shows that about 3% to 4% of adults and about 6% of children have an immune-induced allergic reaction to food (Sicherer & Sampson, 2006). For children with atopic disease, however, the incidence of food allergies can be as high as 35% (Sampson, 2004). Only a few foods—cow's milk, hen's eggs, peanuts, soya, wheat, fish, Crustacea, and tree nuts (including almonds and cashews)—account for nearly 90% of actual IgE-mediated allergic reactions. Any food, however, can cause reactions in a specific individual, and food is the most common cause of anaphylaxis in children (Clark & Ewan, 2003). Factors contributing to adverse food reactions include the following:

- *Heredity.* A child with one parent with a food allergy has a 30% to 35% chance of developing the condition; if both parents have food allergies, the child's chances increase to 65%. Children born with a metabolic disorder (e.g., deficient lactase enzyme) can have adverse reactions to specific foods.
- *Immature gastrointestinal tract.* Before 7 months old, the infant gastrointestinal tract is more permeable to large molecules, including most food proteins. Allergies to milk and eggs are more common in younger infants and are often "outgrown" with age.
- *Compromised gastrointestinal tract.* As a result of injury or illness, the gastrointestinal system can be more permeable to allergens, such as large proteins.
- *Type of food.* Some foods are more allergenic than others, and some individuals have greater sensitivity to certain

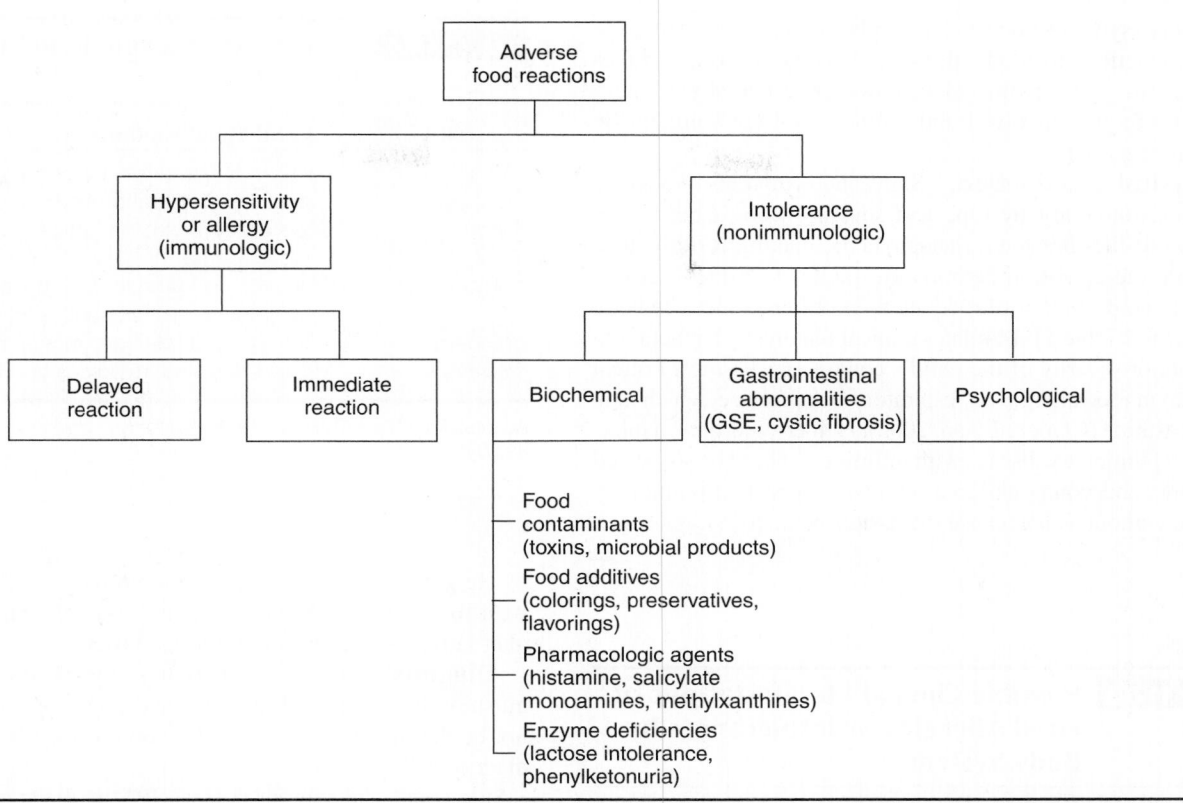

FIG. 11-2 Adverse food reactions. (From Davis J, Sherer K: *Applied nutrition and diet therapy for nurses*, Philadelphia, 1994, WB Saunders.)

foods. Commercial baby foods that may appear to be only one fruit or vegetable can have eggs or milk added, sometimes under an unfamiliar name.

- *Allergic load or tolerance level.* Conditions, such as illness, stress, surgery, or trauma, can place excessive metabolic demands on the body. An individual who is susceptible to food intolerance or allergy can have a reaction when these conditions are present. Additionally, individuals may be allergic to more than one food.

Clinical Assessment and Findings

The goals of clinical assessment are to determine whether an allergic reaction has occurred, whether it is related to food, to which food is it related, and how serious is the problem. This process is extremely challenging and can require referral to a registered dietitian or use of a team approach with primary provider, dietitian, and allergist for a more in-depth diagnostic work-up. The basic examination includes the history, physical examination, laboratory studies, and food elimination and challenge.

History. The history should assess the following:

- Age of child
- Suspected food
- Route of exposure: Ingested? Skin touched? Food dust inhaled?
- Amount of exposure

- Onset of symptoms relative to exposure
- Description of symptoms (look, too, for change over the course of the reaction)
- Description of other factors that are present and may contribute to or aggravate an allergic response (e.g., stress, environment, exercise)
- Treatment given and child's response
- Does child have previous history of symptoms following exposure to this food?
- What is the child's diet history? When and what types of foods were introduced into the diet?
- Does the child have a history of symptoms frequently seen in food allergies (e.g., respiratory distress, eczema, urticaria, rashes, colic, vomiting, diarrhea), unaccompanied by other signs of illness or history of exposure to infectious agents?
- Is there a family history of allergies, especially a history of reaction to certain foods?

Describe the child's usual intake. A food diary is an excellent mechanism for obtaining these data and includes the following:

- All foods and fluids ingested for at least 3 days
- How food is prepared (e.g., commercially, at home, fried, baked)
- How food is stored and fed to the child
- All medications

A food-symptom diary can also be maintained, listing the child's reactions to foods ingested. This can become a time-consuming, cumbersome task, however, especially if more than one food is involved and requires real commitment on the part of parents.

Physical Examination. Signs and symptoms of adverse food reactions vary by type and severity, from a mild local reaction to life-threatening anaphylaxis, making it difficult to diagnose the condition definitively. Table 11-13 lists possible clinical manifestations of food allergies or intolerances by body system, and Table 11-14 relates clinical features of a reaction to the level of severity of the child's condition. The most critical problem in food allergies is respiratory compromise, which may mimic asthma (Clark & Ewan, 2003). Heiner syndrome, a milk-induced pulmonary disease with infiltrates, should be suspected in infants and young children who have persistent pulmonary disease without a clear cause (Moissidis et al, 2005).

TABLE 11-14 **Severity of Allergic Reactions to Foods**

Severity	Clinical Manifestations
Mild	Localized cutaneous erythema, urticaria, angioedema, oral pruritus
Mild	Generalized erythema, urticaria, angioedema
Mild	At least 1 or 2 (above) plus gastrointestinal symptoms, rhinoconjunctivitis
Moderate	Mild laryngeal edema/mild asthma
Severe	Marked dyspnea; hypotension

Adapted from Clark AT, Ewan PW: Food allergy in childhood, *Arch Dis Child* 88:79-81, 2003.

TABLE 11-13 **Possible Clinical Manifestations of Food Allergies or Intolerances by Body System**

System	Symptoms
Respiratory system	Chronic rhinitis
	Asthma
	Croup
	Cough
	Serous otitis media
	Bronchitis
Gastrointestinal system	Tingling and swelling of lips, mouth, throat
	Nausea, vomiting
	Diarrhea
	Colic
	Protein-losing enteropathy
	Bloating, flatulence
	Constipation
	Gastrointestinal blood loss
	Malabsorption
Integumentary system	Eczema
	Pruritus
	Atopic dermatitis
	Rashes
	Urticaria
Central nervous system	Headaches (sinus, migraine)
	Fatigue
	Drowsiness, listlessness
	Irritability
	Depression
	Excessive sweating
Circulatory system	Hypotension
	Cardiac arrhythmias
	Anaphylaxis
	Pallor

Height and weight should be monitored closely in children with food allergies because growth may be compromised as alternatives to the offending food are tried.

Diagnostic Tests. Laboratory studies assist in distinguishing between food allergies and intolerances. They may not be definitive, however, and a good history is often key to diagnosis. Tests include:

- Skin tests. The skin prick test (SPT) is the standard and is very sensitive. Cutaneous response may not correlate with systemic response, however. Antihistamine medications must be discontinued 3 to 20 days before the test, and the test should be avoided in children who have generalized skin lesions, dermographism, or a severe reaction to food following skin contact or inhalation.
- Serum IgE and eosinophil count (elevated serum IgE and eosinophilia greater than $400/mm^3$ are usually related to allergies). This test is done if the child cannot have an SPT done, but it can be expensive, especially if more than one food is suspected. Also results must be interpreted carefully by an allergist since findings can reflect exposure to other allergens.
- Radioallergosorbent tests
- Metabolic screening tests (e.g., PKU)

Food Elimination and Challenge. When a food has been identified as a potential source of the problem, the process of elimination and challenge is used to confirm the diagnosis. This process should be managed by an allergist or immunologist. Medical supervision during the elimination and challenge is essential.

The suspected foods are completely eliminated from the child's diet for at least 2 weeks and then gradually reintroduced, one at a time. With older children, a single- or double-blind with placebo challenge is most reliable. The initial reintroduction dose should be small, then increased until either the reaction recurs or the amount normally eaten is given. During the elimination and challenge, the child should receive no treatment medications for symptoms of reaction (e.g., antihistamines), and if exercise is thought to contribute to the initial allergic reaction, then exercise must be part of the challenge. An allergy or intolerance is confirmed if symptoms cease when the food is eliminated and then reappear as it is reintroduced. Approximately one-third of individuals are able to replicate signs and symptoms of a problem when challenged (Knight & Bahna, 2006).

If the potential reaction to a food is severe (e.g., anaphylaxis), the child should be hospitalized with emergency cardiovascular support available for the challenge part of this process. Allergy to peanuts or tree nuts can be lifelong, and children with allergies to nuts should never be challenged.

Differential Diagnosis

The differential diagnoses for food allergy and food intolerance include:

- Reactions related to other environmental allergens
- Asthma as a result of other causes
- Immunodeficiency
- Psychological reactions to feeding
- Malabsorption syndromes (e.g., celiac disease), cystic fibrosis
- Lactose intolerance
- Chronic diarrhea

Management

Care of children with adverse food reactions aims to maintain nutrition levels adequate for normal growth and development, prevent nutritional deficits, avoid exposure to offending food or foods, and respond promptly and appropriately to episodes of exposure. Achieving these goals requires the coordinated efforts of pediatric allergists, dietitians, the primary care provider, and teachers or child care providers, in addition to children and their families. Once a child has been assessed as to the cause and severity of the condition (see Table 11-14), a treatment plan can be made (Fiocchi & Martelli, 2006). First, the offending food or foods must be avoided. Doing this raises several challenging issues:

- The foods to which most individuals are allergic are very common and very nutritious—difficult to avoid and difficult to replace.
- The food may contaminate other foods or be found in minute amounts in other, often processed, foods.
- Skin or inhalant contact may take place (e.g., breathing peanut dust) even if food is not eaten.
- Sometimes the individual is allergic to the food in its raw form, but could eat it in a cooked (heat-treated) form; completely eliminating it means unnecessary loss of a good source of nutrients.
- Extensive use of elimination diets can lead to malnourishment; these diets should be used for as short a time as possible.
- Cross-reacting allergens may further limit diets.

Restricted foods need to be replaced with those of equivalent nutrient value in the context of a well-balanced diet. Additionally, the physical problems caused by allergies (e.g., diarrhea, vomiting, dehydration, eczema) can create a need for extra nutrients to maintain health and foster growth. The provider, family, and child should work with a dietitian to structure dietary care looking at nutritional substitutes. The child's eating habits should be reevaluated periodically to ensure nutritional needs are being met and the child is growing well.

The child's allergic status should be reevaluated regularly. Because food allergies and intolerances are often outgrown, the child may be challenged with most offending foods every year or two. Cow's milk allergy is usually outgrown by 2 years; eggs by 4 to 5 years (Fiocchi & Martelli, 2006). Some foods appear to remain allergenic for longer periods (e.g., seafood). If the child's reaction has been serious or even life threatening, the parents may decide to continue to avoid the food; as noted previously, children with allergies to nuts should never be challenged. Even if the child is able to clinically tolerate the food, there is evidence that physiologic changes in the gastrointestinal system may continue (Assa'ad, 2006). Many fatalities related to food allergies occur among older children, teenagers, and young adults.

Self-administered epinephrine is prescribed for children with moderate or severe allergies. Children, their parents, and other caregivers should be educated on intramuscular injection using preprepared EpiPens™. Antihistamines are prescribed for children with mild allergies, unless there is a history of a reaction to trace amounts of the allergen or the child has asthma from another cause. In these cases, epinephrine is appropriate (Clark & Ewan, 2003). Children with food allergies should wear a medical-alert (Medic Alert™) bracelet or necklace. School personnel should be informed of the child's allergy, and a medical plan put in place for the time the child is in school.

Education of families, children, and adults who are responsible for the child's well-being is critical; the provider can do outreach to teachers, schools, and day care centers with information about how to understand and safely manage the child's condition and be an ongoing source of suggestions, support, and advocacy for parents.

Management of food intolerances secondary to metabolic disorders is discussed earlier in this chapter (see Disorders Requiring Restricted or Supplemental Diets).

Complications

Complications of adverse food reactions include the following:

- Anaphylaxis
- Convulsive coughing and sneezing, leading to aspiration or choking
- Asthma
- Malnutrition
- Gastrointestinal dysfunction
- Secondary skin infections
- Disruption of family processes

Prevention

The best treatment for food allergies and intolerances is prevention. Ideally, all infants should be breastfed for a minimum of 4 to 6 months and for 12 months if possible; infants who have been identified as being at high risk for adverse reactions, especially allergies, should be exclusively breast-fed until they are 6 months old (Chandra, 1997). If formula is used preventively for high-risk children, soy-based formulas are often the first substitute, but there is about a 10% possibility (greater in infants under 6 months old) that the infant will also be allergic to soy. Extensively hydrolyzed, heat-treated, ultrafiltered cow's milk-based preparations are well tolerated, but can be expensive, and the infant may not accept the taste; elemental formulas, synthesized free amino acids with vitamin and mineral supplements, can be used. The first foods introduced should be hypoallergenic (e.g., rice cereal, squash, bananas). At least 3 to 5 days are allowed between each new food introduced so that any adverse reaction has time to occur. Cow's milk, wheat, corn, and citrus fruits should be avoided completely before children are 12 months old. If an allergy to cow's milk or egg is diagnosed, peanuts, tree nuts, fish, and seafood should be avoided until at least 3 years old.

Breastfeeding mothers of infants at high risk for allergies should avoid allergenic foods as well (e.g., cow's milk, nuts, fish) because the proteins from these foods may be passed to the infant via breast milk. Garlic, onions, cabbage, and broccoli also have been noted to cause gastrointestinal reactions in infants.

EFFECT OF MEDICATIONS ON NUTRITIONAL STATUS

Description

Medications are designed to alter the body's biochemistry in an effort to produce a healing effect. Biochemical processes inherent in drug therapy have implications for the individual's nutritional status. Some medications deplete essential nutrients from the body; others interfere with the body's ability to metabolize nutrients; still others have an adverse effect on the appetite or cause nausea. Although a medication can have an immediate effect on an individual, adverse changes in nutritional status are most often seen after prolonged therapy.

Epidemiology

Drug-induced malnutrition results from drug-related alterations in the body's ability to absorb, distribute, metabolize, use, or excrete nutrients and their metabolites (Wynne et al, 2002). Absorption is affected by characteristics of the molecule being absorbed (size, ionization, lipid solubility), gut motility (too rapid as with diarrhea or too slow as with Hirschsprung's disease), and environment of the gastrointestinal tract (e.g., gastric pH, lack of intrinsic factor). As medications change gastrointestinal motility or environment, they influence the absorption of nutrients.

Distribution of nutrients is affected by plasma protein-binding capabilities, total body water content, and relative fat content in the body. For example, if a drug that binds highly with plasma protein is taken for long periods of time or if a child has low serum albumin, nutrients have to compete for protein-binding sites.

Metabolism occurs primarily in the liver, and drugs can either inhibit or stimulate hepatic enzyme activity, thus influencing the body's ability to metabolize nutrients for use at the cellular level. The relationship of medications and nutrients in terms of excretion is less marked than with absorption, distribution, and metabolism, but drugs can have an effect on renal function, especially tubular reabsorption, which then affects nutritional status.

Clinical Assessment

Nutritional assessment of children on medication includes the general parameters discussed earlier, such as anthropometric measures, physical examination, and diet history. Specific attention should be paid to those nutrients for which drug therapy places the child at risk of deficiency.

Management

Management involves ongoing assessment and anticipatory intervention to prevent nutritional problems for children on drug therapy. Referral to a dietitian can be helpful. General interventions include the following:

- Alter dietary intake to include more foods containing nutrients affected.
- Supplement diet with required vitamins or minerals, or both.
- Administer medications in a manner that minimizes their impact on nutrition.
- Consider alternative medications and treatment modalities.

Table 11-15 provides dietary suggestions related to specific classes of medication. This list is limited, and a comprehensive pharmacology reference should be consulted for specific drugs.

Complications

Malnutrition, slowed growth, delayed healing, and drug toxicity are complications of the effects of medication on nutritional status.

TOXIC EXPOSURES IN FOODS

Exposure to toxins and chemicals through the food chain contribute to many health problems in children. Chapter 41 examines more closely the relationship between toxic exposure in foods and children's health.

CONTROVERSIES IN PEDIATRIC NUTRITION

Cow's Milk in Children's Diets

During the first year of life, the use of unmodified cow's milk is contraindicated because of its high protein content, its inappropriate nutrient composition, and the risk of gastrointestinal bleeding and allergic reactions. Instead, infants should receive breast milk or an approved iron-fortified infant formula that closely matches the composition of breast milk. Although most pediatric providers agree on this recommendation, there is some debate about the use of cow's milk in the toddler's diet.

TABLE 11-15 **Nutritional Risk of Selected Drugs***

Drug Category or Name	Nutritional Risk	Nutritional Intervention
Antibiotic (e.g., chloramphenicol)	Inhibits vitamin K–producing intestinal microflora Increases excretion of riboflavin Nausea, vomiting, diarrhea Decreases absorption of calcium, fat, and protein Decreases lactase activity Suppresses bone marrow (chloramphenicol) May cause aplastic anemia	Use acidophilus tablets, acidophilus milk, or yogurt to replace gastrointestinal organisms Supplement with vitamin C, B-complex vitamins, vitamin B_{12}, biotin, vitamin K, or well-balanced vitamin and mineral supplement Use lactose-reduced milk
Barbiturate (e.g., phenobarbital)	Breaks down vitamin D May cause calcium deficiency, rickets, or osteomalacia May decrease serum folate, vitamin B_{12}, pyridoxine (vitamin B_6), magnesium May cause nausea, vomiting, constipation	May need vitamin D and calcium supplements Give drug with meals Give high-fiber and high-fluid diet If folic acid supplementation is indicated, administer cautiously
Antihistamine (e.g., cimetidine, diphenhydramine)	Decreases gastric acid secretion, increases pH Decreases absorption of iron, folate, vitamin B_{12} May lead to hyperglycemia May disrupt vitamin D metabolism	
Corticosteroid	Increases protein catabolism and gluconeogenesis; decreases protein synthesis, contributing to nitrogen wasting Stimulates appetite May cause hypokalemia, hyperglycemia, hypernatremia, hypocalcemia associated with osteoporosis May elevate serum lipids	If edema occurs, restrict sodium intake High doses require calcium and vitamin D supplements Supplement with vitamin B_6, vitamin C, and folic acid Increase dietary protein Monitor weight and restrict calories if there is excessive weight gain
Digoxin	May cause anorexia and nausea, weight loss May cause hypokalemia May increase urinary excretion of magnesium and calcium	Increase dietary potassium Evaluate need to increase dietary magnesium and calcium
Isoniazid	Interferes with enzyme pathway for creation of niacin Increases excretion of vitamin B_6 and folic acid May cause nausea and vomiting Decreases absorption of vitamin E Increases absorption of iron May cause hyperglycemia	Give vitamin B_6 supplement Increase foods high in folate, niacin, vitamin B_6, and magnesium Avoid foods with histamine and tyramine, such as tuna, mackerel, sardines, dry sausages and meats, imitation and hard cheeses, meat and protein extracts, and excessive amounts of caffeine (Davis & Sherer, 1994)
Methotrexate	Folate antagonist, contributes to folate deficiency May cause stomatitis, anorexia, diarrhea Decreases absorption of vitamins A, D, E, and K, β-carotene	Give mineral oil Supplement with multivitamin given midway between times mineral oil is administered Give folate
Oral contraceptive	Increases vitamin A and calcium absorption Causes low serum vitamin C; possibly contributes to low levels of vitamins B_1, B_{12}, B_6, B_2, folate, magnesium, zinc	Increase intake of vitamins C, B_1, B_{12}, B_6, B_2, folate, magnesium, zinc
Phenothiazide	Increases excretion of riboflavin	
Hydantoin, phenytoin	May cause nausea, vomiting, constipation May cause hyperglycemia Impairs metabolism and absorption of folate; may lead to megaloblastic anemia Inactivates vitamin D; can lead to osteomalacia Decreases serum vitamin K	Supplement with vitamin D, vitamin K, folate, but excessive folate levels can decrease action of anticonvulsants Administer drug with, or immediately after, a meal

Continued

TABLE 11-15 Nutritional Risk of Selected Drugs*—Cont'd

Drug Category or Name	Nutritional Risk	Nutritional Intervention
Supplements		
Calcium	If taken with iron supplement, only calcium carbonate does not affect iron absorption; if taken with fluoride, absorption of both is decreased	
Zinc	>1500 mg/day: decreases copper absorption, possibly leading to anemia-related fatigue	
Iron	Causes nausea, possibly anorexia	
Theophylline	May cause vitamin B_6 deficiency	Give pyridoxine supplements

*See Appendix A, *Medications*, for additional information related to interaction between drugs and foods.

In most cases, children older than 1 year old can safely drink cow's milk, and it can be recommended as a rich source of protein, calcium, riboflavin, and vitamin D. The calcium and vitamin D are present in highly absorbable forms, and the protein is highly bioavailable. Cow's milk is an easy and sure way for children to receive these essential nutrients. For some children, true allergy to cow's milk causes gastrointestinal, respiratory, or skin problems; parents may wonder whether the nutritional benefits of cow's milk are worth possible health risks. If the protein and nutrients found in milk are included in the child's diet with other foods, milk may not be necessary.

Lactose intolerance, a condition caused by a lack of the enzyme lactase, normally present in the small intestine, can also limit dairy product intake by children. Lactose intolerance is rare in infants but common in older children and adults from Asian, Native American, black, and Hispanic ethnic groups. Acquired lactose intolerance may follow an episode of viral gastroenteritis in children. The condition causes symptoms of bloating, flatulence, abdominal cramps, and diarrhea between 15 minutes and 2 hours after the consumption of foods containing lactose. Children with low lactase levels may be able to digest small amounts of milk and other dairy products. Yogurt, aged cheese, and fermented dairy products, which are much lower in lactose than milk, are usually better tolerated. Commercial preparations are also available (e.g., Lactaid) that break down the lactose in milk.

Effects of Sugar

Many parents, teachers, and even children believe that sugar intake causes behavior problems, primarily hyperactivity. An extensive review of controlled scientific studies failed to find evidence of a link between sugar and behavior or cognitive performance (Cruz & Bahna, 2006). An association between soft drinks and hyperactivity has recently been demonstrated in teenagers (Lien et al, 2006), but the researchers acknowledge the possibility that other components of the soft drink (e.g., caffeine), not sugar, may be the cause of symptoms. The misconception of an association between sugar and hyperactivity may stem from the fact that sugar consumption is often related to activities (e.g., birthday parties, Halloween) that result in excited behavior among children. An elimination diet (no sugar) can be tried; if symptoms improve, a double-blind, placebo-controlled challenge should be used to confirm a relationship.

The role of the provider is to educate and reassure parents that moderate sugar consumption rarely results in adverse behavior. High-sugar diets are to be avoided, however, because these foods tend to replace more nutrient-dense foods and contribute to overweight and dental caries if eaten frequently throughout the day. Current dietary recommendations are that 10% or less of calories should come from sugar. If the average child who consumes 2000 calories daily, this amounts to 50 g or the equivalent of 10 teaspoons each day.

NURSING DIAGNOSES

Related to Nutrition: Functional Health Pattern

Diagnoses are related to the concepts of infant feeding pattern, swallowing, nutrition, fluid volume.
- Anorexia (not a NANDA diagnosis)
- Bulimia (DSM-IV diagnosis)
- Ineffective infant feeding pattern
- Impaired swallowing
- Imbalanced nutrition: less than body requirements
- Imbalanced nutrition: more than body requirements
- Readiness for enhanced nutrition
- Deficient fluid volume
- Risk for deficient fluid volume
- Excess fluid volume
- Risk for fluid volume imbalance
- Readiness for enhanced fluid balance
- Nausea
- Risk for unstable blood glucose

From NANDA International: *NANDA-I nursing diagnoses: definitions & classification 2007–2008*, Philadelphia. 2007, Author.

RESOURCE BOX

Nutrition Issues

ALLERGIES

Allergy Information and Referral Hotline
800-822-2762

Asthma and Allergy Foundation of America
www.aafa.org

Food Allergy Center
www.nutramed.com/foodallergy
Program of Alpha Nutrition, Division of Environmed Research Inc.

The Food Allergy and Anaphylaxis Network
www.foodallergy.org

EATING DISORDERS

Anorexia Nervosa and Related Eating Disorders (ANRED)
www.anred.com
Affiliated with National Eating Disorders Association (NEDA)

National Association of Anorexia Nervosa and Associated Disorders (ANAD)
www.anad.org

National Eating Disorders Association (NEDA)
www.edap.org

National Eating Disorder Information Centre (NEDIC) (Canada)
www.nedic.ca

Shapedown
www.shapedown.com
Child and adolescent obesity weight control program

FOR PARENTS AND ADOLESCENTS

Fletcher AM: *Weight loss confidential: how teens lose weight and keep it off—and what they wish parents knew*, Boston, 2007, Houghton Mifflin.

BAM! Body and Mind
www.bam.gov

Powerful Girls Have Powerful Bones
www.cdc.gov/powerfulbones

DIABETES

American Diabetes Association
www.diabetes.org
English and Spanish-speaking assistance

Juvenile Diabetes Research Foundation International
www.jdrf.org

GASTROINTESTINAL DISEASES

Canadian Celiac Association
www.celiac.ca

Celiac Disease Foundation
www.celiac.org

Celiac Sprue Association/United States of America, Inc.
www.csaceliacs.org

Crohn's and Colitis Foundation of America
www.ccfa.org

Gluten Intolerance Group
www.gluten.net

The North American Society for Pediatric Gastroenterology, Hepatology, and Nutrition
www.naspghan.org

PULMONARY DISEASES

Cystic Fibrosis Foundation
www.cff.org

GROWTH CHARTS FOR CHILDREN WITH SPECIAL CONDITIONS

In Hall J, Frostr-Iskenius UG, Allanson JE: *The handbook of normal physical measurements*, Oxford, 1989, Oxford University Press.

- Achondroplasia height and head circumference, male and female
- Marfan syndrome height
- Noonan syndrome height
- Prader-Willi height
- Williams syndrome height
- Arthrogryposis-amyoplasia, height and distal heights, male and female
- Multiple pterygium height, male and female
- Diastrophic dysplasia height
- Pseudoachondroplasia height
- Spondyloepiphyseal dysplasia congenita height
- Turner syndrome

From Child Development and Rehabilitation Center, Genetics Clinic, 503-494-8307
- Myelomeningocele height and weight, male and female, 2–18 old years
- Asian children, height and weight, male and female, 0–6 years old (also see *www.fwcc.org*)

From Cystic Fibrosis Foundation: *Cystic fibrosis growth chart.* Available at *www.cff.org.*

From Platt OS: Sickle cell anemia, *N Engl J Med* 311:7, 1984. Sickle cell anemia growth chart.

OTHER

About Face USA
www.aboutfaceusa.org
Craniofacial conditions

Continued

RESOURCE BOX

Nutrition Issues—Cont'd

American Cleft Palate Association
www.cleftline.org

American School Food Service Association
www.asfsa.org
School Nutrition Association

National Agricultural Library/USDA
www.nutrition.gov

National Association of Pediatric Nurse Practitioners (NAPNAP)
www.napnap.org
Healthy Eating and Activity Together (HEAT)

National Association of School Nurses
www.nasn.org

Pediatric/Adolescent Gastroesophageal Reflux Association (PAGER)
www.reflux.org

The American Dietetic Association
www.eatright.org

☑ DISCUSSION FORUM

1. What is the rationale regarding the use of infant formula with ARA and DHA? What is the evidence regarding the benefits and risks of these formulas?
2. The mother of a toddler asks what she should be feeding her child. What advice will you give her? What resources will you use and why?
3. When taking a diet history from a family, you realize that you are unfamiliar with most of the foods they are feeding their child. What information do you need to ensure the child is well nourished? How will you get that information? What is your approach to the family?
4. A 15-year-old states that she feels she is "fat." Her BMI is on the 10th percentile and has fallen from the 35th percentile in the past year. What are key points in the history and physical for this 15-year-old? What would be your management? What community resources are available for the family?
5. As the primary care provider for a 10-year-old with cystic fibrosis, what goals will you set for the child's nutrition? What management plan and strategies will you use to achieve those goals?

REFERENCES

The American Academy of Pediatrics (AAP) Work Group on Breastfeeding: Breastfeeding and the use of human milk, *Pediatrics* 115:496-506, 2005.

American Dental Association: *Fluoridation facts*, Chicago, 2002, American Dental Association.

American Dietetic Association: Position of the American Dietetic Association: dietary guidance for healthy children aged 2 to 11 years, *J Am Diet Assoc* 104(4):660-677, 2004a.

American Dietetic Association: Position of the American Dietetic Association: nutrition intervention in the treatment of anorexia nervosa, bulimia nervosa, and other eating disorders, *J Am Diet Assoc* 106(12):2073-2082, 2006.

American Dietetic Association: Position of the American Dietetic Association: providing nutrition services for infants, children, and adults with developmental disabilities and special health care needs, *J Am Diet Assoc* 104(1):97-107, 2004b.

American Dietetic Association, Dietitians of Canada: Position of the American Dietetic Association and Dietitians of Canada: vegetarian diets, *J Am Diet Assoc* 103(6):748-765, 2003.

American Medical Association (AMA): *Recommendations for physician and community collaboration on the management of obesity* (A-05), 2005. Available at *www.ama-assn.org/ama/pub/category/15495.html#recommendations* (accessed Jan 15, 2007).

American Psychiatric Association (APA): *Diagnostic and statistical manual of mental disorders*, ed 4, Washington, DC, 1994, American Psychiatric Association.

Assa'ad AH: Gastrointestinal food allergy and intolerance, *Pediatr Annals* 35(10):718-726, 2006.

Bergmann KE et al: Early determinants of childhood overweight and adiposity in a birth cohort study: role of breast-feeding, *Int J Obes Relat Metab Disord* 27:162-172, 2003.

Briefel R et al: Feeding Infants and Toddlers Study: do vitamin and mineral supplements contribute to nutrient adequacy or excess among US infants and toddlers? *J Am Diet Assoc* 106(Suppl 1):S52-S65, 2006.

Caro et al: Decreased cerebrospinal-fluid/serum leptin ratio in obesity: a possible mechanism for leptin resistance, *Lancet* 348(9021):159-161, 1996.

Carter JC et al: The impact of childhood sexual abuse in anorexia nervosa, *Child Abuse Negl* 30(3):257-269, 2006.

Centers for Disease Control and Prevention (CDC): Youth Risk Behavior Surveillance–United States, 2005, *MMWR* 55(SS-5):1-108, 2006.

Centers for Disease Control and Prevention (CDC): *Overweight and obesity: defining overweight and obesity*. Available at *www.cdc.gov/nccdphp/dnpa/obesity/defining.htm* (accessed Aug 6, 2007).

Chan GM et al: Effects of dietary calcium intervention on adolescent mothers and newborns: a randomized controlled trial, *Obstet Gynecol* 108(3 Pt 1):565-571, 2006.

Chandra RK: Five-year follow-up of high-risk infants with family history of allergy who were exclusively breast-fed or fed partial whey hydrolysate, soy, and conventional cow's milk formulas, *J Pediatr Gastroenterol Nutr* 24:380-388, 1997.

Clark AT, Ewan PW: Food allergy in childhood, *Arch Dis Child* 88:79-81, 2003.

Croll JK et al: Adolescents involved in weight-related and power team sports have better eating patterns and nutrient intakes than non-sport-involved adolescents, *J Am Diet Assoc* 106(5):717-718, 2006.

Cruz NV, Bahna SL: Do foods or additives cause behavior disorders? *Ped Annals* 35(10):744-745, 748-754, 2006.

Dagnelie PC: Some algae are potentially adequate sources of vitamin B-12 for vegans, *J Nutr* 127:379, 1997.

Davis J, Sherer K: *Applied nutrition and diet therapy for nurses*, ed 2, Philadelphia, 1994, WB Saunders.

Dennison BA et al: Rapid infant weight gain predicts childhood overweight, *Obesity (Silver Spring)* 14(3):491-499, 2006.

Dubois L, Girard M: Early determinants of overweight at 4.5 years in a population-based longitudinal study, *Int J Obes (Lond)* 30(4):610-617, 2006.

Dunham L, Kollar LM: Vegetarian eating for children and adolescents, *J Pediatr Health Care* 20(1):27-34, 2006.

Ekvall SW, Ekvall V: Early intervention and nutrition. Manual IV, MCHB. In Stevens F, Ekvall S, editors: *Empowering children through early intervention with good nutrition—focusing on culturally diverse children with special health care needs*, Rockville, MD, 2001, Health Resources and Service Administration.

Expert Committee on the Assessment, Prevention, and Treatment of Child and Adolescent Overweight and Obesity: *Recommendations on the assessment, prevention, and treatment of child and adolescent overweight and obesity*. Available at www.ama-assn.org/ama/pub/category/11759.html (accessed Aug 6, 2007).

Farrow C, Blissett J: Does maternal control during feeding moderate early infant weight gain? *Pediatr* 118(2):e293-298, 2006.

Fiocchi A, Martelli A: Dietary management of food allergy, *Pediatr Annals* 35(10):755-763, 2006.

Fleith M, Clandinin MT: Dietary PUFA for preterm and term infants: review of clinical studies, *Crit Rev Food Sci Nutr* 45(3):205-229, 2005.

Food and Nutrition Board, Institute of Medicine (IOM): *Dietary reference intakes for energy, carbohydrate, fiber, fat, fatty acids, cholesterol, protein, and amino acids*, Washington, DC, 2005, The National Academies Press.

Fox MK et al: Sources of energy and nutrients in the diets of infants and toddlers, *J Am Diet Assoc* 106(Suppl 1):S28-S42, 2006.

Gable S, Chang Y, Krull JL: Television watching and frequency of family meals are predictive of overweight onset and persistence in a national sample of school-aged children, *J Am Diet Assoc* 107(1):53-61, 2007.

Greene-Finestone LS et al: Dietary intake among young adolescents in Ontario: associations with vegetarian status and attitude toward health, *Prev Med* 40(1):105-111, 2005.

Guenther PM et al: Most Americans eat much less than recommended amounts of fruits and vegetables, *J Am Diet Assoc* 106(9):1371-1379, 2006.

Hahn NI: When food becomes a cry for help: how dietitians can combat childhood eating disorders. Interview with Monika M. Woolsey, *J Am Diet Assoc* 98:395-398, 1998.

Haines J et al: Weight teasing and disordered eating behaviors in adolescents: longitudinal findings from Project EAT (Eating Among Teens), *Pediatrics* 117(2):e209-215, 2006.

Hourihane JO'B: Prevalence and severity of food allergy–need for control, *Allergy* 53(suppl):84-88, 1998.

Inge TH, Xanthakos SA, Zeller MH: Bariatric surgery for pediatric extreme obesity: now or later? *Int J Obes* 31(1):1-14, 2007.

Joint Working Group of the Canadian Paediatric Society (CPS) and Health Canada: *Nutrition recommendations update: dietary fat and children*, Ottawa, reaffirmed Feb 2001.

Joy EA, Wilson C, Varechok S: The multidisciplinary team approach to the outpatient treatment of disordered eating, *Curr Sports Med Rep* 2(6):331-336, 2003.

Kay JP et al: Beneficial effects of metformin in normoglycemic morbidly obese adolescents, *Metabolism* 50(12):1457-1461, 2001.

Knight AK, Bahna SL: Diagnosis of food allergy, *Pediatr Annals* 35(10):709-714, 2006.

Kral TVE, Faith MS: Child eating patterns and weight regulation: a developmental behavior genetics framework, *Acta Paediatr Suppl* 96(454):29-34, 2007.

Lien L et al: Consumption of soft drinks and hyperactivity, mental distress, and conduct problems among adolescents in Oslo, Norway, *Am J Public Health* 96(10):1815-1820, 2006.

Litt IF: Anorexia nervosa and bulimia. In Behrman RE, Kliegman RM, Jenson HB, editors: *Nelson textbook of pediatrics*, ed 17, Philadelphia, 2004, WB Saunders.

Lustig RH: The "skinny" on childhood obesity: how our Western environment starves kids' brains, *Pediatr Annals* 35(12):899-907, 2006.

Lytle LA et al: Nutrient intake over time in a multi-ethnic sample of youth, *Public Health Nutr* 5:319-328, 2002.

Manz F, Wentz A, Sichert-Hellert W: The most essential nutrient: defining the adequate intake of water, *J Pediatr* 141:587-592, 2002.

Messina V, Melina V, Mangels AR: A new food guide for North American vegetarians, *J Am Diet Assoc* 103(6):771-775, 2003.

Moissidis I et al: Milk-induced pulmonary disease in infants (Heiner syndrome), *Pediatr Allergy Immunol* 16(6):545-552, 2005.

Nader PR: Frequency and intensity of activity of third-grade children in physical education, *Arch Pediatr Adolesc Med* 157:185-190, 2003.

Nader PR et al: Identifying risk for obesity in early childhood, *Pediatrics* 118(3):e594-601, 2006.

National Association of Pediatric Nurse Practitioners (NAPNAP): *Healthy Eating and Activity Together (HEAT): clinical practice guideline, identifying and preventing overweight in childhood*, Cherry Hill, NJ, 2006, NAPNAP.

National Center for Health Statistics: *Health, United States, 2006 with chartbook on trends in the health of Americans*, Hyattsville, MD, 2006, US Government Printing Office.

Neumark-Sztainer D et al: Obesity, disordered eating, and eating disorders in a longitudinal study of adolescents: how do dieters fare 5 years later? *J Am Diet Assoc* 106(4):559-568, 2006.

Nielsen JN et al: Interventions to improve diet and weight gain among pregnant adolescents and recommendations for future research, *J Am Diet Assoc* 106(11):1825-1840, 2006.

Niinikoski H et al: Growth until 3 years of age in a prospective, randomized trial of a diet with reduced saturated fat and cholesterol, *Pediatrics* 99:687-694, 1997.

O'Connor TM, Yang SJ, Nicklas TA: Beverage intake among preschool children and its effect on weight status, *Pediatrics* 118(4):e1010-1018, 2006.

Oregon Dairy Council: *Pyramid Plus*, Portland, OR, 2006, Nutrition Education Services/Oregon Dairy Council.

Orenstein S et al: The esophagus. In Behrman RE, Kliegman RM, Jenson HB, editors: *Nelson textbook of pediatrics*, ed 17, Philadelphia, 2004, WB Saunders.

Padwal RS, Majumdar SR: Drug treatment for obesity: orlistat, sibutramine, and rimonabant, *Lancet* 369(9555):71-77, 2007.

Painter J, Rah J-H, Lee Y-K: Comparison of international food guide pictorial representations, *J Am Diet Assoc* 102(4):483-489, 2002.

Perry CL et al: Adolescent vegetarians: how well do their dietary patterns meet the *Healthy People 2010* objectives? *Arch Pediatr Adolesc* 156:431-437, 2002.

Perry CL et al: Characteristics of vegetarian adolescents in a multiethnic urban population, *J Adolesc Health* 29:406-416, 2001.

Pollan M: Unhappy meals: thirty years of nutritional science has made Americans sicker, fatter and less well nourished. A plea for a return to plain old food, *The New York Times Magazine*, Jan 28, 2007.

Preeyasombat C et al: Racial and etiopathologic dichotomies in insulin hypersecretion and resistance in obese children, *J Pediatr* 146(4):474-481, 2005.

Preti A et al: Sexual abuse and eating disorder symptoms: the mediator role of bodily dissatisfaction, *Compr Psychiatry* 47(6):475-481, 2006.

Ramacciotti A et al: Attachment processes in eating disorders, *Eat Weight Disord* 6:166-170, 2001.

Rathbun JM, Peterson KE: Nutrition in failure to thrive. In Grand RJ, Sutphen JL, Dietz WH, editors: *Pediatric nutrition*, Boston, 1987, Butterworth.

Reinhardt WC, Brevard PB: Integrating the Food Guide Pyramid and Physical Activity Pyramid for positive dietary and physical activity behaviors in adolescents, *J Am Diet Assoc* 102:596-599, 2002.

Rezvani I: Phenylalanine. In Behrman RE, Kliegman RM, Jenson HB, editors: *Nelson textbook of pediatrics*, ed 17, Philadelphia, 2004, WB Saunders.

Rosenbaum M et al: Low dose leptin administration reverses effects of sustained weight reduction on energy expenditure and circulating concentrations of thyroid hormones, *J Clin Endocrinol Metab* 87(5):2391-2394, 2002.

Royo-Bordonada et al: Saturated fat in the diet of Spanish children: relationship with anthropometric, alimentary, nutritional and lipid profiles, *Public Health Nutr* 9(4):429-435, 2006.

Rudolph CD et al: Pediatric GE reflux clinical practice guidelines, *J Pediatr Gastroenterol Nutr* 32(suppl 2):S1-S31, 2001.

Sakurai K et al: Bisphenol A affects glucose transport in mouse 3T3-F442A adipocytes, *Br J Pharmacol* 141(2):209-214, 2004.

Sampson HA: Update on food allergy, *J Allergy Clin Immunol* 113(5): 805-819, 2004.

Sanchez A et al: Patterns and correlates of physical activity and nutrition behaviors in adolescents, *Am J Prev Med* 32(2):124-130, 2007.

Sicherer SH, Sampson HA: 9. Food allergy, *J Allergy Clin Immunol* 117 (2 Suppl Mini-Primer):S470-S475, 2006.

Sinha et al: Prevalence of glucose intolerance among children and adolescents with marked obesity, *N Engl J Med* 346(11):802-810, 2002.

Spruijt-Metz D et al: Longitudinal influence of mother's child-feeding practices on adiposity in children, *J Pediatr* 148(3):314-320, 2006.

Stice E et al: Age of onset for binge eating and purging during late adolescence: a 4-year survival analysis, *J Abnorm Psych* 107:671-675, 1998.

Stice E, Fisher M, Martinez E: Eating disorder diagnostic scale: additional evidence of reliability and validity, *Psychol Assess* 16(1):60-71, 2004.

Stice E, Presnell K, Spangler D: Risk factors for binge eating onset in adolescent girls: a 2-year prospective investigation, *Health Psychol* 21:131-138, 2002.

Stice E, Telch CF, Rizvi SL: Development and validation of the Eating Disorder Diagnostic Scale: a brief self-report measure of anorexia, bulimia, and binge-eating disorder, *Psychol Assess* 12(2):123-131, 2000.

Story M, Holt K, Sofka D, editors: *Bright Futures in practice: nutrition*, ed 2, Arlington, VA, 2002, National Center for Education in Maternal and Child Health.

Suitor CW, Gleason PM: Using dietary reference intake-based methods to estimate the prevalence of inadequate nutrient intake among school-aged children, *J Am Diet Assoc* 102:530-536, 2002.

Sukalich S, Mingione MJ, Glantz JC: Obstetric outcomes in overweight and obese adolescents, *Am J Obstet Gynecol* 195(3):851-855, 2006.

Taylor CB et al: Prevention of eating disorders in at-risk college-age women, *Arch Gen Psychiatry* 63(8):881-888, 2006.

Tyrka AR et al: Prospective predictors of the onset of anorexic and bulimic syndromes, *Int J Eat Disord* 32:282-290, 2002.

US Department of Health and Human Services (USDHHS), US Department of Agriculture (USDA): *Dietary guidelines for Americans, 2005*, ed 6, Washington DC, 2005, US Government Printing Office.

US Preventive Services Task Force (USPSTF): Screening and interventions for overweight in children and adolescents: recommendation statement, *Pediatrics* 116(1):205-209, 2005.

Vandewater EA et al: Digital childhood: electronic media and technology use among infants, toddlers, and preschoolers, *Pediatrics* 119(5): e1006-1015, 2007.

Van Horn L et al: A summary of results of the Dietary Intervention Study in Children (DISC): lessons learned, *Prog Cardiovasc Nurs* 18:28-41, 2003.

Vereecken CA et al: Television viewing behaviour and associations with food habits in different countries, *Public Health Nutr* 9(2):244-250, 2006.

Wosje KS, Specker BL, Giddens J: No differences in growth or body composition from age 12 to 24 months between toddlers consuming 2% milk and toddlers consuming whole milk, *J Am Diet Assoc* 102:53-56, 2002.

Wynne AL, Woo TM, Millard M: *Pharmacotherapeutics for nurse practitioner prescribers*, Philadelphia, 2002, FA Davis.

CHAPTER 12

Breastfeeding

Pamela J. Hellings

Breast milk is the ideal food for newborns and infants and supports infant nutrition essential for optimal growth and development. In addition to healthy nutrition, breastfeeding gives parents and infants physical, psychological, and emotional benefits that last a lifetime. A high priority should be placed on promoting and supporting breastfeeding whenever possible.

Health care providers have an important role in the promotion of breastfeeding. This role includes assessment, education, support, outreach, and advocacy. As breastfeeding is a learned skill for both the mother and the infant, providers must assess the mother's knowledge level and provide information and guidance to increase the skills of the mother-infant dyad as the breastfeeding experience develops. They can teach about the benefits of breast milk so that families can make educated choices about infant feeding. They can provide classes to increase knowledge in order to prevent common problems or assist in the decision to seek consultation for problems. Support for breastfeeding occurs when providers take the time required to determine the cause of a breastfeeding problem, to develop a plan to address the problem, and to guide the family through difficulties; these interventions can make the difference in the decision to continue breastfeeding. Outreach and advocacy for breastfeeding is demonstrated when providers contribute to hospital, clinic, and community committees, advisory boards, and task forces to develop policies that promote and support breastfeeding; when they advise and educate colleagues on breastfeeding issues, teach breastfeeding content to students in the health professions, and serve as an expert contact for the media on issues related to breastfeeding. In all these activities, the health care provider serves an important leadership function in promoting and supporting breastfeeding.

BREASTFEEDING RECOMMENDATIONS

Major health professional organizations, including the National Association of Pediatric Nurse Practitioners (2007) and the American Academy of Pediatrics (AAP) (2005), recommend breastfeeding for the first year of life.

Although breastfeeding rates have increased in the U.S. (Table 12-1), they continue to be well below *Healthy People 2010* goals (CDC, 2007). Much work remains to be done, and providers can make a major contribution to the success of efforts to support breastfeeding.

HOSPITAL-BASED SUPPORT
THE BABY-FRIENDLY HOSPITAL INITIATIVE

In 1991, a worldwide effort to recognize hospitals that provide optimal lactation support was developed by the World Health Organization (WHO) and the United Nations International Children's Emergency Fund (UNICEF) (UNICEF, 2007). This effort, known as the Baby-Friendly Hospital Initiative, bases assessment of the quality of a lactation program on ten steps for successful breastfeeding, delineated in a joint WHO-UNICEF statement (WHO/UNICEF, 1989). Every facility that provides maternity services and care for newborn infants should:

- Have a written breastfeeding policy that is routinely communicated to all health care staff.
- Train all health care staff in skills necessary to implement this policy.
- Inform all pregnant women about the benefits and management of breastfeeding.
- Help mothers initiate breastfeeding within one half hour of birth.
- Show mothers how to breastfeed and how to maintain lactation even if they are separated from their infants.
- Give newborn infants no food or drink other than breast milk, unless medically indicated.
- Practice rooming in (i.e., allow mothers and infants to remain together) 24 hours a day.
- Encourage unrestricted breastfeeding.
- Give no artificial teats or pacifiers (also called dummies or soothers) to breastfeeding infants.
- Foster the establishment of breastfeeding support groups and refer mothers to them on discharge from the hospital or clinic.

Currently, 19,250 hospitals have been designated "baby-friendly" internationally. Most are in developing countries, with fewer than 500 located in industrialized nations (Philipp & Radford, 2006). As of August 2007, only 61 hospitals and birthing centers in the U.S. held a "baby-friendly" designation, so much work remains for U.S. health care providers (Baby-Friendly Hospital Initiative [BFHI] USA, 2007).

BENEFITS OF BREASTFEEDING

With rare exception, breast milk is the ideal food for the human infant. Each mammalian species provides milk uniquely suited to its offspring, and milk from the human breast is no exception. It is a living fluid rich in vitamins, minerals, fat, proteins

TABLE 12-1 *Healthy People 2010* Objectives: Initiation and Duration of Breastfeeding for Children Born in 2004

Healthy People 2010 Objective	Actual % of Total Population Breastfeeding By Age of Infant	Number of States Meeting *Healthy People 2010* Objective	States That Met First Three Objectives
75% of mothers will initiate breastfeeding (breastfeeding at 7 days)	71.2%	21	
50% of mothers will be breastfeeding 6-month-old infant	39.1%	9	
25% of mothers will be breastfeeding 12-month-old infant	20.1%	12	Alaska, California, Hawaii, Montana, Oregon, Utah, Washington, Vermont
Exclusive breastfeeding to 3 months old: ≥60% of months	30.5%	—	
Exclusive breastfeeding to 6 months old: ≥25% of mothers	11.3%	—	

Data from Centers for Disease Control and Prevention (CDC) National Immunization Program: *Breastfeeding: data and statistics: breastfeeding practices–results from the National Immunization Survey.* Available at *www.cdc.gov/breastfeeding/data/NIS_data/data_2004.htm* (accessed Aug 3, 2007).

(including immunoglobulins and antibodies), carbohydrates (especially lactose), enzymes, and cellular components, including macrophages and lymphocytes, in addition to many other constituents that offer ideal support for growth and maturation of the human infant. Amazingly, as the infant grows and develops, the properties of the breast milk change. The sequence of colostrum, transitional milk, and mature milk meets the changing nutritional needs of the newborn and infant. Thus the milk of a mother of a 9-month-old has different concentrations of fat, protein, and carbohydrate and different physical properties, such as pH, when compared with the milk of the mother of a newborn or 1-month-old. In addition, some of the constituent properties in the milk are different from one time of the day to another.

In addition to providing optimal nutrition for growth and development, breastfeeding confers many short- and long-term health benefits to infants. In the short term, studies show that breastfed babies have added protection against bacterial, viral, and protozoan illnesses during infancy. The incidence of respiratory and gastrointestinal infections, especially diarrhea, is significantly lower among breastfed infants (Quigley et al, 2006; Chantry et al, 2006). Hospitalization for these diseases is also lower for the breastfed infant (Paricio-Talayero et al, 2006). The human-milk glycans and immunoglobulins appear to inhibit pathogens from adhering to intestinal mucosa, replicating, and causing disease (Correa et al, 2006; Morrow et al, 2005). Breast milk also supports the growth of *Lactobacillus bifidus* in the intestine of the breastfed infant; this, in conjunction with lactoferrin, an iron-binding protein found in breast milk (50 times more than in cow's milk), creates an environment that discourages growth of pathogens.

The long-term benefits of breastfeeding include a decreased incidence of atopic diseases and an association with lower rates of asthma in breastfed infants (Oddy, 2001; Schack-Nielsen & Michaelsen, 2006). Breastfeeding may also be protective against obesity and has been associated with lower cholesterol and blood pressure (Mayer-Davis et al, 2006).

Initiating breastfeeding is crucial; the infant enjoys health benefits with every day of breastfeeding. Maintaining breastfeeding is also crucial; there is evidence, for example, that infants who are breastfed for 6 months have less risk for infection that those breastfed for 4 months (Chantry et al, 2006). However, exclusive, prolonged breastfeeding may actually contribute to health problems. In a recent study, infants exclusively breastfed for 9 months or longer had an increased incidence of atopic dermatitis and food hypersensitivity in childhood (Pesonen et al, 2006). Complementary foods should be added to the infant diet by 6 months of age (see Chapter 11); breastfeeding provides important nutritional and health-related benefits and should be continued to at least 1 year.

There are also benefits for the mother that include more rapid return to her nonpregnant state, establishment of the strong bond associated with successful nursing, and decreased risk for premenopausal ovarian cancer and breast cancer (Collaborative Group on Hormonal Factors in Breast Cancer, 2002; Schack-Nielsen et al, 2005).

Breastfeeding also provides an economic incentive as a free and plentiful source of excellent infant nutrition. The cost of formula and other necessary supplies easily exceeds $1000 to $1200 each year.

CONTRAINDICATIONS TO BREASTFEEDING

In addition to all the beneficial nutrients that are provided to the infant during breastfeeding, certain infections and many drugs or medications can be passed to the infant via breast milk.

Although rare, contraindications to breastfeeding occur in some of these situations. In addition, a small number of infant conditions also preclude breastfeeding. Contraindications to breastfeeding include the following:

- Herpetic lesions on the mother's nipples, areolas, or breast
- Maternal diagnosis and treatment of cancer
- Infant with galactosemia

SPECIAL SITUATIONS

Additional circumstances require special consideration regarding the advisability or management of breastfeeding. These circumstances include the following:

- Significant maternal or infant illness affecting the ability to feed
- Maternal illness, such as tuberculosis, chickenpox, or hepatitis B
- Invasive breast surgery, in particular breast reduction in which the areola is removed and reattached
- Documented history of milk supply problems

▬▬ CHARACTERISTICS OF HUMAN MILK
COMPONENTS OF HUMAN MILK

The uniqueness of human milk to support the growth and development of the human infant cannot be overestimated. Scientists continue to find new components and to clarify the purposes of known components. More than 200 constituents of milk have been identified (Lawrence & Lawrence, 2005).

Colostrum

Colostrum production begins at about 20 weeks of gestation. The pregnant woman may notice a small amount of yellow discharge on her nipple or clothing. After delivery of the baby, production of colostrum increases, but is still of low quantity. This thick, rich, yellowish fluid has fewer calories than mature milk does (67 versus 75 kcal/100 mL) and is lower in fat (2% versus 3.8%). It is rich in immunoglobulins, especially IgA, and other antibodies. In addition, it is higher in sodium, chloride, protein, fat-soluble vitamins, and cholesterol than mature milk, and it facilitates the passage of meconium. Because of the outstanding contribution to the infant's immunologic status, colostrum is often referred to as the infant's "first immunization." Colostrum provides everything that a normal term newborn needs for the first few days of life. No supplementation is needed.

Transitional Milk

Transitional milk appears several days after delivery. Significant variability is seen in the constituent properties of transitional milk between mothers and within samples from the same mother. However, as a general rule, transitional milk has more lactose, calories, and fat and less total protein than colostrum.

Mature Milk

Mature milk gradually replaces transitional milk by about the second week after delivery and provides, on average, 20 kcal/oz.

Water. Approximately 90% of human milk is water. Breast milk can meet the fluid needs of the infant without any supplementation, even in tropical and desert climates.

Lipid (Fat) Content. Various lipids (fats) make up the second greatest percentage of constituents of human milk. They are also the most variable component, with differences noted within a feeding, between feedings, in feedings over time, and between different mothers. On average, the fat content is approximately 3.8% and contributes 30% to 55% of the kilocalories in human milk. During feeding, the fluid content of the mammary gland becomes mixed with droplets of fat in increasing concentration. Thus, the fat content is higher at the end of the feeding (hindmilk) than it is at the beginning (foremilk). The type and amount of fat in the maternal diet are thought to affect the type of lipid but not the total amount of fat found in the mother's breast milk.

The cholesterol content varies little in human milk and is approximately 240 mg/100 g of fat. Changes in the maternal diet do not produce changes in these cholesterol values. Breastfed infants have higher plasma cholesterol levels than do formula-fed infants. Recent research suggests, however, that breastfeeding may have a protective effect against cardiovascular disease because adolescents and adults tend to have lower cholesterol levels if they were breastfed (Singhal et al, 2004; Owen et al, 2002).

Recent research on how fatty acids, such as docosahexaenoic acid (DHA) and other long-chain polyunsaturated acids (e.g., LC-PUFA), are regulated during breastfeeding, and the role they play in brain and retinal growth has shown equivocal results. Early evidence does suggest that DHA has a beneficial effect on an infant's neurobehavioral functioning, especially in preterm infants (Heird & Lapillonne, 2005; Hart et al, 2006). If infants are not breastfed, formula should be supplemented with DHA.

Protein. Approximately 0.9% of the content of human milk is protein. When milk is heated or exposed to enzymes as in digestion, a clot, or casein, is formed. The clear portion that remains is known as whey. In human milk, 60% to 70% of the protein is whey, which primarily consists of α-lactalbumin and lactoferrin, and 30% to 40% is casein. In contrast, cow's milk is 20% β-lactalbumin and 80% casein, with distinct chemical differences between the casein found in cow's milk and that found in human milk. The curds of human milk are more easily digested by the infant. Other proteins include immunoglobulins, nonimmunoglobulins, and lysozyme—a nonspecific antibacterial factor.

Carbohydrates. The primary carbohydrate of human milk is lactose, which is synthesized by the mammary gland from glucose. Lactose is highly concentrated in human milk (6.8 versus 4.9 g/100 mL in cow's milk) and appears to be essential for growth of the human infant. In addition, lactose enhances the absorption of calcium, a potentially important role because of the relatively low level of calcium in human milk.

Vitamins and Minerals. Human milk has more than adequate amounts of vitamins A, E, K, C, B_1, B_2, and B_6. However, the level of vitamin D intake may not be adequate in breastfed infants who lack exposure to sunlight. Thirty minutes per week of unprotected exposure to the sun while dressed in a diaper only or 2 hours per week clothed (as long as the head is not covered) provides adequate vitamin D for a white breast-fed infant (Konek & Mascarenhas, 2006). Sunscreen blocks vitamin D absorption. The AAP recommends a supplement of 200 IU/day for all breastfed infants unless they are weaned to at least 500 mL/day of vitamin D-fortified formula or milk (Gartner & Greer, 2003).

Iron is found in low levels in human milk. However, iron absorption from human milk is highly efficient, with 49% of the available iron absorbed in contrast to 4% from formula. A full-term infant who is exclusively breastfed for 4 to 6 months is not at risk for iron deficiency anemia. Zinc is readily available in human milk and has an absorption rate of 41% versus 31% from cow's milk protein formulas and 14% from soy formulas.

ANATOMY AND PHYSIOLOGY

Pregnancy brings about the final stage of mammogenesis—growth and differentiation of the mammary gland and development of the structures to support breast milk production. Estrogen, progesterone, placental lactogen, and prolactin all play a role in mammogenesis. By approximately 20 weeks, the breast is capable of milk production. The actual production of breast milk is triggered by the fall in progesterone concentration after birth of the baby. Placental retention inhibits milk production because of the influence of progesterone and other hormones.

Suckling by the infant is essential to establish and maintain lactation. The amount of milk produced depends on stimulation of the breast, removal of milk from the breast, and release of hormones. The concept of "supply and demand" is an important one for providers and parents to understand. Suckling stimulates the hypothalamus to decrease prolactin-inhibiting factor, permits release of prolactin by the anterior pituitary, and leads to a rise in the level of prolactin. Prolactin levels are directly proportional to the level of suckling by the infant and are more important to the initiation than to the maintenance of lactation. The hypothalamus also stimulates the synthesis and release of oxytocin by the posterior pituitary (Fig. 12-1). Oxytocin reacts with receptors in the myoepithelial cells of the milk ducts to initiate a contracting action that results in forcing milk down the ducts. This action increases milk pressure called the *letdown reflex* or *milk ejection reflex*. Oxytocin also aids in maternal uterine involution.

Under the influence of the hormones mentioned previously, the mammary gland undergoes a dramatic change with an increase in size and rapid growth of the lobuloalveolar tissue. The alveoli are the site of milk production and combine in numbers of 10 to 100 to form lobuli. Twenty to 40 lobuli combine into lobes, and 15 to 25 lobes empty into a lactiferous duct. The ducts transport the milk to the nipple (Fig. 12-2).

The nipple and surrounding areola serve as a visual and tactile target to assist with latch-on. The size and shape of the woman's breast and areola vary greatly. Fortunately the size of the breast is not a predictor of breast milk volume. Women with very small breasts can successfully breastfeed. The provider should be alert, however, for the occasional presence of insuffi-

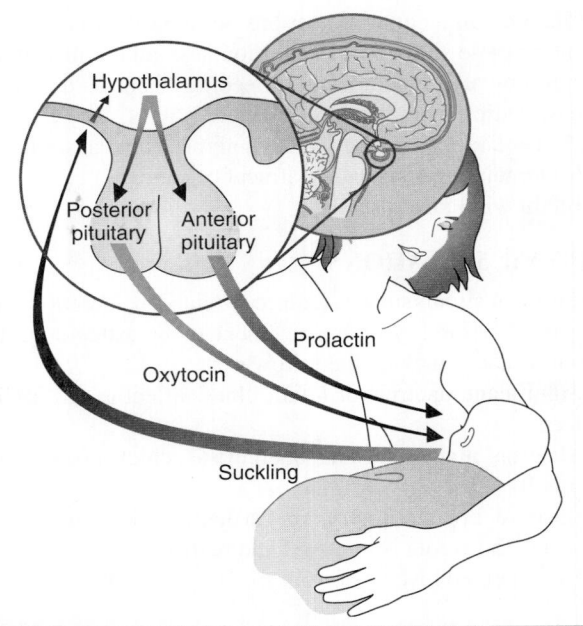

FIG. 12-1   Neuroendocrine loop.

cient glandular tissue, which is characterized by the absence of breast changes associated with pregnancy, a unilaterally underdeveloped breast, or conical-shaped breasts.

The size, shape, and position of the nipple also vary among women. The nipple may be everted (protuberant from the breast), flat, or inverted. It is not always possible to detect an inverted nipple by observation only. The "pinch test" may be needed to identify nipples that invert with tactile stimulation to the areola. To do the pinch test, place the thumb and forefinger on opposite sides of the areola about 1 to 1.5 inches back from the nipple-areolar junction. Gently

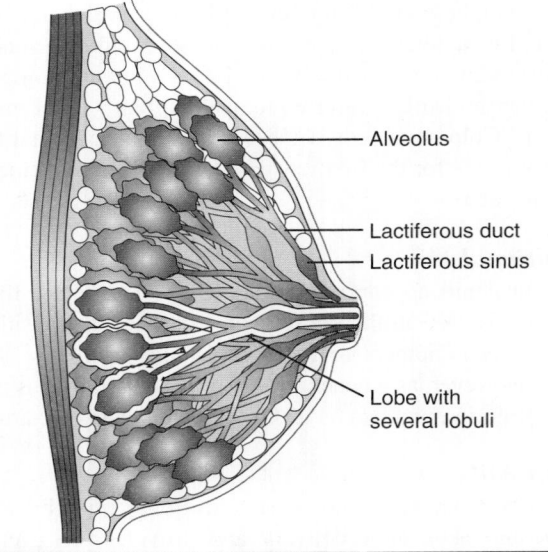

FIG. 12-2   Anatomy of the breast.

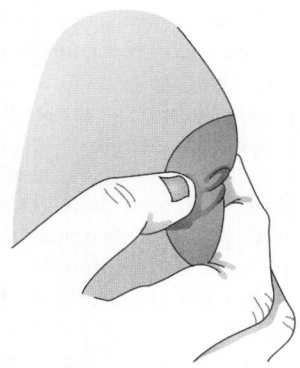

FIG. 12-3   Pinch test.

compress as though bringing the two fingers together, causing the nipple to become more everted or inverted. This assessment should be conducted prenatally on every patient (Fig. 12-3). Management of inverted nipples is discussed later in this chapter.

Despite the complexity of the anatomic and physiologic processes, the great news is that breastfeeding can proceed for the mother and the baby with little or no awareness on their part of these considerations.

■ ASSESSMENT OF THE BREASTFEEDING DYAD

Prenatal assessment focuses on maternal expectations for breastfeeding; knowledge about breastfeeding, especially techniques for getting off to a good start; and identification of any contraindications to breastfeeding. A nipple evaluation should be completed. All pregnant women should be assessed, not just *primigravidas*. In the early postpartum period, assessment focuses on the transition to breastfeeding and should include *close* observation of a feeding. In addition, signs of progress for successful breastfeeding should be reviewed, and the names and phone numbers of contact persons should be given to mothers for follow-up or questions.

MATERNAL HISTORY

In general data should be collected about the following areas:
- Overall health, including documentation of any chronic illnesses or allergies
- Previous breastfeeding experience
- Routine use of over-the-counter, prescribed, or recreational or street drugs, including tobacco
- Surgical interventions, especially to the breast or thoracic region
- Nutritional status
- Family and community support for breastfeeding
- Pregnancy history, especially any complications or need for medications
- Labor and delivery history, including medications, procedures, or complications

INFANT HISTORY

Data are gathered on the infant in the following areas:
- Overall health status
- Congenital conditions, such as cardiac, respiratory, or orofacial conditions
- Trauma or complications during delivery
- Medications received during labor and delivery or in the early postpartum period
- Activities including circumcision, use of bilirubin lights, or use of bottle, cup, or tube feeding
- Gestational age
- Early responses to feeding attempts

MATERNAL EXAMINATION

Examination of the mother should focus on an evaluation of the breast in the following areas:
- Type of nipples—everted, flat, or inverted
- Presence of surgical scars on the breast or thoracic area
- Any nipple bruising or bleeding

INFANT EXAMINATION

Evaluation of the infant's oral-motor skills and structures is the basis for the examination. The examiner's finger should be inserted beyond the gum line nearly to the soft palate. The infant should be able to suck smoothly and evenly in a wavelike motion of the tongue as the finger is drawn in for suckling. The hard and soft palate should be intact, without palpable clefts or submucosal clefts. The infant should be able to extend the tongue over the lower gum with no evidence of a tight frenulum. In the process of the examination, the infant's state of alertness and readiness for feeding are also observed.

■ POSITIONS FOR BREASTFEEDING

Getting off to a good start begins with positioning the baby at the breast in a way that is comfortable for both the mother and baby and that allows for good latch-on. The three most common positions are the cradle, side-lying, and football-hold positions.

PRINCIPLES OF CORRECT POSITIONING

Several principles are common to all of the various positions for breastfeeding, including the following:
- Both the mother and the baby should be comfortable.
- The infant should be positioned "face on" at nipple height so that no head turning or tilting is required. The nipple should be directed toward the center of the infant's mouth.
- The infant should be lying on the side, not the back.
- The infant's body should be in good alignment, with a straight line from the ear to the shoulder to the hips.
- The infant's top and bottom lips should be flanged out (Fig. 12-4).
- The infant's tongue should extend forward over the lower gum line and cup around the nipple and areola.
- Good latch-on results in quiet feedings. No "clicking" or "popping" sounds should be heard from the infant. After mother's milk is in, audible swallowing, such as a "glug" or air blowing out the baby's nose, should be heard.

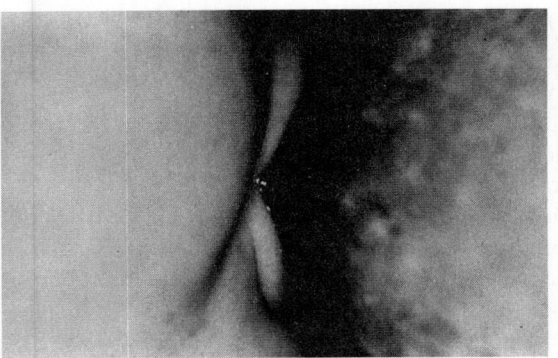

FIG. 12-4   Lip position. (Courtesy UNICEF.)

CRADLE POSITION

The cradle position (also called the Madonna or cuddle position) and its variation, known as the cross-cradle position, begin with the mother sitting upright or leaning slightly forward with her feet on the floor or stool or her legs crossed in front of her. The infant is held with the mouth at nipple height, and the mother and infant are in a tummy-to-tummy arrangement. The mother uses her free hand to support the breast, if needed, while keeping her fingers well back from the areola so that she does not interfere with latch-on. The "cigarette hold," or pinching of the breast tissue, should not be used. In the regular cradle position, the baby's head is supported in the crook of the elbow on the same side as the breast being suckled (Fig. 12-5). In the cross-cradle position, the opposite hand supports the baby's head and shoulders. This position often works well for a premature infant because it provides extra support to the head and trunk.

After positioning the baby, the mother should touch the baby's lower lip with her nipple to stimulate mouth opening.

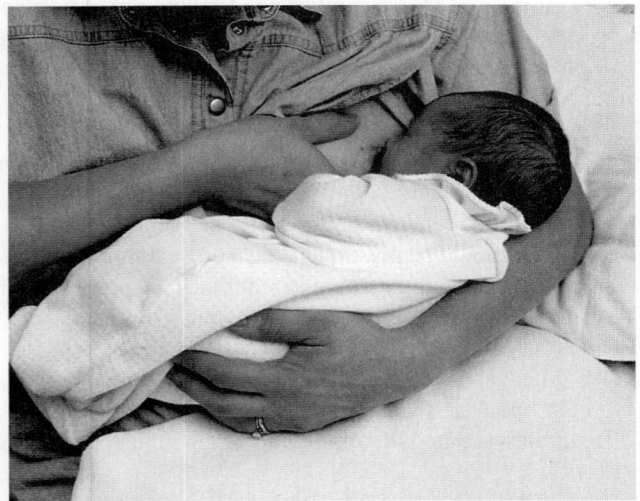

FIG. 12-5   Cradle hold. The mother positions the infant's head at or near the antecubital space and level with her nipple with her arm supporting the infant's body. Her other hand is free to hold the breast. Once the infant is positioned, pillows or blankets can be used to support the mother's arm, which may tire from holding the baby. (From McKinney ES et al: *Maternal-child nursing,* Philadelphia, 2002, WB Saunders.)

As the mouth opens, the mother should bring the baby close so that the lips come up and over the nipple and back onto the areolar tissue and the nipple rests on top of the baby's tongue. Once the baby appears latched on, the mother can check the lips for a flanged, open placement. At this point, the baby is very close to the breast, with the tip of the infant's nose touching it. Mothers often need to be shown that the baby is able to breathe without a need to press down on the breast tissue. If the baby appears to be pushed into the breast, the infant's buttocks should be brought closer into the tummy-to-tummy position. As the mother looks down at her baby, she should see a straight line from the baby's ear to the shoulders to the hips. Once the baby is suckling well, the mother can usually remove the hand that was supporting her breast and use it to cradle the baby in her arms. She can also relax back from the forward-leaning position that she used at the beginning.

SIDE-LYING POSITION

The side-lying or other lying-down variations are often helpful when the mother is uncomfortable sitting up or wishes to nap or sleep with her baby. In the early days of learning to achieve latch-on, the side-lying position is not easy to use because the mother cannot see her breast and nipple quite as well. In the hospital, a nurse should be available to help the mother and infant. At home and with practice, the mother and infant can achieve latch-on without assistance.

In the side-lying position, the mother lies on her side, cradles her infant in her elbow, and supports the infant's back and neck. The mother or the nurse should arrange one to two pillows under the mother's head and shoulders and a rolled towel or blanket along the infant's back to keep the infant in a side-lying position. As in the cradle position, the mother may support her breast with her upper hand (Fig. 12-6).

FOOTBALL HOLD

In the football hold, the infant is supported off to the side of the mother. This position is often used by a mother who has had a cesarean delivery because it does not require that the infant be positioned along her abdomen or by a mother of multiples when she would like to feed two babies at once. Finally, mothers with flat or inverted nipples are often able to achieve latch-on more easily with this position.

One or two firm pillows should be placed at the mother's side to help support the infant. The baby is in a side-lying position and flexed at the hips, with the buttocks back against the chair or couch. As in other positions, the mother may support her breast to assist with latch-on and remove her hand once the baby is suckling well (Fig. 12-7).

▄▄▄ DYNAMICS OF BREASTFEEDING
EARLY FEEDINGS

The first breastfeeding should take place as soon after birth as possible. Full term neonates often have an alert period for 30 to 60 minutes after delivery that is ideal for the first feeding practice. This first feeding can take place in the delivery

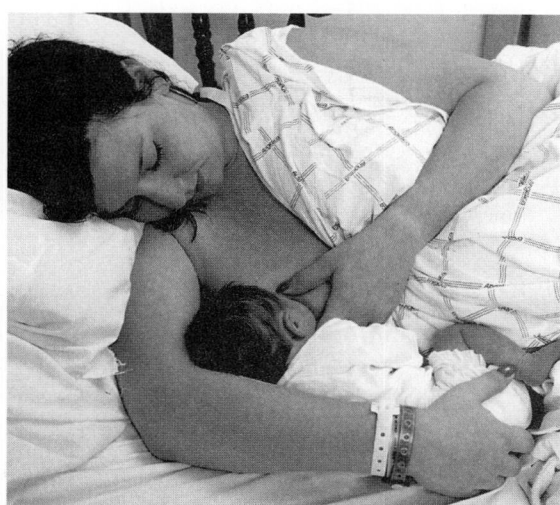

FIG. 12-6   The side-lying position prevents pressure on episiotomy or abdominal incisions and allows the mother to rest while feeding. She lies on her side, with her lower arm supporting her head or placed around the infant. A pillow behind her back and between her legs provides comfort. Her upper hand and arm are used to position the infant on the side at nipple level and hold the breast. When the infant's mouth opens to nurse, the mother leans slightly forward or draws the infant to her to insert the nipple into the mouth. (From McKinney ES et al: *Maternal-child nursing*, Philadelphia, 2002, WB Saunders.)

area, if necessary, and should be encouraged by all in attendance. It will not delay, to any significant extent, any procedures required, such as weighing and measuring the infant, instilling ointment or drops in the infant's eyes, and giving vitamin K injections. These procedures can be done one at a

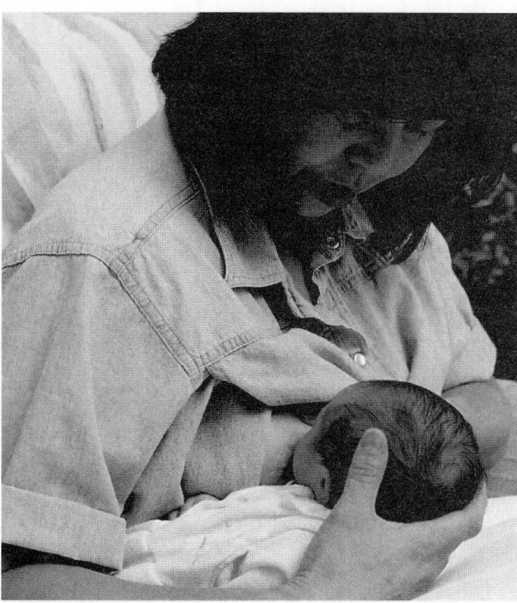

FIG. 12-7   Football hold. The mother supports the infant's head in her hand, with the infant's body resting on pillows alongside her hip. This method allows the mother to see the position of the infant's mouth on the breast, helps her control the infant's head, and is especially helpful for mothers with heavy breasts. This hold also prevents pressure against an abdominal incision. (From McKinney ES et al: *Maternal-child nursing*, Philadelphia, 2002, WB Saunders.)

time in the delivery room or at the bedside after return to the room. The mother and infant should remain together as much as possible, with rooming-in preferable. The family needs to be encouraged and supported to make their desire to promote close contact and initiate breastfeeding known to the staff. In addition, the health care provider should advocate changes in institutional policy to support the needs of breastfeeding families.

The infant usually goes into a deep sleep after the initial alertness and is difficult to wake for feeding practice. Parents should be instructed to watch for any awakening behavior, such as opening eyes or movement in the bed. Many newborns will not cry at this point, so parents need to be alert for these signs of feeding readiness. Full term infants are born with stores of fluid and energy to carry them through this early transition to the nonuterine environment, a time of infrequent feeding and low volume of colostrum. The infant's stomach, liver, and kidneys are gearing up for the larger volumes of higher-fat food that will come in a few days. It is not necessary to provide any supplement, including water, to a healthy, full term neonate. In addition, feeding with a rubber or silicone nipple may lead to nipple confusion because it does not work like the breast in delivering milk.

During this transition time, assistance and support from an individual knowledgeable in breastfeeding can be helpful to the mother and infant as they practice latch-on and suckling. The infant should be encouraged to go to each breast for at least 10 to 15 minutes of active suckling, although some infants may spend even longer. The infant's behavior is much more important during this time than the clock. However, an infant who falls asleep in 5 minutes should be stimulated to continue active suckling. Attention to proper positioning and technique becomes important as the frequency and duration of the suckling behavior increase. A mother is unlikely to get sore or cracked nipples when her infant is latched on correctly. These early feedings are excellent "practice" sessions both for the mother, who gains confidence in her breastfeeding ability, and for the infant, who gets first colostrum and then milk for the efforts at suckling.

The goal of discharge planning is to maintain successful breastfeeding and includes the following:

- Review proper positioning.
- Review signs of good latch-on.
- Review signs of infant progress indicating adequate nutrition (Table 12-2).
- Arrange daily follow-up for 2 to 3 days after discharge.
- Provide a phone contact for questions and concerns.
- Encourage the mother to contact breastfeeding resources whenever she has questions.

These early efforts to provide contact and support during the transition to home can make all the difference in maintaining breastfeeding. Problems encountered during engorgement, sleep deprivation, and times of uncertainty or lack of confidence can be addressed quickly and directly rather than after a bottle has been introduced or the mother's nipples are cracked and bleeding.

TABLE 12-2   Signs of Infant Progress: A Handout for Parents

	First 8hr	8-24hr	Day 2	Day 3	Day 4	Day 5	Day 6 on
Milk supply	You may be able to express a few drops of milk.		Milk should come in between the second and fourth day.			Milk should be in. Breasts may be firm or leak milk.	Breasts should feel softer after nursing. Baby should appear satisfied after feeding.
Baby's activity	Baby is usually wide awake in first hr of life. Put to breast within ½hr of birth.	Wake your baby. Babies may not awaken on their own to feed.	Baby should be more cooperative and less sleepy.	Look for early feeding cues: rooting, lip smacking, hands to face. Note that baby swallows regularly while nursing.			
Feeding routine	Baby may go into a deep sleep 2-4hr after birth.	Feed your baby every 1½-3hr or as often as wanted.	Feedings should be at least 8-10 times each day.			May go up to 5hr between feedings (once in a 24-hr period).	
Breastfeeding	Baby will wake up and be alert and responsive for several more hours after the initial deep sleep.	Nurse at both breasts as long as baby is actively suckling and mother is comfortable.	Try to nurse on both breasts at each feeding, aiming for 10-15 min each side. Expect some nipple tenderness.	Consider hand expressing or pumping a few drops of milk to soften the nipple if the breast is too firm for the baby to latch-on.	Nurse at least 10-15 min each side every 2-3hr for the first few months of life.		Mother's nipple tenderness is decreased or gone.
Baby's urine output		Baby must have at least 1 wet diaper in first 24hr.	Baby should have at least 1 wet diaper every 8hr.	Wet diapers should increase to 4 to 6 in 24hr.	Baby's urine should be light yellow.	Baby should have 6 to 8 wet diapers per day of colorless or light yellow urine.	
Baby's stools		Baby should have a black-green stool (meconium stool).	Baby may have a second very dark (meconium) stool.	Baby's stools should be changing from black-green to yellow.		Baby should have 3 to 4 yellow, seedy stools per day.	The number of stools may slowly decrease after 4-6wk.

hr, Hour(s); *min*, minute(s); *wk*, week(s).
From Thilo EH, Townsend SF: Early newborn discharge: have we gone too far? *Contemp Pediatr* 13:29-46, 1996.

FREQUENCY AND DURATION OF FEEDINGS

After the first 24 hours, the infant should be going to the breast 8 to 12 times (or every 2 to 3 hours) in 24 hours for approximately 20 to 45 minutes at each feeding. Frequent suckling stimulates milk production and establishes a regular routine. Exclusive breastfeeding for the first month should be encouraged to ensure the establishment of adequate milk supply and prevent any nipple confusion. Parents need to be alert for an infant who sleeps for 4 to 5 hours at a time or who goes to sleep at the breast in 5 minutes. These infants must be actively wakened and stimulated for feeding.

If the mother and infant must be separated for one or more feedings or supplements are medically necessary, they may be given with a dropper, a cup, or a 5-French feeding tube placed at the breast. Proper instructions, close supervision, and follow-up are needed for each of these methods, and they should not be used routinely.

URINE AND STOOL OUTPUT GUIDELINES

Urine

In the first 2 days of life as the volume of breast milk is increasing, the infant may urinate only one to three times in 24 hours. By day 3, the infant should have 4 or more wet diapers in 24 hours and then, by day 4, four to six wet diapers per 24 hours. Over time, the infant should have a minimum of six to eight wet diapers in a 24-hour period. The urine should be light yellow with no strong odor. If the parents are anxious or if they have a question about breastfeeding progress, a diary of wet diapers can be kept to aid in the accurate assessment of progress. Parents need to be alerted, however, to the difficulty of doing accurate diaper counts with disposable diapers and may elect to insert a tissue liner into the diaper or to use cloth diapers for the first few weeks. Ultraabsorbent diapers should be avoided when close monitoring of output is necessary.

Stool

In the first 24 hours after delivery, the baby should have at least one meconium stool followed by another on the second day of life. By day 3, stools are beginning to make the transition to the characteristic loose, yellow, seedy stools of breastfeeding, and the infant should begin having two to three stools in 24 hours. That number may continue to increase in the first few weeks of life. Some infants stool with every feeding. After the first month, the pattern may change again because some infants begin to stool less frequently and may go several days between stools. As long as the infant is healthy and gaining weight, there is no problem. However, infrequent stooling, especially in the first month, should stimulate a feeding history and possibly a weight check to make sure that the infant is getting enough breast milk.

PUMPING

Routine pumping is unnecessary for mothers who are available for a feeding every 2 to 4 hours. However, if the mother and infant must be separated for more than one or two feedings, pumping should be part of the plan to assist with milk production.

If the mother and infant are separated right after birth, pumping should begin as soon as possible, within the first 24 hours. The mother should pump 6 to 8 times in 24 hours for 15 minutes if she is using a double-pump setup or 10 minutes per breast if she is using a single-pump setup. She should be encouraged to save even the smallest amounts of colostrum to be given to her infant.

Hand expression and manual pumps work well for infrequent or short-duration pumping. However, a hospital-grade, piston-style pump that permits pumping both breasts at the same time is ideal for a mother who will have to pump for several weeks or months. No pump works as well as an infant in stimulating production, but frequent pumping goes a long way toward establishing a milk supply and provides the mother a concrete, healthful contribution to her sick or preterm infant. As the volume of milk goes up over the first few days, the mother can see the success of her efforts. She should be counseled about the increase in production in contrast to the small volume of colostrum produced in the first few days.

COLLECTION AND STORAGE OF BREAST MILK

A mother who is pumping should be reminded to wash her hands well before she begins pumping and to use clean containers for collection and storage. In addition, the pump parts should be thoroughly cleaned after each use. Many of the pump parts can go through a dishwasher, but the directions that come with the pump should be consulted for specific instructions on cleaning.

Milk collected from pumping should be stored in clean plastic bottles or disposable milk bags. It is preferable to store breast milk in small amounts so that only the amount that is needed is defrosted and used. Milk that has been defrosted and not used within 24 hours should be discarded. Pumped breast milk should be refrigerated as soon after pumping as possible and can be stored there for up to 8 days. It can be stored on "blue ice" in a cooler for about 24 hours. If it is not going to be used in that time, it should be frozen. In a refrigerator freezer that maintains a steady temperature, breast milk can be stored for 3 months. Breast milk can be stored for up to 12 months in a freezer where 0° F is routinely maintained (Jones & Tully, 2005). The bottles or bags should be labeled with the date of collection so that the oldest milk can be used first. If the milk must be transported to the hospital or day care facility, it should be placed in ice or on a blue ice unit to minimize the amount of warming or thawing.

INFANT WEIGHT GAIN

Normal newborn infants lose 5% to 8% of their birth weight in the first few days of life. It is helpful for parents to be aware of both the birth and discharge weights. Once the maternal milk volume increases, the infant begins to gain weight in the range of 0.5 to 1 oz/day or 4 to 7 oz/wk. Most breastfed infants have regained their birth weight by 2 weeks. One criterion for failure to thrive is lack of return to birth weight by 3 weeks. Breastfed infants usually double their birth weight by 5 to 6 months old and triple it by 1 year old.

An early study of the growth patterns and nutrient intake of a cohort of breastfed and formula-fed infants has presented evidence that breastfed babies gain at a slower rate after the first 3 months (Dewey et al, 1992). More recent research indicates that breastfed infants may grow more rapidly initially, then slow their weight-for-age gain between 3 and 12 months, but catch up by 12 months. Head circumference showed no significant difference at any age (Kramer et al, 2002).

An infant who has followed the growth grid curves until 3 or 4 months and then falls slightly may be growing at a normal rate for a breastfed infant. In the absence of growth grids specifically designed for breastfed infants, an important consideration in assessing an apparently slowly gaining infant is developmental progress and other measures of growth. Characteristics of a healthy, but slowly growing, breastfed infant include the following:

- Active and alert state
- Developmentally appropriate progress
- Age-appropriate height and head circumference
- Good skin turgor and color
- Sufficient output of at least six wet diapers and several stools per day
- Contented and satisfied behavior after feeding

GROWTH SPURTS

Just when the parents begin to think that breastfeeding is going well, the first growth spurt occurs and can once again arouse their concern. The term *growth spurt* is often used to describe those recurring times during breastfeeding when the baby's growth exceeds the breast milk supply at that moment. For 2 to 4 days, the infant feeds more frequently to increase milk production. However, an inexperienced parent may interpret this behavior as a sign of inadequate milk production and begin supplementation. This practice leads to inadequate breast milk volume, whereas allowing and even encouraging more frequent breastfeeding results in an appropriate increase in milk production. Once the level of milk production has risen, the infant returns to the normal feeding pattern. Growth spurts tend to occur every 3 to 4 weeks, but parents seem to notice them less as time goes on. The behavior becomes an expected part of the breastfeeding experience.

WEANING

The decision about the time for weaning is an individual one. Breastfeeding should be encouraged for at least 1 year, but individual circumstances may dictate a different choice for a family. Sometimes weaning is led by the mother and other times by the infant. Typically a natural weaning process occurs as other foods become a part of the infant's diet and the infant begins to participate in self-feeding. When a family inquires about the ideal time to begin weaning, the provider can counsel them to consider factors, such as the following:

- Beliefs and desires of individual family members
- Developmental readiness of the infant
- Nutritional replacements for breast milk
- Social and environmental issues affecting the decision

Whether weaning occurs as a planned or unplanned activity, it is best to implement it gradually. If necessary the mother can use a breast pump to gradually decrease milk production

and prevent breast engorgement, blocked ducts, and discomfort. A good approach is to pump when uncomfortable and to pump only to comfort, not to empty. In situations where weaning was not an anticipated or planned event, the health care provider may help the mother deal not only with the act of weaning but also with her feelings about it. Some mothers grieve the early loss of the breastfeeding experience.

In an effort to prevent premature weaning, the providers should maintain close communication with families, especially those who are more likely to wean early. Early identification and support of these families may assist them to continue breastfeeding for a longer period. Factors associated with early weaning include the following:

- Non-Hispanic black mothers
- Younger, poorer mothers
- Lower maternal education
- Early return of the mother to work outside the home
- Lack of support from family or health professionals
- Previous breastfeeding failure

MATERNAL NUTRITIONAL NEEDS DURING BREASTFEEDING

Maternal nutritional needs increase during lactation. Characteristics of a good diet include the following:

- A minimum of 1800 calories
- An additional 500 calories more than the nonpregnant diet
- Generous intake of fruits and vegetables, whole grain breads and cereals, calcium-rich dairy products, and protein-rich meats, fish, and legumes
- Rich sources of calcium, zinc, folate, magnesium, and vitamin B_6
- Culturally appropriate foods
- Supplementation with calcium or prenatal vitamins or both only if the diet is poor (Lawrence & Lawrence, 2005)

The mother should be encouraged to eat well for her own sake to keep herself healthy and to meet the energy demands of nursing. In addition, an adequate intake of fluid is necessary, but excessive use of fluids does not increase breast milk production. A good guideline for adequate fluid intake is maternal urine that is light yellow and has no strong odor. Eligible mothers and infants should be referred to the Women, Infants, and Children (WIC) special supplemental food program for nutritional counseling and for food supplements. Most WIC programs offer food supplements for the breastfeeding mother's diet because she does not need formula for the infant. Even with a diet that is adequate in nutrients and calories, a gradual maternal weight loss of 1 to 2 lb per month usually occurs. In fact breastfeeding is the ideal way for a mother to return to her prepregnancy weight.

No foods need to be routinely excluded from the maternal diet unless there is evidence that a particular food bothers the infant or the infant appears to be allergic to it. Sometimes the food does not need to be eliminated but merely decreased. Maternal intake of cow's milk products has been associated with colic, and some highly allergic babies are sensitive to their mother's intake of saturated fats (Hoppu et al, 2000). When a mother has markedly decreased or eliminated cow's milk from her diet, she must add another source of calcium.

Certain foods, such as onions and garlic, may change the flavor and odor of the milk, but do not negatively affect its quality. The nutrient characteristics of breast milk are fairly stable. One positive way to look at the variety of foods in the diets of mothers from all over the world is to acknowledge that infants are getting early exposure to the foods of their culture.

Increased alcohol intake does not improve lactational performance, and intake of an amount more than 0.5 g/kg of maternal body weight (2 cans of beer, 8 oz of wine, or 2 to 2.5 oz of liquor) can impair the milk ejection reflex (Institute of Medicine, 1991). The occasional use of small amounts of alcohol need not be avoided, but regular use should be discouraged.

Large amounts of caffeine from coffee, sodas, or chocolate should be discouraged because caffeine is associated with jitteriness in the infant and may have a negative effect on the iron content of the breast milk. However, the equivalent of one to two cups of coffee per day should pose no problem (Institute of Medicine, 1991).

RETURNING TO WORK

Women who return to work outside the home after initiating breastfeeding should be encouraged to continue breastfeeding and be supported in their decision with accurate information about how to manage both work and breastfeeding. The mother can be assisted to investigate her work environment by use of tools, such as a breastfeeding assessment worksheet that reviews type of work performed and where, space for pumping and storing, and individuals and policies that support her intention (Bar-Yam, 1998). The ideal work environment provides the following:

- Breaks or lunchtime (or both) in which the mother can pump or go to the infant
- A private, convenient location for pumping with access to a sink for washing up and a refrigerator for storage
- Supportive colleagues and supervisors

In addition to providing information regarding pumping, storing, and transporting breast milk; introducing the bottle; and handling the challenges of multiple demands (Box 12-1), providers can support community initiatives that promote these conditions in employment settings. Women are more likely to continue breastfeeding if they have workplace support (Ortiz et al, 2004), and employers also benefit from breastfeeding mothers whose infants tend to be healthier (Ball & Bennett, 2001).

■ MEDICATIONS FOR BREASTFEEDING MOTHERS

Frequently, women question whether they can take certain medications while they are breastfeeding. Concerns relate primarily to two areas—the effect of the drug on maternal milk supply and the effect of the drug on the infant. General guidelines for maternal drug recommendations include the following:

- Give drugs that are normally safe for infants or have been tested in infants.
- Avoid long-acting forms of a drug.

BOX 12-1 Advice for Mothers on Returning to Work

Before Delivery
Discuss plans with employer before maternity leave.
Provide employer with information to help in planning (see www.usbreastfeeding.org).
Discuss options with other employees who have continued to breastfeed after returning to work.
Gain support of co-workers.
Investigate pumps, including rental or purchase.
Identify place to pump and to store breast milk at work.

During Maternity Leave
Practice method of breast milk expression that will be used at work.
Begin freezing milk.
Introduce bottle after breastfeeding is well established (usually around 3 to 4 weeks).

After Return to Work
If available use on-site or nearby child care, so you can go to infant during day.
Ask employer if caregiver for child can bring infant on-site once a day to nurse.
If possible arrange work hours to maximize times to nurse infant (e.g., arrive at work at 8:30 instead of 8:00).
Have a picture of your baby at the pump.
Plan on 15 to 30 minutes to complete pumping.
Wear clothes for easy access to breasts and to hide leaks.

Feeding Breast Milk
Warm or thaw milk in warm water.
Do not use microwave because milk heats unevenly and presents a risk for burns.
Refrigerate thawed milk for no more than 24 hours; do not refreeze.
Do not add milk to a bottle that has already been used.

Important Reminders
Wash hands before and after pumping.
Rinse pump parts with cool water, then wash with dish detergent and rinse well after each use.

Tully MR: Working & breastfeeding: helping moms and employers figure it out, *AWHONN Lifelines* 9(3):198-203, 2005.

- Schedule feeding at times when the drug level is lowest. Often breastfeeding immediately after taking the drug is the safest time.
- Observe the infant for changes in feeding pattern, fussiness, vomiting or diarrhea, or rash.
- Consider all appropriate options and select the drug with the lowest level in breast milk.
- Avoid drugs that inhibit prolactin release, such as estrogen, antihistamines, and ergot compounds.
- Be cautious about the use of herbal preparations.

The AAP committee on drugs (2001) has developed eight categories of drugs grouped by their risk factors for breastfeeding. Four of these groups are summarized in Table 12-3, including drugs that:

TABLE 12-3 Medications Affecting Breastfeeding

Contraindicated Drugs	Drugs Requiring Temporary Cessation of Breastfeeding	Drugs Whose Effect Is Unknown	Drugs Associated With Significant Effects: Give With Caution
Amphetamine Bromocriptine Cocaine Cyclophosphamide Cyclosporine Doxorubicin Ergotamine Lithium Methotrexate Phencyclidine (PCP) Phenindione	Radioactive compounds, such as • ^{64}Cu • ^{67}Ga • ^{111}In, ^{123}I, ^{125}I, ^{131}I • Radioactive sodium • ^{99m}Tc, ^{99m}TcO$_4$ Need to stop breastfeeding for a minimum of 5 half-lives of the drug. Milk samples can be screened by radiology departments for radioactivity before resuming breastfeeding	Antidepressants • Amitriptyline • Amoxapine • Bupropion • Clomipramine • Desipramine • Dothiepin • Doxepin • Fluoxetine • Fluvoxamine • Imipramine • Nortriptyline • Paroxetine • Sertraline • Trazodone Antianxieties • Alprazolam • Diazepam • Lorazepam • Midazolam • Perphenazine • Prazepam • Quazepam • Temazepam Antipsychotics • Chlorpromazine • Chlorprothixene • Clozapine • Haloperidol • Mesoridazine • Trifluoperazine Others • Amiodarone • Chloramphenicol • Clofazimine • Lamotrigine • Metoclopramide • Metronidazole • Tinidazole	Acebutolol 5-aminosalicylic acid Aspirin Atenolol Clemastine Phenobarbital Primidone Sulfasalazine

Data from American Academy of Pediatrics (AAP) Committee on Drugs: The transfer of drugs and other chemicals into human milk, *Pediatrics* 108:776-789, 2001.

• Are contraindicated
• Require temporary cessation of breastfeeding
• Have an unknown effect on nursing, but may be of concern
• Have been associated with significant effects on some infants and should be used with caution

A good drug reference should be available to providers. Four excellent resources are shown in Box 12-2. Decisions about drug selection are difficult, especially when contraindicated drugs are being considered, but the consequences of weaning and loss of breast milk for the infant must be included in the deliberations.

BOX 12-2 Drug References

American Academy of Pediatrics (AAP) Committee on Drugs: The transfer of drugs and other chemicals into human milk, *Pediatrics* 108:776-789, 2001.

Hale TW: *Medications and mothers' milk*, Amarillo, TX, 2006, Pharmasoft Medical Publishing. Updated and reprinted every other year. Order from 800-378-1317 or *www.ibreastfeeding.com*.

Lawrence RA, Lawrence RM: *Breastfeeding: a guide for the medical profession*, ed 6, St. Louis, 2005, Mosby.

Wynne AL, Woo T, Millard M: *Pharmacotherapeutics for nurse practitioner prescribers*, Philadelphia, 2002, FA Davis.

■ COMMON BREASTFEEDING PROBLEMS

FLAT OR INVERTED NIPPLES

Description

A nipple can look as though it is inverted, but a "pinch test" is necessary to determine what happens to the nipple during breastfeeding (see the previous description and Fig. 12-3 for the technique). If the nipple pulls in, it is considered to be inverted. If the nipple does not pull in, as happens most often, or everts with compression, it is considered to be flat.

Inverted nipples can make it more difficult for the infant to latch-on in the early days because it is harder to pull the nipple into the mouth for suckling. As the baby continues to breastfeed, the nipple tissue elongates, and with time the problem usually becomes less severe, and successful breastfeeding is possible. Flat nipples do not generally change over time, but the infant develops a style to more easily latch-on successfully.

Epidemiology

Adhesions cause retraction or inversion of the nipples. Flat nipples are often found in women with larger breasts.

Differential Diagnosis

The differential diagnosis for flat or inverted nipples is dimpled, fissured, or unusually shaped nipples.

Management

Prenatal. If the patient is not at risk for preterm labor, breast shells can be used during the third trimester for inverted nipples. The obstetrician or nurse-midwife should be notified before their use. Shells are plastic, dome-shaped devices with small holes for ventilation. An opening in the portion that lies against the skin fits over the nipple, and gentle suction during use helps stretch the nipple tissue (Fig. 12-8). The bra cup holds the shell comfortably in place, and the use of shells during the last trimester generally helps stretch out adhesions in preparation for breastfeeding.

Postpartum. The provider should stay with the mother during early feeding attempts; give extra praise, reassurance, and support; and emphasize the need for extra patience and persistence. Encourage use of the football-hold position during feedings and have the mother lean slightly forward as she latches the baby on.

The mother should do the following:
- Wear breast shells between feedings.
- Manually pull or roll the nipple immediately before latch-on.

- Use a breast pump for 1 or 2 minutes before latch-on.
- Put a cold cloth or ice on the nipple for a few seconds.
- Avoid pacifiers and bottle nipples until the infant is 4 to 6 weeks old.
- If supplementation is medically indicated, use a syringe, dropper, feeding tube, or supplemental nutrition system (Fig. 12-9).

Although there are arguments against the use of nipple shields, in some cases their use may prevent premature weaning (Chertok et al, 2006), and they have been shown to increase milk intake by preterm infants (Meier et al, 2000). Every mother-infant dyad should be uniquely assessed and managed, and for some infants, use of a thin, silicone nipple shield may ensure continued breastfeeding. Cleansing and drying both the shields and breast after feeding is important to prevent skin breakdown and infection.

Complications

Complications of flat or inverted nipples include the following:
- Frustration
- Loss of self-confidence
- Inadequate infant nutrition and its sequelae
- Severe maternal engorgement, plugged ducts, or mastitis
- Discontinued breastfeeding

SORE NIPPLES

Description

Soreness of the nipples is pain caused by irritation or trauma to the nipples and areola, often accompanied by a breakdown in skin integrity.

Epidemiology

Sore nipples have many causes, including the following:
- Improper latch-on and positioning at the breast
- Prolonged negative pressure
- Inappropriate suction release from the breast
- Use of or sensitivity to nipple creams and oils
- Incorrect use of breastfeeding supplies (e.g., pumps, shells, shields)
- Thrush (candidiasis)
- Leaking nipples that are not properly air-dried

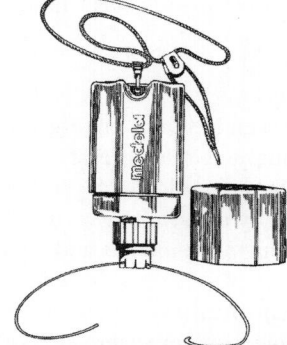

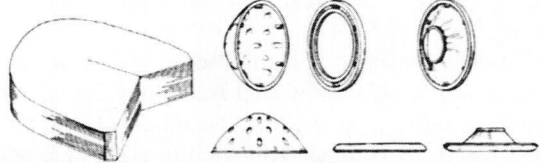

FIG. 12-8   Breast shells. (Courtesy Medela.)

FIG. 12-9   Supplemental nursing system. (Courtesy Medela.)

Clinical Findings

The nipples, areolae, and breasts are tender, bruised, raw, cracked, bleeding, blistered, discolored, swollen, or traumatized.

Differential Diagnosis

The differential diagnoses for sore nipples include the following:

- Mild tenderness, which is sometimes described by new mothers as they are getting used to the infant's suckling
- Breast or nipple trauma from another cause
- Thrush (candidiasis)
- Mastitis
- Abscess
- Milk plugs at the nipple pores

Management

The following measures can be taken to manage sore nipples:

- Assess breastfeeding at an early feeding. Prevent the problem by demonstrating and reinforcing the proper latch-on technique and positioning of the infant.
- Counsel mothers to seek help early for more than mild tenderness. Nipples can be damaged by constant high negative pressure and do not "toughen up" as breastfeeding progresses. Cracking and bleeding are not normal.
- Rub a few drops of colostrum or hindmilk onto the nipple and areola after every feeding and let it air-dry.
- Expose the nipples to air for short periods several times a day.
- Use breast shells to prevent the bra or clothing from rubbing against the nipple.
- Nurse from the least sore side first.
- Use short, frequent feedings.
- Pump the affected breast if pain is too severe to allow nursing.
- Use mild analgesics, as necessary.
- Refer to a lactation specialist as appropriate.

SEVERE ENGORGEMENT

Description

Severe engorgement is characterized by extremely full, sore, and swollen breasts, beyond the normal fullness experienced as the milk comes in.

Epidemiology

Engorgement is caused by milk stasis in the breast from inadequate emptying.

Clinical Findings

The following are seen in severe engorgement:

- Painful, hard, lumpy, swollen breasts
- Breasts usually warm to the touch
- Nipples flattened by the swelling
- Bruising or trauma to the nipples and areolae

Differential Diagnosis

The differential diagnosis for severe engorgement is bilateral mastitis.

Management

The following measures can be taken to manage engorgement:

- Take a hot shower or wrap the breasts with warm, wet compresses for 5 to 10 minutes before nursing. Disposable diapers can be wet with hot water and then wrapped around each breast and "tabbed" to hold them in place. The plastic liner holds the heat in longer than an ordinary washcloth or towel does.
- Gently massage the entire breast or use an electric pump with intermittent suction on the minimal setting for several minutes after using wet heat.
- Manually express milk before feeding to soften the areola and make it easier for the infant to latch-on properly.
- Nurse frequently and make certain that latch-on and position are correct, and audible swallowing is heard.
- Avoid long stretches between feedings in the early weeks as the milk supply is being established. Pump the breasts if a feeding will be missed.

MASTITIS

Description

Although rarely seen in the postpartum hospital setting, mastitis is an infection of the breast that can occur at any time during lactation. Occasionally, it has been identified during the third trimester of pregnancy.

Epidemiology

Staphylococcus aureus is most commonly associated with mastitis, but *Escherichia coli* and, more rarely, various streptococci are also found (Foxman et al, 2002). Predisposing factors include the following:

- Stress, fatigue
- Cracked nipples, plugged ducts
- Constricting, improperly fitting bra
- Inadequate emptying of the breast
- Sudden weaning or a significant decrease in the number of feedings
- Using a manual pump

Clinical Findings

The following are seen in mastitis:

- Malaise
- Breast tenderness or pain
- A reddened, warm lump in any quadrant, sometimes associated with red streaking
- Flulike symptoms, including fever, chills, and body aches

An old adage is that the "flu" in a breastfeeding woman is mastitis until proved otherwise.

Management

Recommendations for treatment of mastitis include the following:

- Penicillinase-resistant penicillin or a cephalosporin that covers *S. aureus*. Currently, dicloxacillin is most commonly recommended to treat mastitis. Treatment should be maintained for 10 to 14 days. Amoxicillin-clavulanic acid and cefuroxime have been found to be effective with few adverse effects, though more studies are recommended (Benyamini et al, 2005).

- Fluconazole has been used for candida-caused mastitis (Chetwynd et al, 2002).
- Rest (extremely important).
- Nurse frequently, or if pain is severe, pump milk carefully from the affected breast. Breast milk is not infected and is fine for the infant.
- Do not wean abruptly because of the possibility of mastitis progressing into an abscess.
- Take warm showers or use warm wet compresses.
- Increase fluids.
- Use analgesics as necessary (Foxman et al, 2002; Lawrence & Lawrence, 2005).

Complications
Abscess and septicemia are complications of mastitis.

NIPPLE CONFUSION
Description
Nipple confusion occurs when an infant is accustomed to nursing from a bottle and is introduced to the breast. When offered the breast, these babies use the same sucking pattern as with a bottle, which makes it difficult to obtain adequate nourishment and may contribute to maternal sore nipples. They may cry, fuss, or push away with their arms during attempts to nurse.

Epidemiology
Different oral-motor skills are used in breastfeeding and bottle feeding, and infants who have been given a bottle or pacifier sometimes attempt to breastfeed as though they were bottle feeding. Use of pacifiers or bottles, especially in the neonatal period, are detrimental to breastfeeding (Howard et al, 2003). Thus, unless absolutely necessary, early bottlefeeding and pacifier use should be avoided in the breastfeeding infant.

Clinical Findings
The following are seen in nipple confusion:
- Ineffective suckling at the breast
- Breast refusal
- Sore, red, or bruised maternal nipples

Differential Diagnosis
The differential diagnoses for nipple confusion are other causes of fussiness and refusal to feed.

Management
The following are recommended to manage nipple confusion:
- Avoid all rubber bottle nipples and pacifiers for the first 4 to 6 weeks.
- Retrain the infant to suck correctly at the breast by correct positioning at the breast, proper latch-on technique, suck training to repattern tongue movements, and supplementation via alternative methods if required.
- Consult with a lactation specialist as indicated.

- If supplements are medically indicated, give with an eye-dropper, spoon, syringe, or cup or through a 5-French feeding tube (attached to a 20- or 30-ml syringe) taped to the areola or breast. The end of the tubing protrudes slightly past the end of the nipple so that the tube, nipple, and areola are in the infant's mouth.

As with management of inverted nipples, some infants who experience nipple confusion may continue to refuse the breast despite the best efforts of mothers and lactation specialists. When confronted with a decision of whether to continue to attempt to offer the breast (and maintaining a conflictive and frustrating interaction between the mother and baby), discontinue breastfeeding altogether or use a thin, silicone nipple shield and encourage the infant to suckle at the breast; mothers may decide to try the nipple shield. In some cases they are successful at getting latch-on and suckling until the breastfeeding difficulties can be resolved. Some mothers continue to breastfeed using the nipple shield for months or years. Infant weight gain must be monitored to ensure continued growth.

Complications
The following are complications of nipple confusion:
- Failure to thrive
- Hyperbilirubinemia
- Colic and crying
- Prolonged feedings
- Sore and cracked nipples
- Plugged ducts
- Mastitis
- Frustration

BREAST MILK JAUNDICE
Description
Breast milk (late onset) jaundice is an elevated serum indirect bilirubin concentration with the peak level occurring on or after the seventh to tenth day of life in an infant drinking an adequate amount of breast milk with no other signs of liver abnormality.

Epidemiology
The exact cause of breast milk jaundice is unknown; however, an enzyme may be present in some mothers' milk that inhibits the action of glucuronyl transferase and increases intestinal absorption of bilirubin. Breast milk jaundice is more common in Asian and North American Indian infants. Siblings with the same mother are often affected. True breast milk jaundice is uncommon and estimated to occur in less than 1 in 200 births (Lawrence & Lawrence, 2005).

Clinical Findings
Physical Examination. The following are seen with breast milk jaundice:
- Healthy and thriving infant
- Adequate stooling and voiding
- Appropriate weight gain
- Appearance of elevated bilirubin levels between the seventh and tenth day of life

- Bilirubin peaks around day 10 to 15
- Persistence into the third month of life

Diagnostic Tests. The following tests are usually indicated:

- Serum bilirubin
- Urine and other cultures, which are sometimes necessary to rule out infection

Differential Diagnosis

The differential diagnosis for breast milk jaundice is pathologic jaundice.

Management

In breast milk jaundice, breastfeeding should be continued unless clinical signs of pathologic jaundice are observed. See Chapter 38 for a discussion of pathologic jaundice. The family should be reassured that breast milk jaundice is not harmful.

THRUSH

When oral candidiasis is diagnosed in the infant or found on the nipple or areolae of the nursing mother, both members of the dyad should be treated. See Chapter 33 for a discussion of thrush.

POOR WEIGHT GAIN

Description

Problems associated with poor weight gain occur at two different times and represent different challenges for management. During the newborn period, initiation of breastfeeding may not proceed normally, and the infant may actually continue to lose weight or, at best, gain very slowly. After the newborn period, infants may gain weight more slowly than expected given normal parameters for their age.

Epidemiology

Poor weight gain has a number of contributing factors, including the following:

- Infrequent or inadequate feeding because of poorly managed breastfeeding or environmental or social circumstances in the family system
- Inadequate milk production
- Genetic predisposition
- Infection
- Organic disease
- Physical anomaly that prevents good suckling or swallowing

Clinical Findings

The following may be seen in poor weight gain:

INFANT FACTORS

- Continued weight loss after 5 to 7 days old
- Failure to regain birth weight by 2 to 3 weeks old
- Failure to maintain an ongoing weight gain of 0.5 to 1 oz/day
- Weight below the 3rd percentile for age (this finding can be a pattern over time or a sudden change)
- Lethargic, sleepy, inactive, unresponsive infant

- Newborn or young infant sleeping longer than 4 hours between feedings
- Dry mucous membranes
- Poor skin turgor

TECHNIQUE FACTORS

- Ineffective latch-on or sucking
- Short time at the breast (the infant is removed before nursing is finished, thus reducing access to hindmilk and total consumption)
- Infant kept on a preset schedule despite cues for more feeding
- Infant given water between feedings to "get through" to the next feeding
- Infant encouraged or allowed to sleep through the night before 8 to 12 weeks old
- Fewer than eight f eedings in 24 hours
- Infant fed in a distracting environment
- In older infants, breastfeeding offered after solids are given
- Infant in a day care setting that does not facilitate breastfeeding

MATERNAL FACTORS

- Does not initially respond to infant's cues for feeding or does not recognize that waking is needed to establish feeding
- Uses nipple shields
- Hectic schedule with limited time for breastfeeding
- Recent illness or significant weight loss
- Uses oral contraceptives or other hormones

Differential Diagnosis

The differential diagnoses for poor weight gain are a pattern of slower but normal weight gain in healthy breastfed infants and failure to thrive.

Management

The following measures should be taken to manage poor weight gain:

- Complete a thorough history to elicit information regarding infant and maternal factors.
- Conduct a thorough assessment of breastfeeding techniques to accurately determine the extent to which mismanagement is a cause.
- Provide instruction, encouragement, and reinforcement for correct breastfeeding techniques.
- Refer for treatment of physical or organic causes.
- Be alert for any infant who has lost too much weight and is unable to feed with vigor at the breast; such infants require an immediate infusion of calories for energy.
- Use a supplemental system at the breast if supplementation is required (see Fig. 12-9).
- Encourage and reassure the parents.

Complications

Complications of poor weight gain include developmental delay, poor bonding, and severe dehydration. In situations of early failure to establish breastfeeding, some infants may appear to be in a septic state and require hospitalization for rehydration and further evaluation.

NURSING DIAGNOSES

Related to Breastfeeding

- Effective breastfeeding
- Interrupted breastfeeding
- Ineffective breastfeeding

From NANDA International: *NANDA-I nursing diagnoses: definitions & classification 2007–2008*, Philadelphia, 2007, Author.

☑ DISCUSSION FORUM

1. Only 50% of women in your community breastfeed beyond 1 month postpartum. Discuss measures you could initiate to improve rates of breastfeeding in your community.
2. A 25-year-old mother of a 2-month-old is upset because she has to stop breastfeeding for 2 weeks as a result of her medical problems. She is doing well with nursing her thriving infant. How can you help her?
3. A mother of a 22-month-old states that she is still breastfeeding. She wants to stop, but does not know how. What additional information do you need? What advice would you give her?
4. You see a couple for a prenatal visit at 8 months gestation. You will be their primary pediatric provider. The woman states that she wants to breastfeed, but both members of the couple tell you that the father's family feels the baby should be fed formula. Discuss how you will approach this issue. What information and advice will you give to the couple?

RESOURCE BOX

Breastfeeding

Ameda-Egnell
www.hollister.com/us/mbc/breastfeeding
Breast pumps and breastfeeding products

Breastfeeding and Human Lactation Study Center
Department of Pediatrics
University of Rochester Medical Center
ruth_lawrence@urmc.rochester.edu

Centers for Disease Control and Prevention
www.cdc.gov/ncbddd/meds/
Information on medications and breastfeeding

Human Milk Banking Association of North America
www.hmbana.org
Guidelines and information on human milk banking; as a clearinghouse for member milk banks; currently lists 10 regionally located human milk banks in U.S.; 1 in Mexico; 1 in Canada

International Board of Lactation Consultant Examiners (IBLCE)
www.iblce.org
International board certification program for lactation consultants

International Lactation Consultant Association (ILCA)
www.ilca.org
Annual conference with continuing education programs and peer-reviewed professional journal, *Journal of Human Lactation*

Lactation Education Resources
www.leron-line.com
Education materials and training course; parent handouts

Lactation Institute
www.lactationinstitute.org
Programs for lactation consultant preparation, educational materials for families and health care providers, lactation educator program, specialized treatment center

La Leche League International
www.lalecheleague.org
Educational materials for breastfeeding families, annual workshops for lactation consultants and primary care providers

Medela, Inc.
www.medela.com
Breast pumps and breastfeeding products, referral hotline for consumers, corporate lactation program

National Alliance for Breastfeeding Advocacy
www.naba-breastfeeding.org
Continuing education programs, educational materials for families and health care providers; links to other breastfeeding resources and advocate groups

Nursing Mothers Counsel
www.nursingmothers.org
Support group for mothers

Rocky Mountain Poison and Drug Center
www.rmpdc.org
Pharmaceutical and over-the-counter medication and drug information and consultation services for health care providers; information on poisoning; link to other regional poisoning centers

Wellstart
www.wellstart.org
International educational programs, curricula, materials, speakers, conferences on breastfeeding

WHO Global Data Bank on Breastfeeding and Complementary Feeding
www.who.int/nutrition/databases/infantfeeding/en/index.html
International information and links on infant, child, and maternal nutrition; links to WHO-UNICEF Baby-Friendly Hospital Initiative

REFERENCES

American Academy of Pediatrics (AAP): Breastfeeding and the use of human milk, *Pediatrics* 115:496-506, 2005.

American Academy of Pediatrics (AAP) Committee on Drugs: The transfer of drugs and other chemicals into human milk, *Pediatrics* 108:776-789, 2001.

Baby-Friendly Hospital Initiative (BFHI) USA: *Baby-friendly hospitals and birth centers, as of August 2007.* Available at *www.babyfriendlyusa.org/eng/03.html* (accessed Oct 12, 2007).

Ball TM, Bennett DM: The economic impact of breastfeeding, *Pediatr Clin North Am* 48(1):253-262, 2001.

Bar-Yam N: Workplace lactation support, part I: a return-to-work breastfeeding assessment tool, *J Hum Lact* 14:249-254, 1998.

Benyamini L et al: The safety of amoxicillin/clavulanic acid and cefuroxime during lactation, *Ther Drug Monit* 27(4):499-502, 2005.

Centers for Disease Control and Prevention (CDC) National Immunization Program: *Breastfeeding: data and statistics: breastfeeding practices–results from the National Immunization Survey.* Available at *www.cdc.gov/breastfeeding/data/NIS_data/data_2004.htm* (accessed Aug 3, 2007).

Chantry CJ, Howard CR, Auinger P: Full breastfeeding duration and associated decrease in respiratory tract infection in US children, *Pediatrics* 117(2):425-432, 2006.

Chertok IR, Schneider J, Blackburn S: A pilot study of maternal and term infant outcomes associated with ultrathin nipple shield use, *J Obstet Gynecol Neonatal Nurs* 35(2):265-272, 2006.

Chetwynd EM et al: Fluconazole for postpartum candidal mastitis and infant thrush, *J Hum Lact* 18:168-171, 2002.

Collaborative Group on Hormonal Factors in Breast Cancer: Breast cancer and breastfeeding: collaborative reanalysis of individual data from 47 epidemiological studies in 30 countries, *Lancet* 360:187-195, 2002.

Correa S et al: Human colostrum contains IgA antibodies reactive to colonization factors I and II of enterotoxigenic *Escherichia coli*, *FEMS Immunol Med Microbiol* 47(2):199-206, 2006.

Dewey KG et al: Growth of breast-fed and formula-fed infants from 0 to 18 months: the DARLING study, *Pediatrics* 89:1035-1041, 1992.

Foxman B et al: Lactation mastitis: occurrence and medical management among 946 breastfeeding women in the United States, *Am J Epidemiol* 155:103-114, 2002.

Gartner LM, Greer FR: Section on Breastfeeding and Committee on Nutrition: Prevention of rickets and vitamin D deficiency: new guidelines for vitamin D intake, *Pediatrics* 111:908-910, 2003.

Hart S et al: Brief report: newborn behavior differs with decosahexaenoic acid levels in breast milk, *J Ped Psych* 31:221-226, 2006.

Heird WC, Lapillonne A: The role of essential fatty acids in development, *Annu Rev Nutr* 25:549-571, 2005.

Hoppu U, Kalliomaki M, Isolauri E: Maternal diet rich in saturated fat during breastfeeding is associated with atopic sensitization of the infant, *Eur J Clin Nutr* 54:702-705, 2000.

Howard et al: Randomized clinical trial of pacifier use and bottle-feeding or cup feeding and their effect on breastfeeding, *Pediatrics* 111(3):511-518, 2003.

Institute of Medicine Subcommittee on Lactation: *Nutrition during lactation*, Washington, DC, 1991, National Academies Press.

Jones F, Tully MR: *Best practice for expressing, storing, and handling human milk in hospitals, homes, and child care settings*, Raleigh NC, 2005, Human Milk Banking Association of North America.

Konek S, Mascarenhas MR: Vitamin deficiencies and excesses. In Burg FD et al, editors: *Current pediatric therapy*, ed 18, Philadelphia, 2006, WB Saunders.

Kramer MS et al: Breastfeeding and infant growth: biology or bias? PROBIT study group, *Pediatrics* 110:343-347, 2002.

Lawrence RA, Lawrence RM: *Breastfeeding: a guide for the medical profession*, ed 6, St Louis, 2005, Elsevier-Mosby.

Mayer-Davis EJ et al: Breast-feeding and risk for childhood obesity: does maternal diabetes or obesity status matter? *Diabetes Care* 29(10):2231-2237, 2006.

Meier PP et al: Nipple shields for preterm infants: effect on milk transfer and duration of breastfeeding, *J Hum Lact* 16:106-114, 2000.

Morrow AL et al: Human milk glycans that inhibit pathogen binding protect breast-feeding infants against infections diarrhea, *J Nutr* 135(5):1304-1307, 2005.

National Association of Pediatric Nurse Practitioners: NAPNAP position statement on breast-feeding, *J Pediatr Health Care* 21(2):A39-A40, 2007.

Oddy WH: Breastfeeding protects against illness and infection in infants and children: a review of the evidence, *Breastfeed Rev* 9:11-18, 2001.

Ortiz J, McGilligan K, Kelly P: Duration of breast milk expression among working mothers enrolled in an employer-sponsored lactation program, *Pediatr Nurs* 30(2):111-119, 2004.

Owen CG et al: Infant feeding and blood cholesterol: a study in adolescents and a systematic review, *Pediatrics* 110:597-608, 2002.

Paricio-Talayero JM et al: Full breastfeeding and hospitalization as a result of infections in the first year of life, *Pediatrics* 118(1):e92-99, 2006.

Pesonen M et al: Prolonged exclusive breastfeeding is associated with increased atopic dermatitis: a prospective follow-up study of unselected healthy newborns from birth to age 20 years, *Clin Exp Allergy* 36(8):1011-1018, 2006.

Philipp BL, Radford A: Baby-Friendly: snappy slogan or standard of care? *Arch Dis Child Fetal Neonatal Ed* 91(2):F145-149, 2006.

Quigley MA et al: How protective is breastfeeding against diarrhoeal disease in infants in 1990s England? A case control study, *Arch Dis Child* 91(3):245-250, 2006.

Schack-Nielsen L, Michaelsen KF: Breast feeding and future health, *Curr Opin Clin Nutr Metab Care* 9(3):289-296, 2006.

Schack-Nielsen L, Larnkjaer A, Michaelsen KF: Long term effects of breastfeeding on the infant and mother, *Adv Exp Med Biol* 569:16-23, 2005.

Singhal A et al: Breast milk feeding and lipoprotein profile in adolescents born preterm: follow-up of a prospective randomized study, *Lancet* 363(9421):1571-1578, 2004.

United Nations International Children's Emergency Fund (UNICEF): *Baby-friendly hospital initiative*. Available at *www.unicef.org/programme/breastfeedingbaby.htm* (accessed Oct 12, 2007).

World Health Organization/United Nations International Children's Emergency Fund (WHO/UNICEF): *Protecting, promoting and supporting breastfeeding: the special role of maternity services: a joint WHO/UNICEF statement*, Geneva, 1989, World Health Organization.

CHAPTER 13

Elimination Patterns

Ardys M. Dunn

Patterns of elimination include skin, bowel and bladder habits, and excretory function. These serve as indicators of how well the gastrointestinal (GI), renal, urinary, and integumentary systems are functioning. This chapter discusses normal bowel and bladder function, normal developmental activities, such as toilet training, and behaviors that are often self-limited in young children but that can require intervention (e.g., encopresis and enuresis). Problems related more directly to GI and renal pathophysiology are presented in Chapters 32 and 34. Dermatologic conditions are discussed in Chapter 36.

Healthy children demonstrate an extremely wide range of "normal" elimination behavior, and primary care providers have a responsibility to help parents understand what is typical of normal behavior and what constitutes a problem. This can be a challenge because cultural and social expectations about elimination vary greatly, causing some parents to believe that their child has a problem when none exists. Also, developmental processes, such as toilet training, can lead to problems if not appropriately managed. Providers must conduct thorough and accurate assessments, provide anticipatory guidance for parents about what to expect as their child develops, help parents facilitate healthy bowel and bladder function, and refer for more complicated conditions.

■ STANDARDS

The American Academy of Pediatrics (AAP) recommends routine urinalysis for asymptomatic children at 5 years old and again in adolescence at about 16 years old. A dipstick test for leukocytes is recommended annually for all sexually active male and female adolescents (AAP, 2000). Otherwise, screening urinalysis should be conducted based on a specific clinical symptom or condition (Bock, 2006). The U.S. Preventive Services Task Force (1996) does not recommend "routine screening for asymptomatic bacteriuria in … persons (other than pregnant women)." The guidelines for adolescent preventive services (GAPS), from the American Medical Association (AMA), recommend screening for urine leukocyte esterase in adolescent males as one way to assess for sexually transmitted diseases (AMA, 1997). The AAP recommends that toilet training begin when the child is ready, which is not before 18 to 24 months old (Wolraich & Tippins, 2003).

■ NORMAL PATTERNS OF ELIMINATION: BOWEL AND URINARY

INFANTS

Bowel Patterns

Bowel patterns of infants are related to the frequency and amount of feeding and differ between formula-fed and breast-fed babies. Breastfed infants commonly have many small stools per day in the first weeks of life; frequent stooling in the neonate is an indicator of adequate breast milk intake (Shrago et al, 2006). As children grow, fewer stools are typical, with some older breastfed infants having a stool once a day or as infrequently as once every 8 to 10 days. In exclusively breastfed infants, this infrequent stooling is not a problem; if the infant is thriving, happy, and has no clinical signs (e.g., abdominal distention, irritability), parents can be reassured that it is transient (Eggermont, 2004; Choe et al, 2004). The stools of breastfed infants are usually soft, sticky, or watery with a curdlike texture, light yellow, and have a "sour" but not unpleasant odor. Iron supplements can darken the stool and make it firmer.

Formula-fed babies have 2 to 4 stools each day in the first month. As patterns become established, the number of stools decreases and older formula-fed infants may have 1 to 3 soft, semiformed stools each day. Stools of formula-fed infants are firmer, darker, and smellier than those of breastfed infants. They may be brown, greenish, or dark yellow, depending on the type of formula and whether it is iron-fortified or if the child is given iron supplements. The stools of both breastfed and formula-fed babies become firmer and darker as solid foods are introduced.

Urinary Patterns

Urination is associated with fluid intake, increasing as infants take more fluids. Healthy, well-hydrated infants, whether breastfed or formula-fed, should urinate a minimum of 6 times a day but can void, in small amounts, 15 to 20 times a day. Fever in infants can quickly lead to dehydration, with less frequent urination.

Infants are not capable of voluntary bowel and bladder control because these functions are dependent on myelination of the pyramidal tracts in the spinal cord, a process probably completed between 12 and 18 months old. Infants 9 to 12 months old generally have regular patterns; they may have a bowel movement early in the morning or after feeding or stay dry for several hours and urinate immediately after waking from a nap.

TODDLERS AND PRESCHOOLERS
Bowel Patterns
Toddlers and preschoolers usually have a regular pattern of elimination. Although they typically have 1 to 3 stools a day, it is not unusual for children in this age group to defecate every other day or every third or fourth day. It is a myth that healthy children must have a bowel movement every day. Normal stools have an unpleasant odor and are soft, formed, and various shades of brown, depending on the child's diet.

Urinary Patterns
By the time children are 2 years old, renal function is fully developed. Fluid intake, environmental conditions, perspiration, fever, and diarrhea with significant fluid loss influence the urinary pattern of toddlers and preschoolers. They typically urinate 8 to 14 times a day. Cold weather, excitement, and stress lead to increased frequency. Children generally do not void during sleep after 18 months (Jansson et al, 2000).

SCHOOL-AGE CHILDREN
Bowel Patterns
Elimination patterns in school-age children approximate those of adults. Depending on a child's intake, bowel movements occur from 1 to 3 times a day to once every 2 to 3 days. Stool is soft, formed, and brown and has an odor. School-age children should be completely toilet trained, although occasional soiling of underwear occurs as a result of poor hygiene or because children do not respond quickly to cues to defecate. It is important to remember children's increasing needs for independence and privacy during the school-age years and incorporate consideration of those needs into management of toileting.

Urinary Patterns
School-age children have essentially the same capacity as adults to produce urine—between 650 and 1500 mL in a 24-hour period—but the kidneys are still small and accommodate a smaller urine volume at any one time than those of adults. Children normally void 5 to 6 times a day. Girls appear to have slightly larger bladder capacity than boys. Dysfunctional voiding (too little means 1 to 3 times a day; too much means 8 to 12 times a day), daytime incontinence, or nocturnal enuresis warrant further evaluation, especially because these conditions can be associated with infection, dehydration, constipation, or sexual abuse.

ADOLESCENTS
Bowel and Bladder Patterns
GI and renal function is at adult levels in adolescents, and patterns of elimination are similar to those of adults. Abnormal variation can occur in teenagers who have eating disorders. Adolescents are also susceptible to the demands of schedules, stress, and irregular eating patterns. The need for privacy and personal space can inhibit normal elimination in public places, such as school or dormitory restrooms

(Lundblad & Hellström, 2005). Sexual activity can contribute to changes in bowel or bladder function, including infections or constipation.

◼ ASSESSMENT OF PATTERNS
Assessment of elimination patterns begins with a thorough health history with questions being asked of the parent or the child, depending on the child's age and ability. As variations of normal behavior become evident, relevant follow-up questions should be asked to clarify and complete the patient's health picture.

HEALTH HISTORY
Description of Current Status
The patient's current elimination status can be assessed with the following questions:
- How often does your child urinate? How many wet diapers does your baby have in a 24-hour period?
- How often does your child have a bowel movement? Describe what the stools look and smell like. How does your child act when having a bowel movement?
- Describe anything unusual about your child's elimination habits. Does your child resist going to the bathroom?
- Describe your child's toileting habits. For example, at what time of day does your child have a bowel movement?
- Do you use any medications, including over-the-counter preparations or home remedies, to help your child with bowel movements?
- How do you think the process of toilet training will happen? (Ask parents of a 9- to 12-month-old child.)
- Is your child toilet trained? When did training begin? Describe the process. How often do "accidents" happen? How do you (parent) feel toilet training is progressing?
- What names do you use in your family for stool and urine, for body parts, and for the process of using the toilet?

Birth History
Determine whether any problems with the child's urine or stool were present at birth. For example, did the baby pass a meconium stool within 48 hours after birth? How soon after birth did the baby urinate?

Review of Systems
The review of systems should include the following questions:
- Has your child ever been constipated or had diarrhea? (Box 13-1 summarizes the criteria for functional constipation). Is it chronic or only occasional? Did it start after a particular incident (e.g., illness, during toilet training, with a certain food or change in diet)? How does the parent define constipation and diarrhea?
- Has your child ever had a urinary tract infection (UTI)? Describe. Any work-up (e.g., ultrasonography, urethrogram)?
- Has your child had any illness, injury, or operation related to the bowel or bladder? Describe.

Rome III Criteria for Functional Constipation: Infants and Children

Child must have at least two of the following criteria, at least once a week, for at least 1 month (infants to 4 years old) or for at least 2 months (children >4 years old); with no evidence of structural, metabolic, or endocrine disease:
- Two or fewer defecations per week
- One episode of fecal incontinence per week (after child is toilet trained)
- History of excessive stool retention
- History of painful bowel movements
- History of large diameter stools, could obstruct toilet
- Presence of large fecal mass in rectum

Data from Hyman PE et al: Childhood functional gastrointestinal disorders; neonate/toddler, *Gastroenterology* 130(5):1519-1526, 2006; Rasquin A et al: Childhood functional gastrointestinal disorders: child/adolescent, *Gastroenterology* 130(5):1527-1537, 2006.

- Does your child have a physical condition or chronic illness that affects voiding or bowel movements?
- What medications, including over-the-counter preparations, does your child take?

Family History

Determine whether any family members, including parents, have had problems with urination or bowel movements and describe them (e.g., chronic constipation or diarrhea, bed-wetting). Has there been any travel or residence outside the U.S.? Does the family residence use well water?

Environment and Psychosocial Issues

Environmental and psychosocial issues should be assessed, using questions such as:
- How do you, as a parent, feel about the issue of toileting?
- How do you interact with your child around toileting issues?
- How do you deal with toileting "accidents"?
- What plans do you have for managing toilet training?
- Describe your child's typical diet.
- Tell me about the toileting facilities at your child's house, day care, and school. How do you think they affect your child's toileting habits?

PHYSICAL EXAMINATION

The physical examination includes external examination of the perineum, anus, and urinary meatus and auscultation and palpation of the abdomen for bowel sounds, softness, masses, peristalsis, and tenderness.

LABORATORY AND DIAGNOSTIC TESTS

- Urinalysis as indicated based on symptoms
- Routine asymptomatic screening once at about 5 years old and again during adolescence, at about 16 years old
- Annual urinalysis for leukocytes for all sexually active adolescents (AAP, 2000)

■ MANAGEMENT STRATEGIES FOR NORMAL PATTERNS

TOILET TRAINING

Toilet training occurs in the toddler and preschool years and is usually complete by 4 years old. Successful toilet training requires sensitivity, understanding of development, good communication, hope, humor, and patience. In addition to becoming self-sufficient in their toileting, children should also learn that elimination is a natural and necessary process. As self-toileting is mastered, both parents and children should experience pride and satisfaction in having worked together to accomplish an important developmental task.

The health care provider plays an important role in providing anticipatory guidance to parents. The topic of toilet training should be introduced at the 9-month visit and again at 12, 15, and 18 months; parents' expectations and plans should be assessed, and ample opportunity for discussion of realistic toileting outcomes should be provided at these visits. In the U.S., parents from different racial and socioeconomic groups have been noted to have differing beliefs about the appropriate age to begin toilet training, with higher income Caucasian parents viewing 25.4 months as an appropriate age, in contrast to African Americans (18.2 months) and other racial groups (19.4 months) (Horn et al, 2006). In some cultures, early *assisted* toilet training (in contrast to *independent* toilet training where the child learns self-management) may be the norm, with Asian and African families often beginning to train their children between 1 and 3 months old. The parent takes responsibility for placing the child on the toilet when necessary. As the child matures, he or she takes more self-responsibility (Sun & Rugolotto, 2004). As families from these non-Western groups immigrate to the U.S., health care providers need to understand the cultural differences and be open to developing mutually agreed-upon approaches to toilet training.

Because true voluntary sphincter control is a function of psychological and social, in addition to physiologic development, children are not usually ready for independent toilet training until 18 to 24 months or even older. Every child is unique, and readiness cues should ultimately be used to decide when to begin training. If begun too early, the process can be very stressful, and at least one study has shown that children with primary encopresis had more difficult and disruptive toilet-training experiences than those without (Fishman et al, 2002). In contrast, a study by Bakker and associates (2002) found that children with bed-wetting problems tended to be trained later than those without problems; this study suggests, however, that a structured yet flexible approach to training that is responsive to the child's cues is likely to be most successful. Guidelines for assessing toilet-training readiness include physical, cognitive, interpersonal or psychological, and parental skills (Table 13-1).

Typically, children are trained first for nocturnal bowel control, then daytime bowel control, daytime bladder control, and finally nocturnal bladder control. Average times for being fully trained are around 3 to 4 years old, with a range of up to a year for individual children as normal. Average ages for

TABLE 13-1	Guidelines for Assessing Readiness to Toilet Train
Child's physical skills	Has voluntary sphincter control
	Stays dry for 2 hours, may wake from naps still dry
	Is able to sit, walk, and squat
	Assists in dressing self
Child's cognitive skills	Recognizes urge to urinate or defecate
	Understands meaning of words used by family in toileting
	Understands what the toilet is for
	Understands connection between dry pants and toilet
	Is able to follow directions
	Is able to communicate needs
Child's interpersonal skills	Demonstrates desire to please parent
	Expresses curiosity about use of toilet
	Expresses desire to be dry and clean
Parental skills	Expresses desire to assist child with training
	Recognizes child's cues of readiness
	Has no compelling factor that will interfere with training (e.g., new job, move, family loss)

BOX 13-2   Management of Toilet Training

- Keep child as clean and dry as possible:
  - Change diapers frequently.
  - Use training pants or underwear when child stays dry for several hours during the day; use diaper at night.
- Talk to child about toilet training:
  - Praise child for asking to have diaper changed.
  - Explain connection between being clean and dry and using toilet.
  - Provide opportunity for child to use toilet, especially before going out to play, going on a trip, before naps, and at bedtime; set an example with adult behavior.
  - Do not constantly remind child to use the toilet; avoid "nagging."
- Teach child how to use toilet:
  - Allow child to observe while parents or older siblings use toilet.
  - Demonstrate how to sit on toilet, use toilet paper, flush, and wash one's hands.
- Provide practice time for child:
  - Provide a potty chair or portable toilet seat.
  - Allow child to sit on potty chair with clothes or diaper on.
  - Encourage child to use potty chair while parent uses regular toilet.
  - Have child sit on potty chair without diapers for 5-10 minutes at a time.
  - Practice at times the child usually urinates or defecates.
- Provide a comfortable, safe-feeling environment:
  - Seat child facing backward on a regular toilet or provide a footstool to rest the feet on.
  - Never flush the toilet when child is sitting on it.
  - Stay with child for safety reasons.
- Give consistent, positive feedback:
  - Praise child for trying and for success.
  - Be understanding of child's refusal to use toilet.
  - Never demand performance.
  - Never make child sit on toilet if child resists.
  - Ignore or minimize undesired behavior.
  - Never scold or punish if a child wets or soils.
  - Use star chart or other reward for success.
  - Do not praise excessively.

---

girls and boys to accomplish other tasks of toilet training are as follows (Schum et al, 2002):

- Showing an interest in using the toilet: girls, 24 months; boys, 26 months
- Telling parents of their need to use the toilet: girls, 26 months; boys, 29 months
- Staying dry for at least 2 hours: girls, 26 months; boys, 29 months
- Staying dry during the day: girls, 32.5 months; boys, 35 months

When children and parents are ready to begin toilet training, several management techniques are helpful (Box 13-2). If children resist training, the project should be put on hold for a few weeks before trying again. If toddlers seem to be toilet trained for a brief period and suddenly regress to wetting and soiling consistently, they should be placed back in diapers and the process begun again within a few weeks. It is extremely important that parents and children do not become engaged in a "battle for control" over toilet training. Ultimately, it is the child's responsibility to control his or her bowel and urinary function, and toilet training is only one of the tasks toddlers master on their way to independence. Parents have the responsibility of assisting in the process by providing a positive environment and opportunities, teaching the techniques, and setting a positive example.

Parents can become extremely frustrated if their expectations do not match the abilities and performance of their children,

and the incidence of child abuse related to toilet training is high. Berkowitz (2000) notes that issues around toileting are the second most prevalent factor precipitating fatal child abuse. Health care providers can play a crucial role in making the experience a positive one and preventing abuse by giving parents information about child development, techniques for managing the process, and support and encouragement for their efforts.

ALTERED PATTERNS OF ELIMINATION

The following discussion focuses on four relatively common conditions of childhood related to elimination: stool toileting refusal (STR), encopresis, enuresis, and dysfunctional voiding. These conditions are considered here as developmental problems of normal urinary and bowel habits. If assessment reveals indication of a pathologic condition, further investigation and different management, including referral, are necessary.

STOOL TOILETING REFUSAL

Description

STR is present when a child demonstrates a pattern of successfully using the toilet to urinate, but refuses to use the toilet for bowel movements. These children will usually defecate in a diaper, training pants, or "pull-ups." In some cases, children will retain stool or defecate outside the toilet. Encopresis without constipation also fits this description: the child defecates outside the toilet when beyond the age of expected training.

Epidemiology

The incidence of STR has not been recently documented. Taubman (1997) found that 22% of healthy children between 18 and 30 months old experienced at least 1 month of STR. The cause of STR is unknown, but the presence of younger siblings in the household and the parents' inability to set limits for the child may be related. Although children who displayed STR tended to have "a more difficult temperament" than did children who were toilet trained, they did not have any more behavior problems (Blum et al, 1997). Constipation and painful bowel movements appear to precede rather than follow the problem (Blum et al, 2004).

Clinical Findings

History. Parents or caregivers report that the child demonstrates the following:
- Bladder control but refusal to defecate on the toilet
- A regular pattern of bowel movements
- Signs that a bowel movement is imminent
- May have a history of hiding when defecating, either before or after toilet training begins (Blum et al, 2003)

Physical Examination. The physical examination will be unremarkable if the child has a pattern of regular bowel movements.
- Examine the anus for fissures or irritation that may cause a child to refuse to defecate.
- Check for signs of stool retention:
  ○ Abdominal distention
  ○ Abdominal tenderness on palpation
- Palpation of a mass in the sigmoid colon or at the midline in the suprapubic area (impaction).

Differential Diagnosis

The differential diagnosis includes stool withholding, constipation, and encopresis.

Management

When parents refrain from expressing negative messages about stooling or fecal matter and praise the child for defecating in the diaper, the duration of STR appears to shorten (Taubman et al, 2003). Behavioral management is appropriate for younger children. Return them to diapers and reintroduce toilet training in about a month or when the child indicates interest. Some children prefer not to wear diapers all the time, but will ask to have one put on when they feel the urge to defecate. After having a bowel movement, they ask to be changed and return to wearing training pants. This pattern may continue for several weeks or months. For older children, schedule daily times for the child to sit on the toilet for 5 to 10 minutes; have these times be positive, never punitive or forced. Never flush the toilet while the child is sitting on it. Provide incentives and give positive feedback when the child successfully uses the toilet for bowel movements (e.g., the parent can use star charts). If the child has constipation, fecal impaction, or both, initial bowel clean-out is necessary, in conjunction with increased fiber and fluid in the diet. Mineral oil, suppositories, or medication may be useful. Table 13-2 outlines the management of a child with encopresis with constipation.

Complications

Refusal to use the toilet for bowel movements may lead to stool withholding, constipation, and impaction, conditions that result in primary encopresis. Psychological complications include embarrassment, shame, conflict, and stress between children and parents, especially as the child becomes older. Child abuse can be a significant complication (Berkowitz, 2000).

Patient Education and Prevention

Prevention through appropriate toilet training is key (see Box 13-2). If a child refuses to defecate on the toilet, use of punishment or force can complicate the problem. Parents should be alert for signs of constipation (hard stools, fewer than 3 bowel movements per week) and should encourage fluids, fiber, and exercise to facilitate bowel movements and prevent encopresis.

ENCOPRESIS AND CONSTIPATION

Description

Encopresis is defined as stool incontinence after an age when children should be able to control bowel movements, usually 4 years old. Primary, or continuous, encopresis is present in children who have never been toilet trained. Secondary, or discontinuous, encopresis is seen in those who were previously trained but who begin to soil. There are two subtypes of encopresis: encopresis with constipation, associated with stool retention, constipation, and incontinence overflow, and encopresis without constipation. In encopresis with constipation, stool retention over time leads to distention of the colon and stretching of the rectum, ineffective peristalsis, decreased sensory threshold in the rectum, and weakened rectal and sphincter muscles. Stool becomes dry, hard, and difficult to evacuate (can be impacted), and bowel movements can be painful. Soft, semiformed, or liquid stool from higher in the colon can leak around retained stool and pass through the rectum, causing soiling. Soiling with encopresis with constipation is involuntary, and the child is often unaware of the actual incontinence. Children with encopresis with constipation may either refuse or be willing to use the toilet.

Those few children with encopresis without constipation have voluntary bowel movements, but in their clothing or other inappropriate places.

Epidemiology

Encopresis may be more common than believed because many families hesitate to inform their health care provider about it. In the school-age child, it is more common among boys than girls (Boris & Dalton, 2004a). The cause of encopresis

---

TABLE 13-2   Management of Children With Encopresis With Constipation

Treatment Phase	Treatment Program	Comments
Catharsis	In the home: four 3-day cycles (12 days total): • Day 1, 4, 7, 10: Fleet enema (adult size) • Day 2, 5, 8, 11: Bisacodyl suppository • Day 3, 6, 9, 12: Bisacodyl tab (children >3 yr old) • Day 13: Bisacodyl tab Return to clinic Follow-up abdominal radiograph to confirm catharsis	Goal of catharsis is to empty the bowel; there are no absolute best ways to achieve this. Catharsis may need to occur in the hospital if • Retention is severe. • Home compliance is poor. • Parents prefer admission. • Parents should not administer enemas for psychological reasons. Enema should be fully expelled to prevent hypertonic dehydration. The child may have watery or soft stools for several days after catharsis; parents and patient should be informed that ongoing maintenance is essential for the bowel to return to fully normal functioning (see Fig. 13-1). Initial improvement can be falsely reassuring and may contribute to poor compliance with maintenance regimen.
Maintenance	**Medications** Stool softener: Mineral oil, titrate dose starting at 2 tbsp bid, increase until there is leakage from the rectum; then decrease just until leakage stops. Docusate sodium or docusate calcium Daily multivitamin to counteract possible decreased absorption of fat-soluble vitamins Oral laxatives: Polyethylene glycol 3350 (PEG) 0.5 g/kg tid (max 24 g tid) (Schmitt, 2006) titrated up or down to maintain soft stools Milk of magnesia, 6-12 yr: 15-30 mL/day **Behavioral changes** Toilet sitting 3-4 times a day for 10 min; at least twice a day for 10 min each time Increased physical activity **Dietary changes** Increased fluids (other than milk), increased fiber in diet, consider limiting constipating foods **Other** Document every bowel movement: time, quality, amount, location Regular visits to provider at 2 wk, 1 mo, 3 mo, 6 mo	Goals of maintenance: • No soiling; prevent reimpaction. • Regular, soft bowel movements (at least every other day; >3 per wk). • Increased ability to sense the urge to defecate; sensation may not reappear until rectum has been emptied for 2-3 wk, and the urge to defecate might not be consistent for 6-9 mo after treatment. Laxatives may be substituted for or used alternately with stool softeners. PEG has been shown to be effective in treatment of constipation when used alone (Pashankar & Bishop, 2001) and more effective than lactulose (Gremse et al, 2002). Use of senna is not recommended. Toilet sitting should be scheduled at times the child is most likely to have a bowel movement (e.g., on wakening, after meals). Use a foot stool to help give child leverage and relax pelvic floor. Plan on 6 mo of treatment before bowel regains full function.
Follow-up	Regular visits (about every 4-10 wk) depending on severity and need of family Telephone availability to discuss progress and adjust doses Counseling or referral as appropriate for psychosocial and developmental issues Continued education of normal bowel function (see Fig. 13-1)	Goals of follow-up visits: • Monitor compliance. • Provide encouragement and support. • Detect and treat relapse early if it occurs.

tid, Twice a day; *min*, minute(s); *mo*, month(s); *wk*, week(s); *yr*, year(s).
Data from Levine MD, Carey WB, Crocker AC: *Developmental-behavioral pediatrics*, ed 3, Philadelphia, 1999, WB Saunders;
Felt B et al: Guideline for the management of pediatric idiopathic constipation and soiling, *Arch Pediatr Adolesc Med* 153:380-385, 1999.

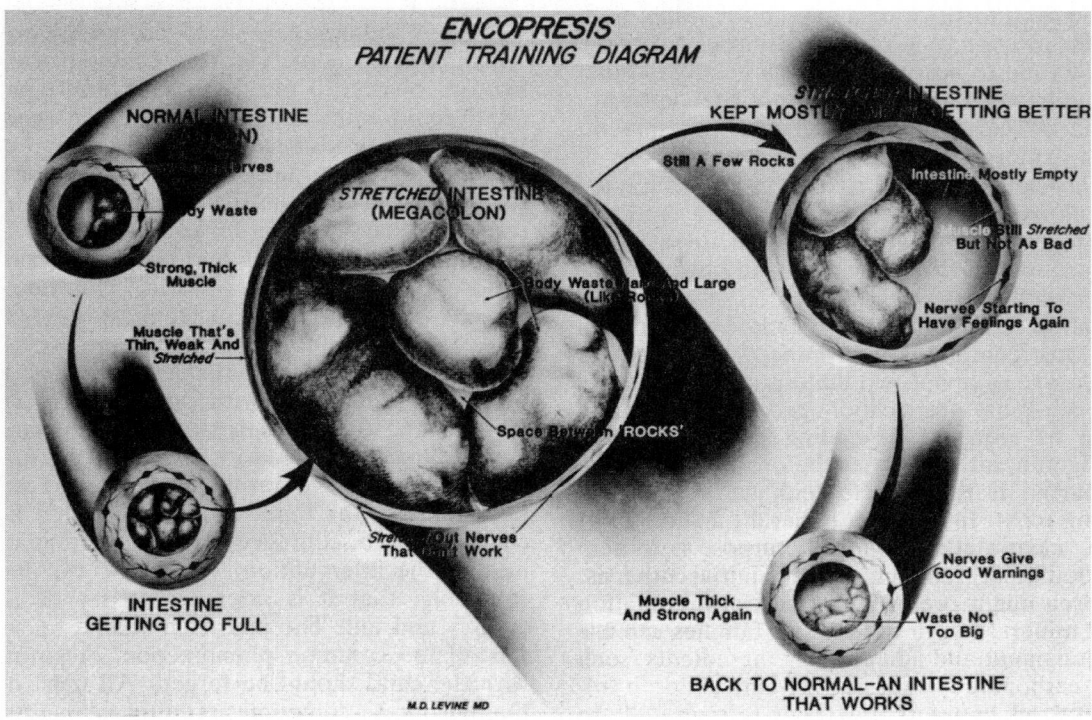

FIG. 13-1 Encopresis: patient training diagram. (From Levine MD, Carey WB, Crocker AC: *Developmental-behavioral patterns*, ed 3, Philadelphia, 1999, WB Saunders.)

is unclear and appears to differ among children. Both physiologic and psychosocial factors are involved. Often there is a history of an acute stool problem (e.g., child had an illness that caused dehydration and constipation) that was not adequately managed, leading to a cycle of constipation—painful defecation—stool retention—more severe constipation—more painful defecation—more stool retention and so on. Children with nonretentive encopresis appear to have more behavioral problems and externalizing behavior than those without stooling problems, though it is unclear which causes which (Benninga et al, 2004). Some of these children may also have delayed or faulty perception of the need to stool and as a result will have soiling (Pakarinen et al, 2006).

Physiologic. Physiologic factors related to constipation and encopresis include the following:
- Inadequate fluid intake
- Dehydration caused by illness and fever or during active play in hot weather
- A change in diet, such as the introduction of solids or increased carbohydrates and decreased fiber
- Inappropriate use of laxatives, suppositories, or enemas by parents who do not understand normal bowel patterns in children and infants
- Stool retention and constipation secondary to the following:
  - Painful bowel movements
  - Anal fissures
  - Paradoxic constriction of the external anal sphincter muscle during attempted defecation
  - Neurogenic conditions (e.g., aganglionic colon [Hirschsprung disease], cerebral palsy, myelomeningocele)
  - Endocrine and metabolic conditions (e.g., hypothyroidism)
  - Medications (e.g., opioids, iron supplements)

Psychosocial. Psychosocial factors related to constipation and encopresis include the following:
- Major family or life adjustments, such as loss of a parent, sibling, or other significant person
- Inappropriate toilet-training techniques leading to a power struggle; children who are pushed might rebel in the only way they can, by refusing to cooperate
- Irregular toileting patterns, often caused by travel, unfamiliar or unpleasant bathrooms, lack of regular routine, or child being absorbed in play or activities
- Physical abuse and sexual abuse

Clinical Findings
History. The history can include the following:
- Stained underwear
- Report of fewer than three bowel movements per week
- Difficult or painful defecation
- Large-caliber or hard stool
- Child suddenly becoming still during play, attempting to hide when urge to defecate is felt
- Child attempting to retain stool (e.g., crossing legs, grimacing, or shifting from one foot to another)
- Reports of a bloated sensation, abdominal pain, or both
- Odor of stool from leakage into underwear
- Streaks of bright blood on toilet paper or underwear
- Enuresis
- UTIs
- Anorexia

Physical Examination. The physical examination should assess for the following:

- Overflow soiling
- Abdominal distention
- Abdominal tenderness on palpation
- Impactions felt on digital rectal examination (rectal examination may be deferred if the history and other signs allow for a clear diagnosis because it can be traumatic for the child)
- Mass felt at the midline in the suprapubic area
- Anal fissures
- Neurologic signs: absent or diminished abdominal, cremasteric, anal wink reflexes, and deep tendon reflexes (DTRs) in lower extremities may indicate a neurologic cause

Laboratory and Diagnostic Tests. X-rays and laboratory tests to identify structural or organic causes of constipation are not routinely necessary, but can be appropriate if clinical suspicion is high or primary treatment for encopresis is unsuccessful. Results of an abdominal radiograph can indicate accumulation of stool in the sigmoid colon (see Chapter 32).

Differential Diagnosis

The differential diagnoses for encopresis with constipation are as follows:

- Anorectal stenosis
- Spina bifida occulta, spinal cord dysplasia
- Hirschsprung disease
- Mental retardation
- Hypothyroidism
- Hypercalcemia
- Cerebral palsy
- Other organic causes of constipation (e.g., cystic fibrosis)
- The normal red-faced grunting and straining of infants on defecation

Management

Treatment of children with encopresis differs depending on whether they have impactions, are constipated, or have normal bowel movements but defecate in places other than the toilet. In all cases, the goals of treatment are to establish a regular bowel routine, "demystify" the problem, alleviate blame, and gain cooperation for treatment plans (Schonwald & Rappaport, 2004).

Box 13-3 outlines approaches to treating a child with encopresis without constipation. (Also see management of stool toileting refusal earlier in this chapter.)

Children who have encopresis with constipation present a greater challenge. Education of parents and children is vital to successful treatment (Schonwald & Rappaport, 2004). A clear message to children and parents should be that the dynamics of encopresis (retention, stretching, decreased peristalsis, impaction, leaking) are not voluntary—no one is to blame; they can, however, be reversed through bowel rehabilitation. Correcting them will take hard work, cooperation, and time, and the provider will work with the family to ensure success. Fig. 13-1 can be used to educate parents and children about the bowel rehabilitation process involved in the treatment plan.

BOX 13-3 **Management of Children With Mild Encopresis Without Constipation**

- Monitor diet:
  - Ensure adequate fiber and water intake (cereals, oatmeal, breads, fruits, and vegetables).
  - Decrease milk to 16 oz/day; limit cheese, rice, applesauce, bananas.
  - Provide 2 to 4 oz prune juice daily (high-sorbitol content).
- Avoid use of stool softeners or laxatives.
- Give child all responsibility for own toilet habits. Stop parental reminders to use toilet. Stop all encouragement and criticisms.
- Use incentives or rewards to reinforce positive behavior. Give incentives immediately after child defecates in toilet. Put time limit on use of incentive (e.g., can watch a video for 30 minutes, can ride a bike for 15 minutes). Parent controls incentive; child controls defecation (Schmitt, 2006).
- Establish a regular toileting routine.

Figs. 13-2 and 13-3 present algorithms primary care providers can use to manage constipation in children younger and older than one year. Table 13-2 provides guidelines to treating a child with encopresis with constipation, including appropriate medications. Retentive encopresis without impaction may not require such extensive intervention; polyethylene glycol 3350 (PEG) and mineral oil may be used for catharsis in children under 7 years old or those who are unable to tolerate enemas or suppositories.

Management of encopresis is often multidisciplinary, and adding behavioral interventions to medical treatment appears to reduce incontinence slightly more effectively than medical treatment (i.e., laxatives) alone (Brazzelli & Griffiths, 2006). Psychological counseling of both the child and family may be necessary. In some cases, referral to a psychologist or behavioral pediatrician is appropriate. Because this problem often occurs in school-age children, medical providers may need to consult with the school nurse to ensure that the child receives appropriate medications, hygiene management, and essential psychological and emotional support.

Complications

Persistent encopresis is an unpleasant condition, and children with encopresis often experience ridicule and shame. Age-group peers frequently treat children with scorn, hostility, and rejection. Teachers and other adults might be disgusted by children with encopresis, and parents, dealing with anger, guilt, embarrassment, and helplessness, find their children and the condition extremely difficult to manage. Social, interpersonal, and family relations are at grave risk.

Patient Education and Prevention

The best treatment of encopresis is prevention. If constipation or encopresis is caused by an underlying anatomic or organic cause (e.g., Hirschsprung disease, occult spina bifida,

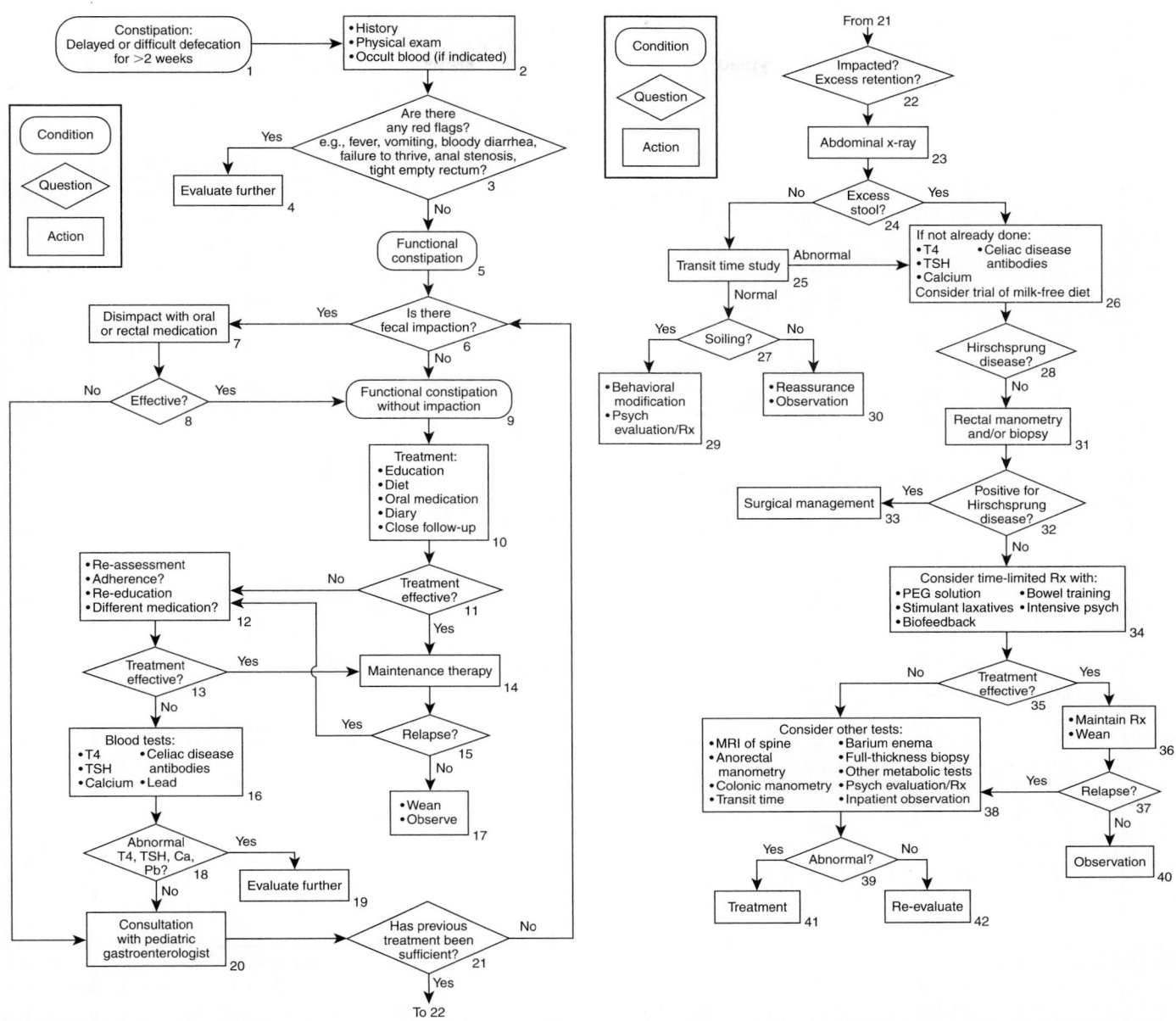

FIG. 13-2 An algorithm for the management of constipation in children 1 year and older. *Ca,* Calcium; *MRI,* magnetic resonance imaging; *Pb,* lead; *Rx,* prescription. (From Baker SS et al: Clinical practice guideline. Evaluation and treatment of constipation in infants and children: recommendations of the North American Society for Pediatric Gastroenterology, Hepatology and Nutrition, *J Pediatr Gastroenterol Nutr* 43:e1–e31, 2006.)

hypothyroidism), early diagnosis and referral is essential. It is important for the pediatric provider to understand the relationship between constipation and encopresis, recognize conditions that may contribute to each, and provide parents with anticipatory guidance related to dietary and toileting management of their children to prevent their occurrence. It is equally important to provide support during treatment. Although parents should be informed that treatment may be required for months or years, providers should emphasize that by following a clear, consistent, aggressive treatment protocol the condition can be managed. Finally, providers, parents, and the child must work together to prevent recurrence of symptoms after successful treatment.

ENURESIS

Description

Enuresis is defined as involuntary urination or intentional urination into bed or clothes at an age when toilet training should be complete. Children who have never established control have primary enuresis. Secondary enuresis is present when children have been dry for more than 6 to 12 months and begin wetting. Nocturnal enuresis, also called monosymptomatic nocturnal enuresis (MNE), is incontinence during sleep; wetting appears to occur most frequently in the first two-thirds of the night (Wolfish, 2001). Diurnal enuresis occurs during waking hours. There is no consensus on what frequency of wetting justifies a diagnosis of enuresis. The DSM-IV specifies

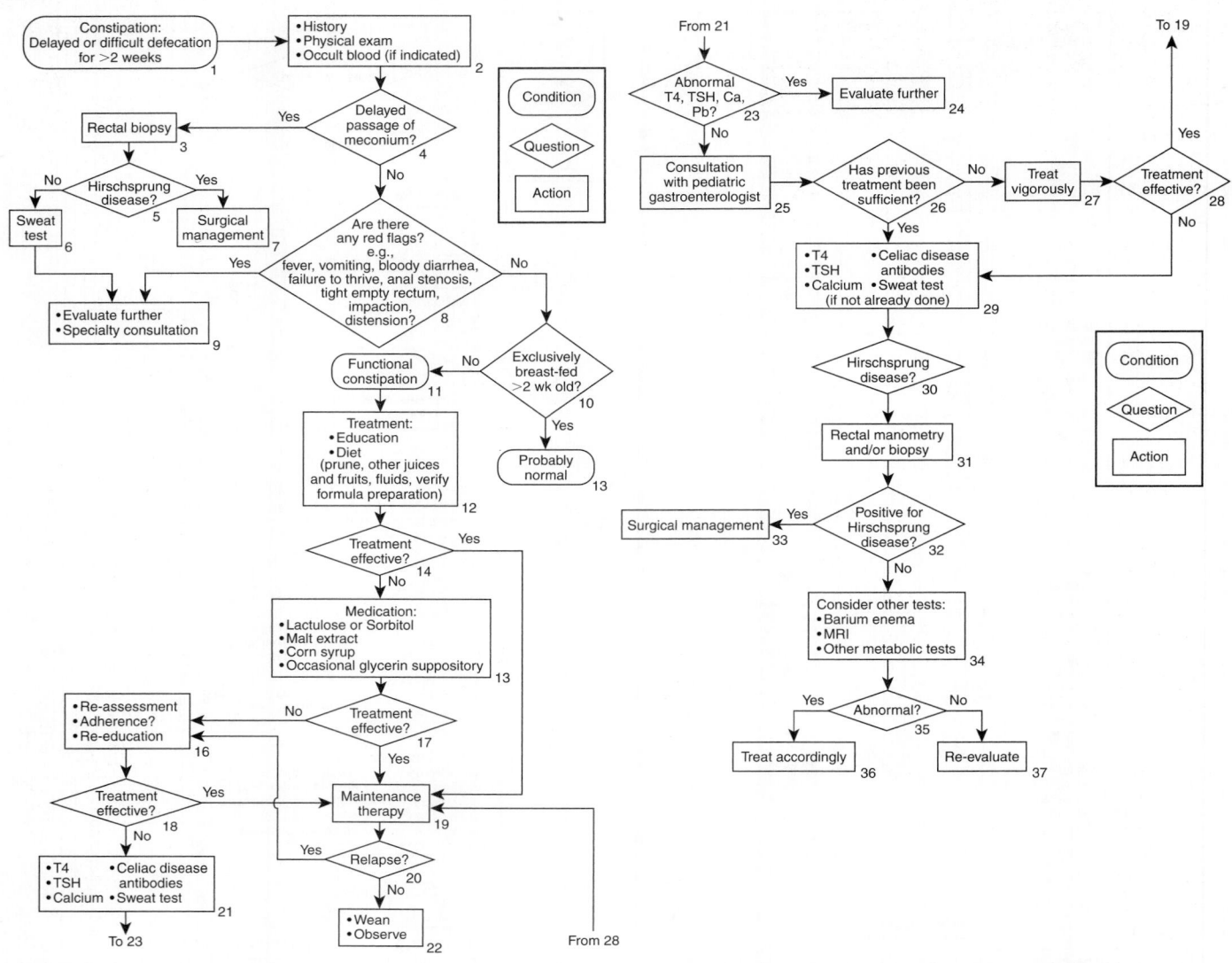

FIG. 13-3 An algorithm for the management of constipation in infants less than 1 year old. *Ca*, calcium; *MRI*, magnetic resonance imaging; *Pb*, lead; *wk*, week(s). (From Baker SS et al: Clinical practice guideline. Evaluation and treatment of constipation in infants and children: recommendations of the North American Society for Pediatric Gastroenterology, Hepatology and Nutrition, *J Pediatr Gastroenterol Nutr* 43:e1–e31, 2006.)

2 wet nights per week, and the International Classification of Diseases (ICD) specifies 1 night per month as the threshold for enuresis. Parents may ask for help if their child has as few as 1 to 3 wet nights per month, a number that some use as a standard for "cure or full response to therapy" (van Gool, 2002).

Epidemiology

The age at which urinary continence is normally achieved varies greatly. As a result, the prevalence of enuresis is difficult to assess. Boys are more likely to have nocturnal enuresis than girls, and black children have a greater incidence of enuresis than white children. Generally, enuresis is not considered to be outside the range of normal limits before 5 to 6 years old. Approximately 7% of 5-year-old boys and 3% of 5-year-old girls have enuresis; 3% of 10-year-old boys and 2% of 10-year-old girls. At 18 years old, 1% of boys have enuresis, but it is rarely seen in girls (Boris & Dalton, 2004b). Although the numbers of children with enuresis decrease with age (suggesting that most

children "grow out" of the problem), for those who continue, the problem is severe. In one large study, nearly half of the affected 19-year-olds were wet 7 nights a week (Yeung et al, 2006).

Approximately 95% of voiding problems are functional, whereas the remainder may represent an organic condition. Primary nocturnal enuresis has an organic cause in only about 1% of cases (Sulkes & Dosa, 2002). The actual cause of enuresis varies among children and can be difficult to determine. A number of factors have been found to be associated with enuresis, including the following:

- Familial disposition. Chromosomal studies suggest a genetic linkage for enuresis, but the exact placement is unclear (Loeys et al, 2002; Bayoumi et al, 2006). It is estimated that 77% of children with enuresis have two parents with a history of enuresis; 50% of children have one parent with a history of enuresis; and for 15% of children with enuresis, neither parent has a history of enuresis.
- Neurologic developmental delay (Freitag et al, 2006).

- Small bladder capacity. A bladder capacity of 300 to 350 mL is necessary for a child to sleep through the night without incontinence. In some children, bladder capacity appears normal during the day, but is functionally reduced at night (Yeung et al, 2002).
- Sleep arousal patterns. Difficult arousal has been found to be more common in children with nocturnal enuresis (Chandra et al, 2004)).
- Stress and family disruptions, such as a divorce, move, or a new member.
- Detrusor instability, in which the child has learned to inhibit sphincter relaxation and prevent complete emptying of the bladder, combined with delayed arousal from sleep and polyuria can be a factor in nocturnal enuresis (Chandra et al, 2004).
- Hormonal regulation. Some children with enuresis may have lower levels of antidiuretic hormone (ADH), contributing to nocturnal polyuria (Pomeranz et al, 2000; Tomasi et al, 2001).
- Chronic constipation or fecal impaction.
- Stress incontinence.
- Inappropriate toilet training, especially when parents are overly demanding or punitive of the child.

Clinical Findings

History. With daytime enuresis, parents often report that the child:

- Demonstrates an immediate urgency to void
- Becomes restless or jiggly, crosses the legs, or holds the penis or pubic area
- May smell of urine

Nocturnal enuresis is characterized by the following:

- Spot urination (the child wakes after beginning to urinate and is able to stop the stream)
- Bed-wetting

Parents should be asked about the following:

- History of enuresis, treatment, and age of resolution for other family members, including parents
- Frequency of wetting
- Time of wetting (daytime or nighttime)
- Volume of urine voided
- Type of urinary stream
- Any urgency, dysuria, polyuria, or dribbling
- History of toilet training; age began, how handled (Was child ever dry? For how long?)
- Presence of other behavior problems
- Changes in the home, family, or school environment
- Effect on child and parents
- Manner in which family deals with the enuresis (e.g., is child punished?)

Physical Examination. The physical examination includes the following:

- Assess the external genitalia for signs of irritation, infection, labial fusion, meatal stenosis.
- Assess for bladder capacity; parents can collect and measure urine over 3 days.
- Observe the size and velocity of the urine stream.
- Check for fecal impaction.

- Examine the abdomen for masses, especially at the suprapubic midline and in the left lower quadrant.
- Examine the lower back for dimples, hair tufts.
- Assess for neurologic function, DTR.

Laboratory and Diagnostic Tests. A urinalysis, with culture, is recommended in all children with enuresis. More sophisticated testing is usually not necessary.

Differential Diagnosis

The differential diagnosis includes daytime or extraordinary urinary frequency syndrome, a benign condition of excessive (more than 8 to 12 per day, often as frequent as every 15 to 30 minutes) urination seen in previously toilet-trained children. Daytime urinary frequency syndrome has no known cause, but may be associated with viral cystitis or urethritis, stress, and hypercalciuria. Though considered self-limited because it does not typically respond to medication, daytime frequency syndrome can persist for months or even years. Treatment of urge syndrome and voiding dysfunction with pelvic floor exercise (Kegel), electrical stimulation, and bio-feedback has shown promise (in one study more than 85% of children improved), but further research is indicated (Barroso et al, 2006). Organic causes of enuresis must be identified; the most common is UTI, which occurs in 1% to 2% of cases. UTIs may be related to encopresis, and a child with enuresis should be examined for fecal impaction and a history of soiling. Other organic causes to consider are listed below, and worsening incontinence, development of neurologic signs (e.g., weakness in legs), increased urine volumes or dilution warrant referral to specialists for further evaluation.

- Diabetes mellitus
- Diabetes insipidus
- Sickle cell disease, in which treatment by means of forced fluids may lead to increased urine output
- Chronic renal failure, in which the kidneys are unable to concentrate urine
- Structural anomalies such as vesicoureteral reflux, ectopic ureter (constant leakage is noted)
- Neurologic abnormalities, including neurogenic bladder
- Hypercalciuria
- Obstructive uropathy
- Vaginitis
- Sleep apnea

Management

Although most children maintain urinary continence after toilet training is established, wetting is a common phenomenon, and parents should be reassured that it rarely indicates disease. A thorough examination to distinguish between organic and nonorganic causes is the first step in treatment. Treatment is then based on the underlying cause and involves behavioral modification, medication, treatment of comorbid or organic conditions, or a combination of these modalities. Referral to a pediatric urology specialist may be necessary. Nontraditional or experimental measures also have been used. Hypnosis, self-hypnosis, and acupuncture may have promise, but require more clinical research (Yuping et al, 2006; Glazener et al, 2005a). Although not yet approved for use in pediatrics, sacral nerve stimulation may be appropriate for children with severe voiding dysfunction that has not responded to aggressive medical or behavioral treatment (Humphreys et al, 2006).

A "full-spectrum" treatment plan, combining alarms, behavioral and motivational therapy, and medication is highly effective (Van Kampen et al, 2002). Successful treatment has been correlated to family functioning and requires committed involvement of both parents and children. Families should be active in deciding what treatment is most appropriate and when it should be implemented.

Outcomes of treatment are categorized as full response (greater than 90% reduction in wet nights), partial response (50% to 90% reduction in wet nights), or no response (less than 50% reduction in wet nights). A cure is a full response that continues 6 months or longer after treatment has ended (van Gool, 2002).

Because functional enuresis is largely self-limited, there is consensus to delay aggressive treatment until the child is 6 to 8 years old. Treatment strategies for children 6 years old or older include the following:

- *Enuresis alarm.* Use of an enuresis alarm has a significantly higher success rate than desmopressin or tricyclic drugs and should be a first line of therapy (Glazener et al, 2005b). Behavioral modification results when an electric alarm with a bell or buzzer is triggered as the child begins to wet. Reflexively, urination stops and the child must then use the toilet. Initially, children may not rouse, and parents must take them to the toilet, even though the child may not be fully awake. Wet bed linens and pajamas are then changed and the alarm is reset. Subsequently, as the alarm is triggered and the child is roused, the child learns to associate a full bladder and the beginning of urination with waking and toileting. Once the child has achieved 2 consecutive weeks of dryness, the alarm is used every other night for another 2 weeks. The effect of alarm therapy is reinforced if the child "overlearns" (is given extra fluids at bedtime) and has "dry bed training" (is taken to toilet repeatedly and changes his or her own sheets when they get wet). Use of alarms takes longer than medication to have an effect (on average, 12 weeks), but is more effective, has no serious side effects, and shows a significantly lower relapse rate. Low functional bladder capacity and difficulty arousing the child have been found to limit the success of alarms (Butler & Robinson, 2002). Some children, especially older children, may object to continued use, others may relapse without the external stimulus, and parents must be committed to getting up with the child for up to 3 months of treatment.
- *Bladder control training (urotherapy).* Because many children with enuresis have low functional bladder capacities, the goal of urotherapy is to increase children's awareness of the need to urinate and to give them more control of the urination process. Urotherapy involves increasing daytime urination by encouraging children to urinate frequently, *not* holding urine until the micturition urge is felt. Urotherapy trains children through visualization exercises to imagine what it feels like to have the urge to urinate and encourages

them to practice urinating. Proper posture (sitting upright, feet on floor; standing erect) while urinating is important to be more sensitive to cues of a full bladder and to control urination. This approach has been used effectively for children with hyperactive bladders, may make medication unnecessary for many children, and warrants further clinical research (Robson & Leung, 2002).

- *Motivational therapy.* This strategy assumes that children will take responsibility for the problem and for learning how to resolve it. The family is expected to provide supportive reinforcement for positive behavior such as use of a "star chart," rewards, and praise. Children are taught to be increasingly sensitive to their body's cues to urinate, encouraged to void in the toilet, and reinforced, either emotionally, materially, or both, for success. This therapy is emotionally time-consuming and requires a high level of healthy communication between parents and children. Provider support of both parents and children is essential, and the provider should see children every 2 weeks; 70% to 90% show improvement.
- *Drug therapy.* Drug therapy (Table 13-3) is often used in conjunction with other strategies and usually has high initial success rates. Unfortunately, it is expensive and extremely high relapse rates can occur when the drug is discontinued. However, it can be very useful for overnight stays (e.g., camp) when staying dry is important to the child. Medications used for children with MNE include antidiuretic analogs (desmopressin), tricyclic antidepressants (imipramine), and muscarinic acetylcholine receptor blockers (oxybutynin, more often used for urge incontinence) (see also Appendix A). Medications used for adults may be found to have pediatric application as well (Humphreys & Reinberg, 2005).

Desmopressin has an antidiuretic effect and appears to be effective in children with large nocturnal urine production and normal nocturnal bladder capacity. Some researchers suggest that desmopressin, combined with use of an enuresis alarm, could lead to nearly 100% correction of nocturnal enuresis (Mellon & McGrath, 2000). There is a high relapse rate associated with short-term therapy, but long-term oral therapy has been found to be safe and more effective (Wolfish et al, 2003). Desmopressin nasal spray is NOT indicated for use with nocturnal enuresis, as it can lead to hyponatermia, seizures, and death (Waknine, 2007).

Imipramine is a tricyclic antidepressant whose action related to enuresis is not entirely clear. Because of serious side effects, most significantly cardiac death, high failure rate when the drug is discontinued, and a low long-term response rate, imipramine is not considered a first-line medication and is not used by most providers. The panel of the First International Consultation on Incontinence, sponsored by the World Health Organization (WHO) and the International Union Against Cancer (UICC), does not recommend use of imipramine in the treatment of enuresis (Abrams et al, 1998). If all other treatments are ineffective, especially in older children, imipramine can be effective (Gepertz & Neveus, 2004).

Oxybutynin chloride is an anticholinergic drug that relaxes the smooth muscle of the bladder, allows increased urine retention, and reduces frequency. It is sometimes used in conjunction with desmopressin, and it appears to be most effective as a treatment for MNE if the child also has daytime incontinence (Robson & Leung, 2006).

Children taking medications on a regular basis should have a drug "holiday" every 3 to 6 months to assess the need for continued pharmacotherapy. If wetting recurs, medication can be continued at the effective dosage for another 3 to 6 months. After 1 month without wetting, medications can be tapered over a 2- to 4-week period, decreasing the dose (e.g., from 0.6 to 0.4 mg/day of desmopressin), decreasing dosing by 1 day a week, then to every other day. Some providers discontinue medication abruptly without apparent problems (Brunell et al, 2001).

Complications

Enuresis contributes to poor self-esteem and disrupted family interactions and threatens the child's ability to establish strong peer relationships. Children with nocturnal and diurnal enuresis tend to demonstrate a higher level of problem behaviors than children without enuresis (Van Hoecke et al, 2006). Self-concept is lower in girls than boys and in older children, and more treatment failures are related to lower self-concept (Theunis et al, 2002; Wolanczyk et al, 2002).

Patient Education and Prevention

Supportive education of parents and positive reinforcement of children's efforts can help prevent enuresis. For 3- to 5-year-old children, a nonjudgmental attitude of "benign neglect" in the face of accidents is the best approach.

DYSFUNCTIONAL VOIDING

Description

Dysfunctional voiding, or pediatric unstable bladder, is characterized by poor initiation of micturition, poor inhibition of voiding (incontinence), or incomplete emptying of the bladder.

Epidemiology

The cause of dysfunctional voiding is unknown, but it is believed to be primarily related to voiding immaturity. Detrusor instability or overactivity may be a factor. Children may learn to inhibit relaxation of the external sphincter. Constipation, UTI, structural abnormalities, stress, and abuse must be considered. It is more common in girls and is usually seen in children 4 to 8 years old, after toilet training but before puberty.

Clinical Findings

History.   Because of the varied problems associated with dysfunctional voiding, children have a history of differing symptoms, including the following:
- Infrequent voiding
- Sudden daytime incontinence after having been dry
- Urgency
- Frequency
- Inability to stop the voiding stream
- Occasional nocturnal enuresis, but usually daytime wetting

TABLE 13-3   **Drug Therapy for Children With Monosymptomatic Nocturnal Enuresis**

Medication	Dosing	Comments
Desmopressin acetate (DDAVP)	Oral: 0.2 mg tab once daily at bedtime; can be adjusted up to max of 0.6 mg/day	Not recommended in children younger than 6 yr. Caution must be used with patients who are hypertensive or have a potential for fluid-electrolyte imbalance (e.g., children with cystic fibrosis susceptible to hyponatremia). Use least amount effective. Take on empty stomach; avoid caffeine, chocolate, NutraSweet, and carbonated beverages. Children must be wakened to urinate within 10 hr of taking the medication.
Imipramine hydrochloride	Dosing: 0.9-1.5 mg/kg/day (Zaontz & Welch, 2002) Initially, 10-25 mg daily 1 hr before bedtime. After 1 wk can increase by 25 mg/day to max of 50 mg for children 6-12 yr, 75 mg for children older than 12 yr	Not recommended in children younger than 6 yr. Administer with great care. Use least amount effective. Has serious side effects and a high level of toxicity; has been fatal to patient or siblings in some cases. Requires electrocardiogram before and after treatment has started to rule out cardiac conduction disorder (long QT syndrome).
Oxybutynin chloride Immediate release Oxybutynin chloride Extended release	5 mg once daily; increase as tolerated in 5 mg increments to max of 20 mg daily	Effective in children with daytime enuresis. Not recommended in children 5 yr old or younger.

hr, Hour(s); *min*, minute(s); *wk*, week(s); *yr*, year(s).

- Constipation or enuresis
- UTI

The history should also include information about the child's general development (achievement of developmental milestones), pattern of toilet training and elimination (frequency and volume of voiding and timing of episodes of incontinence), any stressors experienced following toilet training, family history of dysfunctional voiding, and the child's behavioral patterns.

Physical Examination.   A complete physical examination should be done.

Laboratory and Diagnostic Tests.   Urodynamic diagnostic procedures are not routinely necessary. The following tests are indicated:

- Urinalysis
- Urine culture and sensitivity
- Renal and bladder ultrasound if structural abnormalities are suspected; an abnormal ultrasound can show a normal upper renal system and a thick-walled bladder
- Voiding cystourethrogram (VCUG) in boys and radionuclide cystogram:
  - In girls if there is a history of recurrent or febrile UTI and a thickened bladder wall on ultrasound (US)
  - In boys more than 5 years old with nocturnal and diurnal enuresis
  - In children at puberty with persistent enuresis (Feldman & Bauer, 2006).

Differential Diagnosis

The differential diagnoses for dysfunctional voiding are as follows:

- UTI
- Structural abnormality, such as abnormal sphincters, ectopic ureter, duplicated urethra, or urethral valves
- Neurogenic bladder
- Vesicoureteral reflux
- Trauma or abuse
- Urethritis (may be caused by chemicals in soaps, bubble baths)

Management

The goal of management is to prevent or break the cycle of urinary dysfunction, infection, and/or irritable bladder. Intervention includes the following:

- Treat any UTI if present (see Chapter 34 for a discussion of infections).
- Retrain the bladder. This process works well with 6- to 8-year-olds, but requires a motivated child (see Box 13-4 for suggestions on bladder retraining).
- Treat pelvic floor dysfunction, if appropriate (e.g., Kegel exercises with biofeedback) (Vasconcelos et al, 2006)).
- Treat constipation if present. This may correct the entire problem.
- Treat symptoms with anticholinergics, such as oxybutynin chloride. Oxybutynin chloride is not recommended for use in children younger than 5 years old; the dose in children older than 5 years is 2.5 to 5 mg every day or twice a day,

---

BOX 13-4   Bladder Retraining for Dysfunctional Voiding

Establish a schedule for voiding. Have child go to the bathroom every 2-4 hours, whether urgency is felt or not.

Void with relaxation. Have child take a deep breath and relax sphincter when exhaling; use a straw to breathe through. Have child try grasping fingers together and pulling them apart.

Void to completion. Teach child to use Credé maneuver or manual pressure over suprapubic area to complete voiding.

Double void. After voiding completely, have child wait on toilet several minutes and attempt to void again.

---

to a maximum of 20 mg in 24 hours. Recently, tolterodine has been used effectively and with fewer side effects than oxybutynin in children with detrusor instability (Kilic et al, 2006). Tolterodine dosage in children 5 to 10 years old is 1 mg twice a day; in older children, up to 4 mg twice a day (Hjalmas et al, 2001; Munding et al, 2001).

- Teach parents or child to perform intermittent catheterization if appropriate. Self-catheterization has been effective in decreasing dysfunctional voiding and promoting continence (Pohl et al, 2002).
- Treat skin breakdown if present.

Patient Education and Prevention

Effective toilet training can prevent urinary retention, especially if children learn to be sensitive and responsive to cues to urinate. Parents should be instructed to be alert to signs of dysuria. If urination is painful, children often struggle to retain urine or void incompletely. Early treatment for UTIs is essential to prevent renal dysfunction.

NURSING DIAGNOSES
Related to Elimination

Urinary Function

- Enuresis (not a NANDA diagnosis)
- Urinary incontinence: total, functional, stress, urge, reflex, risk for
  - Risk for overflow urinary incontinence
- Readiness for enhanced urinary elimination
- Impaired urinary elimination
- Urinary retention

Gastrointestinal Function

- Bowel incontinence
- Diarrhea
- Constipation
- Risk for constipation
- Perceived constipation
- Encopresis (not a NANDA diagnosis)

From NANDA International: *NANDA-I nursing diagnoses: definitions and classification 2007-2008*, Philadelphia, 2007, Author.

RESOURCE BOX

Elimination

ENURESIS
National Kidney Foundation/National Enuresis Society
www.kidney.org/patients/bw/

National kidney and urologic diseases information clearinghouse
www.kidney.niddk.nih.gov/kudiseases/pubs/uichildren

Enuresis alarms
www.wetbuster.com/alarms.htm
www.bedwettingstore.com
General information and list of alarm options, with prices, available from a variety of local pharmacies and corporations in countries around the world

Malem ultimate alarm
www.malem.co.uk
Malem Medical

Nite Train'r alarm
www.nitetrain-r.com
Koregon Enterprises

Nytone enuretic alarm
www.nytone.com
Nytone Medical Products

PottyMD WET-STOP2 alarm
www.pottymd.com
PottyMD

Potty pager
www.pottypager.com
Ideas for Living, Inc.

ENCOPRESIS
Keep kids healthy
www.keepkidshealthy.com
General information for providers and parents about pediatric conditions, including encopresis and enuresis

Nemours Foundation
www.kidshealth.org

North American Society of Pediatric Gastroenterology, Hepatology, and Nutrition
www.naspghan.org

National Digestive Diseases Information Clearinghouse, National Institutes of Health
http://digestive.niddk.nih.gov/ddiseases/pubs/constipation/index.htm

✓ DISCUSSION FORUM

1. What are the dietary and medical options for treating constipation in a 1-year-old? Consider various causes. How would the treatment vary for a 5-year-old or a 15-year-old? Explain the pathophysiology of the relationship between constipation and UTIs.
2. What are key points in the history and physical examination of a school-age child with dysfunctional voiding? Outline a plan to work with the family and child to treat this problem. When do you refer to a urologist?
3. A mother reports that despite following your advice about toilet training, her 4-year-old son insists on using diapers and has never urinated in the toilet. She states she is concerned. What will you review in the history and the physical exam? What suggestions do you have for this mother?
4. An adolescent with recurrent UTIs reports that she cannot void in school because the bathrooms are unsafe. What can you do to advocate for her?

REFERENCES

Abrams P, Khoury S, Wein A, editors: *Conservative management in children.* Proceedings from the First International Consultation on Incontinence, June 28-July 1, 1998, St. Helier, Jersey, United Kingdom, 1998, Health Publication, Ltd.

American Academy of Pediatrics Committee on Practice and Ambulatory Medicine: Recommendations for preventive pediatric health care, *Pediatrics* 105:149-150, 2000.

American Medical Association: *Guidelines for adolescent preventive services (GAPS): recommendations monograph,* Chicago, 1997, American Medical Association.

Baker SS et al: Clinical practice guideline. Evaluation and treatment of constipation in infants and children: recommendations of the North American Society for Pediatric Gastroenterology, Hepatology and Nutrition, *J Ped Gastroenterol Nutr* 43:e1-e13, 2006.

Bakker E et al: Results of a questionnaire evaluating the effects of different methods of toilet training on achieving bladder control, *BJU Int* 90: 456-461, 2002.

Barroso U Jr et al: Nonpharmacological treatment of lower urinary tract dysfunction using biofeedback and transcutaneous electrical stimulation: a pilot study, *BJU Int* 98(1):166-171, 2006.

Bayoumi RA et al: The genetic basis of inherited primary nocturnal enuresis: a UAE study, *J Psychosom Res* 61(3):317-320, 2006.

Behrman RE, Kliegman RM, editors: *Nelson essentials of pediatrics,* ed 4, Philadelphia, 2002, WB Saunders.

Benninga MA et al: Colonic transit times and behaviour profiles in children with defecation disorders, *Arch Dis Child* 89(1):13-16, 2004.

Berkowitz CD: *Pediatrics: a primary care approach,* ed 2, Philadelphia, 2000, WB Saunders.

Blum NJ, Taubman B, Nemeth N: During toilet training, constipation occurs before stool toileting refusal, *Pediatrics* 113(6):e520-522, 2004.

Blum NJ, Taubman B, Nemeth N: Children who hide while defecating before they have completed toilet training: a prospective study, *Arch Pediatr Adolesc Med* 157(12):1153-1154, 2003.

Blum NJ, Taubman B, Osborne ML: Behavioral characteristics of children with stool toileting refusal, *Pediatrics* 99:50-53, 1997.

Bock GH: Screening UA should be based on specific conditions, *AAP News* 27(12):18-19, 2006.

Boris NW, Dalton R: Encopresis. In Behrman RE, Kliegman RM, Jenson HB, editors: *Nelson textbook of pediatrics,* ed 17, Philadelphia, 2004a, WB Saunders.

Boris NW, Dalton R: Enuresis (bedwetting). In Behrman RE, Kliegman RM, Jenson HB, editors: *Nelson textbook of pediatrics*, ed 17, Philadelphia, 2004b, WB Saunders.

Brazzelli M, Griffiths P: Behavioural and cognitive interventions with or without other treatments for the management of faecal incontinence in children, *Cochrane Database of Systematic Reviews*, 2006, Issue 2 Art. No. CD002240, DOI: 10.1002/14651858.CD002240.pub3.

Brunell PA et al: Taking a closer look at primary nocturnal enuresis, *Monograph: infectious diseases in children*, sponsored by Aventis Pasteur, 2001.

Butler RJ, Robinson JC: Alarm treatment for childhood nocturnal enuresis: an investigation of within-treatment variables, *Scand J Urol Nephrol* 36: 268-272, 2002.

Chandra M et al: Prevalence of diurnal voiding symptoms and difficult arousal from sleep in children with nocturnal enuresis, *J Urol* 172(1):311-316, 2004.

Choe YH et al: The infrequent bowel movements in young infants who are exclusively breast-fed, *Eur J Pediatr* 163(10):630-631, 2004.

Eggermont E: Transient, infrequent bowel movements in the exclusively breast-fed infant, *Eur J Pediatr* 163(10):632-633, 2004.

Feldman AS, Bauer SB: Diagnosis and management of dysfunctional voiding, *Curr Opin Pediatr* 18(2):139-147, 2006.

Fishman L et al: Early constipation and toilet training in children with encopresis, *J Pediatr Gastroenterol Nutr* 34:385-388, 2002.

Freitag CM et al: Neurophysiology of nocturnal enuresis: evoked potentials and prepulse inhibition of the startle reflex, *Dev Med Child Neurol* 48(4):278-284, 2006.

Gepertz S, Neveus T: Imipramine for therapy-resistant enuresis: a retrospective evaluation, *J Urol* 171(6 pt 2):2607-2610, 2004.

Glazener CMA, Evans JHC, Cheuk DKL: Complementary and miscellaneous interventions for nocturnal enuresis in children, *Cochrane Database of Systematic Reviews*, 2005a, Issue 2, Art. No. 1 CD005230, DOI: 10.1002/14651858.CD005230.

Glazener CMA, Evans JHC, Peto RE: Alarm interventions for nocturnal enuresis in children, *Cochrane Database of Systematic Reviews*, 2005b, Issue 2, Art. No.1 CD002911, DOI: 10.1002/14651858.CD002911.pub2.

Gremse D, Hixon J, Crutchfield A: Comparison of polyethylene glycol 3350 and lactulose for treatment of chronic constipation in children, *Clin Pediatr* 41:225-229, 2002.

Hjalmas K et al: The overactive bladder in children: a potential future indication for tolterodine, *BJU Int* 87:569-574, 2001.

Horn IB et al: Beliefs about the appropriate age for initiating toilet training: are there racial and socioeconomic differences? *J Pediatr* 149(2):151-152, 2006.

Humphreys MR, Reinberg YE: Contemporary and emerging drug treatments for urinary incontinence in children, *Paediatr Drugs* 7(3):51-62, 2005.

Humphreys MR et al: Preliminary results of sacral neuromodulation in 23 children, *J Urol* 176(5):2227-2231, 2006.

Jansson UB et al: Voiding pattern in healthy children 0 to 3 years old: a longitudinal study, *J Urol* 164:2052-2054, 2000.

Kilic N et al: Comparison of the effectiveness and side-effects of tolterodine and oxybutynin in children with detrusor instability, *Int J Urol* 13(2): 105-108, 2006.

Loeys B et al: Does monosymptomatic enuresis exist? A molecular genetic exploration of 32 families with enuresis/incontinence, *BJU Int* 90:76-83, 2002.

Lundblad B, Hellström A: Perceptions of school toilets as a cause of irregular toilet habits among school children aged 6 to 16 years, *J Sch Health* 75(4):125-128, 2005.

Mellon MW, McGrath ML: Empirically supported treatments in pediatric psychology: nocturnal enuresis, *J Pediatr Psychol* 25:193-214, 2000.

Munding M et al: Use of tolterodine in children with dysfunctional voiding: an initial report, *J Urol* 165:926-928, 2001.

Pakarinen MP, Koivusalo A, Rintala RJ: Functional fecal soiling without constipation, organic cause or neuropsychiatric disorders? *J Pediatr Gastroenterol Nutr* 43(2):206-208, 2006.

Pashankar DS, Bishop WP: Efficacy and optimal dose of daily polyethylene glycol 3350 for treatment of constipation and encopresis in children, *J Pediatr* 139:428-432, 2001.

Pohl HG et al: The outcome of voiding dysfunction managed with clean intermittent catheterization in neurologically and anatomically normal children, *BJU Int* 89:923-927, 2002.

Pomeranz A et al: Night-time polyuria and urine hypo-osmolality in enuretics identified by nocturnal sequential urine sampling–do they represent a subset of relative ADH-deficient subjects? *Scand J Urol Nephrol* 34: 199-202, 2000.

Robson WL, Leung AK: An approach to daytime wetting in children, *Adv Pediatr* 53:323-365, 2006.

Robson WL, Leung AK: Urotherapy recommendations for bedwetting, *J Natl Med Assoc* 94:577-580, 2002.

Schmitt B: *Encopresis*, Presentation: TCH Encopresis-Enuresis Clinic, June 2006.

Schonwald A, Rappaport L: Encopresis: assessment and management, *Pediatr Rev* 25(8):278-283, 2004.

Schum TR et al: Sequential acquisition of toilet training skills: a descriptive study of gender and age differences in normal children, *Pediatrics* 109 (3): e48-e55, 2002.

Shrago LC, Reifsnider E, Insel K: The Neonatal Bowel Output Study: indicators of adequate breast milk intake in neonates, *Pediatr Nurs* 32(3):195-201, 2006.

Sulkes SB, Dosa NP: Developmental and behavioral pediatrics. In Behrman RE, Kliegman RM, editors: *Nelson essentials of pediatrics*, Philadelphia, 2002, WB Saunders.

Sun M, Rugolotto S: Assisted infant toilet training in a Western family setting, *J Dev Behav Pediatr* 25(2):99-101, 2004.

Taubman B: Toilet training and toileting refusal for stool only: a prospective study, *Pediatrics* 99:54-58, 1997.

Taubman B, Blum NJ, Nemeth N: Stool toileting refusal: a prospective intervention targeting parental behavior, *Arch Pediatr Adolesc Med* 157(12):1193-1196, 2003.

Theunis M et al: Self-image and performance in children with nocturnal enuresis, *Eur Urol* 41:660-667, 2002.

Tomasi PA et al: Decreased nocturnal urinary antidiuretic hormone excretion in enuresis is increased by imipramine, *BJU Int* 88:932-937, 2001.

US Preventive Services Task Force: *Guide to clinical preventive services*, ed 2, Baltimore, 1996, Williams & Wilkins.

van Gool JD: Enuresis and incontinence in children, *Semin Pediatr Surg* 11:100-107, 2002.

Van Hoecke E et al: Internalizing and externalizing problem behavior in children with nocturnal and diurnal enuresis: a five-factor model perspective, *J Pediatr Psychol* 31(5):460-468, 2006.

Van Kampen M et al: High initial efficacy of full-spectrum therapy for nocturnal enuresis in children and adolescents, *BJU Int* 90:84-87, 2002.

Vasconcelos M et al: Voiding dysfunction in children. Pelvic-floor exercises or biofeedback therapy: a randomized study, *Pediatr Nephrol* 21(12):1858-1864, 2006.

Wolanczyk T et al: Attitudes of enuretic children towards their illness, *Acta Paediatr* 91:844-848, 2002.

Wolfish NM: Sleep/arousal and enuresis subtypes, *J Urol* 166:2444-2447, 2001.

Wolfish NM et al: The Canadian Enuresis Study and Evaluation–short- and long-term safety and efficacy of oral desmopressin preparation, *Scand J Urol Nephrol* 37(1):22-27, 2003.

Wolraich ML, Tippins S: *American Academy of Pediatrics guide to toilet training*, NY, 2003, Bantam Books.

Yeung CK et al: Reduction in nocturnal functional bladder capacity is a common factor in the pathogenesis of refractory nocturnal enuresis, *BJU Int* 90:302-307, 2002.

Yeung CK et al: Differences in characteristics of nocturnal enuresis between children and adolescents: a critical appraisal from a large epidemiological study, *BJU Int* 97(5):1069-1073, 2006.

Yuping W, Runfang L, Hua K: Acupuncture treatment of children nocturnal enuresis: a report of 56 cases, *J Tradit Chin Med* 26(2):106-107, 2006.

Zaontz M, Welch V: *Enuresis: state of the art*. Presentation at National Association of Pediatric Nurse Practitioners Annual Educational Conference, Mar 16, 2002.

CHAPTER 14

Activities and Sports for Children and Adolescents

Catherine G. Blosser

Maintenance of activity is a basic health need of all people, including infants, children, and adolescents. Activity promotes motor and cognitive development and physical health. It is essential for optimal functioning of the body; body systems are influenced by the metabolic, physical, and neurologic responses needed to execute and maintain a healthy level of activity. Activity also fosters psychological development by promoting self-esteem as the child masters new skills and learns to interact with others in mutual activities. Further, activity patterns become long-term lifestyle habits that either promote or compromise the health of the individual in the future.

The trend toward obesity in youth is one staggering consequence of inactivity. Cardiovascular heart disease, depression, diabetes, musculoskeletal pain and strain, and breathing disorders are imminent long-term consequences of inactivity and obesity (Hendrickson, 2003).

The increase in chronic global disease rates caused by energy-dense, nutrient-poor foods and inactivity is also a concern of the World Health Organization (WHO). A 2003 WHO report cited that the epidemic of childhood obesity affected 17.6 million children worldwide. In 2004, WHO developed a population-wide, global strategy on diet, physical activity, and health and in 2006 published a framework for member countries to implement and monitor their progress (WHO, 2004a; WHO, 2006).

Results of health-related surveys illustrate the magnitude of the problem in the U.S. The number of students enrolled in daily school physical education (PE) showed: (a) children spent less time participating in PE as they progressed from ninth through twelfth grade; (b) vigorous physical activity declined for adolescents; and, (c) of the six main indicators of physical activity and fitness in the *Healthy People 2010* objectives, five showed little or no change (one could not be assessed because of limited data; National Center for Health Statistics [NCHS], 2004; CDC, 2006a). Meanwhile 15.8% of children 6 to 11 years old and 16.1% of children 12 to 19 years old were defined as being overweight (USDHHS, 2005).

The *Healthy People 2010* progress review also showed that the greatest increase in prevalence of overweight was in the 12- to 19-year-old age group (NCHS, 2004). The DHHS summarized the NCHS progress review data on the indicators for nutrition and overweight in children as showing "a trend for the worse" (USDHHS, 2004). Not only does the U.S. have one of the higher rates of obesity of countries belonging to the WHO, but it also has one of the highest rates of dieting among girls (almost 30%) and boys (20% [rate is less than 11% in all other countries]; WHO, 2004b).

The percentage of males who participate in PE class grades nine through twelve exceeds that of females. The average nationwide prevalence rate for *daily* PE attendance in these grade levels for both sexes is 33%, whereas attendance prevalence rates for *one or more days* average 54.2% (CDC, 2006a). Studies have demonstrated that a lower body satisfaction in adolescents is related to lower physical activity and more hours of TV watching (Neumark-Sztainer et al, 2004), and that those greater than 85th percentile in weight do fewer minutes of physical activity (less than 60 min/day moderate to vigorous activity) and consume less fiber per day than those of normal weight (Norman et al, 2004). A recent study done in Europe concluded that children needed to achieve at least 90 minutes of daily physical activity (versus a previous norm of 60 minutes/day) to prevent insulin resistance (Andersen et al, 2006).

The activity pyramid is adapted from the United States Department of Agriculture Food Pyramid and is being used to engage children, adolescents, and adults in efforts to increase their activity levels. An example of the youth activity pyramid is provided (Fig. 14-1).

A survey in 1995 showed that 30% of nurse practitioners (NPs) asked their patients about exercise, and 14% discussed an exercise plan (Clark & Ferguson, 2000). A 1999 survey of pediatricians showed that 41% to 59% reported always discussing physical activity with children from 2 to 18 years old (Galuska et al, 1999). A more recent survey of adults 18 years and older revealed a statistically significant decline in such counseling between 1994 and 2000 (from 42% to 40%). Declines were reported greatest in women, in the younger (18 to 29 years old) and older (greater than 70 years) age groups, in those whose BMIs were between 30 and 34.9, and in those not diagnosed with diabetes. The results further showed that of those who had received counseling from their health provider, 80% attempted to lose weight (CDC, 2000). Although the most recent U. S. Preventive Services Task Force (USPSF) review concluded that the "evidence is insufficient to recommend for or against behavioral counseling in primary care settings to promote physical activity" (USPSTF, 2002, p. 2), we believe that counseling about the health benefits of physical activity is an efficacious use of time for all clinicians.

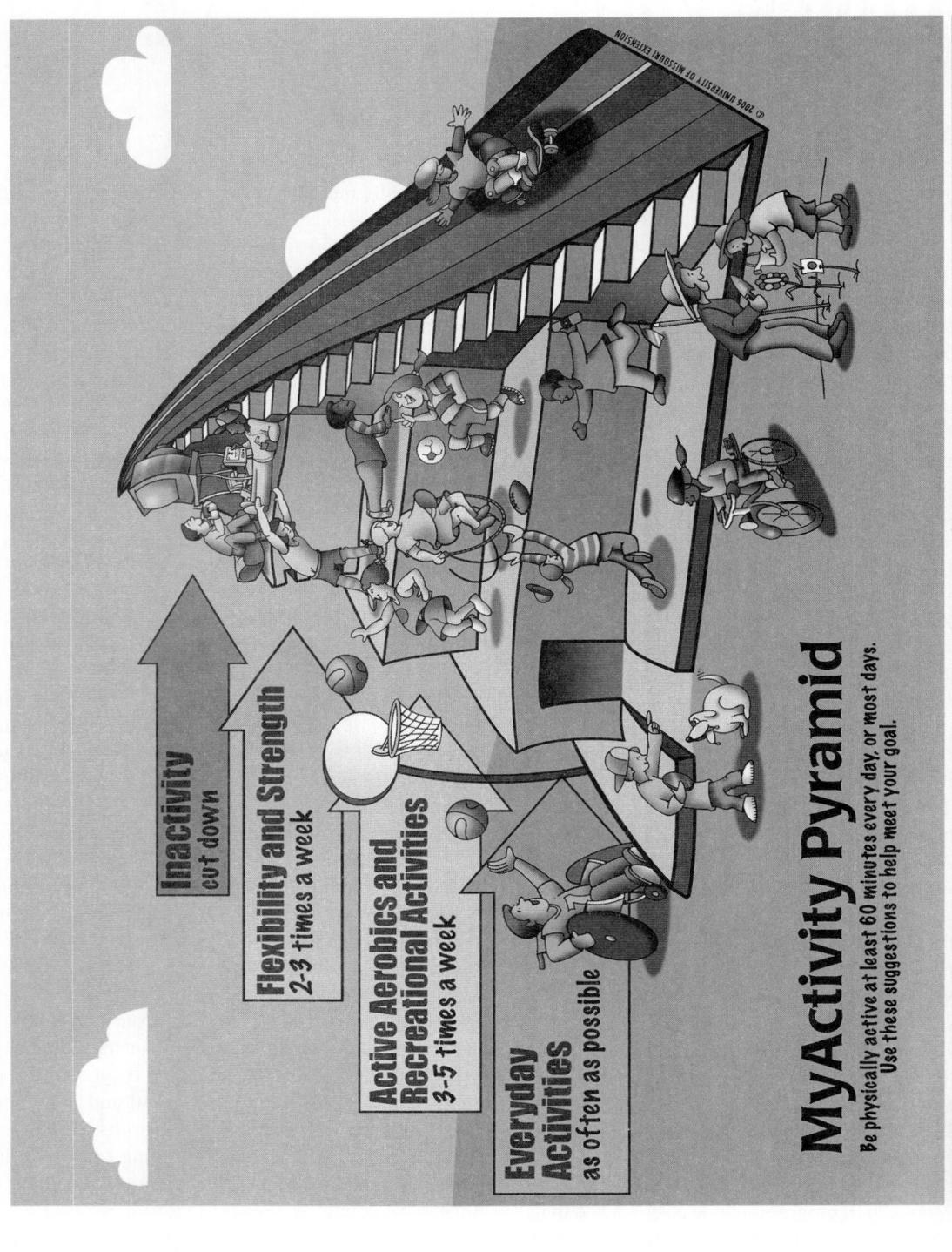

FIG. 14-1 Youth activity pyramid. (From University of Missouri Extension: *MyActivity Pyramid*, 1999, Columbia, MO. Adapted from USDA's MyPyramid. Available at www.extension.missouri.edu/explore/hesguide/foodnut/n000386.htm [accessed Oct 10, 2007].)

MyActivity Pyramid

Be physically active at least 60 minutes every day, or most days.
Use these suggestions to help meet your goal:

Everyday Activities

As often as possible

- Playing outside
- Helping with chores around the house or yard
- Taking the stairs instead of the elevator
- Picking up toys
- Walking

Active Aerobics and Recreational Activities

3-5 times a week

- Playing basketball
- Biking
- Playing baseball or softball
- Rollerblading
- Skateboarding
- Playing soccer
- Swimming
- Playground games
- Jumping rope

Flexibility and Strength

2-3 times a week

- Practicing martial arts
- Rope climbing
- Stretching
- Practicing yoga
- Doing push-ups and pull-ups

Inactivity

Cut down

- Watching television
- Playing on the computer
- Sitting for too long
- Playing video games

Find your balance between food and fun:

- Move more. Aim for at least 60 minutes every day, or most days.
- Walk, dance, bike, rollerblade – it all counts. How great is that!

This publication is adapted from USDA's MyPyramid and was funded in part by USDA's Food Stamp Program.

UNIVERSITY OF MISSOURI ■ Issued in furtherance of Cooperative Extension Work Acts of May 8 and June 30, 1914, in cooperation with the United States Department of Agriculture. L. Jo Turner, Interim Director, Cooperative Extension, University of Missouri, Columbia, MO 65211. ■ University of Missouri Extension does not discriminate on the basis of race, color, national origin, sex, sexual orientation, religion, age, disability or status as a Vietnam-era veteran in employment or programs. ■ If you have special needs as addressed by the Americans with Disabilities Act and need this publication in an alternative format, write: ADA Officer, Extension and Agricultural Information, 1-98 Agriculture Building, Columbia, MO 65211, or call (573) 882-7216. Reasonable efforts will be made to accommodate your special needs.

⊞ Extension

FIG. 14-1   cont'd.

■ CLINICAL PREVENTIVE SERVICES, GUIDELINES, AND STANDARDS FOR PHYSICAL ACTIVITY AND FITNESS IN CHILDREN

HEALTHY PEOPLE 2010 GUIDELINES FOR PHYSICAL ACTIVITY AND FITNESS

Healthy People 2010 includes objectives for physical activity and fitness in children (USDHHS, 2000). These include the following:

1. Increase the proportion of adolescents who have engaged in moderate physical activity for at least 30 minutes on 5 or more of the previous 7 days.
2. Increase the proportion of adolescents who engage in vigorous physical activity that promotes cardiorespiratory fitness 3 or more days per week for 20 or more minutes per occasion.
3. Increase the proportion of the nation's public and private schools that require daily physical education for all students.
4. Increase the proportion of adolescents who participate in daily school physical education.
5. Increase the proportion of adolescents who spend at least 50% of school physical education class time being physically active.
6. Increase the proportion of adolescents who view television 2 or fewer hours on a school day.
7. Increase the percentage of children from 5 to 15 years old who walk (if less than 1 mile) or bicycle (if less than 2 miles) to school; children who walk or cycle to school are more likely to be active on all days and weekdays versus irregular or nonactive commuters (Sirard et al, 2005).

AMERICAN ACADEMY OF PEDIATRICS GUIDELINES

The American Academy of Pediatrics (AAP) policy statement addresses the issue of physical activity for young people and includes the following recommendations (AAP, 2006a):

1. Physicians and health care professionals should participate with schools in implementing and setting goals to develop wellness policies for healthy nutrition, physical activity, and other strategies that promote wellness of students.
2. Advocate for school curricula that emphasize the health benefits of regular physical activity and for recreational programs that allow for the use of community and school facilities after hours by children and youth at reasonable costs.
3. Advocate for the reinstatement of compulsory, quality, daily PE classes K through 12 that are enjoyable and help students develop attitudes and skills for lifelong active lifestyles; maintain school recess, and promote extracurricular physical activity programs before and after school hours.
4. Promote recreational facilities, parks, playgrounds, bicycle and walking paths, sidewalks, and marked crosswalks.
5. During office visits, inquire about nutritional intake, plot BMIs, promote healthy eating and physical activity, note and discuss the limitation of sedentary activities.
6. Encourage children and adolescents to be moderately physical for 60 minutes/day (not necessarily contiguous minutes).
7. Encourage a culture of family physical activity by advocating that parents act as role models, incorporate physical activity in their own lives, and support their children in age-appropriate sports and recreational activities.
8. Suggest that overweight children initially participate in activities that place less stress on weight-bearing joints, such as swimming, water polo, strength training, and cycling.

SPORTS INJURIES

An estimated 35 million children, adolescents, and young adults participate in some manner of sport, whether organized or recreational. Though relatively safe in children, athletic participation becomes more high risk for serious injury in adolescents. A Centers for Disease Control and Prevention survey in 2005 revealed that of the 78.8% of students nationwide who exercised or played sports, 22.2% needed medical evaluation for an injury during the preceding 30 days. The prevalence rate was higher for males than females and highest for black and Hispanic males. By the time they reached twelfth grade, females were injured less than they were in the lower high school grades (CDC, 2006a).

An estimated 4.2 million nonfatal sports- and recreation-related injuries were evaluated in nationwide hospital emergency departments in a one-year period; hospitalization was required for 2.3% of those injured (CDC, 2002). Traditionally, football, gymnastics, and wrestling have involved the most injuries, but since the increase in popularity of pole vaulting and cheerleading (especially for females), these sports have produced catastrophic head and spinal injuries (Hergenroeder, 2002).

One of the goals of this chapter is to provide information to help young people engage in healthy and age-appropriate fitness activities and sports while minimizing the risks of injury. The preparticipation physical examination (PPE) plays an important role in identifying those at most risk for injury. Preparticipation examinations, however, are not required for many recreational activities of children and adolescents. Consider the risks of injury to youngsters participating in nonorganized recreational activities, such as in-line skating, skateboarding, cycling, skiing, swimming, and off-road vehicle and motorcycle riding.

CHOOSING AGE- AND PHYSICALLY APPROPRIATE FITNESS ACTIVITIES

Although the focus of this chapter is on sports for older children and adolescents, it is recognized that younger children also need daily activity and play to promote their growth and development. Table 14-1 provides the clinician with information to counsel parents on age-appropriate physical activities by age groups. All children, regardless of disability or chronic health conditions, benefit from fitness activities.

For school-age youth and adolescents with health problems wanting to participate in organized sports, the process for decision-making about the appropriateness of various sports is more complex. The young person's overall health needs to be assessed, then reviewed in the context of the recommendations for participation in various sports for given health conditions, and a decision made about the client's participation (Fig. 14-2 and Table 14-2). Consultation with the appropriate

TABLE 14-1 Appropriate Fitness Activities by Age Group

Age-Group	Strengths/Development Factors	Fitness Activities	Family Fitness Fun
Infant-toddler	Enjoys playing with family and others Enjoys moving Enjoys playing with objects Is curious and explores environment Moves in new ways when challenged with interesting activities Mastering basic motor milestones	5 min of "tummy time" for young infants. Provide safe spaces to crawl, roll, pull, stand, cruise, climb, walk, run, and explore.	Walking, playing, running
2-3 years	Participates in and enjoys many physical activities Enjoys playing with family and others Fundamental skills developing: throwing, catching, running, jumping, skipping, hopping	Unstructured play that focuses on participation not competition: running, swinging, climbing, playing in sandbox, supervised water play, tumbling, tag.	Walking, playing, and running
4-5 years	Mastering more complex motor activities—running, jumping, skipping, throwing, climbing, kicking, balancing	Most children are not ready for organized or competitive sports. Roll large balls, play catch, ride bike with training wheels away from traffic, swimming, dancing, jumping rope, skiing, skating, hopscotch, Frisbee, walking, kickball. Judgment, safety awareness, and coordination skills are limited. Enroll in swimming lessons.	Walking, playing, running, tennis, skiing, dancing, ice skating, hiking, bike riding
6-12 years	Participates in and enjoys many physical activities Develops a positive attitude toward physical activity Wants to improve motor skills Is developing a sense of responsibility for own health Has positive role models for physical activity Has opportunities for participation in physical activities 5-6 years: mastering fundamentals of skilled movements 7-9 years: refining skills, such as distance 10-11 years: beginning complex skills (e.g., basketball); integrating cognitive skills with motor skills for sports (e.g., rules, strategy, team roles)	Abilities developed sufficiently for participation in organized sports, but muscles and tendons are short, tight, and easily injured as a result of growth. Noncompetitive sports include swimming, cycling, netball, gymnastics, dance, and martial arts. Competitive sports: netball, baseball, tennis, table tennis, soccer. Avoid sports specialization until older than 10 years. Weight lifting at 11 years old (with supervision) helps build muscles to minimize later injury. Monitor for eating disorders for those in gymnastics, wrestling, or dance. Number of pitches should be limited (<75 per game) among 9- to 12-year-olds to prevent shoulder or elbow injury (Lyman, 2001). May start actual "exercise" program (i.e., aerobic or resistance training) as long as supervised and employs full-range, multijoint exercise not more than twice weekly with 8-12 repetitions per set, no more than 2 sets of 8-10 different exercises (Luebbers, 2003).	Walking, bike riding, camping, himing, tennis, skiing, dancing, ice skating, swimming Do not use trampolines
13-18 years	Participates in physical activities Enjoys physical activities Wants to improve skills, but feels competent Takes responsibility for own health Has positive role models for physical activity Mastering complex skills for some sports or recreational activities	Any activity, including competitive sports, skateboarding, in-line skating, power walking, rock climbing, snowboarding, rowing, weight training (with supervision); exercise at least 60 min, 3 times a wk.	Walking, cycling, camping, hiking, tennis, skiing, dancing, ice skating, swimming

min, Minute(s); *wk,* week(s).

Data from American Medical Association: *Fitness,* 1999. Available at *www.medem.com;* Faigenbaum A, Micheli L: Preseason conditioning for the preadolescent athlete, *Pediatr Ann* 29(3):156-161, 2000; Patrick K: *Bright Futures in practice: physical activity,* Arlington, VA, 2001, National Center for Education in Maternal and Child Health; Luebbers PE: The right time for kids to exercise. In American College of Sports Medicine: *Fit society: youth sports and health,* Spring 2003. Available *www.acsm.org.search* under Luebbers *(fitsc203.pdf)* (accessed July 31, 2006).

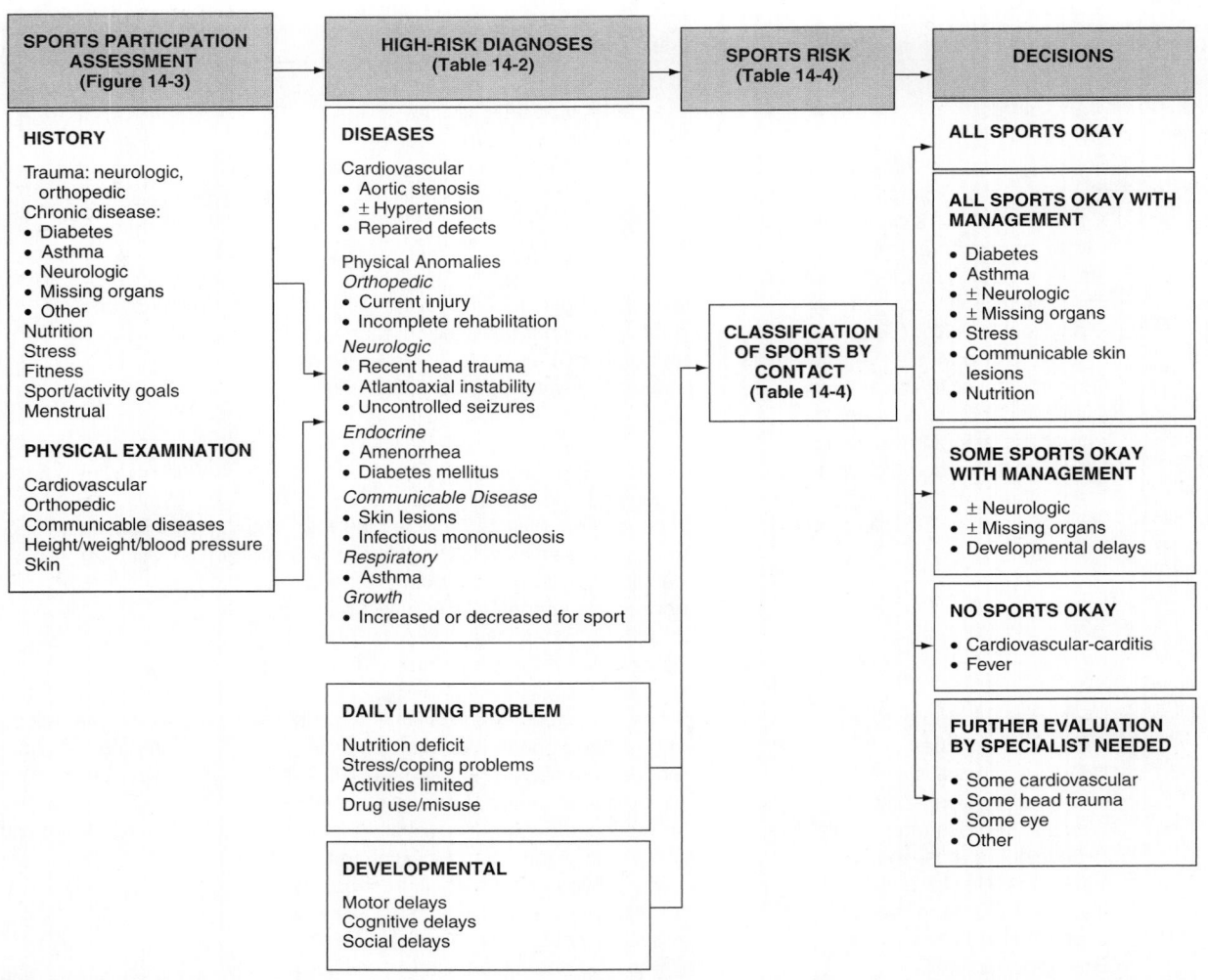

FIG. 14-2 Decision-making for sports participation.

specialist working with the patient's particular health condition is needed before recommending any specific modification or adaptation to a fitness regimen.

■ ASSESSMENT

THE PREPARTICIPATION SPORTS EXAMINATION

The PPE is one of the most common reasons for youth and adolescents to seek primary health care. Approximately 1% to 8% of patients will have findings that need further evaluation or referral before participation, and less than 1% will have significant enough findings (neurologic, musculoskeletal, or vascular) to warrant exclusion from sports participation (Hergenroeder & Chorley, 2004). For the majority of youth, this examination is their only health assessment for the year. The American Heart Association (AHA) recommends a sports examination before starting any organized high school sport and every 2 years thereafter through high school, once upon starting a college sport, and, thereafter, yearly blood pressure and interim history. The examinations should be done at least 6 weeks before the season begins

to allow time for follow-up of problems before engagement (Madden et al, 2003).

For the health care provider to avoid any malpractice liability, it is important that the PPE be done according to customary and standard practices for this type of examination; all history and physical findings must be fully documented, particularly cardiovascular in case of sudden death occurrences. Should the athlete, athlete's family, or guardian disagree with the provider's advice against participation in a certain chosen sport, the provider needs to obtain the athlete's, parent's, or guardian's signed informed consent statement acknowledging understanding of the advice and potential dangers of participation. It is acknowledged that data on the exact risks of a known sport are often limited, but providers must exercise their best assessment skills using such data as that provided in this chapter and/or in consultation with a sports medicine specialist. Counseling about more appropriate alternative sports may be indicated (AAP, 2001a).

The PPE historically served as a vehicle to provide liability protection, satisfy insurance regulations, and detect cardiovascular risks for sudden death. Over the years, other objectives

TABLE 14-2 **Medical Conditions and Sports Participation***	
Condition	**May Participate?**
Atlantoaxial instability (instability of the joint between cervical vertebrae 1 and 2)	Qualified yes
Explanation: Athlete needs evaluation to assess risk of spinal cord injury during sports participation.	
Bleeding disorder	Qualified yes
Explanation: Athlete needs evaluation.	
Cardiovascular diseases: carditis (inflammation of the heart)	No
Explanation: Carditis may result in sudden death with exertion.	
Hypertension (high blood pressure)	Qualified yes
Explanation: Those with significant essential (unexplained) hypertension should avoid weight lifting and power lifting, bodybuilding, and strength training. Those with secondary hypertension (hypertension caused by a previously identified disease) or severe essential hypertension need evaluation.	
Congenital heart disease (structural heart defects present at birth)	Qualified yes
Explanation: Those with mild forms may participate fully; those with moderate or severe forms or those who have undergone surgery, need evaluation.	
Dysrhythmia (irregular heart rhythm)	Qualified yes
Explanation: Athlete needs evaluation because some types of dysrhythmia require therapy or make certain sports dangerous, or both.	
Mitral valve prolapse (abnormal heart valve)	Qualified yes
Explanation: Those with symptoms (chest pain, symptoms of possible dysrhythmia) or evidence of mitral regurgitation (leaking) on physical examination need evaluation. All others may participate fully.	
Heart murmur	Qualified yes
Explanation: If the murmur is innocent (does not indicate heart disease), full participation is permitted. Otherwise the athlete needs evaluation (see "congenital heart disease" and "mitral valve prolapse" previously).	
Cerebral palsy	Qualified yes
Explanation: Athlete needs evaluation.	
Diabetes mellitus	Yes
Explanation: All sports can be played with proper attention to diet, hydration, and insulin therapy. Particular attention is needed for activities that last 30 min or more.	
Diarrhea	Qualified no
Explanation: Unless disease is mild, no participation is permitted because diarrhea may increase the risk of dehydration and heat illness (see "fever" discussed later).	
Eating disorders: anorexia nervosa, bulimia nervosa	Qualified yes
Explanation: These patients need both medical and psychiatric assessment before participation may be allowed.	
Eyes: functionally one-eyed athlete, loss of an eye, detached retina, previous eye surgery, or serious eye injury	Qualified yes
Explanation: A functionally one-eyed athlete has a best corrected visual acuity of 20/40 in the worse eye. These athletes would suffer significant disability if the better eye was seriously injured, as would those with loss of an eye. Some athletes who have previously undergone eye surgery or had a serious eye injury may have an increased risk of injury because of weakened eye tissue. Availability of eye guards approved by the American Society for Testing Materials (ASTM) and other protective equipment may allow participation in most sports, but this must be judged on an individual basis.	
Fever	No
Explanation: Fever can increase cardiopulmonary effort, reduce maximal exercise capacity, make heat illness more likely, and increase orthostatic hypotension during exercise. Fever may rarely accompany myocarditis or other infections that may make exercise dangerous.	
Heat illness: history of	Qualified yes
Explanation: Because of the increased likelihood of recurrence, the athlete needs individual assessment to determine the presence of predisposing conditions and to arrange a prevention strategy.	
Human immunodeficiency virus (HIV) infection	Yes
Explanation: Because of the apparent minimal risk to others, all sports may be played that the state of health allows. In all athletes, skin lesions should be properly covered, and athletic personnel should use universal precautions when handling blood or body fluids with visible blood.	
Kidney: absence of one	Qualified yes
Explanation: Athlete needs individual assessment for contact, collision, and limited-contact sports.	

Continued

TABLE 14-2   **Medical Conditions and Sports Participation*—Cont'd**

Condition	May Participate?
Liver: enlarged	Qualified yes
Explanation: If the liver is acutely enlarged, participation should be avoided because of risk of rupture. If the liver is chronically enlarged, individual assessment is needed before collision, contact, or limited-contact sports are played.	
Malignancy	Qualified yes
Explanation: Athlete needs individual assessment.	
Musculoskeletal disorders	Qualified yes
Explanation: Athlete needs individual assessment.	
Neurologic disorders: history of serious head or spine trauma, severe or repeated concussions, or craniotomy	Qualified yes
Explanation: Athlete needs individual assessment for collision, contact, or limited-contact sports and also for noncontact sports if there are deficits in judgment or cognition. Research supports a conservative approach to management of concussion.	
Convulsive disorder: well controlled	Yes
Explanation: Risk of convulsion during participation is minimal.	
Convulsive disorder: poorly controlled	Qualified yes
Explanation: Athlete needs individual assessment for collision, contact, or limited-contact sports. Avoid the following noncontact sports: archery, riflery, swimming, weight lifting, power lifting, strength training, or sports involving heights. In these sports, occurrence of a convulsion may be a risk to self or others.	
Obesity	Qualified yes
Explanation: Because of the risk of heat illness, obese persons need careful acclimatization and hydration.	
Organ transplant recipient	Qualified yes
Explanation: Athlete needs individual assessment.	
Ovary: absence of one	Yes
Explanation: Risk of severe injury to the remaining ovary is minimal.	
Respiratory: pulmonary compromise, including cystic fibrosis	Qualified yes
Explanation: Athlete needs individual assessment, but generally all sports may be played if oxygenation remains satisfactory during a graded exercise test. Patients with cystic fibrosis need acclimatization and good hydration to reduce the risk of heat illness.	
Asthma	Yes
Explanation: With proper medication and education, only athletes with the most severe asthma have to modify their participation.	
Acute upper respiratory infection	Qualified yes
Explanation: Upper respiratory obstruction may affect pulmonary function. Athlete needs individual assessment for all but mild disease (see "fever" previously).	
Sickle cell disease	Qualified yes
Explanation: Athlete needs individual assessment. In general if status of the illness permits, all but high-exertion, collision, or contact sports may be played. Overheating, dehydration, and chilling must be prevented.	
Sickle cell trait	Yes
Explanation: It is unlikely that individuals with sickle cell trait (AS) have an increased risk of sudden death or other medical problems during athletic participation except under the most extreme conditions of heat, humidity, and, possibly, increased altitude. These individuals, like all athletes, should be carefully conditioned, acclimatized, and hydrated to reduce any possible risk.	
Skin: boils, herpes simplex, impetigo, scabies, *Molluscum contagiosum*	Qualified yes
Explanation: While the patient is contagious, participation in gymnastics with mats, martial arts, wrestling, or other collision, contact, or limited-contact sports is not allowed. Herpes simplex virus probably is not transmitted via mats.	
Spleen: enlarged	Qualified yes
Explanation: Patients with acutely enlarged spleens should avoid all sports because of risk of rupture. Those with chronically enlarged spleens need individual assessment before playing collision, contact, or limited-contact sports.	
Testicle: absent or undescended	Yes
Explanation: Certain sports may require a protective cup.	

*This table is designed to be understood by medical and nonmedical personnel. In the "Explanation" section, "needs evaluation" means that a physician with appropriate knowledge and experience should assess the safety of a given sport for an athlete with the listed medical condition. Unless otherwise noted, this is because of the variability of the severity of the disease or of the risk of injury among the specific sports listed in Table 14-4.
Used with permission of the American Academy of Pediatrics (AAP). From American Academy of Pediatrics Committee on Sports Medicine: Medical conditions affecting sports participation, *Pediatrics* 107(5):1205-1209, 2001a. Copyright 2001 by the American Academy of Pediatrics.

have been identified that include the following (Glover et al, 1999; Madden et al, 2003):

- Evaluation of health status, including fitness level
- Detection of injuries and illnesses that might limit competition and lead to significant morbidity or mortality and require further evaluation and treatment
- Opportunity to recommend alternative sports activities, as appropriate, or to exclude the person from certain sports
- Identification of lifestyle risk factors and promotion of healthy choices
- Documentation of an athlete's age, grade-level eligibility, and emotional maturity level
- Collection of medical data for emergencies
- Opportunity to recommend ways to improve athletic performance
- Interaction with youth for a variety of health-related issues

Ideally, the sports physical examination should be an individually scheduled appointment with the child's primary care provider. However, mass screenings are common in many school districts as an efficiency measure or because some youth may not be able to afford the examination or may have difficulty getting to such appointments. The mass screenings can be designed with stations for each part of the examination or organized with one-station visits for each child. However, with mass screenings, there is a loss of continuity from history to physical examination, lack of privacy for consultation, lack of provider and patient familiarity, and minimal opportunity to use the visit for health-promotion purposes. For clinicians working in school-based clinics, the sports physical can provide an opportunity to introduce clinic services to the students and to encourage them to return for other health-related services. Communication with parents, coaches, and trainers is essential, whichever process for conducting the examinations is selected.

The psychosocial implications of sports participation need to be clearly identified both for practitioners and for the children and families with whom they work (Table 14-3).

Risk Factors

When assessing the young person for participation in sports, any history or physical findings in the following areas should be of special concern:

- Previous trauma, especially musculoskeletal or central nervous system injuries
- Cardiovascular disease, hypertension (greater than 90th percentile), or exertional syncope
- Prior heat-intolerance episodes
- Asthma or other allergic reactions
- Seizure disorder
- Infectious mononucleosis
- Skin infection
- Anatomic abnormalities, Down or Marfan syndrome, or history of Marfan syndrome in the family
- Obesity
- Medications, immunization status
- In females: menstrual history and eating habits

If there are concerns in any of the above areas, recommendations for sports participation are discussed later in this chapter. Specific conditions that put a child at risk for injury are listed in Table 14-2. Table 14-4 classifies various sports by risk.

TABLE 14-3 Psychosocial Implications of Sports Activities

Positives	Negatives
Fitness	Stress
Social skills	Meeting adult goals
Family activity and involvement	Potential for injuries
Self-esteem	Child may be made to feel
Confidence	inadequate; negative
Coordination and physical skills	attributes may be
Fun and recreation	emphasized

TABLE 14-4 Classification of Sports by Contact

Contact/Collision	Limited Contact	Noncontact
Basketball	Baseball	Archery
Boxing*†	Bicycling*	Badminton
Diving	Cheerleading	Bodybuilding
Field hockey	Canoeing and	Canoeing and
Football*	kayaking	kayaking
• Flag	(white water)	(flat water)
• Tackle	Fencing	Crew, rowing
Ice hockey*	Field	Curling
Lacrosse*	• High jump	Dancing
Martial arts*	• Pole vault*	Field
Rodeo	Floor hockey	• Discus
Rugby*	Gymnastics*	• Javelin
Ski jumping	Handball	• Shot put
Soccer*	Horseback riding	Golf
Team handball	Racquetball	Orienteering
Water polo	Skating*	Power lifting
Wrestling	• Ice	Race walking
	• In-line	Riflery
	• Roller	Rope jumping
	Skiing	Running
	• Cross-country	Sailing
	• Downhill	Scuba diving
	• Water	Strength training
	Softball	Swimming
	Squash	Table tennis
	Ultimate Frisbee	Tennis
	Volleyball	Track
	Windsurfing and	Weight lifting
	surfing	

*Most hazardous for head and spinal injuries.
†Participation not recommended.
Cantu RC: Head injuries. In DeLee JC, Drez Jr D, Miller MD, editors: *DeLee and Drez's orthopaedic sports medicine: principles and practice*, Vol 1, ed 2, Philadelphia, 2003, WB Saunders.
Used with permission of the American Academy of Pediatrics (AAP). From American Academy of Pediatrics Committee on Sports Medicine: Medical conditions affecting sports participation, *Pediatrics* 94:757-760, 1994. Copyright 1994 by the American Academy of Pediatrics.

History

Coaches and others need to be aware of the athlete's health status in case problems arise during participation. Many medical history forms are available that are used to identify children with health conditions that might be adversely influenced by participation in a sport. A health history and physical examination form is illustrated in Fig. 14-3. Many of the questions on the form relate to the risk factors listed earlier.

Many children and adolescents with mild to moderate intellectual and developmental disabilities (e.g., those with Down, fragile X, Turner, Klinefelter, or autism) are capable of performing exercise or strenuous activities as do their peers without disabilities. However, fewer children with such disabilities participate fully in school physical education activities; many do not have the capacity and motor skills to participate, and as a result, they have lower levels of physical fitness (Pitetti, 2001; Special Olympics, 2006). These children are at particular risk for obesity, which in turn leaves them susceptible to developing chronic diseases, including heart disease, stroke, hypertension, and diabetes. Though the Special Olympics has highlighted global competitive games, the enduring focus has been to educate those with disabilities to make healthy lifestyle choices that will improve their overall long-term health. The Special Olympics provides guides for healthy nutrition, lifestyle choices, and entertaining ways to increase one's level of physical fitness. The provider can help families advocate for "adapted" PE in schools, can urge families to regularly involve, encourage, and advocate for their children in a sports activity that is interesting for the child and makes use of his or her physical strengths. The Special Olympics Healthy Athletes program (held in communities throughout the world) sponsors clinics staffed by volunteer health care providers and students to conduct health screenings of people with disabilities. This organization also serves as a resource for community professionals to learn about the physical activity opportunities for children with disabilities that will enable them to participate and compete at high levels.

When performing the history portion of the PPE, providers should assume a more holistic view about the planned activity by asking about the following:

- The particular sports activity planned
- Extent of participation
- Level of competition
- Training schedule
- Coaching and supervision; is there a team physician?
- Hazardous playing and field conditions
- Plans for the activity in the future
- Health promotion and preventive strategies planned
- Planned nutrition
- Preparticipation conditioning
- Risk behaviors, such as increased alcohol consumption, driving while intoxicated, lack of seat-belt use; lack of helmet use during extreme recreational sports activities, such as in-line skating, skateboarding, snowboarding (children 13 to 18 years old underuse protective equipment in these sports as a result of discomfort and lack of perceived need) (American College of Sports Medicine [ACSM], 2005a); use of drugs or performance-enhancing substances (including steroids [dehydroepiandrosterone or DHEA, androstenedione] creatine, gamma-hydroxybutyrate [GHB], gamma-hydroxybutyrolactone [GBL], 1,4-butanediol [BD]); smoking; unprotected sexual activity; and numbers of sexual partners
- Family involvement and support (athletes participating in extreme sports who do use protective equipment do so because of parental and peer influence, rules and requirements [ACSM, 2005a])
- Psychological issues
- Stress management during the competitive season
- Measures for success
- Recent life changes
- Strategies to maintain schoolwork

Physical Examination

The physical examination (PE) should consist of two parts, the musculoskeletal examination and the general physical examination. The 90-second musculoskeletal screening examination is recommended (Fig. 14-4). It is standardized to detect 90% of significant injuries, has 51% sensitivity and 97% specificity (McCarthy, 2006). The examination focuses on musculoskeletal alignment, flexibility, and proprioception, which are effective measures of abnormalities and injury sequelae. Table 14-5 describes the components that should be included for different organ systems. It is important for the provider to include a genital exam, especially for counseling reasons. Testicular torsion can occur during or after sports activities. In addition, sexually transmitted infections, testicular cancer, and varicoceles are important topics to consider and discuss during the PE (McCarthy, 2006).

Laboratory Studies

Urinalysis and hematocrit or hemoglobin are not recommended as part of the sports preparticipation examination. Although these can be useful for evaluation of a specific disease, there is no true indication from a health screening perspective. For adolescent girls, iron deficiency anemia is common enough that it may be appropriate to screen for the condition. Urine drug screening and human immunodeficiency virus (HIV) testing may be required by certain elite amateur or professional organizations. Voluntary testing should be encouraged if the athlete has any risk factors.

Classification of Sports for Risk

The AAP has classified the most common sports activities into three types: contact and collision, limited contact, and noncontact (see Table 14-4). When used with Table 14-2, the clinician can make specific recommendations as to which sports are appropriate for young people with identified health problems.

Recommendations for Participation in Sports for Children With High-Risk Conditions

Table 14-2 summarizes the AAP's recommendations for sports for youth with specific health conditions. Tables 14-2 and 14-4 should be available in the clinic setting. They lend credibility to sports participation recommendations and should serve as guidelines for recommendations made to students and their families. Although families and schools will make their own

Text continued on p. 285.

Ohio High School Athletic Association
Preparticipation Physical Examination Form

(Please type or print)

Student's Name _____ Birth Date _____ Sex _____ Grade _____

Last   First   Middle

City _____ School _____ Place of Birth _____

Student's Address _____

Street   City   Zip   Telephone

Parent(s) or Guardian(s) Name _____

Address (if different than student) _____

Street   City   Zip   Telephone

Family Physician's Name, Address, Telephone _____

History

This section is to be carefully completed by the student and his/her parent(s) or legal guardian(s) before participation in interscholastic athletics in order to help detect possible risks.

Explain "YES" answers below. Circle questions you don't know the answer to.

	Yes	No
1. Have you had a medical illness or injury since your last checkup or sports physical?	☐	☐
Do you have an ongoing or chronic illness?	☐	☐
2. Have you ever been hospitalized overnight?	☐	☐
Have you ever had surgery?	☐	☐
3. Are you currently taking any prescription or nonprescription (over-the-counter) medications or pills or using an inhaler?	☐	☐
Have you ever taken any supplements or vitamins to help you gain or lose weight or improve your performance?	☐	☐
4. Do you think you are in good health?	☐	☐
5. Do you have any allergies (for example, to pollen, medicine, food, or stinging insect)?	☐	☐
6. Have you ever had a rash or hives develop during or after exercise?	☐	☐
Have you ever passed out during or after exercise?	☐	☐
Have you ever been dizzy during or after exercise?	☐	☐
Have you ever had chest pain during or after exercise?	☐	☐
Do you get tired more quickly than your friends do during exercise?	☐	☐
Have you ever had racing of your heart or skipped heartbeats?	☐	☐
Have you had high blood pressure or high cholesterol?	☐	☐
Have you ever been told you have a heart murmur?	☐	☐
Has any family member or relative died of heart problems or of sudden death before age 50?	☐	☐
Is there a family history of heart problems in a close relative younger than age 50 (examples are enlarged heart, cardiomyopathy, long QT interval, abnormal EKG, abnormal heart rhythm)?	☐	☐
Have you had a severe heart infection (for example, myocarditis or pericarditis)?	☐	☐
Is there a family history of Marfan's Syndrome?	☐	☐
Has a physician ever denied or restricted your participation in sports for any heart problem?	☐	☐
7. Have you ever had a severe viral infection within the last month (for example, mononucleosis)?	☐	☐
8. Do you have any current skin problems (for example, itching, rashes, acne, warts, fungus or blisters)?	☐	☐
9. Have you ever had a head injury or concussion?	☐	☐
Have you ever been knocked out, become unconscious or lost your memory?	☐	☐
Have you ever had a seizure?	☐	☐
Do you have frequent or severe headaches?	☐	☐
Have you ever had numbness or tingling in your arms, hands, legs or feet?	☐	☐
Have you ever had a stinger, burner or pinched nerve?	☐	☐

	Yes	No
10. Have you ever become ill from exercising in the heat?	☐	☐
11. Do you cough, wheeze or have trouble breathing during or after activity?	☐	☐
Do you have asthma?	☐	☐
Do you have seasonal allergies that require medical treatment?	☐	☐
12. Do you use any special protective or corrective equipment or devices that aren't usually used for your sport or position (for example, knee brace, special neck roll, foot orthotics, retainer on your teeth, hearing aid)?	☐	☐
13. Have you had any problems with your eyes or vision?	☐	☐
Do you wear glasses, contacts or protective eyewear?	☐	☐
14. Have you ever had a sprain, strain or swelling after injury?	☐	☐
Have you broken or fractured any bones or dislocated any joints?	☐	☐
Have you had any other problems with pain or swelling in muscles, tendons, bones or joints?	☐	☐

If yes, check the appropriate box and explain below.
☐Head ☐Upper Arm ☐Hand ☐Knee
☐Neck ☐Elbow ☐Finger ☐Shin/calf
☐Back ☐Forearm ☐Hip ☐Ankle
☐Chest ☐Wrist ☐Thigh ☐Foot
☐Shoulder

	Yes	No
15. Do you want to weigh more or less than you do now?	☐	☐
Do you lose weight regularly to meet weight requirements for your sport?	☐	☐
16. Do you feel stressed out?	☐	☐

17. Record the dates of your most recent immunizations (shots) for:
Tetanus _____ Measles _____
Hepatitis B _____ Chickenpox _____

18. FEMALES ONLY
When was your first menstrual period? _____
When was your most recent menstrual period? _____
How much time do you usually have from the start of one period to the start of another? _____
How many periods have you had in the last year? _____
What was the longest time between periods in the last year? _____

19. ALL PARTICIPANTS
Explain "Yes" answers here: _____
_____
_____
_____
_____
_____
_____
_____
_____

We consent to the participation of the above-named student in the interscholastic program of his/her school including practice sessions and travel to and from athletic contests. We also agree to emergency medical treatment as deemed necessary by the physician(s) designated by school authorities. **We have read and understand the OHSAA Athletic Eligibility Information Bulletin.**

Student Signature _____ Parent or Guardian Signature _____ Date _____

The student has family insurance ___ Yes ___ No; If yes, family insurance co. name, policy #: _____

NOTE: History and Consent Must be Completed Prior to Physical Examination

Modified from the form approved by the American Academy of Family Physicians, the American Academy of Pediatrics, the American Medical Society for Sports Medicine, the American Orthopaedic Society for Sports Medicine and the American Osteopathic Academy of Sports Medicine.

FIG. 14-3 PPE form. Available at *www.ohsaa.org* (accessed Aug 8, 2002).
(Modified from the form approved by the American Academy of Family Physicians, the American Academy of Pediatrics, the American Medical Society for Sports Medicine, and the American Osteopathic Academy of Sports Medicine. Used with permission from Ohio High School Athletic Association [OHSAA]).

Physical Examination

(Please type or print)

Student's Name _____　Birth Date _____

　　　　　　　　Last　　　　　　　　First　　　　　　　Middle

Height _____　Weight _____　% Body Fat (optional) _____　Pulse _____　BP _____/_____

Vision R 20/ _____　L 20/ _____　　Corrected:　Y　　N　　Pupils: Equal _____　Unequal _____

	Normal	Abnormal Findings	Initials*
MEDICAL			
Eyes/Ears/Nose/Throat			
Lymph Nodes			
Heart			
Pulses			
Lungs			
Abdomen			
Genitalia (males only)			
Skin			
MUSCULOSKELETAL			
Neck			
Back			
Shoulder/Arm			
Elbow/Forearm			
Wrist/Hand			
Hip/Thigh			
Knee			
Leg/Ankle			
Foot			

*Station-based examination only

Clearance

☐ **Cleared**

☐ **Cleared after completing evaluation/rehabilitation for:** _____

_____

_____

_____

☐ **Not cleared for:** _____　**Reason:** _____

　　Recommendations: _____

_____

_____

_____

I certify that I have on this date examined this student and that, on the basis of the examination requested by the school authorities and the student's medical history as furnished to me, I have found no reason which would make it medically inadvisable for this student to compete in supervised athletic activities **(Note exceptions above).**

_____

Physician's Name and Address (stamp or print)
If the Physician's Assistant (P.A.) or Advanced Nurse Practitioner (A.N.P.) performed the exam, name and address of collaborating physician or physician group:

_____

Examiner's Signature　　　　　　　　**Date**

_____

Examiner's Telephone Number

NOTE: History and Consent Must be Completed Prior to Physical Examination

FIG. 14-3　cont'd.

• Appropriate for interscholastic, intramural, and extramural sports activities.

• A screening evaluation created to direct attention to problems but not evaluate the problems.

• Identifies the following conditions that might be adversely affected by athletic participation:

a. Congenital problems

b. Acquired problems

Questions such as the following are to be answered by the athlete and signed by BOTH the athlete and parent:

• Have you ever had an illness, condition, or injury that required you to go to the hospital, either as a patient overnight or in the emergency room or for x-rays; required an operation; caused you to see a doctor; caused you to miss a game or practice?

• Are you now or have you been under the care of a physician for any reason?

• Do you currently have any medical problems or injuries?

• Have you ever had a broken bone, joint sprain or ligament tear, muscle pull, head injury, neck injury or nerve pinch, dislocated joint, back trouble or problems?

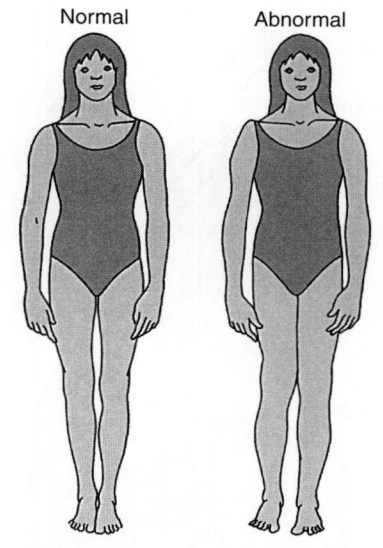

ACTIVITY 1

Normal   Abnormal

Instructions to patient:
  "Stand up straight and face me."

What is screened:
  Acromioclavicular joints, symmetry of extremities

ACTIVITY 2

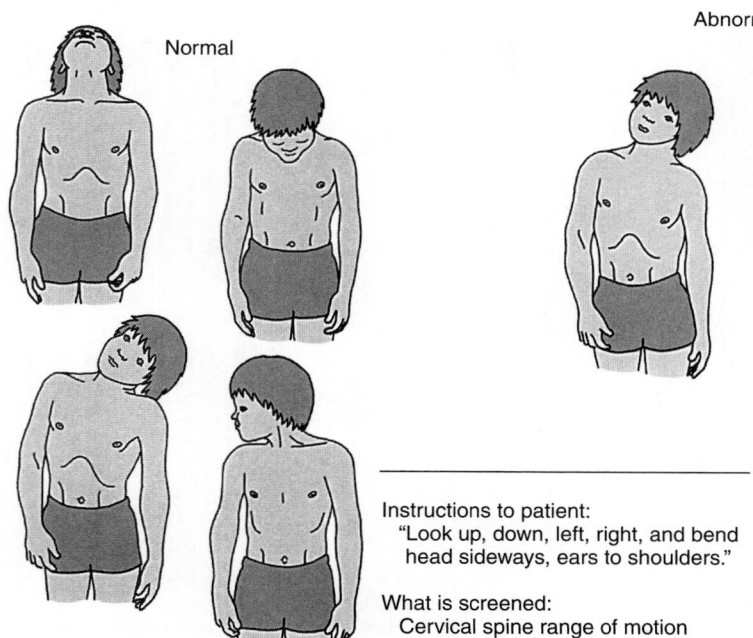

Normal

Abnormal

Instructions to patient:
  "Look up, down, left, right, and bend head sideways, ears to shoulders."

What is screened:
  Cervical spine range of motion

FIG. 14-4   Illustration of the 90-second sports musculoskeletal examination. (Adapted from Ross Products Division, Abbott Laboratories, Columbus OH 43216. From *For the practitioner: orthopaedic screening examination for participation in sports.* ©1981 Ross Products Division, Abbott Laboratories. Text adapted from Garrich JG: Sports medicine, *Pediatric Clin North Am* 24:737-747, 1977.)

ACTIVITY 3

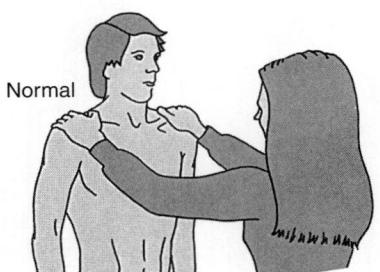

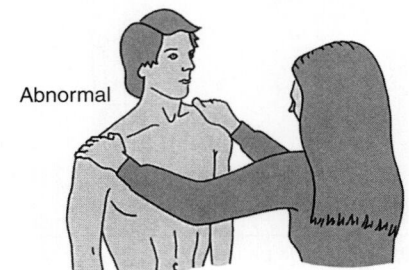

Instructions to patient:
   "Shrug your shoulders." (Against resistance
   by examiner)

What is screened:
   Trapezius strength

ACTIVITY 4

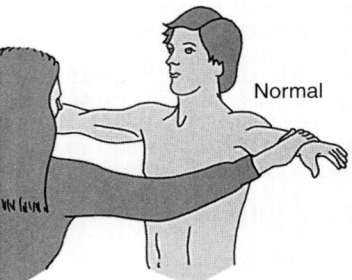

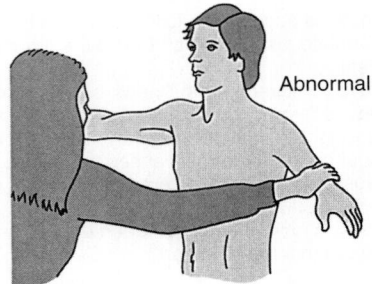

Instructions to patient:
   "Hold arms outstretched from your sides and lift
   them." (Against resistance as examiner pushes
   down)

What is screened:
   Shoulder range of motion

ACTIVITY 5

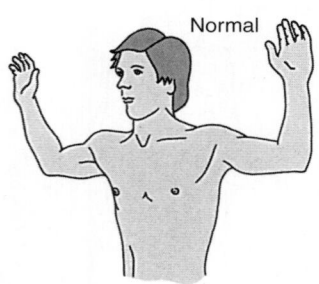

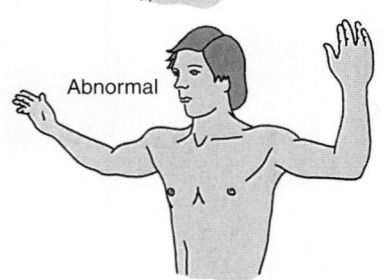

Instructions to patient:
   "Raise your elbows at your sides 90 degrees.
   Rotate your hands backwards."

What is screened:
   Deltoid strength
   Shoulder rotation

ACTIVITY 6

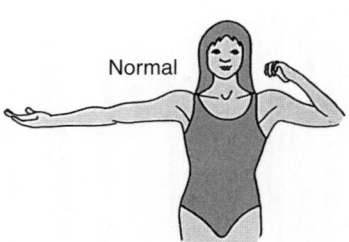

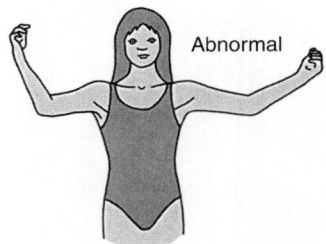

Instructions to patient:
   "Hold arms straight out from sides, palms up.
   Flex and extend your elbows."

What is screened:
   Elbow range of motion

FIG. 14-4   cont'd.

ACTIVITY 7

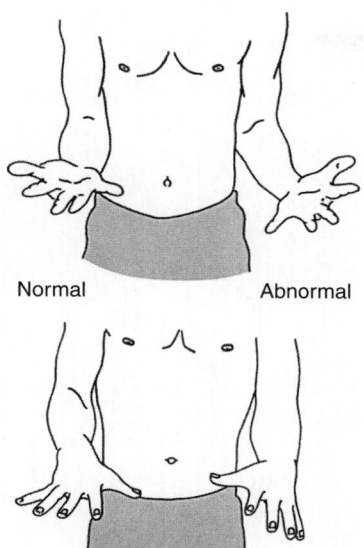

Normal   Abnormal

Instructions to patient:
 "Let your arms down again. Flex your elbows so that your hands reach straight out. Rotate your wrists, palms facing up, then down."

What is screened:
 Wrist range of motion (pronation/supination)

ACTIVITY 8

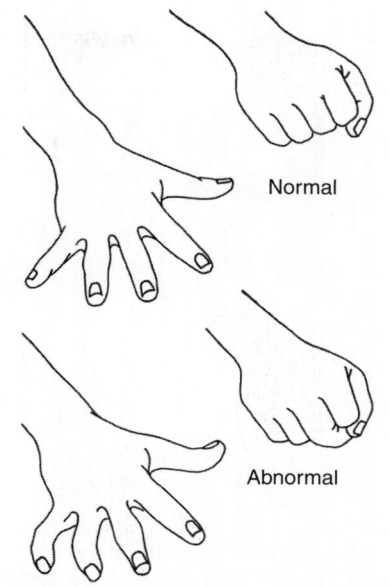

Normal

Abnormal

Instructions to patient:
 "Show me your hands. Spread your fingers out (examiner resists spreading). Make a fist and squeeze."

What is screened:
 Hand/finger range of motion and strength

ACTIVITY 9   Normal   Abnormal

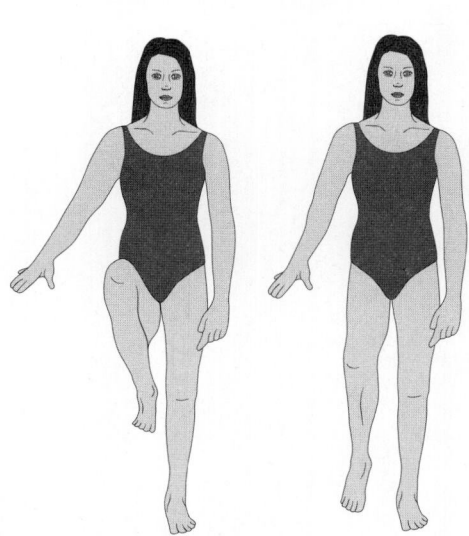

Instructions to patient:
 "Lift your right leg up, bent at the knee. Repeat using the other leg."

What is screened:
 Leg symmetry, knee or ankle effusion

Normal

ACTIVITY 10

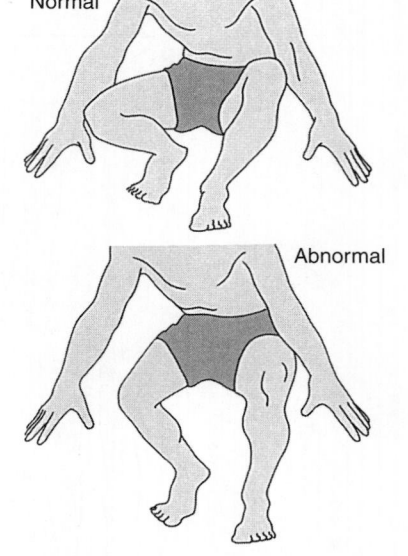

Abnormal

Instructions to patient:
 "Squat like a duck, and walk four steps away from me."

What is screened:
 Hip, knee, and ankle range of motion

FIG. 14-4   cont'd.

ACTIVITY 11

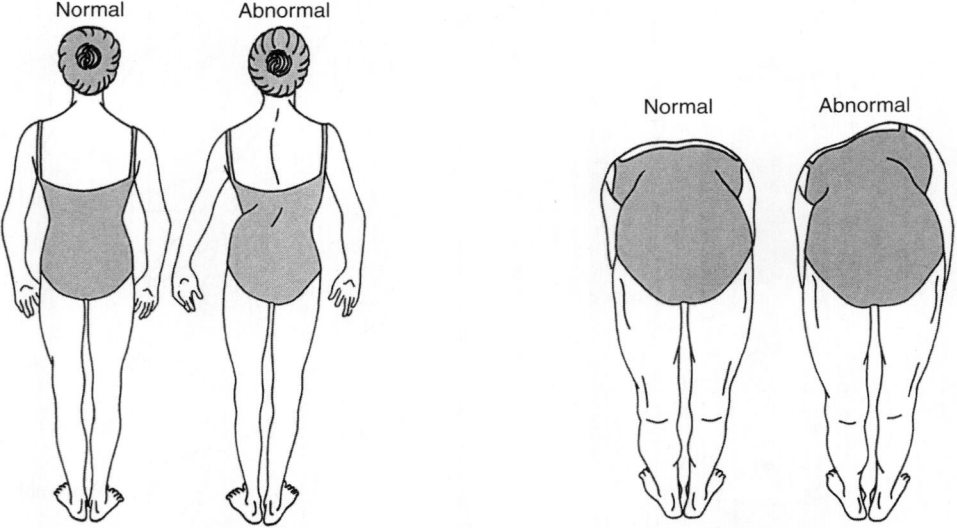

Instructions to patient:
   "Stand up straight. Keep your knees as straight as you can, and
   try to touch your toes. Straighten slowly."

What is screened:
   Shoulder symmetry, scoliosis, hip range of motion, hamstring tightness

ACTIVITY 12

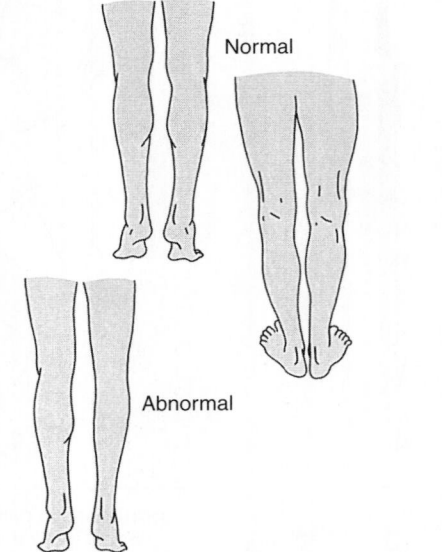

Instructions to patient:
   "Stand up on your tiptoes."

What is screened:
   Calf symmetry, leg strength

FIG. 14-4   cont'd.

TABLE 14-5   Example of an Appropriate Preparticipation Physical Examination

Examination Feature	Comments
Height and weight	Establish baseline and monitor for eating disorders, steroid abuse.
Blood pressure	Assess in the context of participant's age, height, and sex.
General appearance	Excessive height and excessive long-bone growth (arachnodactyly, arm span greater than height, pectus excavatum) suggest Marfan syndrome.
Eyes	Important to detect vision defects that leave one of the eyes with <20/40 corrected vision. Lens subluxations, severe myopia, retinal detachments, and strabismus are associated with Marfan syndrome. Note any anisometropia for the record. Absence of one eye will limit some sport choices.
Cardiovascular	Palpate the point of maximal impulse for increased intensity and displacement, which suggest hypertrophy and failure, respectively. Note heart rate, rhythm. Check for murmurs. A murmur that worsens with standing or Valsalva suggests hypertrophic cardiomyopathy. Perform auscultation with the patient supine and again with the patient standing or straining during Valsalva maneuver. Check femoral against radial pulses; femoral pulse diminishment suggests aortic coarctation.
Respiratory	Observe for accessory muscle use or prolonged expiration and auscultate for wheezing. Exercise-induced asthma will not produce manifestations on a resting examination and requires exercise testing for diagnosis.
Abdominal	Assess for masses, tenderness, organomegaly (especially liver and spleen). In females assess for any pain, enlargement over hypogastric area or pelvis that might suggest pregnancy or gynecologic problem; proceed with further work-up as indicated.
Genitourinary	Hernias and varicoceles do not usually preclude sports participation. Check for single, undescended testicle, masses. Discuss testicular cancer and provide information about the self-testicular exam.
Musculoskeletal	Use the 90-second orthopedic examination (see Fig. 14-3). Consider supplemental shoulder, knee, and ankle examinations as indicated specific to the chosen sport's injury-prone areas.
Skin	Evidence of *Molluscum contagiosum*, herpes simplex, impetigo, tinea corporis, or scabies would temporarily prohibit participation in sports where direct skin-to-skin competitor contact occurs (e.g., wrestling, martial arts).
Neurologic	Gross motor assessment with attention to equality of strength, especially with a history of recurrent stingers or burners, head injury. Usually sufficiently grossly assessed during the 90-second musculoskeletal exam.

From Kurowski K, Chandran S: The preparticipation athletic evaluation, *Am Fam Physician* 61:2683-2690, 2696-2698, 2000.

choices, the recommendations should be recorded in both the student's permanent record and the form returned to the school or sports facility. The goal is to find safe, healthful activities for all children, not to restrict their activities unnecessarily. Several high-risk conditions are discussed in the following section.

■ HIGH-RISK CONDITIONS FOR SPORTS PARTICIPATION

PREVIOUS TRAUMA

Musculoskeletal

All musculoskeletal injuries require individual assessment and decision-making. Sprains, subluxations, dislocations, muscle contusions, and overuse injuries can result in pain and changes to joints, ligament stability, range of motion, strength, and endurance. Referral to an orthopedist may be required. Before returning to sports participation, the athlete must be able to demonstrate the following (Magee, 2006):

• Minimal swelling or joint effusion; some mild discomfort, swelling, and/or stiffness can be expected during initial reentry into activity, which should respond to icing

• Pain-free full range of motion
• At least 90% to 95% of normal strength
• Ability to perform all motions and actions of the required sport
• Confidence in ability to do the activity at requisite level for the sport

If these conditions are not met, repeated injury can be anticipated from residual musculoskeletal deficiencies (Hergenroeder, 2002). Successfully returning to sport participation does not solely depend on the absence of pain; correct rehabilitation, which includes regaining strength and coordination of the injured area, is a more important factor (Metzl, 2002; Magee, 2006).

Neurologic

An estimated 300,000 sports- or recreation-related traumatic brain injuries occur annually in the U.S. (Brain Injury Association, 2004). Head and neck injuries cause 70% of sports-related traumatic deaths and 20% of permanent disabilities (Cantu, 2003). Football injuries are considerably more serious (fractures, dislocations, concussions) and occur more often (Radelet et al, 2002). One study found that a child was six times more likely to acquire a severe concussion during an organized sport than from other recreational activities (Browne & Lam, 2006). Central nervous system trauma is important to assess because repeated concussions are often progressively more serious. Various neurologic assessment and concussion management protocols have evolved (the gold standard is the American Academy of Neurology Quality Standards Subcommittee, 1997; Tables 14-6 and 14-7). For the young person with a history of any serious head injury or intracranial surgery, consultation with a neurosurgeon should occur before participation.

Athletes may suffer from *second-impact syndrome*, which can arise when a second brain injury occurs before symptoms

TABLE 14-6	Recognizing a Concussion in Athletes

Symptoms	Signs Frequently Observed (Note If Early vs. Late)
Early (minutes to hours) • Headache • Dizziness or vertigo • Unawareness of surroundings • Nausea or vomiting **Late** (days, weeks to months) • Lightheadedness • Persistent, mild headache • Poor attention and concentration • Memory dysfunction • Fatigue • Irritability, low frustration tolerance • Sleep disturbance	Vacant stare (befuddled facial expression) Delayed verbal and motor responses (slower to answer questions or follow instructions) Confusion, distractibility (easily distracted and unable to follow through with normal activities) Disorientation related to time, place, date (walking in wrong direction; unaware of time, date, place) Slurred, incoherent speech (making disjointed or incomprehensible statements) Gross incoordination (stumbling, unable to walk tandem or straight line) Emotions out of proportion to situation (appearing distraught, crying for no apparent reason) Memory deficits (asking same question repeatedly; cannot remember words, numbers for 5 min) Any period of loss of consciousness (paralytic coma, unresponsive to stimuli)

Note: Approximately 2%-6% of children after traumatic brain injury will have a seizure; these are generally short lived and self-limiting.
Adapted from American Academy of Neurology Quality Standards Subcommittee: Practice parameter: the management of concussion in sports (summary statement), *Neurology* 48:581-585, 1997; Stevenson K, Adelson PD: Pediatric sports-related head injuries. In DeLee JC, Drez Jr D, Miller MD, editors: *DeLee and Drez's orthopaedic sports medicine: principles and practice*, vol 1, ed 2, Philadelphia, 2003, WB Saunders.

TABLE 14-7	Sideline Evaluation for Assessment of Head and Neck Trauma

Mental Status Testing

Orientation	Time, place, person, activity, situation before and after the trauma
Concentration	Digits said backward, or able to repeat numbers: 3-1-7, 4-6-8-2, 5-3-0-7-4 Months of year said backward
Memory	Names of teams in prior contest Details of contest, such as plays or strategies used Recall of 3 words and 3 objects at 0 and 5 minutes Recent newsworthy events

Exertional Provocative Tests

Exercises*	40-yard sprint 5 push-ups, 5 sit-ups, 5 knee bends

Neurologic Tests

Pupils	Symmetry and reaction
Coordination	Finger-nose-finger Tandem walk
Sensation	Finger-nose with eyes closed Romberg test

*Any associated symptoms are abnormal, including headache, dizziness, nausea, unsteadiness, photophobia, blurred or double vision, emotional lability, or mental status changes.
From American Academy of Neurology Quality Standards Subcommittee: Practice parameter: the management of concussion in sports (summary statement), *Neurology* 48:583, 1997.

of a prior head injury have resolved. Recovery can take days, weeks, or months. Massive brain swelling and herniation with significant risk of mortality (approximately 50%) or morbidity can result within minutes, even though the second blow may have seemed minor (e.g., a blow to the chest or back) (Cantu, 2003; Stevenson & Adelson, 2003).

Approximately 20% of athletes suffer from postconcussive syndrome after any grade of concussion; such sequelae can take several months to resolve. Symptoms include headache, irritability, minor personality changes, decreased ability to concentrate, fatigue, and dizziness. Rest and a nonsteroidal antiinflammatory drug are usually sufficient while awaiting remission. It is critical to properly identify the concussion (see Table 14-6) and accurately exclude the athlete from competition based on set criteria (Box 14-1) to prevent early reinjury.

After neck injuries, the athlete should be free of neck and arm pain, have a full range of neck motion, and have full neck strength. Neck radiographs and magnetic resonance imaging (MRI), if done, should not reveal abnormal position, disk disease, or spinal stenosis (Cantu, 2003).

Burners and stingers are nerve root or brachial plexus compression or traction injuries and generally cause unilateral symptoms. This is a common injury in contact or collision

BOX 14-1   Recommendations for Management of Concussion* in Sports

Definition	First Concussion	Second Concussion	Third Concussion
Grade 1 No LOC; transient confusion, duration of mental status abnormalities[†] of <30 minutes	No sports activities for 7 days; RTP if asymptomatic on mental status parameters after resting and exerting self. *Should be taken to the ED if mental status abnormalities[†] last more than 1 hour.*	No sports activity for 4 weeks; RTP if asymptomatic after resting and exerting self on the last 7 days of the 4 weeks off.	No further sports activity in current season.[‡] May RTP after the third season.
Grade 2 LOC < 5 minutes; duration of mental status abnormalities[†] ≥30 minutes but <24 hours	No sports activity for 4 weeks; RTP if asymptomatic on mental status parameters after resting and exerting self in the last 7 days of the 4 weeks off.	No sports activity for rest of season; RTP following season if asymptomatic in all parameters.	Terminate contact sports for 1 year; RTP in non-contact sports after that.
Grade 3 LOC greater than 5 minutes; mental status abnormalities >24 hours	No sports activity for 4 weeks; RTP if asymptomatic on mental status parameters after resting and exerting self in the last 7 days of the 4 weeks off.	No sports activity for rest of season. No further contact sports after following season; may participate in noncontact sports.	Terminate contact sports for 1 year; RTP in noncontact sports after that.

*A *concussion* is defined as head-trauma-induced alteration in mental status that may or may not involve loss of consciousness. Concussions are graded in three categories. Definitions and treatment recommendations for each category are presented.
[†]Mental status abnormalities include impairment in orientation, memory, concentration, or delayed recall.
[‡]Season refers to a playing season, not a year. Examples: football season is one season. If followed by a baseball season, that is the second season, etc.
LOC, Loss of consciousness; *RTP,* return to play.
Question: Can the athlete return to the field in the same game? In collegiate sports: YES, if the athlete meets the criteria of (a) Grade 1 concussion, (b) has no headache, dizziness, posttrauma amnesia, and can recall events of the game and, (c) the athlete, after doing exertion testing with sprints and push-ups on the sidelines, still has no symptoms as assessed by the team physician. **NO, if in middle or high school sports.**
Adapted from Stevenson KL, Adelson PD: Pediatric sports-related head injuries. In DeLee JC, Drez Jr D, Miller MD, editors: *DeLee and Drez's orthopaedic sports medicine: principles and practice,* Vol 1, ed 2, Philadelphia, 2003, WB Saunders, pp 775-787.

sports, notably football and wrestling. The names derive from the sensation of a burn, stinging, electric, or "lightening bolt" sensation down an arm to the hand. The sensation can last seconds to minutes, but up to 10% can last hours, days, or longer. They may require a more extensive evaluation if:

- Weakness lasts more than a few days
- There is a symptom of neck pain, or burners or stingers occur in both arms
- There is prior history of recurrent burners or stingers

Transient quadriplegia is a much more significant problem and generally appears with bilateral symptoms. It is a contraindication for contact and collision sports until fully evaluated or if any objective structural problems are found. Youth with mild to moderate burners, stingers, or transient quadriplegia symptoms need careful evaluation and must be free of all symptoms before sports clearance; they should never be allowed to play in the presence of neck pain or arm weakness. Rehabilitation may be needed to regain function if symptoms persist for longer than several days (American Academy of Orthopaedic Surgeons [AAOS], 2006).

CHRONIC MEDICAL CONDITIONS
Cardiac Disease
Most grade I to II systolic murmurs without significant cardiovascular history do not need further evaluation. However, diastolic murmurs, unusual loudness, wide splitting of S_2, or increased loudness with Valsalva maneuver or standing require further evaluation. The following warrant a complete cardiac exam, including 12-lead ECG, ECHO, event capture monitor, and stress test with cardiology consultation: a history of presyncope or syncope with exertion, palpitations, exertional chest pain or discomfort, right ventricular dysplasia, prolapsed mitral valve, or exertional shortness of breath, a family history of Marfan syndrome, hypertrophic cardiomyopathy (formerly called idiopathic hypertrophic subaortic stenosis), prolonged QT, atherosclerosis (especially premature), or sudden unexpected death in the young or middle-aged (Hergenroeder & Chorley, 2004).

Hypertrophic cardiomyopathy is the primary cause of sudden death; the incidence is rare at approximately 8 to 12 deaths per year with 65% occurring in athletes with either no prior symptoms or in those with prior histories of congenital heart problems (corrected, palliative, or uncorrected;

Dubin, 2004). Other cardiovascular causes of sudden death among children and teenagers engaged in athletic events are listed in Box 14-2. Anabolic steroids can alter the myocardial texture and produce cardiotoxic effects (Hergenroeder, 2002). The gold standard, *Twenty-Sixth Bethesda Conference: Recommendations for Determining Eligibility for Competition in Athletes With Cardiovascular Abnormalities* (Mitchell et al, 1994), may serve as a useful reference for the clinician. Specific exercise prescriptions can be developed under a cardiologist's direction for children with known cardiac disease.

Hypertension

Hypertension should be diagnosed only after elevated blood pressures have been demonstrated on three separate occasions with use of proper technique. Children with: (a) mild hypertension (less than 90th percentile for normal blood pressure ranges for age) or (b) greater than 90th but less than 99th percentile without target organ damage should not be restricted from any sport, but a thorough evaluation (including a pregnancy test in sexually active females) to determine the cause of the hypertension is necessary. Those with severe hypertension (greater than 99th percentile for age) should not be cleared for participation until the condition is evaluated and treated, which may require pharmacologic therapy (Working Group, 2004). Hypertensive youth need to be counseled to adopt healthy lifestyle behaviors, including avoidance of anabolic steroids, growth hormone, alcohol, tobacco, and high sodium intake. For some athletic governing bodies, use of diuretics and β-blockers is prohibited.

BOX 14-2 **Screening the Athlete for Potential Sudden Death: Key Warning Signs, Especially When Under Exertion**

Syncope
Near syncope
Lightheadedness or dizziness
Palpitations
Exertional dyspnea
Excessive, unexplained shortness of breath
- Fatigue
- Orthopnea
- Paroxysmal nocturnal apnea
Chest pain
- Long QT wave
- Heart murmur
- Increase in systolic blood pressure
History of death or significant heart disease in family member younger than 50 years old

Adapted from Greene P: Pearls for practice: recognizing young people at risk for sudden cardiac death in preparticipation sports physicals, *J Am Acad Nurse Pract* 12(1):11-14, 2000.

Asthma

Children with asthma should be encouraged, not discouraged, from participation in sports. Properly managed asthma should not cause respiratory problems with exertion, as were common in the past. The great majority of patients with asthma can engage in sports, even though many may experience exercise-induced asthma (EIA).

EIA (aka, exercise-induced bronchospasm) is found in up to 90% of children with asthma and in approximately 20% of elite athletes (American Academy of Allergy, Asthma, and Infections [AAAAI], 2004). Symptoms can occur after 6 to 8 minutes of near maximal activity. Progressive airway obstruction generally occurs after physical activity ceases, with peak airway resistance occurring 5 to 20 minutes after activity stops and resolving within 20 to 60 minutes. There is a refractory period for 50% of people that lasts up to 2 hours after an EIA episode. This period either allows the person to exercise without recurrence or to experience a lessened EIA event. Doing warm-up drills just to the point of wheezing, then cooling down to an asymptomatic state before vigorous exercise can help athletes use this refractory period to resume vigorous exercise without experiencing EIA. Breathing cold, dry air is more irritating than warm, humid air. Thus swimmers are known to experience less EIA, whereas hockey players and figure skaters have high incidences of the condition. EIA is generally not life threatening.

A spirometer test remains the gold standard for testing for EIA. A reading that shows a 15% decrease in peak expiratory flow or FEV1 (initial reading is made, then repeated every 5 minutes over the next 20 to 30 minutes after exercise) is diagnostic. It has been suggested that a free-run challenge test for 5 to 8 minutes be part of the PPE to identify at-risk youth. Bronchospasm generally will occur within 15 minutes of the challenge. This running test can also be useful and more predictive than peak expiratory flow rates in detecting such risk (Hammerman et al, 2002). EIA will cause the following symptoms: persistent coughing, wheezing, chest tightness or shortness of breath after participating in physical activity, avoidance or reluctance to participate (because of poor conditioning or lack of interest), or a low stamina level (AAP, 2005).

Recommended management includes using both pharmacologic and nonpharmacologic regimens. The use of a short-acting β2-agonist bronchodilator (inhaled albuterol, levalbuterol, pirbuterol, or terbutaline ideally taken 15 minutes [range of 5 to 30 minutes] before exercise) or an antiinflammatory (e.g., inhaled cromolyn sodium or nedocromil sodium) 20 to 30 minutes before exercise is needed by most. Inhaled steroids and leukotrienes may be necessary for general asthma control and usually decrease the frequency and severity of EIA (AAP, 2005). The inhaled β2-agonists are effective in 80% to 90% of users for up to 4 to 6 hours; long-acting bronchodilators (salmeterol, formoterol fumarate) can act for up to 12 hours. Cromolyn and other mast cell release inhibitors are effective in some but not all users.

The warm-up drills maintain airway warmth and moisture. Covering the mouth and nose with a scarf or mask when exercising in cold air achieves the same purpose. Athletic conditioning also helps improve muscle and exercise efficiency. Warming down, or gradually decreasing exercise at the end of a session, also seems to help decrease the magnitude of the attack. Teachers and coaches should be aware of EIA. A written school management plan should be in place (AAAAI, 2006).

Two recent study results are of interest and may serve as diagnostic nuggets for the health care provider when treating and advising children about their asthma symptoms during sports activities. One concerns the link between obesity and asthma, finding that the more overweight a child is, the greater the likelihood of developing asthma (Sheerin, 2005). The other study demonstrated worsening asthma symptoms and an increase in bronchodilator use in female athletes when in the midluteal phase (day 21 of a 28-day cycle) of their menstrual cycles (Stanford et al, 2006).

EIA is less likely to be triggered by:
- Swimming, walking, leisure cycling, hiking, free downhill skiing, team sports requiring short burst of energy (baseball, football, wrestling, golf, gymnastics, short-distance track and field)

It is more likely to be triggered by:
- Sports that required continuous activity or that may be performed in cold weather (soccer, basketball, ice and field hockey, long-distance running, cross-country skiing)

Seizures

Children and adolescents with seizure disorders should be encouraged to participate in the majority of sports. In fact, the psychological benefits generally outweigh risks caused by acute stress, hyperventilation, or the occasional altered pharmacokinetics of drug therapy that may occur during activity. Benefits of participation include some evidence of a reduction in number of seizures, in addition to improved cardiovascular health, enhanced self-esteem, independence, improved social interactions, and increased physical fitness (Fountain & May, 2003).

Children should be excluded from certain sports only if having a seizure would put them at significant risk. Special consideration needs to occur when the person wishes to hang glide, free climb, sky-dive, bungee jump, high dive, or rock climb. Horseback riding needs to be supervised. If the seizures are poorly controlled, the person should be excluded from contact or collision activities or hazardous sports until controlled (e.g., archery, riflery, swimming [discourage or closely supervise], weight lifting). Other water sports (scuba diving, underwater swimming, and diving) should be avoided or warrant considerable discussion. Contact sports have not conclusively been shown to provoke seizures; though head injury is always a risk, especially in football (Fountain & May, 2003). The child with seizures should be discouraged from participating in motor sports, secondary to potential injury to self and others; and many state laws prohibit such activity. Flotation devices should always be worn when participating in rowing, fishing, or boating activities.

A decision about participation in a specific sport should be made with information about the type of seizure, likelihood of having a seizure, and any comorbid conditions present. Discussions ought to include the participant, parents, coaches or trainers, and neurologist (Howard et al, 2004).

Diabetes Mellitus

Children with diabetes, whether insulin dependent or not, should be the least restricted of all those with chronic diseases. Exercise is an essential component of management as it often improves insulin sensitivity, leading to decreased levels of needed insulin, and glycemic control. The child should be well-controlled before entering a sports program and should have immediate access to a home blood glucose monitoring system. Assistance from a diabetic educator is important because a carbohydrate snack may be necessary before exercise to prevent hypoglycemia resulting from exercise.

Children with diabetes should not participate in high-risk contact sports if they have a current retinal hemorrhage, HTN, peripheral neuropathy, if they are ill, or have an infection (see Table 14-2). They should take a blood sugar before, during, and after a period of physical exertion. Adjustment either to their insulin dosage or carbohydrates is then made according to the timing of activity and meals (Kamboj & Draznin, 2006). Medical identification, proper nutrition, injection of insulin into body parts that are less active, consideration of timing of insulin, and adjustment of the dosage will help prevent diabetic problems. Keep high-carbohydrate foods available for the athlete to prevent hypoglycemia. Provision of fluids for adequate hydration is also advised.

ACUTE INFECTIONS

Infectious Mononucleosis

The risk of splenic rupture with mononucleosis needs to be considered. The incidence is approximately 0.1% to 0.5% with an increased risk after 4 to 21 days of symptom onset. Ultrasonography may reveal splenomegaly that is not clinically palpable. Splenic rupture is rare 6 to 7 weeks after onset of clinical symptoms. This can be a good guideline to follow for deciding when the young person can return to contact sports, assuming that splenomegaly is not present on examination.

Skin Infections

Skin infections are a special consideration for wrestlers and rugby players. The incidence of a wrestler contracting *Herpes gladiatorum* (or a rugby player contracting *H. rugbiaforum* or serum pox) from exposure to a person with a herpes simplex infection ranges from 20% to 50%. Lesions should be healed before wrestling is resumed. For other sports, bandaging may be sufficient to prevent transmission. Athletes with impetigo or other streptococcal or staphylococcal infections should be on antibiotics for at least 48 hours or until significant improvement is seen before participating in contact or collision sports. Scabies, lice, and *Molluscum contagiosum* preclude participation in contact or collision sports, especially in sports in which mats are used and in sports, such as baseball, in which equipment is shared.

Tinea infections (*Tinea gladiatorum*) can also be passed from athlete to athlete; headgear and mats do not harbor the dermatophyte. Treatment with topical ointments for 2 to 4 weeks is indicated. Oral treatment is only indicated if topical therapy fails to clear the lesions. The athlete should be instructed to cease participation until he/she has been on treatment for 48 to 72 hours; covering lesions is not acceptable practice.

Human Immunodeficiency Virus and Other Blood-Borne Viral Pathogens

The transmission of HIV infection via skin or mucous membrane exposure to blood or other infectious body fluids during a contact or collision sport has never been documented (CDC, 2006b). If bleeding occurs, the participant needs to cease playing until the bleeding has stopped. Thus, infected athletes should be allowed to participate in all sports. Their health status is to be treated with confidentiality, and universal precautions should be practiced in all sports. Hepatitis B virus (HBV) immunizations should be encouraged. The *Red Book* (AAP, 2006d) provides additional measures for the protection of all.

PHYSICAL ANOMALIES

Hernia

Hernias should be repaired. However, the teen with a hernia need not be restricted from sports participation, but should be aware of the symptoms of incarceration.

Absence of Paired Organs

Sports that involve objects, sticks, or racquets, or aggressive play, such as football or basketball, have greater risks for eye injuries. Baseball is the most dangerous eye sport. Face shields are now required for hockey, and the incidence of serious injuries in this sport has dramatically decreased. Eyewear is available for all sports except those, such as boxing and full-contact martial arts.

The child with one eye or best-corrected vision in one eye worse than 20/40 should be required to wear molded polycarbonate sport frames with 3 mm-thick polycarbonate lenses for all sports involving rapidly moving objects, bats, or racquets. For collision sports involving headgear, such as football, hockey, or lacrosse, the same frames and lenses should be worn under the cage shield or mask. These children should not participate in sports in which the use of eye protection is not possible. A history of detached retina is significant, and participation should be limited to nonstrenuous sports until consultation with an ophthalmologist is complete.

Those with a single polycystic or abnormally located kidney should be excluded from contact or collision sports.

Young men with a single testicle can be adequately protected with the use of a hard-cup athletic supporter for contact and collision sports and those in which objects are projected at high speed. Although somewhat uncomfortable to wear, the clinician is obliged to explain the risks of sterility. Females with one ovary are not restricted because of the protected

location of the organ (National College Athletic Association, 2000).

Atlantoaxial or Atlantooccipital Instability

Children with Down syndrome can have a bony anomaly and ligament laxity that causes instability where the skull and the first and second cervical vertebrae articulate. The incidence of this atlantoaxial instability is between 10% and 30%. Routine radiographic screening has traditionally been recommended for these children; those with atlantoaxial separation greater than 4.5 mm or a neural canal width less than 14 mm were excluded from certain sports. Removal of this recommendation, by the American Academy of Pediatrics Committee on Sports Medicine and Fitness (AAP, 1995) proved to be contentious. The current AAP policy statement still recommends radiographic screening once during the preschool years (AAP, 2001b). Clearance for Special Olympics still requires such screening. Any other youths with known problems in the cervical area should not engage in contact or collision sports, limited-contact or impact sports, or in diving (see Table 14-2). They may, however, engage in most of the noncontact sports listed in Table 14-4. An MRI is done if instability is detected by radiograph. Surgical fusion may be indicated. The risk of spinal cord injury cannot be minimized.

RISKS FOR THE FEMALE ATHLETE

Females are less likely to suffer sudden death than males. However, there are some issues specific to females that the clinician needs to be aware of because of environmental, anatomic, hormonal, biomechanical, and neuromuscular factors. Such awareness affords the opportunity to provide vital preventive health care.

The *female athlete triad* (anorexia, amenorrhea, and osteoporosis) refers to a progressive array of symptoms that is becoming a common finding as more females participate in sports. The symptoms of the triad occur along a continuum rather than in unison; therefore, the identification of the early existence of an eating disorder or weight loss from a PPE history or examination should alert the provider to take a more thorough history and initiate early treatment (Metzl, 2002).

Amenorrheic female athletes can suffer from osteoporosis. Primary or secondary amenorrhea or stress fractures are also good clues to the possible existence of the *triad*. Stress fractures are twelve times more likely to occur in female runners than in male runners. Highly active impact sports, such as running, cheerleading, and gymnastics, place females at greater risk for these fractures (Loud et al, 2005).

Females participating in running and aesthetic sports, such as gymnastics, cheerleading, dance or ballet, and figure skating, seem more prone to eating disorders. Competitive cheerleading is a more continuous sport throughout the year than that of sideline cheerleading. Upon diet analysis, both groups have shown insufficient caloric and nutrient intakes (ACSM, 2003a).

The female athlete is at increased risk for anterior cruciate ligament (ACL) injury that typically occurs during deceleration, landing, or contact with another athlete. Sports that leave them particularly vulnerable to this injury include basketball, field hockey, lacrosse, skiing, and soccer. Other injuries common in the female athlete include those of the patellofemoral joint and shoulder (sustained during diving, gymnastics, swimming, throwing, and volleyball) (ACSM, 2003b).

Maffulli and Baxter-Jones (2002) disproved the notion that intensive sport training delays the growth and sexual maturation of young female athletes. This concern has been repeatedly raised at every world Olympics in regard to female gymnasts. However, the aforementioned report credits the differences in growth and maturation more to the genetic makeup of the individual rather than to extended, intensive training.

■ MANAGEMENT STRATEGIES TO SUPPORT ACTIVITY PATTERNS FOR CHILDREN AND ADOLESCENTS

Health care providers can address a variety of health-oriented issues to support children and adolescents participating in physical activities. Injury management should not be the goal. These are summarized in Box 14-3 and discussed in greater depth in this section. Injury management is addressed in Chapter 39.

BOX 14-3   Primary Care Sports Participation Management

Diseases
- Control symptoms of specific diseases or conditions
- Rehabilitate injuries
- Prevent injuries, heat illnesses
  - Hydration
  - Protective equipment
  - Correct footwear
  - Proper training
  - Safe environment
  - Educated coaching

Daily Living
- Nutrition
  - Balanced diet
  - Adequate calories
  - Hydration
- Stress management
  - Realistic expectations
  - Stress reduction for performance
  - Supportive coaching
  - Supportive parenting
- Balanced home, school, recreation goals, and outcomes
- Drug-free performance

Development
- Sports and activities are selected for success within capacity
- Supportive training and coaching

COUNSELING FAMILIES ABOUT SPORTS FOR THEIR CHILDREN

Physical activity needs to be encouraged from infancy. Playing outside and engaging in family physical activities serve important developmental needs. When children enter school, sports opportunities become organized, so children and their families need to make specific decisions and choices about the sports in which they want to participate. At this time, it is important to identify the parent who has sports goals for the child that may be meeting the parent's needs more than the child's. For the prepubertal child entering sports, the goals should be healthful activity, learning basic skills, and mastering the rules of the game. All children do not mature at the same rate. The skills of several children of the same age can be widely discrepant, and the performance of a 16- or 17-year-old is very different from that of the same child at 12 years old. Refer to Table 14-1 for further information.

The following are some basic concepts to keep in mind for counseling:
- Noncontact team sports participation can begin at about 7 years old but should be guided by the child's motor development and individual interest. Organized sports should be delayed until 10 years old (Luebbers, 2003). Competitive sports can be emotionally stressful to a child; it is important to keep the focus on participation rather than on winning.
- The child who is an exceptional athlete may still have maturation difficulties in social and psychological areas. Finding a balance in supporting the development of an athletically gifted child can be difficult given the stress this child may face in the competitive arena.
- Parents need to wear bicycle helmets when riding with their children to model injury prevention.
- Children with handicaps can participate in sports. With the clinician and their parents, they can make the choice of which sport best fits their limitations. Advice about the health effects that can result and the conditioning that may be necessary should be included in the counseling.
- Children with academic problems should not be denied participation in sports. Studies have concluded that an increase in PE time at school does not negatively impact academics (AAP, 2006a). Sports can be the best arena for boosting self-esteem for the child who does not experience success in the classroom. Helping the child find a balance between academic work and sports participation is essential.
- Boys and girls can play together, especially in the prepubertal years. Differences in height and weight can make it unsafe for smaller girls to compete in contact sports with boys after puberty.
- Injuries occur in some sports more often than in others. Refer to Table 14-2 when discussing potential injuries with a family. Good supervision and appropriate equipment can help minimize some of the risks.
- Families need to support physical activity for children, provide opportunities for children to engage in a variety of activities, role model healthy physical activity, and supervise to ensure safety and a positive experience for each child.

- Children who maintain high levels of everyday physical activity increase their whole body and trochanter bone mineral content (Janz, 2006). One study recommended that children get 40 minutes of exercise in their prepubertal through pubertal years for the greatest increase in bone mass (Clinical Advisor, 2005).
- Females are more likely to actively engage in exercise and sports if competition is deemphasized, participation is in small groups rather than in group or team activities, and emphasis is placed on activities they favor and that achieve a stated goal. They are also more likely to be physically active if their fathers model physical activity and their mothers provide logistical support (ACSM, 2003c and 2005b).
- Children can play sports when they have a common upper respiratory infection without compromising their immune function (ACSM, 2001a).
- Use of nasal dilators does not aid performance (ACSM, 2001b).
- Children may overtrain or, when pushed to their physical and mental abilities, get "burned out." Symptoms include repeated injuries (particularly overuse injuries), participation becomes a chore, and a lack of joy and enthusiasm is expressed (Metzl, 2003).
- Supportive athletic footwear should be advised.

INJURY PREVENTION

A variety of strategies can be used to reduce the incidence and severity of injuries. Safety rules for games are designed to reduce injuries, especially for contact sports. Safety factors include: protective equipment, such as head and mouth protection; maintenance of playing fields, floors, and equipment; coaches that teach good techniques and guide athletes through adequate warm-up and stretching exercises before and after the game; support personnel who are qualified to administer first aid, recognize and manage spinal and head injuries and other acute trauma; and cardiopulmonary resuscitation. Heat-related illnesses and dehydration can be prevented. Many injury-prevention interventions are best considered in terms of the specific sport or recreational activity at hand.

Proper Use of Bicycle Helmets

More children and adolescents visit emergency departments for cycling injuries than for any other recreational activity. Two thirds of all brain injury fatalities result from such incidences (AAP, 2001c). Despite preventing from close to 70% of head injuries, only 25% of children 5 to 14 years old reported wearing a helmet (AAP, 2001c). The use of bicycle helmets can prevent or reduce the severity of brain trauma. Proper use starts with proper fitting:

- Try on several sizes and models to find the best fit which:
  - Places the helmet low on the forehead
  - Positions the brim so that it is parallel to the ground when the head is upright (child should be able to see the brim when looking up)
  - May require removing or installing inside pads to enable a snug fit

- Securely fastens the chin strap to the point where the helmet will not shift over the eyes or come off when the child shakes the head.
- Helmet needs to carry a U.S. Consumer Product Safety Commission (CPSC) sticker.
- A helmet should be thrown away if it has been involved in any substantial blow that resulted in marks on the outer surface; do not purchase secondhand helmets.
- Replace helmets every 5 years or sooner, depending upon manufacturer recommendations.
- Children are more likely to wear helmets if a parental rule exists, parents wear helmets during cycling activities, and if there is a mandatory state helmet law, though these usually only apply to children younger than 16 years old.

Preventing Injury: the Readiness Factor

Readiness can be addressed from two perspectives, developmental readiness and preseason conditioning readiness. Of course physical and cognitive development for play begins in infancy and should continue throughout the life span. Patel and others (2002) discuss developmental readiness for organized sports participation, an issue for many children and their parents. They note that children are not able to compare their abilities with those of others until 6 years old, do not understand the competitive nature of sports until 9 years old, and do not understand the complex nature of tasks involved in a given sport until 12 years old. Sports participation involves not only physical but also cognitive and social readiness.

Preseason conditioning (examples: preparatory muscle conditioning and plyometric training [exercises that combine strength with speed of movement to enhance power, such as hops and jumps. The central nervous system becomes conditioned to react quickly to stretching and shortening]) is a method for decreasing overall injuries. One study showed a 51% decrease in knee and ankle injury incidence and the severity of injuries (Olsen et al, 2005). Conditioning also lessens overuse injuries (stress fractures, bursitis, tendonitis) and the amount of time needed for rehabilitation, helps strengthen bone, facilitates weight control, enables the nervous system to react more quickly to the stretch-shortening cycle, and improves performance (Faigenbaum & Chu, 2001). When started in players as young as 10 to 12 years old, warm-up programs help them establish overall motion patterns (Olsen et al, 2005). Such conditioning is not sport specific, but entails activities geared toward improving strength, flexibility, and endurance; it is not intended to be confused with weight lifting or bodybuilding. Coaches and fitness instructors should be certified and be knowledgeable about age-specific training techniques and safety; adult training techniques should never be applied to children.

Traumatic Injury Prevention

Muscle Soreness.   Soreness should be minor, resulting from microscopic muscle or connective tissue damage; it is a normal result in muscles that are adapting to a new exercise program. Providers should explain this soreness ahead of time so that new exercisers do not use this condition as an excuse to stop their fitness regimen.

- Warm up body temperature before gentle stretching to maintain flexibility.
- Start with lighter weights and fewer repetitions when starting a new regimen.

Strains and Sprains.   These injuries are most related to pivoting sports, such as basketball, football, and volleyball.

- Do preseason stretching.
- Tape site of previous injury.
- Warm up body temperature before stretching.
- Maintain playing surfaces.
- Use proper footwear.
- Limit practice time.

Knee braces do not have sufficient scientific evidence to recommend them for pediatric athletes. However, their use seems to provide subjective relief, and thus they are prescribed clinically. They should not replace rehabilitation and surgery, if required (AAP, 2001d).

Fractures.   These injuries most commonly involve the upper extremities, as when falling on an outstretched hand. Lower extremity fractures can occur with such sports as soccer.

- Do strength-conditioning exercises.
- Use proper techniques.
- Take safety precautions.
- Use protective gear that fits well, such as wrist guards.

Lacerations, Contusions, and Abrasions.   These injuries are most related to baseball (contusion and abrasion), soccer, cycling, and ice hockey (lacerations).

- Protective equipment is essential.

Head and Neck.   Greatest risks for injury are from cycling, diving, equestrian sports, football, gymnastics, ice hockey, wrestling, trampolines, rugby, and cheerleading. Risks increase with age (Luckstead & Patel, 2002; Luke, 2003).

- Have appropriate supervision and coaching that teaches proper skills, such as tackling.
- Adhere to safety rules of the game.
- Strengthen neck muscles.
- Use appropriate equipment—helmets, face and mouth gear.
- Follow management of concussion guidelines for return to sport after injury.

Eye.   Eye injuries are most commonly related to baseball and ice hockey.

- Use headgear and protective glasses.

Overuse Injury Prevention
Stress Fractures
- Use soft running and playing surfaces.
- Use proper footgear.
- Do strengthening exercises.
- Stop activity when pain occurs.

Anterior Leg Pain Syndrome (Shin Splints)
- Stretch before and after activity.
- Pronate and supinate feet while standing.
- Use soft playing surface.
- Use proper footwear—proper fit, impact-absorbing sole, support for hindfoot

- Avoid sudden increase in activity.
- Limit forceful, extensive use of foot flexors.
Plantar Fasciitis
- Use proper footwear (cushioned with fitted heel counters or lifts).
- Stretch calf and Achilles tendon.
- Do ice massage after event.
- Correct biomechanical errors.
- Limit hills and speed work; increase soft-surface running.
Blisters
- Wear socks.
- Wear properly fitted shoes.
- Use powder, petroleum jelly, or a product, such as Second Skin, on reddened or at-risk areas.

HEAT AND HUMIDITY

Muscular contractions produce heat 75% of the time; 25% goes into muscle work. This can result in an increase of core body temperature of $1\,^\circ$ C in 5 minutes. An exercising muscle produces 10 to 20 times the heat produced by a resting muscle. Unless the usual heat dissipation mechanisms are properly working, heat stroke can result within 15 to 20 minutes. Heat is dissipated through evaporation (20% to 25%), convection (15%), and radiation (60%). It is dissipated only through evaporation when environmental temperature exceeds body temperature and, thus, only when humidity is 75% or less. There is no evaporation at 90% to 95% humidity.

Because children have a higher metabolic rate at a given submaximal walking or running speed, they produce more heat per mass unit. This higher metabolic load, in addition to several other pediatric physiologic factors, including poor sweating capacity, larger surface-to-mass ratio, and an immature cardiovascular system, results in a shorter tolerance for exercising in hot climates and greater susceptibility to heat stress for children. They dehydrate sooner and have higher core temperatures than adults do under the same conditions. Therefore, they are at greater risk for heat illness, heat exhaustion, and heat stroke. Heavy uniforms or sweat suits can reduce evaporation further.

Acclimatization requires gradual heat exposure over a period of 8 to 12 days. Acclimatization allows the individual to dissipate more heat through evaporation with decreased sodium concentration in sweat and thus exercise longer and harder in heat without loss of excessive electrolytes. Children require more time to acclimatize and may need 8 to 10 exposures of 30 to 45 minutes per day to make the adjustment.

Very young children with a higher surface-to-mass ratio, those with fever, and those who are dehydrated are at greater risk for heat illnesses. Children with a variety of chronic illnesses are also at risk. Fever, vomiting, diarrhea, diabetes insipidus, and diabetes mellitus may increase risk through fluid losses. Decreased sweat production may occur with spina bifida, quadriplegia, scleroderma, severe eczema, and sunburn, among other conditions. Excessive sweating as with cystic fibrosis, sweat gland dysfunction, and some cardiac conditions can increase fluid losses. Diminished thirst sensation increases the likelihood of dehydration, and obesity, especially related to lack of conditioning, predisposes to heat illness. Certain drugs can also increase heat production or decrease sweating (e.g., amphetamines, LSD, alcohol, thyroid hormone, antihistamines, anticholinergics, haloperidol, phenothiazines, diuretics, laxatives, monoamine oxidase inhibitors, tricyclic antidepressants).

Heat Illnesses (Hyperthermia)

Heat Cramps. Prickly heat, heat edema of hands and feet, and heat syncope are early indicators of the body's responses to excessive heat. Heat cramps are one of the mildest forms of heat illness. Symptoms include painful muscle spasms, usually of the calf and hamstrings (can occur in the abdomen, shoulders) during or after strenuous exercise with profuse sweating. The cramps are brief (less than 1 minute), intermittent, and painful. They may occur after intense exercise and are thought to be related to electrolyte depletion. The subject is thirsty but well oriented and alert. Oral rehydration with an electrolyte solution (a sports drink, or 0.5 to 1 teaspoon of salt in 1 quart of water), gentle stretching, and resting in a cool area is generally sufficient treatment. Heat cramps occur most commonly when athletes are not adequately conditioned for participation at high temperature and/or humidity and fail to hydrate properly. Intravenous saline solution may be needed in more severe situations.

Heat Exhaustion. Heat exhaustion is the most common heat illness of athletes. It occurs with excess sweating in a hot, humid environment. It is a reversible condition, whereas heat stroke causes irreversible damage to tissues. Symptoms include headache, fatigue, weakness, dizziness, orthostasis, nausea, anorexia, and possibly syncope and diarrhea. The core temperature may rise above 38° C, but is usually less than 40° C (99° to 104° F). Mentation is generally normal; dry tongue and mouth and weight loss may occur. Cardiovascular symptoms may result from volume loss and include tachypnea and orthostatic hypotension. Malaise, myalgias, vertigo, chills, visual disturbances, and cutaneous flushing may also occur. The skin is ashen, cold, and clammy because of sodium depletion or hot and dry from water depletion. Mild shock may be present, but there are no major central nervous system dysfunctions. Management includes rest in a cooler environment; cooling measures, such as removing clothing, fanning, spraying and sponging the skin with water, applying ice to the groin and axilla areas; and oral or intravenous fluids. The child should be allowed unrestricted access to salty foods. Emergency department monitoring is preferred. If the athlete is confused or refuses to drink, intravenous fluids are needed. A patient with the latter symptoms may need hospitalization.

Heat Stroke. Heat stroke is a medical emergency with a mortality rate of 10% to 50% (Hergenroeder & Chorley, 2004; AAP, 2006b). It can occur over several days as with a heat wave or rapidly with exertion. In either case, rapid cooling is essential because the high body temperature damages tissues and alters heart, lung, brain, kidney, and other organ system functions. Persons participating in intense exertion experience the symptom of excessive sweating, whereas heat stroke seen in the elderly or chronically ill occurs during heat waves, evolves over several days, and is typified by hot, dry skin. High core temperature (greater than 104.9° F and can be greater than 107° F or greater than 40.5° C), shock or coma, circulatory abnormalities, disseminated intravascular coagulation, rhabdomyolysis, arrhythmias, and seizures can result. Sweating may or may not be present, depending on the degree of depletion of fluids that has occurred. Rapid transport to an emergency department is essential for administration of intravenous fluids; rapid cooling with ice water immersion or lavages and monitoring and supporting respiratory, cardiovascular, and renal functions are indicated. While waiting for transport, the patient should be placed in a cool environment, clothing should be removed, and water should be applied to the body with fanning to increase evaporation. Fluids should be given orally if the athlete is alert; antipyretics will not be useful. The patient may need cardiopulmonary resuscitation until emergency transportation arrives.

Preventive Measures. Preventive measures for heat illnesses are listed in Box 14-4. They include efforts to decrease metabolic effort, increase evaporation, and increase hydration. Children are also at risk in hot water, such as saunas. Acclimatization is helpful for young athletes.

NUTRITION

Adolescents are growing at a rate second only to that of infants. Thus, the nutritional intake of adolescent athletes must

---

BOX 14-4 **Strategies to Prevent Heat Illnesses**

- Athletes should wear lightweight, dry, permeable clothing.
- Athletes should be fully hydrated before activity begins.
- Athletes should drink cool water (more efficiently absorbed than warm water) every 20 minutes at a rate of 5 oz if <40 kg; 9 oz if 60 kg; 10-12 oz >60 kg.
- Water is adequate if exercise lasts <1 hour; if available, oral rehydration solutions should be used if activities exceed 1 hour.
- Athletes should have scheduled rest periods in the shade every 20-30 minutes, with helmets removed.
- Athletes should be gradually acclimatized to heat over 8-12 days, if possible.
- Athletes at greater risk should be observed carefully. Risk factors include cystic fibrosis; hyperthyroidism; obesity; previous heat stroke; general health problems; poor conditioning; diabetes; kidney disorders; and medications, such as diuretics, antihistamines, antidepressants, and others.
- Activities should be scheduled in early morning or evening to avoid direct sunlight and hottest time of day.
- Activity should cease if any signs and symptoms of heat illness develop.
- **Salt tablets should not be used.**

meet both growth and activity needs. The AAP Committee on Nutrition (2006c) recommends the following:

- Calories to support energy requirements for the sport, in addition to normal growth
- A balanced diet using the food guide pyramid (no particular dietary constituents should be emphasized)
- Adequate iron to provide adequate stores for growth and oxygen transport during activity
- Calcium following recommendations for all youth—1200 to 1500 mg/day

Depending on the sport, calorie requirements for active teenagers exceed baseline needs by 1500 to 3000 calories. The recommended diet for the athlete is the same as for all people—high in carbohydrates (6 to 8 g/kg of body weight/day; 55% to 75% of total calories), fats (25% to 30% of total calories/day), and protein (1 g/kg of body weight; 15% to 20% of total daily calories). Normal growth of children requires an intake of 60 kcal/kg of ideal body weight per day (see Chapter 11). Vitamins and minerals do not need to be supplemented except in women who have a diet low in both calcium (less than 1200 mg/day) and iron. Neither increased muscle mass nor decreased body fat result from amino acid supplementation.

Short-term, high-intensity activities, such as high jumping or diving, involve use of anaerobic fuel sources, whereas longer-term activities, such as running or cross-country skiing, involve use of aerobic sources. Carbohydrates are used in both anaerobic and aerobic metabolic states, but fats and proteins are used only aerobically. Most of the carbohydrate intake should come from nutritional foods, such as fruits and vegetables, grains, and milk sugars, rather than refined sugars. Nutrition recommendations are summarized in Table 14-8.

In general, ingesting carbohydrates before activities has no effect on performance, and carbohydrate loading has not been studied in children. Carbohydrate intake during physical activity lasting more than 1 hour improves performance. After competition, carbohydrate intake is again important to improve muscle glycogen resynthesis, which is most rapid in the first few hours after exercise. Consuming carbohydrates in the first 30 minutes and again in 2 hours after performance will achieve this resynthesis. This can be in the form of snacks or liquids. Weight gain of mostly muscle mass occurs primarily through eating extra carbohydrate calories and exercising. Carbohydrate intake must meet basic needs plus replacement for exercise energy expenditure to ensure normal growth.

Protein requirements are easily met with normal diets of 1 g/kg of body weight. No protein supplements are needed. In fact, hypercalciuria with calcium loss and dehydration can occur if protein intake is too high because the excess nitrogen, and hence water, is excreted. Intense endurance sports and

TABLE 14-8   Nutrition Recommendations for Athletes

Nutrient	Recommendations
Calories from carbohydrates, fat, protein	Maintain same as for all people: 50%-75% carbohydrate, 25%-30% fat, 15%-20% protein.
	Do not decrease caloric intake during sports season.
	May need 1500 to 3000 calories more than recommended daily allowance to meet activity requirements.
	Allow appropriate vegetarian diets.
Vitamins and minerals	Same as for all people, unless an increase is medically indicated.
	Adolescent girls may need to bring calcium and iron intake up to recommended range.
	Do not take salt tabs because hypernatremia and delayed gastric emptying can result.
Carbohydrates	6-8 g/kg body weight.
	Use nutritious foods, such as fruits, vegetables, grains, and milk sugars.
	Carbohydrate intake during prolonged activity may increase performance.
	Carbohydrate intake of 100 g in first 30 minutes after performance is recommended to promote muscle glycogen resynthesis and rapid reloading.
Protein supplements	None needed; hypercalciuria with calcium loss and dehydration can occur if protein intake is too high.
Fluids	Plain water before, during, and after activity.
	Athletic drinks containing electrolytes may be helpful for endurance athletes and those who sweat heavily; avoid carbonated drinks (can delay gastric emptying and intestinal absorption).
	Fluid every 15-20 minutes (5 oz in those weighing <40 kg; 9 oz for 60 kg; 10-12 oz if >60 kg).
	Replace water loss after activity at 16 oz or ½ L/lb of weight lost (determined by prepractice and postpractice weights).
	Avoid caffeine drinks because they can increase diuresis.

Adapted from American Academy of Pediatrics (AAP) Committee on Nutrition: Guidelines for pediatricians: nutrition and sports. In *Sportshorts*, issue 6. Available at *www.aap.org/family/sportsshorts_06.pdf* (accessed July 30, 2006).

strength training probably require an additional 1500 to 3000 kilocalories above the recommended daily allowance (RDA). Youth who eat too much protein may not consume adequate carbohydrates and fats; excess protein may be stored as fat.

Weight loss by adolescent athletes can be a dangerous practice. Wrestlers may try to make weight or be eligible to compete in a lower weight class; runners sometimes vomit to run lighter; and female gymnasts may practice significant nutritional control to maintain weight and size. Dancers, divers, figure skaters, and cheerleaders also control weight for appearance advantages. Bodybuilders, rowers, distance runners, and swimmers often try to control their weight. Starvation can lead to suppressed growth hormones, can interfere with pubertal gonadal hormone changes, and may result in eating disorders. Nutritional counseling is essential, with a reminder that muscle weighs more than fat and that weight gain during adolescence with growth is normal.

Wrestlers often engage in repeated bouts of excessive weight loss or weight cycling. Such transient weight cycling can deplete electrolytes, decrease glycogen stores, affect hormones, diminish nutritional status, impair mental and academic performance, reduce immune function, and lead to pulmonary emboli and pancreatitis (Housh, 2001). Studies have demonstrated that this temporary weight cycling generally does not lead to long-term adverse effects or altered growth patterns in weight and height. However, the practice is to be discouraged because of the risk for long-term dysfunctional eating and short-term effects discussed above. Measurements of body composition before and during the wrestling season can help coaches and parents stay alert to risky behavior; any planned weight loss should involve appropriate dietary changes and exercise training. Wrestlers, coaches, and parents may elect to sign a contract requiring that the child eat 3 meals a day, that fluid be available at all times, and that no artificial means be employed to remove fluids from the body (e.g., sauna or sweat suit, laxatives, diuretics, diet pills, licit or illicit drugs, nicotine, prolonged fasting, overexercising, or vomiting).

DEHYDRATION

The young person can prevent dehydration by drinking cool, flavored water before, during, and after activities. Performance and normal thermoregulation can decrease with as little as 1% dehydration. The first sensations of thirst are initiated at the 2% to 3% level of dehydration; drinking needs to begin before the need is felt (Hergenroeder & Chorley, 2004). After competition, rehydration is important. Small amounts of sodium and carbohydrates, such as are found in sports drinks, enhance rehydration; additional sodium supplements are not recommended. Drinking fluids with caffeine should be avoided because these beverages increase urine output, causing further dehydration. Use of separate fluid containers for each child participating may help monitor the intake of each while decreasing the risk of disease spread (See Table 14-8 for fluid intake recommendations for athletes). Scheduling fluid breaks and rotating players more frequently may also help prevent dehydration.

STRESS AND SPORTS: KEEPING ACTIVITIES FUN

Children and adolescents need to enjoy sports and to find that they reduce rather than induce stress if they are going to include vigorous physical activity in their lifestyles. The athletic environment should foster psychological and physical well-being. It is part of the provider's role to assess the psychological dimensions of sports participation and intervene when problems appear. Most children will benefit from participation in a variety of sports and recreational activities, both in terms of reducing repetitive movements that can increase overuse injury risks and to avoid premature commitment to a sport for excellence. Children should experience happiness and success from their sports participation (Metzl, 2002).

Athletic stress arises as a result of the interactions between situational factors, personality factors, and motivational factors. Situationally, athletes need to have sufficient developmental and psychological resources to meet the demands of the event. Cognitively, athletes make an appraisal of the situation. They assess the demands and their resources, the consequences of success or failure, and their personal interpretation of the consequences. A person with low self-confidence might assess a particular event as more stressful than would a person with high self-confidence even if both have equal skills. Stress occurs when the assessment yields perceived negative outcomes. There is also a physiological component to stress. When the athlete becomes overexcited, performance decreases. Finally, stress is related to the coping and behavioral responses the athlete uses. In part these will be related to his or her developmental level.

The consequences of excessive athletic stress can be withdrawal from sports, decreased enjoyment, decreased performance, and negative physical effects, including interference with eating and sleeping or possible increase in injuries.

Management of Athletic Stress

Cognitive interventions can be taken to manage athletic stress. The following are key points that may be helpful to youngsters and their families:

- Winning is not everything.
- Failure is not the same thing as losing.
- Success is not winning, but rather striving for victory (the effort) and participation.
- Preferred goals include the following:
  ○ Regular physical activity to promote health
  ○ Participation in organized sports to acquire basic motor skills, learn social skills for teamwork, learn sportsmanship, and have fun

The organization and administration of sports programs can make a difference in the pleasure experienced by young athletes. Some positive strategies include the following:

- Establishing different skill and competition levels
- Organizing homogeneous groups by age and size
- Not scoring games, keeping season records, or calculating individual statistics
- Altering games to increase opportunities for success, such as playing T-ball instead of pitched softball, lowering the

basket, decreasing the length of games, using a smaller playing field, and changing some rules, such as no press defense in basketball or no stealing in baseball.

Coaching roles and relationships can be modified. Coach-effectiveness training has been shown to positively influence athletes' feelings of self-esteem, player attitudes, appreciation of the coach, and relationships among the players. Coaches should use positive control techniques, reframe winning into success for effort, and work on team cohesion and development of positive desire. Coaches may also need to support the injured athlete's need for reduced training and rehabilitation. Coaches should not overtrain athletes because this results in fatigue and a sense of being "stale."

Parents need to focus on supporting their children rather than identifying with them. Parental success and feelings of self-worth should not derive from having a child who wins at sports. Neither should the family build its identity around the young athlete to the extent that poor performance becomes a family catastrophe. Parents need to stay alert to signs of "burnout," discussed earlier in this chapter. Finally, stress management training can be recommended for the child who anticipates giving a significant amount of energy and commitment to a sport over several years.

ERGOGENIC DRUGS AND SUPPLEMENTS

Ergogenic drugs refer to legal and illicit substances used to enhance athletic performance. They encompass the anabolic-androgenic steroids, steroid precursors (androstenedione and DHEA), growth hormone, creatine, and ephedra alkaloids. Some of these are marketed as nutritional supplements; the precursors, growth hormone, and ephedra substances have not been proven to enhance performance, yet they can have serious side effects of which the young are often unaware. Street names include gym candy, pumpers, weight trainers, stackers, and Arnolds.

The preponderance of ergogenic drug use can be attributed to many modern influences. These include: the message by top athletes and sports icons that ergogenic drugs are acceptable because of their own use; the emphasis, and status placed, on sports by society that produces greater incentive for parents to advocate for—and children at younger ages to desire—excelling and competing at a sport; canvassing ever younger players by sports scouts; and pressure to fund college education via sports scholarships. Impressionable youngsters are manipulated by an aggressive media and product industry. Alluring advertising techniques, such as flashy, catchy labels on supplements and "used-by-the-pros" proclamations, capitalize on immature developmental levels that make youth more vulnerable to peer pressure and the need for success and self-esteem. The written information that discusses the warnings and side effects of ergogenic aids are often above the reading levels of middle schoolers (Calfee & Fadale, 2006).

Anticipatory guidance and education are essential in this area. Education needs to include both benefits and risks, and the educator needs to be well informed to be credible. Schools and colleges need to issue and enforce no-tolerance policies

and endorse the U.S. Anti-Doping Agency regulations and world anti-doping code. "Clean" team members can provide leadership by disavowing performance-enhancing drugs and emphasizing the integrity (fair play) of sports competition. Parents and coaches should intervene whenever necessary. The Adolescents Training and Learning to Avoid Steroids program first described in 1996 (Goldberg et al, 1996) is a model for such interventions. Nutrition and strength-training techniques are important aspects of athletic performance enhancement programs (ACSM, 2003d). It is imperative that parents adhere to the directives given previously under "Stress and Sports: Keeping Activities Fun."

Anabolic-Androgenic Steroids

The anabolic-androgenic steroids (AASs) are Class III controlled substances. Endogenous AASs start adolescent development in the prepubertal male. The exogenous AASs used by males and females are derivatives of testosterone. These steroids naturally produce changes in nonreproductive tissues, such as closure of bony epiphyses, changes in the larynx, increases in muscle bulk and strength, and aggressiveness.

Reports of anabolic steroid use by Olympic athletes first appeared in the 1950s; since then the prevalence has increased as athletes as young as fifth graders have donned a "win-at-all-costs" mentality. Current use rates among high school students range from 4% to 11% in boys and up to 3.3% for girls. Up to one-third of those taking AASs are non-athletes who use them to enhance their appearance (Calfee & Fadale, 2006).

Those taking the risk of using steroids also exhibit other high-risk activities, including driving while under the influence, carrying weapons, practicing unsafe sexual behavior, and having an increased use of marijuana and alcohol. Twenty-five percent to 33% who use the injectable form report sharing needles, which puts them at risk for HIV, hepatitis B, and hepatitis C (Calfee & Fadale, 2006).

Steroid users may use the substance in three preparations: oral, injected, or transdermal. The oral forms are shorter acting and excreted over days; the injectables are longer acting and can take months to eliminate from the body. Generally used in the off-season (to gain strength and prevent detection), these drugs are taken in cycles of use lasting 4 to 12 weeks each. Sometimes more than one type of steroid is used at a time ("stacking"), or the steroids are dosed incrementally and then tapered at the end of a cycle ("pyramiding"). Newer, "designer" steroids are being produced. They are designed to prevent detection by doping tests; they pose the same serious threats to the health of those taking them. Tetrahydrogestrinone (THG) is one such drug.

Clinical effects can be irreversible in both males and females. Up to 30% of users experience some mild subjective effects, which can include acne, seborrhea, weight gain, deepening voice, precocious puberty, or premature balding. With sustained use, some of the more serious side effects include cardiac failure, impotence, edema, testicular atrophy, liver dysfunction, and tendon or muscle injuries (as a result of the development of dysplastic collagen fibrils). Premature epiphyseal closure can leave the immature athlete shorter than expected. Hepatotoxicity is most related to the 17-alkylated derivatives. In females AASs can cause irreversible menstrual irregularities and breast atrophy, enlargement of the clitoris, hirsutism, male pattern baldness, amenorrhea (may be partially reversible after termination of use), and deepening of the voice with larynx changes.

Approximately 50% of steroid users meet the mental health illness standards for drug dependence or abuse. Mood swings, violent behavior, heightened aggression, and depression severe enough to be linked with suicide have been described (Calfee & Fadale, 2006).

Androstenedione and Dehydroepiandrosterone

Androstenedione ("andro") and related DHEA are prohormones that are converted to either testosterone or estrone. Androstenedione is the more potent of the two and is a Class III controlled drug. DHEA may be purchased over the counter. Usage data is scant, but studies have shown that up to 4% of high school athletes and nonathletes used precursors, and 5.3% of college athletes reported use (Calfee & Fadale, 2006).

Steroid precursors are used because of the mistaken belief that they will increase testosterone and produce the same effects on muscles and performance as seen with anabolic steroids. Studies, however, have demonstrated no convincing measurable changes in athletic performance. Rather than show increases in testosterone levels, steroid precursors significantly increase estrone and estradiol levels to the point of causing adverse changes in lipid levels, male gynecomastia, virilization in females, priapism, possible hyperplastic prostatic changes, and affect the regulation of normal endogenous testosterone over time. Additionally, potential impurities in the products can produce positive drug screens (Calfee & Fadale, 2006).

Growth Hormone

Growth hormone (available in a biosynthetic, injectable form) is often used one or more times a month with a cost approaching $5000 per month, is banned by sporting leagues, and is so far immune from any doping detection tests. It is taken in the mistaken belief that it will enhance athletic performance. It will, however, produce premature epiphyseal closure, jaw enlargement, hypertension, slipped capital femoral epiphysis, and (rarely) papilledema with intracranial hypertension. Athletes who take it report a "feel-good" sensation (probably caused by fluid shifts within tissues) and decreases in subcutaneous fat for a fit appearance. There is risk of hepatitis B and C and HIV because of needle-sharing practices. Incidence rates approached 5% in one study of high school students, with half of them combining it with steroids. A National Collegiate Athletic Association (NCAA) study revealed an incidence use of 3.5% (Calfee & Fadale, 2006).

Creatine and Other Supplements

Creatine occurs naturally in the body, is an amino acid, and 95% is stored in muscle as phosphocreatine (the rest goes to the brain and heart). Synthetic creatine is an over-the-counter supplement used in the belief that it enhances athletic endurance. Supplementation does produce an increase in muscle strength and performance in short-duration, anaerobic events. It produces this effect by increasing (by approximately 20%) stores of muscle phosphocreatine that in turn release initial energy for muscle contraction in short, high-intensity activities (e.g., wrestling), quickening phosphocreatine replenishment during recovery, and delaying fatigue onset. The exercise must be maximal and anaerobic and last long enough to deplete the stores nonusers would have. If the duration of the activity is too long, however, other sources of energy supplant the creatine effects, and benefit is not seen. The normal daily body requirement is about 2 g for a 70-kg person. Half comes from meat and fish, and half is synthesized by the body.

Athletes generally take a cycle of 5 g, four times daily for 4 to 6 days and then a maintenance dose of 2 g/day for the following 3 months. A month of abstinence then is practiced. It is important for those taking creatine to drink 6 to 8 oz. of water to prevent dehydration. Carbohydrate-rich fluids increase the absorption, and caffeine impairs uptake.

Athletes have reported poorer performance, muscle cramps, mild gastrointestinal distress, and renal disease (rare) as side effects. There is no data showing the effects of long-term use, the effect of supplementation on the other creatine storage organs (brain or heart), or effects in those younger than 18 years old.

Creatine supplementation is not encouraged in those less than 18 years old. However, incidence studies have reported a usage range of 5.6% to 8.2% in 10- to 18-year-olds; the majority did not know how much they consumed or that they were, in fact, consuming beyond the recommended amounts. The use in twelfth graders (44%) and college athletes (25% to 78%) are similar (Calfee & Fadale, 2006).

Ephedra

Ephedrine has a chemical structure similar to amphetamine. It enhances the release of norepinephrine and stimulates the central nervous system. The herbal form is ma huang. Metabolife 356 and Ripped Fuel were brands that were previously sold, but were banned in 2004 by the FDA. A subsequent ruling in 2005 placed this ban in jeopardy and left many to think that the sale of these products might yet resume. However, because of the 2006 nationwide effort to curb the retail sale of pseudoephedrine, the whole issue of ephedrine products is yet to be resolved.

Athletes use ephedra to provide quick energy and help in losing body fat, thereby enhancing speed and appearance. Studies have demonstrated no actual boost in performance but have shown an increase in quadriceps strength.

Adverse reactions include tachycardia (most often), hypertension, arrhythmias, anxiety, tremors, insomnia, seizures, paranoid psychoses, cerebral vascular accident, myocardial infarction, and death.

The incidence of use is up; it is used by more high school females (26%) than males (12%). Pseudoephedrine in cold tablets is often used. The product is sometimes combined with the herbal form or caffeine (Calfee & Fadale, 2006).

Nutritional Supplements

Nutritional supplements are readily available to aspiring athletes who believe that they will perform better if using them. They generally are composed of one or more of the following: a vitamin, a mineral, an herb or other botanical, an amino acid, a dietary supplement that raises the total daily intake or a concentrate, metabolite, constituent, extract, or a combination of the last four ingredients. The concern with these products is that studies have shown a broad inconsistency in the accuracy of labeling ingredients and amounts and/or contamination and/or the inclusion of dangerous substances (e.g., steroids). They are to be discouraged because of their listing as an unregulated dietary supplement under the 1994 Dietary Supplement Health and Education Act (Calfee & Fadale, 2006).

RECREATIONAL ACTIVITY SAFETY

All-Terrain Vehicles (ATVs)

Of the 5791 ATV-related deaths between 1982 and 2003, 32% were children less than 16 years old (CDC, 2006c). Helmets can help prevent head trauma, but not the other causes of ATV morbidity including spinal cord, thoracic, and abdominal injuries and asphyxiation.

The following age and size recommendations differ, depending upon whether they come from the ATV industry or from the AAP and other agencies.

They include:

- No operation for children less than 6 years old (industry and AAP agree on this.)
- ATV engine producing 50 to 70 cc, for children 6 to 11 years old (yes, per industry; no, per AAP and other agencies)
- ATV engine producing 70 to 90 cc, for children 12 to 15 years old (yes, per industry; no, per AAP and other agencies)
- ATV engine greater than 90 cc, for 16 years and older (industry, AAP, and other agencies agree on this.)

ATVs should not be driven on public roads, only on designated trails and at safe speeds. Drivers should not carry passengers, should take an ATV safety course, and wear helmets and other protective gear (Oregon Department of Human Services, 2006).

Bicycling

Bicycling can be an excellent aerobic activity. However, children need to wear helmets, learn to handle their bicycles with skill, and know the rules of the road for cyclists. Wearing a helmet decreases the severity of injury (refer to Proper Use of Bicycle Helmets under Injury Prevention in the preceding section).

Golfing

Approximately 3.3 million children play golf; one third are from 5 to 11 years old. Tiger Woods' playing and popularity are largely credited with the 30% increase in players from 5 to 17 years old since 1997. In 2002, more than 11,000 golf-related injuries were reported in children 14 years old and younger; 86% involved the head, face, eye, ear, or mouth (Brian & Glazer, 2005). Golf is categorized as a high-risk sport because it: (a) has the third highest incidence of ocular enucleation per injury, and (b) injury results in a preponderance of depressed skull fractures. The injuries largely occur during unsupervised play, when a child is hit by another child's swinging club. Preventive measures include: supervision at all times if a child has a golf club in hand, proper education about the rules of golf (standing at least four club lengths away from a swinging club; "stop-look-and-swing" before swinging), and storing golf clubs out of reach of children because they can become lethal weapons (Brian & Glazer, 2005).

Nonpowder Guns

Nonpowder guns include ball-bearing (BB) guns, pellet guns, air rifles, and paintball guns. In 2000, there were more than 21,000 injuries; 39 nonpowder gun-related deaths were reported of which more than 80% were children less than 15 years old. Eye, skin, internal organs, and bones are the most vulnerable body sites for injury. The popularity of war games and paintball guns has contributed to the attractiveness of "playing" with these types of guns. They should not be regarded as toys because both the low- and high-velocity nonpowder guns cause serious injuries (Laraque & AAP, 2004). Protective eyewear, ear protection, supervision, training, and the developmental and maturity levels of participants need to be appreciated as preventive measures.

Playground Equipment

There are approximately half a million children medically treated for injuries sustained on playground equipment yearly (AAOS, 2004a). The AAOS program, Prevent Injuries America! provides the following safety guidelines for parents:

- Playground surfaces should be regularly inspected for hazards (sharp protrusions, intact matting, no exposed concrete footings) and be constructed out of shock-absorbing, single-unit materials (e.g., rubber mats and loose fill double-shredded bark mulch, wood fibers, sand, fine or medium gravel). Under no circumstance should children be allowed on equipment that is over a hard surface (concrete, asphalt, grass and soil [soil can become hard packed]).
- Playgrounds should be properly designed for safety: swings should be away from sandboxes, separate areas for preschoolers and older children; widely spaced for popular activities; good sight lines for supervision; barriers between playground and street.

Roller Sports

The roller sports include in-line skating, skateboarding, and riding scooters. Combined, these sports account for more than 290,000 visits annually for medical treatment of musculoskeletal injuries. These sports allow aerobic fitness, independent transportation, cross-training for other sports, and are relatively low cost, but they can be risky. Inexperience, losing one's balance, poor equipment, trying tricks beyond one's skill level, lack of protective equipment, homemade ramps, riding near traffic, and irregular riding surfaces are the most common etiologic factors for the accidents. Some statistics are in order:

- Thirty-seven percent of all in-line skating injuries involve the wrist, the majority of which are fractures.
- There are more than 50,000 hospital emergency department visits as a result of skateboard accidents. Sixty percent of injuries occurred in male children less than 15 years old (AAOS, 2004b). Injuries range from minor cuts and abrasions to fractures to severe head injuries. Fractures to the ankle, forearm, wrist, and face (nose and jaw) are the most common injuries.
- Scooter injuries often occur on the street or sidewalk, from collisions with motor vehicles, and are related to poor braking or mechanical problems (Mankovsky et al, 2002).

Preventive measures include: riding in skateboarding parks; riding on smooth surfaces away from traffic; using quality skateboards (shorter decks are best for beginners; fit to weight of child); keeping all equipment in proper shape (inspect for broken, cracked parts, sharp edges; slippery board top with nicks or cracks; lubricate parts); learning basic skills of slowing, turning, and falling safely; practicing tricks and jumps only in controlled parks; keeping in good physical shape by stretching and conditioning before and after activity; not wearing headphones while riding; not putting another rider on the same skateboard or scooter; knowing rules of the road (stopping at stop signs, etc.); knowing what to do in emergencies; not riding at night; and wearing proper safety equipment (properly fitted helmet, wrist guards, kneepads and elbow pads, shoes). Replace a helmet if damaged, outgrown, or older than 5 years. The AAP advises that skateboards not be ridden by children less than 6 years old; 6- to 10-year-olds should be closely supervised by knowledgeable adults or adolescents.

Swimming

All children should learn to swim. This is essential to their safety near water environments because an estimated 500,000 significant emersions occur annually in the U.S. (approximately 500,000 people drown worldwide each year) (Kallas, 2004). Swimming is an excellent sports activity that can be engaged in throughout life.

Trampolines

Although the AAP recommended that trampolines be banned from schools and competitive sports in 1977, trampolines are still popular for home recreational use by children and adults. Injury rates almost tripled from 1991 to 1999. There are annually more than 240,000 medically treated injuries resulting from trampoline use with more than half in children 14 years old or younger. Injuries include fractures (extremities and other body parts [e.g., necks]), dislocations, muscle damage, spinal cord injuries, head traumas; some of these result in permanent paralysis or death (Foundation for Spinal Cord Injury Prevention, 1999).

Trampolines cannot be recommended for home use. However, the clinician can offer the following advice to those using this equipment:

- Children should only be allowed on the trampolines under the close instruction and supervision of adults who are prepared to respond to medical emergencies.
- The jumping surface should be at ground level.
- Netting around the trampoline perimeter will help keep the jumper confined to the jumping surface, but will not reduce accidents caused by the surface itself.
- Do not allow jumpers to jump onto trampoline from a higher level, object, or surface.
  - Pad all bars, strings, landing surfaces
  - One person rule on trampoline at any given time
  - Proper education, use of protective equipment [e.g., harness], and trained spotters should be part of any acrobatic maneuvers

Winter Sports

Approximately 12% of ski injuries occur in children less than 18 years old, with a fracture of the lower extremity (spiral fracture of the tibia) being most common. Fifty-eight percent of injuries occur when the skier hits a stationary object. The efficacy of helmet use for young recreational skiers has not been studied (Suresh, 2006), but they are highly advocated by the National Ski Areas Association and such winter sports programs as Lids on Kids (see Resource Box). Much of the decrease in injury rates over the past 20 years has been the result of improvements in equipment. Children should have formal training, not be outfitted in hand-me-down equipment, and have well-fitting boots and poles with bindings appropriately adjusted.

Snowboarders have higher fracture rates than skiers. The most common injuries involve the upper limbs (notably the wrist), head, and lower limbs. Fewer knee injuries occur than found in skiing, whereas ankle injuries are more frequent because soft-shell boots protect the ankle less well than ski boots do. Most injuries occur in adolescent males who have had no training or professional lessons (Langran, 2006).

Sledding often involves small children; because of their head size and higher centers of gravity, they are at the highest risk for head traumas. Head injuries occur three times as often in children younger than 6 years old as in those more than 12 years old (Finnegan & Tongue, 2003).

Snowmobiling accounts for approximately 14,000 accidents and 200 deaths per year; 12% of all injuries occur in children younger than 17 years old (Suresh, 2006).

Cross-country skiing is relatively safe. Back-country skiers assume more risk because of environmental factors (e.g., avalanches, hypothermia). Medial collateral ligament knee sprain, acute inversion ankle sprain, and shoulder separation are the most common injuries.

Measures to prevent winter sporting accidents include: fitness training to reduce fatigue, going slower, choosing terrain that fits skill levels, making two to three warm-up runs when skiing or snowboarding, checking snow conditions, wearing helmets, staying within the boundaries of the ski areas, and staying alert and in control. Lessons can help all sports enthusiasts learn proper techniques (especially jumping) and principles of safety.

RESOURCE BOX

Activities and Sports for children and Adolescents

Academy of Sports Dentistry (ASD)
www.sportsdentistry-asd.org
Organization dedicated to the prevention of sports-related injuries to the head, face, mouth, and related oral structures

Adolescents Training and Learning to Avoid Steroids (ATLAS) prevention program
www.ohsu.edu/hpsm/about.cfm
Drug prevention program geared towards male high school athletes.

American Academy of Pediatrics
www.aap.org
Pediatric health care focus with a committee on sports medicine that sets standards for children and sports

American Alliance of Health, Physical Education, Recreation and Dance
www.aahperd.org
Promotes school physical activities

American College of Sports Medicine
www.acsm.org
Diagnosis, treatment, and prevention of sports-related injuries and advancement of research related to exercise

American Orthopaedic Society for Sports Medicine (AOSSM)
www.sportsmed.org
Provides a variety of pamphlets on nutrition for sports, heart and athletic performance, flexibility, designing weight programs, and PPE; provides a resource directory for disabled athletes from their committee on athletes with disability

American Sport Education Program
www.asep.com
Provides on-line courses on sports coaching for coaches and parents

Athletes Targeting Healthy Exercise & Nutrition Alternatives (ATHENA)
www.ohsu.edu/hpsm/athena.cfm
Program that addresses young female athletes, eating disorders, and drug use

International Society of Sports Nutrition (ISSN)
www.sportsnutritionsociety.org
Association to stimulate research related to nutrition and human performance

Lids on Kids
www.lidsonkids.org
Advocates and has programs that promote the use of helmets for children participating in winter sports; includes proper fitting of ski helmets

National SAFE KIDS Campaign
www.safekids.org

Sports, Cardiovascular and Wellness Nutritionists (SCAN)
www.scandpg.org
Nutrition professionals with expertise in the role of nutrition in sports, cardiovascular health, health promotion, fitness, and the prevention and treatment of eating disorders; associated with the American Dietetic Association and Centers for Disease Control and Prevention

NURSING DIAGNOSES

Related to Activity and Exercise: Functional Pattern

- Activity intolerance
- Deficient diversional activity
- Impaired physical mobility
  - Impaired bed mobility
  - Impaired wheelchair mobility
  - Impaired transfer mobility
  - Delayed surgical recovery
  - Sedentary lifestyle

From NANDA International: *NANDA-I nursing diagnoses: definitions & classification 2007-2008*, Philadelphia, 2007, Author.

☑ DISCUSSION FORUM

1. What physical assessment techniques should be done during a sport physical to screen for hypertrophic cardiomyopathy?
2. What role can the primary care provider play in ensuring that daily physical activities are part of the school curriculum?
3. How are PPEs done in your local community?
4. How can you impact the safety issues around organized and nonorganized sports in your community?
5. A 15-year-old is not wearing a bike helmet. The state law only mandates bike helmets until 14 years old. What can you do in the office to encourage bike helmet use? What impact can you have at a community and state level?
6. What are the signs and symptoms of steroid use in children and adolescents? How do you screen for them? What impact does screening athletes have on steroid use?

REFERENCES

American Academy of Allergy, Asthma and Immunology (AAAAI): *Topic of the month: winning with exercise induced asthma*, Aug 2004. Available at *www.aaaai.org/patients/topicofthemonth/0804/* (accessed Aug 4, 2006).

American Academy of Allergy, Asthma and Immunology (AAAAI): *Tips to remember: exercise-induced asthma*. Available at *www.aaaai.org/patients/publicedmat/tips/exerciseinducedasthma.htm* (accessed Aug 4, 2006).

American Academy of Neurology Quality Standards Subcommittee: Practice parameter: the management of concussion in sports (summary statement), *Neurology* 48:581-585, 1997.

American Academy of Orthopaedic Surgeons (AAOS): *10 common questions about playground safety*, Dec 2004a. Available at *www.orthoinfo.aaos.org/fact/thr_report.cfm?thread_ID=443&topcategory=children* (accessed Aug 7, 2006).

American Academy of Orthopaedic Surgeons (AAOS): *Skateboarding safety*, June 2004b. Available at *www.orthoinfo.acos.org/fact/thr_report.cfm?thread_ID=373&topcategory=children* (accessed Aug 7, 2006).

American Academy of Orthopaedic Surgeons (AAOS): *Burners and stingers*, 2006. Available at *www.orthoinfo.acos.org/fact/thr_report.cfm?thread_ID=226&topcategory=shoulder* (accessed July 30, 2006).

American Academy of Pediatrics (AAP) Committee on Sports Medicine and Fitness: Atlantoaxial instability in Down syndrome: subject review, *Pediatrics* 96:151-154, 1995.

American Academy of Pediatrics (AAP): Practice guideline: medical conditions affecting sports participation, *Pediatrics* 107(5):1205-1209, 2001a.

American Academy of Pediatrics (AAP): Health supervision for children with Down syndrome, *Pediatrics* 107(2):442-449, 2001b.

American Academy of Pediatrics (AAP) Committee on Injury and Poison Prevention: Bicycle helmets, *Pediatrics* 108(4):1030-1032, 2001c.

American Academy of Pediatrics (AAP) Committee on Sports Medicine and Fitness: Technical report: knee brace use in the young athlete, *Pediatrics* 108(2):503-507, 2001d.

American Academy of Pediatrics (AAP): *Guideline for pediatricians: exercise induced asthma*, issue 13, 2005. Available at *www.aap.org/family/sportsshort.13.pdf* (accessed Aug 4, 2006).

American Academy of Pediatrics (AAP): Policy statement: active healthy living: prevention of childhood obesity through increased physical activity, *Pediatrics* 117(5):1834-1842, 2006a.

American Academy of Pediatrics (AAP): Guidelines for pediatricians: exertional heat-related illness. In *Sportshorts*, issue 2. Available at *www.aap.org/family/sportsshorts_02.pdf* (accessed Aug 4, 2006b).

American Academy of Pediatrics (AAP) Committee on Nutrition: Guidelines for pediatricians: nutrition and sports. In *Sportshorts*, issue 6. Available at *www.aap.org/family/sportsshorts_06.pdf* (accessed July 30, 2006c).

American Academy of Pediatrics (AAP): *Red book: 2006 report of the committee on infectious diseases*, ed 27, Elk Grove, IL, 2006d, American Academy of Pediatrics.

American College of Sports Medicine (ACSM): Does exercise help or harm a cold? *News Release*, Oct. 18, 2001a. Available at *www.acsm.org/publications/newsreleases2001/exercold.htm* (accessed July 29, 2006).

American College of Sports Medicine (ACSM): Nasal dilators do not enhance performance during exercise. *News Release*, April 9, 2001b. Available at *www.acsm.org/publications/newsreleases2001/nasaldilators.htm* (accessed July 29, 2006).

American College of Sports Medicine (ACSM): High school cheerleaders demonstrate athleticism; but may need nutritional counseling. *News Release*, May 28, 2003a. Available at *www.acsm.org/publications/newsreleases2003/cheerleaders060103.htm* (accessed July 14, 2006).

American College of Sports Medicine (ACSM): *Female athlete issues for the team physician: a consensus statement*, 2003b. Available at *www.acsm.org/Am/Template.cfm?Section=clinicians&Template=/cm/ContentDisplay.cfm&content ID=1617* (accessed July 30, 2006).

American College of Sports Medicine (ACSM): Girls more likely to be active when parents participate. *News Release*, Sept 4, 2003c. Available at *www.acsm.org/publications/newsreleases2003/activegirls090903.htm* (accessed July 29, 2006).

American College of Sports Medicine (ACSM): Steroids threaten health of athletes and integrity of sports performance. *News Release*, Oct 23, 2003d. Available at *www.acsm.org/publications/newsreleases2003/Steroids102403.htm* (accessed July 29, 2006).

American College of Sports Medicine (ACSM): Young "extreme" athletes underuse protective equipment: injuries, high-risk behaviors linked to infrequent usage. *News Release*, June 1, 2005a. Available at *www.acsm.org/publications/news-releases* (accessed July 14, 2006).

American College of Sports Medicine (ACSM): Girls more active with exercise and sports they enjoy. *News Release*, March 21, 2005b. Available at *www.acsm.org/publications/news-releases* (accessed July 14, 2006).

Andersen LB, et al: Physical activity and clustered cardiovascular risk in children: a cross-sectional study (The European Youth Heart Study), *Lancet* 368(9532):299-304, 2006.

Brain Injury Association: *Fact sheet: sports and recreation*, 2004. Available at *www.biausa.org/BIAUSA.ORG/word.files.to.pdf/good.pdfs/factsheets/sportsandrec.pdf* (accessed Aug 20, 2007).

Brian R, Glazer G: Taming the little tigers: golf-related head injuries in children, *Adv Nurse Pract* 13(6):59-60, 2005.

Browne GJ, Lam LT: Concussive head injury in children and adolescents related to sports and other leisure physical activities, *Brit J Sports Med* 40:163-168, 2006.

Calfee R, Fadale R: Popular ergogenic drugs and supplements in young athletes, *Pediatrics* 117:577-589, 2006.

Cantu RC: Head injuries. In DeLee JC, Drez Jr. D, Miller MD, editors: *DeLee and Drez's orthopaedic sports medicine: principles and practice*, vol 1, ed 2, Philadelphia, 2003, WB Saunders.

Centers for Disease Control and Prevention (CDC): *Behavior risk factor surveillance system 2000*. Available at *www.cdc.gov/brfss* (accessed Aug 9, 2006).

Centers for Disease Control and Prevention (CDC): Nonfatal sports-and recreation-related injuries treated in emergency departments—United States, July 2000-June 2001, *Morb Mortal Wkly Rep* 51-MM33:736-740, 2002.

Centers for Disease Control and Prevention (CDC): Youth risk behavioral surveillance, US, 2005, *Morb Mortal Wkly Rep* 55:SS-5, 2006a.

Centers for Disease Control and Prevention (CDC): *Can I get HIV while playing sports*? Available at *www.cdc.gov/HIV/AIDS* (accessed July 30, 2006b).

Clark M, Ferguson S. The physical activity and fitness of our nation's children, *J Pediatr Nurs* 15(4):250-252, 2000.

Clinical Advisor, editorial staff: Newsline: childhood exercise increases bone mass, *Clin Advisor* 8(11):21, 2005.

Dubin A: Cardiac arrhythmias. In Behrman RE, Kliegman RM, Jenson HB, editors: *Nelson textbook of pediatrics*, ed 17, Philadelphia, 2004, WB Saunders.

Faigenbaum AD, Chu EA, American College of Sports Medicine (ACSM): Plyometric training for children and adolescents. In *Current Comment*, Dec 2001. Available at *www.acsm.org/health+fitness/pdf/currentcomments/plyometr.pdf* (accessed July 28, 2006).

Finnegan MA, Tongue JR: The hidden dangers of winter sliding, *Clin Orthop* 409:73-77, 2003.

Foundation for Spinal Cord Injury Prevention, Care and Cure: *Trampoline injuries, 1999*. Available at *www.fscip.org/tramp* (accessed Aug 7, 2006).

Fountain NB, May AC: Epilepsy and athletics, *Clin Sports Med* 22:605-616, 2003.

Galuska DA et al: Are health care professionals advising obese patients to lose weight? *JAMA* 282(16):1581-1582, 1999.

Glover D, Maron B, Matheson G: The preparticipation physical examination: steps toward consensus and uniformity, *Physician Sportsmed* 27(8), 1999. Available at *www.postgradmed.com/back_iss.htm* (accessed Aug 20, 2007).

Goldberg L et al: The Adolescents Training and Learning to Avoid Steroid (ATLAS) Prevention Program: background and results of a model intervention, *Arch Ped Adol Med* 150(7):713-721, 1996.

Hammerman S et al: Asthma screening of high school athletes: identifying the undiagnosed and poorly controlled, *Ann Allergy Asthma Immunol* 88(4):380-384, 2002.

Hendrickson K: Making exercise a family affair. In American College of Sports Medicine (ACSM): *Fit society, youth sports and health*, Spring 2003. Available at *www.acsm.org.Search for Hendrickson (fitsc203.pdf)* (accessed July 14, 2006).

Hergenroeder AC: Sports medicine. In Finberg L, Kleinman R, editors: *Saunders manual of pediatric practice*, ed 2, Philadelphia, 2002, WB Saunders.

Hergenroeder AC, Chorley JN: Sports medicine. In Behrman RE, Kliegman RM, Jenson HB, editors: *Nelson textbook of pediatrics*, ed 17, Philadelphia, 2004, Saunders.

Housh TJ, Johnson GO, American College of Sports Medicine (ACSM): Growth in young wrestlers, *Current Comment*, Nov 2001. Available at *www.acsm.org/content/contentFolders/publications/currentcomment/2001/wrestler/3101.pdf* (accessed July 28, 2006).

Howard GM, Radloff M, Sevier TL: Epilepsy and sports, *Curr Sports Med Rep* 3(1):15-19, 2004.

Janz KF: Physical activity augments bone mineral accrual in young children: the Iowa Bone Development Study, *J Pediatr* 148(6):793-799, 2006.

Kallas HJ: Drowning and near drowning. In Behrman RE, Kliegman RM, Jenson HB, editors: *Nelson textbook of pediatrics*, ed 17, Philadelphia, 2004, WB Saunders.

Kamboj MK, Draznin MB: Office management of the adolescent with diabetes mellitus, *Prim Care Clin Office Pract* 33:581-602, 2006.

Langran M: *Snowboarding injuries: injury rates*. Available at *www.ski-injury.com* (accessed Aug 6, 2006).

Laraque D, American Academy of Pediatrics (AAP) Committee on Injury, Violence, and Poison Prevention: Technical report: injury risk of non-powder guns, *Pediatrics* 114(5):1357-1361, 2004.

Loud KJ et al: Correlates of stress fractures among preadolescent and adolescent girls, *Pediatrics* 115(4):e399-406, 2005.

Luckstead E, Patel D: Catastrophic pediatric sports injuries, *Pediatr Clin North Am* 49(3):581-591, 2002.

Luebbers, PE: The right time for kids to exercise. In American College of Sports Medicine: *Fit society: youth sports and health*, Spring 2003. Available at *www.acsm.org.Search for Luebbers(fitsc203.pdf)* (accessed Aug 20, 2007).

Luke A: Common injuries in young athletes. In American College of Sports Medicine: *Fit society: youth sports and health*, Spring 2003. Available at *www.acsm.org.Search for Luke(fitsc2003.pdf)* (accessed July 31, 2006).

Lyman S et al: Longitudinal study of elbow and shoulder pain in youth baseball pitchers, *Med Sci Sports Exerc* 33(11):1803-1810, 2001.

Madden CC, Walsh WM, Mellion MB: The team physician: the preparticipation examination and on-field emergencies. In DeLee JC, Drez Jr D, Miller MD, editors: *DeLee and Drez's orthopaedic sports medicine: principles and practice*, vol 1, ed 2, Philadelphia, 2003, WB Saunders.

Maffulli N, Baxter-Jones A: Intensive training in elite young female athletes: effects of intensive training on growth and maturation are not established, *Br J Sports Med* 36(1):13-15, 2002.

Magee LM, American College of Sports Medicine: *Return to play: a common sense guide for coaches*. Available at *www.acsm.org.Search for Magee (RTP brochure.pdf)* (accessed July 30, 2006).

Mankovsky AB et al: Evaluation of scooter-related injuries in children, *J Pediatr Surg* 37(5):755-759, 2002.

McCarthy VM: Getting to the big game: keys to performing an efficient sports physical, *Adv Nurse Pract* 14(6):67-69, 2006.

Metzl JD: Expectations of pediatric sports participation among pediatricians, patients, and parents, *Pediatr Clin North Am* 49(3):497-504, 2002.

Metzl JD: Overtraining in children and adolescents. In American Academy of Sports Medicine: *Fit society: youth sports and health*, Spring 2003. Available at *www.acsm.org.Search for Metzl (fitsc203.pdf)* (accessed Aug 3, 2006).

Mitchell J, Haskell W, Raven P: Classification of sports. Twenty-Sixth Bethesda Conference: recommendations for determining eligibility for competition in athletes with cardiovascular abnormalities, *Med Sci Sports Exerc* 26(suppl):S242-S245, 1994.

National Center for Health Statistics (NCHS): *Healthy people 2010: progress review focus area 22, physical activity and fitness*, 2004. Available at *www.cdc.gov/nchs* (accessed July 28, 2006).

National College Athletic Association: *NCAA guideline 3a: participation by the impaired student-athlete*, 1976, revised 2000. Available at *www.ncaa.org/library/sports_sciences/sports_med_handbook/2003-04/3a.pdf* (accessed Aug 20, 2007).

Neumark-Sztainer D et al: Associations between body satisfaction and physical activity in adolescents: implications for programs aimed at preventing a broad spectrum of weight-related disorders, *Eat Disord* 12(2):125-137, 2004.

Norman PK et al: Diet, physical activity, and sedentary behaviors as risk factors for overweight in adolescence, *Arch Pediatr Adolesc Med* 158(4):385-390, 2004.

Olsen O-E et al: Exercises to prevent lower limb injuries in youth sports: cluster randomized controlled trial, *BMJ* 330:449-452, 2005.

Oregon Department of Human Services: Children and all-terrain vehicles: one size does not fit all, *CD Summary* 55(10):1-2, 2006. Available at *Oregon.gov/DHS/Ph/cdsummary* (accessed Aug 20, 2007).

Patel D, Pratt H, Greydanus D: Pediatric neurodevelopment and sports participation. When are children ready to play sports? *Pediatr Clin North Am* 49:505-531, 2002.

Pitetti K: Exercise important for children and adolescents with mental retardation. In American College of Sports Medicine: *Fit society: youth sports and health*, Fall 2001. Available at *www.acsm.org.search for Pitetti (fitsc401.pdf)* (accessed Aug 3, 2006).

Radelet MA et al: Survey of the injury rate for children in community sports, *Pediatrics* 110(3):e28-30, 2002.

Sheerin KA: The link between asthma and obesity. In American Academy of Allergy, Asthma, and Immunology: *Asthma and advocate*, 2005, p 3. Available at *www.aaaai.org/patients/advocate/2005/summer/obesity.stm* (accessed Aug 4, 2006).

Sirard JR et al: Physical activity and active commuting to elementary school, *Med Sci Sports Exerc* 37(12):2062-2069, 2005.

Special Olympics: *Healthy athletes initiative*. Available at *www.specialolympics.org* (accessed Aug 4, 2006).

Stanford KI et al: Influence of menstrual cycle phase on pulmonary function in asthmatic athletes, *Eur J Appl Physiol* 96(6):703-710, 2006.

Stevenson K, Adelson PD: Pediatric sports-related head injuries. In DeLee JC, Drez Jr D, Miller MD, editors: *DeLee and Drez's orthopaedic sports medicine: principles and practice*, vol 1, ed 2, Philadelphia, 2003, WB Saunders.

Suresh S: Winter sports injuries: patterns of injury-preventive measures, *Consultant Pediatricians* 5(3):168-175, 2006.

US Department of Health and Human Services (USDHHS): *Healthy People 2010: understanding and improving health*, ed 2, Washington, DC, 2000, US Government Printing Office.

US Department of Health and Human Services (USDHHS): *Health, United States, 2005: with chartbook on trends in the health of Americans*, DHHS publication No. 2005-1232, Washington, DC, 2005.

US Department of Health and Human Services (USDHHS): *Summary Report of the Healthy People 2010 Progress Review*, Jan 21, 2004. Available at *www.healthypeople.gov/data/2010progress/focus19/Nutrition_Overweight* (accessed July 28, 2006).

US Preventive Services Task Force (USPSTF): Behavioral counseling in primary care to promote physical activity: recommendations and rationale. In *Guidelines from guide to clinical preventive service (2000-2003)*, ed 3, Washington, DC, 2002, US Department of Health and Human Services.

Working Group of the Preparticipation Evaluation: Determining clearance during the preparticipation evaluation, *Phys Sportsmed* 32(11), 2004. Available by search engine for physician and sportsmedicine.

World Health Organization (WHO): *Global strategy on diet, physical activity and health*. Presented to the World Health Assembly. 2004a. Available at *www.who.int/dietphysicalactivity/strategy/ebr1344/strategy_english_web.pdf* (accessed July 28, 2006).

World Health Organization (WHO): *Young people's health in context: selected key findings from the health behaviour in school-aged children study*, 2004b. Available at *www.euro.who.int/mediacentre/PR/20040603_1* (accessed July 28, 2006).

World Health Organization (WHO): *Framework to monitor and evaluate the implementation of the WHO global strategy on diet, physical activity and health*, 2006. Available at *www.who.int/dietphysicalactivity/DPASindicators/en/* (accessed July 28, 2006).

CHAPTER 15

Sleep and Rest

Catherine E. Burns

Every child needs adequate sleep for good health. Without it, serious health and developmental problems may appear. Sleep disturbances may manifest as bedtime resistance, inability to fall asleep, nighttime waking, arousal difficulties, or excessive daytime sleepiness.

Sleep problems represent one of the most common concerns of parents, and children's sleep is currently receiving much needed attention, both clinically and in research. Sleep will be an extremely frequent topic for discussion with parents. A variety of studies begin to highlight some of the issues and significant prevalence of sleep problems in children. In their review of sleep studies, Howard and Wong (2001) note that 20% to 30% of children experience sleep problems. Twenty percent of 1- to 3-year-olds and 10% of 4- to 5-year-olds experience night awakenings and difficulty initiating sleep (Ramchandani et al, 2000). Canadian researchers, Touchette and colleagues (2005), found that 23.5% of 5 month-old-children did not sleep 6 consecutive hours. Further, 33% of children who did not sleep 6 consecutive hours at 5 months or 17 months continued to be unable to sleep 6 hours at 2.5 years old. Stein et al (2001) found that 10.8% of parents reported sleep problems in their school-age children. Problem areas of sleep—night awakening, bedtime resistance, and excessive daytime sleepiness—were common; the best predictor of a current sleep problem was a history of prior sleep dysfunction. Similarly, Owens and colleagues (2000) reported that 37% of their school-age sample described significant sleep problems in at least one sleep area, and 10% had significant daytime sleepiness with problems in all sleep areas measured.

Insufficient sleep affects and is affected by many areas of child and family well-being, including both physical and mental health issues. School failure, irritability, hyperactivity, distractibility, and accidents are all related to sleep problems. It is also important to recognize that sleep problems of infants and children can be interrelated with family problems, such as those stemming from maternal depression, social stresses, child abuse, or a combination of these. Pediatric sleep problems may also produce sleep deprivation and stress in the caregiver(s).

Sleep problems may result from a variety of other problems, including the following:
- Physical factors
  - Ear infections
  - Neurologic disorders
  - Hypothyroidism
  - Obesity
  - Tonsillar and adenoid hypertrophy
  - Pain
  - Blindness
  - Orofacial anomalies
  - Asthma
  - Down syndrome and other genetic conditions
  - Chronic diseases, such as cystic fibrosis
- Psychological factors
  - Developmental stage
  - Separation anxiety
  - Depression, anxiety, or other mental health problems
  - Stress
  - Learning and behavior problems
  - Attention-deficit/hyperactivity disorder (ADHD)
  - Mental retardation
  - Autism
- Family factors
  - Parental mismanagement of sleep routines
  - Maternal depression
- Environmental and temperamental factors
  - Temperament characteristics, including low sensory threshold, negative mood, and decreased adaptability
  - Environmental factors, including sleeping arrangements, altered daily routines, and feeding practices
  - Caffeine, medications, toxins, or substance abuse

As with all other primary care problems in pediatrics, the provider must be vigilant for a myriad of potential causes and recognize that the family disruption caused by a rebellious or noisy non-sleeper in a household may be significant.

Attention to cultural definitions of normal sleep habits also is essential. "Sleep can be considered a biologically driven behavior that is strongly shaped and interpreted by cultural values and beliefs of the parents" (Jenni & O'Connor, 2005, p. 3). Not all cultures expect children to sleep in separate beds or rooms, nor is it expected that most sleep will occur during the nighttime hours in an uninterrupted fashion.

NORMAL SLEEP STAGES AND CYCLES

The essential functions of sleep are not fully understood. Sleep is traditionally considered a time of renewal for the mind and body, but it is not simply a state of rest. At times the brain is more active in sleep than in wakefulness and, because infants and young children spend the majority of their time in sleep, it is considered a time for essential brain development. Growth and healing, learning and processing of information, and many other functions are facilitated by the sleep state.

Fewer studies have been done with children, but sleep deprivation in adults has negative effects on concentration, cognition, and emotional functioning (Davis et al, 2004).

CIRCADIAN RHYTHMS AND ESTABLISHMENT OF NORMAL SLEEP PATTERNS

Many biologic activities are set on a 24-hour cycle. These include sleep and wakefulness; body temperature regulation; hormonal activity; and respiratory, cardiac, renal, and intestinal functions. Circadian rhythms are not established in the newborn, and homeostatic mechanisms are also poorly developed. Thus, sleep can occur around the clock with ease though patterns are irregular. Circadian rhythms emerge at about 2 to 3 months old (Sheldon, 2004).

Melatonin secreted by the hypothalamus is responsible for the timing of physiologic processes, including the sleep-wake cycle. Light suppresses melatonin production, and darkness is associated with the highest melatonin levels. In normal humans, melatonin begins to rise when the sun sets, peaks at 2 AM, and falls to almost undetectable levels in the daytime. The day-night melatonin cycle is established between 4 and 6 months old. Levels peak at 1 to 3 years old and then decline with age. Maternal melatonin crosses the placental barrier and is secreted in breast milk.

SLEEP CYCLE

Normal sleep can be divided into two distinct phases: rapid eye movement (REM) sleep and nonrapid eye movement (non-REM) sleep. Each phase has distinctive levels of arousal, autonomic response, brain activity, and muscle tone. Non-REM sleep can be further divided into four distinct stages as defined by changes in electroencephalographic (EEG) patterns.

Rapid Eye Movement Sleep

REM sleep is considered to be the dreaming phase. EEG waves are similar to those of the awake state, suggesting that higher levels of brain activity are at work. The function of REM sleep is unclear. Although nerve impulses to the spinal cord and muscles are blocked, leaving the body paralyzed except for minor twitching, the respiratory, eye, and middle ear muscles remain active. The child may smile in a transitory way or make short utterances. Breathing and heart rates become irregular and relatively rapid. Reflexes, kidney function, hormonal secretions, and auditory sensitivity are all altered. The rapid eye movements of this phase are of particular interest. People awakened during REM sleep may report dreams at the time. Children as young as 2 years old have reported dreams during REM sleep. Newborns enter the sleep cycle with REM sleep (sometimes called "active sleep" in neonates), but by 6 months, non-REM sleep occurs first. Because REM sleep is associated with arousals and is preponderant in the first year of life, infants are likely to have problems with maintenance of sleep. Some mothers are concerned about their infants' restless sleep when it is only REM sleep that they are observing.

REM sleep occurs in approximately 90-minute periods with the longest REM episode occurring just after the body temperature reaches its lowest point during the night,

around 5 AM. Thus, in older children and adults, most REM sleep occurs later in the night. The proportion of REM sleep decreases from 55% in infancy to about 25% by the time the child is 5 years old.

Nonrapid Eye Movement Sleep

The four stages of non-REM sleep become distinguishable within 6 months of birth. In the preschool and school-age years, non-REM stages III and IV are preponderant. These stages end with a REM phase. The parasomnias, including nightmares and sleepwalking, which are related to this transition from non-REM to arousal or REM phases, occur most commonly in children in these age groups.

Stage I. Stage I sleep is a state of drowsiness and transition to sleep. There may be eye-rolling movements, decreased body movements, and perhaps opening and closing of the eyelids. Individuals may believe that they are awake, but they cannot report accurately events that occurred during this time. In mature individuals, stage I accounts for about 5% of sleep.

Stage II. Stage II sleep is somewhat deeper than that of stage I, although the person can still be easily aroused. Eye movements, breathing, and heart rate slow. Muscles weaken, though the child can reposition. If aroused, the person may report thinking about things and may report dreams. Mature sleepers spend about 50% of their sleep in this stage, generally in the last half of the night.

Stages III and IV. These two stages are nearly identical and sometimes called delta, deep, or slow-wave sleep. Stage III sleep is deeper than that of stage II. The body is deeply relaxed, breathing is shallow, and heart rate is slow. Stage IV is defined by the EEG pattern it produces. When the delta waves occupy 50% of the EEG pattern, stage IV sleep has begun. Growth hormone appears to be secreted in larger amounts during stages III and IV of sleep (Owens, 2004).

During both stages III and IV, the sleeper is hard to arouse. If awakened, the individual feels confused and disoriented. About 15% to 20% of sleep takes place in stages III and IV, occurring earlier in the night. Stages III and IV sleep seem to develop at about 3 to 4 months old; by 4 months stages III and IV comprise more than half of the total sleep. The transition from stage IV to waking is related to several common pediatric sleep disorders, such as night terrors and sleepwalking.

Sleep Cycle Processes

Two main processes are theorized to regulate sleep and wakefulness. The circadian process dictates sleep and wakefulness based on an internal rhythm related to a light-dark cycle. The homeostatic process requires the body to build a need for sleep while awake and as the sleep need is satisfied through sleeping, to build a need for wakefulness. The longer one is awake, the greater the drive for sleep and vice versa.

Sleep onset is the time when the person enters stage I non-REM sleep. The sleep period begins with sleep onset and continues until full arousal occurs. The sleep cycle includes the repeated episodes of non-REM and REM sleep of the sleep period. Waking involves full alert and recall after the sleep period. Semiwakefulness or alerting to the immediate environment

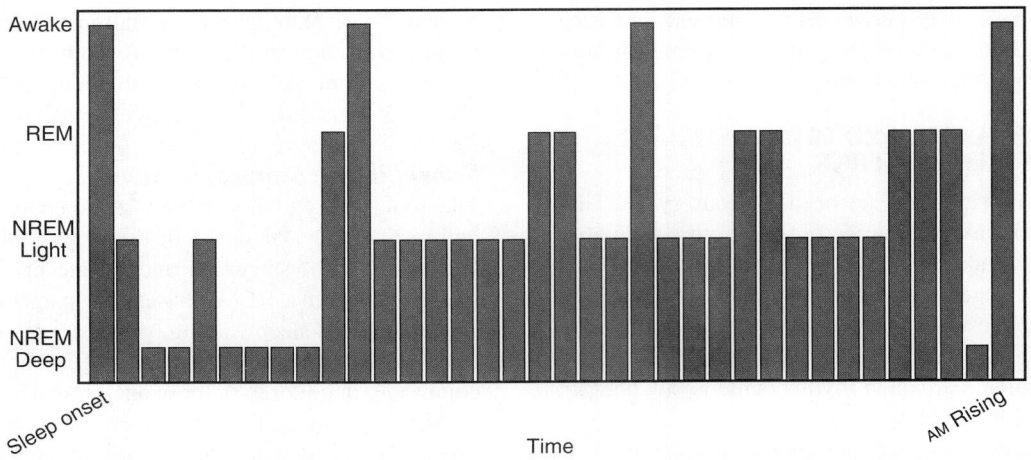

FIG. 15-1   Schema of typical night sleep pattern of sleep states and stages. *REM,* rapid eye movement; *NREM,* nonrapid eye movement. (From Adair R, Bauchner H: Sleep problems in childhood, *Curr Probl Pediatr* 23[suppl 4]1:150, 1993.)

occurs easily in REM sleep or stages I or II in non-REM sleep. The child cycles between REM and non-REM phases throughout the night (Fig. 15-1). Both total amount of sleep and proportion of REM sleep decrease with age (Table 15-1).

REM sleep usually precedes a brief period of semiwakefulness, after which the individual descends again through the non-REM stages to REM, followed by another brief awakening. Later in the evening, the REM phase becomes more pronounced. In older children and adults, the periods of semi-wakefulness may last for a few seconds to a few minutes. It may be the time when one turns over, looks at the clock, or adjusts the covers. The infant sometimes has difficulty returning to the next sleep cycle from this normal waking episode. Young infants have more sleep cycles per night than older individuals do, and each cycle has a brief waking that precedes the next sleep period. Therefore, more opportunities for sleep disturbance can arise with infants. Children generally achieve adult sleep patterns by 3 years old, and each cycle will last from 70 to 100 minutes (Howard & Wong, 2001).

Knowledge of the sleep cycle pattern is helpful for the clinician. Most of the non-REM deep sleep occurs in the early night so associated problems, such as night terrors and sleepwalking, occur then. Most REM sleep occurs in the second half of the night, so problems associated with REM sleep, such as night-mares, occur more in this phase. The short periods of wakefulness throughout the night are times when problems of night waking or difficulty entering the next sleep cycle may occur.

DURATION OF SLEEP

The typical neonate sleeps 16.5 hours each day, but some may require up to 20 hours of sleep per day. Half of this is daytime sleep. The longest neonate sleep period is 2.5 to 4 hours and can occur at any time during the 24-hour day. By 3 months, the baby sleeps almost 15 hours, but the sleep times are more clearly organized into daytime wakefulness and nighttime sleep. Most 6-month-old infants sleep through the night and have morning and afternoon naps. At 1 year old, most children sleep about 13.9 hours. The morning nap is generally given up between 12 and 24 months, but the afternoon nap may persist until the child is 4 or 5 years old. By 2 years old, the child is probably sleeping 11 to 12 hours at night with a 1- to 2-hour nap after lunch. Six-year-olds sleep 10.75 hours per night on average. The average sleep requirement for adolescents is believed to be about 8 to 9 hours per night (see Table 15-1) (Iglowstein et al, 2003).

People use a variety of cues to set the cycle, including daylight, darkness, meals, and activities. Parents need to make these cues clear to infants and children to help them establish healthful bedtime and sleep patterns. *Sleep hygiene* is a term used to define healthful sleep behaviors. Exposure to bright light of even 1 minute at night will suppress melatonin for at least 40 minutes. Use of aspirin, ibuprofen, and other nonste-roidal anti-inflammatory drugs during the night also suppresses melatonin synthesis. These drugs inhibit the lowering of body temperature during the night, another factor in melatonin production. The cues of darkness and cool temperature should

TABLE 15-1   **Average Sleep by Age**

Age (hr)	Nighttime Sleep (hr)	Daytime Sleep (hr)
1 wk	8.25	8.25
1 mo	8.5	7
3 mo	9.5	5.5
6 mo	11	3.4
9 mo	11.2	2.8
12 mo	11.7	2.4
18 mo	11.5	2
2 yr	11.5	1.8
3 yr	11.4	1.7
4 yr	11.2	1.5
6 yr	10.9	
9 yr	10.2	
12 yr	9.3	
15 yr	8.3	

Adapted from Howard B, Wong J: Sleep disorders, *Pediatr Rev* 22: 327- 341, 2001, p. 335.

enhance sleep. Lights should not be turned on brightly at night (for both mother and infant sleep support), but the child may nap in a lighter room during the day (DiLeo et al, 2002).

Sleep in the Newborn and Feeding Effects on Sleep

Normal neonates require 16 to 20 hours of sleep per 24 hours (Glaze, 2004). Three types of sleep are recognized: quiet, active, and indeterminate sleep. These correspond to non-REM sleep, REM sleep, and a period that is neither of these as measured by polysomnography. In the first weeks, sleep cycles consist of equal periods of active and quiet sleep with active sleep initiating each cycle. Because the neonate's sleep is inefficient, it is easily interrupted. As the infant matures, consolidation of sleep cycles occurs and awake periods lengthen during the day. REM sleep decreases and social cues, such as feeding and nighttime routines, begin to influence sleep-wake cycles as the circadian rhythms emerge at 2 to 3 months old (Davis et al, 2004). In a classic study, Anders found that, on average, infants less than 12 months old awaken three times per night regardless of whether their parents are aware of these awakenings (Anders, 1979).

Breastfed infants need to eat more frequently than babies fed formula. Probably this is due to the shorter emptying time for breast milk. Because of this, breastfed babies probably wake more frequently in the night. Bed sharing by mother and infant increases both the length and frequency of breastfeeding episodes in 3- to 4-month-old infants (McKenna et al, 1997). By 6 months, most babies can go for a 6- to 12-hour period without being fed. This extended period coincides with the longest sleep period. Thus, after 6 months, feeding in the night can be considered a learned behavior. Starting solids early to increase length of nighttime sleeping is a myth. Several studies have shown that solids do not help the baby sleep for longer periods. The most common complaints are prolonged night and early morning awakenings (Glaze, 2004).

Sleep in Older Children and Adolescents

Sleep needs steadily decrease with the child's age. The percentage of stage II sleep increases and REM sleep decreases with age (Ohayon et al, 2004). Nighttime sleep should increase somewhat when naps are eliminated from the child's schedule. The circadian timing system changes with puberty (Carskadon et al, 2004). These changes, including phase, period, melatonin secretory pattern, light sensitivity, and phase relationships, have the potential to alter sleep patterns substantially, putting the adolescent at risk for sleep problems.

Indicators of Sleep Problems in Children and Adolescents

Sleepiness in infants is especially difficult to notice since they sleep so many hours normally. They should not have sleepiness that is severe enough to interfere with feeding. Toddlers and preschoolers may have increased activity levels when sleepy. Hyperactivity, emotional lability, irritability, and aggressiveness are all symptoms. Alternately, the child may fall asleep during activities when alertness would be expected, such as at mealtimes.

School-age children are usually considered to be good sleepers. Taking naps or sleeping at school are not normal behaviors. Some other symptoms may include inattention, restlessness, emotional lability, or daydreaming at school. There is considerable overlap of symptoms with ADHD, and indeed the two problems are often related. However, there are some children who, with adequate rest, will resolve their ADHD behaviors.

Adolescents have many problems with sleep that may manifest as excessive sleepiness, difficulties with mood regulation, impaired academic performance, and increased risk for accidents. These may be related to adolescent changes in sleep physiology and lifestyle habits of the teen years. Middle adolescents (14- to 16-year-olds) seem to have more sleep disturbances than younger or older teenagers. Chronic sleep deprivation is a common reason for sleepiness in adolescents (Given, 2004). Sleep loss or disturbances have been associated with increased risk of future suicidal action in adolescents (Liu & Buysse, 2006).

Co-sleeping Issues

Sleep habits are strongly influenced by culture (Jenni & O'Connor, 2005; Liu et al, 2005). Co-sleeping is common in many cultures and has been the human norm for many thousands of years. Co-sleeping by family members is probably more common worldwide than is separate sleeping as advocated in the U.S. Warmth, protection, and a sense of well-being are undoubtedly facilitated by having babies sleep with their mothers or siblings. It is most common in black and Hispanic families. Co-sleeping is also common with absence of one parent from the home. Co-sleeping is not, in itself, a reason for sleep problems, although it is associated with increased risks of sudden infant death syndrome (SIDS). However, some families allow the child to sleep with the adults because of problems with enforcing bedtimes, anxiety about leaving the child alone, problems with the quality of daytime interactions, or a desire to avoid the spouse. Sexual abuse of the child also needs to be considered. In these cases, intervention may be helpful to the family (Howard & Wong, 2001). The hours of sleep, methods of helping child to initiate the sleep cycle, and expectations for normal sleep behavior are also culturally driven.

The American Academy of Pediatrics (AAP) Task Force on Sudden Infant Death Syndrome (AAP, 2005) states that bed sharing should not be considered as a strategy to reduce SIDS risk. Rather, there is some evidence that bed sharing is a SIDS risk factor. The task force recommends "a separate but proximate sleeping environment" in which the young infant sleeps in the same room but in a separate bed, crib, bassinet, or cradle. If a mother chooses to sleep with her infant, care should be taken to avoid using soft sleep surfaces. Quilts, blankets, pillows, comforters, or other similar materials should not be placed under the infant. The bed sharer should not smoke or use substances that impair arousal. Finally, parents should understand that safety standards are in place for the design of infant cribs, but there are no standards for adult beds, so entrapment might be possible. Parents who plan to co-sleep should have an "exit plan," such as ending the practice at 6 months, before the child will protest excessively (Howard & Wong, 2001).

School-age children who want to co-sleep may have significant emotional problems, such as separation anxiety, which may require counseling.

Sleep Positioning

Studies have provided strong evidence that positioning young infants on their backs significantly decreases the incidence of SIDS. The current recommendation of the AAP (2005) is to have all infants sleep in a supine position unless there is some specific medical contraindication to that position. Side sleeping is not recommended. The AAP also recommends use of a crib and avoidance of soft materials in the sleep environment, bed sharing, smoking during pregnancy and afterwards, and overheating the infant. Offering a pacifier at sleep times seems to have some effect in reducing SIDS risks.

The AAP also recommends that parents place the baby on its stomach sometimes while awake to encourage upper body motor development and to prevent positional plagiocephaly (AAP, 2005).

■ ASSESSMENT

Assessment of sleep patterns requires an understanding of the developmental progression of sleep patterns, a comprehensive history, and a physical examination. Assessment of sleep patterns should be included in all well-child visits. Before a decision is made that a sleep problem exists, the provider must be sure to determine whether the child's sleep pattern is: (a) problematic for the caregiver and/or (b) results in daytime sleepiness with disruption to the child's health and well-being. The clinician must be careful not to impose his or her ideas of the best sleep habits onto the family and remember that cultural patterns are very strong in this area of childrearing. Late bedtimes, early rising, night waking, and co-sleeping may be upsetting to some parents but not to others. Of course, preventive counseling is always in order.

HISTORY

Pediatric sleep has become a topic of interest in the recent past with much more research and attention to sleep issues in children with a variety of health problems. Several child sleep screening tools have appeared in the literature (Sadeh, 2004; Lee & Ward, 2005, Howard & Wong, 2001). Items from these three questionnaires can be used by clinicians in everyday practice to assess sleep hygiene (Box 15-1). Because sleep problems are so common and tend to persist, it is recommended that sleep be addressed at well-child visits, as a component of care of sick children where sleep is likely to be interrupted, and with all children with chronic conditions since so many have associated sleep problems. The normal

---

BOX 15-1   Sleep Screening Tool

1. Does your child attend day care or school?
   Starts at_____AM/PM, Ends at_____AM/PM
2. In the past week, has your child taken a medication, alcohol, or herbal remedy for sleep?
   If yes list name_____, frequency of use_____.
3. Rate your child's sleep quality.
   _____ Good (sleeps through the night most nights)
   _____ Poor (has problems sleeping most nights)
   _____ Very bad (has problems sleeping every night)
4. Bedtime routine and child response:
   ◆ What time does your child typically go to bed? weeknights_____, weekends_____.
   ◆ Where does child sleep?
   ◆ How difficult is it for your child to settle and fall asleep after bedtime rituals?
   _____Not difficult
   _____Somewhat of a struggle
   _____A constant struggle
   ◆ Length of time between going to bed and sleep onset?
   _____min
   ◆ Does your child fall asleep by himself or herself? yes/no
   If no what is the child's routine? (Needs body contact, bottle or pacifier, television or radio noise, or other stimuli to induce sleep)
5. What is the nap(s) routine?
   ◆ What are typical hours for naps? AM:_____, PM:_____
   ◆ Repeat other questions for bedtime routine: place, difficulties, routines.

6. How difficult is it for the child to get up in the morning?
   _____Not difficult
   _____Somewhat of a struggle (15-30 minutes some mornings)
   _____A constant struggle (more than 30 minutes every morning
7. Night waking: In the past week, how many times did your child wake up during the night?
   _____never or once,_____ 2-3 times,_____4 or more times
   What was the main reason for waking?_____thirst,_____ bladder,_____other reason (please describe)
   How much time does the child spend awake between 10 PM and 6 AM?_____hr_____min
8. In the past week, how sleepy was your child during the day?
   _____Not at all sleepy
   _____Naps or falls asleep some days
   _____Naps or falls asleep most days
   _____Falls asleep in class most days
9. Risk factors for sleep problems: Does your child have:
   _____Other behavioral or emotional problems?
   _____Health or developmental problems?
   _____Take substances that might affect sleep—medicines, caffeine drink intake, street drug use, smokes?
10. Do you consider your child's sleep to be a problem?_____yes,_____no
   _____Serious problem
   _____A small problem
   _____Not a problem at all

Data from Howard & Wong, 2001; Lee & Ward, 2005; Sadeh, 2004.

sleep pattern, the general health history, sleep habits of the parents and family, and the sleep environment are assessed for factors that may affect sleep and rest. Significant sleep problems need to be referred to sleep centers or other specialists.

Normal Sleep Pattern

1. Nighttime and daytime sleep hygiene patterns include the following:
   - Quality and quantity of sleep
   - Sleep hours, including naps and awake time when parents are also awake
   - Number and frequency of feedings (for infants less than 3 months old), day and night
   - Description of the state changes of the child, moving from wakefulness to sleep and then to waking again
   - Cues given by the infant or child to indicate need for sleep or rest
   - Daytime sleepiness indicators—napping, falling asleep in class, inattention, behavioral problems, accidental injuries in adolescents (Fallone et al, 2002)
   - Factors that might mask daytime sleepiness, such as sensory input, exercise, psychoactive substances, such as caffeine, emotional state, motivation, or competing physiologic needs, such as hunger
   - The routines used for getting the child to sleep and the child's behavior at these times, especially sleep resistance and sleep latency

2. Sleep problem history questions generally focus on normal sleep habits and then sleep onset, maintenance of sleep through the night, arousal, and daytime sleepiness issues. Factors which might affect sleep need to be identified. For each problem, the clinician needs to know:
   - Age when problem began and circumstances
   - Aggravating and relieving factors
   - Effects on daily living for child and family
   - Effects on the child's health and well-being

   Additionally the environment should be assessed for noise, light, temperature, safety, and co-sleeping pattern. Schedules that affect sleep are also assessed (e.g., shift work, school hours, night work, child care schedules). A sleep activity record (Fig. 15-2) should be completed.

General Health History

1. Indicators of the health and well-being of the child: Energy and alertness for daily activities need evaluation. The child with chronic inadequate sleep may appear to the parents to be functioning well. However, with more sleep, the parents will notice a decrease in irritability and better performance in many arenas.

2. Past medical history and review of systems: Medical problems of the child are often associated with sleep difficulties. Ear infections; medications, such as bronchodilators; neurologic problems, such as ADHD, Rett syndrome, and cerebral palsy (Newman et al, 2006);

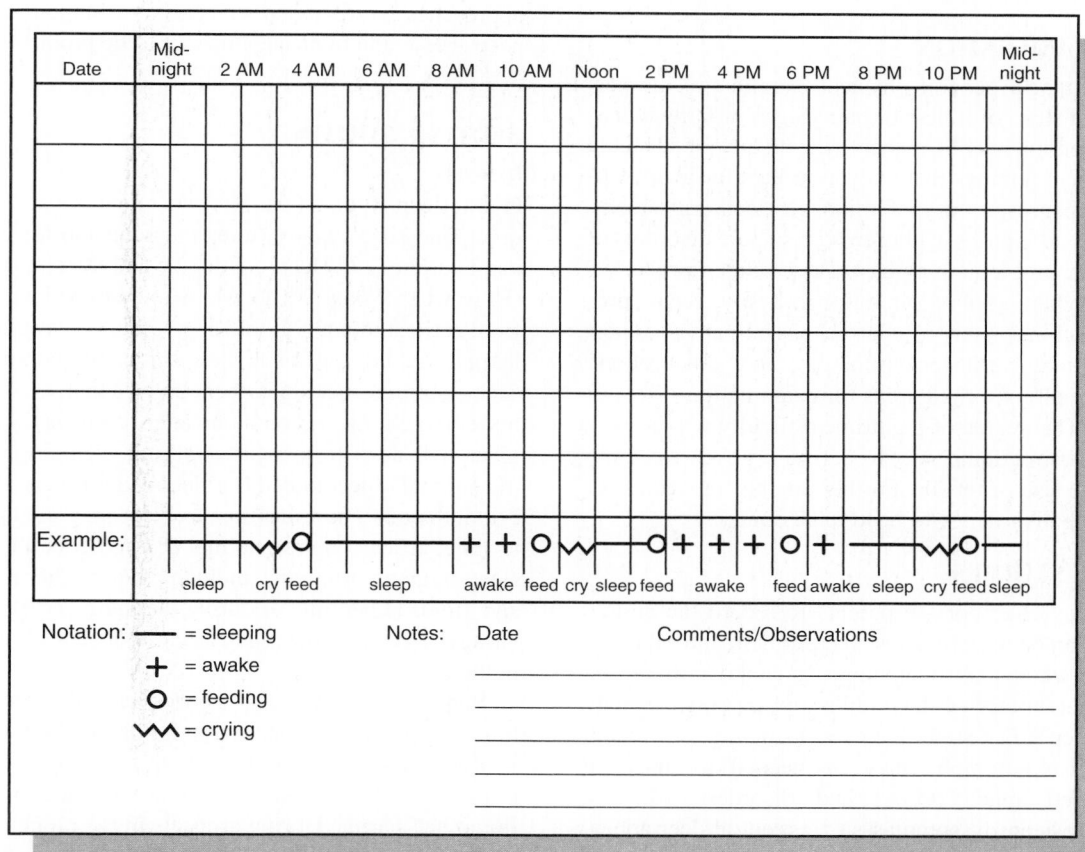

FIG. 15-2   Example of sleep–activity–feeding record.

respiratory conditions; atopic conditions; gastroesopha-geal reflux; cardiac conditions; or anything that causes pain can affect sleep. Consider all the physical factors identified earlier in this chapter.

3. Developmental problems can affect the child's ability to learn appropriate sleep behaviors.
4. Depression, anxiety, or other psychiatric problems may be significant in older children with sleep problems.
5. Psychoactive Substance/medication/tobacco use, including caffeine drinks and alcohol, can affect sleep.
6. School performance or peer relationships can contribute to disrupted sleep.

Parental and Family Assessment

1. Indicators of the health and well-being and rest of the care-giver. Maternal depression has been clearly associated with children's sleep disruptions.
2. Parental knowledge and beliefs about infant and child sleeping patterns. Parental understanding of the relationships between illness, temperament, and sleep should be explored.
3. Parental ability to modulate the child's sleep and rest state and stress in doing so.
4. Family sleep routines and expectations.
5. Recent changes in family living arrangements.
6. Divorce, separation, or other family stresses.
7. Extent of disparity of problem with family's cultural expectations.
8. Family history of sleep disorders.

PHYSICAL EXAMINATION

It is important that a general physical examination be per-formed to detect signs of illness or pain. Signs of fatigue, irri-tability, or inattention may be associated with lack of adequate rest. Other clinical findings that may contribute to sleep prob-lems include upper respiratory infection, gastroenteritis, teeth-ing, pinworms, and injuries. Children with seizure disorders or other neurologic problems may have sleep-related problems. Vital signs, oxyhemoglobin saturation, obesity, facial pro-file, mouth breathing, signs of allergies, nasal patency, chest wall configuration, cardiac examination, and a neurologic examination are all important areas for examination (Ward & Mason, 2002). The degree of nighttime difficulty with airway resistance and obstruction cannot be accurately evaluated only by assessing the size of tonsils. Further diagnostic studies for obstructive sleep disorders will need to be done.

DIAGNOSTIC STUDIES

A 24-hour, 7-day chart for the parents to record the child's sleep patterns can be used to assess the problem and establish a baseline from which to evaluate improvement over time (see Fig. 15-2). An audiotape of the child's snoring episodes may be helpful. Sleep EEG studies are occasionally warranted. Nocturnal polysomnography may be needed to diagnose obstructive sleep apnea (OSA) and disorders affecting breathing during sleep; dyssomnias, such as central sleep apnea, or central hypoventilation syndrome; narcolepsy; sleep move-ment disorders; sleep-related seizures; and gastroesophageal

reflux. Nocturnal polysomnography requires study in a sleep laboratory and is not helpful for evaluation of children with parasomnias. Actigraphy is another current methodology that measures the child's state of activity. It is helpful in understanding patterns of sleep-wake activity over time. The child wears a wrist or ankle bracelet for several days that monitors movement patterns.

■ STRATEGIES FOR PREVENTION AND MANAGEMENT OF SLEEP PROBLEMS

Prevention of sleep problems is always best. Management of sleep problems is not easy. Clinicians need to be aware of their own cultural biases and avoid assumptions about family sleep values and practices before deciding that a problem exists. If the family identifies sleep as a problem or the child's health and well-being are affected, then a sleep problem diagnosis may be made. Usual management strategies include counsel-ing parents, modifying diet, ignoring nocturnal crying, and scheduling awakenings. Deeper fears, depression, or family stresses may require counseling. Parenting tips for managing the infant's state changes are helpful, and successful parenting strategies should be supported (Table 15-2). Evidence-based information should be used, and acknowledgement of the lack of data in some areas needs to be discussed openly (Riter & Wills, 2004).

For sleep disorders, both parental and child behavioral approaches are discussed with each condition. Parental compli-ance is essential to management of sleep problems in children.

BEDTIME ROUTINES

Infants

Good sleep hygiene requires an environment that is dark, quiet, and slightly cool; a regular schedule for waking, naps, and bedtime; and sleep-conducive activities in the child's life (Howard & Wong, 2001). Many authors believe that children from earliest infancy should be put into bed awake so that they learn to put themselves to sleep with self-soothing behaviors, such as thumb sucking. Others believe that self-soothing does not emerge until 3 months or later; until that time, the care-giver will need to provide soothing. Bringing an inanimate transitional object to bed is a sleep aid for many children from 3 months on. The transitional object may change from time to time, at least among infants (Burnham et al, 2002). Other sleep hygiene principles include avoiding hunger and exces-sive fluids at bedtime or during the night and avoiding stimu-lating drugs and foods, such as caffeine, coffee, and chocolate in the evening.

Some sleep problems, such as trained night feeding and trained night crying, are learned. For instance, the child who is always rocked to sleep in mother's arms and then moved to the crib when asleep learns that the place to go to sleep is in mother's arms. During arousals in the night, the child then looks for those arms and not the sides of the crib to move into the next sleep cycle. Parent education about the development

TABLE 15-2	**Prevention of Sleep Problems: Highlights for Parental Counseling**
Newborn	
During the day	Respond to crying; hold the baby when fussy.
	Hold the baby frequently to prevent fussy episodes.
	Schedule feedings at least 2 hours apart.
During the night	Put the baby to bed while drowsy but still awake.
	Feed the baby at the parents' bedtime and then let the baby awaken for feedings and feed with little stimulation, dim lights, no play.
	Avoid bringing the baby into the parents' bed, but sleeping in the same room is recommended.
Age 2-4 months	
During the night	Move the baby to a separate bedroom unless this is not the cultural norm for the family.
	Try to delay and then discontinue middle-of-the-night feedings.
	No bottles in the crib.
	Continue to keep middle-of-the-night feedings (if they are still occurring) as nonstimulating occasions.
Age 6-12 months	
During the night	Keep soft toy animal, doll, or blanket in the crib for snuggling.
	Leave the bedroom door open and respond to any fears quickly and with reassurance.
Age 1 year and older	
During the night	Keep bedtimes friendly and predictable occasions. Establish a routine.
	Always respond to nighttime fears with reassurance and comfort.
	Allow the child to take increasing responsibility for self-management of body functions, including sleep.
	Expect the child to remain in bed during the night.
	Do not send the child to bed hungry.
	Keep the bedroom quiet, cool, and dark.
During the day	Avoid products containing caffeine for at least several hours until bedtime.
	Be sure the child has had some active play time, preferably outdoors everyday.
	Keep televisions out of the child's bedroom.
	Do not use the bedroom for timeout punishment.

of normal sleep patterns in children and sleep hygiene patterns they need to teach their children are helpful.

Children

After the neonatal period, for most infants and children, establishing a bedtime routine is probably the most important thing that parents can do. Often this routine includes "stepping-down" activities to provide cues for sleep: a bath (if this can be a quiet activity); changing into pajamas; brushing teeth; and sharing a story, song, or prayer. Getting ready for nighttime should be a pleasant time that the child looks forward to. If the child responds with a tantrum, the pleasant activities are stopped, and the child is immediately put to bed. It may be difficult for parents to maintain consistent responses.

The room temperature should be less than 75° F. Lights should be turned out, although a hall light or nightlight may be reassuring to the child. Establishing consistent wake-up and naptime routines and schedules are also useful strategies. The wake-up time is the most powerful time for setting the sleep-wake cycle. Avoidance of caffeine during the afternoon and evening is important.

Sleep Management for Difficult Children

Helping parents to understand their child's temperament can be a useful intervention. A variety of studies have associated intense or difficult temperament patterns with sleep difficulties (Riter & Wills, 2004). For example, for the child who is less adaptable or who has tendencies to withdraw from new situations, changing the sleep routine in any way may be particularly difficult. For children who are "difficult" (irregular, intense, with frequent negative moods), parents should be informed that sleep schedules and needs will be unpredictable, and reactions to parental interventions may be intensely resistant. Strategies parents have used with success in the past should be identified, and similar parenting activities adapted for managing sleep difficulties. Children with low sensory thresholds also have more problems with night waking because they are more sensitive to light, sound, temperature, and tactile stimulation (Carey, 1974). All these stimuli must be considered by parents who are trying to promote sleep onset and maintenance behaviors in their children.

Sleep and Television Viewing

In a study of more than 2000 children 4 to 35 months old, Thompson & Christakis (2005) found that 34% had irregular naptime schedules and 27% had irregular bedtime schedules. The number of hours of television watched per day was positively correlated to both the irregular nap and bedtime schedules. Another study by Johnson et al (2004) found that teens who watched 3 or more hours of television per day were at significantly higher risk for frequent sleep problems by early adulthood. Further, teens who reduced their television viewing to less than 1 hour per day experienced a significant reduction in subsequent sleep problems. Viewing television for more than a short time daily affects sleep routines and the likelihood of sleep problems across the pediatric age range.

Family Issues

Family stressors need to be recognized and dealt with. Posttraumatic stress disorder, abuse, domestic violence issues, or other psychological problems in children may also be factors requiring family and individual counseling.

Comorbidities

The outcomes of sleep problems, such as poor school performance and behavioral problems, need to be addressed as do the precursors, such as chronic pain. As many as 50% to 60% of children with ADHD have been reported to have sleep problems. Sleep-disordered breathing; restless legs syndrome (RLS); medication effects; and comorbid psychiatric conditions, such as depression and anxiety, may all be associated with difficulties falling asleep. Targeted positive reinforcement, good sleep hygiene, and other behavioral interventions may help (Meltzer & Mindell, 2004).

Medications

Medications are not generally recommended for childhood sleep problems. The recent *Pharmacologic Management of Insomnia in Children and Adolescents: Consensus Statement* (Mindell et al, 2006) specifically notes that the treatment of pediatric insomnia is an unmet medical need. However, "before appropriate pharmacologic management guidelines can be developed, rigorous, large-scale clinical trials of pediatric insomnia treatment are vitally needed to provide information to the clinician on the safety and efficacy of prescription and over-the-counter agents for the management of pediatric insomnia" (p. e2). Hypnotic drugs, such as benzodiazepines, are discouraged because of the problems with dependence and because they are used for their sedative adverse effects rather than for primary effects on sleep-wake cycles or hyperarousal. Antihistamines have not been studied for effectiveness when used for long periods. Tricyclic drugs are sometimes used, especially for arousal disorders where other treatments are inadequate. Clonidine, antidepressants, mood stabilizers, and antihistamines are being used for children with ADHD but without data related to efficacy or safety (Mindell et al, 2006).

Ineffective management strategies include use of diphenhydramine medication, which will provide moderate improvement, but the sleep problems can be expected to return when medication is stopped.

■ COMMON SLEEP PROBLEMS

The line between normal and problematic sleep may be somewhat fuzzy. The clinician needs to determine that the child's sleep patterns are problematic for the caregivers and family or are resulting in problems for the child's health and well-being. The *International Classification of Sleep Disorders, Revised (ICSD-R)* (American Academy of Sleep Medicine, 2001) is more complex than the system used in this chapter and refers to both adult and child sleep problems. It classifies sleep problems as *dyssomnias,* or problems of insufficient, excessive, or inefficient sleep; *parasomnias,* or problems that intrude on the sleep state; and medical or psychiatric sleep disorders. This section discusses the problems summarized in Table 15-3.

DYSSOMNIAS

Dyssomnias are disorders of sleep related to the process of going to sleep, putting oneself back to sleep from an arousal, and sleeping on a regular basis at a reasonable time. Causes may be intrinsic, such as narcolepsy, obstructive sleep apnea, restless legs syndrome, or extrinsic, such as adjustment to a new environment (Glaze, 2004).

Sleep-Onset Association Disorder (Night Waking)

Description. The child is unable to enter the sleep cycle easily unless a particular routine is carried out. For the infant, the problem results in frequent night waking and crying, most often between midnight and 5 AM.

Epidemiology. This is most commonly a learned behavior, often seen in infants who fall asleep while being rocked or fed and who are then put in their beds. For the child older than 6 months who feeds at night, night feeding in volume, frequent daytime feedings (grazing), feeding until asleep, and leaving a bottle in the bed are all causes of this sleep disturbance.

Sleep-onset association problems are common. The frequency of night waking in a variety of studies was found to be 20% to 25% of children 1 to 5 years old and was more common in infants. Ward and Mason (2002) cite studies indicating that 95% of infants cry after a nighttime awakening and require parental help to return to sleep. This number falls to 30% to 40% by the time the child is 1 year old.

Clinical Findings. The history reveals a baby or child who has frequent night awakenings. When the parent goes to the child and repeats a particular intervention, the child falls asleep promptly. The history needs to assess why the child has difficulty falling asleep or awakens during the night, in addition to the parental response and bedtime routine. With this disturbance, middle-of-the-night feedings occur in a child older than 4 months.

Differential Diagnoses. The differential diagnoses for sleep-onset association problems are pain or a medical condition affecting sleep, fear in an older child, and inappropriate expectations related to the amount of sleep the child needs. Day-night reversal and gastroesophageal reflux are other possible causes to be addressed. OSA, nightmares, RLS, and mood disorders can all cause night waking (Howard & Wong, 2001).

Management. The infant or child must learn to independently transition from the arousal phase into the next sleep cycle throughout the night. The parent must learn to change the responses given during the night. Two strategies have been recommended in the literature:

TABLE 15-3   Summary of Common Pediatric Sleep Problems and Interventions

Sleep Problem	Clinical Findings	Differential	Intervention
Dyssomnias			
Night waking	Needs help during the night to enter the next sleep cycle	Medical problem, pain, hunger, trained night feeder Depression	Always put the child to bed while still awake; keep day and nighttime cues very clear; do not reinforce calling out or crying behavior; try scheduled wakening technique
Sleep refusals	Toddler or preschooler refuses to settle down when put to bed	Fears, separation anxiety, sleep needs less than parents' expectations Temperament irregular or low sensory threshold Emotional stress	Maintain consistent sleep routine and expectations; use transitional objects
Trained night feeder	Infant awakens predictably to be fed after 4 months old	Night wakening, pain or medical problem, feeding needs	Move the child onto a 3-4 hour feeding schedule in the day; at first feed the infant only once after the parents' bedtime; then either eliminate the feeding or progressively decrease the volume of that feeding
Delayed sleep phase	Child goes to bed late and awakens late	Sleep refusal Depression	Have the child awaken progressively 15 minutes earlier until appropriate bedtimes and waking times result
Advanced sleep phase	Child goes to bed early and awakens early		Progressively have child stay up later; awakening will occur later
Unpredictable schedule	Child goes to bed and awakens at random times	Family on erratic schedule; inconsistent parent expectations; excessive naps	Keep predictable eating, activity, and sleeping schedules for the family; maintain consistent expectation for bedtime and awakening but allow child to stay awake in bed if not disruptive to others
Parasomnias			
Nightmares	Child awakens in fear, crying, has memory of event; is interactive while upset; occurs in latter half of the night; slow return to sleep	Night terrors; seizures; stress if nightmares occur frequently	Soothe and reassure the child; a nightlight or flashlight child can use may help if afraid of the dark
Night terrors and sleepwalking (variant)	Child awakens screaming, crying, but is not interactive with the parent at the time; has no memory of the event; occurs in the first third of night; rapid return to sleep; sleepwalking is variant	Nightmares; seizures; physical exhaustion	Protect the child from injury if he or she is thrashing about or walking; help the child to lie down to return to sleep; protect child from stairways and other unsafe places sleepwalker might go
Medical/psychiatric problems			
Depression	Insomnia or hypersomnia or both with other symptoms of depression	Other psychiatric disorder; dyssomnia or parasomnia disorder	Manage the psychiatric condition first
OSA	Snoring with apneic periods against increased respiratory efforts, restless sleep, daytime sleepiness, fatigue	Central apnea, benign snoring, seizure disorder	Refer to sleep studies and then to ENT for possible adenotonsillectomy if OSA is diagnosed

OSA, Obstructive sleep apnea; *ENT,* ear, nose, and throat.

1. Extinction and graduated extinction. Put the child down to sleep at night while he or she is awake. When the child awakens and cries in the night, the parent should go to him or her briefly to give comfort and reassurance but not to hold, rock, or feed. The parent's response must be supportive and comforting but should not reinforce a return to old patterns of infant behavior or parental response. This technique is termed *extinction*. Going "cold turkey" (not going to the child at all from the very beginning) is difficult for parents to do, although children learn to return to sleep alone within a few nights, crying for shorter periods each time. Results should be seen in 3 to 5 days and will be maintained over time for extinction. With extinction, a mild increase in problem behaviors may recur 15 to 30 days after treatment begins. Parents must maintain the extinction behaviors at this time (Meltzer & Mindell, 2004).

   Waiting for progressively longer intervals before going to the child over several nights may work if the parents can maintain compliance (graduated extinction). Parents' behaviors, such as the amount of touch, the proximity to the child, the duration of time between and the duration of the check in are faded (Meltzer & Mindell, 2004). Graduated extinction results will be evident in a few days to a few months.

2. Scheduled awakenings. Alternatively, use a planned or scheduled awakening approach. The first night, the parent should go to the child 15 minutes before night awakening is expected. The child is awakened, rocked for a few minutes, and then left again. When spontaneous awakenings stop, scheduled awakenings are gradually delayed 15 to 30 minutes more each night. If the child then awakens spontaneously, he or she learns to wait for the parents to come, knowing it will happen, and gradually learns to return to sleep (Meltzer & Mindell, 2004). Difficulties with this method include the requirement that parents waken their child once or several times during the night. Also it can take several weeks for effects to be seen. The awakenings do not address bedtime resistance or independent sleep initiation (Meltzer & Mindell, 2004).

   It may be easier to work on development of self-sleep during naps first and then transfer this behavior to nighttime. Most infants use sleep aids, such as a blanket or stuffed animal, to assist with self-soothing (Burnham et al, 2002).

   Complications.   Night feedings should not be withheld from children who are not thriving for other reasons and who need the nutrition of another night time feeding.

Sleep Refusal (Behavioral Insomnia)

   Description.   In toddlers and preschoolers, the problem is one of difficulty with bedtime settling. A child needs to learn to sleep alone and put himself or herself to sleep. The child may experience an inability to make the transition from daytime activities to nighttime sleeping.

   Epidemiology.   A variety of studies report that approximately 20% of children between 15 and 48 months old engage in bedtime resistance. Bedtime resistance was identified in 25% of patients 2 to 13 years old, with 29% of preschoolers experiencing the problem (Archbold et al, 2002). Separation anxiety is a problem for some, as are nighttime fears.

   Clinical Findings.   The child makes repeated attempts to obtain parental attention (e.g., demanding snacks, asking for a drink, requesting another story, leaving bed to return to family activities, watching activities from afar).

   Differential Diagnoses

   Infant: Sleep association problem, hunger, circadian rhythm disorder

   Preschooler: Sleep association problem, circadian rhythm disorder, limit setting, bedtime fears

   School age and adolescent: Sleep association problem (TV or radio on); circadian rhythm disorder; anxiety at bedtime related to daytime stresses, exposure to violence, chaotic household, family stresses, sexual or physical abuse (Howard & Wong, 2001).

   Management.   For the toddler or preschooler who exhibits sleep refusal, try the following regimen:

1. Use a sleep log to chart the child's pattern initially. It can then be used to mark progress toward the goal.
2. Maintain the bedtime routine and use transitional objects and a quiet environment for sleep. The routine should not be longer than 30 minutes (Mindell, 2006).
3. Positive routines may be helpful for children having difficulty falling asleep at bedtime. The parents develop a set of bedtime routines that the child enjoys. Four to seven activities are included. If a tantrum occurs, the routine is terminated, and the child is told that it is time for bed (Meltzer & Mindell, 2004).
4. Set limits on the child's demands for attention. The parent should leave the room at the end of the bedtime routine, expecting good behavior. If the child arises, return the child to bed, saying, "It is time for bed," each time the child gets up. Tantrums of up to 45 minutes may occur the first night and perhaps longer the second but then should decrease on succeeding nights (Meltzer & Mindell, 2004).
5. Be sure that the child is not being expected to sleep earlier or for longer periods than expected for his or her age.

   For children older than 3 years, positive rewards, such as sticker charts, may help. Payoffs need to occur frequently.

   Stresses and fears must be addressed. If the child has bedtime fears, leaving may increase the problem. In these cases, the parent may sit quietly in the room until the child falls asleep. When the child can fall asleep easily this way, the parent should move to the bedroom door and eventually out of sight. The child needs to understand that the parent will only remain in the room if there are no tantrums and the child stays in bed.

Insomnia and Hypersomnia and Comorbid conditions in Adolescents

Adolescents may have problems with difficulty falling asleep, sleeping less than usual, sleep quality, waking up with difficulty, sleeping more than usual, napping during the day, and trouble waking up. These conditions are considered significant if they persist more than 2 weeks.

For adolescents with diagnosed depression, 53% had insomnia, 9% had hypersomnia, and 10% had both. Those with more severe depression had more reported sleep difficulties. Sleep problems should be considered a marker of more significant depression. Some of the associated mental health symptoms may include greater depressed mood, irritability, sadness, psychomotor agitation, fatigue, anhedonia, inappropriate guilt, weight loss, diurnal variation, and anxiety disorders (Liu, 2007).

SLEEP-CYCLE PROBLEMS (CIRCADIAN RHYTHM DISORDERS)

Delayed Sleep Phase

Description. The sleep cycle begins at a late hour and is followed by a late awakening. This is commonly an adolescent problem.

Etiology. The child's internal clock for sleep and rest is not consistent with appropriate hours for sleep. Excessive naps or late morning waking may be related factors, especially for school-age children and adolescents.

Differential Diagnoses. The diagnoses are prolonged bedtime routine and oppositional disorder, which both involve active resistance to going to bed rather than inability to fall asleep.

Management. Three approaches are suggested:
1. Keep the nighttime routine in place but awaken the child earlier each morning in 15-minute increments.
2. For the adolescent or older child who is off schedule by many hours (e.g., at the end of summer, when beginning the school year will require getting up earlier), it could take weeks to back up the cycle appropriately using 15-minute increments. In this case, it is better to go forward in time. In other words, have the child remain awake until the next evening and then go to bed at the desired hour, beginning the desired routine from that point.
3. Have the child or family keep a sleep log to document gradual change (Howard & Wong, 2001).

Advanced Sleep Phase

Description. The sleep cycle begins too early with correlated early rising.

Management. Meals, naps, and bedtime should be delayed until the desired times. The early waking resolves itself.

Inappropriate or Unpredictable Schedules

Description. Some people have a poorly organized sleep-wake cycle. This is described by some as a temperament problem of rhythmicity.

Management. The routines of eating, activities, and sleeping should be kept as regular as possible. The older child may need to learn to play quietly in bed until others awaken or until a clock radio begins to play. At night the child may need to learn to read or listen to music in bed when bedtime comes.

PARASOMNIAS: NIGHT TERRORS, SLEEPWALKING, AND NIGHTMARES

In parasomnias, behaviors intrude upon ongoing sleep rather than representing disruptions of the sleep process, such as going to sleep, waking in the night, or sleeping on an inappropriate schedule. Parasomnias are divided into arousal disorders, sleep-wake transition disorders, REM parasomnias, and miscellaneous. The arousal disorders include sleep terrors and sleepwalking. A nightmare is a REM parasomnia, and enuresis and bruxism are miscellaneous parasomnias. Parasomnias usually do not result in excessive daytime sleepiness or insomnia but are disruptive to a sleeping household.

Positive family histories are common. In general they are more common in males, and children with one type of parasomnia are more likely to exhibit symptoms of another at some point. A study by Guilleminault and colleagues (2003) sampled 84 children, 2 to 11 years old, with parasomnias and found that 51 (61%) had an additional sleep disorder; 49 (96%) of these were sleep-disordered breathing diagnoses, and two were RLS. When the associated problem was managed, the parasomnias disappeared.

Arousal Disorders

Night Terrors or Sleep Terrors

Description. Night terrors are defined as a partial awakening during the transition from non-REM sleep stage III or IV in which the child is not fully conscious and aware of surroundings. Confusional arousals are similar to night terrors although the child does not express fear, terror, or panic. Rather the child has marked mental confusion (Ward & Mason, 2002).

Epidemiology. These disorders are related to the transition from the stage IV non-REM sleep to the REM sleep cycle and are not psychological or developmental problems. Excessive fatigue or unusual daytime stresses may precipitate attacks in some children, but they are not considered mental health problems. A full bladder, fever, pain, and environmental factors, such as noise, are also considered trigger factors. Family history is often positive. Night terrors are most common in 3- to 6-year-olds, although they occur in children from 18 months to adolescence. Incidence has been reported at 3% of children, mostly from 18 months to 6 years.

Clinical Findings. Episodes occur 60 to 90 minutes after onset of sleep and may last from less than a minute to 5 minutes or more. The child usually sits up screaming but cannot be reasoned with or consoled. Indeed, the child does not even seem to hear the caregiver. The child can have pallor, pupil dilation, piloerection, tachycardia, and sweating, all symptoms of an autonomic discharge (Sheldon, 2004). The child may speak incoherently and may thrash about. The child is not awake or aware of the surroundings and does not remember the episode in the morning. It is the caregiver who is disturbed, not the child. Episodes may occur in bouts of up to twenty per night for a few weeks and then disappear, with possible later recurrences.

Differential Diagnosis. The differential diagnosis is nightmares or seizures with stiffening, jerking, or drooling. Consider sleep-disordered breathing as a secondary sleep disorder.

Management. Reassurance that the child is mentally and developmentally normal should be provided. Interventions should focus on preventing injury and guiding the child back to bed. Emptying the bladder at bedtime should be routine. Waking the child 30 minutes before the expected episode each night for about a week may interrupt the pattern. The child should be protected from injury, and baby sitters should be prepared for these episodes. An afternoon nap may change the sleep stages at night (Howard & Wong, 2001).

If sleep-disordered breathing is identified through polysomnography, referral to an otolaryngologist for consideration of tonsillectomy with or without adenoidectomy and/or turbinate treatment is indicated. 100% of children with parasomnias and sleep-disordered breathing treated surgically were cured of their parasomnia postoperatively (Guilleminault et al, 2003) in a well-designed and monitored study.

For severe cases (frequent or with safety problems), benzodiazepines are the most commonly prescribed medication. Clonazepam, lorazepam, or diazepam can be effective in small doses. However, prolonged use can result in significant side effects (Sheldon, 2004).

Sleepwalking (Somnambulism)

Description. Sleepwalking is a variation of night terrors in which the manifestation is walking rather than sitting up and screaming. It occurs with arousal from stage IV sleep, usually 1 to 2 hours into sleep. Episodes usually last less than 15 minutes and vary in frequency.

Epidemiology. The cause is the same as that for night terrors; it is an arousal disorder in stage IV. It can be triggered by excessive fatigue, changes in routines, or daily stress. Consider sleep-disordered breathing as a second sleep disorder (see night terrors above). Family history is often positive. Sleepwalking is more common in boys and tends to be outgrown. It occurs in 15% of children at one time or another. It is most common in children between 4 and 6 years old.

Clinical Findings. The child arises and walks about without being fully alert and responsive. The child may fall or bump into things, wander in illogical places, or urinate outside the toilet. He or she does not remember the incident in the morning.

Differential Diagnosis. The differential diagnoses are dissociative state and seizure.

Management. The child needs to be led back quietly to bed. A gate may need to be placed across the bedroom door if the sleepwalking becomes frequent. Doors may need to be secured to ensure that the child does not wander into unsafe areas. Stairways are particularly dangerous to the sleepwalking child (Howard & Wong, 2001). An afternoon nap may also be helpful in altering the stage IV pattern.

As with sleep terrors, consider tonsillectomy for children with associated documented sleep-disordered breathing.

Nightmares, Monsters, and Other Nighttime Fears

Description. A nightmare is classified as a REM parasomnia disorder. Nightmares occur as the child awakens from REM sleep, remembering dreams that are disturbing. Occasional nightmares are normal and benign. The child is awake, frightened, and able to describe the fears.

Differential Diagnosis. The differential diagnosis for nightmares is night terrors, in which the child is not fully conscious. The significance and severity of other nighttime fears need to be assessed. Separation anxiety in toddlers, domestic violence, or a scary event may make nighttime frightening. They are rare before 3 years old. Certain drugs, such as L-dopa and beta-adrenergic blockers, may trigger nightmares (Ward & Mason, 2002).

Management. Parents should give comfort, reassurance, and a sense of security and not dismiss the fear as imaginary. The child may need to have the parent lie down with him or her for a period of time, or the child may even get into bed with the parent. However, this should not become habitual. Monsters may be kept away by keeping on a nightlight, by using a flashlight, or pantomiming actions to "sweep them away," or by keeping the bedroom door open. Behavioral strategies or counseling may be required if nighttime fears are frequent or the degree of fear is exceptionally severe or associated with daytime behavioral or performance problems (Sheldon, 2004).

Restless Legs Syndrome (RLS) and Periodic Limb Movements (PLMs)

Description. RLS has long been identified as a parasomnia in adults. It has recently been identified in multiple studies of children (Maheswaran & Kushida, 2006).

RLS is a sensory and motor disorder characterized by an uncontrollable sensation in the legs accompanied by an irresistible urge to move the legs, usually with immediate resolution of the noxious sensations. The syndrome is clinical and difficult for children to describe and thus has been considered to be underdiagnosed (Maheswaran & Kushida, 2006). Children with RLS have been shown to frequently have aggression, inattention, hyperactivity, and daytime sleepiness caused by an inability to sleep or difficulty maintaining sleep (Chervin et al, 2002b). The following criteria must be met for diagnosis:

1. An urge to move the legs, usually accompanied by unpleasant sensations in the legs that:
   - Begin or worsen with rest or inactivity, such as lying or sitting
   - Are worse or only occur at night
   - Are partially or totally relieved by movement, such as walking or stretching, at least as long as the activity continues
2. If the child cannot describe the sensations discussed above, the child should meet at least two of the following criteria:
   - Sleep disturbance not typical for age
   - Biologic parent or sibling with documented RLS

PLMs are repetitive jerks, typically of the legs, that are found by polysomnography to occur every 5 to 90 seconds. They occur most often during stages I and II of non-REM sleep. RLS and PLMs usually occur together, but PLMs may occur without RLS.

Epidemiology. Central dopaminergic systems are involved since dopaminergic medications improve symptoms.

There is an inherited tendency. Iron deficiency is a common cause of secondary RLS. Peripheral neuropathy and uremia are also causes of secondary RLS. Medications, such as antidepressants, SSRIs, sedating antihistamines, and dopamine receptor antagonists may worsen or precipitate cases. One study showed a prevalence of almost 6% in children younger than 18 years. PLMs are related to RLS.

Differential Diagnoses.   Other differential diagnoses include pain for an identifiable physiologic reason, sleep-disordered breathing, such as OSA, growing pains, muscle tics, ADHD, muscle pain, leg cramps, Osgood-Schlatter disease, chondromalacia patellae, and arthralgias (Maheswaran & Kushida, 2006).

Management.   No medications have been approved for children with RLS. Clonidine and clonazepam have been used, but it is recommended that these be managed by a sleep specialist because clonazepam may exacerbate problems of children with sleep-disordered breathing (including respiratory collapse). Dopaminergeric agents and benzodiazepines have been used (Ward & Mason, 2002). Reducing conditions that worsen the RLS should be tried, including management of iron deficiency, good sleep hygiene practices, and limiting medications that make it worse.

Head Banging and Bruxism

Sleep-wake transition disorders include sleep talking, nocturnal leg cramps, and rhythmic movement disorders, such as head banging and body rocking, which usually occur with sleep onset. Rhythmic sleep disorders are common and reported in two thirds of normal children, with a male-to-female ratio of 4:1 (Sheldon, 2004). Bruxism is seen in 8.2% of the population (Wills & Garcia, 2002). Most of these disorders disappear by 5 years old. No interventions are considered necessary aside from ensuring the child's safety.

Sleep bruxism is stereotypic grinding or clenching of the teeth during sleep. There may be some relationship to stress. It frequently appears between 10 and 20 years old, although there is a short-lived infant version. Seizure disorder would be a differential diagnosis. A dental referral may be useful.

SLEEP-DISORDERED BREATHING AND OBSTRUCTIVE SLEEP APNEA (OSA)

Description

OSA syndrome is a serious problem for some infants and children because it is an indicator of severe airway obstruction. It is "a disorder of breathing during sleep characterized by prolonged partial upper airway obstruction and/or intermittent complete obstruction (obstructive apnea) that disrupts normal ventilation during sleep and normal sleep patterns" (American Thoracic Society, 1996). Sleep-disordered breathing is considered to be a continuum of problems ranging from partial obstruction of the airway (snoring) to increased upper airway resistance syndrome to continuous episodes of complete upper airway resistance (Goldstein et al, 2004). The conditions without obstructive apnea, frequent arousals from sleep, or gas exchange abnormalities are not of concern.

Etiology

Collapse of the pharyngeal airway with increased airway resistance above the collapsing segment causes sleep apnea. The child makes repeated vigorous attempts to breathe. Snoring is associated with these efforts, but will not be heard if obstruction is complete. Arousal may occur, and with it upper airway muscle tone improves. The cycle may repeat many times during the night. The condition may also be partial, called *obstructive hypoventilation*. Other causal factors may include the following:

- Large adenoids or tonsils or both
- Nasal deformities
- Abnormally small oropharyngeal structures as in Pierre Robin syndrome
- Craniofacial structural problems, such as midface hypoplasia
- Factors affecting neural control, such as generalized hypotonia, central nervous system injury, and brainstem dysfunction, which includes cerebral palsy and muscular dystrophy (these conditions relate to incoordination of upper airway muscles)
- Idiopathic or genetic cause—Prader-Willi syndrome, sickle cell disease, mucopolysaccharidosis, Down syndrome
- Obesity

Epidemiology

Prevalence estimates vary from 0.7% to 3% for sleep apnea in children (Rosen, 2004). Sleep-disordered breathing among adolescents has been estimated at 20% with snoring at least a few nights per month, 6% with snoring every or nearly every night, and 2.5% to 6% of adolescents with apnea-like symptoms. Rates are higher among African Americans and those with a higher body mass index (Johnson & Roth, 2006).

Clinical Findings

History.   Sleep screening should be a part of all routine health care visits (AAP, 2002). The following signs and symptoms are associated with OSA:

- Disrupted sleep patterns (timing, restlessness, positions, diaphoresis, behavior while asleep)
- Snoring (pitch, periods of silence, intensity, onset, frequency, duration)
- Observed increased breathing effort (rib cage retraction, paradoxic chest wall movement) or apnea
- Decreased alertness and functioning when awake
- Associated conditions (e.g., craniofacial syndromes, tonsillar hypertrophy, atopy)
- Impaired growth and development
- Factors indicating high-risk patient: infant, patient with craniofacial disorder, Down syndrome, cerebral palsy, neuromuscular disorder, chronic lung disease, sickle cell disease, central hypoventilation syndromes, or genetic-metabolic storage disease.

Physical Examination.   The physical examination should include the following:

- Vital signs, including evaluation for hypertension
- Height and weight for failure to thrive or obesity
- Complete ear, nose, and throat examination, including tonsils and adenoids, midfacial hypoplasia, retrognathia or

micrognathia, patency of nasal passages, tongue size, signs of cleft palate

- Cardiac functioning for evidence of cor pulmonale, to include increased pulmonic component of the second heart sound indicating pulmonary hypertension
- Observation for digital clubbing, pectus excavatum
- Muscle tone

Laboratory Evaluation. Tape-recording the apneic episodes may be helpful in assessing the problem. The child needs to be referred for a variety of sleep studies, in addition to electrocardiogram and echocardiogram if the problem is severe. Nocturnal pulse oximetry, videotaping, and daytime nap polysomnography are useful if the results are positive, but they do not rule out OSA syndrome if negative. Nocturnal polysomnography is the gold standard diagnostic technique and should be used initially or if the pulse oximetry, videotaping, and daytime nap polysomnography results are negative. Radiographs of the head and neck are usually not helpful. (AAP, 2002).

Differential Diagnosis. The differential diagnoses are seizure disorder and central apnea, which are characterized by no airflow and no respiratory effort. Central apnea is a brainstem problem that is more commonly seen in premature or newborn infants. Primary snoring (without obstruction) also needs to be considered.

Management. The child should be referred for sleep studies and possible adenotonsillectomy (the first-line treatment) or other surgical strategies. Tonsillectomy with or without adenoidectomy is considered to be 85% to 90% effective. (Goldstein et al, 2004). Nasal continuous positive airway pressure (CPAP) has also been used. Drugs are ineffective. Avoidance of indoor pollutants may be helpful. Weight loss may help if the child is overweight. Oxygen therapy does not prevent the problems of the condition and may worsen hypoventilation. Patients undergoing surgical intervention should be reevaluated as recommended by the sleep clinic. High-risk children need to be referred to a pediatric specialist because they are at increased surgical risk and require more complex management (AAP, 2002).

Complications. Cardiac problems, including cor pulmonale resulting from hypoxic episodes, right ventricular hypertrophy, pulmonary hypertension, heart failure, systemic hypertension, and polycythemia can occur (AAP, 2002). Neurologic problems, including failure to thrive, developmental delay, learning problems, hyperactivity, excessive daytime sleepiness, and morning headache, have been reported. However, some studies have not been well controlled, including snoring children without objective evaluation, control groups, or sleep studies to distinguish those with apnea from those without sleep-disordered breathing (AAP, 2002; Chervin et al, 2002a).

ℛESOURCE BOX

Resources for Sleep Disorders

National Sleep Foundation
www.sleepfoundation.org

☑ DISCUSSION FORUM

1. How are the causes and presentations of dyssomnias and parasomnias similar? How are they different?
2. How might a primary care provider's personal beliefs and values about childhood sleep hygiene and patterns impact the clinician's ability to assess and treat sleep disturbances? What strategies might the clinician use to overcome the impact of those biases?
3. The mother of a healthy 6-month-old has a complaint that her son is awakening two or three times each night. What are the likely causes of his night awakening, and what advice would you give her? How would your advice change if he were 3 years old? What if he were 9 years old?
4. Develop a nursing intervention for a family with a child that has nightmares and night terrors once or twice a week. Make sure you consider cultural, physiologic, and psychological interventions.

𝒩URSING DIAGNOSES

Related to Sleep and Rest Functional Health Pattern

- Disturbed sleep pattern
- Sleep deprivation
- Fatigue
- Readiness for enhanced sleep
- Risk for sudden infant death syndrome (SIDS)

From NANDA International: *NANDA-I nursing diagnoses: definitions & classification, 2007-2008,* Philadelphia, 2007, Author.

REFERENCES

American Academy of Pediatrics (AAP) Section on Pediatric Pulmonology, Subcommittee on Obstructive Sleep Apnea Syndrome: Clinical practice guideline: diagnosis and management of childhood obstructive sleep apnea, *Pediatrics* 109:704-712, 2002.

American Academy of Pediatrics (AAP) Task Force on Infant Position and Sudden Infant Death Syndrome: Changing concepts of sudden infant death syndrome: implications for infant sleeping environment and sleep position (RE9946), *Pediatrics* 105:650-656, 2000.

American Academy of Pediatrics (AAP) Task Force on Sudden Infant Death Syndrome: The changing concept of sudden infant death syndrome: diagnostic coding shifts, controversies regarding the sleeping environment, and new variables to consider in reducing risk, *Pediatrics* 116:1245-1255, 2005.

American Academy of Sleep Medicine: *International classification of sleep disorders, revised: diagnostic and coding manual (ICSD-R),* Westchester, IL, 2001, The Academies.

American Thoracic Society: Standards and indications for cardiopulmonary sleep studies in children, *Am J Respir Crit Care Med* 153:866-878, 1996.

Anders T: Night waking in infants during the first year of life, *Pediatrics* 63:860-4, 1979.

Archbold K et al: Symptoms of sleep disturbances among children at two general pediatric clinics, *J Pediatr* 140:97-102, 2002.

Burnham M et al: Use of sleep aids during the first year of life, *Pediatrics* 109:594-601, 2002.

Carey W: Night waking and temperament in infancy, *J Pediatr* 84:756-758, 1974.

Carskadon MA, Acebo C, Jenni OG: Regulation of adolescent sleep: implications for behavior, *Ann NY Acad Sci* 1021:276-291, 2004.

Chervin R et al: Inattention, hyperactivity, and symptoms of sleep-disordered breathing, *Pediatrics* 109:449-456, 2002a.

Chervin R et al: Associations between symptoms of inattention, hyperactivity, restless legs, and periodic leg movements, *Sleep* 25:213-218, 2002b.

Davis K, Parker K, Montgomery G: Sleep in infants and young children: part 1: normal sleep, *J Pediatr Health Care* 18:65-71, 2004.

DiLeo H, Reiter R, Taliaferro D: Chronobiology, melatonin, and sleep in infants and children, *Pediatr Nurs* 28:35-39, 2002.

Fallone G, Owens J, Deane J: Sleepiness in children and adolescents: clinical implications, *Sleep Med Rev* 6:287-306, 2002.

Given D: The sleepy child, *Pediatr Clin N Am* 51:15-31, 2004.

Glaze D: Childhood insomnia: why Chris can't sleep, *Pediatr Clin N Am* 51:33-50, 2004.

Goldstein N et al: Clinical assessment of pediatric obstructive sleep apnea, *Pediatrics* 114:33-43, 2004.

Guilleminault C, Palombini L, Pelayo R: Sleepwalking and sleep terrors in prepubertal children: what triggers them? *Pediatrics* 111:e17-25, 2003.

Howard B, Wong J: Sleep disorders, *Pediatr Rev* 22:327-341, 2001.

Iglowstein I et al: Sleep duration from infancy to adolescence: reference values and generational trends, *Pediatrics* 111:302-307, 2003.

Jenni O, O'Connor B: Children's sleep: an interplay between culture and biology, *Pediatrics* 115:204-216, 2005.

Johnson EO, Roth T: An epidemiological study of sleep-disordered breathing symptoms among adolescents, *Sleep* 29(9):1135-1142, 2006.

Johnson JG, Cohen P, Kasen S: Association between television viewing and sleep problems during adolescence and early adulthood, *Arch Pediatr Adolesc Med* 158:597-598, 2004.

Lee K, Ward T: Critical components of a sleep assessment for clinical practice settings, *Issues Ment Health Nurs* 26:739-750, 2005.

Liu X et al: Sleep patterns and sleep problems among schoolchildren in the United States and China, *Pediatrics* 115:241-249, 2005.

Liu X et al: Insomnia and hypersomnia associated with depressive phenomenology and comorbidity in childhood depression, *Sleep* 30:83-90, 2007.

Liu X, Buysse D: Sleep and youth suicidal behavior: a neglected field, *Curr Opin Psychiatry* 19:288-293, 2006.

Maheswaran M, Kushida C: Restless legs syndrome in children, *Medscape Gen Med* 8:79, 2006.

McKenna J, Mosko S, Richard C: Bed-sharing promotes breastfeeding, *Pediatrics* 100:214-219, 1997.

Meltzer L, Mindell J: Nonpharmacologic treatments for pediatric sleeplessness, *Pediatr Clin N Am* 51:135-151, 2004.

Mindell J et al: Pharmacologic management of insomnia in children and adolescents: consensus statement, *Pediatrics* 117:e1223-1232, 2006.

Newman CJ, O'Regan M, Hensey O: Sleep disorders in children with cerebral palsy, *Dev Med Child Neurol* 48:564-568, 2006.

Ohayon MM, Carskadon M, Guilleminault C: Meta-analysis of quantitative sleep parameters from childhood to old age in healthy individuals: developing normative sleep values across the human lifespan, *Sleep* 27:1255-73, 2004.

Owens J: Sleep disorders. In Behrman R, Kliegman R, Jenson H, editors: *Nelson textbook of pediatrics,* ed 17, Philadelphia, 2004, WB Saunders, pp. 75-80.

Owens JA, Spirito A, McGuinn M: Sleep habits and sleep disturbance in elementary school-aged children, *J Dev Behav Pediatr* 21:27-36, 2000.

Ramchandani P et al: A systematic review of treatments for settling problems and night waking in young children, *BMJ* 320:209-213, 2000.

Riter S, Wills L: Sleep wars: research and opinion, *Pediatr Clin N Am* 51:1-13, 2004.

Rosen C: Obstructive sleep apnea syndrome in children: controversies in diagnosis and treatment, *Pediatr Clin N Am* 51:153-167, 2004.

Sadeh A: A brief screening questionnaire for infant sleep problems: validation and findings for an internet sample, *Pediatrics* 113:e570-e577, 2004.

Sheldon SH: Parasomnias in childhood, *Pediatr Clin N Am* 51:69-88, 2004.

Stein M et al: Sleep and behavior problems in school-aged children, *Pediatrics* 107:e60, 2001.

Thompson DA, Christakis DA: The association between television viewing and irregular sleep schedules among children less than 3 years of age, *Pediatrics* 116:851-856, 2005.

Touchette E et al: Factors associated with fragmented sleep at night across early childhood, *Arch Pediatr Adolesc Med* 159:242-9, 2005.

Ward T, Mason T: Sleep disorders in children, *Nurs Clin N Am* 37:693-706, 2002.

Wills L, Garcia J: Parasomnias: epidemiology and management, *CNS Drugs 2002* 16:803-810, 2002.

Cognitive-Perceptual Problems: Attention-Deficit/Hyperactivity Disorder, Blindness, Deafness, and Autism

Kathleen C. Shelton and Bridget O'Boyle-Jordan

Cognition and perception are interrelated activities engaged in by all humans. Gordon (1987) describes the cognitive-perceptual functional health pattern to include "the adequacy of sensory modes, such as vision, hearing, taste, touch, or smell, and the compensation or prostheses utilized for disturbances. Also included are the cognitive functional abilities, such as language, memory, and decision-making." Gordon notes that "to hear, see, smell, taste, and touch are human functions taken for granted until deficits arise." Little has been written about children in terms of the cognitive-perceptual pattern per se. However, attention-deficit/hyperactivity disorder (ADHD), deafness, blindness, and autism are all pediatric problems that involve use of sensory modes and are related to cognition, language, and the functional abilities of day-to-day life; (that is, they represent problems within the cognitive-perceptual pattern).

Facilitating the developmental progress of children should be an overriding concern for families and health care providers. Cognition is an essential component of development. Assisting children and families to minimize the effects of perceptual problems on cognition, and thus development as a whole, is an important role of the pediatric primary care providers. In this chapter, selected cognitive-perceptual problems of children are addressed as they relate to functioning in daily life.

◼ STANDARDS FOR CARE

Healthy People 2010: Health Promotion and Disease Prevention Objectives for the Year 2010 (U.S. Department of Health and Human Services, 2001) supports the need for primary care for children with cognitive and perceptual problems. The American Academy of Pediatrics recommends developmental screening and surveillance for all children; such screening should identify children with cognitive and perceptual problems needing further assessment.

The American Medical Association (AMA) Guidelines for Adolescent Preventive Services (GAPS) (Elster & Kuznets, 1994) recommend "all adolescents should be asked annually about learning or school problems." Learning disabilities, ADHD, medical problems, and other factors are identified as areas for further assessment if the young person is not successful in school. GAPS provides a structured and successful model for including relevant screening in pediatric and adolescent health practices (Gadomski et al, 2003; Low, 2003).

◼ CONCEPTUAL BACKGROUND
NORMAL COGNITIVE-PERCEPTUAL PATTERNS

Cognition and general knowledge represent the accumulation and reorganization of experiences that result from participating in a rich learning setting with skilled and appropriate adult interventions. From these experiences, children construct knowledge of patterns and relations, cause and effect, and methods of solving problems of everyday life.

For children to develop, they must perceive and process information from varied stimuli. External stimuli include visual, auditory, proprioceptive, tactile, and other modalities, whereas internal stimuli include emotions, associations, fantasies, visceral-autonomic sources, and memory sources (Levine et al, 1999). When children experience problems perceiving their environment, both animate and inanimate, development is at risk. For example, the deaf child who fails to hear sounds or learn a communication system early in life can develop faulty language and experience decreased knowledge acquisition and storage skills, reading difficulties, and social difficulties.

Learning requires feedback related to behaviors exhibited. Feedback provides information to the child, positive reinforcement for correct responses to stimuli, and negative reinforcement for behaviors that are not appropriate. Parents, peers, and others provide important feedback to the child. For the child with perceptual problems, not only is the initial cue missed but also the feedback cues, which the child needs to know whether his or her response was appropriate. This feedback is an essential component of the learning process.

INFORMATION-PROCESSING THEORIES

Information processing is thinking or problem-solving. The collection of information-processing theories can serve as a useful framework for understanding learning from the perspective of cognitive and perceptual processes. The theories collectively focus on information presented, processes used to transform information, and memory limits that constrain the amount of information that can be represented and processed. Unlike Piaget's learning model, information-processing theories try to develop a complete theory of cognition, are relatively specific, and are testable. Information-processing theorists sometimes use computer models to develop and test their ideas.

Atkinson and Shiffrin (1968) provided a broad theory of information processing. They proposed a system with structural and process components. Structural features include a sensory store with both visual and auditory registers, a short-term store, and a long-term store. There are also several processes or actions essential to the system. Rehearsal activity is used to keep information in the short-term store—the working memory. Automatic processing activities transform information outside the direct control of the individual to retain information not consciously remembered. One can see immediately that blind or deaf children will have difficulty with the two registers, visual and auditory, with deficits in one and the necessity for greater skill in the other. Children with ADHD or autism can have serviceable visual and auditory registers, but have difficulty screening input from the registers appropriately or have problems using the processes of rehearsal and automatic processing effectively and efficiently, or both.

The task environment or the context in which the child acts is also important. For example, a particular solution to a problem may create moral conflicts and thus alter the child's options. Encoding is also important. It involves identification of critical information in a situation and use of it to create internal representations (Kelly, 2004). If children fail to identify or comprehend critical elements or do not know how to encode them efficiently, they do not learn from potentially useful experiences. A key role of parents and teachers is to help children learn to identify critical cues and encode and process the information so that it becomes useful knowledge.

Levine and colleagues (1999) and Kelly (2004) applied information-processing concepts to the clinical understanding and management of pediatric learning disorders. Their information-processing model (Fig. 16-1) asserted that selective attention is a gateway between the availability and perception of stimuli and the representational and storage processes the child mobilizes to use the information. A great deal of information in the form of various stimuli may be available to the child. Selective attention begins the processes of information management—taking in, manipulating, storing, and responding.

Perception and attention are closely related phenomena. Perception is awareness of stimuli, whereas attention serves as a filtering process to focus on the most important perceptions at the moment. The primary care provider needs to assess both perceptual and selective attention skills of cognition.

COGNITIVE-PERCEPTUAL DEVELOPMENTAL PATTERNS

Infants

The infant uses perceptions in a highly literal way to develop cognition as explained by Piaget's sensorimotor stage. The infant watches, listens, tastes, smells, and manipulates objects in the environment to learn. Eye-hand coordination is important; achieving object permanence as a concept is essential.

Toddlers and Preschoolers

Toddlers continue to develop cognitively in the sensorimotor stage, whereas preschoolers, sometime after 2 years old, move into the preoperational stage. In this egocentric phase, they continue mentally to construct models that explain how the world works. However, they are unable to do several critical operations, including the following: considering several variables at once; recognizing that others have different perceptions; classifying proficiently; and understanding that some objects are inanimate, without intention and ability to act. Visual and auditory perceptions and selective attention are key factors in toddler learning. Language development assists them to encode and store information for retrieval and use.

School-Age Children

School-age children have increased perceptual skills. They have mastered the concept that others may have a different perception of the world from theirs, an especially important step that helps them understand the world from psychosocial perspectives. Piaget described their thought processes as concrete operations. For school success, they must have efficient memory use—both short and long term, excellent language skills, the ability to perceive and order the world in space, awareness of time and sequencing, and neuromotor dexterity—both fine motor and gross motor. They must also be able to use concepts, problem-solve, and think critically (Kelly, 2004). Reading becomes another type of coded language that allows further broadening of experience beyond that which is directly observable. Social cognition is also important to their developmental success.

Adolescents

Most adolescents can use formal operational thinking, including the capacity to reason from hypotheses and to identify various possible outcomes. Cognitive and perceptual skills are considered mature. (Of course, both adolescents and adults do not always use formal operational reasoning.)

The developmental milestones for children with cognitive-perceptual problems are altered from these normal patterns. A summary of some of the differences in blind and deaf children is found in Table 16-1. Children with ADHD often achieve motor milestones on time, but may experience delays in speech, social, and emotional areas of development.

Delays or Alterations in Cognitive-Perceptual Developmental Patterns

Although most children develop according to normal patterns, developmental delays, specific deficits, and alterations in cognitive-perceptual patterns sometimes occur. Developmental

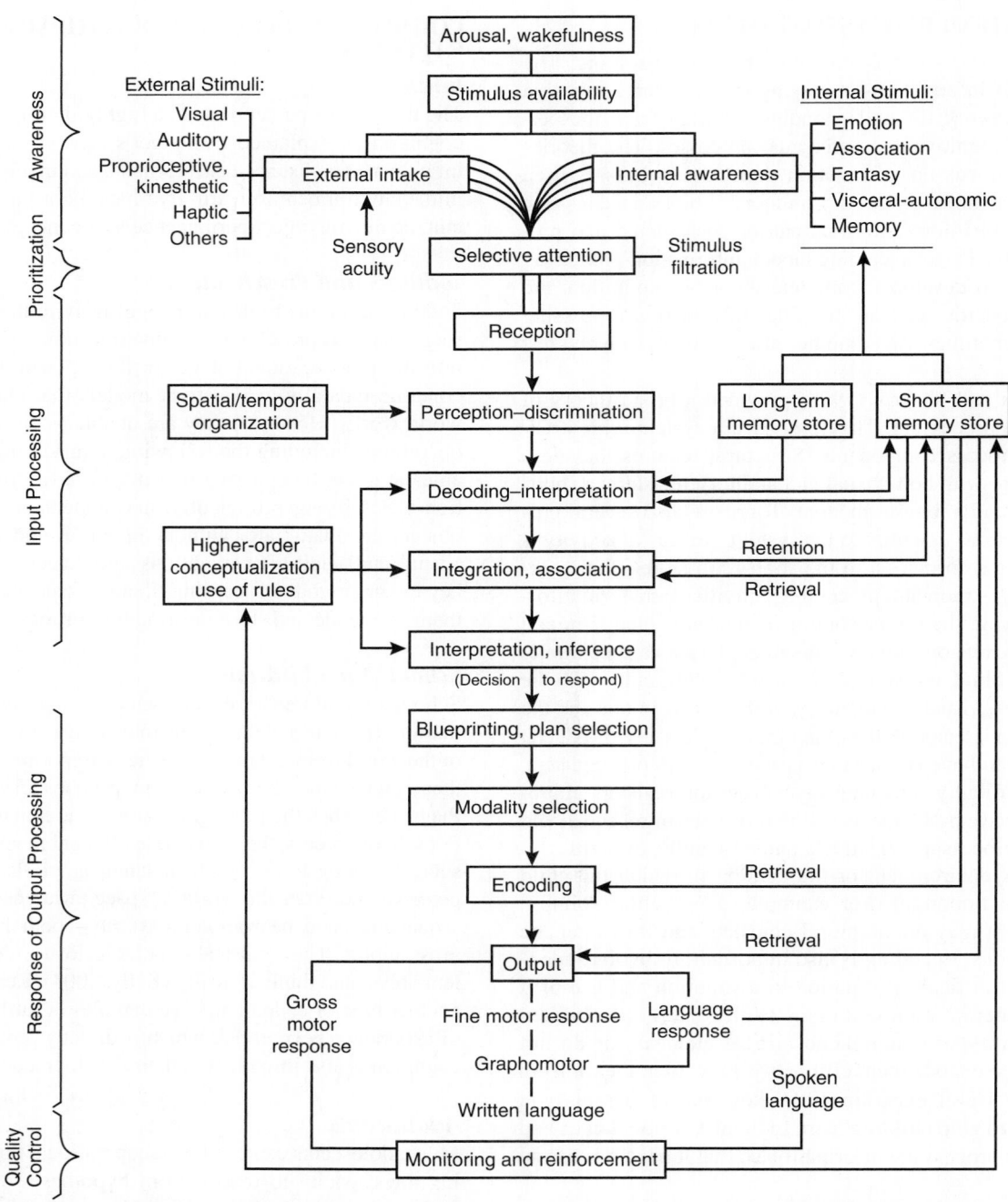

FIG. 16-1 Information-processing model. (From Levine M, Brooks R, Shonkoff J: *A pediatric approach to learning disorders,* New York, 1980, Wiley, p 480.)

delays from environmental deprivation or neglect are frequently reversible once identified. Other forms of developmental delays may result from prenatal or perinatal events, genetic dispositions, environmental toxins, trauma, or other insults to normal developmental patterns. Mental retardation results in mild, moderate, or severe cognitive deficits. The spectrum of learning disabilities may mimic alterations in cognitive-perceptual development; however, learning disabilities do not necessarily indicate lower intelligence. Instead, the challenge is to identify how the child can learn and to provide adequate experiences. It is not within the scope of this text to address the many disabling conditions involving cognitive-perceptual patterns; however, the provider can play an active role on an interdisciplinary team for diagnosis and management of developmental delays by providing care coordination, health maintenance monitoring, and family education and support (Gedaly-Duff et al, 2000).

EFFECTS OF COGNITIVE-PERCEPTUAL PATTERN PROBLEMS ON THE FAMILY

Family caregiving of children with impairments of all types is a related area that the primary care provider must understand.

TABLE 16-1	Developmental Milestones of Blind and Deaf Infants and Children	
	Blind (Without Associated Handicaps)	**Deaf**
Infants (0-1 yr)	◆ Tend to lie quietly in crib. Attachment problems possible as a result of decreased social cues and visual following. ◆ Decreased use of hands and bringing hands to midline, decreased prone position, decreased facial expressions. ◆ Gross motor: Head control 3-6 mo, sit 10.3 mo, pull to sit 15.6 mo, creep 15 mo, stand 15.3 mo and walk independently 19.8 mo. Creeping delayed until "reach on sound" cue is achieved. ◆ Fine motor: hands to midline 4.8 mo, reaches 5.5 mo, ulnar grasp 6 mo, transfers 8.5 mo, pincer grasp 12.6 mo. ◆ "Reach on sound": turns toward sound 6 mo, tries to reach 9.1 mo, reaches for sound nearby 12.2 mo. Uses sound for orientation 18.2 mo (Fazzi et al, 2002). ◆ Social: Increased separation anxiety may begin by 6 mo. Increased echolalia (Ryan, 1988). ◆ Cognitive: Sensorimotor delays common. Delayed object permanence.	◆ Sensorimotor stage normal. ◆ Language development: deaf children exposed early to sign language develop language similarly to hearing children exposed to spoken language (Meadow-Orlans, 1990). ◆ Deaf children exposed to both spoken and sign language learn both and progress as hearing children (Meadow, 1980). Deaf children exposed only to spoken language have language delays (Gregory & Mogford, 1981). ◆ Language output decreased around 6-9 mo old.
Toddlers (12 mo-2 yr)	◆ Decreased aggression but increased tantrums and motor behavior when frustrated. Continued delayed object permanence. Walks at 17 mo on average. "Blindisms" appear—rocking, swaying, head turning (Phillips & Hartley, 1988).	◆ Sensorimotor stage normal. ◆ Language output decreased.
Preschoolers (3-5 yr)	◆ Decreased social skills, decreased self-help skills. "I" sense of self delayed to 4 yr (Phillips & Hartley, 1988).	◆ May have preoperational delays (Quigley & Kretschmer, 1982). Symbolic play may be delayed if language skills are decreased.
School-age children (6-12 yr)	◆ Reading and mobility delays. Conservation delayed to 9 yr (Tobin, 1972).	◆ May have concrete operations delays (Quigley & Kretschmer, 1982). Decreased self-concept.
Adolescents (13-19 yr)	◆ Delays may continue or adolescent may finally achieve developmental level with achievement in academic and social maturity areas.	◆ Increased adjustment problems and decreased social maturity (Meadow, 1980). Decreased self-concept. ◆ May have formal operations delays.

mo, Months; *yr*, year(s).

Families adapt to achieve caregiving demands while trying to maintain family integrity. This adaptation is sometimes stressful. Because children with chronic conditions are rarely institutionalized, society relies on families to provide complex and time-consuming care.

How families cope with chronic disabling conditions and developmental delays is of interest to nursing researchers. Knafl and colleagues (Knafl et al, 1996; Knafl et al, 2001) identified the following family management styles when a child had a chronic or disabling condition: thriving, accommodating, enduring, struggling, and floundering. Each management style described how parents perceived the child (normal, problematic, tragic), the parenting philosophy and view of illness, and their perception and approach to managing the illness. For example, parents who embraced a thriving

family management style viewed the illness from a "life goes on" perspective and normalized the child's illness as best they could. They had a parenting philosophy that was able to accommodate the illness into parenting activities and a confident mind-set, and they were proactive in their management approach.

Other typologies have been described for families with children with other cognitive-perceptual problems. Kendall (1998) described four types of families of children with ADHD along a trajectory: the chaotic family, the ADHD-controlled family, the surviving family, and the reinvested family. Other studies of families living with ADHD indicate considerable disruption to family routines and an inability to achieve some sense of "normalcy"; some families describe family life as a "nightmare," despite outward indicators (intact marriage, stable residence, adequate income, resources to manage the ADHD, etc.) that the family is doing well (Shelton, 2001). Families of learning-disabled children have been described as healthy, split, chaotic, and blaming (Ziegler & Holden, 1988).

ASSESSMENT OF COGNITIVE-PERCEPTUAL PATTERNS

NORMAL PATTERNS

Assessment of normal cognitive-perceptual patterns is discussed earlier in this book. Developmental assessments appropriate to the age of the child and hearing and vision screening are the usual modes of assessment.

ASSESSMENT OF CHILDREN WITH COGNITIVE-PERCEPTUAL PROBLEMS

No matter what the particular type of problem, an assessment should include three aspects:
1. Diagnosis or monitoring, or both, of the child's health from a primary care perspective
2. Evaluation of parent and family responses to the problem
3. Evaluation of the child's development

The details of these assessments vary with the condition. A variety of special assessment tools are available and are generally administered by experts. Some assessment tools for children with ADHD are listed in Table 16-2. Mislabeling of children can occur when tools for sighted or hearing children, for instance, are adapted intuitively for children with visual or auditory disabilities.

MANAGEMENT STRATEGIES

Children and families with problems in this domain generally need support in four areas: social and adaptive skills, education, social support, and multidisciplinary health care team consultations. Many families find this support lacking from their primary care providers. Satisfaction with primary care received by families of children with developmental disabilities including both physical and mental problems was studied by Liptak and colleagues (2006). They found that most families felt satisfied with physicians' abilities to keep up with new aspects of care and with their sensitivity to the needs of the children. They indicated dissatisfaction with the ability of physicians to put them in touch with other parents, understand the impact of the condition on the family, answer questions about the condition, and provide information and guidance. They rated physicians' knowledge about complementary and alternative medicine and their qualifications to manage children with developmental disabilities most negatively. Families with a child with autism rated primary care physicians worse on several factors than did other families.

SOCIAL AND ADAPTIVE STRATEGIES

Social and adaptive care relates to helping children achieve maximal independence in living and learning to get along with family and others in a variety of social environments. The family delivers most of this care, but some parents need help with knowing what social and adaptive developmental steps children should master at various ages. Sorting out what "normal" children do at given ages versus what the handicapped child is doing requires thoughtful analysis. Particular strategies to help the impaired child learn new skills are often learned by trial and error or can be gleaned from parents of children with similar handicaps. Physical therapists, occupational therapists, and teachers with special education and skills to help children with cognitive-perceptual impairments can be important resources. The primary care provider can serve as case manager; help parents explore other ideas, or act as a conduit to help parents find others who have solved similar problems.

TABLE 16-2 **Assessment Instruments Specific to Attention-Deficit/Hyperactivity Disorder**

The following scales have been recommended by the American Academy of Pediatrics Committee on Quality Improvement and Subcommittee on Attention Deficit Hyperactivity Disorder (2000) as clinical options for evaluating children with ADHD. Use of broadband scales is not recommended in the diagnosis of children with ADHD, although they may be useful for other purposes.

Study	Scale	Age (In Years)
Connors (1997)	Connors Parent Rating Scale—1997 Revised Version: Long Form, ADHD Index Scale	6-17
Connors (1997)	Connors Teacher Rating Scale—1997 Revised Version: Long Form, ADHD Index Scale	6-17
Connors (1997)	Connors Parent Rating Scale—1997 Revised Version: Long Form, DSM-IV Symptoms Scale	6-17
Connors (1997)	Connors Teacher Rating Scale—1997 Revised Version: Long Form, DSM-IV Symptoms Scale	6-17
Connors & Wells (1997)	Connors Wells Adolescent Self Report Scale	12-17
Breen & Altpeter (1991)	Barkley School Situations Questionnaire—Original Version, Number of Problem Settings Scale	6-11
Breen & Altpeter (1991)	Barkley School Situations Questionnaire—Original Version, Mean Severity Scale	6-11

EDUCATIONAL STRATEGIES

Children with ADHD, deafness, blindness, and other problems are entitled to special education opportunities to maximize their learning potential. Infant stimulation opportunities are extremely important for blind and deaf children and early-intervention preschool programs are essential. Two federal laws, the Americans with Disabilities Act (ADA), passed in 1990, and the Individuals with Disabilities Education Act (IDEA), reauthorized in 1997, provide mandates for services for children with cognitive-perceptual problems. These laws provide mechanisms for parents and teachers to use to facilitate optimal learning opportunities for students with cognitive-perceptual difficulties.

- The Individualized Educational Plan (IEP) is designed for children who demonstrate a gap between learning potential and actual academic performance. The IEP is mandated for children with medical conditions that interfere with academic success and arises from the IDEA. The current IDEA program also provides for mental health services for children with learning problems.
- The "Section 504 Plan" provided within the ADA is a civil rights protection to facilitate academic success in students whose disability might otherwise make them ineligible for a public education. Many children with ADHD and learning disabilities who do not have cognitive deficits but do have significant behavioral or emotional problems that interfere with learning are eligible for the Section 504 Plan.

School programs need to be individualized. When children reach school age, decisions are made collaboratively between parents and school personnel about the best placement of the child, whether in a mainstream classroom, in a special classroom, or in a combination of settings. Blind and deaf children sometimes attend special schools designed to meet their needs in either residential or day programs. Children with ADHD or learning problems are usually managed in regular schools. Annual planning of the educational program is often a frustrating experience for parents because school resources and teacher experience vary from year to year.

Information for parents about these legal rights and provisions can be found on websites about ADHD and learning disabilities and governmental websites at the Centers for Disease Control and Prevention (CDC), National Institutes of Health (NIH), and National Institutes of Mental Health (NIMH) (also see Resource Box at the end of the chapter).

SOCIAL SUPPORT STRATEGIES

Living with a child with a cognitive-perceptual problem, whether the problem is blindness, deafness, ADHD, learning difficulties, or some other problem, generally requires that the family develop a structure and organization to support the child without becoming overprotective or intrusive and that they develop an environment that offers consistency for the child. For many families, maintenance of family organization and consistency is difficult.

Social support has been shown to provide significant benefits to families with children with health problems of all sorts. National organizations provide information and expert advice, and local groups can facilitate direct help. Connecting families to others with similar experiences is helpful. Further, the extended family, especially grandparents, can provide significant tangible support to families working to cope with the stresses (financial, temporal, energy, and emotional) of caring for a child with special needs. Siblings may also need support. Providers can be helpful in organizing, supporting, and providing referrals to community support groups. Often national support groups provide expertise to communities that wish to establish a local chapter.

MULTIDISCIPLINARY TEAM STRATEGIES

The use of a variety of specialists can provide the best resources for children with special needs. Generally, these include medical specialists, physical and occupational therapists, social workers, and specially educated teachers. The primary care provider helps families identify appropriate teams, serves as a case manager among the parties, and ensures that primary health care needs are integrated with the special services provided.

■ COGNITIVE-PERCEPTUAL PROBLEMS OF CHILDREN

ATTENTION-DEFICIT/HYPERACTIVITY DISORDER (ADHD)

Description

ADHD is the most commonly diagnosed behavioral problem in childhood. The cardinal features of this disorder are inattention, distractibility, impulsivity, and overactivity (American Psychiatric Association [APA], 2000). These primary behaviors and their secondary manifestations have an impact on every aspect of life for affected children. The intensity and effect of ADHD behaviors vary widely among children. Behaviors can also change over time in response to normal maturational influences. ADHD is now regarded as a chronic condition that continues into adulthood. ADHD in adolescence requires particular attention because of the increased demands on students at school and the decreasing abilities of adolescents with ADHD to succeed in school without interventions (Schonwald, 2005; Wolraich et al, 2005).

In an attempt to unify the understanding about ADHD, Barkley (1997) outlined a theoretical model of ADHD. The essential impairment is a deficit in behavioral inhibition, disrupting the developmental process of learning to self-regulate behaviors. Instead, external behaviors of inattention, distractibility, impulsivity, and hyperactivity, which may be age-appropriate in young children, persist into school age and adolescence and result in the inability to regulate behavior internally as the child matures.

Attention.   Attention includes the ability to maintain concentration for an appropriate period of time and to resist attending to competing stimuli. Without these abilities, children and adolescents appear distracted at times when they are expected to concentrate. Attention also implies skill at picking out salient versus trivial information and choosing effective problem-solving strategies. Lacking this component of attention leads to missing the point in academic and social situations and doing things the hard way without careful thought about how to plan and solve a problem.

Distractibility. Distractibility is a by-product of inattention that results when one pays attention to multiple stimuli at one time or in rapid succession. Difficulty maintaining enough mental effort to complete a task is related to distractibility. These characteristics lead to inconsistent performance in school and lost interest in activities and social plans.

Impulsivity. Impulsivity, acting before thinking, is described in the *Diagnostic and Statistical Manual of Mental Disorders,* edition 4, text revision (DSM-IV TR) (APA, 2000), in part by the behaviors manifested: impatience; difficulty delaying responses, such as blurting out answers in class or interrupting conversations; and blundering without following directions.

Hyperactivity. Hyperactivity describes the cluster of overactivity behaviors, including fidgeting, an inability to remain seated when expected, and moving "as though driven." These behaviors interfere with attention. They are also regarded as disruptive to group activities and create negative social consequences for the child with ADHD.

Epidemiology

ADHD has multiple etiologies. Faraone (2006), using data from 20 twin studies, reports the mean heritability across these studies to be 76%. Thus, it is among the most heritable of all psychiatric disorders with a polygenic cause including the dopamine receptor D4 gene among others. It is believed that genes and environment work in a multifactorial process so that only genetically susceptible people are affected (Faraone, 2006). However, there are a variety of environmental risk factors that play a role. Elevated lead levels, cigarette smoking, and ingestion of alcohol or drug use during pregnancy are three environmental factors implicated with ADHD (Braun et al, 2006). Most findings appear to be correlational rather than causal. A variety of antecedent factors seem to cause a disturbance in a final common pathway in the nervous system. Neurologic and physiologic factors associated with ADHD include perinatal hypoxic and anoxic insults, other injuries at birth, delayed brain maturation, imbalances in neurotransmitter functions, and differences in cerebral blood flow patterns.

Psychiatric studies give the incidence of ADHD as 7.5% of children (Schonwald, 2005; MMWR, 2005). ADHD is more commonly diagnosed in boys than girls, with a ratio of 3:1 found in several studies. Debate persists if girls are less frequently diagnosed because they are truly fewer in number or because girls are less likely to demonstrate the more problematic, hyperactive symptoms. Confusion around diagnostic criteria and the unique manifestation of symptoms in each child contributes to wide discrepancies in reported incidence.

ADHD has been well documented outside of the U.S. Studies show that similar rates of incidence occur internationally (Buitelaar et al, 2006). Although there is agreement across cultures about the presence of ADHD, perceptions often vary by culture (Norvilitis & Fang, 2005). For example, the Chinese teachers and adults surveyed by Norvilitis and Fang focused more frequently on hyperactivity than inattentiveness compared with American peers. Kendall and colleagues (2005b) found that whites used more support services and resources than Hispanics. Hispanics were also less likely to use traditional child services than whites or African Americans.

Attention-Deficit/Hyperactivity Disorder and Family Functioning

The effects of ADHD often produce stress in families, day care, and school environments. At home, family functioning and activities of daily living are most disrupted. Parents are often frustrated and exhausted. Frequently, there is increased physical fighting between the child with ADHD and his or her siblings or parents. Tolerance for this aggressive behavior results in the absence of successful family interventions. A cycle develops whereby families minimize the degree of aggression and violence as a coping strategy. Correlational studies indicate that increasing age and severity of ADHD symptoms are associated with more negative effects on family functioning (Robin, 2002). Of course, some families cope better than others.

Several common themes have been found through interviews with mothers of children with ADHD. First, they thought the children were different, sometimes from birth or before. Despite the differences, however, they hoped to develop the child as an ideal adult. Medication was viewed as crucial to management of children with ADHD though they understood it was not a cure, nor the only thing necessary to manage the child. Managing the children was very difficult as contingencies, parental authority, and other measures for controlling behavior usually were ineffective. The mothers had high expectations that their work with the child would improve his/her behavior. Finally, they found little community support to help them (Bull & Whelan, 2006).

A family study has identified developmental trajectories for the child with ADHD, the parents, and other family members (Kendall, 1998) and indicates that early interventions are necessary to prevent the escalation of family violence, the deterioration of family functioning, and negative effects on all family members. Even when families appear to be "doing well," parents still report that family life with an ADHD child is frequently a "nightmare" (Shelton, 2001). Specialized services are needed by most families of children with ADHD and should be tailored to each family's need for counseling, support services, school services, and auxiliary services (Kendall et al, 2005a).

Children With Attention-Deficit/Hyperactivity Disorder at School

Children with ADHD may be unsuccessful in developing meaningful relationships with peers and other adults. Social interactions at school may involve aggressive behaviors, leading to exclusion from group activities or isolation and withdrawal on the part of the child with ADHD. Developmental tasks of adolescence frequently are negatively affected by ADHD.

The school experience comprises both educational and social aspects. Inattention, distractibility, and hyperactivity can interfere with learning directly by disrupting the child's ability to concentrate and complete work. Indirectly, the social consequences of the disruption produced by ADHD symptoms may alienate and frustrate the child, the teacher, and classmates, which reinforces the cycle of difficulty with learning, low self-esteem, and lack of satisfying friendships.

Adolescents With Attention-Deficit/Hyperactivity Disorder

Most children do not appear to outgrow ADHD as once thought. As many as 65% of children diagnosed with ADHD in childhood will continue to have difficulties related to the disorder into adolescence. Some teens will be first diagnosed as adolescents (Wolraich et al, 2005). Some clinical manifestations change over time. Hyperactivity will be less apparent and often academic problems increase. Peer relationships also become more difficult. Unhappiness, anxiety or depression, and signs of emotional immaturity emerge along with a tendency for co-occurring oppositional defiant or conduct disordered behavior (25% to 75%). Sleep disturbances may be significant. New risks with dating, sexual activity, and driving emerge (Barkley, 2004; Wolraich et al, 2005).

Assessment

The AAP recommends gathering data using DSM-IV criteria, parent assessment, and teacher assessment with consideration of coexisting conditions (Schonwald, 2005). DSM-IV criteria must be met and differential diagnoses ruled out to confirm the diagnosis and to plan treatment for this highly individualized problem. If problems have been identified by different observers and noted since early childhood, ADHD is more likely to be diagnosed. Children who display impulsive and hyperactive behaviors are more likely to be evaluated at a younger age than children who display inattentive and distractible behaviors. The American Academy of Pediatrics (AAP) published practice guidelines for the diagnosis and treatment of ADHD (AAP Committee on Quality Improvement and Subcommittee on Attention Deficit Hyperactivity Disorder, 2000, 2001). The American Academy of Child and Adolescent Psychiatry (AACAD) has reaffirmed and updated these guidelines (Pliszka, 2007).

Proper diagnosis of ADHD is labor-intensive and cannot be done adequately in a short office visit. Frequently, during the office visit, parents express concerns about ADHD characteristics. Information must then be gathered from other settings, such as school or other structured activities, and a detailed medical, social, and family history is taken from the parents at a follow-up visit. After this information is gathered, the child should be examined and, in some cases, referred for further testing by a psychologist, an occupational therapist, or a learning specialist before a final diagnosis is made. Structured interviews may be helpful in discriminating ADHD from other comorbid conditions.

A variety of evaluations are helpful in clarifying the diagnosis of ADHD. Cognitive testing provides information about the child's ability to process information and may screen for some language-based disabilities. Most standardized cognitive assessments also give insight into the child's processing speed and working memory. Academic testing provides further information about learning disabilities. This is important because a child with dyslexia may appear inattentive, particularly in the school setting. Psychoeducational evaluations may be obtained through the school psychologist. Unfortunately, resources are limited and getting the child tested may take months to years depending upon the child's academic success. Furthermore, school psychologists and teachers may identify learning or cognitive difficulties, but are often restricted from giving parents specific diagnoses.

The use of clinical pathways may be helpful in guiding the assessment for ADHD in the primary care setting. Assessment domains should include the physical condition of the child, psychological condition of the child, family assessment, and educational performance and behaviors (Magyary et al, 1999). Clinical pathways also provide guidance through diagnosis, goal setting, and monitoring.

History. Questioning in a direct and nonjudgmental way often invites children and parents to share sensitive information. DSM-IV criteria for ADHD signs and symptoms are found in Table 16-3. Suggestions for a complete history of the child who may have ADHD are found in Table 16-4. The history must include assessment of a broad range of health-related areas. These will include family history, birth history, general health, development, behavioral history, and social and environmental history. Parents are interviewed. The child is also interviewed separately.

Physical Examination. The physical examination should include the following:

- Complete health history and physical examination
- Neurologic examination
- Minor congenital anomalies (e.g., fetal alcohol syndrome features)
- Auditory screening
- Visual screening
- Growth parameters
- Signs of anemia, chronic illness, or allergy

Other Studies. Additional studies may be needed, including the following:

- Neurodevelopmental examination with fine and gross motor skills test
- Brief mental status examination and screening for learning disabilities
- Laboratory work, including tests for anemia and lead, in addition to a thyroid screen and levels of anticonvulsants if indicated by history and physical examination
- Behavior checklists completed by parents and teachers (see Table 16-2 for suggested tools)
- Psychoeducational tests to identify children with cognitive, language, or visual-spatial-motor problems

It is difficult to diagnose children with ADHD who are younger than 4 years old when the characteristic features of ADHD may still be age-appropriate. Often, the diagnosis is made in these young children only when behaviors are extreme.

TABLE 16-3 DSM-IV Criteria for Attention-Deficit/Hyperactivity Disorder

Domain	Criteria
Essential features	Symptoms occur in two or more settings (home, work, school, in public) *and* there is clear evidence of significant impairment in social, school, or work settings Symptoms have persisted for more than 6 months Symptoms have been present before 7 years old
Inattention traits	At least six of the following symptoms of inattention are present: • Fails to tend to details, makes careless mistakes routinely in work and schoolwork • Has difficulty sustaining attention on a task at work or at play • Does not seem to listen when spoken to • Fails to follow instructions or fails to complete tasks (not as a result of oppositional behavior or failure to understand instruction) • Has difficulty organizing tasks and activities • Often avoids or puts off tasks requiring sustained mental effort • Often loses things necessary for performing tasks • Is easily distracted by extraneous stimuli • Is often forgetful in daily activities
Hyperactivity, impulsivity traits	At least six of the following symptoms of hyperactivity and impulsivity are present: • Often squirms in seat or fidgets with hands or feet • Often leaves seat when remaining in seat is expected • Often runs, climbs, or moves restlessly in situations when it is inappropriate • Often has difficulty playing or enjoying quiet leisure activities • Is often described as "on the go" or "driven" • Often talks excessively • Often answers before question is completed or blurts out answer • Has difficulty taking turns • Often interrupts or intrudes in others' activities

Differential Diagnosis

Other diagnoses to consider include normal variation; giftedness; language disorder; mental retardation; migraines; lead poisoning; hearing loss; thyroid dysfunction; visual disturbance; genetic disorders, such as fragile X syndrome; seizure disorder; Tourette's syndrome; psychological disorders, such as anxiety, bipolar disorder, oppositional defiant disorder, conduct disorder, posttraumatic stress disorder, or depression; substance abuse; pervasive developmental disorder; environmental disorders (e.g., child abuse, family stress, domestic violence, parenting disruptions, parental psychopathology; inappropriate educational setting); sleep disorder; and learning disabilities. Careful differentiation is needed to identify proper pharmacologic and psychotherapeutic interventions (Jensen et al, 2001).

Primary ADHD can exist simultaneously with family situations that predispose children to exhibit behaviors similar to those seen in children with ADHD. With increased evidence that domestic violence, family dysfunction, and child abuse can mimic ADHD, it is important to do an in-depth family assessment to ensure accuracy of the diagnosis and to intervene when domestic violence and child abuse are occurring. Primary ADHD is the only form that is properly treated with medication; therefore it is important to make an accurate diagnosis of ADHD to develop an appropriate management plan.

Primary Attention or Behavioral Problems. These children have attention problems that are chronic, permeate most areas of the child's life, and meet the DSM-IV diagnostic criteria (see Table 16-3). ADHD characteristics represent maladaptation and are often not consistent with age-specific developmental expectations. This type of inattention is also associated with concurrent difficulties with planning, self-monitoring, and completing tasks. Medication used to treat ADHD is targeted to this category of attention problems and works well in about 70% to 80% of children in this group (Greenhill et al, 2001).

Situational Attention or Behavioral Problems. These problems develop in specific situations and often reflect inappropriate environmental expectations. They do not permeate all settings. Problems with boredom, distractibility, and hyperactivity can be traced or related to family social problems; difficult temperament leading to a poor fit between child, parent, and school; parent-child relational problems; environmental overstimulation; and inappropriate reward systems. These children are still able to accomplish age-specific developmental tasks despite inattention and hyperactivity and do not meet the DSM-IV criteria for an ADHD diagnosis. Stimulant medication is not recommended when attention or behavioral problems are situational.

Secondary Attention or Behavioral Problems. These problems result from underlying deficits in cognitive

TABLE 16-4   Attention–Deficit/Hyperactivity Disorder History

Assessment Area	Suggested Topics to Explore
Chief complaint and history of present problem	Major areas of concern
	First awareness of problem
	Beliefs about causation of problem
	Previous evaluations and results
	Medication history for behavioral, emotional, or learning problems
Birth history*	Prenatal history; maternal health; use of medications, recreational drugs, alcohol, and tobacco during pregnancy
	Birth anoxia, difficult delivery
	Postpartum complications, birth defects
	Neonatal behavior: feeding, sleep, temperament problems
General health*	Neurologic status, vision, hearing, chronic diseases
	Hospitalizations, prolonged illness
	Frequent injuries
	Poisoning or lead or environmental exposures
	Outbursts of uncontrollable sounds or words
	Tics, habit spasms, uncontrollable twitches
	Ongoing medications
ADHD history	Attention: paying attention, sustaining attention, listening, following through, organization, reluctant to engage in activities that need sustained attention, loses things, distracted, forgetful
	Activity: fidgets, leaves seat, runs or climbs when inappropriate, has difficulty with quiet games, talks excessively, has problems waiting turn, interrupts, "on the go"
Developmental history*	Milestones: motor, personal-social, language, cognitive
	Strengths (e.g., personality, activities, friendliness)
	Weaknesses
Behavioral history*	Frequency with which child complies when told to do something
	Methods used at home to improve behavior and effectiveness
	Parenting skills training
	Parental agreement about child management
	Counseling history for child or family (or both)
Academic history	Child's progress at each grade level
	Adjustment problems at school
	Difficulties with specific skills: reading, writing, spelling, math, concepts
	Performance problems—attention, grades, participation, excessive talking, disturbing others, fighting, abusive language, not completing work
	School assistance: tutoring, counseling, special help
Functional Health Patterns	
Feeding	Not able to sit through a complete meal
	Messy and clumsy with utensils, dishes, and glasses
	Inadequate caloric intake can be result of symptoms and further exacerbated by medications used to treat ADHD
	Gastric distress may be a side effect of stimulant medication
Sleeping	Difficulty falling asleep, night waking, needs less sleep than other family members
	Complains about fatigue interfering with completion of tasks
Activity	Difficulty maintaining routines for activities of daily living
Cognitive	Level of performance is below potential for achievement
	Tends to miss the point of conversations and activities
	Often does things the hard way in absence of established routines
Self-concept	Struggles with low self-esteem, moodiness
Role relationships	Inadequate social and relational skills
	Lies, steals, plays with fire, hurts animals, is aggressive with other children, talks back to adults

Continued

TABLE 16-4   **Attention-Deficit/Hyperactivity Disorder History—Cont'd**

Coping and stress tolerance	Low tolerance for frustration
	Outbursts of temper
	Moody, worried, sad, quiet, destructive, fearful or fearless, self-deprecating
	Somatic complaints
Social and environmental history*	Family stress and coping patterns
	Home, day care, and school environments
	Family social risk factors: recent moves, financial stress, parental job losses, births, deaths, divorces, remarriages, alcohol and drug use, involvement with law enforcement, weapons in the home
Family history*	ADHD, neurologic problems, learning difficulties
	Mental health history of close family members, health or behavior problems in other family members
Teacher history	Obtain information from school about child's problems, strengths, weaknesses, academic management of issues

*These must be included in the assessment.

abilities; specific learning disabilities; undetected vision and hearing problems; medical problems, such as mild cerebral palsy, seizure disorders, allergies, and asthma; and side effects to medications used for such conditions. The gifted child who is bored may also fit some of the behavioral patterns listed here. Other significant and perhaps undiagnosed emotional problems, including unresolved anger, depression, anxiety, oppositional defiant disorder, conduct disorder, autism, and abuse, may exist. These children do not meet the DSM-IV criteria for ADHD and should be diagnosed according to their other diagnostic features.

Comorbidity

A number of children with ADHD also have a concurrent diagnosis for learning disabilities (35%) or a psychiatric disorder, such as anxiety (25%), depression (25%), bipolar (10%), oppositional defiant disorder (60%), tic disorder (11%), or conduct disorder (50%) (Schonwald, 2005). Substance use is more common in adolescents and adults with ADHD (Olfson, 2004; Wilson & Levin, 2005). A mental health specialist should evaluate children for comorbid conditions. The management of ADHD needs to include strategies for prioritizing needs and interventions in concert with these other conditions. If more than one health care provider is involved because of comorbid conditions, the primary care provider may serve as case manager to keep family members and other health care professionals informed and to coordinate treatment plans and services.

Management

ADHD should be considered a chronic illness (AACAP, 2007). The clinical practice guideline (AAP Committee on Quality Improvement and Subcommittee on Attention-Deficit/Hyperactivity Disorder, 2001) provides the rationale and strategies for careful management of children with ADHD. It acknowledges the lack of in-depth education on ADHD that primary care providers may have and stresses the importance of continuing education in this area. A toolkit was developed and is available from AAP to assist primary care providers in the diagnosis and management of ADHD in an office practice. The AAP guideline stresses the importance of regular monitoring and suggests that monitoring should be focused on specific outcomes and that information regarding these outcomes be regularly obtained from parents, the child, and teachers. See Fig. 16-2 for the AAP algorithm. The AACAP (2007) parameter focuses more on the role of child psychiatric specialists.

Medication.   Medications should be used in conjunction with behavioral, family, cognitive-behavioral, and other interventions (Table 16-5). The landmark MTA Cooperative Group study (1999) has supported the use of combined medications and behavioral therapy.

Careful monitoring of children on medications for ADHD is necessary to minimize side effects. Antidepressants, stimulants, and allergy and asthma medications (especially over-the-counter preparations) should not be taken simultaneously without proper education; moreover, physicians should prescribe each medication with awareness of the other drugs the patient is taking. All medications for acute illnesses should be prescribed only with full knowledge of potential interactions with medications for ADHD and concurrent problems. Even with monotherapy, ongoing monitoring is recommended. This may include intermittent reassessments for psychological disorders and regular vital signs and body mass index tracking.

It is common for medication regimens to need periodic adjustment or complete change as the child grows. Increase in body weight or other medical conditions requiring medication may indicate the need to reassess the medication plan for ADHD. Social and emotional maturation may decrease or eliminate the need for medication in late childhood and adolescence. Changes in family or school schedules may necessitate a long-acting preparation or an adjustment in the timing of doses. For example, once a medication regimen has been established in early elementary grades, the plan may be successful for several years. As the child approaches middle school, the symptoms of greatest concern to the school and family may have changed, or the child may decide he or she no longer wants to take medication.

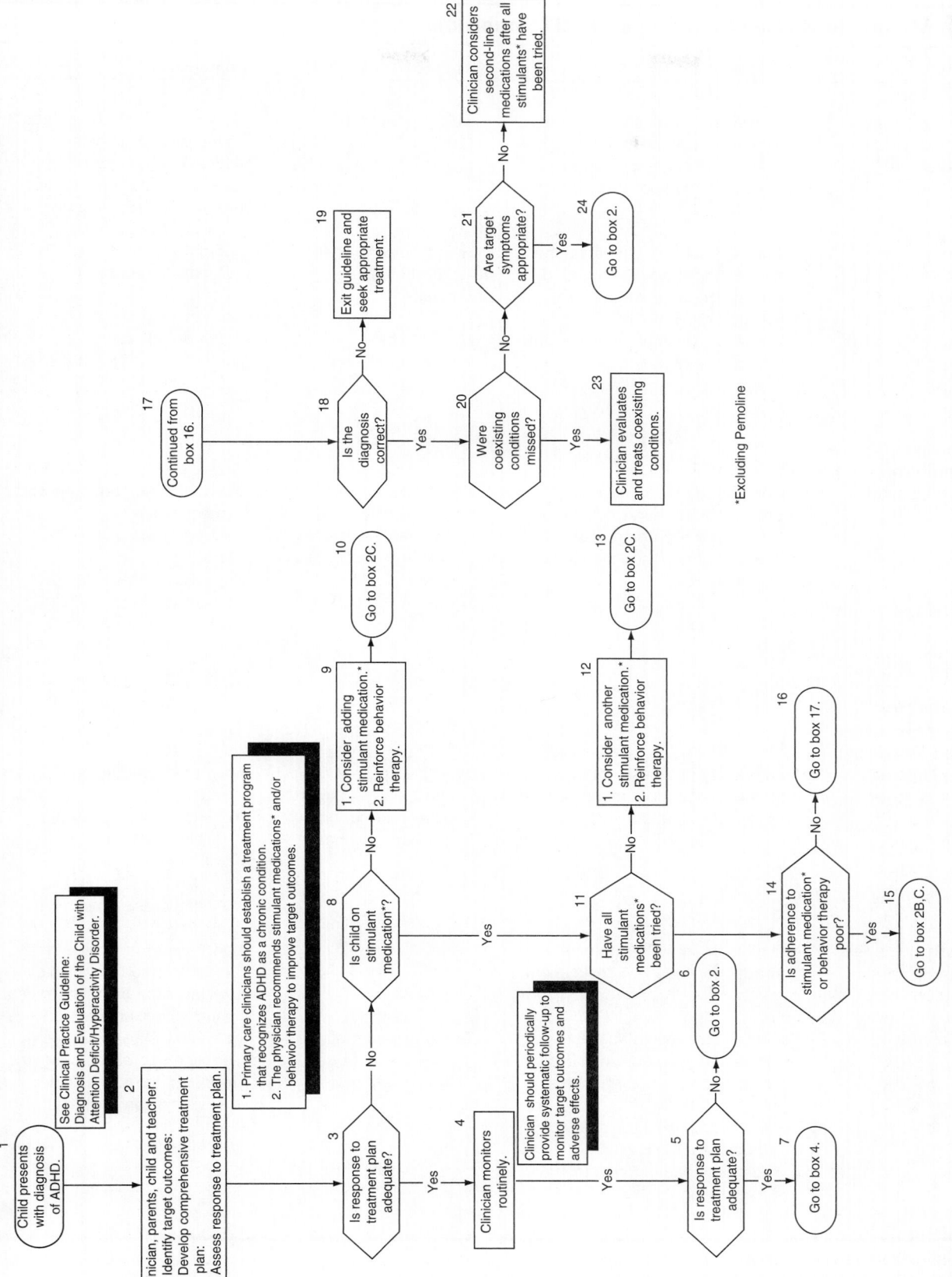

FIG. 16-2 Algorithm for the treatment of the school-age child with ADHD. (From American Academy of Pediatrics [AAP]: Clinical practice guideline: treatment of the school-aged child with attention–deficit/hyperactivity disorder, *Pediatrics* 108:1035, 2001.)

TABLE 16-5 **Medications Used to Manage ADHD Symptoms**

Medication	Side Effects	Monitor	Comments
Stimulants			
Methylphenidate (Ritalin [Ritalin LA], Metadate CD, Concerta, Daytrana, Focartin, Methylin)*	Anorexia, insomnia, stomachache, headache, irritability, "rebound," flattened affect, social withdrawal, crying, tics, weight loss, reduced growth rate	Height, weight, BMI, blood pressure, pulse	Do not chew or cut sustained-release tabs in half Avoid decongestants Capsules may be sprinkled Daytrana patch must be removed after 9 hours
Dextroamphetamine (Dexedrine, Dextrostat)*	Anorexia, insomnia, stomachache, headache, irritability, "rebound," tics, stereopathy, weight loss, reduced growth rate	Height, weight, BMI, blood pressure, pulse	Avoid decongestants Potential for abuse
Four mixed amphetamine salts (Adderall, Adderall XR)*	Same as dextroamphetamine, rare occurrence of sudden cardiac failure	Consider baseline ECG and repeat yearly	8-10 hour effect Tablet can be split, capsule may be sprinkled Potential for abuse
Selective Norepinephrine Reuptake Inhibitor			
Atomoxetine (Strattera)	Slight diastolic blood pressure and heart rate increase FDA cautions regarding possible liver impairment and increased risk of suicide Slight decrease in appetite, stomach upset Headaches	Weight decreases significantly in first 9-12 weeks, then expect catch-up and parallel growth curve Consider yearly liver studies Monitor for suicidal thinking	Nonstimulant, nonadrenergic mechanism Once or twice-daily dosing Do not open capsule Monitor closely for suicidal thinking and behavior Greatest effect at 6 weeks
Nonstimulants (Try behavior therapy before these second-line drugs)			
Desipramine (Norpramin)	Tachycardia, dizziness, fatigue, upset stomach, dry mouth, blurry vision, constipation	Baseline ECG, ECG and blood level with dose change, blood pressure and heart rate	May affect cardiac conduction rate Increased blood pressure levels and heart rate with methylphenidate Use with ADHD-related tics, enuresis, and anxiety
Bupropion (Wellbutrin [Wellbutin SR, Wellbutrin XL])	Agitation, dry mouth, insomnia, headache, nausea, constipation, tremor		Lowers seizure threshold Contraindicated in patients with eating disorders or tics, current seizure disorders
Clonidine (Catapres)	Sedation, dizziness, nausea, orthostatic hypotension, clinical major depression, nightmares	Blood pressure at baseline, after dose adjustment and follow-up	Not first-line agent Sedation decreases over time Rebound hypertension if stopped abruptly; follow-up
Guanfacine (Tenex)	Sedation, dizziness, nausea, orthostatic hypotension, insomnia, agitation, headache, stomach ache	Blood pressure at baseline, after dose adjustment and follow-up	Not first-line agent May need 3 times a day dosing Superior to placebo at 1.2 to 1.8 mg/day studies

*Approved by U.S. Food and Drug Administration for ADHD treatment.
ADHD, Attention-deficit/hyperactivity disorder; *BMI*, body mass index; *ECG*, electrocardiogram.

- Ask the parents and the child at regular intervals about how the medication is working and if they perceive a need to make adjustments.
- Assess the need to adjust medication at the beginning of each school year and at times when major changes are occurring in the family that affect the family system (e.g., births, deaths, divorces, remarriages, residential moves, death of pets, significant illness or injury).

Stimulant medication is often the most effective intervention. Stimulants have been shown to increase attention span, gross and fine motor coordination, and compliance while decreasing impulsiveness, hyperactivity, and aggression. Methylphenidate and amphetamines are the most commonly used and researched drugs for treating children with ADHD (Schonwald, 2005; Simms, 2004).

New formulations of these two basic classes of stimulant medications are now available and provide more flexibility and individual tailoring of medications for children and adolescents. Both short- and long-acting medications are available. The short-acting forms provide greater flexibility to maximize positive behaviors at important times of the day. Usually, they are given at breakfast and again at lunch. The long-acting forms last 6 to 12 hours, getting a child through the school day. The potencies may differ between the two forms. Some families mix the forms, giving, for instance, the long-acting form for the day and then a short-acting dose to last until bedtime (Olfson, 2004).

Atomoxetine (Strattera) is a nonstimulant drug that may be used as a first-line medication for children older than 6 years. Other nonstimulant medications may help children who respond poorly to an adequate trial of stimulants. This may be due to their comorbid conditions. These medications are used cautiously because some are not yet approved by the Food and Drug Administration (FDA) for these uses, but controlled studies and clinical data support their trial. Current research reports that desipramine is more effective than placebo in treating ADHD symptoms (Brown et al, 2005). The studies for other tricyclic antidepressants are less supportive. Bupropion is an antidepressant that has been used. Antihypertensives, such as clonidine and guanfacine, have also been used (Adesman, 2002). Clonidine plus a stimulant have been used with greater success to treat conduct symptoms but not hyperactivity (Olfson, 2004).

Parents are often in a dilemma regarding the use of stimulant medication for ADHD management. They need to weigh the medication's desirable versus undesirable effects in various settings. They may worry about the role of medications in their child's future (Hansen & Hansen, 2006). A variety of studies demonstrate that adolescents often stop taking medications despite their continued effectiveness (Wolraich et al, 2005).

Family Education About Diagnosis. Families need to be well educated about the disorder because a large part of the treatment for ADHD involves parent-management techniques. The chronic nature of ADHD has a tremendous impact on family functioning. Conversely, family factors play a part in the outcomes for children with ADHD. Parents often have to educate others about the special needs of their child. Because children with ADHD manifest a great variety of behaviors, parents become the experts who ultimately manage the problems and affect the outcome for their child.

Family education must be ongoing and reflect the developmental maturation of the child and unique expression of ADHD within each child and family. When the diagnosis is shared with parents, it is best to arrange for adequate time to educate families about ADHD, parenting strategies, community resources, and medication management. Parents are better able to pay attention to this information when the child is not present in the room; it is helpful if parents arrange a separate appointment for this discussion or bring a family helper to stay with the child in the waiting area. Educational needs at the time of diagnosis usually emphasize the broad scope of ADHD and address the parents' most pressing concerns. As parents and children adjust to the progression of this condition, their needs for education become more individualized to reflect the particular needs of the family. In addition, features of ADHD appear differently in early and middle childhood and adolescence. Parents and the children themselves need periodic assessment to ascertain which developmental tasks are being met and how education and support to accomplish those tasks should be focused.

Another perplexing but predictable situation arises when behavioral modifications that have worked for a period of time seem to become ineffective. Education about how normal growth and development interacts with the symptoms of ADHD should be updated as children move through developmental stages.

- Designate at least one visit (or more) per year to assess developmental milestones, acknowledge gains in skills and abilities, and plan strategies with the family to address any developmental lags.
- Routinely ask how the child's behavior is affecting the family. Plan with the family how to address the needs of the child with ADHD without eclipsing the needs of other family members.
- Routinely ask about significant changes within the family that may affect general family functioning. Individualize behavioral modifications for all family members to facilitate adjustment to changes within the family.

Family Support. Support is necessary initially to help parents understand the complexity of the diagnosis, to deal with feelings of shock or confusion, and to cope with guilt. The diagnosis of a child is often the first clue to the eventual diagnosis of an older sibling or a parent who is experiencing similar difficulties. ADHD symptoms can impact the already complex relationships within a family. Child behavior problems, maternal distress, and family conflicts all should be assessed within the family context. Evidence is mounting regarding the need to support the mothers in these families because they often mediate the relationship between the child who has distressing behaviors and family conflict (Kendall et al, 2005a).

National support groups with local affiliates can offer understanding and specific expertise in managing daily problems that come from living with a diagnosis of ADHD (see

Resource Box at the end of the chapter). Support groups are often helpful around the time of the initial diagnosis. Many families use these support group services initially and then stop attending. Families need to know that they may return to such groups during times of increased stress as children move through developmental stages or other family stressors appear. Family therapy is sometimes useful and is frequently used for short terms with goals specific to the family's current situation. With that in mind, the care provider should:

• Periodically assess the need for family support.
• Ask families if there is aggressive behavior toward family members.
• Encourage family members to offer support to other families experiencing ADHD.
• Make referrals to professionals who are experienced with clients who have ADHD and their families.

Nutrition. Monthly height, weight, body mass index, and blood pressure checks may be needed to monitor growth and potential weight loss as side effects of stimulant medications. When possible, give the morning dose before breakfast. Saltines offered with the morning dose of stimulant medication can decrease complaints of stomachaches. Providing instant breakfast drinks and other high-calorie foods to supplement calories when the child has low calorie intake because of difficulty sitting through meals or side effects of medications may be helpful.

Ask the child about his or her favorite foods and level of appetite. Diet therapy has not proven to be effective, and ADHD children should not be put on special diets. Efforts to control the child's diet can put strains on the family. Guilt can result when inevitable indiscretions occur. If the whole family goes on the diet, some members may become resentful of the affected child. Further, once the child enters school, it is very difficult for the family to fully control the child's diet.

Sleep. Many children and adults with ADHD do not require as much sleep as other people. It is important to periodically ask if the child is sleeping well and staying in bed the entire night. Ritualized bedtime routines are important to ADHD families; detailed instruction in massage, deep breathing, and relaxation techniques is sometimes helpful. It is necessary to ascertain the safety of children with ADHD who remain awake after other family members go to bed. Sleepwalking and night prowling sometimes cause safety concerns; a safety plan is needed for night prowling. Sleep problems should be addressed in a comprehensive assessment and a parent-training program.

Academic Functioning. When ADHD affects a student's academic performance, schools have a role in the management of ADHD (Hannah, 2002). IEPs are usually necessary for ADHD children. Special accommodations at school are provided by the 1997 reauthorization of the IDEA. These plans should always include academic learning objectives and behavior modification objectives. Providers who are familiar with state and federal laws and local educational resources can guide parents as they work with the school to develop the child's plan.

Frustration is common in ADHD students, their families, and school personnel. Inform parents that special assessments and evaluations can take 6 to 8 months of a school year, and children may be without special services during this entire time. IEP objectives are written in educational terms and may need to be restated in behavioral terms that children, parents, and classroom teachers can readily understand and implement. A helpful suggestion for parents is to ask that they be given a list of who is responsible for each aspect of the IEP. This spells out what is expected of the parents and individual teachers over the course of the year. Midterm or midyear monitoring of the IEP objectives is advised. A case manager may be helpful for children and adolescents who are not succeeding in school by the first grading period of each school year. School nurses and NPs in clinical settings often are well positioned to coordinate the medical, behavioral, and educational needs of children with ADHD.

• Ask parents what the IEP objectives are for the current school year and if they understand and support them. Help them identify whom to contact for clarification.
• Make sure that medication slips and medical examination forms required by schools are completed and available at the time prescriptions are renewed. This simple office routine can provide significant help to parents and schools. Keep in mind that learning and language problems can coexist with ADHD. Therefore psychoeducational testing is essential to develop an appropriate educational plan. (Box 16-1 provides suggestions for classroom adaptations.)
• When a child must take medication at school, routinely ask if there are any problems.

Psychological Interventions. The MTA Cooperative Group study (1999) supports behavioral therapy along with medications. Social skills training and cognitive-behavioral training are helpful when social skills deficits exist. However, recent reconceptualizations of ADHD suggest that this disorder is not caused by lack of knowing what behavior is appropriate, but by lack of ability to act on what is known. In addition, counseling may help with problems related to anxiety, self-esteem, and depression.

Children with ADHD may be overwhelmed by the number of adults involved with managing their symptoms. When this situation occurs, professionals should prioritize treatment recommendations in the following ways:

• Ask parents whether there is confusion or conflict about the management strategies of the professionals involved with their child to determine the best way to address these problems.
• Ask about daily and weekly schedules to determine whether the child has plenty of time for normal activities of childhood, including time to do nothing and daydream.
• Periodically assess the child and adolescent for anxiety or depression. Ask if other family members are in need of psychological assessment or support.

Advocacy. Families often need assistance in accessing educational services. Primary care providers are often in a position to exercise some influence in the local schools when services are not forthcoming. Some specialize in the care and support of ADHD children and families. Those who monitor medications and provide family support should undertake these tasks only with adequate knowledge and experience and the availability of consultation with ADHD experts.

BOX 16-1   Suggestions for Classroom Adaptations for Children With Attention-Deficit/ Hyperactivity Disorder

Memory and Attention
- Seat the child close to the teacher away from heavy traffic areas (e.g., doorways).
- Keep oral instructions brief with repetitions.
- Provide written directions.
- "Walk" the child through assignments to be sure they are understood.
- Break tasks and homework into small tasks.
- Use visual aids, hands-on, and experiential teaching methods rather than strict lecture style.
- Teach active reading with underlining and active listening with note taking.
- Provide remedial help in small sessions.
- Teach subvocalization to aid memorizing.
- Establish a hand gesture that reminds the child to focus and return to task.
- Allow nondistracting motor activity during tasks requiring concentration (e.g., squeezing a ball or fingering Velcro to replace pencil tapping).

Impulse Control
- Allow for freedom of movement as much as possible (e.g., classroom helper).
- **Never** punish the child by taking away physical education, recess, or other physical outlets.
- Teach the child to monitor quality of work before turning it in.

Classroom Atmosphere
- Provide a structured classroom with clear expectations.
- Use moderate, consistent discipline.
- Rely on positive reinforcement for good behavior.
- Provide a quiet place to work in the classroom (headsets with select music may block out distractions).

Organizational Skills
- Establish a daily checklist of tasks.
- List homework assignments in a special notebook with the due date and needed resources.
- Follow up on homework not turned in.
- Allow extra time for gathering necessary items, packing backpack, etc.
- Provide an extra set of textbooks for use at home.
- Teach strategies for time management and basic study skills.

Productivity Problems
- Divide work sheets into sections.
- Reduce the amount of homework and written class work.
- Cut down on the number of math problems to be completed.

Written Expression
- Give extra time to complete written tests and assignments.
- Provide help with handwriting.
- Allow child to dictate reports and take tests orally.
- Reduce the quantity of written work required.
- Do not reduce grades for untidy work, spelling errors, poor handwriting.

Self-Esteem
- Reward progress.
- Encourage performance in areas of child's strength.
- Avoid humiliation.
- Give hand signals only the child can see as private reminders of appropriate behavior.

Social Relationships
- Provide feedback about behavior involving other children.
- Make sure other children do not believe that the child with ADHD is doing less or is allowed unacceptable behavior; change the rules for all children, if necessary.

Adapted from Baren M: Managing ADHD, *Contemp Pediatr* 11:33, 1994; Connors S: *Catalog of accommodations for students with Tourette's syndrome, attention deficit hyperactivity disorder, and obsessive compulsive disorder*, Bayside, NY, 2005, Tourette's Syndrome Association.

Case Management Issues. Primary care providers may be in a unique position to offer case management services to ADHD families. Coordination of medical supervision, school programs, and family therapy or parent training programs is necessary for families to manage ADHD successfully.

- Ask whether the family thinks that the efforts to manage their child's ADHD are coordinated.

Complications

Children with ADHD can develop depression, problems with self-esteem, and failure to meet school educational expectations. Medication interactions and side effects are also potential complications for children with ADHD. Children with concurrent diagnoses of emotional disorders and chronic illness are at greatest risk for complications involving medication interactions. Often, different physicians prescribe medications; side effects can be missed because they mimic symptoms already present in a confusing and complicated disorder.

A cumulative effect can be seen when relationships at home, school, and in the community deteriorate, putting the child or adolescent with ADHD at risk for engaging in delinquent or socially unacceptable behaviors. High school dropout rates for adolescents with ADHD are significantly higher than those in the general population, as are rates for juvenile offenses, underemployment, and imprisonment in adulthood (Wolraich et al, 2005). By young adulthood, children with ADHD are at greater risk for addictive, mood, and anxiety disorders (Biederman et al, 2006). Illegal drug use and abuse rates are also higher among young adults with ADHD (Flory et al, 2003; Barkley, 2004; Wolraich et al, 2005; Wilson & Levin, 2005). Automobile accident rates also increase (Wolraich et al, 2005).

LEARNING DISORDERS

Description

Learning disorders, or learning disabilities as psychologists prefer, are diagnosed when an individual's achievements on individually administered standardized tests in reading, writing, or mathematics are below the expected performance based on age, education, and intelligence level (Gottesman & Kelly, 2000).

A group of disorders characterized as learning disorders share the following factors:

- The disorders are manifested by significant difficulties in acquiring and using listening, speaking, reading, writing, reasoning, and mathematic skills.
- The problems are always present in the individual and are assumed to be caused by central nervous system dysfunction.
- The disorders may occur with other handicapping conditions, such as sensory impairment, mental retardation, or emotional disturbance; cultural differences; or educational deficits, but are not caused by those conditions or influences.

Epidemiology

Learning disorders may result from a variety of genetic, constitutional, or neurodevelopmental factors. Any factor that disrupts central nervous system function may result in a learning disorder. The incidence is thought be 10% to 15% of the population.

Clinical Findings

Language processing, visual and auditory processing, memory, motor coordination, and spatial and temporal orientation difficulties are hallmarks of the condition, although a given child will probably not have difficulties in all areas.

- Reading: difficulty decoding unfamiliar words, poor comprehension and retention, slow reading rate
- Mathematics: difficulty remembering number facts, solving practical problems
- Writing: poor and labored handwriting, faulty spelling, grammar and syntax errors

Assessment

The assessment is similar to that for children with ADHD. It will include identification of risk factors, observation for characteristics of learning disorders, and consideration of other causes for the learning problems.

History

- Parent interview:
  - Functioning at home versus school
  - Coping with school
  - Birth and past medical history for risk factors
  - Developmental history
  - Family history of learning problems and level of academic achievement
  - Ability to attend to and complete tasks
  - Strengths and weaknesses of the child
  - Psychological, behavioral, and stress responses to the problems
- School review:
  - Teacher's report of academic performance, behavioral information
  - Any academic test results
- Patient assessment:
  - Child's description of the problems
  - Child's perception of the cause of the problems
  - Child's experiences at school with teachers, peers, homework

Physical Examination

- Behavioral observations
- Hearing and vision evaluation
- Physical examination, especially for neurologic problems

Differential Diagnosis

Visual or hearing problems, school absence, environmental deprivation in preschool, ADHD, fetal alcohol syndrome, lead or other toxic exposure, mental retardation, and emotional disturbance are included in the differential diagnosis.

Management

- *Educational:* In 1997, the IDEA mandated that all public schools assess and educate children with learning disabilities. The school should have a multidisciplinary team available to evaluate the child's needs and develop an IEP. The team should include a school psychologist, an educator, a special educator, a social worker, and a language specialist.

- *Parent support:* Community agencies and national organizations can provide assistance and support (see Resource Box at the end of the chapter). Parents may also need advocacy help and sometimes legal help.
- *Assistive technologies:* Read-aloud devices from text and computer programs to help remediate deficiencies may be helpful. Calculators and word processors may help circumvent handwriting problems.

DEAFNESS

Description

Deafness as a cognitive-perceptual problem is discussed here. Other information related to hearing screening and ear problems is found in Chapter 29. Deafness is classified as conductive or sensorineural. Conductive deafness is caused by a mechanical interruption of the sound waves from the external ear to the inner ear. It can sometimes be corrected through medical or surgical management. Hearing aids can be useful in assisting transmission of sound waves. Sensorineural deafness indicates inability of the inner ear or nerve to respond to sound waves. Sensorineural deafness can involve some frequencies more than others, resulting in a distortion of sound that is not helped by amplification. Central deafness is the least common hearing condition seen in children and is a problem between the brainstem and cortex in which sounds are heard but not understood. Mixed types also occur.

Epidemiology

Deafness is categorized as profound, severe, or less-than-severe. Profound deafness is deafness in which only sounds higher than 90 dB are perceived (41% of deaf children). Severe deafness is deafness to sounds 71 to 90 dB (19% of deaf children). Less-than-severe deafness is deafness to sounds less than 71 dB (33% of deaf children). The prevalence rate of newborns and infants with profound hearing loss is estimated to range between 1 and 3 per 1000 live births (AAP, 1999; Van Naarden et al, 1999).

Conductive deafness results from damage, inflammation, obstruction, or malformation of the outer or middle ear, or a combination of these. Sensorineural hearing loss is caused by damage or malformation of the inner ear or auditory nerve and accounts for 90% of all cases of serious and profound hearing loss in children (Van Naarden et al, 1999). Heredity, encephalitis, intrauterine infections, exposure to loud noise, ototoxic drugs, and premature birth with anoxia, severe jaundice, or intraventricular hemorrhage are also causes of both conductive and sensorineural hearing loss. Syndromes involving renal, cardiac, musculoskeletal, dermatologic, neurologic, and ophthalmologic systems can include deafness. Approximately 30% of prelingual deafness is related to a genetic syndrome (Jeng & Robin, 2002).

Assessment

The AAP (1999) recommends universal hearing screening of all neonates. Methods may include evoked otoacoustic emissions (EOAE) and auditory brainstem response (ABR), either alone or in combination (Haddad, 2004). Because health care professionals treat infants and toddlers on multiple occasions, there are many opportunities for screening and paying close attention to parental concerns about their child's hearing. Early identification and intervention in children with hearing impairments significantly affects the child's development, language acquisition, and academic achievement (Johnson, 2002; Haddad, 2004).

- For children with possible deafness, the provider should do a thorough assessment as described in Chapter 29 for hearing loss.
- A variety of hearing tests are described in Chapter 29.
- Vision screening should be done because deaf persons need good sight. Also Usher's syndrome, which includes deafness and later retinitis pigmentosa, may need to be identified.
- Development needs to be monitored regularly, especially in linguistic and cognitive areas.

Differential Diagnosis

Cerumen impaction, otitis media with effusion, and chronic suppurative otitis media with perforation of tympanic membrane are differential diagnoses. Consider tumor with sensorineural loss. For the child with significant hearing loss, comorbidities may exist, including developmental and communication problems, family disruptions, depression, genetic disorders, and others.

Management

Multidisciplinary Team. The use of a multidisciplinary team working with the family provides the best support for the child with a hearing impairment. The team should include a primary care provider, a physician, an audiologist, a speech and language pathologist, a sign language specialist, a teacher of the deaf, and others as needed. From an information-processing perspective, much of the management of the deaf child is directed at providing stimuli that the infant and child can use to understand and interact with the environment. Visual stimuli are used as the primary substitute for auditory deficits. Language serves not only as a communication device but also as a system for storing and using information.

Amplification Devices and Their Care. Identification and amplification before 6 months old makes a significant improvement in speech and language abilities of hearing-impaired children (Haddad, 2004). Different types of hearing aids have different purposes. The body box is used for children younger than 3 years old and for those in need of more powerful or durable amplification. Postauricular devices are used for older children. Ear molds need a good fit (sometimes revised every 3 to 6 months with growth) and careful cleaning to avoid clogging. By 4 to 6 years old, ear molds are changed yearly. Batteries last only about 100 to 150 hours and are toxic if ingested.

External otitis media can be avoided with use of petroleum jelly to decrease friction and adjustment of molds to reduce irritation. Ear molds should be washed with soap and water each night. If an infection occurs, it can usually be managed by using an antibiotic ointment and leaving the molds out for

1 to 2 days. For fungal infections, antifungal drops should be used and molds left out for 3 to 5 days.

Cochlear implants are used with some children who will not benefit from traditional hearing aids. They help children access some sounds in the environment, but positive outcomes involve multidisciplinary teams of specialists (Arts et al, 2002). Cochlear implants provided to infants who had exhibited normal hearing, even if only for a brief period in life, can result in better speech and language proficiency at 5 years old (Geers, 2004). Children with cochlear implants have been found to have better motor development, verbal development, and attention at 5 to 9 years old (Schlumberger et al, 2004).

Communication Needs. Communication needs can be supported by the use of text telephone devices, smoke alarms and doorbells with lights instead of alarms, a hearing ear dog, and other communication systems in the child's environment.

Family Support. Often there is stress for the family when the diagnosis is made. Siblings may need support as they cope in a family with a child identified as having a disabling condition (Bat-Chava & Martin, 2002). Parents often need counseling, support, and information related to their acceptance and parenting of the identified child. Grandparents and extended family can also need information and support.

Children with hearing impairments are at higher risk than the general population for child maltreatment and neglect (Sullivan & Knutson, 1998). The most prevalent form of maltreatment among deaf children is child neglect (Sullivan et al, 2000). Children with hearing impairments often demonstrate more behavior problems than their peers and need mental health services with professionals experienced in treating children with disabilities. Periodic screening for family stress and child maltreatment is an important part of well child care.

Education. Children identified with hearing loss by 6 months old who received early intervention services had better language development than children identified later (Yoshinaga-Itano et al, 1998). Deaf children need opportunities to learn by using their strongest modalities. Language and communication needs are paramount. There are several schools of thought related to education of the deaf. Oralists focus on amplification, speech reading, and speech training. They do not support exposure to sign language. Those who believe in the total communication approach counter that the use of sign language links the deaf to the deaf community and increases their acquisition of language and functioning in adulthood. Total communication methods include amplification, sign language, finger spelling, speech reading, and speech training. Parents are sometimes pressured by professionals or other deaf people to accept one approach over the other.

Parents also need education to communicate with their child effectively. One study indicates that two-thirds of children learn sign language, but only one-half of parents learn the same language. Lederberg and Everhart (1998) found that mothers of deaf 2-year-olds primarily communicated with their children by speech, even though the children did not visually attend. Thus, in some families, parents and children cannot fully communicate with one another. Early education for deaf children should begin in infancy. Educational services

need to be family centered and culturally sensitive. American Sign Language (ASL) is the language the deaf use with one another, and it provides the strongest link with the deaf community for the child.

Interpreter Services. If children sign, they should be provided with an interpreter during health care visits. Deaf children may have inadequate health care information and knowledge because of poor communication between provider and child.

Genetic Counseling. Refer families for genetic counseling if the problem is inheritable.

BLINDNESS
Description
Blindness varies from inability to distinguish light from darkness to *partial vision,* defined as visual acuity between 20/70 and 20/200 best corrected. *Legal blindness* is defined as distant visual acuity of 20/200 in the better eye or a visual field that includes an angle not greater than 20 degrees.

Children with visual impairments experience developmental delays. Children with blindness plus other handicapping conditions will have greater developmental delays. Blindness affects bonding, wakefulness, balance, gross and fine motor functions, spatial concepts, language, and learning. Children with blindness have a tendency to develop stereotyped motor behaviors. In one study, all 9 children with blindness alone walked independently at a mean of 19.8 months old, whereas only 1 of 11 children with blindness and associated handicaps walked independently. The remaining 10 of that group displayed an absence of almost all neuromotor skills (Fazzi et al, 2002). Refer to Table 16-1 for a summary of some developmental milestones to be expected.

Epidemiology
Blindness is caused by a variety of pathologic conditions, including congenital cataracts, congenital glaucoma, high refractive errors, retinopathy of prematurity (ROP), detached retina, neurologic conditions involving cranial nerve II, cortical blindness, and optic atrophy. ROP is the most common cause of severe visual impairment. Retinoblastoma, trauma, infection, hydrocephaly, and genetic conditions are also etiologic factors. Abruptio placentae is a strong risk factor for blindness. Increased risks also exist for low birth-weight, small-for-gestational age and large-for-gestational age babies. Preeclampsia and breech deliveries also increase risks (Tornqvist & Kallen, 2004). See Chapter 28 for more information.

About 1 in 500 children in the U.S. has partial vision, whereas about 35,000 children are legally blind (Olitsky & Nelson, 2004). Up to 30% to 70% of visually handicapped children have additional handicaps, including mental retardation, deafness, seizures, and cerebral palsy (Mervis et al, 2000).

Assessment
Primary care providers need to remember that the blind child needs special cues to understand the environment. Talk softly to the infant or child before touching and look for a variety of body cues rather than visual or facial signals. Be gentle in touching because the child has no warning that contact is coming.

For older children, address the child by name, describe what you plan to do and how, warn the child of contacts or discomforts anticipated, and let the child touch or examine instruments when possible.

Signs and Symptoms of Blindness. Characteristics to assess include the following:
- History of failure of the infant to follow a moving object or wandering eyes
- Poking the eyes or waving the hands in front of the face
- Nystagmus
- Failure to blink at a camera flash in front of the face
- Failure to fix and follow by 6 weeks
- Photophobia or chronic tearing
- History of prematurity with diagnosis of ROP
- Fixed strabismus or intermittent strabismus persisting longer than 6 months
- Lack of smiling in response to visual stimuli
  The following should also be assessed:
- Family history of genetic visual impairments
- Family issues and environment
- General medical history
- Developmental history (attachment, midline play, reaching, gross motor skills, language skills)

Physical Examination. The physical examination should include a search for the following:
- Enlarged or cloudy cornea
- Abnormal or absent red reflex
- Lack of pupillary reflex
- Nystagmus
- Neurologic disorder

Other Tests. Regular ophthalmologic examinations and developmental testing are also recommended.

Differential Diagnosis

See the etiologic factors discussed earlier. Complex ophthalmologic studies are often needed to diagnose the cause of blindness. These are best done by specialists.

Management

Multidisciplinary Team. The primary care provider, ophthalmologist, special certification teacher, and orientation and mobility specialist are among important team members for visually impaired children and their families. Genetics counselors, social workers, and other specialists can also be useful.

Family Support. As noted, families with blind children adapt in a variety of ways. Because visual cues are so important in language and social interactions, the family of the blind child may experience difficulties with attachment resulting from failure of eye contact and facial expressiveness. For instance, smiling is not recognized or imitated by the blind infant. Families of children with visual impairment may benefit from specialized anticipatory guidance designed to facilitate development throughout childhood. One hospital found that designating a health care worker to accompany families and patients to key diagnostic visits and serve as a first contact person with support and information about educational,

social, and multidisciplinary health care services had positive outcomes for families (Rahl et al, 2004).

Parent support groups are valuable, and national organizations provide reading materials that are very helpful (see Resource Box). Sometimes families benefit from counseling.

Education. Public school educational programs for the visually impaired child include several distinct models. Infant early education and developmental preschool programs are essential. When children are ready to enter elementary school, full-time classes for blind children are sometimes available. These are taught by teachers with special certification to work with the blind. Some schools have resource-room programs where the child spends part of the day with a specially trained teacher and the remainder of the day in a regular classroom. Some school districts provide itinerant programs in which a specially trained teacher works with several teachers in regular classrooms, consulting with them about the learning needs of the visually handicapped children involved. Schools for the blind are generally reserved for children with multiple handicaps.

IEPs need to be developed annually, with input from both parents and school officials. When the child enters school, psychological assessments need to be done using tests designed for blind children to ensure correct educational placement and appropriate educational support systems.

Educational programs for visually handicapped children need to include some extra components. Blind children begin learning Braille when sighted children learn to read. They learn to write Braille in the early elementary grades by using a special typewriter. By fourth grade, blind children should also learn to use a regular typewriter. Developing additional listening skills and gaining proficiency in the use of computers with aids are also essential skills. The Optacon is a hand-held device that translates printed text into tactile displays. Children are ready to use this device at about 10 years old. The ViewScan can be used by partially sighted individuals to enlarge type size for reading text on a screen.

Daily living skills include dressing, eating, hygiene, use of the telephone, and handling money. An orientation and mobility specialist teaches the visually handicapped child to travel with a sighted guide, use a cane, and use public transportation.

Physical education and fitness are as important to visually impaired children as to other children. Generally, individual sports, such as gymnastics and swimming, are more successful endeavors for a blind child than team sports, even if the child is partially sighted.

Developmental Interventions. Some strategies that parents can use to promote development in their visually impaired infant or child are found in Table 16-6.

AUTISTIC SPECTRUM DISORDER (ASD): AUTISM, ASPERGER SYNDROME, PERVASIVE DEVELOPMENTAL DISORDERS

Description

Autism is a "complex neurodevelopmental disorder characterized by impaired reciprocal social interaction, impaired communication, and restricted, repetitive, or stereotyped behaviors" (Barbaresi et al, 2006, p 1167). It is a lifelong disability

TABLE 16-6   Developmental Interventions for Visually Impaired Infants and Children

Age	Psychosocial	Cognitive	Motor
Birth-4 months	Hold and talk to the infant to promote recognition through tactile and auditory modalities.	Stimulate the hands and mouth. Provide a cradle gym so that reaching and touching give feedback. Provide toys with feedback, such as sound, interesting textures, or tastes.	Encourage the prone position at times while awake, a position that blind children do not generally like, because they have no reinforcement visually for lifting the head. Also encourage head turning. Bring the hands into midline. Exercise the legs and massage during baths and diaper changes. Put bells on booties.
5-8 months	Stranger anxiety occurs early. Parents need to be available. Provide predictable routines.	Provide finger foods. Provide new temperatures, textures, toys with various sounds and sensations. Talk to the child. Call attention to music and other sounds in the environment.	Encourage play out of doors and on the floor. Dance and move the child actively.
9-12 months	Provide predictable routines. Touch and voice are all important. Cuddle.	Encourage reaching to find a sound source. Provide toys that respond to the actions of the child to develop cause-and-effect concepts. Name and describe the activities and items in the environment.	Encourage creeping about, which will occur after the child can reach for a sound. Help to stand and cruise. Touch and name body parts.
13-24 months	Stranger anxiety continues. Reassure toddler of return. Regression and tantrums are frustration responses. Guide behavior into more appropriate responses. Reduce frustrations when possible.	Continue to work on object permanence concept, which is delayed. Noncontingent sounds, such as television or radio, are not helpful.	Walking should begin. Crab walking is a common problem that needs to be eliminated. Walking with the child's feet on the adult's can help develop the reciprocal pattern. "Blindisms" may appear and can be altered with teaching. Walk together both indoors and outdoors.
2-5 years	Interactions with peers and sighted children. Establish behavioral limits as with sighted children. Teach self-help skills—hygiene, feeding, dressing.	Teach games with directional concepts Provide experiences in a variety of settings—park, grocery, etc.	Develop motor skills— walking, concepts. climbing, swimming.
6-10 years	Continue to develop social skills and develop self-esteem through opportunities to be successful in activities. Provide opportunities to be with other children. Continue to develop self-help skills.	School with additional supports for the visually impaired. Braille and computer education.	Specific mobility training.

Data from Lewis V: *Development and disability,* Philadelphia, 2003, Blackwell; Teplin S: Visual handicaps. In Green M, Haggerty R, editors: *Ambulatory pediatrics,* Philadelphia, 1999, WB Saunders.

that usually becomes apparent in the first 3 years of life. Development is uneven, with occasional talent in a limited area, such as music or mathematics, coupled with severe deficits in other areas. Many autistic children have other impairments, such as mental retardation (60% to 75%) or seizures. The disorder varies considerably in severity.

The diagnostic criteria for autism require the presence of six symptoms from three categories. Box 16-2 lists these categories. In general, they encompass problems with social interactions, communication, and language skills with abnormal ways of relating to people, objects, and events; abnormal responses to sensory stimuli, usually sound; and restricted, repetitive, or stereotyped behaviors and echolalic speech. Sleep disturbances are also common among children with autism.

Milder forms of autistic spectrum disorder (ASD) are Asperger syndrome and pervasive developmental disorder—not otherwise specified (PDD-nos). Asperger syndrome consists of qualitative impairments in development of social interactions. Language is not as severely impaired as it is with autism. Clinical findings include repetitive movements and restricted, obsessional interests. The person with Asperger syndrome may appear "eccentric" to others.

Whether this condition is a distinct diagnosis or a milder form of autism with higher functioning has not been determined (Dalton et al, 2004). See Box 16-3 for "red flags" for autism screening.

Epidemiology

There is good evidence of a genetic link for some types of autism (10%). Other causes include prenatal infections, such as congenital rubella or cytomegalovirus, and neonatal infections. The cause is unknown for most cases. A hypothesized relationship with measles-mumps-rubella (MMR) vaccine has not been supported (AAP Committee on Children with Disabilities, 2001; Nelson & Bauman, 2003).

The incidence rate for autism is about 6.7:1000 children. The ratio of male to female children is 2.8 to 5.5:1(CDC, 2007).

Assessment

When behavior difficulties are first addressed by health care professionals, fewer than 10% of children with autism are diagnosed, and most families report little help after multiple visits (Report of the Quality Standards Subcommittee, 2000).

BOX 16-2   **Diagnostic Criteria for Autistic Disorders**

A. A total of more than six items from the following criteria with at least two from criterion 1 and one each from criteria 2 and 3:
  1. Qualitative impairment in social interaction as manifested by at least two of the following:
    a. Marked impairment in the use of multiple nonverbal behaviors, such as eye-to-eye gaze, facial expression, body posture, and gestures to regulate social interaction
    b. Failure to develop peer relationships appropriate to developmental level
    c. Lack of spontaneous seeking to share enjoyment, interests, or achievements with other people (lack of showing, bringing, or pointing out objects of interest)
  2. Qualitative impairments in communication as manifested by at least one of the following:
    a. Delay in or total lack of development of spoken language (not accompanied by an attempt to compensate through alternative modes of communication, such as gesture or mime)
    b. In individuals with adequate speech, marked impairment in the ability to initiate or sustain a conversation
    c. Stereotyped and repetitive use of language or idiosyncratic language
    d. Lack of varied, spontaneous make-believe play or social imitative play appropriate to developmental level
  3. Restricted, repetitive, and stereotyped patterns of behavior, interests, and activities as manifested by at least one of the following:
    a. Encompassing preoccupation with one or more stereotyped and restricted patterns of interest that is abnormal either in intensity or focus
    b. Apparently inflexible adherence to specific, nonfunctional routines or rituals
    c. Stereotyped and repetitive motor mannerisms (e.g., hand or finger flapping or twisting, or complex whole-body movements)
    d. Persistent preoccupation with parts of objects
B. Delay or abnormal functioning in at last one of the following areas with onset before 3 years old:
  1. Social interaction
  2. Language as used in social communication
  3. Symbolic or imaginative play
C. Disturbance not better accounted for by Rett disorder or childhood disintegrative disorder

Data from the American Psychiatric Association (APA): *Diagnostic and statistical manual of mental disorders,* ed 4, text revision, Washington, DC, 2000, American Psychiatric Association.

| BOX 16-3 | Red Flags for Autism Screening |

- Failure to meet childhood developmental milestones
- Sibling with autism
- Problems with eye contact
- Child does not respond to his or her name
- Not babbling or gesturing by 12 months old
- No single words by 16 months old
- No two-word (not echolalic) phrases by 24 months old
- Loss of any language or social abilities at any age

Data from Report of the Quality Standards Subcommittee of the American Academy of Neurology and the Child Neurology Society: Practice parameter: screening and diagnosis of autism, *Neurology* 55:468-479, 2000.

Early identification is important because intervention services may be more effective if started early in the child's life. A two-step early identification process should be followed in which children who fail routine developmental screening (step 1) should be screened for autism (step 2). Diagnosis should be made by experts in the field.

Signs and Symptoms by Age

Infants. An autistic infant may be a passive, nonengaging, quiet, floppy infant or a difficult, colicky, stiff baby with poor eye contact. Attachment problems appear. There is failure to respond to name or gestures. Usually, autism is not identified in infancy although some development problems, especially in the social arena, are emerging.

Toddlers. During the toddler stage, parents are convinced that something is wrong with their child. Language delays, lack of social relatedness, and severe behavior problems are common. Expressive language is delayed. Socially the child exhibits detachment, decreased eye contact, a lack of fear, and poor creative play skills. Tantrums that persist; repetitive movements; a preference to line, stack, or spin toys; and insistence on routines are commonly observed behaviors. Use of echolalia is persistent. Children will have relative strengths in visual-motor problem-solving and delays in language (Barbaresi et al, 2006). The Modified Checklist for Autism in Toddlers (M-CHAT) is one of several scales developed to identify autism in 24-month-old children.

Preschoolers. Language delays include lack of meaningful speech, decreased gestures, and gaze disturbances. Social interaction disturbances, such as lack of fear of strangers, invasion of the territory of others, preference to be alone, and lack of social awareness, are often seen. Persistent and insistent behaviors are common. Symbolic play is limited. The child may have precocious or average development of rote memory skills but often without comprehension of concepts.

School-Age Children. School-age children with autism often lack reciprocal friendships and continue with language, social, and behavioral problems. Transitions from place to place and activity to activity are difficult. Behaviors are ritualistic.

Adolescents. Adolescents usually continue with similar behaviors. Rote learning is possible, but comprehension lags. It should be noted, however, that some high-functioning autistic children are mainstreamed and do very well in regular classrooms. Mildly affected persons may have social relationship problems.

History. Developmental history is essential. A family history may reveal other members with pervasive developmental disorder, autism, speech delay or language deficits, mood disorders, or mental retardation. The review of systems should investigate seizures, hearing loss, head injury, and meningitis.

Physical Examination. The child should be checked for general appearance of genetic syndromes and neurologic findings of focal abnormalities.

Other Tests. Evaluation of the child for autism is best done at a specialty center. It is a diagnosis by exclusion. Testing should include the following:

- Developmental and IQ testing
- Behavioral assessment
- Audiologic evaluation
- Periodic lead screening because the children have a high prevalence for putting things in their mouths
- DNA analysis for fragile X syndrome and high-resolution chromosome analyses, especially in those with mental retardation, dysmorphic features, congenital anomalies, or a family history of autism or mental retardation. Fluorescence in situ hybridization (FISH) testing for specific chromosome problems should follow if first DNA analyses are negative.
- Metabolic testing if there is a history of developmental plateauing or deterioration, decompensation with illnesses, unusual odors, food intolerances, failure to thrive, seizures, cyclic vomiting, questionable newborn screening results, or other indicators of metabolic disease.
- Electroencephalogram (EEG) if needed for seizures (Barbaresi et al, 2006).
- Computed tomography scans and magnetic resonance imaging are not routinely indicated (Barbaresi et al, 2006; AAP Committee on Children with Disabilities, 2001).

Differential Diagnosis

Two levels of diagnosis are required: the first in primary care for screening and early identification; the second, by specialists, to investigate identified children and differentiate autism from other developmental disorders (Report of the Quality Standards Subcommittee, 2000).

Gifted child, elective mutism, obsessive-compulsive disorder, Tourette syndrome, schizophrenia of childhood, conduct disorder, mental retardation, Rett syndrome, hearing impairment, lead poisoning, phenylketonuria, tuberous sclerosis, and fragile X syndrome are all differential diagnoses for autism. Asperger syndrome includes characteristics of mild autism but without language or developmental delays. Children with ADHD may appear rigid, whereas children with autism may seem poorly focused.

Management

Management of children with ASD is complex and will require a multidisciplinary approach. A focus on interactive patterns is the mainstay of management of autism. Children need social skills training, early and intense developmental work, and assistance with learning. Early intervention programs offer diverse approaches for autistic children; it is important to match the aim of interventions to the individual needs of each child for optimal outcomes (Erba, 2000).

Behavior. The most important aspect of management is behavioral training. The target behaviors vary according to age, developmental level, and disruptiveness of behaviors. Reasonable goals need to be set (AAP Committee on Children with Disabilities, 2001). The applied behavior analysis (ABA) approach to development of appropriate behaviors in autistic children is considered an optimal strategy. It involves teaching new behaviors using operant conditioning while using data to modify interventions to promote specific learning objectives. Another well-researched model is TEACCH (Treatment and Education of Autistic and Related Communication Handicapped Children) though TEACCH has relatively less well-documented outcomes (Barbaresi et al, 2006).

Education. Extensive assessment and early, intense intervention are necessary to maximize educational abilities and enhance learning for children with autism. Planning for care requires cognitive testing to identify the child's strengths and weaknesses, in addition to social, behavioral, and language assessment. Early intervention programs for preschoolers, school-based special education, and information and assistance for school personnel are essential.

When special abilities are discovered in children with autism, attempts should be made to encourage opportunities for success in these areas. Although these children may not be successful in many educational activities, this should not preclude their participation in areas where they have talents or excel. A child with musical or mathematical gifts, for example, may not be able to complete other grade-level work or tolerate the social demands required to demonstrate his or her special abilities. Accommodations to advance children in the areas of their unique abilities are necessary, and parents and school personnel will need to become skilled advocates for the child. Protection from unrealistic expectations of social competence is often necessary to help the child with autism to succeed. "The long-term goal should be to permit the child to function as effectively and comfortably as possible in the least restrictive environment" (Bauer, 1995, p. 32).

Medication. None works well. Haloperidol is sometimes used, but it can have serious side effects, including dyskinesias. Usually, autistic children do not benefit from stimulant medications. Fluoxetine (Prozac) may be helpful for some if they are also depressed. Because 25% of autistic children also have seizures, they may be given anticonvulsants. Atypical antipsychotics, such as risperidone, are sometimes used for aggression and other difficult behaviors (FDA, 2006). Medication should never be used in isolation to treat autism.

Diet. No significant effects result from special diets.

Family Counseling and Support. Families need a great deal of support and training to manage children with autism. They may benefit from assistance from members of the Autism Society of America (see Resource Box).

- The family and siblings may need supportive counseling and referral because of the considerable stress found in families with children with autism.
- Long-term care needs to be addressed because few autistic children become fully independent, employed adults, although the prognosis for children with autism is highly variable and very difficult to predict. Those who are highly functioning as children will do best as adults.

Alternative Therapies and Sensory Integration Therapy. Autism is a chronic disorder. To date, there is no cure. Neither is there scientific evidence that supports alternative interventions, such as restricted gluten and casein-free diets to minimize opioid-like peptide absorption (the leaky gut hypothesis), or an autoimmune disorder that would benefit from intravenous immunoglobulins (AAP Committee on Children with Disabilities, 2001). There is no support for mercury causation from vaccines, bacterial or fungal contamination, and the pancreatic enzyme, secretin, has not been shown to be effective in treating autism. Clinicians should counsel parents that they will be confronted with some of these theories. Parents should be sure that they only consider evidence from randomized, double-blind, placebo-controlled clinical trials published in peer-reviewed journals and realize that "such treatments may take time, effort, and financial resources away from effective, evidence-based interventions" (Barbaresi et al, 2006, p. 1171).

There is no empirical support for sensory integration therapy, and it should not be routinely recommended nor viewed as a primary intervention strategy for autistic children. Facilitated communication, auditory integration training, and music therapy are also not supported as effective interventions (Barbaresi et al, 2006).

RESOURCE BOX

Resources for Cognitive-Perceptual Problems of Children

ADHD
ADD WareHouse
www.addwarehouse.com
Distributors for all ADHD literature published for children, parents, professionals, and educators

Children and Adults With Attention Deficit Hyperactivity Disorders (CHADD)
www.chadd.org
Six hundred local chapters, educational literature, newsletter available with membership

National Attention Deficit Disorder Association
www.add.org

DEAFNESS
Alexander Graham Bell Association for the Deaf and Hard of Hearing (AGBAD)
www.agbell.org

American Association of Deaf-Blind
www.aadb.org

American Society for Deaf Children (ASDC)
www.deafchildren.org

Cochlear Implant Association
www.listen-up.org/ci/ci-information.htm

Imagery Language and Visual Communication
www.handspeak.com

Laurent Clerc National Deaf Education Center Gallaudet University
www.clerccenter.gallaudet.edu

National Association of the Deaf (NAD)
www.nad.org

S.E.E. (Signing Exact English) Center for Advancement of Deaf Children
www.seecenter.org

Telecommunications for the Deaf and Hard of Hearing
www.tdi-online.org

BLINDNESS
American Council of the Blind (ACB)
www.acb.org

American Foundation for the Blind (AFB)
www.afb.org

Blind Children's Fund (BCF)
www.blindchildrensfund.org

National Association for Parents of Children with Visual Impairments (NAPVI)
www.spedex.com/napvi
A national organization that enables parents to find information and resources for their children who are blind or visually impaired, including those with additional disabilities

National Federation of the Blind—Division for Parents of Blind Children
www.nfb.org

AUTISM
Autism Research Institute
www.autism.com/ari

Autism Society of America
www.autism-society.org

Treatment and Education of Autistic and Related Communication-Handicapped Children (TEACCH)
www.teacch.com

ALL CHILDREN WITH DISABILITIES
Family Voices
www.familyvoices.org
Advocacy for children and youth with special health care needs

National Disseminated Center for Children and Youth With Disabilities
www.nichcy.org
Source for age-appropriate books

National Family Association of the Deaf-Blind
www.nfadb.org

National Institute on Deafness and Other Communication Disorders
www.nidcd.nih.gov

NURSING DIAGNOSES

Nursing Diagnoses Related to Cognitive-Perceptual Functional Health Pattern

Diagnoses are related to the concepts: environmental interpretation, sensory perception, and cognition—knowledge, memory, thought processes.

- Confusion (acute or chronic)
  - Risk for acute confusion
- Deficient knowledge (specify)
- Readiness for enhanced knowledge
- Disorganized infant behavior
  - Risk for disorganized infant behavior
  - Readiness for enhanced organized infant behavior
- Disturbed sensory perception (specify sense)
- Disturbed thought processes
- Impaired environmental interpretation syndrome
- Impaired memory

From NANDA International: *NANDA-I nursing diagnoses: definitions & classification 2007-2008,* Philadelphia, 2007, Author.

✓ DISCUSSION FORUM

1. How would a visual or auditory deficit impact a child's cognitive-perceptual development? Cite specific examples for infants, toddlers, preschoolers, school age, and adolescents.
2. Make a list of agencies in your community that provide services to help meet the educational, social, or physical needs of children with ADHD, visual deficits, auditory deficits, or pervasive developmental disorders.
3. You see a 7-year-old who was told by his teacher that "he needs treatment for ADHD." What assessment strategies will you use to establish this possible diagnosis? Create a plan of care to manage a child with ADHD that includes this child's physical, developmental, social, and family needs.
4. You see a 2-month-old for a well-child check. She has been blind since birth as a result of congenital cataracts. What anticipatory guidance related to this infant's visual deficit do you give this family? How will the anticipatory guidance change during the first and second year of life?
5. You are asked to speak to a mothers of preschoolers group about how to distinguish behaviors that indicate ADHD and pervasive developmental disorder from normal preschool behavior. What information will you provide this group? What will you tell these parents about the comorbidities associated with these disorders?
6. The mother of a 4-year-old who was diagnosed with autism at 3 years old comes in for a well-child exam for her 2-year-old. She is concerned that her younger child may have autistic-like behaviors and wants her second child evaluated for a pervasive developmental disorder. What screening is appropriate for a child this age? What pharmacologic and nonpharmacologic interventions would be appropriate for a newly diagnosed 2-year-old with PDD? Make sure you include guidelines for referral and consultation and follow-up.

REFERENCES

Adesman AR: New medications for treatment of children with attention deficit hyperactivity disorder: review and commentary, *Pediatr Ann* 31:514-521, 2002.

American Academy of Pediatrics (AAP): Newborn and infant hearing loss: detection and intervention, *Pediatrics* 103:527-530, 1999.

American Academy of Pediatrics (AAP) Committee on Quality Improvement and Subcommittee on Attention Deficit Hyperactivity Disorder: Clinical practice guideline: treatment of the school age child with attention deficit hyperactivity disorder, *Pediatrics* 108:1033-1044, 2001.

American Academy of Pediatrics Committee (AAP) on Quality Improvement and Subcommittee on Attention Deficit Hyperactivity Disorder: Diagnosis and evaluation of the child with attention deficit hyperactivity disorder, *Pediatrics* 105:1158-1170, 2000.

American Psychiatric Association (APA): *Diagnostic and statistical manual of mental disorders,* ed 4, text revision, Washington, DC, 2000, American Psychiatric Association.

Arts HA, Garber A, Zwolan TA: Cochlear implants in young children, *Otolaryngol Clin North Am* 35:925-943, 2002.

Atkinson R, Shiffrin R: Human memory: a proposed system and its control processes. In Spence K, Spence J, editors: *Advances in the psychology of learning and motivation research and theory,* vol 2, New York, 1968, Academic Press.

Barbaresi WJ, Katusic SK, Voight RG: Autism: a review of the state of the science for pediatic primary health care clinicians, *Arch Pediatr Adoles Med* 160:1167-1175, 2006.

Barkley RA: *ADHD and the nature of self control,* New York, 1997, Guilford Press.

Barkley RA: Adolescents with attention deficit/hyperactivity disorder: an overview of empirically based treatments, *J Psychiatr Pract* 10(1):39-56, 2004.

Bat-Chava Y, Martin D: Sibling relationships of deaf children: the impact of child and family characteristics, *Rehabil Psychol* 47:73-91, 2002.

Bauer S: Autism and the pervasive developmental disorders: part 2, *Pediatr Rev* 16:168-176, 1995.

Biederman J et al: Adult outcome of attention deficit hyperactivity disorder: a controlled 10-year follow-up study, *Psychol Med* 36:167-179, 2006.

Braun J et al: *Exposures to environmental toxicants and attention deficit hyperactivity disorder in US children* (2006). Available at *www.ehponline. org/docs/2006/9478/abstract.html* (accessed Oct 13, 2006).

Breen MJ, Altpeter TS: Factor structures of the home situations questionnaire and the school situations questionnaire, *J Ped Psych* 16:59-67, 1991.

Brown R et al, American Academy of Pediatrics Committee on Quality Improvement, American Academy of Pediatrics Subcommittee on Attention-Deficit/Hyperactivity Disorder: Treatment of attention-deficit/hyperactivity disorder: overview of the evidence, *Pediatrics* 115:749-757, 2005.

Buitelaar J et al: Comparison of North American versus Non-North American ADHD study populations, *Eur Child Adolesc Psychiatry* 15:177-181, 2006.

Bull C, Whelan T: Parental schemata in the management of children with attention deficit-hyperactivity disorder, *Qualitative Health Res* 16(5):664-678, 2006.

Centers for Disease Control and Prevention (CDC): Prevalence of autism spectrum disorders-autism and developmental disabilities monitoring network, six sites, United States, 2000, *MMWR* 56(SS01):1-11, 2007.

Dalton R et al: Pervasive developmental disorders and childhood psychoses, In Behrman R, Kliegman R, Jenson H, editors: *Nelson textbook of pediatrics,* ed 17, Philadelphia, 2004, WB Saunders.

Elster A, Kuznets N: *AMA guidelines for adolescent preventive services (GAPS),* Baltimore, 1994, Williams & Wilkins.

Erba HW: Early intervention programs for children with autism: conceptual frameworks for implementation, *Am J Orthopsychiatry* 70:82-94, 2000.

Faraone SV: The genetics of attention-deficit/hyperactivity disorder: current status and clinical implications, *Medscape Psychiatry Mental Health* 11(2), 2006. Available at *www.medscape.com/viewarticle/546469* (accessed Nov 8, 2006).

Fazzi E et al: Gross motor development and reach on sound as critical tools for the development of the blind child, *Brain Dev* 24(5):269-275, 2002.

Food and Drug Administration (FDA): *FDA approves the first drug to treat irritability associated with autism, Risperdal* (2006). Available at *www.fda. gov/bbs/topics/NEWS/2006/NEW01485.html* (accessed Nov 11, 2006).

Flory K et al: Relation between childhood disruptive behavior disorders and substance use and dependence symptoms in young adulthood: individuals with symptoms of attention-deficit/hyperactivity disorder and conduct disorder are uniquely at risk, *Psychol Addict Behav* 17: 151-158, 2003.

Gadomski A et al: Guidelines for adolescent preventive services, *Arch Pediatr Adolesc Med* 157:426-432, 2003

Gedaly-Duff V, Stoeger S, Shelton K: Working with families. In Nickel RE, Desch LW, editors: *The physician's guide to caring for children with disabilities and chronic conditions,* Baltimore, 2000, Brookes.

Geers A: Speech, language, and reading skills after early cochlear implantation, *Arch Otolaryngol, Head Neck Surg* 130:634-638, 2004.

Gordon M: *Nursing diagnosis: process and application,* New York, 1987, McGraw-Hill.

Gottesman R, Kelly M: Helping children with learning disabilities toward a brighter adulthood, *Contemp Pediatr* 17:42-61, 2000.

Greenhill L et al: Impairment and deportment responses to different methylphenidate doses in children with ADHD: the MTA titration trial, *J Am Acad Child Adolesc Psychiatry* 40:180-187, 2001.

Gregory S, Mogford K: Early language development in deaf children. In Kyle WJ, Deucher M, editors: *Perspectives on British sign language and deafness,* London, 1981, Croon Helm.

Haddad J: Hearing loss. In Behrman R, Kliegman R, Jenson H, editors: *Nelson textbook of pediatrics,* ed 17, Philadelphia, 2004, WB Saunders.

Hannah JN: The role of schools in attention deficit hyperactivity disorder, *Pediatr Ann* 31:507-513, 2002.

Hansen DL, Hansen EH: Caught in a balancing act: parents' dilemmas regarding their ADHD child's treatment with stimulant medication, *Qualitative Health Res* 16(9):1267-1285, 2006.

Jeng L, Robin N: Progress in understanding the genetics of impaired hearing, *Contemp Pediatr* 19:79-96, 2002.

Jensen P et al: ADHD comorbidity findings from the MTA study: comparing comorbid subgroups, *J Am Acad Child Adolesc Psychiatry* 40:147-158, 2001.

Johnson AN: Update on newborn hearing screening programs, *Pediatr Nurs* 28:267-270. 2002.

Kelly D: Neurodevelopmental dysfunction in the school-aged child. In Behrman R, Kliegman R, Jenson H, editors: *Nelson textbook of pediatrics,* ed 17, Philadelphia, 2004, WB Saunders.

Kendall J: Outlasting disruption: process of reinvesting in families with ADHD children, *Qualitative Health Res* 8:839-857, 1998.

Kendall J et al: Service needs of families with children with ADHD, *J Fam Nurs* 11:264-288, 2005a.

Kendall J et al: Modeling ADHD child and family relationships, *West J Nurs Res,* 27:500-518. 2005b.

Knafl K et al: Family response to childhood chronic illness: description of management styles, *J Pediatr Nurs* 11:315-326, 1996.

Knafl K, Dietrick J, Kirby A: Normalization promotion. In Craft-Rosenberg M, Denehy J, editors: *Nursing interventions for infants, children, and families,* Thousand Oaks, CA, 2001, Sage.

Lederberg A, Everhart V: Communication between deaf children and their hearing mothers: the role of language, gesture, and vocalizations, *J Speech Lang Hear Res* 41:887-899, 1998.

Levine M, Brooks R, Shonkoff J: *A pediatric approach to learning disorders,* New York, 1980, Wiley.

Levine M, Carey W, Crocker A: *Developmental-behavioral pediatrics,* ed 3, Philadelphia, 1999, WB Saunders.

Liptak GS et al: Satisfaction with primary health care received by families of children with developmental disabilities, *J Pediatr Health Care* 20(4):245-52, 2006.

Low LK: Guidelines for adolescent preventive services (GAPS), *J Midwifery Womens Health* 48:321-233; 2003.

Magyary D, Brandt P, Kovalesky A: *Children with ADHD: a manual with decision tree and clinical path,* Seattle, 1999, University of Washington.

Meadow K: *Deafness and child development,* Berkeley, CA, 1980, University of California Press.

Meadow-Orlans KP: Research on developmental aspects of deafness. In Moores DE, Meadow-Orlans KP, editors: *Educational and developmental aspect of deafness,* Washington, DC, 1990, Gallaudet University Press.

Mervis C, Yeargin-Allsopp M, Winter S: Aetiology of childhood visual impairment, metropolitan Atlanta, 1991-93, *Paediatr Perinat Epidemiol* 14:70, 2000.

MMWR: *Mental Health in the United States: Prevalence of Diagnosis and Medication Treatment for Attention-Deficit/Hyperactivity Disorder-United States, 2003* (2005). Available at *www.cdc.gov/mmwr/preview/mmwrhtml/ mm5434a2.htm* (accessed Jan 31, 2006).

MTA Cooperative Group: A 14-month randomized clinical trial of treatment strategies for attention-deficit hyperactivity disorder. The MTA Cooperative Group. Multimodal treatment study of children with ADHD, *Arch Gen Psychiatry* 56:1073-1086, 1999.

Nelson KB, Bauman ML: Thimerosal and autism? *Pediatrics* 111:e277-282, 2003.

Norvilitis J, Fang P: Perceptions of ADHD in China and the United States: a preliminary study, *J Atten Disord* 9:413-424, 2005.

Olfson M: New options in the pharmacological management of attention-deficit/hyperactivity disorder, *Am J Managed Care* 10:S117-S123, 2004.

Olitsky S, Nelson L: Disorders of the eye. In Behrman R, Kliegman R, Jenson H, editors: *Nelson's textbook of pediatrics,* ed 17, Philadelphia, 2004, WB Saunders.

Phillips S, Hartley JT: Developmental differences and interventions for blind children, *Pediatr Nurs* 14(3):201-204, 1988.

Pliszka S: Practice parameter for the assessment and treatment of children and adolescents with attention-deficit/hyperactivity disorder, *I Am Acad Child Adolesc Psychiatry* 156:504-511, 2007.

Quigley S, Kretschmer R: *The education of deaf children: issues, theory, and practice,* Baltimore, 1982, University Park Press.

Rahl JS et al: Meeting the needs of parents around the time of diagnosis of disability among their children: evaluation of a novel program for information, support, and liaison by key workers, *Pediatrics* 114:e477-82, 2004.

Robin AL: Attention deficit/hyperactivity disorder in adolescents, *Pediatr Ann* 31:485-491, 2002.

Report of the Quality Standards Subcommittee of the American Academy of Neurology and the Child Neurology Society: Practice parameter: screening and diagnosis of autism, *Neurology* 55:468-479, 2000.

Ryan: Hearing and speech assessment. In Ballard R, editor: *Pediatric care of the ICN graduate,* Philadelphia, 1988, WB Saunders.

Schonwald A: Update: attention deficit/hyperactivity disorder in the primary care office, *Curr Opinion Pediatr* 17:265-274, 2005.

Schlumberger E et al: Non-verbal development of children with deafness with and without cochlear implants, *Dev Med Child Neurol* 46:599-606, 2004.

Shelton K: *The family experience with school when an adolescent has ADHD,* Unpublished doctoral dissertation, Oregon Health & Science University, 2001.

Simms M: Attention-deficit/hyperactivity disorder. In Behrman R, Kliegman R, Jenson H, editors: *Nelson textbook of pediatrics,* ed 17, Philadelphia, 2004, WB Saunders.

Sullivan P, Brookhouser P, Scanlan J: Maltreatment of deaf and hard of hearing children. In Hindley P, Kitson N, editors: *Mental health and deafness,* London, 2000, Whurr.

Sullivan PM, Knutson JF: Maltreatment and behavioral characteristics of youth who are deaf and hard of hearing, *Sexuality Disability* 16:295-319, 1998.

Tobin MJ: Conservation of substance in the blind and partially blind, *Br J Edu Psychol* 142:192-197, 1972.

Tornqvist K, Kallen B: Risk factors in term children for visual impairment without a known prenatal or postnatal cause, *Paediatr Perinat Epidemiol* 18(6):425-430, 2004.

US Department of Health and Human Services: *Healthy People 2010: health promotion and disease prevention objectives for the year 2010,* Washington, DC, 2001, US Government Printing Office.

Van Naarden K, Decouflé P, Caldwell K: Prevalence and characteristics of children with serious hearing impairment in metropolitan Atlanta, 1991-1993, *Pediatrics* 103:570-575, 1999.

Wilson J, Levin F: Attention deficit/hyperactivity disorder and early-onset substance abuse disorders, *J Child Adolesc Psychpharm* 15(5):751-763, 2005.

Wolraich M et al: Attention deficit/hyperactivity disorder among adolescents: a review of the diagnosis, treatment, and clinical implications, *Pediatrics* 115(6):1734-1746, 2005.

Yoshinaga-Itano C et al: Language of early- and later-identified children with hearing loss, *Pediatrics* 102:1161-1171, 1998.

Ziegler R, Holden L: Family therapy for learning disabled and attention deficit disordered children, *Am J Orthopsychiatry* 58:196-210, 1988.

CHAPTER 17

Self-Perception Issues

Nancy Barber Starr

All people—children and adults—have mental pictures of themselves that steer the course of their lives. This mental picture, or self-perception, begins to develop at birth, emerges in childhood, and is refined and crystallized in adolescence, but it continues to evolve throughout life. Significant relationships, attachment, temperament, heredity, and experiences in life are some of the factors that influence self-perception (Fig. 17-1). Self-perception has to do with how individuals act, think, and feel about themselves, their abilities, and their bodies. It is also influenced by the response of others to them. This perception, in turn, influences the attitudes each person takes and the choices each person makes throughout life. Children's self-concept will powerfully impact their happiness, academic performance, relationships, creativity, healthy risk-taking, perseverance, resilience, and problem-solving (Neifert, 2005). A positive self-perception is a precious gift that provides the confidence and energy to take on the world, to withstand crises, and to focus outside one's self. It enhances the building of relationships and giving to others. People with a negative self-perception tend to focus on their own needs, trying to get and prove their self-worth. A negative self-perception drains energy, interferes with building relationships, and often leaves the person feeling like a victim.

Over the last several decades, much research has focused on self-esteem and its potential effect on "a host of social ills, from poor academic performance and marital discord to violent crime and drug abuse" (Goode, 2002). Recent research, however, debunks the idea that positive self-esteem prevents many of these behaviors and cites other psychological factors, such as narcissism or self-absorption and the use of external measures (e.g., academic performance or appearance) as much more important in determining or predicting negative behaviors or outcomes (Goode, 2002). An extensive review of objective evidence in the self-esteem literature looked at the effects of self-esteem. Baumeister and colleagues (2003) found that the "benefits of high self-esteem are far fewer and weaker than proponents...had hoped (p. 38)." The authors recommend "a new emphasis on self-esteem that accurately reflects capabilities and interpersonal characteristics," not just "indiscriminate praise (p. 39)." Linking self-esteem to lifelong learning (academically, socially, culturally, and occupationally) and improvement provides praise along with correction and results in enhanced rather than inflated self-esteem.

Assessment of self-perception is not a straightforward task but is interwoven with other data that the provider collects. It may be helpful to think of self-esteem as including cognitive, affective, and behavioral aspects (Reasoner, 2002).

The *cognitive* element emerges as an individual thinks about the discrepancy between the ideal self and the perceived self. The *affective* component refers to the feelings that emerge when considering the discrepancy between the two selves. The *behavioral* aspect is seen in traits, such as assertiveness, resilience, and being decisive and respectful of others. Routine anticipatory guidance, education, and counseling, individualized to the child and family, give the provider the opportunity to facilitate the development of positive self-perception and to assist in preventing potential problems. Self-perception problems are often hidden within somatic complaints and require an awareness and sensitivity to the child or adolescent to identify and deal with them. If done successfully, the child's life can be significantly affected.

■ STANDARDS OF CARE

Bright Futures in Practice: Mental Health (Jellinek et al, 2002) focuses on prevention of psychosocial problems and early recognition of mental disorders. The comprehensive practice guide and tool kit have a section in each developmental chapter that focuses on self-functioning and its appropriate assessment and management. Goals in *Healthy People 2010* (U.S. Department of Health and Human Services, 2002), the *Guide to Clinical Preventive Services* (U.S. Preventive Services Task Force, 2006), the *AMA Guidelines for Adolescent Preventive Services (GAPS)* (Elster & Kuznets, 1994) all address screening for depression and potential suicide. These are potential complications of negative self-esteem and should be considered by the provider working with children and adolescents (see Chapter 20 for an in-depth discussion of these topics).

■ NORMAL PATTERNS OF SELF-PERCEPTION

COMPONENTS OF SELF-PERCEPTION

The term *self-perception* may be used interchangeably with terms such as *self-concept, self-esteem,* and *self-image.* The term *body image* refers to one's picture of and feelings regarding the body.

Self-perception, being personal and subjective, includes both a description of the self and an evaluation of that description. The description a person draws and the evaluation a person makes come from thoughts and feelings, beliefs and convictions, observations, understanding, insight, and awareness received both from the self and from others. The three key components of self-perception are significance, worthiness, and competence (Box 17-1).

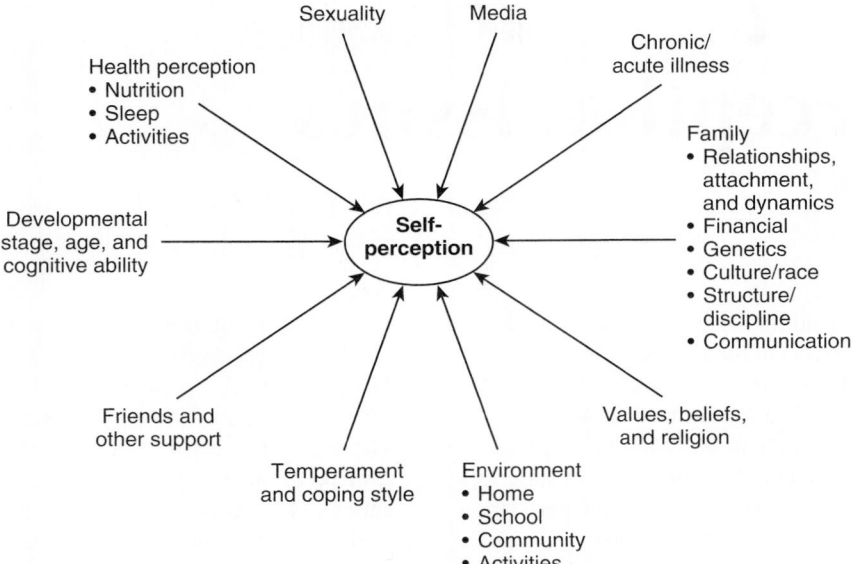

FIG. 17-1   Factors that influence self-perception.

Significance comes from having a sense of belonging; feeling loved and lovable; feeling secure, cared for, and supported; and being accepted and understood unconditionally for who one is, not what one does. This is the most important component in developing and maintaining a healthy self-esteem. Some people believe that females are more likely to channel their self-perception into feeling desirable especially through relationships (Slattery, 2005).

Worthiness comes from understanding that as an individual you have a purpose in life. It is feeling valuable, acceptable, meeting personal moral standards, and respecting and feeling good about oneself. It also has to do with being respected and accepted by others. Feeling unconditional love, "no strings attached," is the cornerstone of self-worth.

Competence comes from feeling capable, confident, adequate, in control, and able to approach new tasks and deal with life optimistically, hopefully, and with courage. Males are more likely to channel their self-perception into feeling capable especially through significance and achievement (Slattery, 2005). Competence is one part of resilience—the inner strength to cope with any challenge one faces in life (Brooks, 2002). Competence is measured in terms of cognitive, physical, or social skills.

Children who feel significant, worthy, and competent confidently initiate activities, explore the environment, take risks,

and rebound from disappointments. Appreciating themselves, they are able to reach out to and interact with others, accepting and offering love, respect, and encouragement. Perry (2001) describes an active learning process beginning with a child's natural curiosity that leads to mastery and accomplishment, thereby growing a child's self-esteem and resilience (Box 17-2).

Children who do not feel significant, worthy, and competent look increasingly to *external measures,* such as those listed in Box 17-3, to try to create a positive self-perception. Physical attractiveness, financial status, and intelligence are three measures frequently used in society to evaluate people. State of physical health, temperament, coping style, and an overly protective environment are other factors that affect self-perception. However, undue or excessive emphasis on external measures causes children to compare themselves with others, adopting the description and evaluation others make of them. "Most of us are what we think others think we are" (Dobson, 1999) or "If you think you can't, you can't" (Neifert, 2005). Children whose self-perception is based on a comparison of themselves with others feel and describe themselves as insecure, inferior, and

---

BOX 17-1   Key Components of Self-Perception

Significance: "I am loved." (Parent: "I love you, no matter what.")
Worthiness: "I am OK. I like and respect myself." (Parent: "I accept and respect you.")
Competence: "I can do it." (Parent: "I believe in you. You can do it.")

BOX 17-2   Enhancing Self-Perception: The Cycle of Learning

- Curiosity results in exploration.
- Exploration results in discovery.
- Discovery results in pleasure.
- Pleasure leads to repetition.
- Repetition results in mastery.
- Mastery results in new skills.
- New skills lead to confidence.
- Confidence contributes to self-esteem.
- Self-esteem increases sense of security.
- Security results in more exploration.

From Perry BD: Creating novelty, *Scholastic Parent Child* 9:67–68, 2001.

BOX 17-3 **External Measures Used to Build Self-Perception**

Physical appearance or attractiveness: How do I look?
Intelligence: What do I know?
Performance: How do I do?
Importance: Who do I know? Who knows me?
Financial status: What and how much do I have?
Control: What and who do I control?

inadequate. Attempting to prove themselves, they often become both bossy and aggressive or people pleasers and approval seekers. Red flags for self-perception are listed in Box 17-4.

DEVELOPMENTAL STAGES

The development of children's self-perception is closely tied to normal growth and development. Each stage of growth and development provides opportunities to learn about the self and interact with and observe others and the environment. Transient periods of low self-esteem can occur when a child is working on mastering new skills or sets new goals and are a normal part of development. Self-perception can change as a result of relationships or experiences or can be maintained in spite of contrary evidence (e.g., the adolescent cheerleader who is loved and is successful in school and relationships, yet is anorexic and feels she is never "good enough").

One theoretic perspective that can be useful clinically is to view the development of self-perception as occurring in two stages (Box 17-5). The *first stage, emergence of the self,* occurs in infants, toddlers, and preschool-age children. Parents and caretakers play a key role during this stage. Infants as early as 4 months old learn that they are separate individuals who affect others by their behavior, thus laying the foundation for self-development (Rochat & Striano, 2002). This is best accomplished in a supportive environment where the infants come to view the world (their parents and caretakers) as responsive to their needs, both physical and emotional. Toddlers, with their new motor, cognitive, and language skills, learn to explore their capabilities and limits and make others aware of their needs, desires, and concerns. They thrive with positive acceptance, praise, and guidelines that set limits while allowing them to make choices. As preschoolers develop

BOX 17-4 **Red Flags for Self-Perception Problems**

- Constantly asking for reassurance: Do I look OK? Am I fat?
- Constantly showing a bravado: Do you know I know so and so? Do you know I'm involved with such and such?
- Depression or suicide: You are better off without me.
- Obsessive disorders, such as eating disorders, alcohol or drug use

Data from Slattery J: Self-esteem. In *Discovery Years, Focus on Your Child* CD, 2005.

BOX 17-5 **Developmental Stages of Self-Perception**

Emergence of Self (first stage)
- Infants—view the world as responsive or unresponsive to their needs and learn that they are separate individuals who affect others by their behavior.
- Toddlers—explore their capabilities and limits and make others aware of their needs, desires, and concerns.
- Preschoolers—begin to use personal pronouns and pretend play, become aware of discrepancies in abilities, discover their bodies, move from seeing themselves as the center of the world, categorically describe themselves.

Refining the Self (second stage)
- School-age children—become more confident of their own self-evaluation, evaluate self on the basis of external evidence, compare themselves with others, increasingly depend on peers for self-evaluation, criticize and ridicule deviations from normal, use comparative self-evaluation.
- Early adolescents—"try-on" images, finalize body image, focus on physical and emotional changes with peer acceptance determining self-evaluation, use interpersonal self-description.
- Late adolescents—refine and crystallize self-perception (physical, social, spiritual) with values, goals, and competencies guiding their future in place.

Data from Dixon S, Stein M: *Encounters with children,* ed 2, St Louis, 1992; Kump T: Self-esteem: why little kids need BIG egos, *Healthy Kids* Oct/Nov 1998, pp. 53-58; Hunsberger M: Fostering self-esteem. In Betz CL, Hunsberger M, Wright S, editors: *Family centered nursing care of children,* ed 2, Philadelphia, 1994, WB Saunders; Sieving RE, Zirbel-Donisch ST: Development and enhancement of self-esteem in children, *J Pediatr Health Care* 4:290-296, 1990.

better self-recognition, they demonstrate increasing use of personal pronouns and pretend play (Lewis & Ramsay, 2004). They become aware of discrepancies in abilities and discover their whole body, including the differences in sexes. Feelings of competence begin to emerge, and preschoolers can be coached through early problem-solving. Preschoolers internalize parents' demands and move away from seeing the self as the center of the world. Siblings and peers play an increasingly important role in the preschooler's life. When 4- to 7-year-old children are asked to describe themselves, they give *categorical identification,* describing themselves according to basic features with concrete, often external facts (Dixon & Stein, 2000).

Refining the self, the second stage of self-development, occurs in school-age children and adolescents as they developmentally become more self-aware. Friendships, peers, and the time spent in various activities play increasingly larger roles in shaping the child's character and personality and thus self-perception. As early as 5 to 10 years old, children will cite themselves, not adults, as the authority on self-knowledge (Burton & Mitchell, 2003). Cultural stereotypes, such as those found in magazines, television, billboards, and the Internet, all influence the child's perception of society's "ideal" self.

School-age children are preoccupied with evaluating themselves on the basis of external evidence: cognitive and physical skills, achievements, physical appearance, social abilities and acceptance, and a sense of control. They are particularly prone to comparing themselves with others, making them more vulnerable to social pressure. Any deviation from what society considers "normal" is subject to criticism and ridicule. From 8 to 11 years old when asked to describe themselves, school-age children give *comparative assessments* detailing linear, often rigid and rule-based descriptions that compare self with peers (Dixon & Stein, 2000). Recent studies stress the importance of assessing peer perception hand in hand with self-perception in determining social functioning (Salmivalli et al, 2005; Troop-Gordon & Ladd, 2005). Studies of children having chronic difficulties with peers show a more negative self-belief development, often leading to psychological adjustment problems (loneliness, internalizing and externalizing problems) (Salmivalli & Issacs, 2005; Troop-Gordon & Ladd, 2005; Ladd & Troop-Gordon, 2003).

Self-perception continues to be refined during early adolescence, solidifying in later adolescence. Early adolescents, from 12 to 15 years of age, provide descriptions of themselves with *interpersonal implications* that lack flexibility and detail their sense of self based upon relationships, with personal characteristics as the basis and reason for relationships (Dixon & Stein, 2000). Early adolescents are still highly dependent on cultural stereotypes and peer acceptance, with physical and emotional changes being the main focus of self-evaluation. Body image formation, a crucial element in shaping identity, is finalized at this stage. Any defect, disability, or discrepancy between what is seen and what is visualized as ideal is magnified and significant in the adolescent's eyes. Part of the development of body image includes developing a sense of sexual self or becoming comfortable with one's sexuality, assuming culturally defined sexual roles, behaviors, and activities (Dixon & Stein, 2000). Teens "try on" different images as they attempt to reach their own self. Self-esteem, shown to have low stability during childhood, is increased throughout adolescence (Trzesniewski et al, 2003). By late adolescence, a more established view of the self should be in place, with acceptance of personal identity—physical, social, and spiritual. At this stage, adolescents may begin to develop their own life story with important memories that help to make sense of their past, present, and future (McLean, 2005). Teenagers with positive self-perception have values, goals, and competencies that guide them into adulthood.

Areas to be evaluated in the adolescent include academic achievements, athletic achievements, peer acceptance, physical attributes, interpersonal acceptance (close friendships, romantic appeal), moral behaviors as compared with internal standards, sense of control over personal accomplishments, relationships, and participation in activities.

One study of adolescent self-esteem examined eight domains identified across a number of instruments: personal security, home and parents, peer popularity, academic competence, attractiveness, personal mastery, psychological permeability, and athletic competence (Quatman & Watson, 2001). Of the eight domains, only peer popularity and academic competence showed no significant difference between genders, though boys still exceeded girls in all eight. Parents and home life, personal security, academic competence, and personal mastery were the four domains that strongly influenced global self-esteem. Low priority was assigned to athleticism. The authors concluded that boys seem to have an "at homeness" in the world, both in the home and outside, where they feel confident and masterful, not undone by adversity. In contrast, girls felt significantly less confident and masterful and more psychologically vulnerable.

DEVELOPMENTAL ASSETS

Developmental assets are basic life skills and attributes that are critical building blocks to help a child or adolescent grow into a caring, competent, contributing, and responsible adult. Developmental assets have been shown to promote positive attributes and behaviors including exhibiting leadership, maintaining good health, valuing diversity, and success in school. The assets have also been shown to be protective against high-risk behaviors, such as alcohol use, violence, illicit drug use, and sexual activity (Search Institute, 2006a). The more assets a young person has, the more likely he or she is to make wise decisions and choose positive lifestyles while avoiding risky behaviors or dangerous activities. Developmental assets have been identified and revised by the Search Institute based on nationwide surveys of more than 100,000 young persons in 200 communities (Benson et al, 1998a). There are two categories of assets: (1) external assets, things in the environment (home, school, community) that support, nurture and empower, set boundaries and expectations, and make constructive use of time and (2) internal assets, attitudes (commitment to learning and a positive identity), positive values, and social competencies that belong in the head and heart of every child (Benson et al, 1998a). Forty developmental assets have been described (Table 17-1). Most children and adolescents have only 18. Girls tend to have more assets than boys do in a ratio of 19.5 to 16.5, and younger children have more assets than older ones do (Benson et al, 1998a). The Search Institute believes that young people should have at least 31 assets. Those with low levels are two to four times more likely to use alcohol, tobacco, and other drugs (Search Institute, 2006b).

Building on the initial research to develop the list of youth assets, the Search Institute has now completed research and created 40 developmental assets for both middle childhood (Table 17-2) and for early childhood (3 to 5 years old) (Table 17-3). Common threads and unique features for each developmental age group are reflected in these new assets lists. The middle childhood assets include the transition toward emerging selfhood and self-regulation. The early childhood assets respond to early childhood issues with essential ingredients that relate to school readiness, school success, and a happy productive life (Search Institute, 2006c).

Ten developmental deficits, or roadblocks to building assets, have also been identified by the Search Institute (Benson et al, 1998a). The more deficits a child has, the more likely he or she is to make negative choices and decisions. The deficits are as follows:

TABLE 17-1   40 Developmental Assets for Youth

Category	Asset Name and Definition
External Assets	
Support	Family support—Family life provides high levels of love and support.
	Positive family communication—Young person and her or his parent(s) communicate positively, and young person is willing to seek advice and counsel from parent(s).
	Other adult relationships—Young person receives support from three or more nonparent adults.
	Caring neighborhood—Young person experiences caring neighbors.
	Caring school climate—School provides a caring, encouraging environment.
	Parent involvement in schooling—Parent(s) are actively involved in helping young person succeed in school.
Empowerment	Community values youth—Young person perceives that adults in the community value youth.
	Youth as resources—Young people are given useful roles in the community.
	Service to others—Young person serves in the community 1 hour or more per week.
	Safety—Young person feels safe at home, at school, and in the neighborhood.
Boundaries and expectations	Family boundaries—Family has clear rules and consequences and monitors the young person's whereabouts.
	School boundaries—School provides clear rules and consequences.
	Neighborhood boundaries—Neighbors take responsibility for monitoring young people's behavior.
	Adult role models—Parent(s) and other adults model positive, responsible behavior.
	Positive peer influence—Young person's best friends model responsible behavior.
	High expectations—Both parent(s) and teachers encourage the young person to do well.
Constructive use of time	Creative activities—Young person spends 3 hour or more per week in lessons or practice in music, theater, or other arts.
	Youth programs—Young person spends 3 hours or more per week in sports, clubs, or organizations at school or in the community.
	Religious community—Young person spends 1 hour or more per week in activities in a religious institution.
	Time at home—Young person is out with friends "with nothing special to do" two or fewer nights per week.
Internal Assets	
Commitment to learning	Achievement motivation—Young person is motivated to do well in school.
	School engagement—Young person is actively engaged in learning.
	Homework—Young person reports doing at least 1 hour of homework every school day.
	Bonding to school—Young person cares about her or his school.
	Reading for pleasure—Young person reads for pleasure 3 hours or more per week.
Positive values	Caring—Young person places high value on helping other people.
	Equality and social justice—Young person places high value on promoting equality and reducing hunger and poverty.
	Integrity—Young person acts on convictions and stands up for her or his beliefs.
	Honesty—Young person tells the truth even when it is not easy.
	Responsibility—Young person accepts and takes personal responsibility.
	Restraint—Young person believes it is important not to be sexually active or to use alcohol or other drugs.
Social competencies	Planning and decision-making—Young person knows how to plan ahead and make choices.
	Interpersonal competence—Young person has empathy, sensitivity, and friendship skills.
	Cultural competence—Young person has knowledge of and comfort with people of different cultural, racial, and ethnic backgrounds.
	Resistance skills—Young person can resist negative peer pressure and dangerous situations.
	Peaceful conflict resolution—Young person seeks to resolve conflict nonviolently.
Positive identity	Personal power—Young person feels that he or she has control over "things that happen to me."
	Self-esteem—Young person reports having a high self-esteem.
	Sense of purpose —Young person reports that "my life has a purpose."
	Positive view of personal future—Young person is optimistic about her or his personal future.

TABLE 17-2 40 Developmental Assets for Middle Childhood

Category	Asset Name and Definition
External Assets	
Support	Family support—Family life provides high levels of love and support.
	Positive family communication—Parent(s) and child communicate positively. Child feels comfortable seeking advice and counsel from parent(s).
	Other adult relationships—Child receives support from adults other than her or his parent(s).
	Caring neighborhood—Child experiences caring neighbors.
	Caring school climate—Relationships with teachers and peers provide a caring, encouraging environment.
	Parent involvement in schooling—Parent(s) are actively involved in helping the child succeed in school.
Empowerment	Community values youth—Child feels valued and appreciated by adults in the community.
	Children as resources—Child is included in decisions at home and in the community.
	Service to others—Child has opportunities to help others in the community.
	Safety—Child feels safe at home, at school, and in his or her neighborhood.
Boundaries and expectations	Family boundaries—Family has clear and consistent rules and consequences and monitors the child's whereabouts.
	School boundaries—School provides clear rules and consequences.
	Neighborhood boundaries—Neighbors take responsibility for monitoring the child's behavior.
	Adult role models—Parent(s), other adults in the child's family, and nonfamily adults model positive, responsible behavior.
	Positive peer influence—Child's closest friends model positive, responsible behavior.
	High expectations—Parent(s) and teachers expect the child to do his or her best at school and in other activities.
Constructive use of time	Creative activities—Child participates in music, art, drama, or creative writing two or more times per week.
	Child programs—Child participates two or more times per week in cocurricular school activities or structured community programs for children.
	Religious community—Child attends religious programs or services one or more times per week.
	Time at home—Child spends some time most days both in high-quality interaction with parents and doing things at home other than watching TV or playing video games.
Internal Assets	
Commitment to learning	Achievement motivation—Child is motivated and strives to do well in school.
	Learning engagement—Child is responsive, attentive, and actively engaged in learning at school and enjoys participating in learning activities outside of school.
	Homework—Child usually hands his homework in on time.
	Bonding to school—Child cares about teachers and other adults at school.
	Reading for pleasure—Child enjoys and engages in reading for fun most days of the week.
Positive values	Caring—Parent(s) tell the child it is important to help other people.
	Equality and social justice—Parent(s) tell the child it is important to speak up for equal rights for all people.
	Integrity—Parent(s) tell the child it is important to stand up for one's beliefs.
	Honesty—Parent(s) tell the child it is important to tell the truth.
	Responsibility—Parent(s) tell the child it is important to accept personal responsibility for behavior.
	Healthy lifestyle—Parent(s) tell the child it is important to have good health habits and an understanding of healthy sexuality.
Social competencies	Planning and decision-making—Child thinks about decisions and is usually happy with results of her or his decisions.
	Interpersonal competence—Child cares about and is affected by other people's feeling, enjoys making friends, and when frustrated or angry, tries to calm himself or herself.
	Cultural competence—Child knows and is comfortable with people of different racial, ethnic, and cultural backgrounds and with his or her own cultural identity.
	Resistance skills—Child can stay away from people who are likely to get him or her in trouble and is able to say no to doing wrong or dangerous things.
	Peaceful conflict resolution—Child seeks to resolve conflict nonviolently.
Positive identity	Personal power—Child feels he or she has some influence over things that happen in his or her life.
	Self-esteem—Child likes and is proud to be the person that he or she is.
	Sense of purpose—Child sometimes thinks about what life means and whether there is a purpose for his or her life.
	Positive view of personal future—Child is optimistic about his or her personal future.

TABLE 17-3	40 Developmental Assets for Early Childhood (3–5 years old)

Category	Asset Name and Definition
External Assets	
Support	Family support—Parent(s) and/or primary caregiver(s) provide the child with high levels of consistent and predictable love.
	Positive family communication—Parent(s) and/or primary caregiver(s) express themselves positively and respectfully, engaging young children in conversations that invite their input.
	Other adult relationships—With the family's support, the child experiences consistent, caring relationships with adults outside the family.
	Caring neighbors—The child's network of relationships includes neighbors who provide emotional support and a sense of belonging.
	Caring climate in child care and educational settings—Caregivers and teachers create environments that are nurturing, accepting, encouraging, and secure.
	Parent involvement in child care and education—Parent(s), caregivers, and teachers together create a consistent and supportive approach to fostering the child's successful growth.
Empowerment	Community cherishes and values young children—Children are welcomed and included throughout community life.
	Children seen as resources—The community demonstrates that children are valuable resources by investing in a child-rearing system of family support and high-quality activities and resources to meet children's physical, social, and emotional needs.
	Service to others—The child has opportunities to perform simple but meaningful and caring actions for others.
	Safety—Parent(s), caregivers, teachers, neighbors, and the community take action to ensure children's health and safety.
Boundaries and expectations	Family boundaries—The family provides consistent supervision for the child and maintains reasonable guidelines for behavior that the child can understand and achieve.
	Boundaries in child care and educational settings—Caregivers and educators use positive approaches to discipline and natural consequences to encourage self-regulation and acceptable behaviors.
	Neighborhood boundaries—Neighbors encourage the child in positive, acceptable behavior and intervene in negative behavior, in a supportive and nonthreatening way.
	Adult role models—Parent(s), caregivers, and other adults model self-control, social skills, engagement in learning, and healthy lifestyles.
	Positive peer relationships—Parent(s) and caregivers seek to provide opportunities for the child to interact positively with other children.
	Positive expectations—Parent(s), caregivers, and teachers encourage and support the child in behaving appropriately, undertaking challenging tasks, and performing activities to the best of his or her abilities.
Constructive use of time	Play and creative activities—The child has daily opportunities to play in ways that allow self-expression, physical activity, and interaction with others.
	Out-of-home and community programs—The child experiences well-designed programs led by competent, caring adults in well-maintained settings.
	Religious community—The child participates in age-appropriate religious activities and caring relationships that nurture his or her spiritual development.
	Time at home—The child spends most of his or her time at home participating in family activities and playing constructively, with parent(s) guiding TV and electronic game use.
Internal Assets	
Commitment to learning	Motivation to mastery—The child responds to new experiences with curiosity and energy, resulting in the pleasure of mastering new learning and skills.
	Engagement in learning experiences—The child fully participates in a variety of activities that offer opportunities for learning.
	Home-program connection—The child experiences security, consistency, and connections between home and out-of-home care programs and learning activities.
	Bonding to programs—The child forms meaningful connections with out-of-home care and educational programs.
	Early literacy—The child enjoys a variety of prereading activities, including adults reading to him or her daily, looking at and handling books, playing with a variety of media, and showing interest in pictures, letters, and numbers.

Continued

TABLE 17-3	40 Developmental Assets for Early Childhood (3–5 years old)—Cont'd
Category	**Asset Name and Definition**
Positive values	Caring—The child begins to show empathy, understanding, and awareness of others' feelings.
	Equality and social justice—The child begins to show concern for people who are excluded from play and other activities or not treated fairly because they are different.
	Integrity—The child begins to express his or her view appropriately and to stand up for a growing sense of what is fair and right.
	Honesty—The child begins to understand the difference between truth and lies and is truthful to the extent of his or her understanding.
	Responsibility—The child begins to follow through on simple tasks to take care of himself or herself and to help others.
	Self-regulation—The child increasingly can identify, regulate, and control his or her behaviors in healthy ways, using adult support constructively in particularly stressful situations.
Social competencies	Planning and decision-making—The child begins to plan for the immediate future, choosing from among several options and trying to solve problems.
	Interpersonal skills—The child cooperates, shares, plays harmoniously, and comforts others in distress.
	Cultural awareness and sensitivity—The child begins to learn about his or her own cultural identity and to show acceptance of people who are racially, physically, culturally, or ethnically different from him or her.
	Resistance skills—The child begins to sense danger accurately, to seek help from trusted adults, and to resist pressure from peers to participate in unacceptable or risky behavior.
	Peaceful conflict resolution—The child begins to compromise and resolve conflicts without using physical aggression or hurtful language.
Positive identity	Personal power—The child can make choices that give a sense of having some influence over things that happen in his or her life.
	Self-esteem—The child likes himself or herself and has a growing sense of being valued by others.
	Sense of purpose—The child anticipates new opportunities, experiences, and milestones in growing up.
	Positive view of personal future—The child finds the world interesting and enjoyable and believes that he or she has a positive place in it.

Copyright 2005 by Search Institute, Minneapolis, MN 55415, 800-888-7828. Available at *www.search-institute.org* (accessed Sept 14, 2007).

1. Spending 2 hours or more a day alone at home without an adult
2. Putting a lot of emphasis on selfish values
3. Watching more than 2 hours of television a day
4. Going to parties where friends drink alcohol
5. Feeling stress or pressure most or all of the time
6. Being physically abused
7. Being sexually abused
8. Having a parent with an alcohol or drug problem
9. Feeling socially isolated from people who provide care, support, and understanding
10. Having numerous close friends who often get into trouble

ENVIRONMENTAL INFLUENCES

Significant relationships in a child's life, attachment, temperament, traits endowed by heredity, race, and experiences in everyday life are all environmental factors that influence the development of self-perception.

Significant relationships include parents or parent figures, siblings and other family members, and ongoing caretakers. Studies have shown that first-born children have higher levels of self-worth (Shebloski et al, 2005). As children get older,

peers and authority figures also have an influence. Constant unconditional acceptance and love, empathy, and an attitude of understanding, coupled with appropriate limits and boundaries, are the most important interactions these significant others offer. Time spent with and encouragement given to the child, both in being together and in doing things, in addition to sharing life's happenings (listening, talking, and problem-solving), are also essential ingredients (see the Parenting Pyramid discussed in Chapter 4). The sturdy base built by positive relationships is a key component in the child's developing positive self-esteem. By feeling, seeing, and hearing these continual reinforcements, children internalize or know that they are significant, worthy, and competent. In contrast Neifert (2005) has identified six common errors that parents unintentionally make that chip away at their child's self-esteem (Box 17-6). A study of French-Canadian children who experienced verbal aggression from parents (rejection, demeaning, terrorizing, criticizing, or insulting) showed significantly lower self-esteem. These children perceived themselves as less competent, less comfortable, less worthy, and more prone to depression (Solomon & Serres, 1999). In general peers and authority figures serve to confirm or deny what is taught at home.

BOX 17-6 **Common Errors That Erode Self-Esteem**

Although no parent deliberately undermines their child's self-esteem, many unintentionally chip away at their youngster's self-worth by committing the following common errors.

- **Negating a child's feelings.** A child's feelings are an important part of their identity, and when we reject their emotions, it feels like we are rejecting them.
- **Frequent criticism and dwelling on negatives.** Your disappointment in your child makes her disappointed in herself. Whereas parents may forget their critical remarks, children often take such comments literally and internalize them.
- **Using put-downs and derogatory labels.** Negative labels damage a child's self-image and often become self-fulfilling prophecies. Chose positive nicknames that convey affection and your high opinion of your child, "Ace, champ, precious, pal."
- **Typecasting or stereotyping.** Although children enjoy having a unique identity, typecasting can restrict their sense of possibility and narrow their expectations.
- **Expecting too much.** Unrealistic expectations create excessive pressure and feelings of inadequacy. "Just a little bit better" gets translated as "not good enough." Praise a child for what he does well, instead of focusing on what could be better.
- **Tying a child's character or personal worth to her performance or behavior.** Verbal blasts, such as "I'm so disappointed in you," make your love feel conditional and subject to cancellation when the child's behavior does not measure up. Focus on the problem behavior rather than criticizing your child. Unconditional love means that nothing your child could ever say or do would cause you to withdraw your love.

From Neifert MA: Self-esteem and emotional health, *A Dr Mom Presentation,* Denver, 2005.

Neurobiologic studies of brain development are confirming and expanding the important role that *attachment* plays in a developing child's brain, mind, and emotions. The right brain specifically deals with self-awareness, self-recognition, and processing "self-related material" (Schore, 2005). Attachment and right-brain development in turn have a significant impact on the development of a child's self-perception. Rees (2005) describes attachment as observed patterns of relationships. A child's attachment may be described as follows (Zuckerman et al, 2005; Rees, 2005):

- *Secure*—These children value relationships, but are independently confident of their own self-worth.
- *Insecure avoidant*—These children appear emotionally independent, but often have difficulty relating to peers and a poorly developed sense of self; these children's skills lie with inanimate objects rather than personal and social.
- *Insecure anxious*—These children often depend on the attention and approval of others for their self-worth, use physical symptoms for attention, and become uncertain and anxious in social situations.

- *Insecure ambivalent or resistant*—These children depend on relationships and are fairly organized in life circumstances, but may also be wary of their safety.
- *Insecure disorganized*—These children are neither effectively self-sufficient nor able to use relationships; they tend to have more associated social and emotional developmental problems.

Insecure attachment is not in and of itself pathologic but is on a continuum of attachment styles that may or may not present a problem (Rees, 2005). Because attachment has to do with a secure, confident, basic connection to a caring adult and the adult's ability to foster a positive attachment to their child, the role of the adult's or parent's attachment must also be considered. Adult attachment has been categorized into four categories (Zuckerman et al, 2005), with as high as an 85% predictive correlation between the adult assessment and the actual parent attachment to their children. The four categories identified by Zuckerman et al (2005) are:

- Free or secure in adult relationship and attachment extending to their children
- Dismissive of early attachment—minimizing the importance of attachment with subsequent emotional disconnection from their own children
- Preoccupied with their own early attachment—past issues interfere with current functioning and often lead to ambivalent attachment of parent and child
- Disorganized with unresolved trauma or loss—overwhelming issues from the past intrude unpredictably often causing disorganized attachment in the child

Temperament may also play a role in the child's development of self-perception. This is particularly the case when there is a mismatch of temperaments, especially between parent and child, or when a child has traits that are labeled difficult or challenging. If these traits are understood and managed correctly, the child's self-esteem can be positively affected (see Kurcinka [1998] for an in-depth discussion of temperament). However, if temperament is not understood, the child may carry negative perceptions and labels that adversely affect his or her self-perception (see Chapter 20 for further discussion of temperament).

The role that *heredity* plays in the development of self-perception is due to family traits over which the child has no control. Appearance, intelligence, and family characteristics, including alcoholism, mental illness, and disfiguring disease, are to be considered. Teasing that occurs when a child is obese is consistently associated with low self-esteem, depression, and potential suicide (Eisenberg & Newmark-Sztainer, 2003). Conditions, such as poverty and homelessness, also are important (Costello et al, 2003). Family traits and attributes either contribute to a positive self-perception or may become barriers to overcome.

The effect of *race* on self-esteem has been much studied over the last 50 years. One study reported that self-identified mixed-race adolescents have higher health and behavioral risk (Udry et al, 2003). In 2000, Chapman and Mullis, studying racial differences in adolescent coping and self-esteem, found no difference between the self-esteem of white and black adolescents. Additionally, Gray-Little and Hafdahl (2000) performed a meta-analysis of 261 studies on self-esteem. Comparisons based on more than one-half million respondents showed that black children, adolescents, and young adults had higher self-esteem scores than their comparable Caucasian counterparts. The authors, however, caution against using race as an independent variable in assessing self-esteem.

Children's *social experiences* provide opportunities to observe the world, test skills and abilities, interact with others, and try various roles. Positive experiences, such as success in solving problems, working out difficulties, and learning to carry on after setbacks, contribute to significance, self-worth, and competence, encouraging further exploration and risk-taking. Negative experiences cause children to retreat or attempt to compensate through other means. The effects of the Internet and role-playing fantasy games are just emerging. Beneficial outlets include forging a sense of identity apart from one's family ("experience of a virtual community, amelioration of social anxiety and loneliness and 'trying on' of new identities") (Allison et al, 2006) must be weighed against the addictive, all-consuming nature of the games that interfere with an adolescent's interaction with the real world.

■ ASSESSMENT OF SELF-PERCEPTION

The goal of assessing self-perception is to know how children describe and evaluate themselves and to identify the sources that provide the input they use to develop their sense of self. These assessments then lay the groundwork for planning interventions for the child and family. Corresponding assessments of the parents', caretaker's, and peer's perception of the child is important. Assessment of self-perception is not a simple task. It cannot be observed directly or obtained from questioning alone, but must be inferred from observed behavior, self-statements or self-ratings, and other relevant information. Self-rating, observational scales, draw-a-person tests, and puppet interviews are possible means of assessment. The puppet interview is an indirect interview with a large hand puppet for 5- to 7-year-olds (Verschueren et al, 2001). The draw-a-person test, used with younger children, asks the child to draw a picture of himself or herself and also a picture of another child. A comparison of the two drawings often gives an idea of the child's self-perception. Somewhere between fourth and sixth grades, self-esteem inventories can be considered. A comprehensive meta-analysis of measures of self-esteem for young children offers helpful information if the reader is interested in tools for young children (Davis-Kean & Sandler, 2001). A variety of measures are available for adolescents (see Schott & Bellin, 2001 for an example).

HISTORY

Although there are a variety of tools or questionnaires available to assess self-perception at various ages, the following questions may be considered in assessing a child's self-perception in the clinical setting.

General Questions (Spratt, 2002)
- What does your child think she or he does well?
- How does your child respond to failure?

- Does your child have close friends?
- How does your child respond to new challenges?
- How does your own style (e.g., personality, patience, energy level, talents) compare with your child's?
- Are you setting reasonable or attainable expectations for your child?

Components of Self-Perception
Significance
- Does the child feel loved, lovable, cared for, secure, supported, accepted, and understood?
- Is this love conditional or unconditional? Is this based on who the child is or what the child does?

Worthiness
- Does the child feel valuable, acceptable?
- Are self-respect and self-liking evident?
- What beliefs or convictions does the child have about himself/herself? Are these beliefs or convictions realistic? Do they match the child's lifestyle?

Competence
- Does the child feel capable, adequate, optimistic overall?
- Does the child approach new tasks with confidence?
- What are the child's cognitive, physical, and social strengths?

Developmental Stage
Infant
- Does the infant recognize self as separate from others?
- Does the infant realize his or her effect on others?

Toddler
- Does the toddler explore capabilities and limits?
- Does the toddler make others aware of needs, desires, and concerns?

Preschooler
- "How do you describe yourself in two or three words?"
- Does the child use personal pronouns? Participate in pretend play? Describe activities? Discover his or her body?
- Is the child internalizing parental demands? Moving away from self as center of world?
- Are siblings and peers increasingly important? How does the child think, feel, and act about self?

School-Age Child
- "How do you describe yourself in two or three words?" (home, sports, school, activities may be clue words)
- How does this view compare with the child's perceptions of peers' evaluation of him or her?
- What cognitive and physical skills and achievements are described?
- What friends, social abilities, and activities are described?
- Is there a sense of control over life? Confidence in self?

Early Adolescent
- "How do you describe yourself in two or three words?" (home, sports, school, activities may be clue words)
- What role do peers play in how the adolescent feels about himself/herself?
- How are physical attributes described (body image)?

- What are academic, physical, and social activities and achievements?
- How do moral behaviors compare with internal standards?
- Is there a sense of control over personal activities, accomplishments, and relationships?

Late Adolescent

- "How do you describe yourself in two or three words?" (home, sports, school, activities may be clue words)
- What lifestyle choices are being made? What values, goals, and plans are expressed? Is there a sense of optimism about that direction?

Developmental Assets

To determine how many and what assets a child has, appropriate-aged (early, middle, or youth) asset lists can be used as checklists. The Search Institute has compiled checklists for both parents and children (see Resource Box). It is suggested that parents and children complete the lists separately, then sit down and share each other's responses. These checklists become helpful tools for parents and children to compare their perceptions, identify strong and weak areas, and plan for areas of growth.

Environmental Influences

Family Structure

- Who makes up the family? Significant others? Caretakers? What is the family like?
- What is the family's social and financial status?
- What is the physical living situation?
- Does anyone in the family have any physical disease? Any mental or social problems (e.g., mental illness or retardation, alcoholism)?

Parental Influences

- Who plays the parental role? How do parents describe themselves? Perceive their role?
- How does the parent describe the child? How valued is the child? How is that shown?
- What are parental expectations for the child? Is the child given age-appropriate guidance, responsibilities, and freedoms?

Significant Others Outside Family

- Who are they? Peers? Teachers? Neighbors? Authority figures? Social supports? Networks? Mentors?
- What are the relationships like?

Attachment

- "How does the child relate to adults?" (Rees, 2005)
  - Secure—seeks closeness and attention appropriately?
  - Insecure, avoidant—seeks closeness and attention too little?
  - Insecure, anxious—seeks closeness and attention too much?
  - Insecure, ambivalent—seeks closeness and attention, but is not calmed by it? Seeks closeness and attention inconsistently?
  - Insecure, disorganized—interpersonal behavior chaotic and ineffective?
- What is the parental attachment style? Free? Dismissive? Preoccupied? Disorganized?

Temperament Issues

- What temperament traits does the child have?
- How does the parent describe the child? React to the child? Interact with the child?

Environment

- What is the child's environment like? What experiences or opportunities are there? Within the family? In the neighborhood? More formally (e.g., play groups, extracurricular activities)?
- What experience or opportunities are there both within the family and in the community to test skills and abilities? Interact with others? Try new roles? Is this encouraged?
- How protected is the child?

Discipline

- How is the child disciplined? What methods are used? Is guidance given?
- Are limits and consequences clear?
- Is the child allowed to try without unrequested assistance provided too soon and not be rescued?

Communication

- What messages is the child receiving (e.g., "you are a helper," or "you are a bad boy")?
- Is he or she listened to? Are feelings acknowledged?
- What does the child say about himself or herself (e.g., describes self as "good" or "bad," "smart"or "dumb")?

OBSERVATIONS DURING THE HISTORY AND EXAMINATION

Direct questioning about all the areas previously listed gives the provider information about the child. However, equally important is observation of the child and interactions between the child and the accompanying person throughout the office visit.

- What is the relationship between the two?
- What actual words are said? With what tone of voice?
- What kind of nonverbal interaction occurs? What kind of physical interaction?
- Is the child encouraged to answer questions and perform tasks? Is rescuing occurring? Is guidance given?
- What expectations are voiced?
- How is discipline conducted within the examination setting? What limits are set?

Box 17-7 lists risk factors for low self-perception.

■ MANAGEMENT STRATEGIES FOR DEVELOPING POSITIVE SELF-PERCEPTION

Anticipatory guidance, education, and counseling are strategies the provider uses to guide and direct the family, child, and adolescent in developing healthy self-perception. If problems are significant and the child or family is in distress, refer for more in-depth counseling (see Chapter 20).

When working with the child and family, specific strategies to improve self-perception are chosen, keeping in mind that familial, generational, ethnic and cultural practices, and chronic illness influence the choice and use of strategies. A multitude of books on developing children's self-esteem are

---

BOX 17-7 Risk Factors for Low Self-Perception

1. *Physical alterations, including body image:* chronic illness (visible or not), disfiguring disabilities, sensory disabilities, obesity, anorexia
2. *Mental and emotional alterations:* school problems, such as slow learner, semiliterate, underachiever, culturally deprived, late bloomer, difficult temperament, emotional or mental illness or abuse
3. *Environmental and relational alterations:* disrupted families and family relationships or inability to meet basic needs, unrealistic expectations or faulty thinking, temperament or personality misfits, attachment disorders, social disorders, stress, past experiences of failure, rejection, criticism

---

available, a few of which are listed in the references at the end of the chapter. See also Suggested Readings and Resource Box at the end of this chapter.

FACILITATE GOOD PARENTING

- "Know yourself." Parental self-perception, either positive or negative, has a significant effect on the child's self-perception. "If Mama ain't happy, ain't nobody happy." Parents should be encouraged to understand and accept themselves, acknowledge their strengths and accept their uniqueness, take care of themselves, treat themselves with respect, and be aware of their own feelings.
- "Know your child." See what they see; feel what they feel; hope what they hope. This provides needed empathy. Children have their own personality, temperament, dreams, and opinions and need to be known, loved, accepted, and respected for who they are.
- Value your child. Appreciate and praise who they are rather than what they do. Show belief in their ability to learn, improve, and grow. Look in their eyes when you talk to them. Recognize their unique means of self-expression. Delight in their discoveries. Contribute to their collections. Identify their strengths, focus on their efforts, structure situations for success, and offer thanks for what they do. Avoid shame, criticism, and humiliation.
- Avoid comparing children. Children are individuals who grow and develop in their own way and at their own rate. Celebrate their accomplishments. Tell them how terrific they are. Their individuality needs to be respected, and comparisons with siblings or peers should be avoided.
- Be available to the child both physically and emotionally, teaching the child, modeling behavior, and helping the child learn to relate to others. A sense of security and belonging occurs as you meet basic needs and spend time together, enjoying the child, having fun, touching, talking, and watching.
- Make them believe you are always on their team. Do things with them, not just for them. Show up at their concerts, games, and events. Visit their schools. Presence endorses the child's involvement and reinforces the importance of their efforts.

- Take time; avoid being hurried, especially during times of transition. Schedule times to be together. Play with your children, and let them chose the activity and set the pace. Spend at least 20 minutes each day giving them undivided attention. Consider whether dawdling, acting out, or feeling bad may be related to being hurried and feeling lack of emotional support (Jellinek et al, 2002).
- Know their friends. Encourage positive involvement with friends and activities. Help find the right niche (e.g., length of time, type of activity) that fits the child. Show an interest in friends (e.g., host a sleepover, take a group to the zoo). Steer them away from less constructive friends and activities.
- Let go. Empower them to make decisions. Trust them. Give them responsibility. Develop a gradual, planned granting of freedom and responsibility, beginning in infancy and ending in late adolescence. Letting go offers trust, provides opportunities, gives choices, instills confidence, and refrains from rushing to aid a struggling child. As part of this process, each year the child should make more decisions and assume more routine responsibilities than during the prior 12 months (Dobson, 1999).

MAINTAIN APPROPRIATE EXPECTATIONS OF THE CHILD

- Keep expectations involving tasks, toys, and roles appropriate to the child's age. Expectations that are too high lead to pressure on children and a constant feeling of failure even when children are doing their best. Expectations that are too low diminish children's value and make them feel as if the parent has no faith in them. Expecting their best can even be overly demanding because no one can consistently "do their best" all the time (Spratt, 2002).
- Set expectations that are appropriate to the child's unique qualities. Each child's individual personality, temperament, strengths, and weaknesses must be considered. Parent-driven versus child-driven expectations need to be identified. Although this is a sensitive issue, knowing where expectations begin (with parent or child) and how they fit the child and family is important. Recognize differences between the parent's style and abilities and the child's.
- Clearly stating expectations so that both the child and parent understand can prevent frustration, distrust, and further problems.
- Develop resilience in children by learning to view failure or mistakes as chances to learn. Mistakes are accepted and expected. Realistically assessing performance, emphasizing strengths, and discussing strategies that could lead to success prepare children to approach future obstacles and disappointments (Spratt, 2002).

USE DISCIPLINE TECHNIQUES THAT ENHANCE SELF-PERCEPTION

- The goal of discipline is to teach children, not punish them. The manner and intent of providing discipline are as important as the techniques used. See Chapter 4.
- Identify limits and consequences clearly and follow through. Knowing clearly what is expected provides security for the

child. Encourage flexible limit setting (e.g., "You have to wear a coat, but you can choose the blue or red one")

- Help the child learn to choose acceptable behaviors and learn self-control. Establish house rules. Catch the child being good and offer praise. Be sincere.
- Foster problem-solving to build confidence. Begin by providing opportunities to make choices and decisions. Teach the steps to problem-solving (stating the problem, expressing needs, considering alternatives, agreeing on a solution, and implementing and following through with the agreed-on solution). Take time and let the child work through the process.
- Provide guidance, but avoid rescuing children. Respect their choices, allowing them to persevere, learn, and work through frustration. This helps them learn independence and empowers them for further success. Rescuing (providing unrequested assistance too soon) must be differentiated from guiding, encouraging, and being an ally to the child. Guidance helps children understand themselves and the surrounding world, develop a conscience, and steer clear of potential problems.

COMMUNICATE POSITIVELY AND WITH RESPECT

- Listen to children. Good listening means taking them seriously, being interested, and letting them finish what they are saying. Show love in the way the child most appreciates. This may be through touch (giving hugs and back rubs), verbally (encouraging words and tone of voice), or nonverbally (positive facial expressions or high-fives). Say "I love you" often and in a variety of ways.
- Be aware of the words used, in addition to the tone of voice, the intent of the words, and body language. Avoid negative messages that are sent in comparisons, put-downs ("You are such a baby"), humiliation ("You can't do anything right"), labeling ("You're such a slob"), and fault finding.
- Praise and encourage children often, especially as they undertake new challenges or roles. Say "thanks" for their cooperation. Catch them doing well (e.g., "I like the way you…"). Acknowledge their help (e.g., "I appreciate…"). Love their person (e.g., "I love being with you…")
- Use communication techniques that convey respect. Ask open-ended questions to encourage dialogue. Listen with empathy. Apologize and ask forgiveness when appropriate (Neifert, 2005).
- Help children identify, handle, and express their feelings by accepting and acknowledging them. Avoid trying to change them or stop them by denial or reassurance. Listen. Parents should share their own feelings and failures. Intervention may take place at the thought and behavior level after feelings are brought forward.
- Use "I" statements, not "you" judgments. This separates performance from worth and validates children's behavior while still allowing the behavior to be modified. "I like your drawings *and* I need you to color on the paper, not on the wall." Use "and" which tends to connect words instead of "but" which tends to negate what was said before (Neifert, 2005).

- Be aware of children's "self-talk." What children say to themselves not only reflects what they believe, but also gives further definition to who they are. Positive statements enhance self-perception and minimize stress children feel. "Stinkin' thinking" (Hart, 1990) or negative statements reflect low self-perception and require intervention.
- Nurture curiosity and exploration to encourage mastery of new skills and help children reach their potential (Perry, 2001).

PROVIDE HELPFUL STRATEGIES FOR THE CHILD AND ADOLESCENT

- Support early and ongoing self-assertions as means of children expressing themselves (Kump, 1998). For example, allow a preschooler to wear the outlandish outfit chosen unless it is totally inappropriate (a bathing suit in November) or a school-age child to create the menu one night a week.
- Offer genuine encounter moments (GEMs) (Hall, 1998). GEM is a mutually agreed-on time that is set apart for 100% attention and love, focused attention, or direct involvement. The child takes the lead in how the time is spent.
- Assume the best in your child and focus on the positives. Make a list of positive attributes and strengths, and let your child hear you speak positively about him (Neifert, 2005).
- Encourage a healthy connectedness. Children need to belong to and feel that they are a part of their family and groups outside their family through social activities and links within their community, ethnic group, or geographic area.
- Find and build on the "island of competence" (Brooks, 2002; Kump, 1998). Every child has interests and abilities that can be developed and displayed to provide the child with a sense of success and a defense from failure. Identify what the child is interested in and good at and encourage and praise those skills, talents, efforts, and achievements. Seven kinds of intelligence have been identified: linguistic, mathematic, spatial, musical, bodily, interpersonal, and intrapersonal, and any or all can be used to build and affirm the child's island of competence.
- Help your child compete (Dobson, 1999). A child needs encouragement to develop skills, opportunities to use the skills, and second chances when failure occurs. A child is empowered by having an ally in these endeavors.
- Help your child develop a sense of purpose, knowing that he or she can affect the outcome of events in life. Children feel more effective and less bored and resentful if they feel they are contributing. Provide opportunities to make choices, solve problems, and develop responsibilities (Spratt, 2002).
- Promote a sense of ownership. Children who are given responsibility for themselves and their actions are also given a sense of control over their life.
- Keep a close eye on the classroom (Dobson, 1999). Problems in the classroom are often symptoms of other problems in a child's life. Temporary rough spots are normal and must be distinguished from more pervasive problems that require intervention.
- Defuse feelings of inferiority (Dobson, 1999). Throughout the school years and adolescence, comparisons are the norm, and feelings of inferiority often result. Children aware of

this fact who have learned to compete and compensate are more likely to believe in themselves despite feelings of inferiority.

- Prepare for adolescence (Dobson, 1999). A special time set aside to talk with preadolescents about the coming physical, social, and hormonal changes helps prepare them to handle the transitions with greater ease.

ENCOURAGE ASSET BUILDING

Fostering developmental assets can positively change a young person's life. Because all young people need assets and building assets is an ongoing process, everyone (child, parents, teachers, health care providers, and community members) can be involved in developing assets in the young people around them. Relationships are critical to building assets. Consistent messages about what is important in life and what is expected from the young person are essential. *Intentional redundancy,* hearing the same positive messages over and over again from many different people, is also important. One way for anyone to start developing assets in a young person is to use the asset lists (see Tables 17-1, 17-2, and 17-3) to help identify areas in which to begin to build one or more assets. The Search Institute has many resources and programs to assist individuals and communities to build assets in young people (see the Resource Box). Two particularly helpful books, *What Kids Need to Succeed* and *What Teens Need to Succeed* (Benson et al, 1998a and 1998b, also available in Spanish), define each asset and give ideas for building that asset in the home, school, community, and congregational setting.

It is possible to overcome the deficits in a young person's life. Five areas identified by the Search Institute (Benson et al, 1998a) that are helpful in overcoming deficits are:

1. Getting involved in structured, adult-led activities
2. Setting boundaries and limits
3. Nurturing a strong commitment to education
4. Providing support and care in all areas of life, not just the family
5. Cultivating positive values and concern for others

■ SPECIFIC SELF-PERCEPTION PROBLEMS IN CHILDREN

SELF-ESTEEM PROBLEMS

Description

When a child's sense of significance is disturbed, self-esteem problems arise. The child has a loss of confidence, and feelings of insecurity are evidenced, "Am I loved?"

Etiology

Self-esteem problems arise when children are unsure of belonging and of being loved, cared for, and accepted. Love is often conditional, with acceptance coming for what they do rather than who they are. Attachment problems may be found in the family system. Emotional maltreatment (abuse or deprivation) is an extreme example of this (see Chapter 18). Self-esteem problems may be situational or transient, or they

may be chronic. Girls with low self-esteem are three times more likely to initiate sexual intercourse than girls with high self-esteem (Spencer et al, 2002). Interestingly, neither children with idiopathic short stature (Theunissen et al, 2002) nor adolescents who were extremely low birth weight (less than 1000 g) (Saigal et al, 2002) showed significant difference in self-esteem from controls.

Assessment

The child with self-esteem problems seeks attention, importance, and security. There may be a history of rejection or a dysfunctional family. Parental insensitivity, fatigue and time pressure, guilt, and rivals (e.g., siblings) may all contribute. Self-destructive behaviors (e.g., suicide, eating disorders, teen pregnancy) may be present (Goode, 2002). Self-absorption or obsession with external markers of self-worth may be evident (see Box 17-3).

Because of the desire for acceptance and love, these children are often people pleasers. Position and status are attempts to prove importance. Counterproductive coping strategies may be used (Table 17-4). Disruptive behavior, social withdrawal, poor academic achievement, anxiety, depression, and delinquency are associated with poor self-esteem. Attention seeking may be extreme, causing aggression and leading to behavior problems.

Differential Diagnosis

Differential diagnoses include personal identity problems, role performance problems, and body image problems.

Management

Unconditional love, acceptance, belonging, and security are needs that are not being met. Refer to the management strategies section for specific ideas to achieve these, especially

TABLE 17-4	**Counterproductive Coping Strategies: Signs of Low Self-Esteem**
Behavior	**Example**
Quitting	Ending a game before it is over to avoid losing
Avoiding	Not even trying something for fear of failure
Cheating	Copying answers from someone else on a test
Clowning around	Acting silly to minimize feeling like a failure
Controlling	Telling others what to do
Bullying	Putting others down to hide feelings of inadequacy
Denying	Minimizing the importance of a task
Rationalizing or making excuses	Blaming the teacher for failing a test

From Brooks R: Self-esteem. In Parke S, Zuckerman B, editors: *Behavioral and developmental pediatrics,* Boston, 1995, Little, Brown.

"parental roles," "know your children," and "limits and consequences." The 10-20-10 strategy (spending 10 uninterrupted minutes in the morning, 20 uninterrupted minutes after school or in the afternoon, and 10 uninterrupted minutes in the evening) (Forbes & Post, 2006) may be especially helpful with these children. Children with chronic illness may be assisted by participating in groups with others dealing with similar issues.

Complications
Anxiety, attachment disorders, behavior problems, depression, suicide, eating disorders, teen pregnancy, aggression, and violence are complications of self-esteem problems.

PERSONAL IDENTITY PROBLEMS
Description
When children are uncertain of their worth, personal identity is shaky, and feelings of inferiority are manifested. Children may feel confusion about who they are, "Am I OK?"

Etiology
Personal identity problems arise when children do not receive respect as individuals and are not valued for who they are. This results in their questioning their worth and makes them wonder if they truly are OK. The child relies on others to define self, never knowing for sure who he or she is. This leads to internalizing others' negative perceptions. Potential parental factors that contribute to these feelings of inferiority include insensitivity to the child in words or attitude, fatigue and time pressure, guilt, and rivals for love. Attachment problems may be found in the family system.

Assessment
Children with personal identity problems do not feel good about themselves and often lack evidence of self-respect and self-liking, feeling as if they have not lived up to adult expectations. They may talk about themselves in degrading terms. There is a struggle to prove "I am OK." Coping may take the form of withdrawal, fighting, clowning, denying there is a problem, or striving for conformity (Dobson, 1999). There may be a history of the child being criticized, embarrassed, shamed, or humiliated, or a history of familial mental illness or abuse.

Differential Diagnosis
Self-esteem problems, role performance problems, and body image problems are differential diagnoses for personal identity problems.

Management
Self-respect, self-value, and feeling good about oneself are aspects of self-perception that are not developed. See the section on management strategies for specific ideas to work on these aspects of self-perception, especially "value children," "maintain appropriate expectations of the child," and "defuse feelings of inferiority." Helping the child learn to compensate can conquer low self-esteem (see section on finding the "island of competence"). Time must be made to spend with the child

in one-on-one interaction. The 10-20-10 strategy (described in Self-Esteem Problems, Management) should be especially helpful with these children. Nondirective or experiential play therapy may be useful to help the child discover self and experience growth (Galligan, 2000).

Complications
Anxiety, depression, guilt, anger, and hostility are complications of personal identity problems.

ROLE PERFORMANCE PROBLEMS
Description
When children are unable to perform expected activities or behaviors because of physical, mental, or cognitive disability or if they feel incompetent, role performance problems emerge and feelings of inadequacy often result, "I can't do it." A typical scenario involves a child with school problems.

Etiology
Role performance problems arise when children do not feel adequate, confident, and in control and can occur in cognitive, social, and physical arenas.

Assessment
Children with role performance problems may retreat and be hesitant to approach new opportunities and experiences, or they may be perfectionists, always striving to prove competence. A history of "failure," or being a slow learner, semiliterate, an underachiever, a late bloomer, or culturally deprived may be found.

Differential Diagnosis
Self-esteem problems, personal identity problems, body image problems, and actual physical, mental, learning, or cognitive problems are differential diagnoses for role performance problems.

Management
Since feelings of competence, confidence, adequacy, and being in control are inadequate, strategies to develop these are needed. See management strategies section for specific ideas to work on these aspects of self-perception, especially "find and build on the 'island of competence'" (a key) and "help your child compete." Working with the school and the parents to achieve these goals is helpful.

Complications
Complications of role performance problems include anger, anxiety, behavior problems, depression, withdrawal, and somatic complaints.

BODY IMAGE PROBLEMS
Description
Discrepancy between how children's bodies are and how they want them to be results in body image problems. The discrepancy may be temporary or permanent, seen or unseen,

occurring in terms of size, function, appearance, or potential. Attitudes, feelings, and fantasies all play a role in body image. Eating disorders are one example of a body image problem.

Etiology

Disturbance in body image arises from sources as varied as physical illness or disability, chronic illness, emotional disturbances, abuse, or attitudes conveyed by others. Body image problems are most common in adolescence, when teenagers are most concerned about physical appearance in comparison with that of their peers, but they also occur in younger children. An example of a younger child's body image disturbance can be seen when a child is unable to cope with the inability to master his or her environment because of a fracture and the subsequent immobilization.

Assessment

Children with disturbed body image may have concerns related to body size, function, appearance, or potential. These may be noted by questioning or techniques such as puppet interview or draw-a-person. A body esteem questionnaire for adolescents is available (Mendelson et al, 2001).

Possible behaviors include the following:

- Lack of maternal identification (aspiring to be like one's mother). Maternal identification positively correlates with self-esteem and negatively correlates with eating problems and body dissatisfaction in girls (Hahn-Smith & Smith, 2001)
- Refusing to look at or touch an altered or missing body part
- Preoccupation with the loss or change
- Feeling shame and embarrassment
- Distorted perception of a normal body
- Fear of rejection or unwanted attention from others
- Overexposure or hiding of body part
- Actual or perceived change in structure and function of body or body part

Differential Diagnosis

Self-esteem, personal identity, or role performance problems are differential diagnoses for body image problems.

Management

The discrepancy between the real and the desired body, in addition to the cause of the discrepancy, must be identified. Severity and cause of the discrepancy guide the intervention. If the discrepancy is developmental and not severe, education and counseling should help. If the problem is significant, referral for mental health care is often necessary.

Practices to develop appropriate ideas about appearance and value include the following (Hostetler, 2001):

- Explore parental feelings about appearance. Look for ways to broadcast healthy attitudes.

- Prompt children to determine where attitudes originate. Appreciate concern about physical appearance, but discuss extremes. Favorite television shows or movies are good starting points.
- Teach that happiness and beauty do not go hand in hand. Discuss feeling beautiful (outward changes) and being beautiful (inward growth).
- Celebrate each family member's uniqueness. Focus on personality traits and attitudes about life, school, and people, not on externals.

Other interventions that are helpful include the following:

- Encourage regular physical activity. One study (Ransdell et al, 2001) showed improved physical self-perception in adolescent girls and their mothers when they participated in a physical activity intervention together.
- Point out ways the child or adolescent is on target developmentally and identify what can be expected over the next year. Emphasize the fact that there is a high degree of variability in development.
- Identify areas where assistance is needed.
- Refer to counselors, dietary therapy, occupational therapy, or physical therapy as appropriate.
- Visit school or social arenas before a child with health problems returns to that setting to educate and prepare the setting for the child.
- Involve the child in a peer group with similar problems.
- Provide ongoing support and encouragement as a primary care provider with focus on positive aspects of body and functioning.
- Verbalize acceptance.
- Use play therapy to encourage verbalization.
- Teach new ways of handling situations to accommodate for loss or change.
- Discuss ways to camouflage (e.g., wig or scarf for hair loss).
- Compliment behaviors that indicate acceptance.

BOX 17-8 | **Suggested Readings**

Jones A, Jones AE: *104 activities that build self-esteem, teamwork, communication, anger management, self-discovery, and coping skills,* Richland, WA, 1998, Rec Room Publishing.

Kvols KJ: *Redirecting children's behavior,* ed 3, Seattle, 1997, Parenting Press.

Rosemond J: *Parent power and the six point plan for raising happy, healthy children,* Kansas City, MO, 2001, Andrews McMeel Publishers.

Webster-Stratton C: *The incredible years: a trouble-shooting guide for parents of children aged 3-8,* Toronto, 1997, Umbrella Press.

*R*ESOURCE BOX

Resources for Building Self-Perception

Arthur M. Blank Family Foundation
www.blankfoundation.org
Supports programs and organizations that create and enhance self-esteem and increase awareness about cultural and community issues among young people

Bright Futures
www.brightfutures.org
A national initiative to promote and improve the health and well-being of infants, children, and adolescents; volume 1: Mental Health Series; *Practice Guide;* volume 2: *Tool Kit*

Campaign for Real Beauty
www.campaignforrealbeauty.com
Campaign for Real Beauty aims to change the status quo and offer in its place a broader, healthier, more democratic view of beauty

Free Spirit Publishing, Inc.
www.freespirit.com
Publishes books and other learning materials for children and teens, parents, educators, counselors, and everyone else who cares about kids

Kids-Health
www.kidshealth.org
Kid's and teen link has information about self-esteem, feelings, and emotions

Kid Source Online
www.kidsource.com
Provides information about self-esteem and how to help children

Marsh Media
www.marshmedia.com
Books and videos to help kids grow up safe, healthy, and with a sense of self-worth

Ms. Foundation for Women
www.ms.foundation.org
From the creators and sponsors of Take Our Daughters to Work, an "empowering" GirlWorld site with information on organizations, publications, and websites for girls and their parents

MV-Parent
www.mvparents.com
A resource for parents using the developmental assets to assist in raising smart, strong, responsible kids

National Association for Self-Esteem (NASE)
www.self-esteem-nase.org
Includes a book list, links to other sites, and lots of information on self-esteem

Raising Resilient Children Foundation
www.raisingresilientkids.com
Disseminates information that assists adults to raise, support, and develop stress-hardy children; books, videos, articles, and a resiliency quiz

Redleaf Press
www.redleafpress.org
Books, videos, and resources for early childhood that are developmentally and culturally appropriate and free of stereotypes

Resilience, Self-Esteem, Motivation, and Family Relationships
www.drrobertbrooks.com
Monthly newsletter, books, and online articles

Search Institute
www.search-institute.org
These researchers of developmental assets have multiple resources for individuals, schools, communities, and congregations; includes books, handouts, newsletter, and programs

Soy Unica! Soy Latina!
www.soyunica.org
Bilingual initiative for Hispanic girls 9 to 14 years old (and their mothers and other caregivers) by the Substance Abuse and Mental Health Services Administration (SAMHSA) designed to help build and enhance self-esteem, mental health, and decision-making and assertiveness skills, and to prevent the harmful consequences of alcohol, tobacco, and illicit drugs

Verb™ It's what you do
www.cdc.gov/youth campaign
From the U.S. Department of Health and Human Services, Centers for Disease Control and Prevention; geared toward keeping 9- to 13-year-olds active and increasing their self-esteem

Winners on Wheels
www.wowusa.com
Provides an innovative learning environment to promote academic, social, and emotional development for children in wheelchairs

BOOKS THAT TEACH SELF-ESTEEM
- *Brave New Girls* by Jeanette Gadeberg (Fairview Press, 1997) for 9 years and older.
- *Corduroy* by Don Freeman (Viking, 1968) for 3 to 8 years old.
- *I Like Being Me: Feeling Special, Appreciating Others and Getting Along* by Judy Lalli (Free Spirit, 1997) for 4 to 8 years old.
- *Leo the Late Bloomer* by Robert Kraus (Harper Collins, 1971) for 4 to 8 years old.

Continued

RESOURCE BOX

Resources for Building Self-Perception—Cont'd

- *On the Day You Were Born* by Debra Frasier (Harcourt Brace, 1991) for 2 years and older.
- *Those Can-Do Pigs* by David McPhail (Dutton, 1996) for 5 to 9 years old.
- *A-Z Child's Guide to Self-Esteem* by Bonita Blazer. (Available at UCB Pharma or *www.bblazer.org*) for 5 to 9 years old.
- *I Like Myself!* by Karen Beaumont (Free Spirit Press) for 3 to 7 years old.

- *Stick Up For Yourself!* by Gershen Kaufman, Lev Raphael, & Pamela Espeland (Free Spirit Press) for 8 to 12 years old.
- *I'm Gonna Like Me: Letting Off a Little Self-Esteem* by Jamie Lee Curtis.
- *Incredible You!* by Wayne Dyer.
- *Don't Feed the Monster on Tuesdays! The Children's Self-Esteem Book* by Adolph Moser for 4 to 10 years old.

NURSING DIAGNOSES

Related to Self-Perception Functional Health Pattern

Diagnoses are related to the concepts: identity, loneliness, self-esteem, and body image.
- Disturbed personal identity
- Powerlessness
  - Risk for powerlessness
  - Readiness for enhanced power
- Hopelessness
  - Readiness for enhanced hope
- Risk for loneliness
- Chronic low self-esteem
- Situational low self-esteem
- Risk for situational low self-esteem
- Disturbed body image
- Readiness for enhanced self-concept
- Risk for compromised human dignity

From NANDA International: *NANDA-I nursing diagnoses: definitions & classification 2007-2008,* Philadelphia, 2007, Author.

✓ DISCUSSION FORUM

1. Compare and contrast the strategies used to assess a 5-year-old, an 11-year-old, and a 16-year-old's self-perception. Identify at least four developmentally appropriate questions for each child.
2. Do a developmental asset evaluation on a child of your choosing. Pay special attention to identify family and environmental influences that impact the child's self-perception.
3. Create a plan of care to teach a parent parenting skills that promote a child's healthy self-perception. Focus on communication and discipline skills.
4. You identify altered self-perception and role performance problem in an adolescent female. Create a plan of care that addresses these issues and maximizes her developmental assets.

REFERENCES

Allison SE et al: The development of the self in the era of the Internet and role-playing fantasy games, *Am J Psychiatry* 163(3):381-385, 2006.

Baumeister RF et al: Does high self-esteem cause better performance, interpersonal success, happiness, or healthier lifestyles? *Psych Sci Public Interest* 4(1):1-44, 2003.

Benson PL, Galbraith J, Espeland P: *What kids need to succeed,* Minneapolis, 1998a, Free Spirit Publisher.

Benson PL, Galbraith J, Espeland P: *What teens need to succeed,* Minneapolis, 1998b, Free Spirit Publisher.

Brooks R: *What is resilience?* 2002. Available at *www.raisingresilientkids. com* (accessed Feb 5, 2007).

Burton S, Mitchell P: Judging who knows best about yourself: developmental change in citing the self across middle childhood, *Child Dev* 74(2):426-443, 2003.

Chapman PL, Mullis RL: Racial differences in adolescent coping and self-esteem, *J Genet Psychol* 161(2):152-160, 2000.

Costello EJ et al: Relationships between poverty and psychopathology, *JAMA* 290(15):2023-2029, 2003.

Davis-Kean PE, Sandler HM: A meta-analysis of measures on self-esteem for young children: a framework for future measures, *Child Dev* 72(3):887-906, 2001.

Dixon SD, Stein MT: *Encounters with children: pediatric behavior and development,* ed 3, St Louis, 2000, Mosby.

Dobson J: *The new hide or seek: building self-esteem in your child,* Grand Rapids, MI, 1999, FH Revell.

Eisenberg ME, Newmark-Sztainer D, Story M: Associations of weight based teasing and emotional well-being among adolescents, *Arch Pediatr Adolesc Med* 157:733-738, 2003.

Elster AB, Kuznets NJ: *AMA guidelines for adolescent preventive services (GAPS),* Baltimore, 1994, Williams & Wilkins.

Forbes HT, Post BB: *Beyond consequences, logic and control,* Orlando, FL, 2006, Beyond Logic Consequences Institute.

Galligan AC: That place where we live: the discovery of self through creative play experience, *J Child Adolesc Psychiatr Nurs* 13(4):169-176, 2000.

Goode E: *Deflating self-esteem's role in society's ills.* Available at *www. nytimes.com/2002/10/01/health/psychology/0125TE.html?ei=1&en= d2809ed774* (accessed Oct 2, 2002).

Gray-Little B, Hafdahl AR: Factors influencing racial comparisons of self-esteem: a quantitative review, *Psychol Bull* 126(1):26-54, 2000.

Hahn-Smith AM, Smith JE: The positive influence of maternal identification on body image, eating attitudes, and self-esteem of Hispanic and Anglo girls, *Int J Eat Disord* 29(4):429-440, 2001.

Hall H: *Ways to enhance your child's self-esteem.* Presentation at the NAPNAP National Conference, Chicago, 1998.

Hart L: *The winning family: increasing self-esteem in your children and yourself,* Oakland, CA, 1990, LifeSkills Press.

Hostetler B: Looking beyond looks: helping your child look beyond their physical appearance, *Focus Fam* July 2001.

Jellinek M, Patel BP, Froehle MC, editors: *Bright futures in practice: mental health,* vol 1, *Practice guide,* vol 2, *Tool kit,* Arlington, VA, 2002, National Center for Education in Maternal and Child Health.

Kump T: Self-esteem: why little kids need BIG egos, *Healthy Kids,* Oct/Nov 1998.

Kurcinka MS: *Raising your spirited child,* New York, 1998, Harper Perennial.

Ladd GW, Troop-Gordon: The role of chronic peer difficulties in the development of children's psychological adjustment problems, *Child Dev* 74(5):1344-1367, 2003.

Lewis M, Ramsay D: Development of self-recognition, personal pronoun use, and pretend play during the 2nd year, *Child Dev* 75(6):1821-1831, 2004.

McLean KC: Late adolescent identity development: narrative meaning making and memory telling, *Dev Psychol* 41(4):683-691, 2005.

Mendelson BK, Mendelson MJ, White DR: Body esteem scale for adolescents and adults, *J Pers Assess* 76(1):90-106, 2001.

Neifert, MA: Self-esteem and emotional health. *A Dr Mom Presentation* Denver, 2005.

Perry PD: Creating novelty, *Scholastic Parent and Child* 9:67-68, 2001.

Quatman T, Watson CM: Gender differences in adolescent self-esteem: an exploration of domains, *J Genet Psychol* 162(1):92-117, 2001.

Ransdell LB et al: Daughters and mothers exercising together (DAMET): a 12-week pilot project designed to improve physical self-perception and increase recreational physical activity, *Women Health* 33(3/4):101-116, 2001.

Reasoner R: *The true meaning of self-esteem,* 2002. Available at *www.self-esteem-nase.org/whatisselfesteem.shtml* (accessed Sept 14, 2007).

Rees CA: Thinking about children's attachments, *Arch Dis Child* 90:1058-1065, 2005.

Rochat P, Striano T: Who's in the mirror? Self-other discrimination in specular images by four- and nine-month-old infants, *Child Dev* 73(1):35-46, 2002.

Saigal S et al: Self-esteem of adolescents who were born prematurely, *Pediatrics* 109(3):429-433, 2002.

Salmivalli G, Isaacs J: Prospective relations among victimization, rejection, friendlessness, and children's self- and peer-perceptions, *Child Dev* 76(6):1161-1171, 2005.

Salmivalli C, Ojanen T, Haanpaa J: "I'm OK but you're not" and other peer-relational schemas: explaining individual differences in children's social goals, *Dev Psychol* 41(2):363-375, 2005.

Schore AN: Attachment, affect regulation, and the developing right brain: linking developmental neuroscience to pediatrics, *Pediatr Rev* 26(6):204-211, 2005.

Schott ER, Bellin W: The relational self-concept scale: a context specific self-report measure for adolescents, *Adolescence* 36(141):85-103, 2001.

Search Institute: *Asset power,* 2006a. Available at *www.search-institute.org/research/assets/assetpower.html* (accessed Sept 26, 2006).

Search Institute: *Insights and evidence,* 2006b. Available at *www.search-institute.org/whatsnew* (accessed Sept 26, 2006).

Search Institute: *The positive human development,* 2006c. Available at *www.search-institute.org/research/HDindex.html* (accessed Sept 26, 2006).

Shebloski B, Conger KJ, Widaman KF: Reciprocal links among differential parenting, perceived partiality, and self-worth: a three-wave longitudinal study, *J Fam Psych* 19(4):633-642, 2005.

Slattery J: Self-esteem, *Discovery Years, Focus Your Child CD,* Dec 2005.

Solomon CR, Serres F: Effects of parental verbal aggression on children's self-esteem and school marks, *Child Abuse Negl* 23(4):339-351, 1999.

Spencer JM et al: Self-esteem as a predictor of initiation of coitus in early adolescents, *Pediatrics* 109(4):581-584, 2002.

Spratt E: Assessing and reinforcing your child's self-esteem. In Jellinek M, Patel BP, Froehler MC, editors: *Bright Futures in practice: mental health,* vol 2, *Tool kit,* Arlington, VA, 2002, National Center for Education in Maternal and Child Health.

Theunissen NCM et al: Quality of life and self-esteem in children treated for idiopathic short stature, *J Pediatr* 140(5):507-515, 2002.

Troop-Gordon W, Ladd GW: Trajectories of peer victimization and perceptions of the self and schoolmates: precursors to internalizing and externalizing problems, *Child Dev* 76(5):1072-1091, 2005.

Trzesniewski KH, Donnelan MB, Robins RW: Stability of self-esteem across the life span, *J Pers Soc Psych* 84(1):205-220, 2003.

Udry JR, Li RM, Hendrickson-Smith J: Health and behavior risks of adolescents with mixed-race identity, *Am J Public Health* 93:1865-1870, 2003.

US Department of Health and Human Services: *Healthy People 2010.* Available at *http://healthypeople.gov/document/htm/volume2/18mental.htm* (accessed Sept 15, 2007).

US Preventive Services Task Force: *The guide to clinical preventive services 2006,* Baltimore, 2006, Agency for Healthcare Research and Quality AHRQ Pub. No. 06-0588, June 2006 (accessed Sept 14, 2007).

Verschueren K, Buyck P, Marcoen A: Self-representations and socioemotional competence in young children: a 3-year longitudinal study, *Dev Psychol* 37(1):126-134, 2001.

Zuckerman B, Zuckerman PM, Siegel DJ: Promoting self-understanding in parents—for the great good of your patients, *Cont Ped* 22(4):77-90, 2005.

CHAPTER 18

Role Relationships

Margaret A. Brady and Ardys M. Dunn

Understanding family dynamics and role relationships is essential to the delivery of health care services to children and adolescents in all pediatric settings. However, advising parents on how to effectively handle relationship issues with children at home, in school, and in the community is an essential responsibility of nurse practitioners (NPs) working in primary care settings. Parents and other family members are solely responsible for the health and welfare of their young children and must learn key communication and interaction skills to effectively parent their child. The pediatric provider must be sensitive to the roles that parents or caregivers, siblings, extended family members, and peers have in shaping the developing child. Likewise the community is an extension of the family and serves as a major component in the widening circle of influence that affects children's and adolescents' lives. Chapter 2 outlines important considerations and appropriate tools to be used when assessing family systems. This chapter discusses the family life cycle and family variations, in addition to the assessment and management of situations or events that the provider is likely to encounter in a primary care setting related to family relationship problems, sibling rivalry, child maltreatment or neglect, and violence. Preventive interventions for role-relationship problems that are directed at the population as a whole (universal interventions) and specific individuals or groups at risk (selective interventions) are identified. Advice about securing nurturing, safe, and developmentally appropriate child care is discussed.

FAMILY RELATIONSHIPS AND DYNAMICS

FAMILY LIFE DYNAMICS

The family is a dynamic social system that is usually the most powerful influence in a child's development and life both in depth and sphere of influence. The family unit creates unique emotional bonds between its members and is the training ground for teaching children how to become competent members of society (Berk, 2006). Changes in one family member's behavior affect everyone else in the family unit.

Healthy families are cohesive and adaptable, with positive communication patterns (Friedman et al, 2003; Berk, 2006). Family cohesion is an indication of the strength of the emotional bonding between family members and can range from the extremes of very low (disengaged) to very high (enmeshed) bonding, with moderate to high (connected) bonding representing the middle ground. Family adaptability is the ability of a family system to change its power structure, role relationships, and relationship rules in response to situational and developmental stress. The range of adaptability varies from very rigid (very low) to chaotic (very high), with a middle ground between structured and flexible. A key element in adaptability is the ability to change when appropriate. Communication patterns range from positive communication skills that convey messages, such as empathy, reflective listening, and supportive comments, to negative communication skills that reflect double messages, double binds, or criticism and that minimize opportunities to share feelings. Communication is one of the most crucial elements within any interpersonal relationship. Family cohesion and adaptability are threatened and thwarted with negative communication patterns. The end result of negative communication is a chaotic household marked by high levels of family distress.

Each family has its own unique pattern of growth and development, and family systems evolve and change, demonstrating different dynamics depending on the stage of the family's life cycle. Just as a child goes through stages of development, so do family units. Family life with young infants and preschool children is vastly different from family life with school-age children, with early versus late adolescents, or with young adults. Also, different types of family units—nuclear, single-parent, divorced, or blended—will express different styles or patterns of family life.

DIMENSIONS OF FAMILY FUNCTIONING

Regardless of how a family is classified or typed, common themes exist within all families, and six key dimensions have a significant impact on family functioning, contributing to cohesiveness, adaptability, and positive communication. To assist parents and children across the family life cycle and during times of stress, the provider must carefully assess these elements, which include family:

- Resources
- Stresses
- Child-rearing styles
- Values
- Structures
- Coping styles

Family resources include a social support network of extended family members, friends, and community, in addition to financial and other material assets. Families with limited resources or social support networks are more vulnerable to stressful life events than are families with resources and support systems in place.

Potential family stresses and changes are numerous and include financial strains, illness, marital strain, family transitions, losses, and lack of effective coping strategies. Life brings transitions that necessitate change. Many transitions are normal, some are anticipated, and others are unexpected; all can have a significant impact. Child-rearing styles are composed of parenting behaviors and beliefs that influence the environmental milieu in which the child learns about the world. Certain child-rearing styles (e.g., an uninvolved, overindulgent or permissive, or strict authoritarian parenting style) are ineffective and have dire consequences for the emotional health of a child.

Values shared by family members provide a framework to guide, explain, and understand events being experienced and within which to find comfort, joy, and solace. Spiritual beliefs are one example of values that can support a family in its everyday life and in times of challenge.

Family roles and structures vary greatly from one family to another, within an individual family, and as family members grow and develop. Role responsibilities and structures often change in response to external demands experienced by the family, and shifts in the role of one family member will affect the role functions of other family members.

The ways that demands are met, transitions handled, and concerns resolved all depend on the family's ability to cope. Positive or effective coping is characterized as a creative response to a change or stressor that results in a new behavior or attitude. Coping styles reflect habitual patterns of action. In contrast, coping efforts refer to specific actions taken as a direct result of a specific situation.

THE INTERACTIVE FAMILY

The family is interactive, both within the family circle and between the family and its community. Within the family, each member influences all others in the family and is likewise affected by them. Maladaptive patterns of interaction among family members can place a child and family at risk for negative outcomes. For example, if the family unit does not provide a protective, warm, responsive, attentive, sensitive, supportive, and loving environment to nurture the child or fails in its responsibility to help the child learn self-discipline and the ability to socialize with others, the child often develops maladaptive behaviors.

A child-rearing style that is authoritative is best because it makes reasonable demands based on the child's level of maturity (Berk, 2006). An authoritative style grants autonomy that is age-appropriate and permits the child to make decisions based on readiness factors; encourages the expression of feelings, thoughts, and desires; and promotes joint decision-making when appropriate as the young child matures and develops throughout childhood and adolescence.

In addition, children are at risk for developing mental health problems as a result of environmental factors, such as living in poverty, living in a community with a high crime rate, living in a home marked by marital conflict or domestic violence, living in a home in which they or their siblings are the victims of child maltreatment or neglect, or having a parent who abuses alcohol or other substances or has mental illness.

In contrast to at-risk factors, there are factors that are protective and foster child resiliency. Certain temperaments, a caring relationship and/or social support outside the immediate family, community resources and opportunities, and effective parenting can counter the negative effects of adverse risk factors and contribute to a child's positive mental health. The degree of satisfaction as a married couple and as parents is an important outcome measure of how well the family is functioning as a family unit. Single-parent households may face many challenges that can have a negative impact on the family unit, but are enhanced by developing nurturing relationships in both the parent's and the child's life.

ASSESSMENT OF FAMILY RELATIONSHIPS AND DYNAMICS

In addition to issues that may arise with "typical" family relationships, pediatric providers are likely to encounter parent- or child-initiated concerns, situations, and events related to relationship problems, child maltreatment or neglect, and violence. Families and children who are either experiencing or who are at risk for these stressful situations must be identified. Also, family strengths and attributes that sustain and help families effectively deal with stress are important factors to evaluate in the assessment process. In an assessment of family dynamics, the health care provider must investigate the relationships among child, parent or caretaker, and social and environmental factors. Each factor must be analyzed separately, with its various component parts identified. The interactive effect of these factors must then be explored. The goal of assessment is to determine factors that have a negative impact on the child's ability to achieve his or her optimal level of physical, social, cognitive, or emotional growth and development, in addition to factors that support healthy growth.

The following list of significant child, parent or caregiver, and social and environmental factors is not exclusive, but can be used to alert the provider to areas that need further investigation.

Significant points to identify as part of the child factor are the following:

- Chronologic age and developmental level
- Present or past history of physical, emotional, or cognitive problems
- Personality traits and characteristics and temperament
- Prior maltreatment or significant negative life events
- Special care needs
- School performance

Significant points to identify as part of the parent or caregiver factor are these:

- Physical, intellectual, or emotional abilities, illnesses, or limitations
- Level of involvement in child care and life events of child
- Awareness of, responsiveness, and availability to the child
- Level of parenting skills and pattern of communication
- Parental role—two-parent family, single-parent household, or other patterns
- History of maltreatment as a child

- A victim or perpetrator of domestic violence
- Previous parental history of child neglect or maltreatment
- Current drug use in the home or previous history of substance abuse (drugs or alcohol, or both)
- Financial resources, especially if poverty or limited finances are an issue
- Child-rearing practices experienced as a child
- Child-rearing style and beliefs about discipline and corporal punishment

Significant points to identify as part of social and environmental factors are the following:

- Type and strength of family social support network or social isolation
- Peer group relationships
- Sibling assessment
- Cultural belief system
- Environmental condition of home
- Community characteristics—both needs and assets
- Availability and accessibility of community support systems and partnerships
- Stresses, crises, or conflicts in the home environment
- Stresses in neighborhood environment

■ MANAGEMENT FOR HEALTH PROMOTION AND DISEASE PREVENTION

Primary care providers are often approached by parents with concerns about developmental or role-relationship issues that can be managed with healthy parenting and good communication (see Chapters 4 through 8 and Chapter 17). The NP, as a supportive health care professional, is in a strategic position to prevent problems and empower parents and children by providing anticipatory guidance, education, motivational support, resources, and opportunities for counseling. Pediatric providers must always take a proactive approach in promoting health and remember to emphasize the need for preventive services for children and their parents and families.

The pediatric provider is typically involved in universal preventive interventions related to both physical and mental health issues and, depending on background and education, can be involved in selective and indicated preventive interventions. Universal preventive interventions are directed at enhancing the parent-child relationship and are an essential part of routine pediatric health care supervision. Universal interventions address the population as a whole and stress wellness promotion, improving communication, and strengthening relationships. Selective preventions are directed at individuals or groups at risk for the development of mental health or relationship problems, or both. Indicated preventions are for high-risk individuals who are experiencing symptoms or who have biologic markers for mental illness. Selective and indicated preventions often employ a multidisciplinary approach, with community resources and other professionals from various social fields joining together. The provider must develop a plan of action with goals and outcome measures and specific criteria that indicate when there is need for referral to a mental health or other professional.

Healthy People 2010: Understanding and Improving Health addresses issues of violence and abusive behavior and their negative effect on children, families, and society (U.S. Department of Health and Human Services [USDHHS], 2000). Child maltreatment is recognized as a significant public health problem. The target goal of *Healthy People 2010* for maltreatment of children is 10.3 per 1000 children under 18 years old and for child maltreatment fatalities, 1.4 per 100,000 children under 18 years old (USDHHS, 2000). Sadly, recent statistics reveal a rate of 2.03 deaths per 100,000 children from abuse or neglect and a victim rate of 11.9 per 1000 children. Data continue to indicate that the vast majority of child abuse (75%) is perpetrated by parents—mother only, father only, or both (USDHHS, Administration on Children, Youth and Families, 2006). National, state, and local efforts must be dedicated to reducing preventable death and disability and to enhancing the quality of life for all children. Health professionals in their individual practice settings and as a collective group must commit time and talents to improving the quality of life by incorporating health promotion and disease prevention as integral components of health care for children and their families. Identification of at-risk families and referral for intervention must always be viewed as a priority issue.

■ CHALLENGES TO FAMILY RELATIONSHIPS

SEPARATION AND DIVORCE

Description

Divorce or the separation of parents has a profound effect on family life and can lead to major emotional disruption and disequilibrium in the lives of children who typically perceive divorce as a dramatic, painful, and challenging event in their life. Behavioral changes are an expected reaction as the child attempts to adjust to the changing family situation. Custodial and visitation arrangements for children are variable. Joint custody is an option that allows both parents the opportunity to participate in mutual decision-making about their child's life and welfare. Various living arrangements and visitation rights are possible with joint custody. There are instances in which single custody is in the best interest of the child, however, and the noncustodial parent may have sporadic contact with the child and limited involvement in the child's life.

Research studies investigating the psychological consequences of divorce on children have reported varying data on its negative effect. Divorce per se has not been specifically related to psychopathology in children. Rather, it is a factor of vulnerability (McMahon et al, 2003; Vangyseghem & Appelboom, 2004; Pilowsky et al, 2006). Although children from divorced families have more adjustment problems and depressive symptoms than children whose parents do not divorce (Ge et al, 2006), those problems may arise from the conflictive relationships existing before the divorce, rather than the divorce per se (Kelly, 2000). Data have also suggested that in divorce situations children's adjustment problems (internal and external behavioral issues) at home and school are influenced by depressive and/or withdrawn parenting (Wood et al, 2004).

Children's fear of abandonment may be a critical factor in their degree of successful adaptation to divorce (Wolchik et al, 2002b). There also are data to support that children can adapt to and successfully cope with marital separation and divorce with no long-term negative effect, especially if family conflict is minimized or they have significant nurturing support, such as with a grandparent (Cohen, 2002; Lussier et al, 2002; Wolchik et al, 2002a).

Incidence

In recent years, the rate of divorce has decreased slightly in the U.S. The Centers for Disease Control and Prevention (CDC) reported a provisional divorce rate of 3.6 per 1000 marriages in 2005, down slightly from the 3.8 and 3.7 per 1000 reported in 2003 and 2004 (CDC, 2006). Parents who marry at younger ages are more likely to experience divorce. Approximately 40% of first marriages will end in divorce with about half of these marriages ending within the first 7 years (Christian & Blum, 2006). Thus, though divorce occurs in marriages with children of all age groups, the children in divorcing families tend to be younger. Also, many marriages end in legal separation but not divorce (Bramlett & Mosher, 2002).

Assessment

The goal of assessment of the family experiencing separation or divorce is to determine the needs and strengths of the family and use that information to assist them to healthy coping. Areas to investigate include the following:
- Developmental stage of the children
- Common psychosocial reactions to divorce likely at that stage
- The psychosocial impact of the divorce on the parents
- The economic consequences of divorce on the family unit
- Family assets and resources, both internal and external to the family unit (Boxes 18-1 and 18-2)

Management

Anticipatory guidance given to parents who are in the process of separating and divorcing should cover five main topics:
- The need to prepare the child for the impending separation, if possible
- The need to reassure the child that the divorce was not his or her fault
- The need to give ongoing explanations about the divorce and custody issues plus assurances that the child will be taken care of and is loved
- Suggestions about self-help measures
- Indications when referral for mental health counseling is needed (Table 18-1)

Patient Education and Prevention

The goal of health education for children and parents experiencing divorce is to help restore a sense of wholeness and integrity in children's lives. Providers must stress those factors that have been shown to significantly affect whether the child will experience a healthful adjustment to the divorce (Box 18-3).

BOX 18-1 **Child-Related Assessment Factors in Divorce**

Developmental Stage of Children
- Age and developmental stage of children greatly affect their response to separation and divorce of parents.
- Common reactions of children to divorce by age group:
  - 2-5 yr: Regression, irritability, sleep disturbances, aggression
  - 6-8 yr: Open grieving and feelings of rejection or being replaced; whiny, immature behavior, sadness, fearfulness
  - 9-12 yr: Fear and intense anger at one or both parents
  - ≥13 yr: Worried about own future, depressed, or acting-out behaviors (e.g., truancy, sexual activity, alcohol or drug use, suicide attempts)

Common Issues for Children of Divorcing Parents
- Continued tension, conflict, and fighting between parents
- Litigation disputes over custody and visitation arrangements
- Abandonment by one parent or sporadic visitation (decreased availability) vs. denial of visitation
- Diminished parenting resulting from such factors as availability issues or emotional inaccessibility, distress, or instability
- Limited social support system outside nuclear family
- Feelings of loneliness or emotional abandonment, or both

BOX 18-2 **Parental and Family Unit Assessment Factors in Divorce**

Impact of Divorce on Parent
Psychological functioning of parent and availability to child are often negatively affected.
Feelings of bitterness and acrimony toward divorcing spouse are common.
Feelings of helplessness and depression can overwhelm parent, who may no longer be able to maintain household standards or standards of behavior for child.

Economic Consequence of Divorce
Often devastating economic hardships and decline in living standards are problems that families (especially women) face as a result of divorce.
Nonpayment or delinquency in payment of child support is a widespread problem.

Successful efforts implemented during initial periods of disequilibrium and reorganization will strengthen normal development and prevent future psychological trauma. In an early research study, Wallerstein (1983) identified six psychological tasks that children of divorce must master beginning from the time of parental separation and culminating in young adulthood. These tasks continue to be relevant for children whose parents

TABLE 18-1 Key Anticipatory Guidance Issues for Families Experiencing Divorce or Separation

Anticipatory Guidance Issue	Discussion Points With Parents
Advise parents to prepare the child for the impending breakup	If possible tell the child in advance of the breakup. Children who are told before the separation occurs handle the situation more calmly than those who are given no preparation and wake up to find the parent gone. Discussions should focus on supporting the child's needs for reassurance and stability, not on blame, recriminations, or the parent's needs.
Explain to parents the need to discuss the following key issues with their children	Assure children they will continue to see the departing parent if this is true. Explain what divorce means in language appropriate to the child's cognitive and developmental level; offer an explanation of reasons for the divorce in the same terms. Reassure children (particularly important for preschoolers) that they did not cause the divorce or separation, that they cannot correct their parents' unhappiness in the marriage, and that the divorce is the parents' decision. Explain what the family structure will look like afterward and what imminent changes will be necessary in the way the family functions. Explain the visitation arrangements as soon as they are established. Reassure children that they will be cared for, and they are not being abandoned by either parent, unless a parent has disappeared or refuses involvement. Tell children that feelings of sadness, anger, and disappointment are normal; that they should not "take sides," but love both parents.
Discuss the need for consistency	As much as possible maintain routines or rituals that the child is familiar with; if appropriate encourage the use of security items that the child may depend upon (favorite blanket, toys, objects) during the transitional period. Be consistent in disciplinary practices.
Suggest self-help measures	Children and parents may benefit from attending divorce recovery workshops, classes about families in transition, or peer support groups. School counselors, religious groups, or community and social service agencies may be resources for children and parents.
Acknowledgement of grief	Provider should separately acknowledge to both the parent and child the grief that they are experiencing and provide support.
Discuss when referral for mental health counseling might be indicated	Children often demonstrate internalized or externalized psychosocial problems (e.g., sadness, depression, acting-out behaviors, drug use, promiscuous sexual behavior, anger, violence) in response to divorce. Professional counseling can be an essential part of the recovery process, depending on the nature of symptoms, their severity, and how long they continue without improvement. Referral to individual or family counseling with mental health providers may be appropriate.

are divorced. If these psychological tasks are not achieved, the child's mastery of normal developmental tasks associated with growing up is negatively affected. Long-range and preventive interventions need to focus on helping the child to achieve these tasks or goals:

- Acknowledge the reality of the marital breakup.
- Disengage from parental conflict and distress and resume customary pursuits.
- Resolve loss of familiar daily routine, traditions, and symbols and the physical presence of two parents.
- Resolve anger and self-blame.
- Accept the permanence of the divorce.
- Achieve realistic hope regarding relationships—the capacity to love and be loved.

The pediatric provider should offer support and may schedule additional visits or telephone contacts with the family to

---

| BOX 18-3 | **Factors Affecting a Child's Ability to Achieve Healthy Adjustment to Divorce in His or Her Family** |

The opportunity for continued participation of the noncustodial or visiting parent in the child's life on a regular basis

Custodial parent attempts to make visits with the other parent a routine event so there is consistent contact (phone, visiting, e-mail)

The ability of the custodial parent to handle and successfully parent the child

The ability of parents to separate their own feelings of anger and conflict and resolve their own hostility toward the other parent so that the child's need for a relationship with both parents is met; divorced parents do not put the child in the middle

The child does not become involved in parental conflict and does not feel rejected

The availability of a social support network

The ability of parents to meet the child's developmental needs and to help the child master the developmental tasks before him or her

The child's overall personality and personal assets and deficits

---

monitor their adjustment. Be careful not to use terminology that is offensive, such as "broken home," "intact family," and "child of divorce." In addition, look at each family as unique and avoid negative stereotyping (e.g., "deadbeat dad" or "angry mom"). In addition, help the family cope by focusing on their positive strengths and ability to be resilient.

SINGLE-PARENT FAMILIES

Description

A *single-parent family* is defined as a household in which there is one parent only (no spouse) and one or more children under 18 years old. In some cases, other people related by birth (e.g., a brother or sister), marriage (e.g., a sister-in-law), or adoption may live in the household; unrelated (e.g., a friend) adults or children may also live with the family. Single-parent families are distinguished from *multigenerational families,* which are defined as families with a single parent or a married couple living with their children, their parents, their in-laws, or their grandchildren. Being a single parent is often a difficult, challenging role. Children living in single-parent households generally experience significantly lower standards of living and family income than children in two-parent households.

Incidence

The traditional two-parent family has gradually declined over the past few decades, although it is still the norm for non-Hispanic white, Hispanic, and Asian families with children (Child Trends Data Bank, 2006). According to the 2000 census, 51% of all U.S. households are headed by a married couple, and 23.5% consist of a married couple with children under 18 years old. Just more than 7% of all households (7.2%) have a female head of household (no spouse present) with children under 18 years old, and 2.1% are single-parent families with a male head of household (Simmons & O'Neill, 2001). These data represent an increase from 1990 when 6.6% of households with children were headed by single mothers. The incidence of single-parent families varies by geographic, racial, and ethnic demographics.

In 2005, the percentages of black and Hispanic children who lived in single-parent households were 55% and 30% respectively compared with 21% of white children. Similarly, the overall reported percentage of children under 18 years old living at home with two married parents (whether biologic, adoptive, or stepparents) was 67% in 2005. This continues to reflect a leveling off of the trend toward single parenting first seen in the 1990s as opposite to 1969 data where 85% of children lived in two-parent households (Child Trends Data Bank, retrieved Sept 20, 2006).

Resiliency in single-parent families occurs and is associated with individual characteristics of optimism, perseverance, faith, expressions of emotions, and self-confidence (Greeff & Ritman, 2005). The percentage of births to unmarried women has steadily increased in the U.S. In 2003 more than 34% of woman 25 to 29 years old who gave birth were unmarried, in sharp contrast to 5.3% in that age group in 1960. More than half of women, 20 to 24 years old, giving birth in 2003 were unmarried (Child Trends Data Bank, 2006).

Numerous circumstances lead to single-parent households, including unemployment, divorce, births to unmarried mothers, abandonment of the family by a parent, incarceration of a parent, or death of a parent. Studies demonstrate higher levels of depressive symptoms and problematic substance use in children living in single-parent families compared with mother-father families (Barrett & Turner, 2005). Barrett and Turner (2006) report that this relationship probably is linked more with exposure to stress and association with deviant peers. Likewise, living in a single-parent household is strongly associated with poorer child health, largely as a factor of an associated accumulation of social disadvantage (Bauman et al, 2006).

Assessment

Several key areas are important to assess when working with single parents and their children. They can be divided into parent- and child-related factors.

Parent-related factors include the following:

- Availability of emotional support from a social network, such as extended family members, friends, or church and community groups
- Presence of financial difficulties and economic hardships, which are often major concerns
- Living situation and insurance coverage
- Availability and quality of child care for parents who must work
- Opportunities for the single parent to have a social life and relationships or personal time
- Emotional and physical well-being of the parent; the capacity to parent when exhausted or overwhelmed
- Ability of the parent to maintain consistency in discipline, in addition to a positive outlook and commitment to parenting

(e.g., does the parent have the energy and temperament to parent in a consistent fashion?)

- Availability of financial and emotional support from a noncustodial parent

Child-related factors to assess include the following:

- Availability of emotional support from a social network, such as extended family members and friends
- Role of the child in the family; responsibilities to care for siblings, and opportunities to participate in activities outside of home
- Relationships with custodial parent (e.g., is the child the single parent's primary source of emotional support or contact?)
- Location of and relationship with the noncustodial parent (e.g., is it supportive or conflictive?)
- Availability of opportunities to accomplish age-appropriate developmental tasks (e.g., is child doing well in school? Does he or she have friends? Is child participating in sports or club activities?)
- Signs of problem behavior at school, at home, or with social activities or the presence of children in the home with special needs (e.g., developmental disability, cognitive delay, or chronic illness)

Management

Many single families cope well with the demands they face, benefiting from advice, anticipatory guidance, encouragement, and support of the pediatric provider. On an individual level, several critical factors promote successful child rearing in single-parent homes. They involve the availability of a social support network and positive communication patterns (Box 18-4). Social organizations, such as Big Brothers and Big Sisters, offer a supportive role model for children in single-parent families. Parents Without Partners is a national organization that offers social activities and support for single parents (see Resource Box at the end of the chapter).

Two issues that single parents commonly seek advice about involve dating situations and explaining money problems to their children. Dating can present challenges depending on the age of the child or children. Suggest that the parent meet his or her date outside the home until a decision is made as to the direction of the adult relationship. Young children tend to quickly attach to individuals who are kind and spend time with them, whereas an older child may become jealous or see the individual as a threat. Financial concerns frequently are issues in single-family homes. Urge the parent to explain the family's money situation in a way the child can understand based on age. When money is limited or tight, simply and briefly tell the child that the family may have to wait to buy or limit buying "extras" or that some activities may have to be limited. Then talk with the child about the value of saving up money for special treats.

If parents request specific help or demonstrate signs of being exhausted, depressed, overwhelmed, burdened, or socially isolated, a referral to more specialized services, such as counseling, may be appropriate. Similar signs in children plus deviant behaviors, emotional adjustment problems, or school disciplinary, academic, or behavioral problems can be indicators for mental health referral. The type of referral depends on the nature of the problem, the severity of symptoms, and the continuance of symptoms or problems without signs of improvement. Referrals can include individual or family counseling with mental health practitioners (see Management section under Separation and Divorce).

Patient Education and Prevention

Although individual families may be helped to gain better coping skills, significant positive change in the quality of life of single-parent families depends on restructuring and increasing economic, educational, and family support resources in the community. Primary care providers should become informed of the impact that social service legislation has on the families they serve and provide information to policy makers to help them make appropriate decisions. Legislation regarding health insurance coverage including mental health coverage is a key topic providers should monitor.

REMARRIAGE: THE BLENDED FAMILY

Description

The *blended family* is a term used to describe family reorganization or reconstitution associated with remarriage. Often children from two families are involved in becoming one "blended" household. Because of past negative connotations of the term *stepfamily*, the currently preferred term is *blended family*.

Incidence

The majority of women and men who divorce or are widowed remarry. Children whose parents are divorced spend an average of 5 years in single-parent households. With remarriage, children become members of blended families. Blended families

---

BOX 18-4 **Significant Determinants for Successful Child Rearing in a Single-Parent Home**

- Support persons in the child's life who:
  - Collaborate with the single parent
  - Develop quality relationships with the child
  - Are available for the child
- Adults in child's community who provide support, including:
  - Teachers
  - School officials
  - Health care providers
  - Support person(s) for the parent
- Capacity of parent to communicate with child in open, direct, and understanding manner
- Ability of parent to recognize child's need for opportunities for enjoyment and accomplishment outside the home and to provide for them
- Economic stability and well-being that is adequate to meet family's needs

can present unique parenting challenges in family adaptation, cohesiveness, coping, and role relationships.

Assessment

The introduction of a stepparent and possibly stepsiblings can be beneficial for a child or can be a time of difficult adjustment. The majority of children within blended families gradually adjust well to their new family situations. However, role-relationship problems do arise related to the special needs of reconstituted families. The pediatric provider must remember several important points when assisting blended families during times of transition or problems. They include the developmental stage of the children, the common psychosocial issues that these children experience, and characteristics of problem behaviors in blended families (Box 18-5).

Management

The goal of primary care interventions is to foster positive parenting behaviors, protect the development of the stepchild, and enhance family functioning. A careful assessment of any behavioral concern should be done. Whether the family is given guidance and followed closely by the primary care provider or given a referral to mental health services depends on the presence of significant behavioral or mental health problems. Providers should investigate community services that assist blended families, such as a self-help group for stepparents or a parenting group. Written information including telephone numbers of community resources should be maintained in a handbook or resource guide kept in the practice setting.

Patient Education and Prevention

Counseling and guidance before remarriage that look at coping with transition in a blended family should be explored with parents. Relationships develop and are created over time. Many children go on to develop strong and meaningful attachments to their stepparents if the relationship is cultivated over time with careful sensitivity to the needs of the child.

BOX 18-5   **Assessment of and Counseling Tips for Children in Blended Families**

Assessment
Developmental stage of child
Age and developmental stage of child greatly affect child's response to the remarriage and ability of child to cope with change and new family relationships.
Early adolescence is often a time of greatest difficulty in adjustment to remarriage.
A mother's subsequent pregnancy is often a time of increased frequency and intensity of problems with young children.

Common issues for children in blended families
Complex relationship with new family members
Altered relationships with own family members and possible feelings of betraying other biologic parent or being torn between parents
Possible relocation and separation from family members and friends
Continued or new tensions between parents and tensions between stepparents; rivalries between parents and stepparents
Jealousy among stepsiblings
Establishing new family traditions and values
Continuing to respect earlier family history, traditions, and loyalties that may be in conflict with new family ties
Unrealistic expectations by child of stepparent
Unrealistic expectations by stepparent for instant love, respect, and obedience from child
Tensions within blended family household, creating anxiety and fear of another family breakup

Characteristics of problem behaviors in blended families
Problems can occur both at home and at school.
Children in divorced and blended families experience more behavioral, social, emotional, and educational problems than do children from nondivorced families.
Parental conflict more than family structure is the critical factor that influences both marital and family adjustment.

Counseling tips
Discuss upcoming changes with your child before remarriage and address possible fears, feelings, and expectations.
Keep the marriage strong by a nurturing husband-and-wife relationship.
Blended family parents need to agree on discipline issues, how to set limits, and type of discipline; remember to be consistent.
Start new family traditions, such as weekly family meetings.
Be patient and as flexible as possible; do not expect your child(ren) to have an immediate positive relationship with the new stepparent.
Spend quiet, alone time with your child as much as possible and preferably every day.
Do not force your child to align with the new parent and remember that a second parent does not replace the first; support and help maintain the relationship of your child with the other birthparent.

ADOPTION

Description

Adoption is the legal process that gives individuals who are not birth parents legal and permanent parental responsibility for children. Birthparents terminate their rights, and the adoptive parent(s) are awarded legal custody. Thus, a new nuclear family is created. The adoption process has changed greatly from that of the traditionally married couple adopting a newborn. Single-parent adoption; intrafamily adoption; subsidized adoption of children with special needs; independent, identified, and international adoptions; surrogacy arrangements; and open adoptions are examples of various forms of adoption. Public and private agencies, independent adoption through attorneys, and foreign adoption services are potential avenues to assist in the placement of children.

Incidence

Since 1975, with the dissolution of the National Center for Social Statistics, there have been no federal agencies or nonprofit organizations collecting data on the annual number of total adoptions in the U.S. Statistics are kept on the adoption of foster children. It is known that adoption rates have declined markedly as more unwed women elect to keep their babies. Adoption of children from minority backgrounds continues to be a problem because of the limited availability of adoptive parents of the same race or ethnic group as the child.

Assessment

Important information that the provider should attempt to ascertain when assisting adoptive families includes the following:

- Legal arrangements and circumstances surrounding adoption process
- What, if any, contact will the birthparent or parents have with the child?
- When will the adoption be finalized? How long is the waiting period?
- Are there support services available for the adoptive family if an agency is arranging the adoption?
- Knowledge of medical and psychosocial history of birthparents and child
- Was the presence of any inherited diseases or mental illnesses reported about the birthparents? Does the child have any known or suspected medical problems?
- Is information about the pregnancy, delivery, and neonatal period or subsequent medical problems available?
- Children adopted from foreign countries can be at risk for medical problems. Routine recommended screening tests are outlined in Box 18-6. If the reliability of prior vaccination history is questionable, an acceptable practice is to repeat the vaccinations (Peter, 2004; Christian & Blum, 2006)
- Availability of social supports for adoptive parents and older child
- The presence of a social support network is important. Adoptive parents face the same parenting challenges as biologic parents do when their child passes through the various developmental stages of childhood. In addition, adoption is a special circumstance and can present special challenges to parents.

BOX 18-6   **Recommended Screening Tests for Children Adopted from Foreign Countries**

- Newborn metabolic screening panel (all infants)
- Complete blood count with differential, platelet count, and indices
- Thyroid function tests (if not done as part of newborn screen)
- Urinalysis
- Lead level
- PPD, despite any previous BCG vaccination; if positive result obtain, chest x-ray
- Stool for ova and parasites and Giardia antigen
- Hepatitis B panel, including surface antibody and antigen and core antibody
- Hepatitis C antibody
- Syphilis serology
- Cytomegalovirus (may need to consider)
- HIV-1, HIV-2 enzyme-linked immunosorbent assay (ELISA), with confirmatory Western blot; if positive result for children under 18 months old, further evaluation is necessary
- Developmental, dental, hearing, and vision screening
- Hemoglobin electrophoresis (Asian, Latin-American, and African children)
- G-6-phosphate dehydrogenase assay (Asian, Mediterranean, and African children)
- Malaria (peripheral blood smear) (children from tropical or subtropical regions and those with fever of unknown origin)
- Polycythemia, familial or congenital (central European and Russian children)
- Rickets (radiograph) (Chinese children)
- Lactose intolerance (black, Latino, American-Indian, and Asian children)

BCG, Bacille Calmette-Guérin; *HIV,* human immunodeficiency virus; *PPD,* purified protein derivative.

Management

Often parents will request a preadoption consultation. This is an ideal time to review many of the identified issues. Other families may be in a foster-care situation, considering adoption. Support through this process, before adoption is finalized, is crucial because there may be many hurdles with which to contend. Once adoption is finalized, close monitoring and support by the primary care provider during the initial adoption period are important. Scheduling of additional or more frequent health supervision visits is appropriate even when all appears well, but especially if high-risk situations or conditions are identified. If problems arise, prompt referral to mental health or social service agencies is imperative. Children with known special needs who are adopted are often eligible for federal and state financial support and services. Excellent books about adoption for adults and children are available in local bookstores. The provider should select and recommend those books that best fit the needs of the parents and children in the practice.

Patient Education and Prevention

In considering adoption, parents often benefit from a pre-adoption visit to the health care provider who will take care of their child. Parents often have many questions about the initial adoption period and the establishment of a family relationship. Adoption is a lifetime commitment. Issues that the provider should address with parents include the following:

- There should be a gradual disclosure of the adoption to the child. Such disclosure should be done earlier rather than later, and children should always be told the truth about where they came from and why they were adopted.
- Discussions of the adoption should be open, keeping in mind the child's developmental stage, cognitive abilities, and emotional needs. It is important for adoptive parents to reassure the child in words and actions that he or she is loved and the adoptive parents will always be there for the child.
- Discussions with the parents should address any myths, concerns, or fears that the parents might have about adoption and their adopted child.
- Parents need to understand that their child's wish to know about or seek out the biologic parents is not a rejection of them.
- Adolescence can be difficult for adoptive children as they seek their own identity and deal with the fact that they are adopted. If teenagers wish to seek out their biologic parents, they should be encouraged to wait until they are older.
- Adoption of an older child may present an extra challenge, especially if the child has been shuffled between homes or emotionally scarred by abuse or neglect. Telling parents about such challenges can help them to be better prepared to handle some of the difficulties that may lie ahead for their family and, hopefully, seek counseling early if needed.

TEENAGE PARENTS

Description

Teens who become pregnant and give birth face the challenge of raising an infant at a period in their lives when they are seeking to learn who they are and what they are about. The phrase often used to describe teen mothers is "children having children." Adolescent pregnancy is linked with lower self-esteem and poor educational and vocational outcomes for the mother, which in turn are associated with socioeconomic disadvantage. Often adolescent mothers feel isolated, exhausted, and depressed. Their children are at high risk for cognitive delays, behavioral problems, and difficulties in schooling (Christian & Blum, 2006). Some teens can successfully parent their infant if given support. Maternal age is an important predictor of successful parenting; however, preexisting family and individual factors that lead a teenager to become a mother before completing the educational and developmental tasks necessary for adult life are more relevant predictors of successful parenting.

Incidence

The birth rate for teenagers 15 to 19 years old in 2004 was 1 per 1000 population, the lowest rate ever reported in the U.S. This represents a decline of nearly one third since 1991 (Child Trends Data Bank, 2006). Pregnancy rates for white and black non-Hispanic teenagers fell by about one third each in 2000 with rates for Hispanic teens falling by about 15% that same year. Declines in teen pregnancy have been steeper for younger (15 to 17 years old) than older teens (National Center for Health Statistics, 2006).

Assessment

Key issues to address in assessment of at-risk status vary depending on the stage of the teen. Assessment issues related to each of these stages are separately addressed.

Before-Pregnancy Issues Adolescent sexuality is an issue that should be discussed routinely at every health care encounter (see Chapter 19). Early identification and targeting of at-risk teens (both female and male) for intervention is an important role of the provider. Predictors of teen motherhood include the following:

- Sexual molestation as a child
- Abuse or neglect in childhood
- Being a child of an addicted parent or family history of mental illness
- Lack of family involvement; an intolerable home situation
- Poor academic achievement or school dropout
- Loss of a parent by death, separation, divorce, or foster placement
- Living in an impoverished social environment where adolescent pregnancy is commonplace and accepted

Addressing issues that arise during pregnancy, at birth, and postpartum can contribute to a more successful pregnancy outcome and prevent problems from appearing later in the child or teen parent's life.

Pregnancy

- Disclosure of pregnancy to family, the baby's father, peers, or other significant people. Who has the teen told about the pregnancy? Are they supportive? Many teens and their families are in turmoil during the pregnancy.
- Access to prenatal care and adherence to pregnancy health supervision guidelines. Does the teen need to access federal- and state-sponsored programs for medical financial coverage and general assistance?
- Adjustment to the emotional and physical changes of pregnancy.
- Preparation and plans for the delivery and after the baby is born: current living arrangements; plans for future living and child care arrangements, returning to school or work, and financial support.

Birth and Postpartum

- Preparation for childbirth and postpartum care
- Identification of people available to give emotional support and physical help at this critical time

Infancy

- Adolescent mother–infant attachment. Is there evidence of healthy attachment or emotional or physical neglect?
- Confidence of teen mother to care for her infant.
- Conflicts between the teen's needs and those of her infant. Is the mother more interested in reestablishing her adolescent lifestyle or caring for her infant?

- Living arrangements. With whom and where are the teen mother and baby living?
- Plans for birth control.
- Degree of involvement of the social support network in the mother's and infant's life. Is the baby's father invested in the child? Is the teen mother's or father's family supportive, overprotective, or not involved?
- Return to school or the workforce. What are the child care arrangements? How has this affected the teen mother and baby?
- Adequacy of financial resources.

Later Years. Toddler years are challenging, particularly for teens who themselves are survivors of abuse or neglectful parenting. Typically, the teen mother and young child, if living with family, move out on their own or move in with the mother's partner. The provider needs to assess the following:
- Mother's ability to cope with the normal inquisitive and provocative behaviors of her toddler
- How well the family unit is functioning
- Progress made by the mother toward reaching her life goals

As the child gets older, the teen mother is thought of as a young mother. Children of these mothers, especially those who are poor and living in urban settings, are more likely than their peers to have behavioral problems. When their own children are adolescents, they find this a particularly difficult period, and often they become young grandmothers as the teen pregnancy circle is perpetuated.

Management. Key points in management include the following:
- Maintain regular and frequent contact with the teen mother during her pregnancy and during the child's infancy and early childhood.
- Refer to a community health nurse for home visits early in pregnancy and postpartum. This intervention has proven most successful in delaying subsequent pregnancy and improving healthy parenting and family life (Olds, 2002).
- Provide referrals for resources and community agencies that can assist teen mothers (e.g., parenting classes or literature; support groups; special clinic programs that see both infants and teen mothers; Women, Infants, and Children [WIC] program; early child intervention programs provided by school districts and Head Start).
- Remember that both the teen mother and the infant or child have their own separate needs for health supervision and guidance.
- Provide a supportive environment for the teen mother. Have a plan for follow-up so that teen mothers do not get lost in the system.
- Involve other family members (e.g., grandparents, the father) in discussions about child-rearing issues depending on the teen's wishes.
- Emphasize the strengths of the teen mother and praise her positive efforts.
- Intervene early when warning signs of potential neglect or abuse are evident.
- Facilitate further education to minimize effects of poverty on child rearing.

OTHER VARIATIONS IN THE FAMILY UNIT

There are a number of variations in the family unit that reflect changes in American family life and the diversity of parental experiences. Each of these situations is unique and requires a thorough assessment. Key issues to consider when working with these families follow.

Children Living With Grandparents or Extended Family Members

In 2005, approximately 5.6% of children under 18 years old lived with their grandparents, some in multigenerational households (approximately 3.5% of children) that included their parents as well (Child Trends Data Bank, 2006). The first time that large-scale census data were collected on the number of grandparents caring for their grandchildren was in the 2000 census. Approximately 2.4 million grandparents were responsible for their own grandchildren under 18 years old; nearly half of 1 million of these grandparents lived below the poverty level; 38.5% of these grandparents (many 60 years or older) had cared for their grandchild or grandchildren 5 or more years, and 19% had incomes below the 1999 poverty level (Simmons & Dye, 2003). Providers should be alert to the following factors as they work with grandparents who are primary caregivers:
- Often children have lived with one or two biologic parents before either voluntary or court-ordered placement with the grandparent. Such children frequently bring with them a history of significant stress, hardship, and emotional turmoil.
- Children can be involved in continuing conflict with their biologic parent or parents and may experience emotional reaction to separation from or abandonment by the parent or parents.
- Children can experience the loss of friends, schoolmates, and familiar surroundings.
- Caring for children can be an overwhelming responsibility, especially for older relatives or grandparents; the parenting experience can be physically, emotionally, and financially draining on relatives.
- Children need a supportive environment and consistency in discipline.
- Such families need significant support from social service agencies, the educational system, and health care providers.

Children Living in Foster or Group Homes

The number of children in foster homes is increasing, and meeting their psychosocial needs is a growing problem in the U.S. About half of all foster children live in family foster homes with nonrelatives. Data collected in late 2005 by the Administration for Children and Families (ACF) noted that on September 30, 2004 there were 518,000 children in foster-care placements in the U.S. compared with 552,000 children at the same time in 2000 (ACF, 2006). Foster family care numbers are more meaningful when broken down. For instance, in 2004, there were 283,000 children who exited out of foster family placement, 51,000 who were adopted, 304,000 who entered care that year (a fairly stable number since 2000), 118,000 waiting to be adopted, and 65,000 whose parental rights had been terminated.

Thus, in that one year, there were approximately 800,000 children involved in the foster-care system.

- Children are generally placed in protective custody because of concerns of neglect, physical abuse, sexual abuse, or other forms of child maltreatment or because their parents are unable to care for them.
- Children frequently have a history of significant stress, hardship, and emotional turmoil in their family life.
- Children can experience multiple placements and separation from siblings—40% of children in foster-care placement for more than 1 year experience three or four placements (Christian & Blum, 2006).
- Foster children are often involved in family reunification programs and are placed back with their parents under the supervision of the child protective services, with home-based family preservation services available to monitor the situation, assist the parents, and safeguard the children.
- Foster children are placed under legal mandates in foster homes that mirror the children's ethnic, racial, and cultural identities as much as feasible.
- Foster children often receive erratic health care before and after their placement; a medical passport can be used as a means to keep track of medical problems, treatments, and special needs.
- Foster children have special needs, should be followed closely, and should receive preventive health services.
- Children are emancipated from the foster-care system at 18 years old and need to be prepared for this major life change.

Children Living With Homosexual Parents

- Children living with homosexual parents may be the "biologic products" of former heterosexual relationships, or they may have been adopted, or they may have been conceived by artificial technology (planned lesbian or homosexual family). These families reflect every ethnic, racial, and socioeconomic group in the U.S.
- Many studies have demonstrated that children of homosexual parents show no significant differences in their emotional and social adaptation, self-esteem, gender identity, sexual behavior, or sexual orientation than their counterparts raised with heterosexual parents (Anderssen et al, 2002; Golombok et al, 2003; Hunfeld et al, 2002; Gartrell et al, 2005). In contrast Cameron (2006) in a study of 77 adult children of homosexual parents reported findings that suggested that a parent's sexual inclination influences their children's sexual inclination.
- Children can experience problems because of teasing or social isolation and stigmatization by peers, secrecy of parents, or negative reaction of the noncustodial, biologic parents; this may be problematic for some children especially adolescents.
- Children do well if parents are committed to their children, are sensitive to the children's needs, and are patient.
- Children do well if the homosexual stepparent is supportive of the other parent and the child or children. Some states allow adoption by the nonbiologic parent; this is called *coparent adoption.*
- Children find it easier to deal with questions posed about their parents if they learn about their parents'

sexual orientation during childhood rather than during adolescence.

- Children are not at risk to develop a homosexual identity based on their living situation.

Children Living With Two Parental Figures Who Are Unmarried

- Children can be the biologic children of two adults who decide not to marry but live together (cohabitation), the biologic children of one of the adults but not the other, or children who live with their guardian and the guardian's unmarried partner.
- In each of these family situations, the development of a high-quality parent-child relationship, consistency in discipline, and a continued commitment to the child are hallmarks of successful parenting and child rearing.
- Children face significant developmental risks if they sense a lack of permanence or certainty in their lives; if family life is characterized by conflict or poverty; or if there is inconsistency in who lives in the home, frequent breakups, new adult relationships, or frequent changes in living arrangements.
- Children can be torn emotionally if other significant adults in the children's lives (other biologic parents, grandparents, or other extended family members) express distress about the relationship between the unmarried adults.
- Many families who cohabit live in poverty, and the outcome for children may be no better or even worse than living in low-income single-parent families (Acs & Nelson, 2002; Lerman, 2002).

Homeless Children and Their Families

The homeless family and homeless children are an increasing special-need population. In 2003, approximately 39% of the homeless population was under 18 years old with 42% of these children under 5 years old. The results of a 2005 survey of 24 American cites with populations more than 30,000 noted children accounted for 33% of the homeless population. In rural areas, the proportion of homeless families is typically higher. With the decrease in affordable housing units, the average stay of families in shelters reported in this 2005 study was 7 months compared with an average 5-month stay in the mid-1990s. Sadly, this same survey reported that as a result of lack of adequate shelter resources, 32% of requests for shelter by homeless families were denied in 2005 (National Coalition for the Homeless, 2006; U.S. Conference of Mayors, 2005).

Characteristics of these homeless children include the following:

- Living in poverty because of low income and inadequate social support services (e.g., housing, job training, educational opportunities)
- Families with a history of substance abuse, domestic violence, mental illness, or unexpected family or economic crisis
- A significant minority representation, with the majority of these children being younger than 5 years old
- A teen population composed of runaway and "throwaway" adolescents who are often victims of physical and sexual abuse and neglect or teens alienated from their parents for multiple reasons

- Living in a variety of environments, such as a car, motel, makeshift shelters of cardboard or tents, or homeless shelters; often children and parents in families are separated
- Only 77% of homeless children attend school regularly; lack of school attendance has a significant negative effect (National Coalition for the Homeless, 2006b)

Health care problems for which these children are at high risk include the following:

- Early initiation of and sustained substance abuse
- Diseases linked to poverty, including tuberculosis, multiple caries, impetigo
- Sexually transmitted infections (STIs) for runaway teens who prostitute themselves
- Emotional health problems; social isolation
- Those who attend school may be ostracized by other children because of their unkempt appearance, poor hygiene, or substandard living conditions

Children With Chronic Illnesses

Common chronic illnesses in children include allergies (e.g., asthma and eczema) and neurologic conditions (e.g., seizure disorders or cerebral palsy). The incidence of type 2 diabetes is increasing, and celiac disease may be more common than once thought. Nevertheless, pediatric chronic illnesses tend to cover a wide range of conditions. Approximately 15% to 18% of children seen in health care facilities have some level of a chronic condition, causing mild to severe disability or illness (Perrin, 2004). Demands on families of children with chronic illnesses are constant and challenging. The pediatric provider can be a resource as families develop ways to maximize family function and enhance the growth of all family members. Providers can also assess family systems for the risk of stress and its consequences, such as maltreatment of the child. The Family Impact of Childhood Disability (FICD) scale has been found to predict future parenting stress of both mothers and fathers (Trute & Hiebert-Murphy, 2002). Chapter 22 provides a discussion of critical issues for primary care providers to consider when working with families of children with chronic disease.

◾ OTHER CHALLENGES TO THE FAMILY UNIT

Sibling rivalry, multiple births, and death are challenges to the family unit that can cause a period of disequilibrium. Sibling rivalry is a familiar problem, with tales of sibling rivalry recorded in early historical writings. With advances in reproductive technology and the use of fertility drugs, multiple births of two or more infants are much more common, particularly to women older than 30 years. Many families are faced with death of grandparents, parents, siblings, and others in the child's social network.

SIBLING RIVALRY

Birth or Adoption of a New Infant

The birth or adoption of a sibling is often an occasion marked by some degree of unrest and distress for an older sibling. Many parents dread the possibility of jealousy on the part of an older

child and frequently voice concern about transient behavioral regressions occurring after a new infant is brought home. The developmental stage of the older sibling at the time of the new sibling's arrival is an important consideration in helping parents prepare their older child for the new sibling and in dealing with rivalry behaviors afterward. For example, the 2-year-old who is working on developing autonomy often feels highly vulnerable with the appearance of a new sibling. However, many school-age children experience feelings of sibling rivalry, which may continue in varying degrees as the children grow and develop. Sibling rivalry involves the realization by the child that he or she must share his or her parents' attention and affection. The child may feel threatened or displaced.

Anticipatory guidance about this common challenge is critical. The provider needs to prepare parents before the arrival of the new sibling for the possibility of sibling rivalry and guide them in managing this situation.

Assessment. Key issues to discuss with parents about sibling rivalry after the arrival of a new infant are whether the older child has:

- Manifested regressive behaviors since the new sibling arrived (e.g., bed-wetting, return to the bottle, temper tantrums, deliberate naughtiness, clingy behaviors) and, if so, what they are
- Made negative comments about the new sibling or become more demanding of the parents
- Voiced psychosomatic complaints

In addition, the provider should ask parents to describe how they have reacted to the older sibling's behaviors or verbal comments and if and how they have disciplined the child.

Management

Management strategies include the following:

- Before delivery or adoption:
  - Explain to parents that sibling rivalry is a common, probably universal, response of older siblings at the time of the arrival of a younger sibling and continues throughout childhood.
- Encourage parents to do the following:
  - Tell child about pregnancy or adoption and new baby, using time frame and language appropriate to child's developmental stage.
  - Investigate possibility of sibling preparation classes for older siblings.
  - Be honest with older child (e.g., tell child that it will be a long time before the baby can play with him; mom will be tired and busy).
  - Include older child in preparations for new baby and in excitement of the event (e.g., have child visit mother and baby in hospital if possible).
- After the infant or child comes home:
  - Help parents plan ways to spend special time with the older sibling so that he or she feels appreciated and valued (e.g., plan to do simple activities around the house or amusing outdoor activities, such as going to the park).
  - Emphasize the need to see the individuality of each child and his or her uniqueness.

- Explain the need for tolerance when a child younger than 4 years old exhibits regressive behaviors, such as toileting accidents; wanting the bottle or pacifier again; willful destruction of toys, books, or valuables; or temper tantrums.
- Reassure the parents that regressive behavior associated with the arrival of a new sibling is not a reflection of poor parenting.
- Educate parents about teaching children to distinguish between acceptable and unacceptable behaviors.

See Box 18-7 for additional suggestions for parents.

Sibling Rivalry Between Older Children

To assess sibling rivalry, ask parents to:
- Describe sibling behaviors that concern them—fighting, verbal abuse, bickering.
- Identify any precipitating events or situations that seem to elicit negative behaviors between the siblings.
- Identify how rivalry behaviors between siblings were handled in the past.

In advising parents, tell them that older siblings have fewer struggles when allowed to work their sibling issues out themselves rather than have a parent always trying to resolve the issues. Parents should assure their older children that they can work it out rather than the parent trying to figure "who started it."

MULTIPLE BIRTHS

There are several important points to cover in anticipatory guidance for parents who experience multiple births. Typically, twins or triplets multiply the behavioral challenges that the parents face. Characteristically, these children:
- Often develop a special sibling relationship marked by loyalty and cooperative play
- Have periods in which they get along well or quarrel with each other just as other siblings do

---

BOX 18-7   Clues for Parents for Coping With Rivalry Between Siblings

Do

Allow children to vent negative feelings.

Encourage children to develop solutions for problems with siblings.

Anticipate problem situations.

Foster individuality in each child.

Spend time with children individually.

Compliment children when they are playing together.

Tell children about the conflict you had with your siblings when you were a child.

Define acceptable and unacceptable behaviors for sibling interactions.

Do Not

Take sides.

Serve as a referee.

Foster rivalry by comparing siblings or their accomplishments.

Use derogatory names.

Permit physical or verbal abuse between siblings.

- Work out relationships among themselves and function more independently, needing less parental attention
- May develop their own language among themselves as young children
- Display sibling rivalry, especially if they are fraternal rather than identical twins

Advise parents who have multiple births to do the following:
- Breastfeed if possible. Twins can be breastfed at the same time or one right after the other. Develop a plan to rotate breastfeeding if the mother has more than two infants.
- Organize the home for daily activities and plan ahead to have sufficient supplies, such as bottles, diapers, and car seats.
- Attempt to get twins or triplets on the same schedule (awake, sleep, feeding) as much as possible.
- Schedule daily activities to accomplish all that needs to be done—this is crucial.
- Take time out for themselves and as a couple.
- Keep a sense of humor.
- Promote individuality of each child (e.g., discipline and praise as individuals, build a one-to-one relationship with each child).
- Seek out support people to help (e.g., enlist the aid of extended family members) during early infancy when the tasks of physically caring for multiple infants can be overwhelming.
- Contact support groups, such as the National Organization of Mothers of Twins Clubs, Inc. (see Resource Box at the end of the chapter).

Dressing alike when older should be an individual child's choice. Likewise if twins or triplets want to be in the same classroom and the school allows this placement, this should be an option if it is in the best interest of the children. However, school-age children of multiple births may find it easier to have their own, separate, and unique identities if in separate classrooms and if they have separate friends. If an older sibling or siblings are in the family, be cognizant of their needs and feelings during this time of major family transition. Suggestions for strategies to handle this are discussed in the section on arrival of a new sibling.

A DEATH IN THE FAMILY

Death in families is traumatic and disruptive. If the death is natural and "expected" (e.g., an elderly, ill, or frail grandparent), families may be more prepared and able to cope more effectively. Nonetheless, loss of a loved one who has been special to the child, even if expected, can be devastating. If a parent or sibling dies, the remaining children and parent may be unable to cope well. Parents, however, need to incorporate caring for their children into their own grieving of a family loss. This responsibility can be overwhelming and requires sensitive and intensive support from health care professionals. The primary care provider can help parents understand and respond to their children's needs and support parents in their own grief. The provider can explain the following to parents:
- Children's perceptions of death vary by age and developmental stage.
- Children's responses to death depend on both their understanding of death and the cues they receive from adults and other children around them.

- Children must grieve their loss and often are disruptive, "acting out" their anger, fear, and sense of loss or guilt.
- The grief process is a long-term one, with both parents and children needing to "reprocess" their feelings about the loss at subsequent stages of development (e.g., parents often will become saddened when they reflect that their child would "be starting first grade this fall").

Parents should be encouraged to do the following:
- Give clear, honest, age-appropriate information to their children; correct misconceptions.
- Encourage children to express and share their feelings about the person who has died and about their response to the death (e.g., they may be angry or feel guilty). Drawing, painting, or making collages are all ways children can express their feelings of loss.
- Comfort their children and empathize with their feelings.
- Permit children to participate in rituals, funerals, memorials, or other ceremonies; prepare them for what they can expect.
- Keep as consistent a family routine as possible (e.g., school, meals, bedtimes).
- Take time for themselves.
- Seek out support and counseling as appropriate.

Although the primary care provider can be an invaluable resource for support to the family, referral for grief counseling is often helpful. A mental health referral also may be appropriate, and many books are available to help children understand and cope with a family death.

▆ CHILD CARE

Selecting a child care provider and a setting that offers safe, nurturing, and developmentally appropriate child care are challenges for many parents. The individual needs of the child together with parental needs for work coverage and flexibility must be matched with the philosophy and constraints of the child care setting. The primary care provider is often called on to advise parents about how to select a suitable provider. The four-step approach developed by the Administration for Children and Families, USDHHS, is recommended as a guideline for parents (Box 18-8; also see Resource Box at the end of the chapter).

▆ ROLE-RELATIONSHIP PROBLEMS
VIOLENCE
Description
Violence is the outcome of aggressive behavior that becomes destructive and results in physical injury to people or damage to property. Violence has been acknowledged as a major social and public health problem, and it has become a way of life for many of today's youth, who are either perpetrators, victims, or witnesses of violent acts (see Chapter 20 for additional discussion).

Certain key features are characteristic of violence:
- *Continuity:* Once it is used as a coping mechanism, violence becomes a habit that is hard to break.
- *Reciprocity:* Violence generates violent behavior in others, increasing tension and eliciting negative responses.

- *Sameness:* One form of violence becomes as acceptable as another. As its use becomes more common, violence permeates all of one's life.
- *Addiction:* Violence gives a sense of power and control that, though temporary, is addictive.
- *Limitations of options or alternative actions:* Reasoning is difficult in violent situations, and problem-solving abilities are not used.
- *Escalation:* Violence begets more frequent and more intense violence, with potential for serious sequelae.

Five main categories of violence can have an impact on children and their families:
- Domestic violence, including child abuse, corporal punishment, sibling violence, and spousal abuse
- Predatory violence (e.g., a crime or assault)
- Peer violence, such as fighting, gang violence, and bullying (that can become violent)
- Sexual assault and rape
- Dating violence including date rape

Primary health care providers are likely to become involved with young people who are involved as witnesses, victims, or perpetrators of crime related to one or more of these five categories.

There is no one cause of violent behavior. Violence has certain antecedents, such as a situational crisis, and risk factors have been identified that increase the likelihood of violent behavior (e.g., abuse of alcohol). There are developmental and environmental factors that contribute to violence (e.g., impulsivity in young children; poverty and limited resources). Not all individuals exposed to such factors resort to violence, however. Violence is, in large part, a learned behavior, and what children are taught, by example and instruction, will become part of their methods of social interaction.

Effective management of violence in families and communities depends on understanding major influences and key risk factors that contribute to or sustain violence. These include the following (Commission for the Prevention of Youth Violence, 2000; National Center for Injury Prevention and Control, 2006; Bauer et al, 2006; Borowsky et al, 2002):
- *Family influences:* The following family risk factors are associated with violent behavior by youths: authoritarian child-rearing attitudes; harsh, lax, or inconsistent disciplinary practices; low parental involvement and/or education; low emotional attachment to parents or caregivers; poor family functioning or high levels of family disruption; poor monitoring and supervision of children; and parental substance abuse or criminality.
- *Individual influences:* Youths who demonstrate violent behavior are more likely to have low IQ; poor behavioral control; deficits in social, cognitive, or information-processing abilities; antisocial beliefs and attitudes; high emotional distress; history of treatment for emotional problems; exposure to violence and family conflict; involvement with drugs, alcohol, or tobacco; history of early aggressive behavior, attention deficits, hyperactivity, or learning disorder; history of violent victimization or involvement. They may become easily frustrated, have difficulty making transitions, and have no sense of a future or hope for a better life.

BOX 18-8   **Guidelines for Selecting a Child Care Provider: a Four-Step Approach**

Step 1:   Interview Potential Child Care Providers and Observe the Program or Setting
Start early in your search for an appropriate child care facility.

Ask questions about:
1. Cost—cost calculation per hr, daily, weekly, monthly; any late fees; policy about fee structure and rules (e.g., if the child is absent)
2. Enrollment—number of children enrolled in the program, the max daily capacity of setting, adult to child ratio, number of children in a group
3. Child factors—age of the children served in the setting or program
4. Daily activities or program plan—structured vs. unstructured activities
5. Accreditation and licensing regulations related to the provider or setting; review copy of any license or certificate
6. Caretaker issues—credentials and experience and turnover rates (e.g., academic degrees, course, cardiopulmonary resuscitation certification)
7. Policies—open visiting, illness in the child, emergency care, nutrition and feeding policies
8. Illness prevention—immunization requirements for child and staff

Carefully observe the environment:
1. Look at provider-child interactions—check for evidence of nurturing, responsive, comforting interactions
2. Look at safety issues of the physical environment—the play areas, toileting and diaper changing areas, outdoor environment, napping and eating areas
3. Assess the quality of the learning materials and toys (from an educational and safety perspective)

Step 2:   Check References
1. Talk to parents with children enrolled in the program or being cared for by the provider; ask about their experience relative to how the providers handled the care (discipline) and whether they were nurturing and responsive to parents and the child; ask about reliability and consistency of the providers.
2. Talk to local child care resource and referral program or licensing office; Child Care Aware (1-800-424-2246) provides information about the nearest child care resource and referral programs.

Step 3:   Make a Decision Based on Specific Criteria
1. The child will be happy with this care provider and have a safe, nurturing, and developmentally appropriate environment.
2. If the child has special needs, these will be met.
3. The values of the provider and parents are compatible.
4. The child care is affordable.

Step 4:   Be an Involved Parent
1. Regularly talk to the provider about how the child is doing.
2. Talk to the child daily about activities and experiences at the facility.
3. If possible visit the setting unannounced and observe at various times of the day.
4. Communicate with other parents and become involved in child care events as much as possible.
5. Join in special events (e.g., field trips, holiday activities)

Data from *Child care aware, 5 steps to choosing quality child care.* Available at *www.childcareaware.org/en/5steps* (accessed Sept 25, 2006).

- *Economic influences:* The child poverty rate in the U.S. is among the highest in the developed world. In 2004, approximately 18% of children were poor, up from 17% in 2000. There is great disparity in the poverty rates based on ethnic group with black children at a 36% poverty rate compared with non-Hispanic white children at 11% (2006 Kids Count Data Book Online, 2006). Factors associated with poverty (poor housing, malnutrition, transience, and lack of connectedness to schools and community) are also risk factors for aggressive behavior.
- *Societal and environmental influences*: Exposure to violence in the media and at school, easy access to weapons, alcohol and other drugs, and lead poisoning are some of the social and environmental factors that contribute to aggressiveness and

violence in children and youth. Other community risk factors include diminished economic opportunities, high level of transience, high concentration of poor residents; low levels of community participation, socially disorganized neighborhood.

Key factors that interact with the above influences to increase the risks of youth violence include the following:
- Alcohol and other drug use
- Child maltreatment
- Gang membership
- Access to guns
- Media violence
- Violence among peers and intimate family members

Boys are more likely to perpetrate violence and are more often victims of violence, except for sexual assault, though more girls are engaging in aggressive behaviors (Simmons, 2002; Christian & Blum, 2006)). Aggressiveness, bullying, and violent behavior increase with age, peaking around 15 years old.

Epidemiology

Homicide and injury to another are typically the end results of violence. Although murders of children have decreased significantly in the past few years (the good news), they continue to be the fourth leading cause of death for 1- to 4-year-olds and for 5- to 14-year-olds and the second leading cause of death among 15- to 24-year-olds. In 2003, firearm-related death rates, including homicides, suicides, and accidents for children 5 to 14 and 15 to 19 years old, were 0.8 and 12.1 per 100,000 resident population, respectively (National Center for Health Statistics, 2005). There are major differences in firearm-related death rates between males and females 15 to 19 years old (21.2 versus 2.4 per 100,000, respectively). Although there are major differences in rates of violence-related injuries and death by ethnic groups, the majority of homicides involve people who know each other and are of the same race. The typical scenario is played out as follows: an argument occurs, alcohol or drugs have been consumed, a weapon is available and used, and a homicide is the end result.

Youth are often the innocent victims of a crime or assault and, at the same time, are perpetrators of crime; most know the other person or persons involved. In 2005, the number of reported nonfatal assault injuries for youths 15 to 19 years old was approximately 1411 per 100,000 population (age-adjusted rate using the year 2000 as the standard population) (National Center for Injury Prevention and Control, 2006a). The direct and indirect costs in medical expenses, loss of productivity, and decreased quality of life are immense.

Assessment

The assessment of youths who are victims or perpetrators of violent crime should focus on certain key pieces of historical information and the presence of risk factors to help determine the potential for future violence. Table 18-2 outlines risk factors for youth violence by age of onset. If possible the youth and parent(s) should be interviewed separately.

- History of the episode
  - What seemed to cause the incident?
  - Did the child or family know who was involved, or was this a random event?
  - Were alcohol and/or drugs involved?
  - Did either the victim or the perpetrator have or threaten to use a weapon? If yes what type of weapon?
- Past history
  - Have there been prior incidents of violence or assault?
  - What is the usual pattern of drug or alcohol use?
  - Does the child have a history of mental health problems, or was the youth a victim of child abuse?
  - Does the youth have a criminal or police history?

TABLE 18-2   Risk Factors for Serious Youth Violence

Factor	Early Onset (<12 years old)	Later Onset (>12 years old)
Individual	Male	Male
	Substance use*	Aggression (males only)
	General offenses*	General offenses
	Low IQ	Low IQ
	Antisocial behavior and attitude	Substance abuse
	Aggression and dishonesty (males only)	Criminal activity (directed at people)
	Hyperactivity	Risk-taking behaviors
	Exposed to TV violence or video games	
Family	Low SES or poverty	Low SES or poverty
	Antisocial parents	Antisocial parents
	Single-parent home	Single-parent home
	Poor parent-child relationship	Antisocial or abusive parents
	Abusive, neglectful parents	Lack of parent involvement
School	Poor attitude and performance	Poor attitude and performance
		Academic failure
Peer	Weak social ties (the loner)	Weak social ties*
	Antisocial peers	Antisocial delinquent peers*
		Gang membership*
Community		Neighborhood crime, drugs, violence, and disorganization

*Factors with strongest effect.
Adapted from Christian CW, Blum NJ: Violence. In Kliegman RM, et al, editors: *Nelson essentials of pediatrics,* ed 5, Philadelphia, 2006, Elsevier, p. 125.

- Is he or she a loner with weak social ties? Do the youth's friends engage in antisocial or delinquent behavior?
- Is there gang involvement or membership, or do friends carry weapons?
- Does the youth have access to or carry a weapon or weapons?
- Family and social history
  - Does the youth feel safe at home and in his or her neighborhood? How is the youth supervised by his or her parent(s)?
  - Is there a family history of child abuse, substance abuse, domestic violence, mental illness, fighting at home, or a criminal record?
  - Are there handguns or rifles in the home?
  - Does anyone in the home use drugs or have a problem with alcohol?
  - Is the youth attending school? If yes, have there been any academic or behavioral problems?
  - Does the youth have a job? How is free time spent? Are the youth's friends in gangs or in trouble with the law? Gang involvement and association with antisocial delinquent peers is a major risk factor for involvement in violent behavior.
  - Are siblings involved in gangs? Do they have criminal histories? Have any family members ever been victims, witnesses, or perpetrators of crime?

Management

The primary care provider is likely to become involved with (1) the health care management of minor trauma resulting from assault, (2) counseling after an incident of violence or threat of violence, and (3) the prevention of youth violence. In brief, the following are the key points in the management of minor assaults:

- Treatment of minor trauma or referral
- Alcohol and drug screening
- Reporting the incident to law enforcement
- Referral to social worker or mental health professional and to community programs as appropriate

Protective factors have been identified that are associated with decreased violent behaviors in youths. Examples of these factors include some of the following: frequent shared activities with parents; the ability to discuss problems with parents; connectedness to family or adults outside of the family; perceived parental expectations for school performance that are high; religiosity; positive social orientation; commitment to school and involvement in social activities with peers; and consistent presence of parents during one of any of the following times—when awakening, arriving home from school, at evening mealtime, or bedtime. Providers should discuss how parents can incorporate such protective factors in their family life.

Prevention of Youth Violence

Prevention of youth violence requires use of a public health model that addresses the complexity of causes and risk factors behind the problem. Some suggested approaches follow. Primary care providers are able to address many of these issues as they give individual family and child care in the primary care setting.

Others require more active involvement in the community as a child and family advocate.

Primary Prevention

- Strengthen families:
  - Provide parents with skills for effective parenting (see Chapters 4 through 8 and 17).
  - Support parents to be actively involved with their children, to supervise youths and their activities, and to monitor the child's peer group (having friends who engage in conventional, nonviolent behaviors is a protective factor).
  - Connect families to needed community service resources.
  - Educate parents about the impact of violence on their children; discuss ways to minimize exposure; teach about gun safety.
- Strengthen developmental competencies of youth:
  - Educate youths about violence at an early age.
  - Teach anger management and strategies for preventing a fight (role-playing).
  - Teach self-defense strategies, such as teaching youths martial arts and the use of mace.
  - Discuss ways to manage a difficult or potentially violent situation (Boxes 18-9 and 18-10).
- Improve the environment:
  - Support diversity training and bullying prevention programs in public schools.
  - Support after-school programs for youth and work for community commitment to youth programs.
  - Make neighborhoods and schools safe places for youth.
  - Involve the community in a commitment to preventing violence.
  - Address the issues of media violence and of condoning violence as a way of life.

BOX 18-9 **Practical Hints for Talking With Teens About How to Keep Out of Trouble**

Do not carry a weapon; instead, "fight clean" (i.e., discuss the issue in conflict). Carrying weapons only makes one less safe; pulling out a weapon begins a cycle of retaliation.

Do not go into harm's way. Avoid being around fights because the cycle of escalation and retaliation often involves innocent people.

Avoid being caught alone; stay with friends.

Do not be provoked into fighting. Words are said and names are called, not because the names are true, but rather to provoke anger and a fight.

If one becomes involved in a fight, try to end the incident on equal ground; that way anger is more likely to be diffused. The person who wins often takes on the aggressor role; the loser then becomes the scapegoat. Thus violence continues and becomes cyclic.

Suggest discussions with friends about ways to handle potential situations in which a gun or knife might be brandished.

Do not join gangs or associate with individuals who turn to violence as a way of settling differences.

Report threats of school violence to adults.

BOX 18-10 **Talking With Teens About Date or Gang Rape**

Both males and females can be victimized.

Alcohol intoxication or the use of drugs is a major factor in date rape. Prevention includes not placing oneself in harm's way by using such substances.

Manipulative verbal threats and physically trapping the victim are common tactics used by perpetrators.

Reluctance to report gang or date rape is common. However, keeping the rape a secret only leads to self-doubt and delays healing. The teen should report the rape immediately and seek professional counseling.

- Regulate alcohol sales and use to youth.
- Support legislation to control handguns.
- Limit access to and carrying of weapons.

Secondary Prevention

- Care for children exposed to or threatened by violence:
  - Treat any physical or emotional problems resulting from violence in the primary care setting. Early intervention can prevent more serious problems later; referral may be necessary.
  - Provide home visits for mothers of new babies, especially those in low-income and teen-mother families.
  - Create support groups for children who have suffered trauma or loss (e.g., school counseling for traumatic experiences).
  - Refer families to community support programs, such as Big Brothers Big Sisters of America (see Resource Box).
- Screen for potential problems:
  - Assess for violence risk factors at all health supervision and illness visits.
  - Screen for alcohol abuse problems.
  - Ask about weapons in the home—their presence, use, storage, and access.

Tertiary Prevention. Treatment and rehabilitation programs for offenders and treatment for victims and their families can be difficult and costly and yield only mixed results. It is essential to prevent violence by strengthening families and communities so that violent behavior is no longer an acceptable option.

CHILD MALTREATMENT

Description

Child maltreatment or child abuse includes physical abuse, physical neglect, sexual abuse, mental injury or emotional maltreatment, and threat of harm. The acts of inflicting injury (commission) and allowing injury to occur (omission) are key determinants in defining abuse. Children may be maltreated in more than one way; thus reporting by type of abuse for a single child may include one single category or any combination of two or more maltreatment types.

Epidemiology

In 2004, child protective services agencies in the U.S. investigated reports of suspected child abuse and neglect on 3,503,000

children. An estimated 872,000 children were found to be victims. The rate of victimization of children in 2004 was 11.9 per 1000 children, with young children (birth to 3 years old) experiencing the highest rate of maltreatment. Nearly three quarters of these maltreated children were first-time victims. The victimization rate by type of maltreatment has been fairly stable from 1999 to 2004 (USDHHS, Administration on Children, Youth, and Families [ACYF], 2006).

As children become older, abuse decreases. In 2004 there were 16.1, 13.4, and 10.9 cases of abuse per 1000 children in the age groups of birth to 3 years old, 4 to 7 years old, and 8 to 11 years old. Percentages for overall abuse of boys and girls were similar: 43.8% and 51.7%, respectively. The majority of victims were white (53.8%); 25.2% were African American; and 17% were Hispanic. The rate of victimization per 1000 children of the same race was 10.7, 19.9, and 10.4 for white, African-American, and Hispanic races or ethnicities, respectively. Disparity in rate of victimization based on race is evident (USDHHS, ACYF, 2006).

Abuse, as with violence, can be a multigenerational, learned means of coping or disciplining children. Situational stress, drug or alcohol use, poverty, and limited social supports can aggravate the problem. Sadly, more than 75% of child fatalities in 2004 were caused by one or both parents, with almost one third of fatalities caused by the child's mother acting alone. Male partners of a parent were implicated in 3.3% of child fatalities in this same year (USDHHS, ACYF, 2006).

Furthermore, today the Internet poses multiple risks for children and adolescents with predators using sexual solicitation via chat rooms and instant messaging. Protecting children is a mandate for all pediatric health care providers. Identification of at-risk children and families before injury or neglect has occurred is of paramount importance.

Assessment

Box 18-11 lists behavioral signs that should be investigated in a child suspected of having been abused.

BOX 18-11 **Behavioral Signs Associated With Child Maltreatment**

- Overly compliant or exhibits exaggerated fearfulness
- Clingy and indiscriminate attachment
- Extremes in behavior (aggressive or passive)
- Apprehensive when other children cry
- Wary of physical contact with adults
- Frightened of parents and/or of going home
- Exhibits drastic behavioral changes in and out of parental or caregiver presence
- Depressed, hypervigilant, withdrawn, apathetic, antisocial; exhibits destructive behavior
- Suicidal (suicide attempts or plans) or engages in self-mutilation
- Overprotective of parents or caregivers
- Displays sleep or eating disorders

Management

All categories of child abuse endanger the child's physical or emotional health and development. Although the severity of injury is always an important consideration in treatment and disposition of the child, it does not determine, per se, whether intervention should occur. The burden to report minor injury or emotional maltreatment is just as great as the burden to report significant trauma resulting in grave bodily injury.

Pediatric primary care providers are in a unique position to identify children who are maltreated and to institute strategies for primary prevention aimed at high-risk families. Each state has its own laws related to the various categories of child maltreatment. All health care providers are mandated to report known or suspected child abuse. Both civil and criminal immunity is ensured to mandated reporters who are acting within their professional role when making a required or authorized report. If the history or physical examination is suspicious for child abuse and the child is not in acute danger, the pediatric provider only need notify the child abuse registry. If the child requires protection and is in imminent danger, both the police and the child abuse registry must be called. Most states have a system of cross reporting cases with their social service agency, usually referred to as child protective services, responsible for child abuse investigations and law enforcement. Providers should contact the department of social services or the office of the attorney general in their state for written guidelines about individual state reporting laws and procedural policies related to child abuse. The telephone number for reporting suspicion of child abuse should be readily available in each practice setting. In addition, consultation with experts in the field of child maltreatment is appropriate for those situations that are problematic or questionable.

Children who are maltreated are at risk for revictimization and are prone to psychological and behavioral difficulties across their life span. This is especially true for children who are sexually abused or experience physical abuse and aggression (Wekerle et al, 2006). The importance of early identification and intervention cannot be emphasized enough. It has been pointed out that the philosophy "I am not my brother's keeper" should never be applied to children. Children are a vulnerable, easily traumatized, powerless group, and it is the responsibility of all those who work with them to provide protection and care and to be our children's keepers. Pitfalls that pediatric providers must be alert to include:

- Missing significant injury or findings by not doing a complete evaluation
- Failing to consider the possibility of child abuse as one of the differential diagnoses
- Not recognizing abuse or neglect as the source of a behavioral problem
- Assuming that a family is not abusive (i.e., "a good family")
- Keeping inadequate records of the encounter and evaluation (Stirling, 2006)

PHYSICAL ABUSE

Description

Any act that results in nonaccidental physical injury to a child is physical abuse. Physical abuse often occurs when the parent or caregiver is frustrated or angry. In these instances, the injury is frequently a result of shaking, striking, or throwing the child and can involve unreasonably severe corporal punishment or unjustifiable punishment. Physical injury also can represent intentional, deliberate assault, such as burning, biting, cutting, poking, twisting limbs, or torturing. Children who suffer physical abuse are usually younger. Children reported as disabled are more likely to be victims of maltreatment than are children without disabilities (USDHHS, ACYF, 2006).

Incidence

In 2004, approximately 17.5% of victims of child abuse suffered physical injury for a rate of 2.1 per 1000 child victims; approximately 1490 children died that year of child abuse or neglect (USDHHS, ACYF, 2006).

Assessment

Determining the presence of physical abuse can be difficult. A child or parent may disclose a history of an inflicted injury, or there may be suspicious behavioral or physical findings. Behaviors are not definitive signs of physical abuse, but are important areas to investigate for additional information. Specific physical findings are often the key to a diagnosis of nonaccidental injury resulting from physical abuse. The provider should have a high level of suspicion if there are discrepancies in the history of the injury, the child's age and developmental capabilities, and the type and severity of injury. For example, young infants who do not cruise rarely bruise.

History. The history should assess for the following:
- Child states that injury was caused by abuse.
- Injury is unusual for a specific age group.
- Injuries are unexplained or implausible (e.g., parent or caregiver cannot explain injury, is vague about how the injury occurred, gives discrepant accounts of what happened, or blames someone else); explanation does not match the type or mechanism of injury; or child is not developmentally capable of reported injurious behavior.
- Parent or caregiver delays seeking care for child or seeks inappropriate care, or age of injury is inconsistent with the history.
- Child, parent or caregiver, or both, hides injury (e.g., child wears excessive layers of clothing), or child is kept out of school.
- There is presence of triggering behaviors, such as inconsolable, colicky crying in an infant, toilet-training accidents, or sleeping or discipline problems that may have led to a violent response by a caregiver.
- There is a report of a crisis or stressful time for the family (e.g., financial difficulties) or domestic violence.
- There is a problem with substance abuse in the family.

Physical Findings. Key considerations of abuse that should guide the physical examination include the following:
- Location of the physical injury
- Pattern of bruises, abrasions, lacerations (i.e., does it resemble a known object?)
- Type of injury: bruising, burns, inflicted fractures, or head trauma (Tables 18-3 and 18-4)

TABLE 18-3 Common Sites of Injury in Physical Abuse of Children	
Location of Injury*	**Common Physical Finding**
Head area	Eyes—bilateral black eyes Earlobe—pinch and pull marks Cheek—slap marks, squeeze marks Upper lip and frenulum—lacerations or bruises Scalp—bare and broken hair, bruises
Neck	Choke marks
Trunk	Chest—bite marks, fingertip encirclement marks Buttocks and lower back—paddling and strap marks
Genitals	Pinch marks, penile wrapping with constrictive materials
Extremities	Upper arms—grab marks Ankles or wrists—tethering, friction burn marks Feet—pin or razor tattoo marks

*The shins, elbows, and knees are the most typical sites of accidental, non–child abuse, injuries. Bruises, cuts, and abrasions are most commonly seen. The back surface of the body, from knees to neck, is the most common site of intentional, abusive injuries.

- Presence of multiple injuries, particularly in different stages of healing
- Multiple mechanisms of injury (burns, fractures, bruises)
- Signs of concurrent medical, hygienic, supervisory, or nutritional neglect (Hymel & Hall, 2005)

Diagnostic Studies. These should include (1) blood coagulation studies (platelet count, bleeding time, prothrombin time, and partial thromboplastin time) on any child who is severely bruised or has a history of "easy bruising" and suspicious bruises (see Table 18-5 for general dating of contusion injuries) and (2) radiographic studies. A child with limited range of motion or bony tenderness on examination should have a local radiologic evaluation. A radiologic skeletal survey should be ordered for any child with soft tissue findings who is nonverbal or unable to give a clear history (usually younger than 4 to 5 years old) or for infants suspected of failure to thrive (FTT). The minimal radiologic survey is a skull series, long bones, and ribs. Bone scan, computed tomography scan, and a magnetic resonance imaging study should be ordered on the basis of physical findings or symptoms. Serum calcium, phosphorus, and alkaline phosphatase levels are useful measurements if bone disease is suspected. Ultrasonography is useful if visceral injury is suspected. Other studies are ordered depending on physical findings.

Differential Diagnosis

Differential diagnoses are identified by type of intentional physical injury:

- Soft tissue injuries:
- Normal bruising from accidental injuries that typically involve the knees, anterior tibia, and forehead
- Mongolian spots and allergic shiners
- Bleeding disorders
- Cultural practices, such as "coining (cao gio) or spoon rubbing (quat sha)," sometimes practiced by Southeast Asian groups
- Burns: impetigo, bullous impetigo, or toxic epidermal necrolysis (scalded skin syndrome)
- Fractures: osteogenesis imperfecta and rare bone diseases, such as scurvy, congenital syphilis, and neoplasms
- Head injuries: bruising from falls
- Bruising: hematologic disorders, such as Vitamin K deficiency and hemophilia

Most infant falls do not result in head injury. Falls from beds or sofas do not cause skull fractures, and less than 1% of infants in a large study suffered concussion or skull fracture because of a fall (Warrington et al, 2001).

Management

Medical treatment of specific types of injuries is discussed in Unit 4 of this text under the appropriate illness-related heading. If physical abuse is suspected, certain general management strategies should be followed. The provider must:

- Report suspicions of child maltreatment to child protective services or law enforcement agencies, or both.
- Carefully document findings and any statements made by parent or caregiver or child, or both.
- Secure photographic documentation of soft tissue injury or burn injury; this can be done by law enforcement personnel or health care providers, as appropriate.
- Refer for appropriate medical treatment of injuries depending on type and severity of injury.
- Refer for psychological counseling; this is generally handled by child protective services. The need for long-term or intermittent therapy often depends on the individual child, the severity of the physical and emotional injuries, and other life events.

Patient Education and Prevention. Prevention of physical abuse involves the following steps:

- Screen for parental history of abuse during childhood, history of domestic violence, and absence of a social support network in the family. Pursue positive results from screens.
- Identify at-risk families and children. At-risk families include those with any of the following characteristics:
  - Prior history of child maltreatment, drug abuse, violent behavior, or serious mental illness
  - Evidence that the mother is not showing attachment to her infant, makes negative remarks about the child, or lacks basic parenting knowledge, skill, and motivation
  - Evidence of spanking of young infants
  - Isolated parent who lacks social support network
  - History of infant or child death resulting from child maltreatment (categorized as extremely high risk)
- Make early referrals for supportive service, including social service referrals, parenting classes, self-help groups

TABLE 18-4 **Common Characteristics of Physical Abuse by Type of Injury**

Type of Injury	Key Considerations
Bruises—surface and soft tissue	Pattern, shape, outline or image of the object (e.g., hand print, cord or buckle shapes) Location Number Stages of coloring
Burns—superficial or deep	Location: burns on palms, soles, flexor surface of thighs or perineum are pathognomonic for abuse; positive image of the shape of the object used to burn the child (e.g., curling irons, cigarette lighters, cigarettes, irons) Patterns, such as sharply demarcated or circumferential (e.g., sock, glove, zebra, branding, doughnut or cigarette shape) Cigarette burns—7.5- to 10-mm round lesion, raised edges and deep eschar
Human bite marks	Oval-shaped pattern, such as doughnut or double-horseshoe shape; adult >3 cm between canine teeth; can be on any part of the body; can have discrete tooth marks within the arcs or central ecchymosis between the arcs
Abrasions and lacerations	Location Number "C" or "U" shape typical of belt buckle mark
Ligature marks	Typically, around neck or extremities; linear image at site where tool placed
Central nervous system trauma	Radiographic findings (e.g., subdural hematomas, subarachnoid hemorrhages, skull fractures, suture spread), retinal hemorrhages; head trauma can have symptoms of irritability, lethargy, seizures, apnea, or coma
Shaken infant syndrome	Retinal hemorrhage, subdural hematoma, posterior rib and metaphyseal fractures
Internal organ trauma	Liver, bowel, spleen, pancreas, kidney damage consistent with blunt-force trauma May be no visible marks or bruises on abdomen May have symptoms of shock Internal injury is second leading cause of death in child abuse
Skeletal fracture	Spiral fractures of long bones, avulsion of metaphyseal tips, multiple rib fractures in different stages of healing, subperiosteal proliferation reaction, unexplained fracture, especially in a young, nonambulatory child; fractures from birth injuries heal by 4 mo
Poisoning or ingestion of medication	Deliberate poisoning or exposure to substance abuse via breast milk, passive inhalation of marijuana
Munchausen syndrome by proxy	Creates a fictitious illness or induces illness in child; signs and symptoms stop when perpetrator no longer has unsupervised contact with child

(e.g., Parents or Alcoholics Anonymous plus battered women's services), respite care, public health nurse visits, or a combination of these.

- Provide close primary care supervision and ill-child follow-up visits of at-risk families and children.
- Use a multidisciplinary team approach to manage at-risk or high-risk families. A team approach gives objectivity to a situation.
- Report immediately to child protective services if abuse is suspected.
- Gain the support of community child abuse prevention programs.

NEGLECT

Description

Physical neglect refers to the negligent treatment or maltreatment of a child that can harm or threaten harm to a child's health or welfare. Neglect by the parent or caregiver can be severe or more subtle in its effects. Severe neglect includes instances in which the parent or caregiver fails to protect the child from dangers, such as severe malnutrition (may be seen clinically as medically diagnosed nonorganic FTT); willfully places the child in a situation in which the child's health is endangered (e.g., exploitation requiring a child to engage in criminal behavior); or intentionally fails to provide adequate clothing, shelter, education, or medical care. General neglect refers to failure to meet the child's basic needs, such as adequate food, clothing, shelter, medical care, or supervision where no obvious physical injury to the child occurred as a result. A key factor in neglect is the extreme or persistent presence of these conditions in the child's home.

Incidence

In 2004, approximately 62.4% of child victimizations were due to neglect; another 2.1% experienced medical neglect.

TABLE 18-5　Bruising: General Dating of Contusion Injury and Other Key Points

Bruise Characteristic	Age of Bruise
Swollen, tender	0-2 days
Red, purple, blue	0-5 days
Green	5-7 days
Yellow	7-10 days
Brown	10-14 days
Clear	2-4 weeks

Key points to consider	Suspicious findings
Pattern	Resembles an object that might inflict injury
	• Hand slap—typically a negative image with white area of palm and fingers outlined with rim of petechiae
	• Pinch mark—small paired, oval bruises the size of a fingertip
	• Belt mark or other objects
Aging	Multiple bruises in various stages of aging
Site(s) of injury—location on body	Sites other than knees, shins, elbows, or forehead
	In the anogenital region, buttocks, earlobes
	Central location on trunk is more suspicious vs. overlying boney prominences
Extension	More than one body surface or plane

This represented a general neglect victimization rate of 7.4 per 1000 child victims (USDHHS, ACYF, 2006).

Assessment

Assessment should focus on the key issue of whether the child's safety and welfare are threatened. General indicators of neglect are divided into child, home, and supervision factors (Box 18-12). In the primary care setting, providers can more accurately assess child factors (i.e., child's appearance and general status, in addition to access to needed dental and health care) than they can assess home factors or the degree of adult supervision provided. Questions and discussion about the home situation, however, can be included in the history.

Referral to a public health nurse for home assessment may be necessary, and a report of child neglect to child protective services may lead to an investigation. Child protective workers look at home factors with a focus on a safe and sanitary environment. To determine degree of adult supervision, factors, such as the child's age and level of functioning, the length of time the parent was away, where the parent went, whether the parent left a plan of supervision (e.g., relative or adult living next door or nearby who was readily available to the child), and how often the child has been left alone, are investigated. Most child protective services hold parents to the standard of a "reasonable or prudent" parent. Economic factors are also considered when making judgments about parents' efforts to provide adequately for their children.

BOX 18-12　General Indicators of Neglect: Child, Home, Supervision Factors

Child
Dirty, malnourished, poor hygiene, inadequately dressed for weather
Inadequate medical and dental care (has multiple caries)
Always sleepy (chronic fatigue) or hungry

Home
Fire hazards or other unsafe conditions
No heating or plumbing
Nutritional quality of the food inadequate
Meals not prepared; food spoiled in refrigerator or cupboards

Supervision
Child has history of repeated physical injuries or ingestion of harmful substances with evidence of poor supervision by adult caregiver
Child cared for by another child
Child left alone in the home, car, or anywhere without supervision (typically defined as a child younger than 12 years old who is left unsupervised during the daytime or child 16 to 18 years old left unsupervised by an adult at night)

Differential Diagnosis

Differentiating willful neglect from neglect resulting from poverty, mental retardation, or mental illness is necessary. Educational neglect differs from truancy (i.e., child is sent to school, but never arrives) in that the parent makes no provisions for the child to attend school.

Management

Referral to child protective services is needed in cases of neglect. Pediatric providers can also refer families to public health and social service agencies.

EMOTIONAL MALTREATMENT

Description

Emotional maltreatment or mental injury is harm to a child's ability to think, reason, or feel. Emotional maltreatment may take two forms: emotional abuse or emotional deprivation. Parents who subject children to cruel statements and acts or who reject, terrorize, ridicule, isolate, and corrupt the child are perpetrating emotional abuse. Torture, confinement, exposure to violence (witnessing domestic violence), and deprivation of food and water are extreme examples.

Failure to adequately nurture children with support and affection so that the child can develop a healthy personality is an example of emotional deprivation. Parents or caregivers who do not provide the normal experiences necessary for a child to feel loved, wanted, secure, or worthy are depriving their child of the emotional security that is critical for positive self-esteem.

Emotional maltreatment may contribute to psychological FTT, speech or sleep disorders, or a wide range of behavioral and emotional problems in children (e.g., withdrawal, aggressiveness, neediness, conduct disorders). The issue of consistency or recurrence of negative parental behaviors and willful cruelty or unjustifiable emotional punishment is a key indicator of emotional maltreatment.

Epidemiology

Parents or caregivers can ignore or reject their child for any number of reasons, including drug use, psychiatric disturbances, personal problems, or other preoccupying situations. Poor coping skills, high stress levels, a history of emotional maltreatment, and poor parenting can contribute to the parent's behavior. Children with chronic illness or those who are "different" than their siblings may become scapegoats in the family system.

Approximately 7% of all abused children in 2004 suffered emotional maltreatment for a psychological maltreatment rate of 0.9 per 1000 child victims (USDHHS, ACYF, 2006).

Assessment

Behavioral indicators often lead to suspicions of emotional maltreatment, but can also be due to other causes; therefore a careful history is important. Interviewing both parent or caregiver plus any child older than 3 years is essential. A range of behavioral indicators can be exhibited by children who are emotionally deprived or abused. Physical indicators of emotional maltreatment, such as psychosocial FTT, are assessed for degree of severity, in addition to cause. The assessment includes the history, physical examination, and diagnostic studies.

History.   The history can include the following:
- Past health history—might be suggestive of neglect (e.g., little or no health care supervision, immunizations not up to date, earlier removal of a sibling for neglect)
- Interview with mother—might reveal mother's negative feelings toward child, a state of feeling overwhelmed or depressed, plus feelings of being deprived or unloved; mother may be cognitively delayed

- Behavior problems with child in school, among peers (e.g., bullying, being picked on, withdrawal)
- Feeding and dietary history—can be helpful in distinguishing accidental feeding or formula-preparation error from neglect and organic or psychological causes; dietary history should be obtained, but might not be truthful
- Inquire about financial hardships related to inability to provide for basic needs, especially food

Physical Findings.   Physical assessment of emotional maltreatment can be difficult. Assessment of psychosocial or nonorganic FTT is one means of assessing emotional maltreatment. *Psychosocial FTT* is defined as a condition in which children younger than 5 years old have growth persistently and significantly below the norms for their age and sex with no organic cause. Infancy is the major period of time when FTT as a result of nonorganic causes is diagnosed. Children older than 2 years can often get their own food. However, purposeful starvation in older children by their caregiver does happen. FTT can be related to both physical and psychosocial factors; and both should be considered because they may be concurrent. The physical assessment in FTT includes the following (see Chapter 32):

- *Weight-for-height ratio:* Will be less than normal in FTT; short stature with a proportional weight can reflect chronic malnutrition or a genetic or endocrine-based problem.
- *Growth trajectory:* Child fails to maintain normal growth trajectory.
- *Signs of general neglect:* Poor hygiene, such as filthy fingernails, clothes, body, rampant diaper rash, or untreated impetigo. Child may have flattened occiput from lying in one position; however, this is commonly seen with supine positioning now recommended for infant sleep.
- *Appetite:* Child may be ravenous; the pediatric provider should try to observe the caregiver feed the infant.
- *Child's behavior:* Child may avoid eye contact, resist being cuddled, or have an expressionless face.
- *Mother-child interaction:* Parent may indicate a lack of attachment or presence of anger or dislike of child; may belittle, tease, or verbally abuse child.
- *Associated developmental delays:* Results from little psychosocial stimulation.

Diagnostic Studies.   Diagnostic evaluation by a mental health professional is needed to determine whether the behaviors or psychopathology, or both, in the child are due to parental emotional abuse or deprivation.

If the child has FTT, dietary management should be undertaken for 1 week to determine whether there is significant weight gain before laboratory studies are ordered to rule out organic causes of FTT (see Chapter 32).

Differential Diagnosis

Intentional mental injury should be distinguished from that caused by parental deficits, such as cognitive, psychological, and economic limitations. Psychopathology in the child resulting from other causes is also in the differential diagnosis.

The differential diagnoses for emotional maltreatment resulting in FTT include accidental feeding or formula errors and organic causes of FTT, such as endocrine, metabolic, gastrointestinal, cardiovascular, genetic, neurologic, infectious, and renal conditions.

Management

Because emotional maltreatment is generally difficult to prove, the provider must carefully document what was said in the interview and what behavioral indicators were found. Referral to a community health nurse for in-home assessment is appropriate if the provider has concerns. Referral to a mental health professional for evaluation should be considered. Reporting concerns to the appropriate child protective services agency is essential, as is close supervision of these families. Family therapy may be necessary, and parents can benefit from parenting support and education, in addition to social service support to cope with demands on the family system (e.g., child care, nutritional education, access to economic resources). The child may need to be placed in foster care.

If a child has FTT, the condition must be treated clinically. Hospitalization may be required. Demonstration of adequate weight gain while out of the home (either in hospital or foster care) is diagnostic. Dietary management should include an appropriate diet for age that generally provides 150 kcal/kg (ideal weight) per 24 hours for 1 week; ideal weight is median weight in kilograms for measured length. Most infants with nonorganic FTT gain more than 2 oz every 24 hours for 1 week or at least more weight than achieved in the same period of time at home (Behrman et al, 2004). Close and long-term health care supervision and follow-up plus psychosocial intervention and local case management by child protective services are needed.

Patient Education and Prevention

Prevention of emotional maltreatment and psychosocial FTT generally involves the same prevention strategies as identified in the section on physical abuse and neglect. Early recognition and intervention are key to preventing subsequent mental health problems. The importance of frequent health visits to monitor height and weight for infants who are falling behind is essential to prevent significant growth and development problems.

SEXUAL ABUSE

Description

Sexual abuse or *sexual maltreatment* is defined to include acts of sexual assault or sexual exploitation of minors, or both. These acts can occur over an extended period of time or involve a one-time incident; they may or may not involve force; they can involve threats of physical harm to a child or others in the family or involve emotional entrapment of the child; and they can often involve a secret between the victim and the perpetrator. The perpetrator is usually known to the child and is often a "trusted" adult. A growing group of perpetrators are adolescents who commit sexually aggressive acts on young children.

Sexual assault of children includes a range of acts including rape, rape in concert, incest, sodomy, lewd or lascivious acts on a child younger than 14 years old (e.g., fondling or touching of genital areas and breasts or inappropriate kissing), oral copulation, and penetration of genital or anal openings by a foreign object. Sexual exploitation includes activities, such as pornography depicting minors and promoting prostitution by minors. Proving sexual abuse in young children is difficult.

Incidence

In 2004, the incidence of sexual abuse made up 9.7% of the total number of child abuse and neglect cases. The percentage of sexual abuse cases increases with age. For example, in 2004, approximately 9% of child maltreatment in children 4 to 7 years old involved sexual abuse as compared with 16.5% in 12- to 15-year-old child abuse victims. Reported abuse among girls is more prevalent than among boys (USDHHS, ACYF, 2006). Multigenerational abuse is common in cases of child sexual abuse.

Assessment

Chapter 35 discusses the examination of the genitalia in girls. The child or adolescent who has been sexually assaulted by a stranger usually discloses the abuse and comes in for an immediate evaluation. This type of assessment is straightforward and involves the usual taking of a history and performing the medical examination with collection of possible evidence. If the incident occurred within 72 hours, evidence (e.g., semen, nail scraping, and pubic hair) is collected, and testing for sexually transmitted diseases should be done. These children are often seen in the emergency department of a local hospital or, ideally, at a special center that treats victims of child sexual abuse.

The pediatric provider in a primary care setting is likely to become involved in a child sexual abuse case in any of the following circumstances: there is a spontaneous disclosure by the child; a parent voices concerns about the possibility of abuse or reports a disclosure by the child; there are suspicious physical or historical findings, or both; or laboratory tests indicating sexually transmitted infections (STIs) are positive. In many instances, sexual abuse occurs over several years before the child discloses.

If possible, the assessment of the child should be done by a health care provider who is an expert in the field of sexual abuse of children. The assessment of a child who has been molested in the past but whose molestation has only recently been disclosed, or who is suspected of being sexually abused, should focus on three areas: behavioral indicators, physical indicators, and the interview of the child.

Behavioral Indicators

- Loss of bowel and bladder control
- Regressive behaviors, such as newly manifested clinging and irritability in young children, thumb sucking, renewed need for a security object
- Night terrors, inability to sleep alone, bed-wetting after having been dry at night

- Overeating or lack of appetite; compulsive behaviors or unusual fears and phobias
- Change in school performance; loss of concentration or easy distractibility
- Sexualized behavior or play inappropriate for developmental level
- Depression or inactivity, poor peer relationships, poor self-esteem, acting out, excessive anger
- Runaway, suicide attempts, prostitution or promiscuity, substance abuse, teen pregnancy, psychosomatic gynecologic and gastrointestinal complaints

Behavioral indicators per se are not diagnostic of sexual molestation, but indicate a need for a thorough investigation.

Physical Indicators–Nonspecific

- Pain on urination; vaginal or penile discharge; vaginal, rectal, or penile bleeding; enuresis and encopresis
- Urethral or lymph gland inflammation; genital or perianal rashes; labial adhesions
- Pain in anal, gastrointestinal, pelvic, and urinary areas
- Genital injuries or signs, such as bruising, scratches, bites, grasp marks, swelling of the genitalia that are unexplained or inconsistent with history

Physical Indicators–Specific

- Blunt-force trauma (lacerations, bruising, abrasions, tears) to the genital or rectal areas, or both, that is inconsistent with the history or these same findings with a history of sexual contact or penetration
- Commonly encountered STIs (by probability of sexual abuse in prepubertal infants and children):
  ○ Diagnostic of sexual abuse—gonorrhea (by culture) and syphilis if not perinatally acquired and nondelivery-related or nonpregnancy-related chlamydia (culture is the only reliable diagnostic method), HIV, and herpes type II
  ○ Probably diagnostic—condyloma acuminatum (appearing after 3 years old and not perinatally acquired) and *Trichomonas vaginalis*
  ○ Possible—herpes type 1 and nonvenereal warts (may be due to autoinoculation in the genital or anogenital area)
  ○ Uncertain—bacterial vaginosis and *Mycoplasma*

Pregnancy, sperm, and semen are certain indicators of sexual abuse in young children (Behrman et al, 2004).

Lack of Significant Physical Findings

- Most child victims of sexual abuse do not have any significant physical findings.
- Lack of findings is often the result of delayed disclosure and the nature of the abuse.
- Most sexual abuse of young children does not involve penetrating trauma.

Interview of the Child. The purpose of the health provider interview with the child is to collect adequate information to decide whether to report the case. A social worker, psychologist, or law-enforcement person with experience in evaluating sexually abused children will conduct a detailed interview after the case is reported.

When talking with a child who is disclosing sexual abuse, or whom you suspect was or is being sexually abused, the provider needs to be nonjudgmental, use language that the child understands, identify the words the child uses for the genital and rectal areas, have the child report what happened in his or her own words, and ask open-ended questions. Leading questions should not be used.

If the child gives a spontaneous or clear disclosure of sexual abuse during a primary care visit, report the case. Children rarely lie about such matters. Always think, "How would a child that age know about such sexual details?" Consider separate questioning of the child and parent or caregiver if the child is 4 years old or older.

Recanting a disclosure of sexual abuse is not uncommon because of fear of what disclosure can bring to the family or child.

Diagnostic Studies. Any sexual abuse of children that involves oral, genital, rectal, or penile contact or penetration within the previous 72 hours requires that appropriate forensic specimens be collected. In addition, the rectal, throat, urethral, or endocervical areas should be cultured for *Neisseria gonorrhoeae* and *Chlamydia trachomatis*. Blood testing for syphilis should be obtained. In selected cases, additional diagnostic tests for human immunodeficiency virus (HIV), hepatitis B, herpes simplex, bacterial vaginosis, human papillomavirus, and *T. vaginalis* can be performed if indicated.

Testing for STIs in children who were molested in the past (more than 72 hours previously) is a judgment call. Recent exposure and the possibility of penile contact are key indicators for whether specimens need to be collected for possible STIs. Testing for *N. gonorrhoeae, C. trachomatis,* and syphilis should be considered in all children with a history of sexual abuse. A colposcopic examination of the genital and rectal areas by an expert in the field is often requested by law-enforcement agencies to determine whether there is evidence of acute traumatic or past healed injury to the genital or rectal areas.

Differential Diagnosis

Differential diagnoses include straddle injury to the genitalia or rectal area, which produces labial ecchymosis, abrasions, or tears; penetrating vaginal trauma from accidental injury, such as jumping from dresser onto bedpost (needs careful investigation); perinatally acquired STIs or STIs acquired through close contact but not sexual abuse; lichen sclerosus, poor hygiene, and pinworm infestation, resulting in vulvar skin irritation; and foreign body (frequently toilet paper) and other nonsexually transmitted bacteria causing vaginal discharge.

Management

An immediate forensic examination for a chain of evidence is required if the child gives a history that sexual abuse including ejaculation occurred within 72 hours. Specimen collection for semen, STI, pregnancy, and other evidence is done according to the local law-enforcement protocol for child or adolescent rape. If possible the child should be referred to health providers who are skilled in performing this special examination on children and adolescents. An expert in the medical examination of children suspected of being sexually abused should evaluate the child if the incident or incidents occurred more than 72 hours before the disclosure. A psychosocial interview with an expert in the field of child sexual abuse is often part of the evaluation.

If the primary care provider is the first health care provider to see the child, he or she is likely to become involved in the following management issues:

- Careful documentation of the history and physical examination findings for medical-legal purposes
- Reporting of the case to law-enforcement and social service agencies as required by law
- Referral for medical and psychosocial evaluation by experts in the field of child sexual abuse
- Referrals for crisis counseling of the child and other family members as needed
- Prescribing medication for treatment of STI; follow-up STI cultures or blood work as indicated
- Referrals for therapy, in addition to support and encouragement, for the child and family

Patient Education and Prevention

Prevention of later psychological problems related to child sexual abuse and revictimization are key issues. Prevention of sexual abuse involves the following steps:

- Instruct parents and caregivers about the need for early and consistent education of their children about good, bad, and questionable touching of private parts; how to say no or the use of self-defense techniques (e.g., yelling, kicking, or fighting back) if someone inappropriately touches them; to tell a responsible adult; and not to keep secrets. Parents should again bring up this subject as their child progresses through the various developmental stages. Young children who have been molested by a trusted adult often do not disclose for many years because they were threatened not to tell anyone or they interpreted the sexual activity (if it is not painful) as a sign of affection from the trusted adult and not as molestation. Later feelings of guilt, fear, and betrayal can emerge when children realize they were molested.
- Emphasize to parents that they must not place their child in high-risk situations (e.g., a parent who was abused by her father may have kept this a secret, blaming herself for what happened; she may erroneously believe that the perpetrator will not sexually abuse her child and leaves her daughter with him). Counsel that children are never safe around a pedophile.
- Provide families with information and educational reading materials about the topic of sexual abuse of children. Teaching should be tailored to the child's cognitive and learning abilities.
- Report promptly any suspicion of sexual abuse.
- Refer for individual and family counseling if sexual abuse is confirmed or suspected.
- Support efforts to target high-risk groups for intervention to prevent the continued spread of child abuse (e.g., adolescents who have exhibited sexual curiosity beyond the bounds of normal or have experimented with but not yet victimized

younger children; hence they become a juvenile perpetrator acting out the sexual activity or violence done to them).
- Support public education efforts and community child sexual abuse prevention programs.
- Educate parents about the need to talk to their children about their daily activities, especially what their children did during the time they were not with the parents.

NURSING DIAGNOSES

Related to Role Relationships: Functional Health Pattern

Nursing diagnoses are related to the following concepts: caregiving, parenting, family processes, role performance, and social interaction.
- Risk for impaired parent, infant, or child attachment
- Ineffective role performance
- Impaired social interaction
- Readiness for enhanced communication

Nursing diagnoses related to families
- Ineffective role performance
- Impaired parenting and risk for impaired parenting
- Readiness for enhanced parenting
- Risk for impaired parent/infant/child attachment
- Interrupted family processes
- Readiness for enhanced family processes
- Caregiver role strain and risk for caregiver role strain
- Dysfunctional family processes: alcoholism
- Parental role conflict
- Disabled family coping, compromised family coping, readiness for enhanced family coping
- Ineffective family therapeutic regimen management
- Impaired social interaction
- Relocation stress syndrome

From NANDA International: *NANDA-I nursing diagnoses: definitions & classification 2007-2008*, Philadelphia, 2007, Author.

✓ DISCUSSION FORUM

1. Conduct a family role assessment on the family of your choice. Be sure to identify each individual's roles, strengths, and weakness within the family. Which individual(s) is most critical to maintaining the family's dynamic?
2. After a careful assessment of family dynamics and strengths, what key anticipatory guidance issues should the pediatric provider address with the mother at this time related to the developmental needs of her children?
3. Parents of a 6-year-old child with terminal cancer seek counseling about how to best address this child's imminent death with her younger (3 years old) and older (14 years old) siblings. Discuss the areas of guidance you would provide and identify referrals to specific agencies in their community.
4. List three strategies that can be used by a pediatric provider to identify victims of child maltreatment. What biases and beliefs must the provider overcome to identify at-risk children? What are the local or regional resources available for abused or neglected children?

*R*ESOURCE BOX

Role Relationships

ADOPTION

Casey Family programs

www.casey.org/Home

Promotes advances in child-welfare practice and policy and collaborates with foster, kinship, and adoptive parents to provide safe, loving homes to children

Community Directory of International Adoption Medical Clinics

www.comeunity.com/adoption/health/clinics.html

Resource list of clinics and physicians in the U.S. and Canada specializing in international adoption health

International Adoption Clinic

www.peds.umn.edu/iac/

Clinic at the University of Minnesota; provides counseling and expert advice for parents and providers and clinical screening for recently arrived children

Medical passports for adopted children

www.in.gov

The state of Indiana has legislation providing for medical passports for adopted children; search the state website for "medical passport"

National Adoption Center

www.adopt.org

CHILD ABUSE

American Professional Society on the Abuse of Children

www.apsac.org

Professional education and resources

Child Welfare Information Gateway

U.S. Department of Health and Human Services, Children's Bureau, Administration for Children and Families

www.childwelfare.gov

Services formerly provided by the Clearinghouse on Child Abuse and Neglect Information and the National Adoption Information Clearinghouse have been combined under this heading. This website provides access to information and resources to help protect children and strengthen families

National Children's Advocacy Center

www.ncac.hsv.org/

Focuses on prevention and treatment options for physically and sexually abused children and their families

The Kempe Center For the Prevention and Treatment of Child Abuse and Neglect

www.kempecenter.com

Resources for professionals and families working with child abuse

CHILD CARE

Child Care Aware

www.childcareaware.org

Information on child care resources

National Child Care Information Center

www.nccic.org

Project of Child Care Bureau, a national resource for information regarding child care delivery system; links to other resources

CHRONIC CARE

Administration on Developmental Disabilities

www.acf.hhs.gov/programs/add

Federal government site with links to information, advocacy, and policy related to children with special needs

Brave Kids

www.bravekids.org

Support for families with children with chronic illness; links to resources for health professionals on a wide range of chronic illnesses; material in Spanish

DEATH

The Dougy Center for Grieving Children and Families

www.dougy.org

National center for grieving children and families; counseling, therapy, informational resources

VIOLENCE

American Medical Association

www.ama.org

Knox L: *Connecting the dots to prevent youth violence: a training and outreach guide for physicians and other health professionals*, 2002, AMA

Brady Campaign to Prevent Handgun Violence

www.handguncontrol.org

National lobbying and activist group

OTHER TOPICS

Big Brothers Big Sisters of America

www.bbbsa.org

Youth service organization whose website connects to state programs

Kids Health

www.kidshealth.org

Support group, information for parents, kids, and adolescents

Mothers of Supertwins (MOST)

www.mostonline.org

Resource for parents with triplets and more

National Center on Secondary Education and Transition

www.ncset.org

Educational and occupational opportunities for youth with disabilities; links to other resources

National Coalition for the Homeless

www.nationalhomeless.org

Excellent resource for information about the homeless population

REFERENCES

Acs G, Nelson S: *The kids are alright? Children's well-being and the rise in cohabitation,* Washington, DC, 2002, The Urban Institute. Available at *www.urban.org/url.cfm?ID =5 310544* (accessed Oct 20, 2003).

Anderssen N, Amlie C, Ytteroy EA: Outcomes for children with lesbian or gay parents. A review of studies from 1978 to 2000, *Scand J Psychol* 43:335-351, 2002.

Barrett AE, Turner RJ: Family structure and mental health: the mediating effects of socioeconomic status, family process, and social stress, *J Health Soc Behav* 46:156-169, 2005.

Barrett AE, Turner RJ: Family structure and substance abuse use problems in adolescence and early adulthood: examining explanations for the relationship, *Addiction* 101:109-120, 2006.

Bauer NS et al: Childhood bullying involvement and exposure to intimate partner violence, *Pediatrics* 118:e235-e242, 2006.

Bauman LJ, Silver EJ, Stein RE: Cumulative social disadvantage and child health, *Pediatrics* 117:1321-1328, 2006.

Behrman RE, Kliegman RM, Jenson HB: *Nelson textbook of pediatrics,* ed 17, Philadelphia, 2004, WB Saunders.

Berk LE: *Child development,* ed 7, Boston, 2006, Pearson Education.

Borowsky IW, Ireland M, Resnick MD: Violence risk and protective factors among youth held back in school, *Ambul Pediatr* 2:475-484, 2002.

Bramlett MD, Mosher WD: Cohabitation, marriage, divorce, and remarriage in the United States, *Vital Health Stat* 23(22): 1-34, 2002.

Cameron P: Children of homosexuals and transsexuals more apt to be homosexual, *J Biosoc Sci* 38:413-418, 2006.

Centers for Disease Control and Prevention (CDC): *National Vital Statistics Reports*: *Births, marriages, divorces, and deaths: provisional data for 2005,* 54, 20, 2006. Available at *www.cdc.gov/nchs/data/nvsr/nvsr54/ nvsr54_20.pdf* (accessed Sept 20, 2006).

Child Trends Data Bank. Available at *httpo://www.childtrendsdatabank.org/ indicators/59FamilyStructure.cfm* (accessed Sept 20, 2006).

Christian CW, Blum NJ: Psychosocial issues. In Kliegman RM et al, editors: *Nelson essentials of pediatrics,* ed 5, Philadelphia, 2006, Elsevier.

Cohen GJ, American Academy of Pediatrics Committee on Psychosocial Aspects of Child and Family Health: Helping children and families deal with divorce and separation, *Pediatrics* 110:1019-1023, 2002.

Commission for the Prevention of Youth Violence: *Youth and violence: medicine, nursing, and public health: connecting the dots to prevent violence,* Chicago, 2000, American Medical Association. Available at *www. ama-assn.org/ama/upload/mm/386/ fullreport.pdf* (accessed Oct 20, 2003).

Friedman MM, Bowden VR, Jones E: *Family nursing: research, theory and practice,* ed 5, Upper Saddle River, NJ, 2003, Prentice Hall.

Gartrell N et al: The National Lesbian Family Study. 4. Interviews with the 10-year-old children, *Am J Orthopsychiatry* 75:518-24, 2005.

Ge X, Natsuaki MN, Conger RD: Trajectories of depressive symptoms and stressful life events among male and female adolescents in divorced and nondivorced families, *Dev Psychopathol* 18:253-273, 2006.

Golombok S et al: Children with lesbian parents: a community study, *Dev Psychol* 39:20-33, 2003.

Greeff AP, Ritman IN: Individual characteristics associated with resilience in single-parent families, *Psychol Rep* 96:36-42, 2005.

Hunfeld JA et al: Child development and quality of parenting in lesbian families: no psychosocial indications for a-priori withholding of infertility treatment. A systematic review, *Hum Reprod Update* 8:579-590, 2002.

Hymel KP, Hall CA: Diagnostic pediatric head trauma, *Pediatr Ann* 34(5): 358-370, 2005.

Kelly JB: Children's adjustment in conflicted marriage and divorce: a decade review of research, *J Am Acad Child Adolesc Psychiatry* 39:963-973, 2000.

2006 Kids Count Data Book Online. Available at *www.aecf.org/kidscount/sid/ summary/13.isp* (accessed Sept 24, 2006).

Lerman RI: *How do marriage, cohabitation, and single parenthood affect the material hardships of families with children?* Washington, DC, 2002, The Urban Institute. Available at *www.urban.org/url.cfm?ID =5 410539* (accessed Sept 21, 2006).

Lussier G et al: Support across two generations: children's closeness to grandparents following parental divorce and remarriage, *J Fam Psychol* 16:363-376, 2002.

McMahon SD et al: Stress and psychopathology in children and adolescents: is there evidence of specificity? *J Child Psychol Psychiatry* 44:107-133, 2003.

National Center for Injury Prevention and Control: *Assault all injury causes: nonfatal injuries and rates per 100,000,* 2006a. Available at *http:// webappa.cdc.gov/cgi-bin/broker.exe* (accessed Oct 2, 2006).

National Center for Injury Prevention and Control: *Youth violence: fact sheet,* 2006b. Available at *www.cdc.gov/ncipc/factsheets/yvfacts.htm* (accessed Oct 2, 2006).

National Center for Health Statistics: *NCHS data on teenage pregnancy (2006),* 2006b. Available at *www.cdc/gov/nchs/data/factsheets/teenpreg. pdf* (accessed Sept 21, 2006).

National Center for Health Statistics: *Health, United States, 2005, with chartbook on trends in the health of Americans,* Hyattsville, MD, 2005, US Department of HHS.

National Coalition for the Homeless: *Homeless families with children NCH fact sheet #12,* 2006a. Available at *www.nationalhomeless.org/ publications/facts.html* (accessed Sept 21, 2006).

National Coalition for the Homeless: *Education of homeless children and youth. NCH fact sheet no 10,* June 2006, 2006b. Available at *www. nationalhomeless.org/publications/facts/acts/education.pdf* (accessed Sept 21, 2006).

National Coalition for the Homeless: *Homeless families with children. NCH Fact Sheet no 12,* June 2006, 2006c. Available at *www.nationalhomeless. org/publications/facts/families.pdf* (accessed Sept 21, 2006).

Olds DL: Prenatal and infancy home visiting by nurses: from randomized trials to community replication, *Prev Sci* 3:153-172, 2002.

Perrin, JM: Developmental disabilities and chronic illness. In Behrman RE, Kliegman R, Jenson HB, editors: *Nelson textbook of pediatrics,* ed 17, Philadelphia, 2004, WB Saunders.

Peter G: Immunization practices. In Behrman RE, Kliegman R, Jenson HB, editors: *Nelson textbook of pediatrics,* ed 17, Philadelphia, 2004, WB Saunders.

Pilowsky DJ et al: Family discord, parental depression, and psychopathology in offspring: 20 year follow-up, *J Am Acad Child Adolesc Psychiatry* 45:452-460, 2006.

Simmons R: *Odd girl out: hidden culture of aggression in girls,* New York, 2002, Harvest Book Harcourt Brace.

Simmons T, Dye JL: *Grandparents living with grandchildren 2000: census 2000 brief,* Washington, DC, 2003, US Census Bureau, US Department of Commerce.

Simmons T, O'Neill G: *Households and families: 2000 census,* Washington, DC, 2001, US Census Bureau, US Department of Commerce.

Stirling J: Child maltreatment. In Burg FD et al, editors: *Current pediatric therapy,* ed 18, Philadelphia, 2006, Elsevier.

Trute B, Hiebert-Murphy D: Family adjustment to childhood developmental disability: a measure of parent appraisal of family impacts, *J Pediatr Psychol* 27:271-280, 2002.

US Department of Health and Human Services (USDHHS): *Healthy People 2010: understanding and improving health,* Washington, DC, 2000, US Government Printing Office.

US Department of Health and Human Services (USDHHS), Administration for Children and Families (ACYF): *Child maltreatment 2004,* Washington, DC, 2006, US Government Printing Office.

US Conference of Mayors 2005, SODEXHO, Inc: *A status report on hunger and homelessness in America's cities: a 24-city survey,* December, 2005, Available at *www.usmayors.org/uscm/hungersurvey/2005/HH2005Final. pdf* (accessed Sept 9, 2007).

Vangyseghem S, Appelboom J. Psychological repercussions of parental divorce on child, *J Rev Med Brux* 25:442-448, 2004.

Wallerstein JS: Children of divorce: the psychological tasks of the child, *Am J Orthopsychiatry* 53:230-243, 1983.

Warrington SA, Wright CM, Team AS: Accidents and resulting injuries in premobile infants: data from the ALSPAC study, *Arch Dis Child* 85: 104-107, 2001.

Wekerle C et al: *Childhood maltreatment,* Cambridge, MA, 2006, Hogrefe & Huber Publishers.

Wolchik SA et al: Six-year follow-up of preventive interventions for children of divorce: a randomized controlled trial, *JAMA* 288:1874-1881, 2002a.

Wolchik SA et al: Fear of abandonment as a mediator of the relations between divorce stressors and mother-child relationship quality and children's adjustment problems, *J Abnorm Child Psychol* 30:401-418, 2002b.

Wood JJ, Repetti RL, Roesch SC: Divorce and children's adjustment problems at home and school: the role of depressive/withdrawn parenting, *Child Psychiatry Hum Dev* 35:121-142, 2004.

CHAPTER 19

Sexuality

Teral Gerlt, Catherine G. Blosser, and Ardys M. Dunn

Children and adolescents are sexual beings throughout life. Sexuality is a multidimensional process that begins at birth. Despite what parents may think, children will become sexual people "with or without their involvement" (Thornton & Collins, 2004, p. 802). The primary care provider can play a crucial part in educating parents to anticipate, recognize, and guide their children through the stages of sexual development. At age-appropriate times, the primary care visit provides children and adolescents with opportunities to explore questions they have about their sexuality. Much of the literature on sexuality deals with problems. This chapter focuses on health promotion, emphasizing that sexual development is a normal and healthy part of human growth.

■ STANDARDS

The *Guidelines for Adolescent Preventive Services (GAPS)*, developed by the American Medical Association (AMA, 1997), still offer the best evidence- and consensus-based strategies concerning clinical preventive counseling and screening for adolescents between 11 and 21 years old. These guidelines include many interventions that address the promotion of healthy adolescent sexual development and the prevention of negative consequences of sexual behaviors. Strategies include:

- Ensuring a confidential environment in which the adolescent and health provider can freely exchange information
- Health guidance to promote a better understanding of physical, sexual, and emotional development
- Supporting parental behaviors that promote healthy adolescent adjustment
- Health guidance regarding responsible sexual behaviors, including abstinence
- Education about the use of latex condoms to prevent sexually transmitted infections (STIs), including infection with human immunodeficiency virus (HIV), and appropriate methods of birth control with instructions on how to use them effectively
- Annual interviews about involvement in sexual behaviors that may result in unintended pregnancy and STIs, including HIV infection
- Questions that explore the adolescent's sexual orientation, number of sex partners in the previous 6 months, if they have exchanged sex for money or drugs, pregnancy, and STI history
- Screening sexually active adolescents for STIs, pregnancy

- Confidential HIV screening of adolescents at risk for HIV infection
- Annual screening of sexually active females or females older than 18 years for cervical cancer by use of a Papanicolaou (Pap) test
- Annual interviews about a history of emotional, physical, and/or sexual abuse
- Initiating the series of hepatitis B vaccinations for those 11 years and older

The Advisory Committee on Immunization Practices has recommended the Centers for Disease Control and Prevention extend the recommended immunizations for adolescents to include:

- Human papillomavirus (HPV) vaccination for females 9 to 26 years old or before first sexual encounter, if possible

■ NORMAL PATTERNS OF SEXUALITY

Clinicians need to be well versed and comfortable using the multiple definitions involved in the term "sexuality" to be credible when providing comprehensive sexuality education and answering questions of parents, children, and adolescents. The following discussion will lay the groundwork for understanding the initial theoretical forays into longitudinal sexual development. Many of the definitions used today were coined in the nineteenth century, but they continue to play a part in the contemporary age-relevant framework of sexual development.

HISTORICAL AND CULTURAL CONTEXT OF SEXUALITY

The term *psychosexual* development is often used to describe the continuum of sexual development from infancy to adulthood. Historically, however, Freud first used this term as an integral concept in his theories of personality development— and eventually psychoanalysis. His concern was focused on the "sexual desires" he believed were intrinsic formative drives, instincts, and appetites that led to one's behaviors and beliefs. The interplay between expressing these sexual desires and the perceived need to repress them led to his five psychosexual stages of normal sexual development (*oral:* 0 to 18 months old; *anal:* 18 to 36 months old; *phallic:* 3 to 6 years old; *latency:* 6 years old to puberty; *genital:* puberty and beyond). The developmental characteristics and the ages at which he assigned the stages varied as Freud advanced his theory throughout his career.

Among others, Erik Erikson furthered the discussion of sexual development by maintaining that children developed in predetermined stages. The stages were based upon socialization and the effect this had on a child's personality, interactions with others, and self-esteem. Unsuccessfully fulfilling one stage prevented one from progressing to the next, until resolved. Successful completion of Erikson's stages related to the eventual healthy development of sexuality in terms of one's gender-role socialization, body image, social relationships, attitudes, values, and self-esteem (Schultz & Schultz, 1987).

Societal socialization norms and values provide males and females with rules about how they should behave. In Western cultures (though this is becoming less absolute), a person's sexual orientation is often used to summarize their total personality and identity. Other cultures and societies differ markedly on this last point. They allow for greater gender diversity, viewing sexual roles, sexual assignment, and sexual behaviors on a continuum with female and male at opposite ends of the spectrum (Ahmed et al, 2004).

Contemporary Definitions

Sexuality has been defined by the Sexuality Information and Education Council of the United States (SIECUS, 1990, p. 10) as encompassing:

> the sexual knowledge, beliefs, attitudes, values, and behaviors of individuals. It deals with anatomy, physiology, and biochemistry of the sexual response system; with roles, identity, and personality; with individual thoughts, feelings, behaviors, and relationships. It addresses ethical, spiritual, and moral concerns, and group and cultural variations.

Murphy and Elias (2006, p. 398) summarize that:

> sexuality extends beyond genital sex to include gender-role and socialization, physical maturation and body image, social relationships, and future social aspirations.

Both definitions illustrate the multidimensional process of sexual development. The complexity of sexuality hinges upon the key notion of gender. The following contemporary definitions explore this notion more fully:

- *Gender identity:* The knowledge of oneself as being male or female. It is believed to evolve from a combination of genetic, prenatal and postnatal endocrine influences, and postnatal psychosocial and environmental experience (Ahmed et al, 2004; Frankowski, 2004; Murphy & Elias, 2006). It usually relates to anatomic sex, but not always (e.g., transgendered persons). One's gender identity is regarded as developing in stages according to age-stage and cognitive development, which will be discussed later. Many theorists argue that gender identity is not fully established until a child has mastered the concept of gender permanency (5 to 7 years old). Others believe gender identity is achieved in the toddler and preschool years. Research of children with complex genital anomalies suggests that genital appearance alone may not be as crucial a determinant in the formation of gender identity. In males, genital appearance does not necessarily predetermine their gender identity. In females, prenatal androgen exposure, rather than the degree of evident virilization, proved to be more causal in atypical gender identity (Ahmed et al, 2004).

- *Gender role:* The outward expression of maleness or femaleness; it usually relates to anatomic sex, but not always, such as with transvestites (Frankowski, 2004). This process begins at preschool age and continues into adulthood. It is characterized by the emergence of behaviors, attitudes, and feelings that are labeled as male, female, or neutral. Ahmed et al (2004) suggest that gender role behavior is dependent on testosterone and estradiol exposure.

- *Gender assignment:* Gender assignment generally occurs at birth, based upon genital appearance and is the keystone, in many societies, for future gender socialization (i.e., gender identity). In most cases, genital appearance is determined from conception and is based on the 46XX and 46XY chromosome karyotypes and the appropriate masculinization effect of prenatal steroid exposure (testosterone and dihydrotestosterone). In approximately 1 in 4500 births, gender assignment may be difficult to assign at birth as a result of complex genital anomalies. In these cases, chromosomal analysis may be only one step in the process of assigning gender, because gonadal dysgenesis can lead to karyotype variations. In these cases, gender assignment is done after careful consideration of the pathologic conditions of the clinical syndrome (fetal exposure to prenatal steroids and degree of masculinization), long-term psychosexual and psychosocial functional outcome of surgical correction, and androgen support. See Chapter 25.

- *Gender attribution:* This is a subjective perception of person based upon a number of cues (e.g., manner of dress, hairstyle, gait, mannerisms, choice of occupation).

- *Gender, or sexual, orientation:* ("Whom do I love?") refers to an individual's feelings of sexual attraction and erotic potential. For most people, their gender identity, role, and gender behaviors are congruent (heterosexual), and they are attracted to the opposite sex. For others, their gender manifestations do not match their gender orientation, and they are attracted to the same sex (homosexual). As discussed previously, many cultures accept more ambiguity between gender role, gender assignment, and symbolic behaviors, allowing permutations of the expression of sexuality.

One's sexual orientation is not necessarily the same as their sexual activity or their sexual feelings. Effects of defects in androgen biosynthesis on brain tissue may alter the perception of body image and influence sexual behavior (Ahmed et al, 2004). Adolescents may express different sexual behaviors, including short-term homosexual experiences. Teens may actually not be sexually active, but label themselves gay, lesbian, or bisexual because of to whom they are physically or emotionally attracted.

Sexual Health

Sexual health has been defined in a holistic perspective by the World Health Organization (1975) as the positive integration of somatic, emotional, intellectual, and social aspects of sexual being in ways that are positively enriching and that enhance personality, communication, and love. Sexual health also involves having the opportunity to make decisions to control one's life to the extent of being able to build meaningful and fulfilling sexual relationships, to be able to express a wide range of feelings and emotions while feeling safe within the environment.

Sexual function incorporates the biologic component of the human sexual response cycle and refers to the ability to give and receive sexual pleasure. Sexual self-concept is the psychological component of sexuality, the image one has of oneself as a man or a woman, and the evaluation of one's adequacy in masculine and feminine roles. Sexual relationships refer to the social domain of sexuality and include the interpersonal relationships in which one's sexuality is shared with others.

STAGES OF DEVELOPMENTAL PATTERNS OF SEXUALITY

The primary care provider is in a unique position to incrementally educate parents about their child's sexual maturation starting from infancy. Such anticipatory guidance will not only enable parents to accurately understand their child's normal sexual development but also provide a structure for healthy parent-child sexual discussions in an ongoing, open manner throughout the child's life. Table 19-1 discusses the components of development related to sexuality.

Infancy to 2 Years Old

Newborn infants are reflexive beings, responding to their physical environment without hesitation or cognition. Sexual reflexes are present prenatally and are easily stimulated in the infant. It is not uncommon to observe a penile erection in prenatal ultrasounds or in the nursing child, for example. Just as infants are fascinated by and explore their hands and feet, they explore their genitalia. Touching the genitalia—even masturbating—is pleasurable and soothing, is a natural part of exploring their environment, and begins as early as 3 to 5 months old. The provider should point out the spontaneity of this reflexive behavior so that a parent does not assign an adult sexuality interpretation to it.

Healthy parent-infant bonding requires physical contact and social interaction. Parents must hold, cuddle, stroke, talk to, look at, and respond to children if children are to develop a sense of trust, on which intimacy will be based in later years, and a positive self-image.

By the end of the first year, the child can differentiate between the sexes; some may even discriminate between sex-assigned toys. As society furthers its influence, children form their identities early and learn about their gender roles from the reinforcement of behaviors expected of males and females.

Two to 5 Years Old

Toddlers are able to recognize and pronounce themselves "I'm a girl" or "I'm a boy," but they can easily confuse gender in others and sometimes in themselves. Changing one's style of clothes, for example, can be perceived as a change in gender. Children cannot integrate gender identity into their self-concept until they understand that gender is a permanent condition. The age at which this notion occurs is around 4 or 5 years old. Theorists argue that gender identity is fully attained between 5 to 7 years old, at which time this identity truly motivates sex-appropriate gender behavior (Ahmed et al, 2004).

Children in this age group are extremely curious about their environment; they love to explore and experiment. They have a cognitive awareness of the pleasure self-stimulation gives them and frequently masturbate, but, as with infants, they attribute no erotic or sexual meaning to their actions. This is a good time for parents to discuss the notion of "private parts" and begin to teach the child that self-stimulation is acceptable, but done in private.

The combination of curiosity and lack of self-consciousness characteristic of toddlers can contribute to embarrassing social incidents for their parents. They may be curious about what others look like under their clothes, they may explore other children's bodies, "play doctor," pretend to be mommy and daddy, and they may enjoy running around naked. By 4 years old, children may attach themselves more to the parent of the opposite sex. Sexual behavior among 3- to 6-year-olds has been found to be more open at home than in a more structured preschool setting (Larsson & Svedin, 2002).

Parents should be encouraged to use the appropriate names for body parts and bodily functions, even though they may also be using slang words. This will enable children to better comprehend discussions with health providers, teachers, and/or health educators when the anatomic and physiological terms are used.

The ways in which parents communicate about sexuality are important for the toddler and preschooler. Because children at this age interpret statements literally and have "magical" thinking, their understandings of the physical self can be distorted, and lengthy explanations about body functions can be misunderstood. Parents should help children understand that they and their bodies come in different shapes, sizes, and colors; that all of these are equally important; that boys and girls also share the same parts, but different genital parts; and that sharing and respect are important aspects for developing friendships. It is appropriate for parents to introduce the notion of germs and hygiene, such as washing hands. This will help establish a framework for parents to advance the discussion to include sexually transmitted infections later in life.

Five to 9 Years Old

School-age children continue to have a high level of curiosity about sexuality and their bodies and their environment. They are aware of the pleasure stimulation gives and continue to actively seek autoerotic arousal for enjoyment. Again reassure parents that this behavior is not associated with sexual fantasies. Contacts with other children may give them new ideas about sex, and sex games are typical (e.g., playing house or doctor) between same-aged children, either of the same or opposite sex. This is normal behavior, as long as a child is not emotionally distraught by the encounter or if it involves one child who is older than the other. Parents should avoid being overly alarmed if they witness this play. It is appropriate for

TABLE 19-1 **Sexual Function, Self-Concept, and Relationships During Childhood Through Young Adulthood**

	Sexual Function	Sexual Self-Concept	Sexual Role and Relationship
Infancy	Orgasmic potential present Erectile function present	Gender identity reinforced	
Toddler	Genital pleasuring and exploration Sensual activity (e.g., hugging, stroking)	Association of sexuality and good and bad Distinction between self and others	Sex role differences learned Discrimination between male and female role models Sexual vocabulary learned
Preschool	Sex play—exploration of own body and those of playmates Self-pleasuring (masturbation) especially when tired	Gender identity understood as a permanent condition	Sex roles learned Parental attachment and identification
School age	Same as preschool	Curiosity about sex Sexual fears and fantasies Interest in aspects of sexual development Self-awareness as sexual being	Same-sex friends Off-color humor related to sexuality
Adolescence, prepubertal	Menarche (female) Seminal emissions (male)	Concerns about body image	Same-sex friends Sexual experiences as part of friendship
Adolescence, early	Awkwardness in first sexual encounter Masturbation, petting May or may not be sexually active	Anxiety over inadequacy, lack of partner, virginity	Appropriate sex friendships Dating
Adolescence, late	May or may not be sexually active	Responsibility for sexual activity	Intimacy in relationships learned
Young adult	Experimentation with sexual positions, expressions Exploration of techniques	Responsibility for sexual health (e.g., contraception, STI prevention) Development of adult sexual value system, tolerance for others	Giving and receiving pleasure learned Long-term commitment to relationship developed

parents to redirect the play to other activities. They should then discuss the situation later with their child to explore the experience, ascertain if the child was uncomfortable, and again emphasize the notion of privacy and respect for one's body. Box 19-1 discusses sexual actions beyond self-stimulation and sex play that can indicate possible sexual abuse.

By 5 to 7 years old, the use of sexual or "potty" language becomes evident, often to test parental reaction. Children at this age identify more with the same sex parent; they tend to cluster into same sex groups if given the opportunity. They are curious about where babies come from.

By the time children are about 8 years old, they begin to understand the significance of sexuality. They learn more about their body and body functions, "giggle" with children of their same sex when talking about sexuality, perhaps because they conceive that sex is a secretive topic. Unless parents actively communicate with their children, sexual lessons will be learned from peers, the media, jokes, and movies.

Some children may begin pubertal changes during this time and may be embarrassed by them. Acne, oily skin, and sweating may occur. As their bodies change, they become curious and want to see others' bodies. Masturbation is still a normal

way for them to explore their bodies. Sexual language is often used more to insult others or appear smart in front of their friends.

Parents and teachers are in key positions to teach children that their sexual curiosity and feelings are normal, to help both boys and girls better understand how sexual development is an integral part of growing up, to use respectful language, and to reinforce that they are always available for questions. Simple discussions about the body can introduce discussions about hormones and reproductive systems. Establishing a good history of communication about sexuality and other subjects lays the groundwork for being accessible to update information as the child matures. This is also a good time for parents and others to reinforce the notion that there is diversity in families within which parents and adults love and care for children.

Preadolescence

Preadolescence is marked by the onset of pubertal changes. About this time, children understand sexuality as a normal part of life. Both males and females understand the changes that are occurring in each others' bodies and by 10 to 12 years old

| **BOX 19-1** | **Signs That Sexual Play May Go Beyond Normal** |

- The behavior is not age-appropriate.
  - *Example*: A 5-year-old walks around the house with his or her hands in his or her underwear.
- The behavior is prolonged.
  - *Example*: Child frequently engages in sexual play and rarely moves on to other activities.
- The child looks anxious or guilty or becomes extremely aroused.
  - *Normal behavior*: Most sexual play is accompanied by laughter and lightheartedness (the little girl who giggles when lifting her skirt; the little boy who laughs when he shows you his penis wrapped in a towel).
- Child is being forced into sexual play through bribes, name-calling, physical force.
- Child knows more about sexual matters than age-appropriate.
  - *Example*: Mimicking sexual intercourse.

Adapted from Todd CM: Responding to sexual play, *Child Care Center Connections* 3(5):1-3, 1994. University of Illinois Cooperative Extension Service. Available at *www.nncc.org/guidance/cc35_respond.sex.play* (accessed Aug 29, 2006).

are ready to discuss sexual behavior and reproduction. Self-stimulation as a result of sexual reflexes may now become connected to sexual fantasies, sexual behavior, and sexual relationships. It is still common for preadolescents to socialize and develop close relationships mostly with members of the same sex. Both sexes often become uncomfortable or embarrassed about the changes in their bodies, particularly girls because breast development is more obvious to others. Privacy becomes more important.

Parents should discuss menstruation before it occurs so as not to cause undue alarm and have the child be caught "off guard." Being mindful of their values and beliefs, parents should discuss abstinence, sexually transmitted infections (including HIV), birth control, consequences of early sexual activity (including teen pregnancy), and the influence of peer pressure. This is also a good time to discuss sexual orientation.

Adolescence

Adolescence is a period of rapid physical, emotional, and social change that presents a developmental challenge to both children and parents. In terms of sexuality, adolescents fit their sense of sexual being into their evolving self-image and personal identity; they learn about their bodies' (sometimes unexpected and embarrassing) sensual and sexual responses to stimulation, and they develop a sense of the moral significance of sexuality. The average age of first intercourse, or sexual debut, is 17 years for females and 16 years for males in the U.S. (Klein, 2005), with a median age of 16.5 years (Thornton & Collins, 2004).

Privacy is essential for the adolescent to explore this emerging self. Activities, such as group social functions, dating, participation in sports, and interactions at work and school,

provide opportunities to learn social and interpersonal skills of intimacy.

Learning how to communicate about sex, how to set limits, how to prevent misunderstandings, and how to say yes or no are important skills for adolescents. Equally important is the process of developing a set of sexual values. Whether the adolescent practices abstinence, has a double standard for men's and women's sexual behavior, or is exploitative or nurturing in close personal relationships is a reflection of the adolescent's sexual values.

Sexuality in Individuals With Intellectual and Developmental Disabilities

The sexual development of youth with intellectual and physical developmental disabilities (I/P/DD) is the same as those without such physical or cognitive limitations. The clinician needs to recognize that these individuals have the same desires to make decisions and foster fulfilling relationships with others. Their abilities to develop healthy sexual identities and engage in sexual behaviors often largely hinge upon society's comfort and proactive support concerning their right for healthy sexual expression. Individuals with I/P/DD are frequently seen by society (including health providers, teachers, and parents) as being childlike, asexual, sexually inappropriate, having uncontrollable sexual urges, or being sexual deviants. Institutional isolation, overprotection, lack of awareness by others of their sexual needs, and pessimism about their potential often ends up inhibiting the healthy sexual and psychosocial development of these individuals. As a consequence, many people with disabilities are vulnerable to sexual abuse and exploitation by those who house, employ, and take care of them. This victimization can lead to low self-esteem, anxiety, depression, and adjustment disorders (Murphy & Elias, 2006).

People with I/P/DD largely acquire their sex education from formal educational programs and the media, rather than from family or friends. Females may obtain such education in the form of abuse. These individuals are less likely to share their thoughts, feelings, and experiences with family and friends (Ailey et al, 2003); "the whole topic of sexuality is less likely to be normalized, because it is not discussed" (McCabe, 1999). Unless healthy sexuality is taught and supported, unhealthy and abusive sexuality can occur. Sex education can be effective for those with I/P/DD, and topics should include: body parts, concepts of privacy and choice, masturbation, sexual abuse prevention, menstruation, homosexuality, marriage, sexual interaction, dating and intimacy, appropriate social behaviors, birth control, pregnancy, STIs, self-esteem, attitudes and values, sexual responsibility and privileges, and consent (Ailey et al, 2003). The depth and length of discussion should vary depending upon the type of disability (e.g., sex education taught to a child with autism would have a different focus than that taught to a child with Down syndrome). Excellent resources and books are available to parents, teachers, and clinicians from Planned Parenthood, the SIECUS, and the National Dissemination Center for Children and Youth With Disabilities (NICHCY).

ASSESSMENT OF NORMAL PATTERNS OF SEXUAL DEVELOPMENT

Sexual development, questions, and concerns are present throughout childhood, although for many children the onset of their first sexual intercourse is the cornerstone of their "sexuality." Assessment of sexuality and sexual maturation should be integrated into the health history, interview and discussion, and physical examination at all health maintenance visits.

CONFIDENTIALITY

Research has shown clear evidence that sexuality education leads to a reduction in early onset of sexual intercourse and risky sexual behaviors (Alexander, 2001).

The AMA (1997), American Academy of Pediatrics, Society for Adolescent Medicine (SAM), American College of Obstetricians and Gynecologists, Association of Women's Health, Obstetric and Neonatal Nurses (AWHONN), National Medical Association, and the American Academy of Family Physicians have endorsed policies advocating confidential medical visits for adolescents (AWHONN, 2000; SAM, 2004). The National Association of Pediatric Nurse Practitioners (NAPNAP) supports confidentiality regarding sexual orientation and gender identity in accordance with state regulations regarding confidentiality of minors (NAPNAP, 2006). Despite these outstanding policies, a survey found that confidential services for adolescents are limited in pediatric, family, and internal medicine primary care settings. The limitations were largely due to unwritten office policies that led to a discrepancy in understanding—between providers and office staff—about the availability of confidential appointments for adolescents (Akinbami et al, 2003). Another study showed that 69% to 80% of adolescents who met with a health care provider did not even receive the screening or counseling interventions recommended by GAPS (Klein et al, 2001). Equally worrisome, only 45% of teens surveyed perceived confidentiality would be accorded to them (Thrall et al, 2000).

Generally, adolescents, especially females, are less likely to seek health care about sexuality unless they can depend upon a confidential environment in which to do so (Reddy et al, 2002). This lack of confidentiality can have serious repercussions. One study found that requiring parental consent for contraceptives apparently raised the incidence of pregnancies and births among teens (Zavodny, 2004).

Health providers need to be clear about their policy of confidentiality with both the youth and parent before the need arises. This discussion needs to include confidentiality boundaries (i.e., severe mental health issues and safety) and billing statements that may be sent to parents.

HISTORY

Functions of the Sexual History

The sexual history achieves several purposes. Not only is it a tool to collect information, but the process itself gives permission to the child, adolescent, or parent to ask questions

and receive reliable information regarding issues of sexual concern. In this way, it sets the stage to incorporate accurate, sexuality-specific education as a normal component of anticipatory guidance.

Types of Sexual History

The sexual history can be either comprehensive or problem-oriented. The comprehensive sexual history is detailed, encompassing all aspects of sexual information about individuals, their family of origin, siblings, and peer relationships. It includes information about each phase of sexual development, body image, masturbation, learned attitudes, feelings about sexuality, sexual debut, sexual orientation, and a range of sexual behaviors. A comprehensive history is lengthy and may not be accomplished at the first visit or in a single interview; it can be anxiety producing to have the client disclose such a level of detail during early visits, and clients can become fatigued by one lengthy interview.

In contrast, the problem-oriented sexual history usually focuses on the current complaint or assessment of specific behaviors such as the risk of exposure to pregnancy or the acquisition of STIs. Problem-oriented sexual histories are shorter, more direct, and specific to the issue at hand.

Approach to Taking a Sexual History

Taking a sexual history should be integrated as one part of the health history. In taking a sexual history, the interviewer should do the following:
- Reassure the client that asking sexual questions is a normal part of clinical practice: "I'm going to ask you a few questions that I ask all my young-adult patients about their health and relationships" (Rakel, 2002).
- Give appropriate, factual information; use medical-sexual terminology rather than slang, unless the client cannot relate to medical terms.
- Create an accepting environment.
- Use language that validates the client's understanding of terms and concepts. For example, when talking with adolescents, the question "Are you sexually active?" seeks information regarding current activity on a planned and regular basis. The adolescent who has concrete cognitive abilities may respond negatively. However, the question "Have you ever had a romantic relationship with a boy or a girl?" allows for a more inclusive description of sexual activity.
- Use open-ended questions. For example, phrases, such as "explain how that happened," "what happened next," or "tell me about a typical date," elicit more complete information than do closed-ended questions. Questions that contain "why" can require a level of analysis beyond the capabilities of children operating at a concrete level of cognition.
- "When you think of people to whom you are sexually attracted, are they males, females, both, neither, or are you not sure yet?" is a useful question that opens up a conversation for youth struggling with their sexual orientation (Murphy & Elias, 2006).
- Phrase questions that may be emotionally laden in a way that lets clients know that their experience may not be

exceptional (e.g., "Many people have been sexually abused or molested as children; did this happen to you?" (Rakel, 2002).

- When asking sensitive questions, phrasing the question in a way that implies that everybody does it makes answering the question easier: "How often do you masturbate?" is better than "Do you masturbate?" (Rakel, 2002).

Content of a Sexual History

The content of a comprehensive adolescent sexual and reproductive history is contained in Box 19-2. Box 19-3 lists questions for a problem-oriented sexual history.

Questions for parents about their children follow. As the child grows, these same questions can be reworded to be more age-appropriate and asked directly of the child or adolescent.

- Does your child have meaningful interactions with men and women who have positive self-images?
- Do you have positive feelings about your child's gender?
- Is your child aware of physical sexual differences between men and women?
- What does your child know about his or her body parts? Does he or she know the correct terminology for body parts?
- What does your child know about sexuality? About gender differences?
- What does your child know about how babies are born and cared for (e.g., pregnancy, childbirth, breastfeeding)?

BOX 19-2 Comprehensive Adolescent Sexual and Reproductive History

Background Data

Adolescent
 Age (birth date)
 Sex
 History of risky behaviors (e.g., drug history: onset, duration, and frequency of use of cigarettes, alcohol, other illicit drugs)
Parents
 Ages
 Religions
 Educational levels
 Occupations
 Marital status
 Affectional relationship (parent to parent)
 Child's feelings toward parent(s)

Childhood Sexuality

What were your parents' attitudes about sexuality when you were a child?
How did your parents handle nudity?
When do you first recall seeing a nude person of the same sex? Opposite sex?
Who taught you about sex, sex play, pregnancy, intercourse, masturbation, homosexuality, STIs, birth?
How often did you play doctor or nurse or have other sex play with another child?
Tell me about any other sexual activity or experience that had a strong effect on you.

Adolescent Sexuality

Girls
 Onset of breast development?
 When did pubic hair appear?
 Onset of menstruation (age, regularity of periods [initially, now])?
 When was your last normal menstrual period (LNMP)?
 What hygienic methods are used (pads, tampons)?
 How were you prepared for menstruation? By whom?
 What were feelings about early periods? Later periods?
 Have you had unusual bleeding or pains?
Boys
 How were you prepared for adolescence? By whom?
 Age of first orgasm (ejaculation)?
 What were "wet dreams" like? How did they make you feel?
 When did pubic hair appear?
Body image
 How do you feel about your body? Breasts? Genitals?
 How much time do you spend nude in front of a mirror?
Masturbation
 How old were you when you began?
 What are others' reactions to your masturbation?
 What methods do you use?
 What are your feelings about it?
Necking and petting
 How old were you when you began? How often?
 How many partners do you currently have?
Intercourse
 How often have you had intercourse?
 How many partners?
 How often do you initiate sex?
 How often do you currently have sex?
 How often have you had oral sex?
 Are your partners male, female, or both?
 Type of intercourse: penile-vaginal, orogenital, penile-anal, oral-anal
Contraceptive use
 What kinds of contraceptives have you used?
 What are you using now?
 Do you have any problems with contraceptives?
 Do you use condoms?
 How do you communicate about contraception with your partner?
Homosexuality
 What does it mean to be lesbian, gay, or bisexual?
 Do you think you might be lesbian, gay, or bisexual?
 Do you think you need to have sex to find out? (Ryan & Futterman, 2000)
 Have you known any homosexual individuals?

Continued

BOX 19-2 **Comprehensive Adolescent Sexual and Reproductive History—Cont'd**

Adolescent Sexuality—Cont'd

How often have you had homosexual feelings?
How often have you been approached?
How often have you had homosexual experiences? What kinds of experiences? What were the circumstances?

Seduction and rape

When have you seduced someone sexually?
When has someone seduced you?
Have you been raped?
Have you raped someone? How often have you forced someone to have sex?

Incest and abuse

What kinds of touching did you receive in your home?
From your mother? Father? Brother(s)? Sister(s)? Other relatives? Others?

Prostitution

What feelings do you have about prostitution?
Have you ever accepted money for sex?

Have you ever had sex with a prostitute?

STIs

How old were you when you learned about STIs?
Have you ever had an STI? Gonorrhea? Syphilis? Chlamydia?
Do you have any signs or symptoms now of STIs?

Pregnancy

Have you ever been pregnant? At what age?
How was it resolved—miscarriage, abortion, adoption, marriage, single parenthood?
Do you think there is a chance you are pregnant now?
Have you caused a pregnancy?

Abortion

What are your feelings about abortion?
Have you (or a partner) had an abortion? If yes, at what age? What were your feelings?
What about your feelings now? What about your feelings immediately afterward? What about your feelings after 1 year?

Adapted from Laube HH: The use of a sexual history with adolescents. In Blum RW, editor: *Adolescent health care: clinical issues,* New York, 1982, Academic Press; Neinstein L, editor: *Adolescent health care: a practical guide,* Philadelphia, 2002, Lippincott Williams & Wilkins.

- What does your child know about STIs and acquired immunodeficiency syndrome (AIDS)?
- Does your child (older than 8 years) have a healthy awareness of alternative sexual preferences?
- How do members of your family demonstrate affection?
- Does your child seek and receive positive touching from others?
- Does your child experience a variety of sensory stimuli?
- Does your child have friends (same or opposite sex)? In what types of interactions do they engage? Is exploration (e.g., masturbation, playing "doctor") occurring? How is it handled?
- How does your child express sexuality? In play? By touching? Verbally?
- What sorts of questions does your child ask about sex?
- How do you respond to your child's sexual behavior and questions?
- What do you know about human sexuality? What are your feelings and attitudes about it?
- Does the child's school provide appropriate information about sexuality and reproduction?
- Is your child at risk for sexual abuse?

PHYSICAL EXAMINATION

The physical examination serves to identify normal variations of sexual anatomy, the stage of sexual development (Tanner stages), and any pathologic condition. The physical examination should include examination of the breasts, pattern of body hair growth, and external genitalia. In sexually active adolescents or when an abnormality is suspected, a pelvic and/or rectal exam may be indicated. Laboratory studies are performed as needed, which may include a Pap smear (see Chapter 35 for current guidelines); cervical, urethral, rectal,

and/or pharyngeal cultures; urine-based nucleic acid amplification test (NAAT); blood work for STIs (see Chapter 35); or genetic studies if indicated.

The physical examination should be performed with care and sensitivity to the child's or adolescent's feelings. Very young children and toddlers make no distinction between examination of external genitalia and other body parts; young school-age children can be extremely modest, act embarrassed, and resist taking off their clothes for the examination. Older school-age children and adolescents can misinterpret the examination procedures and may feel violated or abused. The child needs to feel an element of control during the exam. By taking the time to provide clear explanations of procedures, using straightforward techniques, and involving the child in the examination (e.g., asking if the child wishes to have the parent or another adult present), the clinician can better achieve the fine balance necessary to perform a thorough, respectful examination.

■ MANAGEMENT STRATEGIES OF NORMAL PATTERNS

The health provider has two primary goals related to management of sexual development in children: first, to help children achieve a healthy sexual identity and function and second, to provide support for parents to enable them to guide their children through the process. By counseling parents about children's sexual development, both goals can be achieved. Anticipatory guidance about sexual development and maturation that is age-appropriate should be provided to parents and their children as a matter of course. In particular the provider must:

- Assess the parent's level of understanding regarding normal physical and psychosocial sexual development in children.

BOX 19-3   Problem-Oriented Adolescent Sexual History

Describe the sexual concern, problem, issue, or difficulty that you have. Include:
History:
- Condoms—consistency of use, for which sexual practices
- Previous STIs; medication allergies
- Most recent sexual encounter; number partners in past 2 months
- Use of illegal drugs and alcohol by self and partner (include which drugs, frequency, route)
- Does patient and/or partner have sex with men, women, or both?
- Recent travel and location
- Any symptoms of: dysuria, frequency, hematuria; adenopathy; fatigue; weight loss; nights/sweats; unexplained diarrhea; fever; rectal discharge, bleeding, constipation, pain?
- Women only: additional symptoms of:
  ○ Vaginal discharge, bleeding, color of discharge; skin rashes, lesions, sores and location; pruritus (vulvar, anal, oral, other); pain (abdominal, vaginal, vulvar, anal, headache, joints)
  ○ LNMP, description, changes
- Birth control method(s), consistency of use
- Men only: symptoms of:
  ○ Penile discharge; lesions and/or pruritus (penis, scrotum, urethra, oral cavity); pain in testes
How do you feel about discussing this problem?
How long have you had it? When did this problem begin?
What do you think caused you to have this problem?
What might be contributing to this problem?
What kinds of things have you done to treat or solve this problem?
What health professionals have you seen?
What, if any, medication have you taken or are you taking?
Have you talked to a friend or relative?
Have you read any books to solve this problem? What books?

STI, Sexually transmitted infection; *LNMP*, last normal menstrual period.
Adapted from Laube HH: The use of a sexual history with adolescents. In Blum RW, editor: *Adolescent health care: clinical issues,* New York, 1982, Academic Press. Additional information from Buttaro TM et al: *Primary care: a collaborative practice,* ed 2, Philadelphia, 2003, Mosby, p 695, Box 160-3.

- Provide or clarify information as needed.
- Provide strategies and support for teaching children about sexuality.
- Assist the parent to connect to community-based resources.

SETTING THE STAGE

When working with children, the provider focuses on establishing and maintaining a positive relationship based on mutual trust and respect, and in which the child is validated and feels comfortable revealing concerns and asking questions. In addition to using a constructive approach to taking a sexual history, a positive relationship can be achieved by:

- Asking questions to give the message that the child is expected to be changing and is aware of and curious about those changes (e.g., "How are you feeling?" "How's your body?" "Do you notice that you're getting taller?")
- Asking questions to give the message that sexual changes are to be expected and are as normal as other body changes (e.g., "Have you noticed your breasts getting any bigger?" "Boys' penises begin to get longer and wider as they become teenagers. Have you noticed any changes in yours?")
- Asking questions to give the message that you care about the child's feelings (e.g., "How does that make you feel?" "Do you wonder sometimes about what's happening to your body?")
- Listening thoughtfully and carefully to the child's input
- Responding positively by answering the child's questions as fully as possible; being nonjudgmental, calm, friendly, and open; and having a sense of humor, yet taking the child seriously
- Using appropriate teachable moments during the health visit (e.g., when examining a 3-year-old for inguinal hernia, the clinician can discuss appropriate and inappropriate touching with the child and his or her parent)
- Providing accurate information and referral resources as appropriate
- Respecting the child's need for privacy (e.g., knocking before entering the examination room, providing appropriate gowns, examining the child semiclothed)
- Maintaining confidentiality as appropriate, especially with an adolescent; however, children of any age may give information that need not be shared with the parent

SEX EDUCATION

For the child, developing healthy sexuality means gaining knowledge about physical changes; shaping a positive gender identity; clarifying one's sexual identity as a boy or a girl; establishing close, intimate relationships with others; and demonstrating the ability to make healthy judgments about sexuality and sexual activity. It is the parents' responsibility to facilitate this learning. Human sexuality, however, is an emotionally charged issue for many parents, and they can find it difficult to be comfortable with their child's normal, innocent curiosity about sex, gender, and body parts and functions.

The questions a child asks and the behaviors displayed can embarrass some parents, who may respond in a manner that frightens, shames, or confuses the child. Children are born as sexual beings, and parents, whether or not they are aware of it, are constantly providing lessons in sex education. The way parents respond to a child's innate sexuality and allow it to unfold is the core of a child's sex education. This response does more to mold that child's mature sexual behavior than all the information or misinformation parents may provide.

Parents should be encouraged to take advantage of teaching opportunities in normal childhood sexual play and to answer questions simply and directly at the child's level of understanding (Box 19-4). Box 19-5 outlines what children should know about sexuality at different ages.

| BOX 19-4 | Approaches to Teaching Your Child About Sex |

Find out what your child already knows.

Understand the question before answering.

Check to be sure your answer is understood. Make sure you answer the question that is asked, and give your child a chance to ask more questions.

If your child asks a question about sexuality at an inconvenient time, set a time and place as soon as possible to answer the question.

Discuss sex in a matter-of-fact way.

Use correct terminology when talking about body parts; use dolls and books as guides.

Keep the topics short and to the point, remembering the child's attention span.

Do not worry about telling children too much about sex. They tune out what they do not understand.

Encourage questions. Never embarrass children or tell them they are too young to understand or that they will learn that when they grow up.

Include values, emotions, feelings, and decision-making in your discussion. Do not focus only on biologic facts.

Let your child know that people have different beliefs about sexuality, and these differences are OK.

Bring up topics of STIs, including AIDS.

Discuss anticipated changes of puberty before they occur. Do not wait until your child is a teenager.

Discuss menstruation with boys and with girls.

If you do not know the answer to your child's question, say so, and then look it up. Ask your pediatric primary care provider.

If your child is masturbating in public or engaging in sex play, redirect them to other activities. At a later time, discuss where a more appropriate private place is for the child to masturbate.

When your child uses "four-letter words," calmly explain what they mean, why it is not appropriate to use them, and that use of certain words can be insulting (e.g., "gay"). Do not laugh or joke about your child's four-letter words because this can serve as encouragement.

STI, Sexually transmitted infection; *LNMP*, last normal menstrual period. Information from Masters WH, Johnson VE, Kolodny RC: *Human sexuality*, ed 5, New York, 1995, HarperCollins College Publishers; Dunn J, Myers-Walls JA: *Tips for providers*. Written for Provider-Parent Partnerships, Purdue University. Available at *www.ces.purdue. edu/providerparent/Health-Safety/tips* (accessed Aug 29, 2006).

Research has shown clear evidence that comprehensive sexuality education leads to a reduction in early onset of sexual intercourse and risky sexual behaviors (Alexander, 2001; Kirby, 2001; National Campaign to Prevent Teen Pregnancy, 2006). Yet, sex education in the schools remains controversial and subject to federal, state, and local mandate as to content. The federal government, through Section 510 of the Social Security Act, funds "abstinence only" education programs whose " 'exclusive purpose' [is] the promotion of abstinence outside of marriage for people of any age and may not in any way advocate contraceptive use or discuss contraceptive

methods except to emphasize their failure rates" (Dailard, 2002). Current evidence shows that these programs do not reduce teen sex and its untoward consequences (As-Sanie et al, 2004; Kirby, 2002; Santelli et al, 2006). Comprehensive sex education programs do (Kirby, 2001; National Campaign to Prevent Teen Pregnancy, 2006).

The research brief called Putting What Works to Work (National Campaign to Prevent Teen Pregnancy, 2003) outlined the ten criteria of effective curriculum-based programs as proposed by Kirby (2001):

1. Have a specific, narrow focus on behavior
2. Are based on theoretical approaches that have been effective in influencing other risky health-related behavior
3. Provide clear messages about sex and protection against STIs or pregnancy
4. Provide basic, not detailed, information
5. Address peer pressure
6. Teach communication skills
7. Include activities that are interactive
8. Reflect the age, sexual experience, and culture of the young people in the program
9. Last longer than several hours
10. Carefully select leaders and train them

The SIECUS (2004) published *Guidelines for Comprehensive Sexuality Education: Kindergarten—12th Grade*. The guidelines are organized around six key concepts, and content is divided into four developmental levels. The six key concepts are human development; relationships; personal skills; sexual behavior; sexual health; and society and culture (Table 19-2). This curriculum is broad based yet meets the majority of Kirby's criteria.

Many professional nursing and medical organizations have policy statements or position papers that support comprehensive sex education in the schools and at home (American Academy of Family Physicians [AAFP], 2005; American Academy of Pediatrics [AAP], 2001; American College of Obstetricians and Gynecologists [ACOG], 2005; American Nurses Association [ANA], 1991; SAM, 2006; and Society of Pediatric Nurses, 2004). They encourage abstinence as the adolescents' best choice to prevent pregnancy and STIs; they also encourage parental involvement. However, all state that counseling and education on contraception, STIs, and HIV/AIDS are essential.

COUNSELING OF THE ADOLESCENT

Today's adolescents face multiple influences, including: societal expectations at odds with the media's portrayal of sexuality; cultural norms, beliefs, and attitudes of the family of origin; peer group pressure to conform; and the individual's own values and belief system (AAP, 2001; Brown & Brown, 2006). All these influences need to be considered and addressed when counseling.

The health care provider should use the answers given by the adolescent in the sexual history to further guide the counseling and educational needs of that individual. Trust, honesty, mutual respect, an open nonjudgmental attitude, and confidentiality are extremely important to the adolescent (Burgis &

BOX 19-5   Sexual Development: What Should Children Know?

By 5 Years Old, Children Should:
Use correct words for all sexual body parts.
Be able to understand what it means to be male or female.
Understand that their bodies belong to themselves, and they have a right to say "no" to unwanted touch.
Know where babies come from; how they "get in" and "get out."
Be able to talk about body parts without feeling "naughty."
Be able to ask trusted adults questions about sexuality.
Know that "sex talk" is for private times at home.

Elementary School Children (6–9 Years Old) Should:
Be aware that all creatures grow and reproduce.
Be aware that sexuality is important at all ages, including at their parents' and grandparents' ages, and that it changes over time.
Know and use proper words for body parts—their own and those of the opposite sex.
Understand that there are many kinds of caring family types so that they do not see a single model of family as the only possible one.
Be aware that sexual identity includes sexual orientation: lesbian, gay, heterosexual, or bisexual.
 Understand the basic facts about AIDS.
Take an active role in managing their body's health and safety.

Nine- to 13-Years-Olds Should:
Be informed about human reproduction
Be aware of changes they can expect in their bodies before puberty (9-11 years old)
Know how normal developmental changes begin, including normal differences and when those events occur for males and females.

Know how male and female bodies grow and differ.
Understand the general stages of the body's growth.
Understand the facts about menstruation and wet dreams.
Know that emotional changes are very common during this time.
Understand that human sexuality is a natural part of life (12-13 years old).
Be aware of how behavior can be seen as sexual and how to deal with sexual behavior (by 12-13 years old)
Be aware that sexual feelings are normal and OK.
Know how to recognize and protect themselves against potential sexual abuse, and how to react to such dangers.
Be able to recognize male and female prostitution and its dangers.
Know how babies are made and what behaviors are likely to lead to pregnancy.
Know that it is possible to plan parenthood.
Understand that having a child is a long-term responsibility, and every child deserves mature, responsible, loving parents.
Be aware that contraceptives (birth control methods) exist (and should be able to name some).
Know what abortion is.
Know what STIs are.
Understand how a person can get STIs
Be aware of how a person can protect himself or herself from STIs
Know how STIs are treated.
Look for more detailed information and information about what older teens should know and understand about sexuality: *www.plannedparenthood.org*. Search: "What children should know." Or *www.plannedparenthood.org/educational-resources/for-parents/human-sexuality-what-children-need-to-know.htm.*

STI, Sexually transmitted infection.
From Purdue University Provider-Parent Partnerships, Human Development Extension: *Sexual development: what should children know?* Prepared by Dunn J, Myers-Walls J, 2003. Available at *www.ces.purdue.edu/providerparent* (accessed Aug 10, 2006).

Bacon, 2003). It may take several visits for the trust relationship to grow before the adolescent is willing to divulge certain aspects of their sexual self. The provider's job is to assure the adolescent of the confidential nature of the relationship and provide opportunities for trust to develop.

Adolescents should be counseled that abstinence is the most effective strategy for the prevention of pregnancy, STIs, and HIV/AIDS (AAFP, 2005; AAP, 2001; ACOG, 2005). Further they need to know that they have choices. It is a choice to remain abstinent and a choice to become sexually active, not just something that happens; with that choice come responsibilities. Open communication and respect for self and their partner will lead to choices that include protection from STIs and pregnancy.

The approach taken when counseling the adolescent needs to be appropriate for their psychosocial developmental stage (Burgis & Bacon, 2003; Clark, 2003). Using Piaget's stages of development as the basis, counseling may

be tailored accordingly. Early adolescents, 12 to 14 years old, are concrete thinkers and cannot get to the abstract thought of "what if." Counseling language needs to be in simple concrete terms. Using pictures and direct questions and statements will help facilitate this. Middle adolescents, 15 to 17 years old, are starting to understand abstract concepts, but will often regress to concrete thinking in stressful situations. An adolescent at this age may demonstrate mature thought processes at one point in time yet revert to concrete thinking at another. The provider needs to adjust the approach to the middle adolescent accordingly, help them to identify the inconsistencies in their thought processes, and guide them through to the logical consequences. Late adolescents, 18 to 21 years old, generally have abstract thought more firmly established and are future oriented. However, this ability will vary, as with the general adult population.

TABLE 19-2 Comprehensive Sexuality Education

Content Area	Examples
Human development	Differences in anatomy between the sexes Puberty, menstruation Pregnancy and where babies come from
Relationships	Families Dating Respect for others and self Marriage and lifetime commitments
Personal skill	Communication How to say no How to be affectionate Importance of responsible behavior Judgment and decision-making How to talk with parents about sexual questions
Sexual behavior	Appropriate limits on behavior Abstinence Masturbation Sexuality throughout life
Sexual health	STIs Contraception Reproductive health Sexuality in the law and religion Sexual diversity Sexuality in the arts and media

STI, Sexually transmitted infection.
From Sexuality Information and Education Council of the United States (SIECUS), National Guidelines Task Force: *Guidelines for comprehensive sexuality education: kindergarten-12th grade.* Reprinted with the permission of the Sexuality Information and Education Council of the United States (SIECUS), 130 W. 42nd Street, Suite 350, New York, NY, 10036. Copyright 1996.

CONTRACEPTIVE AND SAFER SEX COUNSELING

It is important to use gender-neutral phrasing when discussing safer sex and contraception and not assume heterosexuality. Providers who provide contraceptive and safer sex counseling to adolescents should understand that the successful use of any method requires a complex process of knowledge, decision-making skills, and public behaviors. To use contraceptives and/or protective barriers successfully, an individual must master the following:

- *Knowledge.* The person must acquire, process, and retain accurate information regarding the specific methods of birth control under consideration. For most adolescents, this means mastery of a barrier method (such as male or female condoms) to prevent an STI, in addition to a variety of hormonal methods for contraceptive purposes.
- *Ability to plan for the future.* Planning for the future requires self-admission that the adolescent will have sex in the future and the ability to take the steps necessary to use a method consistently and correctly. Adolescents must be willing to use the chosen method of protection consistently, not just when it is convenient to do so.
- *Willingness to acquire needed contraceptive and/or barrier methods publicly.* The adolescent must be willing and able to be public with requests for contraceptive and/or protective devices (e.g., to purchase condoms at a local pharmacy or to seek services at the local clinic, school-based health facility, or private practice) (see Chapter 35 for more in-depth information on contraceptive methods).
- *Communication skills.* Adolescents must have the ability to communicate with another person, such as their partner, health care provider, pharmacist, or salesperson, about their individual contraceptive and/or protective barrier needs. Communication also involves adolescents' willingness and ability to articulate how they feel about sexual activity, how it affects them, and the thinking behind their decision to be sexually active.

■ SPECIAL COUNSELING NEEDS

Sexual development is an integral part of children's whole development. Children's sense of self; personality; relationship to others and to the physical world; cognitive, emotional, and spiritual abilities; perceptions; and expressions are all influenced by and, in turn, influence their sexual development. If children experience difficulties with sexuality, all other aspects of development are affected. Issues of major concern include child sexual abuse (see Chapter 18) and adolescent pregnancy (see Chapter 35). The counseling and support needs of gay, lesbian, bisexual, transgendered, and questioning (GLBTQ) youth is another issue.

SEXUAL MINORITY YOUTHS

Description

Sexual orientation refers to a person's sexual responsiveness to partners of the same gender, homosexual; the opposite gender, heterosexual; or both, bisexual. The concept of sexual orientation includes at least three distinctive components: sexual imagery (fantasies or attraction), actual sexual behavior, and the person's self-identification as heterosexual, bisexual, or homosexual. Transgendered individuals identify themselves as the gender opposite of their biologic sex. Their sexual orientation may be heterosexual, homosexual, or bisexual.

Epidemiology

Sexual orientation received considerable attention after the release of data from the Kinsey studies of comprehensive sexual histories (Kinsey et al, 1949). Kinsey concluded that 4% of men in the cohort born between 1920 and 1930 were exclusively homosexual throughout their lives, and 10% were more or less exclusively homosexual for at least 3 years. The estimates of the prevalence of homosexuality for American women were half those of corresponding male rates (Kinsey et al, 1953). Criticism has been raised as to whether Kinsey's data can be generalized because the small convenience samples of students and tradesmen in the studies may have skewed findings. Adolescent-specific data on sexual orientation are sparse. Remafedi et al (1992) surveyed a representative sample of 34,706 Minnesota junior and senior high school youths and reported that 10.7% were unsure of their sexual orientation, 88.2% described themselves as exclusively heterosexual, and 1.1% described themselves as bisexual or primarily homosexual. Random-probability nationally based survey data on adolescent sexual orientation are absent.

The etiology of sexual orientation is unknown. Sexual orientation appears to develop in phases, from the prenatal period through latency. Although the dynamics of its evolution are unknown, sexual orientation tends to be fixed by the end of the child's prepubertal years.

Currently, there is no scientific evidence to explain this development of sexual orientation, and many theories have been postulated. Some postulate that it is a purely biologic phenomenon, largely determined in utero, as evidenced by the high concordance of homosexuality among monozygotic twins. Researchers have studied prenatal androgen exposure, loci on the X chromosome, and neuroanatomic differences in the brain (Frankowski, 2004; Gooren, 2006). The work of Bell and colleagues (1981) served to rule out many psychosocial components when the researchers concluded that homosexuality does not result from a cold, distant father; poor peer relationships; sexual abuse; or sexual experimentation in childhood. The development of sexual orientation is probably multifaceted and a combination of genetic, hormonal, and environmental factors (Frankowski, 2004).

Assessment

The development of a nonheterosexual orientation involves a process of acknowledging and integrating one's sexual identity. The gold standard model of homosexual identity formation includes sensitization, identity confusion, identity assumption, and commitment (Troiden, 1988).

- Sensitization occurs during childhood when individuals identify themselves as feeling different from others of the same gender. Girls describe themselves as "unfeminine," whereas boys often report feelings of disinterest in sports and a proclivity for artistic endeavors. Boys state that they are often called "sissies."
- Identity confusion usually occurs during adolescence when individuals begin to question whether they may be homosexual. On average, this occurs for males at 17 years old and for females at 18 years old. Feelings of inadequacy, insecurity, self-deprecation, poor self-esteem, and depression can result from unresolved identity confusion.
- Identity assumption is the stage at which the child assumes a homosexual identity that is shared with others. The age at which this occurs varies by gender, with males reporting an average age of 19 to 21 years and females 21 to 23 years. Exploration of the homosexual role can lead to multiple sexual experiences with accompanying risks of acquiring STIs, including HIV infection. In contrast, close, long-term relationships can develop. The sexually active, late adolescent-young adult homosexual, is at risk for having the same relationship problems as his/her heterosexual counterpart.
- Commitment is an internalized pledge to live as a homosexual and enter into a same-sex relationship. This process can be referred to as "coming out." External disclosure to others who are not homosexual may vary, depending on what is perceived to be safe to the individual. A stigma management strategy of blending, or acting in a "gender-appropriate" manner, may be adopted in an attempt to be safe in environments that are not tolerant or accepting of homosexuality.

Management

The goal of the provider working with adolescents who are GLBTQ is the same as with any adolescent: promote healthy sexual development, assess social and emotional well-being, and encourage physical health through healthy lifestyle choices (Frankowski, 2004). It is important to support and validate the adolescent throughout the process of developing his or her awareness of and commitment to a nonheterosexual orientation and provide a safe environment in which to access health care (Frankowski, 2004; Garofalo & Katz, 2001). Specific interventions include the following:

- Ensuring confidentiality
- Using gender-neutral nonjudgmental language
- Displaying information that is important to GLBTQ youth
- Provide information about available resources for support

Sexual minority adolescents have indicated that there are qualities of the primary care provider that they find most helpful in supporting their health needs (Ginsburg et al, 2002). These include the following:

- Cleanliness
- Confidentiality
- Respect
- Competence
- Honesty
- Good listener
- Nonjudgmental attitude

The counseling needs of GLBTQ youth are much the same as with any adolescent. All adolescents need to be assessed for risky behaviors, depression, suicidal thoughts, and personal violence. Providers need to encourage abstinence, promote safer sex for those who are sexually active, and counsel about the association between substance abuse and unsafe sexual practices (Frankowski, 2004). However, one needs to remain cognizant of the special mental health needs and risk behavior profile of the GLBTQ population (Garofalo & Katz, 2001).

Sexual minority youth are at increased risk of poor health outcomes secondary to their nonheterosexual status. Society as a whole and family, friends, and peers in particular may not be supportive of a GLBTQ youth. These adolescents can be subject to prejudice, verbal and/or physical abuse, and ridicule. Internalizing these messages may result in drug and alcohol abuse, risky sexual practices, depression, suicidal ideation, and other risk-taking behaviors (Garofalo & Harper, 2003; Garofalo & Katz, 2001).

Complications

Garofalo and Harper (2003) list the top ten threats to the health and well-being of gay and bisexual male youth; many are applicable to all GLBTQ youth:

1. HIV/AIDS
2. Stigma and heterosexism
3. Suicide
4. Club drugs and circuit parties
5. STIs
6. Cigarettes, alcohol, and substance abuse
7. Body image and disordered eating
8. Homelessness
9. Violence and victimization
10. Access to care

It is beyond the scope of this text to do justice to the many management issues facing the primary care provider working with sexual minority youth. Several professional resources are available to guide the clinician including the AAP Clinical Report on Sexual Orientation and Adolescents (Frankowski, 2004); Garofalo & Harper, 2003; Meininger et al, 2002; NAPNAP, 2006.

NURSING DIAGNOSES

Related to the Sexuality Functional Health Pattern

- Sexual dysfunction
- Ineffective sexuality patterns

From NANDA International: *NANDA-I nursing diagnoses: definitions & classifications 2007-2008*, Philadelphia, 2007, Author.

RESOURCE BOX

Resources for Building Self-Perception

SEXUALITY
American Academy of Pediatrics
www.aap.org

American College of Obstetricians and Gynecologists
www.acog.org

Association of Reproductive Health Professionals
www.arhp.org
Interdisciplinary organization, research, and advocacy

ETR Associates
www.etr.org
Provides leadership, educational resources, training and research in health promotion, especially in sexuality and health education

National Dissemination Center for Children and Youth with Disabilities
www.nichcy.org
Provides guidelines on sex education for people with disabilities

Purdue University Cooperative Extension Service
www.ces.purdue.edu
Provides an extensive array of information, guidelines, and handouts for professionals and parents on childhood sexuality

ReproLine
www.reproline.jhu.edu
Information and training for health professionals; maintained by JHPIEGO, an organization affiliated with Johns Hopkins University

Sexuality Information and Education Council of the United States (SIECUS)
www.SIECUS.org
Education and policy related to sexuality issues across the life span; English and Spanish

The Society for Adolescent Medicine
www.adolescenthealth.org

PREGNANCY
Planned Parenthood Federation of America
www.plannedparenthood.org

HOMOSEXUALITY
Family Pride Coalition
www.familypride.org
Resources and links to legal and medical support

Parents, Families and Friends of Lesbians and Gays, Inc. (PFLAG)
www.pflag.org
The national organization can provide referrals to local chapters

SEXUAL ASSESSMENT AND HISTORY TAKING
Davis CM et al: *Handbook of sexuality-related measures*, Thousand Oaks, CA, 1998, Sage Publications. Includes 197 standardized measurement tools or questionnaires that measure 50 sexuality-related states, traits, behaviors, and outcomes with discussion of their use, reliability, and validity in research, educational, and clinical settings

☑DISCUSSION FORUM

1. How will you as a health care provider resolve any conflicts between your personal views and professional practice in discussing sexuality or birth control?

2. A mother of 16-year-old refuses to leave the room during the well-child check. How are you going to handle a situation like this?

3. A father of 17-year-old wants to know whether his child is sexually active. What will you tell him? What if the child was 14 years old? What if the child was 11 years old? What is your state law regarding parental notification?

4. A mother confides that she thinks her 8-year-old is going to be homosexual since he likes playing with dolls. What topics do you need to explore? How would you educate a mother who believes that homosexuality is a disease and can be changed?

5. Discuss what questions you could use to illicit parents' attitudes and ability to teach their children about sexuality as part of their child's life cycle?

6. How would you counsel the parents of a developmentally disabled 18-year-old who is going into a sheltered work and living environment about pregnancy prevention?

REFERENCES

Ahmed SF, Morrison S, Hughes IA: Intersex and gender assignment; the third way? *Arch Dis Child* 89:847-850, 2004.

Ailey SH et al: Promoting sexuality across the life span for individuals with intellectual and developmental disabilities, *Nurs Clin N Am* 38:229-252, 2003.

Akinbami LJ, Gandhi H, Cheng TL: Availability of adolescent health services and confidentiality in primary care practices, *Pediatrics* 111:394-401, 2003.

Alexander EA: Adolescents and young adults. In Noble J, editor: *Textbook of primary care medicine,* ed 3, Philadelphia, 2001, Mosby.

American Academy of Family Physicians (AAFP): *Policy & advocacy, adolescent health care,* (2005). Available at *www.aafp.org/online/en/home/policy/policies/a/adolescent.html* (accessed July 26, 2006).

American Academy of Pediatrics (AAP), Committee on Psychosocial Aspects of Child and Family Health and Committee on Adolescence: Sexuality education for children and adolescents, *Pediatrics* 108:498-502, 2001.

American College of Obstetricians and Gynecologists (ACOG), Committee on Adolescent Healthcare: Resource guide, adolescent sexuality and sex education, 2005. Available at *www.acog.org/departments/dept_notice.cfm?recno=7&bulletin=3271* (accessed July 15, 2006).

American Medical Association (AMA): *Guidelines for adolescent preventive services (GAPS): recommendations monograph,* Chicago, 1997, American Medical Association.

American Nurses Association (ANA): *Position statement, HIV infection and U.S. teenagers,* 1991. Available at *http://nursingworld.org/readroom/position/blood/blteen.htm* (accessed Sept 10, 2007).

Association of Women's Health, Obstetrics and Neonatal Nurses: *Confidentiality in adolescent health care: policy position statement reaffirmed 2000.* Available at *www.awhonn.org.* health policy and legislation (accessed Nov 20, 2006).

As-Sanie S, Gantt A, Rosenthal M: Pregnancy prevention in adolescents, *Am Fam Physician* 70:1517-24, 2004.

Bell AP, Weinberg MS, Hammersmith SK: *Sexual preference,* Bloomington, IN, 1981, University Press.

Brown RT, Brown JD: Adolescent sexuality, *Prim Care* 33:373-390, 2006.

Burgis JT, Bacon JL: Communicating with the adolescent gynecology patient, *Obstet Gynecol Clin North Am* 30:251-260, 2003.

Clark LR: Tips for clinicians: approaching the adolescent patient from a psychodevelopmental framework, *J Pediatr Adolesc Gynecol* 16:327-330, 2003.

Dailard C: *Abstinence promotion and teen family planning: the misguided drive for equal funding,* Washington, DC, 2002, The Alan Guttmacher Institute. Report No. 5(1). Available at *www.guttmacher.org/pubs/tgr/05/1/gr050101.html* (accessed Aug 12, 2006).

Frankowski BL: Committee on adolescence of the American Academy of Pediatrics: Sexual orientation and adolescents, *Pediatrics* 113:1827-1832, 2004.

Garofalo R, Harper G: Not all adolescents are the same: addressing the unique needs of gay and bisexual male youth, *Adolesc Med* 14:595-611, 2003.

Garofalo R, Katz E: Health care issues of gay and lesbian youth, *Curr Opin Pediatr* 13:298-302, 2001.

Ginsburg KR et al: How to reach sexual minority youth in the health care setting: the teens offer guidance, *J Adolesc Health* 31:407-416, 2002.

Gooren L: The biology of human psychosexual differentiation, *Horm Behav* 50(4):559-501, 2006.

Kinsey AC, Pomeroy WB, Martin CE: *Sexual behavior in the human male,* Philadelphia, 1949, WB Saunders.

Kinsey AC, Pomeroy WB, Martin CE: *Sexual behavior in the human female,* Philadelphia, 1953, WB Saunders.

Kirby D: *Do abstinence-only programs delay the initiation of sex among young people and reduce teen pregnancy?* Washington, DC, 2002, National Campaign to Prevent Teen Pregnancy. Available at *www.teenpregnancy.org/resources/research/reports.asp* (accessed July 29, 2006).

Kirby D: *Emerging answers: research findings on programs to reduce teen pregnancy (summary),* Washington, DC, 2001, National Campaign to Prevent Teen Pregnancy. Available at *www.teenpregnancy.org/resources/data/report_summaries/emerging_answers/default.asp* (accessed Aug 12, 2006).

Klein JD et al: Improving adolescent preventive care in community health centers, *Pediatrics* 107:318-327, 2001.

Klein JD: Adolescent pregnancy: current trends and issues, *Pediatrics* 116:281-286, 2005.

Larsson I, Svedin CG: Teacher's and parent's reports on 3- to 6-year-old children's sexual behavior–a comparison, *Child Abuse Negl* 26:243-245, 2002.

McCabe MP: Sexual knowledge, experience and feelings among people with disability, *Sex Disabil* 17:157-170, 1999.

Meininger E et al: Gay, lesbian, and bisexual adolescents. In Neinstein L, editor: *Adolescent health care: a practical guide,* Philadelphia, 2002, Lippincott Williams & Wilkins.

Murphy NA, Elias ER: Sexuality of children and adolescents with developmental disabilities, *Pediatrics* 118:398-403, 2006. Available at *http://aappolicy.aappublications.org/cgi/content/full/pediatrics;118/1/398* (accessed Aug 10, 2006).

National Association of Pediatric Nurse Practitioners (NAPNAP) Executive Board: Position statement on health risks and needs of gay, lesbian, bisexual, and transgender (GLT) adolescents, *J Pediatr Health Care* 20:29A-30A, 2006.

National Campaign to Prevent Teen Pregnancy: *Putting what works to work, science says research brief: characteristics of effective curriculum-based programs,* Washington, DC, 2003. Available at *www.teenpregnancy.org/works/default.asp#briefs* (accessed Aug 12, 2006).

National Campaign to Prevent Teen Pregnancy: *What works: curriculum-based programs that prevent teen pregnancy,* Washington, DC, 2006. Available at *www.teenpregnancy.org/works/default.asp* (accessed Aug 8, 2006).

Rakel RE: *Textbook of family practice,* ed 6, Philadelphia, 2002, WB Saunders.

Reddy DM, Fleming R, Swain C: Effect of mandatory parental notification on adolescent girls' use of sexual health services, *JAMA* 288:710-714, 2002.

Remafedi G et al: Demography of sexual orientation, *Pediatrics* 89:714-721, 1992.

Ryan C, Futterman D: Homosexuality. In Coupey S, editor: *Primary care of adolescent girls,* Philadelphia, 2000, Hanley & Belfus, Inc.

Santelli J et al: Abstinence-only education policies and programs: a position paper of the Society for Adolescent Medicine, *J Adolesc Health* 38:83-87, 2006.

Schultz DP, Schultz SE: *A history of modern psychology,* Orlando, FL, 1987, Harcourt-Brace.

Sexuality Information and Education Council of the United States (SIECUS): *Position statements 1990,* SIECUS Report, 18(2):1-310, Available at *www.SIECUS.org.Positionstatements1990* (accessed Nov 8).

Sexuality Information and Education Council of the United States (SIECUS) National Guidelines Task Force: *Guidelines for comprehensive sexuality education: kindergarten-12th grade,* ed 3, New York, 2004, Sexuality Information and Education Council of the United States. Available at *www.siecus.org/pubs/pubs0004.html* (accessed July 29, 2006).

Society for Adolescent Medicine (SAM): Protecting adolescents: ensuring access to care and reporting sexual activity and abuse, *J Adol Hlth* 35: 420-423, 2004.

Society of Pediatric Nurses Position Statement: *The role of the pediatric nurse working with sexually active teens, pregnant adolescents, and young parents,* prepared by Herrman JW, 2004. Available at *www.pedsnurses.org/all.php?l=positions* (accessed Aug 12, 2006).

Thrall JS et al: Confidentiality and adolescents' use of providers for health information and for pelvic examinations, *Arch Pediatr Adolesc Med* 154:885-892, 2000.

Thornton AC, Collins JD: Teaching parents to talk to their children about sexual topics, *Clin Fam Pract* 6:801-819, 2004.

Troiden RR: Homosexual identity development, *J Adolesc Health Care* 9:105-113, 1988.

World Health Organization: *Education and treatment in human sexuality: the training of health professionals,* Technical Report Series, no 372, Geneva, 1975, World Health Organization.

Zavodny M: Fertility and parental consent for minors to receive contraceptives, *Am J Public Health* 94(8):1347-1351, 2004.

Coping and Stress Tolerance: Mental Health Problems

Mary Margaret Gottesman and Gail M. Houck

The twentieth century saw tremendous progress in preventing and treating infectious diseases and unintended injury, both of which are major causes of childhood disability and death. Remarkable progress occurred also in the management of childhood chronic illnesses allowing children to live into adulthood who would not have done so at an earlier time. Puberty begins earlier now than ever before in history, without a concomitant earlier maturing of cognition and emotional control. These physically mature younger children are less able to handle the effects of changes in body and changes in feelings and behavior. As Dahl (2004) notes, the effect is one of an inexperienced driver sitting inside a Formula One racing car.

Not only has physical health changed, but, just as importantly, psychosocial stressors for children have changed. Mental health issues have emerged as a major focus in pediatric primary care in the U.S. In a study of children on the west coast and in Ohio, Ryan-Wenger and colleagues (2005) identified children's top stressors as distress over family discord, feeling overwhelmed with sports and schoolwork, and difficulty coping with boy-girl relationships. A national survey of youth by Melnyk and colleagues (2003) found that the top worries and stresses for school-age and adolescent children in descending order of frequency were uncertainty over how to cope with stress, anxiety, depression, self-esteem problems, and difficulties in their relationships with parents. Concerns of parents were similar but in a slightly different order of frequency: uncertainty over how to cope with stress, anxiety, self-esteem problems, depression, and difficulties in their relationships with their children. Parents (90%) were more likely to report talking to their child about the child's problems at least some of the time compared with the number of children (60%) who report talking with their parents. Not only were parents and children not talking often with one another, but the vast majority of children (78%) and adults (66%) never discussed communication issues with their child's pediatric primary care professional. Dramatic changes in the U.S. have occurred in family structure with increases in the number of divorces and single-parent families, in addition to increases in childhood poverty rates and the number of international adoptions (Bledsoe & Johnson, 2004; Bosch et al, 2003; Hass & Cauther, 2006). According to Hass and Cauther (2006), nearly 13 million children (18%) in the U.S. live in families with incomes at or below the federal poverty level, up 12% in the past 5 years. The largest increase occurred among children living in the Midwest (Koball & Douglas-Hall, 2006).

In the U.S., there are complex interrelationships among poverty, race and ethnicity, foster care, homelessness, and mental health disorders. White children are least likely to be poor (10%), with African-American children (35%), Latino children (28%), and American-Indian children (29%) disproportionately affected by poverty. The rate of mental health problems among poor children is double that of the general child population in the U.S. (Masi & Cooper, 2006). At the same time, white children (31%) are more likely to receive mental health services than ethnic minority children (13%) (Masi & Cooper, 2006).

Among poor children in the U.S., 500,000 are homeless on any given day (Karr & Klein, 2004). Children under 5 years old make up the largest number of homeless children (41%) with the majority of homeless families headed by single mothers (85%). Developmental (54%) and mental health problems (46% to 57%) affect many homeless children at all ages. Child abuse investigations involve 24% to 35% of homeless children (Karr & Klein, 2004).

Abuse and neglect are also more common among low income families regardless of ethnicity; however, African-American children are more likely to be removed from their homes to foster care than are white or Hispanic children (Pecora et al, 2003). African-American youth also are represented disproportionately in the juvenile justice system (Showyra & Cocozza, 2006). Estimates are that 50% of children and youth in the child welfare system have mental health problems; 67% to 70% of youth in the juvenile justice system have mental health disorders (Masi & Cooper, 2006).

Happiness and a secure sense of being loved are critical elements for child mental health. Yet by the time children are 4 years old, 1 in 5 will have a mental health disorder and 1 in 10 will have a serious emotional disturbance. The Substance Abuse and Mental Health Services Administration (SAMHSA) defines mental health problems for children and adolescents as "the range of all diagnosable emotional, behavioral, and mental disorders." These definitions and numbers do not include the mental health problems now recognized as occurring among the very young—infants, toddlers, and early preschool-age children (Furman & O'Riordan, 2005).

There are many reasons for mental health problems in children, ranging from environmental toxins, such as lead and mercury that alter behavior and cognition, to exposure to violence in homes and neighborhoods leading to posttraumatic stress disorder (PTSD). Anxiety and depression stem from inherited predispositions and the stresses and strains of modern family life. Stress related to poverty and discrimination impairs both parenting ability and child self-esteem. The loss of significant people in children's lives through death, divorce, and entry into foster care are particularly stressful experiences for children.

The 2006 America's children report of leading health indicators for children 4 to 17 years old (Forum on Child and Family Statistics, 2006) showed that 5% of responding parents identified their children as having a definite or severe emotional or behavioral problem. Significant problems were identified for 5.8% of males and 4.8% of females and were more likely to occur for children living in families with incomes at 100% of the federal poverty level (7.1%) than those with incomes at or above 200% of the federal poverty level (5.3%). Children without parents (9.4%) or those living with their mother only (7.8%) were more likely to be identified as having significant problems compared with children living in two-parent families (4%). Hispanic children were least likely to have a definite or severe emotional or behavioral problem (3.3%) compared with 6% of white children and 6% of black children.

The current number of child psychiatric professionals (about 6700 in the U.S.) is far below the estimated number needed (30,000) to deal with an increasing prevalence in childhood mental health problems or at least better recognition of them (Melnyk et al, 2003). In addition, health insurance coverage for mental health services has declined, and more restrictions on access to mental health care have occurred in an attempt to control costs. Consequently, primary care professionals now manage approximately 75% of children with mental health disorders, and only 2% of children receive care from child mental health professionals (Melnyk et al, 2003).

■ THE FOUNDATIONS OF MENTAL HEALTH

NEUROBIOLOGIC CONTEXT

The foundation for mental health begins at conception with the genetic endowment of the child and the influence of the maternal intrauterine environment on the developing fetus (Field et al, 2006). Maternal nutrition and stress hormone levels are among the most well-documented influences on the structure and function of the evolving central nervous system (Reiger et al, 2004). This collaborative influence of genetic endowment and environmental experiences on central nervous system development and function continue throughout infancy, childhood, and adolescence (Goodman et al, 2004). Risks and protective factors for psychopathologic conditions emerge from the interaction of genetic endowment and environmental experiences within the context of developmental changes and challenges (Als et al, 2003; 2005). As noted by Spessot and colleagues (2004), the number and particular combination of risk and protective factors for any individual are likely to determine the behavior patterns, comorbidities, severity, and course of psychopathologic conditions across the childhood, adolescent, and adult years.

Advances in neuroimaging, such as functional magnetic resonance imaging (fMRI) and positron emission tomography (PET) scans, have allowed researchers to identify and describe patterns of developmental change in brain structure and function in normal children and adolescents (Eluvathingal et al, 2006). These imaging techniques have begun, as well, to document altered patterns of structure and function in children and adolescents diagnosed with psychopathologic conditions. From infancy through early adulthood, changes in the limbic system, specifically the amygdala and hippocampus, are strongly implicated in emotional development and in the emergence of affective disorders, substance abuse, and high-risk behaviors (De Kloet & Derjik, 2004). As researchers are quick to point out, however, none of these brain differences appear to be necessary or sufficient for psychopathologic conditions to occur (Dahl, 2004). Rather, environmental strengths and vulnerabilities and accumulated life experiences influence the number and severity of symptoms and the adaptive competencies the child displays at any age (Dahl, 2004; Gunnar & Cheatham, 2003).

Research has demonstrated the profound effects of stress and environmental deprivation on the young child's brain architecture (Carmody et al, 2006; Gunnar & Cheatham, 2003). Activation of the hypothalamic-pituitary-adrenal (HPA) axis triggers release of cortisol, feeding the fight-or-flight response (Gunnar & Cheatham, 2003). Elevated serum cortisol levels act as a toxin on neurons in the central nervous system, inhibiting the growth of dendrites and neuronal growth and causing the death of neurons. Research has also demonstrated the profound effects of the use-it-or-lose-it phenomenon on the number of neurons and dendritic growth and interconnections. In the final phase of brain growth, differentiation, the brain prunes away unused neurons and dendritic connections (McEwen, 2004). Imaging of the brains of children exposed to the chronic stress of emotionally and materially deprived environments show markedly reduced brain volumes compared with the brain size of age- and sex-matched children from nondeprived environments. In short, all forms of material and interactive experiences actively shape children's brain architecture.

In addition, chronic triggering of the HPA stress response hones the speed and intensity of a response. In children, chronic stress leads to swift, strong expressions of distress to even minor stressful stimuli. For example, preterm infants respond with a strong cry to even minor chilling or discomfort. Infant and child crying have profoundly negative effects on normal adults, triggering the adult's own stress response. Thus excessive and prolonged crying is a significant risk factor for child abuse and the development of problems in the parent-child relationship (Freund et al, 2005). Normal developmental changes add an important layer of influence and complexity to the interaction between the genetically driven biology of the child and his or her interaction with the environment.

THE SOCIAL DEVELOPMENTAL CONTEXT

Those who value the challenges of pediatrics know that normal development cannot be taken for granted. Normal development depends upon the presence of effective regulation either by oneself or by others. It is marked by periods of significant qualitative change from infancy to adolescence. Consistent monitoring of the direction of developmental change and progress is critical. Departures from normal achievements at early points in development often have negative consequences for later developmental achievements, making it more difficult to overcome deviations in later development (Lloyd & Rosman, 2005).

The Newborn Period

The newborn period is a highly vulnerable time in development. The newborn infant faces tremendous changes in physiological function and is completely dependent on others for nutrition and physiological and emotional regulation. The first social developmental task is to effectively guide caregivers to meet the newborn's needs; newborns do this by providing clear behavioral, vocal, and emotional cues (Zero to Three, 2005). From the start, newborns use all of their fully functioning senses for learning and their temperaments for responding to handling and stimulation (Als et al, 2005).

The goal for parents is to successfully read their babies' cues and provide the nutrition, warmth, and calming measures that facilitate growth and adaptation. Difficulties in feeding and high levels of irritability are among the most frustrating challenges parents encounter (Zero to Three, 2005). Negative perceptions of the baby, disappointment in the baby, disinterest in and unresponsiveness to the baby are red flags for problems in the parent-newborn relationship (Jellinek et al, 2002).

Early Infancy

In the normally developing infant, a major developmental step occurs at 2 to 3 months old with the appearance of social smiling. Longer periods of alertness and an enhanced ability to make eye contact with others and follow their movements multiply opportunities for interacting with others and learning about the world. Intact young infants skillfully convey distress, happiness, interest, and distaste (Gross, 2007). Although young infants recognize and prefer their primary caregivers, they easily accept care from others. Temperament patterns are also now clearly displayed. Attentive parents are able to describe their baby's preferences and dislikes, sensitivities, and signals (Jellinek et al, 2002). Many babies are now able to comfort themselves for brief periods. Babies who receive prompt responses to their needs typically provide less intense distress signals and develop the ability to wait for care (Melendez, 2005). Parents face the challenge of becoming effective, adaptive teachers for their changing baby.

Ongoing excessive irritability and lack of infant social smiling are red flags for disorders in the parent-infant relationship (Jellinek et al, 2002). Limited responsiveness to infant bids for interaction, parent depression, inability to describe the infant's strengths, perception of the baby as difficult, and frustration with the baby are also cause for concern about the quality of the parent-infant relationship (Rosenblum, 2005).

Middle Infancy

At 5 to 8 months old, tremendous changes have occurred in the infant's ability to control the head, back, arms, and hands, allowing ever greater levels of exploration and learning. When caregivers have been consistent, the infant now shows the onset of focused attachment to primary caregivers (Rosenblum, 2005). Separation and stranger anxieties make their appearance as well. The older infant is an active play partner with the caregiver, able to recall how to play simple games, such as peek-a-boo, anticipating the joy of these interactions, and remembering familiar people and objects not within view. New emotions appear—anger, fear, and sadness (Gross, 2007). Crying may increase as infants struggle to convey their desires. Parents are challenged to provide a safe learning environment and to cope with the broader range of negative emotions displayed by their infants (Jellinek et al, 2002).

Social developmental concerns occur when the infant makes limited or no vocalizations or shows no caregiver preference. Negative attributions about infant behavior, frustration with infant self-feeding, lack of mutual enjoyment in interaction, and parent discomfort with the broader range of infant emotions signal a poor quality parent-infant relationship (Rosenblum, 2005).

Late Infancy

Around 10 to 13 months old, many older infants begin to walk, greatly expanding their abilities for exploration. This also leads to new experiences with protective limit setting by parents that often lead to meltdowns of distress for the thwarted explorer (Jellinek et al, 2002). Interestingly, Emde and colleagues (2005) have noted that early milestone achievers tend to experience more distress with restraints and limitations than do on-time or late milestone achievers. Parents who enjoyed the dependency of earlier infancy may feel frustrated with their active, independent child and need guidance in balancing the provision of safety with the provision of new opportunities for learning. They also may need assistance with handling the broader range of potent cues of distress exhibited by their child.

Infant behaviors of concern include marked clinginess to the parent, the persistence of irregular sleep and feeding patterns, and failure to use the parent as a safe base from which to explore. Parent behaviors of concern include laxity about setting limits, failure to allow the child to separate, frustration with emerging negativity behaviors, and a poor fit between the infant's developmental needs and the parent's ability to meet them (Rosenblum, 2005).

Transition from Infancy to Early Childhood

Eighteen to 22 months old brings the major transition from infancy to early childhood. Multiword speech appears as does self-awareness and recognition by the child that he or she is truly separate from the major caregiver. New emotions appear—pride, possessiveness (Mine!), affection, generosity, and anxiety (Gross, 2007). Adherence to routines and meeting the child's established expectations help the toddler to regulate the tendency to negativity. Violations of routines and expectations often lead to distress. Empathy and the ability to comfort the distress of others appear if the child has received sensitive empathetic care (Emde et al, 2005). Toddlers are challenged by their parents' new expectations for compliance with rules and emotional self-regulation. Parents are challenged to begin the initiation of their child to their culture's manners and mores and to cope calmly with the toddler's negativity and limited ability to express feelings in words rather than behavioral meltdown (McDonough, 2005).

Limited or absent speech, failure to engage in eye contact with parents, self-abusive behaviors, failure to explore, and frequent tantrums indicate the need for a more detailed social developmental and mental health evaluation. Parental behaviors of concern include difficulty with limit setting, frustration and negativity with toddler behavior, limited or absent verbal communication with the child, hurtful teasing, and multiple bruises and injuries suggesting inadequate supervision, abuse, or neglect of the child (Jellinek et al, 2002; Rosenblum, 2005).

Transition to the Preschool Years

Verbal fluency expands at 3 to 4 years old allowing children to share their experiences and feelings with others. Imagination flowers, reflected in fantasy play, as well as the emergence of fears (e.g., the fear of monsters). As children move into the larger world of the neighborhood and preschool, they are challenged to develop the social skills necessary to deal with separation from the parent and a wide range of situations and people. They begin to learn more about their abilities in comparison with those of other children and their performance in comparison with the expectations of other adults. The new emotions of shame, envy, and embarrassment appear, as may behavior problems (Gross, 2007).

Concerns about the child include poorly understood speech, lack of fantasy play, deliberately hurting other children or animals, and behavior with others that is withdrawn, aggressive, anxious, or defiant (Jellinek et al, 2002). Parent behaviors of concern continue to include failure to set appropriate limits on behavior or excessively restrictive limits, disparagement and criticism of the child, use of corporal punishment, overt or covert encouragement of aggression, and evidence of abuse or neglect of the child (McDonough, 2005).

Transition to the School-Age Years

Significant neural maturation occurs in the brain at 5 to 7 years old. Significant strides occur in cognitive, perceptual, and social capacities rendering children ready to meet the challenges for starting their formal education in kindergarten. Normal children at this age have significant ability to control their emotions, behavior, and attention. The child's social roles and behavior expectations change dramatically at home, at school, and among peers. The child's self-concept and self-esteem face daily challenges in comparisons with peers' performance in academics, sports, and social interactions. Parents are challenged to support their child's self-esteem and exploration of a wide range of interests and to protect the child from early engagement in competition for which they are not emotionally ready (Jellinek et al, 2002).

Concerns for the child include inability to pay attention and participate appropriately in class, problems getting along with other children either because of shyness or aggression, failing academically, difficulty separating from parents (defiant or hostile behavior toward the parent or siblings), frequent visits to the health office, refusal to participate in previously enjoyed activities, and frequent complaints of stomach pain and headaches (Jellinek et al, 2002). Failure of the parent and child to establish eye contact with each other, failure of the parent to limit child behavior appropriately and provide appropriate responsibilities, and anger and negativity toward the child all signal difficulties in the parent-child relationship.

Transition to Adolescence

The onset of puberty brings dramatic changes to the body and mind (Dahl, 2004). Large pulses in sex hormones change feelings and interests as well as the body. Major brain growth, reorganization, and interconnectedness occur within multiple regions of the brain that will extend into young adulthood (Giedd, 2004). Adolescents' cravings for strong emotional experiences are reflected in their enjoyment of loud music, horror movies, and extreme amusement park rides. Although their cognitive skills are nearly at adult levels, their ability to make good decisions under the influence of strong emotions is poor (Dahl, 2004). Girls especially become vulnerable to affective disorders. Social roles and behavior expectations change dramatically with sexual maturation. On the positive side, altruism and idealism emerge, leading many adolescents to significant achievements. Parents are challenged to provide accurate and timely information, sensitive support, and appropriate limits to their adolescent.

Concerns for the adolescent include engaging in high-risk behaviors, such as sex, alcohol and drug use, driving while intoxicated, and using tobacco products, in addition to aggressive or hostile behavior, depressed mood, and school absenteeism or academic failure (Jellinek et al, 2002). Failure to set appropriate limits and expectations, lack of pride in the adolescent's achievements, negative affect towards the adolescent, frustration or anger with the normal level of adolescent mood lability, and failure to support the adolescent's positive engagement in the community and school signal problems in the parent-adolescent relationship (Gutgesell, 2004).

ROLE OF TEMPERAMENT IN COPING

Temperament serves as a foundation for coping. Temperament involves an individual's characteristic style of emotional and behavioral response across situations and has generally come to be accepted as inborn. Although biologic in origin, temperament characteristics evolve and develop over time and are influenced by and patterned in significant ways by the social environment. This view of temperament is clinically important because both short- and long-term psychosocial adjustments are shaped by the goodness-of-fit between the individual's temperament and the social environment. Goodness-of-fit refers to the congruence of a child's temperament with the expectations, demands, and opportunities of the social environment, including those of parents, family, and day care or school setting.

Infants' first coping efforts are determined by temperament and linked to reactivity and self-regulation. Physiologic reactivity includes individual differences in the threshold, dampening, and reactivation of autonomic arousal, and it varies across different emotions (Compas et al, 2001). Individual differences in temperament and reactivity affect the individual's initial automatic response to stress and thereby constrain or facilitate certain types of coping responses. Infants are also capable of regulating aspects of their autonomic arousal, behavior, and emotions, initially through involuntary, biologically based processes that are augmented by responses acquired through learning and experience in accordance with contextual cues. Coping continues to be influenced by the emergence of cognitive and behavioral capacities for regulation of the self in response to stress. Nonetheless, temperament is foundational and relatively stable from infancy through toddlerhood. Overall, there appears to be consensus for three factors inherent in temperament: sociability (reactivity), activity, and emotionality (mood) (Jellinek et al, 2002).

Temperament Types

Three types of temperament have clinical utility and can be generalized cross-culturally: difficult, easy, and slow-to-warm-up. Children with difficult temperaments tend to be characterized by an intense and negative mood, slow adaptability, withdrawal from new situations, and irregularity in biologic functions. Children with easy temperaments typically exhibit a prevailing positive mood, low intensity, ready adaptability, and regularity and predictability of biologic and behavioral patterns. In other words, these children are easygoing. Children with slow-to-warm-up temperaments are characterized by initial quiet alertness and subdued emotionality. This reserve in the face of new situations and stimuli gives way to features of an easy or difficult temperament. There is no absolute standard for any of these classifications, and all features of temperament must be considered in the context of the parents' evaluations.

Temperament as a Risk Factor

Temperament predicts behavioral disturbance in preschool, elementary school (Mesman & Koot, 2002), and adolescence and young adulthood. Difficult temperaments seem to be most consistently related to behavior disorders, although temperament alone is not a risk factor for maladjustment. Rather, temperament exerts an influence on children's psychosocial adjustment by way of its effect on caretaker-child interactions. Difficult temperamental features tend to engender parental criticism and irritability, in addition to coercive interactions and restrictive parenting. Critical mediators of the role of temperament in the development of behavioral disorders include parental psychological functioning, marital adjustment, child-rearing attitudes and practices, and social support factors. Although temperament is unrelated to intelligence quotient (IQ), it affects academic outcomes, and some children are clearly disadvantaged by their more difficult temperaments in the majority of school environments.

Temperament Management

The goal for the primary care provider is to help parents achieve goodness-of-fit for their children. Specific strategies for intervening with temperament issues have been developed for parents. Strategies for helping parents respond effectively to their child's temperament at each developmental phase are outlined in *Bright Futures in Practice: Mental Health Practice Guide* (Jellinek et al, 2002) and can be readily integrated into well child care. Those who care for children (e.g., parents, teachers, other caregivers) should be helped to:

- Recognize the child's innate behavioral qualities as expressions of temperament. Perceptions about the child can be obtained through an interview about typical situations (e.g., changes in activities, new situations, changes in routines, new people) or by completing a standard temperament questionnaire.
- Understand how temperament is related to behavior and is not amenable to change. This means allowing parents, for example, to express their feelings about their child or their child's behavior and assisting them to reframe their assessment more positively. Members of the extended family who often advise parents may need to be included to help alleviate feelings of failure.
- Develop temperament-based management strategies, especially ways to deal with the more challenging areas of temperament. Such strategies can be applied to new situations as the child develops and becomes more autonomous, including those that occur in toddlerhood and preschool, such as mealtime and bedtime, or during school-related activities, such as doing homework.

■ ASSESSMENT OF MENTAL HEALTH DISORDERS

Because mental health problems cover a broad range of behavioral, emotional, and psychological disorders and have genetic bases, assessment necessarily encompasses a broad array of data about both the child and the family (Guerro et al, 2003). In addition, a thorough physical exam assists the primary care provider to identify any physical illnesses underlying changes in behavior and emotional well-being. This is critical at every age because children at many ages, not just preverbal children, often lack awareness that physical symptoms are out of the ordinary and signal illness. Their behavior and affect change to reflect their lack of wellness, but without a fever or other observable symptoms, parents may assume these changes signal a mental health problem.

During all health visits, the primary care provider should be attentive to the quality of the verbal and nonverbal exchanges of infants, children, and adolescents with their parents and with the health care provider (Strine et al, 2006; Sullivan & Lewis, 2003), specifically looking at the emotions and energy the child displays and the presence or absence of interaction among those present in the exam room.

How the provider conducts the history and physical is as important as the content of the evaluation itself. Many parents share their concerns only after a long period of trying to solve the problem themselves. They are frequently upset, worried, and frustrated. Providers are more likely to get a clear picture of what is happening and gain the family's trust if they take the time to sit down and actively listen at length to the parent's concerns and perceptions. When children are old enough, their concerns and perceptions should be solicited (Green et al, 2002). It is critical to avoid rapidly firing questions, restrict the history to a preprinted schedule of questions, or take notes that detract from giving full attention to the child and family. If possible, an hour should be blocked out for the history and physical. If a potentially significant, but nonemergent, problem is uncovered in the course of an episodic visit, a lengthier appointment should be scheduled to avoid hurrying the assessment and potentially missing important data.

Mental health, behavioral, social, and emotional expressions always occur in a relational context (Hacker et al, 2006). It is essential to obtain information from the child's perspective. How the primary care provider does this differs depending upon the age of the child.

Infants. Observations of babies and toddlers with their parents in structured and unstructured situations offer valuable clues to the strengths and limitations of each partner in the interaction (Squires & Nickel, 2003). The Nursing Child Assessment Satellite Training (NCAST) Parent-Child Interaction Feeding and Teaching Scales allow the observer to identify specific areas of parental skill and weakness in interacting with their babies, in addition to ways infants respond to the parents and convey their needs (Sumner & Spietz, 1994a, 1994b). This provides guidance in developing a plan of care for any identified problems and also is a way to follow progress in the relationship over time. Even unstructured observations allow the observer to appreciate the emotional exchanges and the presence or absence of sensitive and contingent interactions between the infant and parent. Use and interpretation of the NCAST scales require training, but the scales are at the level of an assessment rather than a simple screening.

Toddlers and young preschoolers. Playing with figures, dolls, and toys gives older toddlers and young preschoolers a way to express their feelings and emotions. Having a variety of dolls and toys on hand and allowing the child to play spontaneously provides the opportunity for the professional to ask questions within the nonthreatening context of play. This will also help to direct probing with parents. If the parent has already identified situations or people who provoke troubled behavior, the provider may select toys that are likely to elicit the child's story in play. For example, if the concerning behaviors began shortly after the birth of a new sibling, a baby doll, mother and father dolls, and a doll the age and sex of the child could be selected.

School-age children. Effective strategies to use with older preschoolers and young school-age children include offering them the opportunity to draw a picture of themselves and their family. When it is complete, the child is asked to tell a story about their picture. This allows the professional the opportunity to evaluate the child's feelings and emotions and, if problems and concerns become apparent, clarify details from the child's perspective in a nonthreatening and familiar way.

Adolescents. The primary care provider should have a separate interview with the school-age child and adolescent. Allow 20 to 30 minutes for the school-age child and 30 minutes or more for the adolescent to share their perspectives and feelings. Most children are comfortable talking about their feelings and experiences if they have a supportive listener. Tailor questions to the child's or adolescent's level of understanding, keeping questions simple and providing examples to younger children. Sample questions might include:

- "Tell me about some of the things you do very well. What type of things do you have a hard time doing?"
- "You look very sad to me. Would you share with me what is making you sad?"
- "Many children have things they worry about. What worries you most?"
- "How are things going in your family?"
- "Everyone feels angry at times. What makes you angry? What do you do when you are angry?"
- "If you could change one thing in your life, what would it be?"
- "Tell me what you think the problem is from your point of view."

HISTORY

The accurate identification of emotional, social, behavioral, and mental health status requires a thorough history, with the physical exam serving to confirm findings from the history. Correctly pinpointing problems requires a more wide-ranging history than does the diagnosis of many physical health problems (Green et al, 2002). Common stressors that should be identified through the history are discussed in this section. Questions and specific examples of stressors are found in Table 20-1.

Common Stressors

Recent Changes. When inquiring about recent changes in the home, it is frequently helpful to review specific changes since parents may not perceive some changes as potential sources of stress for their child. For example, parents may welcome a promotion that includes the need for travel and a significant pay increase. However, this same change may stress the child, who is old enough to worry about how life will change with a traveling parent. It is important to consider the developmental context of events and whether or not most children of a similar age would find the incident threatening or upsetting.

Contextual Changes Within the Family. Contextual changes are more enduring changes in life circumstances, either for better or worse, that provoke changes in the child's perception of self, family, or feelings of relationship security. These changes may also stem from the child's behavior and may result in self-blame or stem from the actions of other family members, especially parents, creating a sense of betrayal.

Parenting and Temperament. It is important to explore the experiences that reflect the quality of everyday parenting in which the child grows and develops. Parents face a tremendous challenge to adapt their parenting skills to

TABLE 20-1   **History Taking: Areas for Assessment of Mental Health**

Topic	Sample Question	Potential Stressors
Recent changes	"What events or changes have occurred in your family in the past year?"	• Moves of any type, even within the same neighborhood or city • Recent severe illness or hospitalization of the child or close family members • Changes in parents' work (e.g., promotions, job loss, change in working hr, addition of or increase in travel requirements) • Changes in school (e.g., new teachers, new class, new school, transition to a different level of schooling, such as to middle school or high school, academic difficulties, bullying) • Recent major traumatic incidents (e.g., involvement of child or other close family members in a motor vehicle accident, witnessing violence) • Recent exposure to a natural disaster • Changes in routines (e.g., a new after-school caregiver)
Contextual changes within the family	"Let me make sure I understand who all of the family members are in your home and also any changes among family members or family relationships."	• Changes in household composition (e.g., births, expansion of household to include elders) • Risk of loss or loss of attachment figure(s) • Changes in family relationships (e.g., death, separation, divorce, older sibling moving away) • Separation from the usual caregiver for foster care or care by others to assist the parent • Return to the biologic family from kinship care or foster care • Family violence • Witness to trauma or violence • New role or responsibilities presenting a psychological challenge (e.g., birth of a new sibling) • Social isolation of the family • Sibling with special health care needs • Mental health problems of parents, especially maternal depression • Child's chronic illness or handicap
Recurring experiences	"Tell me about the things you find difficult or stressful as a parent, especially in caring for this child."	• Parental overprotection • Restrictive parenting • Control struggles • Ineffective conflict resolution • Lack of effective parental supervision • Parental failure to protect child in risky situations • Ineffective limit-setting strategies • Use of harsh discipline practices • Reliance on the child by the parents for emotional comfort and support
Behavioral manifestations	"Tell me about your child's behavior problems. When did you first notice the problem? How have you tried to help your child? How does the behavior make you feel? How do think your child feels?"	• Parental description of undesirable and desired behaviors • Parental perceptions about the nature of the child's problems, including cause and severity as measured by frequency and duration • Situational context that elicits or maintains problem behavior (setting, timing, who is present, triggers) • Situational contexts in which the problem behavior does not occur • Parent, peer, and teacher responses to and consequences of problem behavior • Parent's feelings engendered by the behavior • Parent's thoughts about how the child feels • Parents thoughts about what the parent needs and what the child needs to improve the situation
Parent's personal history of being parented	"Tell me about your most favorite and least favorite memories of growing up. How is your parenting similar to and different from the parenting you received	• Parent abused or neglected as a child • Parent adopted or in foster care as a child • Unhappy parent childhood, poor role models • Poor family communication patterns in family of origin • Any indicators of parental psychopathologic condition, particularly maternal depression

Continued

TABLE 20-1	History Taking: Areas for Assessment of Mental Healh—Cont'd	
Topic	**Sample Question**	**Potential Stressors**
	as a child? What are your expectations for your child?"	• The parents' perception of the child, especially temperament, poor fit with parent • The parents' knowledge and beliefs about harsh discipline or coercive parent-child interactions • The parents' knowledge and beliefs about the development of autonomy and self-esteem, especially in relation to parenting strategies (e.g., praise and affection) and conflict resolution • Parental strategies to facilitate the child's coping, given developmental level and temperament • Unrealistic academic, athletic, or social expectations of the child

the individual behavioral style of each child in their family. Also important is the goodness-of-fit between the parent and child's temperament (e.g., a high activity level child may be difficult to handle for a parent who has a naturally quiet temperament). Further, some parenting behaviors are clearly not functional for most children (e.g., lack of appropriate and consistent limit setting).

Behavioral Manifestations

Parents are keen observers of their children, so it is wise to listen carefully to their observations and concerns. Behaviors that concern a parent may include those that are developmentally normal for the child, or they may represent extremes of the range of normal behavior, both too little or too strong. By obtaining a clear idea of the parent's concerns, the provider is able to assess the parent's level of knowledge about child development and behavior, clarify which behaviors are developmentally normal (but distressing to the parent), and confirm which behaviors fall outside the range of normal.

Parent's Personal History of Being Parented

A significant body of research confirms the impact of the parent's personal history of being parented on the quality of parenting provided to children (Schore, 2005). These "ghosts in the nursery" are powerful influences on the perceptions of child behavior, beliefs about children and child rearing, and ultimately the parenting behaviors employed in the home (Lieberman et al, 2005). It is important to have the parent share memories, good and bad, of their childhood, what they liked and disliked about the parenting they experienced. See Table 20-1.

Family Health History

A thorough history of mental and developmental disorders in family members should be conducted, including: school failure, delinquency, substance abuse, learning disorders, reading problems, bipolar disorder, attention-deficit/hyperactivity disorder (ADHD), autism, genetic syndromes, and birth defects.

Prenatal History

Planned and wanted pregnancy; illnesses and discomforts during the pregnancy; problems with the pregnancy; when

prenatal care began; maternal alcohol, drug, and tobacco use; results of prenatal testing; maternal weight gain during pregnancy; response of significant others to the pregnancy; maternal depression during pregnancy.

Birth History

Spontaneous or induced labor, length of labor, complications or medical conditions arising during labor, type of delivery, complications.

Postnatal History

Gestational age, birth weight and length, problems after delivery, problems in the first 2 weeks of life, maternal postpartum depression.

Past Medical History

Childhood illnesses and traumatic injuries, especially neurologic injuries, soft neurologic signs of developmental significance (e.g., delayed speech).

Developmental Progress

Achievement of milestones, level of social skills, relationships with peers.

PHYSICAL EXAMINATION

The practitioner should complete a thorough physical examination with particular attention to recognition of physical anomalies and evaluation of the neurologic system. A structured developmental screening or assessment, depending on one's level of preparation, should be included in the assessment. If warranted by suspicious or ambiguous findings, a referral for a thorough developmental evaluation by a skilled psychologist or multidisciplinary developmental assessment team is appropriate.

DIAGNOSTIC STUDIES

Laboratory

Pertinent laboratory tests (hemoglobin, blood lead level, or urinalysis) can rule out physical health problems with behavioral manifestations. The family history and findings on the physical exam may warrant chromosomal studies as well.

Imaging

Imaging of the central nervous system may be recommended depending on family history, developmental, and neurologic findings.

STRUCTURED PARENTAL REPORTS

Behavioral rating scales or checklists are valuable screening tools, especially those with established reliability and validity that provide norms as a basis for comparison. Screening instruments with sound reliability and validity include The Ages & Stages Questionnaire for developmental screening; the Ages & Stages Socio-Emotional Screen for social and emotional concerns; the 10-minute Brief Infant-Toddler Social-Emotional Assessment (BITSEA) screen and its companion in-depth assessment, Infant-Toddler Social-Emotional Assessment (ITSEA), for use as a follow-up assessment if problems arise on the BITSEA screen. The Achenbach Child Behavior Checklist has excellent reliability and validity and has been used successfully with a wide variety of clinical populations. Available in English and Spanish, it provides separate checklists for assessment of children 2 to 3 years old and 4 to 16 years old, with norms provided by age and gender, and separate report forms for parents and teachers. Other checklists with clinical utility include the Eyberg Child Behavior Inventory (ECBI) (Eyberg & Ross, 1978) for 2- to 16-year-olds and the Pediatric Symptom Checklist (PSCL) for 6- to 12-year-olds (Jellinek et al, 2002). Even if children's scores do not reach a clinical level by normative standards, attention must be paid to notably high scores, stable problem behavior, and attending circumstances (see the Resource Box for a list of assessment tools).

An assessment of temperament can be useful for infants, toddlers, preschoolers, and school-age children (Tuecki, 2003). Parent reports of temperament reflect the parent's perception, which may not accurately reflect objective reality. However, accurate or not, the parents' perceptions influence their behavior and feelings toward the child and must be taken seriously.

A behavioral diary or log kept by parents, by the school-age child, and by the teacher informs the practitioner and family about the situational context for and severity of the behavior problem or problems. Often, this monitoring process itself serves as an effective intervention.

▒ STRATEGIES FOR MANAGEMENT

Pediatric primary care providers manage more mental health problems than ever before, largely as a result of the lack of mental health services or insurance coverage that places mental health care out of reach for many families. However, many primary care providers lack adequate education to manage complex problems. In addition, it is financially difficult for many busy primary care practices to offer the extended appointments needed for high-quality mental health care.

As a general rule, if the cause of the problem is a life event with acute, short-term consequences, such as the death of a pet or a friend moving away, or a common developmentally normal but troublesome behavior (e.g., temper tantrums or sibling rivalry), it can be managed in the primary care setting. More enduring problems, such as loss of a parent or major depression, require referral to a pediatric mental health specialist. Strategies that primary care providers can use effectively include primary, secondary, and tertiary prevention of social, emotional, and behavior problems.

PRIMARY PREVENTION

Primary prevention of mental health problems occurs through positive, nurturing parent-child relationships. It is crucial for children to experience a secure attachment relationship, with a sense of worth and being lovable, as a foundation for developing social, emotional, and cognitive competence (Lieberman et al, 2005; Paulson et al, 2006).

It is critical for pediatric providers to screen consistently for parent depression at health visits beginning with the prenatal visit since maternal depression threatens healthy parenting. A large body of research supports the significant negative effects of maternal depression, including prenatal depression, on the behavior and development of infants and young children (Minkovitz et al, 2005). The U.S. Preventive Services Task Force (2006) states that the two-question depression screen (i.e., persistent feelings of sadness or the blues and lack of pleasure in things previously enjoyed) is as effective as longer screening tools commonly used with adults to identify maternal depression.

Healthy parenting strategies are positive in tone and regard for the child, responsive to the child's autonomy and individuality, neutral in response to unwanted behavior, and attentive to the child's needs (see Box 20-1 and Chapters 4 and 17). Parents who have not experienced this type of nurturance often need education and coaching in positive parenting behaviors from the pediatric provider (McDonough, 2005).

The development of trust and a sense of security in the world begins with effective, timely parental response to the helpless infant's needs (Melendez, 2005). Contrary to popular belief, responsive parenting results in children who are able to self-regulate their behavior and who are confident and competent rather than clingy. As children become more mobile and autonomous late in the first year, parental use of teaching-based limit-setting strategies, with reasoning, explanations, and distractions are more effective for behavior control and the development of self-regulation than are power-based strategies (Houck & LeCuyer-Maus, 2001; Houck & Stember, 2002; Houck & LeCuyer-Maus, 2004). Effective use of discipline and a teaching-based style enhances the development of self-regulation and fosters a strong self-concept and social competence (see Chapters 4 and 17). Through anticipatory guidance, pediatric providers can assist parents to handle predictable life events that are likely to influence children, such as changes in day care, moves, or changes in schools. Increasing the parent's awareness of the child's developmental and temperamental needs helps identify strategies to effectively facilitate transitions. Providers should work with parents to find ways to facilitate children's use of developmentally appropriate coping strategies. For example, parents can encourage

---

BOX 20-1 Positive Parenting Strategies

Attending to the Child Individually
Allow the child to make reasonable choices.
Respond to child's bids for attention with eye contact, smiles, and physical contact.
Comment on child's appropriate and desirable behavior frequently and positively throughout the day.
Provide guaranteed special time daily: no interruptions, no directions, no interrogations.
Prevent secondary gains for the child's minor transgressions by having no discussion, physical contact, perhaps even eye contact; be neutral and simply state the preferred behavior.

Listening Actively
Paraphrase or describe what child is saying.
Reflect the child's feelings.
Share the child's affect by matching the child's body posture and tone of voice.
Avoid giving commands, judging, or editorializing.
Follow the child's lead in the interaction.

Conveying Positive Regard
Communicate positive feelings (e.g., love) directly.
Give directions positively, firmly, specifically.
Provide notice before requiring child to change activities.
Label the behavior, not the child.
Praise competency and compliance; say thank you.
Apologize when appropriate.
Avoid shaming or belittling the child.
Strive for consistency.

---

symbolic play in preschoolers, or use discussion about developmentally appropriate books or movies with older children to help children express feelings and worries and gain control of their situation.

SECONDARY PREVENTION

Secondary prevention, or early detection and intervention, addresses unanticipated life events. Social, emotional, or behavioral problems may emerge even in the context of positive parenting approaches. At the level of secondary prevention, pediatric providers work collaboratively with parents to identify and implement appropriate management strategies or to explain and reinforce the value of recommendations from mental health specialists if a referral has been made.

Medication may be necessary to manage some mental health problems in children. It is important that primary care providers help parents and children understand that most mental health problems require a combined approach of psychotherapy and medication. There are no studies showing medication alone to be superior to medication combined with psychotherapy.

Use of medication to treat mental health problems in children is increasing, but there are concerns about pharmacologic interventions of which primary providers must be aware.

There continues to be a lack of adequate randomized control trials involving children, both in terms of efficacy and safety. Existing research shows that medications that are effective in the management of adult mental health conditions are less effective or may be completely ineffective in children with similar diagnoses, likely due to differences in the organization and function of the developing brain of children at different ages. Drugs used to treat mental health conditions have serious adverse side effects and require ongoing physiologic monitoring (Table 20-2). It is critical for primary care providers to assess for interactions between medications used in treating mental health conditions and commonly prescribed medications also used in primary care, such as antibiotics and contraceptives, that may result in impaired drug effectiveness or toxic side effects.

Tertiary Prevention

Tertiary prevention and intervention address major losses and trauma (e.g., victimization through sexual or physical abuse, parental marital problems, divorce, substance abuse, and parental psychopathologic conditions). Even in the absence of behavioral manifestations of distress, a referral to a mental health specialist for further assessment and intervention is fruitful given the difficulties that often result from these significant problems in both the short and long term (Lilienfeld, 2005). In these cases, parents may not understand the need for referral. It is most helpful for the pediatric provider to frame the behavior problem as a "normal response to an unusual or stressful situation" with the goal of referral being to maximize the child's development and growth. A release of information allows direct contact with the consultant to ensure follow-through. Ongoing follow-up is essential with children, families, and other professional providers.

COMMON MENTAL HEALTH PROBLEMS
SPECIAL PROBLEMS OF INFANCY AND EARLY CHILDHOOD

For many years, infants and young children were believed not to have mental health problems. It was as though pediatric health care providers believed that young children were magically protected from even the most adverse experiences. Research since the 1940s has clearly demonstrated that this was not the case. Today, despite a growing body of knowledge about children's mental health problems, frameworks used to identify and treat disorders in older children, adolescents, and adults still provide little guidance in the care of the very young. In 1994, Zero to Three, the National Center for Infants, Toddlers, and Families, sought to fill this void by releasing *The Diagnostic Classification of Mental Health and Developmental Disorders of Infancy and Early Childhood (DC:0-3)*. Following 10 years of clinical research in using the classification system in countries around the world, a revision (DC:0-3R) was released in 2005 (Zero to Three, 2005).

At first glance, the diagnoses seem to address familiar issues in infant and early childhood development, commonly addressed in pediatric primary care. Closer examination of the

TABLE 20-2 Evidence-Supported Drug Therapy for Common Mental Health Conditions in Childhood

Drug Class and Examples	Conditions Treated	Primary Care Drug Interactions	Common Side Effects
SSRIs			
Fluoxetine (Prozac) (only FDA-approved drug for depression in children)	Anxiety; major depressive disorder, OCD, selective mutism	Multiple drug interactions. Contraindicated drugs: MAOIs, tryptophan, and St. John's wort, thioridazine, TCAs. Increased risk of bleeding: NSAIDs, aspirin, warfarin	Headache, nervousness, insomnia or sedation, fatigue, nausea, diarrhea, dyspepsia, appetite loss. Diet: Avoid tryptophan supplements, grapefruit juice, and alcohol
Fluvoxamine (Luvox) (not approved for children under 18 years old)	OCD		
Sertraline (Zoloft) (only approved for OCD)	OCD		
Mood stabilizer			
Lithium (Lithobid)	Bipolar disorder, CD	Multiple drug interactions. Risk for toxic drug levels: NSAIDs, metronidazole, and a wide range of antihypertensives	Weight gain, acne, sedation, tremors, GI upset, hair loss. Diet: Limit caffeine, alcohol; ensure good fluid intake; maintain salt intake
Anticonvulsants used as mood stabilizers			
Carbamazepine (Tegretol)	Bipolar disorder	Multiple drug interactions. Decreased effectiveness: corticosteroids, oral and subdermal contraceptives, and doxycycline. Risk for toxic drug levels: clarithromycin, cimetidine, erythromycin, ketoconazole, itraconazole, and loratadine	Drowsiness, restlessness, nausea, vomiting, diarrhea, dyspepsia, tremor. Diet: Avoid alcohol and grapefruit juice
Valproic acid (Depakene)	Bipolar disorder	Multiple drug interactions. Risk for toxic drug levels: Aspirin-containing products	Drowsiness, irritability, restlessness, headache, ataxia, dizziness, nausea, vomiting, diarrhea, dyspepsia, weight gain, pancreatitis, hyperammonemia and hyperammonemic encephalopathy, thrombocytopenia, carnitine deficiency, tremor, liver failure, diplopia, blurred vision. Diet: Increase foods high in carnitine (red meats and dairy products)
Second-generation antipsychotic			
Risperidone (Risperdal)	Aggression, CD, ODD, Schizophrenia, Tourette's syndrome	Multiple drug interactions. Avoid: St. John's wort. Potentiates: Antihypertensives	Hypotension, syncope, tachycardia, insomnia, agitation, headache, dizziness, seizures, rash, weight gain, nausea, vomiting, diarrhea, polyuria, rhinitis, sinusitis, coughing, abnormal vision. Diet: Oral solution not compatible with cola or tea

CD, Conduct disorder; ODD, oppositional defiant disorder; OCD, obsessive-compulsive disorder; TCAs, tricyclic antidepressants; MAOI, monoamine oxidase inhibitors; NSAIDs.
Information in the table drawn from AACAP: Practice parameters for the assessment and treatment of children and adolescents with anxiety disorders, 2006. Available at www.aacap.org; AACAP: Practice parameters for the assessment and treatment of children and adolescents with bipolar disorders, J Am Acad Child Adolesc Psychiatry, 46:107-125, 2007a; AACAP: Practice parameters for the assessment and treatment of children and adolescents with oppositional defiant disorder, J Am Acad Child Adolesc Psychiatry 46:126-141, 2007b; Cohen D et al: Pharmacological treatment of adolescent major depression, J Child Adolesc Psychopharmacol 14:19-31, 2004; Hudson JL, Deveney C, Taylor BA: Nature, assessment, and treatment of generalized anxiety disorder in children, Pediatr Ann 34:97-106, 2005; March J et al: The Treatment for Adolescents with Depression Study (TADS): methods and message at 12 weeks, J Am Acad Child Adolesc Psychiatry 45:1393-1403, 2006; Ruths S, Steiner H: Psychopharmacologic treatment of aggression in children and adolescents, Pediatr Ann 33:318-327, 2004; and Taketomo CK, Hodding JH, Kraus DM: Pediatric dosage handbook, ed 13, Hudson OH, 2007, LexiComp.

diagnostic criteria demonstrates that the diagnoses address a more serious degree of maladaptive behavior, often with a significant degree of parental dysfunction and distress. These issues are beyond the management abilities of most primary care providers who do not have extensive preparation in the field of infant mental health. Three of the most common classifications are presented here, and the remaining DC:0-3R diagnoses are summarized in Table 20-3. The purpose of including them in this discussion is to increase the primary care provider's awareness of the range of conditions that are best treated by the infant mental health specialist.

Feeding Disorders

Feeding the infant and young child successfully is a key task for parents. Parents feel successful and competent when their infant or young child feeds vigorously and grows well (Sumner & Spietz, 1994a). Conversely, feeding problems resulting in parental frustration and failing child growth provoke feelings of failure in many parents. Feeding problems are among the most stubborn challenges primary care providers encounter (see Chapter 11). A serious problem exists when an infant or young child fails to establish a regular feeding pattern based on hunger and satiety. The potential diagnoses cover problems in:

- State regulation that interfere with the infant's ability to feed well
- Lack of reciprocity between the caregiver and infant during the feeding
- Infantile anorexia associated with a very active infant or young child who refuses food
- Sensory food aversions that are so numerous and extreme they result in nutritional deficiencies (Zero to Three, 2005)

Sleep Behavior Disorder

Sleep problems are very common in the first year of life. Research over the past decade has demonstrated the beneficial effects of good quality sleep on child behavior and learning from infancy through adolescence (Blair et al, 2005; Stockton, 2002). The converse is also true. Insufficient and poor quality sleep is consistently associated with behavior problems and learning difficulties at all ages (Holditch-Davis et al, 2004). DC:0-3R (Zero to Three, 2005) offers two sleep diagnoses for children 1 to 3 years old. Sleep-onset disorder addresses the child who has difficulty for more than 1 month in falling asleep. Night-waking disorder addresses the child who needs parental intervention on a nearly nightly basis to cope with night awakenings (see Chapter 15).

TABLE 20-3 **Summary of the Diagnostic Classification of Mental Health and Developmental Disorders of Infancy and Early Childhood: Revised Edition**

Major Clinical Disorders	Subclassifications
PTSD	
Deprivation/maltreatment disorder	
Disorders of affect	
Prolonged bereavement/grief reaction	
Anxiety disorders	Separation anxiety disorder
	Specific phobia
	Social anxiety disorder
	Generalized anxiety disorder
	Anxiety disorder not otherwise specified
Depression	Major depression: Type I
	Depressive disorder: Type II
Mixed disorder of emotional expressiveness	
Adjustment disorders of sensory processing	
Hypersensitive	Type A: Fearful/cautious
	Type B: Negative/defiant
Hyposensitive/underresponsive	
Sensory stimulation seeking/impulsive	
Sleep behavior disorder	Sleep-onset disorder
	Night-waking disorder
Feeding behavior disorder	Feeding disorder of state regulation
	Feeding disorder of caregiver-infant reciprocity
	Infantile anorexia
	Sensory food aversions
	Feeding disorder associated with concurrent medical condition
	Feeding disorder associated with insults to the gastrointestinal tract
Disorders of relating and communicating	
Multisystem developmental disorder	

PTSD, Posttraumatic stress disorder.

Regulation Disorders of Sensory Processing

Regulation disorders of sensory processing focus on constitutionally based responses to stimuli that provoke problems regulating emotions, behaviors, and motor abilities that subsequently impair development and functioning (Gomez et al, 2004). These problems exist across settings and relationships. Three major patterns of problems emerge: hypersensitivity, in which sensory input experiences are aversive to the child; hyposensitivity, in which the quiet child requires high-intensity sensory experiences to mount a response; and sensory stimulation seeking or impulsivity in which the very active child aggressively seeks high-intensity, frequent, or prolonged sensory experiences. Some occupational therapists have preparation to manage these problems and may be a helpful resource to the primary care provider.

FEARS, PHOBIAS, AND ANXIETIES

Fears and Phobias

Description.   Fear is the occurrence of various avoidance responses to particular stimuli; it is a state of apprehension or response to threatening situation (Jellinek et al, 2002). In contrast, a phobia is a persistent, extreme, and irrational fear triggered by the presence or anticipation of the presence of a specific person, object, or situation. The onset of fears occurs during the transition to toddlerhood and is normally reflected in separation anxiety and stranger anxiety (Egger & Angold, 2006).

Epidemiology.   Childhood fears are a part of normal development. Fears have a developmental function, and the nature of predominant fears varies with age. Specific phobias occur in about 5% of the population and in 15% of children referred for anxiety-related problems. Phobias are determined by multiple factors, with genetic influences, temperament, parental mental health problems, and individual conditioning histories converging in specific phobias (Egger & Angold, 2006).

Clinical Findings.   Infants typically react fearfully to loss of support, height, and unexpected stimuli. Toddlers experience separation anxiety and fear physical injury and strangers. Preschoolers fear imaginary creatures, animals, darkness, and being alone, and they also demonstrate some persistent separation anxiety. Fear of animals and darkness extends into school age, but safety, natural events, and school- and health-related fears dominate. In preadolescence and adolescence, fears of bodily injury, economic and political catastrophes, and social fears are central. Fear and phobic reactions typically involve symptoms of autonomic arousal. In phobias, the symptoms of autonomic arousal may evolve into panic attacks or phobic-avoidant reactions.

Differential Diagnosis.   Distinction must be made between abnormal fears and normal developmental fears that encourage the acquisition of boundaries, caution, and safety. Clinical phobias are defined on the basis of persistence, magnitude, and maladaptiveness.

Management.   Most fears are short-lived, are not serious, and do not predict adult mental health problems. Parents absolutely must be cautioned against using fears as a form of behavioral control (e.g., threats of abandonment with toddlers) or as a discipline strategy (e.g., leaving a preschooler alone in a dark room). When the fear negatively impacts the child's functioning, developmental progress, learning experiences, and level of comfort, referral is necessary. Treatment for fearful and phobic infants, toddlers, and preschoolers focuses on improving parent mental health, parental child behavior management skills, and the quality of the marital relationship. Various management strategies are available for treatment of phobias in children older than 5 years, including systematic desensitization, contingency management, cognitive-behavioral procedures, and family interventions (American Academy of Child and Adolescent Psychiatry [AACAP], 2006).

Anxiety

Anxiety is distinguished from fear on the basis of diffuse apprehension in response to less specific stimuli. It is a normal developmental phenomenon that is experienced by nearly every person at some point. Anxious responses include somatic symptoms mediated through the autonomic system, with physiologic changes, such as increased heart rate and blood pressure, tremor, sweating, and enhanced vigilance and reactivity. Anxiety that persists at high levels and is reflected in maladaptive behavior warrants diagnosis and treatment. Children diagnosed with anxiety disorders tend to have multiple problems, are impaired in important areas of social functioning, and live with parents who experience symptoms of anxiety or mood disorders. Anxiety disorders typically appear earlier than behavior disorders, which, in turn, appear earlier than mood disorders.

Risk factors include the following: (1) genetics, (2) temperamental disposition for behavioral inhibition, and (3) social environment or life circumstances (e.g., parental distress or dysfunction or trauma), especially during vulnerable developmental periods (e.g., attachment or separation-individuation) (Stafford et al, 2004). Youngsters with anxiety disorders are at high risk for subsequent anxiety disorders, for comorbid mood disorders, and for adolescent substance abuse. Anxiety disorders show distinct clustering in families (AACAP, 2006).

Separation Anxiety Disorder

Description.   The essential feature of separation anxiety disorder is abnormal reactivity to real or imagined separation from major attachment figures, home, or familiar surroundings (Hanna et al, 2006). Separation anxiety is a normal developmental phenomenon from about 7 months old through the preschool years. However, some infants and toddlers experience excessive levels of distress with separation from the major caregiver (Jursberg & Ledley, 2005). These children may cry persistently and cannot be comforted or refuse to be cared for and comforted by a competent, substitute caregiver. Alternatively, older infants, toddlers, and preschoolers may act aggressively toward the substitute caregiver or intentionally injure themselves (Zero to Three, 2005).

Separation anxiety disorder, in which reactivity to separation interferes with daily activities and developmental tasks, manifests from 5 to 16 years old; the mean age for clinical presentation is 9 years (Hanna et al, 2006). Although the diagnosis has been reserved for children and not included in adult epidemiologic studies, there is growing evidence that adults with histories of school refusal exhibit a range of anxiety and depressive disorders and that adult separation anxiety is associated with a history of childhood separation anxiety disorder (Silove et al, 2002). This diagnosis can be a precursor for panic disorder in adolescence or adulthood (Stafford et al, 2004).

Epidemiology. Separation anxiety disorder is thought to evolve from a poor attachment relationship or the interaction among physiologic, cognitive, and overt behavioral factors in response to life events that threaten safety or primary relationships, or both (Egger & Angold, 2006). It is probably the most common anxiety disorder from older infancy through the school-age years and the most common mental health reason for referral (Zero to Three, 2005). Among infants and young children, only about 10% of those affected by separation anxiety are referred for care despite the concerns of the majority of parents. Older children are usually brought to the health care provider when the disorder results in school refusal or somatic symptoms. About 80% of children with school refusal are thought to have separation anxiety disorder, many of these with comorbid depression (Stafford et al, 2004).

Clinical Findings. The following are found in separation anxiety disorder:

- Developmentally inappropriate or excessive anxiety about separations
- Unrealistic worry about harm to self or attachment figures or about abandonment during periods of separation
- Reluctance to sleep alone or sleep away from home
- Persistent avoidance of being alone
- Nightmares about separation
- Physical complaints and signs of distress in anticipation of separation
- Social withdrawal during separations
- Environmental stress, parental dysfunction, and maternal depression are risk factors for separation anxiety disorder, especially with panic disorder or agoraphobia

The Spielberger State-Trait Anxiety Inventory for Children (STAIC) is a twenty-item, self-report scale useful with children 9 to 12 years old; it can also be used with high reading–skill younger children and low reading–skill adolescents.

Differential Diagnosis. Anxiety disorder not associated with separation is a differential diagnosis. Anxiety may occur as a response to trauma or a manifestation of posttraumatic stress disorder (PTSD) (AACAP, 2006). It is essential to attend to cues that a traumatic experience or situation (e.g., sexual or physical abuse) is the source of the symptoms of anxiety. From 30% to 70% of children and adolescents with an anxiety disorder have a depressive disorder, and 15% to 25% of children and adolescents with an anxiety disorder also meet the diagnostic criteria for ADHD (AACAP, 2006). Common comorbidities with separation anxiety include social phobia and overanxious disorder (Jellinek et al, 2002). In adolescence, comorbid substance use disorder (SUD) increases in prevalence (Dias, 2002).

Management. Anxiety disorder is preferably treated as a family system or relationship-based problem (Hudson et al, 2005). Relief of symptoms is the first priority in school-age children. Identifying and treating the sources of the problem is the first line of treatment for infants through preschoolers and a secondary focus of treatment for school-age children (Egger & Angold, 2006). Note the role of attachment figures and refer the child to a child therapist for early intervention. Among school-age children, psychoeducational, behavioral, and cognitive-behavioral approaches have been effective (In-Albon & Schneider, 2007). In general, pharmacotherapy is used only if the child fails to respond to nonpharmacologic intervention and considerable impairment in function is experienced.

Before beginning a medication regimen, it is a good idea to refer the patient to a child psychiatrist or child and adolescent mental health primary care provider for a medication evaluation. Selective serotonin reuptake inhibitors (SSRIs) are the first-choice medications in separation anxiety disorder, in part because of their limited adverse effects (Stafford et al, 2004). Until the SSRI becomes effective, benzodiazepines may be used if a rapid reduction of symptoms is necessary; this class of drugs has an adverse effect profile and potential for abuse and dependence.

Generalized Anxiety Disorder

Description. Generalized anxiety disorder, or overanxious disorder, is cognitive and obsessive in nature. The child experiences excessive anxiety, worry, and apprehensive expectations generalized to a number of events or activities. These anxieties do not focus on a specific person, object or situation, nor are they the result of a recent stressor. Children with generalized anxiety disorder are characterized as "worriers." The exact onset is not known, but the diagnosis occurs most often among older children and adolescents 9 to 18 years old.

Epidemiology. There is a familial association for generalized anxiety disorder that suggests a genetic vulnerability to anxiety; twin studies suggest that shared environment is far less important than genetic factors (AACAP, 2006). Five percent to 18% of all children are thought to have anxiety disorders of one type or another (Stafford et al, 2004).

Clinical Findings. Major symptoms of generalized anxiety disorder are (Ginsburg et al, 2006):

- Worry about future events
- Poor quality sleep
- Irritability and tantrums in young children
- Preoccupation with past behavior
- Overconcern about competence
- Marked self-consciousness
- Restlessness
- Difficulty concentrating
- Somatic complaints without a physical basis
- Fatigue
- Need for reassurance

Comorbidity with other anxiety disorders or mood disorder is common.

Differential Diagnosis. Differential diagnoses are separation anxiety, adjustment disorder associated with a specific stressor, and attention-deficit disorder; the last does not involve worry about the future. It is important to attend to cues that might point to traumatic experiences or conditions as the source of anxiety symptoms. It is important to rule out the presence of pediatric autoimmune neuropsychiatric disorders associated with streptococcal infections (PANDAS); these are induced disorders that are effectively treated with antibiotics.

Management. The treatment of preschool children and toddlers generally focuses on behavioral and family intervention. Preschoolers may also receive play therapy. Although clinicians have administered SSRIs and other psychotropic medications to children as young as 2 years old, there is no efficacy data, and long-term developmental sequelae of such treatment are unknown. Refer the older child or adolescent to a pediatric mental health therapist for treatment of symptoms using relaxation techniques or cognitive-behavioral therapy (CBT). Individual and/or family counseling can be used to identify the source of anxiety. Treatment outcomes are more positive when parents are involved in interventions that target familial contextual processes. Younger school-age children especially seem to benefit from a combination of cognitive-behavioral strategies and family intervention (AACAP, 2006). Individual and group treatments or child- and family-focused treatments are equally effective, and follow-up data demonstrates that treatment gains are maintained up to several years after treatment (In-Albon & Schneider, 2007).

Pharmacologic intervention is advisable, especially if there is comorbid social phobia or separation anxiety disorder. Evidence points to the safety and efficacy of the SSRIs, especially fluvoxamine and fluoxetine or buspirone (Stafford et al, 2004). Although effective, tricyclic antidepressants have adverse cardiotoxic effects, and benzodiazepines have not been shown to be superior to placebo in RCTs, while also carrying the potential for the development of tolerance and dependency (AACAP, 2006).

Obsessive–Compulsive Disorder

Description. Obsessions are recurrent thoughts, images, or impulses that are disturbing to the child and difficult to dislodge. They often involve a sense of risk or fear of harm to the child or family members; concerns for contamination are common. Compulsions are repetitive behaviors or mental acts that the child feels driven to perform to prevent harm or remove contaminants, such as washing (e.g., hands, objects, or body), counting, or arranging objects. Recurrent worries, rituals, and superstitious games are common in children at various stages of development. These behaviors are attended by mild anxiety but do not cause distress. Abnormal compulsive behavior is distinguished by a sense of urgency or a profound discomfort until the ritual is completed. Children often deny the fear and lack recognition of the "senselessness" of the ritual and seem to hide their illness. Obsessive thoughts are intrusive, recurrent, and disturbing and, unlike anxious worries, are generally unrelated to events or situations.

Epidemiology. Obsessive-compulsive disorder (OCD) is more common than previously thought. Neurobiologic underpinnings include a role for serotonin and involve abnormalities in the basal ganglia and functionally related cortical structures (Lewin et al, 2005). OCD appears to affect primarily preado-

lescents and adolescents, with boys more likely to have onset in preadolescence and girls more likely to have onset in puberty. OCD is increasingly diagnosed in younger children, some as young as 2 years old, manifested in play or interests that have a compulsive or ritualistic quality (e.g., playing with objects in only one certain sequence, with interruption producing intense distress). Approximately 2% to 4% of children are affected with other children not diagnosed or misdiagnosed (Merlo et al, 2005). Familial transmission is evident, and 10% have a poststreptococcal autoimmunity response apparently causing onset (Stafford et al, 2004). OCD is a chronic condition, with high rates of comorbidity, typically with some other anxiety disorder, major depression, or SUD. Tic disorders, disruptive behavior disorders, and learning disorders are also common comorbid diagnoses.

Clinical Findings. OCD is characterized by obsessions and compulsions, as previously defined. Children do not recognize that the obsessions or compulsions are excessive or unreasonable. They derive no pleasure from their ritualistic activity. The obsessions and compulsions are time consuming and may significantly interfere with the child's or adolescent's normal routine, academic performance, and social functioning. Washing, checking, and ordering rituals are more common in children (American Psychiatric Association [APA], 1994).

Differential Diagnosis. A diagnosis of OCD is warranted if the content of the obsessions and compulsions is unrelated to another disorder (e.g., social phobia, trichotillomania, body dysmorphic disorder). If the obsessions or compulsions are a direct physiologic consequence of a specific medical condition, the diagnosis is anxiety disorder caused by a general medical condition. If a substance causes the obsessions or compulsions, a diagnosis of substance-induced anxiety disorder is assigned. A major depressive episode is diagnosed if the obsessions are mood congruent (e.g., guilt), and generalized anxiety disorder is diagnosed if the obsessions are experienced as excessive worry about real-life circumstances (APA, 1994). In the case of acute onset or exacerbation of OCD, a thorough assessment of recent medical illnesses, including upper respiratory infections, is warranted.

Management. Clinical and empirical evidence suggests that CBT, alone or in combination with pharmacotherapy, is effective treatment for OCD in children and adolescents. Anxiety management training and OCD-specific family interventions play an adjunctive role, especially in preventing the avoidant behavior that is a complication of OCD (AACAP, 2006). Recent findings support the efficacy of CBT with a structured family component. SSRIs are first-line pharmacologic agents.

RESPONSES TO TRAUMA: POSTTRAUMATIC STRESS DISORDER

Description

Childhood trauma is the result of one sudden, traumatic event or exposure to repeated trauma over time, such as physical or sexual abuse. A single trauma is an unanticipated solitary event directed at the child or witnessed by the child, such as an act of violence that involves threat, injury, or death. It includes learning about unexpected or violent death, harm, or threat experienced by a family member or close friend. Repeated trauma or repeated exposure to a painful event, usually maltreatment (physical or sexual abuse, or both) or community violence is long standing. Other family dysfunctions, including emotional abuse, neglect, and substance abuse typically accompany ongoing maltreatment. Exposure to trauma constitutes the first criterion for PTSD (AACAP, 1998).

PTSD describes a characteristic set of symptoms that develops following exposure to a severe stressor or trauma. A decade ago, stress responses were conceptualized according to whether the trauma was a single event ("one sudden blow" trauma) or variable, multiple, long-standing traumas, such as ongoing maltreatment. Distinct symptoms distinguish between acute and chronic types of PTSD. According to the *Diagnostic and Statistical Manual of Mental Disorders, edition 4 (DSM-IV)*, the duration of the symptoms distinguishes three subtypes:
- Acute stress disorder—symptoms appear within 1 month of exposure to extreme stressor; last less than 1 month
- Acute PTSD—symptoms last less than 3 months
- Chronic PTSD—symptoms last longer than 3 months

According to the practice parameters for children and adolescents with PTSD (AACAP, 1998), the child's response to trauma must include a specific number of symptoms from each of three broad categories for a diagnosis:
- Reexperiencing the trauma in some way (one symptom)
- Avoidance or numbing (three symptoms)
- Increased arousal (two symptoms)

Epidemiology
Exposure to trauma is a key feature of the diagnosis of PTSD. Unfortunately, there has been skepticism that children suffer from PTSD (Ziegler et al, 2005). Parents and teachers frequently minimize traumatic impact, perhaps to relieve themselves of vicarious distress or to reassure themselves that their children have not suffered harm. Others—including mental health professionals—have rationalized that children are too young to remember the trauma or too immature to be affected. However, the clinical descriptive and empirical literature has expanded, documenting PTSD symptoms and other psychological difficulties experienced by children in various catastrophic situations and in situations of maltreatment.

Substantial rates of PTSD have been documented for children in foster care who were sexually abused and who were physically abused, leading to a better understanding of the clinical manifestations of PTSD in children. Three factors consistently influence the severity of the response: severity of the trauma exposure, parental distress related to the trauma, and temporal proximity to the event.

Retrospective reports of adults with mental health problems indicate that PTSD is more common than previously believed. Prevalence rates of 13% to 45% for children exposed to traumatic stressors are reported (Ziegler et al, 2005). The rate of PTSD is high among those who have been physically and sexually abused, with estimates ranging from 25% to 75% of sexual abuse victims, depending on the perpetrator. The closer the perpetrator is in relation to the victim, the greater the trauma (e.g., PTSD is more likely when the perpetrator is a member of the immediate family as opposed to an extended family member, family friend, or stranger) (Zero to Three, 2005).

Clinical Findings
A diagnosis of PTSD requires that the child demonstrate specific behaviors following trauma, as follows:
1. The child repeatedly reexperiences a set of symptoms from each of three categories (APA, 1994), including the following:
   - Recurrent and intrusive memories of the trauma
   - Nightmares of monsters or threats to self or others or distressing dreams about a specific event
   - Distress at exposure to cues that symbolize or resemble an aspect of the trauma, including physiologic reactivity
2. The child demonstrates three of the following symptoms reflecting avoidance of stimuli associated with the traumatic event(s) and numbing of general responsiveness. These symptoms must not have been present before the trauma:
   - Avoidance of reminders of the trauma
   - Efforts to avoid thoughts, feelings, or conversations linked to the trauma
   - Amnesia for an important aspect of the trauma
   - Detachment or estrangement from others
   - Emotional constriction (restricted range of affect)
   - Diminished interest in or participation in usual activities
   - A sense of a foreshortened future
3. Two persistent symptoms of increased arousal must be new to the child, present for at least 1 month, and cause clinically important distress or negatively affect functioning. These symptoms include the following:
   - Sleep disturbances
   - Hypervigilance
   - Difficulty concentrating
   - Exaggerated startle response
   - Agitated or disorganized behavior
   - Irritability or angry outbursts, extreme fussiness or tantrums

Among infants, toddlers, and preschoolers, symptoms must be understood within the context of the trauma itself, the child's temperament and personality, and the caregiver's ability to support the child and provide a sense of safety and protection. Infants, toddlers, and preschoolers retain fragments of memories to the extent that they have the verbal capacity to articulate them. PTSD may present in infancy as failure to thrive; feeding problems; sleep disturbance; aggression in older infants in response to distress; preoccupation with certain words or symbols or avoidance of situations that may or may not have an obvious connection to the event; or as generalized anxiety symptoms, such as separation fears, stranger anxiety, fear of monsters or animals (Scheeringa, 2006; Zero to Three, 2005). In early childhood, PTSD may appear as recurrent nightmares, as a repetitive trauma theme in play, sleep problems, hypervigilance, failure to progress developmentally, or developmental regression. Other symptoms to consider include play reenactment that is not especially repetitive or constriction of play. Another presentation may be disturbed social relationships marked by social withdrawal, indifference to caregivers, extreme ambivalence, failure to have a preference for a specific caregiver, or a combination of these behaviors (Zero to Three, 2005). Sexualized (i.e., seductive) behavior is a hallmark sign of sexual abuse, and preschoolers can display behavioral or physical symptoms that prompt the caregiver's or other adults' suspicions of sexual abuse.

As children mature, especially adolescents, they are more likely to exhibit adult-like PTSD symptoms. School-age children may not become amnesic for the event or certain aspects of it; they may retain full, detailed memories. They may not have avoidant or numbing symptoms or visual flashbacks. Anxiety with sleep disturbances tends to characterize responses to exposure to a single traumatic event. Reenactment of the trauma through play, drawings, or verbalizations is typical for this developmental stage. Disclosures by school-age children tend to be purposeful and unrelated to a precipitating event. However, repression and dissociation often preclude disclosure until adulthood. Adolescents with chronic PTSD who have experienced prolonged or repeated traumatic stressors (i.e., maltreatment) may experience depersonalization and dissociative episodes, sadness and thoughts that life is too hard, rage directed against self or others, and internalizing or externalizing behavior problems. PTSD symptoms are also related to adolescent suicidal ideation and behavior.

Differential Diagnosis

The stressor must be of an extreme nature to warrant a diagnosis of PTSD, whereas the stressor can be of any severity in an adjustment disorder (e.g., moving, starting a new school, birth of a sibling, divorce); the clinician has some latitude in this determination. Acute stress disorder is distinguished by the symptom pattern occurring and resolving within a 4-week period after the traumatic event. Recurrent intrusive thoughts occur in OCD but are experienced as inappropriate and are not related to an experienced trauma as they are in PTSD. Flashbacks also connect to the event and involve a feeling of reliving the event in PTSD, whereas hallucinations and other perceptual disturbances are unrelated to exposure to trauma. With depression or externalizing disorders, such as conduct disorder (CD) unrelated to trauma, memory is intact and psychic numbing and dissociation are absent. The most typical differential diagnosis is an anxiety disorder, which is distinguished by not being precipitated by a traumatic event.

Among preschoolers, comorbid conditions differ from those of adults and older children. Oppositional defiant disorder (ODD) is most common, followed by separation anxiety disorder and ADHD. Major depressive disorder is very unlikely (Scheeringa, 2006).

Management

Assessment of PTSD in children requires careful and direct clinical interviews with the child and parents. If the identified traumatic event involves a parent as the perpetrator of child maltreatment or domestic violence, the nonoffending parent or other caretaker should be interviewed. During assessment, do not use prompting or leading questions. Instead, ask questions about whether someone has invaded the child's privacy, how it may have happened, and how the injuries came to be. Specific guidelines for such an interview can be found in AACAP (1998). Enough of an assessment should be conducted to ascertain that a trauma has occurred, the nature of the trauma, and the consequent symptom pattern. A report to social service agencies is essential for children younger than 18 years old. Referral to a pediatric mental health specialist is crucial, even in the absence of a disclosure.

Crisis intervention is often necessary for both the child and parents. The primary care provider should educate parents about trauma and PTSD. Most pediatric psychiatrists use medications to treat PTSD, preferring SSRIs and alpha-adrenergic agonists. Child psychiatrists tend to additionally prefer psychodynamic or cognitive-behavioral approaches, and nonmedical therapists tend to prefer the modalities of cognitive-behavioral, family, and nondirective play therapy. Symptom patterns persist, so consistent follow-up assessment is important. Emergency department staff are being alerted to the issue of preventive counseling for PTSD when children and families are treated in that arena (Ziegler et al, 2005).

MOOD DISORDERS
Depression

Description. There are three categories of depression that may be assigned regardless of age: major depressive disorder, dysthymic disorder, and adjustment disorder with depressed mood (APA, 1994). A major depressive disorder is defined as a depressed or irritable mood or a markedly diminished interest and pleasure in almost all of the usual activities for a period of at least 2 weeks, or both. A dysthymic disorder is characterized by a depressed or irritable mood for the majority of days in the past year and other symptoms but not to the extent of a major depressive episode. Adjustment disorder with depressed mood typically occurs within 3 months after a major life stressor, involves less severe symptoms, and is relatively mild and brief.

Epidemiology. Like that of other disorders, the rate of depression increases with age. Although depression occurs in children under 5 years old, the true incidence is unknown given the limits of cognitive and language skills to communicate feelings. Depression is estimated to affect 1% to 3% of school-age children; the rate increases up to 17% by late adolescence. Twenty percent to 50% of adolescents report significant, subsyndromal levels of depression (Hankin, 2006). This rate increase for adolescents is thought to be linked to biology (e.g., sexual maturation), social environment (e.g., greater social and academic expectations, greater exposure to negative events), and developmental factors (e.g., increased autonomy and abstract thinking). Vulnerability to depression involves an interplay of genetic, biologic, biochemical, and psychosocial forces. Genetic factors underlie the risk for major depression, especially for childhood onset. The offspring of depressed parents are three times as likely to be diagnosed with depression, with a peak incidence at 15 to 20 years old (Boris et al, 2004).

Three biologic theories of depression are used to understand the psychopharmacology of depression: impaired neurotransmission, endocrine dysfunction, and biologic rhythm dysfunction. Given a biologic predisposition, certain life events may trigger the onset of depression. These include loss of a parent or significant other, losses that attend a disability or injury, family dysfunction, and physical or sexual abuse. There is a high risk of recurrent depression in diagnosed children and adolescents that appears to persist into young adulthood. Cognitive vulnerabilities have also been implicated as factors related to depression. These include negative inferential styles about causes, consequences and the self, the tendency to ruminate in response to depressed mood, and self-criticism (Hankin, 2006).

An important feature of early-onset depressive illness is a switch from unipolar depression to bipolar depression. Psychiatric comorbidity with depression is to be expected. The most common comorbidity with depression is an anxiety disorder (up to 70%), which co-occurs two to three times more often than CD. Other disorders most frequently found with major depression include dysthymia, disruptive behavior disorders, eating disorders, substance abuse and/or dependence, and ADHD (Hankin, 2006). Comorbidity may also occur with a variety of medical conditions, especially those with a neurologic component, such as brain injury, learning disorder, migraine headaches, and epilepsy.

Clinical Findings. Infants and toddlers present with a new pattern of depressed affect, altered behavior, and lack of pleasure in previously pleasurable activities occurring independent of any negative events (McLearn et al, 2006; Zero to Three, 2005). These changes should represent a persistent change that occurs across settings, activities, and relationships and causes the child distress, impaired functioning, or developmental alteration. Other symptoms may include failure to thrive, speech and motor delays, repetitive self-soothing behaviors, withdrawal from social interaction, poor attachment, and loss of developmental skills. Infants may not respond to extra efforts to sooth or engage them.

Toddlers and preschoolers may lack energy, be too eager to please others, be excessively or unusually clingy or whiney, and have problems with separation, with a persistence and intensity atypical for toddlerhood (Luby & Belden, 2006). Common symptoms of major depression in preschoolers include sad or grouchy mood (98%), lack of pleasure in play or activity (98%), poor appetite and weight loss, sleep problems (80%), low levels of energy and activity (80%), low self-esteem (78%), and increased death or suicide play or talk (74%). Regression in development affects 37% of preschoolers with 51% evidencing physical complaints and 55% showing increased whining and crying (Luby & Belden, 2006).

School-age children may manifest irritability, anger, or hostility in addition to externalizing behavior, such as hyperactivity, difficulty handling aggression, or reckless behavior. Frequent absences from school, perhaps because of school phobia, or poor performance and other school problems are common. On the other hand, school-age children may have internalizing symptoms, such as boredom, lack of interest in playing with friends, social withdrawal, somatic complaints (e.g., stomachaches, headaches, muscle aches, or tiredness), eating or sleeping disturbances, and enuresis or encopresis. Some children who are depressed describe themselves in negative terms, whereas others, in an effort to compensate for feelings of poor self-worth, become preoccupied with attempting to please others. Depressive symptoms in adolescents additionally include impulsivity, fatigue, and hopelessness. Social withdrawal with the appearance of shyness, boredom, or a lack of motivation is common (Jellinek et al, 2002). Substance abuse is a problem for about 20%.

Children and young adolescents with depression typically have difficulty in identifying or describing their emotional or mood states and are more likely to be irritable or act out behaviorally. Tearfulness and depressed affect, observable psychomotor agitation or retardation, and somatic complaints are common. Talking directly with the child or adolescent is essential because it is thought that half of depression cases are missed when parents alone are interviewed. The following depressive symptoms may exist:

- Depressed mood: sad, "blue," down, angry, bored
- Loss of interest and pleasure in usual activities
- Change in appetite or weight (loss or increase)
- Insomnia or hypersomnia
- Low energy and fatigue
- Difficulty concentrating; indecision
- Feelings of worthlessness or inappropriate or excessive guilt
- Recurrent thoughts of death or suicidal ideation

A diagnosis of major depressive disorder is made if there have been at least 2 weeks of depressed mood or loss of interest and at least four additional symptoms of depression. The symptoms cause considerable distress and impairment in social and academic functioning. Therefore, it is important to assess the following:

- Recent life events and losses
- Family history of depression or other psychiatric disorders
- Family dysfunction
- Changes in school performance
- Risk-taking behavior, including sexual activity and substance use
- Deteriorating relationships with family
- Changes in peer relations, especially social withdrawal
  Possible warning signs for suicide are listed in Table 20-4.

Depression Scales. Both patient self-report and clinician-completed rating scales are available. The following are used in pediatrics:

- Child Behavior Checklist (CBCL; 4 to 18 years old)
- Children's Depression Rating Scale-Revised (CDRS-R; 6 to 12 years old)
- Reynolds Child Depression Scale (RCDS; 6 to 12 years old)
- Children's Depression Inventory (CDI; 6 years old to adolescent)
- Beck Depression Inventory (BDI; adolescents)

TABLE 20-4	Warning Signs for Suicide
Area of Functioning	**Signs***
Changes in behavior	Accident prone
	Drug and alcohol abuse
	Physical violence toward self, others, or animals
	Loss of appetite
	Sudden alienation from family, friends, co-workers
	Worsening performance at work or school
	Putting personal affairs in order
	Loss of interest in personal appearance
	Disposal of possessions
	Writing letters, notes, or poems with suicidal content
	Taking unnecessary risks
	Buying a gun
Changes in mood	Expressions of hopelessness or impending doom
	Explosive rage
	Dramatic swings in affect
	Crying spells
	Sleep disorders
	Talk about suicide
Changes in thinking	Preoccupation with death
	Difficulty concentrating
	Irrational speech
	Hearing voices, seeing visions
	Sudden interest (or loss of interest) in religion
Major life changes	Death of a family member or friend (especially by suicide)
	Separation or divorce
	Public humiliation or failure
	Serious illness or trauma
	Loss of financial security

*These signs must be interpreted in context. Many of them are common outside the realm of presuicidal behavior.
Data from Oregon Health Division: Suicidal thoughts, suicidal deaths, *CD Summary* 46:24, 1997.

- Reynolds Adolescent Depression Scale (RADS; adolescents)
- Center for Epidemiologic Studies-Depression Scale (CES-D; adolescents)
- Depression Self-Rating Scale (adolescents)

From a review of depression rating scales for children and adolescents, the RCDS and the RADS were recommended for screening purposes. For clinical assessment, a combination of the clinician-administered CDRS-R along with the self-report CDI is recommended as the optimal approach (Myers & Winters, 2002). Although the CDRS-R was originally developed for children, it has been used widely with adolescents. The BDI and the CES-D are both good screening tools for adolescents.

Differential Diagnosis.   Some medications (steroids, phenobarbital, antihypertensives) and certain chronic illnesses (hypothyroidism, multiple sclerosis, inflammatory bowel disease, and type 1 diabetes) predispose children and adolescents to mood disorder. If a substance (e.g., medication, toxin, or drug of abuse) is related to the mood disturbance, a substance-induced mood disorder is diagnosed. Medications commonly causing depressive symptoms include beta-blockers, benzodiazepines, clonidine, corticosteroids, oral contraceptives, and isotretinoin. Infections, lead intoxication, anemia, eating disorders, mitral valve prolapse, premenstrual syndrome, and neurologic disorders can also mimic depression in children and adolescents. In general, a physical examination and screening laboratory tests are necessary to rule out potential organic causes.

Depressive symptoms in response to a psychosocial stressor are diagnosed as adjustment disorder, which has a good short-term prognosis and does not predict later dysfunction. With separation anxiety disorder, depressive symptoms usually arise only in the context of separation and resolve quickly with reunion; however, concomitant depressive disorder is not uncommon. A depressive episode with irritable mood can be difficult to distinguish from a manic episode with irritable mood; careful evaluation of the presence of manic symptoms (e.g., excessive activity, inflated self-esteem, little need for sleep, talkativeness) is required. Many adolescents and adults who develop mania had preponderantly depressive symptoms in childhood. Family history of bipolarity is an important risk factor. Mood disturbance that reflects irritability rather than sadness or loss of interest must be differentiated; mood disorder can be overdiagnosed in youths with ADHD (APA, 1994). Children with mood disorder do not usually manifest impulsivity. In addition, they typically have a normal attention span before the onset of symptoms.

Management.   The first goals of management are to determine suicidal risk and intervene to prevent suicide. For young people, 15 to 24 years old, suicide is the third leading cause of death, behind unintentional injuries and homicide (Catallozzi et al, 2001). Acute suicidal intent, which includes a plan, requires immediate psychiatric evaluation. Cumulative suicidal risks—prior suicidal behavior or attempts, depression, and alcohol or drug use—require psychiatric intervention as well, and immediate referral must be made. Attention must also be paid to the establishment of a safe environment (e.g., removal of firearms and lethal medications). Families of depressed adolescents may frequently be noncompliant with recommendations to remove guns from the home in spite of compliance with other aspects of treatment. Vigilant follow-up in this regard is crucial. Other management strategies by the primary care provider include provision of community resources, such as hotlines, and commitment to a no-suicide agreement by which the adolescent agrees to refrain from harming himself or herself and promises to notify the caretaker or health care professional if suicidal ideation returns (March et al, 2006).

A major depressive episode requires intervention by a mental health specialist (primary care provider or psychiatrist). Therapies typically include cognitive-behavioral strategies in a group or individual psychotherapy format. There is a growing body of evidence for the effectiveness of CBT in groups for adolescence (Stein et al, 2006). Often, family therapy or psychoeducation is indicated.

A central issue in psychopharmacologic approaches is that children and adolescents are not usually included in clinical drug trial research; safety and efficacy data from the literature about adults are often extrapolated to children. Available studies do not support the efficacy of tricyclic antidepressants for depression in young children, and they may actually be harmful (Cohen et al, 2004). Although a recent "black box" warning has been attached to SSRIs in view of the number of adolescents who have committed suicide while taking SSRIs (Ferren, 2006), fluoxetine (Prozac) has been shown to be most effective in treating moderate to severe depression in adolescents when combined with CBT (Hankin, 2006). Preliminary findings from the recent Treatment for Adolescents with Depression Study (TADS) support the superior efficacy of fluoxetine in combination with CBT. CBT appears to have a protective effect against suicide. Suicidal events were twice as common among adolescents treated with medication alone (Ferren, 2006). Currently, fluoxetine is the only SSRI with FDA approval for use in children 12 years and older. The FDA recommends specifically against the use of paroxetine in children and adolescents because of the 3.5-fold increased risk for suicide.

Prognosis. More than 90% of depressed children and adolescents recover in 1 to 2 years. However, recurrences are common, from 40% to 70%. Comorbidities are common with 30% to 80% of depressed children and adolescents also having an anxiety disorder, 20% to 30% having a substance abuse problem, and 10% to 80% with disruptive conduct of ODD. Many will also complain of physical symptoms not associated with a medical condition or mental health problem.

Bipolar Disorder

Description. Bipolar disorder is characterized by unusual shifts in mood, energy, and functioning and may begin with manic, depressive, or a mixed set of manic and depressive symptoms. There is evidence that depression precedes mania early in the course of bipolar disorder in children and adolescents (Lansford, 2005), with bipolar disorder developing in 20% to 40% of depressed children and adolescents (AACAP, 2007a). It is a recurrent disorder in which nearly all of those (90%) who have a single manic episode will have future episodes.

A characteristic pattern usually evolves for a particular person, with manic episodes preceding or following major depressive episodes. Most individuals with bipolar disorder return to a full level of functioning between episodes; 20% to 30% experience persistent mood lability and interpersonal difficulties (APA, 1994). Sometimes psychotic symptoms develop after several days or weeks of manic symptoms. Such features tend to predict that the individual with subsequent manic episodes will again experience psychotic symptoms.

Epidemiology. There is evidence of a genetic influence for bipolar disorder from twin studies and adoption studies; bipolar disorder tends to cluster in families. Parents who are bipolar are at greater risk for having bipolar children (AACAP, 2007a). Nearly one third of bipolar adults identify significant psychiatric symptoms before 14 years old, most notably

depression. There is no differential incidence based on race, ethnicity, or gender. Children with ADHD seem to be vulnerable to bipolar illness, or it may be that attention-deficit disorder or ADHD is a misdiagnosed early sign of the mania to come. If children are also bipolar, treatment of ADHD with psychostimulants or antidepressants may precipitate a manic episode. Antidepressants in depressed children (6 to 12 years old) may also precipitate mania and the onset of bipolar illness (Jellinek et al, 2002).

Clinical Findings. Bipolar disorder in childhood or early adolescence appears to be a different, more severe form of the illness than occurs with late adolescent or adult onset. The early-onset form is typically characterized by irritability and continuous, rapid-cycling, and mixed-symptom state that may also co-occur with disruptive behavior disorders (e.g., ADHD or CD); features of ADHD or behavior disorder are often early symptoms. This prepubertal and early adolescent bipolar disorder is a fairly homogeneous phenotype, with no differences according to gender, puberty, or comorbid ADHD. In the later-onset form, the hallmark features are a classic manic episode, a more episodic pattern of mania and depression, and more stability between episodes. Symptoms include the following:
- Severe mood changes—extreme irritability or overly elated and silly
- Inflated self-esteem or grandiosity
- Increased energy
- Decreased need for sleep (sleeps few hours or no sleep for days without tiring)
- Talkativeness or compulsion to talk; frequent topic changes or cannot be interrupted
- Distractibility, with attention moving constantly from one thing to another
- Increase in goal-directed activity (socially or at school)
- Physical agitation
- Risk-taking behaviors or activities; taking "more dares"
- Hypersexuality in talk, thoughts, feelings, or behaviors (for those who have reached puberty)

In the context of a family history of bipolar disorder, these symptoms should definitely raise concerns for bipolar disorder in the child. The child or adolescent who has depression but also manifests symptoms of ADHD that seem severe (e.g., extreme temper outbursts and mood changes) should be evaluated by a child psychiatrist with experience in bipolar disorder. Symptoms are manifested in relatively age-specific ways (AACAP, 2007a).

With mania, children appear to the happiest of people and, as with adults, the happiness and laughter must be examined in the context of their history (usually negative). Grandiosity may manifest in efforts to correct teachers or critique their efforts, seeing themselves as above rules and laws, or devoting time to an activity for which they have no talent. Children's sleep difficulties are reflected in high activity levels before bed (e.g., rearranging the furniture), whereas adolescents need little sleep at all. Risk-taking behavior ranges from children climbing excessively high trees or hopping between rooftops to adolescents driving recklessly and speeding. In adolescents, manic episodes are more likely to include psychotic features and may be associated with school truancy, school failure, substance use, or antisocial behavior. No laboratory findings diagnostic of a manic episode have been identified, so a careful history and a thorough assessment are crucial.

Assessment for comorbid conditions often associated with bipolar disorder is important (AACAP, 2007a). Anxiety disorders affect about 30% of prepubertal patients and 10% of adolescent patients with bipolar disorder. CD occurs in 20% of children and adolescents with bipolar disorder as does substance abuse in 10% of school-age bipolar children and 40% of bipolar adolescents (AACAP, 2007a).

Differential Diagnosis.   A manic episode must be distinguished from a mood disorder caused by a medical condition (e.g., brain tumor) and a substance-induced mood disorder (e.g., laughing fits with marijuana, amphetamine highs followed by withdrawal "crashes," perceptual distortions or hallucinations of hallucinogens). ADHD is also characterized by excessive activity, poor impulse control and judgment, and denial of problems that are found with a manic episode. ADHD is distinguished from a manic episode by its lack of clear onset or episodes, absence of mood disturbances, and lack of psychotic features. However, recent evidence that children with ADHD are vulnerable to bipolar disorder and that pharmacologic treatments may precipitate manic episodes points to the need for very careful evaluation and referral to the provider who is treating the ADHD or, preferably, to a child psychiatrist or psychiatric–mental health primary care provider who has experience working with bipolar disorder in youth.

Management.   Referral to a child psychiatrist or child mental health primary care provider is critical. Current recommendations for pharmacologic treatment include the use of mood stabilizers, such as lithium and valproate alone or in combination with the atypical antipsychotics, such as risperidone. Neither antidepressants nor stimulants have proven effective. The use of lithium must be carefully monitored, especially given data that strongly support long-term maintenance on lithium to prevent relapse of bipolar symptoms (AACAP, 2007a).

In combination with pharmacotherapy, psychoeducation and counseling for the entire family are recommended to facilitate the understanding and management of this episodic disorder. This is especially important in light of research findings that living with an intact family improves the recovery rate for children and adolescents with bipolar disorder (Geller et al, 2001).

THE AGGRESSIVE CHILD
Social Aggression
Description.   Social aggression is a pattern of social behavior based primarily on aversive control of situations and others. Onset may occur as early as toddlerhood.

Epidemiology.   Approximately 5% to 6% of U.S. children have behavioral problems with aggression (Copelan, 2006). Acute, stressful life events or transitions can precipitate a brief period of social aggression. A range of antecedents have been found, including a history of maltreatment; inconsistent or harsh discipline, or both; lack of maternal responsiveness; separations from parents, shifts in parent figures, or parental

rejection; and other enduring circumstances. Social aggression can be a precursor to CD or oppositional disorder.

Clinical Findings.   During preschool, social aggression manifests as oppositional or defiant behavior and is considered clinically significant if it interferes with normal developmental functioning (Ruths & Steiner, 2004). The pervasiveness, intensity, and persistence of irritable, argumentative, defiant, and easily annoyed behaviors identify a pathologic condition in contrast to losing one's temper as an expression of developmentally appropriate self-assertions and frustration. The former may be precursors to ODD. In the preschool period, children have a beginning understanding of the impact of their behavior on others and can control their behavior on the basis of internalized norms and developing self-regulation (Keenan & Wakschlag, 2002). When social aggression becomes a pattern, peer rejection is common. Aggressive behavior involves the following:

- Destruction of property
- Name-calling
- Physical pestering and deliberately annoying others
- Hitting, biting, kicking, fighting
- Frequent conflict with peers
- Temper tantrums
- Carrying expectations of others' hostility
- Misinterpreting social cues and responding aggressively
- Lack of problem-solving in social situations
- Use of bad language, swearing, obscene language and gestures
- Arguing for long periods
- Inappropriately suggestive or aggressive sexual behaviors

Differential Diagnosis.   Oppositional disorder is directed primarily toward parents and teachers and is more defiant than aggressive in nature. CD is a clear pattern of behavior established over a 6-month period, typically diagnosed at school age. However, there is growing evidence that preschool children manifest clinically significant disruptive behavior problems, and valid diagnoses of oppositional defiant and CD can be made even in young children. Typical and atypical problems can be differentiated, and, with a developmentally based DSM framework, children with these problems can be identified (Keenan & Wakschlag, 2002).

Management.   It is important to ascertain whether a difficult temperament underlies the behavioral difficulty, especially in conjunction with a lack of fit with parental temperament. A difficult temperament may account for a child's being harder to discipline, having social behavior problems in school (e.g., poor fit with the teacher), or having poor academic achievement. In these situations, the use of positive parenting strategies does not have to change, but supportive counseling for the parents should be provided regarding temperament, its manifestations, and strategies for managing transitions and other difficult times or behaviors. A conference with the teacher may be valuable to provide similar information and to explore strategies to facilitate the child's learning and positive behavior.

When social aggression is a response to acute stress, the problem usually resolves if parents employ positive parenting strategies and facilitate developmentally appropriate coping efforts. If peer-relationship development is hampered, close monitoring of and intervention with peer interactions by day care, preschool, and school personnel, especially with the parents present for observation, enhances appropriate social behavior and competence. Changing schools in an effort to ameliorate problems is not advised because children have been found to carry their social difficulties with them and assume the same roles in new groups. Teachers need to be supportive and facilitative.

When social aggression becomes a pattern of social behavior, referral for intervention is critical. Negative behavior in preschool playgroups is predictive of externalizing behavior problems in the classroom when children are in kindergarten. Substantial research literature supports the stability and persistence of disruptive behavior and aggression from toddlerhood to school age (Keenan & Wakschlag, 2002). Early intervention is essential.

Conduct Disorder

Description. Conduct disorder (CD) is a repetitive and persistent pattern of behavior in which either the basic rights of others or major age-appropriate societal norms and rules are violated (APA, 1994). The onset of aggressive behavior is observed in toddlerhood. Early-onset conduct problems are diagnosed from 4 to 6 years old; a formal diagnosis is typically made when the child is 7 years or older.

Epidemiology. The cause of the disorder rests in chronic negative circumstances, as described for social aggression. CD is frequently associated with a history of harsh discipline, abuse, or neglect. Prevalence rates vary according to the age groups and assessments used for classification. The rates range from 9.3% to 15.8% of boys from 10 to 18 years old and from 3.8% to 9.2% of girls in that age range. Several studies have found that CD was three to four times higher for boys than girls (Loeber et al, 2000). CD accounts for one third to one half of adolescent psychiatric clinic appointments (Boris et al, 2006). However, it is thought that the prevalence data do not accurately reflect the occurrence of CD for females because the diagnostic criteria emphasize physical aggression.

The expression of behavioral dysregulation tends to become notable during the transition from early to middle childhood and is mediated by changes in the structure and demands of the social environment—peers and school settings. There is a high rate of comorbidity with major depression, and the joint presence of CD and depression increases the risk for substance abuse and suicide. ADHD is found to influence the development, course, and severity of CD.

Clinical Findings. In assessment, several factors are relevant to practitioners for their prognostic importance: how atypical the behaviors are for age or gender, how overt versus covert the behaviors are, the nature of any aggression, and the presence of early antisocial or psychopathy-related symptoms. Most common referrals for clinical treatment are for aggressive behavior patterns. Physical aggression toward others includes the following:

- Hitting, kicking, fighting
- Physical cruelty to animals or people
- Physical destruction (including fire setting)
- Frequent temper tantrums
- A high rate of annoying behavior, such as yelling, whining, or threatening

- Disobedience to adult authorities
- Lying, cheating
- Covert stealing
- Truancy and running away from home
- Blaming others for mistakes
- Use or selling of illegal drugs
- Engaging in deviant sexual behaviors (e.g., sexual assault)
- Academic problems

There is growing evidence that preadolescent and adolescent girls manifest CD more indirectly, using verbal and relational aggression, including alienation, ostracism, and character defamation directed at the relational bonds between friends. With CD, social role functioning tends to be impaired, with poor academic performance, poor family and peer relationships, and poor self-management. For adolescent girls, CD is predictive of medical problems and substance abuse in early adulthood.

Differential Diagnosis. Oppositional disorder is characterized by more disobedience than aggressiveness and is evidenced in preschool or early school age. Attention-deficit disorder, with which there is considerable overlap, is characterized by inattention, impulsiveness, and hyperactivity. CD is distinguished from isolated acts of aggressive behavior by the repetitive and persistent pattern over at least 6 months (APA, 1994). A thorough physical examination is essential to rule out organic causes of behavior and to identify evidence of abuse, neglect, and substance abuse disorders.

Management. If aggressive behavior is identified before a CD develops, preventive efforts can be implemented. Successful programs typically address multiple-risk domains, including a parent-directed component (e.g., parent education and support for positive parenting strategies and healthy, consistent approaches to discipline), social-cognitive skills training, proactive classroom management and teacher training, and group therapy (Burke et al, 2002). Once a CD is evident, referral for child and family intervention is crucial.

Safety is a priority in caring for children with aggressive and oppositional disorders. Because of the strong association of child abuse and neglect with CD, it is critical to determine if the child is in safe living conditions. If there is evidence of abuse or neglect, prompt referral to child protective agencies is mandatory. The practitioner must also determine whether other family members are safe from the child's or adolescent's aggressive behavior. Potential interventions when family safety is at risk include referral for inpatient psychiatric evaluation, notification of the police of criminal activity, supporting the family to petition the juvenile court for services, and referral to community health services.

Among the most effective treatments are parent management training (Burke et al, 2002). Videotaped parent training programs, such as those developed by Webster-Stratton in the parenting clinic at the University of Washington School of Nursing, have been found to be effective in the treatment of CD. In a comparison of interventions, a combination of child training groups and parent training was found to produce the most significant improvements in child behavior 1 year later (Webster-Stratton et al, 2004).

For adolescents, the results are generally supportive of family therapy for CD, although there were some negative findings (Lilienfeld, 2005). Collaboration between the family and the school is of critical importance, and the primary care provider can assist with strategies in this regard. Isolated individual treatment has not been found to be superior to parent intervention programs, and, in fact, the results are thought to be rather modest (Burke et al, 2002). In conjunction with parenting interventions, problem-solving skills training as a way of building prosocial behavior has been found to be effective (Lilienfeld, 2005).

Psychopharmacologic intervention tends to be reserved for explosive aggression and includes mood stabilizers, typical and atypical antipsychotics, clonidine, and stimulants; however, few randomized controlled trials have been performed. Effectiveness is not well established, and, given the high risk for substance abuse in those with CD, caution should be exercised in prescribing medications.

Prognosis.   CD in childhood may predict antisocial personality disorder in adulthood. The prediction is stronger among lower socioeconomic status families (Lahey et al, 2005).

Oppositional Defiant Disorder

Description.   Oppositional defiant disorder (ODD) is a pattern of negative, hostile, and defiant behavior that is excessive compared with other children of the same age (AACAP, 2007b; Jellinek et al, 2002). Precursors appear in early childhood, from 3 to 7 years old. The disorder typically begins by 8 years old.

Epidemiology.   Etiologic factors include many of the parenting and family dysfunctions identified for social aggression (AACAP, 2007b). Precursors to the disorder are common in early childhood, especially defiance and negativism. More common in boys before puberty, the gender distribution is approximately equal thereafter. Estimates range from 10% of girls and 14% of boys 10 to 13 years old to 12% of 17- to 20-year-olds. Data on gender differences in ODD during middle childhood and adolescence are inconsistent across studies, with most suggesting either slightly higher rates in boys or no gender differences (Loeber et al, 2000).

Clinical Findings.   The essential feature of ODD is a recurrent pattern of behavior that is negative, defiant, disobedient, and hostile toward authority figures. Behavior is typically directed at family members, teachers, or peers whom the child knows well. The child manifests the following behaviors to an extent that leads to impairment:

- Actively defies or refuses adult requests or rules
- Is argumentative, angry, resentful, touchy, or easily annoyed
- Easily loses temper
- Blames others for own mistakes or difficulties
- Deliberately does things to annoy others

Children often see their own behavior as justifiable, not oppositional or defiant (APA, 1994).

Differential Diagnosis.   CD involves more serious violations of the rights of others.

Management.   Attend to the early signs of defiant and oppositional behavior or aggression, or both, by educating parents about positive parenting strategies and by exercising consistent, healthy discipline, as with the management of CDs.

Because these children typically do not perceive themselves as having a problem and the cause rests with the family system, referral for intervention is indicated. As described for CD, parent training programs are more successful, especially if multiple-risk domains are targeted for intervention. Child training groups provide added benefit if combined with parent training groups. Again, collaboration with the school is important. These multiple approaches, conducted simultaneously, are most effective.

The Shy Child

Description.   Shyness is a pattern of social inhibition with unfamiliar people, with novel objects, or in unfamiliar situations. Inhibition is evident in infancy as an inborn bias to respond to unfamiliar events with anxiety, distress, or disorganization. Shyness appears as a social behavior pattern in toddlerhood, with stability by early school age (Theall-Honey & Schmidt, 2006). Although most shy children do not develop later internalizing disorders, extremely shy toddlers may be at risk for becoming socially withdrawn in later childhood and for developing an anxiety disorder in adolescence (Cox et al, 2005).

Epidemiology.   Shyness is caused by a rather stable temperamental disposition toward withdrawal that is linked to family factors. Shyness is common. Behavioral inhibition in social situations may be adaptive if handled effectively by the parent and can be indicative of optimal self-regulation and development of conscience.

Clinical Findings.   Retreat and withdrawal from social stimulation are noted in infancy. In toddlerhood, general inhibition persists, evidenced by irritability, withdrawal, and clinging to the mother in new situations. Shy children are slower to approach peers or initiate play with an unfamiliar child and often spend more time observing the situation and other children in play before engaging. School-age shy children continue to make fewer social approaches. They usually "warm up slowly" or may engage in solitary but appropriate play. Viewed by their peers as likable but shy, these children may be neglected by their peers. One or both parents usually identify themselves as shy (Burgess et al, 2006).

Differential Diagnosis.   Children with social withdrawal rather than shyness have a lower rate of social interaction overall and do not warm up to social situations.

Management.   Parenting strategies that provide warmth, sensitivity, and responsiveness to the child's inhibition and shyness will foster security in attachment relationships and facilitate social competence. In preschool and school-age children, insensitivity and a lack of responsiveness foster a sense of insecurity and predict social withdrawal, with associated internalizing disorders, including depression and adolescent anxiety. It is helpful to have parents prepare shy children for new situations by visiting new settings, identifying a sensitive adult to whom they may turn with requests or concerns, and negotiating for them to be allowed to watch and observe before engaging in play or other activities.

Social Withdrawal

Description.   Social withdrawal is a pattern of social behavior characterized by a low rate of social interaction with peers. Onset occurs in school-age children. Some withdrawn children avoid peers because of their own fearfulness, some simply prefer to play alone, and some are socially unskilled and are rejected by their peers (not allowed to play).

Epidemiology. A rather stable inhibited temperament is usually antecedent and linked to a lack of family sensitivity and warmth, with consequent insecurity, or to a highly stressful experience or an exacerbation of stressful life events. Social withdrawal is less common than shyness.

Clinical Findings. Socially withdrawn children have low interaction with peers; they make few social approaches and demonstrate limited or compliant (or both) responses to initiations by peers. These children tend to engage more often in solitary play. In group play, they are less communicative, deferential, submissive, and immature. Initially, socially withdrawn children may appear shy, but, unlike shy children, they do not warm up to social situations. Preschoolers are described as anxious and fearful. In early school age, similar patterns persist with poor social functioning. By middle childhood, social anxiety and low self-esteem are more prominent, and, by late childhood, depressive symptoms become evident. Peer rejection is common, and social problem-solving skills are poorly developed.

Differential Diagnosis. A differential diagnosis is depression, which is usually not diagnosed until the child is 10 years old. Anxiety is another differential diagnosis and has been found in children as young as 6 years old in relation to poor social functioning. The severity of symptoms may warrant a diagnosis of social phobia.

Management. The key is to intervene as early as possible to prevent the negative consequences of poor social development. Addressing any acute or chronic life events alleviates the source of the problem. In addition, parent education and positive parenting strategies support efforts to restore social behavior. Confidence-boosting social experiences can be developed, such as opportunities to interact with or help younger playmates. Such situations provide opportunities for self-assertion and successful play. Similarly, assigning responsibilities in the social setting can serve to enhance the withdrawn child's social behavior (e.g., introducing and orienting a new child). Finally, structured intervention, such as assertiveness training and social skills training, might be necessary. Friendships have been found to mediate social withdrawal, especially in late childhood (10 years and older) (Guerro et al, 2003). Small-group interventions with socially withdrawn girls have been effective for developing social skills and friendships (Houck & Stember, 2002).

BEREAVEMENT

Description

Bereavement is the sad or lonely state resulting from loss or death. Grief is the effect of bereavement and typically involves distress, sorrow, and painful regret. Mourning is the psychological process set in motion by loss of a loved one. The death of someone important to a child is considered one of the most stressful events to be experienced. For children and adolescents, death of a parent or sibling is the most profoundly disturbing.

Epidemiology

The clinical picture of bereavement and grief depends, to some extent, on the concept of death. In infancy and toddlerhood, death is perceived as separation or abandonment, with no real cognitive understanding of death or the emotional resources to deal with loss; the central issue is the sense of loss or abandonment resulting from disruption in caretaking or an attachment relationship (Cerel et al, 2006). Preschoolers, up to 6 years old, tend to perceive death as a continuation of life under different circumstances. Death is personified and perceived as a punishment (AAP, 2000). From 6 to 11 years old, children grasp the irreversibility and finality of death, akin to the adult concept, although they struggle with understanding the specific loss of the loved one. Preadolescents and adolescents are able to be more abstract and philosophic about death. At any given developmental stage, a child can resolve the impact of the death only at that developmental level. Thus bereavement resurfaces, and the significance of the loss needs to be reworked at each subsequent developmental stage. It is expected that most children and adolescents experience at least one significant loss before they reach adulthood. It is estimated that 5% of children lose one or both parents to death before 15 years old.

Clinical Findings

Infants and toddlers cry out or search for the absent caregiver, refuse the attempts of others to soothe them, withdraw emotionally, appear sad, and no longer engage in age-appropriate activities. Sleep and feeding are disturbed; they display developmental regression and demonstrate extreme reactions to reminders of the missing caregiver through apathy, anger, or crying.

For a child, grief is a process that unfolds over time. Initially, children may seem emotionally unmoved, but the initial shock and denial will give way to depressive symptoms that can last for weeks or months. A normal reaction to loss, depressive symptoms include sadness, feeling depressed, poor appetite, weight loss, insomnia, crying, anxiety, guilt, and idealization of the person who died. Rage is a common reaction to the death of a parent, typically directed at the surviving parent and others in the immediate family. Angry behavior may be directed at peers as well, compounding a sense of inferiority and alienation. Fears of dying, disease, and growing old are often stimulated. Identification with the deceased is common and needs to be assessed to determine whether this furthers or inhibits development. Similarly, a fantasy connection to a dead parent can develop and may be helpful. Guilt and responsibility are typical issues for children but are less problematic for adolescents. Adolescents often manifest a sudden "maturity" along with numbness, regrets, disorganization, and despair before closure and reorganization are achieved. It is not unusual for adolescents to develop stronger ties with friends and to distance from family while grieving.

Differential Diagnosis

Children at high risk for pathologic bereavement or depression generally have a previous history of individual and family problems. Symptoms of bereavement that should concern the provider include the following:

- Long-term denial and avoidance of feelings
- Suicidal wishes
- Preoccupation with death
- Distressing guilt about actions taken or not taken
- Preoccupation with worthlessness
- Persistent anger
- Decline in school performance
- Social withdrawal
- Persistent sleep problems
- Hallucinations beyond transitory experience of hearing the voice of, or seeing the image of, the deceased

Management

Parent education can facilitate effective management of bereavement in children and adolescents. A first question is typically whether children and adolescents should attend the funeral or memorial service. Children need to be allowed to participate in the rituals around death as much as they choose. Such services and rituals provide even young children with an important way to grieve, especially if such involvement is supportive, appropriately explained, and congruent with the family's values.

Children need parental help to understand the facts of death and to correct misunderstandings as they develop; children cannot understand, however, beyond their cognitive level. Parents often need to be reassured that their showing of feelings (e.g., disbelief, guilt, sadness, anger) is normal and helpful to children; sharing feelings about and memories of the family member who died is helpful as well (AAP, 2000). Sensitivity to the child's reactions of grief and restlessness is important, as is support for the child's assimilation and mastery of the loss and emotional experience. Children need to express and work through feelings and fantasies related to the loss; open communication is a must.

There are many books about death, loss, and grieving available for children and adolescents that are geared to the various developmental levels. It is critical for children to have an attachment to an adult who can be an effective source of support and involvement, as well as a focus for reactions to loss (AAP, 2000). The child must be sensitively prepared for any changes occurring at the same time as the death, with the family advised to minimize these as much as possible. Any parental loss before 5 years old probably warrants treatment. Because bereavement resurfaces at subsequent developmental phases, early parental loss should be determined and current symptoms assessed as a possible manifestation of recurring bereavement issues.

SUBSTANCE ABUSE

Description

Substance use is a precursor to abuse or dependence, and regular use clearly increases the risk for developing a substance use disorder (SUD). However, the use of substances per se is not sufficient for a diagnosis of SUD (AACAP, 2005). Substance abuse is a maladaptive pattern of the use of alcohol or drugs manifested in significant impairment or distress. The criteria for substance dependence in adults include tolerance, withdrawal, and compulsive drug use. For children and adolescents, tolerance and loss of control are not good indicators for a diagnosis. Instead, alcohol-related blackouts, craving, and impulsive sexual or risk-taking behavior tend to be more important criteria (AACAP, 2005). Twenty-five percent of students had drunk alcohol for the first time before 13 years old, and about 25% reported episodic heavy drinking in the 2005 Youth Risk Behavior Surveillance report (Eaton et al, 2006). However, nearly half of problem drinkers are thought to have tried alcohol by 10 years old and two thirds by 13 years old. The percentage of students reporting lifetime use of alcohol, marijuana, steroids, methamphetamines, and hallucinogenic drugs has decreased since 2001 to 2003, although those reporting current use of cocaine and amphetamines has not changed significantly (Eaton et al, 2006).

Epidemiology

The cause of SUD is multifaceted (AACAP, 2005). Many contributing factors exist, including the following:

- Genetic vulnerability (family history)
- Parental substance use
- Dysfunctional family relationships, such as rigidity, distant relationships, neglect, or lack of supervision
- Negative life events
- Psychiatric conditions (e.g., CD, ADHD, depression)
- Low self-esteem, poor body image
- Ineffective coping (poor emotional regulation, poor problem-solving skills)
- School failure
- Rigid, teetotaler, ultraconservative families
- Latchkey child
- Poor sleep hygiene
- Low religiosity
- Sexual activity
- Homosexuality, bisexuality
- Competitive athleticism

Precipitating life events tend to center around loss of relationships (e.g., parental separation, divorce, or death; death of a close friend) and chronic negative circumstances (e.g., parental substance abuse, maltreatment).

There is no question that primary care providers see children and adolescents with SUDs given that 1 in 5 teens is a current alcohol user and 1 in 10 adolescents 12 to 17 years old is a current illicit drug user. Approximately 32% of 18- to 25-year-olds binge drink. By the end of high school, 90% of students have tried alcohol and more than 40% have tried an illicit substance (AACAP, 2005). The majority of adolescents who use drugs do not progress to abuse or dependence. Peer influence seems to be less significant to the cause of substance abuse than previously thought. Boys tend to be more involved in use of both alcohol and drugs of all kinds than girls are at the same age. It is estimated that, for both boys and girls, abuse of alcohol and other drugs is negligible from 10 to 13 years old, but doubles between midadolescence (12 to 16 years old) and late adolescence (17 to 20 years old), peaks between 18 and 25 years old, and declines thereafter (Eaton et al, 2006).

Clinical Findings

Identifying an adolescent's problem with substance abuse requires a careful assessment, conducted with an accepting, nonjudgmental, nonthreatening, matter-of-fact attitude. The covert nature of substance abuse and the dynamic of denial make it crucial to avoid a critical tone (see Chapter 8 for discussion of adolescent risk behavior). Research shows that fewer than 50% of pediatricians screen adolescent patients for substance abuse (Kulig et al, 2005).

History.   Interviewing the adolescent with the parents is a key strategy for obtaining information about etiologic factors and behavioral, cognitive, emotional, and physical changes they have observed in the adolescent. However, it is essential that the adolescent also be interviewed alone at every visit to assess mental health and family issues.

When talking about substance use with an adolescent, it is important to begin with general questions that are not overly personal. Begin by asking the adolescent about acquaintances or friends who smoke, drink, or use drugs; whether anyone in the family has had problems with these; and what the adolescent does with friends when they get together. It is helpful to ask about experimentation, under what circumstances it occurs, and the adolescent's feelings about it. To obtain a chronologic history of tobacco, alcohol, or drug use, it may be helpful to approach the subject by inquiring about prescription drugs and moving to illicit substances. The key is to remain nonjudgmental to elicit information that will indicate whether the adolescent is experimenting, a regular user, or dependent on substances. A helpful question asks about the adolescent's source of drugs or alcohol; the adolescent who uses substances provided by a friend or acquaintance is less advanced than one who purchases them directly. The practitioner should ask: What? How much? How often? When? How? Where? With whom? Does the patient use substances at parties, home, school, alone, or with friends?

A two-item conjoint screening test (TICS) for alcohol and other drug problems has been developed for adults, including 18- to 20-year-olds (Dias, 2002). The TICS asks:
- "In the last year, have you ever drunk or used drugs more than you meant to?"
- "Have you felt you wanted or needed to cut down on your drinking or drug use in the last year?"

In a primary care setting, respondents who replied to both items with "no" had a 7.4% chance of having a current SUD, those with one positive response had a 45.5% chance of having a current SUD, and those with positive responses to both items had a 75% chance of having a current SUD (Dias, 2002). This may also be helpful for screening adolescents because such assessments typically do not account for developmental differences in substance use patterns.

Significant behavioral changes that may reflect drug use include the following:
- Lethargy, hyperactivity or agitation, hypervigilance
- Disinhibition; deviant or risk-taking behavior
- Repeated absences from school; suspensions from school
- Decline in academic performance
- Loss of interest in previously enjoyed activities
- Withdrawal from family and usual friends
- Change in friends to those involved in drugs and alcohol
- Angry or violent outbursts
- Early sexual activity

Parents may also be able to report on changes in personal habits, such as the following:
- Altered sleep pattern (lack of or excessive sleep)
- Loss of appetite
- Less attention to hygiene
- Use of eyedrops

Cognitive changes may include the following:
- Impaired concentration
- Changes in attention span
- Perceptual and overt changes in thinking (e.g., paranoia, delusions)

Mood changes include swings from depression to euphoria, nervousness, unreasonable anger, and frequent expressions of hopelessness or failure. Low self-esteem typically characterizes those who abuse substances.

Physical Examination.   Physical signs that indicate a substance use problem include the following:
- Weight loss
- Red eyes are associated with marijuana use
- Hoarseness, chronic cough, wheezing occur with use of inhalants and cocaine
- Frequent "colds" or "allergy" symptoms, epistaxis, and perforations of nasal septum occur with cocaine and inhalant use
- Accidents, trauma, injuries
- Intoxication
- Complete or partial amnesia for events during intoxication occur with alcohol and date rape drug use
- Dilated or constricted pupils
- Gynecomastia, irregular periods, small testes occur with marijuana
- Needle tracks occur with IM steroids or IV heroin use
- Generalized pruritus occurs with opiate use
- Reflux, diarrhea, gastritis, and constipation occur with opiate and alcohol use
- Perioral sores or pyodermas occur from huffing and bagging

Laboratory Studies

Urine toxicology can be helpful to verify adolescent truthfulness, although a positive drug screen result does not indicate substance abuse or dependence, but only indicates substance use. A negative drug screen result does not rule out an SUD. The approximate duration that drugs can be detected in the urine is as follows (AACAP, 2005):
- Stimulants—1 to 2 days
- Cocaine and its major metabolite—1 to 3 days
- Sedative-hypnotics—1 day to 1 week
- Barbiturates—2 to 4 weeks
- Quaaludes—2 to 3 weeks
- Opiates—1 to 2 days
- Marijuana—up to 30 days

Duration of detection from last substance use varies according to the laboratory and type of test used. The AACAP recommends that, to obtain a valid result, a positive result on immunoassay should be followed by confirmation with a more sensitive method, such as gas chromatography or mass spectrometry.

Differential Diagnosis

Substance abuse is distinguished from social drinking or non-pathologic substance use by the presence of compulsive use, craving, or substance-related problems (AACAP, 2005). SUDs are comorbid most often with CD, depression, and anxiety.

Management

Exposure to tobacco and alcohol and illicit substances begins in early childhood. The pediatric primary care provider should discuss parental modeling for the use of alcohol, tobacco products, and other substances in early childhood during routine well-child visits (Joffe, 2006). It has become more important to provide education to school-age children and their parents about substance use and its consequences. For adolescents, a direct assessment and an interview about substance use are essential. Parents should be advised not to involve their child in their own substance use. Something as seemingly innocuous as "getting dad a beer from the refrigerator" gives the child practice in alcohol use.

Substance abuse must be treated, and referral to a substance abuse program is crucial. However, the initial goal may be best defined as helping adolescents take positive steps toward changing their substance use and abuse behavior (Levy et al, 2002). If the adolescent denies any problem, efforts should focus on helping the adolescent acknowledge problems. Clarifying reported negative consequences, creating doubts about substance use, and raising awareness of the risks related to current use are motivational interviewing strategies that may be helpful. It is important to remain empathetic and yet emphasize the adolescent's responsibility to make healthy choices. If the adolescent has not reached a level of chronic use, prevention of harm is the goal of the intervention. Guide the adolescent to examine his or her substance use responsibly and identify ways to prevent harmful consequences.

If the adolescent has progressed to chronic substance use, a number of options exist. Outpatient or day treatment programs are effective for those who can live and be managed at home. For adolescents with more serious addiction, comorbid psychiatric conditions, or suicidal ideation, residential treatment or hospitalization may be necessary. Given the prominence of family dysfunction and family life events in the cause of the problem, family-based treatment programs are essential. Family treatment, rather than family psychoeducation or family support groups, has been shown to be superior to other modalities. Follow-up assessments should include substance use issues and other predictors of use: stress or negative life events, depression or negative affect regulation, and the presence of positive support within or outside of the family. Self-help or 12-step groups are thought to be an essential element in the recovery process.

■ SUMMARY

The prevalence of social, emotional, and mental health disorders among children has increased with primary care professionals providing a large portion of care for these disorders. High-quality care depends on an accurate assessment and diagnosis for direction. A Resource Box with websites is provided at the end of this chapter to assist primary care providers in caring for this important dimension of pediatric health.

New resources include the release of the completely revised third edition of the *Bright Futures Health Supervision Guidelines*. Special emphasis on the promotion of mental health is evident throughout the text and accompanying resources. Work has begun on a revision of DSM criteria. Health professionals may sign up for a newsletter update on anticipated changes at *www.dsm5.org*.

NURSING DIAGNOSES

Related to the Coping–Stress Tolerance Functional Health Pattern

Diagnoses are related to the concepts: posttrauma responses, rape-trauma, posttrauma response, fear, anxiety, sorrow, denial, adjustment, coping, self-mutilation, and violence.

- Anticipatory grieving
- Anxiety
- Chronic
  - Compromised family coping
  - Disabled family coping
  - Readiness for enhanced family coping
- Death anxiety
- Defensive coping
- Depressive episode (DSM-IV diagnosis)
- Dysfunctional grieving
- Fear
- Impaired adjustment
- Ineffective coping
- Readiness for enhanced coping
- Ineffective community coping
  - Readiness for enhanced community coping
- Ineffective denial
- Rape-trauma syndrome—silent reaction or compound reaction
- Relocation stress syndrome
- Risk for suicide
- Risk for violence (other-directed or self-directed)
- Self-mutilation
  - Risk for self-mutilation
- Substance misuse or abuse (not a NANDA diagnosis)
- Posttrauma syndrome
  - Risk for posttrauma syndrome
- Disorganized infant behavior
  - Readiness for enhanced organized infant behavior

From NANDA International: *NANDA-I nursing diagnoses: definitions & classification 2007-2008*, Philadelphia, 2007, Author.

*R*ESOURCE BOX

Internet Resources for Infant, Child, and Adolescent Mental Health

NATIONAL ORGANIZATIONS
American Academy of Child and Adolescent Psychiatry
www.aacap.org

American Academy of Pediatrics
www.aap.org

Bright Futures: Mental Health
www.brightfutures.org/mentalhealth

National Institute of Mental Health
www.nimh.nih.gov

INFANT AND EARLY CHILDHOOD MENTAL HEALTH
Ounce of Prevention Fund
www.ounceofprevention.org

Zero to Three
www.zerotothree.org

CHILD AND ADOLESCENT MENTAL HEALTH
About Our Kids
www.aboutourkids.org

KidsHealth
www.kidshealth.org

Substance Abuse and Mental Health Services
Administration
www.family.samhsa.gov

Talking With Kids About Tough Issues
www.talkwithkids.org

CHILDREN WITH SPECIAL HEALTH CARE NEEDS
Bright Futures for Families
www.brightfuturesforfamilies.org

Family Voices
www.familyvoices.org

☑ DISCUSSION FORUM

1. Conduct a mental health assessment on a school-age child of your choice. Be sure to include stressors, parent-child interaction, and social, emotional, and behavioral development assessment. How would your assessment be different if the child was an adolescent?

2. A concerned parent brings in her 3-year-old daughter because the child is "terrified of dogs." Further questioning reveals that the child cries and clings to the parent anytime she sees a dog. There is no prior history of dog bite or attack, and the parents "can't figure where this came from" since they are both dog lovers. The child's growth and development are normal. The child's fears have become so intense that the family no longer visits the grandmother's home since she owns two dogs. What management will you provide? Would the management be different if the child were 8 years old, and her fear kept her from playing outside or taking the school bus because of fear of encountering a dog? If so, how?

3. You see a 7-year-old child, MJ, in your office for a well visit. During the last 12 months, the parent reports that MJ has become more "clingy." He will separate from his parents as long as he can see them near by. For example, his mother reports that MJ will play soccer, but will turn around every 3 to 5 minutes to make eye contact with his mother and becomes quite agitated if he cannot find her in the crowd. Despite earlier excitement about the plans, MJ declined going to Boy Scout camp because his mother could not attend the overnight session. Lastly, his mother reports that MJ has begun to have significant nightmares approximately four times a week, and MJ has moved from his bedroom to a pallet at the floor of the parent's bed because he is now afraid to go to sleep. What management do you suggest? Be sure to include pharmacologic and nonpharmacologic interventions where appropriate.

4. You are asked to speak to a Parent Teacher Association at a local elementary school following a recent, well-publicized traumatic event in the community (weather-related, terrorism, child abduction, etc.). Specifically the group is interested in learning about how children between first and eighth grade respond to trauma and how parents can help their children to cope. Create an educational plan for this meeting, making sure you identify normal and dysfunctional responses.

5. SH is a premenarchal 12-year-old female who has a 6-week complaint of difficulty concentrating, loss of appetite, and insomnia. Her mother notes that SH has stopped talking to her friends and seems "very withdrawn." There are no recent changes in the family and no history of trauma. What are the appropriate steps to evaluate this child for depression? What management will you recommend?

6. You receive a phone call from the parent of a 3-year-old child who has been asked to leave his preschool because of fighting with the children and teachers, biting his classmates, and "dramatic" temper tantrums that often result in him throwing objects at others. His mother reports that he has "always been a difficult child" and does not respond to verbal redirection and time outs "like his older brother does." In addition, he has always been a "physical child" and will often hit and push older children when angered. What disorder do you suspect, and what will be your management of this child?

REFERENCES

Akin LK: Pediatric and adolescent bipolar disorder: medical resources, *Med Ref Ser Q* 20:31-44, 2001.

Als H et al: The assessment of preterm infants' behavior (APIB): furthering the understanding and measurement of neurodevelopmental competence in preterm and full-term infants, *Mental Retard Develop Disab Res Rev* 11:194-102, 2005.

Als H et al: A three-center, randomized, controlled trial of individualized developmental care for very low birthweight preterm infants: medical, neurodevelopmental, parenting, and caregiving effects, *J Devel Behav Pediatr* 24:399-408, 2003.

American Academy of Child and Adolescent Psychiatry (AACAP): *Practice parameters for the assessment and treatment of children and adolescents with anxiety disorders,* 2006. Available at *www.aacap.org* (accessed Dec 27, 2006).

American Academy of Child and Adolescent Psychiatry (AACAP): Practice parameters for the assessment and treatment of children and adolescents with bipolar disorders, *J Am Acad Child Adolesc Psychiatry* 46:107-125, 2007a.

American Academy of Child and Adolescent Psychiatry (AACAP): Practice parameters for the assessment and treatment of children and adolescents with oppositional defiant disorder, *J Am Acad Child Adolesc Psychiatry* 46:126-141, 2007b.

American Academy of Child and Adolescent Psychiatry (AACAP): Practice parameters for the assessment and treatment of children and adolescents with PTSD, *J Am Acad Child Adolesc Psych* 37(10S):4S-26S, 1998.

American Academy of Child and Adolescent Psychiatry (AACAP): Practice parameters for the assessment and treatment of children and adolescents with substance use disorders, *J Am Acad Child Adolesc Psychiatry* 44:609-621, 2005.

American Academy of Pediatrics, Committee on Psychosocial Aspects of Child and Family Health: The pediatrician and childhood bereavement, *Pediatrics* 105:445-447, 2000.

American Psychiatric Association (APA): *Diagnostic and statistical manual of mental disorders,* ed 4, Washington, DC, 1994, American Psychiatric Association.

Blair C, Granger C, Peters R: Cortisol reactivity is positively related to executive function in preschool children attending head start, *Child Dev* 76:554-567, 2005.

Bledsoe JM, Johnson BD: Preparing families for international adoption, *Pediatr Rev* 25:242-249, 2004.

Boris N, Dalton R, Forman M: Mood disorders. In Behrman R, Kliegman R, Jenson H, editors: *Nelson textbook of pediatrics,* Philadelphia, 2004a, WB Saunders.

Boris N, Dalton R, Forman M: Disruptive behavioral disorders. In Behrman R, Kliegman R, Jenson H, editors: *Nelson textbook of pediatrics,* Philadelphia, 2006, WB Saunders.

Bosch J et al: Promoting a healthy tomorrow here for children adopted from abroad, *Contemp Pediatr* 20:69-70, 73-74, 77, 2003.

Burgess KB et al: Social information processing and coping strategies of shy/withdrawn and aggressive children: does friendship matter? *Child Dev* 77:371-383, 2006.

Burke JD, Loeber R, Birmaher B: Oppositional defiant disorder and conduct disorder: a review of the past 10 years, part II, *J Am Acad Child Adolesc Psychiatry* 41:1275-1293, 2002.

Carmody DP et al: Early risk, attention, and brain activation in adolescents born preterm, *Child Dev* 77:384-394, 2006.

Catallozzi M et al: Prevention of suicide in adolescents, *Curr Opinion Pediatr* 13:417-422, 2001.

Cerel J et al: Childhood bereavement: psychopathology in the 2 years postparental death, *J Am Acad Child Adolesc Psychiatry* 45:681-690, 2006.

Cohen D et al: Pharmacological treatment of adolescent major depression, *J Child Adolesc Psychopharmacol* 14:19-31, 2004.

Compas BE et al: Coping with stress during childhood and adolescence: problems, progress, and potential in theory and research, *Psychol Bull* 127:87-127, 2001.

Copelan R: Assessing the potential for violent behavior in children and adolescents, *Pediatr Rev* 27:e36-e41, 2006.

Cox BJ, MacPherson PSR, Enns MW: Psychiatric correlates of childhood shyness, *Behav Res Ther* 43:1019-1027, 2005.

Dahl RE: Adolescent brain development: a period of vulnerabilities and opportunities, *Ann NY Acad Sci* 1021:1-22, 2004.

De Kloet ER, Derjik R: Signaling pathways in brain involved in predisposition and pathogenesis of stress-related disease, *Ann NY Acad Sci* 1032:14-34, 2004.

Dias PJ: Adolescent substance abuse: assessment in the office, *Pediatr Clin N Am* 49:269-300, 2002.

Eaton DK et al: Youth risk behavior surveillance—United States, 2005, *Morbidity and Mortality Weekly Rep* 55(SS-5), June 9, 2006.

Egger HL, Angold A: Anxiety disorders. In Luby JL, editor: *Handbook of preschool mental health,* New York, 2006, Guilford Press.

Eluvathingal TJ et al: Abnormal brain connectivity in children after early severe socioemotional deprivation: a diffusion tensor imaging study, *Pediatrics* 117:2093-2100, 2006.

Emde RN, Everhart KD, Wise BK: Therapeutic relationships in infant mental health and the concept of leverage. In Sameroff AJ, McDonough SC, Rosenblum KL, editors: *Treating parent-infant relationship problems,* New York, 2005, Guilford Press.

Eyberg SM, Ross AW: Assessment of child behavior problems: the validation of a new inventory, *J Clin Child Psychol* 7:113-116, 1978.

Ferren PM: Demystifying the black box warning on antidepressants, *Contemp Pediatr* 23:28-35, 2006.

Field T, Diego M, Hernandez-Reif M: Prenatal depression effects on the fetus and newborn: a review, *Infant Behav Dev* 29:445-455, 2006.

Forum on Child and Family Statistics: *America's children report,* 2006. Available at *Childstats.gov/americaschildren* (accessed Feb 14, 2007).

Freund PJ et al: Healthcare and early intervention collaborative supports for families and young children, *Infants Young Child* 18:25-36, 2005.

Furman L, O'Riordan MA: Mothers' feelings about their very low birth weight infants, *Infant Ment Health J* 26:153-172, 2005.

Geller B et al: Adult psychosocial outcome of prepubertal major depressive disorder, *J Am Acad Child Adolesc Psychiatry* 40:673-677, 2001.

Giedd JN: Structural magnetic resonance imaging of the adolescent brain, *Ann NY Acad Sci* 1021:77-85, 2004.

Ginsburg GS, Riddle MA, Davies M: Somatic symptoms in children and adolescents with anxiety disorders, *J Am Acad Child Adolesc Psychiatry* 45:1179-1187, 2006.

Gomez CR, Baird S, Jung L: Regulatory dysfunction disorder: identification, diagnosis, and intervention planning, *Infants Young Child* 17:327-339, 2004.

Goodman M, New A, Siever L: Trauma, genes, and neurobiology of personality disorders, *Ann NY Acad Sci* 1032:104-116, 2004.

Green M, Sullivan P, Eichberg C: Avoid a "Swiss-cheese" history when psychosocial complaints are on the menu, *Contemp Pediatr* 19:115-125, 2002.

Gross JJ: *Handbook of emotion regulation,* New York, 2007, Guilford Press.

Guerro PS, Derauf C, Nguyen MAK: Early detection and intervention for common causes of psychosocial morbidity and mortality in children and adolescents, *Pediatr Ann* 32:408-412, 2003.

Gunnar MR, Cheatham CL: Brain and behavior interface: stress and the developing brain, *Infant Ment Health J* 24:195-211, 2003.

Gutgesell ME: Issues of adolescent psychological development in the 21st century, *Pediatr Rev* 25:70-884, 2004.

Hacker KA et al: Mental health screening in pediatric practice: factors related to positive screens and the contribution of parental/personal concern, *Pediatrics* 118:1896-1906, 2006.

Hankin B: Adolescent depression: description, causes, and interventions, *Epilepsy Behav* 8:102-114, 2006.

Hanna Gl, Fischer DJ, Fluent TE: Separation anxiety disorder and school refusal in children and adolescents, *Pediatr Rev* 27:56-62, 2006.

Hass S, Cauther NK: *Who are America's poor children: the official story,* 2006. Available at *www.nccp/publications/pub_684.html* (accessed Dec 10, 2006).

Holditch-Davis D, Belyea M, Edwards LJ: Prediction of 3-year developmental outcomes from sleep development over the preterm period, *Infant Behav Dev* 28:118-131, 2004.

Houck GM, LeCuyer-Maus EA: Maternal limit-setting patterns and toddler development of self-concept and social competence, *Issues Compr Pediatr Nurs* 25:21-41, 2001.

Houck GM, LeCuyer-Maus EA: Maternal limit-setting during toddlerhood, and delay of gratification and behavior problems at age five, *Infant Ment Health J* 25:28-46, 2004.

Houck GM, Stember L: Small group experience for socially withdrawn girls, *J Sch Nurs* 18:206-211, 2002.

Hudson JL, Deveney C, Taylor BA: Nature, assessment, and treatment of generalized anxiety disorder in children, *Pediatr Ann* 34:97-106, 2005.

In-Albon T, Schneider S: Psychotherapy of childhood anxiety disorders: a meta-analysis, *Psychother Psychosom* 76(1):15-24, 2007.

Jellinek M, Patel BP, Froehle MC, editors: *Bright Futures in practice: mental health,* vol 1, *Practice guide,* Arlington, VA, 2002, National Center for Education in Maternal and Child Health.

Joffe A: Your role in curbing prescription and OTC drug abuse by adolescents, *Contemp Pediatr* 23:97-101, 2006.

Jursberg N, Ledley DR: Separation anxiety disorder, *Pediatr Ann* 34:108-115, 2005.

Karr C, Kline S: Homeless children: what every clinician should know, *Pediatr Rev* 25:235-240, 2004.

Keenan K, Wakschlag L: Can a valid diagnosis of disruptive behavior disorder be made in preschool children? *Am J Psychiatry* 159:351-358, 2002.

Koball H, Douglas-Hall A: *The new poor: regional variation in child poverty since 2000.* Available at *www.nccp.org/publications/pub_672.html.* (accessed Dec 10, 2006).

Kulig J, Committee on Substance Abuse, American Academy of Pediatrics: Tobacco, alcohol and other drugs: the role of the pediatrician in prevention, identification, and management of substance abuse, *Pediatrics* 115:816-821, 2005.

Lahey B et al: Predicting future antisocial personality disorder in males from a clinical assessment in childhood, *J Consulting Clin Psychol* 73:389-399, 2005.

Lansford AH: The importance of recognizing a child with bipolar disorder, *Contemp Pediatr* 22:69-78, 2005.

Levy S, Vaughan BL, Knight JR: Office-based intervention for adolescent substance abuse, *Pediatr Clin North Am* 49:329-343, 2002.

Lewin et al: Current directions in pediatric obsessive-compulsive disorder, *Pediatr Ann* 34:129-134, 2005.

Lieberman A et al: Angels in the nursery: the intergenerational transmission of benevolent parental influences, *Infant Ment Health J* 26:504-520, 2005.

Lilienfeld SO: Scientifically unsupported and supported interventions for childhood psychopathology: a summary, *Pediatrics* 115:761-764, 2005.

Lloyd CM, Rosman E: Exploring mental health outcomes for low income mothers of children with special needs, *Infants Young Child* 18:186-100, 2005.

Loeber R et al: Oppositional defiant and conduct disorder: a review of the past 10 years, part I, *J Am Acad Child Adolesc Psychiatry* 39:1468-1484, 2000.

Luby JL, Belden AC: Mood disorders. In Luby JL, editor: *Handbook of preschool mental health,* New York, 2006, Guilford Press.

March J et al: The Treatment for Adolescents with Depression Study (TADS): methods and message at 12 weeks, *J Am Acad Child Adolesc Psychiatry* 45:1393-1403, 2006.

Masi R, Cooper JL: *Children's mental health: facts for policymakers,* 2006. Available at *www.nccp/publications/pub_687.html* (accessed Dec 10, 2006).

McDonough SC: Interaction guidance: promoting and nurturing the caregiving relationship. In Sameroff AJ, McDonough SC, Rosenblum KL, editors: *Treating parent-infant relationship problems,* New York, 2005, Guilford Press.

McEwen BS: Protection and damage from acute and chronic stress, *Ann NY Acad Sci* 1032:1-7, 2004.

McLearn KT et al: The timing of maternal depressive symptoms and mothers' parenting practices with young children: implications for pediatric practice, *Pediatrics* 118:e174-e182, 2006.

Melendez L: Parental beliefs and practices around early self-regulation, *Infants Young Child* 18:136-146, 2005.

Melnyk BM et al: Improving the mental/psychosocial health of U.S. children and adolescent: outcomes and implementation strategies from the national KySS summit, *J Pediatr Health Care* 17:S1-S24, 2003.

Mesman J, Koot HM: Common and specific correlates of preadolescent internalizing and externalizing psychopathology, *J Abnorm Psychol* 109:428-437, 2002.

Merlo LJ et al: Assessment of pediatric obsessive-compulsive disorder: a critical review of current methodology, *Child Psychiatry Human Dev* 36(2):195-214, 2005.

Minkovitz CS et al: Maternal depressive symptoms and children's receipt of health care in the first 3 years of life, *Pediatrics* 115:306-314, 2005.

Myers K, Winters NC: Ten-year review of rating scales. II. Scales for internalizing disorders, *J Am Acad Child Adolesc Psychiatry* 41:634-659, 2002.

Paulson JF, Dauber S, Leiferman JA: Individual and combined effects of postpartum depression in mothers and fathers on parenting behavior, *Pediatrics* 118:659-668, 2006.

Pecora PJ et al: *Assessing the effects of foster care: early results from the Casey National Alumni Study,* 2003. Available at *www.casey.org/Resources/Publications/NationalAlumniStudy.htm* (accessed Dec 10, 2006).

Reiger M et al: Influence of stress during pregnancy on HPA activity and neonatal behavior, *Ann NY Acad Sci* 1032:228-230, 2004.

Rosenblum KL: Defining infant mental health. In Sameroff AJ, McDonough SC, Rosenblum KL, editors: *Treating parent-infant relationship problems,* New York, 2005, Guilford Press.

Ruths S, Steiner H: Psychopharmacologic treatment of aggression in children and adolescents, *Pediatr Ann* 33:318-327, 2004.

Ryan-Wenger NA, Sharrer VW, Campbell KK: Changes in children's stressors over the past 30 years, *Pediatr Nurs* 31:282-288, 2005.

Scheeringa MS: Posttraumatic stress disorder. In Luby JL, editor: *Handbook of preschool mental health,* New York, 2006, Guilford Press.

Schore AN: Attachment, affect regulation, and the developing right brain: linking developmental neuroscience to pediatrics, *Pediatr Rev* 26:204-217, 2005.

Showyra KR, Cocozza JJ: *Blueprint for change: a comprehensive model for the identification and treatment of youth with mental health needs in contact with the juvenile justice system,* 2006. Available at *www.ncmhjj.com/Blueprint/default.shtml* (accessed Dec 27, 2006).

Silove D, Manicavasagar V, Drobny J: Associations between juvenile and adult forms of separation anxiety disorder: a study of adult volunteers with histories of school refusal, *J Nerv Ment Dis* 190:413-415, 2002.

Spessot AL, Plessen KJ, Peterson BP: Neuroimaging of developmental psychopathologies, *Ann NY Acad Sci* 1021:86-104, 2004.

Squires J, Nickel R: Never too soon: identifying social-emotional problems in infants and toddlers, *Contemp Pediatr* 20:117-125, 2003.

Stafford B, Boris N, Dalton R: Anxiety disorders. In Behrman R, Kliegman R, Jenson H, editors: *Nelson textbook of pediatrics,* Philadelphia, 2004, WB Saunders.

Stein REK, Zitner LE, Jensen PS: Interventions for adolescent depression in primary care, *Pediatrics* 118:669-682, 2006.

Stockton L: Sleep and adjustment in preschool children: sleep diary reports by mothers relate to behavior reports by teachers, *Child Dev* 73:62-74, 2002.

Strine et al: The associations among childhood headaches, emotional and behavioral difficulties, and health care use, *Pediatrics* 117:1728-1735, 2006.

Sullivan MW, Lewis M: Emotional expressions of young infants and toddlers, *Infants Young Child* 16:120-142, 2003.

Sumner G, Spietz A: *NCAST caregiver/parent-child interaction feeding manual,* Seattle, 1994a, NCAST Publications.

Sumner G, Spietz A: *NCAST caregiver/parent-child interaction teaching manual,* Seattle, 1994b, NCAST Publications.

Theall-Honey LA, Schmidt LA: Do temperamentally shy children process emotion differently than non-shy children? Behavioral, psychophysiological, and gender differences, *Dev Psychobiol* 48:187-196, 2006.

Tuecki S: The behavioral complaint: symptom of a psychiatric disorder or a matter of temperament? *Contemp Pediatr* 20:111-119, 2003.

U.S. Preventive Services Task Force: *The guide to clinical preventive services,* ed 2, Rockville MD, 2006, Agency for Healthcare Research and Quality. Available at *www.ahrq.gov/clinic/pocketgd.htm* (accessed Sept 11, 2007).

Webster-Stratton C, Reid MJ, Hammond M: Treating children with early-onset conduct problems: intervention outcomes for parent, child, and teacher training, *J Clin Child Adolesc Psychol* 33:105-124, 2004.

Zero to Three: *Diagnostic classification of mental health and developmental disorders* of *infancy and early childhood: revised edition (DC: 0-3R),* Washington, DC, 2005, Zero to Three Press.

Ziegler M et al: Posttraumatic stress responses in children: awareness and practice among a sample of pediatric emergency care providers, *Pediatrics* 115:1261-1267, 2005.

CHAPTER 27

Values and Beliefs

Ardys M. Dunn

Children's health and well-being are not determined by physical measures only. As discussed in previous chapters, being part of a family and community, being valued and nurtured by others, belonging and *mattering* to other individuals give children a strong sense of self and the foundation to establish healthy relationships and face life's challenges positively. The child's values and beliefs and expression of spirituality and faith are integral to this process of development. Pediatric primary health care providers must be aware that beliefs, faith, religion, and spirituality affect children's health. The use of meditation, prayer, relaxation, and other mind-body therapies is known to facilitate healing (Sibinga et al, 2006; Williams et al, 2006; Wright, 2006), and there is growing recognition of the importance of attending to matters of spirituality, morality, and religion in health care (Josephson & Dell, 2004; Carnevale et al, 2006; Ventegodt et al, 2006). Holistic pediatric care includes assessment of social, cultural, and spiritual dimensions. It considers the impact of values and beliefs on health care decisions and explores ways to support values, beliefs, and subsequent actions that promote health.

▰ STANDARDS OF PRACTICE

Primary care providers are expected to give comprehensive care, which includes examining and treating all aspects of the individual—physical, emotional, psychosocial, and spiritual. Nursing, as a discipline, has incorporated spirituality into caregiving more than other health disciplines (Kilpatrick et al, 2005). Overall, however, health care in the U.S. has tended to focus on physical health and illness rather than the integration of mental, emotional, and spiritual health. As a result, there are currently few standard guidelines related to spiritual issues in the care of children.

The American Medical Association's (AMA's) *Guidelines for Adolescent Preventive Services (GAPS)* (Elster & Kuznets, 1994) includes the following points related to values and beliefs:

- Preventive services should be appropriate for age and development and sensitive to individual and sociocultural differences.
- All adolescents should receive health guidance annually to promote a better understanding of their physical growth, their psychosocial and psychosexual development, and the importance of being actively involved in decisions regarding their health care.

- All adolescents should be asked annually about behaviors or emotions that indicate recurrent or severe depression or risk of suicide.

The U.S. Preventive Services Task Force (1996) places emphasis on the importance of being alert to behavioral disorders, parent and family dysfunction, signs of child abuse or neglect, abnormal bereavement, and, among adolescents, depressive symptoms and suicide risk factors. Problems in these areas may reflect emotional or spiritual dysfunction.

The spiritual and child health initiative developed by the Department of Pediatrics, Boston Medical Center and Medical Anthropology (Barnes et al, 2000), articulated guidelines for practice, suggesting that providers:

- Anticipate patients will have spiritual or religious concerns.
- Develop a self-awareness of their own spiritual and religious history and perspective.
- Become broadly familiar with the religious worldview of the patient groups for whom they care.
- Work with individual families and children to learn their specific values and beliefs.
- Develop strategic interviewing skills.
- Develop a resource list and network of local consultants.
- Refer patients to appropriate spiritual care providers.

The above guidelines emphasize the importance of including discussions of spiritual and religious concerns in the provider-patient interaction, primarily in an effort to reach understanding, not necessarily agreement. Much of the focus on spiritual needs of children and families has been related to critical care or end-of-life decisions, and addressing spiritual beliefs may be particularly important for families facing illnesses that seem unfair or that have no reasonable explanation. However, these discussions should be part of well-child visits as well as care of children who are acutely and/or chronically ill. Spirituality is essential to all human life and is a critical part of a child's healthy development.

▰ NORMAL PATTERNS OF BEHAVIOR
DEFINITIONS AND RELATIONSHIP TO BEHAVIOR

Values have been defined as perceptions held about the worth or importance of a certain thing, person, or idea. *Beliefs* are attitudes representing whether one holds something to be true. Values and beliefs influence actions, both consciously and unconsciously. They are guides that individuals use as they make decisions. Values and beliefs are learned phenomena, and recognition and acceptance of shared values and beliefs are fundamental to the integrity of the individual, the family, and the social group (see Chapter 3). Although perceptions, attitudes, values, and beliefs are transmitted from one generation to another, they remain open to change and are responsive to social contexts and situations. Values clarification is the process by which one examines behavior in light of values and changing circumstances and asks why a certain action is taken or whether that action is consistent with the values one claims to have. Change in values, beliefs, and behavior can result from the process of values clarification. *Faith,* according to Fowler and Dell, is the basis for developing beliefs, values, and meaning. Faith "(1) gives coherence and direction to persons' lives; (2) links them in shared trusts and loyalties with others; (3) grounds their personal stances and communal loyalties in a sense of relatedness to a larger frame of reference; and (4) enables them to face and deal with the challenges of human life and death, relying on that which has the quality of ultimacy in their lives" (Fowler & Dell, 2004, p. 17). In this broad conceptualization, faith encompasses a wide range of religious and spiritual expression.

Spirituality has been defined as a unifying force that gives meaning to life or "the feelings, thoughts, experiences, and behaviors that arise from a search for the sacred" (Larson et al, 1997). It is the recognition of a nonmaterial higher power that encompasses all of life's affairs and is mediated through the individual's relationships to others, to the community, and to the environment. Although integral to religion, spirituality should not be confused with religious activities, rituals, and behaviors. Characteristics of spirituality are listed in Table 21-1 (Howden, 1993).

EXPECTED PATTERNS OF BEHAVIOR RELATED TO VALUES AND BELIEFS

Children's values and beliefs are related to their developmental stage and are reflected in different behaviors at different ages. In general, healthy behaviors are expressions of positive values. In particular, the development of moral integrity (or conscience) and spirituality (or faith) is expected of the healthy child. As they develop moral and spiritual values, healthy children achieve a positive sense of self, learn to value themselves and their contribution to the family and larger social system, and feel a sense of understanding and belonging to their community.

DEVELOPMENT OF MORAL INTEGRITY OR CONSCIENCE

Moral and spiritual values are grounded in cultural, social, and family dynamics, but moral judgments appear to apply across cultures (Comunian, 2004) (see Chapter 3 for a discussion of the cultural dynamics that shape children's growth; Chapter 17 presents stages and factors influencing the development of healthy self-perception in children). Moral integrity involves demonstrating an understanding of right and wrong; engaging in reflection on ethical issues of justice and fairness; and expressing a sense of responsibility to oneself, others, and the environment. Moral virtues include things such as honesty, openness, fairness, self-control, constancy, unity, and dedication. The development of moral integrity is enhanced if children believe that they and their contributions to the family and community are valued; if they are rewarded emotionally, psychologically, and intellectually for their participation in the community; and if their peer groups support positive behavior. Simply stated, children must believe that they make a difference and have a future.

Research on the ways children gain moral judgment has primarily been based in developmental theory. Kohlberg's moral phases (based on the intellectual stages of children) are probably the most well known of these theories (Kohlberg, 1969). The following developmental theorists have presented several perspectives on moral development in children:
- Freud asserted that children develop a conscience through identification with a significant caregiver and the processes of guilt and shame.
- Piaget claimed that children's moral development parallels their intellectual development and ability to reason.
- Kohlberg theorized that moral development proceeds sequentially through phases related to intellectual development and social interactions and that mature moral reasoning did not appear until postconventional stages 5 and 6.
- Social learning theory (e.g., Vygotsky) states that positive role modeling teaches moral behavior.

TABLE 21-1 Characteristics of Spirituality

Inner resources and identity	Those who possess inner resources have a sense of wholeness, competence, and direction. They are capable of responding to crises or turmoil and draw on inner strengths to maintain a sense of stability and control. They have values that give them courage and hope.
Interconnectedness	Interconnectedness is the sense of being an integral part of the world, attached to others, to one's environment, and to a universal or supreme being.
Purpose or meaning of life	A sense of direction and meaning and a reason for existence are developed in the relationships individuals have with others and their world.
Transcendence	The ability to go beyond, or transcend, the experiences of daily life is evident in the expression of hope, meaning, and direction when an individual is faced with fear, inability to effect change, uncertainty, and ambiguity.

From Howden J: Development and psychometric characteristics of the Spirituality Assessment Scale, *Dissertation Abstracts Int* 54:166, 1993.

Developmental theories suggest that younger children have little sense of right and wrong and are often concrete in their thinking, whereas older children and adolescents are more likely to be reflective as they examine moral dilemmas and are able to articulate and understand motivation or conditions that influence behavior. In contrast to Kohlberg, Gibbs and associates (1992) argued that mature moral reasoning can appear as early as stage 3 and 4 (early school-age children), as children develop friendships, learn to care about others, and understand rights and responsibilities as essential to societal functioning.

Other theorists have suggested that gender plays a significant role in the way children interpret situations and make choices based on moral judgment (Gilligan, 1990); that moral judgment and decisions are guided more by a pragmatic desire to achieve a cooperative social system in which individual and group goals can be achieved (Krebs & Denton, 2005); and that even very young children demonstrate a moral awareness, though it may be primarily experiential rather than reflective (Johansson, 2001).

Finally, recent research explores the importance of prefrontal cortical development on behavior. The prefrontal cortex continues to develop into the third decade of life, so adolescents and young adults are still expanding their capacity for moral judgment (Sapolsky, 2004). Studies of individuals with brain damage support the conclusion that long-term "cognitive, social-emotional, and moral development" is directly influenced by early cortical lesions (Eslinger et al, 2004; Anderson et al, 2006).

DEVELOPMENT OF SPIRITUALITY

Although it has been argued that children are intrinsically spiritual, the development of spiritual expression in children is largely seen as paralleling cognitive and moral development. Table 21-2 presents a developmental perspective of faith and outlines age-specific interventions to enhance healthy growth (Stilwell et al, 1998; Walker et al, 2000; Wolf, 2000). Infants and toddlers are engaged in the processes of gaining trust and establishing autonomy or separateness of self from the parent. They are becoming a part of a bigger culture (i.e., the family). Preschool and early school-age children gain an understanding of the meaning of life through fantasy play, active engagement with their environment, strong attachments to their parents, and growing relationships with their peers. Although they have achieved the task of defining themselves as separate individuals, the thinking and behavior of preschool and early school-age children in relation to faith issues is still largely an expression of the family's faith and practice. School-age children and adolescents define life's meaning within the context of their "self-sufficiency, competence, and role differentiation" and in their relationship to both peers and adults. Children at this age need to explore their understanding of the ultimate questions in life (Pasupathi et al, 2001). They are interested in issues such as life, death, war, evil, good, and creation, and develop increasing wisdom as they discuss and think about these important matters.

ASSESSMENT

The goals of assessing values and beliefs include the following:

- Determine the nature of the child's and family's belief system.
- Identify ways that the family interacts to support these beliefs.
- Clarify how beliefs affect decisions and behaviors related to health care.

Because children are in the process of developing values and beliefs and because much of their development depends on their interaction with the parent or caregiver, assessment questions are often directed to or focused on the parent or caregiver. This can give a wealth of information, but it may not accurately or completely assess the child's needs or understandings. Children may not be able to understand what is happening to them; they cannot always express themselves clearly or use the words or symbols related to values, beliefs, faith, or spirituality that are more familiar to adults. Interpreting and understanding the emotional and spiritual meaning a given experience has for a child is a significant challenge to even the most skilled health care provider.

Measures of spirituality are necessarily subjective, and spirituality is often included in the psychosocial assessment. Use of a broad framework, including culture, religion, and spirituality is recommended to guide assessment (McEvoy, 2003). Many of the tools used to assess spirituality in health care are focused on older adults who are confronted with end-of-life issues (King et al, 2006; Daaleman & Frey, 2004). Some of these tools can be adapted in work with children and families. One assessment model uses the mnemonic HOPE to focus clinical questions on the client's sources of **H**ope, peace, and comfort; participation in **O**rganized religion; **P**ersonal spiritual practices; and the **E**ffect these behaviors have on the client's medical care or end-of-life decisions (Anandarajah & Hight, 2001). Another model uses the mnemonic BELIEF: **B**elief system; **E**thics or values; **L**ifestyle behaviors (e.g., diet, rituals); **I**nvolvement in a spiritual community; religious **E**ducation; and **F**uture events, especially decisions about health that will be affected by religious beliefs (McEvoy, 2000). As the relationship between spirituality and health is investigated further, more valid and reliable measures, applied to both children and adults, are likely to be developed. The following discussion provides guidelines that incorporate elements from the models mentioned above. These guidelines can be used for assessment in pediatric primary and acute care settings and, if not directly applicable to children, may be useful when working with parents and families. Assessment questions should look at subjective spiritual understandings and objective religious practices.

HISTORY

Moral Integrity or Conscience

The following points can guide the assessment:

- How does the child define right and wrong? How does the child's behavior reflect his or her moral understanding? How does the child demonstrate moral reasoning?

TABLE 21-2 Developmental Outcomes and Appropriate Interventions Related to Values and Beliefs

Area of Development	Infant (0-12 months old)	Toddler and Preschooler (1-5 years old)	School-Age Child (6-12 years old)	Adolescent
Moral integrity and conscience (right and wrong; sense of responsibility to oneself, others, and the environment)	Develops sense of trust in caregivers (Erikson, 1963); learns to adjust to family routine (e.g., sleeping, eating)	Believes rules are absolute; behaves well for fear of punishment or to receive rewards (Kohlberg, 1969); develops sense of autonomy, initiative, and purpose; differentiates self from others (Erikson, 1963)	Believes rules exist to keep order and protect people and that everyone benefits from them; behaves well to please others, to avoid guilt, and to maintain status of "good" child (Kohlberg, 1969); develops sense of industry, faith in self-competence; explores, creates, collects; understands cause and effect (Erikson, 1963)	Rules are based on ethical judgment; believes individual answers to personal conscience, has moral obligation to a social contract; behaves to maintain respect of self, peers, and larger community (Kohlberg, 1969); integrates personality and develops sense of identity, loyalty to group and significant others (Erikson, 1963)
Faith development	Primal or undifferentiated faith based on trust in relationships with parents and caregivers (Fowler & Dell, 2004); infant develops object permanence, sense of trust, attachment, and sense of being nurtured	Intuitive-projective faith based on images, feelings, and symbols; children make meaning of their world using imagination and forming images to "hold and order…feelings and impressions" of threats and protective elements in their world (Fowler & Dell, 2004); egocentric thinking may contribute to misconceptions; child begins to participate in family's religious practices and rituals	Mythic-literal faith, with more concrete beliefs, more rigid system of order and activities, of good and bad (Fowler & Dell, 2004); faith as assent, as child learns to master environment and become competent (Aden, 1976); child begins to explore ultimate issues, develop understanding of the meaning of life, understand and manage strong feelings, develop and express moral decision-making	Synthetic convention stage—ideas about spirituality are synthesized in process of interpersonal relations with peers, parents, and other significant adults, and life experiences; adolescent explores identity and personal meaning of faith (Fowler & Dell, 2004); faith as identity (Aden, 1976) as child seeks identity, understanding of self in the world; child demonstrates self-reflection, insight, sense of inner spiritual process and presence in the world, and continues to more fully develop understanding of ultimate questions, life's meaning
Experienced faith (infancy through early adolescence)	Children experience faith through relationships with others and others' faith traditions			
Affiliative faith (late adolescence)				Adolescent actively participates in a faith community, feels a sense of belonging, awe, and wonder; acknowledges authority of faith community

Parental Interventions to Foster Healthy Development

Respond to infant's physiologic and emotional needs promptly and adequately; demonstrate loving, gentle approach in communication and interaction

Treat child with respect and acceptance; provide security, love, and companionship; set realistic limits on behavior, using positive discipline rather than punishment; remove temptation from environment; provide positive role model; provide guided opportunities to interact with adults and other children and active play alone; be patient; involve child in family religious practices; begin to establish regular tasks for child in family activities

Treat child with respect and acceptance; set realistic limits on behavior; provide opportunities for active play alone and with other children; encourage peer group activity; allow children to make decisions as appropriate, helping them to explore meanings of feelings, events, and interactions; choose narrative stories related to children's experience of moral dilemmas to explore right and wrong and to help child develop values; establish regular tasks for child as member of family; help child be successful in the family; teach family values and standards; encourage continued participation in family religious practices

Treat adolescent with respect and acceptance; set realistic limits on behavior; model and encourage family's moral standards; encourage involvement in family activities; allow children to make more of own choices regarding values and beliefs; allow experimentation in dress, hair, makeup as child develops sense of self; do not overreact to adolescent "crises;" provide opportunities to discuss values, ethics, and moral behavior; provide support and encouragement for successes and failures in school, social, athletic, and work activities; encourage continued participation in family religious practices

- What are family attitudes about right and wrong?
- How are parents teaching the child about right and wrong?
- What other influences affect the child's concept of right and wrong (e.g., day care, teachers and counselors, peer group)?
- How do parents set limits on the child's behavior?
- How does the child respond to discipline and limits?
- What messages do parents give about the value and importance of the child's contribution to the family and the community?
- What messages do parents give about the value of respecting other people, ideas, property, and the environment?
- What opportunities do parents give the child to make independent, age-appropriate decisions?
- What traditions and activities does the family have? How is the child included in these activities?

Spirituality

The following information should be identified in relation to spirituality:

General. Tell me about your religious beliefs related to the following issues:

- Family relations, gender roles, and children's and parents' responsibilities
- Sexuality issues (e.g., homosexuality, premarital sex)
- Dietary restrictions
- Rituals (e.g., at mealtime or bedtime)
- Use of drugs, alcohol, or tobacco
- Medical treatment

Inner Resources and Identity

- What are your child's goals in life? Your family's goals?
- What are your child's strong points? Your family's strong points?
- What do you like about yourself? Your child? Your family?
- How important is faith in your child's life? In your life?
- What brings you, your child, and your family joy and peace? Where do you find hope and comfort?

Interconnectedness

- How do you feel about your child? About yourself? About your family?
- What do you do as a family to show love for each other?
- Who are significant people in your child's and your family's life?
- Whom do you ask for support when your family needs help?
- How do members of your family share feelings with others?
- Do you feel that you and your family are part of a community? Of a larger world or universe?
- Does the family belong to a religious or spiritual group?

Purpose or Meaning of Life

- What are your family's religious and cultural beliefs? What ethics or values are important in your family's life?
- What gives life meaning? What is the most important thing in life?
- How does your family express religious and cultural beliefs? How is your child involved?

- What religious rituals or practices contribute to a sense of spiritual fulfillment or peace?
- How do you teach your child about values and beliefs? How else does your child learn about values and beliefs?
- Are you comfortable talking about your beliefs with your child?

Transcendence

- How do members of your family deal with spiritual distress during a crisis?

PHYSICAL EXAMINATION

Objective assessment of values and beliefs is largely based on observation, and, though subject to interpretation, these observations can indicate the child's sense of valuing others, self, and the environment. Observe the child's behavior, especially noting interaction with parents, other adults, and peers. The child exhibits the following behavior:

- Appears at ease, although behavior may vary (e.g., shy, quiet, active, talkative, engaging) depending on developmental level and temperament
- Engages actively, spontaneously, and affectionately with parent or caregiver
- Responds to parent or caregiver cues; follows directions and conforms to limits set without demonstrating guilt or fear of punishment
- Shares toys, depending on age
- Respects people and property
- Is not physically aggressive, depending on age
- Is able to articulate moral reasoning (older child)
- Is able to articulate a faith statement, depending on spiritual, religious, and cultural background (older child)

■ MANAGEMENT OF NORMAL PATTERNS

Parents should function in the following ways:

- Be a loving, responsive, and accepting presence in their children's lives. This responsibility cannot be overemphasized; children's understandings and expressions of self-concept, spirituality, and moral integrity derive in large part from the quality of their interactions with significant adults.
- Set realistic standards or limits for right and wrong behavior.
- State what is acceptable and what is unacceptable behavior.
- Provide a rationale for limits set; the explanation varies depending on the cognitive and developmental level of the child.
- Articulate personal values, beliefs, and faith statements for the child. Give clear, age-appropriate explanations of God and spiritual lessons.
- Be a role model for constructive and positive behavior.
- Reinforce positive behavior and attempts at positive behavior.
- Hold children accountable for negative behavior.
- Teach children strategies to avoid misbehavior; teach constructive coping skills.

- Use creative parenting strategies (e.g., distraction, diversional activities) to help children avoid misbehavior.
- Provide a developmentally appropriate environment to minimize children's misbehavior. It is usually easier to remove a breakable object from a table than to keep saying no or to discipline a child for breaking it.
- Provide opportunities for children to make age-appropriate decisions independently.
- Praise children in front of others.
- Do not give false praise.
- Articulate and reinforce messages that children belong and are valued for themselves, not just for their behaviors.
- Establish family traditions and projects that actively involve children (e.g., family outings, family value sessions, during which family members share a meal with directed conversation). Do not expect perfection.
- Involve children in the family's religious and cultural practices.
- Provide opportunities for the child to explore moral and ethical dilemmas and to develop possible solutions.
- Discuss moral and spiritual implications of events in the child's life (e.g., death of a grandparent, birth of a sibling, sharing, stealing, violence portrayed in media).
  Primary health care providers should do the following:
- Be aware of their own values and beliefs.
- Distinguish between moral and medical advice. Be willing to offer both, while recognizing that personal proselytizing is inappropriate in the provider-patient relationship.
- Recognize and appreciate differences between own and client's values.
- Provide an opportunity for parents to express values and beliefs and to discuss their child's moral and spiritual development.
- Provide information about parenting strategies, discipline, and effective communication between child and parents.
- Assist parents and child in values clarification as appropriate.
- Provide a role model of positive behavior.
- Offer an understanding, compassionate, and accepting presence.
- Modify the treatment plan as appropriate to meet spiritual needs.
- Refer the family for religious or spiritual counseling as indicated or requested.

■ ALTERED PATTERNS
LACK OF MORAL INTEGRITY OR CONSCIENCE
Description
Although lack of moral integrity is not a clinically defined condition, some children demonstrate a lack of an age-appropriate capacity to respect others or the environment, to judge behavior as right or wrong, and to express empathy or remorse.

Epidemiology
The complexity of moral judgment or conscience makes it likely that a multitude of factors contribute to poor moral reasoning and antisocial behaviors. Research indicates that the development of a conscience is mediated by a child's socialization in the family, temperament (Kochanska & Aksan, 2006; Kochanska et al, 2005), and early development of trust, in which the child feels a strong sense of security in his or her relationship with the mother (Kochanska et al, 2004). Research also indicates that children whose mothers used power-assertive discipline (e.g., critical comments and physical coercion) tend to show less guilt when confronted with a hypothetical moral dilemma (Kochanska et al, 2002) and have more child conduct problems (Webster-Stratton et al, 2001).

Clinical Findings
Many behaviors seen are typical of normal children, depending on age, developmental, and cognitive levels (e.g., lying, hitting, refusing to share), but the child expresses little or no remorse for negative behavior; demonstrates no internalization of a sense of justice, fairness, or right and wrong; and fails to develop an ability to self-regulate behavior.

Differential Diagnosis
Attention-deficit/hyperactivity disorder, conduct disorder, oppositional defiant disorder, and depression are differential diagnoses.

Management
In addition to strategies listed here, see the earlier discussion of management strategies for normal moral development. In extreme cases, referral for psychiatric management may be necessary.
- Tell stories to younger children.
- Use storytelling to explore moral and ethical issues (Binnendyk & Schonert-Reichl, 2002).
- Encourage interaction with older children who demonstrate higher levels of moral reasoning (Leman, 2002).
- Watch films and discuss books with adolescents.
- Assist child in values clarification process.

Complications
Antisocial behavior and delinquency are behavioral disorders in which lack of moral integrity is a key component.

SPIRITUAL DISTRESS
Description
Spiritual distress is "a disruption in the life principle that pervades a person's entire being and integrates and transcends one's biological and psychosocial nature" (North American Nursing Diagnosis Association [NANDA], 2007). For children, issues of death and dying and serious illness are major reasons for seeking spiritual counsel. They are fearful and threatened and often ask "why?" Comprehensive care involves support of a child's—and the family's—spirituality to prevent spiritual distress (Hufton, 2006).

Epidemiology

Because of the complex nature of spirituality, spiritual distress can result from a number of factors. These factors challenge the child's or family's belief system or contribute to separation from spiritual ties and can include the following:

- Trauma or violence
- Loss of significant other, especially parent or sibling
- Debilitating disease
- Chronic disease
- Separation of child from his or her family
- Isolation
- Homelessness
- Recommended medical therapies in conflict with child's or family's religious or spiritual beliefs (e.g., Christian Science)
- Barriers in the health care setting to practicing spiritual rituals (e.g., hospital routines that ignore patient's need to worship)
- Beliefs of health care providers, family members, or peers that conflict with those of child or parent

Clinical Findings

The following may be seen in spiritual distress:

- Depressive behavior (may be suicidal)
- Withdrawal
- No participation in usual religious practices
- Disparaging family's spiritual beliefs and values
- Questioning one's own value, meaning, and purpose of life
- Expressions of anger, resentment, fear of God, suffering, death
- Expressions of inner conflict and doubts about beliefs
- Expressions of sense of spiritual emptiness
- Sleep disturbance
- Behavior changes with mood swings
- Request for spiritual assistance

Differential Diagnosis

Depression, poor coping mechanisms, conduct disorders, and antisocial behavior are differential diagnoses for spiritual distress.

Management

The primary care provider should take the following management steps:

- Identify situational factors that contribute to distress.
- Consult with parents as appropriate to identify family values and belief system.
- Assist parents to help their child process experiences contributing to distress. Referral may be necessary in cases in which child is experiencing significant psychological trauma. An integrated team composed of psychologist, clergy, and parish nurse can be appropriate. Use of hospital chaplains can be especially helpful to families (Robinson et al, 2006), and crisis response play therapy can be effectively used when individuals are unable to verbally express their distress (McPherson, 2004).

- Provide comfort and security to allay fears and reassure child.
- Encourage child to participate in spiritual practices as desired. Adolescents who have a relationship with a religious institution, in particular, tend to have healthier attitudes and behaviors (Wong et al, 2006).
- Encourage child to express feelings about spiritual distress.
- Encourage child to talk about beliefs and understandings of stressors such as death and illness.
- Answer questions honestly, according to the child's age and developmental level.
- Advocate for the child and parent when they express beliefs in conflict with those of other health care providers or other family members.
  If parents refuse treatment for their child:
- Consider use of alternative methods of care.
- Provide opportunity for parents to discuss implications of decision and possible court order for a temporary guardian who will give consent to treat the child.
- Provide opportunity for parents to express negative feelings.

Complications

Depression, suicide, and conduct disorders can be complications of spiritual distress.

⋀URSING DIAGNOSES

Related to Values and Beliefs Diagnoses

- Spiritual distress and Risk for spiritual distress
- Readiness for enhanced spiritual well-being
- Decisional conflict (specify)
- Moral distress
- Noncompliance (specify)
- Impaired religiosity and Risk for impaired religiosity
- Readiness for enhanced religiosity.

From NANDA International: *NANDA-I nursing diagnoses: definitions & classification, 2007-2008,* Philadelphia, 2007, Author.

✓ DISCUSSION FORUM

1. How might a pediatric health care provider's own values, beliefs, and spirituality impact the ability to care for children and their families? Examine your own values, beliefs, and spirituality.
2. Discuss how health care providers can interact with children and their families to effectively include this component of health into their care.
3. What are unique issues related to values, beliefs, and spirituality of preschoolers? School-age children? Adolescents? How can assessment of values and beliefs be incoporated into the preventative care of each of these age groups?
4. Conduct a values and beliefs assessment on a child. What anticipatory guidance strategies and family education strategies will you use in your wellness plan for this child that are based upon your findings?

REFERENCES

Aden L: Faith and the developmental cycle, *Pastoral Psychol* 24:215-230, 1976.

Anandarajah G, Hight E: Spirituality and medical practice: using the HOPE questions as a practical tool for spiritual assessment, *Am Fam Physician* 63:81-88, 2001.

Anderson SW et al: Impairments of emotion and real-world complex behavior following childhood- or adult-onset damage to ventromedial prefrontal cortex, *J Int Neuropsychol Soc* 12(2):224-235, 2006.

Barnes LL et al: Spirituality, religion, and pediatrics: intersecting worlds of healing, *Pediatrics* 106:899-908, 2000.

Binnendyk L, Schonert-Reichl KA: Harry Potter and moral development in pre-adolescent children, *J Moral Education* 31:195-201, 2002.

Carnevale FA et al: Daily living with distress and enrichment: the moral experience of families with ventilator-assisted children at home, *Pediatrics* 117(1):e48-e60, 2006.

Comunian AL: Construction of a scale for measuring development of moral judgement, *Psychol Rep* 94(2):613-618, 2004.

Daaleman TP, Frey BB: The spirituality index of well-being: a new instrument for health-related quality-of-life research, *Ann Fam Med* 2:499-503, 2004.

Elster AB, Kuznets NJ: *AMA guidelines for adolescent preventive services (GAPS): recommendations and rationale,* Baltimore, 1994, Williams & Wilkins.

Erikson EH: *Childhood and society,* ed 2, New York, 1963, Norton.

Eslinger PJ, Flaherty-Craig CV, Benton AL: Developmental outcomes after early prefrontal cortex damage, *Brain Cogn* 55(1):84-103, 2004.

Fowler JW, Dell ML: Stages of faith and identity: birth to teens, *Child Adolesc Psychiatr Clin N Am* 13(1):17-33, 2004.

Gibbs JC, Basinger KS, Fuller RL: *Moral maturity: measuring the development of sociomoral reflection,* Hillsdale NJ, 1992, Erlbaum.

Gilligan C: *Mapping the moral domain,* Cambridge, MA, 1990, Harvard University Press.

Howden J: Development and psychometric characteristics of the Spirituality Assessment Scale, *Dissertation Abstracts Int* 54:166, 1993.

Hufton E: Parting gifts: the spiritual needs of children, *J Child Health Care* 10(3):240-250, 2006.

Johansson E: Morality in children's worlds—rationality of thought or values emanating from relations? *Stud Philosophy Education* 20:345-358, 2001.

Josephson AM, Dell ML: Religion and spirituality in child and adolescent psychiatry: a new frontier, *Child Adolesc Psychiatr Clin N Amer* 13(1):1-15, 2004.

Kilpatrick SD et al: A review of spiritual and religious measures in nursing research journals: 1995-1999, *J Relig Health* 44(1):55-66, 2005.

King M et al: Measuring spiritual belief: development and standardization of a Beliefs and Values Scale, *Psychol Med* 36(3):417-425, 2006.

Kochanska G et al: Guilt in young children: development, determinants, and relations with a broader system of standards, *Child Dev* 73:461-482, 2002.

Kochanska G et al: Maternal parenting and children's conscience: early security as moderator, *Child Dev* 75(4):1229-1242, 2004.

Kochanska G et al: Pathways to conscience: early mother-child mutually responsive orientation and children's moral emotion, conduct, and cognition, *J Child Psychol Psychiatry* 46(1):19-34, 2005.

Kochanska G, Aksan N: Children's conscience and self-regulation, *J Pers* 74(6):1587-1617, 2006.

Kohlberg L: Stage and sequence: the cognitive-development approach to socialization. In Gastin D, editor: *Handbook of socialization: theory and research,* New York, 1969, Rand McNally.

Krebs DL, Denton K: Toward a more pragmatic approach to morality: a critical evaluation of Kohlberg's model, *Psychol Rev* 112(3):629-649, 2005.

Larson DB, Swyers JP, McCullough ME: *Scientific research on spirituality and health: a consensus report,* Rockville, MD, 1997, National Institute of Healthcare Research.

Leman PJ: Argument structure, argument content, and cognitive change in children's peer interaction, *J Genet Psychol* 163:40-58, 2002.

McEvoy M: An added dimension to the pediatric health maintenance visit: the spiritual history, *J Pediatr Health Care* 14:216-220, 2000.

McEvoy M: Culture and spirituality as an integrated concept in pediatric care, *Matern Child Nurs* 50(1):39-43, 2003.

McPherson K: Pastoral crisis intervention with children: recognizing and responding to the spiritual reaction of children, *Int J Emerg Ment Health* 6(4):223-233, 2004.

North American Nursing Diagnosis Association (NANDA) International: *NANDA-I nursing diagnoses: definitions & classification, 2007-2008,* Philadelphia, 2007, NANDA.

Pasupathi M, Staudinger UM, Baltes PB: Seeds of wisdom: adolescents' knowledge and judgment about difficult life problems, *Dev Psychol* 37:351-361, 2001.

Robinson MR et al: Matters of spirituality at the end of life in the pediatric intensive care unit, *Pediatrics* 118(3):e719-729, 2006.

Sapolsky RM: The frontal cortex and the criminal justice system, *Philos Trans R Soc Lond B Biol Sci* 359(1451):1787-1796, 2004.

Sibinga EM et al: Pediatric patients with sickle cell disease: use of complementary and alternative therapies, *J Altern Complement Med* 12(3):291-298, 2006.

Stilwell BM et al: Moral volition: the fifth and final domain leading to an integrated theory of conscience understanding, *J Am Acad Child Adolesc Psychiatry* 37:202-210, 1998.

US Preventive Services Task Force: *Guide to clinical preventive services,* ed 2, Baltimore, 1996, Williams & Wilkins.

Ventegodt S et al: Human development II: we need an integrated theory for matter, life and consciousness to understand life and healing, *Sci World J* 6:760-766, 2006.

Walker LJ, Hennig KH, Krettenauer T: Parent and peer contexts for children's moral reasoning development, *Child Dev* 71:1033-1048, 2000.

Webster-Stratton C, Reid J, Hammond M: Social skills and problem-solving training for children with early-onset conduct problems: who benefits? *J Child Psychol Psychiatry* 42:943-952, 2001.

Williams PD et al: Symptom monitoring and dependent care during cancer treatment in children: pilot study, *Cancer Nurs* 29(3):188-197, 2006.

Wolf AD: How to nurture the spirit in nonsectarian environments, *Young Child* 55:34-36, 2000.

Wong YJ, Rew L, Slaikeu KD: A systematic review of recent research on adolescent religiosity/spirituality and mental health, *Issues Ment Health Nurs* 27(2):161-183, 2006.

Wright LD: Meditation: a new role for an old friend, *Am J Hosp Palliat Care* 23(4):323-327, 2006.

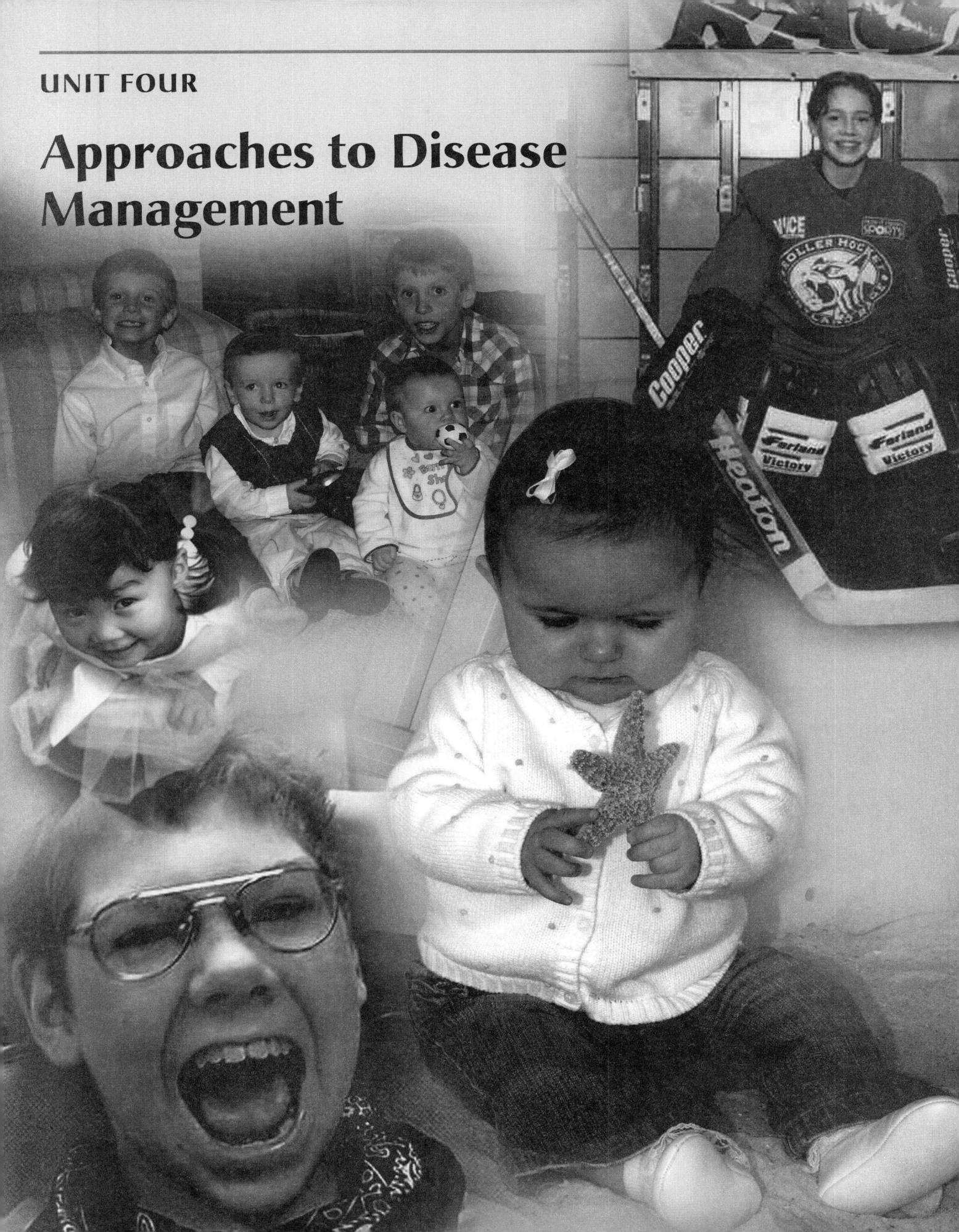

UNIT FOUR

Approaches to Disease Management

CHAPTER 22

Introduction to Disease and Pain Management

Margaret A. Brady

■ APPROACHES TO ACUTE DISEASE IN CHILDREN

A major role of the primary care provider in pediatrics is to arrive at a diagnosis and to treat common illnesses of childhood with a management plan that is consistent with the community standard of practice. This process begins with a thorough assessment of the child and the presenting complaint. In caring for children with acute illnesses, health care providers must always remember that an accurate assessment of the ill child is contingent on the following six points:

1. Careful observation of the child
2. Attention to pertinent positive and negative historical and physical findings
3. Knowledge of physiologic functions and developmental considerations that vary by age
4. Consideration of the trajectory of the problem over time
5. Inclusion of the parents or caretakers and, if appropriate, the child as participants in the evaluation process
6. Assurance that the parent understands medical terminology used in questions that are asked or advice given. Similarly, it should not be assumed that any medical term used by the parent means the same to providers. For example, a parent's definition of fever may be any temperature above 99° F, or wheezing to a parent may in fact be rhonchi. A parent who is told that the management needed for the child's problem is some "tincture of time" may go to the local pharmacy looking for that "medication."

When satisfied that these six parameters have been given adequate attention, an action or management plan is formed that can include ordering basic laboratory and imaging studies and other special testing, if needed, to arrive at a final diagnosis. Extensive laboratory and other diagnostic tests are often not in the best interest of children, especially for those who would be best served by being referred to a pediatrician or pediatric specialist for diagnosis or treatment of their disease.

Like other providers, nurse practitioners (NPs) are responsible for the assessment and management of children with common pediatric illnesses or conditions. The NPs' effectiveness in primary care is due largely to their ability to educate patients and their families about the prevention of disease and the management of common illnesses. The patient-parent educational component of the management plan must be individualized but should always include the following essential points:

- Information about the length of time it can take before the child improves and symptoms wane; description of what the course of the disease or illness is likely to be and signs of improvement
- Written information about specific signs and symptoms that indicate worsening of the illness, the need for immediate medical attention or for a return visit sooner than planned (examples for parents include a sick newborn, severe lethargy, tender abdomen, labored breathing, stiff or injured neck, bluish lips, purple "dots" on the skin, severe pain, child who cannot walk, or fever above 105° F [40.6° C])
- Specific instructions about when to return for a follow-up visit or telephone conference if needed. A clinic tickler file is particularly useful for tracking patients whose diagnostic studies or follow-up appointments are crucial to successful management or treatment. This tickler file can be a simple card file, divided by months. For example, a card would list the patient's name, date, clinic number, medical problem, and contact information and be placed in the file in the month when follow-up is needed.
- Written instructions about any special treatment or therapy that is required or how to use adaptive devices and perform home monitoring tests
- Careful instructions about medication, both prescription and over-the-counter (OTC) drugs (see Use of Medication, later in this chapter)
- Issues related to administration of medications at school— appropriate forms completed and school personnel instructed on key issues related to pharmacologic therapy
- Specific information about any dietary needs or changes, special hydration needs, such as electrolyte solutions or increase in fluid intake, plus any changes in eating patterns that can be expected
- The rationale for and procedures involved with diagnostic testing including laboratory, radiographic, or imaging tests (e.g., in and out urine catheterization for urine cultures) and the meaning of results
- Estimations of length of time frame for lab or imaging results, especially when there will be long waiting periods (long waiting times are particularly frustrating for parents)
- Information about the cause, transmission, and communicability of an infectious disease

- Information about the cause if known and epidemiology of infectious or noninfectious illnesses or medical condition, communicability issues, and prevention guidelines if applicable
- Information about prevention and recurrence risk
- Determination of impediments that prevent the parent or the child from complying with the management plan (e.g., limited financial resources, inability to read, dysfunctional family, transportation problems) and discussion about steps to correct these difficulties
- Recognition and discussion of cultural practices and beliefs about illnesses. Discuss the potential benefit or harm from specific folk medicine or complementary and alternative medicine (CAM) practices (including herbal, dietary supplements, or botanical preparations) if used either alone or concurrently with prescribed or OTC medications
- Information for the working parent about resources for sick care in the community, which are both convenient (accessible) and affordable.

If at all possible when discussing the management plan with parent(s) and/or child, sit down and have eye contact with them. It is a sign of respect and should be a standard of care. In many situations, giving written information to parents about what signs and symptoms to expect with an illness or what warrants further evaluation and a return visit is essential. The parents' or caregivers' understanding of instructions should always be assessed by asking them to repeat what they have been told. By doing this, any misunderstandings can be addressed. Be sure to have the family's current or contact telephone number in case a telephone contact needs to be made regarding the results of diagnostic tests that come back or to monitor the course of the child's condition.

It is important to allow time for the natural defense system of the body to fight disease. Premature and excessive pharmacologic therapy can result in needless iatrogenic disease and often serves to confuse the clinical picture. The drug of first choice—the one that is least harmful—should be given time to work. Prematurely changing to a new drug, adding additional drugs, and using more toxic drugs are dangerous practices.

For the most part, parents are alert to subtle changes in their children, so it is important to listen attentively when parents voice concerns about their children. Any sick child who is at high risk because of physical or social problems merits closer observation and follow-up than does the average thriving child who becomes ill. Finally, if the child returns and is not significantly improved or is more symptomatic, the initial evaluation and diagnosis should be revisited by carefully analyzing the symptoms, investigating problems related to compliance issues, repeating the physical examination, reviewing likely differential diagnoses, and confirm the diagnosis before deciding on another management plan.

Management of an ill child also can include a short stay in an outpatient clinic, private office, or emergency or prompt care department for intravenous hydration, pulmonary therapy, medication, and close observation. Hospitalization might not be needed if the child's condition stabilizes, the parent is reliable, the child can be monitored closely at home, the home has a telephone, and the parent has transportation available to return for follow-up or an emergency visit. However, before discharging an ill infant or child to home rather than admitting the child to the hospital, the provider must carefully assess the parent's ability to cope with a significantly ill child and to identify signs or symptoms of increasing illness.

The number of infants and young children in group day care is expanding as the number of women in the workforce increases. The disease pattern in this cohort of children is often related to group exposure to illnesses. The issue of multiple caregivers can complicate history taking. In these situations, obtaining accurate information about the manifestation or pattern of an illness can be difficult. Often, parents express feelings of guilt about being a poor parent because their child has been exposed at day care and they must work. Addressing these issues during the health encounter is often helpful for parents.

With the diversity of dialects spoken in the U.S., language issues can be barriers to providing optimal health care. If a practice setting does not have access to an interpreter or native speaker, interpreter services can sometimes be obtained from local telephone services as a last resort. It is important that both the health care provider and the parent or caretaker can communicate with and understand each other.

Emergency department (ED) visits are often used for the treatment of minor illnesses by families without insurance or by those whose employment precludes visits to a primary care provider during regular clinic or office hours. Data about ED visits in 2003 revealed that 12.9% of children under 6 years old classified as poor had two or more ED visits compared with 6.4% of nonpoor children in that same period of time (National Center for Health Statistics, 2005). NPs employed in EDs must adhere to illness assessment and management protocols and provide critical documentation outlining their assessment findings and management strategies and their educational plan and counseling regarding follow-up.

APPROACHES TO CHRONIC DISEASE IN CHILDREN

It is estimated that between 15% to 18% of children and adolescents have some type of chronic physical, mental health, developmental, or learning condition. These figures do not include children with speech defects, visual and hearing disabilities, chronic ear infections, chronic skin conditions, and dental decay. Approximately 6% to 7% of children experience illness or disability that interferes with the child's usual daily activities. Some chronic conditions are not permanent, serious, or obvious, whereas other conditions are nonreversible, serious, and readily apparent. The health care provider may be faced with providing care to a child with a rare disease or disorder or be concerned with the management of a child with a much more common chronic condition, such as asthma or cerebral palsy. Furthermore, the number of children with severe, long-term illness reaching young adulthood continues to grow with advances in medical and surgical technology, and the percentage of children with certain chronic conditions, such as asthma and obesity, is also escalating (Perrin, 2004). Of note, an increasing number of NPs are involved in the specialty care of children with chronic conditions.

There can be great variability in both the presentation and the course of illness among children. Children with chronic medical or psychiatric conditions have special health needs. They and their families often face a range of problems that are as diverse as the conditions that cause these difficulties. A variety of genetic, congenital, and acquired conditions can lead to permanent or persistent problems that have a significant impact on the child's and family's lifestyle. Health care providers must remember that family members are the ones who must bear the major daily burden of care. Hence, to serve these children and their families well, a multidisciplinary team approach to management is essential. There are several key points to keep in mind when working with these children and their families:

- Prevention of special health problems is a primary goal of care and includes the following:
  - Early prenatal care for all pregnant women.
  - Genetic counseling as indicated.
  - Elimination of environmental triggers or toxins.
  - Early identification of the condition or disease is of paramount importance.
- Amelioration of any functional problem that is treatable is as essential as prevention of secondary complications.
- Early intervention from birth and whenever possible to prevent secondary psychosocial difficulties is crucial; the developmental aspects of long-term illness must be addressed.
- Counseling may be needed for the child and family to handle psychosocial and behavioral problems or to discuss their emotions and feelings.
- The child, the family, and school personnel must be consulted to ensure that the child is able to attain realistic developmental milestones.
- Appropriate educational support in school is a right.
  - Public law 94–142, the Education for All Handicapped Children Act of 1975, mandates an appropriate education for all school-age children with developmental disabilities in the least restrictive environment.
  - Public law 99–457 (1986) provides states with the opportunity to extend benefits of public law 94–142 to children from birth to 2 years old.
  - Prevention of discrimination is a right and is mandated under legislation related to individuals with disabilities. The Americans with Disabilities Act (1990) is a law that provides federal protection in the areas of employment, transportation, public accommodations, and communication for individuals with disabilities. The scope of protection covers both private and public sectors. The Individuals with Disabilities Educational Act (IDEA) Amendments were signed into effect in 1997 to bridge the gap between what children with disabilities learn and what is required in regular curriculum (IDEA-public law 105–17). It provides for the least restrictive environment for educating all children with disabilities.

  - IDEA Section 504 of the Rehabilitation Act for students with disabilities in regular education/inclusive settings provides safeguards and support for reasonable accommodations in the school settings, such as altered test schedules and settings, therapies, and support for medical issues.
- Each state has programs (Title V) to assist children with special health needs with medical care and linkage to social services, in addition to state vocational rehabilitation programs and state school-to-work projects.
- Social service support is essential to assist parents who need special services for their child and to help determine financial eligibility for Supplemental Security Income (SSI) or state program benefits (e.g., Medicaid) for individuals with physical, mental, or developmental disabilities or specific chronic diseases.
- Advocacy for children with chronic conditions and their families includes assisting them to secure coordinated and comprehensive health care and community-based services as needed.
- Provision of primary care services—regular health maintenance supervision and anticipatory guidance—must not be overlooked.
- Recognizing that parents commonly seek cures by using alternative treatments or medications, some of which can potentially cause harm or have no proven effectiveness is important.
- The time of diagnosis and periods of exacerbations of illness are viewed as times of crisis and added stress.
- Chronic sorrow is a phenomenon that involves feelings of sadness, anger, guilt, or failure that parents of a child with a chronic condition may experience at various times during their child's life. The term was coined by Olshansky in the 1960s to describe cyclical, recurring feelings of sadness during one's lifetime that are of differing degrees of intensity. It involves grieving without finality. It is not pathologic and does not occur uniformly within families (Hobdell, 2004; Roos, 2002; Shepard & Mahon, 2002).
- Developing a trusting relationship with these children and their families involves being respectful and accepting of their varied emotional needs.
- Engaging parents and their children in the treatment plan is a major and essential task.
- Research has demonstrated that more paternal involvement in illness-related support is associated with better family and maternal outcomes in families of children with chronic illness; hence in a two-parent household, participation by both parents in their child's care and health care visits should be encouraged (Gavin & Wysocki, 2006).
- Partial or poor adherence to complex treatment regimens is a frequent issue in caring for pediatric patients with chronic conditions. It should be dealt with in a collaborative, "blame-free" problem-solving approach.
- Parents of children with chronic diseases are more likely to think about using, or are using, CAM practices. It is not common for parents to reveal this to their conventional pediatric providers, so it is important that the health care provider ask about such practices. See Chapter 42 for a full discussion on

engaging the parents in a discussion about CAM, for being an advocate for the patient, and becoming a collaborative agent with the family.

Although chronic illnesses are diverse in their severity and effect on the child, certain issues are often common concerns for children with chronic conditions and their families. They include the following:

- The high cost of treatment—the potential need for financial assistance
- Lack of, or difficulties and barriers in, acquiring health care insurance coverage
- Family lifestyle alterations that may be required of parents or siblings, or both, in caring for the child
- The need to overcome system barriers that families may face navigating through the maze of agency paperwork
- The need for supervised care by multiple health care providers and the frequent lack of coordination of services in providing continuity of care
- Unpredictability of the condition and the potential for complications, frequent medical visits, hospitalizations, and death
- The desire to be kept informed of their child's condition and progress
- Often daily treatments or procedures are required that may be embarrassing, painful, or time consuming
- The developmental impact that chronic disease can have on a child, especially during adolescence and early adulthood (periods of increased vulnerability)
- Longevity concerns—ability to live and function independently as an adult, including the need for career and vocational counseling
- The level of knowledge parents need about the pharmacologic management of pain and the disease process or other therapeutic treatments, including nutritional support for the at-home care of the child
- The impact of stress on emotional and psychological well-being of the child and family members—parents or caregivers, siblings, and possibly the extended family support network
- Acceptance by peers
- Parental striving to successfully normalize their child's life—by acknowledging the child's condition and its impact on family lifestyle while actively engaging in accommodations to focus on the child and not the condition
- Dealing with feelings (e.g., anger, sorrow) while attempting to cope with chronic illness
- Developing advocacy skills for these children to access services through schools, state and community agencies, or special federally sponsored programs
- Securing special illness-related equipment (e.g., movement and mobility aids, such as walkers, wheelchairs, or braces) or acquiring communication aids, such as hearing aids or special computers with voices
- Finding respite care
- Legal conservatory issues and the concern about who will care for the child as an adult when parents are no longer capable of providing physical care or are deceased

Medically fragile and technology-dependent children are living longer than in the past and are reaching adulthood mainly as a result of improved technology and major advances in medical and surgical care. These children require a multidisciplinary team approach to their care. In addition, a multidisciplinary team approach is also the best for children with complex chronic diseases. These teams offer the expertise of many individuals in a united approach. Involvement of a clinical social worker, a community health nurse, or a nurse case manager is important to secure essential community resources for child and family. The family should be part of the team and not viewed as only the recipient of interventions. All team members must remember to respect the knowledge that parents or caregivers have about their child, their child's condition, and how the child is likely to respond both physically and emotionally to new therapeutic interventions or treatments, situational changes, or exacerbations of illnesses.

Empowerment of the child and family is a key concept that should be emphasized. Parents who have infants and young children with chronic conditions should be viewed as therapeutic partners in the management plan. Communications with parents should be open and honest. They should be treated with respect and dignity and allowed to vent their emotions and to use coping mechanisms that work for them. Likewise as the older child and adolescent mature, their partnership role emerges. Relapses in adherence behavior are problematic but not unusual in situations involving complex treatment plans. Problems of adherence to the management plan can lead to serious medical complications, increased rates of hospitalization, greater length of hospital stay, and increased health care costs. Therefore, the provider must vigilantly assess adherence factors and seek ways to improve adherence for children and adolescents living with chronic illnesses. Table 22-1 outlines categories and key factors to consider when addressing concerns about adherence. Training in motivational interviewing, where the interviewer seeks to ascertain the individual's level of readiness to change, is a promising technique to use in situations of less than optimal adherence. The key tenets of motivational interviewing are to establish and express empathy; to provide the choice to change or not; to work with patients and families to identify their own personal treatment goals; to work with resistance; to assist in the removal of barriers to change; to provide feedback; and to advocate for the development of patient self-efficacy (Fielding & Duff, 2006). See Chapter 9 for more information.

Family support groups are often beneficial; they offer an opportunity to interact with others who have experienced many of the same challenges, difficulties, sorrows, and triumphs. Sibling issues and feelings, such as anger, embarrassment, a sense of being overwhelmed with added responsibilities, or believing they need to be the protector for their brother or sister also must be addressed.

The critical issue in health promotion and disease management for children with special health needs is to ensure an organized and coordinated approach to provide appropriate treatment for the child's specific chronic disease or condition and to ensure that the child's primary health care needs

TABLE 22-1	**Key Factors That Affect Treatment Adherence in Children and Adolescents**			
Illness	**Management**	**Family**	**Patient**	**HCP and Environment**
Severity of the illness and its predictability	Complexity of treatment plan	Support network and size of family	Age	Communication style of HCPs with child, family, and other HCPs; belief in patient empowerment
Length of illness and prognosis	Length of time for each treatment, how often, and for what length of time must continue such treatments	Financial resources; knowledge base and the understanding of illness or condition; overall cognitive skills; communication style	Cognitive, social, and emotional level of development; temperament	Organization of clinic or office setting to be child, teen, and family friendly; need for adaptive modifications in their environment
Impact of illness on functional and social activities of daily living	Visibility of equipment	Coping ability and skills; Problem-solving skills Family's belief system and spiritual base	Peer group; coping ability	Number of HCPs involved in the child's care; team member collaboration and partnership among themselves and with the family Open and "blame-free" approach when compliance issues arise

HCP, Health care provider.

are met. Health care management for children with special health needs includes: (1) assessing their needs; (2) planning comprehensive health care to provide for both physical and psychosocial needs; (3) facilitating and coordinating services; (4) following up and monitoring services given and the child's progress; and (5) empowering the child and family through education, counseling, and support. Addressing issues upfront about quality of life should always be part of the assessment process in chronic pediatric illness management. Child and parent perceptions about quality of life issues, such as physical and emotional pain and discomfort, may not be the same as those held by the health care provider. Child, parent, and health care provider may each have different perceptions. It is vitally important to determine how the child and the parent feel—physically, emotionally, and socially—by listening to them and asking for their input, rather than assuming that all is going well based on outward appearances (Janse et al, 2005). Health care management of children with chronic disease is about empowering them to live their lives to the fullest potential.

The level or type of involvement in the treatment and management of a child with a specific chronic disease may vary depending on the unique situation of the child and family and the health care provider's subspecialty training and education. Strategies related to fostering the child's psychosocial development should be addressed at each health care encounter. Certain situations may require additional advocacy, such as when children with special needs and their families are in a particularly vulnerable position (e.g., if the parent of a child with special needs loses his or her job or suffers significant illness or injury and cannot adequately provide for the child). Children with chronic conditions do well when family functioning is high and there is positive family adaptation.

Finally, to promote effective child and family functioning, primary health care providers need to design a flow of care that is based upon a chronic care model, such as the one described by Bodenheimer and colleagues (2002). Optimal chronic care management must take into consideration the following six elements: linkages with community resources, an integrated or organized approach to health care delivery (chronic care management is viewed as a priority in the health care organization and setting), a focus on and support for self-management by patients and families, a delivery system design that provides for planned care not scattered episodic visits, decision support that is based upon evidence-based guidelines, and a clinical information system of documentation that promotes easy access to important information (e.g., individual and population-based registries that document care including laboratory results and key measurements—blood pressures, peak flow readings, etc).

■ ASSESSMENT
HISTORY AND PHYSICAL EXAMINATION

Chapter 2 discusses the complete history and physical examination of children from infancy through adolescence. In addition, each of the pediatric disease management chapters in this unit focuses on key questions to ask in history taking and highlights significant findings to be alert to if found on physical examination. Careful attention must be given when analyzing the signs and symptoms of a child's illness, including the presentation of clinical findings, the course of the disease process, and its associated manifestations. A clear history of the illness is essential.

The physical examination is often a challenge when a young child is ill and uncooperative. Patience is important when examining children who are sick. The sick child should be carefully assessed so that significant physical findings are not missed during a hurried or cursory examination. The parts of the physical examination that are especially bothersome or frightening to a child, based upon either historical information, observation, or age factors, should be performed last. Often times examining the child on the parent's lap can be a helpful practice in these situations. Repeating parts of the examination or observational reassessment is sometimes useful (e.g., after a febrile child is given acetaminophen and the fever abates somewhat).

Chapter 23 discusses an overall assessment and management plan for sick, febrile children. It also identifies specific infectious diseases and assessment criteria for illnesses or problems commonly seen in childhood. In general, with infectious diseases, the age of a child is a significant factor to consider when doing an assessment and creating a management plan. The immune response in infants birth to 90 days old, for example, is particularly poor because of their immature immune system. Infants and young children are at increased risk for overwhelming bacteremia with any infection. Similarly, in other noninfectious diseases and conditions, age often continues to remain a key factor in the assessment of the child.

To assess the severity of illness in infants and young children, careful attention must be given to judging six key indicators during both the history and the physical examination (Box 22-1). These indicators are an important part of the assessment and judgment when determining management and include level of consciousness, hydration, color, reaction to stimulation, sleep-to-awake or awake-to-sleep state, and response to social clues. The child should be noted to have either a normal (NL), moderately impaired (MI), or severely impaired (SI) response in each of the six key areas (McCarthy, 2004).

DIAGNOSTIC STUDIES

When deciding whether to order diagnostic tests, the provider should keep the following goals in mind. Order only those tests that give the most information for the least money, are crucial in the establishment of a concrete diagnosis, or are critical elements in the development of the treatment plan. If radiographic or imaging tests are necessary, order the test that is the least invasive. There are several useful points to remember about common imaging tests:
- Conventional radiographs are:
  - Useful diagnostic tools

BOX 22-1 Critical Indicators for Assessing Severity of Illness in Pediatric Patients and a Scoring Guide*

1. Level of consciousness or quality of cry:
   - Strong cry with normal tone or content and not crying (NL)
   - Whimpering or sobbing (MI)
   - Weak or moaning or high pitched (SI)
2. Hydration:
   - Skin normal; eyes and mouth moist (NL)
   - Skin and eyes normal and mouth slightly dry (MI)
   - Skin doughy or tented and eyes may be sunken, dry eyes and mouth (SI)
3. Color:
   - Pink (NL)
   - Pale hands, feet, or acrocyanosis (MI)
   - Pale or blue or ashen gray or mottled (SI)
4. Reaction to stimulation by parent or health care provider (HCP) (How a crying child reacts when held, patted on back, jiggled on lap, or carried):
   - Strong cry and normal tone or content and not crying (NL)
   - Crying on and off (MI)
   - Cries continuously or minimal response (SI)
5. Sleep to awake or awake to sleep state:
   - If awake then stays awake or, if asleep and stimulated, wakens quickly (NL)
   - Eyes close briefly then awakens or awakens but needs prolonged stimulation (MI)
   - Not able to arouse or falls to sleep (SI)
6. Response to social cues (being held, kissed, hugged, touched, quietly talked to, or comforted)—For infants 2 months or less use alert ratings:
   - Smiles or alerts (NL)
   - Either briefly smiles or alerts to cue (MI)
   - No smile, face anxious, dull look, expressionless, or no alerting (SI)

*NL, Normal; MI, moderately impaired; SI, severely impaired.

- ○ The least expensive of the imaging tests
- ○ Readily available
- Computed tomography (CT) imaging:
  - ○ Provides excellent bone and soft tissue detail and can image bone, soft tissue, and blood vessels at the same time
  - ○ Can be used with contrast material (taken by mouth, rectum, or injected via vein) for special evaluations, such as abnormalities affecting blood vessels; check for allergies to iodine or seafood, kidney disease, or prior reaction to contrast materials
  - ○ Shows relationships well; images can be presented in the frontal, transverse, or sagittal planes or obtained in three-dimensional imaging
  - ○ May require sedation or anesthetic for infants and young children
  - ○ Requires radiation exposure
  - ○ Is costly
- Magnetic resonance imaging (MRI):
  - ○ Provides excellent images of soft tissue without exposure to ionizing radiation; bone imaging is poor
  - ○ Is expensive
  - ○ Often requires sedation or anesthetic in infants and young children because immobilization is necessary
- Ultrasonography:
  - ○ Gives two-dimensional images and measurements of internal organ systems; however, air-filled lungs and gas-filled bowel loops are impenetrable to ultrasound
  - ○ In the form of Doppler ultrasound, blood flow direction and velocity can be measured; a still picture of the image can be recorded as a permanent record, or sonography can be viewed as the image is being projected on a video screen
  - ○ Is highly dependent on operator skill and experience
  - ○ Does not require sedation
  - ○ Involves no radiation exposure

Chapter 26 contains a detailed discussion of the complete blood count (CBC) and provides insight as to the information that can be gained from a CBC, in addition to indications for ordering this basic laboratory study. Coagulation studies are also discussed. Chapter 23 discusses the laboratory work-up for young children with a fever of undetermined origin. All disease entities or conditions addressed in this text include information about diagnostic studies and laboratory tests. Diagnostic studies and tests are valuable but are only one part of the entire database. Tests should be ordered only when the results are necessary to guide clinical decision-making.

▰ USE OF MEDICATION

Pediatric patients are at increased risk for adverse drug reactions for numerous reasons, such as the need for individualized doses based on patient's age, weight, and clinical condition and changing pharmacokinetic parameters at various ages and stages of maturational development. Selecting the appropriate pharmacologic agent to adequately treat an illness or condition and minimizing the risk of medication errors are important factors to consider. List current medications and dosages for both prescription and OTC drugs, herbals, dietary supplements, and botanical preparations in a standard place in the patient's chart. Allergies to medications, with the identified adverse response, should be highlighted in a place that is easily visible.

Several key principles serve as guides in the use of prescription drugs and OTC medications.

SAFE PRESCRIPTION-WRITING PRACTICES

Prescriptions should be written in a manner that conveys accurate information to the pharmacist and the patient or parent. The following suggestions are made to ensure safe prescription writing for children (Taketomo et al, 2007):

- Never place a decimal and a trailing 0 (zero) after a whole number, because the decimal point might not be read correctly (e.g., 3.0 mL can be mistaken for 30 mL).
- Place a leading 0 (zero) before fractions less than 1 (one). For example, write 0.3 mL rather than .3 mL, which can be confused with 3 mL if the decimal point is inadvertently missed.
- Insert a space between the last number and its units (e.g., 15 mg not 15mg). Do not place a period after mL or mg when writing a prescription.
- Never use dangerous abbreviations, such as q.d. or qd (daily) or U or u (unit), which may be misinterpreted for q.i.d. or qid (4 times daily) or 0 (zero), respectively. Write out in full the words "daily" or "unit." The abbreviation O.D. means right eye; never use O.D. as an abbreviation for once daily.
- Do not use the abbreviation μg; instead use mcg.
- Use the metric system only.
- Write legibly.
- Issue a complete prescription that contains all of the following:
  - ○ Patient's full name, age (date of birth), and weight (for infants and young children)
  - ○ Name of the drug, dosage, and strength
  - ○ Instructions if a brand name drug is to be used rather than the generic drug option
  - ○ Total amount or quantity (number of pills, milliliters of liquid) to be dispensed
  - ○ Route of administration (e.g., take by mouth, instill in both ears, insert in rectum, instill in right eye)
  - ○ General instructions to the patient or parent about indications for or the purpose of taking the medication, how frequently, and for how long (e.g., take three times a day until completed, take every 4 to 6 hours as needed for pain for 3 days)
  - ○ Special instructions to the patient or parent about the drug (e.g., give with food, do not give with dairy products) or other instructions (e.g., translate to the primary language of the parent if English is not spoken or read)
  - ○ Number of refills
  - ○ Instructions to fill with a measuring device or other essential delivery devices (e.g., spacer or Aerochamber for an aerosolized medication)

In addition, some prescription plans or health care settings may require that a diagnosis and allergies to medication be listed on the prescription form. Do a SCRIPT analysis after you have written a prescription for any medication to review the pharmacologic management plan. SCRIPT is a useful acronym to remember and stands for the following:

- **S**ide effects
- **C**ontraindications
- **R**ight medication, dosage, frequency, route, and duration
- **P**ediatric considerations
- **T**ransmittal of all necessary information on the prescription

PRESCRIBING PHARMACOLOGIC AGENTS

When prescribing pharmacologic agents or recommending OTC drugs, it is important to be knowledgeable of the pharmacodynamics and pharmacokinetics of the drug, the usual dosage, adverse reactions, and the indications and contraindications for its use in children. The provider must have a clear purpose in mind for using a particular drug and should not prescribe or recommend agents because of pressure from a parent or any other individual. Keep the following points in mind when prescribing drugs or OTC medications:

- Lack of compliance in taking medications can be a major problem. Factors that affect compliance include the following:
  - The more often a drug must be given per day the greater the chance that a dose or doses will be missed.
  - Drugs that have a bitter or repulsive taste are difficult and sometimes impossible to get a child to take. For an extra cost, some pharmacies will sell flavoring products that increase palatability (e.g., FLAVORx).
  - The greater the number of drugs that a child is given, the greater the potential for a drug dose to be missed, drug interactions, or the wrong drug to be taken. Be sure to check for interactions between pharmacologics and any herbal, botanical, or dietary supplements.
  - Waking a child to take a medication is difficult for parents; prescribe round-the-clock dosing only when it is essential to maintain tight therapeutic drug levels.
- Poorly given or inadequate instructions increase the risk that the prescribed agent will be misused.
- Children with renal or hepatic dysfunction require dosing adjustments.

EDUCATING PARENTS AND CHILDREN ABOUT PHARMACOLOGIC AGENTS

The success of any pediatric health care encounter depends on the ability of the health provider to educate parents or children, or both. Before patients and their parents or caregivers leave the health care setting, they should have a basic understanding about the pharmacologic effect of any medication or OTC drug that is prescribed or recommended. Points of information that should be emphasized include the following:

- The purpose of the drug, how much should be given, and the frequency of administration
- Instructions about the indications for using a drug that is given on an "as necessary" basis or under specific circum-

stances (e.g., a rescue plan for the child with asthma whose symptoms are worsening)
- Signs or symptoms that indicate that a drug is either effective or not producing the desired effect or effects
- Possible drug-drug or drug-nutrient interactions, precautions, or adverse reactions that can occur
- Information about drug stability, such as the need for refrigeration or storage and compatibility issues (not exposed to light or mixing with foods or other drugs)
- If applicable, any monitoring parameters that are required for safe administration of the drug or to maintain effective therapeutic blood levels (e.g., blood levels)
- Pregnancy risk factor of a drug (refers to the Federal Drug Administration's A, B, C, D, or X categories that indicate the potential of a systemically absorbed drug causing birth defects) and the need to screen for pregnancy when giving specific drugs to female teenagers
- For children who take multiple medications, the importance of always carrying with them an up-to-date list of medications (prescription, OTC, herbal products, vitamins, and minerals), their strengths, and dosages, in addition to a list of medications the child cannot take in case of an emergency or if the child is seen by another health care provider
- Tips to help parents administer medications that may be difficult to get the child to take (e.g., how to hold an infant or small child when administering a medication)

Some medications can be safely mixed to mask the flavor of unpleasant medications. However, be sure to counsel about any medication that may have untoward interactions with foods or that should be administered on an empty stomach. The following is a listing of liquids or solid foods that may be suggested: chocolate or strawberry syrup, ice cream, applesauce, frozen juice concentrates (orange, grape, lemonade), chocolate pudding, regular or frozen yogurt, and jelly. Other suggestions are to have the child eat peanut butter crackers before taking a medicine, eat part of a flavored ice pop before and after taking medications, or chew on ice chips before or after the dose. Be sure to tell parents that they need to check with the pharmacist to determine whether the medication can be taken with a food.

Return demonstration can be a useful adjunct to evaluate the ability of the parent or child to administer a drug or drugs in the desired fashion. Return demonstration is a desired teaching tool in many situations. Examples of such circumstances include the following:

- Administering oral suspensions to infants and young children
- Measuring small or exact dosages (e.g., when a syringe is needed to measure amounts)
- Giving injectable, intravenous, gastrostomy, or nasogastric tube medications
- Instilling ophthalmic drops or ointments or nasal sprays or drops
- Using a metered-dose inhaler (MDI), spacers, or inhalation equipment
- Ensuring that parents with limited cognitive abilities can safely administer medication to their children

- Administering multiple medications to ensure that the correct dose of the correct medication is given (e.g., 3 mL of amoxicillin suspension and 1 mL of metoclopramide syrup and not the reverse)

PRESCRIPTIVE AUTHORITY FOR NURSE PRACTITIONERS

NPs must be knowledgeable about the individual state regulations that govern their prescription-writing privileges. Some states do not use the term *prescribe* to identify what NPs do when writing medication prescriptions for patients. For example, in California the term *furnish* is used to describe this activity. The individual state board of registered nursing identifies the terminology to be used for this activity and regulates (either as a single state regulatory entity or jointly with medicine or pharmacology state boards) the activities and procedures related to this particular function. Regulations about prescriptive activity vary from state to state. NPs are governed by individual state guidelines and are legally obliged to follow all state regulations and mandates related to any prescriptive authority granted to them.

■ EDUCATIONAL STRATEGIES

The severity of the illness or disease and the child's age, maturity, and cognitive level are key factors that determine the child's degree of involvement in self-care activities related to acute illness and chronic disease management. Children should be taught basic health promotion and disease prevention behaviors from early childhood. Likewise, they should be involved in the management of their illness to the fullest extent possible considering their developmental capabilities. Health professionals frequently ignore or forget to include the school-age child or adolescent as a partner in the management plan. Children should be consulted regarding their responsibilities for self-care. The pediatric provider also might be called on to be a liaison with the school nurse by educating other school district personnel about the child's illness or medical condition so that the child's educational and social experience at school can be optimized.

Written instructions and easy-to-read handouts are useful for parents, caregivers, and children, whether the instructions deal with common illness management, complex treatment needs, or information about developmental milestones and anticipatory guidance issues. An excellent resource for parents is *Immunizations and Infectious Diseases: an Informed Parent's Guide* (Fischer, 2005). *Patient Education for Children, Teens and Parents* (American Academy of Pediatrics [AAP], 2006) and *Health Care Advice: Patient Education for Children, Teens and Parents* (AAP, 2004) contain useful guidelines for parents or caretakers and are available in both English and Spanish versions. Whether a practice setting develops its own instruction sheets or uses information sheets from other resource texts, important issues are that the instructions should be written in the family's native language and at a reading level appropriate for the individual family.

There are a number of textbooks written for the lay public that are excellent resources to suggest to parents. The care providers should develop a list of appropriate textbooks and websites to give to parents based on the parent's literacy level and unique characteristics. Select books that offer guidance about common infections of childhood, preventive pediatrics, common behavioral problems, and other frequently encountered pediatric concerns. Each practice setting should have its own list of books and supply of handouts, brochures, pamphlets, and other printed resources to share with families in their practice. All written materials either recommended or given to families should be congruent with the reading level of the family and their primary spoken language.

■ PREVENTION OF ILLNESS

Prevention of illness and communicable diseases is a significant goal when providing primary health care services for children or managing the care of children with chronic diseases or conditions. Health care providers must be vigilant in their practice settings to prevent or reduce the possibility of exposure to communicable diseases and to control the spread of infectious diseases that are a threat to infants, children, and youth. Adherence to the following guidelines will further the goal of prevention:

- All children should be appropriately immunized against vaccine-preventable diseases according to the recommendations of the Advisory Committee on Immunization Practices (ACIP), the American Academy of Pediatrics (AAP), and the American Academy of Family Physicians (AAFP).
- Communicable diseases need to be identified and treated appropriately and reported in a timely fashion to public health departments as required by law.
- Develop practice setting policies about the following: segregating infected children from well children as quickly as possible; avoiding crowded waiting rooms, shorten waiting times, and minimize sharing of toys; washing of hands before and after patient contact; wiping the body of otoscopes or ophthalmoscopes regularly; and cleaning of ear curettes after each use and disinfecting with bleach solution or alcohol if contaminated with blood.
- Health practices to prevent or control the spread of infectious disease are carried out in home care programs, out-of-home child care programs, schools and health care settings, and hospitals. Key practices include the following:
  - Use effective personal hygiene—hand washing for 10 seconds to prevent fecal-oral and person-to-person skin contact spread of disease. Teach children the importance of washing their hands, especially after toileting and blowing their nose and before eating.
  - Ensure appropriate environmental sanitation—disposing of waste (e.g., blood, urine, feces, vomit, saliva) together with proper cleaning and disinfection of equipment, toys, toilets, eating areas, and diaper-changing surfaces. There should be a regular schedule of cleaning, in addition to cleaning when contaminated.

○ Reduce respiratory spread of disease—cough into one's sleeve and minimize use of handkerchiefs; cover mouth when sneezing or coughing, dispose of tissue after wiping nose, and wash hands immediately; discourage habits of touching the mouth, nose, and eyes; eliminate passive smoke and provide adequate ventilation.

○ Do not serve raw or undercooked eggs or meats.

○ Promote appropriate handling, preparation, sanitation, and storage of food.

○ Reduce exposure to communicable disease by separating sick children from well children.

• Educate youth about the prevention of sexually transmitted infections.

• Educate young children and teenagers to not share food, liquids, personal hygiene products, cosmetics, hair coverings, grooming products, or towels with others.

• Discourage children from kissing pets.

• Provide preventive health guidance about avoiding second-hand smoke, especially in cars and other confined areas.

Out-of-home day care is a risk factor for the spread of infectious diseases. Day care in a small day care home is associated with less spread of infectious disease than is day care provided in a larger day care center. The American Public Health Association and the AAP, as part of a collaborative project, published *Caring for Our Children. National Health and Safety Standards: Guidelines for Out-of-Home Child Care Programs* (2002). This book outlines preventive health practices that promote a safe environment for infants and children and addresses the issues of disease prevention and management in family and group day care homes and child care centers. Preventing and controlling the spread of illness in these group settings are important issues in maintaining health.

■ PAIN IN CHILDREN

Health care providers must be familiar with the assessment and effective management of pain in the pediatric and adolescent population. Unrelieved pain has both negative physiologic and negative psychological consequences. Pain can result from injury or disease processes or as a side effect of diagnostic or therapeutic procedures or surgery. Early pain stimuli and experiences can produce long-term consequences for the child. Likewise, inadequate pain relief during initial procedures can decrease the effect of adequate analgesia during subsequent procedures. Neonates and pediatric oncology patients who had inadequate analgesia experiences have been shown to suffer long-standing alterations in their pain perceptions and responses to later painful procedures (Zempsky et al, 2004). Accordingly, best practice standards for pediatric care necessitate that pain management be part of all treatment plans for even minor painful procedures and when it is associated with more serious illness or injury. Therefore, the elimination of preventable pain and the reduction of unpreventable pain should be management goals for all health care treatment plans. The importance of effective pain management in children cannot be overemphasized. To this end, a joint statement was issued by the AAP and the American Pain Society (2001) reinforcing the need for health care providers to treat pain and suffering in all infants, children, and adolescents. This statement continues to be a relevant document in today's health management of children.

Assessment and management of minor pain in primary and emergency care settings is the focus of this section. The pediatric provider should seek other references for a more in-depth discussion of the treatment of chronic pain in pediatric patients.

Key factors that can influence effective pain management in children include the following:

• Established pain is difficult to control; therefore, prevention of and quick action in response to pain are essential goals of pain management.

• Pediatric and adolescent patients and their families should be involved in pain education, its assessment and management as much as possible. Parents must be educated about their role in engaging and providing distraction and comfort to their child during and after painful procedures (e.g., needle sticks, ear exams, vaccinations).

• Culture and family learning patterns must be considered (e.g., beliefs about pain, folk remedies, how pain is expressed verbally, and language barriers).

• Genetic stressors may be responsible for differing levels of neurotransmitters or responses to medication.

• Physiologic and psychological differences between individuals, memories, and possible prenatal and perinatal stressors can influence a child's perception of pain.

• Chronic pain is rarely associated with sympathetic nervous system arousal. Therefore, children with chronic pain may not appear to be in pain, which may negatively affect their evaluation and treatment. However, to effectively treat chronic pain in children, the physical and psychological manifestations of chronic pain must be considered.

• Developmental issues (e.g., cognitive, emotional, and physical), age, and temperament significantly affect how pain is interpreted, expressed, and controlled. Therefore, pain management must be tailored to the child's age and developmental level.

• Cognitive issues that influence pain perception include the child's memory and level of understanding, ability to control what will happen, attachment of a meaning to the situation with regard to pain, and expectations of the intensity of the pain.

• Emotional issues that affect a child's pain perception include anxiety, fear, frustration, anger, and depression.

• Social issues, such as how others react (their behaviors) to the child in pain, can influence the treatment plan. Likewise family harmony or conflict can influence a child's pain.

• Pain perception involves complex neural interactions that send out impulses or noxious stimuli generated by tissue damage. The physiologic process associated with pain is termed *nociception* and includes the following (Golianu et al, 2000):

- ○ Transduction—painful stimuli are translated into electrical signals at sensory nerve endings and forwarded to the spinal cord.
- ○ Transmission—the electrical impulses are forwarded through the sensory nervous system.
- ○ Modulation—alteration of information by endogenous mechanisms results in lessening or amplification of the initial signal.
- ○ Perception—the emotional and physical experience of pain.
- For a variety of reasons (e.g., fear of getting a shot), some children do not report pain to health care providers.

The goal of acute pain management in pediatrics is to effectively control pain with minimal therapy side effects. Positive outcomes of effective pain control are decreased suffering, increased satisfaction for the child and parents, and an enhanced recovery process.

PAIN ASSESSMENT

A systematic approach to the assessment of pain in children and adolescents begins by obtaining a pain history from the child or the parent. When talking with younger children, ask the parent what words the child uses for pain (e.g., "owie," "boo-boo," "ouchie," "hurting," "uncomfortable," "warm," or "stinging") and use these words with the child. Behavioral observations and physiologic findings provide additional information to complete a comprehensive pain assessment. The evaluation of pain in children needs to be multidimensional. The provider must collect data about what children say about their pain, assess for physiologic and emotional manifestations of pain, and investigate other pertinent factors that can contribute to the child's pain as listed earlier.

CLINICAL FINDINGS

History

A careful history is necessary and requires a systematic approach to history taking. An interval history and examination is always needed when pain does not abate as expected or there is a change in the quality, intensity, duration, or location of pain. In assessing pain, the following information should be obtained:

- Pain history (symptom analysis):
  - ○ Intensity (mild, moderate, severe, overwhelming)
  - ○ Location (areas with pain and without pain)
  - ○ Quality—how pain is described by child or parent (e.g., stinging, burning, "big ouchie") and any pain behaviors noted
  - ○ Duration (how long has the pain been present)
  - ○ Temporal features or chronology (when and how did the pain start, precipitating factors, any variations in intensity and quality)
  - ○ Previous treatments or procedures
  - ○ What makes the pain worse or better
  - ○ Other associated symptoms, such as anxiety
- Past experience with pain, including child's memory of the painful experience and how the pain was treated
- Cultural beliefs about pain and its treatment

- Self-reports of pain in the verbal child (if possible obtain pain history as noted). Identify a tool that is reliable, valid, sensitive, and simple for the child to understand and use the tool consistently. The use of self-report tools, patient pain diary or journal, and other objective pain measures helps to objectively quantify pain before treatment and serves to evaluate the outcome of treatment (Table 22-2).

Pain can be categorized into five types: acute, chronic persistent, recurrent, neuropathic, and psychogenic (Table 22-3). Choice of treatment depends upon these types, in addition to the intensity: fair, moderate, or severe. Table 22-4 provides management guidance using pharmacologic drugs.

Behavioral Indicators

Behavioral observations include vocalizations (e.g., crying, whimpering, whining); social withdrawal; changes in sleep patterns (more or less); verbalizations; facial expressions of guarding, grimacing, tightly closed eyelids, vigilance, or anger; motor responses; body posture; and activity, such as rubbing or touching the painful site, avoiding the painful site, or guarding the affected area (e.g., not letting anyone touch the abdomen or withdrawal of an injured limb). These may be the only cues of pain in preverbal or nonverbal children. Infants in pain sleep less, are irritable and agitated, do not feed as well or refuse to feed, and have increased muscle tone (Schechter, 2006).

Physiologic Indicators

Physiologic parameters (e.g., alterations in heart rate, SpO_2 reading, respiratory rate and pattern, and blood pressure) are neither sensitive nor specific indicators of pain, particularly in children who experience chronic pain. Other physical indicators include such findings as diaphoresis and pallor. Pulse-oximetry readings may be decreased because of increased oxygen consumption. Other physiologic responses to pain can include changes in metabolic functioning (e.g., hypermetabolism, hyperglycemia, or lipolysis), decreased gut motility, sodium and water retention, and cytokine production.

MANAGEMENT

If there is a known etiology or underlying disease causing the pain, treat its causes. Other measures may be needed to control pain symptoms. Principles of effective office-based pain management include the use of a combination of pharmacologic and nonpharmacologic measures. Other elements should also be considered within the practice setting environment that can contribute to anxiety and its resultant effect on patients' perceptions of pain. The environment should be child-friendly, calming, with colorful walls that have pictures, together with a collection of toys and games to minimize fear associated with an unfamiliar setting. There can be interactions between herbal preparations and common pain relievers and anesthetics (see Table 42-2). For postoperative surgical pain, when the surgery was elective, certain herbal preparations need to be discontinued 1 week before the procedure (see Table 42-2). Should the provider and family or patient wish to consider nonpharmacologic management of pain as an option, Table 42-5 provides some guidance.

TABLE 22-2 **Common Pain Rating Scales Used to Measure Pain in Pediatric and Adolescent Patients**

Pain Scale/Description	Instructions	Recommended Age/Comments
FACES Pain Rating Scale* (Wong, 1996; Wong & Baker, 1988): Consists of six cartoon faces ranging from smiling face for "no pain" to tearful face for "worst pain."	*Original instructions:* Explain to the child that each face is for a person who feels happy because he has no pain (hurt) or sad because he has some or a lot of pain. Face 0 is very happy because he does not hurt at all. Face 1 hurts just a little bit. Face 2 hurts a little more. Face 3 hurts even more. Face 4 hurts a whole lot. Face 5 hurts as much as you can imagine, although you do not have to be crying to feel this bad. Ask the child to choose the face that best describes how he or she is feeling. Record the number under the chosen face on the pain assessment record. *Brief word instructions:* Point to each face using the words to describe the pain intensity. Ask the child to choose the face that best describes his or her own pain and record the appropriate number.	Children as young as 3 years Using original instructions without affect words, such as *happy* or *sad,* or brief words resulted in same pain rating, probably reflecting child's rating of pain intensity. For coding purposes, numbers 0, 2, 4, 6, 8, 10 can be substituted for 0-5 system to accommodate 0-10 system. The FACES Pain Rating Scale provides three scales in one: facial expressions, numbers, and words.
Oucher (Beyer et al, 1989): Consists of six photographs of child's face representing "no hurt" to "biggest hurt you could ever have"; also includes a vertical scale with numbers from 1-100; scales for African-American and Hispanic children have been developed (Villarruel & Denyes, 1991).	*Numeric scale:* Point to each section of scale to explain variations in pain intensity: • "Zero means no hurt." • "This means little hurts" (pointing to lower part of scale, 1-29). • "This means middle hurts" (pointing to middle part of scale, 30 to 69). • "This means big hurts" (pointing to upper part of scale, 70-99). • "100 means the biggest hurt you could ever have." Score is actual number stated by child. *Photographic scale:* Point to each photograph on Oucher and explain variations in pain intensity using the following language: first picture from the bottom is "no hurt," second is "little hurt," third is "a little more hurt," fourth is "even more hurt than that," fifth is "pretty much or a lot of hurt," and the sixth is the "biggest hurt you could ever have." Score pictures from 0-5, with the bottom picture scored as 0. *General:* Practice using Oucher by recalling and rating previous pain experiences (e.g., falling off a bike). Child points to number or photograph that describes pain intensity associated with the experience. Obtain current pain score from the child by asking, "How much hurt do you have right now?"	Children 3 to 13 years. Use numeric scale if child can count to 100 by ones and identify larger of any two numbers or by tens (Jordan-Marsh et al, 1994). Determine whether child has cognitive ability to use photographic scale; child should be able to seriate six geometric shapes from largest to smallest. Determine which ethnic version of Oucher to use. Allow the child to select a version of Oucher or use the version that most closely matches the physical characteristics of the child.
Poker chip tool† (Hester et al, 1998): Uses four red poker chips placed horizontally in front of the child.	Say to the child: "I want to talk with you about the hurt you may be having right now." Align the chips horizontally in front of the child on the bedside table, a clipboard, or other firm surface. Tell the child, "These are pieces of hurt." Beginning at the chip nearest the child's left side and ending at the one nearest the right side, point to the chips and say, "This (first chip) is a little bit of hurt and this (fourth chip) is the most hurt you could ever have." For a young child or for any child who may not fully comprehend the instructions, clarify by saying, "That means this one (first chip) is just a little hurt, this (second chip) is a little more hurt, this (third chip) is more yet, and this one (fourth chip) is the most hurt you could ever have." Do not give children an option for zero hurt. Research with the poker chip tool has verified that children without pain will so indicate by responses, such as "I don't have any." Ask the child, "How many pieces of hurt do you have right now?" After initial use of the poker chip tool, some children internalize the concept of "pieces of hurt." If a child gives a response, such as "I have one right now," *before* you ask or before you lay out the chips, record the number of chips on the pain flow sheet. Clarify the child's answer by words, such as, "Oh, you have a little hurt? Tell me about the hurt."	Children as young as 4 years.

TABLE 22-2   **Common Pain Rating Scales Used to Measure Pain in Pediatric and Adolescent Patients—Cont'd**

Pain Scale/Description	Instructions	Recommended Age/Comments
Word-Graphic Rating Scale[‡] (Tesler et al, 1991): Uses descriptive words (may vary in other scales) to denote varying intensities of pain.	Explain to the child, "This is a line with words to describe how much pain you may have. This side of the line means no pain and over here the line means the worst possible pain." (Point with your finger where "no pain" is and run your finger along the line to "worst possible pain," as you say it.) "If you have no pain, you would mark like this." (Show example.) "If you have some pain, you would mark somewhere along the line, depending on how much pain you have." (Show example.) "The more pain you have, the closer to worst pain you would mark. The worst pain possible is marked like this." (Show example.) "Show me how much pain you have right now by marking with a straight, up-and-down line anywhere along the line to show how much pain you have right now." With a millimeter rule, measure from the "no pain" end to the mark and record this measurement as the pain score.	Children 4 to 17 years.
Numeric Scale: Uses straight line with end points identified as "no pain" and "worst pain" and sometimes "medium pain" in the middle; divisions along line are marked in units from 0-10 (high number may vary).	Explain to the child that at one end of the line is a 0, which means that a person feels no pain (hurt). At the other end is usually a 5 or 10, which means the person feels the worst pain imaginable. The numbers from 1-5 or 10 are for a very little pain to a whole lot of pain. Ask the child to choose a number that best describes his or her own pain.	Children as young as 5 years, as long as they can count and have some concept of numbers and their values in relation to other numbers. Scale may be used horizontally or vertically. Number coding should be same as other scales used in a facility.
Visual Analogue Scale (Cline et al, 1992): Defined as a vertical or horizontal line that is drawn to a certain length, such as 10 cm, and anchored by items that represent the extremes of the subjective phenomenon, such as pain, that is measured.	Ask the child to place a mark on a line that best describes the amount of his or her own pain. With a centimeter ruler, measure from "no pain" end to the mark and record this measurement as the pain score.	Children as young as 4.5 years, preferably 7 years. Vertical or horizontal scale may be used.
Color tool (Eland, 1993): Uses markers for child to construct own scale that is used with body outline.	Present eight markers to the child in random order. Ask the child, "of these colors, which color is like …?" (the event identified by the child as having hurt the most). Place the marker (represents severe pain) away from the other markers. Ask the child, "Which color is like a hurt, but not quite as much as …?" (the event identified by the child as having hurt the most). Place the marker next to the marker chosen to represent severe pain. Ask the child, "Which color is like something that hurts just a little?" Place marker with the others. Ask the child, "Which color is like no hurt at all?" Show the four marker color choices to the child in order from worst to the no-hurt color. Ask the child to show on the body outlines where he or she hurts, using the markers. After the child has colored in the hurts, ask if they are current hurts or hurts from the past. Ask if the child knows why the area hurts if it is not clear to you why it does.	Children as young as 4 years, provided they know their colors, are not color blind, and are able to construct the scale if in pain.

From Hockenberry-Eaton M et al: *Wong's nursing care of infants and children,* ed 7, St Louis, 2001, Mosby, pp 1052-1053.
Wong-Baker FACES Pain Rating Scale Reference Manual, describing development and research of the scale, is available from the Mayday Pain Resource Center, City of Hope National Medical Center, 1500 East Duarte Road, Duarte, CA 91010; phone: 626-301-8941.
[†]Developed in 1975 by NO Hester, University of Colorado Health Sciences Center, School of Nursing, Denver, CO 80262. Also available in Spanish and French.
[‡]Instructions for Word-Graphic Rating Scale from Acute Pain Management Guideline Panel: *Acute pain management in infants, children, and adolescents: operative and medical procedures; quick reference guide for clinicians,* AHCPR pub no 92-0020, Rockville, Md, 1992, Agency for Health Care Policy and Research (now the Agency for Healthcare Research and Quality [AHRQ]), Public Health Service, US Department of Health and Human Services. Word-Graphic Rating Scale is part of the Adolescent Pediatric Pain Tool and is available from Pediatric Pain Study, University of California, School of Nursing, Department of Family Health Care Nursing, San Francisco, CA 94143-0606; phone: 415-476-4040.

TABLE 22-3 **Five Kinds of Pain**

Type	Description	Examples
Acute	Brief; associated with tissue damage or inflammation; intensity steadily diminishes over days to weeks	Surgical pain, burns, fractures
Chronic persistent	Persistent or near-persistent pain over a period of 3 months or longer	Arthritis, sickle cell crisis
Recurrent	Repetitive painful episode alternating with pain-free intervals	Headache; abdominal, chest, or limb pain
Neuropathic	Persistent pain related to persistent or abnormal excitability in the peripheral or central nervous system with no ongoing tissue injury; often described as "burning," "strange," or "pins and needles"	Amputation pain syndromes, plexus injuries, reflex sympathetic dystrophy
Psychogenic	Persistent pain that is a manifestation of a psychiatric disease	Somatization disorder, somatoform pain disorder, conversion disorder

From Betz CL, Sowden LA: *Mosby's pediatric nursing reference,* ed 5, Philadelphia, 2004, Mosby.

TABLE 22-4 **Common Oral Pain Medications and Doses Used With Children (<50 kg)**

Pain Medication	Dose (mg/kg)	Frequency	Comments
Acetaminophen	10-15	Every 4-6 hr (do NOT exceed five doses/24 hr)	Nonopiod No inflammatory activity 24-hr maximum limit: infants (80-90 mg/kg); neonates (60-75 mg/kg); preterm (45 mg/kg); children (90-100 mg/kg)
Ibuprofen	10	Every 6 hr	Nonsteroidal antiinflammatory (NSAID)
Codeine	0.5-1	Every 4 hr; max dose for children 60 mg/dose	Opiod Decreased incremental analgesic effect with doses higher than 65 mg; 10% of individuals cannot metabolize this drug, so does not always work well
Naproxen	5	Every 12 hr	NSAID Oral liquid available
Acetaminophen with codeine	0.5-1 (by codeine) and a safe dose of acetaminophen	Every 4-6 hr	
Acetaminophen with hydrocodone (moderate to severe pain)	Dose in children has not been well established. Dose is limited by appropriate dose of acetaminophen and hydrocodone (0.2 mg/kg).	Every 4 hr	Used for moderate pain; preferred over acetaminophen with codeine, as it causes fewer side effects; consider if acetaminophen or ibuprofen are not effective
Oxycodone	0.05-0.15	Every 4-6 hr	Opioid
Acetaminophen with oxycodone	10-15 (by acetaminophen) or 0.05-0.15 (by oxycodone)	Every 4-6 hr	
Methadone	0.05-0.1	Every 6 hr	Opioid Half-life is up to 96 hr; useful in chronic pain and with opioid-tolerant people
Aspirin	10-15	Every 4 hr	NSAID Inhibits platelet aggregation; may cause postoperative bleeding; do not administer to children with suspected or confirmed viral infection—used only in limited conditions

hr, Hour(s).
Data from Taketomo CK, Hodding JH, Kraus, DM: *Pediatric dosage handbook,* ed 13, Hudson, OH, 2007, Lexi-Comp.

An essential consideration in giving analgesics is whether there is a need to maintain certain serum concentration levels. In situations that require a steady-state serum concentration for pain relief (e.g., following same-day surgery, fractures), around-the-clock dosing of pain medications for 48 to 72 hours is preferable to "as needed" or "prn" dosing. "As needed" dosing is associated with drops in serum concentration levels. When the child is then given a "prn" dose of medication, a significant period of time may elapse before adequate analgesic effect occurs.

Acute Care Pain Management

Common nonpharmacologic measures used with acute pain include the following:

Infants

- Sensorimotor techniques for infants, such as pacifiers, swaddling, holding, singing or calming music, and rocking
- Sucrose solution via pacifier or gloved finger. Administer 2 minutes before a procedure is started. Analgesic effect may last for 8 minutes and may repeat (Bursch & Zeltzer, 2004).

Children and Adolescents

- Cognitive-behavioral strategies, such as relaxation procedures, music and play therapy, and preparatory information before painful procedures or surgeries
- Physical strategies, such as application of heat (if muscle spasm) or cold (if swelling, bleeding, or pain), pressure, massage, acupuncture, exercise, rest, or immobilization
- Distraction techniques, such as having the child watch a video, practice imagery, perform self-hypnosis, look out the window, or play with a toy; use an etch-o-sketch; praising the child; giving the child a party blower or pinwheel and asking the child to blow the pain away; providing stickers or stamps; gently stroking the child; or giving multiple injections (e.g., immunizations) at the same time

Pharmacologic measures used in primary care settings for acute pain include the following (see Table 22-4):

- Analgesic for mild to moderate pain: acetaminophen—10 to 15 mg/kg every 4 hours. Use of an antiinflammatory agent is more effective if inflammation is a key factor causing pain because acetaminophen has limited peripheral antiinflammatory action. Acetaminophen is potentially hepatotoxic so avoid in children with hepatic disease or dysfunction. Because it is a component in many OTC preparations, be alert to the potential for overdose if several drugs with acetaminophen are taken by the patient.
- Oral nonsteroidal antiinflammatory drugs (NSAIDs): The usual pediatric dosage for children weighing less than 50 kg and dosages for children and adolescents 50 kg or more are listed in pediatric drug texts (Schechter, 2006; Taketomo et al, 2007). See Appendix A for additional information about drugs, such as their availability in liquid, tablet, or gel form and the corresponding concentration (milligrams per dose) of the various preparations:
  - Aspirin—10 to 15 mg/kg every 4 hours up to a maximum of 90 mg/kg/day for children or 4 g/day for adults. However, because its use is contraindicated in most children because of its association with Reye syndrome, use

only in the management of selected pediatric conditions (e.g., juvenile rheumatoid arthritis and Kawasaki disease). Because of bleeding issues, 10 to 14 days between discontinuance and major invasive procedures or surgeries is recommended.
  - Ibuprofen—10 mg/kg every 6 hours for infants and children; adolescent and adult, 200 to 400 mg/dose 3 to 4 times/day with 3.2 g/day maximum. Avoid if there is an aspirin allergy, anticipated surgery, bleeding disorder, hemorrhage, or renal disease.
  - Naproxen (Naprosyn)—older than 2 years, 5 to 7 mg/kg every 8 to 12 hours; adolescents and adults for mild to moderate pain or dysmenorrhea; initial 500 mg dose and then 250 mg every 6 to 8 hours, maximum 1250 mg/day.
- Opioid agonists for moderate or severe pain:
  - Codeine—oral, 0.5 to 1 mg/kg every 3 to 4 hours. For younger patients, it is typically given as an acetaminophen and codeine elixir. It is a highly constipating drug and associated with vomiting.
  - Hydromorphone (Dilaudid)—oral, young children 0.03 to 0.08 mg/kg/dose every 4 to 6 hours, maximum 5 mg/dose; older children and adults, 2 to 4 mg/dose every 4 to 6 hours with a maximum of 8 mg/dose.
  - Hydrocodone (in Lorcet, Lortab, Vicodin)—oral, children 2 to 13 years old or less than 50 kg, 0.135 mg/kg/dose every 4 to 6 hours, not to exceed 6 doses/day or the maximum recommended dose of acetaminophen; children and adults greater than 50 kg hydrocodone 5 to 10 mg, four times/day, the dosage of acetaminophen not to exceed 4 g/day (maximum). Dose range of hydrocodone is 2.5 to 10 mg every 4 to 6 hours, maximum 60 mg hydrocodone/day or if limited by acetaminophen maximum dose. Is available in fixed combinations with acetaminophen.
  - Oxycodone—oral, 0.05 to 0.15 mg/kg every 4 to 6 hours (available in liquid 1 mg/mL) for children. Initial dose 5 mg every 6 hours for children greater than 50 kg and adults. For moderate to severe pain usual initial dose is 10 mg every 3 to 4 hours. It comes in 5 mg tablets and a controlled-release product. Available alone or in fixed combinations with acetaminophen.
  - Morphine—oral, 0.3 mg/kg every 3 to 4 hours; intravenous (IV) bolus, 0.05 to 0.1 mg/kg every 2 to 4 hours. Adult dosage is 10 to 30 mg orally every 4 hours as needed. IV, IM, or subcutaneous 2.5 to 20 mg/dose every 2 to 6 hours as needed; typically 10 mg/dose every 4 hours as needed. This drug is not used commonly in primary care settings for the management of acute pain. IV necessitates close monitoring of vital signs and pulse oximetry.
- Topical analgesic creams, such as eutectic mixture of local anesthetics (EMLA) and iontophoresis delivery of drugs, are used with procedures involving skin punctures. Topical liposomal 4% lidocaine creams (LMX$_4$) provides effective analgesia in 30 minutes, whereas EMLA takes 1 hour for full effectiveness. Lidocaine iontophoresis provides anesthesia in 10 minutes, but about 5% of children view the resultant sensation as unpleasant (Zempsky et al, 2004). Subcutaneous injection of combinations of local anesthetics,

such as lidocaine, epinephrine, and tetracaine (LET), is useful in suturing lacerations. Never use epinephrine-containing local anesthetics for digits or the penis because of end artery adverse effect.

- The use of benzodiazepine may play a role in the treatment of pain if spasms are a contributing factor to the pain experienced by a child (Schechter, 2006). Again check for drug and herbal interactions with benzodiazepines (Table 42-2).

Chronic Pain Management

Pharmacologic measures and nonpharmacologic techniques are used in primary care settings for chronic pain management.

Pharmacologic measures include:

- NSAIDs, acetaminophen, and tricyclic antidepressants (TCAs) are the primary treatments used to treat chronic pain unrelated to disease or trauma. Assess for the efficacy of the pharmacologic therapy as follows:
  - Have the child or parent use a pain intensity rating scale and keep a diary of the child's activities and pain.
  - On follow-up visits, question whether symptoms have improved.
- Selective serotonin reuptake inhibitors, opioids, certain anticonvulsants, and other selected medications may be needed. The pain dosage for tricyclic antidepressants (more commonly used in children with chronic pain) is lower than the dosage prescribed in the treatment of depression. Gabapentin is the anticonvulsant most frequently used to treat neuropathic pain associated with burning, stabbing, or aching. Children requiring these agents for the management of their chronic pain are best handled by referral.

Nonpharmacologic techniques issues:

- Frequently used as adjuvants to pharmacologic therapy of chronic pain. They include physical therapy, relaxation, massage, guided imagery, biofeedback, hypnosis, heat and cold, distraction, transcutaneous electrical nerve stimulation (TENS), music therapy, acupuncture, and psychological therapy. Invasive techniques, such as neuroablative procedures and spinal cord stimulation, are occasionally used as a last resort.
- Assessment of the level of distress the child and family are experiencing (including their level of anxiety, depression, and feelings of hopelessness) and their perception of the pain are critical factors that need to be explored when chronic pain is a problem.

Table 22-4 identifies common oral pain medications used in pediatrics and their doses to use as a quick guide. Table 22-5 outlines specific pain problems commonly seen in pediatrics, in addition to their pain relief strategies.

■ FEVER IN CHILDREN

Fever is a common phenomenon seen in children and involves neurologic, endocrine, and metabolic functions. It is a complex systematic inflammatory response that involves modification of the body's thermoregulatory center (hypothalamus)

set point. Cytokines are a critical factor in the fever and the inflammatory response. Viral infections are responsible for most fevers in children. Bacterial infection, malignancy, reaction to immunizations, and connective tissue disease are other known etiologic factors. Most pediatric sources define *fever* as a rectal temperature higher than 100.4° F (38° C) (Feld, 2006). In infants and young children, unless contraindicated for a medical reason, a rectal temperature should be obtained when critical clinical decisions must be made because it more closely approximates body core temperature readings than do axillary, oral, or tympanic measurements. Because environmental conditions (e.g., swaddling an infant) may produce transient elevated temperatures, it may be necessary to take several readings to verify whether an elevated temperature is due to an environmental or a pathologic cause.

Those parents who have "fever phobia" need reassurance because they believe that temperatures greater than 104° F to 104.2° F (40° C to 40.1° C) cause brain damage or, if not treated, will go higher. Cellular damage does not occur until temperatures reach above 105.8° F to 107.6° F (41° C to 42° C). Fevers below 105.8° F (41° C), per se, are not associated with brain damage. Parents need to know that, except for temperatures more than 104° F (40° C), fevers are a body defense mechanism. Fevers are thought to impart a beneficial effect by enhancing immunologic responses, such as increasing phagocytosis and leukocyte migration, and interfering with viral replication and virulence of some microbes. However, there are potential adverse effects from fevers, including increased metabolic rate with associated fluid loss, oxygen consumption, and increased caloric needs. High temperature can precipitate seizures in susceptible infants and young children. Associated symptoms of headache, malaise, anorexia, and irritability are uncomfortable for the child and always worrisome to parents (Powell, 2004).

Health care providers generally treat fevers depending on the severity of the fever or to provide comfort to the child. Parental concern can be a factor in a decision to use an antipyretic. Likewise, suppressing a fever in a young child who is ill can also assist in clinical decision-making if the irritability, tachypnea, and tachycardia associated with a fever resolve after administration of an antipyretic. However, a febrile child's response to antipyretics should not be the sole criterion used to decide whether a pediatric patient is bacteremic or not. Many health care providers treat fevers to provide comfort to a child and use pharmacologic agents when a temperature exceeds 102° F (38.9° C) and the child is uncomfortable or if the child has a persistent temperature above 101° F (38.3° C). Some clinicians use temperatures greater than 101.5° F (38.7° C) as their guide to treatment.

Management strategies for fever control include the following:

- Nonpharmacologic measures:
  - Provide adequate hydration.
  - Provide reassurance to parents and advice that not all fevers need to be treated.
  - Provide appropriate clothing—not bundled in additional clothing or coverings.

TABLE 22-5 **Common Pediatric Pain Problems and Pain Relief Strategies**

Pediatric Pain Problems	Pain Relief Strategies
Otalgia	Acetaminophen or ibuprofen Auralgan otic drops Warm oil in the ear Warmed compresses pressed against the ear
Pharyngitis	Acetaminophen or ibuprofen Antibiotics if GABHS Saltwater gargles Anesthetic lozenges for older child
Stomatitis	Ibuprofen Bland diet Saline mouth rinses for older children Benadryl-Maalox (in a 1:1 preparation) to coat the mucous membranes Viscous lidocaine (remember the potential for aspiration and toxicity) Sucralfate
Musculoskeletal injury	RICE—**R**est, **I**ce, **C**ompression, and **E**levation Immobilization of affected area Cold for the initial 48-72 hours NSAIDs
Fractures and sprains	NSAIDs Narcotic analgesics if severe fracture or sprain Topical ibuprofen, ketoprofen, and felbrimac have been shown to give relief in situations of soft tissue trauma, strains, and sprains; however, studies have involved only adults
Injection pain	Distraction and relaxation techniques EMLA cream (maximum recommended dose based on application area and is also age and weight dependent)* Ice Spot pressure (press down into muscle where shot is to be given)
Neonate and infant procedural pain	Sucrose orally Sucrose pacifier Acetaminophen
In ED or urgent care settings: Intravenous line placement or venipuncture, lumbar puncture, abscess drainage, joint aspiration	EMLA/LMX₄ (prevent mucous membrane contact or ingestion)†
Laceration	Lidocaine, epinephrine, and tetracaine (LET) Procedure: Use on open wounds that are simple lacerations of head, neck, extremities, or trunk that are <5 cm in length; use 3 mL max; place LET mixed with cellulose on open wound and cover with occlusive dressing or place two cotton balls soaked with LET in the wound Contraindications: allergy to amide anesthetics, gross contamination of wound. Do not use on mucous membranes, digits, genitalia, ear, or nose.

*EMLA (eutectic mixture of local anesthetics) is contraindicated in patients with congenital or idiopathic methemoglobinemia or in infants <12 months old who are being treated with sulfas, acetaminophen, benzocaine, chloroquine, dapsone, nitrofurantoin, phenobarbital; phenytoin or quinine.
†EMLA/LMX₄ (liposomal 4% lidocaine cream) contraindicated with nonintact skin, allergy to amide anesthetics or in emergent situations.
GABHS, Group A β-hemolytic streptococci; NSAIDs, non-steroidal antiflammatory drugs.
Data from Zempsky WT, Schechter NL: Office-based pain management, *Pediatr Clin North Am* 47:601-615, 2000; Zempsky WT, Craver JP, Committee on Pediatric Emergency Medicine and Section on Anesthesiology and Pain Medicine: Relief of pain and anxiety in pediatric patients in emergency medical systems, *Pediatrics* 114:1348-1354, 2004; Taketomo CK, Hodding JH, Kraus DM: *Pediatric dosage handbook,* ed 13, Hudson, OH, 2007, Lexi-Comp.

○ Provide ambient environment temperatures of around 72° F (22° C).
○ Sponge with tepid water for temperatures above 104° F (40° C). Sponging should be stopped if the child starts to shiver. Ice-water baths and alcohol sponging should not be done.

• Pharmacologic measures—antipyretic agents (Table 22-6) (Feld, 2006; Taketomo et al, 2007):
• Acetaminophen, PO, 10 to 15 mg/kg/dose every 4 to 6 hours, not to exceed five doses in 24 hours; temperature generally is reduced by 1° C to 2° C within 2 hours. Rectal dosage is 10 to 20 mg/kg/dose. At an oral dose of 15 mg/kg/dose, it is

TABLE 22-6   Antipyretics: Infants and Young Children

Drug	Dose	Comments
Acetaminophen	PO, 10 to 15 mg/kg every 4-6 hr (not to exceed 5 doses/24 hr) Rectal, 10-20 mg/kg	Temperature reduced by 1.8° F to 3.6° F (1° C to 2° C) within 2 hr; 15 mg/kg/dose as effective as ibuprofen at 10 mg/kg/dose; drug of first choice.
Ibuprofen	<102.5° F (39° C), 5 mg/kg every 6-8 hr; ≥102.5° F (39° C), 10 mg/kg every 6-8 hr	Use in children 6 mo-12 yr; max daily dose of 40 mg/kg; temperature stays lower for a longer period of time with ibuprofen vs. acetaminophen.

hr, Hour(s); *mo,* months(s); *yr,* year(s).

as effective as ibuprofen at 10 mg/kg/dose. Acetaminophen is the drug of first choice.

○ Ibuprofen in children 6 months to 12 years old: for temperature less than 102.5° F (39° C), 5 mg/kg/dose every 6 to 8 hours; for temperature greater than or equal to 102.5° F (39° C), 10 mg/kg/dose every 6 to 8 hours with a maximum daily dose of 40 mg/kg/day. The duration of fever response with ibuprofen may be longer than with acetaminophen. Thus the temperature remains lower for a longer period of time with ibuprofen.

○ Naproxen sodium is marketed as a "fever reducer." However, it has not been well studied as an antipyretic in children and should not be used for this purpose.

○ Alternating acetaminophen and ibuprofen has not proven to be clinically beneficial in the management of fevers (Koch, 2002; Mayoral et al, 2000). The best approach is to use acetaminophen and switch to ibuprofen if the child fails to respond. Studies by Nabulsi and colleagues (2006) and Sarrell and colleagues (2006) indicate alternating is more effective. Similarly a randomized clinical trial by Erlewyn-Lajeunesse (2006) demonstrated that the combination of acetaminophen and ibuprofen was marginally better than acetaminophen alone, but the effect was less than one half a degree centigrade. The "community standard," however, seems to still be to use only one, that the safety of alternating the two has not been adequately determined, and using them alternately may actually be dangerous.

■ TELEPHONE MANAGEMENT OF ILLNESSES

Several excellent resources address telephone management of illnesses in children (Schmitt, 2004, 2006, 1998a, 1998b). Many daytime telephone calls represent routine questions about common pediatric problems and can be effectively managed by office nurses with special training. NPs, with their specialty education and background in primary care, are frequently called on to give advice to parents over the telephone or are assigned to take telephone calls either during the daytime or after regular office hours. All primary care providers should ensure that their practice settings have developed a safe system for managing ill-child calls and follow-up calls on patients seen by the primary care providers.

Nonemergency calls to a practice about a sick child during the day are usually routed through a telephone receptionist, who can make an appointment, if appropriate, or transfer the call to a triage nurse or primary care provider, who can determine the urgency of the need to see the child, give home care advice, or refer to the primary care provider for care. If home care advice is given, the triage person should use standards of care or telephone advice protocols addressing a particular set of symptoms, complaints, or a diagnosis that is agreed on for use in that particular setting.

TRIAGE CATEGORIES

Schmitt's (1998b, 1998c) triage categories for sick calls are as follows:

• Life-threatening situation—call 911.
• Emergent—see patient immediately.
• Urgent—see patient within 4 hours.
• Urgent or uncomfortable patient—see the patient that day.
• Nonurgent—see the patient that day or the next day.
• Recurrent or persistent—see the patient within 2 weeks.
• Mildly ill—give home care advice.

The development of telephone protocols is a key factor to ensure an effective telephone management system for a busy practice setting. Schmitt's (2004) excellent quick reference for pediatric telephone protocols can be reviewed for ideas about how to develop office protocols. Management-by-telephone protocol in an individual practice setting should accomplish the following objectives:

• Allow the telephone triage person to manage ill-child calls safely.
• Provide a standard of care.
• Prevent omissions resulting from forgetfulness or fatigue.
• Prevent harmful triage or recommendations.
• Improve quality of care.

The provider who is doing telephone triage must be a perceptive, conscientious, and calm individual who carefully listens to the caller, asks selected questions, processes the information, determines the correct management protocol to use for a particular situation, gives the necessary instructions to parents, and writes notes in a logbook. In addition, all these activities must be performed in a relatively short period of time. The sequence of steps that one must go through in using telephone protocols includes the ability to do all of the following:

- Collect data about the symptoms through open-ended and direct questioning.
- Identify the problem or main symptom.
- Determine a diagnosis or working assessment.
- Decide on a triage category for the patient.
- Select the correct protocol.
- Educate the parent about the plan of care.

DOCUMENTATION

Documentation of the telephone call and disposition is an important element in a successful system for managing telephone calls for sick children. A documentation system, whether it consists of a log sheet or notepad, should be simple and brief. Written documentation serves several purposes, including the following:

- A medicolegal defense
- A method to review charts for quality improvement and assurance purposes
- An avenue to assist in complaint resolution if parents are upset about the advice given to them
- A tool to use when making follow-up calls to the family

Important items to include in any telephone log are:

- Date and time
- Patient data—name, age, sex, telephone number—and history of chronic disease or condition
- The chief complaint and a brief list of symptoms and signs, including their duration and frequency
- Diagnosis or working assessment
- Triage category
- Instructions given about follow-up
- List of medications and their dosage if prescribed by the health care providers
- An "other" section for any additional comments that are deemed important information

When using telephone protocols in a practice setting, training of all individuals who are doing telephone triage is essential and is the best method to ensure consistency in the use of the system. Staff sessions, designed to review the written documentation, are also useful teaching tools and should be encouraged. Perhaps the most important point to emphasize in training and about the use of any telephone management system is the need to assess the comfort of the parent with the advice given. Parents should be asked at the end of the telephone contact whether they are comfortable with the advice and plan. If the parent is not satisfied or is uneasy about the plan, primary care provider consultation should be an option. Finally, parents should be told to call back if their child's condition worsens or the problem persists too long.

RELATING TO PARENTS VIA THE TELEPHONE

There are several critical points about telephone management of common pediatric illnesses, conditions, or concerns. These include method of interaction, screening questions to ask, and points at which intervention is necessary. The individual should be receptive to the parent's call, using language and taking the necessary time to give the message that the call is as important to the provider as it is to the parent. Parents can be anxious and find it difficult to calmly state the problem. The individual also must be calm, direct, and comforting to help parents manage their child's illness.

Screening questions that should be asked of parents include the following:

- *Duration:* How long has the problem been present?
- *Description:* Tell me about the problem. What signs and symptoms are present?
- *Clinical changes:* How has the child's behavior or activity level changed (e.g., eating, sleeping, playing, interaction with peers and family members)?
- *Environmental problems:* Has there been any recent exposure, change, or stress in the child's environment?
- *Cause:* What does the parent believe is contributing to or causing this condition?
- *Management:* What has the parent done for the condition, and with what effect?
- *Feelings:* Does the parent feel anxious about how the child is behaving?

Questions should be asked in an effort to narrow the problem clinically and to assist the parent to be clear and focused. Questions should be clustered by area of concern, should move from most to least serious, and should follow a logical sequence based on initial data obtained.

After-hours or call centers are another avenue that pediatric practices use for handling sick calls after office hours. These centers employ nurses and NPs who use telephone protocols to guide parents in the management of their child's illness until their regular health provider is available. These call centers alleviate the burden of night call and are set up to use telephone protocols and a software program for documentation. It is incumbent on the pediatric health care providers within their practice setting to evaluate whether such a center would effectively meet their standards of care for after-hours management of children.

EDUCATING PARENTS ABOUT TELEPHONE MANAGEMENT OF ILLNESS

Practice settings should have a telephone call policy about sick calls and should acquaint parents with this policy. The policy should cover basic information about the office protocol for handling calls about sick children during office hours, well-child questions, prescription refills, nighttime (after-hours) calls, and weekend and holiday calls. Who screens calls, when calls are returned (e.g., during the noon hour or from 4 to 5 PM), and after-hours coverage are points to cover in the policy.

Parents should be encouraged to handle minor illnesses at home without unnecessary calling in for advice. Home instruction sheets for managing fevers (including dosage charts) and common childhood illnesses or books on common pediatric illnesses designed for parents are excellent resources to provide to parents (Schmitt, 2005). Pamphlets can be given to parents at anticipatory guidance visits. During illness visits, parents should be told what to expect when their child is ill, preparing them for the increasing temperature, vomiting, or diarrhea, in addition to what to do if they occur.

Parents need to know what type of situations require a call for emergency medical services or the poison control center. If sick care is necessary after scheduled office hours, parents will need to give the following information about their child:

- The main symptoms
- Any chronic disease or health problem
- Temperature (and route it was taken)
- Approximate weight
- Names and dosages of current medications
- Type of insurance coverage
- Preferred name of pharmacy and phone number

Box 22-2 provides general rules for parents when calling a health care provider. Box 22-3 gives parental guidelines for deciding when to call.

▪ REFERRALS AND CONSULTATIVE SERVICES

On many occasions, primary care providers identify clinical or behavioral problems that they are uncomfortable managing for any number of reasons, such as being out of the scope of their practice parameters or a problem that requires the expertise of a provider in a subspecialty practice. In these instances, patients should be referred to other providers for management

of that problem. In other situations, the primary care provider may wish to continue to manage the patient's care, but seek consultation with other experts in the field about particular aspects of the case. Whether the primary care provider refers the patient and family out to or consults with another health care expert, certain information must be shared with the referral or consultant provider in an organized, logical fashion. Guidelines for presenting this information are as follows:

- Give the patient's name, age, and actual or tentative diagnosis or chief clinical findings.
- Briefly discuss, in a sentence or two, why the patient or family is being referred to another provider or the reason that a consultation is being requested.
- Give a synopsis of the patient's history, clinical findings, prior management plan, and outcome of treatment if applicable.
- Identify any pertinent past medical history, such as chronic illnesses or conditions.
- Provide pertinent family, educational, or social information, including insurance coverage if this is problematic.

If the primary care provider is referring the patient out for problem-focused care, this should be made clear to the referral provider. In addition, guidelines should be established for when the patient should be seen again for primary care supervision and how information about the child's progress will be shared with the primary care provider. If the child is to be

---

BOX 22-2 **General Rules When Calling the Nurse Practitioner or Physician: Guidelines for Parents**

When calling for **nonurgent** matters, such as well-baby advice, prescription refills, or appointments, call during office hours whenever possible.

When calling for an **emergency,** tell the receptionist or answering service that your call is an emergency call.

Give the following **information on every call:** your child's name, age, sex, major problem, and telephone number where you can be reached.

Be ready to give **information related to your child's problem** as briefly and clearly as possible:

- What are signs and symptoms?
- How long has the problem existed?
- What have you done for the problem?
- How did your child respond to what was done?
- How do you feel about your child's condition? What is your intuition? Is your child getting better or worse?

Be ready to give information about your **child's general health:**

- Does your child have any chronic illnesses that need to be considered?
- Is your child receiving medications for this problem or another problem? Has your child recently received immunizations?
- Does your child have any allergies?

If you do not talk to your provider directly, **before hanging up,** ask when your call will most likely be returned.

If you do not receive a return call within a reasonable amount of time, **call back** to make sure your message was taken correctly.

If your provider decides not to examine your child, **before hanging up,** make sure you determine the following:

- The most likely cause of your child's condition.
- Which medicines or treatments should be given.
- What signs or symptoms to watch for.
- When you should call back for more advice or to report changes in your child's condition.

If you do not **understand the instructions** given, ask to have them repeated or call back for clarification.

If you are instructed to come to the office or go to an emergency department, make sure you have **clear directions** on how to get there. If you are too anxious to drive, ask a friend or neighbor to drive or call a taxi. If an ambulance is necessary, the provider may be able to call it for you.

BOX 22-3   Deciding When to Call the Nurse Practitioner or Physician: Guidelines for Parents

When to call immediately for an infant younger than 3 months:
Baby has the following symptoms:
- Is lethargic (very sleepy or difficult to arouse), has poor color, or appears limp and unresponsive
- Has a rectal temperature of 100.4° F (38° C) or higher
- Refuses to eat three or four times in a row
- Has repeated bouts of diarrhea or vomiting
- Has a labored, wheezing, or grunting breathing pattern that lasts longer than ½ hr
- Has an illness associated with a rash that looks like bleeding under the skin
- Baby's eyes, hands, or feet have a yellow, jaundiced color or if the baby develops pumpkin-colored skin
- You feel very nervous about your baby's illness or general condition

When to call immediately for an older child:
Child has the following symptoms:
- Seems unresponsive, does not make eye contact with you, or has cold and clammy skin that is not associated with vomiting
- Looks much sicker than usual with a routine illness
- Has an illness associated with a rash that looks like bleeding under the skin
- Has any symptom that you believe to be unusual or frightening; this includes labored breathing, severe headache, or very high fever

When to call immediately after trauma or injury:
- Child has struck his or her head and has lost consciousness, has nausea or vomiting, or complains of severe headache; also call if there is mental confusion, unbalanced walking, poor coordination, loss of memory, or a discharge coming from one or both ears
- There is persistent swelling, tenderness, or deformity of the injured part
- Child refuses to use an injured extremity for more than ½ hour
- There is a deep puncture wound, a cut longer than ½ inch, or your child has not received a tetanus shot within the past 5-10 years
- There is injury to an eye that causes redness, pain, or tearing for more than 15 minutes
- Child has been bitten by an animal, and the bite has gone through the skin
- You need first aid instructions for uncontrolled bleeding or other problems
- You believe that your child may have swallowed a toxic or poisonous substance

When to call about symptoms:
- You are concerned about your child's general appearance
- Symptoms seem to be getting progressively worse or last longer than expected
- Fever of more than 101° F has persisted for longer than 24 hours
- Cough, cold, sore throat, or runny nose has lasted longer than 48 hours
- Vomiting has lasted longer than 8 hours or diarrhea longer than 24 hours or when there is blood in the stool or vomit
- Child has severe stomach pains lasting longer than 4 hours
- Symptom seems more severe than it has in the past
- Child has a rash or other problem, and you are not sure what is causing it
- You are not certain whether the child needs to be seen by the health care provider

seen for primary care services and at the same time by the referral provider for specialty care, coordination of responsibilities between the two providers relative to the need for follow-up testing, monitoring, treatments, or therapy should be identified.

The primary care provider should maintain a listing of specialty providers in the local area who take referrals from the primary care provider's work setting. The child's insurance coverage is often a major factor in referral, and often prior authorization from an insurance carrier is needed for a referral. If the provider is employed in a large health maintenance organization, he or she should maintain a list of pediatric specialty providers in the organization. Important information to

gather about these individuals includes their specialty or subspecialty practice area, evaluation of their effectiveness (can be an informal notation, such as "great resource person"), and, if applicable, their fees for service (e.g., full fee or sliding scale) or which insurance plans will reimburse for their services.

Whether consulting formally or informally with another provider about the care of a particular patient, the primary care provider should present information about the patient, as listed previously, and discuss potential management options. At the end of the consultation, the primary care provider should summarize in the patient's chart the key areas that were discussed and the recommendations that were agreed on.

A notation about the consultation, the main discussion points, and the recommendations should be included.

Often overlooked sources of free consultation are state and local public health departments or agencies and health-related professional organizations and some major medical centers that provide telephone consultation about patients for providers in their service area. Again a notation should be placed in the child's chart if the case is discussed with a consultant in such an agency. Connecting with colleagues on the Internet is another option. Real-time chat sessions and e-mail exchanges are possible sources of consultation; however, information secured from unknown sources or not documented or referenced should be verified for accuracy.

When a patient is referred to another provider, the primary care provider must explain the reason for the referral to the child and parent, how the transfer of care will be managed, and when the patient is to return to see the primary care provider. The information should be presented in such a manner as to dispel fears of abandonment or giving up. The bond between the child, the parent, and the primary care provider is a strong relationship that individuals rely on. If the primary care provider plans to seek a consultation, the child and parent should be informed by explaining the need for a second opinion or the desire to collaborate with others to ensure that nothing has been missed. After the consultation, parents should be informed about what was decided. Finally, the parent may seek consultation with another health care provider. If so, treat this as the parent's need to collaborate in the child's care and listen to the recommendation by this consultant. Be sure that the consultant's reports are filed in the child's chart.

■ TIPS REGARDING DOCUMENTATION: PATIENT VISIT AND FOLLOW-UP

There are several important rules for the primary care provider to remember regarding documentation when charting. Many malpractice claims against care providers are because of a lack of documentation. The old adage, "If it isn't in writing, then it wasn't done" has been used more than once to find care providers liable and render a judgment in favor of the plaintiff. Good documentation practices include:

- Being alert to a complaint or combination of complaints that are red flags for more serious illness (e.g., abdominal or chest pains, headache, syncope). Be sure to note pertinent positive and negative history and physical findings relative to these complaints when charting.
- Identifying differential diagnoses and ruling out the worst possible illness first. Be sure to gather enough data to either rule in or out the diagnosis based on history, physical findings, or diagnostic studies.
- Conveying the seriousness of the issue to the family or caretaker if there is the probability of a serious illness and the patient needs to return for additional visits or have diagnostic studies done. Be sure to document that conversation.
- Knowing patient or family risk factors and screening for them through diagnostic tests or history.

- Ensuring that there is a system in place in the practice setting to follow up and secure the results of diagnostic tests that were ordered. There should be a mechanism to ensure that the test or procedure was done and that the provider was given the results and documented reviewing them.
- Following up all abnormal test results. There should be a note placed in the patient's chart that the abnormal results were discussed (and with whom) and what the plan of action would be.
- Following up on referrals to other health care professionals or agencies and documenting the recommendations or treatments implemented from these referral sources.
- Revisiting an unresolved problem until it is resolved. This can be accomplished by:
  - Rescheduling a follow-up examination.
  - Telephone contact with the family to determine if the complaint or illness has been resolved.

Chart audits should be a regular part of practice quality improvement. Look for such things as omissions of information, whether problems identified in earlier visits were addressed at subsequent visits until resolved, and compliance with routine health maintenance screenings.

■ NATIONAL AND LOCAL ORGANIZATIONS AND RESOURCES

Parents and their children with specific disease entities or health conditions can benefit from the educational materials, resources, and support that national health organizations provide. Learning to live with a chronic disease or handicapping condition presents a special challenge to families. Most national organizations provide written materials that parents and children can easily understand about the cause, management, and treatment of the particular disease in question. These materials also help parents explain their child's condition to teachers and others. Many of these national organizations can guide parents and children to support groups with other families and children who are similarly challenged and to health professionals and other related groups who specialize in the treatment of a particular disease entity. Likewise these organizations can assist parents in accessing unique services to benefit their children (e.g., enrolling in special camps and sports activities, learning about the various legal rights of children with disabilities or handicapping conditions, and acquiring special adaptive equipment).

Many national and local health organizations and foundations provide educational materials and valuable information designed for health professionals about a variety of subjects related to their target population of children. For children with rare disorders, the National Organization for Rare Disorders (NORD) may be able to assist parents and offer information about the child's condition or disease. Often these national organizations can provide up-to-date information about new treatment modalities or management strategies. Health care providers should take advantage of the services that national health organizations and local chapters offer and inform parents about national organizations and local chapters that can assist them in meeting their child's special needs. In addition, every clinical or practice setting should have a listing of local community resources. One can make up a personal local resource guide and keep this information along with a listing of national organizations. Many such resources are listed at the end of each chapter in this textbook.

RESOURCE BOX

Pain Assessment and Management

American Academy of Pain Management
www.aapainmanage.org/links/Links.php

American Pain Society: Pediatric Chronic Pain
www.ampainsoc.org/advocacy/pediatric.htm

Doses of Tylenol for children
www.musc.edu/dfm/Home%20Health%20Handbook/tylenol.htm

Pediatric Pain–science helping children
www.pediatric-pain.ca/links.html

UCLA pain assessment tools
www.anes.ucla.edu/pain/assessment_tools.html

U.S. Food and Drug Administration: how to give medicine to children
www.fda.gov/fdac/features/196_kid.html

Wong on Web: Links to websites related to pain and end-of-life care
www3.us.elsevierhealth.com/WOW

Yale Anesthesiology, Yale University School of Medicine–pediatric pain management
http://anesthesiology.yale.edu/clinical/ped_pain.html

CHRONIC CARE ISSUES
Medication administration
www.kidsmeds.com/admin.ccml

National Organization for Rare Disorders (NORD)
www.rarediseases.org

Pediatric Pain Sourcebook of Protocols, Policies, and Pamphlets
http://painsourcebook
Comprehensine website that provides easy access to pediatric pain management information

Tips for Providers
www.ces.purdue.edu/providerparent/Health-Safety/Tips.htm
Parent instructions for giving medications to children

✓ DISCUSSION FORUM

1. Using each of the essential points on patient education, create a comprehensive education plan for an acute disorder treated by primary care providers.
2. Compare and contrast the primary care health care needs of a child with normal growth and development with a child with a chronic physical or developmental condition.
3. List at least five strategies a pediatric provider can use to coordinate a multidisciplinary team to provide care for a chronically ill child. Develop at least one strategy that addresses advocacy for the parents, family, and siblings.
4. Explain how the pain assessment of a 9-month-old differs from that of a 7-year-old. How are they similar? How does pain assessment of a 15-year-old differ from that of a school-age child, if so how?
5. Develop a pain management plan for the following children: an 18-month-old with an ear infection; a 3-year-old with toxic synovitis of the hip; a 9-year-old after a tonsillectomy, and a 12-year-old with juvenile arthritis. Include both pharmacologic and nonpharmacologic interventions.

NURSING DIAGNOSES

Related to Comfort

Acute pain
Chronic pain
Nausea
Readiness for enhanced comfort

From NANDA International: *NANDA-I nursing diagnoses: definitions & classification 2007-2008,* Philadelphia, 2007, Author.

REFERENCES

American Academy of Pediatrics (AAP): *Health care advice: patient education for children, teens and parents,* ed 2, Elk Grove Village, IL, 2004, American Academy of Pediatrics.

American Academy of Pediatrics (AAP): *Patient education for children, teens and parents,* ed 3, Elk Grove Village, IL, 2006, American Academy of Pediatrics.

American Academy of Pediatrics (AAP), American Pain Society: Policy statement: the assessment and management of acute pain in infants, children, and adolescents (0793), *Pediatrics* 108:793-797, 2001.

American Public Health Association, American Academy of Pediatrics (AAP): *Caring for our children. National health and safety standards: guidelines for out-of-home child care programs*, ed 2, Elk Grove Village, IL, 2002, American Academy of Pediatrics.

Beyer JE: *The Oucher: a user's manual and technical report*, Denver, 1989, University of Colorado.

Bodenheimer T, Wagner EH, Grumbach K: Improving primary care for patients with chronic illness, *JAMA* 2888:1775-1779, 2002.

Bursch B, Zeltzer LK: Pediatric pain management. In Behrman RE, Kliegman RM, Jenson HB, editors: *Nelson textbook of pediatrics*, ed 17, Philadelphia, 2004, WB Saunders.

Cline ME et al: Standardization of the visual analogue scale, *Nurs Res* 41:378-380, 1992.

Eland J: Children with pain. In Jackson OB, Saunders RB, editors: *Child health nursing*, Philadelphia, 1993, JB Lippincott.

Erlewyn-Lajeunesse MD et al: A randomized controlled trial of combined acetaminophen (paracetamol) and ibuprofen for fever, *Arch Dis Child* 91:414-416, 2006.

Feld LG: Fever in infants and children from birth to 3 years. In Burg FD et al, editors: *Current pediatric therapy*, ed 18, Philadelphia, 2006, WB Saunders-Elsevier.

Fielding D, Duff AJ: Adherence to treatment in children and adolescents living with chronic illness. In Burg FD et al, editors. *Current pediatric therapy*, ed 18, Philadelphia, 2006, WB Saunders-Elsevier.

Fisher, MC, editor: *Immunizations & infectious diseases: an informed parent's guide*, Elk Grove Village, IL, 2005, American Academy of Pediatrics.

Gavin L, Wysocki TJ: The association between paternal involvement and maternal and family outcomes in families of children with chronic illness, *Pediatr Psychol* 31:481-489, 2006.

Golianu B et al: Pediatric acute pain management, *Pediatr Clin North Am* 47:559-587, 2000.

Hester NO et al: Putting pain measurement into clinical practice. In Finley GA, McGrath PJ, editors: *Measurement of pain in infants and children*, vol 10, Seattle, 1998, International Association for the Study of Pain Press.

Hobdell E: Chronic sorrow and depression in parents with children with neural tube defects, *J Neurosci Nurs* 36(2), 82-88, 94, 2004.

Janse AJ et al: Quality of life in children with chronic illness: differing perceptions of parents and pediatricians, *Arch Dis Child* 90:486-491, 2005.

Jordan-Marsh M et al: Alternate Oucher form testing gender, ethnicity, and age variations, *Res Nurs Health* 17:111-118, 1994.

Koch WC: Fever. In Burg FD et al, editors: *Gellis and Kagan's current pediatric therapy*, ed 7, Philadelphia, 2002, WB Saunders.

Mayoral CE et al: Alternating antipyretics: is this an alternative? *Pediatrics* 105(5):1009-1012, 2000.

McCarthy PL: Evaluation of the sick child in the office and clinic. In Behrman RE, Kliegman RM, Jenson HB, editors: *Nelson textbook of pediatrics*, ed 17, Philadelphia, 2004, WB Saunders.

Nabulsi et al: Alternating ibuprofen and acetaminophen in the treatment of febrile children: a pilot study, *BMC Med* 4:4, 2006.

National Center for Health Statistics: *Health, United States, 2005 with chartbook on trends in the health of Americans*, Hyattsville, MD, 2005.

Perrin JM: Chronic illness in childhood. In Behrman RE, Kleigman RM, Jenson HB, editors: *Nelson handbook of pediatrics*, ed 17, Philadelphia, 2004, WB Saunders.

Powell K: Fever. In Behrman RE, Kliegman RM, Jenson HB, editors: *Nelson textbook of pediatrics*, ed 17, Philadelphia, 2004, WB Saunders.

Roos S: *Chronic sorrow: a living loss*, New York and London, 2002, Brunner-Routledge.

Sarrell EM, Wielunsky E, Cohen HA: Antipyretic treatment in young children with fever: acetaminophen, ibuprofen, or both alternating in a randomized, double-blind study, *Arch Pediatr Adoles Med* 160(2):197-202, 2006.

Schechter WS: Pediatric pain management. In Burg FD et al, editors: *Gellis and Kagan's current pediatric therapy*, ed 18, Philadelphia, 2006, WB Saunders.

Schmitt BD: Calls about sick children: a triage system for the office, *Contemp Pediatr* 15(7):138-152, 1998a.

Schmitt BD: Calls about sick children: launching your own triage system, *Contemp Pediatr* 15(8):49-71, 1998b.

Schmitt BD: *Pediatric telephone protocols: the quick reference*, ed 2, Littleton, CO, 1998c, Decision Press.

Schmitt BD: *Pediatric telephone advice*, ed 3, Littleton, CO, 2004, Lippincott Williams & Wilkins.

Schmitt BD: *Pediatric telephone protocols: office version*, ed 11, Elk Grove Village, IL, 2006, American Academy of Pediatrics.

Schmitt BD. *Your child's health: the parents' one-stop reference guide to symptoms, emergencies, common illnesses, behavior problems and healthy development*, New York, 2005, Bantam Dell Publishing Group.

Shepard MP, Mahon MM: Family considerations. In Hayman LL, Mahon MM, Turner JR, editors: *Chronic illness in children*, New York, 2002, Springer.

Taketomo CK, Hodding JH, Kraus DM: *Pediatric dosage handbook*, ed 13, Hudson, OH, 2007, Lexi-Comp.

Tesler MD et al: The word-graphic rating scale as a measure of children's and adolescent's pain intensity, *Res Nurs Health* 14:361-371, 1991.

Villarruel AM, Denyes MJ: Pain assessment in children: theoretical and empirical validity, *ANS Adv Nurs Sci* 14:32-41, 1991.

Wong DL: The Wong-Baker FACES pain rating scale, *Home Health Focus* 2(8):62, 1996.

Wong D, Baker C: Pain in children: comparison of assessment scales, *Pediatr Nurs* 14:9-14, 1988.

Zempsky WT, Cravero JP, Committee on Pediatric Emergency Medicine and Section on Anesthesiology and Pain Medicine: Relief of pain and anxiety in pediatric patients in emergency medical systems, *Pediatrics* 114:1348-1354, 2004.

CHAPTER 23

Infectious Diseases and Immunizations

Catherine G. Blosser, Margaret A. Brady, and William K. Muller

Infections are among the most common reasons for children to be brought to medical attention. Although viruses are the most frequent cause of childhood infectious illness, bacterial infections (particularly of the skin and mucosal surfaces) are also common. The ability to distinguish serious infections from those that will resolve with minimal or no intervention is an important skill for primary care providers. Nearly as important as the medical care provided to the sick child is the ability to effectively communicate with, educate, and support their often frustrated and anxious parents.

PATHOGENESIS OF INFECTIOUS DISEASES

Bacteria are virtually everywhere in the environment, and humans become colonized with bacteria on the skin and mucosal surfaces (including the upper respiratory and gastrointestinal tracts) shortly after birth. These bacteria are generally harmless and may be beneficial because many normal flora can minimize colonization by potentially pathogenic organisms (Relman, 2004). Refer to Table 23-1. Infectious agents cause disease when the balance between harmless colonization and protective immunity is disrupted in favor of the microorganism. The human immune system is complex and provides many layers of protection from disease. Skin and mucosal surfaces provide a barrier to invasion by microorganisms, and antibodies and immune cells allow the body to defend itself in both general and specific ways against invasion by pathogens. Microorganisms may breach the immune barrier provided by skin and mucosa by binding to cell surface structures; for example, the influenza virus uses its hemagglutinin protein to attach to cell membranes and invade respiratory mucosa. Disease caused by microbial pathogens can result from destruction of infected cells and tissues and from disruption of normal cell functions. Some disease symptoms are caused by the immune system response to infection, which can result in local or systemic inflammatory responses. An example of this is the local redness, swelling, and tenderness at the site of a bacterial cellulitis, which result from the production of cytokines by immune system cells that leads to capillary leak, recruitment of more immune cells, and destruction of infected tissue cells. Fever associated with an infectious illness is an example of a systemic inflammatory response.

CLINICAL FINDINGS

Most infectious illnesses in pediatrics are diagnosed solely based on history and physical examination. Laboratory testing is generally reserved for unusual, serious, or difficult to diagnose cases.

HISTORY

As with all medical encounters, an accurate history of the patient's presentation is the key to a comprehensive and efficient evaluation when an infectious disease is suspected. The goal of a comprehensive history is the generation and prioritization of a differential diagnosis for that particular individual. Crucial aspects of the history that help distinguish infectious illnesses from other diseases include:

- *The nature of the presenting symptoms as gathered when eliciting the history of present illness.* When did the symptoms start? What other symptoms were associated with the illness? Were there periods when the patient seemed improved or even back to normal? Details about the presenting history are critically important and can help narrow the differential diagnosis from a broad list of possibilities. As an example, fever is most commonly associated with infectious illnesses, but also occurs with rheumatologic or oncologic diseases.
- *A comprehensive past medical history.* Careful questioning makes certain diagnoses more or less likely. A history of asthma in a teenager with fever and cough may raise suspicion for atypical pneumonia, for example.
- *Current and recent medications.* Recent antibiotic use may affect your ability to interpret negative culture results or be important information to know in the case of methicillin-resistant *Staphylococcus aureus* (MRSA) tissue infection. Included in the medication history should be questions regarding any nonprescription, herbal, or natural health products that may have been used recently.
- *Immunizations.* Adherence to recommended vaccine schedules (including spacing of vaccines) is an important consideration if the child's symptoms suggest a disease usually prevented with vaccines. For example, a preschool-age child with diarrhea and jaundice who has been correctly immunized against hepatitis A (HA) is unlikely to have that disease.
- *Family history, particularly regarding infectious illness.* Important information includes a history of any relative

TABLE 23-1	Common Distribution Sites of Normal Microflora* Found in Humans	
Bacterium	**Very Commonly or Commonly Found in These Locations**	**Notes**
Aerobic Bacteria		
Gram-positive		
Staphylococcus		
S. aureus	Skin, hair, nasooropharynx, colon, cerumen	Rarely found in the vagina and conjunctiva; trachea, bronchi, lungs, and sinuses are normally sterile
S. epidermidis	Skin, hair, nasooropharynx, adult vagina, urethra, conjunctiva, ear (including cerumen)	Occasionally found in the vagina of prepubertal females; found in low numbers in "normal" urine, probably as result of contamination from urethra and skin areas
Streptococci		
S. saprophyticus	Skin, hair, nasooropharynx, colon, cerumen, mouth, nasal passages, nasopharynx	Occasionally found in urethra and conjunctiva; Group B uncommonly found in oropharynx and postpubertal vagina
S. faecalis (Streptococcus Group D, Enterococcus faecalis)	Colon, postpubertal vagina; occasionally found in mouth, urethra	
S. mitis	Skin, conjunctiva, nasooropharynx; less commonly in adult vagina and urethra	Uncommon in GI tract
S. mutans	Mouth; less common in pharynx	Has the potential of being a pathogen
S. pneumoniae (Pneumococcus, Diplococcus)	Conjunctiva, ear, mouth; rarely found in conjunctiva, ear; 20%-40% of population also have in nasopharynx	Has the potential of being a pathogen
S. pyogenes (Group A)	Skin, conjunctiva, ear, adult vagina	<10% also have in oropharynx as normal flora
S. viridans	Nasopharynx, mouth, skin	
Bifidobacterium bifidum	Colon	
Propionibacterium acnes	Skin	
Gram negative		
Acinetobacter johnsonii	Skin, urethra, adult vagina	
Corynebacteria	Skin, cerumen, nasooropharynx, mouth, colon, urethra, adult vagina	
Citrobacter diversus	Colon	
Enterobacter	Colon, prepubertal vagina, mouth, axillary area	Has the potential of being a pathogen
Escherichia coli	Colon, vagina, mouth, urethra	Has the potential of being a pathogen
Haemophilus influenzae	Conjunctiva, ear, nasopharynx, but not commonly	Has the potential of being a pathogen
Klebsiella pneumoniae	Nose, colon, axillary area	
Lactobacillus spp.	Skin, ear, mouth, colon, adult vagina	
Moraxella catarrhalis	Nasopharynx	
Morganella morganii	Colon	
Mycobacterium spp.	Conjunctiva, ear, genital and axillary areas	
Mycoplasma	Nasooropharynx, colon, vagina	
Neisseria spp. (e.g., N. mucosa)	Nasopharynx (90%-100% of population)	*N. meningitidis* occurs in 5%-20% of the population as normal flora in anterior nares area
Proteus spp.	Colon, vagina, skin	
Pseudomonas aeruginosa	Nasopharynx and colon, but not common; lungs of patients with cystic fibrosis (CF)	Has the potential of being a pathogen
Anaerobic Bacteria		
Bacteroides spp.	Skin, nasooropharynx, colon, adult vagina	Has the potential of being a pathogen
Clostridium spp.	Colon	Less commonly found in adult vagina, skin; can be found in small numbers in urine, but is probably a contaminant
Streptococci	Mouth, colon, adult vagina	
Fungi		
Actinomyces spp.	Mouth, colon, skin	
Candida albicans	Skin, conjunctiva, mouth, colon, adult vagina	Can be found in voided urine, but is a contaminant

| | Very Commonly or Commonly | |
Bacterium	Found in These Locations	Notes
Cryptococcus spp.	Skin	
Protozoa	Mouth, colon, adult vagina	
Viruses		500 species have been identified; the role of viruses as normal flora is undetermined

TABLE 23-1   Common Distribution Sites of Normal Microflora* Found in Humans—Cont'd

*Normal microflora in humans consist of environmental organisms that colonize human body tissues. An individual's microflora depends upon genetics, age, sex, stress, nutrition, and diet. More than 200 species of bacteria are known to comprise the normal microflora. Skin microflora can also include yeast (*Malassezia furfur*), molds (*Trichophyton mentagrophytes* var. *interdigitale*), and mites (*Demodex folliculorum*). The spinal fluid, blood, and tissues are normally sterile; the cervix is normally sterile, but can demonstrate flora similar to those in the upper area of the vagina. Antibiotics can have a minor to major impact on the microflora (e.g., ampicillin has a major effect; erythromycin a moderate effect; and sulfonamides and penicillins minor effects).
Data from Burton GR, Engelkirk PG: *Microbiology for the health sciences*, ed 5, Philadelphia, 1996, Lippincott Williams & Wilkins, p 177; Mikat DM, Mikat KW: *A clinician's dictionary guide to bacteria and fungi*, ed 4 (revised), 1983, distributed by Eli Lilly and Company, pp 60-64; Tannock GW, editor: *Medical importance of the normal microflora*, Boston, 1999, Kluwer Academic Publishers, pp 3-5; University of Wisconsin-Madison Department of Bacteriology: *Bacteria 303—the bacterial flora of humans*, 2002. Available at *www.bact.wisc.edu/Bact303* (accessed Feb 24, 2007).

(first or second degree) with a known immune deficiency, with numerous infections or difficulty recovering from infections, or with a history of recurrent miscarriages. Any of these may raise suspicion for an immune deficiency. A strong history of autoimmune disease in the family may suggest possible rheumatologic diagnoses as opposed to an infectious process.

- *Social history*. Attendance at day care, school, or living in a crowded setting is associated with increased exposure to viral infections. A history of travel to areas with endemic illnesses is important to obtain. Such diagnoses as Lyme disease, malaria, or parasitic illnesses may be suggested from a history of travel to certain parts of the world. A sexual history obtained under confidential conditions is very important for accurate assessment of the adolescent.
- *Exposure history, including any known contacts with individuals with similar symptoms*. In addition to suggesting a presentation consistent with epidemic illness (e.g., as occurs with viruses, such as influenza or enterovirus), a comprehensive, in-depth exposure history can provide important clues in diagnosis of infections that might otherwise not be considered. Specific questions include any contact with individuals with known illnesses, such as tuberculosis (TB) or human immunodeficiency virus (HIV), contact with individuals in high-risk groups for certain illnesses, contact with animals or animal by-products (e.g., hides, waste, blood), and a travel history. Other exposures of importance include environmental tobacco smoke or mold, which increase susceptibility to viral respiratory infection.
- *Complete review of symptoms*. Some presenting features of the illness may be discounted or forgotten by parents or patients and are recalled only when direct questions are asked.
- *Diet history*. Any ingestion of raw milk or undercooked or raw meats and/or fish; history of pica.

PHYSICAL EXAMINATION

A complete physical examination is necessary for all patients for whom there is concern about infectious illness. However, the differential diagnosis generated during the process of taking the history can stimulate the examiner to provide extra focus on certain aspects of the exam. Details of the elements of the physical examination are discussed in other chapters.

Physical findings that may be encountered with infectious diseases include:

- Abnormal vital signs. In addition to fever as a sign of possible systemic infection, tachypnea is common in children with pneumonia. Low blood pressure is very concerning for dehydration and/or septic shock.
- Irritability is nonspecific in ill children, but may raise concern for meningitis or Kawasaki disease. Lethargy raises concern for meningitis, particularly in younger children and infants.
- A stiff or painful neck is often associated with meningitis.
- A new murmur may herald the possibility of endocarditis or rheumatic fever.
- Refusal to walk is never normal in a child and can be a manifestation of deep tissue infections (such as pyomyositis) or meningitis.
- Skin or mucous membrane changes (exanthema or enanthema, respectively) are common with viral illness, and characteristic rashes are typically associated with specific illnesses (e.g., chickenpox).

DIAGNOSTIC AIDS
LABORATORY STUDIES

As noted earlier in this chapter, the history and physical examination are usually all that are needed for the diagnosis of most infectious illnesses in children. In selected circumstances, however, laboratory evaluation can help clarify a diagnosis and/or rule out a serious illness that may be under consideration.

The following factors should be kept in mind when determining which diagnostic test(s) to order if an infectious disease is suspected (Brooks et al, 2004; Mitchell, 2002):

- The quality of the specimen sent to the lab will strongly affect the reliability of the results. For example, pus aspirated from a skin infection is generally more likely to grow the pathogen of concern than is a surface swab and has the added advantage of allowing the specimen to undergo a Gram stain. The collection site of the microbiologic specimen needs to be appropriately cleansed to minimize possible contamination.
- The timing of sample collection affects the degree to which the results help in diagnosis. Bacterial cultures collected after the administration of antibiotics may remain negative, even with active infection. Acute and convalescent titers or certain blood chemistries can help in a diagnosis or monitor response to treatment.
- The amount of any specimen can affect the laboratory's ability to process the sample correctly.
- Microbiologic samples can require special handling and should be transported to the laboratory promptly. The laboratory should be contacted if there is any question regarding the collection and transport of samples.

Specific laboratory tests commonly used in the evaluation of possible infectious diseases are discussed below.

Complete Blood Count

A complete blood count (CBC) provides information on the relative amount of different cell types in the circulation. From an infectious disease standpoint, the white blood cell (WBC) count is generally the most useful piece of information obtained from the CBC. It is often elevated (*leukocytosis*) in bacterial infections and may be decreased (*leukopenia*) in some viral infections. A differential white cell count is often obtained along with a CBC; bacterial infections often (but not always) cause increases in the neutrophil (or polymorphonuclear cell) count and may cause an elevation in bands (immature neutrophils). It is important to keep in mind that normal values for total white cell count and the differential vary with age (see Appendix C, Table C-1). Medications may also commonly affect the WBC count. Steroids can increase the white count, for example, and the long-term use of medications can decrease the white count. The clinical state of the patient may also require careful interpretation of the white count; as an example, overwhelming bacterial sepsis can lead to a decreased WBC.

Other components of the CBC include the hemoglobin, hematocrit, and platelet count. Although acute infection generally does not affect the hemoglobin or hematocrit levels (both measures of circulating red cell levels), chronic disease processes commonly cause low red cell levels (*anemia*). The platelet count is often elevated (*thrombocytosis*) during acute infection.

C-Reactive Protein

The C-reactive protein (CRP) is among the serum measures known as "acute phase reactants," referring to parameters found in blood that increase in the setting of acute inflammation. Serious bacterial infections are more likely to lead to an increased CRP than other types of infections (Maheshwari, 2006). Although the optimum value above which CRP is most highly predictive of bacterial rather than viral infection has not been established, it is generally uncommon for a viral infection to result in a CRP above about 10 mg/dL in young children (Hsiao & Baker, 2005). In addition, CRP is sometimes a beneficial tool for monitoring the body's response to treatment in certain infections. For example, the CRP often is elevated in osteomyelitis before antibiotic treatment, but usually falls rapidly with effective therapy.

Inflammatory processes other than infection may lead to an elevated CRP, including trauma, rheumatologic diseases, and oncologic diseases. Of note, different laboratories may report CRP in different units (usually either mg/L or mg/dL; 10 mg/L equals 1 mg/dL).

Erythrocyte Sedimentation Rate

The erythrocyte sedimentation rate (ESR) is another measure of inflammation and reflects the observation that red blood cells (RBCs) settle more rapidly when acute phase proteins (such as fibrinogen) are present in serum than when they are not. Although the ESR is not a specific test for infection, it is useful in helping evaluate fever of unknown origin and, like CRP, can be used to monitor response to therapy. A low sedimentation rate (less than 10 mm/hr) is unlikely if the cause of prolonged unexplained fever is a bacterial infection. Thus, *Bartonella* infection, mycobacterial infection, or abscesses are typically associated with an elevated ESR. Similarly, viral infection rarely raises the ESR above 20 mm/hr, with the exception of adenovirus, which may be associated with higher values (Long & Nyquist, 2003).

During the waxing and waning period of infection, the ESR tends to both increase and resolve more slowly as compared with CRP values. ESR is considered a useful marker to evaluate the effectiveness of therapy when long-term antibiotics are needed. Thus, it is used when managing diseases (such as osteomyelitis) whereby effectiveness of treatment is judged, in part, by the normalization of the ESR.

Like CRP, the ESR is often elevated in noninfectious conditions causing inflammation, particularly rheumatologic diseases, for which ESRs above 100 mm/hr are not uncommon. Anemia also causes a nonspecific increase in the ESR.

Cultures, Stains, and Antimicrobial Susceptibility Testing

Microbiologic testing is critically important and can be an extremely valuable diagnostic resource. However, the usefulness of such testing is absolutely dependent on the quality of the sample obtained for evaluation and on the correct choice of test for the given clinical situation. Details of appropriate tests for given infections are discussed in the individual sections on those infections.

Bacterial infections occurring in an otherwise normal child typically result in migration of WBCs to the site of infection, especially neutrophils. The presence of pus can assist in the diagnosis of some infections. Sending a specimen of aspirated pus to the laboratory often leads to isolation of the specific bacteria causing the infection. In those cases, Gram stain of the aspirated fluid may reveal the organism. For example, aspirates of pus taken from joint infections (before antimicrobial treatment) may show gram-positive organisms in clusters, suggesting *S. aureus* as the cause of the infection. Although one should not rely on a Gram stain to narrow antimicrobial coverage, it may suggest adding additional coverage in certain situations.

Other staining methods can be useful in certain clinical situations, such as when fungal or other infections are suspected. Fluorescent antigen testing is often used in the diagnosis of viral infections and is commonly done on nasopharyngeal wash specimens. Details of the different available diagnostic staining methods are beyond the scope of this text, although some specific tests are covered in more detail when specific infections are discussed.

Specimens from fluids or tissue can be sent for bacterial, viral, or fungal cultures, although the laboratory may need to be notified of the suspected pathogens for the most accurate evaluation of the sample. Additional testing of bacteria may be done on cultured samples to evaluate susceptibility to the more common antibiotics that could be used. Of particular importance is the growing emergence of MRSA, an increasingly common isolate from cellulitis and other skin structure infections (Kaplan, 2006). In some communities, MRSA may be susceptible to clindamycin; however, susceptibility testing for a given isolate is needed to be sure that an appropriate antibiotic has been chosen.

DNA Testing

DNA testing has become increasingly common in the inpatient setting and is now being used more frequently in clinical practice. These tests generally rely on polymerase chain reaction (PCR) to amplify pathogen-specific DNA, followed by detection using labeled DNA or RNA probes. Specimens of fluid or tissue may be evaluated by PCR. Pathogens that are commonly detected by PCR include *Bordetella pertussis,* herpesviruses, and enteroviruses.

Serologic Tests

For some infections, diagnosis by culture is difficult or impractical. In specific situations, tests that rely on the generation of an antibody response may be useful. Various methods can be used to detect the presence of antibodies to specific infectious organisms, though cross-reactivity may cause false-positive and false-negative test results. Specific organisms that often rely on serologic diagnosis include *Bartonella henselae* and *Mycoplasma pneumoniae.*

Imaging Techniques

Plain Films. Radiographs remain a common modality to assist in the diagnosis of many infections including bone, sinus, and lung infections.

Computed Tomography (CT) Scans. Deeper infections, such as abscesses, often require evaluation via CT scanning.

Magnetic Resonance Imaging. Magnetic resonance imaging (MRI) is the most sensitive imaging modality used in the evaluation of osteomyelitis. It is also often used for brain imaging in cases of encephalitis.

Ultrasound. Ultrasonographic imaging can be used to evaluate the visceral organs, including the liver, spleen, and kidney, for fluid collections suspicious for abscess. It is also commonly used in evaluating kidney anatomy in patients with initial urinary tract infections (UTIs). Echocardiography is a specialized ultrasonographic technique used in the diagnosis, evaluation, and monitoring of endocarditis or Kawasaki disease.

Nuclear Imaging. Several nuclear imaging techniques have been used in evaluating possible infections, including indium-labeled WBC scans ("tagged white cell scans"), gallium scans, bone scans, and positron emission tomography (PET) scans. Some of these techniques may have limited use in pediatrics, although the bone scan remains useful in the diagnosis of osteomyelitis (Lee & Worsley, 2006).

■ GENERAL MANAGEMENT STRATEGIES
PREVENTING THE SPREAD OF INFECTION

Thorough and frequent hand washing is the most effective means of preventing the spread of infection. In addition to educating parents and patients on the importance of proper hand washing, it is crucial that health care providers demonstrate proper hand washing during the care of their patients. There is no excuse for not properly cleaning hands before the examination of a patient. Alcohol-based hand rubs are the preferred alternative to adequate soap and water in most cases (Pittet et al, 2006). Such gels are ineffective against controlling the spread of *Clostridium difficile*. The Centers for Disease Control and Prevention (CDC) recommends using gloves and washing hands with soap and water after being in contact with individuals with *C. difficile*–associated disease (CDC, 2002).

Specific guidance that should be given to children and parents includes:

- Hands should be washed after using the bathroom, before meals, and before preparing foods. The proper technique includes scrubbing with soap and water for at least 20 seconds (the time it takes to sing the "happy birthday" song twice), rinsing with warm water, and drying completely.
- Avoiding finger-nose and finger-eye contact, particularly when there is exposure to someone with a cold (Gwaltney, 2005).
- Using a tissue to cover the mouth and nose when coughing or sneezing may help prevent the spread of pathogens. If a tissue is unavailable, the upper sleeve should be used (not the hands).

USE OF ANTIBIOTICS

It is generally known that antibiotics are often prescribed for conditions that do not require their use and that such inappropriate prescribing patterns are likely to contribute to the emergence of resistant bacteria (McCaig et al, 2002;

Gums, 2004). One of the risk factors associated with inappropriate prescriptions in children is pressure from the parents to provide antibiotics (Bauchner et al, 1999). Studies have demonstrated a decrease in antibiotic prescribing patterns in children from 1989 to 2000 for bronchitis, pharyngitis, otitis media, and upper respiratory infections (URIs) (Steinman et al, 2003; McCaig, 2002). The percentage of decrease ranged from between 11% to 47%, depending upon the illness treated. However, the overuse of broad-spectrum agents increased in children by 13%; they were prescribed principally to treat illness of viral etiology (common cold, unspecified URIs, and acute bronchitis) (Steinman et al, 2003). Providers are encouraged to continue to educate patients and parents about the role and efficacy of antibiotics and to assume a more "targeted therapy" approach when prescribing. Knowledge about emerging resistance patterns, local epidemiology, and susceptibility patterns of bacterial agents within their practice communities will better arm the provider to appropriately prescribe (Gums, 2004).

■ PREVENTION OF INFECTION THROUGH THE USE OF VACCINES

Immunization is the process by which the body is artificially induced to mount a defense against certain foreign antigens. In this way, the immune system is primed to provide future protection with the next exposure to these same antigens. This is achieved by either (a) *active immunization* that involves introducing either a vaccine or toxoid (inactivated toxin) or by (b) *passive immunization* that involves administering an exogenous antibody, such as an immune globulin (IG). The specific agents employed in each type of immunization are discussed in the following sections.

Active immunization has been achieved by the administration of live attenuated and inactivated forms of vaccines. Childhood immunization is the second most valuable, cost-effective preventive service that can be offered in health care (Maciosek et al, 2006). Vaccines now exist to combat 16 childhood and adolescent diseases (*Haemophilus influenzae* type b [HIB], meningococcus, diphtheria, pertussis, tetanus, polio, measles, mumps, rubella, human papillomavirus [HPV], hepatitis A and B [HA and HB], influenza, varicella, rotavirus, and pneumococcus), though primary care providers still see some of these illnesses.

Providers must continue to educate parents and patients about keeping current with necessary immunizations because parents may question their need since many of these diseases have low rates of occurrence in the U.S. Furthermore, the high incidence of global travel leaves underimmunized populations vulnerable to reintroduction of preventable diseases from endemic countries. Preventable epidemics may result.

BARRIERS TO VACCINATION

Primary care providers are frequently faced with immunization issues: shortages of vaccines, vaccine refusal, vaccine schedule changes, and unique immunization needs of special populations of patients. Shortages of vaccine have resulted from manufac-

turing pitfalls. Recent efforts by the Department of Health and Human Services (DHHS) include increasing manufacturing capacity to respond to both seasonal and pandemic influenza vaccines by securing adequate egg supplies year round; providing better guidance for and contracts with vaccine manufacturers; and focusing on cell-based vaccines. In cases of shortages, the CDC provides tiered guidelines for priority administration (see Resource Box at the end of the chapter).

The addition of new vaccines (e.g., HPV in 2006), and/or recommendations for changes and/or substitutions in the vaccine schedule (e.g., Hep A, Tdap use), cautionary pronouncements regarding certain vaccines (meningococcal vaccine, RotaTeq)), and delays in Vaccines For Children (VFC) funding decisions (e.g., RotaTeq) can contribute to provider confusion that can lower or lead to inadequate immunization rates and levels of disease protection. Medical providers also report inadequate reimbursement, storage and stocking issues, documentation hassles, language barriers, inconvenience of counseling, and safety concerns as reasons for not offering vaccinations on site (Riley, 2006).

Immunization rates for 11- and 12-year-old children are below *Healthy People 2010* goals, rendering their immunogenicity subpar by the time these children reach adolescence (Rusk, 2006a). Notably, missing vaccinations include those for HB, MMR, and varicella. The new HPV vaccine is integrated into the schedule, which further complicates compliance. Other compounding factors include the length of time between completion of initial vaccine series, lack of documentation (Hispanic children are more likely to be overvaccinated as a result of language and communication issues) (Darden et al, 2006), and overestimation of vaccination history by parental recall.

Several demonstration and research projects have had success in raising immunization rates including community partnerships that involve school-based immunization programs. Such programs reach a large population of underimmunized children. They also bypass difficulties, such as lack of adequate insurance (the cost of fully vaccinating a child is approximately $1704) (Rodewald & Orenstein, 2006) or lack of priority on the part of families for preventive care measures (Rusk, 2006b).

Strengthening and having consistent school-entry laws may also be a mechanism to increase immunization rates. Moore (2006) extrapolated data from the 2001–2003 National Immunization Survey and showed a positive relationship between state vaccine financing policies and higher immunization rates for completing the heptavalent pneumococcal conjugate vaccine series. Further analysis from this study demonstrated lower vaccination rates for black and Hispanic children. Higher vaccination rates were noted in children who were first born and lived above the poverty level in an urban area.

Parents refuse vaccinations for their children based upon many issues: concerns of vaccine safety; a belief that an excessive amount of vaccinations affect the child's immune system; religious beliefs (7% to 28%); a lack of experience with the ramifications of the diseases; concerns over vaccine side effects; and antigovernment sentiment (8%). One study showed that there were on average approximately 7.2 refusals per 1000 children vaccinated (Fredrickson et al, 2004). The following guidelines may help the provider when faced with parental refusal (Nield & Kamat, 2006a):

- *Listen:* determine the exact reason for the parental refusal and their source of information. Discuss the parent's concerns about vaccine safety, especially at a prenatal or newborn visit.
- *Be open-minded:* Refusals may be overcome by modifying the vaccine schedule to avoid so many vaccinations being given at one time. Be willing to discuss refusals based upon religious beliefs.
- *Educate oneself:* be aware of what the popular press is printing about vaccines and controversies and stay current on evidence-based information. Be aware of state vaccine exemption laws. Should vaccination be required during an epidemic, seek out legal advice of government and professional organizations.
- *Educate parents by discussing:*
  ○ Vaccine safety; vaccines used in the U.S. are thimerosal-free or contain minute amounts, with the exception of some influenza vaccines.
  ○ The immune system's ability to handle multiple vaccines at one time.
  ○ The risk of complications from natural diseases (e.g., encephalitis is more likely to be acquired from wild-type measles than from an MMR); global travel to the U.S. can impact the spread of preventable infectious diseases to those unimmunized or underimmunized.
  ○ That vaccinating their child provides herd immunity for those medically unable to be vaccinated.
  ○ That the majority of complementary-alternative practitioners endorse vaccines (Nield & Kamat, 2006a).
- *Document all refusals and provider-parent discussion:* Have parents sign a vaccine refusal form (available at Childhood Immunizations Support Program, *www.cispimmunize.org*).
- *Do not dismiss the family from clinical practice on the basis of vaccine refusal:* On subsequent visits, respectfully remind parents about vaccination recommendations to keep the topic open.

VACCINES FOR CHILDREN PROGRAM

The VFC program, established in 1994, enabled medical providers to obtain Advisory Committee on Immunization Practices (ACIP)-authorized vaccines without cost. These vaccines are provided free to patients who are uninsured, Medicaid recipients, Native Americans, and Alaska Natives. In addition, children whose insurance does not cover immunizations are eligible to receive vaccines at federally qualified health centers and rural health clinics. All states receive a set level of federal VFC funds. Some states augment that amount to cover more vaccines.

An estimated 40% of all doses of vaccines administered to children in 2004 were furnished by the VFC program (DHHS, 2004). Providers wishing to participate need only to contact their local state Medicaid office to enroll. Free vaccines plus their shipping costs, and an administrative fee, are included in this incentive package; there is a minimum of paperwork for the provider.

VACCINE SHORTAGES

Because of past supply issues, the CDC has an established plan through the VFC program to stockpile 6 months of vaccines to allay shortage problems. The Vaccine Management Business Improvement Project is in charge of addressing all problems related to vaccine shortages including vaccine procurement, ordering, distribution, and management. In addition, there are federal legislative proposals underway to ensure federal-private sector partnerships to provide necessary incentives and protections to quickly bring additional and better vaccines to market.

Medical providers should develop their own tracking system to recall patients whose vaccinations were delayed because of shortages in supply. During such times, providers should check with the website of American Academy of Pediatrics (AAP), ACIP, and National Immunization Program recommendations regarding vaccine deferrals, prioritization of high-risk children, and suspensions of school and child care entry requirements (see Resource Box at the end of the chapter).

VACCINE SAFETY AND RESOURCES FOR PROVIDERS

Informed consent is critical when discussing the benefits and risks of vaccination. The National Childhood Vaccine Injury Act of 1986 (Public Law 99–660, amended by Public Law 101–239) calls for standardized consent forms. All practitioners are required to use these forms to fulfill their duty to warn the public about possible adverse events. The act also requires that the vaccine lot number, site of inoculation, and name of the person administering the vaccine be included in the medical record. Some state laws require a parental signed consent form. People administering vaccines should be knowledgeable about the signs and symptoms of an allergic reaction and be prepared to treat such a reaction.

The National Childhood Vaccine Injury Act also requires health care providers to report vaccine-related adverse events that occur after immunization. The suspected events are to be reported to the DHSS Vaccine Adverse Event Reporting System (VAERS), using their standard confidential form. A VAERS staff member will contact the provider 60 days and 1 year after the report is filed to follow up on the patient's condition. The VAERS telephone number is 800-822-7967. Report forms can be downloaded from *www.vaers.hhs.gov* or from the Food and Drug Administration (FDA) website (see Resource Box at the end of the chapter). VAERS data—minus identifiers—are available from the website. The FDA and CDC use the information to evaluate and detect adverse events, unexpected patterns, and safety concerns. Reportable vaccine-associated events related to all recommended childhood vaccines are identified in Table 23-2. A complete guide to vaccine contraindications is available from the CDC website (*www.cdc.gov/nip/recs/contraindications*).

TABLE 23-2 **VAERS Table of Reportable Events Following Vaccination***

Vaccine/Toxoid	Event	Interval from Vaccination
Tetanus in any combination: DTaP, DTP, DTP-HibB, DT, Td, TT, Tdap	A. Anaphylaxis or anaphylactic shock	7 days
	B. Brachial neuritis	28 days
	C. Any acute complications or sequelae (including death) of above events	Not applicable
	D. Events described in manufacturer's package insert as contraindications to additional doses of vaccine	See package insert
Pertussis in any combination: DTaP, DTP, DTP-Hib, P, Tdap	A. Anaphylaxis or anaphylactic shock	7 days
	B. Encephalopathy (or encephalitis)	7 days
	C. Any acute complications or sequelae (including death) of above events	Not applicable
	D. Events described in manufacturer's package insert as contraindications to additional doses of vaccine	See package insert
Measles, mumps, and rubella in any combination: MMR, MR, M, MMRV, R	A. Anaphylaxis or anaphylactic shock	7 days
	B. Encephalopathy (or encephalitis)	15 days
	C. Any acute complications or sequelae (including death) of above events	Not applicable
	D. Events described in manufacturer's package insert as contraindications to additional doses of vaccine	See package insert
Rubella in any combination: MMR, MMRV, MR, R	A. Chronic arthritis	42 days
	B. Any acute complications or sequelae (including death) of above event	Not applicable
	C. Events described in manufacturer's package insert as contraindications to additional doses of vaccine	See package insert
Measles in any combination: MMR, MMRV, MR, M	A. Thrombocytopenic purpura	7-30 days
	B. Vaccine-strain measles viral infection in an immunodeficient recipient	6 mo
	C. Any acute complications or sequelae (including death) of above events	Not applicable
	D. Events described in manufacturer's package insert as contraindications to additional doses of vaccine	See package insert
Oral Polio (OPV)	A. Paralytic polio	
	In a non-immunodeficient recipient	30 days
	In an immunodeficient recipient	6 mo
	In a vaccine associated community case	Not applicable
	B. Vaccine-strain polio viral infection	
	In a non-immunodeficient recipient	30 days
	In an immunodeficient recipient	6 months
	In a vaccine associated community case	Not applicable
	C. Any sequelae (including death) of above events	Not applicable
	D. Events described in manufacturer's package insert as contraindications to additional doses of vaccine	See package insert
Inactivated Polio (IPV)	A. Anaphylaxis or anaphylactic shock	7 days
	B. Any sequelae (including death) of above event	Not applicable
	C. Events described in manufacturer's package insert as contraindications to additional doses of vaccine	See package insert
Hepatitis B	A. Anaphylaxis or anaphylactic shock	7 days
	B. Any acute complications or sequelae (including death) of the above event	Not applicable
	C. Events described in manufacturer's package insert as contraindications to additional doses of vaccine	See package insert
Hemophilus influenzae type b (conjugate)	A. Events described in manufacturer's package insert as contraindications to additional doses of vaccine	See package insert
Varicella	A. Events described in manufacturer's package insert as contraindications to additional doses of vaccine	See package insert
Rotavirus	A. Intussusception	30 days
	B. Any acute complications or sequelae (including death) of the above event	Not applicable

TABLE 23-2 **VAERS Table of Reportable Events Following Vaccination*—Cont'd**

Vaccine/Toxoid	Event	Interval from Vaccination
	C. Events described in the manufacturer's package insert as contraindications to additional doses of vaccine	See package insert
Pneumococcal conjugate	A. Events described in manufacturer's package insert as contraindications to additional doses of vaccine	See package insert
Hepatitis A	A. Events described in manufacturer's package insert as contraindications to additional doses of vaccine	See package insert
Influenza	A. Events described in manufacturer's package insert as contraindications to additional doses of vaccine	See package insert

**Meningococcal vaccine:* Any case of Guillain-Barré syndrome that results after having Menactra is to be reported to the VAERS system. See Food and Drug Administration: *FDA and CDC update information on Menactra meningococcal vaccine and Guillain-Barré Syndrome,* Oct 20, 2006. Available at *www.fda.gov/cber/safety/gbs102006* (accessed Mar 24, 2007). Available from *vaers.hhs.gov/pdf/*Reportable Events Table (accessed Mar 24, 2007).

In 2001, the CDC established the Clinical Immunization Safety Assessment (CISA) Network. This was in response to the realization that many adverse events became evident only after the prelicensure of vaccines and that many primary care providers would not necessarily be privy to such events. CISA develops research protocols around any given adverse event; helps understand the adverse event at the possible genetic, population, or subpopulation level; establishes risk levels; and serves as a referral source for clinicians. Providers can receive vaccine safety information, including how to manage postvaccine adverse events.

VACCINE CONTROVERSIES

The Institute of Medicine's (IOM's) Immunization Safety Review Committee reported no evidence of a causal relationship between thimerosal-containing vaccines or MMR vaccine and "pervasive developmental disorders," such as autism, attention-deficit/hyperactivity disorder (ADHD), speech/language delays, childhood disintegrative disorder, Asperger syndrome, or Rett syndrome (IOM, 2004). They also reported finding no general connection, no biologic mechanism consistent with a relationship between immunization or an adverse event, or insufficient causal evidence between hepatitis B and demyelinating diseases of the central nervous system (CNS) and peripheral nervous system (multiple sclerosis, acute disseminated encephalomyelitis, optic neuritis, transverse myelitis, Guillain-Barré syndrome [GBS], and brachial neuritis [Stratton et al, 2004]). The IOM also investigated the role that multiple vaccines might play in causing type 1 diabetes or serious infections. After a review of dozens of scientific research studies, a causal relationship was dismissed. However, there was some mixed evidence between studies regarding a possible connection between multiple vaccines and asthma. The Immunization Safety Review Committee concluded that further research in all these areas was warranted given the public concern with vaccine safety, the threat

of increased populations going unvaccinated because of these fears, and the resulting resurgence of preventable diseases.

Vaccines that are thimerosal-free or contain trace amounts are on the CDC's recommended list for childhood immunizations with one exception, inactivated influenza vaccine. Fluzone, Fluvirin, and FluLaval still contain the preservative as of this writing; Fluzone (No Thimerosal), Fluvirin (Preservative Free), Fluarix, and Aluria contain zero or trace amounts of thimerosal. The CDC website regularly updates the list of thimerosol levels in vaccines.

VACCINES ON THE HORIZON

Vaccines under investigation include a shigella conjugate vaccine for children, vaccines for herpes simplex virus types 1 and 2, cytomegalovirus (CMV) (to prevent congenital CMV), Marburg virus (a hemorrhagic fever disease), dengue fever, Hantavirus, HIV, West Nile virus (WNV), and Lassa fever. Other studies are ongoing to develop a conjugate group B streptococcus vaccine for pregnant women to provide passive immunity to their fetuses, a vaccine to cover more serotypes of *H. influenzae,* and live and subunit parainfluenza type 3 vaccines.

New vaccine delivery systems are being researched that include skin-patch vaccines (now undergoing human trials against the flu and travelers' diarrhea), edible vaccines, and needle-free injections. DNA technology is also being explored for use in encoding host immunogenic antigens.

ACTIVE IMMUNITY

Inoculating a child with all or part of a modified product from a microorganism evokes an immune response. Whole organisms (live, attenuated, or killed), modified proteins, and/or sugars are used to prepare certain vaccines. The response to a live attenuated vaccine is often as protective as the natural infection. Antiinvasive, antiadherence, antitoxin, neutralizing antibodies, or other protective responses can be found soon after the vaccination is given. Live attenuated vaccines usually confer broader and longer lived immunity than the inactivated types that require booster vaccines. Killed and inactivated vaccines can provide systemic protection (immunoglobulin G [IgG] antibodies), but may fail to provide local mucosal antibody (IgA). Thus, although protected from systemic illness, a recipient of a killed vaccine can have local colonization or infection that can be a problem during an epidemic. The active and inert vaccine ingredients differ among manufacturers. One must be aware of these components (such as antimicrobials) because of a patient's possible hypersensitivity to the ingredients.

The AAP, the American Academy of Family Physicians (AAFP), and the Advisory Committe on Immunization Practices (ACIP) of the CDC annually approve a new unified recommended childhood immunization schedule (Tables 23-3 and 23-4). The CDC website provides current information regarding specific vaccines, their schedules, administration, and dosages (*www.cdc.gov/node.do/id*).

Maternal antibodies neutralize vaccines; therefore, infants vaccinated in the first year of life require more inoculations than older children. Children who are not immunized in the first year of life should be vaccinated according to the schedule listed in Table 23-5. Missed vaccinations should be given whenever possible, and the entire series does not need to be repeated. Vaccines given outside of the U.S. are acceptable as long as there is strict and reliable written evidence of administration (dates and number of doses), and the age and spacing were the same as CDC recommendations. If in doubt, antibody titers can be checked. Generally, most vaccines used worldwide have been produced with adequate quality control and are reliable, but the handling can be suspect (AAP, 2006). If in doubt, immunize. Children being adopted from overseas generally need all immunizations repeated to account for any inaccuracies in reporting or vaccine potency questions. Proper storage of vaccines and correct immunization technique are critical for optimal results. The manufacturer's package inserts provide this information.

New research has raised questions about the effect of environmental pollutants on the body's immune responses to vaccinations. Increased levels of prenatal and/or postnatal polychlorinated biphenyls (PCBs) have been correlated with lowered antibody response to tetanus and diphtheria vaccines in children at 18 months and 7 years old. Early postnatal exposure to this agent was the primary predictor of decreased response (Heilmann et al, 2006).

The ACIP offers some general vaccination guidelines (*American Journal for NPs*, 2002; AAP, 2006). These include the following:

- Vaccine doses may be given 4 days prior to or later than minimum intervals or ages to provide some 4 days schedule flexibility.
- If two live virus parenteral vaccines are given less than 28 days apart, the vaccine given second should be disregarded; repeat this second vaccine at least 4 weeks later.
- Administering rabies or hepatitis B vaccine in an incorrect site (e.g., gluteus) or via an inappropriate route (e.g., hepatitis

B vaccine not given intramuscularly) decreases immunogenicity; the vaccine(s) should be repeated in such instances.
- Do not aspirate the syringe before injection (unproven necessity).
- Preterm infants whose mothers are hepatitis B surface antigen (HBsAg) positive, or whose status is unknown, should receive both hepatitis B vaccine and hepatitis B immune globulin (HBIG) within 12 hours of birth and three additional doses of hepatitis B vaccine at 1, 2, and 6 months.
- When multiple vaccines are given on the same extremity, the sites of injection should be at least 1 inch apart.
- Parent or guardian recollection of a child's immunization status may not be reliable; use only written, dated records. Reimmunization of an immune individual is not harmful.
- Reduced or divided doses of vaccines should not be given
- Techniques to decrease the pain of immunizations: apply pressure to the injection site for about 10 seconds before vaccination; put sucrose on the tongue or pacifier of an infant; have children blow a pinwheel or bubbles during the procedure.

Inactivated Vaccines

Diphtheria and Tetanus Toxoids With Pertussis Vaccine. Diphtheria and tetanus toxoids with acellular pertussis vaccine (DTaP) is used in the U.S. for children less than 7 years old; the whole-cell product, diphtheria and tetanus toxoids with pertussis vaccine (DTP), is no longer available. Whole-cell vaccines are still used in other parts of the world. The DTaP has fewer side effects than the whole-cell vaccine. If given in another country, DTP is an acceptable alternative to DTaP. Combination vaccines are available that include DTaP, HIB, and other vaccines; however, single conjugated HIB vaccine cannot be mixed with other single DTaP products.

Scheduling for these vaccines is given in Tables 23-3, 23-4, and 23-5. Universal immunization with DTaP (or DTP) is the only effective control measure for these illnesses. The duration of immunity after pertussis infection has not been established, but it is believed to be short (AAP, 2006). Diphtheria and tetanus toxoids are highly effective vaccines as proven by the rarity of these diseases in the U.S. All of the current vaccines available are equally effective, but differ slightly in their components.

- **General guidelines.** Some general guidelines to consider when choosing the appropiate diphtheria, tetanus, pertussis vaccine include:
  - When possible, continue the same brand of vaccine for the first three primary series doses. Guidelines for which brands to use for the fourth and fifth doses are available from the CDC website or the current AAP *Red Book*.
  - If previously vaccinated using the whole-cell vaccine, future vaccines should be DTaP.
  - Children younger than 7 years old must be vaccinated with DT if there are contraindications to giving the pertussis vaccine.
  - Children with a previously documented pertussis infection (or who are seropositive for pertussis) should continue to receive the regular DTaP primary series. At the very least, they should receive the DT vaccine to build their diphtheria and tetanus immunity.

TABLE 23-3 Recommended Immunization Schedule for Persons 0-6 Years Old—U.S., 2008

For those who fall behind or start late, see the catch-up schedule

Vaccine ▼ Age ►	Birth	1 month	2 months	4 months	6 months	12 months	15 months	18 months	19–23 months	2–3 years	4–6 years
Hepatitis B[1]	HepB	HepB		see footnote 1		HepB					
Rotavirus[2]			Rota	Rota	Rota						
Diphtheria, Tetanus, Pertussis[3]			DTaP	DTaP	DTaP	see footnote 3	DTaP				DTaP
Haemophilus influenzae type b[4]			Hib	Hib	Hib[4]	Hib					
Pneumococcal[5]			PCV	PCV	PCV	PCV				PPV	
Inactivated Poliovirus			IPV	IPV		IPV					IPV
Influenza[6]						Influenza (Yearly)					
Measles, Mumps, Rubella[7]						MMR					MMR
Varicella[8]						Varicella					Varicella
Hepatitis A[9]						HepA (2 doses)				HepA Series	
Meningococcal[10]											MCV4

Range of recommended ages

Certain high-risk groups

This schedule indicates the recommended ages for routine administration of currently licensed childhood vaccines, as of December 1, 2007, for children aged 0 through 6 years. Additional information is available at **www.cdc.gov/vaccines/recs/schedules**. Any dose not administered at the recommended age should be administered at any subsequent visit, when indicated and feasible. Additional vaccines may be licensed and recommended during the year. Licensed combination vaccines may be used whenever any components of the combination are indicated and other components of the vaccine are not contraindicated and if approved by the Food and Drug Administration for that dose of the series. **Providers should consult the respective Advisory Committee on Immunization Practices statement for detailed recommendations, including for high risk conditions: http://www.cdc.gov/vaccines/pubs/ACIP-list.htm.** Clinically significant adverse events that follow immunization should be reported to the Vaccine Adverse Event Reporting System (VAERS). Guidance about how to obtain and complete VAERS form is available at **www.vaers.hhs.gov** or by telephone, **800-822-7967**.

1. Hepatitis B vaccine (HepB). *(Minimum age: birth)*
   At birth:
   • Administer monovalent HepB to all newborns prior to hospital discharge.
   • If mother is hepatitis B surface antigen (HBsAg)-positive, administer HepB and 0.5 mL of hepatitis B immune globulin (HBIG) within 12 hours of birth.
   • If mother's HBsAg status is unknown, administer HepB within 12 hours of birth. Determine the HBsAg status as soon as possible and if HBsAg-positive, administer HBIG (no later than age 1 week).
   • If mother is HBsAg-negative, the birth dose can be delayed, **in rare cases,** with a provider's order and a **copy of the mother's** negative HBsAg laboratory report in the infant's medical record.
   After the birth dose:
   • The HepB series should be completed with either monovalent HepB or a combination vaccine containing HepB. The second dose should be administered at age 1–2 months. The final dose should be administered no earlier than age 24 weeks. Infants born to HBsAg-positive mothers should be tested for HBsAg and antibody to HBsAg after completion of at least 3 doses of a licensed HepB series, at age 9–18 months (generally at the next well-child visit).
   4-month dose:
   • It is permissible to administer 4 doses of HepB when combination vaccines are administered after the birth dose. If monovalent HepB is used for doses after the birth dose, a dose at age 4 months is not needed.

2. Rotavirus vaccine (Rota). *(Minimum age: 6 weeks)*
   • Administer the first dose at age 6–12 weeks.
   • Do not start the series later than age 12 weeks.
   • Administer the final dose in the series by age 32 weeks. Do not administer any dose later than age 32 weeks.
   • Data on safety and efficacy outside of these age ranges are insufficient.

3. Diphtheria and tetanus toxoids and acellular pertussis vaccine (DTaP). *(Minimum age: 6 weeks)*
   • The fourth dose of DTaP may be administered as early as age 12 months, provided 6 months have elapsed since the third dose.
   • Administer the final dose in the series at age 4–6 years.

4. Haemophilus influenzae type b conjugate vaccine (Hib). *(Minimum age: 6 weeks)*
   • If PRP-OMP (PedvaxHIB® or ComVax® [Merck]) is administered at ages 2 and 4 months, a dose at age 6 months is not required.
   • TriHIBit® (DTaP/Hib) combination products should not be used for primary immunization but can be used as boosters following any Hib vaccine in children age 12 months or older.

5. Pneumococcal vaccine. *(Minimum age: 6 weeks for pneumococcal conjugate vaccine [PCV]; 2 years for pneumococcal polysaccharide vaccine [PPV])*
   • Administer one dose of PCV to all healthy children aged 24–59 months having any incomplete schedule.
   • Administer PPV to children aged 2 years and older with underlying medical conditions.

6. Influenza vaccine. *(Minimum age: 6 months for trivalent inactivated influenza vaccine [TIV]; 2 years for live, attenuated influenza vaccine [LAIV])*
   • Administer annually to children aged 6–59 months and to all close contacts of children aged 0–59 months.
   • Administer annually to children 5 years of age and older with certain risk factors, to other persons (including household members) in close contact with persons in groups at higher risk, and to any child whose parents request vaccination.
   • For healthy nonpregnant persons (those who do not have underlying medical conditions that predispose them to influenza complications) ages 2–49 years, either LAIV or TIV may be used.
   • Children receiving TIV should receive 0.25 mL if age 6-35 mos or 0.5 mL if age 3 years or older.
   • Administer 2 doses (separated by 4 weeks or longer) to children younger than 9 years who are receiving influenza vaccine for the first time or who were vaccinated for the first time last season, but only received one dose.

7. Measles, mumps, and rubella vaccine (MMR). *(Minimum age: 12 months)*
   • Administer the second dose of MMR at age 4–6 years. MMR may be administered before age 4–6 years, provided 4 weeks or more have elapsed since the first dose.

8. Varicella vaccine. *(Minimum age: 12 months)*
   • Administer second dose at age 4–6 years; may be administered 3 months or more after first dose.
   • Don't repeat second dose if administered 28 days or more after first dose.

9. Hepatitis A vaccine (HepA). *(Minimum age: 12 months)*
   • HepA is recommended for all children aged 1 yr (i.e., aged 12–23 months). The 2 doses in the series should be administered at least 6 months apart.
   • Children not fully vaccinated by age 2 years can be vaccinated at subsequent visits.
   • HepA is recommended for certain other groups of children, including in areas where vaccination programs target older children.

10. Meningococcal vaccine. *(Minimum age: 2 years for meningococcal conjugate vaccine (MCV4) and for meningococcal polysaccharide vaccine (MPSV4))*
   • MCV4 is recommended for children aged 2–10 years with terminal complement deficiencies or anatomic or functional asplenia and certain other high-risk groups. Use of MPSV4 is also acceptable.
   • Persons who received MPSV4 3 or more years prior and remain at increased risk for meningococcal disease should be vaccinated with MCV4.

The Recommended Immunization Schedules for Persons Aged 0–18 Years are approved by the Advisory Committee on Immunization Practices (www.cdc.gov/vaccines/recs/acip), the American Academy of Pediatrics (http://www.aap.org), and the American Academy of Family Physicians (http://www.aafp.org).
DEPARTMENT OF HEALTH AND HUMAN SERVICES • CENTERS FOR DISEASE CONTROL AND PREVENTION • SAFER • HEATHIER • PEOPLE™

CS103164

TABLE 23-4   Recommended Immunization Schedule for Persons 7-18 Years Old—U.S., 2008

For those who fall behind or start late, see the green bars and the catch-up schedule

Vaccine ▼ Age ►	7-10 years	11-12 years	13-18 years	
Diphtheria, Tetanus, Pertussis[1]	see footnote 1	Tdap	Tdap	Range of recommended ages
Human Papillomavirus[2]	see footnote 2	HPV (3 doses)	HPV Series	
Meningococcal[3]	MCV4	MCV4	MCV4	
Pneumococcal[4]	PPV			Catch-up immunization
Influenza[5]	Influenza (Yearly)			
Hepatitis A[6]	HepA Series			
Hepatitis B[7]	HepB Series			Certain high-risk groups
Inactivated Poliovirus[8]	IPV Series			
Measles, Mumps, Rubella[9]	MMR Series			
Varicella[10]	Varicella Series			

This schedule indicates the recommended ages for routine administration of currently licensed childhood vaccines, as of December 1, 2007, for children aged 7–18 years. Additional information is available at **www.cdc.gov/vaccines/recs/schedules**. Any dose not administered at the recommended age should be administered at any subsequent visit, when indicated and feasible. Additional vaccines may be licensed and recommended during the year. Licensed combination vaccines may be used whenever any components of the combination are indicated and other components of the vaccine are not contraindicated and if approved by the Food and Drug Administration for that dose of the series. **Providers should consult the respective Advisory Committee on Immunization Practices statement for detailed recommendations, including for high risk conditions: http://www.cdc.gov/vaccines/pubs/ACIP-list.htm.** Clinically significant adverse events that follow immunization should be reported to the Vaccine Adverse Event Reporting System (VAERS). Guidance about how to obtain and complete VAERS form is available at **www.vaers.hhs.gov** or by telephone, **800-822-7967**.

1. Tetanus and diphtheria toxoids and acellular pertussis vaccine (Tdap). *(Minimum age: 10 years for BOOSTRIX® and 11 years for ADACEL™)*
- Administer at age 11–12 years for those who have completed the recommended childhood DTP/DTaP vaccination series and have not received a tetanus and diphtheria toxoids (Td) booster dose.
- 13–18 year olds who missed the 11–12 year Tdap or received Td only, are encouraged to receive one dose of Tdap 5 years after the last Td/DTaP dose.

2. Human papillomavirus vaccine (HPV). *(Minimum age: 9 years)*
- Administer the first dose of the HPV vaccine series to females at age 11–12 years.
- Administer the second dose 2 months after the first dose and the third dose 6 months after the first dose.
- Administer the HPV vaccine series to females at age 13–18 years if not previously vaccinated.

3. Meningococcal vaccine.
- Administer MCV4 at age 11–12 years and at age 13–18 years if not previously vaccinated. MPSV4 is an acceptable alternative.
- Administer MCV4 to previously unvaccinated college freshmen living in dormitories.
- MCV4 is recommended for children aged 2-10 years with terminal complement deficiencies or anatomic or functional asplenia and certain other high-risk groups.
- Persons who received MPSV4 3 or more years prior and remain at increased risk for meningococcal disease should be vaccinated with MCV4.

4. Pneumococcal polysaccharide vaccine (PPV).
- Administer PPV to certain high-risk groups.

5. Influenza vaccine.
- Administer annually to all close contacts of children aged 0–59 months.
- Administer annually to persons with certain risk factors, health-care workers, and other persons (including household members) in close contact with persons in groups at higher risk.
- Administer 2 doses (separated by 4 weeks or longer) to children younger than 9 years who are receiving influenza vaccine for the first time or who were vaccinated for the first time last season, but only received one dose.
- For healthy nonpregnant persons (those who do not have underlying medical conditions that predispose them to influenza complications) ages 2–49 years, either LAIV or TIV may be used.

6. Hepatitis A vaccine (HepA).
- The 2 doses in the series should be administered at least 6 months apart.
- HepA is recommended for certain other groups of children, including in areas where vaccination programs target older children.

7. Hepatitis B vaccine (HepB).
- Administer the 3-dose series to those who were not previously vaccinated.
- A 2-dose series of Recombivax HB® is licensed for children aged 11–15 years.

8. Inactivated poliovirus vaccine (IPV).
- For children who received an all-IPV or all-oral poliovirus (OPV) series, a fourth dose is not necessary if the third dose was administered at age 4 years or older.
- If both OPV and IPV were administered as part of a series, a total of 4 doses should be administered, regardless of the child's current age.

9. Measles, mumps, and rubella vaccine (MMR).
- If not previously vaccinated, administer 2 doses of MMR during any visit, with 4 or more weeks between the doses.

10. Varicella vaccine.
- Administer 2 doses of varicella vaccine to persons younger than 13 years of age at least 3 months apart. Do not repeat the second dose, if administered 28 or more days following the first dose.
- Administer 2 doses of varicella vaccine to persons aged 13 years or older at least 4 weeks apart.

The Recommended Immunization Schedules for Persons Aged 0–18 Years are approved by the Advisory Committee on Immunization Practices (www.cdc.gov/vaccines/recs/acip), the American Academy of Pediatrics (http://www.aap.org), and the American Academy of Family Physicians (http://www.aafp.org).

DEPARTMENT OF HEALTH AND HUMAN SERVICES • CENTERS FOR DISEASE CONTROL AND PREVENTION
SAFER • HEALTHIER • PEOPLE™

CS103164

TABLE 23-5 **Catch-up Immunization Schedule for Persons 4 Months–18 Years Old Who Start Late or Who Are More Than 1 Month Behind—U.S., 2008**

The table below provides catch-up schedules and minimum intervals between doses for children whose vaccinations have been delayed. A vaccine series does not need to be restarted, regardless of the time that has elapsed between doses. Use the section appropriate for the child's age.

Vaccine	Minimum Age for Dose 1	Minimum Interval Between Doses			
CATCH-UP SCHEDULE FOR PERSONS AGED 4 MONTHS–6 YEARS					
		Dose 1 to Dose 2	Dose 2 to Dose 3	Dose 3 to Dose 4	Dose 4 to Dose 5
Hepatitis B[1]	Birth	4 weeks	8 weeks (and 16 weeks after first dose)		
Rotavirus[2]	6 wks	4 weeks	4 weeks		
Diphtheria, Tetanus, Pertussis[3]	6 wks	4 weeks	4 weeks	6 months	6 months[3]
Haemophilus influenzae type b[4]	6 wks	4 weeks if first dose administered at younger than 12 months of age / 8 weeks (as final dose) if first dose administered at age 12–14 months / No further doses needed if first dose administered at 15 months of age or older	4 weeks[4] if current age is younger than 12 months / 8 weeks (as final dose)[4] if current age is 12 months or older and second dose administered at younger than 15 months of age / No further doses needed if previous dose administered at age 15 months or older	8 weeks (as final dose) This dose only necessary for children aged 12 months–5 years who received 3 doses before age 12 months	
Pneumococcal[5]	6 wks	4 weeks if first dose administered at younger than 12 months of age / 8 weeks (as final dose) if first dose administered at age 12 months or older or current age 24–59 months / No further doses needed for healthy children if first dose administered at age 24 months or older	4 weeks if current age is younger than 12 months / 8 weeks (as final dose) if current age is 12 months or older / No further doses needed for healthy children if previous dose administered at age 24 months or older	8 weeks (as final dose) This dose only necessary for children aged 12 months–5 years who received 3 doses before age 12 months	
Inactivated Poliovirus[6]	6 wks	4 weeks	4 weeks	4 weeks[6]	
Measles, Mumps, Rubella[7]	12 mos	4 weeks			
Varicella[8]	12 mos	3 months			
Hepatitis A[9]	12 mos	6 months			
CATCH-UP SCHEDULE FOR PERSONS AGED 7–18 YEARS					
Tetanus, Diphtheria/ Tetanus, Diphtheria, Pertussis[10]	7 yrs[10]	4 weeks	4 weeks if first dose administered at younger than 12 months of age / 6 months if first dose administered at age 12 months or older	6 months if first dose administered at younger than 12 months of age	
Human Papillomavirus[11]	9 yrs	4 weeks	12 weeks		
Hepatitis A[9]	12 mos	6 months			
Hepatitis B[1]	Birth	4 weeks	8 weeks (and 16 weeks after first dose)		
Inactivated Poliovirus[6]	6 wks	4 weeks	4 weeks	4 weeks[6]	
Measles, Mumps, Rubella[7]	12 mos	4 weeks			
Varicella[8]	12 mos	4 weeks if first dose administered at age 13 years or older / 3 months if first dose administered at younger than 13 years of age			

1. Hepatitis B vaccine (HepB).
- Administer the 3-dose series to those who were not previously vaccinated.
- A 2-dose series of Recombivax HB® is licensed for children aged 11–15 years.

2. Rotavirus vaccine (Rota).
- Do not start the series later than age 12 weeks.
- Administer the final dose in the series by age 32 weeks.
- Do not administer a dose later than age 32 weeks.
- Data on safety and efficacy outside of these age ranges are insufficient.

3. Diphtheria and tetanus toxoids and acellular pertussis vaccine (DTaP).
- The fifth dose is not necessary if the fourth dose was administered at age 4 years or older.
- DTaP is not indicated for persons aged 7 years or older.

4. *Haemophilus influenzae* type b conjugate vaccine (Hib).
- Vaccine is not generally recommended for children aged 5 years or older.
- If current age is younger than 12 months and the first 2 doses were PRP-OMP (PedvaxHIB® or ComVax® [Merck]), the third (and final) dose should be administered at age 12–15 months and at least 8 weeks after the second dose.
- If first dose was administered at age 7–11 months, administer 2 doses separated by 4 weeks plus a booster at age 12–15 months.

5. Pneumococcal conjugate vaccine (PCV).
- Administer one dose of PCV to all healthy children aged 24–59 months having any incomplete schedule.
- For children with underlying medical conditions administer 2 doses of PCV at least 8 weeks apart if previously received less than 3 doses or 1 dose of PCV if previously received 3 doses.

6. Inactivated poliovirus vaccine (IPV).
- For children who received an all-IPV or all-oral poliovirus (OPV) series, a fourth dose is not necessary if third dose was administered at age 4 years or older.

- If both OPV and IPV were administered as part of a series, a total of 4 doses should be administered, regardless of the child's current age.
- IPV is not routinely recommended for persons aged 18 years and older.

7. Measles, mumps, and rubella vaccine (MMR).
- The second dose of MMR is recommended routinely at age 4–6 years but may be administered earlier if desired.
- If not previously vaccinated, administer 2 doses of MMR during any visit with 4 or more weeks between the doses.

8. Varicella vaccine.
- The second dose of varicella vaccine is recommended routinely at age 4–6 years but may be administered earlier if desired.
- Do not repeat the second dose in persons younger than 13 years of age if administered 28 or more days after the first dose.

9. Hepatitis A vaccine (HepA).
- HepA is recommended for certain groups of children, including in areas where vaccination programs target older children. See *MMWR* 2006;55(No. RR-7):1–23.

10. Tetanus and diphtheria toxoids vaccine (Td) and tetanus and diphtheria toxoids and acellular pertussis vaccine (Tdap).
- Tdap should be substituted for a single dose of Td in the primary catch-up series or as a booster if age appropriate; use Td for other doses.
- A 5-year interval from the last Td dose is encouraged when Tdap is used as a booster dose. A booster (fourth) dose is needed if any of the previous doses were administered at younger than 12 months of age. Refer to ACIP recommendations for further information. See *MMWR* 2006;55(No. RR-3).

11. Human papillomavirus vaccine (HPV).
- Administer the HPV vaccine series to females at age 13–18 years if not previously vaccinated.

Information about reporting reactions after immunization is available online at http://www.vaers.hhs.gov or by telephone via the 24-hour national toll-free information line 800-822-7967. Suspected cases of vaccine-preventable diseases should be reported to the state or local health department. Additional information, including precautions and contraindications for immunization, is available from the National Center for Immunization and Respiratory Diseases at http://www.cdc.gov/vaccines or telephone, 800-CDC-INFO (800-232-4636).
DEPARTMENT OF HEALTH AND HUMAN SERVICES • CENTERS FOR DISEASE CONTROL AND PREVENTION • SAFER • HEALTHIER • PEOPLE

CS113897

◦ Children who have progressive developmental delay or a changing neurologic picture should be assessed on an individual basis. Those with stable encephalopathy (e.g., cerebral palsy or cognitive developmental delays) or controlled seizures can be immunized with pertussis. There are no studies that either conclusively prove or disprove a connection that specifically links DTaP (DTP) as a cause of brain damage. However, there can be confusion regarding the cause of some neurologic disorders. Infants and children who have or are suspected to be developing a neurologic disorder or progressive degenerative disease should have the pertussis vaccine deferred until further assessment is complete. The decision to vaccinate should be based on the risk-benefit ratio.

◦ Children with a personal history of seizures are at greater risk for vaccine-related seizures, but this is not a contraindication. If the neurologic condition is stabilized, controlled, or resolved and pertussis vaccination is contraindicated, DT vaccination can be given. However, children under 1 year old whose DTaP immunization has been withheld, should not receive DT; instead they should wait and receive the DTaP when they reach 1 year of age (AAP, 2006).

◦ A family history of adverse immunization reactions should not preclude the use of DTaP in other family members.

- **Contraindications.** There are a few relative contraindications to vaccinating a child with DTaP. The first is an immediate anaphylactic reaction, and the second is encephalopathy within 7 days of receiving DTaP or DTP. Precautions to further administration of DTaP include:
  ◦ Convulsion, with or without fever, within 3 days of immunization
  ◦ Persistent inconsolable screaming (greater than 3 hours) within 48 hours
  ◦ Collapse or shocklike state within 48 hours (referred to as hypotonic-hyporesponsive episodes)
  ◦ Unexplained temperature higher than 104.8° F (40.5° C) within 48 hours

- **Side effects.** DTaP, as previously noted, has a significantly lower probability of vaccine-associated side effects, such as moderate or high fever and local reactions. Most reactions to DTaP occur with the fourth or fifth dose. A reaction to the fourth dose is not predictive of a similar reaction to the fifth. Reactions include swelling, erythema, and pain at the injection site and fever. Reactions occur with mild intensity in 1% to 3% of recipients, usually within the first 48 hours and resolve within days.

Evidence from research studies suggests that controlling pertussis in young infants may depend on older children and adults receiving boosters with DTaP. For this reason, those between 11 and 18 years old needing a booster (or for wound management) should be given Tdap, which contains less diphtheria toxoid and pertussis antigens. If the individual is at an increased risk of complications of pertussis and/or received a Td booster at least 5 years ago, they should still receive a Tdap booster (an interval of less than 5 years between Td and Tdap can be used in cases of pertussis outbreak or other circumstances) (AAP, 2006). The new HPV and meningococcal conjugate (MCV4) vaccines should be given at the same time to bring the adolescent up to date.

Tetanus prophylaxis as part of wound management (Table 23-6) is based upon age, nature of the wound, and prior vaccine reaction history.

Polio Vaccine.   Prior to January 2000, the live oral trivalent polio vaccine (OPV) was the vaccine of choice. However, as the incidence of wild-type polio decreased and the cases of vaccine-associated paralytic polio (VAPP) outnumbered wild virus cases, the recommended vaccine for polio changed to inactivated polio vaccine (IPV) (wild polio outbreaks have occurred sporadically when immunization rates have fallen to between 60% to 80%) (Rusk, 2006c). If mass vaccination is needed to control wild polio outbreaks of paralytic polio, OPV would be considered a public health intervention since IPV does not protect against intestinal infection with wild virus.

The need for booster dosages of enhanced IPV has not been determined; immunity is believed to possibly be lifelong. The contraindication to IPV is an anaphylactic reaction to either neomycin, polymyxin B, or streptomycin; it should be used with caution in pregnant women (AAP, 2006).

Haemophilus Influenzae Type B Vaccine.   Of the six serotypes of *H. influenzae*, type B (HIB) is the most virulent and is spread primarily through respiratory droplets. Until the advent of the first HIB polysaccharide vaccine in 1987, it was the cause of 95% of all *H. influenzae* invasive diseases. Type B disease was the most common cause of bacterial meningitis in children under 5 years old. The mortality rate was 3% to 5%; with neurologic sequelae in 15% to 30% of cases. The issuance

---

TABLE 23-6   **Tetanus Prophylaxis in Wound Management**

Previous Tetanus Immunization	Clean Minor Wound	Dirty Wound
Uncertain or fewer than three doses	Td or Tdap only*	Td or Tdap* and TIG within 3 days
Three doses	Td or Tdap (fourth dose)*	Td or Tdap (fourth dose)*
More than three doses	Td or Tdap* if last dose >10 years ago	Td or Tdap* if last dose >5 years ago

*In children 11-18 years old: Tdap is preferred for prophylaxis; if an adolescent received a Tdap previously and 5 years has elapsed, use Td for prophylaxis rather than tetanus toxoid. For children 7 through 10 years old: use Td. In children younger than 7 years old, use DTaP (DT if pertussis is contraindicated). See text for definitions of abbreviations.
Data from American Academy of Pediatrics (AAP): *Red Book: 2006 report of the Committee on Infectious Diseases,* ed 27, Elk Grove Village, IL, 2006, American Academy of Pediatrics.

of this vaccine has resulted in a phenomenal 99% decrease in the incidence of HIB disease. Most new cases in the U.S. now occur in those underimmunized or in infants who have not completed their primary series (AAP, 2006).

- **General guidelines**. There are some general guidelines and information for this vaccine which include:
  - Adhere strictly to the vaccine schedule as to age and interval between vaccines.
  - Any child younger than 2 years old who had invasive *H. influenzae* disease should be vaccinated with any of the conjugated HIB vaccines according to the schedule recommended for the child's age. Vaccination should occur as soon as possible after the infection but no later than within 1 month of the infection onset. This is because of the decreased natural immunity in this age group.
  - The number of doses of HIB vaccine changes depending on the age at initial immunization. The older the child is, the fewer doses the child receives.
  - The same vaccine should be used for the primary series, but studies have not demonstrated a decline in antibody production if regimens involving different vaccine products are used. Any licensed single HIB vaccine may be used for the booster when the child is 12 to 15 months old.
  - HIB vaccine is not given to children older than 5 years given the rarity of *H. influenzae* infection after this age.
- **Side effects.** Side effects occur in about 25% of cases—mild localized pain, erythema, and swelling that last less than 24 hours (AAP, 2006).
- **Contraindications.** The vaccine has no major contraindications. Follow manufacturer package inserts regarding the schedule for vaccinating children who are receiving chemotherapy or immunosuppressive agents. The caveat concerning use of vaccine during a febrile illness should be observed.
- **Special cases.** Children with immunologic disorders or certain chronic illnesses are at increased risk for invasive HIB. They also may have decreased ability to make HIB antibodies. Children with HIV infection, sickle cell disease, functional or anatomic asplenia, or those who are receiving chemotherapy or immunosuppressive therapy may require additional doses of HIB vaccine:
  - *Asplenia*: If the child has received a complete primary series and booster, no additional vaccinations are needed. A child undergoing elective splenectomy for a medical condition may benefit from an additional dose of vaccine 7 to 10 days before the procedure.
  - *HIV infection, chemotherapy, immunosuppressive therapy, or immunoglobulin G2 subclass deficiency*: There is not enough information at this time to determine whether additional doses of vaccine are helpful. If these children have an incomplete course, they should be vaccinated to finish the series. Unvaccinated or undervaccinated children 12 to 59 months should receive doses of vaccine based on their prior HIB vaccine history (see CDC website for details).

Hepatitis A Vaccine.   Children serve as one of the largest vectors for HA disease. Up to 70% of children under 7 years old can have subclinical signs of infection. This unrecognized illness can then be transmitted to adults in whom the illness is likely to be serious. Therefore, the primary HA vaccine initiatives have focused on children. Current guidelines include universal vaccination for those 1 to 18 years old (CDC, 2006a).

The two inactivated HA vaccines licensed by the FDA for use in persons 1 to 18 years old have seroconversion rates of 94% to 100% after the second vaccine. They are conjectured to provide immunity for up to 20 years. A recommendation for a booster dose has not been determined.

HA vaccine can be administered simultaneously with other childhood vaccines, but should be given at a separate injection site (intramuscular injection in the deltoid). The vaccine is contraindicated in those with an anaphylactic reaction to alum or 2-phenoxyethanol (Havrix only). Seroconversion of immunocompromised patients (including those with HIV) may be suboptimal.

Current recommendations also target the following groups of individuals:

- Those traveling to countries where HA is endemic (countries other than Western Europe, Scandinavia, Austria, Canada, Japan, New Zealand). Children traveling to Latin America are particularly at risk (Brunell, 2006a). Active and passive immunization regimens may be prescribed depending upon the departure date and length of stay.
- Native Alaskans, Native Americans, and those in close contact with people from endemic countries
- Children in diapers in day care centers with high rates of HA virus
- Homosexual and bisexual men
- Severe illness (e.g., chronic liver disease)
- Illicit drug users (using injectable or noninjectable drugs)
- Those with blood clotting disorders (e.g., hemophiliacs)
- Healthy persons who are older than 1 year at the health care provider's discretion

A new combined HA and HB vaccine (Twinrix) was approved for use in 2001 for those older than 18 years. It is recommended for those with similar risk factors as listed above. Studies are ongoing to evaluate the use of HA vaccine (versus IG) as a prophylaxis for preventing infection after exposure. Though the vaccine has not been approved for this use, some researchers view the Twinrix as potentially an effective way to prevent both diseases. The use of postexposure IG and HA vaccine given concurrently at different sites is acceptable.

Side effects to HA vaccine are mild (localized pain). The risk of vaccination to a pregnant woman is considered low to nonexistent (AAP, 2006).

Hepatitis B Vaccine.   Two recombinant hepatitis B (HB) vaccines are currently licensed in the U.S. They are equally immunogenic and interchangeable when used as directed according to manufacturer's guidelines. Seroconversion rate is 90% to 95%. Immunogenicity appears to be 15 or more years. Routine booster doses are not recommended except for patients receiving hemodialysis or for other immunocompromised patients whose annual anti-HBs levels have fallen to less than 10 mIU/mL. Side effects are rare, but pain and soreness at the immunization site are common complaints; it should not be given to individuals who have had an anaphylactic reaction to baker's yeast. Pain at the injection site (3% to 29%) and low-grade fever (1% to 6%) are the most common reactions. Pregnancy and lactation are not contraindicated for vaccination.

Although current recommendations call for universal immunization of all newborns weighing greater than 2100 g, young children, and adolescents not previously vaccinated, there are specific individuals who should also receive HB immunization (AAP, 2006):

- Hemophiliac patients and other recipients of certain blood products
- Intravenous drug users
- Heterosexual persons with a history of multiple sex partners in the previous 6 months or with recent sexually transmitted infections
- Sexually active homosexual or bisexual males
- Household and sexual contacts who are chronic carriers of hepatitis B virus (HBV) or who are HBsAg positive
- Adoptees from foreign countries despite their immunization history. Household members of adoptees and those foreign born from HBV-endemic, high-risk countries or children born to first-generation immigrants from such endemic areas.
- Alaskan Native and Asian-Pacific Islander children
- Specific infants, children, and other household contacts in populations of high HBV endemicity
- Staff and residents of residential institutions for the developmentally disabled
- Staff and attendees of nonresidential day care and school programs for the developmentally delayed if an identified HBV carrier is known to attend or poses risk of infecting others
- Hemodialysis patients
- Health care workers and others with occupational risk
- International travelers who travel to areas of high or intermediate HBV endemicity and who otherwise may be at risk
- Inmates of long-term correctional facilities

Either vaccine can be given with IG to ensure even better protection rates in postexposure vaccination. When used as combination vaccines with DTaP (including Pediarix), the same manufacturer should be used in the first three pertussis series.

Human Papillomavirus Vaccine. Diseases caused by human papillomavirus (HPV) are responsible for approximately 40% to 50% of all annual cases of vulvar and vaginal cancer in the U.S. Cervical cancer, caused by this sexually transmitted virus, carries a lifetime risk of more than 70% (Stephenson, 2006a; Brunell, 2006b).

Vaccination of preadolescent females before the onset of sexual activity is a core goal of the vaccination program surrounding this new vaccine. However, all sexually active women can benefit before they have been exposed to any and all of the different HPVs included in the vaccine.

Gardasil (Merck) is a quadrivalent vaccine that protects against the two strains of HPV known to be associated with cancer (types 16 and 18). There are also two other strains included in the vaccine that cause genital warts (types 6 and 11). Studies have shown antibody levels to the vaccine to exceed those attained by natural infection, even after 3 to 4 years. Clinical trials demonstrated the vaccine to be 99% to 100% effective against cervical dysplasias, genital warts, and/or vulvar and vaginal intraepithelial neoplasias caused by the HPV types targeted by the vaccine. It is unclear about the cross protection against cervical intraepithelial neoplasia types not included in the vaccine. The vaccine should not replace cervical cancer screening. Another vaccine, Cervarix (GlaxoSmithKline) targets HPV types 16 and 18 and is expected to rival Gardasil; in clinical trials it has shown some cross protection against incident infection of HPV types 45, 31, and 52 which also cause cancer (Brunell, 2006c; Paavonen et al, 2007).

Other questions that remain include the duration of protection, need for booster doses, the effect, if any, on acute infection, and the safety and efficacy of the vaccine when given to patients with HIV and other immunocompromising diseases.

ACIP recommends the vaccine be routinely given to females at 11 to 12 years old, though it can be given as young as 9 years old. Studies have involved and shown efficacy in women up to 55 years old. The latest CDC adult vaccine guideline included the HPV vaccine for those under 26 years old, but it can be given up to 49 years old (CDC, 2006b). The vaccine is offered under the VFC program. Men are currently not licensed to receive the vaccine, though this may occur later. Some herd immunity is expected by vaccinating only females. It is contraindicated during pregnancy, but can be given during lactation. Those who become pregnant after starting the series should wait until after childbirth to finish. Primary care providers are expected to be the main administrators and educators for this vaccine.

Influenza Vaccine. Illness from the influenza virus is common, varies by patient age and year of occurrence, and causes approximately 36,000 deaths per year in the U.S. (CDC, 2006c). Children serve as a major vector because of their own high rates of contractility; they shed virus at higher rates and for longer periods of time than adults. After even one influenza illness, people remain susceptible to other influenza strains; severe epidemics have occurred historically.

Two multivalent vaccines are available; each contains three virus strains. The inactivated trivalent vaccine (TIV) is available IM for those 6 months or older, whereas the live-attenuated vaccine (LAIV) is restricted for those 2 years to 49 years. The LAIV is available as an intranasal spray for those age groups (further restrictions available on the CDC website).

The vaccine is formulated yearly based on epidemiologic forecasts. Generally one or two virus strains are changed based upon the anticipated dominant influenza strain(s) projected to infect the population in the approaching flu season. Major changes in viral antigens occur at 10-year intervals. This process is called *antigenic shift*. Minor variations that occur are called *antigenic drift*. These changes within the virus can prevent the body's immune system from recognizing the altered strain and mounting an immunologic response.

Because other common childhood viral agents can lead to diseases that look like influenza, the impact of the vaccine is less likely to be evident in children. The efficacy rate is 70% to 80% in children (higher if the vaccine strain closely matches the circulating wild strain) (AAP, 2006). The vaccine should be given at the beginning of October (it can be started in September if vaccine is available), before the onset of the yearly influenza season. It can be given anytime until the anticipated end of the infective season (including April). Different preparations of the vaccine have different recommendations for administration as to site and concurrent use with live vaccines.

The ACIP has recommended that healthy children between 6 and 23 months old and people in households with infants less than 6 months old be vaccinated for the annual flu season. The recommendation for vaccination has largely been in response to the high influenza infection and hospitalization rates found in young children (Poehling et al, 2006a). Universal influenza vaccination for children 5 to 18 years old and household contacts and caregivers of school-age children is being considered as a future recommendation by ACIP (Rusk, 2006d).

It is especially important that the following individuals receive influenza vaccination:

- High-risk children: children with chronic pulmonary disease (mild to severe asthma, bronchopulmonary dysplasia, cystic fibrosis [CF]) or hemodynamically significant heart disease, immunosuppressed children (should be off chemotherapy 3 to 4 weeks if possible), children with hemoglobinopathies, such as sickle cell anemia
- Children with conditions such as diabetes mellitus, chronic renal disease, severe metabolic illness, symptomatic HIV, rheumatoid arthritis, and Kawasaki syndrome
- Children who are household contacts of high-risk patients
- Pregnant women at any gestation; women in the early postpartum period during flu season
- Children who are on long-term aspirin therapy and who are at risk for developing Reye syndrome
- Residents of nursing homes and those in other chronic care facilities housing patients of any age with chronic medical conditions
- Persons 65 years or older
- Health care workers or others attending or living with high-risk persons
- Siblings and other primary caregivers of children under 24 months old
- Home health or day care workers in contact with children under 6 months old.

Side effects include:

- Young children, 6 to 24 months old, occasionally have fever in the first 6 to 24 hours after vaccination (10% to 35% incidence). Localized skin reactions are more common in adolescents and adults and occur in 10% of recipients.
- Asthmatic children have not demonstrated any increase in airway reactivity after receiving the vaccine. Data demonstrate a small increase in the risk of GBS in adults (approxi-

mately 1 per 1 million recipients), but this estimated risk is small compared with sequelae from severe influenza illness (AAP, 2006).

- Other side effects include tenderness, redness, and pain at the site of injection. Fever, malaise, myalgia, headache, and other flulike symptoms are also reported after immunization.

Contraindications to the influenza vaccine include:

- Children with severe anaphylactic reaction to chickens or egg protein rarely experience a similar type of reaction to TIV. However, because of the risk, the vaccine should not be given even if the person was desensitized (AAP, 2006). Consider the use of chemoprophylaxis instead (oseltamivir, zanamivir, amantadine, rimantadine). However, based upon resistance levels, one or several of these may not be recommended by the CDC in any given flu season. Check the CDC website (*www.cdc.gov/flu*) yearly for current recommendations regarding chemoprophylaxis efficacy.
- Children with a neurologic disorder characterized by progressive developmental delay or a changing neurologic picture should not receive influenza vaccine until the neurologic problem has been stabilized. The occurrence of any neurologic symptom or sign after administration of influenza vaccine is a contraindication to further use.
- The vaccine should not be given to a patient with a febrile illness.
- Children who receive prolonged high-dose corticosteroid therapy (more than 2 mg/kg per dose or 20 mg of prednisone per day) may have impaired antibody response to the vaccine. Immunization should be deferred until the steroid dose is lowered. However, if it is not possible to lower the steroid dose before the influenza season starts, the influenza vaccine should be administered and no longer deferred.
- Immune-deficient individuals should be considered for the vaccine; consult with their subspecialists.

FluMist, the intranasal LAIV, showed an efficacy of 92% against all culture-confirmed influenza cases in clinical trials (CDC, 2007a). It is approved for use in healthy, non-pregnant individuals between 2 and 49 years old and comes in a prefilled nasal sprayer. The number of dosages depends upon the age and vaccine history during any prior influenza season:

The following are contraindications to FluMist:

- Inactivated and live vaccines can be given at the same time; however, live vaccines not administered on the same day should not be given for at least 4 weeks.
- Do not give if patient has history of hypersensitivity to chicken egg protein.
- Do not give to patients receiving aspirin or salicylates, to those who are immunocompromised, those with reactive airway disease, or to those with COPD, cardiac disorders, metabolic diseases, renal, hemoglobinopathies, or on immunosuppressive therapy. Those with a history of GBS also should not receive LAIV.
- Do not administer to pregnant women.

The use of free on-site intranasal FluMist vaccine delivered to those residing in areas of low immunization rates or low socioeconomic levels has been shown to decrease school absence caused by influenza illness (Wiggs-Stayner et al, 2006). Clinical trials of LAIV in children revealed an increased rate of asthma (AAP, 2006).

Lyme Disease Vaccine. Two vaccines previously produced for prevention of Lyme disease caused by the spirochete *Borrelia burgdorferi* were both withdrawn by the manufacturers in 2002.

Meningococcal Vaccine. Most outbreaks of meningococcal meningitis in the U.S. are caused by serogroup C (some outbreaks have been caused by serogroups B and Y). There is no vaccine for serogroup B. Serotypes C and Y account for approximately two-thirds of college-age meningococcal infections.

Two meningococcal vaccines are licensed in the U.S. MPSV4 is a quadrivalent vaccine composed of serogroups A, C, Y, and W-135 *Neisseria meningitidis*. MPSV4 contains bacterial capsular polysaccharides of the respective groups and is not routinely given to children unless there is an epidemic or exposure. It is good for those who only need a brief elevation in immunity, such as college freshman living in dormitories. It is generally given as a single dose and for those who are 2 years and older. It can be given concurrently with other vaccines, but in another injection site. Children 2 to 10 years old who should receive MPSV4 meningococcal vaccine include those with HIV infection, functional or anatomic asplenia, those with terminal complement component or properdin deficiencies, or those who plan to travel to or reside in areas where *N. meningitidis* is endemic. It may be used as an adjunct to chemoprophylaxis. Under epidemic conditions, MPSV4 may be given to children under 2 years old. The most common adverse reaction to MPSV4 is localized erythema lasting 1 to 2 days.

In 2005, Menactra, a conjugate meningococcal vaccine (MCV4) was licensed in the U.S. for routine vaccination of children 11 and 12 years old, for high school and college dormitory freshman, and for those with HIV older than 11 years. It also combines A/C/Y and W-135 serotypes and is preferred over MPSV4 because it induces longer immunogenicity. Pain, induration, and erythema at the injection site are more common after MCV4. Cases of GBS have been reported in adolescents after MCV4; there was concern of a causal affect. However, further analysis showed the number of cases was within the normal range for chance occurrence of GBS in this population. This vaccine is contraindicated in those with a history of prior GBS infection. Any possible cases of GBS following vaccination should be reported to VAERS (Rusk, 2006e).

If vaccine supplies are low for MCV4, the CDC recommends prioritizing adolescents at high school entry and college freshmen living in dorms rather than those 11 and 12 years old (Rusk, 2006e).

Pneumococcal Vaccines. There are 45 known serotypes of pneumococcus. *Streptococcus pneumoniae* is the cause of most bacteremia or sepsis (85%), pneumonia (67%), sinusitis, meningitis (50%), and acute otitis media (AOM) (up to 55%) in children. Two pneumococcal vaccines are available; each is discussed separately.

Heptavalent Pneumococcal Vaccine. The heptavalent pneumococcal conjugate vaccine PCV7 (Prevnar) contains the seven serotypes of pneumococcus most likely causing 80% to 90% of such invasive diseases in children. It has greater immunologic memory than PPV23 (discussed later). It decreases nasopharyngeal carriage of the seven serotypes; there has been no significant evidence of concurrent increase in the nonvaccine serotypes (Black et al, 2006a; CDC, 2005a).

In prelicensure trials, the vaccine proved to have a 94% efficacy; postlicensure studies showed 97.4% efficacy in those fully immunized and 94% in those partially immunized (Black et al, 2006). Cases of invasive pneumococcal disease decreased in neonates (39%), in children under 2 years old (60%), in black infants (11%), adults (46%), and the elderly (32%). Cases in infants 0 to 60 days displayed a 42% decrease in invasive pneumococcal disease, suggesting beneficial herd immunity in neonates and infants too young to receive the vaccine (Poehling et al, 2006b). Studies have also shown that the prevalence of penicillin-resistant *S. pneumoniae* decreased from 15% to 25% to 5% to 12% after three doses of vaccine (Black et al, 2006; Garbutt et al, 2006). Based on this trend, children who have had at least three doses of the vaccine and need treatment for an AOM can be treated with amoxicillin at 40 to 45 mg/kg/day, regardless of age or the child's care situation. Children who did not receive three doses of vaccine or who were recently treated with an antibiotic should be dosed at 80 to 90 mg/kg/day (Garbutt et al, 2006).

The first dose of the vaccine cannot be given before 6 weeks of age; low-birth-weight infants (less than 1500 g) should receive the initial dose when they are 6 to 8 weeks old chronologically, regardless of calculated gestational age (AAP, 2006). There is some serotype priming after two doses, more complete priming after the third dose, but significant response after the booster (fourth) dose. Most reactions have been limited to local reactions (5% to 6%) and fever (up to 13% and depends on concurrent vaccines given). The reactions lessen on the fourth dose. Children younger than 23 months old who did not receive PCV7 before 6 months old should be caught up. It is also recommended for children between 24 and 59 months old who are at greater risk for contracting invasive pneumococcal infection. Children with moderate risk should be evaluated on an individual basis. In making the judgment to vaccinate, the provider may consider such factors as social and/or economic disadvantage, crowded and/or substandard housing conditions or homelessness, excessive tobacco exposure, recurrent otitis media infections, prior tympanostomy tubes, or vaccine shortages necessitating prioritization.

Polysaccharide Pneumococcal Vaccine. The 23-valent pneumococcal vaccine (PPV23, Pneumovax) confers broader coverage against pneumococcal serotypes—23 rather than the 7 in Prevnar. Pneumovax is administered to children 2 years and older and adults at high risk or presumed high risk of pneumococcal disease (e.g., those with HIV). The number of doses varies according to the number of prior PCV7 vaccines given and the age of the child. It can be given concurrently with other vaccines, but administered at a different injection site. Children younger than 2 years old have shown poor immunogenicity to this vaccine because there is poor reduction of overall nasopharyngeal carriage; the vaccine has an efficacy rate of 63% in children 2 to 5 years old.

Anthrax Vaccine. Biothrax is the only vaccine licensed in the U.S. The vaccine is recommended for 18- to 65-year-olds in certain military positions and for laboratory workers working with *Bacillus anthracis*. Not yet determined are its side effects (including birth defects), how many doses are needed, how protective the vaccine is, and how long the protection. In cases of an anthrax outbreak or terrorist attack using anthrax, one of two treatment regimens is recommended, either using the current vaccine (3 doses over a 4-week period) plus antibiotics (for 40 days) or taking antibiotics alone for 100 total days as postexposure prophylaxis. Studies are ongoing regarding alternative vaccines. See further discussion under Infectious Agents Used in Bioterrorism later in this chapter.

Live Vaccines

It is important for providers to consult with infectious disease experts and authoritative reference resources when contemplating administering live vaccines to immunocompromised individuals. Recommendations may differ according to the individual's degree and type of immune compromise. If someone cannot produce antibodies, they are unlikely to respond to a vaccine; if a live vaccine is given while on IVIG, the virus will be neutralized by antibodies in the IVIG product. For example, giving MMR to someone on IVIG is unlikely to do them any good.

An individual with low T-cells or a cellular immune deficiency can be seriously compromised if given a live-attenuated virus vaccine (LAIV). A child with DiGeorge syndrome, HIV infection, cancers, immune suppression, or other cellular immune problems should not receive such viral vaccines until their T-cell function is within an appropriate range. Selected recommendations are discussed under the bulleted point *Special cases* under Measles referenced later under specific live vaccines.

Bacille Calmette–Guérin Vaccine. Bacille Calmette-Guérin (BCG) live vaccine was developed in the early part of the twentieth century to prevent the spread of TB. There are at least seven different locations producing this vaccine in the world; the vaccines differ in composition. All are prepared from attenuated strains of *Mycobacterium bovis*. Two vaccines are licensed for use in the U.S.

The vaccine is recommended at birth as a public health measure in more than 100 countries in order to prevent disseminated and other potentially fatal effects from *Mycobacterium tuberculosis* disease in infants and young children. Well-documented studies have shown that the BCG vaccine is greater than 80% protective against meningeal and miliary TB in children. Newer studies have produced differing conclusions about the protective effect for primary infection or reactivation of latent pulmonary infection (World Health Organization [WHO], 2006; Soysal et al, 2005).

In the U.S., BCG is indicated only for infants and children with negative tuberculin skin testing (TST) meeting the following criteria: (1) live with persons with infectious pulmonary TB who are untreated or ineffectually treated, cannot be removed from those persons, and are without a source of long-term primary treatment; or (2) live with persons who

have drug-resistant forms of TB (to isoniazid and rifampin) and cannot be separated from those persons. Health care workers in high-risk settings also may be candidates for BCG (AAP, 2006).

Before administering BCG in the U.S., pediatric TB experts should be consulted. The vaccine is ideally given to infants at birth. The WHO does not recommend administering it to children after 12 months old because of unknown efficacy. Until 2005, it was routinely administered to children from 10 to 14 years old in the United Kingdom (it is still given to infants at birth). If given properly, a small papule forms at the site of injection. The papule enlarges, crusts, and ulcerates after approximately 2 to 4 weeks; all reactions usually resolve within 2 to 5 months (WHO, 2005). TST testing should be repeated 2 months later. If the second TST is not reactive, repeat the vaccination.

Some general information concerning the use of BCG includes:

- **Side effects.** Where BCG vaccine is part of a standard childhood vaccination program, greater than 80% of newborns and infants are vaccinated each year with minimal side effects (WHO, 2006). One percent to 2% experience localized side effects. These include ulceration, axillary lymphadenopathy, or cervical lymphadenopathy. Osteitis in the long bones can surface years after BCG vaccination. All vaccine complications should be managed by a TB expert. Disseminated infection (meningitis) and death are rare reactions and occur mostly in those that are immunocompromised.
- **Contraindications and special cases.** BCG is contraindicated in patients with immunologic disorders (including symptomatic HIV and those with burns and skin infections). Children who are receiving corticosteroids or other immunosuppressive agents should not be vaccinated. Although no fetal problems have been reported, pregnant women should not be inoculated with BCG. A guideline for the use of BCG is available from the WHO.
- Asymptomatic or suspected HIV-infected children living in areas where the incidence of TB is high should receive BCG as close to birth as possible.
- **Tuberculin skin testing.** BCG vaccine can produce a mild to severe hypersensitivity reaction, giving a false-positive reaction in children who receive TST. However, children with prior BCG vaccination should receive TST. The size of the TST can vary depending upon several factors. These include the age of the BCG vaccine itself, its quality, the strain of *M. bovis* used, the number of doses of vaccine received, nutritional status, immunologic factors, and the frequency of TST.

Measles–Mumps–Rubella Vaccine. Measles-mumps-rubella (MMR) is a trivalent vaccine. It is still possible, but often difficult, to obtain each component individually. Since the monovalent and combined MMR vaccines have been available, the incidence of these diseases (including congenital rubella syndrome) has decreased more than 99% (AAP, 2006). Large studies continue to refute a causal relationship between the development and rise of autism and MMR (Taylor, 2006; D'Souza et al, 2006).

Measles. The Enders' live, attenuated Edmonston strain is the only licensed measles vaccine available in the U.S. It is a chick embryo–prepared virus. Ninety-five percent of vaccinees develop antibodies to measles after the first dose (99% after two doses). The immunity is lifelong in most persons, but a second dose at entry to kindergarten or 4 years old is recommended because immunity wanes in less than 5% of people. Children who do not receive the second dose at kindergarten should be revaccinated at the earliest possible time. Persons vaccinated with killed vaccine, live vaccine and IgG, and those vaccinated before 12 months old should be revaccinated twice more. In children receiving RSV prophylaxis, MMR vaccine can be given any time afterwards.

Information pertinent to measles infection and vaccination includes the following:

- **Side effects.** The measles component is responsible for almost all the adverse reactions to the MMR vaccine. A fever of 103° F (39.4° C) beginning approximately 1 week to 12 days after vaccination occurs in up to 15% of vaccine recipients. Those with fever usually have no other symptoms, and the fever generally resolves within 2 to 5 days. Transient rashes occur about 5% of the time between 5 and 12 days after vaccination. Febrile convulsion is an infrequent occurrence in children after they receive the vaccine. Allergic reactions to trace amounts of one of the components (e.g., neomycin, gelatin) and thrombocytopenia (seen 2 to 3 weeks but up to 2 months after immunization) have been reported, but they are very rare occurrences.
- **Complications.** Encephalopathy and encephalitis are rare complications of the vaccine (less than 1 per 1 million). They occur at a much lower rate than they do after the natural disease. Subacute sclerosing panencephalitis, once a consequence of wild-type measles infection, has declined with measles vaccination.
- **Measles exposure or epidemics.** In cases of exposure to measles infection, the measles vaccine can provide some protection if given within 72 hours. IG can be used within 6 days of exposure to measles infection and prevents or modifies the infection in susceptible people. During measles outbreaks, immunization should begin at 6 to 9 months old. If exposure to measles is imminent, vaccination may be given after a shorter interval and a second dose of the vaccine given after the recommended time period.
- **Contraindications.** Contraindications to measles vaccine include the following:
  - *Measles vaccine can cause anergy to tuberculin skin tests.* Skin testing can be done on the day of measles vaccination or postponed for 4 to 6 weeks.
  - *A child with a history of or who has a first-degree relative with a seizure disorder:* There may be a slightly increased risk for seizures following MMR vaccination. However, the vaccination is still recommended because the benefits outweigh the risks.
  - *Pregnancy:* Women receiving any vaccine containing measles (MR, MMR, MMR-Varicella [MMRV]) should not become pregnant for 28 days after vaccination. If known to be pregnant, the vaccine is contraindicated.
  - *Allergy:* Persons with anaphylactic reaction to gelatin, egg, neomycin, or prior MMR vaccine should not be vaccinated without consulting with an allergist. If vaccination is warranted, it should be done with extreme caution. Persons with nonanaphylactic allergic reactions to egg protein or contact dermatitis from neomycin without anaphylaxis may be immunized. Anaphylaxis is rare in those with egg allergy (AAP, 2006).
  - *Febrile illness:* This is a relative contraindication. If fever suggests a serious illness, the child should not be vaccinated until later.
- **Special cases:** Patients with compromised immune systems should not receive any live vaccine.
  - IG prophylaxis is indicated in case of exposure, regardless of their vaccine history, for children receiving cancer therapy and children with other immunosuppressive disorders. The vaccine can be given to medically suppressed children at least 3 months after the therapy is stopped.
  - Measles vaccine as part of MMR is recommended for HIV-infected children at 12 months old, unless they are severely immunocompromised. Severely symptomatic HIV-infected children should be given IG at the time of exposure to measles (unless they have received immune globulin intravenous [IGIV] within 3 weeks) because they may not be able to manufacture antibodies.
  - Immunocompetent children on high-dose, long-term steroid therapy (longer than 14 days) should wait at least 1 month after discontinuing steroids before being vaccinated.
- **Post-IG.** IG and blood products affect the body's ability to react to measles vaccine. Children who receive IG must be vaccinated according to the following schedule:
  - Children who receive a relatively low dose of IG for tetanus or hepatitis (A or B) prophylaxis may be vaccinated with MMR 3 months after receiving IG.
  - Children who receive rabies IG should wait 4 months before receiving MMR vaccination.
  - Children (especially those who are immunocompromised) who receive large doses of IG in the range of 0.25 to 0.5 mL/kg for the prophylaxis of either varicella or measles should wait 5 to 6 months before being vaccinated with MMR.
  - Children who are receiving replacement therapy for immune deficiencies or therapeutic IG in doses of 300 to 400 mg/kg/mo should wait for approximately 8 months after the last dose of IG before receiving MMR vaccine.
  - Children who receive adenine-saline RBCs, unwashed packed RBCs, whole blood cell transfusions, plasma, or platelets must wait 3, 5, 6, and 7 months, respectively, before being vaccinated with MMR.
  - Children with immune thrombocytopenic purpura (ITP) receiving IG intravenous therapy of 400 to 1000 mg/kg should wait 8 to 10 months before MMR vaccination. With doses of IG of 1600 to 2000 mg/kg, MMR should be withheld for 10 to 11 months (also applies to those with Kawasaki disease).
  - Children who are to receive IG or blood products should receive any scheduled MMR vaccine 2 weeks before these products.
  - After cytomegalovirus (CMV) IG, MMR should not be administered for 6 months.

Mumps. Under experimental conditions, live mumps virus indicated a 95% seroconversion rate. However, recent outbreaks in the U.S. demonstrated efficacy of approximately 80% (Brunell, 2006d). Outbreaks occurred among all ages, but tended to cluster in the range of 18 to 24 years old. Febrile seizures, rash, pruritus, nerve deafness, encephalopathy, encephalitis, purpura, paralysis, and orchitis have been rarely reported. They occur at a much lower rate than they do after the natural disease. Contraindications are the same as for measles. The mumps vaccine can be administered as MMR or MMRV.

Rubella. RA 27/3 is the current vaccine licensed in the U.S. and is used principally to prevent congenital rubella. Seroconversion rate is greater than 95%. Mild reactions to the vaccine include fever (5% to 15%), lymphadenopathy, rash (5%), arthritis (less than 1%) and arthralgia (usually seen more in unvaccinated adolescent females and with onset 7 to 21 days after vaccine), small peripheral joint pain, and paresthesia. Contraindications are the same as for the measles vaccine. Rubella vaccine can be given postpartum with RhoGAM. The vaccine should not be given to pregnant women; if this should occur, it does not serve as an indication for termination of the pregnancy. The fetus is at maximum theoretic risk of 1.4% to exhibit signs of infection.

Children with T-lymphocyte immunodeficiencies, including leukemia and lymphoma, and other malignancies compromising bone marrow or lymphatics and congenital T-cell abnormalities should not be vaccinated with MMR or MMRV. Children with acute lymphoblastic leukemia may be vaccinated using a study protocol available in the current AAP *Red Book*. Children receiving immunosuppressive agents (see current *Red Book* guidelines for dosage of steroids received) need to be free of such agents for 1 month and then vaccination should only be contemplated after consultation with a subspecialist. Others exempt from vaccination include children with a first-degree relative with congenital hereditary immunodeficiency, unless the child is known to be immunocompetent, and children who have received blood products (including IG) within the last 5 to 6 months, depending upon age. Unvaccinated children who are HIV infected should be considered for vaccination but only after consultation with subspecialists.

Measles, Mumps, Rubella, and Varicella. Combination MMR and varicella (ProQuad) vaccine is as safe and effective as when MMR and varicella vaccines are given separately, avoids potentially missing the administration of one of these vaccines, allows fewer vaccinations, and has excellent immunogenicity. There is a slight increase in a measles-like rash (AAP, 2006). It can be given instead of the two individual vaccines at the approved ages.

Varicella Vaccine. An LAIV from the Oka strain of varicella-zoster virus (VZV) is well tolerated and immunogenic. Recent studies have shown seroconversion rates as low as 77% and as high as approximately 87% after one dose; a second dose raises the rate to greater than 99%. One study measured the impact of varicella vaccine in Massachusetts and demonstrated a decreased incidence of infection of 79% (Stephenson, 2006b). Because of the question of the duration of immunity of the vaccine and before a booster dose would be recommended, further surveillance is occurring by the CDC (CDC, 2007b).

A small percentage of vaccinees (20%) develop localized pain, erythema, and tenderness. Others (3% to 5%) may develop a mild, generalized maculopapular rash or a varicelliform eruption (3% to 5%, with a few lesions that are generally nonvesicular) after vaccination. The varicelliform rash generally occurs within 2 weeks of vaccination, and wild-type VZV has been isolated from these lesions. About 5% to 15% of individuals have reported fevers greater than 103° F (39.4° C), generally 6 to 12 days after the vaccine (AAP, 2006).

On rare occasions (5 cases in 10 years with 56 million doses given), secondary transmission of virus to susceptible individuals can occur if vaccinees developed such a rash following vaccination. Given the low risk of secondary transmission, immunocompromised household contacts do not need to be isolated from recently vaccinated individuals. Those that contract varicella infection after being immunized usually have minimal fever, fewer than 50 lesions, and recover more rapidly than if they had not been vaccinated.

If an immunocompromised child has been exposed to wild-varicella disease, the CDC recommends considering the administration of varicella vaccine within 72 hours (possibly up to 120 hours) after exposure to prevent or minimize subsequent disease (AAP, 2006). The vaccine is used in a similar manner to prevent known outbreaks and to modify the severity of disease.

When To Consider Postexposure Prophylaxis for Varicella Disease. Traditionally, postexposure varicella-zoster immune globulin (VZIG) was given to those for whom exposure posed significant risk. However, the only U.S. manufacturer stopped production in 2005. A newer investigational IG became available in 2006, VariZIG (Cangene Corporation of Winnipeg, Canada). It is available 24 hours per day from FFF Enterprises (1-800-843-7477), and participation requires strict compliance to forms and protocols. As a substitute IGIV, acyclovir or varicella vaccine could be used (Rusk, 2005). The indications for prophylaxis include:

- Susceptible unvaccinated children with face-to-face indoor play (5 minutes to 1 hour). In those immunocompromised with no history of varicella and unknown or negative serologic test results, the degree and type of immunosuppression is considered before using prophylaxis.
- Hospitalized patients with face-to-face exposure to varicella or skin-skin contact with a zoster-infected individual.
- Household contacts.
- Newborns whose mothers experience the onset of varicella infection within 5 days before delivery or within 2 days postpartum (does not apply if the mother has zoster infection). If the mother's rash appeared more than 48 hours after delivery, prophylaxis is generally not indicated, unless the mother's skin involvement is severe.

The following individuals would be considered for prophylaxis if significant exposure to varicella or zoster occurred:

- High-risk children and adolescents: immunocompromised children, including HIV-infected children without a history of varicella or varicella immunization
- Pregnant women, particularly in the first and second trimester: subclinical infection is linked to fetal involvement; a "healthy" mother does not rule out congenital disease
- Hospitalized premature infants less than 28 weeks of gestation or less than 1000 g who have been exposed to varicella
- Hospitalized premature infants older than 28 weeks of gestation (with a nonimmune mother) who have been exposed to varicella

In the case of a pregnant woman who has been exposed, the provider should consult with an obstetric specialist before recommending VariZIG or a substitute. Acyclovir may also be considered during pregnancy to decrease risk of complications of maternal infection (Myers et al, 2004). There is limited data on acyclovir as a postexposure prophylaxis measure for healthy children. IGIV may be used in certain people up to 96 hours after exposure or acyclovir if the patient is beyond the 96 hours window.

A negative serologic test result of immune status after natural disease may be unreliable and should not be used to determine susceptibility. A positive history of past varicella infection is considered a reliable indicator (AAP, 2006).

Rotavirus Vaccine. An estimated four out of five children are likely to be infected with a rotavirus before 5 years old. Prior attempts to prevent this disease led to the development of a rotavirus vaccine, RotaShield; this vaccine was withdrawn in 1999 after it was found to be associated with an increased risk of intussusception. The pentavalent rotavirus vaccine (PRV) (RotaTeq, Merck) is a live bovine-human recombinant vaccine that was released in 2006. This bovine strain of rotavirus is less reactogenic than the rhesus virus, which was used in RotaShield. It contains the five human serotypes that cause the most disease worldwide and is part of the VFC program in the U.S.

Prelicensure studies showed the vaccine reduced rotavirus gastroenteritis by approximately 74% in those younger than 8 months old (Kalvaitis, 2006). It decreased emergency department visits by about 94% and hospitalizations (about 96%) that were attributed to the severe diarrheal form of this disease. Side effects were minimal (Brunell, 2006e). Cases of intussusception have been reported, but these may be temporally related to vaccination. Monitoring is ongoing (Rusk, 2006f).

It is recommended for use in infants who were at least 32 weeks of gestation at birth, discharged from the nursery, who are at least 6 weeks old, and stable. The vaccination schedule recommends routine administration at 2, 4, and 6 months old, given at least 2 months apart (referred to as the "strict schedule") and the series completed by 32 weeks old (AAP, 2006). The "free schedule" regimen recommends the doses be given anytime in the first year of life.

RotaTeq has precautions against administering the vaccine to the immunocompromised, to people living with those immunocompromised, or the potential risk of exposure of pregnant women (Brunell, 2006e).

Smallpox Vaccine. There is one smallpox vaccine licensed in the U.S. containing a live vaccinia virus to protect against variola major and variola minor; it differs from Jenner's original variola and cowpox virus vaccine. The vaccine is administered by using a bifurcated needle (vaccine is held between the two needle tines) and inserting it three times into the skin. A telltale blister and subsequent scar at the injection site indicate a "take," or conferred immunity. Adverse effects include lymphadenopathy, fever, headache, arthralgias, inadvert self-inoculation of other body sites, eczema vaccinatum (fatalities have been reported in individuals with a history of eczema), site necrosis, chills, and satellite lesions near the injection area. In some cases, acute illness can occur, notably myopericarditis (incidence in children not determined), postvaccinial encephalitis (seen mostly in children younger than 1 year old and older adults not previously immunized), Stevens-Johnson syndrome, vaccinia keratitis, and vaccinia gangrenosa. Given within 3 to 4 days after exposure (ideally within 72 hours), the vaccine can prevent or lessen symptoms of the disease or prevent death (Unger, 2002). Vaccinia Immune Globulin (VIG) can be useful for certain complications after vaccination.

Smallpox vaccine should not be routinely given. In the case of a smallpox outbreak, high-risk individuals will be vaccinated (e.g., children, those with eczema, pregnant women, immunocompromised, or those with cardiac disease). In the event of such an emergency, current public health wisdom is against a mass, herd vaccination program. Containment will probably rely more on proven methods that entail the rapid identification and vaccination of cases, contacts, and contacts of contacts during incubation. This approach to controlling a wider outbreak is referred to as "search and containment" or "ring" vaccination. Those with smallpox would be isolated as they receive medical care. Vaccination of clinicians will probably be needed to care for the sick and exposed. Other public health measures will focus on eliminating large gatherings of people (including closing public transportation), disseminating public health information, and the isolation of family cohorts or contacts who refused vaccine (CDC, 2006d).

PASSIVE IMMUNITY: THE IMMUNOGLOBULINS

Passive immunization entails immunizing an individual with a solution of preexisting antibodies to prevent or amend an infectious disease. These antibodies are derived from sera of pooled human IG, illness-specific human IG, antibodies formulated from animals, or monoclonal antibodies. Passive immunization is reserved for patients who suffer from immunodeficiencies in whom a live or attenuated vaccine could be dangerous or who have a problem making antibodies. IG is also indicated for nonimmunized or underimmunized patients who have been exposed to an infectious disease and whose incubation period is not long enough to allow complete active immunization. Patients at high risk for developing severe complications from an infectious disease should receive passive immunization when exposed. Some patients who suffer from disease-produced toxins benefit from antitoxin passive immunization. A poisonous snakebite, tetanus, diphtheria, and botulism are examples of this. IG manufactured in the U.S. is screened for HIV-1 and HIV-2, syphilis, human T-lymphotropic viruses (HTLV-1, HTLV-2), West Nile virus (WNV), and hepatitis B and C.

IGs are given either intramuscularly or intravenously (IGIV). Most adverse reactions from IG involve localized pain at the injection site, but can also include flushing, headache, chills, sweating, and shock. It should not be given to people who have had prior adverse reactions to IG. The administrator should be prepared to handle allergic reactions.

There are also some hyperimmune globulin preparations from human donors that provide "superimmunity" because of their high antibody levels to certain infectious diseases. Such products include those for HB (HBIG), rabies (RIG), tetanus (TIG), varicella-zoster (VariZIG, available as an investigational drug from FFF Enterprises 1-800-843-7477), botulinum antitoxin (BIG), cytomegalovirus (CMV-IGIV), and respiratory syncytial virus (RSV). Equine-derived antisera are available for botulism, tetanus, diphtheria, and rabies. These have more severe adverse reactions (including fatal anaphylaxis) associated with them. They should be used with caution and only after hypersensitivity testing to animal sera is completed by a specialist.

IGIV was originally used to provide immunogenicity to individuals with primary immunodeficiencies. Its use has proven effective and is under study for other conditions. In children, these include Kawasaki disease, HIV, and stem cell transplantation. IGIV has also been used with varied efficacy in LBW infants, GBS, toxic shock, severe anemia caused by parvovirus B19 infection, and unresponsive neonatal alloimmune thrombocytopenia. Some of the more routine passive immunizations given to pediatric patients are listed in Table 23-7.

■ ANOTHER PREVENTIVE PROPHYLAXIS AGENT

RESPIRATORY SYNCYTIAL VIRUS PROPHYLAXIS

One product is currently on the market for use in infants at high risk for adverse outcomes after RSV infection: palivizumab (Synagis). Respigam (RSV-IGIV) is no longer available. Palivizumab, a humanized mouse monoclonal antibody, has the benefit of being administered IM rather than IV. It is given in monthly IM injections during RSV season (usually November through March or April) and is generally well tolerated. Palivizumab has been shown to be safe and effective in reducing RSV hospitalizations in high-risk infants. It has a high cost-to-benefit ratio. Consider RSV prophylaxis for the following children (AAP, 2006):

- Infants born at less than 28 weeks of gestation, until they are 12 months old
- Premature infants (less than 32 weeks of gestation) even without a history of chronic lung disease (CLD)
- Children younger than 2 years old with CLD who required treatment for their CLD within 6 months of the onset of RSV season (including oxygen therapy)

- Infants born between 32 to 35 weeks of gestation if RSV season occurs before they are 6 months old, and they have two or more of the following risk factors: in group child care; have school-age siblings; are exposed to environmental toxins (e.g., tobacco smoke); have congenital abnormalities of the airways; or severe neuromuscular disease
- Children younger than 2 years old with hemodynamically significant cyanotic or acyanotic congenital heart disease
- Infants on pharmacologic therapy for congestive heart failure, with moderate to severe pulmonary hypertension, and cyanotic heart disease
- Immunocompromised patients and those with cystic fibrosis (CF).

In clinical trials, there were no statistically significant differences in adverse side effects in infants treated with palivizumab versus placebo. Once opened, a vial of palivizumab must be used within 6 hours (there is no preservative). It can be given concurrently with other vaccines.

Postexposure measures may prevent or lessen the impact of any subsequent contracted disease. Exposure to invasive infection from HIB (now rare), *N. meningitidis,* measles, HA, varicella, and pertussis may include the use of prophylaxis, such as rifampin, IG, antibiotics, or specific vaccines within 24 to 96 hours of exposure. Enteroviruses are a common cause of fever in 1- to 90-day-old infants and up to 40% to 50% of hospital admissions for suspected sepsis in the summer and fall (Byington, 2006). The health care provider can consult with the local public health agency for specific recommendations or consult the *AAP Red Book.*

■ INFECTIONS IN CHILDREN ATTENDING DAY CARE

In the U.S., approximately 13 million children 5 years old and younger and 60% of children under 13 years old spend significant "care time" in settings outside of their homes. (Pickering, 2004). This population is more immunologically susceptible to illness because of their ages, hygiene habits, and close proximity to one another. Transmission depends upon the prevalence in the population, infectivity, and survival characteristics of the organism. The environment enhances easy exposure to many infectious agents, whether spread from diapers, airborne, or from play surfaces. Although any illness can present and spread in a day care setting, the diseases are primarily respiratory and gastrointestinal in nature. Children less than 36 months old and within the first 6 months of child care attendance have a higher incidence of illness. Infections typically spread in day care settings are listed in Table 23-8. With the increase in drug resistance, these infections are eliciting greater concern.

Health care professionals play critical roles in educating parents and day care centers about ways to decrease the incidence and transmission of infectious diseases. Some general guidelines for exclusion are included in Box 23-1. Children should not be excluded simply for yellow or green nasal discharge, nonpurulent conjunctivitis, exanthem without fever or behavioral changes, erythema infectiosum (fifth disease)

TABLE 23-7 **Immunoglobulins Used in Children**

Immunoglobulin	Reference Name	Indications for Use	Comments
Cytomegalovirus immune globulin intravenous	CMV-IGIV	Shows promise for: CMV pneumonia, CMV in children with HIV infection, and CMV transmission to newborns	Used in combination with IV ganciclovir to treat CMV pneumonia
Hepatis A immune globulin	IG	• Household contacts and sexual partners of known cases • Persons accidentally inoculated with a contaminated needle • Newborn infants of infected, jaundiced mothers • Persons with open lesions directly exposed to body secretions of known cases • Children in schools where more than one case is reported • All children and employees of day care centers where a case is reported • Custodial care residents and staff in close contact with an active case • Persons traveling to developing countries for less than 3 months. HA vaccine can be given concurrently with the IG, if warranted, for those traveling internationally.	• Given IM • Is given within 2 weeks of exposure; can be used in children <2 years old; is thimerosal free; >85% effective; dosage for those with continuous exposure to HA virus differs from that given for short term exposure
Hepatitis B immune globulin	HBIG	Prophylaxis for those unvaccinated or incompletely vaccinated who have discrete identifiable exposure to blood or body fluids that contain blood: • Newborns whose mothers are HB surface antigen (HBsAg) positive • Household contacts <12 months old who have received only one prior hepatitis B vaccine and the second dose is not due • Sexual partners of known HBsAg positive cases, including sexual assault or abuse victims • Persons accidentally inoculated with a contaminated needle • Individuals with percutaneous or permucosal exposure to body secretions of known cases	• Newborns receive HBIG and hepatitis B (HB) vaccine within 12 hours after birth at different injection sites. If mother's HB status not known before delivery, infants should receive HB vaccine; HBIG would be given within 7 days of delivery if mother tests positive for HBsAg postpartum. • Sexual partners of known cases: HBIG and HB vaccine up to 14 days after last exposure; repeat vaccine at 1 and 6 months. • Household contacts <12 months: HBIG and three doses of HB vaccine. If >12 months: follow index case's antibody profile (if a carrier, vaccinate all household members). If children and adolescents have documented HB series and unknown seroconversion status, a booster dose is indicated.
Measles immune globulin	IG or IGIV	To prevent or modify infection in unvaccinated children <1 year old, pregnant women, and the immunocompromised who have been exposed to measles	• Not indicated in those who have had one dose of vaccine at ≥12 months old, unless immunocompromised • Given within 6 days after exposure; the dose for those immunocompromised differs according to the degree and type of immune deficiency, if IGIV has been given, and prior dosage amounts of IG.
Mumps immune globulin		Ineffective in preventing infection after exposure	No longer available in the U.S.
Polio	Polio-IGIV	Used for virulent polio outbreaks in the immunocompromised and those with debilitating illnesses	An accelerated IPV schedule is indicated during outbreaks for those underimmunized or unimmunized.

TABLE 23-7 Immunoglobulins Used in Children—Cont'd

Immunoglobulin	Reference Name	Indications for Use	Comments
Respiratory syncytial virus	RSV-IGIV (no longer available)	Reduces risk of RSV bronchiolitis or pneumonia in high-risk children	• Palivizumab (Synagis) is now used. See section in chapter that discusses RSV.

Rubella immune globulin	IG	Modifies or suppresses the clinical manifestations of the disease, urine shedding, and decreases the rate of viremia; for use in:
		• Early pregnancy after confirmed exposure and only if termination of pregnancy is not an option
		• Infants after maternal exposure
			• Given IM.
			• If pregnant woman is exposed to either wild rubella or as a result of being accidentally vaccinated within 3 months of conception, a blood specimen should be obtained as soon as possible. The presence of serum antibodies suggests that the fetus is not at risk (1.4% to 2% theoretic risk). If no antibody is detected, a second maternal sample should be obtained 2-3 weeks later:
			  ○ A positive test indicates recent maternal infection
			  ○ A negative test requires a third sample 6 weeks later. A positive test then indicates recent maternal infection.
			  ○ A negative test at 6 weeks after exposure indicates that maternal rubella infection has not occurred.
			• Administration of IG and the absence of clinical manifestation of maternal rubella infection do not guarantee the infant will be born without congenital rubella syndrome. IgM antibody (not IgG) after IG can be used to determine maternal infection after an exposure.

Tetanus immune globulin	TIG	• For individuals with tetanus-prone wounds who are undervaccinated (fewer than three tetanus toxoid vaccine doses) or whose vaccination status is unknown • For individuals with tetanus infection in concert with antibiotics (metronidazole or penicillin G) • For immunodeficient patients, including those with HIV; they should be considered undervaccinated regardless of actual tetanus toxoid status	• Tetanus-prone wounds include those contaminated with dirt (especially if around horses), feces, or saliva; puncture wounds; avulsions; wounds acquired as a consequence of missiles, burns, crushing, or frostbite. • In infants <6 months old without the initial three-dose series, decision to use TIG depends upon mother's tetanus toxoid immunization history at the time of delivery and if the wound is tetanus prone. • TIG is given IM plus a dose of tetanus toxoid vaccine. • If TIG not available, IGIV may be considered (though not licensed for this use in the U.S.); equine tetanus antitoxin (TAT) is another alternative to TIG (not available in the U.S.)—hypersensitivity testing required before use of TAT. • Smaller dose is administered for tetanus neonatorum
Animal antisera		Considered for use in botulism (other than infant botulism) and diphtheria	• Available from the CDC; used only after careful consideration. • Side effects include fever, serum sickness, anaphylaxis.

Continued

TABLE 23-7	Immunoglobulins Used in Children—Cont'd		
Immunoglobulin	**Reference Name**	**Indications for Use**	**Comments**
Varicella immune globulin	VariZIG—Not presently available in the U.S.	Given to those exposed to varicella infection who are most susceptible to varicella and most likely to develop the disease and in whom complications of the infection would result (household contacts; playmates with face-to-face contact; infant whose mother had varicella onset 5 days or less before delivery or within 48 hours after delivery; immunocompromised children and adolescents without history of varicella, varicella immunization, or known to be susceptible; hospitalized preterm infants (≥28 weeks of gestation) whose mother lacks history of varicella or serologic evidence of protection; hospitalized preterm infants [<28 weeks gestation or ≤1000 g birth weight] regardless of mothers history or varicella-zoster virus serologic evidence)*	• Administered no longer than 96 hours after exposure. • Not indicated in infants whose mother's had zoster infection. • In the absence of VariZIG, IGIV can be used instead.*

*In many of these cases, either VariZIG or acyclovir may be considered, provided significant exposure occurred; consult with an expert in infectious disease or the CDC.
HIV, Human immunodeficiency virus; *IG,* immune globulin; *IM,* intramuscular; *IV,* intravenous; *RSV,* respiratory syncytial virus; >, greater than; <, less than; ≥, greater than or equal to; ≤, less than or equal to.

in an otherwise healthy individual, fever of less than 101° F (38.5° C) without other illness symptoms, HB carrier status, most viral infections, nits if being treated, mononucleosis, or HIV infection. Children should be excluded for scabies until after treatment (Grassia, 2005).

■ SPECIFIC VIRAL DISEASES
ENTEROVIRUSES
Nonpolio Enteroviruses
Epidemiology. These nonpolio ribonucleic acid (RNA) enteroviruses consist of 60 serotypes: A (24 serotypes) and B (6 serotypes), coxsackieviruses, 34 echoviruses, and 5 unnumbered enteroviruses. Eleven serotypes account for most diseases. Hand-foot-mouth, herpangina, pleurodynia, acute hemorrhagic conjunctivitis, myocarditis, pericarditis, viral meningitis, pancreatitis, orchitis, and neonatal sepsis are attributed to enteroviruses.

Enteroviruses are spread by fecal-oral contamination, especially in diapered infants. They are also transmitted via the respiratory route and vertically either prenatally or in the parturition period. They have a worldwide distribution, with increased prevalence in temperate climates during the summer and fall, in tropical climates year round, and in those with poor hygiene. Nonpolio enteroviral infection is not a reportable disease so the overall incidence rate is not known. However, in known cases infants under 12 months have the highest prevalence rate (44.2%) and mortality rate (67%).

The incidence rate in children 1 to 4 years old is 15%. Illness in males under 20 years old occurs more frequently than in females (1:3) (CDC, 2006e).

Infection can range from asymptomatic to undifferentiated febrile illness to severe illness. Young children from 1 to 4 years old are more likely to be symptomatic.

Incubation Period. Incubation period is 3 to 6 days. The virus is shed for several weeks after the infection begins and is viable on environmental surfaces for long periods of time.

Clinical Findings.

History. General symptoms include:
* *Acute respiratory infection:* A mild URI is common and may include complaints of sore throat, fever, vomiting, diarrhea, anorexia, coryza, abdominal pain, rash, and headache.
* *Nonspecific febrile illness of at least 3 days:* In young children, there is an undifferentiated abrupt-onset febrile illness (38.5° C to 40° C; 101° F to 104° F) associated with myalgias, malaise, irritability; fever may wax and wane over several days.

Physical Examination. *General findings:* mild conjunctivitis, pharyngeal injection, cervical adenopathy.
* *Skin:* Rash may be macular, macular-papular, urticarial, vesicular, or petechial. May imitate those of meningitis, measles, rubella.
* *Herpangina:* There is a sudden onset of high fever (up to 41° C; 106° F) lasting 1 to 4 days. Loss of appetite, sore throat, and dysphagia are common, with vomiting and abdominal pain in 25% of cases. Minute vesicles (1 to 2 mm) appear

TABLE 23-8	Pathogens and Modes of Transmission of Infection in Day Care		
Modes of Transmission	**Bacteria**	**Viruses**	**Parasites, Fungi, Mites, and Lice**
Respiratory	*H. influenzae* type b *N. meningitidis* *Group A Streptococcus* *S. pneumoniae* *B. pertussis* *M. tuberculosis*	Adenovirus Coronavirus Influenza A and B Measles Mumps Rubella Varicella-zoster Metapneumovirus Parainfluenza Parvovirus B19 Respiratory syncytial virus Rhinovirus	
Fecal-oral	*Campylobacter jejuni* *Salmonella* species *Shigella* species *C. difficile* *Aeromonas* *Plesiomonas* *E. coli* O157:H7	Enteroviruses Hepatitis A virus Rotavirus Calicivirus Astrovirus Norovirus (Norwalk) Enteric adenovirus	*Cryptosporidium parvum* *Giardia lamblia* *Enterobius vermicularis*
Person to person via skin contact	*Group A Streptococcus* *S. aureus*	Herpes simplex Varicella-zoster Molluscum contagiosum	*Pediculus capitis* *Sarcoptes scabiei* *Trichophyton species* *Microsporum species*

Contact with blood,
  urine, or saliva
		Cytomegalovirus
		Hepatitis B
		Hepatitis C
		Herpes simplex
		Human immunodeficiency
		  virus (HIV)	

Data from Clements DA: Infections in daycare environments. In Burg F et al, editors: *Current pediatric therapy,* ed 18, Philadelphia, 2006, WB Saunders; American Academy of Pediatrics (AAP): *Red Book: 2006 report of the Committee on Infectious Disease,* ed 27, Elk Grove Village, IL, 2006, American Academy of Pediatrics, p. 132.

and enlarge to ulcers (3 to 4 mm) on the anterior pillars of the fauces, tonsils, uvula, and pharynx and the edge of the soft palate. The vesicles commonly have red areolas up to 10 mm in diameter. The entire course usually lasts 3 to 7 days with complete recovery.

- *Acute lymphonodular pharyngitis:* This manifests as an acute sore throat lasting approximately 1 week.
- *Hand-foot-mouth disease:* This is a clinical entity evidenced by fever, vesicular eruption of the buccal mucosa of the mouth, and a maculopapular rash involving the hands and feet. The rash evolves to vesicles, especially on the dorsa of the hands and the soles of the feet, and lasts 1 to 2 weeks. See Color Plate.
- *Aseptic meningitis:* There are the usual signs of fever, stiff neck, and headache. Altered sensorium and seizures are common. Most cases appear in epidemics or as unique cases; most patients recover completely.
- *Paralytic disease:* A Guillain-Barré-type syndrome has been described.

- *Congenital or neonatal infection:* Transplacental infection occurs, and serious disseminated disease can affect the fetal liver, heart, meninges, and adrenal cortex. Symptoms may occur within 2 weeks of birth with an interval history of a viral infection (including fever and abdominal pain). The neonatal infection often manifests as a sudden onset of vomiting, coughing, cyanosis, anorexia, fever or hypothermia, rash, jaundice, irritability, and dyspnea. It is often mistaken for pneumonia. The cyanosis, dyspnea, and tachycardia can progress to myocarditis and congestive heart failure. Infants can go into cardiac collapse, have hepatic and adrenal necrosis, intracranial hemorrhage, and die. For those who survive severe disease, the recovery can be rapid.
- *Acute hemorrhagic conjunctivitis:* Characterized by sudden eye pain, photophobia, blurred vision, tearing, conjunctival erythema and injection, and eye edema. Most patients recover in a few weeks.
- *Pleurodynia* (Bornholm disease or devil's grip): This condition usually occurs in epidemics, but some isolated cases

can occur. It is most often caused by type B disease, but echoviruses have been implicated. There may be a prodrome before the onset of chest pain ushered in by headache, malaise, anorexia, and myalgia.

The onset of chest or upper abdominal pain can be sudden, is pleuritic in nature, and aggravated by deep breathing, coughing, or sudden movements. The pain occurs in waves of spasms that last several minutes to several hours and is described by patients as feeling like being stabbed with a knife or being squeezed in a vise. It can be mistaken for coronary artery disease, pneumonia, or pleural inflammation. Fifty percent of patients have crampy abdominal pain. Low to high fever occurs, and a pleural friction rub often is heard. The disease generally lasts from 3 to 6 days (up to a few weeks).

- *Orchitis:* This type B infection is clinically similar to mumps.
- *Myocarditis or pericarditis:* Type A and B and echoviruses. Symptoms can range from mild to severe (sudden death), and male adolescents and young adults are particularly vulnerable. Respiratory symptoms are frequently reported before the onset of fatigue, dyspnea, chest pain, CHF, and dysrhythmias. It may imitate a myocardial infarction.

Diagnostic Studies. Rapid viral cultures can be obtained from throat, stool, and rectum using centrifugation-enhanced antigen detection available in commercially prepared shell vials. CBC is usually normal. PCR is highly sensitive for most enteroviruses. and results can be available in hours. Serology

for serotype-specific immunoglobulin M (IgM) antibody or other testing is less useful than culture or PCR. Serotype identification is only available in reference labs and used during epidemics.

Differential Diagnosis. The differential diagnosis includes other causes of the aforementioned conditions (e.g., viral, bacterial [pneumonia, meningitis, sepsis], connective tissue diseases).

Management. There is no specific therapy available. Intravenous IgG has been used and proven helpful in some cases. Antiviral therapy is being developed.

Prevention. Enteric precautions and good hand washing are the only efficient control measures.

Poliomyelitis Virus

Epidemiology. The agent is an enterovirus with three serotypes of poliovirus (types 1, 2, and 3). The disease ranges from an asymptomatic illness to severe CNS involvement.

Humans are the only documented source of infection. Transmission is through fecal-oral and respiratory routes. The last North American wild-type polio case occurred in 1979. Since then almost all cases have been associated with oral vaccine-associated use (VAPP). Since the change to all-IPV schedule in 2000, no new cases were reported until 2005 (CDC, 2005b).

Asymptomatic disease occurs in 95% of those infected (AAP, 2006). Communicability is greatest 1 week before the onset of clinical illness and shortly afterward, due to respiratory secretion and high fecal excretion. Contagion exists for approximately 1 week for mouth secretions and for several weeks to months from feces. The incubation period is 3 to 6 days for asymptomatic and nonparalytic forms and 7 to 21 days for the paralytic forms. It is a reportable disease.

Clinical Findings. Poliomyelitis should be considered in any unimmunized or underimmunized child who has a nonspecific febrile illness, aseptic meningitis, or paralytic symptoms.

There are three clinical forms:

1. *Nonspecific febrile illness (abortive polio):* A mild and brief illness. There is an acute onset of fever to 103° F (39.4°C). Malaise, pharyngitis, headache, nausea, vomiting, abdominal pain, constipation, and anorexia are common findings. The entire illness lasts a few hours to 2 to 3 days.
2. *Nonparalytic polio:* The child manifests abortive symptoms, has a symptom-free period of 1 to 2 weeks, and then becomes sicker. Pain and stiffness of the neck, trunk, back, and legs are common. Headache is intense; constipation is common. Hyperesthesia and paresthesia occur. There may be a fleeting bladder paralysis. Reflexes may be increased or decreased 12 to 24 hours before onset of muscular weakness; the superficial reflexes are affected before the deep reflexes. No sensory defects occur.
3. *Paralytic disease:* There are three subtypes of the paralytic forms of the disease. These subtypes are distinguished by which sections of the CNS are involved: *spinal* (upper and lower extremity, single or multiple muscle groups; 5% to

10% mortality); bulbar (respiratory, extraocular, facial, masticatory muscles; 5% to 10% mortality); and polioencephalitis (higher brain centers). The degree of paralysis depends upon the degree of neuronal involvement.

Diagnostic Studies.   The diagnostic test of choice is a viral culture from stool (two stool samples done 24 to 48 hours apart are required if flaccid paralysis is present). The wild-type versus the VAPP type needs to be differentiated. The CSF may be normal or show changes based upon the degree of CNS involvement. Antibody titers vary between the acute phase and 3 to 4 weeks later.

Differential Diagnosis.   Polio is rare. Differential diagnoses include other conditions causing muscular weakness: GBS, peripheral neuritis, transverse myelitis, encephalitis, rabies, tetanus, botulism, demyelinating encephalomyelitis, tick-bite paralysis, spinal cord tumors, familial periodic paralysis, myasthenia gravis, and hysterical paralysis. Conditions that cause decreased limb movement or pseudoweakness are also differential diagnoses and include unrecognized trauma of the sciatic nerve, toxic synovitis, acute osteomyelitis, acute rheumatic fever, scurvy, and congenital syphilitic osteomyelitis.

Management.   There is no antiviral treatment. Management is supportive and directed at minimizing skeletal deformity in the paralytic form of the disease. Both nonparalytic and mild paralytic cases can be managed on an outpatient basis, but otherwise individuals should be hospitalized.

Complications.   The following may be seen:
- Paralysis. If one recovers from paralysis it usually is evidenced within the first 6 months with continued slower progression of function until about 18 months. Male children after puberty are more likely to have paralysis with an increase in disability and mortality (Simoes, 2004).
- Gastrointestinal problems, including bleeding and acute gastric dilation
- Cardiopulmonary problems, consisting of mild hypertension and myocarditis
- Acute pulmonary edema
- Pulmonary embolism
- Metabolic problems (hypercalciuria and renal stones)

Postpolio syndrome can occur 30 to 40 years after initial infection and occurs in up to 30% to 40% of individuals. Symptoms include muscle pain and weakness or paralysis (Simoes, 2004).

Prevention.   Prevention is active and passive vaccination.

Hepatitis A Virus

Epidemiology.   Hepatitis A virus (HAV) is an RNA-containing virus belonging to the Picornavirus family; it causes a primary infection in the liver. It is a highly contagious infection and commonly spreads through person-to-person contact and fecal-oral contamination of food and water; rarely is it transmitted by contaminated blood transfusion. It accounts for approximately 50% of all acute viral hepatitis in the U.S. There is no seasonal variance. It is vaccine preventable.

Transmission occurs readily in households and day care centers. In children under 6 years old, few have symptomatic (icteric hepatitis) or specific illness. Adults tend to have more severe disease. Since the advent of the HA vaccine program for children that targeted high-risk communities in the US, the rate of infectivity has dramatically changed. Children from 5 to 14 years traditionally had the highest rate while currently the highest rate occurs among young adults; the success has produced an overall decrease in HAV of approximately 79% in the US (CDC, 2006a; AAP, 2006). The high anicteric disease incidence allows considerable spread of disease to adult caretakers in child care settings. Infants are protected by maternal antibodies during the first few months of life.

Incubation Period.   The period of contagion is as long as the patient sheds virus and usually lasts 1 to 3 weeks. The patient is most contagious from up to 2 weeks before the onset of illness until 1 week after the onset of jaundice. The incubation period is 15 to 50 days (average 25 to 30 days).

Clinical Findings.   The following two phases may be seen:
1. *Preicteric phase:* This phase manifests as an acute febrile illness. Malaise, nausea, anorexia, vomiting, digestive complaints, and occasional abdominal complaints occur. This phase goes unnoticed in many children. There can be dull right upper quadrant pain during exercise.
2. *Jaundiced phase:* Jaundice appears shortly after the onset of symptoms (70% incidence in older children and adults). Urine darkens, and stools become clay colored. Often these are the only apparent signs of the illness. Diarrhea is common in infants, whereas constipation is more common in older children and adults. Patients feel sick. Infants have poor weight gain during the icteric phase.

Fulminant disease is rare. There is no chronic disease. The icteric phase lasts from a few days to almost a month and may be subtle in children. Complete recovery can be expected within 1 month with occasional relapses lasting up to 6 months.

Diagnostic Studies.   Serologic testing is widely available. IgM-specific antibodies indicate recent infection. These are replaced by IgG-specific antibodies 2 to 4 months later and serve as indicators of past infection. Changes in liver enzymes indicate the degree of injury. There is elevation of serum transaminases (serum glutamic-oxaloacetic transaminase [SGOT], aspartate aminotransferase [AST], serum glutamate pyruvate transaminase [SGPT], alanine aminotransferase [ALT]). Prothrombin time can be elevated.

Differential Diagnosis.   Any cause of jaundice is in the differential diagnosis of HAV.
- *Infancy:* Physiologic jaundice, hemolytic disease, galactosemia, hypothyroidism, biliary metabolic disorders, biliary atresia, α_1-antitrypsin deficiency, and choledochal cysts. Hypervitaminosis A causes a yellow pigmentation (carotenemia) of the skin often mistaken for jaundice in children. Infections, such as toxoplasmosis, rubella, CMV, and herpes (TORCH) also cause hepatitis.
- *Older infants, children, and adolescents:* Hemolytic-uremic syndrome, Reye syndrome, malaria, leptospirosis, brucello-

sis, chronic hemolytic diseases with gallstone development, Wilson disease, CF, Banti syndrome, collagen-vascular disease (e.g., systemic lupus erythematosus [SLE]), infectious mononucleosis (IM), CMV, coxsackievirus, toxoplasmosis, Weil disease, yellow fever, acute cholangitis, amebiasis, and hepatitis B, C, and D. Drugs and poisons, such as pyrazinamide, isoniazid, valproic acid, acetaminophen overdose, zoxazolamine, gold, cinchophen, phenothiazines, and methyltestosterone are among others that also cause hepatitis.

Management.   Therapy is supportive in nature. The use of gamma globulin within 2 weeks of exposure is discussed earlier in this chapter (see Table 23-7).

Complications.   Although patients can become very ill, most cases of HAV resolve completely. Fulminant hepatitis with liver failure is rare.

Hepatitis B Virus

Epidemiology.   Hepatitis B virus (HBV) is a DNA-containing hepadnavirus. It is highly contagious and causes severe liver disease. The most common method of transmission is percutaneous or mucous membrane exposure to contaminated blood or sexual secretions, or both. Saliva contains little virus; it is not spread by the fecal-oral route. HBV can survive in a dried state for more than 1 week, but is highly susceptible to common household disinfectants. Prolonged percutaneous contact with contaminated fomites can be a source of infection. Surface and core antigens are useful markers for epidemiologic studies. Patients are infectious when they are HBsAg positive or if they are chronic carriers of HBV. Hepatitis B e antigen (HBeAg) correlates with viral replication and indicates chronic carriage. Antibodies to core and surface antigen lessen infectivity. The initial infection can be prevented with HB vaccination.

The major reservoirs for HBV are healthy chronic carriers and patients with acute disease. Children who have immigrated to the U.S. from China, Southeast Asia, Africa, and other high endemic areas pose the highest infection and carriage risk. Perinatal transmission during the birthing process (in utero transmission is rare) from female carriers (HBsAg positive or HBeAg positive, or both) to their newborn children has a 70% to 90% infant infection rate unless intervention is undertaken. Whether or not one eventually develops chronic infection depends upon the age one is infected and the rate of loss of HBeAg. Greater than 90% of untreated infants will develop chronic infection after exposure. Approximately 20% to 50% of children who acquire the infection between 1 and 5 years old (versus less than 5% who are exposed as adults) develop chronic HBV infection (Curry & Chopra, 2005). Individuals who abuse IV drugs or who engage in sexual activity with multiple partners or have male-to-male sex have the greatest risk of acquiring HBV. Health care workers who are exposed to blood and blood products or who care for the developmentally disabled are also at a high risk, as are chronic renal dialysis patients. Tattooing or body piercing with contaminated instruments is another route of infection. Breastfeeding is not contraindicated. The prevalence rate of infection in the U.S. is approximately 0.1% to 2% with blacks being infected at four times the rate as whites (Curry & Chopra, 2005). Since the advent of HB vaccinations, the incidence of acute HBV has decreased more than 70% in the U.S. (Suskind & Murray, 2006).

Incubation Period.   The incubation period is 45 to 160 days (average of 90 days).

Clinical Findings.   HBV has a range of illness from asymptomatic seroconversion to fulminating disease and death. HBV usually has a gradual onset. Most children who acquired HBV at an early age are asymptomatic. Some have minimal nonspecific constitutional complaints such as fever, nausea, and minimal hepatomegaly. Arthralgia and skin problems, such as urticaria or other rashes, can be the first apparent signs. Papular acrodermatitis has been described in infants. Acute HB infection is somewhat similar to the icteric phase of HAV, but it is usually more severe. Skin, mucous membranes, and sclerae are icteric. The liver is enlarged and tender.

Diagnostic Studies.   Serologic tests include HBsAg, hepatitis B core antigen (HBcAg), HBeAg, and antibodies to these antigens; the results can be useful in determining the stage of infection (Table 23-9). Positive HBsAg and HBcAg assay results indicate active infection. Changes in liver enzymes indicate the degree of injury. There is elevation of serum transaminases (SGOT, AST, SGPT, ALT). Prothrombin time can be elevated, especially in fulminating disease. Hybridization assays and gene amplification techniques (PCR) are also available.

Differential Diagnosis.   Any cause of jaundice is in the differential diagnosis of HBV. See the section on differential diagnosis of HAV.

Management.   Therapy is supportive in nature. The use of active and passive vaccination has been discussed previously. Interferon alfa-2b and lamivudine have been used with some success (as indicated by the clearance of HBeAg) for chronic HBV in children and are FDA approved. Those older than 18 years have also benefited from interferon alfa-2b and peginterferon alfa-2a, lamivudine, adefovir, or entecavir. Those with chronic infection should receive periodic liver ultrasound, liver function tests, quantitation of viral replication, immunologic response testing, and vaccination for HAV. Liver biopsies are also indicated for accurately monitoring the effects of liver involvement.

Complications.   There are hepatic and extrahepatic complications (e.g., up to 20% of infants and older children with chronic HBV will develop hepatocellular carcinoma or cirrhosis) (Suskind & Murray, 2006).

Fulminating Hepatitis.   The progressive course of hepatitis is distinguished by liver failure and can occur a few days to a month after acute hepatitis. Elevated bilirubin (greater than 20 mg/dl), elevated ammonia levels, marked elevated transaminases, encephalopathy, bleeding, coma, ascites, and abnormal encephalograph (EEG) changes occur. There is a 30% mortality rate.

Extrahepatic Manifestations.   Polyarteritis nodosa, glomerulonephritis, mixed cryoglobulinemia, a serum sickness-like prodrome, and polymyalgia rheumatica are associated with HBV.

| TABLE 23-9 | Interpretation of the Hepatitis B Serologic Panel |

HBsAg*	Anti-HBs	Anti-HBc IgM†	Anti-HBc IgG	Interpretation	Comments
+	–	–	–	Early acute infection	First indicator to appear as early as 1-2 weeks after infection but before clinical symptoms. Usually persists throughout the illness. Ensure household and sexual contacts are vaccinated.
+	–	+	+	Acute infection	Highly infectious, active replication of virus. Ensure household and sexual contacts are vaccinated.
+	–	–	+	Chronic infection	Low replication of the virus, low infectivity, or HbsAg carrier.
–	–	+	–	"Window period" following acute infection	Patient probably not infectious.
–	–	–	+	Remote infection with loss of detectable anti-HbsAg; remote infection with possible low-level HbsAg; possible false-positive test	Patient not infectious to household, sexual, needle-stick exposures.
–	+	+/–	+	Resolved infection	Patient is immune, not infectious.
–	+	–	+/–	Healed infection	Patient is immune, not infectious.
–	+	–	–	Immune following vaccination; resolved infection with loss of detectable anti-HBc	Patient is immune, not infectious.

*The presence of HBsAg alone is insufficient for a diagnosis of acute infection.
†Anti-HBc IgG may also be reported as simply anti-HBc (or HBcAb) and can persist indefinitely.
See text for definitions of abbreviations.
Adapted from State of Alaska Epidemiology Bulletin: *Serologic test for viral hepatitis,* part 2. Available at *www.epi.hss.state.ak.us* (accessed Feb 24, 2007); Centers for Disease Control and Prevention (CDC): *Interpretation of the hepatitis B panel.* Available at *www.cdc.gov/ncidod/diseases/hepatitis/b/Bserology.htm* (accessed Feb 24, 2007d).

Hepatitis C Virus

Epidemiology. Hepatitis C virus (HCV), a single-stranded RNA virus with seven genotypes in the Flaviviridae family, causes the chronic form of what used to be called non-A, non-B hepatitis. The risk factors associated with HCV are illicit IV drug use (60% to 90%), imprisonment, occupational or sexual exposure (1% to 10%), and transfusions (rare). Those with hemophilia treated with blood products before 1987 are at high risk; those on chronic hemodialysis have moderate risk (10% to 20%). Perinatal transmission by non-HIV infected women is approximately 6% to 7%; HIV-positive mothers have four times the likelihood of transmitting the virus to their infants. Vaginal birth and breastfeeding do not contribute to higher rates of transmission, and women with HCV alone should not be discouraged from experiencing either (Borkowsky & Krugman, 2004; Mast et al, 2005). Studies are demonstrating an increased incidence of transmission in female infants. It is postulated that this may be a reflection of hormonal or genetic differences in susceptibility or response to the infection; there is greater mortality in utero for males infected with the virus than for females (Beasley, 2005).

Incidence of persistent hepatitis infection in children is from 50% to 60%, typically asymptomatic. HCV has the highest rate of developing into chronic infection than all of the other hepatitis infections (AAP, 2006). Fifty to 80% percent of adult cases are characterized by chronic infection and liver disease, whereas the incidence of these complications in children is thought to be lower (Snyder & Pickering, 2004).

Incubation Period. HCV has an incubation period ranging from 2 weeks to 6 months (6 to 7 weeks).

Clinical Findings. Onset of symptoms is often insidious, and most children are asymptomatic. Flu-like prodromal symptoms followed by jaundice occur in fewer than 20% of cases. Chronic hepatitis with cirrhosis (a late occurrence, often 20 to 30 years) is associated with hepatosplenomegaly, ascites, clubbing, palmar erythema, spider angiomas, and, uncommonly, hepatocellular cancer. Fulminant hepatitis C is uncommon.

Diagnostic Studies. Confirmation of HCV using IgG assays for anti-HCV or HCV RNA or DNA is diagnostic. The popularly used enzyme immunoassays can result in false-negative results for as long as 1 to 3 months after the onset of illness symptoms; false-positive results are not unusual in low-risk populations and require confirmation using a recombinant immunoblot assay (Snyder & Pickering, 2004). A newborn can be anti-HCV positive from maternal transfer for up to 18 months, so testing should be done after that time. Liver function tests are indicated; liver biopsy is confirmatory.

Differential Diagnosis.   Differential diagnoses include HA and HB and other causes of chronic hepatitis. See section on differential diagnosis of HAV.

Management.   Treatment of acute hepatitis C is supportive; there is no effective treatment to prevent the progression to cirrhosis, liver failure, or hepatocellular cancer. Chronic HCV infections in children respond to therapy with interferon alfa-2 therapy and Ribavirin (Rebetol) (for use in children 3 years and older). HA and HB vaccines should be given to prevent further liver complications. Breastfeeding by an HCV-positive mother is not contraindicated unless she has cracked or bleeding nipples. Children with HCV infection need not be excluded from day care facilities (AAP, 2006).

Individuals with hepatitis C should be discouraged from using alcohol (to prevent further liver injury) and from sharing razors and toothbrushes; condom use should be encouraged.

Prognosis.   The course of HCV is generally mild even with cirrhosis. Liver transplantation is an option, although reinfection is common and gradually progressive. The outcome of chronic HCV disease in children is less known.

Hepatitis D Virus

Hepatitis D virus (HDV) infection is uncommon in children but must be considered in cases of fulminant hepatitis or hepatic failure. It cannot cause infection unless the patient also is infected with HBV. Incubation is 2 to 8 weeks. It is diagnosed most commonly in drug users, individuals with hemophilia, and immigrants from southern Italy and parts of Eastern Europe, South America, Africa, and the Middle East. Mother-to-newborn transmission is uncommon (Snyder & Pickering, 2004). Infection is detected using IgM antibody to HDV. There is no vaccine against HDV. However, HB vaccine is preventive of hepatitis D since HDV requires comorbidity with HBV to be infective. HBIG can be used after known exposure to HDV.

Hepatitis E Virus

Hepatitis E virus is similar to the caliciviruses. It is passed via the fecal-oral route. Contaminated water is the most common reservoir. Endemic areas include India, the Middle East, Southeast Asia, and Mexico. Most cases in the U.S. are found in immigrants or visitors from these locations. Clinical symptoms are similar to HAV, but often more severe; infection has a notably high morbidity rate in pregnant women. Laboratory studies include IgM and IgG assays; IgM antibody is positive about a week after the onset of illness symptoms. There is no treatment or vaccine, but immunoglobulin pooled from individuals from endemic countries may show some usefulness. Chronic infection is not seen.

HERPES FAMILY OF VIRUSES

The herpes family of viruses is large. They have several features in common: all infect humans, the infection is lifelong,

the viruses establish latency, and reactivation is controlled by immune function. Most active infections are self-limited. Infection becomes serious and dangerous when the cellular immune system is not working properly or when it is naïve (newborn). This family of viruses includes herpes simplex virus (HSV), VZV, Epstein-Barr virus (EBV), CMV, roseola (human herpes virus 6 and 7 [HHV-6 and HHV-7, also known as exanthema subitum or sixth disease]), and human herpesvirus 8 (HHV-8, also known as Kaposi sarcoma-associated herpesvirus). HSV, VZV, and roseola are discussed below. The reader should consult other resources for a discussion about herpesvirus 8.

Herpes Simplex Virus

Epidemiology.   Herpes simplex virus (HSV) is among the most widely disseminated infectious agents in humans. HSV has two antigenic types. HSV-1 is associated chiefly with nongenital infections of the mouth, lips, eyes, and CNS. HSV-2 is most commonly associated with genital and neonatal infection. However, there can be mixing and matching of both HSV types in different mucus membrane locations. Type 1 strains can be found in the genital tract (autoinoculation or oral-genital contact). Type 2 lesions found in the mouth or pharynx usually result from oral sexual activity. The spectrum of neonatal HSV infection is changing. Infection can be caused by either type 1 or type 2; both are equally devastating to a newborn.

Primary infection with type 1 virus usually occurs in infants and children between 1 and 4 years old. Distribution is worldwide, but the infection is more frequent in crowded environments. It is spread by intimate, direct contact. The virus can be recovered from stool, urine, skin lesions, saliva, and respiratory secretions. The primary site of clinical infection is gingivostomatitis (12.1%), usually occurring in the second year of life. There is no seasonal variation, and adults are the chief source of infection. Type 2 infections usually occur as a result of sexual activity. Sexual molestation must always be ruled out when the infection is found in non-neonates.

Neonatal HSV infection is primarily transmitted from the mother as the infant passes through an infected birth canal. Viral migration from the vaginal vault to the fetus occurs. Occasionally, a scalp monitor probe becomes contaminated and is the source of infection. Although the majority of neonatal infections are caused by HSV-2, approximately 25% are HSV-1. Risk of infection for an infant born to a mother with a primary genital infection is 33% to 50%. The risk for infants born to mothers with recurrent HSV genital infection is less than 5%. The incidence is 1 in 3000 to 1 in 20,000 live births (AAP, 2006). Most infants with congenital HSV infection are born to women without a history or clinical findings of active infection during pregnancy. Postnatal transmission is described, but is less common. Mothers can inoculate their babies from oral, breast, or skin lesions. Fathers also can inoculate infants with nongenital lesions. There can be lateral transmission from an infected baby in the nursery. Postnatal transmission from nursery personnel with fever blisters is extremely rare.

Incubation Period. Period of communicability for types 1 and 2 (when not in the neonatal period) is 2 days to 2 weeks (AAP, 2006). Some cases of congenital infection occur more than 6 weeks after birth. Infection can be transmitted during either primary or recurrent infections, whether children are clinically ill or asymptomatic.

Clinical Findings. Manifestations are determined by the port of entry of the host, age, state of health, and immune competence. Eczema alone or in combination with other manifestations is also a complicating factor. Specific clinical findings, diagnosis, and treatment of gingivostomatitis, neonatal herpetic infection, eczema herpeticum, herpes vulvovaginitis, and herpes keratoconjunctivitis are discussed in other chapters. It is important to note that many mothers can shed HSV asymptomatically and may not know they have HSV. A history of HSV is helpful, but a negative history does not rule out HSV as an etiology of infection in an infant.

Traumatic Herpetic Infection. This is a localized infection that occurs in a susceptible child because of an abrasion, teething, laceration, or burn that is inoculated with herpesvirus by an orally infected parent who kisses the "booboo." Vesicles appear at the site of the lesion. There may be fever, constitutional symptoms, and regional lymph node involvement.

Acute Herpetic Meningoencephalitis. Primary CNS involvement is an unusual manifestation outside the neonatal period. HSV-1 causes a rapidly progressing infection with a 70% fatality rate. Encephalitis can be focal, mimicking a mass lesion. Diagnosis is made by brain biopsy. In contrast, HSV meningitis is usually a relatively benign disease most often caused by HSV-2.

Recurrent Infections. As with varicella, the body does not truly eradicate the virus, and recurrent infections are common. The usual manifestation of recurrent infections is herpes labialis (aka "fever blister") and involves the skin adjacent to the lips. Some incidence of recurrent aseptic meningitis can be attributed to HSV infection. Constitutional symptoms are rare except in immunocompromised patients.

Diagnostic Tests. Tests may include viral culture, cytology-Papanicolaou smears, Tzanck stains, ELISA, fluorescent techniques, glycoprotein G assay, blood or CSF PCR in neonates, or brain biopsy in cases of encephalitis. Cultures in neonates need to be taken from skin vesicles, mouth, nasopharynx, eyes, urine, blood, stool or rectum, and CSF. Serologic tests are not helpful in neonates. If encephalitis is suspected, an EEG and MRI of the brain are performed.

Differential Diagnosis. The diagnosis is usually not a problem if vesicles are present. Coxsackievirus can cause a vesicular stomatitis.

Management. Treatment is supportive in nature except in life-threatening illness (neonatal infection or immunocompromised patients).

Complications. Usually the infection is mild. Major problems have been discussed. Bacterial superinfection is always a problem. There is an increased incidence of cervical cancer in women with HSV-2 infections.

Prevention. The prevention of neonatal infection is directly tied to the monitoring of women during pregnancy and labor. All pregnant women must be asked about HSV infection in themselves and all sexual partners. Signs and symptoms of HSV should be carefully monitored throughout pregnancy. Again, during labor, all women must be requestioned about HSV. The mother must be carefully examined for signs and symptoms of infection. Cesarean delivery is indicated in women with apparent infection unless membranes are ruptured for more than 4 to 6 hours. Scalp monitoring should be avoided.

After birth, the infant must be carefully examined for vesicular lesions. Any lesion found should be cultured. The child should be started on acyclovir while awaiting culture results if HSV is strongly suspected. Infants born to mothers with a history of HSV but no signs of active disease follow the same protocol. Intrapartum cultures from mother and child should be obtained on the day of delivery (see Chapter 38).

Toddlers and infants with primary gingivostomatitis who are drooling should be excluded from child care centers. Children with "fever blisters" may attend school as long as they have control over their saliva. Covering lesions with a bandage is appropriate for children with active nonmucosal involvement. Wrestlers should be excluded from competition until lesions have healed (AAP, 2006).

Infectious Mononucleosis

Epidemiology. Infectious mononucleosis (IM) is caused by the Epstein-Barr family of herpesvirus 79% of the time; the rest is attributed to acute CMV infection (Johannsen et al, 2005). It is worldwide in distribution. Older children and adolescents in poor urban settings or developing countries are seropositive for EBV. In these children, primary infection tends to produce only mild symptoms and is subclinical. Exposure occurs at any early age. In more developed countries, seroconversion is apparent in 50% to 90% by young adult life (Katz & Miller, 2004). Most symptomatic cases of IM occur during adolescence and in young adults with susceptible college students having an incidence of 5000 per 100,000 persons. Symptoms in college students may be atypical and more suggestive of atypical EBV infections (e.g., thrombocytopenia, hemolytic anemia, pneumonitis, and rash) (Katz & Miller, 2004). The mode of transmission is close personal contact (e.g., kissing). Pharyngeal secretions are the main source of transmission; fomite contamination can be a problem. About 15% to 20% of healthy immune individuals shed EBV at any one time. Up to 50% of patients on immunosuppressive therapy, including those on steroids, shed virus. Blood transfusions laden with EBV-infected lymphocytes can also transmit the infection.

Incubation Period. Because IM virus is found in the saliva and blood of both clinically ill and asymptomatic infected persons for many months, the period of communicability is difficult to assess. The period of incubation is thought to be from 4 to 6 weeks (average 20 to 30 days). It is only mildly contagious.

Clinical Findings. IM is the "great impostor" and can mimic any disease imaginable. It is a disease of the primary lymphoid tissue and peripheral blood. There is enlargement of lymphoid tissue: regional lymph nodes, tonsils, spleen, and liver. Atypical lymphocytes are seen in the peripheral blood. Almost all body organs are involved, including but not limited to the lungs, heart, kidneys, adrenals, CNS, and skin. Symptoms are variable and can last up to 2 to 3 weeks. Clinical presentation can include the following (Johannsen et al, 2005):

- *Fever*: Moderate to high fever (less than 103° F [39.4° C]) lasting 1 to 3 days is common (greater than 90%). In severe cases, fevers can reach 104° F to 105° F (40° C to 40.6° C) and last for several weeks.
- *Sore throat*: Usually begins a few days after the fever. The throat is very painful for 7 to 10 days. There is marked tonsillar enlargement, grayish-colored exudates (in approximately 33%), ulceration, and pseudomembrane formation. Petechiae are found on the palate (in approximately 25% to 60%).
- *Lymphadenopathy*: Both the anterior and especially the posterior cervical nodes are involved; lymphoid tissues commonly are involved as well. Nodes are firm but usually nontender, are discrete in nature, and range from 1 to 4 cm in size (80% to 90% incidence).
- *Splenomegaly*: Occurs in approximately 50% of cases. Rupture is rare.
- *Hepatomegaly*: (10% to 15%); 5% have hyperbilirubinemia.
- *Skin rash*: Occurs in 5% of cases, usually on the trunk, arms, and palms. Can be maculopapular, urticarial, scarlatiniform, hemorrhagic, or nodular (rarely petechial, vesicular, or hemorrhagic) and usually occurs during the first few days of symptomatology onset and lasts 1 to 6 days. The rash occurs more frequently in patients taking ampicillin, probably represents a form of arteritis or vasculitis rather than hypersensitivity to ampicillin, and typically starts 5 to 10 days after the drug has begun.
- *Periorbital edema*: Reported in 25% of cases.

Other systemic manifestations reported as primary disease and not complications include myalgia, arthralgia, chest pain, nausea, anorexia, vomiting, ocular pain, photophobia, conjunctivitis, gingivitis, abdominal pain, orchitis (rare), diarrhea, cough, pneumonia, myocarditis, pericarditis, rhinitis, epistaxis, bradycardia, aseptic meningitis, GBS, Bell palsy, Reye syndrome, and acute cerebellar ataxia (Johannsen et al, 2005).

Diagnostic Studies. The CBC has a classic picture of more than 10% atypical lymphocytes and lymphocytosis. There are a number of serologic tests. Monospot and the serum heterophile test are positive in 80% of infected patients older than 4 years. Children older than 4 years usually must be ill for approximately 2 weeks before seroconverting. Viral culture and Epstein-Barr-specific core and capsule antibody testing are usually used for diagnosis if the primary screening test results are negative, and there is continued suspicion of IM (e.g., in younger children). Depending upon the antibody, levels can be detectable for years after infection. CMV must be considered in patients who have all the symptoms of IM but are negative on primary testing. It is often impossible to differentiate the two clinically, but direct detection of CMV and CMV-specific antibodies should be in evidence.

Differential Diagnosis. IM is in the differential diagnosis of almost every infectious disease. Conditions and infections typically associated with a mononucleosis-like syndrome are gram-positive alpha-beta hemolytic streptococcal pharyngitis, leukemia, lymphoreticular malignancies, adenoviruses, toxoplasmosis, CMV, rubella, HIV, hepatitis, systemic lupus erythematosus (SLE), drug reactions, and diphtheria.

Management. Treatment is supportive, with adequate fluids and calories. Corticosteroids and acyclovir are not recommended for routine uncomplicated disease. Over-the-counter pain relievers can help with discomfort. Contact sports and strenuous exercise should be avoided if the patient has hepatosplenomegaly. Participation is acceptable after the splenomegaly has resolved. Fatigue and weakness may persist for up to 6 to 12 months after severe infection.

Complications. Usually most clinically healthy patients experience few sequelae. Rare complications include splenic rupture, neurologic complications, thrombocytopenia, agranulocytosis, hemolytic anemia, orchitis, myocarditis, and chronic IM. Fatal disseminated disease, or B-cell lymphoma, occurs in patients with congenital or acquired cellular immunity deficiencies. Burkitt B-cell lymphoma and nasopharyngeal carcinoma are also caused by EBV; these conditions are more commonly found in central Africa and Southeast Asia. Death from IM is rare.

Prevention. Persons with a recent history of IM or an infectious mononucleosis-like disease should not donate blood.

Roseola Infantum (Exanthem Subitum)

Epidemiology. Roseola infantum is also known as exanthem subitum or sixth disease. The causative agent is human herpesvirus 6 (and, less commonly, herpesvirus 7 that causes infection later in life).

Humans are the only natural reservoir. The method of transmission is not completely understood but is probably spread via the oral, nasal, and conjunctival routes of other family members or caregivers. Transmission either prenatally or during or after parturition is suspected. The disease is most commonly acquired by children between 6 and 18 months old (mean of 9 months). It is rare in children younger than 3 months old or older than 3 years, but has been documented in infants as young as 8 weeks old (typified by a febrile illness without localized symptoms). Most children are seropositive by 2 years of age. This would indicate that there is asymptomatic illness or roseola without rash. Reactivation of infection can occur in those immunocompromised. Ninety-five percent or greater of adults demonstrate antibodies to HHV-6. Visits to emergency departments are common as a result of the associated fevers, toxicity, and/or seizures associated with this disease (Hall, 2004).

Incubation Period. Incubation period has a mean of 9 to 10 days. The period of communicability is probably greatest during the fever phase before the rash erupts.

Clinical Findings. There is a sudden onset of fever from 101° F to over 103° F (38.3° C to over 39.5° C) for 3 to 6 days, but the child does not seem particularly ill. There may be signs of a URI (rhinitis, sore throat [with small maculopapular lesions on the soft palate and uvula]; lymphadenopathy in the cervical and posterior occipital areas; lethargy; injected palpebral conjunctiva; gastrointestinal complaints (diarrhea, vomiting, anorexia, abdominal pain); reddened TMs (without bulging or effusion); and, occasionally, a febrile convulsion (5% to 10% of cases). As the fever breaks, a diffuse, nonpruritic, discrete, rose-colored, maculopapular rash, 2 to 3 mm in diameter, appears (Fig. 23-1). It fades on pressure and rarely coalesces. The roseola exanthema is similar to the rash of rubella. The rash lasts 1 to 3 days, begins on the trunk, and spreads centrifugally. In the rare case of CNS involvement, the anterior fontanelle may be bulging.

Diagnostic Studies.   The WBC count is distinctive, showing a decrease for age initially, dropping further by the third or fourth day, and then returning into the normal range. It tends to follow the fever pattern. Serologic testing involves isolating HHV-6 for peripheral blood mononuclear cells and documenting a significant rise in antibody titer. A reverse transcriptase-polymerase chain reaction (RT-PCR) assay has been developed that can distinguish between the acute and latent infection, but is not in use clinically.

Differential Diagnosis.   Most viral rashes, scarlatina, and drug hypersensitivity are included in the differential diagnoses. However, the clinical course usually makes this illness easy to diagnose. A roseola-like illness is also associated with parvovirus B19, echovirus 16, other enteroviruses, measles, and adenoviruses. Until the rash develops, fever without focus and bacterial sepsis are in the differential diagnosis. Continued high fever without a ready source usually leads to a septic work-up for some of these children. If a febrile seizure occurs, meningitis is usually added to the differential diagnosis.

Management.   Management is supportive.

Complications.   Rare complications include febrile convulsions, meningoencephalitis, encephalitis, and hemiplegia. Associated diseases include idiopathic thrombocytopenic purpura (ITP), drug sensitivity syndromes, pityriasis rosea, multiple sclerosis (MS), and hepatitis.

Varicella

Epidemiology.   VZV infection is a common, highly contagious virus belonging to the herpesvirus family. Chickenpox is the primary illness. Shingles (herpes zoster) is the reactivation infection of latent VSV acquired during varicella infection (see Chapter 36). It derives its name not from chickens but from the propensity of the lesions to resemble chickpeas.

Humans are the only reservoir of infection, and illness is spread by direct contact, droplets, and airborne transmission. Victims of shingles are also infectious and can cause primary varicella illness. Immunity is usually lifelong. Symptomatic reinfection is rare, but asymptomatic reinfection occurs. Secondary attacks are usually mild. Asymptomatic primary infection is rare. Immunocompromised patients are at risk of developing generalized zoster. Before the varicella vaccine, 90% of varicella patients were younger than 10 years old; now the disease occurs mostly in older adolescents and adults, although their rates have also decreased (AAP, 2006). Chickenpox is worldwide in distribution and endemic in most large cities. Epidemics occur but at irregular intervals; the greatest incidence is in late autumn, winter, and spring. Primary varicella is associated with mortality rates of fewer than 2 per 100,000 cases with the lowest mortality rates now in children 1 to 9 years old. The highest rates occur in infants and adults. Those immunocompromised have a mortality rate of from 7% to 14% (Myers et al, 2004). Since the advent of the varicella vaccine in 1995, there has been a decrease of approximately 85% for varicella disease, and hospitalizations have decreased by about 75% (AAP, 2006; CDC, 2003). Mild varicella infection occurs in approximately 3% of those previously vaccinated. This is due to the efficacy of the vaccine against mild disease (70% to 90%) versus severe disease (95% to 100%) (Orenstein et al, 2005).

Incubation Period.   The incubation period is 10 to 21 days, with a mean of 14 days. The period of communicability is 1 to 2 days before the rash erupts until all lesions have crusted over, which takes about 3 to 7 days. This can be prolonged to 28 days in VZIG recipients (AAP, 2006). Fig. 23-2 shows differences in distribution of the maculopapular eruptions and prodromal symptoms of scarlet fever, chickenpox, and smallpox.

Clinical Findings.   The following two phases are seen in varicella:

1. *Prodrome:* Not always present. It is composed of low-grade fever, listlessness, headache, backache, mild abdominal pain, and occasionally URI symptoms. These symptoms may occur 1 to 2 days before onset of the second phase.
2. *Rash:* Classic appearance. It is centripetal, beginning on the scalp, face, or trunk. Crops of generally highly pruritic lesions progress from spots to "teardrop vesicles" that cloud over and umbilicate in 24 to 48 hours. After a few days, all morphologic forms can be seen simultaneously. Scabs last from 5 to 20 days, depending on the depth of the lesions. There can be high fever, to 105° F (40.6° C). The more severe the rash, the higher the fever. Lesions can develop on all mucosal tissues, mouth, pharynx, larynx, trachea, vagina, and anus.

Other symptoms can include headache, malaise, and anorexia. Vaccinees that exhibit mild varicella infection rarely have greater than 50 lesions (Orenstein et al, 2005).

Diagnostic Studies.   These are of little importance because the clinical picture is easily recognized, except in the case

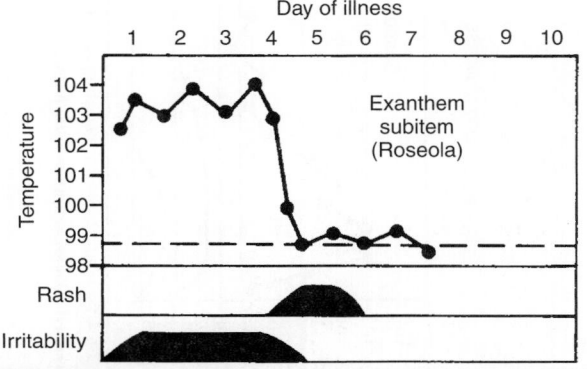

FIG. 23-1   Schematic diagram illustrating the symptoms of roseola. (Adapted from Katz S, Gershon A, Hotez P: *Krugman's infectious diseases of children,* ed 10, Philadelphia, 1998, Mosby.)

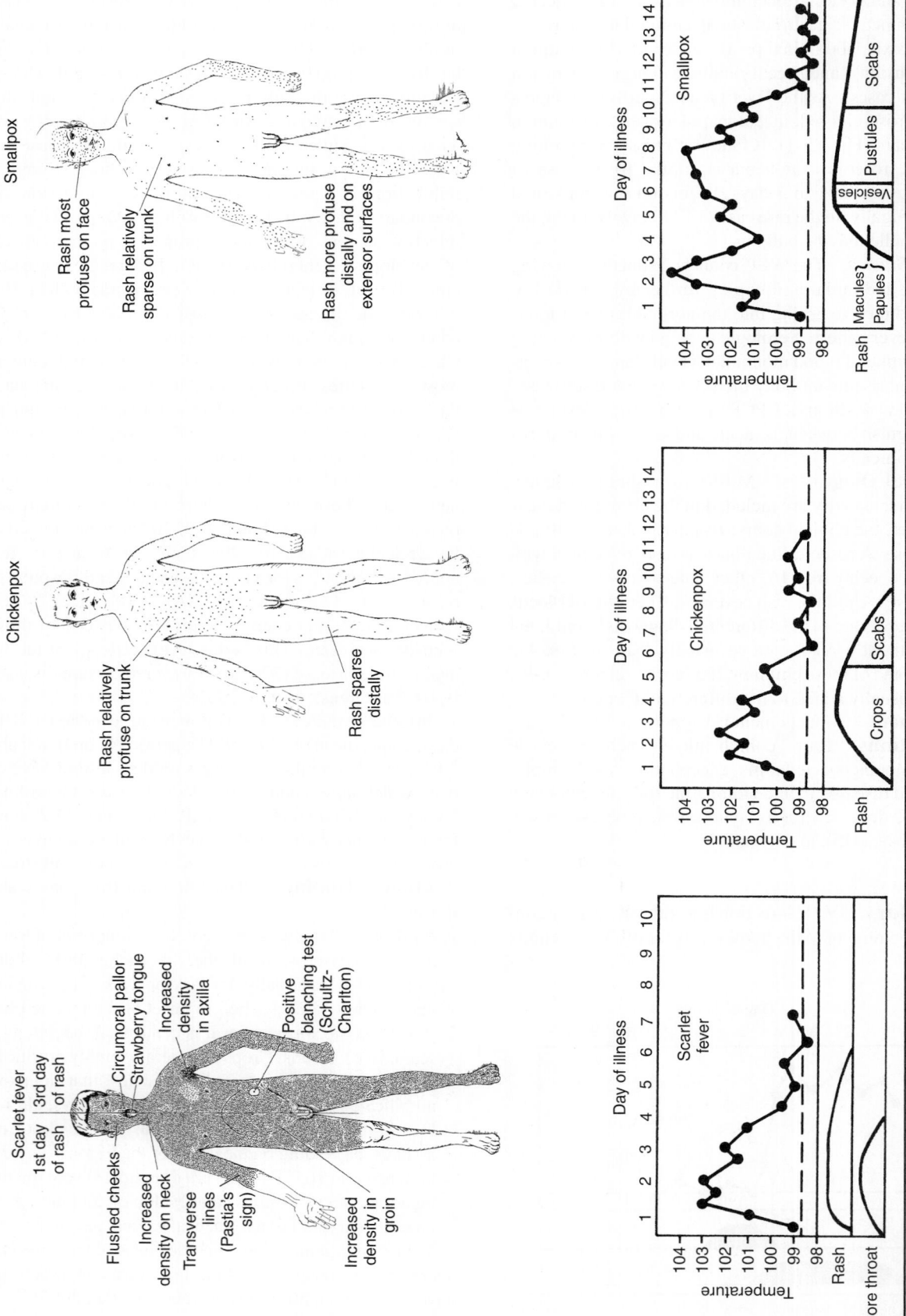

FIG. 23-2 Differences in distribution of the maculopapular eruptions of scarlet fever, chickenpox, and smallpox. (Adapted from Katz S, Gershon A, Hotez P: *Krugman's infectious diseases of children*, ed 10, Philadelphia, 1998, Mosby.)

of exposure of pregnant women. The virus can be cultured. Tzanck smears of lesions demonstrate multinucleated giant cells containing intranuclear inclusion bodies that are diagnostic of herpesviruses (herpes zoster virus or HSV). VZV DNA by PCR of skin lesions or CSF is available. Serologic testing (ELISA) is frequently used to assess antibodies, but lacks specificity and sensitivity to detect immunity from vaccination. The WBC is usually within normal limits.

Differential Diagnosis. The rash is classic; therefore, the diagnosis is usually not a problem. See discussion later in this chapter on differentiating varicella from smallpox. Occasionally, impetigo, cigarette burns, and insect bites can cause some confusion in children with a mild rash. Other infections that can be confused with varicella include eczema herpeticum, HSV, and Stevens-Johnson syndrome.

Management. Chickenpox is usually a benign infection in normal children. Treatment is supportive in nature, including: management of itching with antihistamines or oatmeal baths, acetaminophen for fever, and antistaphylococcal penicillin or cephalosporins for bacterial superinfections until the bacterial agent has been identified. Children with fever for more than several days, or increasing temperatures 4 or more days after the appearance of the rash, should be evaluated closely for invasive disease. Aspirin is contraindicated because of the possibility of Reye syndrome. The use of ibuprofen for fever has been questioned because of a possible causal relationship with bacterial superinfections. Conclusions from studies conflict as to whether ibuprofen is associated with the complication of invasive Group A streptococcal infection after varicella infection (Leroy et al, 2007; Lesko, 2003).

Intravenous acyclovir and vidarabine are effective in treating varicella in immunocompromised patients. VZIG can prevent or modify the course of the infection if given within 48 hours of rash onset or less than 72 hours after exposure. It is not effective after the disease has progressed. Oral acyclovir is expensive and is not routinely recommended for most children (AAP, 2006). When given to otherwise healthy children within 24 hours after eruption of the rash, there is a modest decrease in the symptoms and duration of the illness. Indications for the use of acyclovir include children older than 12 years with chronic pulmonary disorders, those receiving chronic salicylate therapy, or those receiving intermittent or short courses of oral or aerosolized corticosteroids. Dosing information can be found in Appendix A.

Complications. The following complications can occur: pyodermas (about a 5% incidence, causing serious invasive disease with *Streptococcus* and *Staphylococcus*; idiopathic thrombocytopenic purpura (ITP); pneumonia; CNS complications (e.g., encephalitis and Reye syndrome) and, rarely, glomerulonephritis, orchitis, hepatitis, toxic shock, osteomyelitis, necrotizing fasciitis, myositis, myocarditis, arthritis, and appendicitis can result. Morality rates from varicella encephalitis can reach 5% to 20%. For infants exposed perinatally, it can be up to 30%, and for the immunocompromised without treatment, the rate is 15% to 18% (Whitley, 2005).

Prevention. The following are recommended:
- Children exposed to chickenpox can attend school for about 1 week. If they begin to show signs of illness, they must be

kept home for 1 week. If they do not break out in a rash, they can return to school. Children with active disease are to be kept home until all lesions are dry.
- Exposed patients: Use of VZIG has been previously discussed. VZIG is associated with asymptomatic infection. Varicella titers should be obtained 2 months after VZIG is given to assess immune status.
- Chickenpox vaccine has been previously discussed.

Congenital Varicella

Neonatal involvement is directly tied to the timing of the maternal infection. Infection early in pregnancy (between 7 to 20 weeks of gestation) can result in 2% of infants exhibiting significant physical anomalies, CNS complications, and scarring (referred to as congenital varicella syndrome). Fortunately, this syndrome is rare. Maternal infection occurring 5 days or less before delivery results in neonatal varicella-zoster infection 20% to 50% of the time (Myers et al, 2004). There is no time for maternal antibodies to develop and cross the placenta. Infants should be given IGIV (or VZIG if available) as soon as possible if their mothers develop varicella 5 days or less before the delivery or within 2 days postpartum. Despite having received VZIG, 50% of infants may still develop mild varicella infection (Myers et al, 2004).

PANDEMIC INFLUENZA VIRAL INFECTIONS

The influenza virus is an orthomyxovirus of three antigenic types, A, B, and C. Types A and B are responsible for epidemic disease. Type A is further classified into two surface proteins—hemagglutinin (H) and neuraminidase (N). Three hemagglutinin subtypes and two neuraminidase types are known to cause disease in humans (e.g., H3N2, H1N1, HIN2). There are 16 known subtypes of the hemagglutinin and nine of the neuraminidase proteins; all occur in wild waterfowl. Major changes in influenza A subtypes account for global pandemics that result in substantial morbidity and mortality. This process is called *antigenic shift*. Minor variation within a specific subtype is referred to as *antigenic drift* and occurs with both type A and type B; this is what prompts the yearly development of a new "flu" vaccine. Specific antibodies to the virus are important in immunity. Influenza is a highly contagious disease and is spread person to person by direct contact, droplet contamination, and fomites recently contaminated with infected nasopharyngeal secretions.

Both the more typical type of influenza and avian influenza are discussed.

Typical Influenza

Epidemiology. In temperate climates, typical influenza epidemics always occur in the winter months, last approximately 4 to 8 weeks, and peak 2 weeks after the index case. In recent years, some epidemics have lasted 3 months as a result of more than one strain of virus circulating within a community. Children shed the virus longer than adults and, therefore, are particularly prolific transmitters within a community.

After the emergence of a newly shifted subtype, the highest incidence of the illness occurs in infants and children 5 to

14 years old, with an incidence of 15% to 40%. Healthy children under 2 years old (especially infants under 6 months old) and those with chronic diseases have excessively high rates of hospitalization (Zangwill, 2006). Mortality ranges from 4 to 30 per 100,000 cases with the elderly affected to the greatest extent (Alper, 2005).

Incubation Period. The incubation period is 1 to 4 days. Patients become infectious 24 hours before the onset of symptoms. Viral shedding usually ceases 7 days after the onset of illness.

Clinical Findings. Influenza patients are sick! There is a sudden onset of high fever, 102° F to 106° F (38.8° C to 41° C), headache, chills, coryza, vertigo, sore throat, pain in the back and extremities, and dry hacking cough that can resemble pertussis. Vomiting, diarrhea, and croup occur in young children. Infants can appear septic. Conjunctival injection, epistaxis, and myocarditis (evident by weak heart sounds and rapid, weak pulse) are common. In severe infection, there can be involvement of the lower respiratory tract with atelectasis or infiltrates. Severe myocardial involvement can cause distention of the right side of the heart and congestive heart failure,

Diagnostic Studies. Special viral cultures taken from the nasopharyngeal cavity by swab or aspiration within 72 hours of the onset of illness can isolate the virus in 2 to 6 days to confirm the diagnosis. Rapid diagnostic tests have demonstrated low sensitivity (45% to 90%) and specificity (60% to 95%) when compared with viral cultures based upon test and specimen type. Direct fluorescent antibody (DFA) and indirect immunofluorescent antibody (IFA) test results can be obtained within 3 or 4 hours and are available from hospital-based laboratories (AAP, 2006). There are numerous serologic tests: viral agglutination, complement fixation, neutralization, or ELISA. RT-PCR is both sensitive and specific. A CBC shows leukopenia.

Differential Diagnosis. The differential diagnosis includes other viral respiratory infections (common cold, parainfluenza, respiratory syncytial virus (RSV), avian flu based upon risk factors), allergic croup, epiglottitis, and bacterial upper respiratory infections.

Management. Treatment is supportive in nature (bed rest, fluids, antipyretics). Given its expense, antiviral therapy should be reserved for high-risk patients and those in institutions (AAP, 2006). High-risk includes: children immunized less than 2 weeks before influenza circulation; children in whom the influenza vaccine is contraindicated; unimmunized close contacts to children at high risk; immunocompromised children; control of outbreaks in facilities of high-risk children; and cases where the annual vaccine failed to be a good match for the circulating strain. When antivirals are indicated, treatment should be started within 48 hours of symptom onset and continued until the patient is asymptomatic for 24 to 48 hours (AAP, 2006). The effectiveness of the antivirals can vary from year to year based upon the influenza virus in play for that season. Providers should check the CDC website for the antiviral treatment recommendations each influenza season (*www.cdc.gov/flu*). Dosages for different antivirals can be found in Appendix A (see amantidine, rimantadine, zanamivir, oseltamivir).

Complications. Complications include Reye syndrome and respiratory infections (AOM, pneumonia), acute myositis, toxic shock, myocarditis, and CF and asthma exacerbations followed by bacterial superinfection, usually with *H. influenzae*. Do not give aspirin to influenza sufferers!

Prevention.

As previously discussed, influenza vaccine should be widely promoted. Antiviral prophylaxis against specific types of influenza infections may be indicated. The prophylactic doses are the same as for active influenza treatment.

Avian Influenza Strain

The avian influenza A viral strain of H5N1 has the potential to acquire genes from the influenza virus that affects other species. It is spread quickly and has morphed into a more pathogenic virus than when it first emerged in 1996. It was originally found in a goose in China in 1996, but has since been detected in birds in most parts of the world, especially in impoverished rural populations that have unregulated avian flocks. It is also spread by wild, migrating birds. The disease in humans is still restricted, and the virus has not yet mutated to be efficiently transmitted from person to person. To date only humans who have had known contact with poultry or with persons known to have such contact have been infected. However, bird-to-human transmission has been increasing (Nield & Kamat, 2006b). There is concern that it could cause a deadly pandemic. It is postulated that the H5N1 strain could begin sharing genetic material between avian and human influenza virus strains after coinfecting an animal or a human or by mutation in an avian influenza strain.

Humans who acquire the disease are severely ill, in contrast to those who experience mild symptoms with the typical "flu" that occurs in the U.S. Fever, malaise, myalgias, and respiratory symptoms progress to pneumonia, then to respiratory and multiorgan system failure, and then to death. Diarrhea can occur. Those more than 13 years old are expected to experience more severe disease, delay seeking care, have lower respiratory tract involvement, low WBC counts, and lymphopenia. To date, the mortality rate in humans has been greater than 50% (Rosenthal, 2005a).

The current approach of public health officials throughout the world to eradicate the virus is surveillance, the culling of infected domestic fowl, and quarantine. So far this approach has been successful in limiting the human morbidity rate (Rosenthal, 2006a). Vaccines to fight H5N1 and other emerging pandemic threats are in clinical trials. Should infection occur or spread a combination of vaccines and antivirals would be the treatment choices along with measures leading to the protection of the health and safety of citizens, disease control and travel-related risk reduction, plans for employee absenteeism, limiting the economic impact, and ensuring that essential services continue (foods, medicine, power, etc.).

Current guidelines for providers include testing persons with acute respiratory illness who have been in an H5N1-affected area (Cambodia, China, Indonesia, Thailand, Vietnam) within

10 days before illness onset. A nasopharyngeal or throat specimen (swab or aspirate) transported with cold packs are indicated for this. The local or state health department should facilitate the specimen handling, and a rapid, sensitive RT-PCR test for H5 influenza should be ordered. A positive test result will prompt further testing by CDC. Until test results are known, the patient should be masked and kept at home. Travelers to known areas of concern should have their annual flu shot, avoid direct contact with birds and chicken eggs that are not thoroughly cooked, practice good hand hygiene, and seek medical attention if the above symptoms occur within 10 days of returning home. Antiviral prophylaxis before departure is not indicated at this time (Oregon Department of Human Services, 2005a). Providers are encouraged to stay current on their local and state pandemic planning strategies.

OTHER VIRAL DISEASES

Human Immunodeficiency Virus

Epidemiology. Pathogenic human retroviruses include lentiviruses (HIV-1 and HIV-2) and oncoviruses (human T-lymphotropic viruses HTLV-1 and HTLV-2). Both serotypes cause clinically indistinguishable disease. Infection is attributed to RNA human retroviruses HIV-1 and less commonly to HIV-2. Retroviruses integrate into the target cell's genome as proviruses, and the viral genome is copied during cell replication. HIV persists in infected individuals for life, and its protein envelope mutates frequently. This antigenic drift creates havoc with the body's immune system. The body's defense system recognizes only previously encountered immunogenic forms.

Although there are AIDS-like syndromes in other primates and felines, infection cannot be obtained from pets, animals, or insects. Humans are the only known reservoir for HIV. The mode of transmission is intimate sexual contact, sharing of contaminated needles for injection, transfusion of contaminated blood or blood products, perinatal exposure, and breast-feeding. HIV has been isolated from blood (lymphocytes, macrophages, and plasma), CSF, pleural fluid, cervical secretions, human milk, feces, saliva, and urine. However, only blood, semen, cervical secretions, and human milk are implicated in transmission. Without contact from these sources, transmission is practically nonexistent in families, households, hospitals, clinics, schools, or child care settings (Yoger & Chadwick, 2004).

Infectivity is low. The risk of sexual transmission from just one episode of intercourse with an infected person is low. The highest per-act risk for transmission is from blood transfusion, needle sharing between drug users, receptive anal intercourse, and percutaneous needle injuries (CDC, 2006f). Accidental needle sticks in occupational settings rarely account for seroconversion and have a low infectivity rate. Less than 0.3% of the documented cases occurred this way. Transmission from accidental needle sticks from nonoccupational sources is negligible (AAP, 2006). Transmission of HIV from a human bite (even when saliva is contaminated with blood) is extremely rare (Havens & Committee on Pediatric AIDS, 2003).

One of the most rapidly expanding HIV-positive groups is adolescents 13 to 19 years old in the U.S.; the incidence is approximately 0.5%. Adolescents are more likely to acquire the virus from male-male transmission, whereas female adolescents acquire it via sexual transmission and intravenous drug use. The adolescent female incidence is now greater than that of males. An estimated 15% to 20% of HIV infections are acquired between 13 and 19 years old. Because of the long incubation period, these adolescents may not experience symptoms until they are in their twenties or thirties (AAP, 2006). In 2002, the CDC reported a 90% decrease in reported AIDS diagnosis in children as compared with 1992 rates. Less than 5% of cases have no immediately identifiable risk factor, but with further investigation most do fall into an identifiable risk category. Contaminated blood products with HIV is now rare (risk estimated at 1 in 493,000). Injection drug users account for approximately 23% of cases (13.4% were in children 13 to 14 years old) (Brunell, 2006f).

Transplacental infection is well documented. Most babies born to HIV-infected mothers are initially HIV positive owing to the placental transfer of maternal antibodies. If the mother has been infected with HIV during late pregnancy and has not had time to develop antibodies, both mother and child will be antibody negative. Risk of an untreated HIV-infected woman giving birth to an infected infant is 13% to 45% (Borkowsky, 2004; Havens & Committee on Pediatric AIDS, 2003). In vaginal twin deliveries, the firstborn twin has a greater risk of developing HIV than the second. Premature rupture of membranes greater than 4 hours before delivery increases the risk of antiretroviral agent transmission to the newborn. Cesarean delivery appears to reduce the risk of fetal infection by 50%. The mother's age, CD4+ cell percentage, maternal drug use, and viral load are other risk factors for the infant. If women are treated with prophylactic medications during the first trimester, and the infant for 6 weeks antepartum with zidovudine (ZDV), the transmission rate goes from 26% to 8%; this is now standard treatment (Borkowsky, 2004). Another study showed a rate decrease from 12.8% to less than 1% (Magder et al, 2005).

Infection through postpartum human milk transmission depends upon the maternal state of infection and length of time she has been breastfeeding. The transmission rate is greater in women who acquire HIV infection after delivery than in those with chronic infection. Transmission has not been reported in an infant after a single exposure to HIV-infected human milk (Havens, 2003). However, in developing countries where pediatric AIDS is pandemic, treatment regimens—out of nutritional necessity—have traditionally included breastfeeding plus short-term antiretroviral drug treatment for women and infants. Recent research efforts in underdeveloped countries have focused on different ways to prevent transmission via breastfeeding. Strategies studied have included evaluating the acceptance of formula feeding by HIV-infected women, restricting breastfeeding to 4 months, and the long-term use of antiretroviral therapy in both the breastfeeding woman and her infant (Global HIV Prevention Working Group, 2006; Thior et al, 2006; Becquet et al, 2005).

The AAP guidelines (AAP, 2006) for counseling HIV-infected pregnant women and mothers include the following:

- Women and their health care providers need to be aware of the potential risk of transmission of HIV infection to infants in utero and in the postpartum period and through human milk.
- Documented, routine HIV education and routine testing with consent of all women seeking prenatal care are strongly recommended so that each woman knows her HIV status and the methods available to prevent the acquisition and transmission of HIV to her newborn and to document whether breastfeeding is appropriate.
- At the time of delivery, provision of education about HIV and testing with consent of all women whose HIV status is unknown are strongly recommended. Knowledge of the woman's HIV status assists in counseling on breastfeeding and helps each woman understand the benefits to herself and her infant of knowing her serostatus and the behaviors that decrease the likelihood of acquisition and transmission of HIV.
- In general, women who are known to be HIV seronegative should be encouraged to breastfeed. However, women who are HIV seronegative but at particular high risk of seroconversion (e.g., injection drug users) should be educated about HIV with an individualized recommendation concerning the appropriateness of breastfeeding. In addition, during the perinatal period, information should be provided on the potential risk of transmitting HIV through human milk and about methods to reduce the risk of acquiring HIV infection.

Neonatal intensive care units should develop policies that are consistent with these recommendations for the use of expressed human milk for neonates. Current standards of the Occupational Safety and Health Administration (OSHA) do not require gloves for the routine handling of expressed human milk. However, gloves should be worn by health care workers in situations where exposure to breast milk might be frequent or prolonged, such as in milk banking.

Human milk banks should follow the guidelines developed by the FDA, CDC, and AAP. These guidelines stipulate that all donors be screened for HIV and assessed for risk factors that might indicate donor infection and that the breast milk be pasteurized and meet rigid storage requirements.

In addition, providers need to be vigilant regarding maternal compliance with the recommended neonatal HIV prophylaxis. Such compliance has been shown to be lower in women with asymptomatic HIV and in those who have poor social networks (Demas et al, 2002).

Incubation Period. The incubation period is variable. Symptoms of HIV infection in infants untreated perinatally are usually evident during the first 6 weeks of life (median 5.2 months) with lymphadenopathy as the first symptom, then hepatosplenomegaly. Most (approximately 80%) will be symptomatic by 12 months old; those with high HIV loads develop symptoms earlier, including failure to thrive and encephalopathy. Even though HIV infection can have a long latency period (longer than 5 years), 15% to 20% of HIV-infected children

die before 4 years old (median age of death is 11 months) (AAP, 2006). Intrauterine transmission usually occurs by 10 weeks of gestation and is associated with early, severe disease in the newborn. Intrapartum transmission occurs more in premature infants born before 34 weeks of gestation, in low-birth-weight infants, and in mothers who use IV drugs during pregnancy.

Seroconversion usually occurs between 6 and 12 weeks after exposure, and 95% of HIV-infected persons seroconvert within 6 months. In transfusion-associated infection, the time between exposure and clinical disease is months to years, with a mean of 3.5 years. The incubation time of HIV in adolescents and young adults has a median range of 8 to 12 years.

Clinical Findings. Four HIV infection clinical categories for children with HIV infection are based on guidelines established in 1994 by the CDC (available from the CDC website). AIDS in pediatric patients exhibits variable symptoms. Infants are often preterm and of low birth weight; their examinations are usually normal or may demonstrate subtle lymphadenopathy with hepatosplenomegaly, failure to thrive, diarrhea, pneumonia, or thrush. *Pneumocystis carinii* pneumonia (PCP) is the most common cause of death. Once acquired 50% survive less than 2 years. Other opportunistic diseases are candida (15% to 40%), *Mycobacterium avium* infection, severe CMV after 6 months old, EBV, disseminated herpes, disseminated histoplasmosis, RSV, and measles (despite vaccination). Children—other than infants—generally have more recurrent bacterial infections, parotid gland swelling, lymphoid interstitial pneumonitis, or neurologic deficiencies (60%) that progress to encephalopathy (up to 40%). *S. pneumoniae,* HIB, *S. aureus,* and *Salmonella* organisms are common infections in pediatric AIDS patients. Sinusitis, cellulitis, glomerulopathy (especially in those of African descent), cardiac hypertrophy, anemia, congestive heart failure (CHF), and purulent middle ear infections are common. Malignancies are uncommon in pediatric AIDS, but they do occur. Children can have lymphoma, non-Hodgkin B-cell lymphoma (Burkitt type), and leiomyosarcoma. Kaposi sarcoma is rare in children in the U.S. but occurs in children in Africa (Borkowsky, 2004).

Diagnostic Tests. Infants born to HIV-infected, seropositive mothers also are seropositive at birth owing to passive transfer of maternal antibodies. Maternal HIV IgG can persist for as long as 15 to 18 months. HIV proviral DNA testing (PCR) will identify HIV-infected newborns early in the neonatal period and is one of the most sensitive tests. See Table 23-10 for recommended testing times. Assay of IgA subclass HIV-specific antibodies can help identify newborns between 2 and 12 months old. Positive tissue cultures of the virus from blood or CSF and elevated serum immunoglobulin levels are also used to indicate infant infection.

The diagnosis of infection is made serologically in children older than 15 months by ELISA testing, which is generally highly sensitive and specific. The test is repeated, and, if positive, confirmation is made by Western blot or immunofluorescent antibody testing on the same specimen.

Some AIDS patients become seronegative late in the disease because the weakened immune system cannot manufacture anti-

TABLE 23-10 Testing Schedule for Human Immunodeficiency Virus in the Exposed Infant

Test	Time After Birth
First DNA PCR from peripheral blood (not cord blood); confirm if positive with EIA and Western blot analysis	Within 48 hours
Second DNA PCR; confirm if positive	1-3 months
Third DNA PCR; confirm if positive	4 months
*Optional: Enzyme-linked immunosorbent assay (ELISA) followed by Western blot analysis if positive	12 and 24 months
Infection is confirmed if two separate, confirmed samples are positive; infection is excluded if two separate, confirmed assays are negative when performed at the above times.	

*Older literature demonstrates that some children may seroconvert later. See text for definitions of abbreviations.
Data from American Academy of Pediatrics (AAP): *2006 Red book: report of the Committee on Infectious Diseases,* ed 27, Elk Grove Village, IL, 2006, American Academy of Pediatrics.

BOX 23-2 Zidovudine (ZDV) Regimen to Decrease Risk of Perinatal HIV Transmission to Newborns Within 8-12 Hours of Birth

Zidovudine syrup, 2 mg/kg/dose PO 4 times daily* within 8-12 hours of birth[†] and continuing for the first 6 weeks of life*

*For full-term infants unable to tolerate oral intake, IV dosage of ZDV is 1.5 mg/kg every 6 hours. For infants <35 weeks gestation dosage is 1.5 mg/kg/dose IV, or 2 mg/kg/dose orally, every 12 hours, advancing to every 8 hours at 2 weeks of age if >30 weeks gestation at birth or at 4 weeks of age if <30 weeks gestation at birth.
[†]Prophylaxis starting after 48 hours of birth is not likely to prevent the transmission of HIV.
Data from Department of Human Services, Public Health Service Taskforce: *Recommendations for use of antiretroviral drugs in pregnant HIV-1-infected women for maternal health and interventions to reduce perinatal HIV-1 transmission in the United States,* Rockville, MD, 2006, AIDSInfo, Department of Human Services. Available at *www.aidsinfo.nih.gov/guidelines* (accessed Feb 20, 2007); American Academy of Pediatrics (AAP): *Red book: 2006 report of the Committee on Infectious Diseases,* ed 27, Elk Grove Village, IL, 2006, American Academy of Pediatrics.

bodies. Lymphopenia occurs as the disease progresses. There are decreased circulating CD4 cells (T-suppressor, T-helper cells), and the helper-suppressor ratio is less than 1.

Differential Diagnosis. The differential diagnosis includes other causes of immunologic deficiency, such as recent therapy with an immunosuppressive agent, lymphoproliferative disease, congenital immunologic states, inflammatory bowel disease, DiGeorge syndrome, ITP, chronic allergies, CF, graft-versus-host reaction, congenital CMV, toxoplasmosis, ataxia, or telangiectasia.

Management. Any information about HIV is subject to change, and the provider is cautioned to check with the CDC regarding any changes in HIV or AIDS diagnosis or treatment. Current drug regimens include combination therapy with protease inhibitor and nucleoside analogue reverse transcriptase inhibitor (NRTI) agents. Studies are ongoing regarding the use of other new classes of antiretroviral drugs (e.g., fusion inhibitors and ribonucleotide reductase inhibitors).

Primary care providers can manage infants born to HIV-infected women without specialty consultation, though consultation with an HIV or infectious disease specialist is highly recommended (Steele, 2006). Established protocols for the HIV-infected mother and her newborn are available. Box 23-2 outlines the protocol for the HIV-exposed newborn. Treatment of a child infected with HIV should only be undertaken in concert with pediatric HIV specialists because drug regimens are constantly being revised. Treatment of associated conditions with appropriate medical therapy is indicated using IVIG, antifungals, antimycobacterials, antivirals, and nutritional counseling. The CDC is also an excellent source for the latest information regarding treatment. Many centers have ongoing clinical trials for which patients may be eligible. Information about such trials

is available from the AIDS Clinical Trials Information Service (see Resource Box at end of the chapter).

An important role of the primary care provider in HIV treatment is in helping to boost adherence rates. The treatment regimens are highly challenging for parents because of complex dosing schedules and unwillingness of children to take the required medications. Many preparations are not offered in liquid form, or the taste is not attractive to children. To enhance compliance, some clinicians employ several tools: improving information via computer-assisted age-dependent programs; using electronic pillboxes; routinely measuring drug levels; developing simpler drug protocols; studying possible social and economic factors that predict compliance and individualize patient care accordingly; and by referring families to support networks.

Adolescents can present a particular noncompliance risk because of denial and fear of their infection, substance abuse and addiction, misinformation, distrust of and inexperience with the medical system, self-esteem issues, unstable living situations, and lack of familial and social support systems. It is important for the provider to be nonconfrontational, yet discuss risk factors, advocate for family planning services and needle exchange programs, postexposure prophylaxis (PEP) regimens, and prompt involvement in new treatments as they become available.

Complications. HIV becomes a multisystemic illness with multiorgan complications.

Prevention of Complications and Transmission
Recommendations for Childhood Vaccinations. Specific immunization recommendations are included under the vaccine schedule of this chapter.

• Children who live with a symptomatic HIV-infected person: The use of live vaccines is contraindicated with the exception of MMR, since this vaccine does not shed virus. Yearly influenza vaccines should be given to household members who live with infected persons.

- There is no HIV-preventive vaccine.

Reduction of Perinatal Transmission of HIV. The use of combination therapy or monotherapy to reduce perinatal transmission of HIV is recommended. Regimens are available from the CDC; they are being actively researched and altered accordingly. The recommendations may also change depending on the country where treatment is occurring. Developing countries seek the most cost-effective, efficacious, simple, and tolerable regimen. The CDC, WHO, and United Nations AIDS agencies are useful resources for current treatment regimens.

Patient education remains the only method to reduce the risk of acquisition and transmission.

Other control measures

- Adolescent education: Adolescents must be counseled about the risk of HIV transmission (e.g., sexual transmission, sharing of needles or syringes) and the use of condoms.
- School attendance: Children with AIDS or HIV infection should go to school if they are healthy enough to do so. Factors that must be taken into account include the risk to the immunosuppressed child of "normal germs" from "healthy kids and school personnel." The benefit from attendance far outweighs the risks. Because casual transmission is unknown, there is no real risk to other children as long as the infected child can control body secretions. Children who display biting behavior or have oozing wounds should be cared for in a setting that minimizes risk to others. The child's primary care provider is the only person with an absolute need to know the child's primary diagnosis. If the family decides to inform the school, those informed should maintain confidentiality. If the family chooses not to inform the school, parents should get assurance that the school will notify them of any communicable disease outbreaks (e.g., varicella, measles) or physical altercations with others.
- Routine screening of school-age children for HIV antibodies is not indicated.

Control Measures: Postexposure Prophylaxis (PEP) After Nonoccupational Exposure for Children and Adolescents.

The primary care provider may be faced with having to assess and counsel parents after their child has had an accidental puncture wound from a discarded needle found on a street, public transportation, or playground. Other exposures may be from a wound obtained from a bite, a fight, or during a sports activity; from sexual abuse; or from exposure to breast milk from an HIV-infected woman. Though transmission is extremely rare, the provider needs to be able to address the situation with a level of understanding of the risks and current recommendations of the CDC (Fig. 23-3).

The body fluids of an HIV-infected person do not all carry the same amount of viral load or risk. For example, blood of a known HIV-infected person carries the highest risk, whereas blood-free saliva, semen or vaginal secretions, and human milk carry a low risk; urine, feces, and vomitus are unlikely to transmit the virus (CDC, 2005c). Syringes that might have been used and discarded by an HIV-infected, injection-drug

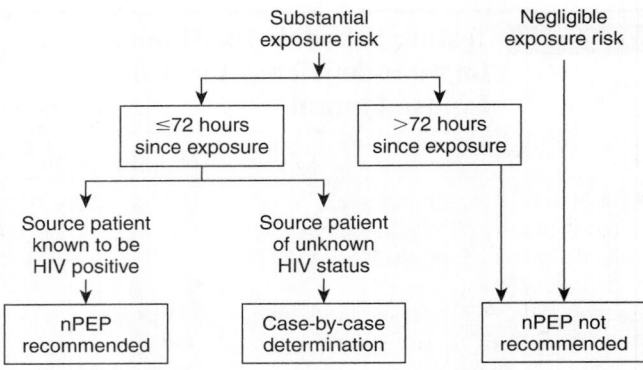

FIG. 23-3 Algorithm for evaluation and treatment of possible non-occupational HIV exposures. (From Centers for Disease Control and Prevention [CDC]: Antiretroviral postexposure prophylaxis after sexual, injection drug use, or other nonoccupational exposure to HIV in the U.S., *MMWR Morb Mortal Wkly Rep* 54 [RR-2]:1-20, 2005. Available at *www.cdc.gov/mmwr/preview/mmwrhtml/rr5402a1.htm* [accessed April 2, 2007].)

user generate the most concern by parents. The following information is useful when counseling parents:

- HIV viability is vulnerable to drying.
- The smaller the needle bore, the more limited the amount of blood present.
- Health care professionals stuck with a needle after withdrawing blood from an HIV-infected individual have a 0.3% HIV transmission risk (Havens & Committee on Pediatric AIDS, 2003). Most syringes (approximately 96%) used for IM or SQ injection by an HIV-infected individual will not have discernible HIV RNA (CDC, 2005c). There has been no documented transmission of HIV from an accidentally found, discarded needle.
- With a bite, one is more likely to face greater risk from biting an individual who is HIV positive (saliva contaminated with HIV-infected blood) than from having been bitten by one infected with HIV (saliva not contaminated by infected blood).

However, the HIV status of the exposure source may not be known or possible to obtain. In that case, the provider and parent must weigh the unproven safety and benefits of participating in the PEP regimen against the significant toxicity of the drugs themselves. If instituted, PEP therapy needs to start within 72 hours after exposure and continue for 28 days. Close follow-up for support, medication monitoring (adherence and toxicity), and serial HIV antibody screening is needed. Box 23-3 provides some management strategies. Should PEP be the most advantageous strategy, the provider is advised to consult the CDC concerning the current PEP prophylaxis antiretroviral drug therapy recommended.

Measles (Rubeola)

Epidemiology. Measles (rubeola) is a *Morbillivirus* in the *Paramyxoviridae* family and is similar to mumps and influenza. There is only one antigenic type. Measles is typified by a rash, indicating viremia. It is a serious illness in children! The disease is associated with high mortality and morbidity rates worldwide.

Humans and primates are the only known reservoir of infection. The source of the infection is respiratory secretions, blood, and urine of infected persons. Virus is transmitted through droplet contact, fomites, and, less likely, aerosol transmission. Peak incidence of infection in susceptible persons occurs during the winter and spring months. The failure rate after the first vaccine at 12 months old is approximately 5%; after the second vaccine the failure rate is about 2% (AAP, 2006).

Incubation Period.   The incubation period is 8 to 12 days. A person is contagious 1 to 2 days before the onset of symptoms, 3 to 5 days before the rash, and 4 days after the appearance of the rash, or roughly 14 days (AAP, 2006). There is no carrier state; disease or two vaccinations usually confers lifelong immunity.

Clinical Findings.   The clinical manifestations are divided into three stages:
1. *Incubation period:* There are no specific symptoms.
2. *Prodromal period:* This is the first sign of the illness and lasts 4 to 5 days. This stage consists of URI symptoms, low to moderate fever (greater than 101° F [38.3° C]), and cough, coryza, and conjunctivitis (the "three Cs" of measles). An enanthem can be found on the oral mucosa opposite the lower molars. These Koplik spots last 12 to 15 hours. They are small, irregular bluish-white granules

---

BOX 23-3   Management of Patients With Possible Exposure to HIV

1. Treat exposure site
- Wash wounds with soap and water; flush mucous membranes with water. Give Td or Tdap booster if appropriate (see Table 23-6).

2. Evaluate exposure source if possible
- Determine the HIV infection status of the exposure source. If unknown, testing with appropriate consent should be offered if possible.

3. Evaluate exposed person
- Perform HIV serologic testing to identify current HIV infection and hepatitis B and hepatitis C serologic testing as appropriate.
- Provide or refer for counseling to address stress and anxiety.
- Discuss prevention of potential secondary HIV transmission.
- Discuss prevention of repeat exposure, if appropriate.
- Report incident to legal or administrative authorities as appropriate to the setting of the exposure and the severity of the incident.

4. Consider PEP
- Explain potential benefits and risks.
- Discuss issues of drug toxicity and medication compliance.
- Measure complete blood cell count, creatinine, and alanine transaminase concentration as baseline for possible drug toxicity.
- Begin prophylaxis as soon as possible after exposure, preferably within 1 to 4 hr; prophylaxis begun more than 72 h after exposure is unlikely to be effective.
- Arrange for follow-up with HIV specialist and psychologist, if appropriate.
- Educate about prevention of secondary transmission (sexually active adolescent should avoid sex, or use condoms, until all follow-up test results are negative).
- Report to PEP registry at CDC.

5. Choose therapy
- Consider drug potency and toxicity, regimen complexity and effects on compliance, and possibility of drug resistance in the exposure source.
- Supply 3-5 days of medication immediately, instructing patients to obtain remainder of medication at follow-up visit.

6. Follow-up
- Perform initial follow-up within 2-3 days to review drug regimen and adherence, evaluate for symptoms of drug toxicity, assess psychosocial status, and arrange appropriate referrals, if needed.
- Continue therapy for 28 days.
- Monitor for drug adverse effects at 4 wk with complete blood cell count and alanine transaminase concentration.
- Evaluate for psychological stress and medication compliance with weekly office visits or telephone calls.
- Consider referral for counseling if needed.
- Repeat HIV serologic testing at 6 weeks, 12 weeks, and 6 months after exposure.

PEP, Postesposure prophylorfis.
PpFrom Havens PL, Committee on Pediatric AIDS: Postexposure prophylaxis in children and adolescents for nonoccupational exposure to human immunodeficiency virus, *Pediatrics* 111 (6): 1475-1489, 2003. Used with permission.

on an erythematous background and are pathognomonic of measles infection.

3. *Rash stage:* The rash of unmodified measles usually appears on the third or fourth day of the illness. As the rash appears, temperature rises, often to 105° F (40.5° C). The rash first appears behind the ears and on the forehead. It is maculopapular in nature. Papules enlarge, coalesce, and move progressively downward, engulfing the face, neck, and arms over the next 24 hours. By the end of the second 24 hours, the rash has spread to the back, abdomen, and thighs. As the legs become more involved, the face begins to clear. The entire process takes approximately 3 days. Respiratory symptoms are most severe on day 3 of the rash. The more severe the rash, the more severe the illness. It can become hemorrhagic. This type of measles can be fatal because of disseminated intravascular coagulation (DIC). After the fourth day of the rash stage, the rash begins to fade. The disease peaks and defervesces. After the rash clears, a residual light pigmentation occurs, lasting approximately 1 week that desquamates. Maternal antibody level and improperly given vaccine can alter the presentation and clinical course of measles.

Modified Measles. This most commonly appears in children who have been passively immunized with IG after exposure to the disease. It can occur in infants with partial maternal immunity. The incubation period can persist as long as 20 days. The illness is an abbreviated version of typical disease. The prodrome period can be as early as 1 to 2 days with normal to low-grade fever. URI symptoms are minimal to absent. Koplik spots usually do not appear. The rash is so mild that it is often missed. There are usually no complications.

Diagnostic Studies. A single measles IgM antibody level is useful if drawn when symptoms suggest this disease; the reactivity is low after more than 30 days. Confirmation of disease can also be made by viral isolation from urine, blood, throat or nasopharyngeal secretions or from serial IgG antibody titers that compare acute and convalescent serum specimens. Measles is a reportable disease in the U.S.

Differential Diagnosis. Any viral rash (e.g., roseola, rubella, echovirus, coxsackievirus, IM, adenovirus, and EBV), toxoplasmosis, scarlet fever, Kawasaki syndrome, meningococcemia, Rocky Mountain spotted fever, drug rashes, and serum sickness are included in the differential diagnosis.

Management. Treatment is supportive (antipyretics, bed rest, adequate fluids, air humidification, warm room, darkened room if photophobia is present). Bacterial superinfections (e.g., ear infections, bronchopneumonia, encephalitis) are treated with appropriate antibiotics. It is recommended that all children with encephalitis, severe pneumonia, or whose immune systems are compromised be managed in consultation with an infectious disease expert (Perry & Orenstein, 2006). Intravenous and aerosol ribavirin treatment of immunocompromised children or in those with severe illness have been used; no controlled studies have been done (AAP, 2006).

Children living in countries where malnutrition is an issue are at greater risk for death with measles infection. These children, and those with severe measles, have low vitamin A levels. Use of vitamin A in infants younger than 6 months old has not been proven efficacious. Guidelines for vitamin A supplementation are outlined in the *Red Book* (AAP, 2006).

Complications. Measles is a severe disease. The measles virus is responsible for a significant inflammatory reaction that extends from the nasopharynx to the bronchi. Death is generally due to respiratory and neurologic sequelae or to bacterial superinfection. One must carefully document complications before specific treatment is undertaken.

Bacterial Superinfection and Viral Complications. These usually manifest as a URI, obstructive laryngitis, otitis, mastoiditis, cervical adenitis, bronchitis, and pneumonia. The causative organism can be the measles virus itself or group A ß-hemolytic streptococci, pneumococci, *H. influenzae,* or *S. aureus.* Infection can exacerbate underlying TB.

Myocarditis. This is a rare but reported complication. Transient electrocardiograph changes are common.

Purpura Fulminans (Black Measles). This is a severe complication with multiorgan bleeding.

Disseminated Intravascular Coagulation. Activation of the coagulation system leads to intravascular fibrin deposit and platelet destruction.

Encephalitis and Neurologic Complications. EEG changes are common, especially during the rash stage, but are usually not significant. However, 1 to 2 per 1000 cases suffer from acute measles encephalitis that more often occurs after the second and fifth day of the onset of the rash (may also occur before the rash) (Maldonado, 2004). The child seems to be either doing well or recovering from the disease. Then there can be a sudden onset of fever, headache, vomiting, drowsiness, convulsions, and possibly coma. Frequently, there are signs of meningeal irritation. The CSF demonstrates increased protein and lymphocytic pleocytosis. An acute demyelinating encephalomyelitis can develop that may be due to an immunologic reaction.

Subacute Sclerosing Panencephalitis. This is a rare condition that is considered a late complication of measles. The incidence increases if the measles disease occurs before 18 months old. It usually occurs 7 to 12 or more years after infection and is considered a "slow virus." The incidence is less than 0.06% per million cases. The infection is slow, progressive, and evidenced by behavioral and intellectual deterioration and seizures, and it may be fatal, frequently within 1 month. The disease is more prevalent in males, in rural and poorer areas, in families with more than two children, and in Hispanic immigrant children living in western states and New York city. Some exposure to birds and animals has shown some unknown correlation (Maldonado, 2004). It is diagnosed by EEG changes, marked elevation of CSF globulin (especially IgG), exceptionally high serum measles antibody titer, and measles antibodies in the CSF.

Care of Exposed Individuals. This is done with active and passive immunization, as discussed previously.

Mumps

Epidemiology. Mumps is an acute generalized viral disease with painful enlargement of one or more salivary glands (usually parotid glands). Mumps is a paramyxovirus. Only one serotype is known, and humans are the only natural reservoir.

The source of infection is the saliva of infected persons. The virus is spread by direct contact, aerosol transmission, fomites, and, possibly, urine from infected persons. Viremia exists, and the virus is found in blood, urine, CSF, saliva, and upper respiratory secretions. Before mumps vaccination, mumps was a disease of childhood in the U.S.; 85% of infections occurred in children 2 to 14 years old. Now, infection is more often seen in young adults born from 1967 to 1977 who lack immunity (Maldonado, 2004). Incidence of this illness has decreased by more than 99% since the advent of the vaccine.

Death from this virus is rare but occurs in about 2% of those who suffer from the complication of meningoencephalomyelitis. Infection occurs during all seasons but is most common during late winter and spring; it affects both genders equally. Mumps virus crosses the placenta, and infection during the first trimester increases the risk of spontaneous abortion. Fetal malformations after prenatal mumps infection have not been demonstrated (AAP, 2006).

Incubation Period. The incubation period is 14 to 24 days (mean of 17 days). The period of communicability is about 1 day before glandular swelling to 3 days after the resolution of the swelling. The virus has been isolated 6 days before to 9 days after the onset of parotid swelling. One third of patients are asymptomatic but infectious. One attack usually confers lifelong immunity. Transplacental antibodies to mumps are protective for 6 months. Maternal infection does not seem to be injurious to the fetus, although infection in early pregnancy does seem to be correlated to spontaneous abortion (Maldonado, 2004).

Clinical Findings. There are two clinical stages:

1. *Prodromal stage:* Rare in children but can cause fever, headache, anorexia, neck or other muscular pain, and malaise.
2. *Swelling stage:* Approximately 24 hours after the prodromal stage, one (in 25% of patients) or both of the parotid glands begin to swell in a characteristic manner. If both glands are affected, one generally swells before the other. The gland fills the space between the posterior border of the mandible and mastoid, pushing downward and forward to the zygoma. The ear is pushed forward and upward. This can take a few hours to a few days. The area becomes swollen and painful. The enlarged glands decrease in size and usually return to normal in 3 to 7 days. Ten percent to 15% of cases involve only submandibular gland swelling. Rarely a maculopapular, pink, discrete rash is seen on the trunk. Pain on the affected side can be elicited by having the patient eat something sour. This is known as the "pickle sign." Stensen's duct is red and swollen. Twenty percent of patients are afebrile during this time. Fever is usually moderate and rarely high. Little pain is associated with submandibular infection. However, the redness subsides more slowly. Wharton's duct is frequently swollen. Sublingual salivary glands are not commonly involved. When they are involved, there is bilateral swelling in the submental region

in the floor of the mouth. Edema caused by lymphatic obstruction of the manubrium and upper chest is reported.

Diagnostic Studies. These include viral isolation and culture, serologic tests (enzyme immunoassay for IgG and IgM antibodies and specific mumps antibody). Leukopenia with relative lymphocytosis and an elevated amylase are typical.

Differential Diagnosis. Cervical or preauricular lymphadenitis, CMV, HIV, enteroviruses, tumor, suppurative parotitis by either bacterial or viral (coxsackievirus, parainfluenza 1 and 3) infection, idiopathic recurrent parotitis, parotid ductal obstruction, Mikulicz syndrome, uveoparotid fever, and cancer (especially lymphosarcoma) are included in the differential diagnosis.

Management. Treatment is supportive (antipyretics, bed rest as needed, diet appropriate for chewing discomfort). Arthritic complications respond better to NSAIDS or corticosteroids rather than to salicylates. Manage orchitis with bed rest and scrotal elevation.

Complications. Complications include meningoencephalitis (approximately 250 per 100,000 cases, mostly males older than 20 years); orchitis and/or epididymitis (14% to 35% incidence in adolescents and adults); oophoritis (7% incidence in postpubertal women without evidence that fertility is impacted); severe pancreatitis (rare); thyroiditis (uncommon in children); myocarditis (13% incidence in adults); deafness (1 in 15,000 cases—transient or permanent); ocular complications (swelling of the lacrimal glands or optic neuritis; complete recovery can be expected within 10 to 20 days); arthritis (rare in children); thrombocytopenia and hemolytic anemia (usually self-limited); mastitis (rare); and glomerulonephritis (rare).

Prevention. School and day care students should be kept home until 9 days after the onset of parotid swelling. Active and passive immunization were discussed previously.

Erythema Infectiosum

Epidemiology. Erythema infectiosum, or fifth disease, is caused by parvovirus B19. The virus is a member of the Parvoviridae family. It is called *fifth disease* because it was the fifth eruptive rash described. These rashes include the following:

- Scarlet fever
- Measles
- Rubella
- Erythema subitum (sixth disease)
- Erythema infectiosum
- Roseola

Humans are the only reservoir. Erythema infectiosum is spread via vertical transmission from mother to fetus, by respiratory tract secretions, and percutaneous exposure to blood or blood products. Distribution is worldwide. Erythema infectiosum is a disease of childhood, highest in 5- to 15-year-olds, but infants and adults are not immune. Secondary spread to household contacts is approximately 50% (Koch, 2004). The disease occurs most commonly in late winter and early spring.

Incubation Period. The incubation period is approximately 4 to 28 days. The rash and symptoms occur between

2 and 3 weeks after exposure. The period of communicability lasts until the rash appears. Chronic infection can occur in those immunocompromised or with most types of hemolytic anemias.

Clinical Findings. The following two phases are seen in erythema infectiosum:

1. *Prodrome:* Consists of mild fever (15% to 30% of cases), myalgias, headache, malaise, URI symptoms.
2. *Rash:* Appears 7 to 10 days after the prodromal stage and occurs in three stages: It first appears on the face and is "slapped cheek" in nature. There is an intense red eruption on the cheeks with circumoral pallor that lasts 1 to 4 days. Next, a lacy maculopapular eruption appears on the trunk and then moves peripherally to the arms, thighs, and buttocks. Palms and soles are generally spared. This phase can last a month. Finally, the rash subsides. Older children may have pruritus. There may be periodic recurrences precipitated by trauma, heat, exercise, stress, sunlight, or cold (see Color Plate). Female adolescents and adults are more likely to complain of arthralgia. Arthralgia most commonly resolves in 2 to 4 weeks. Those with hemolytic anemias or immunocompromised may have fever, pallor, tachycardia, and symptoms of heart failure.

Diagnostic Studies. Laboratory testing is not generally indicated because the diagnosis can be made clinically. Serum B19-specific IgM confirms the presence of infection and persists for 6 to 8 weeks. Anti-B19 IgG confirms past infection. Diagnosis in immunocompromised individuals requires viral DNA testing methods. There are PCR or nucleic acid hybridization tests for B19. The virus is difficult to grow in culture.

Differential Diagnosis. This is not a difficult disease to diagnose. The differential diagnoses include rubella, enterovirus disease, lupus, atypical measles, and drug rashes.

Management. There is no specific antiviral treatment. Those with hemolytic anemia or immunocompromised should be considered for hospitalization. Intravenous IG offers some help for those with immunocompromised conditions.

Complications. These are few and typically not significant. All previously healthy patients usually recover without sequelae. The most frequently reported complications are as follows:

- Arthritis: Symptoms begin 2 to 3 weeks after the onset of initial symptoms. Joint manifestations usually involve the hands, wrists, knees and ankles, are transient, and self-limited.
- Chronic infection: Most common in patients with immunodeficiency. Intravenous IG has been used.
- Aplastic crisis: Most common in patients with chronic hemolytic anemias, including sickle cell anemia, thalassemia, hereditary spherocytosis, or other types of chronic hemolysis.
- Proven maternal infection during pregnancy (especially first 6 months) can cause fetal hydrops and death (5% probability) or intrauterine growth retardation. There are no reports of congenital anomalies.
- Thrombocytopenic purpura or neutropenia.
- Myocarditis: Rare and occurs in fetuses, infants, children, and a few adults

- Papular-purpuric "gloves and socks" syndrome (PPGSS): characterized by fever, pruritus, purpura, painful edema and redness in a glove-and-sock distribution pattern, followed by petechiae and oral lesions. Recovery is spontaneous within a few weeks.

Prevention. Women who are exposed to children with the disease either at home or at work are at increased risk for infection with parvovirus B19. Because B19 has a low risk for fetal infection and there is widespread inapparent infection in children and adults, all women are at some risk of exposure. Because avoidance can reduce but not eliminate the risk of exposure, routine exclusion of pregnant women from the workplace where B19 infection is present is not recommended. Serologic testing for IgG antibody to B19 and fetal ultrasonography can help assess exposure risks if a woman is concerned. The same can be offered to pregnant health care workers caring for aplastic B19 patients or immunocompromised patients with chronic parvovirus infection because they are highly contagious (AAP, 2006).

Children in the rash stage can attend school.

Parainfluenza Virus

Epidemiology. Parainfluenza virus, a paramyxovirus, is similar to the influenza and mumps viruses. Parainfluenza is the major cause of croup. It also is an important cause of bronchitis, bronchiolitis, and pneumonia. There are four antigenic types, classified 1 to 4. Type 4 has two subtypes, A and B, but less is known about them. Most children have been exposed to Type 1, 2, and 3 by the time they are 3 years old. Type 3 is endemic, associated more with illnesses in those under 6 months old, results in shorter immunity (a particular problem for immunocompromised patients), and outbreaks occur more in the spring and summer. Types 1 and 2 usually strike children 2 to 6 years old, and outbreaks are seen more in summer and fall and in odd numbered years; reinfections occur at any age. Type 1 is most frequently associated with croup. Type 4 infections are less well pathologically and clinically understood but are not believed to cause severe illness (Wright, 2004; Burroughs et al, 2004).

This virus is spread by direct contact through infected nasopharyngeal secretions; it is limited to replicating in respiratory epithelium of the upper large airways and eustachian tube environs. Transmission occurs by person-to-person contact and fomite contamination. Infection occurs throughout the year depending on the type.

Incubation Period. The incubation period is 2 to 6 days. Depending upon the serotype, healthy children can shed virus for 4 to 7 days before symptom onset and up to 7 to 21 days after resolution of symptoms.

Clinical Findings. Eighty percent of parainfluenza infections affect the upper airways. This virus accounts for 50% of hospital admissions for croup and 15% of admissions for bronchitis, bronchiolitis, and pneumonia (Wright, 2004). Sore throat is a common complaint in older children. Fever is found in only 20% of cases and is inversely proportional to the age of the child. Discrete maculopapular rashes of short duration can be found if the patient is carefully examined. Rarely has this virus been associated with acute parotitis; the illness is clinically indistinguishable from mumps.

Diagnostic Studies. Routine testing is not needed. The virus can be isolated from nasopharyngeal secretions within 4 to 7 days of being cultured or earlier, depending upon the testing technique available. Confirmation is by rapid antigen detection. Sensitivities vary when rapid antigen identification is done by immunofluorescent assays, enzyme immunoassays, and fluoro-immunoassays. Multiplex RT-PCR may also be available.

Differential Diagnosis. The differential diagnosis includes other viral URIs, allergic croup, and bacterial URIs. The most important clinical differential diagnostic consideration is laryngotracheitis and other acute upper airway obstructive diseases, such as acute angioneurotic edema, epiglottitis, and foreign body aspiration.

Management. The treatment is supportive. Antiviral therapy is not available (AAP, 2006). Oxygen saturation and hypercapnia monitoring in more severely affected children is appropriate. Antibiotics are reasonable in cases of severe infection when secondary bacterial invasion is suspected (e.g., otitis media, pneumonia). See Chapter 31 for more specific treatment recommendations based upon the diagnosis. No vaccine is available. Good hand hygiene is important.

Complications. Complications are infrequent. Secondary bacterial infections, including otitis media and pneumonia, may occur. Immunocompromised hosts can have significant secondary infections, such as bacterial tracheitis, bronchitis, and pneumonia.

Rubella (German or 3-Day Measles)

Epidemiology. Rubella is an acute disease of childhood that occurs in two forms, postnatal and congenital. Rubella is an RNA virus of the genus *Rubivirus,* in the Togaviridae family. Humans are the only reservoir. Infection is spread through nasopharyngeal secretions or transplacentally during either apparent or silent infections. It is worldwide in distribution. The virus has been isolated in blood, stool, and urine of infected individuals. It also has been isolated on fomites for as long as 24 hours.

With the arrival of immunization, the number of epidemics declined. Most cases occur in unvaccinated children, teenagers, and young adults, but by far the highest incidence is now in unvaccinated foreign-born adults (Maldonado, 2004). In closed populations (boarding schools and the military), the attack rate is close to 100%. Males and females are equally affected. Primary maternal infection during the first trimester to the sixteenth week is most associated with congenital defects. Approximately 25% to 60% of infections are subclinical. There is transplacental immunity for approximately 5 to 6 months if the mother is immune. There is probable lifelong immunity for naturally occurring disease. Verified second attacks are rare.

Incubation Period. The incubation period is 14 to 21 days. The period of maximal communicability is approximately 7 days before the rash to 7 to 8 days after its resolution.

Clinical Findings. Postnatal disease is marked by three stages:

1. *Prodrome:* There are mild catarrhal symptoms. This stage is occasionally missed.

2. *Lymphadenopathy:* Usually begins within 24 hours, but can begin as early as 7 days, before the rash appears, and can last for more than 1 week. The postauricular, posterior cervical, and posterior occipital are the primary lymph nodes involved. There is generalized lymph node involvement, and at times splenomegaly is noted.

3. *Rash:* An enanthem can appear in 20% of cases just before the general rash. These Forschheimer spots, which consist of small rose-colored to reddish spots located on the soft palate, were first noted in 1898. They are not considered pathognomonic for rubella and are noted in scarlet fever and other URIs. The rubella rash can be the first obvious sign of illness. It begins on the face and can fade before it spreads to the chest during the next 24 hours. The rash is composed of discrete maculopapules that occasionally coalesce. It spreads caudally, lasting a mean of 3 days. There can be itching without a rash or a fine, branlike desquamation. A low-grade fever can occur during the eruptive phase and continue for up to 3 days. There is no photophobia; anorexia, headache, and malaise are rare. Splenomegaly may be present.

Diagnostic Studies. Diagnosis is usually made by clinical symptoms; however, the only reliable means to check immunity is by antibody testing. Viral cultures and serologic testing of acute and convalescent titers at least 2 weeks apart are done. Hemagglutination inhibition studies are the most widely used method but are being supplanted by latex agglutination enzyme and fluorescent immunoassay, among others. Rubella-specific IgM is an important test in the newborn.

Differential Diagnosis. The disease can be difficult to diagnose unless there is an epidemic. The rash can be confused with scarlet fever, mononucleosis, enterovirus, roseola, rubeola, and drug eruptions.

Management. Treatment is supportive (e.g., antipyretics for fever control) unless complications (e.g., encephalitis) occur; severe thrombocytopenic purpura can be managed with corticosteroid therapy and platelet transfusions.

Complications. Complications in postnatal rubella are rare. They include: ITP, arthritis (most common complication, affecting female adolescents more often than younger children), neuritis (pain and/or paresthesia of arms, wrists, hands, and popliteal area and can occur 1 to 2 months after the infection), and encephalitis (1 in 6000 cases during the eruptive stage with 20% fatality rate).

Prevention. Children with postnatal rubella should be kept home from school or day care for approximately 1 week after the rash erupts. Active and passive immunization has been discussed previously.

Reinfection. There are conflicting studies. Because illness without rash exists, the actual numbers of reinfections are unknown. Rubella virus has many antigenic sites, causing the production of numerous antibodies. Their duration is unknown. In serologically immune persons, the reinfection rate from wild virus is 3% to 10%. The reinfection rate in those immunized is approximately 14% to 18%; in pregnant women reinfection can result in congenital rubella syndrome

(Maldonado, 2004). Many of the reinfections are subclinical. Accidental revaccination of a pregnant woman should not be considered a reason for pregnancy termination alone because surveillance has demonstrated signs of infection in the infant but not congenital rubella syndrome (AAP, 2006).

West Nile Virus

Epidemiology. West Nile Virus (WNV) is an arbovirus (family *Flaviviridae*) and is related to St. Louis and Japanese encephalitis viruses. The virus was previously known to mostly inhabit Africa, West Asia, and the Middle East. Since 1999 it has been identified as occurring and spreading rapidly across the U.S. It recurs yearly when warmer weather occurs, and mosquitoes begin breeding. Temperate weather and drought conditions are also believed to encourage mosquito-borne illnesses.

It is mainly spread to people by bites from infected mosquitoes. The species of mosquito mostly commonly associated with WNV feeds at dawn and dusk and breeds in standing water. Evidence now points to uncommon human-to-human spread via organ transplantation, blood transfusions, prenatally, through breast milk, and possible aerosol transmission. The blood supply has been screened for WNV since 2003.

Mosquitoes become infected by feeding on the blood of previously mosquito-infected birds and then transferring the virus via saliva to other birds, horses, humans, and other animals. A hallmark of the presence of WNV in communities has been the discovery of dead birds (notably crows, jays, and magpies). Bird-to-human transmission is not believed to occur.

Symptoms in immunocompetent humans develop 2 to 14 days after being bitten by an infected mosquito. Approximately 1 in 140 people who develop the infection will have the severe form of the disease (Oregon Department of Human Services, 2005b). The disease causes the highest morbidity and mortality rates in older adults, those with preexisting chronic diseases, those immunosuppressed, and in those having had organ transplants. The mortality rate is approximately 9% in adults and under 1% in children (AAP, 2006).

Clinical Findings. Eighty percent of people bitten by an infected mosquito have minimal symptoms or are asymptomatic. Symptoms of mild infection occur in approximately 20% of people and include fever (102° F to 104° F [38.8° C to 40° C]); headache; muscle aches; eye pain; rash on neck, body, arms, or legs; lymphadenopathy; weakness; anorexia; nausea; and vomiting. Those with mild disease experience symptomatic relief within a week, with fatigue lingering longer.

Those with severe infection may experience the same symptoms as those above plus neuroinvasive involvement. CNS symptoms (severe headache, change in mental status [disorientation], awkward gait or paralysis, stiff neck and nerve abnormalities, tremors or seizures, stupor or coma), and both encephalitis and meningoencephalitis can result. A newborn whose mother was infected with WNV during her pregnancy should be examined for congenital anomalies, neurologic and hearing deficits, and signs of viral infection (AAP, 2006).

Laboratory Studies. The test of choice is the IgM for WNV antibody capture enzyme-linked immunosorbent assay (MAC-ELISA) of serum collected within 8 to 14 days of clinical symptoms onset (or in CSF collected within 8 days). A CBC may be normal or show elevated WBCs, low lymphocytes, anemia; MRI or CT scan (or both) are indicated if the individual has neurologic findings. A newborn exposed in utero to WNV should have either cord or infant serum tested for IgM after delivery. The placenta and umbilical cord should be sent to a histopathologist and tested for WNV infection.

Management. For asymptomatic or mild cases, no treatment is necessary. Hospitalization is indicated for those with symptoms of meningitis or encephalitis. No virus-specific treatment is available for these patients; clinical trials and/or investigations are ongoing to study the use of ribavirin, interferon 2 alpha, anti-WNV immunoglobulin, and other therapies to prevent or treat severe complications. The benefits of organ transplantation, transfusions, and breastfeeding outweigh the risks of acquiring the disease and should not be curtailed.

Most pregnant women who contract WNV deliver infants who show no signs of congenital WNV involvement. However, special management of such a pregnant woman, and subsequently the infant, is required. Guidelines include (AAP, 2006):

- **Pregnant woman:** A detailed ultrasonographic examination of the fetus 2 to 4 weeks after the onset of illness symptoms.
- **Newborn:** If clinical or laboratory evidence suggests congenital WNV infection, the following should occur:
  - Refer the infant for an ophthalmologic examination, CT of the brain, CBC, and liver function tests; consider CSF testing.
  - Refer to a dysmorphologist.
  - Retest infant's serum for WNV-specific IgG and IgM antibodies at 6 months.
  - Closely monitor the head circumference, physical characteristics, and development during the first year.

Complications. With severe infection, complications include: encephalitis, meningoencephalitis, meningitis, cardiac dysrhythmias, optic neuritis, uveitis, chorioretinitis, orchitis, myocarditis, pancreatitis, GBS, respiratory muscle paralysis, and hepatitis.

Prevention. The goal of prevention is to avoid mosquito bites. Mosquito abatement programs have been instituted in communities to reduce mosquito breeding grounds. Providers are encouraged to counsel families about ways to minimize their exposure risk. Counseling should include the following:

- Stay indoors during the mosquitoes' most active times—dawn and dusk; if must be outdoors during these times, wear light-colored, long-sleeved shirts and long pants.
- Apply insect repellent with either N,N-diethyl-3-methylbenzamide (DEET; formerly N,N-diethyl-meta-toluamide), Picaridin, or oil of lemon eucalyptus to exposed skin and clothing (no DEET for children under 6 months old).
- Children 6 months to 3 years old: Apply DEET less than 10% once per day and only if in high-risk areas; do not apply to face or hands; use sparingly. Wash DEET off with soap and water when the child is inside.
- Children 3 to 12 years old: Use DEET less than 10% sparingly and not more than 3 times daily; do not use on face or hands; wash off with soap and water when returned indoors.

- Older than 12 years old: Use DEET less than 30% sparingly; do not spray directly on face, but apply to hands first and then apply to face. Wash off with soap and water when returned indoors.
- Inventory outdoor areas for standing water that can serve as breeding areas for mosquitoes (e.g., old tires, pots or containers, bird bath [change once a week], pool or spa covers). Keep pools and spas clean and chlorinated.
- Use tight-fitting screens on all doors and windows.
- Report any dead birds, especially crows, jays, hawks, magpies, and owls, to local health department or pest control agency.

No vaccine is yet available for humans; however, there are two vaccines in human clinical trials and two others in the investigational stage (National Institute of Allergy and Infectious Diseases, 2006). Equine vaccines are available and strongly recommended for horses.

Hantavirus Pulmonary Syndrome

Epidemiology. Hantavirus pulmonary syndrome (HPS) was formerly referred to as Hantavirus. The causative agent is Sin Nombre virus (SNV) one of 23 hantaviruses. The virus is carried by deer mice (prominent reservoir), white-footed mice, cotton rats, and rice rats. It is spread by aerosolization of the rodent's saliva, urine, and feces excretions. These rodents are distributed equally throughout the U.S.; eradication of rodents is neither feasible nor desirable given their role in biodiversity. Most cases occur in the spring and summer months but can vary depending upon location and rodent population.

HPS, carries a mortality rate of about 30% to 40% (Oregon Department of Human Services, 2006). Human avoidance of infection is the goal in dealing with this disease. The virus is susceptible to common household disinfectants and chlorine.

Incubation Period. Typically, 1 to 6 weeks after exposure to infected rodent body excreta.

Clinical Findings. The illness typically involves a prodromal phase of fever, headache, and myalgia prodrome for 3 to 7 days followed by abrupt onset of pulmonary edema, cardiac decompensation, and hypotension. There is early thrombocytopenia and leukocytosis with a shift to the left. The diagnosis is confirmed by detecting IgM antibodies to SNV using ELISA.

Management. Treatment is supportive.

Prevention. To control outbreaks, the CDC recommends home and work environment modifications and the safe cleanup of rodent waste and nests. Before people work around mouse-infested basements or outbuildings they should endeavor to follow guidelines provided by CDC's campaign "Seal Up! Trap Up! Clean Up!" (available at *www.cdc.gov/rodents*). Other recommendations include:

- Use rubber or latex gloves, goggles, or glasses for all cleanup activities.
- Disinfect areas of infestation with common household disinfectants and chlorine solutions.
- When cleaning out sheds, attics, basements, or other storage areas, aerate the areas first for at least 30 minutes.
- Avoid live or dead wild animals, especially rodents and rodent nesting sites.

Lesser Known Viruses in Circulation

As technology has become more sophisticated, researchers have been able to identify previously unidentified causative agents of infectious diseases. Other factors that have led to the more global emergence of pathogens include drug resistance, exotic travel (exotic diseases), and ownership of exotic pets.

Human Pneumovirus (Metapneumovirus). Metapneumovirus (human pneumovirus; hMPV) is a respiratory pathogen of the Paramyxoviridae family. Its antigenicity is closely related to RSV, as is its symptomatology and epidemiology. In the U.S., it is estimated that 5% to 15% of infant bronchiolitis can be attributed to this virus. Though not a new organism, technologic advances allowed it to be identified and monitored starting in 2001. One study revealed that approximately 25% of children 6 to 12 months old and almost all 5-year-olds tested were seropositive for this agent (Domachowske, 2006). Seventy percent of children hospitalized for respiratory complications caused by this virus were found to harbor only this one virus during their illness. It was detected only between January and April. The role of antiviral agents in treating this virus is unknown.

Enteroviruses. Two enteroviruses (echovirus 13 and echovirus 18) had rarely been seen in the U.S. before 2001. Always circulating in the population, the enteroviruses are the most common cause of aseptic meningitis, and E 13 and E 18 have also associated with paralysis, neonatal sepsis, encephalitis, respiratory, and GI symptoms. They have been isolated from the CSF; E18 has largely been isolated in infants under 12 months old (CDC, 2006e). Antiviral agents currently in use have no benefit. The National Enterovirus Surveillance System (NESS) of the CDC has an ongoing surveillance system and encourages practitioners to test for enterovirus in patients diagnosed with aseptic meningitis. It is currently not a reportable disease in the U.S.

Norovirus (Norwalk-like Virus). Norovirus, also known as Hunter virus and Norwalk-like virus, belongs to the calicivirus family. It has been associated with sporadic epidemics of gastroenteritis in children under 4 years old and is not rapidly inactivated by chlorine. Transmission is person to person by the fecal-oral route, through contaminated water, or food contaminated by infected food handlers. The virus is highly contagious and occurs in closed populations, such as in day care centers, cruise ships, or facilities for the elderly. It is one of several common causative agents of gastroenteritis that affect children who have been exposed to contaminated water in public swimming pools, wading pools, and water parks despite these venues having been chlorine-treated (AAP, 2006). The incubation period is 12 to 72 hours; the duration of illness is 1 to 2 days, but an infected immunocompetent individual can excrete the virus for up to 13 days. Symptoms of infection include nausea, vomiting, diarrhea, and abdominal cramps; some individuals may experience a low-grade fever, chills, headache, muscle aches, and fatigue. Vomiting may be more pronounced in children (CDC, 2007c). Dehydration is a serious complication of this infection.

This illness can recur. Diagnosis can be made with RT-PCR assays and may be available through state and local health department laboratories. There is no antiviral treatment available or vaccine. Preventive measures include good hand washing and other hygienic measures.

Precautions when in public recreational water facilities include not swimming with diarrhea not swallowing the water, washing children's perianal area with soap and water before going in the water, and taking children for frequent bathroom breaks and diaper checks. Individuals known to have been infected should not be in public water facilities for 2 weeks after the illness (AAP, 2006).

Severe Acute Respiratory Syndrome.   Severe acute respiratory syndrome (SARS-CoV) was detected in China in 2003 and spread to 25 other countries during that year. The virus is a coronavirus, a frequent cause of URIs. It is spread by secretions from the respiratory tract or fomites, but the virus has been detected in stool, urine, and blood. The incubation period is not totally known, but is believed to be about 2 to 10 days (AAP, 2006). Transmission of the virus seems most intense during the second week of one's illness. Outbreaks occur during the winter in temperate climates; young children seem particularly vulnerable. Symptoms can include fever (greater than 100.4° F [38° C]), malaise, and myalgias without respiratory tract symptoms. After 2 to 7 days, a dry cough and dyspnea can occur that may then progress to hypoxemia and acute respiratory distress. Recovery occurs in about 21 days.

Diagnostic testing should not proceed unless there are clinical and epidemiologic factors suggestive of SARS. Testing would initially involve antibody assays to rule out RSV and influenza A and B. Testing directly for the CoVs is generally unavailable. If SARS is suggested, the provider is best to consult the CDC website (*www. cdc.gov/ncidod/sars/*) for specimen collection and laboratory guidance. All specimens collected should be saved, including serum. Radiologic findings frequently show focal interstitial infiltrates that progress to generalized, patchy infiltrates and later consolidation. The fatality rate is currently estimated to be between 4% and 50% (Burroughs et al, 2004). Blood tests have demonstrated leukopenia, thrombocytopenia, a platelet count in the low normal range in about half of the infected individuals, and sometimes elevated creatine phosphokinase levels and hepatic transaminases. To date children have exhibited shorter and less severe symptoms than adults. They also have less prominent radiographic findings, and the illness does not progress to respiratory failure and death as it does in adults (AAP, 2006). Management involves strict isolation of the index case, respiratory precautions (hand hygiene, N-95 respirator, gowns and gloves, eye protection); CDC has an infection control guideline that stipulates that those in contact with index cases should stay home until 10 days after all symptoms have resolved in the index case. The patient needs monitoring of pulse oximetry levels, blood cultures, Gram stain and culture of sputum, and should be prescribed antibiotics for both typical and atypical respiratory pathogens. Antivirals have not been useful. For travelers in areas with known SARS, good hand washing and avoiding large crowds is recommended (masks or other protective equipment are not necessary) (WHO, 2003). Research efforts are focused on developing an IG from convalescent serum and the development of an active vaccine against SARS-CoV.

■ TICK-BORNE DISEASES

Lyme disease, Rocky Mountain spotted fever (RMSF), ehrlichiosis, tick-borne relapsing fever, babesiosis, tularemia, and African tick bite fever are common tick-borne diseases in the U.S. African tick bite symptoms may present after a returning traveler has been in East and South Africa. The same tick that causes Lyme disease also can transmit babesiosis, and the tick that transmits RMSF also transmits ehrlichiosis. It is important for providers to be aware of the specific tick vectors and epidemic geographical areas of the vectors. Only the first two diseases are discussed here (tularemia is discussed in the section on bioterrorism agents). A key to including tick-borne diseases in the differential diagnosis is being suspicious when a child complains of influenza-like symptoms (fevers, headache, myalgia) during summer (an unusual time for such symptoms (Richards, 2005).

LYME DISEASE
Epidemiology

Borrelia burgdorferi (Bb), a spirochete, is the causative agent and is carried and transmitted to humans by ticks. Lyme disease is the most commonly reported vector-borne infection in the U.S. and one complicated by differing standards of diagnosis and treatment. The Infectious Diseases Society of America (IDSA) and the International Lyme and Associated Diseases Society (ILADS) have widely divergent views about the nature of transmission, the properties of the spirochete, whether a chronic form of the disease exists, and approaches to treatment.

In the U.S., three clusters (the southern New England and eastern mid-Atlantic states, the upper Midwest [Wisconsin and Minnesota], and the West [Northern California and Oregon]) have reported the most cases. European nations reporting the disease include Scandinavian countries and central Europe (Germany, Austria, Switzerland). In the East, the natural host to *Bb* is the white-footed mouse. The eastern deer tick *(Ixodes scapularis)* becomes infected by feeding on the mouse and then transmits the organism to humans. The size of this tick in the nymphal stage is about 1 mm; in the adult stages from 2.5 to 4 mm. The western deer tick *(Ixodes pacificus)* feeds mostly on lizards. Lyme disease has been reported in habitats that are inhospitable to the tick. The vector in these cases has not been identified. There is varied risk of transmission, depending on the percentage of ticks actually infected with *B. burgdorferi*. In the Northeast and Midwest, 15% to 20% of nymphal and 35% to 40% of adult ticks are infected. In endemic locations, up to 80% or more of adult ticks are infected. In the West, the rate of infected ticks is only 1% to 3% (Shapiro, 2004). Coinfection with other tick-borne pathogens must be considered in endemic regions.

The risk of human infection after a tick bite is related to how long the tick has fed. It takes hours for the tick to fully implant its mouth into the host's skin and days to become fully engorged. Nymphal ticks must feed for equal to or greater than 36 to 48 hours and adult ticks for equal to or greater than 48 to 72 hours before the risk of transmission of *Bb* is significant;

many human victims have removed the tick before this period of time. However, because of the small size of the tick and possible location on the body where it is lodged (e.g., scalp), an engorged tick may not be noticed before it drops off. The disease is not regarded as being teratogenic to fetal development. Incidence is approximately 20 to 1000/100,000 depending upon the geographic area (Shapiro, 2004). Children 5 to 10 years old have a high incidence.

Incubation Period

The incubation period from the bite to the rash stage is approximately 1 to 55 days (median 11 days). Late manifestation of the disease may appear months to more than 1 year later. In the presence of antibiotics *Bb* has been experimentally shown to be able to "hide" intracellularly and change form (Savely, 2006).

Clinical Findings

Lyme disease is hard to diagnosis because the symptoms can be so variable. The classic headache, stiff neck, recurrent rashes, body aches, joint pain, fever, and lymphadenopathy may be nonspecific or mild in the early stages of the disease. They may wax and wane in 4-week cycles. Symptoms in children can vary from those in adults if the infection has disseminated (notably frequent headaches or stomachaches, urinary symptoms, migratory musculoskeletal pains, mood swings, irritability, obsessive-compulsive behavior, new-onset ADHD) (Savely, 2006). Classic Lyme disease can be divided into three stages:

1. *Stage 1 (early localized disease):* Generally, within 1 to 2 weeks after the bite, a typical rash appears at the inoculation site (this time frame can range from 3 to 32 days). Erythema migrans begins as a red, annular macule or papule at the site of the tick bite and progresses into large annular erythematous lesions 5 to 15 cm in diameter. Erythema migrans can vary in morphology. The center of the lesion may be clear, vesicular, or necrotic. The lesion may be pruritic or painful. It typically is located in the axillary, periumbilical, thigh, or groin areas. Organisms are present in the lesions. They may be cultured or seen in biopsy material. The rash remains for a few weeks and fades even if untreated. The patient may experience fever, malaise, headache, arthralgia, and stiff neck during this phase. Without treatment these symptoms, including the rash, may become intermittent, lasting for weeks to months. However, less than half of all individuals demonstrate a rash, and in many cases the rash does not follow the classic erythema migrans description above.
2. *Stage 2 (early disseminated disease):* Through spirochetemia, the organism disseminates through the skin causing multiple skin lesions (1 to 3 cm). These are morphologically similar to, but smaller than, the local lesion. They develop several days to several weeks after the primary lesions. The other systemic manifestations noted in the local disease may return. Infections of eye, bone, heart, synovium, muscle, liver, spleen, and CNS occur because of the hematogenous and lymphatic spread of the organism. The

patient may experience iritis, optic neuritis, conjunctivitis, osteomyelitis, pericarditis, and myocarditis (though rare this may be manifested by varying degrees of heart block), mild arthritis, hepatitis, lymphadenitis, aseptic meningitis, and cranial neuropathies (especially seventh nerve palsy in children that lasts 2 to 8 weeks). Stage 2 can last from weeks to 2 years without treatment. Most of the symptoms (including the rash) wax and wane during this time.
3. *Stage 3 (late disease):* Stage 3 usually begins with pauciarticular or monarticular arthritis that occurs weeks to months after the initial tick bite. The knees are most commonly affected. The joints are red, hot, and swollen, but not as painful as with other types of bacterial arthritis. Untreated, the arthritis initially resolves in a few weeks but becomes recurrent, migratory (but rarely to small joint), and chronic. Lyme arthritis can occur in patients without initial skin lesions. Rarely, adults may suffer late CNS sequelae (progressive encephalopathy), radicular syndrome, chronic leukoencephalitis, and memory impairment.

Diagnostic Studies. Lyme disease is best diagnosed by clinical and epidemiologic history (to give a probability that the patient actually has Lyme disease) and typical physical findings; only if all three exist should one proceed with serologic testing as an adjunct (Shapiro, 2004; AAP, 2006). Serologic tests do not become positive for weeks after a bite; delaying treatment until results are back decreases the chances of successfully treating this disease in the early stages.

Serologically positive results, however, may also indicate prior infection rather than present acute infection because antibodies can remain elevated for years. One medical approach recommends IgM- and IgG-specific antibodies done via the ELISA or IFA assay. Any positive result needs to be followed up with the Western blot test for *Bb* antibodies. IgM antibodies appear in the early stage at 3 to 4 weeks, peak at 6 to 8 weeks, and then decline or persist for years. IgG-specific antibodies appear 6 to 8 weeks after inoculation and peak at 4 to 6 months. They can remain elevated indefinitely. Early antimicrobial intervention may prevent the production of Lyme antibodies. There are many false-positive cross-reactions with other spirochetes, lupus, and varicella organisms.

Another medical approach recommends using the IgM and IgG Western blot as the initial screening tool, using only a reference laboratory that reports all of the bands (e.g., IGeneX, Inc.), and that providers in endemic Lyme disease areas learn to interpret the Western blot bands citing:

> "the CDC's restrictive epidemiologic criteria omit several of the important bands….that are highly sensitive markers for the presence of *Bb*…..the clinician (should) become acquainted with the relative sensitivity and specificity of the various bands. A test with negative results based on epidemiologic criteria may well be a positive test, diagnostically" (Savely, 2006 p 47).

Each band differs as to specificity. By being able to read the 14 to 16 bands, suspicions of *Bb* exposure can be more finely honed and lead to better diagnosis and timely treatment (CDC epidemiologic criteria for Lyme disease considers five out of ten bands as diagnostic; ILADS regards this epidemiologic criteria as a surveillance tool only and one that is inappropriately being applied for clinical diagnosis).

The test kits available commercially are unreliable; their sensitivity is only about 65% (Shapiro, 2004; Savely, 2006). Cultures from a leading-edge biopsy are possible, but the organism is slow growing and may take weeks to isolate. Because *Bb* occurs in such low concentrations, it is often either missed or confused with normal skin structures.

Differential Diagnosis

The rash is characteristic but may not be present in all cases. It may suggest eczema, tinea, granuloma annulare, cellulitis, or an insect bite. Lyme disease should be included in the differential diagnosis of osteomyelitis, West Nile, parvovirus B19, relapsing fever, syphilis, leptospirosis, mycoplasma, septic arthritis, infectious hepatitis, nonresponsive lymphadenopathy, meningitis, multiple sclerosis (MS), amyotrophic lateral sclerosis, Alzheimer disease, juvenile arthritis, Bell palsy, other spirochete-caused diseases, thyroid disease, heavy metal toxicity, and vasculitis. Primary psychiatric disorders, in recalcitrant cases after appropriate treatment for Lyme disease, should also be considered.

Management

The abilities of *Bb* to hide intracellularly, to change form, and to grow slowly are advanced as reasons why the disease is more difficult to diagnose and treat (Savely, 2006). Clinical judgment is crucial in determining whether to treat a patient. The earlier in the migrans stage that treatment is started the better the long-term outcome. As stated in the diagnostic section, false-positive and false-negative test results are frequently reported, and there is an ongoing controversy about the correct way to manage this disease. The primary care provider is best advised to study the literature from the Lyme Disease Association, IDSA, and the ILADS organizations, and consult with infectious disease specialists if uncertain how to proceed. Both organizations agree about the need for early treatment in the erythema migrans stage and the types of drugs; ILADS recommends taking these medications for the full 21 days. The provider can feel confident about using doxycycline or amoxicillin in children when the history includes the following:

- Tick is reliably identified as a nymph or adult *I. scapularis* species (providers in endemic areas should have this expertise of identification).
- Tick was attached for at least 36 hours (as indicated by size of engorgement or known time of exposure).
- Local rate of infection with *Bb* is greater than 20% in the region where the tick was acquired.
- Clinical symptoms fit early stage symptomatology for Lyme disease.

Dosage for Treatment: Early Localized Disease (Stage 1)

Erythema migrans

- Amoxicillin (patients younger than 8 years old): 50 mg/kg/day orally (PO divided into 3 doses a day (maximum dose 500 mg) for 14 to 21 days.
- Doxycycline (patients 8 years or older): 100 mg PO twice daily for 14 to 21 days or 4 mg/kg PO twice daily for 14 to

21 days (maximum 200 mg/day). Give a small snack with doxycycline to reduce nausea.
- For patients unable to take amoxicillin or doxycycline: cefuroxime, 30 mg/kg/day divided twice daily (maximum 500 mg/dose) for 14 to 21 days OR erythromycin, 30 to 50 mg/kg/day PO (maximum 250 mg/dose), divided four times daily for 14 to 21 days.

The IDSA and ILADS differ on the existence of "chronic," "persistent," or "recurrent" Lyme disease. The IDSA postulates that the original diagnosis of Lyme disease was in error and that a patient's failure to respond to treatment was a result of this misdiagnosis. However, the ILADS cites the ability of *Bb* to live intracellularly and avoid antibiotics and encourages the use of long-term combination drug treatment using other drugs not specifically used for Lyme disease (e.g., azithromycin, clarithromycin, metronidazole) to treat chronic disease (Burrascano, 2005). ILADS also regards *Bb* as transmittable by other routes (sexually, in utero, in breast milk from an infected mother, and by other insect vectors). These groups offer current treatment guidelines that are available on their websites (see Resource Box at the end of the chapter).

Both organizations agree that children rarely progress to stage 2 or 3 when treated in the erythema migrans phase; those with arthritic symptoms recover completely. Parental concerns with chronic symptoms after adequate treatment need to be addressed carefully, and other behavioral or organic causes may need to be explored; a Lyme disease infectious disease specialist can be of help in deciding if further treatment is warranted.

Prevention

Avoid tick-infested areas whenever possible. If in such areas, use tick skin repellent with DEET (see recommended DEET percentages based upon age under the prevention section for West Nile Virus). Inspect skin carefully every day during the tick season. Spray permethrin on clothing and wear light-colored long pants (tucked into shoes), long sleeves, and a hat. Chronic absorption of insecticides, however, can produce toxicity, especially in children; however, when used according to directions children older than 2 months can safely use DEET (Wormser et al, 2006). Alternative repellents include permethrin for clothing, Picaridin, and IR 3535.

Post-tick bite prophylaxis with doxycycline (single 200 mg dose) can be effective in preventing the disease. However, this prophylaxis should be given only to those who live in highly endemic areas and when the tick is at least minimally engorged with blood. Otherwise, chemoprophylaxis is probably unwarranted because most ticks are removed before engorgement has occurred.

EHRLICHIOSIS

Three types of this disease occur, all spread by different pathogens transmitted by ticks. Any individual who has a history of tick exposure in an endemic area, a nonspecific febrile illness during the spring or summer, and some of the symptoms listed below should be considered at risk for ehrlichiosis. The southeast, south central, mid-Atlantic states, and the same regions in which Lyme disease occur are common endemic areas. Immunocompromised individuals are at greater risk; males can be affected more, depending upon the pathogen. Children are increasingly acquiring this disease.

All three types produce acute, systemic symptoms with fever, headache, myalgia, malaise, chills, nausea, vomiting, anorexia, acute weight loss, and arthralgia. A rash may or may not occur about 1 week after onset of symptoms and is seen about 60% of the time in children (AAP, 2006). Less common symptoms include diarrhea, abdominal pain, cough, and change in mental status. Leukopenia, neutropenia, anemia, or thrombocytopenia with an elevation in transaminases can be seen on blood tests depending upon the pathogen.

Diagnosis is made by isolating the pathogen from blood or CSF by IFA assay between the acute and convalescent periods (2 to 3 weeks apart) or detecting of the pathogen from a PCR assay in conjunction with an IFA titer. PCR from a peripheral blood sample during the acute phase is showing merit. The CDC can aid in advising the appropriate test.

Treatment of choice is doxycycline (4 mg/kg/day divided twice daily for a minimum of 5 to 10 days and at least 3 days after defervescence; maximum dose 100 mg/dose), even in young children given the potential for this to be a life-threatening illness. Data suggest that discoloration of permanent teeth is not significant if doxycycline is taken for 14 days or less (AAP, 2006). A response to treatment should occur within 1 week. Systemic complications include pulmonary infiltrates, bone marrow hypoplasia, respiratory failure, encephalopathy, meningitis, DIC, spontaneous hemorrhage, and renal failure. The mortality rate ranges from 1% to 3% (Richards, 2005). Recovery is usually complete after 1 to 2 weeks; some neurologic difficulties can remain in children who have had systemic disease.

BACTERIAL INFECTIONS

Although less common overall than viral diseases, bacterial infections allow for interventions (including antibiotics) that can decrease the course of an illness and prevent subsequent complications. Many bacterial infections may be diagnosed clinically and treated empirically. A good understanding of the pathophysiology of common bacterial infections, and knowledge of the most likely organisms involved, allows for efficient and effective implementation of treatment. Bacterial infections of the skin and soft tissue infections, lymphadenitis, osteomyelitis, fasciitis, pneumonia, meningitis, infectious diarrhea, and UTI are discussed in other chapters relevant to the system affected; fungal infections and parasitic infections are likewise found elsewhere.

TACKLING POTENTIAL METHICILLIN-RESISTANT *STAPHYLOCOCCUS AUREUS* (MRSA)

It is increasingly important to recognize a clinical situation in which diagnosis and management of bacterial infections requires consideration of the involvement of community-acquired methicillin-resistant *S. aureus* (CA-MRSA). Knowing the prevalence in one's community of CA-MRSA

is crucial for how a provider should treat severe pneumonia, cellulitis, osteomyelitis, myositis, bacteremia, endocarditis, empyema, meningitis, scalded skin syndrome, toxic shock syndrome (TSS), deep tissue abscesses (especially those that come on quickly), reported spider bites, skin and soft tissue infections, and necrotizing fasciitis. Traditionally health care–acquired MRSA (HA-MRSA) was hospital based. However, CA-MRSA has now reached essentially the same incidence as HA-MRSA and is principally found in the skin and soft tissue areas. It is also increasingly being implicated as the causative agent in pneumonia in the younger age groups and in those without risk factors. One study showed that 22% of children evaluated for skin infections and abscesses that were seen at two emergency departments distant from each other were CA-MRSA positive. Eighty percent of the isolates were cultured from abscesses, and 53% were CA-MRSA positive (Hasty et al, 2007).

CA-MRSA has gone from "simply" a resistant *S. aureus* to an entirely new clone that carries a different gene for Panton-Valentine leukocidin (PVL). This allows it to evade circulating neutrophils and cause leukocyte destruction and tissue necrosis (Voyich et al, 2005). It has a particular affinity for pediatric populations.

There are some clinical clues that MRSA may be involved in the presenting symtomatology or history of an otherwise healthy individual (Rosenthal, 2005b and 2006b; Lewis, 2006; Tufts & Connor Hardman, 2006):

- Child has a boil, furuncle, or abscess without draining pus that is erythematous, warm, painful; onset may have been rapid (key finding) (Hasty et al, 2007).
- Child fails treatment with a β-lactam product.
- Other family members have similar skin infections.
- Child has a recent history of skin infection, even if it was responsive to a β-lactam agent.
- Neonate with skin or soft tissue infection.
- Skin lesion looks like a spider bite; larger lesions are more suspicious for MRSA.
- There is pus present.
- History of recurrent small, nontender, nonpruritic maculopapular lesions that become pruritic or painful; multiple lesions present.
- Child participates in contact sports (wrestling, football) where turf burns and abrasions are common, and athletes share lockers, bars of soap, towels, other equipment.
- Child is an Alaskan native, Pacific Islander, Native American, black, in the military, has traveled to the Middle East, attends day care, or lives in a crowded environment.
- Child has no history in the past year of having been hospitalized, of having had surgery, and has no permanent indwelling medical devices passing through the skin.
- Child has CF or progressive respiratory tract infection.

The provider can safely treat many superficial skin lesions (e.g., impetigo) without a culture using the conventional management strategies of the past. In minor infections, most cases will resolve despite whether or not the antibiotic matched the susceptibility of the organism (Steinberg, 2005). However, providers need to assess each case carefully and diligently provide instructions to parents to return if the child is unresponsive to treatment. Anticipate complications and consider the clinical clues previously mentioned above for skin and soft tissue infection. See Chapters 36 and 39 for other references to MRSA.

Recommended management strategies (Fig. 23-4) include:

- Culture any lesion with purulent exudate or incise and drain nondraining abscesses (especially if 5 cm or larger); when possible express lesions for fluids to culture.
- Send specimens to the laboratory for a Gram stain, culture and sensitivity, and "D-test" (indicates any possible inducible resistance to clindamycin).
- For soft tissue infection without fluid fluctuation, empiric treatment for methicillin-sensitive *S. aureus* is appropriate. After draining an abscess of under 5 cm in size in a healthy older child, observation without an antibiotic is reasonable (John & Schreiber, 2006).
- If CA-MRSA is suspected, Table 23-11 offers antibiotic treatment options. Erythromycin, cipromycin, cephalosporins are not indicated for known CA-MRSA.

Prevention measures for athletes include:

- Bathe with soap and water; athletes should not share bars of soap (recommend that bars be replaced with liquid dispensers) or towels with other teammates.
- Cover all abrasions or skin lesions with clean dressings.
- Do not share possibly contaminated personal items with others (e.g., razors, supportive devices).
- Provide information for coaches and trainers about cleaning shared equipment regularly, recognizing infected wounds, and establishing team protocols for the routine reporting of skin lesions for assessment.

CAT-SCRATCH DISEASE

Epidemiology

Bartonella henselae is the causative organism for cat-scratch disease (CSD). It is the most common cause of chronic persistent (greater than 3 weeks) lymphadenopathy and is a slow-growing, gram-negative bacillus.

CSD is believed to be a common infection, with most cases occurring in patients under 20 years old. Infection occurs after direct, cutaneous contact with a healthy appearing but infected animal. In 90% of the cases, a cat (usually a kitten) is involved (AAP, 2006). Other sources include dog scratches, monkey contact, wood splinters, fish hooks, and other inanimate objects. The disease is most prevalent in fall and winter.

Incubation Period

The incubation period between injury and primary skin lesion is 7 to 12 days. The lymphadenopathy may take 5 to 50 days to develop, but averages 12 days.

Clinical Findings

In approximately one third of cases, patients manifest systemic illness; the rest are not very sick. Greater than 50% have a history of a cat scratch (Stechenberg, 2004). The illness typically presents with cutaneous findings and other key characteristics that include:

- Lesions 3- to 5-mm that arise approximately 1 week after inoculation and can persist for months. The nonpruritic lesions initially begin as vesicles or pustules and evolve into papules. They may follow along a linear pattern that follows the cat scratch. They may be misdiagnosed as impetigo secondary to an insect bite. The cutaneous lesions heal completely without scarring. Up to 10% of patients may have the inoculation lesions present as nonsuppurative conjunctivitis or ocular granuloma (the affected eye is not painful, with little or no discharge, but may be red and swollen).
- Mucous membrane ulcers have been found at the onset of the lymphadenopathy stage.
- One to 4 weeks after the inoculation the axillary, cervical, submandibular, preauricular, epitrochlear, inguinal, and femoral nodes closest to the lesion begin to swell (in that general order). There can be single or multiple nodes involved. The node may swell to 1 to 5 cm. The area around the infected node is usually warm, tender, indurated, and erythematous during the first few weeks. Cellulitis is uncommon, but large nodes may suppurate 10% to 20% of the time. The lymphadenopathy usually lasts approximately 1 to 2 months and up to 1 year in some cases.
- A fever of 38° C to 39° C (100.4° F to 102.2° F), malaise, anorexia, fatigue, and headache also accompany the lymphadenopathy in one third of patients.

Diagnostic Studies. An IFA for serum antibodies is available from many labs, state health departments, or the CDC. CT or ultrasonography may be useful in identifying hepatic or splenic abscesses and granulomas. The CBC may be normal or show mild leukocytosis. The erythrocyte sedimentation rate (ESR) may be elevated early in the disease process. Lymph node biopsy stained with Warthin-Starry silver stain can visualize bacilli, but not specifically *B. henselae*. A cat-scratch antigen skin test is not recommended (AAP, 2006).

Differential Diagnosis

The differential diagnosis includes any cause of lymphadenopathy. The most common of these are bacterial and viral infections (e.g., streptococci [especially Group A ß-hemolytic], staphylococci, anaerobic bacteria, atypical mycobacteria, tularemia, brucellosis, CMV, HIV, EBV, systemic fungal infections, toxoplasmosis, malignancy). Neck masses from other sources (e.g., cystic hygromas, bronchogenic cysts, tumors) are in the differential.

Management

Symptomatic treatment is usually sufficient in most cases because CSD usually spontaneously resolves within 2 to 4 months. Antipyretics can be used if there is moderate fever. Painful nodes can be treated with moist wraps or needle aspiration. Incision and drainage of nonsuppurative lesions should be avoided because of the high risk of chronic draining sinuses. Needle aspiration can yield material for diagnostic testing. Biopsy may be required if neoplasm is in the differential. Antibiotics are not generally used unless there is concern for systemic CSD or bacterial involvement of lesions. Azithromycin, clarithromycin, trimethoprim-sulfamethoxazole,

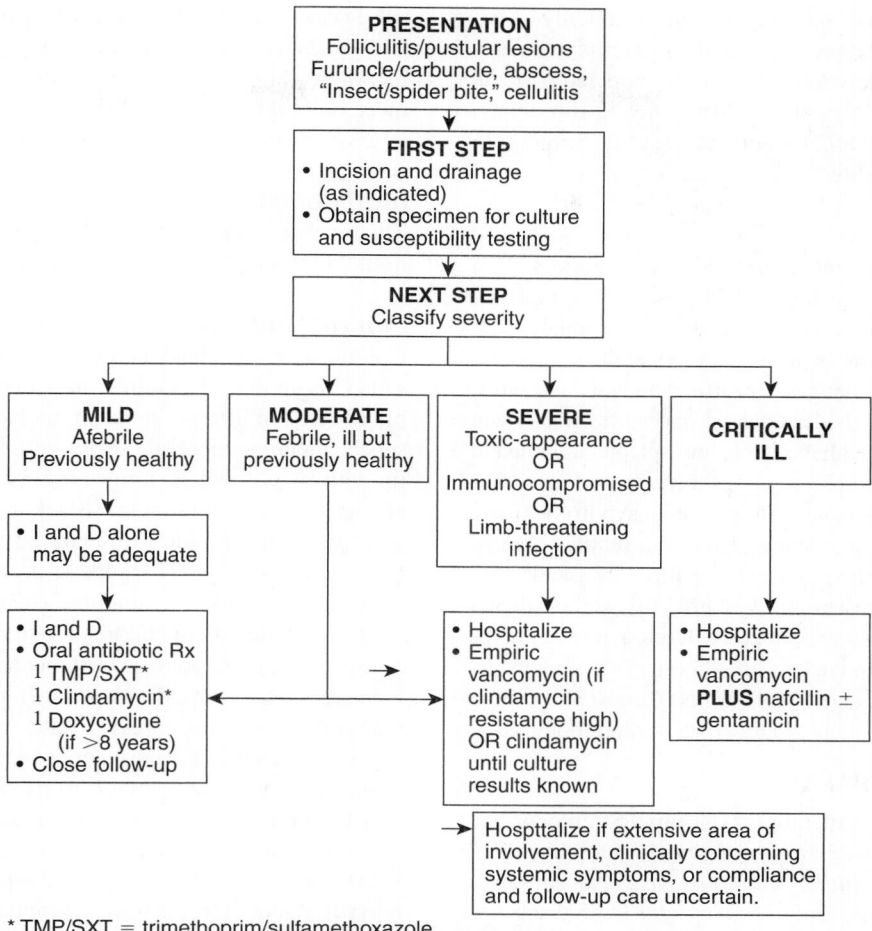

PRESENTATION
Folliculitis/pustular lesions
Furuncle/carbuncle, abscess,
"Insect/spider bite," cellulitis

FIRST STEP
- Incision and drainage
  (as indicated)
- Obtain specimen for culture
  and susceptibility testing

NEXT STEP
Classify severity

MILD
Afebrile
Previously healthy

MODERATE
Febrile, ill but
previously healthy

SEVERE
Toxic-appearance
OR
Immunocompromised
OR
Limb-threatening
infection

**CRITICALLY
ILL**

- I and D alone
  may be adequate

- I and D
- Oral antibiotic Rx
  1 TMP/SXT*
  1 Clindamycin*
  1 Doxycycline
  (if >8 years)
- Close follow-up

- Hospitalize
- Empiric
  vancomycin (if
  clindamycin
  resistance high)
  OR clindamycin
  until culture
  results known

- Hospitalize
- Empiric
  vancomycin
  PLUS nafcillin ±
  gentamicin

Hospttalize if extensive area of
involvement, clinically concerning
systemic symptoms, or compliance
and follow-up care uncertain.

* TMP/SXT = trimethoprim/sulfamethoxazole.
⁺Assume ≥90% prevalence of "D" test negative, erythromycin-resistant CA-MRSA strains.

FIG. 23-4 Algorithm for managing children with suspected CA-MRSA infections suggested by the AAP. Initial outpatient management of suspected CA-MRSA skin and soft tissue infections is schematically illustrated and assumes CA-MRSA strains are prevalent in a community. (Data from Baker CJ, Frenck RW Jr: Change in management of skin/soft tissue infections needed, *AAP News* 2004 25:10, 105-117; Kaplan SL: Implications of methicillin-resistant *Staphylococcus aureus* as a community-acquired pathogen in pediatric patients, *Infect Dis Clin North Am* 19[3]:747-757, 2005.)

TABLE 23-11 Treatment Options for CA-MRSA infections

Antibiotic	Dosage for 10-14 Days	Comments (for Nonsevere Skin/Soft Tissue Infections)
Trimethoprim-sulfamethoxazole (98% efficacy*)	Children ≥2 months old: 8-12 mg/kg/day TMP component (some advocate using up to 15-20 mg/kg/day TMP component) divided into two doses	First-line drug
Clindamycin (92% efficacy*)	10-30 mg/kg/day divided every 6-8 hr	First-line drug; D-test should be done on specimen by lab to ensure clindamycin susceptibility
Doxycycline or minocycline	Children >8 years old: 100 mg twice daily	First-line drug; photosensitivity precautions
Rifampin in combination with one of the above	300 mg twice daily	Alternative to above drugs; not to be used as a single agent because of rapid resistance development; can cause staining of body fluids
Linezolid	400-600 mg every 12 hours	Second-line drug; for complicated skin/soft tissue infections, pneumonia

*Amin NM: What's wrong with this picture? Child with swollen leg and fever, *Consultant* 46(1):45-48, 2006.
Data from Chandy CJ: Therapies and vaccines for emerging bacterial infections; learning from methicillin-resistant *Staphylococcus aureus*, *Pediatr Clin North Am* 53(4):699-713, 2006; Nicolle L: Community-acquired MRSA: a practitioner's guide, *CMAJ* 175(2):145, 2006; Kaplan SL: Implications of methicillin-resistant *Staphylococcus aureus* as a community-acquired pathogen in pediatric patients, *Infect Dis Clin North Am* 19(3):747-757, 2005.

rifampin, ciprofloxin, and gentamycin are commonly used. Oral azithromycin has shown some clinical success in reducing the initial lymph node volume in half the infected patients (500 mg in one dose the first day; 250 mg days 2 through 5; smaller children: 10 mg/kg/24 hours on day 1; 5 mg/kg/24 hours days 2 through 5) (Stechenberg, 2004).

Complications

A small percentage of patients manifest systemic illness. This can be associated with fever up to 106° F (41.2° C), malaise, fatigue, anorexia, emesis, headache, hepatosplenomegaly, sore throat, exanthema, blindness secondary to stellate macular retinopathy, neurologic changes (bizarre behavior), seizures, and arthralgia. Enlarged mediastinal or pancreatic nodes can cause pleurisy, obstructive phenomena, and splenic and hepatic abscesses. Significant weight loss has been reported. Other complications include Parinaud oculoglandular syndrome (from inoculation of the palpebral conjunctivitis from rubbing the eye after touching the cat scratch), encephalopathy (5% incidence), aseptic meningitis, severe chronic systemic disease, erythema nodosa, neuroretinitis, thrombocytopenic purpura, primary atypical pneumonia, relapsing bacteremia, breast mass, endocarditis, angiomatoid papules, and osteomyelitis. Almost all of these problems generally resolve completely over several months.

MENINGOCOCCAL DISEASE

Many organisms can cause meningitis (Group B Streptococcus, *Escherichia coli, Listeria, Monocytogenes,* enterococci, *S. pneumoniae, N. meningitidis, H. influenza*). The causative organism varies with age. Only *N. meningitidis* is discussed here. (Chapter 27 also provides a general discussion of all causative agents of meningitis.)

Epidemiology

N. meningitidis is a gram-negative diplococcus. It is a common commensal organism in the human nasopharynx. It has no animal or environmental reservoirs. There are 13 serotypes identified, and groups A, B, C, W-135, and Y are largely the causes of invasive disease. Groups B and C have traditionally been the most common serotypes in the U.S. and Europe, but Y has more recently emerged as a major cause of disease. Group B is a greater threat to younger children (Krey, 2005).

The organism is spread from person to person via respiratory tract secretions and in most cases causes asymptomatic colonization. This can persist for weeks to months. The asymptomatic carriage rate is approximately 25% in nonepidemic periods. Disease occurs most often during winter and early spring in children, but sporadically (97% of cases) in the U.S. Children less than 5 years old have the greatest incidence. The peak attack rate occurs in children less than 1 year old with 48% of all meningococcal infection occurring in children younger than 2 years old. Epidemics occur in semiclosed communities (e.g., day care centers, schools, college dormitories, and military barracks). Patients with functional or anatomic asplenia, sickle cell disease, agammaglobulinemia, AIDS, and complement deficiency or properdin deficiency are at increased risk for invasive or recurring meningococ-

cal disease (AAP, 2006; Sáez-Llorens & McCracken, 2004). Adolescents have the highest mortality rate as a result of septic complications despite the fact that younger children have more meningitis (Krey, 2005). In children, the risk increases in environments where there is second-hand smoke exposure.

Incubation Period

The incubation period is 1 to 10 days. Patients are contagious until 24 hours after initiation of treatment.

Clinical Findings

Colonization can lead to invasive disease. Bacteremia and sepsis result and, depending on hematogenous spread, multiple patterns of illness can result, including bacteremia without sepsis, meningococcemic sepsis without meningitis, meningitis with or without meningococcemia, meningoencephalitis, and specific organ infection (Black & Shinefield, 2006b).

Presenting symptoms of meningitis can include:
- *Occult bacteremia:* This appears in a febrile child with URI or gastrointestinal-like symptoms. There may be a maculopapular rash. Often these children are treated as having a viral illness. Some have recovered without antimicrobial intervention, whereas others have developed meningococcal meningitis.
- *Meningococcemia:* Fever (characteristic), chills, pharyngitis, headache, purulent conjunctivitis, photophobia, myalgias, weakness, myocarditis, malaise, stiff neck (less in infants), seizures, prostration, irritability, emesis, and a maculopapular or petechial rash (characteristic) that may quickly progress to purpura and septic shock manifested by hypertension, DIC, acidosis, adrenal hemorrhage, renal failure, myocardial failure, and coma. Bacteremia can result in meningitis, purulent pericarditis, myocarditis, pneumonia, or septic arthritis.

Diagnostic Studies. The diagnosis is confirmed with a positive culture or Gram stain from blood, CSF, synovial fluid, sputum, or petechial or purpura lesion scraping. Latex agglutination testing is not recommended. PCR testing is used widely in the United Kingdom and is useful when antibiotics are given before testing, and the organism growth has been suppressed. A CBC shows leukopenia (21%), decreased platelets (14%), and elevated ESR and CRP.

Differential Diagnosis

The list of differential diagnoses is long and includes septicemia caused by other invasive bacteria (e.g., pneumococcus or *H. influenzae,* viral meningitis, TB brain abscess, chronic otitis media, and sinusitis). Collagen-vascular diseases, primary hematologic and oncologic disease, erythema nodosa, erythema multiforme, Rocky Mountain spotted fever, mycoplasma, lead encephalopathy, coxsackievirus, echovirus, rubella and rubeola infections, Henoch-Schönlein purpura, ITP, viral exanthems, and Kawasaki syndrome are also in the differential diagnosis.

Management

If the child is suspected of having meningococcemia, IV antibiotics are started pending culture results. Aqueous penicillin

G (250,000 to 300,000 units/kg/day IV divided every 4 hours for 5 to 7 days) has been the drug of choice for infants and children. An excellent alternative is cefotaxime (200–225 mg/kg/24 hours divided every 8 hours) or ceftriaxone (100 mg/kg once daily). The patient is kept in respiratory isolation until 24 hours after the induction of treatment. Some *N. meningitidis* strains in the U.S. are partially resistant to penicillin, but no treatment failures have been reported. Penicillin resistance is reportedly high in some European countries. In these cases (after susceptibility testing) or if the patient is allergic to penicillin, cefotaxime, ceftriaxone, or chloramphenicol (75 to 100 mg/kg/24 hours IV divided into four doses) may be substituted. Early dexamethasone given within minutes before antimicrobials may reduce the incidence of residual neurologic and audiologic complications (Sáez-Llorens & McCracken, 2004).

Control Measures

Exposed contacts must be carefully monitored. Household, school, or child contacts who develop a febrile illness must be evaluated for invasive disease promptly. High-risk household contacts have 500 to 800 times the risk as do those in the general community.

- *Chemoprophylaxis*: Close contacts (household, day care, nursery school, those who shared oral secretions [kissing, shared utensils or toothbrushes]) of the index case 7 days before the onset of symptoms are at increased risk of invasive disease. Airline travel of greater than 8 hours while sitting next to an infected individual would qualify an individual for prophylaxis (AAP, 2006). Casual contact with the index case, casual contact with a high-risk contact, or medical personnel (unless they performed mouth-to-mouth resuscitation, intubation, or suctioning before antibiotic therapy was instituted) are usually not considered high risk. Oral rifampin, 10 mg/kg/dose (maximum dose 600 mg) PO twice daily for a total of four doses, is the prophylactic treatment of choice for those older than 1 month. Infants younger than 1 month old should be given 5 mg/kg/dose PO twice daily for a total of four doses. Ceftriaxone (125 mg IM for those less than 15 years old; 250 mg IM greater than 15 years old) in a single dose is as effective as oral rifampin; it can be given to pregnant women. Ciprofloxacin (500 mg PO in a single dose) can be given to nonpregnant adults 18 years and older. Azithromycin (500 mg single dose) is effective but warrants more study (AAP, 2006).
- *Vaccine*: Vaccine with serogroups A, C, Y, and W-135, in conjunction with chemoprophylaxis, is advisable to prevent extended outbreaks only if the identified strain is contained in the vaccine. The vaccine MPSV4 is approved for children 2 to 10 years old and MCV4 for those 11 to 15 years old. No vaccine covers serogroup B infection (refer to meningococcal vaccines discussed earlier).

Complications

Complications are caused by inflammation, intravascular hemorrhage, necrosis in multiple organ systems, and shock. Organ abscesses and infarcts cause necrosis of tissue and gangrene. Skeletal deformities and limb amputations are not infrequent. Meningitis can lead to ataxia, seizures, deafness (5% to 20%), arthritis and pericarditis (8% to 24%), visual field defects, palsies and paralysis (10% to 15%), developmental delays, and hydrocephalus. Immune-complex reactions are responsible for arthritis symptoms. The overall mortality rate is 10% to 15% in the U.S. The mortality rate is less than 10% for infants and children; however, there are residual effects in 10% to 30% of children (e.g., seizures, hearing loss, learning and behavioral problems, lower IQ) (Sáez-Llorens & McCracken, 2004).

STREPTOCOCCAL DISEASE

Streptococci are gram-positive spherical cocci that are classified based on their ability to hemolyze RBCs. Complete hemolysis is known as ß-hemolytic. Partial hemolysis is α-hemolytic. Nonhemolysis is γ-hemolytic. Cell wall carbohydrate differences further subdivide the streptococci. These differences are identified as Lancefield antigen subgroups A-H and K-V. Subgroups A-H and K-O are associated with human disease. Group A ß-hemolytic streptococcus is the most virulent, though Group B ß-hemolytic can cause bacteremia and meningitis in neonates.

Group A β-Hemolytic Streptococcus

Epidemiology. There are more than 100 M-protein types of group A ß-hemolytic streptococci (GABHS). Transmission is through infected upper respiratory tract secretions. Fomites and household pets are not vectors. Food-borne epidemics from contamination by food handlers are reported. Most commonly streptococcus microbes involve the respiratory tract, skin, soft tissues, and blood. Both streptococcus pharyngitis and impetigo are associated with crowding, whether at home, school, or other institution. Pharyngitis is rare in infants and children less than 3 years old, but the incidence rises with age until adolescence (commonly from 5 to 15 years old). It is not common in adults unless there is an epidemic. URIs occur year round but are most common in the winter. Temperate climates (especially in colder times of the year, such as autumn, winter, and spring) have greater incidences of pharyngeal infection than tropical climates. Carrier rate is high (20% to 40%) (Todd, 2004). By contrast, streptococcus skin infection (impetigo) is more common in toddlers and preschool-age children and occurs more often during summer, early fall in tropical areas, or in warmer weather in temperate climates. Those at increased risk for invasive GABHS are those with varicella infection, IV drug use, HIV, diabetes, chronic heart or lung disease, infants, and the elderly.

Incubation Period. The incubation period is 2 to 5 days for pharyngitis and 7 to 10 days for skin acquisition to lesions of impetigo. The period of communicability is from the onset of symptoms up to a few months in untreated persons. Transmission rates from a carrier are not high (Todd, 2004).

Clinical Findings. The following may be seen in GABHS:

- *Respiratory tract infection*. Streptococcal tonsillopharyngitis and pneumonia are described in Chapter 31.

- *Scarlet fever.* This is caused by erythrogenic toxin. It is uncommon in children younger than 3 years old. The incubation period is approximately 3 days (the range is 1 to 7 days). There is abrupt illness with sore throat, vomiting, headache, chills, and malaise. Fever can reach 104° F (40° C). Tonsils are erythematous, swollen, and usually covered in exudate. The pharynx also is inflamed and can be covered with a gray-white exudate. The palate and uvula are erythematous and reddened, and petechiae are present. The tongue is usually coated red. Desquamation of the coating leaves prominent papillae (strawberry tongue) (see Fig. 23-2, *A* and *B*).

  The rash appears within 12 to 48 hours. The exanthema is red and finely papular and makes the skin feel coarse, akin to sandpaper. The rash begins in the axilla, groin, and neck, spreads centripetally, is generalized within 24 hours, and blanches on pressure (Schultz-Charlton sign). There is circumoral pallor, and the cheeks are flushed. There is increased rash density on the neck, axilla, and groin. Pastia's lines, transverse linear hyperpigmented areas with tiny petechiae, are seen in the folds of the joints. In severe disease, small vesicles (miliary sudamina) can be found on the hands, feet, and abdomen. Rash, sore throat, and constitutional symptoms resolve in approximately 5 to 7 days. The rash begins to desquamate shortly thereafter. Fine branlike flakes begin on the face and slowly spread to the trunk and extremities. This process may take up to 6 weeks (Todd, 2004).

  Surgical scarlet fever can occur after wound infection, burns, or streptococcus skin infection. The disease manifestations are similar to regular scarlet fever, but there is no pharyngeal or tonsillar involvement.

- *Skin infections.* The characteristic lesion for streptococcal impetigo is a honey-colored scab on an erythematous base (see Color Plate). Localized lymphadenopathy is common. A small, transient, vesicular lesion may precede the scab lesion. Deep soft tissue infection may develop after impetigo. Streptococcal soft tissue abscesses result from puncture wounds contaminated with GABHS. Infants having weepy eczema can have secondary GABHS skin infection. The eczema area develops the typical impetiginous lesions. Erysipelas is an acute cellulitis with lymphadenitis. The skin becomes red and indurated. It begins as a small lesion and spreads marginally for 4 to 6 days. The lesion's borders are firm, raised, and tender. Fever, chills, vomiting, irritability, and other constitutional symptoms are present. These subside when the rash stops spreading. Bacteremia, abscesses, metastatic foci, and death are reported.

- *Bacteremia.* This can occur after respiratory (pharyngitis, tonsillitis, AOM) and localized skin infections. Some children have no obvious source of infection. Meningitis, osteomyelitis, septic arthritis, pyelonephritis, pneumonia, peritonitis, and bacterial endocarditis (acute rheumatic fever caused by a certain "rheumatogenic" strain) are rare but are associated with GABHS bacteremia.

- *Vaginitis.* GABHS causes vaginitis in prepubertal females. Vulvar erythema, serous discharge, and irritation (especially with walking and urination) are common findings. Although the infection is usually the result of autoinoculation, it can be a symptom of sexual molestation if infected saliva is used as a sexual lubricant.

- *Perianal streptococcal cellulitis.* This is uncommon and occurs in either sex. Manifestations include local itching, pain, blood-streaked stools, erythema, and proctitis. Although infection is usually the result of autoinoculation, it can be a symptom of sexual molestation if infected saliva is used as a sexual lubricant.

- *Necrotizing fasciitis.* This occurs in children and often is associated with varicella.

- *Streptococcal toxic shock syndrome.* Toxic shock syndrome caused by GABHS appears as an acute multiorgan disease similar to TSS caused by *S. aureus*. It is more often caused by a nonmenstrual infection (from surgical and gynecologic procedures, and localized and invasive infections, such as bacteremia, pneumonia, cellulitis, myositis, necrotizing fasciitis, osteomyelitis, endocarditis). The overall incidence of TSS is declining. Less than 10% of children with severe invasive streptococcus infection develop TSS (AAP, 2006). Pain at the trauma or surgical site of infection (may look like cellulitis or necrotizing fasciitis) is a common finding. The pain is typically more severe than that suggested by the physical examination. Infection can also be characterized by symptoms suggestive of *S. aureus* TSS infection: fever, rash, asymptomatic pharyngitis, severe diarrhea, severe myalgias, hypotension, respiratory distress, desquamation (palms and soles usually after 7 to 21 days), transient toxic cardiomyopathy, headaches, depressed mentation, and multiorgan dysfunction (especially renal). The rash is similar to that seen with Kawasaki syndrome and scarlet fever. The *S. pyogenes* organism must be isolated to make the diagnosis (unlike that of *S. aureus* TSS infection). The infection can be transmitted by close contact; contact and droplet isolation is recommended.

Diagnostic Studies. Culture of the organism is the most useful method of establishing the diagnosis. A positive throat culture confirms the diagnosis; however, a positive culture may identify a carrier state. Many rapid streptococcal identification tests have poor sensitivity; therefore, a negative rapid test result must be followed up by a culture unless the rapid streptococcal identification test used is highly sensitive (optical immunoassay or chemiluminescent DNA probe). The specificity of most rapid tests is good (95%); therefore, if the rapid test result is positive, the diagnosis of GABHS is confirmed. Documentation of past GABHS infection can be done by drawing a titer for antibodies to various streptococcal enzymes, such as antistreptolysin O (ASO).

Differential Diagnosis. A differential diagnosis is acute pharyngitis caused by viruses, especially adenoviruses or Epstein-Barr (infectious mononucleosis [IM]). Other bacterial upper respiratory diseases in the differential diagnosis, though rare, include diphtheria, tularemia, toxoplasmosis, mycoplasma, tonsillar TB, salmonellosis, and brucellosis. Staphylococcal impetigo must be differentiated from GABHS pyoderma. Septicemia, meningitis, osteomyelitis, septic arthritis, pyelonephritis, and bacterial endocarditis can result from other bacteria causing similar infections. Cultures or serologic testing differentiate the offending organism.

Management. Antimicrobial therapy is the treatment of choice. Tetracyclines, sulfonamides including trimethoprim-sulfamethoxazole should not be used.

- β-lactam drug of choice: providers need to stress the importance of completing the 10-day course.
  - Potassium penicillin V PO at a dose of 250 mg two or three times daily for 10 days for children less than 27 kg; (if equal to or greater than 27 kg, the dose is 500 mg two to three times daily for 10 days). If compliance is good, penicillin PO (500 mg/day twice daily for 10 days) can be given to adolescents and adults. Amoxicillin (40 mg/kg once daily for 10 days) has demonstrated effectiveness (AAP, 2006).
  - Benzathine penicillin G IM (600,000 units if child is less than 60 lb, or 1.2 million units for greater than 60 lb. If given IM, allow mixture to warm to room temperature. Use in those where compliance with oral treatment for 10 days is of concern.
- Oral cephalosporins (cephalexin, cephradine, cefadroxil, cefaclor, cefixime, cefuroxime) are an alternative for penicillin-allergic patients unless they have had an acute onset hyperallergic reaction to penicillin.
- Macrolides
  - Erythromycin estolate (20 to 40 mg/kg/day divided into two or four doses) or erythromycin ethylsuccinate (40 mg/kg/day in two to four divided doses for 10 days), if allergic to penicillin.
  - Clarithromycin for 10 days.
  - Azithromycin dosed at 12 mg/kg/day PO for 5 days (maximum 500 mg/day)
  - Clindamycin (30 mg/kg/24 hours). Clindamycin has proven resistant to CA-MRSA in certain communities.
- Topical antibiotics may be used with simple uncomplicated impetigo (1 to 2 single lesions). See prior discussion about CA-MRSA. Mupirocin ointment is recommended (AAP, 2006). For multiple or migrating lesions, a systemic antibiotic is indicated.
- Asymptomatic carriers generally do not need treatment. If treatment is warranted, clindamycin (20 mg/kg/day divided into three doses; maximum 1.8 g/day) for 10 days is most effective (AAP, 2006). If continued episodes of acute pharyngitis occur, providers should determine carrier status by culturing for GABHS between episodes and checking blood for ASO antigen.
- Supportive care. This includes antipyretics, fluids, and rest. If a clinical relapse occurs, another culture should be done. If positive, a second course of penicillin is indicated, preferably benzathine penicillin IM. If recurrent infection is a problem, simultaneous culturing of the family for chronic carrier state is advised. Children can return to school as soon as they are afebrile and on antibiotics for at least 24 hours.
- Systemic disease. IV penicillin is required often in combination with another drug. Debridement, aggressive hydration, IVIG, and/or steroids may also be employed.

Complications. These are usually caused by the spread of the disease from the localized infection; many have already been discussed. In untreated individuals, other complications include otitis media, sinusitis, peritonsillar and retropharyngeal abscesses, and suppurative cervical adenitis.

Group B ß-hemolytic Streptococcus

Group B ß-hemolytic streptococci (GBBHS or GBS) are a leading cause of perinatal bacterial infection. There are nine serotypes associated with human infection. GBBHS colonizes the GI tract and vagina, with colonization rates in pregnant women and newborns that range from 15% to 40% (AAP, 2006). Early onset infection occurs in approximately 1 to 4 per 1000 live births in exposed infants whose mothers did not receive maternal intrapartum antimicrobial prophylaxis. With prophylaxis the rate drops 81% (AAP, 2006). Transmission occurs by direct contact, mother to child before and during labor, and less commonly after birth by contact with colonized persons, usually through hand contamination. Early-onset disease is more common in high-risk deliveries or premature infants, small-for-gestational-age infants, infants born after prolonged rupture of membranes greater than or equal to 18 hours, and mothers with genital tract infections, intrapartum fever greater than or equal to 38 °C (100.4 °F), GBBHS bacteriuria during pregnancy, or previous birth of an infant with invasive GBBHS infection. Chapter 38 discusses this problem and the management of the disease in infants.

Non-Group A or B Streptococci

These organisms are associated with invasive disease of all age groups. They may cause UTIs, endocarditis, respiratory disease, skin soft tissue infection, pharyngitis, and meningitis in newborns, older children, and adults. The incubation period and communicability times are unknown. Culture and antimicrobial susceptibility are essential. The habitats in humans differ as a result of resistance issues. Generally penicillin G is adequate (AAP, 2006).

TUBERCULOSIS

Tuberculosis (TB) is caused by *M. tuberculosis* and is a very slow-growing organism, taking from 3 to 6 weeks to grow on solid media. This organism is spread primarily by droplet contamination from coughing, sneezing, laughing, and singing. Fomite transmission is uncommon.

Epidemiology

Asymptomatic children and adolescents who are foreign-born account for a large pool of potential transmitters. Individuals with the highest incidence are primarily of low socioeconomic status, have poor nutrition, lack health care, live in crowded living conditions, and have ethnic minority status. Approximately 85% of children in the U.S. with TB are African American, Hispanic, Asian, or Native American. Investigative studies show that infectivity rate is low from children with primary TB (Starke, 2004, AAP, 2006).

The age at the time of infection is predictive of the extent an infection will evolve into disease. Infants and children less that 5 years old account for 60% to 70% of pediatric cases, whereas infection is much less likely to progress to disease in those 5 to 14 years old (Starke, 2004). Male-to-female incidence is the same in preadolescents but changes to a ratio that favors more females in the adolescent years.

Incubation Period

The incubation period is 2 to 12 weeks. Risk for developing tuberculosis disease is highest in the first 6 months to 2 years after infection. Droplets can stay suspended in the air for hours. Infection is defined as converting from a negative to a positive tuberculin skin test. The skin test is reactive within 2 to 12 weeks after initial infection (median 3 to 4 weeks) (AAP, 2006). After appropriate treatment is started, infectivity is believed to cease after several weeks.

Clinical Findings

Table 23-12 describes the stages of TB in children and requisite management strategies.

Primary Pulmonary Tuberculosis. Most children 3 to 15 years old with primary pulmonary TB are asymptomatic when first noted to have a positive TB skin test. However, some may have symptoms that include low-grade fever, cough, malaise, decreased appetite, weight loss, night sweats, chills, erythema nodosum, and phlyctenular keratoconjunctivitis (a hypersensitivity reaction marked by elevated clear nodules with surrounding hyperemia near the limbus). Approximately 25% to 30% of children have extrapulmonary TB symptoms (Munoz & Starke, 2004).

In children under 10 years old, there is usually minimal cough and little expulsion of bacilli; therefore, there is less contagion from these children. There is potential for infection after reactivation of pulmonary TB if cavities or lung infiltrates are present (AAP, 2006).

Enlarging lymph nodes can encroach on mediastinal structures, causing compression, obstruction, or erosion. Compression on the esophagus causes dysphagia or aspiration. Major arteries and veins can also be compressed by enlarging nodes with resulting edema. Superior vena cava syndrome can occur.

Fistulas can occur between the lymph node and the bronchial lumen and cause fibrosis, bronchiectasis, and pneumonia. Recurrent cough, stridor, and wheezing are signs of increasing pulmonary infection. Most children do not suffer significant pulmonary infection, and most reinfections resolve even without chemotherapy. However, progressive primary TB does occur in immunosuppressed children. Instead of resolving, the lesions continue to evolve, often involving an entire lobe. Older children and adolescents suffer from upper lobe infiltrates and cavitation. Calcification and lymphadenitis may be minimal.

Miliary Tuberculosis. Infants and children younger than 3 years old may develop miliary TB. During early stages of the disease, bacilli reach the bloodstream directly from the initial focus or by way of the regional lymph nodes. Necrosis and caseation of multiple organs can occur. Lesions are the size of millet seeds; hence the name "miliary" TB. It is also common in very old and immunosuppressed patients, especially those with AIDS. The disease has a precipitous onset. Moderate to high fever is common. Malaise, decreased appetite, weight loss, and fatigue are constitutional symptoms at the outset. Lymphadenopathy, hepatomegaly, splenomegaly, tachypnea, dyspnea, rales, wheezes, and stridor are often found on physical examination. Other signs and symptoms are present, depending on which organs are involved.

Diagnostic Studies. Generally, chest radiographs are negative or show localized, nonspecific infiltrates. Hilar adenopathy suggest TB, but culture of the organism is essential to establish the diagnosis. Children greater that 5 years old and adolescents can produce sputum after induced to cough with aerosolized hypertonic saline. When age or ability to produce sputum is a factor, an early morning gastric aspirate analyzed by fluorescent staining is an effective and sensitive testing method. Other tests can employ DNA probes, nucleic acid amplification for respiratory tract specimens. Radiography may show calcification (from walled off and caseous lesions), especially in untreated cases and/or a segmental lesion (appears fan-shaped) at the site of the primary pulmonary focus (more common in younger children). Acid-fast bacilli stains and histologic examination for acid-fast bacilli can be helpful. If isolate from the index case is confirmed as TB, culture material does not need to be obtained from the child. However, if the child has HIV infection, is immunocompromised, drug-resistant TB is suspected, or the child has extrapulmonary symptoms, a culture is necessary (AAP, 2006).

TABLE 23-12 The Stages of Tuberculosis in Children			
	Stage		
	Exposure	**Infection**	**Disease**
Skin test	Negative	Positive	Positive (90%)
Physical examination	Normal	Normal	Usually abnormal*
Chest radiograph	Normal	Usually normal†	Usually abnormal‡
Treatment	If <5 years old	Always	Always
Number of drugs	One	One	Three or four

*Up to 50% of older children with pulmonary TB have a normal physical examination.
†Calcification or a small granuloma are considered infection, not disease.
‡Some children with extrapulmonary TB have a normal chest radiograph.
From Starke JR: Tuberculosis. In Gershon AA, Hotez PJ, Katz SL: *Krugman's infectious diseases in children,* St Louis, 2004, Mosby, Table 39-1.

TST is based on the delayed hypersensitivity to *M. tuberculosis* antigens. The test usually becomes positive 2 to 12 weeks after infection with the bacilli. The preparation currently available for skin testing is the Mantoux. This test uses 0.1 ml of 5 tuberculin units (TU) of purified protein derivative (PPD). It is injected intradermally into the volar surface of the forearm, producing a wheal.

Tuberculin skin tests (often referred to as "PPDs") are read 48 to 72 hours later by experienced health care professionals. The induration is measured, not the erythema. Pediatric patients are considered at high risk for TB if they meet any of the following medical risk criteria:

- Contact with adults who have suspected or confirmed TB
- Immigrants and travelers returned from, or in contact with indigenous people, from TB-prevalent parts of the world (Asia, Middle East, Africa, Latin America, countries formally part of the Soviet Union)
- Clinical signs suggestive of TB on chest radiograph or other clinical evidence
- HIV positive or have an immunosuppressive disorder
- Other risk factors, including Hodgkin disease, lymphoma, diabetes mellitus, chronic renal failure, or malnutrition
- Incarcerated adolescents
- Residents of homeless shelters or some medically underserved, low-income populations, such as African, Hispanic, Native Americans
- A Mantoux skin test is defined as positive if the following reactions occur:
- Induration (larger than 15 mm) in children 4 years or older without any risk factors
- Induration (larger than 10 mm) in children younger than 4 years old or with medical risk factors as listed previously
- Induration (larger than 5 mm) in children who are household contacts of active or previously active TB cases and who are themselves suspected of having TB because of either a chest radiograph consistent with active or previously active TB or clinical findings of TB diagnosed with immunosuppressive disorders or HIV infection (AAP, 2006)

Skin testing is not always valid. Ten percent to 15% of children with positive cultures can have a negative skin test. This decreased reactivity can also occur in immunocompromised patients, infants younger than 6 months old, BCG recipients, those with poor nutrition, and those with miliary TB or early TB infection, HIV, or concomitant infection (measles, varicella, influenza). Patients sensitized to nontuberculous mycobacteria can cross-react and have a less than 10-mm sized reaction to the TST. BCG cross-reaction has been discussed previously. High-risk groups and patients living in areas where TB is endemic or on the rise should be skin tested yearly. Low-risk groups do not need to be routinely tested (AAP, 2006).

Differential Diagnosis

The provider should consider TB for patients with symptoms of basilar meningitis, hydrocephalus, cranial nerve palsy, or stroke. Permanent neurologic dysfunction can result and has a worse prognosis in infants than in toddlers and older children. The differential diagnosis includes mycotic infections, staphylococcal pneumonia, sarcoidosis, chronic pneumonia, and Hodgkin lymphoma. Differential diagnosis in lymph node disease includes cat-scratch disease, tularemia, toxoplasmosis, tumor, brachial cysts, cystic hygroma, and pyogenic infection.

Management

A TB specialist should be consulted. The AAP (2006) recommends drugs and treatment regimens based on the disease state, as listed in Tables 23-13 and 23-14. Pyridoxine is not routinely recommended for children and adolescents. It is recommended for use in those individuals whose diets are either limited in meat or milk, in those with HIV, in breastfeeding infants and their mothers, and for pregnant adolescents (AAP, 2006). For children with pleural and pericardial effusion, corticosteroids may be used to decrease the inflammation that is detrimental to organ function; its use also decreases mortality rates and neurologic disability. Prednisone is dosed at 1–2 mg/

TABLE 23-13 Commonly Used Drugs for Tuberculosis

Drug	Daily Dose	Twice-Weekly Dose
Isoniazid (I)	10 mg/kg prevention (max: 300 mg daily); 10-15 mg/kg treatment (max: 300 mg daily); available as syrup or tablets; crushed tablet is more palatable than the syrup	20-30 mg/kg/dose (max: 900 mg/dose)
Rifampin (R)	10-20 mg/kg (max: 600 mg daily); available as syrup or tablets	10-20 mg/kg/dose (max: 600 mg/dose)
Pyrazinamide (Z)	20-40 mg/kg (max: 2000 mg); tablets only	50 mg/kg/dose (max: 2000 mg/dose)
Streptomycin (S)	20-40 mg/kg (max: 1000 mg); IM only	....
Ethambutol (E)	15-25 mg/kg (max: 2500 mg); tablets only	50 mg/kg/dose (max: 2500 mg/dose)
Ethionamide	15-20 mg/kg/24 hours in 2-3 divided doses (max 1000 mg); tablets	....

Isoniazid and rifampin now come in a combination preparation (Rifamate): isoniazid 150 mg/rifampin 300 mg. Another preparation (Rifater) combines isoniazid 50 mg/rifampin 120 mg/pyrazinamide 300 mg.
IM, Intramuscular; *max,* maximum.

TABLE 23-14   Drug Treatment Regimens for Tuberculosis in Infants, Children, and Adolescents

Type of TB Illness	Isoniazid (I)	Rifampin (R)[a]	Pyrazinamide (Z)	Streptomycin (S)
Prophylaxis, no disease				
• Isoniazid susceptible	Daily for 9 mo[b]			
• Isoniazid resistant		Daily for 6 mo[c]		
• If resistant to both I and R, consult TB specialist				
Pulmonary and extrapulmonary disease (miliary, lymph node, bone joint infection)[d] due to *M. tuberculosis* (if due to *M. bovis*, treatment is different)	Daily for 2 mo, then 2-3 times weekly for 4 mo[e] OR 2-3 times/wk for 2 mo under DOT then 2-3 times weekly for 4 mo under DOT[e]	Daily for 2 mo, then 2-3 times weekly for 4 mo[e] OR 2-3 times/wk for 2 mo under DOT then 2-3 times weekly for 4 mo under DOT[e]	Daily for 2 mo 2-3 times/wk for 2 mo under DOT	A fourth drug (ethambutol or an aminoglycoside) may be prescribed until drug resistance is known.
• Hilar adenopathy only	Daily for 6 mo	Daily for 6 mo		
Meningitis (treat for a total of 9-12 mo) due to *M. tuberculosis. M. bovis* requires a different regimen.	Daily for 2 mo, then once daily or twice weekly for 7-10 mo	Daily for 2 mo, then once daily or twice weekly for 7-10 mo	Daily for 2 mo	[f]Daily for 2 mo or can use ethionamide. If suspect drug resistance to streptomycin, substitute with kanamycin, amikacin, or capreomycin.[f]

[a] Rifampin resistance is more likely to occur in those with HIV infection.
[b] DOT twice a week can be used for 9 mo if daily therapy cannot be achieved for prophylaxis.
[c] DOT twice a week can be used for 6 mo if daily therapy cannot be achieved for prophylaxis.
[d] Treatment recommendations are in constant flux; it is advised that providers consult a pediatric TB specialist before initiating treatment for any type of TB infection to ensure that the most current treatment is prescribed; different regimens will be used if child also has concurrent HIV infection.
[e] Directly observed therapy (DOT) is desirable.
[f] This fourth drug is given until drug susceptibility is known.
Boxes indicate that these drug regimens are given concurrently.
mo, Month(s); *wk,* week(s).
Data from American Academy of Pediatrics (AAP): *Red book: 2006 report of the Committee on Infectious Diseases, 2006,* ed 27, Elk Grove Village, IL, 2007, American Academy of Pediatrics, p 686; Munoz FM, Starke JR: Mycobacterial infections: tuberculosis (*Mycobacterium tuberculosis*). In Behrman RE et al, editors: *Nelson textbook of pediatrics,* ed 17, Philadelphia, 2004, WB Saunders; Robinson LG, El-Sadr WM: Tuberculosis. In Burg F et al, editors: *Current pediatric therapy,* ed 18, Philadelphia, 2006, WB Saunders.

kg/24 hours divided into 1 to 2 doses PO for 4 to 6 weeks, then tapered appropriately (AAP, 2006). New combination therapies that could shorten the length of treatment are in clinical trials (Brunell, 2006g).

Complications

The following complications can occur:

Chronic Reactivation Pulmonary Tuberculosis. This complication is a progression of the primary disease. It is most common in those who had their initial infection after 7 years of age. Symptoms include fever, anorexia, malaise, night sweats, weight loss, productive cough, hemoptysis, and chest pain. Full recovery is excellent with appropriate treatment. It can be highly contagious.

Lymph Node Disease. This is an extrapulmonary form of TB affecting the superficial lymph nodes. It can be caused by drinking raw milk contaminated with *M. bovis* or after initial infection with *M. tuberculosis*. The head, trunk, neck, inguinal, and lower extremity nodes are firm (but not hard), fixed to underlying tissue, and nontender. The lymphadenopathy is usually unilateral at first and can progress to multinode involvement. TST is usually positive; a chest x-ray is normal 70% of the time. The diagnosis can be made by culturing node tissue biopsies, but the organism is found in only about 50% of cases.

Pleural Effusion. This frequently occurs in primary disease. It is caused by an extension of the bacillus into the pleural space by subpleural foci or hematogenous spread, or both. It usually occurs 6 months to years after the primary infection. It is infrequent to rare in children under 6 years old (Munoz & Starke, 2004). Symptoms include abrupt onset of low to high fever, shortness of breath, chest pain on deep inspiration, and decreased breath sounds. Response to treatment takes several weeks; radiographic changes can continue to be evident for months following treatment. Scoliosis can be a complication.

Tuberculous Meningitis. This is the most serious complication of TB. It generally follows primary pulmonary disease in 0.3% of untreated infants and young children 6 months to 4 years old. Meningeal infection is also common in miliary TB. Bacilli migrate to the subarachnoid space. Caseous lesions can enlarge, encapsulate, and form a tuberculoma that can act just like any other CNS mass lesion. Symptoms can evolve slowly or rapidly; infants and children generally experience rapid onset. TST is negative in 50% of cases, with 20% to 50% of cases also having negative chest x-rays (Munoz & Starke, 2004). Diagnosis is via CSF culture. Symptoms include fever, malaise, irritability, drowsiness, decreased developmental milestones, nuchal rigidity, positive Kernig or Brudzinski signs, hypertonia, vomiting, seizures, and other neurologic symptoms. The provider should consider TB in the differential diagnosis for any child who has basilar meningitis and hydrocephaly, cranial nerve palsy, or stroke without other apparent cause. Tuberculoma (brain tumor presenting as headache, fever, seizure) is also possible in children.

Skin Tuberculosis. This variant is rare in the U.S. and occurs in 1% to 2% of all TB cases. It occurs in two forms: (1) the TB chancre and (2) multiple skin lesions resulting from hematogenous spread. Those at high risk include those with HIV, those with poor hygiene, and those who are malnourished.

Ocular Tuberculosis. Bacilli usually reach the eye by hematogenous spread. Infected upper respiratory secretions can spread to the cornea, sclera, and conjunctiva by sneezing or by contaminated fingers. Yellow-gray nodules appear at the posterior pole or palpebral conjunctiva. Coalescence of the nodules can form small ulcers. Phlyctenular conjunctivitis, small jelly-like gray nodules seen on the conjunctiva, is the result of a hypersensitivity reaction.

Hematogenous Spread of Tuberculosis to Other Organs or Body Systems. Spread can be to endocrine and exocrine glands, urogenital tract, heart and pericardium, skeleton, abdomen, tonsils, adenoids, larynx, middle ear, and mastoids.

▄▄▄ TEMPERATURE AND FEVER

Fever is defined as an abnormally elevated body temperature with a temperature of 100.4° F (38° C) or higher. Fever results from a resetting of the hypothalamic heat regulatory center or when heat production exceeds heat loss. Peripheral warm and cold neurons and the temperature of blood circulating in the hypothalamus act on the heat regulatory center to keep the human body at a preset core temperature of 98.6° F (37° C). Axillary temperature may be 1° F (36.4° C) lower. Body temperature is lower in the morning and peaks in the late afternoon. In children more than 2 years old, normal temperature fluctuations can range 1.4° F to 2° F (0.8° C to 1.2° C). Those under 2 years old maintain fairly unwavering temperatures.

The human body generates heat by metabolic processes (increased cellular metabolism, muscle activity, and involuntary shivering). Heat conservation is maintained by vasoconstriction and heat preference behaviors. Heat loss occurs by sweating, evaporation, conduction, radiation, convection, vasodilation, and cold preference behaviors. These factor inputs are integrated by the thermoregulatory neurons (Powell, 2004a).

The normal hypothalamic set-point is altered by many different agents. Febrile illnesses in neonates are usually the result of congenital infections, those acquired at delivery (late-onset group B streptococcal infection), those acquired in the nursery (especially premature infants), those acquired at home (pneumococcal or meningococcal infection), or those acquired as a result of anatomic or physiologic dysfunction (e.g., renal). Other causes of fever in children are related to bacterial and viral infections, vaccines, biologic agents, tissue damage, malignancy, drugs, collagen-vascular disorders, endocrine disorders, inflammatory disorders, and other disease states. Temperatures higher than 105.8° F (41° C) are rarely of infectious origin but are due to CNS dysfunction (e.g., malignant hyperthermia, drug fever, heat stroke). Fever-causing agents produce endogenous pyrogens that reset the hypothalamic center. This process takes approximately 90 minutes. Clinically, this means that blood cultures should be obtained before the fever spikes because there would be a greater bacterial or fungal yield.

The incidence of fevers above 106° F (41.2° C) in emergency departments is 0.05%. A temperature of 107° F (41.6° C) or higher is considered a harmful fever and has the potential complication of death or brain damage if not treated (Adam, 2001). The increased metabolic processes can exacerbate problems in children with chronic illness.

Fever is the most common presenting complaint in pediatric practice. There are two situations that are particularly worrisome for any provider: fever without a source or focus in infants and young children, and fever of unknown origin. Each of these situations is discussed separately, and guidelines for their management are given.

FEVER WITHOUT FOCUS IN INFANTS AND YOUNG CHILDREN

Managing fever without an identifiable source in infants and young children is a challenge. The assessment of the child who has an acute fever often involves a careful investigation for a source of infection. Children between birth and 24 months old are at greatest risk for unsuspected bacteremia; it is less common in those older than 36 months.

Etiology

Table 23-15 provides a list of the most common pathogens causing bacteremia in young infants (see also Chapter 38 for management of sepsis).

History

The following should be included in the history of the illness:
- Duration and degree of fever (fever documented at home by reliable caregiver should be considered accurate)

TABLE 23-15 **Age-Related Causes of Serious Bacterial Infections in Very Young Infants***

Bacteremia/Meningitis

<1 mo	Group B streptococcus
	E. coli (and other enteric gram-negative bacilli)
	Listeria monocytogenes
	S. pneumoniae
	H. influenzae
	S. aureus
	N. meningitidis
	Salmonella spp.
1-3 mo	*S. pneumoniae*
	Group B streptococcus
	N. meningitidis
	Salmonella spp.
	H. influenzae
	L. monocytogenes

Osteoarticular Infections

<1 mo	Group B streptococcus
	S. aureus
1-3 mo	*S. aureus*
	Group B streptococcus
	S. pneumoniae

Urinary Tract Infection

0-3 mo	*E. coli*
	Other enteric gram-negative bacilli
	Group D streptococcus (including *Enterococcus* species)

* In decreasing order of frequency.
From Shapiro ED: Fever without localizing signs. In Long SS, Pickering LK, Prober CG: *Principles and practice of pediatric infectious diseases,* ed 2. Philadelphia, 2003, Churchill Livingstone, Table 15-1.

- Possible associated symptoms: vomiting, diarrhea, respiratory symptoms, rash (especially petechiae or purpura)
- Change in play activities
- Irritability, inconsolability
- Lethargy (level of consciousness characterized by poor or absent eye contact or failure to recognize parents or interact with persons or objects in the environment)
- Review of known exposures (family illness, contacts with other ill children, day care contacts)
- Recent vaccination
- Recent travel history
- Past medical history of malignancy, splenectomy, shunt, indwelling catheter, immunologic disorders, recurrent bacterial infections, serious bacterial infection
- Neonatal history of complications, prior antibiotics, prior surgeries, hyperbilirubinemia
- Chronic illness
- Current medications, including antipyretics and antibiotics
- Immunization history with HIB conjugate and pneumococcal conjugate vaccines

Risk Criteria
High Risk (Feld, 2006).
- Any febrile infant younger than 1 month old; any toxic-appearing child regardless of age
- Infant 1 to 3 months old who is toxic appearing
- Infant 1 to 3 months old with a rectal fever of 102.2° F (39° C)
- Infant 1 to 3 months old with a chronic illness or underlying condition with unreliable caretakers, who was premature, with WBC count greater than 15,000 or stool greater than 5 WBCs per high-power field (hpf), or catheterized spun urine sediment with greater than 10 WBC/hpf.

Low Risk (Feld, 2006).
- Infant 1 to 3 months old with a rectal fever greater than 100.4° F (38° C) but less than 102.2° F (39° C) or infant or child 3 to 36 months old with a rectal fever greater than 102.2° F (39° C) who is nontoxic-appearing with a history of previously being healthy and with a nonfocal bacterial infection. Continue with the work-up even if an infant under 3 months old has otitis media.
- Infant 3 to 6 months old with rectal temperature greater than 100.4° F (38° C) but less than 102.2° F (39° C) who does not appear ill.
- Infant or child 3 to 36 months old who appears mildly ill with rectal temperature greater than 102.2° F (39° C) and fewer than 15,000 WBCs; stool fewer than 5 WBCs/hpf if diarrhea present; catheterized urinalysis spun sediment of less than 10 WBC/hpf; negative chest x-ray if cough present.

Laboratory Studies. A negative, low-risk ambulatory work-up is characterized by the following laboratory results:
- CBC with WBC count below 15,000/mm^3, fewer than 1500 bands/mm^3
- Blood culture—no growth in 48 hours (72 hours for those immunocompromised or if fungal infection suspected in the neonate)
- Catheterized urinalysis (fewer than 10 WBCs/hpf spun sediment, negative leukocytes and nitrites)
- When diarrhea is present, fewer than 5 WBCs/hpf in stool
- If cough is present, a negative chest x-ray

Differential Diagnosis
The differential diagnosis includes the following:
- Upper respiratory tract disease, such as viral URI, otitis media, and sinusitis
- Lower respiratory tract disease, such as bronchiolitis and pneumonia
- Gastrointestinal disease, primarily bacterial, or gastroenteritis
- Musculoskeletal infections, such as cellulitis, septic arthritis, and osteomyelitis
- Urinary tract infection
- Bacteremia from pneumococci (11% incidence, which is a decrease of 94% in children less than 5 years old from between 1999 and 2003) (CDC, 2005d), HIB, meningococci (4%), group A and B streptococci, salmonella (5% to 10%), and *S. aureus*.

Management
Research studies and analysis of data have established practice guidelines for the outpatient management of infants and

children from 0 to 36 months old with fever without focus. General practice guidelines include the following management strategies (Fig. 23-5) (Feld, 2006):

- Refer all toxic-appearing 0- to 36-month-old infants and children to an emergency department for lumbar puncture and possible parenteral antibiotic therapy after prompt laboratory work-up.
- Febrile infants younger than 4 weeks old, regardless of whether they meet the low-risk criteria identified previously, should have a sepsis evaluation (culture of CSF, blood, and catheterized or suprapubic urine specimen; a CBC and differential; and

complete analysis of the CSF) and hospitalization for parenteral antibiotics.

- Infants 28 to 90 days old who appear nontoxic and meet the low-risk criteria listed previously can be managed as outpatients using the algorithm illustrated in Fig. 23-5. Febrile infants 28 to 90 days old who do not meet the laboratory low-risk criteria should be hospitalized.
- Infants between 3 and 6 months old with fever greater than 100.4° F (38° C) but less than 102.2° F (39° C) and who appear nontoxic may be managed using the algorithm illustrated in Fig. 23-5.

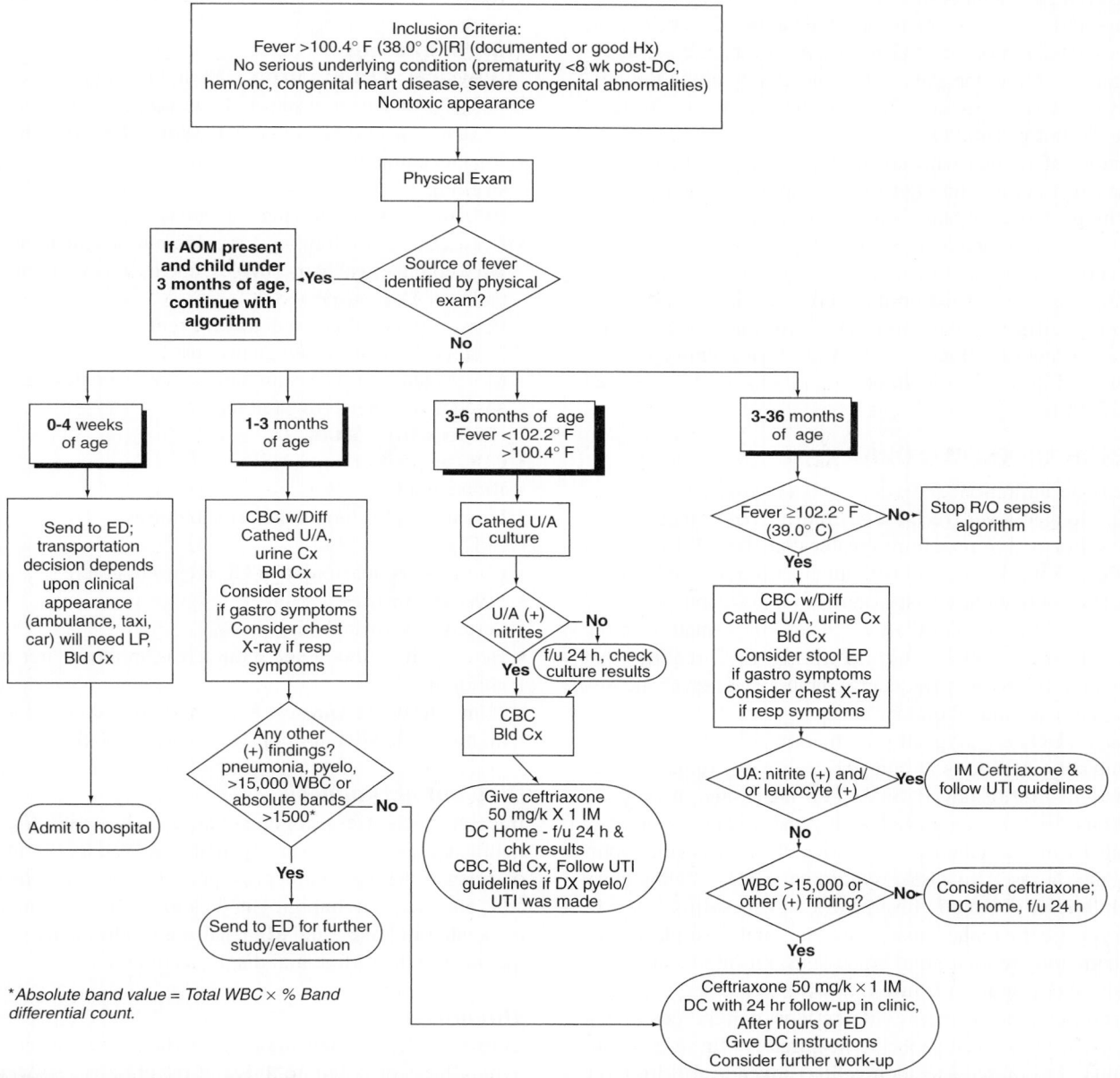

FIG. 23-5 Fever without focus algorithm. *Hx,* History; *R,* rectal; *DC,* discharge; *AOM,* acute otitis media; *ED,* emergency department; *LP,* lumbar puncture; *Bld Cx,* blood culture; *EP,* enteric pathogens (culture); *w/diff,* with differential; *Cx,* culture; *Pyelo,* pyelonephritis; *WBC,* white blood cell count; *Cathed,* catheterized; *U/A,* urinalysis; *f/u,* follow-up; *h,* hours; *IM,* intramuscularly; *chk,* check; *UTI,* urinary tract infection; *Dx,* diagnosis; *Resp,* respiratory; *hem/onc,* hematologic/oncology issue. (Modified from Children's Hospital and Health Center: *R/O sepsis algorithm,* San Diego, 1998, Children's Hospital and Health Center; Meltzer AJ, Powell KR, Avner JR: Fever in infants and children. In Feld LG, Hyams JS, editors: *Consensus in pediatrics,* Evanston, IL, 2005, Mead Johnson.)

- Refer all toxic-appearing children to the emergency department for further work-up and treatment.
- Children 3 to 36 months old with rectal fevers greater than 102.2° F (39° C) and who appear nontoxic can be managed as outpatients using the aforementioned algorithm (Fig. 23-5). Return for visit appointment in 24 hours, if the fever persists longer than 48 hours, or the child is worse.

An important point to remember in treatment is that bacteremia can be an occult infection in young infants and children (i.e., nontoxic-appearing patient whose blood culture is positive for a pathogenic organism). A useful axiom to remember is that the higher the WBC count and the greater the absolute number of neutrophils or bands, the greater the risk of bacteremia in a febrile child. Remember that all toxic-appearing infants under 28 days old need immediate hospitalization. Others require further evaluation or hospitalization. Also remember that the younger the infant, the greater the uncertainty about the possibility of a serious bacterial infection, and the greater the need to rule out this possibility.

Parents of infants who are managed as outpatients need detailed instructions on signs and symptoms that indicate a worsening of their infant's illness. Instruct parents to bring their infant in immediately if any of these signs and symptoms appear: change in or new rash; duskiness, cyanosis, or mottling; coolness of extremities; poor feeding or vomiting; irritability; difficulty in comforting or arousing; seizure activity (eye rolling or jerking of extremities); or bulging anterior fontanelle. Careful follow-up of such infants must be ensured (Feld, 2006).

FEVER OF UNKNOWN ORIGIN

The classic definition of *fever of unknown origin* (FUO) is (1) a prolonged fever (rectal temperature greater than 101° F [38.3° C] or oral temperature greater than 100° F [37.8° C]) for at least 3 weeks or more without an etiology, that includes 3 weeks of outpatient visits, extensive studies, and continued fevers and (2) no etiology after 1 week of evaluation in the hospital (Powell, 2004b). A child with an FUO requires that the health care provider frequently rethink and reevaluate historical, clinical, and laboratory data.

Many FUOs are atypical presentations of common disorders, notably infections or connective diseases (e.g., juvenile rheumatoid arthritis [JRA], SLE). Few are exotic. In the U.S., infectious diseases associated with most diagnoses of FUO are caused by salmonellosis, TB, rickettsial diseases, syphilis, Lyme disease, Kawasaki syndrome, CSD, inflammatory bowel disease, rheumatic fever, IM, CMV, hepatitis, coccidioidomycosis, histoplasmosis, malaria, and toxoplasmosis. Less common are tularemia, brucellosis, rat-bite fever, leptospirosis, and drug fever (Powell, 2004b).

In children under 6 years old, the most common causes of FUO are UTI or pyelonephritis, respiratory illnesses, localized infections (abscess, osteomyelitis), juvenile arthritis (JA), and, rarely, leukemia. In adolescents the most common causes include TB, inflammatory bowel disease, autoimmune disorders, lymphoma, and the causes listed for children under 6 years old (Powell, 2004b).

The approach to evaluating a child with an FUO should include a detailed history, a thorough physical examination, and screening laboratory studies.

History
- Careful analysis of symptoms or signs, a meticulous review of systems, history of the fever pattern, and patient's age
- Past medical history of recurrent infections, surgery, transfusions, and contact with ill individuals or exposure to wild and domestic animals
- Medication use and family medical history, including autoimmune disease or inflammatory bowel disorder
- History of pica; history of travel, returning home with travel souvenirs containing dirt, rocks, or earth-contaminated artifacts

Clinical findings
Physical Examination. Skin findings (e.g., rashes, lesions), presence or absence of sweating
- Local or generalized lymphadenopathy or hepatosplenomegaly
- Joint examination and palpation of bones for tenderness, swelling
- Palpation of sinus and mastoid areas
- Eye examination looking for palpebral or bulbar conjunctivitis, conjunctival hemorrhages, and ophthalmologic examination if JA is suspected
- Pelvic examination in adolescent females
- Rectal examination and guaiac test
- Mouth and throat examination for exudates, erythema, absence of fungiform papillae
  Laboratory Studies.
- CBC with differential, ESR
- Blood and CSF
- Urinalysis plus blood and urine cultures
- PPD
- Chest, sinus, mastoid, and GI tract radiographs
- Liver chemistries
- Serum protein analysis
- Heterophil antibody and antinuclear antibody titer in older children

Other tests may involve bone marrow, radionuclide scans, total body CT, MRI, or biopsies (Powell, 2004b).

Differential Diagnosis
Infectious diseases, collagen-vascular disease (JA, SLE), malignancies, drug fever (typically secondary to ingestion of phenothiazines, antidepressants, atropine, amphetamine, and other anticholinergic medications), nosocomial, HIV-associated illnesses, and Munchausen syndrome by proxy are included in the differential diagnosis of an FUO.

Management
Consider hospitalizing the child if there is evidence of systemic illness or failure to thrive, if the child is very young, or if the parents' anxiety is extreme. Otherwise, the child should be followed up with frequent visits, documented fever pattern, and other specialized tests if screening tests indicate the need or if other physical findings develop. Empirical use of

antibiotics should be avoided unless the child has possible disseminated TB (Powell, 2004b).

HELMINTHIC ZOONOSES

DESCRIPTION

Domesticated dogs, cats, and wild animals kept as pets can be infected with intestinal helminth parasites. Mild to severe illness can result when a helminth is transmitted to children by fecal contamination. With more than half of households in the U.S. having one or more pets, close contact is inevitable (American Veterinary Medical Association, 2002). Helminth zoonoses (transmitted from animal to a human host) are briefly presented, and the most common infections known to occur in children are discussed.

Transmission of zoonotic infections can occur by several routes:

- Direct infection by ingestion of eggs or the penetration of larvae into the body (infections, such as tapeworms and roundworms, are acquired from their eggs; hookworms penetrate the skin)
- Indirect infection by ingestion of larvae in food (e.g., fish, meat, snails, freshwater shrimp, land crabs)
- Exposure to an intermediary vector (e.g., mosquito, flies, fleas, ticks)

Helminth larvae can live for extended periods of time in human and animal organs and tissues, causing an inflammatory condition referred to as toxocariasis or larva migrans (LM). LM can affect many organs and tissues within the body. When LM has been identified, the resulting clinical syndrome produced is classified as visceral, ocular, neural, cutaneous, or covert toxocariasis and noted as asymptomatic or clinically inapparent infection.

The true incidence of LM is unknown because it is not reportable in the U.S. Some studies within the U.S. have shown a range of prevalence rates of *Toxocara canis* (dog) seropositivity in asymptomatic individuals of 3% to 54%. The rates vary depending on location and socioeconomic factors (Nash, 2005).

Different species of roundworms and hookworms found in dogs, cats (as a result of *T. catis*), and raccoons are common causes of LM in humans. Dogs carry the most common cause of zoonotic infection worldwide *(T. canis)*. Young puppies under 3 months old have been known to carry this roundworm; however, dogs of any age can harbor the parasite. Another infection, *Baylisascaris procyonis*, is being increasingly seen in young children who are in contact with raccoons. *T. cati* causes less LM than *T. canis*. The LM from this infestation can lead to a fatal or severe neurologic disease.

Eosinophilia can be a common finding with invasive helminth infections. With migration of the helminth to the intestinal lumen, eosinophil counts are normal or slightly raised. Migration through internal or viscera organs causes the count to be more markedly elevated; the degree of eosinophilia will wane if the helminth completes its migration cycle or is able to wall itself off and prevent provoking a host eosinophilic response (Nash, 2005).

Prevention of zoonotic infections includes identifying possible sources of exposure, referral of pets to veterinarians for testing, decontamination of soiled environments, and prevention of further exposure. The latter intervention includes education about safe pet fecal cleanup, the regular deworming of pets, good hand washing, behavioral modification in cases of pica and geophagia, and covering sandboxes when not in use. Information should be provided to families with pets, especially puppies, kittens, and raccoons, about having them tested for helminth infestations. Communities should be encouraged to promote leash laws and responsible pet ownership (cleaning up pet fecal waste), to disallow dogs from playgrounds and parks where children play, and to restrict open access to sandboxes.

TOXOCARA CANIS

Epidemiology

Infection with *T. canis* can cause zoonotic visceral LM (VLM), ocular LM (OLM), and, in severe cases, neural LM (NLM). Ingestion of these hardy eggs can occur from contact with contaminated soil (in sandboxes, parks, playgrounds, schoolyards, public places where dogs have visited), hands, food, and fomites, such as toys. Once the eggs are ingested and hatched, the larvae can penetrate the intestines and migrate to the liver and lungs and other tissues of the body. With initial or mild infections, the larvae seem to be able to reach other locations, such as the brain and eye, more easily. NLM syndrome can result, which may be mild (subtle neurologic or behavior changes) to severe (CNS involvement). Children under 6 years old (average 2 years old) are most commonly affected by VLM; OLM can occur in children and young adults. Infected patients do not pass eggs or larvae in their excreta.

Clinical Findings

History. Assess for history of pica or geophagia; exposure to dogs, cats, or environments where animals are known to frequent; and recent travel, fever, abdominal pain, hepatomegaly, or respiratory symptoms (cough, wheezing, asthma, pneumonia). In the case of OLM, there may be no history of pica or symptoms of VLM.

Physical Examination.

- OLM: posterior or peripheral subretinal mass, decreased vision, strabismus, or leukokoria; patient may be asymptomatic
- Covert toxocariasis
- Abdominal pain, hepatomegaly, splenomegaly, anorexia, nausea, vomiting
- Lethargy; sleep and behavior changes
- Coughing, wheezing
- Fever
- Cervical adenitis
- Limb pain
- Possible urticaria, nodules

Diagnostic Studies

- CBC reveals leukocytosis, marked eosinophilia, hypergammaglobulinemia, elevated blood group isohemagglutinin titers. In mild disease only eosinophilia may be evident.
- OLM: From a specimen of vitreous-aqueous fluid, elevated *T. canis* antibody titers (ELISA with confirmatory Western blot test) are seen when compared with serum titers.

- Chest x-ray shows radiographic changes in some cases.
- CT and MRI may be used to detect granulomatous lesions in OLM.

Differential Diagnosis

Ascaris lumbricoides, *Baylisascaris procyonis*, schistoso-miasis, and *Fasciola hepatica* are included in the differential diagnoses.

Management

Toxocariasis should be considered in any child with non-specific symptoms, notably recurrent abdominal pain, reactive airway disease, or allergies of unknown cause. A normal eosinophilia count should not predispose the provider from ruling out this infection, if suspected.

Most individuals do not require treatment because they recover spontaneously. A pediatric infectious disease expert should be consulted for treatment recommendations. Management for those with brain, lung, or heart complications is based on controlling inflammatory reactions (corticosteroids and antihistamines) and trying appropriate antihelmintic therapy (rates of successful treatment with antihelmintics are mixed) (Nash, 2005). Antihelmintic medications include albendazole, thiabendazole, mebendazole, diethylcarbamazine and others. OLM may be more responsive to albendazole or thiabendazole. Family pets need evaluation by a veterinarian.

■ INFECTIOUS AGENTS USED IN BIOTERRORISM

Since September 2001, the U.S. has become more aware of a potential threat of infectious diseases acquired through biologic warfare. Most of these diseases have not been seen in clinical practice settings. The most anticipated of these agents are discussed.

Children are at particular risk for exposure to and absorption of biologic agents (e.g., anthrax and botulinum toxin). Factors that predispose them to such risk include being within closer proximity to the ground, having faster ventilation rates and thinner skins, having an increased risk of dehydration, and having greater undeveloped cognition.

Agents of biologic warfare are categorized by the CDC according to their potential for aerosol transmission, susceptibility of the population, degree of person-to-person transmission, expected high morbidity and mortality rates, the likelihood for delayed diagnosis, and the lack of effective and efficacious treatments. Agents at highest risk to the populace are known as *category A weapons of bioterrorism*. These include specific bacteria, viruses, botulinum toxin, *Bacillus anthracis* (anthrax), *Francisella tularensis* (tularemia), variola virus (smallpox), and viruses of hemorrhagic fever (Ebola, Marburg, Lassa fever).

Providers can help their communities in the early detection and prompt large-scale medical response by developing an awareness of syndromes and symptoms that might suggest a biologic warfare agent exposure. They can also join other health care providers in developing pediatric readiness plans. These readiness plans should include: triage; isolation, treatment, and care facilities; transportation; communication; housing; and the establishment of vaccination clinics on a massive scale for children, especially in communities where health departments and/or emergency departments may not have the procedural skills to address a severely ill pediatric population. Health alerts can be requested by e-mail from the CDC. Consult the Resource Box at the end of the chapter.

Table 23-16 includes a full discussion of each agent.

ANTHRAX

Anthrax is found naturally in soil, surviving as long as 40 years in that medium. It has traditionally been known as woolsorters' disease as a result of inhaling the spore-forming gram-positive rod after exposure to hides, wool, or other animal products during processing. It has been largely eliminated in developed countries secondary to the anthrax vaccine for animals. Three forms have been identified: cutaneous, inhalation, and gastrointestinal. Symptoms can appear within 7 days of infectivity with the bacteria (7 to 14 days for the inhalation form). Refer to Table 23-16 for the symptoms associated with each form of anthrax.

If appropriate treatment is not started within 48 hours after the onset of symptoms, the mortality rate can reach 95%. Prophylaxis is effective if administered as soon as possible after exposure. Doxycycline, amoxicillin, penicillin (if the organism is sensitive), levofloxacin, and ciprofloxacin are recommended agents. Amoxicillin is recommended for children younger than 12 years old. Currently, all of the anthrax vaccine is held by the U.S. Department of Defense and cannot be obtained by the private sector; the vaccine might become part of a preventive program in case of a large community exposure (CDC, 2006g). Cephalosporins and trimethoprim-sulfamethoxazole are contraindicated because of known anthrax resistance.

BOTULINUM TOXIN

The poison protein molecules that make up botulinum toxin are secreted by vegetative cells of *Clostridium botulinum* bacteria. These substances are the most toxic poison known to exist in a natural state. There are seven strains designated A through G. Each strain has its own exotoxin; any strain can prove deadly. This gram-positive, spore-forming bacillus occurs naturally in soil and is anaerobic. Infection is generally via a food-borne route. Food is heated high enough to drive off dissolved oxygen but not high enough to destroy all of the *C. botulinum* spores. Any surviving spores germinate and begin producing their exotoxins. Canned vegetables, fish, and marine mammals can serve as such vehicles. Other avenues of infection with *C. botulinum* include the GI tract (because of overgrowth), wound infections, and aerosol exposure from a laboratory accident or terrorism. It is not contagious or spread by person-to-person contact; symptoms are similar despite the mode of exposure. Symptoms begin approximately 12 to 36 hours after exposure but can range from 6 hours to 14 days (CDC, 2006h). See Table 23-16 for symptoms and laboratory analysis.

TABLE 23-16   **Agents of Bioterrorism**

Disease	Signs and Symptoms	Incubation Time (Range)	Person-to-Person Transmission	Isolation	Diagnosis	Postexposure Prophylaxis for Children and Adolescents (see Appendix A for dosing)	Treatment in Children and Adolescents (see Appendix A for dosing)
Anthrax *(B. anthracis)*							
• Inhalation	Flulike symptoms (fever, fatigue, muscle aches, dyspnea, nonproductive cough, headache), chest pain; possible 1-2 day improvement then rapid respiratory failure and shock. Meningitis may develop.	1-6 days (up to 6 weeks)	None	Standard precautions	Chest x-ray evidence of widening mediastinum; obtain sputum and blood culture. Sensitivity and specificity of nasal swabs unknown—do not rely on for diagnosis.	Prophylaxis for 60 days: Amoxicillin* Doxycycline Ciprofloxacin *Alternative:* Ofloxacin or levofloxacin or gatifloxacin	Penicillin G* Amoxicillin* Ciprofloxacin *Alternative:* Ofloxacin or levofloxacin or gatifloxacin
• Cutaneous	Intense itching followed by painless papular lesions, then vesicular lesions, developing into eschar surrounded by edema.	1-12 days	Direct contact with skin lesions may result in cutaneous infection	Contact precautions	Peripheral blood smear may demonstrate gram-positive bacilli on unspun smear with sepsis.		
• Gastrointestinal (GI)	Abdominal pain, nausea and vomiting, severe diarrhea, GI bleeding, and fever.	1-7 days	None	Standard precautions	Culture blood and stool.		
Botulism *(Blostriduim botulinum)*	Afebrile, excess mucus in throat, dysphagia, dry mouth and throat, dizziness, then difficulty moving eyes, mild pupillary dilation and nystagmus, intermittent ptosis, indistinct speech, unsteady gait, extreme symmetric descending weakness, flaccid paralysis; generally normal mental status.	Inhalation: 12-80 hours Food-borne: 12-72 hours (2-8 days)	None	Standard precautions	Laboratory tests available from CDC or Public Health Department; obtain serum, stool, gastric aspirate, and suspect foods before administering antitoxin. Differential diagnosis includes polio, GBS, myasthenia, tick paralysis, stroke, meningococcal meningitis.	Pentavalent toxoid (types A, B, C, D, E) may be available in the future One 10-mL vial trivalent botulism antitoxin IV	Botulism antitoxins Supportive care Ventilation **Avoid clindamycin and amino-glycosides**

Continued

TABLE 23-16 **Agents of Bioterrorism—Cont'd**

Disease	Signs and Symptoms	Incubation Time (Range)	Person-to-Person Transmission	Isolation	Diagnosis	Postexposure Prophylaxis for Children and Adolescents (see Appendix A for dosing)	Treatment in Children and Adolescents (see Appendix A for dosing)
Pneumonic plague (Y. pestis)	High fever, cough, hemoptysis, chest pain, nausea and vomiting, headache. Advanced disease: purpuric skin lesions, copious watery or purulent sputum production; respiratory failure in 1-6 days.	2-3 days (2-6 days)	Yes, droplet aerosols	Droplet precautions until 72 hours of effective antibiotic therapy	A presumptive diagnosis may be made by Gram, Wayson, or Wright stain of lymph node aspirates, sputum, or cerebrospinal fluid with gram-negative bacilli with bipolar (safety pin) staining.	Doxycycline Ciprofloxacin	Streptomycin Gentamycin *Alternatives:* Doxycycline or ciprofloxacin
Smallpox (variola virus)	Prodromal period: malaise, fever, rigors, vomiting, headache, and backache. After 2-4 days, skin lesions appear and progress uniformly from macules to papules to vesicles and pustules, mostly on face, neck, palms, soles, and subsequently progress to trunk.	12-14 days (7-17 days)	Yes, airborne droplet nuclei or direct contact with skin lesions or secretions until all scabs separate and fall off (3-4wk)	Airborne (includes N95 mask) and contact precautions	Swab culture of vesicular fluid or scab, send to BL-4 (Biologic Level 4) laboratory. All lesions are similar in appearance and develop synchronously, as opposed to chickenpox. Electron microscopy can differentiate variola virus from varicella.	Ideally, early vaccine within 3-5 days if available depending upon CDC guidelines	Supportive care, vaccinations within 72 hours of rash; possible use of cidofovir
Tularemia	Fever, headache, acute inflammation, pharyngitis.	2-10 days (average 2-6 days)	No	Standard precautions blood: antibody	Respiratory secretions and titers (>four-fold increase). Light microscopy and fluorescent-labeled antibody.	Streptomycin Gentamicin Amikacin Doxycycline Ciprofloxacin	Streptomycin Gentamicin Amikacin Doxycycline Ciprofloxacin Imipenem-cilastin Chloramphenicol
• Ulceroglandular	Skin papules, granulomatous lesions with necrotic, caseous areas.						

Form	Clinical signs and symptoms	Incubation	Diagnosis	Transmission/Precautions	Vaccine	Treatment
• Oculoglandular	Edematous/inflamed conjunctiva with yellow nodules, ulcers or palpebral conjunctiva/sclera. Cervical/submaxillary/preauricular lymphadenopathy.					
• Typhoidal	Fever >102° F (39.4° C), chills, headache, aches, vomiting, photophobia, hepatosplenomegaly, exanthems on upper extremities (+/− face and neck), diarrhea.					
• Pneumonic	Respiratory symptoms of pneumonia or pleuritis.		Pneumonic: x-ray findings of lobar/subsegmental infiltrates, hilar adenopathy, pleural effusion, atypical infiltrates.			
Hemorrhagic fevers • Crimean-Congo • Dengue • Ebola and Marburg • Hanta pulmonary syndrome • Lassa fever	Generally: fever, muscle aches, dizziness, malaise, weakness. exhaustion, +/− rash, +/− headache. With disease progression: ecchymosis, bleeding from orifices with GI symptoms, can lead to shock, delirium, seizures, renal failure.	Depends on agent Crimean: 2-10 days Ebola/ Marburg: 3-9 days Dengue: 2-7 days Lassa: 6-17 days	Serology of specific viral techniques.	Ebola and Lassa only via blood or body fluids. Mask, contact, and standard precautions, depending on agent; DEET for mosquito-bite resistance	No vaccines available	Supportive: ribavirin therapy may be useful for some agents in certain cases

*If strains are sensitive.

Modified from North Carolina Statewide Program for Infection Control and Epidemiology (SPICE): *Bioterrorist agents, 2002.* Available from University of North Carolina website: *www.unc.edu/depts/spice/chart* (accessed Feb 24, 2007); Centers for Disease Control and Prevention (CDC): *General fact sheets on specific bioterrorism agents.* Available at *www.bt.cdc.gov/bioterrorism/factsheets* (accessed Feb 24, 2007c).

Preventive prophylaxis after exposure and active treatment excludes the use of antibiotics but includes careful use of passive immunization with equine antitoxin for adults. Skin testing before the use of the sera is imperative. Treatment involves administering botulism antitoxin (stored by CDC) and ventilatory support to arrest the progression of paralysis as soon as possible. Prophylaxis consists of the administration of neutralizing antibody in the bloodstream. Equine botulinum antitoxin or specific human hyperimmune globulin can confer passive immunity. Botulinum toxoid can induce endogenous immunity. Any known aerosolized exposure requires the immediate cleaning or disposal of clothes and thorough cleansing and rinsing of skin and hair.

PNEUMONIC PLAGUE

Infection with the *Yersinia pestis* organism manifests in three forms: bubonic, pneumatic, and septicemic. In the fourteenth century, catastrophic epidemics caused by the bubonic form occurred in Europe. The scourge was referred to as the "black death" or "great pestilence." Today, small outbreaks occur around the world. Bubonic is the most common form and is acquired from infected fleas or rats. Pneumonic form is acquired from aerosolized droplets, and septicemic plague results from direct contact with infected animals (hides or secretions) or people (secretions). The pneumonic form is an anticipated biologic warfare agent. The concern is that an antibiotic-resistant strain of pneumonic *Y. pestis* would be used (CDC, 2005e). The pneumonic form is also the most invasive and pathogenic; the mortality rate can be greater than 50% in untreated cases as a result of respiratory failure, shock, and death.

Management depends on rapid diagnosis. Exposure to plague plus either a temperature of 101.2° F (38.5° C) or the new onset of a cough necessitates starting antibiotic therapy. Therapy would preferably begin within 24 hours after the first onset of symptoms or within 7 days after a possible exposure. Asymptomatic people with known exposure should also start antibiotic prophylaxis for 1 week. Unfortunately, the symptoms at the onset of pneumonic plague suggest a respiratory infection. Individuals may not seek treatment until the more advanced symptoms of plague appear.

See Table 23-16 for additional specifics about this agent. There is no vaccine for pneumonic plague. The agent can be successfully controlled with the use of health education and environmental treatment (sunlight and heat, rodenticides). In a known terrorist attack, the CDC would provide guidance as to which antibiotic is to be used after they have tested the implicated agent for sensitivity (results should be back within 24 to 48 hours).

SMALLPOX

There are two virus variants that cause smallpox, variola major and variola minor. Two of the four types of variola minor are particularly fatal (flat and hemorrhagic). The last known naturally acquired case in the world occurred in 1977. The virus is spread from person to person via virus-containing aerosolized droplets from saliva that are then inhaled by exposed persons.

Such droplets can also remain viable for up to 1 week on bedding, clothing, and other surfaces. Those most at risk have been within 6 feet of an infected person.

Historically, unimmunized patients with smallpox suffered an average fatality rate of 30% (AAP, 2006). The disease is not transmittable before the appearance of the rash. The infected person is sometimes contagious in the prodromal stage but fully contagious with the appearance of the rash and for the next week. When the rash reaches the mouth and pharyngeal areas, the transmission rate is especially high. Until all of the scabs have fallen off, the virus has the potential to spread (CDC, 2004a).

Smallpox is anticipated to be a formidable warfare agent because of the propensity for its rash to resemble that of chickenpox and to be dismissed as such. If delivered in an aerosolized form in a terrorist attack, the agent is projected to have a 90% mortality rate within the first 24 hours. However, the astute provider will be able to distinguish the two diseases by the pattern of symptoms preceding the rash. See Fig. 23-2 for the distinguishing differences that aid diagnosis as compared with the features of scarlet fever and varicella.

Laboratory diagnosis can be made by DFA, electron microscopy, or PCR from fluid obtained from the lesions. Management involves interrupting the mode of transmission: isolation of those infected, and isolation and vaccination of contacts and those exposed to the contacts. This approach to epidemiologic control is referred to as "search and containment" or "ring" vaccination. Public health experts are still undecided whether to embrace this more selective ring approach or vaccinate on a mass level if an outbreak should occur. See the prior discussion regarding the smallpox vaccine. Once the rash has occurred, the vaccine would not be helpful to that individual (CDC, 2004b).

There is no known, effective treatment for active smallpox infection. Antibiotics for secondary infections and supportive therapy are the mode of treatment. Antivirals may be attempted (although they are not known to be effective) and include cidofovir, adefovir dipivoxil, cyclic cidofovir, and ribavirin. See Table 23-16.

TULAREMIA

The etiologic agent in tularemia is *F. tularensis*. The organism is a small, aerobic, gram-negative bacterium without toxins. Tularemia is also known as "rabbit fever" and "deer fly fever." Small amounts of the bacteria are highly virulent. Two strains have been identified that occur in the U.S.: strain B (the reservoir includes water-dwelling rodents), and the more virulent strain A (the reservoir includes rabbits, dog, and wood tick). Most cases of tularemia occur in the southern U.S. Without antibiotic treatment, strain A has been known to have a wide-ranging mortality rate (less than 1% to 30%) (Schutze & Jacobs, 2004).

F. tularensis is found in and on soil, water, and vegetation and can be endemic in wild mammals (rabbits, hares, squirrels, voles, mice, water rats). It is spread from animal to animal and animal to human by direct contact with an infected animal or its environment (e.g., nests or sharing an ecologic niche) or by a bite from an infected tick, mosquito, or deer fly that has bitten another infected animal. It is more commonly acquired by hunters and outdoorsmen; it is a particular concern of laboratory workers handling the agent.

The agent enters humans via the cutaneous or mucous membrane routes and invades phagocytes and macrophages. If used as a biologic warfare agent, it may be spread in aerosol form and may be absorbed by the eye or respiratory system. It can also be transmitted by contaminated food or water. Oculoglandular (presents as injected conjunctiva); oropharyngeal (from ingestion and may mimic diphtheria); typhoidal (systemic tularemia with symptoms of fever and sepsis); gastrointestinal (presents as diarrhea and abdominal pain); and pneumonic (rapidly fatal with inhalation) refer to the different forms of the infection.

Successful treatment entails prompt diagnosis of this rare disease. Any suspicious atypical pharyngitis, ulcer at the site of a tick bite, atypical pneumonia, pleuritis, and hilar lymphadenopathy would be clues. Commonly the illness involves fever, headache, chills, myalgia, and fatigue. The differential diagnosis for pulmonary tularemia includes psittacosis, legionellosis, Q fever, mycoplasma and *C. pneumoniae* infections, anthrax, and plague. Laboratory diagnosis is made from blood and respiratory secretions by detecting agglutinating antibodies. PCR analysis may be available. Should a confirmed mass outbreak occur, streptomycin, gentamicin, and amikacin for 7 to 10 days would be the preferred choices for severe disease. Doxycycline, ciprofloxacin, imipenem-cilastin or chloramphenicol may be considered for less severe illness (AAP, 2006). Beta-lactam antibiotics are ineffective. Response is generally seen within 48 hours. The mortality rate is about 3% as a result of pneumonia or to the typhoidal form of the disease. The FDA is reviewing a vaccine against the disease, but it is not currently available in the U.S. See Table 23-16.

VIRAL HEMORRHAGIC FEVERS

There are five families of viral hemorrhagic fevers:
- Arenavirus: Lassa fever, Argentine hemorrhagic fever, Bolivian hemorrhagic fever, Sabia-associated hemorrhagic fever, Venezuelan hemorrhagic fever, lymphocytic choriomeningitis
- Bunyavirus: Crimean-Congo hemorrhagic fever, Hantavirus pulmonary syndrome, hemorrhagic fever with renal syndrome, Rift valley fever
- Filovirus: Ebola, Marburg
- Flavivirus: Tick-borne encephalitis, Omsk hemorrhagic fever, Kyasanur Forest disease viruses
- Paramyxivirus: Hendra virus encephalitis, Nipah virus

Most are spread from infected animal hosts or arthropod vectors (zoonotic); severity of illness ranges from mild to life threatening (23% to 100% mortality rate range). The animal host is often specific to individual viruses. Humans may contract the viruses where these hosts and vectors are found. Infection is usually from contact with the host or vector urine, saliva, or feces. Human-to-human contact can occur from direct contact or indirect contact with bodily fluids or fomites, such as infected needles. If used as a biologic agent (such as with Ebola or Marburg), it is expected to be distributed in an aerosol form to infect the human vascular system. Incubation would show some variation depending upon the agent. Typically, it would be 5 to 10 days (2 to 19 day range) with the development of pleuropneumonitis in the following days. Generally, symptoms would involve fever, headache, myalgia, nausea, vomiting, abdominal pain, diarrhea, cough, chest pain, pharyngitis, maculopapular rash on the trunk (5 days after other symptom onset), petechiae, ecchymoses, and hemorrhages (CDC, 2001).

Prevention focuses on:
- Avoiding direct and indirect contact with those known to be infected
- Employing barrier infectious control techniques
- Isolating infected individuals

In the U.S. the CDC is encouraging control of rodent populations, rapid diagnostic testing, and is stockpiling supportive treatment medications. Further information is available from the CDC website. Diagnosis is anticipated to be from serologic testing or from virologic techniques.

$\mathcal{R}$ESOURCE BOX

Infections Diseases

Advisory Committee on Immunization Practices
www.cdc.gov/vaccines/recs/acip

AIDS information
www.hivatis.org
U.S. Department Health and Human Services

American Academy of Pediatrics
www.aap.org

Association of State and Territorial Health Officials
www.astho.org

CDC Biological Warfare Agent Health Alerts
www.cdc.gov
Available by e-mail request from www.healthalert@cdc.gov

CDC Vaccine Adverse Event Reporting System (VAERS)
www.vaers.hhs.gov
1-800-822-7967

CDC Vaccine Shortages and Prioritization Information
www.cdc.gov/nip/news/shortages

Food and Drug Administration Vaccine Adverse Event Report System (VAERS)
www.fda.gov/cber/vaers/vaers.htm

International Lyme and Associated Diseases Society
www.ilads.org

✓**DISCUSSION FORUM**

1. A new immigrant, who is a healthy 5-year-old, comes for his health care maintenance visit. The family does not have any documentation of prior vaccines. How do you proceed? Are there any vaccines that he no longer needs? Can he be given Pediatrix or is he too old? What resources are available within your community for patients to get vaccines at no cost?

2. A healthy 43-day-old comes in for a health care maintenance visit. What is the minimum age for vaccines. Would you give vaccines today? Why or why not? If the family planned on traveling to Pakistan in 1 week, would that change your decision? How do you respond to a family's concerns about the variety of diseases that are attributed to vaccines?

3. Do all states require prenatal HIV screening? What are the issues about universal screening? How do the new CDC guidelines about HIV screening affect your practice?

4. What is the role of the primary care provider in preventing infections in day care centers?

5. Many viruses have different manifestations. Name at least four viruses and their different manifestations

6. What is the local plan for emergency preparedness within your community? Within your state?

REFERENCES

Adam H: Management of fever. In Hoekelman R: *Primary pediatric care,* ed 4, St Louis, 2001, Mosby.

Alper BS: Influenza, *Clin Adv* 8(11):119-120, 2005.

American Academy of Pediatrics (AAP): *Red Book: 2006 report of the Committee on Infectious Diseases,* ed 27, Elk Grove Village, IL, 2006, American Academy of Pediatrics.

American Journal of Nurse Practitioners Editorial Staff: CDC immunization recommendations, *Am J Nurse Pract* 6(3):9-12, 2002.

American Veterinary Medical Association: *US pet ownership and demographics sourcebook,* Schaumburg, IL, 2002.

Bauchner H, Pelton SI, Klein JO: Parents, physicians, and antibiotic use, *Pediatrics* 103(2):395-401, 1999.

Beasley RP: Nature usually favors females, *J Infect Dis* 192:1865-1866, 2005.

Becquet R et al: Acceptability of exclusive breast-feeding with early cessation to prevent HIV transmission through breast milk, ANRS 12011202 Ditrame Plus, Abidjan, Cote d'Ivoire, *J Acquir Immune Defic Syndr* 40(5):600-608, 2005.

Black SA et al: *Postmarketing assessment of Prevnar, 7-valent pneumococcal conjugate vaccine (PCNV7).* Poster #181. Presented at 2006 Pediatric Academic Societies' Annual Meeting, April 29-May 2, 2006, San Francisco.

Black SA et al: Impact of the use of heptavalent pneumococcal conjugate vaccine on disease epidemiology in children and adults, *Vaccine* 24(Suppl 2):S2-79-80, 2006a.

Black SA, Shinefield H: Meningococcal disease. In Burg FD et al, editors: *Current pediatric therapy,* ed 18, Philadelphia, 2006b, WB Saunders.

Borkowsky W, Krugman S: Viral hepatitis: A, B, C, D, E, and newer hepatitis agents. In Gershon AA, Hotez PJ, Katz SL: *Krugman's infectious diseases in children,* St Louis, 2004, Mosby.

Borkowsky W: Acquired immunodeficiency syndrome and human immunodeficiency virus. In Gershon AA, Hotez PJ, Katz SL: *Krugman's infectious diseases in children,* St Louis, 2004, Mosby.

Brooks GF, Butel JS, Morse SA: *Jawetz, Melnick, & Adelberg's medical microbiology,* ed 23, NY, 2004, The McGraw-Hill Companies, Inc.

Brunell PA, editor: New hepatitis recommendations issued, *Infect Dis Child* 19(7):4-5, 2006a.

Brunell PA, editor: FDA advisory committee recommends Gardasil, *Infect Dis Child* 19(6):1-49, 2006b.

Brunell PA, editor: Cervarix cervical cancer vaccine highly immunogenic in women of all ages, *Infect Dis Child* 19(9):36, 2006c.

Brunell PA, editor: Mumps outbreak 2006: evaluating vaccine efficacy complicated by disease's characteristics, *Infect Dis Child* 19(6):4-5, 2006d.

Brunell PA, editor: Rotavirus vaccine: is it worth doing? *Infect Dis Child* 19(8):4-5, 2006e.

Brunell PA, editor: AAP provides revised recommendations to reduce adolescent HIV caused by illicit drugs, *Infect Dis Child* 19(3):70-71, 2006f.

Brunell PA, editor: New TB therapy offers potential shorter treatment, *Infect Dis Child* 19(2):79, 2006g.

Burrascano JJ: *Advanced topics in Lyme disease; diagnostic hints and treatment guidelines for Lyme and other tick borne illnesses,* Sept 2005. Available from *www.ilads.org/burrascano* (accessed Feb 19, 2007).

Burroughs M et al: Respiratory infections. In Gershon AA, Hotez PJ, Katz SL: *Krugman's infectious diseases in children,* St Louis, 2004, Mosby.

Byington CL: Enteroviruses. In Burg FD et al, editors: *Current pediatric therapy,* Philadelphia, 2006, WB Saunders.

Centers for Disease Control and Prevention (CDC): Recognition of illness associated with the intentional release of a biologic agent, *MMWR Morb Mortal Wkly Rep* 50(41):893-897, 2001.

Centers for Disease Control and Prevention (CDC): Guideline for hand hygiene in health-care settings: recommendations of the Healthcare Infection Control Practices Advisory Committee and the HICPAC/SHEA/APIC/ IDSA Hand Hygiene Task Force, *MMWR Morb Mortal Wkly Rep* 51(RR16):1-44, 2002.

Centers for Disease Control and Prevention (CDC): Decline in annual incidence of varicella-selected states, 1990-2001, *MMWR Morb Mortal Wkly Rep* 52:884-885, 2003.

Centers for Disease Control and Prevention (CDC): *Smallpox disease overview,* last modified Dec 30, 2004a. Available from *www.bt.cdc.gov/agent/anthrax/needtoknow* (accessed Feb 24, 2007).

Centers for Disease Control and Prevention (CDC): *What you should know about a smallpox outbreak,* last modified Dec 29, 2004b. Available from *www.bt.cdc.gov/agent/anthrax/needtoknow* (accessed Feb 24, 2007).

Centers for Disease Control and Prevention (CDC), Advisory Committee on Immunization Practices: Direct and indirect effects of routine vaccination of children with 7-valent pneumococcal conjugate vaccine on incidence of invasive pneumococcal disease-United States, 1998-2003, *MMWR Morb Mortal Wkly Rep* 54(36):893-897, 2005a.

Centers for Disease Control and Prevention (CDC): Poliovirus infections in four unvaccinated children—Minnesota, Aug-Oct 2005, *MMWR Morb Mortal Wkly Rep* 54:1053-1055, 2005b.

Centers for Disease Control and Prevention (CDC): Antiretroviral post-exposure prophylaxis after sexual, injection-drug use, or other non-occupational exposure to HIV in the United States, *MMWR Morb Mortal Wkly Rep* 54(RR2):1-20, 2005c.

Centers for Disease Control and Prevention (CDC): Direct and indirect effects of routine vaccination of children with 7-valent pneumococcal conjugate vaccine on incidence of invasive pneumococcal disease—United States, 1998-2003, *MMWR Morb Mortal Wkly Rep* 54(MM36):893-897, 2005d.

Centers for Disease Control and Prevention (CDC): *Frequently asked questions (FAQ) about plague,* last modified April 5, 2005e. Available from *www.bt.cdc.gov/agent/anthrax/needtoknow* (accessed Feb 24, 2007).

Centers for Disease Control and Prevention (CDC), Advisory Committee on Immunization Practices: Prevention of hepatitis A through active or passive immunization expands hepatitis, *MMWR Morb Mortal Wkly Rep* 55(RR07):1-23, 2006a.

Centers for Disease Control and Prevention (CDC), Advisory Committee on Immunization Practices: Recommended adult immunization schedule—United States, Oct 2006-Sept 2007, *MMWR Morb Mortal Wkly Rep* 55(40):Q1-Q4, 2006b.

Centers for Disease Control and Prevention (CDC), Advisory Committee on Immunization Practices: Prevention and control of influenza, *MMWR Morb Mortal Wkly Rep* 55(RR-10):1-48, 2006c.

Centers for Disease Control and Prevention (CDC): *What you should know about a smallpox outbreak,* last reviewed Feb 21, 2006d. Available from *www.bt.cdc.gov/agent/smallpox/basics/outbreak* (accessed Mar 23, 2007).

Centers for Disease Control and Prevention (CDC): Enterovirus surveillance—United States, 1970-2005, *MMWR Morb Mortal Wkly Rep* 55 (SS08): 1-20, 2006e.

Centers for Disease Control and Prevention (CDC): Epidemiology of HIV/AIDS—United States, 1981-2005, *MMWR Morb Mortal Wkly Rep* 55(21):589-592, 2006f.

Centers for Disease Control and Prevention (CDC): *Anthrax: what you need to know,* last reviewed Feb 22, 2006g. Available from *www.bt.cdc.gov/agent/anthrax/needtoknow* (accessed Feb 24, 2006).

Centers for Disease Control and Prevention (CDC): *Botulism facts for health care providers,* modified April 19, 2006h. Available from *www.bt.cdc.gov/agent/anthrax/needtoknow* (accessed Feb 24, 2007).

Centers for Disease Control and Prevention (CDC): *The nasal-spray flu vaccine (live attenduated influenza vaccine [LAIV].* Last modified Sept 19, 2007a. Available from *www.cdc.gov/flu/about/qa/nasalspray.htm* (accessed Oct 20, 2007).

Centers for Disease Control and Prevention (CDC): *Varicella Active Surveillance Project (RASP).* Available at *www.cdc.gov/nip/diseases/surv/rasp* (accessed Mar 23, 2007b)

Centers for Disease Control and Prevention (CDC): *Noroviruses: Q and A.* Available at *www.cdc.gov/ncided/diseases/submenus/sub_norwalk.htm* (accessed Feb 12, 2007c).

Curry MP, Chopra S: Hepatitis: acute viral hepatitis. In Mandell GL, Bennett JE, Dolin R: *Mandell, Douglas, and Bennett's principles and practice of infectious diseases,* Philadelphia, 2005, Elsevier/Churchill Livingston.

Darden PM, Gustafson KK, Jacobson RM: *Patient-held vaccination records: do they eliminate racial disparities in vaccination?* Abstract #3140.6. Presented at the 2006 Annual Meeting of the Pediatric Academic Societies, April 30, 2006, San Francisco.

Demas P et al: Maternal adherence to the zidovudine regimen for HIV-exposed infants to prevent HIV infection: a preliminary study, *Pediatrics* 110(3):e35, 2002.

Department of Health and Human Services (DHHS): *Vaccines for Children Program,* Dec 2004. Available at *www.cdc.gov/nip/vfc* (accessed Oct 8, 2006).

Domachowske J: *Human metapneumovirus,* updated Feb 24, 2006. Available at *www.emedicine.com/ped* (accessed Feb 12, 2007).

D'Souza Y, Fombonne E, Ward BJ: No evidence of persisting measles virus in peripheral blood mononuclear cells from children with autism spectrum disorder, *Pediatrics* 118(4):1664-1675, 2006.

Feld LG: Fever in infants and children from birth to 3 yrs. In Burg FD et al, editors: *Current pediatric therapy,* ed 18, Philadelphia, 2006, WB Saunders.

Fredrickson DD et al: Childhood immunization refusal: provider and parent perceptions, *Fam Med* 36:431-439, 2004.

Garbutt J et al: Empiric first-line antibiotic treatment of acute otitis in the era of the heptavalent pneumococcal conjugate vaccine, *Pediatrics* 117(6): e1087-1094, 2006.

Global HIV Prevention Working Group: *New approaches to HIV prevention: accelerating research and ensuring future access,* Aug 2006. Available at *www.kff.org/hivaids/hiv081506pkg.cfm* (accessed Mar 25, 2007).

Grassia T: Exclusion from child care recommended for certain diseases, *Infect Dis Child* 18(12):1, 10-11, 2005.

Gums JG: Redefining appropriate use of antibiotics, *Am Fam Physician* 69(1):35, 39-40, 2004.

Gwaltney JM: Upper respiratory tract infections: the common cold. In Mandell GL, Bennett JE, Dolin R: *Mandell, Douglas, and Bennett's principles and practice of infectious diseases,* Philadelphia, 2005, Elsevier/Churchill Livingston.

Hall CB: Human herpesvirus 6,7, and 8. In Gershon AA, Hotez PJ, Katz SL: *Krugman's infectious diseases in children,* St Louis, 2004, Mosby.

Hasty MB et al: Cutaneous community-associated methicillin-resistant *Staphylococcus aureus* among all skin and soft-tissue infections in two geographically distant pediatric emergency departments, *Acad Emerg Med* 14(1):35-40, 2007.

Havens PL and Committee on Pediatric AIDS: Postexposure prophylaxis in children and adolescents for nonoccupational exposure to human immunodeficiency virus, *Pediatrics* 111(6):1475-1489, 2003.

Heilmann C et al: Reduced antibody responses to vaccinations in children exposed to polychlorinated biphenyls, *PLoS Med* 3(8):e11, 2006.

Hsiao AL, Baker MD: Fever in the new millennium: a review of recent studies of markers of serious bacterial infection in febrile children, *Curr Opin Pediatr* 17(1):56-61, 2005.

Institute of Medicine (IOM): *Immunization safety review: vaccines and autism,* Washington DC, National Academies Press, 2004.

Johannsen EC, Schooley RT, Kaye KM: Epstein-Barr virus (infectious mononucleosis). In Mandell GL, Bennett JE, Dolin R: *Mandell, Douglas, and Bennett's principles and practice of infectious diseases,* Philadelphia, 2005, Elsevier/Churchill Livingston.

John CC, Schreiber JR: Therapies and vaccines for emerging bacterial infections: learning from methicillin-resistant S*taphylococcus aureus, Pediatr Clin North Am* 53(4):699-713, 2006.

Kalvaitis K: New rotavirus vaccine well-tolerated in studies, *Inf Dis Child* 19(9):31, 2006.

Kaplan SL: Community-acquired methicillin-resistant *Staphylococcus aureus* infection in children, *Semin Pediatr Infect Dis* 17(3):113-119, 2006.

Katz BZ, Miller G: Epstein-Barr virus infection. In Gershon AA, Hotez PJ, Katz SL: *Krugman's infectious diseases in children,* St Louis, 2004, Mosby.

Koch WC: Parvovirus B19. In Behrman RE et al, editors: *Nelson textbook of pediatrics,* ed 17, Philadelphia, 2004, WB Saunders.

Krey MS, editor: *Meningococcal disease: a new strategy for improved prevention,* Baylor College of Medicine sponsored publication, Haymarket Medical, 2005.

Lee E, Worsley DF: Role of radionuclide imaging in the orthopedic patient, *Orthop Clin N Am* 37(3):485-501, 2006.

Leroy S et al: Ibuprofen in childhood: evidence-based review of efficacy and safety, *Arch Pediatr* 4(5):477-484, 2007.

Lesko SM: The safety of ibuprofen suspension in children, *Int J Clin Prat Suppl* 135:50-3, 2003.

Lewis P: *MRSA and kids.* Lecture presented at the 2nd Annual Pediatric Review and Update series, Oregon Health and Science University, Dec 1, 2006, Portland, OR.

Long SS, Nyquist AC: Laboratory manifestations of infectious diseases: acute-phase response. In Long SS, Pickering LK, Prober CG, editors: *Principles and practice of pediatric infectious diseases,* ed 2, Philadelphia, 2003, Elsevier/Churchill Livingstone.

Maciosek M et al: Priorities among effective clinical preventive services, *Am J Preventative Med* 31(1):52, 2006.

Magder LS et al: Risk factors for in utero and intrapartum transmission of HIV, *J Acq Imm Def Syn* 38(1):87-95, 2005.

Maheshwari N: How useful is C-reactive protein in detecting occult bacterial infection in young children with fever without apparent focus? *Arch Dis Child* 91(6):533-535, 2006.

Maldonado Y: Measles; subacute sclerosing panencephalitis; rubella; mumps. In Behrman RE et al, editors: *Nelson textbook of pediatrics,* ed 17, Philadelphia, 2004, WB Saunders.

Mast EE et al: Risk factors for perinatal transmission of hepatitis C virus (HCV) and the natural history of HCV infection acquired in infancy, *J Infect Dis* 192:1880-1889, 2005.

McCaig LF, Besser RE, Hughes JM: Trends in antimicrobial prescribing rates for children and adolescents, *JAMA* 287(23):3096-3102, 2002.

Mitchell M: Microbiologic diagnosis of infections. In Finberg L, Kleinman R: *Saunders manual of pediatric practice,* ed 2, Philadelphia, 2002, WB Saunders.

Moore J: PCV7 vaccine use contingent on state funding policy, *Inf Dis Child* 19(8):24, 2006.

Munoz FM, Starke JR: Tuberculosis *(Mycobacterium tuberculosis).* In Behrman RE et al, editors: *Nelson textbook of pediatrics,* ed 17, Philadelphia, 2004, WB Saunders.

Myers MG, Stanberry LR, Seward JF: Varicella-zoster virus. In Behrman RE et al, editors: *Nelson textbook of pediatrics,* ed 17, Philadelphia, 2004, WB Saunders.

Nash TE: Visceral larva migrans and other unusual helminth infection. In Mandell GL, Bennett JE, Dolin R: *Mandell, Douglas, and Bennett's principles and practice of infectious diseases,* Philadelphia, 2005, Elsevier/Churchill Livingston.

National Institute of Allergy and Infectious Diseases: *NIAID research on West Nile Virus,* April 2006. Available at *www.niaid.nih.gov/factsheets/westnile.htm* (accessed Feb 11, 2007).

Nield LS, Kamat DM: Vaccine refusal: when parents just say "no," *Consultant Ped* 5(10):55-58, 2006a.

Nield LS, Kamat DM: Avian flu: why all the squawk? *Consultant* 46(2):241-246, 2006b.

Oregon Department of Human Services: Avian influenza: know when the sky is falling, *CD Summary* 54(26):1-2, 2005a.

Oregon Department of Human Services: Why didn't Noah swat those two mosquitoes? *CD Summary* 54(11):1-2, 2005b.

Oregon Department of Human Services: Hanta helper, *CD Summary* 55(13):1-2, 2006.

Orenstein WA et al: Immunization. In Mandell GL, Bennett JE, Dolin R: *Mandell, Douglas, and Bennett's principles and practice of infectious diseases,* Philadelphia, 2005, Elsevier/Churchill Livingston.

Paavonen J et al: Efficacy of a prophylactic adjuvanted bivalent L1 virus-like-particle vaccine against infection with human papillomavirus types 16 and 18 in young women: an interim analysis of a phase III double-blind, randomised controlled trial, *Lancet 369* (9580):2161-2170, 2007.

Perry RT, Orenstein WA: Measles. In Burg F et al, editors: *Current pediatric therapy,* ed 18, Philadelphia, 2006, WB Saunders.

Pickering LK: Child care and communicable diseases. In Behrman RE et al, editors: *Nelson textbook of pediatrics,* ed 17, Philadelphia, 2004, WB Saunders.

Pittet D et al: Evidence-based model for hand transmission during patient care and the role of improved practices, *Lancet Infect Dis* 6(10):641-52, 2006.

Poehling KA et al: The underrecognized burden of influenza in young children, *N Engl J Med* 355(1):31-40, 2006a.

Poehling KA et al: Invasive pneumococcal disease among infants before and after introduction of pneumococcal conjugate vaccine, *JAMA* 295:1668-1674, 2006b.

Powell K: Fever. In Behrman RE et al, editors: *Nelson textbook of pediatrics,* ed 17, Philadelphia, 2004a, WB Saunders.

Powell K: Fever without focus. In Behrman RE et al, editors: *Nelson textbook of pediatrics,* ed 17, Philadelphia, 2004b, WB Saunders.

Relman DA: Introduction to bacterial disease. In Goldman L, Ausiello D, editors: *Cecil textbook of medicine,* ed 22, Philadelphia, 2004, Saunders.

Richards CA: Think tick-borne disease for summertime flu-like symptoms, *Infect Dis Child* 18(7):28-29, 2005.

Riley L: Barriers to best-practice vaccination in rural areas can be modified, *Infect Dis Child* 19(6):26, 2006.

Rodewald L, Orenstein W: Vaccines for Children Program entitling children to protection, *Infect Dis Child* 19(10):4-5, 2006.

Rosenthal M: H5N1 influenza strain raises concern about a pandemic, *Infect Dis Child* 18(10):18-19, 2005a.

Rosenthal M: CA-MRSA becoming fact of life for some athletes involved in contact sports, *Infect Dis Child* 18(11):52-53, 2005b.

Rosenthal M: Pandemic influenza response: dilemmas of preparedness and equity loom large, *Infect Dis Child* 19(4):7, 2006a.

Rosenthal M: Treatment of skin and soft tissue infections changing in an age of MRSA, *Infect Dis Child* 19(4):52, 2006b.

Rusk J: ACIP recommends IGIV as the best alternative for VZIG, *Infect Dis Child* 18(2):22-23, 2005.

Rusk J: More work needed to increase adolescent vaccination coverage levels, research says, *Infect Dis Child* 19(6):37-38, 2006a.

Rusk J: School-based immunizations for adolescents a possibility, *Infect Dis Child* 19(6):23, 2006b.

Rusk J: Polio kills seven so far in Namibia, *Infect Dis Child* 19(7):63, 2006c.

Rusk J: ACIP discusses how best to prime flu vaccine–naïve children, *Infect Dis Child* 19(8):18, 2006d.

Rusk J: CDC recommends MCV4 deferral, *Infect Dis Child* 19(6):1, 2006e.

Rusk J: Cases of intussusception will happen close to vaccination, *Infect Dis Child* 19(8):23, 2006f.

Sáez-Llorens X, McCracken GH: Meningitis. In Gershon AA, Hotez PJ, Katz SL: *Krugman's infectious diseases in children,* St Louis, 2004, Mosby.

Savely GR: Update on Lyme disease, *Clin Rev* 16(4):45-50, 2006.

Schutze GE, Jacobs RF: Tularemia (*Francisella tularensis*). In Behrman RE et al, editors: *Nelson textbook of pediatrics,* ed 17, Philadelphia, 2004, WB Saunders.

Shapiro ED: Tick-borne diseases: Lyme disease. In Gershon AA, Hotez PJ, Katz SL: *Krugman's infectious diseases in children,* St Louis, 2004, Mosby.

Simoes EA: Polioviruses. In Behrman RE et al, editors: *Nelson textbook of pediatrics,* ed 17, Philadelphia, 2004, WB Saunders.

Snyder J, Pickering L: Viral hepatitis. In Behrman RE et al, editors: *Nelson textbook of pediatrics,* ed 17, Philadelphia, 2004, WB Saunders.

Soysal A et al: Effect of BCG vaccination on risk of *Mycobacterium tuberculosis* infection in children with household tuberculosis contact: a prospective community-based study, *Lancet* 366(9495):1443-51, 2005.

Starke JR: Tuberculosis. In Gershon AA, Hotez PJ, Katz SL: *Krugman's infectious diseases in children,* St Louis, 2004, Mosby.

Stechenberg BW: Bartonella: cat scratch disease. In Behrman RE et al, editors: *Nelson textbook of pediatrics,* ed 17, Philadelphia, 2004, WB Saunders.

Steele RW: *Red Book update.* General session, Thursday, Jan 26, 2006. Presented at Masters of Pediatrics 2006 Leadership Conference, Jan 25-30, 2006, Bal Harbour, FL. Lecture available at *www.mastersofpediatrics. com/cme/cme2006/lecture36_1.asp* (accessed May 27, 2007).

Steinberg I: *MRSA therapeutics: dilemmas of preference and amount.* Presented at the Fifth Pediatric Infectious Disease Society Conference, Oct 9-11, 2005, Napa, CA.

Steinman MA et al: Changing use of antibiotics in community-based outpatient practice, 1991-1999, *Ann Intern Med* 138(7):525-533, 2003.

Stephenson M: FDA advisory committee gives green light to Gardasil, Merck's HPV vaccine, *Infect Dis Child* 19(6):49, 2006a.

Stephenson M: Varicella zoster virus vaccine making a big dent in case rates, *Infect Dis Child* 19(6):31, 2006b.

Stratton K et al, editors: *Immunization safety review: influenza vaccines and neurological complications,* Appendix A. Written for Institute of Medicine. Washington DC, National Academies Press, 2004.

Suskind KL, Murray KR: Viral hepatitis. In Burg FD et al, editors: *Current pediatric therapy,* Philadelphia, 2006, WB Saunders.

Taylor B: Vaccines and the changing epidemiology of autism, *Child Care Health Dev* 32(5):511-519, 2006.

Thior I et al: Breastfeeding plus infant-zidovudine prophylaxis for 6 months vs formula feeding plus infant zidovudine for 1 month to reduce mother-to-child HIV transmission in Botswana: a randomized trial: the Mashi Study, *JAMA* 296(7):794-805, 2006.

Todd, JK: Streptococcal infection. In Gershon AA, Hotez PJ, Katz SL: *Krugman's infectious diseases in children,* St Louis, 2004, Mosby.

Tufts G, Connor Hardman ME: Community-acquired methicillin-resistant *Staphylococcus aureus, Clin Rev* 16(1):52-58, 2006.

Unger J, editor: Bioterrorism: what all primary care practitioners need to know, *Nurs Contact Hours NPs* 2:41-52, 2002.

Voyich J et al: Insights into mechanisms used by *Staphylococcus aureus* to avoid destruction by human neutrophils, *J Immunol* 175:3907-3919, 2005.

Whitley RJ: Varicella-zoster virus. In Mandell GL, Bennett JE, Dolin R: *Mandell, Douglas, and Bennett's principles and practice of infectious diseases,* Philadelphia, 2005, Elsevier/Churchill Livingston.

Wiggs-Stayner KS et al: The impact of mass school immunization on school attendance, *J Sch Nurs* 22(4):219-222, 2006.

World Health Organization (WHO): WHO recommended measures for persons undertaking international travel from areas affected by severe acute respiratory syndrome, *Wkly Epidemiol Rec* 78:97-120, 2003.

World Health Organization (WHO): *Model insert, BCG vaccine,* revised Dec, 2005. Available at *www.who.int* (accessed Sept 25, 2006).

World Health Organization (WHO): *BCG vaccine.* Available at *www.who.int* (accessed Sept 25, 2006).

Wormser et al: The clinical assessment, treatment, and prevention of Lyme disease, human granulocytic anaplasmosis, and babesiosis: clinical practice guidelines by the Infectious Diseases Society of America, *Clin Infect Dis* 43:1089-1134, 2006

Wright P: Parainfluenza viruses. In Behrman RE et al, editors: *Nelson textbook of pediatrics,* ed 17, Philadelphia, 2004, WB Saunders.

Yoger R, Chadwick E: Acquired immunodeficiency syndrome (human immunodeficiency virus). In Behrman RE et al, editors: *Nelson textbook of pediatrics,* ed 17, Philadelphia, 2004, WB Saunders.

Zangwill KM: Influenza virus. In Burg F et al, editors: *Current pediatric therapy,* ed 18, Philadelphia, 2006, WB Saunders.

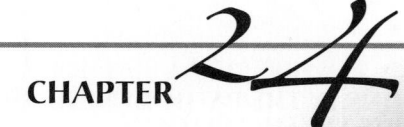

CHAPTER 24

Atopic and Rheumatic Disorders

Catherine J. Goodhue and Margaret A. Brady

Atopic disorders and rheumatic diseases (collagen vascular or connective tissue diseases) of childhood share certain characteristics that lend to their combined discussion in this chapter. Inflammation, chronicity, and genetic predisposition are common to both groups of disorders. The triad of atopic disorders that may or may not coexist consists of atopic dermatitis (AD), allergic rhinitis (AR) (or "hay fever"), and asthma. The two most common childhood rheumatic diseases that primary care providers are likely to encounter are juvenile rheumatoid arthritis (JRA) and systemic lupus erythematosus (SLE). Both are collagen-vascular disorders that have localized or generalized findings marked by inflammation and an autoimmune response.

Fibromyalgia is a rheumatic disease that continues to gain attention in the literature. Brief discussions of this disease, in addition to chronic fatigue syndrome (CFS), are presented. Although the incidence of rheumatic fever has diminished significantly in the U.S., it is still a disease that merits attention by providers. Therefore, a review of its clinical presentation and treatment also is included. The immunopathogenesis and management of Henoch-Schönlein purpura (HSP), the most common vasculitis syndrome of childhood, also are discussed.

◼ PATHOPHYSIOLOGY AND DEFENSE MECHANISMS

ATOPIC OR ALLERGIC DISORDERS

Allergy involves a specific acquired alteration in the body that has an immunologic basis. The union of antigen and antibody creates a cascade of events that culminates in biochemical reactions. There are four types of allergic reactions: I (anaphylactic reactions), II (cytotoxic reactions), III (Arthus-type reactions), and IV (delayed-type hypersensitivity). All four types of allergic reactions are mediated by circulating or cellular antibodies and generally can occur in any individual. Type I involves local and systemic manifestations resulting from an interaction between antigen and tissue cells that have been sensitized with reaginic antibody, generally immunoglobulin E (IgE) (e.g., urticaria and angioedema). Type II involves reactions from antibody interacting with antigenic components on cell surfaces (e.g., hemolytic anemia and transfusion reactions). Type III is characterized by deposition of immune microprecipitates in or around blood vessels. Complement or toxic products are released. A type IV allergic reaction is a delayed-type hypersensitivity interaction involving sensitized lymphocytic cells that results in the release of toxic lymphoid cell products (e.g., tuberculin skin test reactions and contact dermatitis) (Paller & Mancini, 2006).

Atopic disorders are forms of allergic reactivity that occur only in certain susceptible individuals with an unknown and probably genetic predisposition. Environmental factors also play a role in atopy of these individuals who exhibit a hyperresponsiveness in target organs (lungs, skin, or nose). Certain antigens (e.g., cat dander, ragweed) are problematic for atopic individuals but not for others. These atopic individuals become sensitized to the offending allergen, resulting in an atopic disorder.

The development of an atopic disorder or allergic response involves a susceptible individual who is both exposed to an offending antigen and has a predisposition to selective synthesis of IgE when in contact with common environmental antigens. If these conditions are in place and contact with an offending antigen occurs, the following biochemical chain of cascading events unfolds:

- There is a brisk proliferation of T-helper type 2 (Th2) cells that secrete cytokines: interleukin (IL)-3, IL-4, IL-5, IL-9, and IL-13.
- Cytokines are involved in IgE synthesis and activation of eosinophils.
- IgE binds to receptors on mast cells, basophils, and Langerhans cells.
- Chemical mediators that cause biochemical reactions and allergic-related injury to target organs (skin and respiratory tract) are released. Examples of chemical mediators include:
  - Histamine
  - Prostaglandins
  - Leukotrienes
  - Eosinophil chemotactic factor of anaphylaxis
  - High-molecular-weight neutrophil chemotactic factor
  - Platelet-activating factor
  - Arachidonic acid-cyclooxygenase and lipoxygenase products

The end result of this biochemical process is tissue injury of a target organ. Examples of tissue injury include inflammation and hyperresponsiveness, resulting in such symptoms as obstruction, increased mucus discharge, and pruritus.

Immediate allergic reactions can involve sneezing, hives, wheezing, vomiting, or anaphylaxis. Acute reactions can be followed by a late-phase response resulting from the release of toxic mediators by activated eosinophils and mononuclear cells recruited to the site of the acute allergic reaction (Leung, 2004).

The pathogenesis of atopic diseases involves a complex interrelationship of genetic, environmental, and immunologic factors. The main defense mechanism to protect against atopic disorders is the elimination of the offending substance

553

to prevent IgE development and antigen-antibody interaction. For example, if there is a family history of atopic disorders, breastfeeding offers the protection of limited exposure to cow's milk protein and the benefit of maternal immunoglobulin A (IgA) and immunoglobulin G (IgG) antibodies. Once chemical mediators are released, the body's protective responses reduce inflammation and repair tissue damage. Pharmacologic therapy cannot cure atopic disorders, but reduces symptoms and checks the allergic process. For example, drugs may be used to control inflammation (corticosteroids), compete with histamine for receptor sites on target tissues (antihistamines), act as a selective leukotriene receptor antagonist (e.g., montelukast), and prevent mast cell degranulation and mediator release (cromolyn sodium).

RHEUMATIC DISORDERS

Juvenile rheumatoid arthritis is the term currently used in the U.S. to describe a group of conditions involving chronic inflammation of synovial joints in children younger than 16 years old. The British use the term *chronic juvenile arthritis* (CJA) to describe these same conditions. Both JRA and SLE are connective tissue disorders marked by inflammatory changes in connective tissues throughout various parts of the body. The exact cause of these collagen diseases is unknown; however, an autoimmune basis is postulated as a key factor in rheumatic disease.

There are no natural defense mechanisms identified to prevent either of these diseases; however, periods of remission do occur in some children with SLE for unknown reasons, and many children with JRA achieve complete remission with puberty. Because inflammation is a significant factor in these two rheumatic diseases of childhood, administration of corticosteroid preparations is a key therapy to control inflammation responsible for tissue injury and possible permanent tissue changes.

CONSIDERATIONS IN THE PATHOGENESIS OF JUVENILE RHEUMATOID ARTHRITIS

The exact etiology of most forms of JRA is unknown; however, there are two theories about its causation. Genetics is believed to be a predisposing factor. Some genetic factors, such as human leukocyte antigen (HLA) alleles, appear to play a role in influencing the susceptibility to develop disease, and others influence disease severity. Viral agents also have been implicated in JRA and are believed to cause an exaggerated immune response.

The pathophysiology of JRA is marked by proliferation of macrophage-like and fibroblastoid synoviocytes. There is subsequent infiltration of neutrophils and lymphocytes, which is evidence of an autoimmune response, and cytokine production including tumor necrosis factor, interleukin-I, and IL-6. B lymphocytes are activated by T-helper cells and produce autoantibodies that link to self-antigens. The end result is nonsuppurative inflammation of the synovium that can lead to articular cartilage and joint structure erosion. Children with JRA have no demonstrable immunodeficiency (Miller, 2004).

CONSIDERATIONS IN THE PATHOGENESIS OF SYSTEMIC LUPUS ERYTHEMATOSUS

Various immune phenomena are associated with SLE, including altered immunologic reactions in the T- and B-lymphocyte function. There is a strong link between a faulty immune mechanism and SLE because this disease is characterized by inflammatory damage to target organs brought on by autoantibodies attacking self-antigens. The exact etiology of SLE is unknown, but many factors including genetics, hormones, and environment are linked to the immune dysregulation that characterizes this rheumatic disease. Environmental factors that are thought to play a role in its pathogenesis are oral contraceptive use, pregnancy, infectious agents (viral agents mostly), temperate climates, exposure to ultraviolet light, and certain drugs (e.g., hydralazine and procainamide).

There is an association between HLA type and complement deficiency. Characteristic pathologic findings include the production of numerous autoantibodies and impairment in the normal suppression of autoreactive B-cell clones. Immune complexes are abundant, and their clearance may be impaired. In addition, fibrinoid deposits collect in blood vessel walls in many organs that result in ischemic damage (Miller, 2004).

Assessment

History. Key factors to consider in the history of a child who has an atopic disorder include the following:
- A family history or personal history of allergies, asthma, AD (eczema), or AR is frequently found.
- Pruritus is a significant finding in AD and AR.
- The rash of AD is characteristically found in certain locations of the body.
- Coughing or shortness of breath with exercise or exertion and nighttime coughing and wheezing are characteristic of asthma.
- Signs and symptoms of AR and asthma may be associated with certain allergens or key triggering agents and may be seasonal.

Key factors to consider in the history of a child who has a rheumatic disease include the following:
- History of a characteristic rash or joint involvement, or both (common findings)
- Other systemic manifestations of disease

Physical Examination. A detailed physical examination of the cardiovascular, respiratory, integumentary, and musculoskeletal systems may reveal characteristics signs (Chapters 30, 31, 36, and 37).

Diagnostic Studies. Various diagnostic studies or procedures can be used in the outpatient evaluation and management of children with either atopic disorders or rheumatic diseases.

Atopic Disorders. Routine chest radiographs are not indicated in most children with asthma. However, chest radiographs can be useful in selected cases of asthma or suspected asthma. These should be performed with the first episode of asthma or with recurrent attacks; in a child with atypical signs or symptoms; if a secondary infection does not clear with standard therapy; or if there are signs and symptoms of significant pulmonary involvement.

Pulmonary function tests, such as forced vital capacity, forced expiratory volume in 1 second, and forced expiratory flow, are important diagnostic tests in the diagnosis of asthma, especially in young children. Peak expiratory flow (PEF) rate and pulse oximetry measurements can be easily and quickly done in most pediatric settings and provide additional information useful to monitor and manage of asthma.

Eosinophil count, determination of serum IgE concentration, radioallergosorbent test (RAST), ImmunoCAP, and prick test are not needed to confirm the diagnosis or to monitor treatment of the majority of children with an atopic disorder.

Rheumatic Diseases. Laboratory blood studies, including antinuclear antibodies (ANA), anti-DNA antibody, and determination of serum complement levels, are common tests ordered in children with SLE. Other related blood, serologic, and urine laboratory studies are indicated depending on organ involvement (e.g., renal involvement is a frequent complication). A positive rheumatoid factor (RF) by latex fixation, ANA, or erythrocyte sedimentation rate (ESR) may be useful markers in JRA.

Imaging studies (MRI and radiographs) are done to assess and manage joint abnormalities.

Management Strategies

The atopic disorders and rheumatoid diseases tend to be chronic conditions with exacerbation and remission of symptoms. Individual management strategies are based on the specific disease process and are discussed in each of their respective sections. However, certain key concepts apply to these conditions.

General Measures. The following general measures should be part of the management of atopic disorders and rheumatic diseases:

- Encourage self-care and learning about one's disease
- Address issues of living with a chronic disease, such as
  - School, peer, and family dynamics
  - Body image
  - Adolescent adjustment
  - Patient-parent role in management of a long-term illness or chronic condition
- Nutrition and the avoidance of obesity, if activity is limited, or foods if they are triggers

Medications. The control of inflammation associated with atopic disorders and rheumatoid diseases is a key principle in the management of these illnesses. Corticosteroids, whether used topically on the skin, inhaled via the nostrils or throat, taken orally for systemic effect, or taken intramuscularly or intravenously for rapid systemic absorption are a mainstay of treatment. Other pharmacologic agents commonly used are as follows:

- For atopic conditions:
  - Antipruritic agents—to control itching
  - Antihistamines—to control symptoms associated with the release of chemical mediators
  - Anticholinergics—to reduce vagal tone in the airways (may also decrease mucous gland secretion)
  - Bronchodilators—to control bronchospasm
  - Cromolyn sodium and nedocromil—to inhibit mast cell release of histamine

- Leukotriene modifiers—to disrupt the synthesis or function of leukotrienes
- Antibiotics—to treat secondary infections
- Immunomodulators—to inhibit the inflammatory response. They include topical preparations (Protopic to inhibit the inflammatory response) and subcutaneous agents (Xolair for moderate to severe asthmatic with atopy).
- Xolair (omalizumab) is an anti-IgE monoclonal antibody used as a second-line treatment for children older than 12 years who have moderate to severe allergy-related asthma. When used with inhaled corticosteroids, omalizumab has reduced asthma exacerbations (Kinane & Scirica, 2006).
- For rheumatic diseases:
  - Analgesics (salicylates or nonsteroidal agents)—to relieve arthritis or joint pain; to relieve pain in general
  - Other therapeutic agents, such as corticosteroids—to relieve signs and symptoms specific to the disease process and organ system involvement

Parent and Patient Education. Both patients and parents need to be instructed about the following:

- Signs and symptoms necessitating immediate reevaluation.
- Medications—clear instructions are needed on how to administer, how much and when to give, monitoring side effects, and how long medication should be taken. A written plan is highly recommended either based on symptoms or PEF rate.
- Correct administration of inhaled medications. For example, when two puffs or sprays are ordered, the child should activate one puff or spray and then inhale followed in 1 to 2 minutes by a second puff or spray and second inhalation. A parent or child may think incorrectly that being told to take two puffs or two sprays means to activate two puffs or sprays and then inhale.
- Any other measures relevant to the treatment plan (e.g., bathing instructions, monitoring peak flow rate, avoidance of allergens, and environmental control).
- Parent support groups and professional organizations and resource groups.

SPECIFIC IMMUNOLOGIC PROBLEMS OF CHILDREN: COMMON ATOPIC DISORDERS

ASTHMA

Description

Asthma is a chronic respiratory disease and is characterized by the following features (National Heart, Lung, and Blood Institute [NHLBI], 2007):

- Immunohistopathologic responses produce:
  - Shedding of airway epithelium and collagen deposition beneath the basement membrane
  - Edema
  - Mast cell activation
  - Inflammatory infiltration by eosinophils, lymphocytes (Th2-like cells), and neutrophils (especially in fatal asthma)
- Airway inflammation contributes to airflow limitations, including:

○ Acute bronchoconstriction.

○ Airway edema.

○ Mucous plug formation.

• Airflow obstruction is often reversible, either spontaneously or with treatment.

• Persistent inflammation can result in airway wall remodeling and irreversible changes.

• Airway inflammation also triggers hyperresponsiveness (to any of a variety of stimuli, such as physical, chemical, or pharmacologic agents; allergens; exercise; and cold air) and is a factor in disease chronicity.

Asthma in children is classified as intermittent, mild persistent, moderate persistent, or severe persistent depending on symptoms, recurrences, need for specific medications, and pulmonary function measurements (Table 24-1). Children classified at any level of asthma can have episodes involving mild, moderate, or severe exacerbations. Exacerbations involve progressive worsening of shortness of breath, cough, wheezing, chest tightness, or any combination of these symptoms. The degree of airway hyperresponsiveness is usually related to the severity of asthma. Children younger than 5 years old experience greater airway hyperresponsiveness than do older children. Airway remodeling can result from chronic inflammation caused by asthma. Irreversible structural changes take place and result in decreased pulmonary function (Lasley, 2006). A child's classification can change over time.

Many children experience early- and late-phase responses to their asthma episode. The early asthmatic response (EAR) phase is characterized by activation of mast cells and their mediators, with bronchoconstriction being the key feature. EAR starts within 15 to 30 minutes of mast cell activation and resolves within approximately 1 hour if the individual is removed from the offending allergen. The late-phase asthmatic response is a prolonged inflammatory state that usually follows the EAR within 4 to 12 hours after exposure to the allergen, is often associated with airway hyperresponsiveness more severe than the EAR presentation, and can last from hours to several weeks (Liu et al, 2004).

Exercise-induced bronchospasm describes the phenomenon of airway narrowing during or minutes after the onset of vigorous activity. Most asthmatics exhibit airway hyperirritability after rigorous activity and display exercise-induced bronchospasm. However, for some children, exercise is the only stimulus that triggers their asthma. Although asthma is not always associated with an allergic disorder in children, many pediatric patients with chronic asthma have an allergic component.

Epidemiology

It is not known for certain whether hyperresponsiveness of the airways is present at birth in genetically predisposed children or acquired. However, the genetic predisposition for the development of an IgE-mediated response to common aeroallergens, known as atopy, remains the strongest identifiable predisposing risk factor for asthma.

The morbidity and mortality statistics of asthma in childhood demonstrate an alarming increase in the prevalence of asthma and its complications. Asthma has become a lead-

---

TABLE 24-1 **Classification of Asthma Severity in Children: Clinical Features Before Treatment**

Classification and Step	Symptoms*	Nighttime Symptoms	Lung Function
Step 1: Intermittent	Symptoms ≤2 times per wk Asymptomatic and normal PEF between exacerbations Requires SABA 2 days/wk Exacerbations brief (few hr or days); varying intensity No interference with normal activity	≤2 times per mo	FEV_1 >80% predicted Normal FEV1 between exacerbations
Step 2: Mild persistent	Symptoms >2 times per wk but <1 time per day Requires SABA >2 days/wk but not >1/day Exacerbations may affect activity (minor)	3-4 times per mo	FEV_1 >80% predicted
Step 3: Moderate persistent	Daily symptoms Daily use of inhaled short-acting β_2-agonist Some limitations Exacerbations affect activity, ≥2 times per wk; may last days	>1 time per wk but not nightly	FEV_1 >60% but <80% predicted
Step 4: Severe persistent	Continual symptoms Requires SABA several times/day Extremely limited physical activity Frequent exacerbations	Often 7 times per wk	FEV_1 < 60% predicted

*Having at least one symptom in a particular step places the child in that particular classification.
FEV_1, Forced expiratory volume in 1 sec; hr, hours; mo, month; SABA, short-acting β_2-agonist; wk, week
Adapted from National Heart, Lung, and Blood Institute (NHLBI): *Full report of the expert panel: guidelines for the diagnosis and management of asthma,* (EPR-3) NHLBI, 2007, National Institutes of Health.

ing reason for pediatric hospital admissions and accounts for 7 million visits annually to pediatric settings (Centers for Disease Control and Prevention [CDC], 2005). Occupational or environmental exposure can cause airway inflammation associated with asthma. Factors known to precipitate or aggravate asthma in children include the following:

- Atopic individual response to allergens—inhaled, topical, ingested
- Viral infections
- Exposure to known irritants (paint fumes, smoke, air pollutants) and occupational chemicals
- Gastroesophageal reflux
- Exposure to tobacco smoke (for infants, especially smoking by mother)
- Environmental changes—rapid changes in barometric pressure, temperature, especially cold air
- Exercise
- Psychological factors or emotional stresses (e.g., crying, laughter, anxiety attack or panic disorder)
- AR and sinusitis
- Drugs (e.g., aspirin, ß-blockers)
- Food additives (sulfites)
- Endocrine factors

Allergen-induced asthma results in hyperresponsive airways. The majority of children with asthma show evidence of sensitization to any of the following inhalant allergens:

- House dust mites, cockroaches, indoor molds
- Saliva and dander of cats and dogs
- Outdoor seasonal molds
- Airborne pollens—trees, grasses, and weeds

Approximately 5% to 10% of children with asthma have food-induced respiratory symptoms (Sampson & Leung, 2004). The mechanism by which allergens cause asthma is explained in the earlier section on pathophysiology and defense mechanisms.

Clinical Findings

History. The history of a patient being seen for asthma can include the following:

- Family history of asthma or other related allergic disorders (e.g., eczema or AR)
- Conditions associated with asthma (e.g., chronic sinusitis, nasal polyposis, gastroesophageal reflux, and chronic otitis media)
- Complaints of chest tightness or dyspnea
- Cough, particularly at night and in the early morning
- Cough or shortness of breath with exercise or exertion
- Seasonal, continuous, or episodic pattern of symptoms
- Episodes of recurrent "bronchitis" or pneumonia
- Precipitation of symptoms by known aggravating factors (e.g., upper respiratory infections [URIs], aspirin)

Physical Examination. The following may be seen on physical examination:

- Wheezing (may be absent if severe obstruction) or coughing
- Prolonged expiratory phase, high-pitched rhonchi
- Diminished breath sounds

- Signs of respiratory distress, including tachypnea, retractions, nasal flaring, use of accessory muscles, increasing restlessness, apprehension, agitation, drowsiness to coma
- Tachycardia, hypertension or hypotension, pulsus paradoxus
- Cyanosis of lips and nail beds if underlying hypoxemia
- Other possible associated findings include sinusitis, flexural eczema, and rhinitis

Diagnostic Studies. Use of various laboratory and radiographic tests should be individualized to the child and based on symptoms, severity or chronology of the disease, response to therapy, and age. Tests to consider include the following:

- Oxygen saturation by pulse oximetry to assess severity of acute exacerbation. This should be a routine part of every assessment on a patient with asthma. Pulse oximetry measures the oxygen saturation (SaO_2) of hemoglobin—the percent of total hemoglobin that is oxygenated—as follows:
  ○ Greater than 95%, mild
  ○ 90% to 95%, moderate
  ○ Less than 90%, severe lack of oxygen
- A complete blood count (CBC) if secondary infection or anemia is suspected (also check for elevated numbers of eosinophils).
- Chest radiograph for the first episode, and then only if secondary respiratory infection or other pulmonary disorders are suspected or if under 1 year old with persistent wheezing.
- Sinus radiographs may be helpful if sinusitis is suspected; however, computed tomography (CT) scans are more sensitive, specific, and considered the gold standard.
- Allergic work-up, including skin testing, IgE, RAST, or ImmunoCAP.
- Sweat test if cystic fibrosis is a possibility.
- Pulmonary function tests:
  ○ Formal spirometry testing is the gold standard in children older than 4 years for diagnosing asthma.
  ○ Start with PEF assessment in children 4 to 5 years or older; to monitor the effectiveness of ß-agonist treatment (measurements before and after treatments) and assess the severity of airflow obstruction.
  ○ Consider the use of more sophisticated pulmonary laboratory studies for the child with severe asthma.

Pulmonary monitoring and typical findings include the following:

- PEF can be used in some children as young as 4 to 5 years old. Noteworthy is the fact that values are instrument specific. Use child's personal best value as a guideline to help detect possible changes in airway obstruction; can use predicted range for height and age if personal best rate is not available (Table 24-2 and Fig. 24-1).
- Interpretation of PEF reading (see Box 24-1 for use of peak flow meter and interpretation of results)—if PEF is in the:
  ○ Green zone: more than 80% to 100% of personal best signals good control.
  ○ Yellow zone: between 50% to 80% of personal best signals caution.
  ○ Red zone: between 0% to 50% of personal best signals major airflow obstruction.

TABLE 24-2 Predicted Average Peak Expiratory Flow for Normal Children and Adolescents

Height (inches)	Males and Females (Liters/minute)
43	147
44	160
45	173
46	187
47	200
48	214
49	227
50	240
51	254
52	267
53	280
54	293
55	307
56	320
57	334
58	347
59	360
60	373
61	387
62	400
63	413
64	427
65	440
66	454
67	467

Note: It is recommended that PEF rate objectives for therapy be based on each individual's "personal best," which is established after a period of PEF rate monitoring while the individual is under effective treatment.
From National Heart, Lung, and Blood Institute (NHLBI): *Executive summary: guidelines for the diagnosis and management of asthma,* NIH pub no 94-3042A, Bethesda, MD, 1994, National Institutes of Health. Adapted from Polger G, Promedhar V: *Pulmonary function testing in children: techniques and standards,* Philadelphia, 1971, WB Saunders.

- Chest radiograph findings: hyperinflation of the lungs with flattening of the diaphragm on radiograph with or without atelectasis (Greenberger, 2002).

Differential Diagnosis

Numerous conditions can cause airway obstruction and be incorrectly confused with asthma, especially in young children and infants. Examples include the following:

- Acute bronchiolitis, laryngotracheobronchitis, bronchopneumonia
- Bronchial foreign body aspiration
- Congenital malformations of the respiratory, cardiovascular, or gastrointestinal (GI) systems
- Cystic fibrosis (CF)
- Tracheal or foreign body compression (e.g., aortic ring, tumors)
- Chronic lower respiratory tract infections caused by immunodeficiency disorders
- Recurrent aspirations
- Chronic reflux

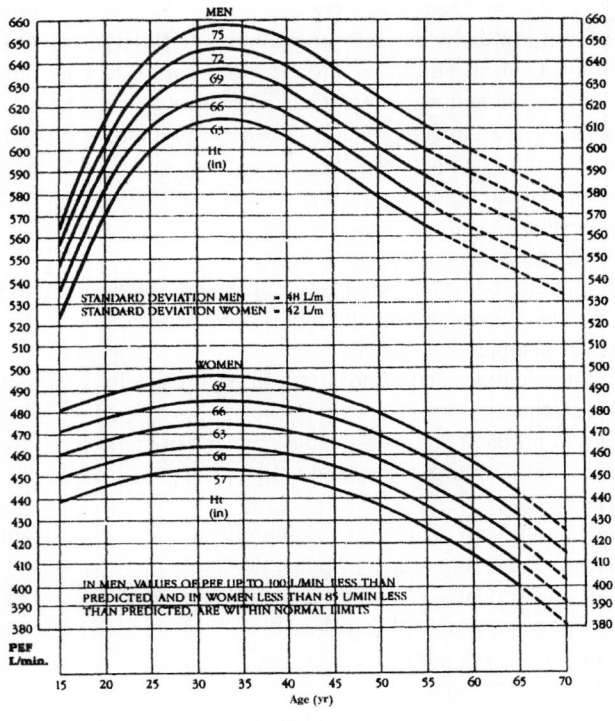

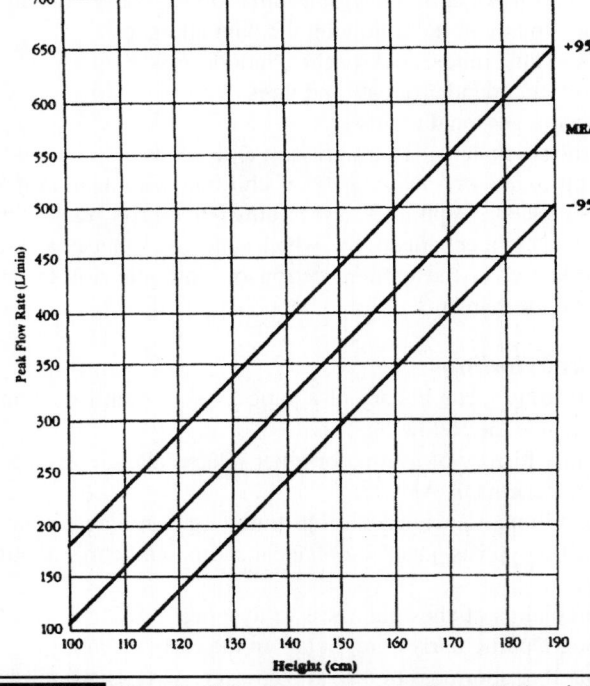

FIG. 24-1 Sample PEF rate nomogram. (From National Heart, Lung, and Blood Institute (NHLBI): *Executive summary: guidelines for the diagnosis and management of asthma,* pub no 94-3042A, Bethesda, MD, 1994, National Institutes of Health. *Top,* Adapted from Nunn AJ, Gregg I: New regression equations for predicting peak expiratory flow in adults, *BMJ* 298:1068-1070, 1989. *Bottom,* Adapted from Godfrey S, Kamburoff PL, Nairn JR: Spirometry, lung volumes and airway resistance in normal children aged 5 to 18 years, *Br J Dis Chest* 64:15-24, 1970.)

BOX 24-1 Use of the Peak Flow Meter and Its Interpretation

Steps to follow in using a peak flow meter:
1. Have child stand up.
2. Make sure that indicator is at the base of the numbered scale.
3. Ask child to take a deep breath.
4. Have the child place the peak flow meter in the mouth with the lips sealing the mouthpiece. Tell the child not to put his or her tongue in the hole of the mouthpiece.
5. Tell the child to blow out as hard and fast as possible.
6. Record the rate, but if the child coughs, do not write down that number.
7. Repeat steps 2 through 6, two more times.
8. Record the highest of the three values.

PEF Rate
The maximum flow rate that is produced during forced expiration with fully inflated lungs

Personal Best Value
The highest value that an individual achieves in measuring PEF rate over a 2-week time period when his or her asthma is under good control is known as one's "personal best" value or rate. Good control is defined as when one feels well without asthma symptoms. To determine personal best, take readings twice daily, in the morning and late afternoon or evening, and 15-20 minutes after taking an inhaled short-acting β_2-agonist. Using the personal best value is the most accurate gauge to use to interpret changes in peak flow measurements because the child's own scores are used as the standard for comparison.

Management

The *Full Report of the Expert Panel: Guidelines for the Diagnosis and Management of Asthma* (ERP-3) (NHLBI, 2007) provides the most recent standards for the treatment of asthma in children. Management strategies are based on whether the child has intermittent, mild persistent, moderate persistent, or severe persistent asthma (see Table 24-1). A stepwise approach is recommended. If control of symptoms is not maintained at a particular step of classification and management, the health care provider first should reevaluate for compliance and administration factors. If these factors do not appear to be responsible for the lack of symptom control, the health care provider should go to the next higher step. Likewise, gradual step-downs in treatment may be considered every 1 to 6 months.

In this chapter, the outpatient management of intermittent, mild persistent, moderate persistent, and severe persistent asthma is discussed, as is the outpatient management of acute exacerbations. The practitioner should refer to other textbooks for management of severe asthma requiring hospitalization.

Chronic Asthma. Treatment of chronic asthma in children is based on general control measures and pharmacotherapy. General control measures include the following:
- Avoid exposure to known allergens or irritants.
- Administer yearly influenza vaccine.
- Control environment to eliminate or reduce offending allergen.
- Provide allergen immunotherapy.
- Treat rhinitis, sinusitis, or gastroesophageal reflux.
- See section on patient education for other measures.

The pharmacologic management of asthma in children is based on the classification of the severity of asthma and the child's age. The stepwise approach to treatment found in Appendix D is based on severity of symptoms and the use of pharmacotherapy to control chronic symptoms, maintain normal activity, prevent recurrent exacerbations, minimize adverse side effects, and maintain nearly "normal" pulmonary function. Also within any classification, a child may experience mild, moderate, or severe exacerbations. NHLBI guidelines for assessing asthma control and initiating and adjusting asthma therapy for the various pediatric age groups are found in Appendix D.

Important considerations to note in the pharmacologic treatment of asthma include the following:
- Control of asthma should be gained as quickly as possible by starting at the classification step most appropriate to the initial severity of the child's symptoms or at a higher level (e.g., a course of systemic corticosteroids or higher dose of inhaled corticosteroid). After control of symptoms, decrease treatment to the least amount of medication needed to maintain control.
- Systemic corticosteroids may be needed at any time and step if there is a major flare-up of symptoms.
- Children with intermittent asthma may have long periods in which they are symptom free; they can also have life-threatening exacerbations, often provoked by respiratory infection. In these situations, a short course of systemic corticosteroids should be used (NHLBI, 2007).
- Variations in asthma necessitate individualized treatment plans.
- The ß$_2$-agonist can be given by nebulization with a compressor (e.g., Pulmo-Aide). Nebulization can be a more effective route than metered-dose inhaler (MDI) therapy for young infants (2 years old or younger) or children who progress to moderate or severe airway obstruction.
- A spacer or holding chamber (Aerochamber or InspirEase) with an attached mask enhances the delivery of MDI medications to the lower airways of a child and should be used. Spacers eliminate the need to synchronize inhalation with activation of MDI. Older children can use the spacer without the mask.
- Dry powder inhalers (DPIs), such as Serevent Diskus, Pulmicort Turbohaler, and Flovent Diskus do not need spacers or shaking before use. Instruct children to rinse their mouth with water and spit after inhalation. DPIs should not be used in children younger than 4 to 5 years old.
- Different inhaled corticosteroids are not equal in potency to each other on a per puff or microgram basis. Table 24-3 compares the daily low, medium, and high doses of the various inhaled corticosteroids used for children. Combination inhaled corticosteroid and long-acting ß$_2$-agonist can now be used in children 5 years and older.
- For treatment of exercise-induced bronchospasm:

| **TABLE 24-3** | Estimated Comparative Daily Dosages for Inhaled Corticosteroids |

Drug	Low Daily Dose		Medium Daily Dose		High Daily Dose	
	Child*	Adult†	Child*	Adult†	Child*	Adult†
Beclomethasone HFA (40 or 80 mcg/puff)	80-160 mcg	80-240 mcg	>160-320 mcg	>240-480 mcg	>320 mcg	>480 mcg
Budesonide DPI (200 mcg/inhalation)	200-400 mcg	200-600 mcg	>400-800 mcg	>600-1200 mcg	>800 mcg	>1200 mcg
Budesonide inhaled suspension for nebulization (child dose)	0.5 mg		1 mg		2 mg	
Flunisolide (250 mcg/puff)	500-750 mcg	500-1000 mcg	1000-1250 mcg	>1000-2000 mcg	>1250 mcg	>2000 mcg
Flunisolide HFA (80 mcg/puff)	160 mcg	320 mcg	320 mcg	>320-640 mcg	>640 mcg	>640 mcg
Fluticasone HFA/MDI						
• MDI: 44, 110, or 220 mcg/puff	88-176 mcg	88-264 mcg	>176-352 mcg	>264-440 mcg	>352 mcg	>440 mcg
• DPI: 50, 100, or 250 mcg/inhalation	100-200 mcg	100-300 mcg	>200-400 mcg	>300-500 mcg	>400 mcg	>500 mcg
Mometasone DPI 200 mcg/inhalation	N/A	200 mcg	N/A	400 mcg	N/A	>400 mcg
Triamcinolone acetonide 75 mcg/puff	300-600 mcg	300-750 mcg	>600-900 mcg	>750-1500 mcg	>900 mcg	>1500 mcg

	Inhaled Corticosteroids in Children 0-4 years		
	Low Daily Dose	Medium Daily Dose	High Daily Dose
Budesonide inhaled suspension for nebulization	0.25-0.5 mg	>0.5-1 mg	>1 mg
Fluticasone HFA/MDI: 44, 110, or 220 mcg/puff	176 mcg	>176-352 mcg	>352 mcg

*Child 5-11 years old.
†Adult ≥12 years old
DPI, Dry powder inhaler; *HFA*, hydrofluoroalkane; *MDI*, metered-dose inhaler; *N/A*, not approved and no data available for this age group.

○ Use either an inhaled short-acting ß$_2$-agonist or a mast cell stabilizer (cromolyn or nedocromil) or both. Combination of both types of drugs is the more effective therapy. A long-acting ß$_2$-agonist can be used in older children.
○ Use two puffs of a ß$_2$-agonist, cromolyn, or nedocromil 5 minutes before exercise.

Table 24-4 identifies the usual dosages for long-term control medications (exclusive of inhaled corticosteroids) used to treat asthma in children. Quick-relief medications are listed in Table 24-5.

Practice parameters are guides and should not replace individualized treatment based on clinical judgment and unique differences in patients.

Acute Exacerbations of Asthma. The treatment of acute episodes of asthma is also based on classification of the severity of the episode. Acute episodes are classified as mild, moderate, and severe. Signs and symptoms are summarized in Table 24-6. Early recognition of warning signs and treatment should be stressed in both patient or parent education, or both.

Characteristics of a *mild acute episode* are:
• Wheezing, usually at the end of expiration
• Increased respiratory rate
• No signs of respiratory distress, cyanosis, or activity restriction

• PEF or forced expiratory volume (PEF or FEV$_1$) greater than 70% of expected value
• Ability to speak in normal sentences between breaths

Children with a *moderate acute episode* of asthma manifest the following:
• Audible wheeze
• Use of accessory muscles
• Increase in respiratory rate
• Unable to walk or utter more than three to five words between breaths

Manifestations of a *severe acute episode* of asthma in children include the following signs of severe respiratory distress:
• Cyanosis
• Use of accessory muscles plus lower rib and suprasternal retractions; nasal flaring
• Agitation and the ability to say only single words between breaths
• Loud wheezing on inhalation and expiration (NHLBI, 2007)

The *initial pharmacologic treatment* for acute asthma exacerbations is inhaled short-acting ß$_2$-agonists, two to six puffs every 20 minutes for three treatments by way of MDI with or without a spacer, or a single nebulizer treatment (0.15 mg/kg; minimum 1.25 mg of 0.5% solution of albuterol in 2 to 3 mL of normal saline).

TABLE 24-4 Long-Term Control Medications for the Treatment of Asthma

Medication	Dosage Form‡	Child Dose‡	Adult Dose**	Comments
Inhaled corticosteroids—see Table 24-5				
Systemic Corticosteroids (applies to all three corticosteroids)				
Methylprednisolone	2-, 4-, 8-, 16-, 32-mg tabs	0.25-2mg/kg daily in a single dose in AM or every other day as needed for control	7.5-60mg daily in a single dose in AM or every other day as needed for control	For long-term treatment of severe persistent asthma, administer single dose in morning either daily or on alternate days (alternate-day therapy may produce less adrenal suppression). If daily doses are required, one study suggests improved efficacy and no increase in adrenal suppression when administered at 3:00 PM.
Prednisolone	5-mg tabs, 5mg/5mL, 15mg/5mL	Same as above	Same as above	
Prednisone	1-, 2.5-, 5-, 10-, 20-, 50-mg tabs; 5mg/mL, 5mg/5mL	Short-course "burst": 1-2g/kg/day, maximum 60mg/day for 3-10 days	Short-course "burst" to achieve control: 40-60mg/day as single or 2 divided doses for 3-10 days	Short courses or "bursts" are effective for establishing control when initiating therapy or during a period of gradual deterioration. The bursts should be continued until patient achieves 80% PEF rate personal best or symptoms resolve. This usually requires 3-10 days, but may require longer. There is no evidence that tapering the dose following improvement prevents relapse.
Cromolyn and Nedocromil				
Cromolyn	MDI 800mcg/puff nebulizer; 20mg/ampule	1-2 puffs tid-qid for 5-11yr;1 ampule tid-qid	2-4 puffs tid-qid 1 ampule tid-qid	One dose before exercise or allergen exposure provides effective prophylaxis for 1-2hr.
Nedocromil	MDI 1.75mg/puff	5-11yr: 2 puffs qid	2 puffs qid	See cromolyn above.
Inhaled Long-Acting β₂-Agonists (should not be used for symptom relief or for exacerbations; use with inhaled corticosteroids)				
Salmeterol	DPI 50mcg/blister	> 5-11yr: 1 blister every 12hr	1 blister every 12hr	Use with inhaled corticosteroid only. Do not use as a rescue inhaler for symptom relief or for exacerbations.
Formoterol	DPI: 12mcg/single-use capsule	>5-11yr: 1 capsule every 12hr for	1 capsule every 12hr	Do not take orally; must be used with Aerolizer.
Sustained-release albuterol	4-mg tab* 8-mg tab†	4mg bid for ≥ 6yr	4-8mg bid	For children 6yr and older.
Methylxanthines				
Theophylline (numerous manufacturers)	Liquids Sustained-release tabs and capsules	Starting dose 10mg/kg/day; usual max dose: <1yr old: 0.2 (age in wk) + 5 = mg/kg/day; ≥1yr old: 16mg/kg/day	Starting dose 10mg/kg/day up to 300mg max; usual max 800mg/day	Routine serum theophylline level monitoring is required (serum concentration 5-15mcg/mL); not commonly used with pediatric patients.

Continued

TABLE 24-4 **Long-Term Control Medications for the Treatment of Asthma—Cont'd**

Medication	Dosage Form	Child Dose[‡]	Adult Dose	Comments
Leukotriene Modifiers				
Montelukast	4- or 5-mg chewable tab, 10-mg tab; granules 4 mg/packet	1-5 yr: 4 mg at bedtime 6-14 yr: 5 mg at bedtime >14 yr: 10 mg at bedtime	10 mg at bedtime	
Zafirlukast	10- or 20-mg tab	7-11 yr: 10-mg tab bid	40 mg daily (20-mg tab bid)	Take zafirlukast at least 1 hr before or 2 hr after meals.
Zileuton	300- or 600-mg tab		2400 mg daily (give tabs qid)	Monitor hepatic enzymes (ALT).
Combined Medication				
Fluticasone/salmeterol DPI	100, 250, or 500 mcg/50 mcg	>4 yr: 1 inhalation bid; dose depends on severity of asthma	1 inhalation bid; dose depends on severity of asthma	
Budesonide/Formoterol HFA MDI	80 mcg/4.5 mcg 160 mcg/4.5 mcg	5-11 yr: 2 puffs bid	2 puffs bid—depends on severity	

*Proventil and Repetabs come in 4 mg only.
†Volmax comes in 4 mg and 8 mg.
‡≤12 yr old
**Adult ≥12 years old
ALT, Alanine aminotransferase; bid, twice daily; DPI, dry powder inhaler; hr, hour(s); max, maximum; MDI, metered-dose inhaler; PEF, peak expiratory flow; qid, four times daily; tab(s), tablet(s); tid, three times daily; yr, year(s).
Adapted from the National Heart, Lung, and Blood Institute (NHLBI): Full report of the expert panel: guidelines for the diagnosis and management of asthma (EPR-3), 2007

TABLE 24-5   Quick-Relief Medications for the Treatment of Asthma

Medication	Dosage Form	Child Dose*	Adult Dose	Comments
Short-Acting Inhaled β₂-Agonists				
Metered-dose inhalers				
Albuterol CFC	90 mcg/puff, 200 puffs	1-2 puffs 5 min before exercise	2 puffs 5 min before exercise	An increasing use or lack of expected effect indicates diminished control of asthma.
Albuterol HFA	90 mcg/puff, 200 puffs	2 puffs every 4-6 hr prn	2 puffs every 4-6 hr prn	Not generally recommended for long-term treatment. Regular use on a daily basis indicates the need for additional long-term control therapy.
Pirbuterol CFC	200 mcg/puff, 400 puffs		1-2 puffs every 4-6 hr	May double usual dose for mild exacerbations.
Levalbuterol HFA	45 mcg/puff	>5 yr: 2 puffs every 4-6 hr prn		
				Nonselective agents (e.g., epinephrine, isoproterenol, metaproterenol) are not recommended because of their potential for excessive cardiac stimulation, especially at high doses.
Nebulizer solution				
Albuterol	5 mg/mL (0.5%) 0.63 mg/3 mL 1.25 mg/3 mL 2.5 mg/3 mL	<5 yr: 0.63-2.5 mg in 3 mL NS every 4-6 hr prn; >5 yr: 1.25-2.5 mg in 3 mL of NS every 4-8 hr prn	1.25-5 mg in 3 mL of NS every 4-8 hr prn	May mix with cromolyn or ipratropium nebulizer solutions; may double dose for mild exacerbations.
Levalbuterol	0.31 mg/3 mL 0.63 mg/3 mL 1.25 mg/3 mL	6-11 yr: 0.31 mg tid every 8 hr max: 0.63 mg tid	0.63-1.25 mg every 8 hr	
Anticholinergics				
Metered-dose inhalers				
Ipratropium-HFA	17 mcg/puff, 200 puff canister	Safety and efficacy not established in children under 12 yr old	2-3 puffs every 6 hr	Evidence is lacking that these drugs produce added benefit to β₂-agonists in long-term asthma therapy.
Nebulizer solution				
Ipratropium	0.25 mg/mL (0.025%)	Safety and efficacy not established in children under 12 yr old	0.25 mg every 6 hr	
Systemic corticosteroids (Dosage applies to all three corticosteroids listed below)				
Methylprednisolone	2-, 4-, 8-, 16-, 32-mg tabs	Short-course "burst": 1-2 mg/kg/day, max 30-60 mg/day, for 3-10 days	Short-course "burst" to achieve control: 40-60 mg/day as single or two divided doses for 3-10 days	Short courses or "bursts" are effective for establishing control when initiating therapy or during a period of gradual deterioration.
Prednisolone	5-mg tabs, 5 mg/5 mL, 15 mg/5 mL			

Continued

TABLE 24-5	Quick-Relief Medications for the Treatment of Asthma—Cont'd				
Medication	**Dosage Form**	**Child Dose***	**Adult Dose**		**Comments**
Prednisone	1-, 2.5-, 5-, 10-, 20-, 50-mg tabs: 5 mg/mL, 5 mg/5 mL				The burst should be continued until patient achieves 80% PEF rate personal best or symptoms resolve; this usually requires 3-10 days, but may require longer; there is no evidence that tapering the dose following improvement prevents relapse.

*<12 yr old.

hr, Hour(s); *max,* maximum; *min,* minute(s); *NS,* normal saline; *PEF,* peak expiratory flow rate; *prn,* as needed; *tabs,* tablets; *yr,* year(s).
Adapted from the National Heart, Lung, and Blood Institute (NHLBI): *Full report of the expert panel: guidelines for the diagnosis and management of asthma* (EPR-3), 2007;Taketomo CK, Hodding JH, Kraus DM: *Pediatric dosage handbook,* ed 13, Hudson, OH, 2006-2007, Lexi-Comp.

If the initial treatment results in a good response (PEF/FEV_1 greater than 70% of the patient's best), the inhaled short-acting ß$_2$-agonists can be continued every 3 to 4 hours for 24 to 48 hours. Consider a 7-to 10-day burst of corticosteroids.

An incomplete response (PEF or FEV_1 between 40% and 69% of personal best or symptoms recur within 4 hours of therapy) is treated by continuing ß$_2$-agonists and adding an oral corticosteroid. The ß$_2$-agonist can be given by nebulizer. Parents should contact their child's health care provider for additional instructions. If there is marked distress (severe acute symptoms) or a poor response (PEF or FEV_1 less than 40%) to treatment, the child should have the ß$_2$-agonist repeated immediately and should be taken to the emergency department. Emergency medical rescue (911) transportation should be used if the distress is severe and nonresponsive.

Children who experience acute asthma exacerbations more than once every 4 to 6 weeks should be reevaluated as to their treatment plan (NHLBI, 2007).

Complications

Complications from asthma can range from mild secondary respiratory infections to respiratory arrest. Unresponsiveness to pharmacologic agents can lead to status asthmaticus and ultimately to death. Chronic high-dose steroid use leads to growth retardation and other related side effects.

Patient and Parent Education and Prevention

The practitioner needs to remember that day-to-day management of asthma is the responsibility of the child or parent. Education should be tailored to meet the patient's individual and family needs. Therefore the primary care provider should provide instruction on the following:
- Factors responsible for asthma symptoms (i.e., inflammation, airway hyperresponsiveness, and obstruction)
- Environmental control of allergens or triggers, such as smoking and dust
- Medication use (when to take, how often to take, side effects)

- Home PEF monitoring
- How to use inhalers, spacer devices, or aerosol equipment (Box 24-2)
- Proper cleaning of aerosol equipment
- What to do if symptoms worsen (what medications to add or increase; how frequently to use inhaled medication; specific indications about when to seek additional medical treatment for worsening of symptoms); development of a written action plan with the child or parent to cover these issues (Fig. 24-2)
- Need to have an adequate supply of all medications (including oral corticosteroids) at home and medications readily accessible to the child at school or other settings where the child frequents
- Management of the child at school, camp, or other places away from home

The primary care provider should stress that asthma is a chronic disease that can be controlled—the goal of therapy is to maintain normal activity. The child should wear a medical alert bracelet. Patients and parents should be acquainted with local asthma education programs and activities, such as asthma camp. Also, written instructions and handouts should be provided for parents, child, and other significant individuals (e.g., school personnel).

Prognosis

Asthma is a chronic disease that, for most children, can be successfully managed with proper pharmacologic therapy, allergen and environmental control, and patient education. Mild asthma is more likely to disappear with increasing age than is moderate or severe asthma.

ALLERGIC RHINITIS

Description

Allergic rhinitis (AR) is a disorder that results in inflammation of the nasal epithelium and other related local manifestations caused by to the release of chemical mediators from the antigen-antibody reaction. It is a clinical diagnosis that

TABLE 24-6 **Classifying Severity of Asthma Exacerbations***

	Mild	Moderate	Severe	Respiratory Arrest Imminent
Symptoms				
Breathless	While walking	While at rest (infant—softer, shorter cry; difficulty feeding)	While at rest (infant—stops feeding)	
	Can lie down	Prefers sitting	Sits upright	
Talks in	Sentences	Phrases	Words	
Alertness	May be agitated	Usually agitated	Usually agitated	Drowsy or confused
Signs				
Respiratory rate	Increased	Increased	Often >30/min	
	Guide to rates of breathing in awake children:			
	Age	*Normal rate*		
	<2 mo	<60/min		
	2-12 mo	<50/min		
	1-5 yr	<40/min		
	6-8 yr	<30/min		
Use of accessory muscles; suprasternal retractions	Usually not	Commonly	Usually	Paradoxic thoracoabdominal movement
Wheeze	Moderate, often only end expiratory	Loud; throughout exhalation	Usually loud; throughout inhalation and exhalation	Absence of wheeze
Pulse/min	<100	100-120	>120	Bradycardia
	Guide to normal pulse rates in children:			
	Age	*Normal rate*		
	2-12 mo	<160/min		
	1-2 yr	<120/min		
	2-8 yr	<110/min		
Pulsus paradoxus	Absent <10 mm Hg	May be present 10-25 mm Hg	Often present >25 mm Hg (adult), 20-40 mm Hg (child)	Absence suggests respiratory muscle fatigue
Functional Assessment				
PEF percent predicted or percent personal best	≥70%	Approximately 40%-69%	<40% predicted or personal best, or response lasts <2 hr	<25%
PaO_2 (on room air) and/or	Normal (test not usually necessary)	>60 mm Hg (test not usually necessary)	<60 mm Hg: possible cyanosis	
PCO_2	<42 mm Hg (test not usually necessary)	<42 mm Hg (test not usually necessary)	≥42 mm Hg: possible respiratory failure	
SaO_2% (on room air) at sea level	>95% (test not usually necessary)	90%-95%	<90%	

*The presence of several parameters, but not necessarily all, indicates the general classification of the exacerbation. Many of these parameters have not been systematically studied, so they serve only as general guides.

hr, Hours; *mo*, months; *min*, minutes; *PaO$_2$*, partial pressure of oxygen in arterial blood; *PCO$_2$*, partial pressure of carbon dioxide; *PEF*, peak expiratory flow; *SaO$_2$*, oxygen saturation in arterial blood; *yr*, years.

From National Heart, Lung, and Blood Institute (NHLBI): *Full report of the expert panel: guidelines for the diagnosis and management of asthma*, (EPR-3), 2007, National Institutes of Health.

BOX 24-2   How To Use a Metered-Dose Inhaler

Using an inhaler seems simple, but most patients do not use it the right way.

Steps for using an inhaler for children under 5 years old

1. The use of a mask chamber, such as the InspirEase, with an MDI allows the delivery of inhaled medications even in an uncooperative child.
2. The child should be placed in the parent's lap, and the mask placed around the child's mouth.
3. Press down on the MDI while firmly holding the mask around the child's mouth. The child will eventually take a deep breath and inhale the medication.

Steps for using an inhaler for children 5 years or older

Getting ready

1. Take off the cap and shake the inhaler.
2. Breathe out all the way.
3. Hold the inhaler the way as shown in A, B, or C below.

Breathe in slowly

1. Start breathing in slowly through mouth, then press down on the inhaler one time. (If a holding chamber is used, first press down on the inhaler. Within 5 seconds, begin to breathe in slowly.)
2. Keep breathing in slowly, as deeply as possible.

Hold your breath

1. Hold breath for a slow count to 10 if possible.
2. For inhaled quick-relief medicine (β_2-agonists), wait about 1 minute between puffs. There is no need to wait between puffs for other medicines.

A. Hold inhaler 1 to 2 inches in front of mouth (about the width of two fingers).	B. Use a spacer/holding chamber. These come in many shapes and can be useful to any patient.	C. Put inhaler in mouth. Do not use for steroids.
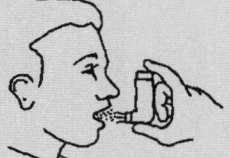	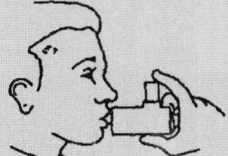	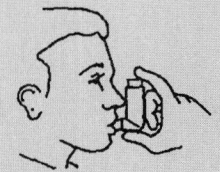

Step A or Step B is best, but Step C can be used if patient has trouble with Step A or Step B.

Clean Inhaler As Needed

Look at the hole where the medicine sprays out from your inhaler. If "powder" can be seen in or around the hole, clean the inhaler. Remove the metal canister from the L-shaped plastic mouthpiece. Rinse only the mouthpiece and cap in warm water. Let them dry overnight. In the morning, put the canister back inside. Put the cap on.

Know When to Replace Inhaler

For medicines taken each day (an example): a new canister has 200 puffs (number of puffs is listed on canister), and child is told to take 8 puffs per day: 8 puffs per day for 25 days equals 200 puffs in canister.

So this canister will last 25 days. If child started using this inhaler on May 1, replace it on or before May 25. Write the date on your canister. For quick-relief medicine, take as needed and count each puff. Do not put canisters in water to see if they are empty. This does not work

Adapted from *Facts about controlling asthma*, NIH pub no 97-2339, National Asthma Education and Prevention Program. National Heart, Lung, and Blood Institute (NHLBI). A reproducible handout.

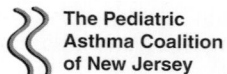

The Pediatric Asthma Coalition of New Jersey

Asthma Action Plan

"Your Pathway to Asthma Control"
www.pacnj.org

(Press Firmly)

Name	Date of Birth	Effective Date / / to / /
Doctor/Nurse Practitioner		Parent/Guardian
Doctor's Office Phone Number		Parent's Phone
Emergency Contact After Parent		Contact Phone

The colors of a traffic light will help you use your asthma medicines.

Green means **Go Zone!**
Use preventive medicine.

Yellow means **Caution Zone!**
Add prescribed yellow zone medicine.

Red means **Danger Zone!**
Get help from a doctor.

Pay Attention to Symptoms.

GO (Green)

You have _all_ of these:
- Breathing is good
- No cough or wheeze
- Sleep through the night
- Can work and play

And/or Peak flow above

Use these medicines every day.

MEDICINE/DOSAGE	HOW MUCH TO TAKE	WHEN TO TAKE IT

COMMENTS:

For asthma with exercise, take:

CAUTION (Yellow)

You have _any_ of these:
- First sign of a cold
- Exposure to known trigger
- Cough
- Mild wheeze
- Tight chest
- Coughing at night

And/or Peak flow from

to

Continue with green zone medicine and ADD:

MEDICINE/DOSAGE	HOW MUCH TO TAKE	WHEN TO TAKE IT
FIRST ➡		
NEXT ➡		

COMMENTS:

➡ IF QUICK RELIEVER/YELLOW ZONE MEDICINE IS NEEDED MORE THAN 2-3 TIMES A WEEK **THEN CALL YOUR DOCTOR.**

DANGER (Red)

Your asthma is getting worse fast:
- Medicine is not helping within 15-20 minutes
- Breathing is hard and fast
- Nose opens wide
- Ribs show
- Lips blue
- Fingernails blue
- Trouble walking and talking

And/or Peak flow below

Take these medicines and call your doctor

EMERGENCY MEDICINE/DOSAGE	HOW MUCH TO TAKE	WHEN TO TAKE IT

COMMENTS:

Get help from a doctor now! It's Important!

Asthma is a potentially life threatening illness. If you cannot contact your doctor, go directly to the emergency room. DO NOT WAIT. Make an appointment with your primary care provider within two days of an ER visit or hospitalization.

Check all items that trigger your asthma and things that could make your asthma worse:

- ❏ Chalk dust
- ❏ Cigarette smoke & second hand smoke
- ❏ Colds/Flu
- ❏ Dust mites, dust, stuffed animals, carpet
- ❏ Exercise
- ❏ Mold
- ❏ Ozone alert days
- ❏ Pests-rodents & cockroaches
- ❏ Pets-animal dander
- ❏ Plants, flowers, cut grass, pollen
- ❏ Strong odors, perfumes, cleaning products, scented products
- ❏ Sudden temperature change
- ❏ Wood smoke
- ❏ Foods: ____
- ____
- ____
- ____
- ❏ Other: ____
- ____
- ____
- ____

❏ This student is capable and has been instructed in the proper method of self-administering the medications named above (or attached prescription).
❏ This student is not approved to self-medicate.

Check asthma severity: ❏ Mild Intermittent ❏ Mild Persistent ❏ Moderate Persistent ❏ Severe Persistent

PHYSICIAN/IPA/APN SIGNATURE_____

PHYSICIAN STAMP

Approved by the New Jersey Thoracic Society, Medical Section of the American Lung Association of New Jersey.

Adapted from the NYC Childhood Asthma Initiative
Adapted from the NHLBI

Funding provided by the New Jersey Department of Health and Senior Services

Printed 2002

WHITE - School Nurse Copy   PINK- Patient Copy   YELLOW- Doctor Copy   Permission to Reproduce Blank Form

FIG. 24-2   Sample asthma action plan. (From the Pediatric Asthma Coalition of New Jersey: *Asthma Action Plan*. Available at *www.pacnj.org* [accessed Jan 17, 2008]).

is based on the presence of rhinorrhea, nasal pruritus and congestion, and sneezing. Manifestations can be seasonal or perennial depending on exposure and subsequent sensitization to the offending allergen.

Epidemiology

AR is second only to asthma as the most common atopic disorder. There is an increased incidence in families with an atopic history. Both genetic (the presence of an abnormal sensitivity that is associated with IgE production) and environmental factors are linked to its cause. Repeated exposure to the offending allergen is an important contributing factor necessary for sensitizing the immune system to produce an allergic IgE response. Many of the allergens that cause asthma produce AR in the same child; AR is postulated to be a distinct feature of the same inflammatory process that results in asthma. Thus, to effectively treat asthma, AR must also be effectively managed.

AR is rare in children under 6 months old and, if present in infancy, is due to foods or household inhalants, not seasonal pollens. Food allergens can occasionally cause rhinitis.

The nasal mucosa is particularly vulnerable to inhaled allergens with a resulting type I, IgE-mediated allergic response. The nasal mucosa of a susceptible individual comes in contact with an allergen that binds to a specific IgE antibody. Superficial mucosal mast cells and basophils then degranulate and release chemical mediators, such as histamine and tryptase, and newly generated mediators including leukotrienes, prostaglandins, and platelet-activating factors. This causes an early-phase reaction of edema, cellular recruitment, and increased vascular permeability with hyperemia and increased serous and mucoid secretions. A late-phase response can occur about 4 to 8 hours later that results in additional release of chemical mediators and nasal obstruction (Lasley, 2006).

AR tends to be seasonal, perennial, or episodic. Seasonal AR (hay fever or seasonal pollenosis) typically occurs after 3 years old. Seasonal AR results from sensitization to airborne allergens, such as pollens of trees, grasses, weeds (ragweed and other weeds), and outdoor molds. There can be geographic variations in seasonal AR depending on climate and when the allergens are released into the environment.

Perennial AR has year-round signs and symptoms that may be more severe in the winter. Onset of manifestations can occur before the second year of life, and offending substances tend to be indoor allergens, including the following:
- Dust mites
- Cockroaches
- Feathers
- Allergens or danders of household pets
- Indoor mold spores

Episodic AR occurs with intermittent exposure to an allergen. Thus, the rhinitis is related to a distinct event, such as visiting a house where a cat dwells.

Clinical Findings

Common nasal symptoms and findings on physical examination include the following:

- Reduced patency from chronic or recurrent bilateral nasal obstruction as a result of congestion and inflammation
- Mouth breathing, snoring, nasal speech
- Pale to purplish color and edema (bogginess) of nasal mucous membranes
- Clear, thin, watery to seromucoid rhinorrhea
- Nasal crease—horizontal crease across the lower third of nose
- Itching, rubbing of nose or "allergic salute"
- Nasal stuffiness, postnasal drip, paroxysms of sneezing, congested cough, or night cough
- Dennie lines, Morgan fold or atopic pleats—extra groove in lower eyelid (Fig. 24-3)
    Associated manifestations include the following:
- Itching of palate, pharynx, or eyes
- High arched palate
- Hoarseness
- Redness of the conjunctiva, tearing, lid and periorbital edema, infraorbital cyanosis or allergic shiners
- Enlarged tonsillar and adenoidal tissue
- "Cobblestone" appearance of the pharynx or palpebral conjunctivae (or both) as a result of increased lymphoid tissue
- Malocclusion if problem is chronic
- May have related sleep disturbances and performance problems at school related to lack of adequate sleep

Diagnostic Studies.   Characteristic symptoms and clinical findings are the key to diagnosis. A history of atopy in the child or family member is helpful in making the diagnosis of AR. The presence of eosinophils on nasal smear can help substantiate the diagnosis, but is a nonspecific, nonuniversal finding. Referrals for skin or serologic testing for IgE antibody to specific allergens should be reserved for the child with significant symptoms who does not respond to traditional management. The RAST or ImmunoCAP, in vitro tests, can be done for suspected allergens.

Differential Diagnosis

Conditions to include as differential diagnoses are the common cold, purulent rhinitis, sinusitis, adenoidal hypertrophy, foreign body obstruction, nasal polyposis of cystic fibrosis,

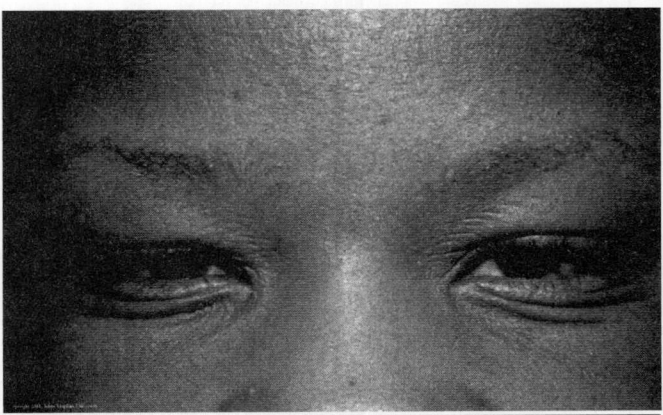

FIG. 24-3   Dennie line or Morgan line.

nasopharyngeal tumors, choanal atresia or stenosis, and vasomotor rhinitis. Overuse of prescription or over-the-counter (OTC) topical nasal decongestants can cause drug-induced rhinitis as can the use of cocaine. Some individuals experience idiopathic rhinitis marked by nasal hyperresponsiveness to nonspecific triggers, such as strong smells (e.g., perfumes, bleach), tobacco smoke, or changes in environmental temperature and humidity. Hormonal rhinitis occurs during pregnancy, puberty, and in hypothyroidism, and food-induced rhinitis is associated with consumption of hot and spicy foods.

Management

There are three strategies for the management of AR: avoidance, pharmacology, and immunotherapy.

Avoidance Strategies.   Avoiding exposure to the offending allergen or irritant as much as possible is essential. Allergens causing seasonal rhinitis are more difficult to avoid than are the indoor allergens, such as molds, because pollens are smaller and lighter and thus remain in the air longer.

Key avoidance measures for indoor allergens and irritants include the following:

- Control house dust, paying special attention to the child's bedroom.
  - Use dust–mite-proof mattress and pillow covers.
  - Wash bed linens in hot water (greater than 130° F [54.4° C]) weekly.
  - Use vertical blinds instead of horizontal blinds or curtains.
  - Remove carpeting from bedroom.
  - Use plastic or wood furniture instead of cloth.
- Eliminate smoking from the child's environment; if household members still smoke despite education, stress that they should smoke outside the house.

- Keep pets outdoors; consider not having pets.
- Reduce mold; avoid damp basements and other sources of moisture from the home environment (see Chapter 41 for further discussion of molds).
- Use dehumidifiers, air conditioners with efficient filters, and air-cleaning devices with an electronic precipitator or with a high-efficiency particulate air (HEPA) filter.
- Eliminate milk, egg, or wheat for infants with perennial AR, if these prove to be offending substances.

Pharmacologic Therapy.   Oral antihistamines, nasal antihistamines, and intranasal corticosteroids are part of the therapy for AR. Pharmacologic agents should be started 1 to 2 weeks before pollen season for children with seasonal AR. For perennial AR, start with maximum recommended dose and then taper to minimum dose needed to control symptoms. Often children with AR benefit from a combination approach; some require only single-line therapy. Antibiotics need to be prescribed for secondary infections (sinusitis). Consult Appendix A for drugs and their administration.

Oral Antihistamines

- Oral antihistamines are especially helpful in seasonal AR. The second-generation antihistamines are particularly effective in controlling symptoms of AR and are often used in the management of this problem.
- Oral antihistamines relieve symptoms of nasal itching, sneezing, and rhinorrhea, but do little to relieve nasal obstruction.
- Oral antihistamines are divided into different classes (Table 24-7).
- Dosage of drug may need to be increased until relief of symptoms is obtained, or side effects are experienced (see Appendix A).

TABLE 24-7   **Antihistamine Classes**

Class	Name	Comments
Ethanolamines	Diphenhydramine (Benadryl)	Sedation, dizziness, thickening of bronchial secretions
	Clemastine (Tavist)	Dry mouth, fatigue, headache, somnolence, bradycardia
	Carbinoxamine (Clistin, Rondec)*	Drowsiness, CNS excitation and difficulty sleeping
Ethylenediamines	Pyrilamine (in Rynatan, Atrohist)	Not used in children
	Tripelennamine	Not used in children
Alkylamines	Chlorpheniramine (Chlor-Trimeton)	Drowsiness, sedation, dry mouth, GI symptoms
	Brompheniramine (in Dimetane, Bromfed)	Palpitations, weight gain, drowsiness, dizziness, headache
Piperazines	Hydroxyzines (Atarax, Vistaril)	Sedation, dizziness, dry mouth
Piperidines	Cyproheptadine (Periactin)	CNS depression, weight gain, dry mouth
Nonsedating antihistamines	Loratadine (Claritin)	Dry mouth, fatigue, headache, somnolence Approved for children ≥2 years old
	Cetirizine (Zyrtec)	Dry mouth, fatigue, headache, somnolence Approved for children ≥2 years old
	Fexofenadine (Allegra)	Dry mouth, fatigue, headache, somnolence, dysmenorrhea, flu-like signs Approved for children ≥6 years old

*The CDC released a report warning about the use of cough and cold medications in children <2 years old. Products containing nasal decongestants (e.g., pseudoephedrine), antihistamines (e.g., carbinoxamine), cough suppressants (e.g., dextromethorphan), and expectorants are often used by parents of children in this age group; however, their use is associated with adverse side effects that may lead to death in children <2yr old.
CDC website: *www.cdc.gov/mmwr/preview/mmwrhtml/mm5601a1.htm;* CDC: Infant deaths associated with cough and cold medications—two states, 2005, *MMWR Morb Mortal Wkly Rep* 56(01):1-4, 2007.

- Patients can develop a tolerance to a particular antihistamine and may need to rotate drugs if tolerance develops.
- If side effects with one antihistamine are experienced, another antihistamine in a different class or one in the same class but with different actions should be prescribed.
- Sedating antihistamines may interfere with daytime activities and negatively affect school performance.

Topical Nasal Antihistamine

- Azelastine is a nasal antihistamine spray approved for use in seasonal AR in children 5 years and older.
- Azelastine acts by competing with histamine for H_1-receptor sites.
- Azelastine has a bitter taste and is associated with sedation.

Decongestants

- Decongestants may help relieve nasal congestion; however, they have limited long-term benefit because of adverse effects associated with their use (Shrime & Keller, 2006).
- Decongestants may be used alone or in combination with an antihistamine.
- Topical decongestants can cause rebound rhinorrhea if used for more than 3 to 5 days; errors in administration can cause systemic absorption and side effects of irritability, nervousness, and insomnia among others.
- Children under 2 years old should not be given decongestants.

Nasal Cromolyn

- Cromolyn is less effective than intranasal corticosteroids.
- Nasal cromolyn can be beneficial and is sometimes used in children when possible dysphonia is problematic with the use of intranasal or inhaled corticosteroids (Shrime & Keller, 2006).

Intranasal Corticosteroids

- Corticosteroids are effective agents to reduce inflammation and subsequent nasal obstruction. The child should clear his or her nasal passages of mucus before use.
- Corticosteroids are considered one of the most effective treatment choices to manage AR. However, parents and health care provides often select second-generation antihistamines because of safety concerns, such as growth suppression (Kaari, 2006).
- Corticosteroids can be effective for relieving symptoms of nasal congestion, rhinorrhea, itching, and sneezing but are less effective for the relief of ocular symptoms, which is rare with usual recommended dose (Lasley, 2006).
- Corticosteroids can take 1 week or more before clinical benefit is observed.
- Side effects can include local burning, irritation, sneezing, soreness, or epistaxis, which is related to improper technique (spraying the nasal septum).
- Table 24-8 lists usual dosages per nostril for intranasal corticosteroid preparations (Taketomo et al, 2006).

Leukotriene Modifiers

- Montelukast (Singulair) is approved for use in seasonal AR.

Antibiotics

- Treat secondary infections (e.g., sinusitis and otitis media) with appropriate antibiotic coverage.

Immunotherapy. Allergen immunotherapy is indicated when symptoms are severe and have not improved with avoidance measures and pharmacologic therapy or when complications of chronic or recurrent sinusitis or otitis media and hearing loss are problematic. It should only be performed in a

---

TABLE 24-8   Intranasal Corticosteroid Preparations Used for Allergic Rhinitis: Usual Doses

Drug	Dose	Number of Inhalations or Sprays and Daily Frequency	Age
Beclomethasone (Vancenase AQ, Beconase AQ)	42 mcg/inhalation	1-2 sprays bid	6-12 yr
		1 bid-qid or 2 bid	≥12 yr
Beclomethasone—aqueous inhalation (Beconase AQ) (Vancenase AQ 84 mcg)	42 mcg/inhalation	1-2 bid	≥6 yr
	84 mcg/spray	1-2 once daily	≥6 yr
Budesonide* (Rhinocort Aqua)	32 mcg/spray	2 sprays	≥6 yr
Flunisolide (Nasalide, Nasarel)	29 mcg/spray	1 spray tid or 2 sprays twice daily; maintenance dose is 1 spray daily	6-14 yr
		2 sprays bid; maintenance 1 spray daily	≥14 yr
Fluticasone (Flonase)	50 mcg/spray	1 spray daily; 2 sprays daily if severe or poor response	≥4 yr
		2 sprays daily	>12 yr
Mometasone (Nasonex)	50 mcg/spray	1 spray daily	3-11 yr
		2 sprays daily	>12 yr
Triamcinolone AQ (Nasacort AQ)	55 mcg/spray	2 sprays daily; maintenance dose 1 spray daily	>12 yr
(Tri-Nasal)	50 mcg/inhalation	2 sprays daily; may increase to 4 sprays daily or 2 sprays bid	>12 yr

*Reduce slowly every 2-4 weeks to smallest effective dose.
bid, Twice daily; *qid*, four times per day; *tid*, three times per day; *yr*, years.
Adapted from Taketomo CK, Hodding JH, Kraus DM: *Pediatric dosage handbook,* ed 13, Hudson, OH, 2006-2007, Lexi-Comp.

facility that has both the necessary equipment and health care professionals who are prepared to treat anaphylaxis.

Complications

Sinusitis may complicate AR owing to associated swelling of the mucosal lining of the sinuses with secondary infection. Likewise eustachian tube dysfunction and its sequela, serous otitis media, are common complications. Malocclusion, the development of a high-arched palate, and the typical allergic facies can result from long-standing AR. In addition, chronic AR may lead to chronic cough and postnasal drip.

Patient and Parent Education and Prevention

Because AR is often a chronic problem, parents and children need to have specific information about control of this disorder.

- Instruct on environmental control. Handouts and a review of ways to individualize this information are essential.
- Review pharmacologic therapy, including the following:
  ○ Indications for and changes in medications
  ○ Frequency of use
  ○ Common side effects and contraindications
  ○ How to use intranasal sprays or inhalers if prescribed

Prognosis

Perennial AR can be a chronic problem unless offending allergens are identified and eliminated from the environment. If this is not possible, pharmacologic therapy is usually helpful in reducing symptoms. As the child grows and the nasal passages increase in size, symptoms may also lessen. Symptoms from seasonal AR often worsen from the adolescent years to mid-adulthood. Moving to a new environment often results in a short respite (1 to 3 years) from symptoms. However, the child frequently becomes sensitized to new airborne pollens, and symptoms of seasonal AR return.

ATOPIC DERMATITIS

Description

Atopic dermatitis (AD) is a common skin disorder of childhood that is characterized by acute and chronic skin eruptions. The term *eczema* is sometimes used interchangeably with *atopic dermatitis*. Eczema means flaring up, which describes the acute symptom complex (erythema, scaling, vesicles, inflamed papules and plaques, and crusts) seen with AD, but does not adequately describe the chronic skin changes that can result from this disorder. AD manifests a typical morphology and distribution of flexural lichenification or linearity in adults and facial and extensor involvement in infants and children. AD is frequently referred to as the "itch that rashes." With AD, the skin's ability to act as a protective barrier is impaired, resulting in dryness, cracking, and susceptibility to skin infection. The skin is then more susceptible to bacterial, viral, and fungal infections (see Color Plate).

Epidemiology

AD affects approximately 17% of the childhood population in the U.S., with higher incidence in other countries. AD develops in 45% of children within the first 6 months of life, and in 60% of children by the first year of life. Approximately 85% of those with AD exhibit this problem by their fifth birthday. AD is often the first manifestation of the "atopic march" with asthma and AR following. Asthma also develops in approximately 50% of those with AD, and AR develops in 50% to 80% of those with AD. The incidence of AD is increasing in the U.S. (Paller & Mancini, 2006).

The exact etiology is unknown and may vary from individual to individual. Although many children have high IgE levels, an exact immune mechanism for this disorder is not evident. Immune dysregulation, epidermal barrier dysfunction, and pharmacophysiologic abnormalities are implicated in its pathogenesis. Abnormalities in histamine production (increased in the skin), chemotaxis, monocytes, and cytokines are associated with AD. T-lymphocyte activation and hyperresponsiveness of Langerhans cells are also thought to be implicated in its expression. The strongest predictor of AD is a positive family history of AD; however, about 25% of those with AD have no personal or family history of atopic disease. Sweating increases itching in atopic skin. A predisposition to development of pruritus is believed to be a key factor with variability in the extent of the skin involvement and severity of presentation (Paller & Mancini, 2006).

Clinical Findings

The following are seen in AD (Paller & Mancini, 2006) (Table 24-9):

- Essential diagnostic features include pruritus and eczematous changes that reflect typical age-specific morphologic patterns and a chronic or relapsing skin condition.
- More than one third of cases begin before 3 months old. Dry skin is the only initial sign. These infants are generally not brought in for health care until pruritus and the itch-scratch-itch cycle develops, generally around 2 to 3 months old.
- Acute manifestations (more common in infants) include the following:
  ○ Intense itching
  ○ Redness
  ○ Papules, vesicles, and edema
  ○ Serous discharge and crusts
  ○ Generalized dry skin (xerosis) with dry hair and scalp; diaper area usually spared
- Chronic manifestations (more common in children and adolescents) include the following:
  ○ Lichenification—thickened, leathery, hyperpigmented skin
  ○ Scratch marks
- Characteristics of infantile phase:
  ○ Begins from birth to 6 months old; may resolve, but can continue into the childhood phase
  ○ Cheeks, forehead, scalp, extending to trunk as symmetric patches or to the extremities; lateral extensor surface of arms and legs
  ○ Tends to be acute with intense itching, erythema, papules, vesicles, oozing crusting, and generalized xerosis; the diaper area and groin are usually spared of lesions

TABLE 24-9	Assessment of Atopic Dermatitis	
Onset	**Signs and Symptoms**	**Comment/Prognosis**
Initial presentation • <3 months old • 2-3 months old	Dry skin first sign Itch-scratch-itch cycle starts	Often not noticed
Infantile phase	Acute presentation—common in infants: intense itching; redness, papules, vesicles, edema; serous discharge and crusts; xerosis, dry hair, scalp; diaper area sparing; cheeks, forehead, scalp, extremities	Two-thirds of cases resolve by 2-3 year
Childhood phase (starts 2 years old to puberty)	Involves wrists, hands, popliteal and antecubital fossa; eyebrows thin and broken off (Hertog sign); some only have feet involved; may have allergic-atopic facies and white dermatographism	One third continue into teenage years
Adolescent phase	Common in children and teenagers; thickened, leathery, hyperpigmented skin; scratch marks	New or recurrent problem

- Characteristics of childhood phase:
  - Beginning around 2 years old and lasting to puberty or may continue from the infantile phase
  - Classic areas of involvement include the wrists (hands), neck, ankles (feet), popliteal and antecubital fossae, commonly of flexural areas; periorbital and perioral areas may also be involved
  - Eyebrows can be thin and broken off (loss of the lateral half of the eyebrow is called Hertog sign)
  - Tends to be chronic; possible lichenification
  - Pruritus is often severe
  - Lesions tend to be dry and papular with circumscribed scaly patches
- Characteristics of adolescent phase:
  - Begins at puberty and can commonly continue into adulthood; often involves the flexural folds (popliteal and antecubital fossae), face, neck, upper arms and back, dorsa of hands, fingers, feet, and toes
  - May be new occurrence or recurrence of a chronic condition
  - Dry skin and lichenification are prominent findings
  - Erythematous, dry-scaling papules and plaques with less exudates
  - Postinflammatory hypopigmentation or hyperpigmentation that disappears
- Other key features of AD:
  - Tendency toward dry skin and a lowered threshold for itching (itch-scratch-itch cycle)
  - Tendency to worsen during dry winter months or with heat in the summer
  - Chronic AD often secondarily infected with *Staphylococcus aureus* (most commonly) or *Streptococcus pyogenes* (occasionally)
  - Hyperpigmentation may be noted especially in areas of lichenification
- Possible associated features:
  - Atopic pleats–extra groove in lower eyelid called Dennie lines or Morgan fold (see Fig. 24-3), crease across upper bulb of nose.
  - Accentuated palmar creases
  - Allergic shiners, mild facial pallor, or dry hair
  - Keratosis pilaris—follicular papules occurring on the extensor aspect of the arms, anterior thighs, and lateral aspects of the cheeks
  - Nummular eczema, dyshidrotic eczema, juvenile plantar dermatitis, nipple eczema, or ichthyosis vulgaris
  - White dermatographism—a red line first appears with firm stroking of the skin, but is replaced by a white line in approximately 10 seconds but without an associated wheal; the normal reaction of skin is to develop a red line at the site of stroking, followed by a red flare, and then later a wheal in 1 to 3 minutes
  - Some with AD have an associated circumoral pallor (thought to be related to local edema and vasoconstriction)

Diagnostic Studies. Diagnosis of AD is based on characteristic historical and physical findings. A chronic or recurring rash that is pruritic and has a characteristic distribution and appearance, together with a family or personal history of atopy, are key in leading to the diagnosis of AD. Histologic examination of the skin is rarely needed and is reserved only for cases that are difficult to diagnose and to exclude other diseases. Serum IgE concentration is elevated in many children with this problem; for the vast majority of children, immunologic testing (e.g., IgE, CAP-RAST, or prick test) is not needed to confirm the diagnosis or to monitor treatment. Skin testing and desensitization are not recommended for children with AD only. If secondary fungal infection is suspected, collect scrapings and use potassium hydroxide (KOH) to look for fungal hyphae.

Differential Diagnosis

Other types of dermatitis, including seborrheic dermatitis, contact dermatitis, allergic contact dermatitis, nummular dermatitis, psoriasis, and scabies, are included in the differential diagnosis. A few genetic conditions are associated with similar skin eruptions (e.g., phenylketonuria, Wiskott-Aldrich syndrome, histiocytosis X, and acrodermatitis enteropathica). Pityriasis alba can also be a differential diagnosis.

Management

Treatment strategy is based on the following key concepts:

- The itch-scratch-itch cycle must be interrupted.
- Dryness of the skin must be corrected; good moisturization is critical.
- If there are known offending agents (irritants and allergic triggers), they must be eliminated.
- Secondary bacterial or viral infections must be treated.

Acute versus chronic care management is also a consideration. The following therapies are key factors in the control of AD.

Pharmacotherapy

- Antihistamine agents have little direct effect on pruritus, but sedating doses at night help children with pruritus fall asleep. They have limited effectiveness as monotherapy in AD. The following agents are often used (Taketomo et al, 2006).
  - Hydroxyzine (Atarax, Vistaril) has excellent antihistaminic qualities, but can cause drowsiness and behavioral changes. If an antihistamine is needed throughout the day, the usual oral dose of Atarax in children is 2 mg/kg/day divided every 6 to 8 hours (Takemoto et al, 2006). This dose may need to be increased.
  - Diphenhydramine hydrochloride (Benadryl) is also a useful antihistamine, especially if sedation is also needed. The usual oral dose of diphenhydramine hydrochloride in children is as follows: 2 to 6 years old, 6.25 mg every 4 to 6 hours with 37.5 mg/day maximum; 6 to 12 years old, 12.5 to 25 mg every 4 to 6 hours with 150 mg/day maximum; children older than 12 years, 25 to 50 mg every 4 to 6 hours with 300 mg/day maximum (Taketomo et al, 2006).
- Nonsedating or low-sedating antihistamines may be considered (see Table 24-9 and Appendix A).
- Topical corticosteroid preparations are a mainstay of therapy. Do not apply topical steroids containing propylene glycol.
  - Gels penetrate well, are somewhat more drying, and are effective in the management of acute weeping or vesicular lesions.
  - Ointments penetrate more effectively than creams or lotions and provide occlusion. They are beneficial in the management of dry, lichenified, or plaquelike areas; however, they may occlude eccrine ducts and lead to sweating.
  - When applied over large areas of dermatitis or if occlusion (covering with plastic wrap) is used, the possibility of significant systemic absorption is greatly increased, especially in infants and young children.
  - Apply a thin layer of 1% hydrocortisone cream (acute stage) or ointment (chronic stage) to affected areas three or four times a day.
  - Use of fluorinated, topical corticosteroid preparations in children should only be done in consultation with a physician or a dermatology specialist. Never use fluorinated, topical corticosteroid preparations on the face; instead use 1% hydrocortisone ointment sparingly two to three times a day until symptoms improve and then withdraw. Do not use for an extended period of time because corticosteroids cause thinning of the skin (see Table 36-1 for a listing of topical corticosteroids by potency rating).
    - Low-potency and mid-potency topical steroids should be used to treat exacerbations in children with mild to moderate severity. Twice daily application is all that is needed. Taper to a less potent topical steroid once the AD is controlled or use it intermittently to control flares. If such steroids are rapidly discontinued, a rebound phenomenon can occur.
- Immunomodulators (tacrolimus 0.03% ointment and pimecrolimus 1% cream) can be used in children 2 years and older and are reserved for severe AD. These nonsteroidal antiinflammatory medications block calcineurin. This results in the inhibition of T-cell activation. The most common side effect is stinging or burning when applied, usually during the first several days of administration and in severe cases of AD. They are safe steroid-sparing agents and work well on thinner skin of the face, neck, groin, and axillae (Cardona et al, 2006; Paller & Mancini, 2006).
- MimyX Cream (Stiefel Laboratories, Inc.) is useful for the management and relief of burning and itching associated with AD in addition to allergic-contact dermatitis, radiation dermatitis, and other dermatoses in pediatric and adult patients.

Skin Care

Hydration is a key element in the treatment of AD.

- Use open wet compresses if there are weeping, oozing lesions and signs of acute skin inflammation. They also help rehydrate the skin (Paller & Mancini, 2006).
  - Aluminum acetate (Burow solution in a 1:20 or 1:40 preparation). Solution should be lukewarm or body temperature.
  - Use a soft cloth that is moderately wet and not dripping; remoisten as needed. Corticosteroid topical preparations can be applied after application of compresses.
  - Apply 2 to 3 times a day and can use up to 5 days; effective during the acute stage of AD.
  - Aveeno or oatmeal baths help soothe acute episodes of pruritus, followed by application of a heavy cream emollient (the thicker and greasier the emollient the more effective).
- Daily bath or shower, 10 minutes, to reduce skin dryness. Excessive soaking in the bathtub depletes the skin of natural moisturizers if not immediately followed with moisturizing topical agents. Use lukewarm, not hot, water. Use mild soap, such as Dove or Basis, for the axilla and groin. Do not use drying or deodorant soaps, bubble-bath products, and oils in bath water. Immediately pat the child and quickly apply occlusive ointments. Some recommend two baths daily, each less than 5 minutes, immediately followed by lubricating oils or ointments as a way to restore water to the skin.
- Cetaphil and Aquanil are nondrying soap-free cleansing agents and can be substituted for bathing. Instruct parents to leave these agents on the skin; they should not be wiped off after applying. Patients with wool or lanolin sensitivity should use glycerine moisturizers, such as Cetaphil.

- Immediately after bath or shower, gently pat dry within 3 minutes; no rubbing or scrubbing. Emolliate with a moisturizer. Lubricants maintain the skin's hydration, and emollients are the treatment of choice for dry skin.
  - An emollient (e.g., petrolatum [Vaseline, Aquaphor]) can be applied just before getting out of the bath water or just after getting out of the bath while still damp. This is also a good time to apply topical corticosteroid preparations because absorption of the agent is more effective if the skin is hydrated.
- Emollients can be applied three to four times a day as needed, such as fragrance-free Eucerin cream, Crisco (plain, not butter flavored), or petroleum jelly (an occlusive agent). If a child is sensitive to fragrances, scented creams, such as Nivea, should be avoided. Other moisturizers include Nouriva Repair, Olay Body Wash, and CeraVe Moisturizing Lotion.
- Children with severe AD may need additional soaking after baths to maintain skin hydration. This should be done at bedtime. Wet gauze and bandage wraps, wrung out to dampness, can be placed on the extremities with a dry dressing over them. Cotton pajamas or soaks can also be used with a wet, wrung-dry pajama or soak next to the skin and then covered with a corresponding dry pajama or sock. For some children with AD (xerotic individuals), frequent bathing may exacerbate their pruritus and thus aggravate their skin problems. Bathing must be limited in these patients and emollients used (Paller & Mancini, 2006).
- Keep fingernails short to decrease additional skin trauma from scratching.

Secondary Infection Management

- Systemic antibiotic agents are essential if secondary skin infection with *S. aureus* or *S. pyogenes* is suspected.
  - First-generation cephalosporins are most commonly used.
  - Be cognizant that community-based methicillin-resistant *S. aureus* has been rapidly increasing (see discussion in Chapter 23 on how to identify and manage).
  - Topical antibiotic preparations are contraindicated, although the use of mupirocin has been demonstrated to reduce colony counts of *S. aureus*. Intermittent application of mupirocin to the nares and hands of patients and their caregivers twice daily for 3 weeks may decrease colonization.
  - Topical antibacterial scrubs are contraindicated because they dry out the skin and cause irritation.
- The addition of ⅛ to ¼ cup of chlorine bleach in a full tub of bath water has been shown to transiently decrease *S. aureus* colonization of the skin (Paller & Mancini, 2006).
- Topical antifungal medication is recommended if KOH positive for hyphae.
- Tar preparations may be added to help manage chronic and lichenified forms of dermatitis.
  - These are topical agents that have limited use.
  - Patients should be cautioned about photosensitivity.
- Systemic corticosteroid agents are rarely needed.

Environmental Management

- A decrease in environmental humidity and an increase in antigen presentation are key causative factors. Therefore increase environmental humidity and decrease exposure to antigens. Cool temperatures (e.g., through the use of air conditioning) help.
- Eliminate or avoid known or suspected offending agents. These include:
  - Nonbreathable fabrics—nylon or wool; wool is irritating whereas soft cotton clothing is not.
  - Overheating and overdressing (heat and perspiration are irritant triggers that increase pruritus).
  - Chlorine, turpentine, harsh soaps, fabric softeners, products with fragrances, and bleach.
  - Allergenic agents, such as feather pillows, fuzzy toys, stuffed animals, pets.
  - House dust mites—careful attention to the child's bedroom is important (e.g., encasing mattresses and pillows, washing bedding in hot water weekly, frequent vacuuming, removing carpets or at least frequent cleaning are recommended).

Dietary Management

- Dietary restrictions may include the elimination of cow's milk from the diet of infants predisposed to atopy. Eggs, fish, chocolate, nuts, and citrus fruits are generally not allowed until 12 months old. In approximately 40% of children with moderate to severe AD, a food allergen may contribute to their problem (Cardona et al, 2006).

Referral. Refer to a dermatologist if child is unresponsive to traditional therapy or has an unusual manifestation (Paller & Mancini, 2006).

Complications

Secondary skin infections are a frequent complication of AD. *S. aureus* is the most frequent bacterial organism associated with skin infection. Treatment of secondary skin infection is imperative in the management of AD. Kaposi varicelliform eruption (eczema herpeticum) is a significant complication that can result in severe illness in children. Lichenification, a secondary skin change marked by thickening of the skin, is associated with chronic itching. Keratoconus is occasionally seen and is associated with chronic rubbing of the eyelids. Individuals with AD may be prone to *Molluscum contagiosum*, tinea, and warts.

Patient and Parent Education and Prevention for Outpatient Management

The provider should stress that AD is often a recurrent disease that can be controlled. The goal of therapy is to prevent the itch-scratch-itch cycle and hydrate the skin. Specific written instructions and handouts should be provided because management is complex.

Parents need to understand:

- The use of medications, (when, how much, and how often to use; side effects; and proper application of topical preparations)
- Care of the skin
- The risks for secondary infection
- The role of environmental controls of allergens or triggers
- Possible dietary management as outlined previously

- What to do if symptoms worsen or signs of secondary skin infection appear and when to seek additional medical treatment
- Precipitating factors:
  - Extreme temperatures or humidity
  - Excess sweat
  - Emotional stress
  - New clothes—wash with mild detergent (with no dyes or perfumes) before wearing them to remove formaldehyde and other chemicals
  - Harsh washing detergents—add second rinse cycle when washing clothes
  - Avoid wearing coarse clothes
  - Excess soap and water
  - Cutaneous or systemic infection

Prognosis

With appropriate treatment, AD can generally be controlled. In two-thirds of children, the symptoms of AD become less severe with complete remission in 25%. However, there is an adolescent and adult stage of the disease. Risk factors for adult AD include widespread dermatitis as a child, family history of AD, early initial childhood age of onset, high serum IgE levels, and a history of asthma or AR (Lasley, 2006). Self-image problems may result if AD is severe.

■ DISEASES WITH AN AUTOIMMUNE BASIS

JUVENILE RHEUMATOID ARTHRITIS (JRA)

Description

JRA is a disease with an autoimmune basis and represents a group of conditions with onset of symptoms in children at or younger than 16 years old that causes chronic inflammation of at least one synovial joint for 6 weeks or more. There are various subtypes of JRA disease in children that are categorized based on differences in their disease onset, severity, duration, and pattern of complications. The three principal types of arthritis are polyarticular (five or more joints involved), pauciarticular or oligoarticular (inflammation of one to four joints), or systemic onset with fever, characteristic rash, and serositis. Some health care providers (generally outside the U.S.) prefer to call this syndrome juvenile idiopathic arthritis instead of JRA; it is also known as juvenile chronic arthritis (Haftel, 2006; Kahn & Imundo, 2006).

Epidemiology

The exact cause of JRA is unknown. In the U.S., approximately 80,000 children are affected. Certain histocompatibility complex antigens are more prevalent in the JRA population. Cytokine production, proliferation of macrophage-like synoviocytes, infiltration with neutrophils and lymphocytes, and autoimmunity are thought to be the major pathologic processes causing chronic joint inflammation (Kahn & Imundo, 2006).

The rate of JRA is significantly higher in girls than in boys in oligoarticular or pauciarticular JRA. This difference is especially noted in younger children and in polyarticular JRA. The female to male ratio in systemic onset is equal. The approximate percentage of occurrence and age breakdown for each of the subtypes follows: systemic—10% and occurs at any age; polyarticular—30% and has a late (greater than 8 years old) or early childhood onset; and oligoarticular—60% with a late or early onset (Kahn & Imundo, 2006).

Clinical Findings

History. The major complaints of the child with JRA are:
- Pain—generally a mild to moderate aching
- Joint stiffness—worse in the morning and after rest

Physical Examination. Associated features of JRA are:
- Nonmigratory monoarticular or polyarticular involvement of large or proximal interphalangeal joints for more than 3 months
- Systemic manifestations—fever, erythematous rashes, leukocytosis, serositis, lymphadenopathy, and rheumatoid nodules

Less commonly seen are ocular disease (e.g., iridocyclitis, iritis, or uveitis), pleuritis, pericarditis, anemia of chronic disease, fatigue, and growth failure, or leg lengths discrepancy if the arthritis is unilateral.

Key physical findings are:
- Swelling of the joint with effusion or thickening of synovial membrane, or both, noted on palpation
- Heat over inflamed joint and tenderness along joint line
- Loss of joint range of motion and function; child typically holds the affected joints in slight flexion and may walk with limp

There are three major patterns of presentation (Haftel, 2006):

1. *Systemic-onset pattern* with spiking fevers once or twice a day that can last for months, an evanescent pale or salmon pink macular rash (occurs with fever), hepatosplenomegaly, leukocytosis, and polyserositis; the arthritis is typically polyarticular and follows the systemic manifestations in 6 weeks to 6 months. This group does not develop iridocyclitis.

2. *Polyarticular pattern (five or more synovial joints involved within the first 6 months of diagnosis)* of chronic pain and symmetric joint swelling; low-grade fever, fatigue, nodules, and anemia of chronic disease may be present, but are not as prominent as in acute form; uveitis occurs in 20% to 30% of children in this group; typically, involves the small joints of the hands, feet, ankles, wrists, and knees. Adolescents who develop this type differ from those with early onset in that they exhibit a positive RF. Adolescents who develop late-onset polyarticular JRA have a course similar to the adult entity.

3. *Pauciarticular pattern* with involvement of few joints, typically the weight-bearing joints within the first 6 months of diagnosis; synovitis may be mild and painless; joint involvement is asymmetric and involves medium-sized joints (commonly the knees) followed by the ankle and wrist; often the laboratory values do not demonstrate

evidence of inflammation; and patients do not tend to have signs of systemic inflammation.

Each of the three principal types of JRA has a typical pattern of presentation. In addition, there are nine distinct course subtypes that have been identified (Miller, 2004). For more information on their specific presentation, the primary care provider should consult other texts on this subject.

Diagnostic Studies. Diagnosis is based on physical findings and history; there is no diagnostic laboratory test for juvenile chronic arthritis. Most children with pauciarticular arthritis have negative laboratory markers. Those with polyarticular and systemic-onset typically have elevated acute-phase reactants and anemia of chronic disease. A positive result for RF by latex fixation may be present, and ANA may be present in up to 60% of children with pauciarticular or oligoarticular disease. A positive ANA helps to identify children at higher risk for uveitis. Other laboratory findings that may be useful include a CBC (to exclude leukemia), ESR, C-reactive protein (CRP), leukocytosis, anemia, hyperglobulinemia, and hypoalbuminemia. Imaging studies (magnetic resonance imaging [MRI]) can help in managing joint pathologic conditions. Analysis of synovial fluid is not helpful in the diagnosis of JRA.

Differential Diagnosis

The various causes of monoarticular arthritis should be considered in the differential diagnosis. These include tumors, leukemia, cancer, bacterial infections, toxic synovitis, rheumatic fever, SLE, Lyme disease, spondyloarthropathies, inflammatory bowel disease, septic arthritis, and chondromalacia patellae.

Management

Children with severe involvement should be followed by a specialist in pediatric rheumatology. Other pediatric subspecialists, such as orthopedists, ophthalmologists, and cardiologists, may be consulted as needed. Therapy depends on the degree of local or systemic involvement.

Aspirin therapy has largely been replaced with the use of NSAIDs. Pharmacologic agents commonly used in the management of JRA include the following (Haftel, 2006; Kahn & Imundo, 2006):
- NSAIDs: Children with oligoarthritis generally respond well to NSAIDs.
  - Ibuprofen: 10 mg/kg/dose qid (maximum 1000 mg/day).
  - Tolmetin: 20 to 30 mg/kg/day divided tid (maximum 2000 mg/day).
  - Naproxen: 10 mg/kg bid (maximum 1000 mg/day).
  - Indomethacin older than 2 years: 1 to 2 mg/kg/day divided in two to four doses (maximum 4 mg/kg/day); adults 25 to 50 mg/dose two to three times/day (maximum 200 mg/day) (Taketomo et al, 2006).
  - Celecoxib (older than 17 years) 100 to 200 mg every day to bid (maximum 400 mg/day).
- Oral or parenteral corticosteroids, sulfasalazine, etanercept (a drug that soaks up tumor necrosis factor, an immune-system protein, and blocks the inflammatory cascade), methotrexate, or cyclosporine A are used in severe forms of JRA. Other possible disease-modifying antirheumatic drugs can

be used and include thalidomide, azathioprine, cyclophosphamide, infliximab, and adalimumab.
- Intraarticular corticosteroid injections are used if there is severe joint involvement.
- Pharmacologic therapy for uveitis is given as indicated by an ophthalmologist. Females with ANA+ oligoarticular JRA are at high risk and require slit-lamp examination every 3 to 4 months. The uveitis often does not correspond to the severity of the arthritis (i.e., uveitis may be present despite quiescent arthritis).
- Physical therapy—range of motion muscle-strengthening exercises and heat treatments—is used for joint involvement, and occupational therapy is beneficial. Rest and splinting are used if indicated.

Complications

Systemic involvement can include iridocyclitis, uveitis, pleuritis, pericarditis, anemia, fatigue, and hepatitis. Residual joint damage caused by granulation of tissue in the joint space can be a problem. Children most likely to develop permanent crippling disability are those with hip involvement, unremitting synovitis, or positive RF test.

Patient and Parent Education and Prevention

The following education and preventive measures are taken:
- For children on aspirin therapy (not typically given)—educate parents about the risk of Reye syndrome and its signs and symptoms.
- Recommend yearly influenza vaccine.
- Offer chronic disease counseling as indicated in Chapter 22.
- Encourage normal play and recreation.
- Educate about side effects of medications, in addition to splinting, orthotics, and bracing requirements.
- Instruct about need to follow up with an ophthalmologist. Frequency of follow-up for uveitis screening is based on subtype of JRA and is determined by the ophthalmologist.
- Ensure that parent and child understand that physical therapy is a mainstay of treatment for chronic childhood arthritis and should be part of the child's daily routine. A daily plan that includes passive, active, and resistive exercises is important.
- Water therapy and the use of heat or cold will reduce pain and stiffness. Swimming is an excellent activity for these children except those with severe anemia and cardiac disease.
- Tricycle or bike riding and low-impact dance are other useful sport activities.
- Refer to the Arthritis Foundation, which has excellent resources for family members and children (see Resource Box).
- Instruct on the need to involve school personnel in the identification of needed school-related services through an individualized education plan (IEP) or a 504.
- Discuss the challenge of pain management and its assessment in children with chronic arthritis and encourage parents to advocate for effective pain control on behalf of their child.

Prognosis

The course of the disease is variable, and there is no curative treatment. After an initial episode, the child may never have another episode, or the disease may go into remission and recur months or years later. The disease process of JRA wanes with age and completely subsides in 85% of children. However, systemic onset, a positive RF, poor response to therapy, and the radiologic evidence of erosion is associated with a poor prognosis. Onset of JRA in the teenage years is related to progression to adult rheumatoid disease.

SYSTEMIC LUPUS ERYTHEMATOSUS

Description

SLE is a chronic systemic disease that can involve many organ systems. Autoantibody formation resulting from activation of B lymphocytes is a key characteristic of this immune complex disease. It is more acute and severe in children than in adults.

Epidemiology

The exact cause is unknown, however, genetics and environment are involved in its pathogenesis. Altered cellular immunity in genetically predisposed individuals is postulated as a key factor in this disease. SLE is an autoimmune disease that is characterized by ANA production. There is widespread multiorgan system inflammation as a result of altered immune regulation. In SLE, immune complexes are deposited in various tissues of the body, and their clearance is impaired. Deposits of immune complexes trigger a generalized inflammatory response that can lead to tissue damage, such as vasculitis and numerous organ system abnormalities (commonly the heart and renal system). There is variety in both the presentation and how it is manifested over time in an individual (Ferguson, 2006).

The mechanism triggering immune complex formation is unknown. Females are preponderantly affected, and most experience symptoms around puberty. Onset before 9 years old is rare; adult onset tends to occur at around 30 to 40 years old. However, SLE tends to be more severe in pediatric patients than in adults (Ferguson, 2006; Haftel, 2006).

Clinical Findings

Clinical findings depend on organ involvement. Its presentation may be abrupt or have a gradual, nonspecific onset.

History.   The history may include the following:
- Joint involvement
  - Most common initial finding
  - Nondeforming arthritis with effusion and tenderness
  - Often symmetric joint involvement
- Arthralgia
- Systemic manifestations
- Low-grade fever—intermittent or sustained
- Fatigue and malaise
- Anorexia and loss of weight
- Malaise

Physical Examination.
The following may be seen on physical examination (Haftel, 2006):

- Malar or "butterfly" rash—scaly erythematous maculopapular rash covering malar areas extending over the bridge of the nose and cheeks; may spread down the face to the chest and extremities; "butterfly" rash and other lesions can be photosensitive
- Discoid rash with plugging of the follicles, hypopigmentation and hyperpigmentation, and scarring
- Lesions may also include small ulcerations in the skin and mucous membranes, indurations, purpura, and erythema nodosum
- Alopecia (as a result of loss of hair follicles from discoid lupus)
- Mucous membrane manifestations of the mouth and nasal septum
- Gingivitis, mucosal hemorrhage, erosions, ulcerations
- Silvery whitening of the vermilion border of the lips or thickening, redness, ulceration, or crusting of the lips
- Raynaud phenomenon is present in some children
- Polyserositis—pleurisy, pericarditis, and peritonitis
- Hepatosplenomegaly and lymphadenopathy
- Signs and symptoms of central nervous system involvement (seizures or psychosis) and cardiac (pleuritis or pericarditis) and renal involvement (e.g., cardiac failure or renal failure)

Diagnostic Studies.   Initial laboratory testing includes CBC, ANA, ESR, CRP, serum chemical analysis (metabolic and protein screen), and urinalysis. The ANA test is positive in 97% of children who have active, untreated SLE; the titers are usually high (Haftel, 2006). A negative ANA excludes SLE from the diagnosis except for the rare false-negative test. A positive ANA test should be followed up with testing for disease-specific types of ANA. Antibodies to double-stranded DNA are present in most patients with SLE. Leukopenia or lymphopenia, hemolytic anemia, and thrombocytopenia are frequent laboratory findings. Other laboratory and radiographic studies depend on organ involvement (e.g., histopathologic studies, urine testing, and serologic testing). Proteinuria and hematuria are a hallmark of lupus nephritis.

Differential Diagnosis

Diseases that resemble SLE include rheumatic fever, rheumatoid arthritis (RA), and viral infections. A temporary, drug-induced SLE can be caused by several pharmacologic agents, including hydantoin compounds, hydralazine, isoniazid (INH), procainamide, and sulfonamides.

Management

Children with SLE need to be followed by a specialist in collagen-vascular disorders. Other pediatric subspecialists may be consulted. Therapy depends on the degree of local or systemic involvement. General measures include avoiding sun exposure and daylight fluorescent light, in addition to applying sunscreen for ultraviolet A (UVA) and ultraviolet B (UVB) protection. The following measures also may be helpful:

- NSAIDs are used for relief of arthritis, arthralgias, serositis, or pain (if nephritis is present, use with caution).
- Oral steroids are prescribed if renal, cardiac, or central nervous system involvement is present. The dose is adjusted depending on clinical and laboratory findings. Cautious tapering of steroids is often needed.

- Antimalarial drugs (e.g., hydroxychloroquine) may be used to treat cutaneous manifestations.
- Immunosuppressant agents may be added if the response to steroids is inadequate.
- Use of other pharmacologic agents or therapies depends on the type and level of organ system involvement.

Complications

Currently, SLE is considered, for the most part, a controllable disease in children. The severity of the illness is variable. A diagnosis of SLE in childhood does not always mean a poor prognosis, especially if renal involvement is not present. Renal failure, central nervous system lupus, myocardial infarction, cardiac failure, and infection are the leading causes of death in children. Exposure to ultraviolet light may bring out or worsen skin lesions and can also result in exacerbation of systemic problems that can cause death. Side effects resulting from chronic use of high-dose corticosteroids (e.g., osteoporosis, avascular necrosis) can be a problem.

Patient and Parent Education

The provider should educate patients and parents about:
- The effect of sun exposure and the need for sunscreen protection
- The need to rest between activities because fatigue is a frequent problem for children with SLE
- The fact that SLE is a chronic disease that can have periods of remission followed by exacerbations

Prognosis

SLE is a chronic disease with periods of exacerbations with waxing and waning of symptoms; however, complete remission can occur. Children with mild disease do well; those with severe major organ involvement have a poor prognosis.

FIBROMYALGIA SYNDROME (FMS)

Description

Fibromyalgia is the term used to describe a condition characterized by widespread myofascial pain and fatigue and multiple trigger points that are discrete painful sites. It is a benign, intermittent, noninflammatory musculoskeletal pain syndrome that is also referred to as myofascial pain syndrome, generalized pain syndrome, fibrositis, and pain amplification syndrome. It is a complex syndrome that involves fatigue and generalized pain involving muscles, ligaments, and tendons. Symptoms are often vague and variable, with no major organ system abnormalities found. Its presentation can range from a generalized increased sensitivity to pain to a more classic pattern of specific symptoms (Imundo, 2006). Fibromyalgia can occur as a primary condition or in conjunction with other rheumatologic disorders (secondary fibromyalgia).

Epidemiology

The cause of fibromyalgia is unknown. It is considered a subset of musculoskeletal pain syndromes. Females are affected more often than males (Imundo, 2006). Fibromyalgia is more common in adults, but can occur in children, generally in those older than 12 years. The prevalence of fibromyalgia in children is estimated at 6% (Haftel, 2006).

Clinical Findings

History. The history may include the following long-standing common symptoms:
- Pain at multiple sites including muscles and in the soft tissues around joints
- Fatigue and malaise
- Insomnia or prolonged night awakenings
- Depression (a significant number exhibit depressive symptoms)

Physical Examination. Local areas of painful (not just tender) trigger points in muscles (usually at areas of tendon insertion) with pressure are characteristic physical findings. Pressure causes pain at the site and also in a circumferential or linear pattern surrounding the site. Common trigger points include: the neck, back, lateral epicondyles, greater trochanter, and knees. Typically, there is no evidence of arthritis or muscular weakness.

Diagnostic Criteria. The criteria for the diagnosis of fibromyalgia are as follows:
- A 3-month or longer history of diffuse pain associated with multiple trigger points
- Pain in 11 of 18 specific tender point sites on digital palpation (using approximately 4 kg of pressure)

Other underlying illness must have been excluded including inflammatory diseases (e.g., SLE, postinfectious fatigue that can follow Epstein-Barr [EBV] or influenza virus infections, or mood and conversion disorders) (Haftel, 2006).

Diagnostic Studies. Laboratory studies are of little benefit. Blood count, liver functions, and muscle enzymes are normal. If secondary fibromyalgia, order appropriate tests to diagnose rheumatoid disorder. However, children with fibromyalgia can have a false-positive ANA as do 20% of normal children (without rheumatoid disorders).

Differential Diagnosis

In CFS, tiredness lasting longer than 6 months rather than pain is the major complaint (Imundo, 2006). Fibromyalgia initially may be mistaken for other rheumatoid diseases, but does not have the associated rashes, weight loss, fever (greater than 101° F [38.3° C]), or joint swelling. Lyme disease is also in the differential.

Management

Children and their parents need reassurance that they do not have a life-threatening disease, but have a chronic condition that can be a lifelong problem. Treatment focuses on relieving symptoms and can include the following:
- Physical therapy for range-of-motion exercises, mild low-impact aerobic exercises (e.g., swimming, bicycling, and walking), and muscle strengthening.
- Amitriptyline (low doses) taken before bedtime has been helpful in stabilizing abnormal sleep patterns and in reducing pain.

- Psychotherapy and relaxation techniques to help cope with this condition and deal with stress.
- NSAIDs can be prescribed for pain control.
- Complementary therapy involves acupuncture.

Patient and Parent Education

The provider should educate patients and parents about:
- Fibromyalgia and that it is not a psychosomatic disorder
- Sleep hygiene
- The possibility that this could be a chronic problem, and there can be periods of remissions followed by exacerbations

Prognosis

The outcome of fibromyalgia in children varies; however, fibromyalgia in children generally has a better prognosis than it does in adults (Haftel, 2006).

CHRONIC FATIGUE SYNDROME

Children can develop idiopathic pain syndromes, which are characterized by the presence of severe disability despite the lack of physical or laboratory findings. Chronic fatigue syndrome (CFS) is one of the subsets of idiopathic pain syndromes as is fibromyalgia (Imundo, 2006). The age of onset is typically 20 years or older; however, it can occur in children from 7 to 20 years old. The presentation of CFS in children and adolescents is similar to that seen with adults. The key patient complaint is fatigue that must have a new onset, is unexplained, not linked to ongoing exertion, and is persistent. This fatigue is not substantially relieved by rest or sleep and results in substantial reduction in activity. Many describe the onset of CFS after a preceding illness with pharyngitis and fever.

In addition to fatigue symptoms as just described, the child needs to have at least four of the following eight symptoms to meet CFS case criteria:
- Impaired memory or concentration (cognitive dysfunction)
- Sore throat
- Painful cervical or axillary lymph nodes
- Muscle pain (myalgia)
- Multiple joint arthralgia with no swelling or redness noted
- Headaches of a new pattern
- Unrefreshing sleep
- Postexertional malaise

Complaints of low-grade fever are noted in about one third of cases, but are generally not documented on examination. There may be a history of neuropsychiatric problems; however, in these cases, a psychiatric illness must first be excluded before a diagnosis of CFS can be made. The debilitating fatigue must have been present for 6 months or longer (Imundo, 2006).

EBV infection has been implicated in the cause of CFS. However, EBV does not explain all the symptoms. No single immunologic abnormality has been consistently identified as the causative factor. The cause of CFS remains undetermined, and treatment is based on symptoms. Care must be taken in diagnosing this disorder in children, and other conditions (e.g., hypothyroidism, sleep apnea, hepatitis B or C, SLE, cancer, alcohol or drug abuse, Lyme disease, and major depressive and other psychiatric disorders) must first be ruled out (Imundo, 2006).

For a definitive diagnosis of CFS once other conditions are ruled out, the child is best referred to a specialist in this area.

Pharmacologic intervention generally is not effective. Psychological support (stressing that this disease is not made up) and exercise are associated with reduced disability. Preliminary studies involving children report improvement in 2 years for the majority of children (Imundo, 2006).

ACUTE RHEUMATIC FEVER

Description

Acute rheumatic fever (ARF) is a nonsuppurative complication following a group A ß-hemolytic streptococcus (GABHS) pharyngeal infection that results in an autoimmune inflammatory process involving the joints, heart, central nervous system, and subcutaneous tissue. ARF is diagnosed based on a set of criteria called the revised Jones criteria (see Box 30-8). Recurrent ARF can follow subsequent GABHS pharyngeal infections.

Epidemiology

The exact pathologic mechanism that is responsible for the inflammatory changes in various organs and tissues is unknown. Abnormalities in the host immune response to streptococcal cell wall proteins are believed to be involved. Greater organism virulence is associated with specific M protein types and a more "mucoid" capsule. There appears to be a strong genetic influence on susceptibility to GABHS infection with a family history of rheumatic fever and a lower socioeconomic status as known risk factors (Schneider, 2006). The latency period from infection with GABHS until symptom onset of ARF is usually 1 to 5 weeks with an average of 2 to 3 weeks (Young & Strong, 2006). Skin infections with GABHS rarely result in ARF. Recurrence of ARF following subsequent episodes of GABHS pharyngitis (symptomatic or asymptomatic infection) is high. The most commonly affected age group is children 5 to 6 years old to 15 years old (Young & Strong, 2006). See Chapter 30 for further discussion of ARF and cardiac involvement.

Clinical Findings and History

The diagnosis of an initial attack of ARF is based on the revised Jones criteria (see Box 30-8) and is as follows:
- Evidence of documented (culture, rapid streptococcal antigen test, or antistreptolysin O [ASO] titer) GABHS pharyngeal infection *and*
- Findings of two major manifestations or one major and two minor manifestations of ARF (Young & Strong, 2006; Schneider, 2006)

Major Manifestations
- Carditis is common (pancarditis, valves, pericardium, myocardium) and can cause chronic, life-threatening disease (i.e., congestive heart failure [CHF]).
- Polyarthritis (migratory and painful) involving large joints and rarely small or unusual joints (e.g., vertebrae); it is the most common manifestation of ARF.
- Sydenham chorea (uncommon).
- Erythema marginatum manifested as pink macules on the trunk and extremities; nonpruritic; this sign is uncommon.

- Subcutaneous nodules associated with repeated episodes and severe carditis; this sign is uncommon.
  Minor Manifestations
- Fever, polyarthralgia, prior history of ARF
  Diagnostic Studies.
- Elevated acute-phase reactants (ESR, white blood cells, CRP)
- Prolonged PR interval on electrocardiogram

Children may be diagnosed with ARF without evidence of a preceding streptococcal infection in the following two situations: a child with Sydenham chorea or with acquired heart disease (commonly mitral valve regurgitation without a congenitally abnormal or prolapsed valve) that can only be linked to ARF. Approximately 80% of children with ARF have an elevated ASO titer. In situations where the ASO titer is normal and ARF is still suspected, titers for anti-DNase B or other group A streptococcal-specific antibodies should be obtained with repeat testing in 2 weeks to look for a fourfold rise in titers (Young & Strong, 2006).

Differential Diagnosis

No single diagnostic test exists for ARF, and many diseases are included in the differential diagnosis (e.g., JA, connective tissue diseases, infective endocarditis, and Lyme disease).

Management

The treatment of ARF includes the following:

- Antibiotic therapy to eradicate GABHS infection. Primary prevention requires that a GABHS infection be treated within 10 days of onset. Benzathine penicillin G is the drug of choice unless there is an allergic history; erythromycin is then the drug of choice. Azithromycin and some oral cephalosporins are also sometimes used (Schneider, 2006; Young & Strong, 2006). A patient with a history of ARF who has an upper respiratory infection should be treated for GABHS whether or not GABHS is recovered because asymptomatic infection can trigger a recurrence.
- Antiinflammatory therapy. Aspirin (ASA) can be used for arthritis after the diagnosis is established; it is usually given only for 2 weeks and then tapered. ASA is also used in the treatment of mild to moderate carditis. ASA and steroids provide symptomatic relief, but do not prevent the incidence of chronic heart disease. However, the use of steroids has been beneficial in the management of severe carditis, reducing its morbidity and mortality.
- Chest radiographs, EKG, and echocardiography are indicated; carditis usually develops within the first 3 weeks of symptoms.
- Referral for treatment of CHF if needed. Medical management or valve replacement may be necessary.
- Bed rest is generally indicated only for children with CHF. Children with Sydenham chorea may need to be kept in bed to protect them until their choreiform movements are controlled. Steroids in the absence of other symptoms are not useful in the treatment of chorea.
- Children with severe chorea may benefit from the use of such pharmacologic agents as phenobarbital, haloperidol, diazepam, or valproic acid (Young & Strong, 2006).

The prevention of ARF includes the following:

- Treat GABHS pharyngeal infections with the appropriate antibiotics. Antibacterial prophylaxis for those with a prior history of ARF is required because of their greatly increased risk of recurrent ARF with subsequent inadequately treated GABHS infections. Intramuscular penicillin G (1.2 million units every 28 days) is more effective than daily penicillin V (Schneider, 2006).
- Antibacterial prophylaxis is continued for 5 years after the last ARF episode in children without carditis and at least until 21 years old. For those with carditis and persistent myocardial or valvular disease, treatment is 10 or more years and may be lifelong (Young & Strong, 2006).
- Children with a history of ARF need bacterial endocarditis prophylaxis treatment for dental or surgical procedures in addition to their regular antibiotic prophylaxis (see Chapter 30).

Complications

Chronic CHF can occur after an initial episode of ARF or follow recurrent episodes of ARF. Residual valvular damage is responsible for CHF. The risk of significant cardiac disease increases dramatically with each subsequent episode of ARF; thus, prevention of subsequent GABHS infections is critical. Intramuscular benzathine penicillin must be given every 4 weeks and not monthly and can be given every 3 weeks in high-risk children. The need for adherence must be stressed to parents (Young & Strong, 2006).

■ VASCULITIS SYNDROME
HENOCH-SCHÖNLEIN PURPURA
Description

Henoch-Schönlein purpura (HSP) is an overwhelming disease of childhood that is marked by acute vasculitis with associated inflammatory change of small blood vessels in various organ systems.

Epidemiology

HSP is the most common systemic vasculitis syndrome seen in children whose cause remains unknown. It can occur anytime from infancy (as early as 6 months old) to adulthood. However, it is primarily a disease of childhood that typically occurs in children 3 to 15 years old. HSP is seen slightly more frequently in males than females and occurs more frequently in winter months than other times of the year. This condition often follows a respiratory infection.

Leukocytic infiltration of tissue, hemorrhage, and ischemia are associated findings. IgA is involved in the immunopathogenesis of HSP. There is widespread leukocytoclastic vasculitis with IgA deposition in vessel walls noted as a common finding. With inflammation of the small blood vessels extravasation of blood occurs into local tissue. Patients with depositions of IgA in their renal mesangium have an associated nephritis. Although unproven, there is some conjecture that HSP may be allergy mediated (Haftel, 2006).

Clinical Findings

Clinical findings are typically characterized by rash (palpable purpura) and arthritis. Signs and symptoms of GI and renal vasculitis are a less frequent occurrence. Arthritis occurs in approximately 80% of patients and has an acute onset. Approximately one half of children develop GI involvement, and one third develop renal involvement. Symptoms of renal involvement can occur as an acute or chronic problem; renal involvement tends to be mild in most cases (Haftel, 2006). HSP is commonly milder and has a shorter duration in younger children, with few recurrences and fewer renal and GI manifestations (Paller & Mancini, 2006).

The diagnosis of HSP is based on the presence of two or more of the following findings:

- Palpable purpura
- Bowel angina
- Diagnostic biopsy (granulocytes found in the walls of arterioles or venules on histologic exam)
- Pediatric age group (less than 20 years old at onset of symptoms)

History.   A history of palpable cutaneous purpura is a hallmark of HSP. The classic presentation is purpura concentrated on the dependent areas of the body below the waist. Palpable purpura on legs and buttocks is a key historical feature; however, the rash may occur anywhere on the body. In addition, the history may include the following:

- Urticarial or small maculopapular rash may precede purpuric lesions, but rapidly progress to purpura with areas of ecchymosis
- Arthritis
  - Typically involves knees and ankles and is migratory, but can occur in any joint
  - May precede the appearance of purpuric lesions
- Colicky abdominal pain
  - Pain typically mild to moderate and may precede the onset of the rash
- Vomiting
- Hematuria (a hallmark of HSP nephritis)
- Gross or occult GI bleeding (bloody diarrhea) or significant abdominal distention—a less common finding

Physical Examination.   The two most common manifestations of HSP are:

- Skin vasculitis: cutaneous purpura—sine qua non for the diagnosis
  - Diameter: 0 to 2 mm
  - Concentrated on the legs and buttocks
  - Can involve trunk, face, and upper extremities
  - Typically lasts 3 days to 1 month
  - May be accompanied by edema typically involving the calves, dorsum of feet, scalp, scrotum, or labia
- Arthritis
  - Initially incapacitates, but is self-limited and nondeforming
  - Commonly is periarthritis and involves the knees and ankles
  - Warmth, swelling, and erythema over the joints

Other common features that may be found include the following:

- Signs of GI obstruction (partial obstruction to intussusception) or bleeding
- Signs of nephritis (can occur within first few months of disease onset, but rarely presents as late renal disease)
  - Hypertension or azotemia
  - Hematuria and proteinuria (classic findings of nephritis)

Other, less common, physical findings are related to complications caused by vasculitis in other body organs (e.g., respiratory, cardiac, and central nervous systems).

Diagnostic Studies.   The diagnosis of HSP is based on clinical findings. A urinalysis must be done to check for hematuria and proteinuria. BUN and creatinine are useful to evaluate renal function. Renal biopsy may be warranted if renal involvement is severe. Checking stools for blood is important in children complaining of abdominal pain. If GI obstruction is a consideration, abdominal radiographs should be ordered. Other diagnostic studies (e.g., chest radiographs, CT scans, or electroencephalographs) are ordered based on the signs and symptoms of complications, such as shortness of breath, seizures, mental status changes, or hypertension. Such studies are useful to identify specific organ system involvement and the severity of the complication.

In HSP, the ESR, CRP, and WBC (nonspecific indicators of systemic inflammation) are elevated. Because this condition is associated with a nonthrombocytopenic purpura, the platelet count is normal or even high.

Differential Diagnosis

Diseases that cause a similar rash with renal abnormalities are part of the differential diagnosis and include poststreptococcal glomerulonephritis, hemolytic uremic syndrome, serum sickness (drug related) and SLE. Other forms of vasculitis, such as Wegener granulomatosis and polyarteritis nodosa, are considerations (Haftel, 2006).

Management

Children with HSP need to be referred to a pediatrician and subspecialists depending on organ system involvement. Hospitalization is necessary with moderate to severe GI and renal system involvement or if pulmonary, cardiac, or central nervous system manifestations are present. Treatment is generally supportive, and careful attention is given to maintaining hydration and electrolyte balance. In addition, the following are key components of the management plan:

- Monitor for GI blood loss.
- Monitor for hematuria and proteinuria.
- Monitor and treat hypertension.
- Prescribe analgesics and NSAIDs for arthritis.
- Prescribe corticosteroids for GI disease (provides significant relief of abdominal pain).
- Acute nephritis typically responds to corticosteroids, but immunosuppressive therapy may be needed in resistant cases.
- Treat complications.

The skin lesions do not require special care and resolve without treatment. Use of other pharmacologic agents or therapies depends on the type and level of organ system involvement.

Complications

Infrequent complications of HSP seen in children include myositis, orchitis, hemorrhagic cystitis, pancreatitis, cholecystitis, bowel infarction, perforation or stricture, intussusception, acute renal failure, seizures, ataxia, pulmonary hemorrhage, carditis, anterior uveitis, and episcleritis. The arthritis associated with HSP does not leave joint damage and typically does not recur (Haftel, 2006).

Patient and Parent Education

The provider should educate patients and parents about:
- The illness, its complications, and the risk of recurrence
- The need to closely monitor for nephritis for at least 3 months, including blood pressure and urinalysis testing

Prognosis

HSP tends to last 3 to 4 weeks and then completely resolves in most cases without significant sequelae. However, the rash can wax and wane for 1 year, and some children have recurrent disease. The presence of nephritis is a potentially serious complication with long-term sequelae, such as hypertension or renal insufficiency. Less than 1% of children with HSP progress to end-stage renal disease. which then requires a kidney transplant (Haftel, 2006).

☑ DISCUSSION FORUM

1. A 12-year-old has recurrent spring time watery nasal discharge with nasal and eye itch. The common OTC medications have not worked. Discuss the following issues related to this child's presenting symptoms: (a) the probable diagnosis and its pathophysiology; (b) which if any diagnostic tests should be considered; (c) the likely offending allergens; and (d) key management issues.
2. A 15-month-old has a recurrent history of erythematous diffuse patches on both cheeks and is unable to sleep at night because of itching. How should this child be managed? Would the management change if a 7-year-old had a similar rash located in the antecubital fossa?
3. A 10-year-old has a painful, nonerythematous swelling in the right knee for 4 days. The pain is worse in the morning and with exercise. The family denies fever or flu-like symptoms. The family history is remarkable for arthritis in the maternal side of the family, and it was noted that they went on a hiking trip in Massachusetts 2 months ago. The rest of history and physical exam is unremarkable. What are the diagnoses that should be considered, and which laboratory studies should be ordered?

ℛESOURCE BOX

National Organizations and Resources

ASTHMA AND ATOPIC DERMATITIS
Allergy and Asthma Network—Mothers of Asthmatics, Inc.
www.aanma.org
www.breatherville.org

American Academy of Allergy, Asthma, and Immunology
www.aaaai.org

American College of Allergy, Asthma, and Immunology
www.acaai.org

American Lung Association
www.lungusa.org

Asthma and Allergy Foundation of America
www.aafa.org

National Asthma Education and Prevention Program
www.nhlbi.nih.gov/health/public/lung/asthma/resolut.htm

National Eczema Association for Science and Education
www.nationaleczema.org

National Heart, Lung, and Blood Institute
National Asthma Education and Prevention Program
www.nhlbi.nih.gov

National Jewish Center Medical and Research Center
www.njc.org

What you need to know about asthma
www.aboutasthma.com

U.S. Environmental Protection Agency
www.epa.gov/iaq/asthma
Information about indoor air quality and information for parents

AUTOIMMUNE DISEASE IN CHILDHOOD (JUVENILE ARTHRITIS AND SYSTEMIC LUPUS ERYTHEMATOSUS)

American Autoimmune Related Diseases Association
1-800-598-4668 (literature requests)
www.aarda.org

American Arthritis Organization
www.arthritis.org

Lupus Foundation of America, Inc.
www.lupus.org

REFERENCES

Cardona I, Boguniewicz M, Leung DYM: Atopic dermatitis. In Burg FS et al, editors: *Current pediatric diagnosis and treatment,* ed 18, Philadelphia, 2006, Saunders Elsevier.

Centers for Disease Control and Prevention (CDC): *National Center for Health Statistics, 2005.* Available at *www.cdc.gov/nchs/data/hus/hus05. pdf* (accessed Feb 13, 2007).

Ferguson PJ: Pediatric systemic lupus erythematosus. In Burg FS et al, editors: *Current pediatric diagnosis and treatment,* ed 18, Philadelphia, 2006, Saunders Elsevier.

Greenberger PA: Asthma. In Grammer LC, Greenberger PA, editors: *Patterson's allergic diseases,* ed 6, Baltimore, 2002, Lippincott Williams & Wilkins.

Haftel HM: Rheumatic diseases of childhood. In Kliegman RM et al, editors: *Nelson essentials of pediatrics,* ed 5, Philadelphia, 2006, Elsevier Saunders.

Imundo L: Idiopathic pain syndromes and chronic fatigue syndrome. In Burg FS et al, editors: *Current pediatric diagnosis and treatment,* ed 18, Philadelphia, 2006, Saunders Elsevier.

Kaari J: The role of intranasal corticosteroids in the management of pediatric allergic rhinitis, *Clin Pediatr* 45(8):697-704, 2006.

Kahn PJ, Imundo L: Juvenile rheumatoid arthritis and spondyloarthropathy syndromes. In Burg FS et al, editors: *Current pediatric diagnosis and treatment,* ed 18, Philadelphia, 2006, Saunders Elsevier.

Kinane TB, Scirica CV: Asthma. In Burg FS et al, editors: *Current pediatric diagnosis and treatment,* ed 18, Philadelphia, 2006, Saunders Elsevier.

Lasley MV: Allergy. In Kliegman RM et al, editors: *Nelson essentials of pediatrics,* ed 5, Philadelphia, 2006, Elsevier Saunders.

Leung DYM: Allergy and the immunologic basis of atopic disease. In Behrman RE, Kliegman RM, Jenson HB, editors: *Nelson textbook of pediatrics,* ed 17, Philadelphia, 2004, WB Saunders.

Liu AH, Spahn JD, Leung DYM: Childhood asthma. In Behrman RE, Kliegman RM, Jenson HB, editors: *Nelson textbook of pediatrics,* ed 17, Philadelphia, 2004, WB Saunders.

Miller ML: Rheumatic diseases of childhood (connective tissue diseases, collagen vascular diseases). In Behrman RE, Kliegman RM, Jenson HB, editors: *Nelson textbook of pediatrics,* ed 17, Philadelphia, 2004, WB Saunders.

National Heart, Lung, and Blood Institute (NHLBI): *Full report of the expert panel: guidelines for the diagnosis and management of asthma.* Available at *www. nhlbi.nih.gov/guidelines/asthma/epr-3/index.htm* (accessed Oct 27, 2007).

Paller AS, Mancini AJ: *Hurwitz clinical pediatric dermatology: a textbook of skin disorders of childhood and adolescence,* ed 3, Philadelphia, 2006, Elsevier Saunders.

Sampson HA, Leung DYM: Anaphylaxis. In Behrman RE, Kliegman RM, Jenson HB, editors: *Nelson textbook of pediatrics,* ed 17, Philadelphia, 2004, WB Saunders.

Schneider DS: The cardiovascular system. In Kliegman RM et al, editors: *Nelson essentials of pediatrics,* ed 5, Philadelphia, 2006, Elsevier Saunders.

Shrime MG, Keller JL: Pediatric rhinitis and acute and chronic sinusitis. In Burg FS et al, editors: *Current pediatric diagnosis and treatment,* ed 18, Philadelphia, 2006, Saunders Elsevier.

Taketomo CK, Hodding JH, Kraus DM: *Pediatric dosage handbook,* ed 13, Hudson, OH, 2006, Lexi-Comp.

Young TW, Strong WB: Acute rheumatic fever. In Burg FS et al, editors: *Current pediatric diagnosis and treatment,* ed 18, Philadelphia, 2006, Saunders Elsevier.

CHAPTER 25

Endocrine and Metabolic Diseases

Melissa L.R. Burchett, Cheryl E. Hanna, and Robert D. Steiner

Endocrine and metabolic disorders affect a large number of children and may be rare (e.g., nephropathic cystinosis) or relatively common (e.g., type 1 and type 2 diabetes mellitus). This chapter begins with an overview of anatomy, physiology, and pathophysiology of the endocrine and metabolic system and general issues related to assessment and management of these disorders. It is then divided into two sections covering endocrine and metabolic disorders, as they are managed by primary care providers in concert with specialists. Although there is a great degree of overlap in these disorders, distinctive processes occur in each, and as such, specific conditions may involve different approaches to assessment and management.

ANATOMY AND PHYSIOLOGY

The endocrine system regulates growth, pubertal development and reproduction, homeostasis of the organism, and the production, storage, and utilization of energy. Classically the endocrine system was understood to function via hormones produced in glands with action at a distant site. It is now understood that hormones may also act in a paracrine fashion affecting cells adjacent to the hormone-secreting cell or in an autocrine fashion in which the hormone affects the secreting cell by diffusion. Many endocrine glands are controlled by the hypothalamic-pituitary axis with regulation by the brain. Many of the hormones of the hypothalamic-pituitary axis (or molecules that are structurally similar to such hormones) are also made in the gut and other tissues.

Hormones are often activated in a feedback loop; e.g., thyrotropin releasing hormone (TRH) from the hypothalamus stimulates pituitary thyrotropin (TSH) secretion, which in turn stimulates thyroid hormone production (T_3 [triiodothyronine] and T_4 [thyroxine]). Thyroid hormone levels feed back to the hypothalamus and pituitary and suppress TRH and TSH secretion so that a balance is reached. In similar fashion, the adrenal glands secrete corticosteroids and the gonads produce progesterone, androgens, and estradiol, all of which influence hypothalamic and pituitary hormone production. For some systems, the set-point changes as individuals develop. Hormone secretion can be regulated by nerve cells and by factors important in the immune system (e.g., cytokines interact with hormones that influence weight homeostasis).

Metabolic function in the body involves complex biochemical processes to transform essential amino acids, carbohydrates, and lipids to substances or energy that can be used at the cellular level; to produce these molecules; and to perform cell functions. These biochemical processes, or metabolic pathways, are driven by enzyme activity.

PATHOPHYSIOLOGY

Endocrine abnormalities occur when there is an alteration in regulation of the normal feedback system that results in hyposecretion or hypersecretion of one or more hormones. Multiple factors cause alterations in hormone production. These include tumors, trauma, infection, systemic disease, genetic disorders, congenital malformation or agenesis of an endocrine gland, idiopathic causes, and iatrogenic causes (e.g., medications). The defect or problem can originate at the pituitary-hypothalamic level, in organ abnormalities, or for unknown reasons that lead to unresponsiveness to endogenous hormone. Hypothyroidism and hyperthyroidism are examples of disease entities in which the interrelationships of the hypothalamic-pituitary-thyroid axis are altered at any one of several possible sites.

Metabolic diseases are inborn errors of metabolism. Alteration in genetic constitution results in disrupted biochemical functioning. In children with phenylketonuria (PKU, a deficiency of the enzyme phenylalanine hydroxylase), for example, phenylalanine, an essential amino acid, accumulates. Type 1 diabetes mellitus is an example of an acquired immune-mediated metabolic disease. In diabetes, a reduction in insulin production or deficiency of its action results in abnormal metabolism of carbohydrate, protein, and fat.

ASSESSMENT

Endocrine and metabolic disorders disrupt various organs throughout the body and can change various body functions. Assessment requires a thorough family history, physical examination, and diagnostic testing for the suspected disorder.

HISTORY

- What is the child's growth pattern since birth?
- Is the child taking any medications that could affect endocrine or metabolic function?
- Have there been signs or symptoms of endocrine or metabolic dysfunction?
- Was there maternal exposure to radioiodine, goitrogens, or iodine medication during pregnancy?

- When did the child show signs of sexual development?
- What is the child's diet and exercise history?
- Is there a family history of endocrine or metabolic disorders?
- Does the child have unusual odors, recurrent vomiting, or unexplained lethargy?

PHYSICAL EXAMINATION

A detailed examination should include the following:
- Measure stature. Supine length is preferred for children under 2 years old. Use a stadiometer for children older than 2 or 3 years. Plot height and weight on a standardized growth chart appropriate to the child (e.g., children with Down syndrome have a different growth chart [see Appendix B]). Serial measures are critical to show growth trends over time.
- Plot rate of weight gain and body mass index (BMI). Measure head circumference.
- Check for proportionate appearance. Measure sitting and standing heights for upper-to-lower segment ratio (see Chapter 32), check for height age, and measure growth velocity.
- Inspect the child's genitalia carefully. Look for signs of either normal or ambiguous genitalia.
- Identify the stage of sexual development using Tanner staging (see Chapter 8).
- Note facial, axillary, and body hair for presence, distribution, and texture.
- Examine the skin for striae and acanthosis nigricans (see Color Plates) of the neck, axilla, breast, knuckles, and skin folds.
- Palpate the neck for thyroid gland enlargement and symmetry.
- Examine for dysmorphic features.

Acquired endocrine disorders are often due to either hyposecretion or hypersecretion of a specific hormone or combination of hormones, and the child may appear ill. Signs of dehydration, exophthalmos, and tachycardia are physical findings associated with endocrine pathology. Newborns with metabolic disorders may initially appear well, but physical signs develop with metabolic activity. Other characteristic physical findings are identified later in this chapter under the specific disease entity.

DIAGNOSTIC TESTS

Laboratory studies measuring hormone levels are key diagnostic tools of endocrine disorders. Specific blood and urine studies that identify end products of abnormal metabolism or elevated or diminished levels of various substances such as glucose, galactose, or amino acids, are important in the diagnosis of metabolic disorders. Accurate interpretation of data requires strict adherence to laboratory protocol for collecting and managing specimens. Additionally, not all laboratories have the ability to conduct tests that are sensitive to the hormone or substance being measured (e.g., measurement of hormones in precocious puberty requires high sensitivity).

Radiographic and imaging studies (e.g., bone age, ultrasonography, computed tomography [CT], and magnetic resonance imaging [MRI]) are also important diagnostic tools in evaluating certain endocrine disorders.

Many of these studies are expensive and can put additional emotional stress on a family that is already uncertain about their child's condition.

■ MANAGEMENT STRATEGIES

GENERAL MEASURES

Clinical consequences for the child affected by an endocrine or metabolic disorder vary from mild to severe. Undiagnosed and untreated, these disorders may lead variably to irreversible mental retardation, physical disability, neurologic damage, and death. Early detection, accurate diagnosis and rapid intervention are necessary to achieve favorable outcomes. Chronic disease issues and the effects of these diseases on lifestyle must also be addressed:
- Family, school, peer, and emotional adjustment
- Body image, self-esteem, and social competence
- Disease understanding, acceptance, and self-care

A successful outcome depends on the patient and family receiving support and encouragement in self-care, learning about the disease, and understanding the patient-parent role in managing a long-term illness or chronic condition.

GENETIC COUNSELING

Genetic counseling is often necessary. There are significant implications for the family of a child with endocrine or metabolic disorders that are genetically linked (see Chapter 40).

MEDICATIONS

Pharmacologic therapy, including hormone replacement, whether temporary or lifelong, is often essential for management of these disorders. Often, medications need to be administered via injection, creating distress in both the child and caregiver. Short, clear instructions about medications are important; how much to give, when to give it, how to give it, possible side effects, and when to make adjustments in medication are key messages to convey.

DIETARY CONSIDERATIONS

Metabolic diseases often require rigid adherence to dietary plans and restrictions. Parents, patients, other caregivers, and school personnel must be informed about the dietary needs and restrictions and the effect of diet on the disease process. They must also be helped to adjust to the economic, social, and psychological demands created by such restrictions.

PATIENT AND PARENT EDUCATION

Close supervision and frequent follow-up are necessary for children with metabolic and endocrine disorders. These children are best evaluated initially and periodically by a multidisciplinary team with expertise in pediatric endocrinology and/or clinical genetics (metabolic disease). Parent and patient education should include:
- The nature of the disorder
- The treatment plan
- Possible complications
- Plan for long-term follow-up

The multidisciplinary team can provide the education and support needed. The primary care provider, as a part of this team, is in an ideal position to reinforce the plan of care. Additionally, it is essential that primary health care needs and anticipatory guidance are not overlooked.

DISORDERS OF ENDOCRINE FUNCTION

An assessment of endocrine pathology most commonly seen in children can be approached by considering the seven following areas:
- Disturbance of growth
- Abnormalities of pubertal development
- Adrenal conditions
- Disorders of sex development
- Thyroid conditions
- Diabetes
- Posterior pituitary gland dysfunction

GROWTH DISORDERS

Children grow in a predictable way, and deviation from a normal growth pattern can be the first sign of endocrine disorders. Every effort should be made to collect serial growth data so a pattern of growth can be seen and a current growth velocity determined. Care must be taken to get accurate supine (for children under 2 or 3 years old) or standing measurements and to plot the child's length or height on the appropriate growth chart (see Appendix B). Children's predicted growth potential is based in large part on genetics and may change with altered nutritional status and illness patterns. An estimate of the expected stature (±2 inches) for a particular child can be made by calculating a "target height":

$$\text{Target height} = \frac{\text{mother's height} + \text{father's height}}{2 + 2\,\frac{1}{2} \text{ inches if a boy; } 2 - 2\,\frac{1}{2} \text{ inches if a girl.}}$$

Growth disorders can be divided into primary growth abnormalities where the defect appears to be in the growth plate itself, genetic or familial short stature, secondary growth disorders resulting from chronic disease or endocrine disorders, and variants of normal growth (constitutional growth delay [CGD]) (Box 25-1). This discussion will focus on growth hormone deficiency (GHD) and CGD (Table 25-1).

BOX 25-1 Classification of Growth Retardation

Primary growth abnormalities
  Osteochondrodysplasia
  Chromosome abnormalities
  Intrauterine growth retardation
  Dysmorphic syndromes
Genetic short stature
  SHOX gene haploinsufficiency
Secondary growth failure
  Malnutrition
  Chronic illness
  Endocrine disorders
  • Hypothyroidism
  • Cushing syndrome
  • Pseudohypoparathyroidism
  • Rickets
  • IGF-1 deficiency
    ◦ GHD
    ◦ Growth hormone insensitivity
    ◦ Defects in IGF 1 synthesis
Variants of normal growth
  CGD and puberty

CGD, Constitutional delay of growth; *GHD,* growth hormone deficiency; *IGF-1,* insulin-like growth factor 1; *SHOX,* short stature homeobox.

TABLE 25-1 Short Stature: Characteristics of Growth Hormone Deficiency (GHD) and Constitutional Growth Delay (CGD) in Children

Condition	Etiology	Onset	Presentation	Endocrine/Metabolic Disturbance
GHD	Most cases are idiopathic; pituitary or hypothalamic disease; trauma; minor organic hypothalamic lesion; infection; radiation	Congenital or acquired	Slow growth rate with normal birth weight; signs and symptoms of increased CNS pressure; microphallus; proportional short stature; delayed bone age	Deficiency or impairment in secretion of growth hormone-releasing hormone
CGD	Variation of normal growth; not a disease	First years of life impaired growth	Growth velocity is normal after 3 years old; delayed puberty and pubertal growth spurt; delayed bone age; positive family history	None—final height is appropriate for parents' height

CNS, Central nervous system.

Growth Hormone Deficiency

Description.   Growth hormone (GH) is an anterior pituitary protein released in response to sleep, exercise, and hypoglycemia. A deficiency is suspected when there are low levels of human growth hormone (hGH) in the serum or when levels of the hormone fail to increase during sleep, exercise, and hypoglycemic states. Growth hormone deficiency (GHD) may be either congenital or acquired. Individuals may also show resistance to GH, and GHD increases with age and immunodeficiency.

Epidemiology.   Estimates of the incidence of idiopathic GHD vary; a recent study in Denmark found an incidence of child-onset GHD of 2.58/100,000 for boys and 1.7/100,000 for girls (Stochholm et al, 2006).

Clinical Findings.

History.   A history obtained to evaluate the short or slowly growing child should include:

- Details of pregnancy, delivery, and newborn period
  - Mother's health
  - Birthing process, type, any problems
  - Birth length and weight
  - Neonatal course, including history of prolonged jaundice, hypoglycemia, microphallus (often diagnostic of congenital GHD)
  - Dysmorphia, especially midline facial defects or eye abnormalities
- Parents' and siblings' height, weight, and growth pattern
- When growth started to slow
- Chronic illness
- Symptoms of hypothyroidism or other known pituitary hormone deficiency
- Trauma or insult to the CNS
- Signs of an intracranial lesion

Physical Examination.   Physical examination of the short or slowly growing child should include:

- Any clinical clues to chronic illness or dysmorphic syndrome (e.g., childlike face with large, prominent forehead)
- Evaluation of the fundi, looking for signs of increased intracranial pressure
- Palpation of the thyroid gland for the presence of a goiter
- Evaluation of the stage of puberty
- Measurement of body proportions to exclude a skeletal dysplasia (dwarfing condition). The measurement of body proportions includes measuring arm span compared with height and upper-to-lower segment ratio (measure from the symphysis pubis to the heel to get the lower segment). Tables exist for children of all ages; some easy ratios to remember are: 1.7:1 as a newborn, 1.3:1 at 3 years old and 1:1 at 10 years old (Gunn & Nechyba, 2002).

Diagnostic Tests.   If growth velocity is slow (or when prior heights are not available), evaluation should include:

- CBC and sedimentation rate (for acute and chronic illness).
- Urinalysis.
- Screen for gastrointestinal illness when appropriate (e.g., celiac disease testing [serum IgA and transglutaminase], irritable bowel disease [ESR], stool for ova and parasites).

- Chemistry panel.
- Growth factors (IGF-1 and IGFBP-3). When both are normal, GHD is unlikely (Badaru & Wilson, 2004).
- Thyroid function tests. Free T_4 and TSH should be obtained to exclude both pituitary TSH deficiency and primary hypothyroidism.
- Bone age x-ray.
- Karyotype to rule out Turner syndrome in girls is necessary when bone age is not very delayed. Turner syndrome is common (1:2000 girls), and half of the girls have none of the typical dysmorphic features (Saenger et al, 2001) (see Chapter 40).

Differential Diagnosis.   Individual children with small size may not fit nicely into a single category, but may have multiple factors contributing to their size. Many chronic illnesses can slow linear growth, likely through a variety of mechanisms including malnutrition, acidosis, anorexia, and deficiencies of minerals (e.g., zinc and iron) and vitamins necessary for growth (Box 25-2). Typically, these children are underweight for height; their weight gain slows before their height does. Thyroid hormones are essential to growth during childhood; sex steroids are important for normal growth in adolescence. Deficiency of these hormones is characterized by subnormal growth velocity, normal to increased weight for height, and extremely delayed bone age depending on duration of the condition. Short stature may be the only sign of hypothyroidism.

Management.   Children should be referred to a pediatric endocrinologist if hypothyroidism, low IGF-1 and IGFBP-3, or other hormone deficiency is discovered or if there is unexplained persistent slow growth and no evidence of chronic illness. The Food and Drug Administration has approved a number of indications for GH therapy (Box 25-3) (Wilson et al, 2003). Reported side effects of GH include insulin resistance, pseudotumor cerebri, edema, growth of nevi, and carpal tunnel syndrome (Cuttler, 2002). The cost of GH may

---

BOX 25-2   Chronic Illness Contributing to Growth Failure

Gastrointestinal disease
   Celiac disease
   Inflammatory bowel disease
   Cystic fibrosis
Cardiovascular disease
   Cyanotic heart disease
   Congestive heart failure
Renal disease
   Uremia
   Renal tubular acidosis
Hematologic disorders
   Chronic anemia
Inborn errors of metabolism
Pulmonary disease
Chronic infection
Anorexia nervosa

BOX 25-3   FDA-Approved Indications for Growth Hormone Therapy

GHD
Growth failure caused by chronic renal failure
Turner syndrome
Prader-Willi syndrome
Intrauterine growth retardation with failure to catch up by 2 years old
Idiopathic short stature
• Unexplained short stature with poor height prognosis

GHD, Growth hormone deficiency.

present a financial burden to the family; cost is based on a weight-dependent dose and, for a 30-kg child, can be as high as $19,000 annually. This may not be covered by insurance. Some states offer assistance through programs for children with special needs, and some manufacturers may also have a program of financial assistance.

Constitutional Growth Delay (CGD)

Description. Constitutional delay of growth and puberty is a common variation in normal growth and should not be considered a disease entity. When there is no evidence of chronic illness, bone age is delayed, and the child is growing at a normal rate for bone age, the likely diagnosis is CGD. These children generally reach normal adult height, although they may be slightly short for their family.

Clinical Findings.

History. The history may include the following:
• Normal length and weight at birth
• Slowed linear growth between 1 to 3 years old and then normal growth velocity; normal height velocity is the most critical factor in diagnosis of constitutional delayed growth
• Growth at or slightly below the third percentile on standardized growth charts
• Delayed pubertal development
• Often male in families where other males have also been late growers

Physical Examination. Findings on physical examination include:
• Delayed bone age, but the rate of growth is normal for bone age
• Final height is within range of target height predicted for family height
• Normal neurologic exam

Diagnostic Tests. The same screening tests as used to evaluate GHD are done to rule out pathologic conditions.

Management. Reassurance and support should be provided to the child and family regarding ultimate height and development. An endocrine referral may be necessary to differentiate CGD from GHD and for possible hormone replacement therapy.

Growth Excess

Just as there are families with CGD, the so-called "late bloomers," there are families of early growers who are tall for their family as young children, enter puberty early, and end up with a height in the normal range for their family. Tall stature in comparison with parents' size or rapid growth velocity in childhood can also, however, represent underlying abnormality. Primary skeletal abnormalities causing tall stature include Marfan syndrome, Klinefelter syndrome, and other overgrowth syndromes. Overnutrition will often accelerate growth and advance the bone age and the timing of puberty. In these children, weight gain occurs first, and weight is further above the growth curve than height. Excess adrenal androgens or gonadal steroids can also accelerate growth. These children will have exam findings of early puberty. Rarely, growth hormone excess can accelerate growth (e.g., pituitary gigantism) that requires referral to a pediatric endocrinologist.

PUBERTAL DISORDERS

The physical changes of puberty occur in response to production of sex steroids by the ovaries or testes (see Chapter 8). Hypothalamic gonadotropin-releasing hormone (GnRH) regulates the release of luteinizing hormone (LH) and follicle-stimulating hormone (FSH) from the pituitary gland, which in turn stimulate gonadal hormone secretion.

The fetus has an intact hypothalamic-pituitary-gonadal axis by midgestation; by term gestation, the production of GnRH, LH, and FSH in this system are at low levels. When placental and maternal hormones are removed at delivery, unrestrained production of these hormones occurs in the newborn, and the infant experiences a "mini puberty" between 2 weeks and 3 months of postnatal life. After infancy, the hypothalamic GnRH pulse generator is more sensitive to feedback inhibition from the brain, and by 1 year old, LH and FSH decrease to the prepubertal range, and the child enters a "latency" period for the next 10 years or so. Puberty occurs when the feedback inhibition is released and GnRH is again produced (Nathan & Palmert, 2005; Greiner & Kerrigan, 2006). The timing of the release correlates better with bone age than chronologic age.

The normal range for entering puberty in girls appears to be earlier now than in past decades. A large epidemiologic study of 17,000 girls found that signs of puberty are present as early as 6 years old in African-American girls and 7 years old in Caucasian girls (Herman-Giddens et al, 1997), and both African-American boys and girls enter puberty earlier than Caucasian or Mexican-American children (Sun et al, 2002). Although girls are starting puberty at a younger age than in past generations, the timing of menarche and reaching Tanner stage 5 has not changed dramatically (Sun et al, 2005). Menarche typically happens within 3 or so years from the start of breast development. Ninety-five percent of girls will have started puberty by 13 years old. Nine years is the lower end of the normal range for boys to begin puberty and 14 years the upper end. The first sign of puberty is increased testicular volume in 85% of boys. Concerns arise with a child's growth when puberty presents early or is delayed.

Early Puberty

Early puberty is divided into four categories; premature thelarche, premature adrenarche, isolated menarche, and true precocious puberty. Premature thelarche occurs in infant and toddler girls and is isolated breast development, sometimes present from birth, without any other features of puberty. It is likely due to estrogens produced during the mini puberty of infancy or increased responsiveness of the breast primordia, can take months or years to resolve, and rarely progresses to true precocious puberty.

Premature adrenarche is the early onset of pubic hair in either boys or girls not associated with other features of true puberty. It may be caused by a mild form of congenital adrenal hyperplasia (CAH), exposure to topical testosterone, or rarely, adrenal tumor. Most often, it is idiopathic. Children with idiopathic premature adrenarche are at increased risk for polycystic ovarian syndrome and metabolic syndrome.

Isolated menarche is an uncommon condition in which girls have one to a few episodes of vaginal bleeding without breast development. In this condition, sexual abuse, vaginal tumor, a functional ovarian cyst that produces estrogen, and primary hypothyroidism all need to be excluded.

Precocious Puberty

True precocious puberty refers to the onset of multiple features of puberty earlier than the normal range. Features may include accelerated linear growth, breast development or penis enlargement, and pubic hair development. Depending on the length of time symptoms have been present, the bone age may be advanced. Precocious puberty can be divided into two broad categories: central, gonadotropin dependent; or peripheral, gonadotropin independent (Box 25-4). Prolonged exposure to exogenous sex hormones (mother's birth control pills or father's topical testosterone) can also cause precocious puberty.

BOX 25-4   **Disorders of Puberty**

Central precocious puberty
- Idiopathic
- CNS disorder
  - Hamartoma
  - Tumor
  - CNS radiation
  - Infection
  - Trauma
- Hypothyroidism
- HCG-secreting tumor

Peripheral precocious puberty
Girls
- McCune-Albright syndrome
- Ovarian cyst
- Estrogen-secreting ovarian or adrenal tumor

Boys
- Severe, non-salt wasting, congenital adrenal hyperplasia
- Testotoxicosis (activating mutation of the LH receptor)
- Testicular tumor

CNS, Central nervous system; *HCG,* human chorionic gonadotropin; *LN,* leutinizing hormone.

Epidemiology.   Any lesion that disrupts the normal connections between the brain and the hypothalamus can cause central precocious puberty. This condition is most often idiopathic in girls. In boys, there is a 30% incidence of central nervous system (CNS) tumors in situations of central precocious puberty.

Clinical Findings.   Children who start with features of puberty at a younger age than normal should have an evaluation as to the etiology. Children who start to develop signs of puberty at the early end of the normal range should be evaluated if they have rapid progression of pubertal signs resulting in a bone age more than 2 years ahead of chronologic age, new CNS-related findings (e.g., headaches, seizures, focal neurologic defects), or behavioral issues suggesting their emotional state is being adversely affected by puberty (Kaplowitz & Oberfield, 1999; Ritzen, 2003).

History.   The history should include details (age of onset, progression, duration) of the symptoms (breast tissue, pubic hair, phallic enlargement, acne, body odor, oily scalp), pattern of growth, any symptoms suggestive of a CNS lesion, and pattern of puberty in family members. Any exposure to topical estrogens or testosterone or oral estrogens should be sought.

Physical Examination.   Physical examination should include:
- Assessment of stature and growth velocity
- Description of the child's Tanner stage
- Breast development
- Pubic and axillary hair (girls)
- Penis size, testicular volume and pubic and axillary hair (boys) (see Chapter 8)

Diagnostic Tests.
- Premature thelarche: no laboratory studies are necessary in the infant or toddler girl unless there are other features of true puberty or continued increase in breast size.
- Premature adrenarche: serum 17-hydroxyprogesterone (17-OHP) to exclude CAH should be done; a 24-hour urine collection for 17-ketosteroids or imaging of the adrenal glands to exclude an adrenal tumor may be indicated.
- Isolated menarche: thyroid function tests to exclude primary hypothyroidism, and pelvic ultrasound looking for an ovarian cyst or pelvic tumor.

Diagnostic tests for children with true precocious puberty include:
- Bone age x-ray.
- LH, FSH, and estradiol or testosterone (use a laboratory with a sensitive assay that will detect early pubertal values at the lower end of the range).
- If LH and FSH are high (in pubertal range: indication of central etiology), do an MRI to exclude CNS tumor.
- If LH and FSH are low (in prepubertal range: indication of peripheral puberty), do a GnRH stimulation test to distinguish central from peripheral puberty.

If etiology is peripheral:
- Pelvic ultrasonography of girls
- Testicular ultrasonography of boys
- Serum 17-OHP to rule out a severe form of CAH

Management.   Treatment of precocious puberty should be done with the guidance of a pediatric endocrinologist.

Management will depend on the underlying disorder, age of the child, degree of advancement of the bone age, and the child and family's emotional response to the condition. Radiation, surgery, or chemotherapy is indicated in the case of CNS tumors. A long-acting GnRH agonist may be used to bring serum sex steroids to prepubertal levels. Treatment of precocious puberty is important to increase final adult height.

Delayed Puberty

Description. Puberty is considered delayed when a boy 14 years or older or a girl 13 years or older has no clinical features of puberty on physical exam.

Epidemiology. Any chronic condition that delays the bone age may cause delayed puberty since the timing of puberty correlates better with bone age than chronologic age (Box 25-5). In addition, failure of any part of the hypothalamic-pituitary-gonadal axis may also delay puberty (Box 25-6). The most common cause of delayed puberty is CGD (Nathan & Palmert, 2005).

BOX 25-5 **Etiology of Delayed Puberty**

Chronic illness
- GI with poor weight gain
- Chronic renal failure
- Anorexia nervosa
- Medication-induced poor weight gain

CGD
- Endocrine diseases associated with delayed bone age
- Hypothyroidism

GHD
- Failure of the hypothalamic-pituitary-gonadal axis

CGD, Constitutional delay of growth; *GHD,* growth hormone deficiency; *GI,* gastrointestinal.

BOX 25-6 **Failure of the Hypothalamic-Pituitary-Gonadal Axis**

Hypothalamic pituitary dysfunction (LH/FSH deficiency)
- Multiple pituitary hormone deficiency
- Isolated gonadotropin deficiency
  - Kallmann syndrome (anosmia and gonadotropin deficiency)
- Hyperprolactinemia
- Functional deficiency associated with ↓ calories or extreme exercise

Gonadal failure
Girls
- Turner syndrome
- Oophoritis
- Galactosemia
- Chemotherapy induced

Boys
- Vanishing testes syndrome (in utero testicular torsion)
- Chemotherapy or radiation

FSH, Follicle-stimulating hormone; *LH,* leutinizing hormone.

Clinical Findings.

History and Physical Examination. History and physical examination should focus on clinical clues indicating a chronic illness, symptoms or signs of hypothyroidism, prior history of CNS insult, or new CNS symptoms suggesting hypopituitarism. Review of systems should include questions about pattern of growth, especially growth velocity, sense of smell, and galactorrhea.

Diagnostic Tests. Laboratory investigation should include:
- Focused screen for acute or chronic illness (CBC, sedimentation rate, urinalysis, liver enzymes, electrolytes [renal function])
- Bone age x-ray
- Free T_4 and TSH
- IGF-1 and IGFBP-3 if GHD is suspect
- Serum prolactin
- LH and FSH (When gonadal failure is present, LH and FSH are abnormally elevated if the bone age is older than 11 years in a girl or 12 years in a boy)

Management. A referral to a pediatric endocrinologist is necessary to determine the etiology and necessary treatment. Hormonal replacement is the treatment of choice for hypogonadism.

ADRENAL DISORDERS

Anatomy and Physiology

Adrenal gland steroid production is under control of the hypothalamic-pituitary axis. The hypothalamus secretes corticotropin-releasing hormone (CRH) in a pulsatile fashion, which stimulates production and secretion of adrenocorticotropin (ACTH) from the pituitary gland. ACTH regulates adrenal glucocorticoid (cortisol) and androgen production. Cortisol is produced in a series of enzymatic steps (see Fig. 25-1) and is highest in the morning, low in the afternoon and evening, and lowest at midnight. It is secreted in response to hypoglycemia, hypotension, pain, or other stressful events. Cortisol has negative feedback on the synthesis and secretion of CRH, vasopressin, and ACTH.

The adrenal gland also produces aldosterone, regulated by renal production of renin interacting with angiotensinogen to create angiotensin. The renin-angiotensin system is involved in regulation of salts, especially sodium; blood pressure; and renal blood flow. Aldosterone production also occurs in enzymatic steps, many of which are common to the cortisol production pathway.

Adrenal insufficiency

Description. Adrenal insufficiency is characterized by a deficiency of hormones produced by the adrenal cortex; deficits of cortisol and aldosterone are perhaps the most important to body function. In primary adrenal insufficiency (hypofunctioning adrenal gland), glucocorticoid (cortisol) and mineralocorticoid (aldosterone) hormones are deficit, whereas in secondary adrenal insufficiency (hypothalamic or pituitary defect), only a glucocorticoid deficit is found. Thus, children with both forms of adrenal insufficiency have hypoglycemia and hypotension caused

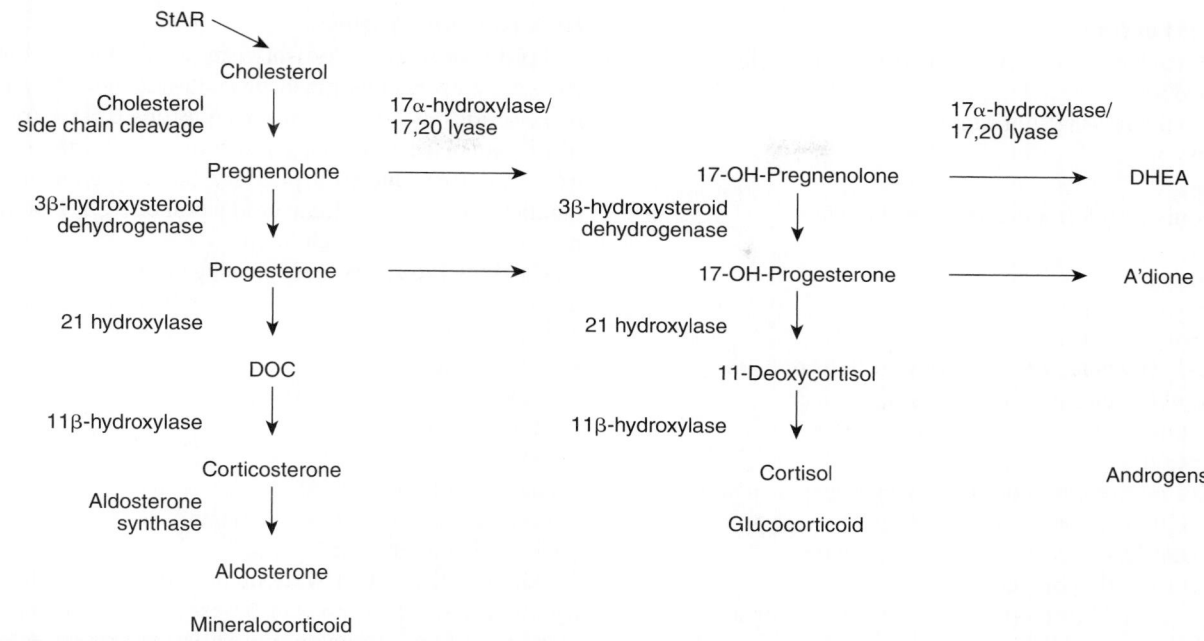

FIG. 25-1 Adrenal steroidogenesis. After the steroidogenic acute regulatory (StAR) protein–mediated uptake of cholesterol into mitochondria within adrenocortical cells, aldosterone, cortisol, and adrenal androgens are synthesized through the coordinated action of a series of steroidogenic enzymes in a zone-specific fashion. *A'dione*, androstenedione; *DHEA*, dehydroepiandrosterone; *DOC*, deoxycorticosterone. (From Stewart PM: The adrenal cortex. In Larsen PR et al, editors: *Williams textbook of endocrinology*, ed 10, Philadelphia, 2003, WB Saunders, p 495.)

by cortisol deficiency. Only those with a primary adrenal insufficiency have a salt-wasting crisis (hyponatremia, hyperkalemia, acidosis, and dehydration) caused by aldosterone deficiency.

Epidemiology. Primary adrenal insufficiency may be due to an enzyme defect in the adrenal steroid pathway to cortisol (termed CAH), hypoplasia of the adrenal gland, or an acquired defect (Box 25-7). Lesions of the hypothalamus or pituitary lead to secondary adrenal insufficiency. Suppression of the hypothalamic-pituitary-adrenal axis secondary to steroid use can also lead to adrenal insufficiency. Infants born extremely prematurely (24 to 28 weeks gestation) sometimes demonstrate symptoms of adrenal insufficiency because of immaturity of the hypothalamic-pituitary-adrenal axis.

Secondary adrenal insufficiency can occur as a result of ACTH deficiency as one of multiple hypothalamic-pituitary deficiencies or rarely as an isolated problem. Most often the infant or child has a syndrome known to be associated with hypopituitarism (for example septo-optic dysplasia), has also been discovered to have idiopathic GHD, has a destructive lesion (e.g., tumor or radiation to the brain), or prior CNS trauma.

CAH is caused by a deficiency of any of the enzymes in the cortisol pathway. Some of the enzymes also control key steps in androgen synthesis and can cause a male fetus to be incompletely masculinized. In addition to interrupting normal cortisol production, the most common enzymatic abnormality, 21-hydroxylase (21-OH) deficiency, causes buildup of cortisol precursors that are shunted into the unblocked androgen pathway causing the female fetus to be exposed to excessive androgens. The fetus with this condition begins to produce abnormal elevated amounts of adrenal androgens in utero so that the female infant is born with an enlarged clitoris and posterior fusion of the labia. About 75% of children with CAH caused by 21-OH deficiency will also have aldosterone deficiency. Many states now have newborn screening for this form of CAH, allowing detection before a salt-wasting crisis.

BOX 25-7 **Adrenal Insufficiency**

Deficiency of CRH or ACTH
- *Isolated deficiency*
  - Congenital
  - Acquired as a result of hypophysitis
- *Multiple pituitary hormone deficiencies*
  - Congenital (septo-optic dysplasia, midline defects, etc.)
  - Acquired (CNS trauma, infection, tumor, radiation)

Primary adrenal
- *Congenital*
  - Congenital adrenal hyperplasia (most common 21-OH deficiency)
  - Adrenal hypoplasia (X-linked, autosomal recessive, ACTH receptor defect)
- *Acquired*
  - X-linked, adrenoleukodystrophy
  - Autoimmune (Addison)
  - Infection

21-OH, 21-Hydroxylase; *ACTH*, adrenocorticotropin; *CNS*, central nervous system; *CRH*, corticotropin-releasing hormone

Clinical Findings.

History. Symptoms of cortisol deficiency include a history of:

- Poor appetite
- Failure to thrive or weight loss
- Weakness
- Vomiting

Symptoms of aldosterone deficiency include:

- Vomiting
- Poor feeding
- Lethargy
- Dehydration

Physical Examination. On physical examination, the infant or child often shows the following signs:

- Dehydration
- Hypotension
- Excessive pigmentation of the skin and mucous membranes (present only with primary adrenal insufficiency)

Diagnostic Tests. Laboratory tests include:

- Serum glucose (hypoglycemia)
- Blood gases and bicarbonate (for metabolic acidosis)
- Electrolytes (low sodium, elevated potassium with aldosterone deficiency)
- Serum cortisol (a cortisol value more than 20 mcg/dL indicates adrenal sufficiency. A value lower than that must be interpreted in the clinical context in which it was drawn. Often an ACTH stimulation test will be necessary to conclusively diagnose both primary and secondary adrenal insufficiency. Consult a pediatric endocrinologist for the best way to do this test.)
- Serum ACTH (elevated in primary adrenal insufficiency)
- Serum 17-OHP (diagnostic in children with suspected CAH caused by 21-OH deficiency)
- Serum renin level (elevated with aldosterone deficiency)
- Aldosterone level (low with aldosterone deficiency)

Plasma renin and aldosterone levels are most easily interpreted if they are drawn at the time when serum sodium levels are low.

Management. Treatment of adrenal insufficiency includes hormone replacement and is best managed by a pediatric endocrinologist. An adrenal crisis is a medical emergency treated with immediate and vigorous administration of intravenous dextrose, normal saline, and stress doses of hydrocortisone. Intravenous stress doses of hydrocortisone vary with age: 25 mg in infants; 50 mg in children; and 100 mg in teens, given every 6 hours. Long-term therapy includes oral hydrocortisone in a dose 8 to 10 mg/M² in children with ACTH deficiency or primary adrenal insufficiency. Children with CAH tend to have higher hydrocortisone needs. If present, aldosterone deficiency must be treated with fludrocortisone.

Treatment of CAH requires a fine balancing act to replace steroids while preventing androgen overproduction. Excess steroid intake can lead to delayed growth; not enough steroids contribute to rapid bone age growth and ultimate short stature. Individual treatment plans are essential to meet the specific needs of individual children. The primary care provider should be familiar with the medical endocrinology treatment plan and reinforce it at routine well- and sick-child visits.

Hyperadrenal States

Epidemiology. Cortisol excess is most commonly caused by exogenous glucocorticoid treatment of an illness (e.g., serious asthma, to prevent rejection after a transplant, or as part of chemotherapy protocols). Endogenous cortisol excess may be due to a pituitary tumor producing ACTH, adrenal tumor, or to ectopic production of ACTH from a non-pituitary tumor (rare in children).

Clinical Findings. Clinical features of cortisol excess include:

- Weight gain
- Growth failure
- Osteopenia
- Hypertension
- Delayed puberty
- Plethora (hypervolemia)
- Skin: acne, purple striae, hirsutism
- Compulsive behavior

Almost all children with simple obesity are tall for their age, and cortisol excess can be excluded on physical exam alone. In situations where growth is slow or growth data is missing and cortisol excess needs to be excluded by laboratory evaluation, a 24-hour urine collection for free cortisol or a late evening serum or salivary cortisol are the best screening tests.

Management. When children receive glucocorticoids for underlying illness for longer than 7 to 10 days, the steroid dose should be weaned rather than abruptly discontinued to allow the hypothalamic-pituitary-adrenal axis to recover normal function and sometimes to prevent a flare of the underlying disease. Procedures for tapering the dose are empiric, but in general, the longer the patient has been on glucocorticoids, the longer the taper. One strategy is to reduce the dose by 50% each week until reaching an equivalent dose of twice normal cortisol production and then taper more slowly. A morning cortisol value of 10 mcg/dL suggests it is safe to wean further or, if the patient is already on half a maintenance dose, discontinue the medication. Even after the steroid has been safely discontinued, the patient may not be able to respond to severe stress for 6 to 12 months.

DISORDERS OF SEX DEVELOPMENT

Description

Abnormalities of sexual differentiation usually present in infancy with ambiguous genitalia. The spectrum of physical examination findings ranges from the appearance of a normal male penis and normal scrotum but with no gonads palpable to an infant who looks mostly female with mild enlargement of the clitoris. True hermaphroditism, in which the infant has both male and female gonadal structures, is rare.

Infants with 46 XY chromosomes who have complete androgen insensitivity (androgen receptor defect) have genitalia that look completely female; these children are not detected in the newborn period unless a karyotype is done for some other reason. They typically are diagnosed when an inguinal hernia is repaired and a testis is discovered or as teenagers when they fail to develop pubic hair or menstruate.

Epidemiology

Disorders of sex development occur when the XX fetus is exposed to excess androgen in utero, the XY fetus is unable to produce or respond to androgens, or rarely true hermaphroditism. The most common cause of a disordered sex development is CAH that exposes an XX fetus to excess androgens during fetal life (see Fig. 25-1). Other much less common virilizing conditions include aromatase deficiency or virilizing tumor in the mother. In an XY fetus, disordered sex development can result from inadequate androgen production or partial androgen insensitivity (Maclaughlin & Donahoe, 2004).

Clinical Findings

All infants should have a careful genital examination before discharge from the nursery. The initial evaluation of an infant with ambiguous genitalia should be under the direction of a pediatric endocrinologist and includes:

- Karyotype. This can be done quickly (within 48 to 72 hours) if the cytogenetics laboratory is alerted to the urgency of the test. Subsequent laboratory studies depend on the chromosome results (Conte & Grumbach, 2003).
- In XY infants, measurement of the precursors of testosterone, testosterone, and dihydrotestosterone.
- In XX infants, serum 17-OHP to establish a diagnosis of 21-OH deficiency.
- Serum müllerian inhibitory substance can also be measured or can be assessed indirectly by obtaining an ultrasound or genitogram.

Management

The family needs to be counseled immediately. The primary health care provider has a responsibility to document the abnormality, refer to a specialist team that includes a pediatric endocrinologist, medical geneticist, and pediatric urologist; send the initial studies; and support and counsel the family in consultation with the specialist team. Families should be educated about the normal process of genital development, the cause of their child's abnormality, what the evaluation of their child will entail, and how the sex of rearing is determined. In concert with the specialist team, the family must come to a decision of the appropriate sex of rearing. Female is the appropriate sex of rearing for XX infants with CAH and for infants with complete androgen insensitivity. Sex of rearing in incompletely masculinized XY infants is complicated, and it is important to wait to assign the sex of rearing until the evaluation is complete (Hughes et al, 2006). Medical treatment for the underlying cause of the condition, if known (e.g., CAH), is essential.

THYROID DISORDERS

Anatomy and Physiology

The hypothalamic-pituitary-thyroid axis begins to function in utero (Fig. 25-2). The hypothalamus produces TRH, which in turn stimulates pituitary production of TSH. TSH stimulates the thyroid gland to secrete primarily T_4. T_4 is converted in peripheral tissues to T_3. Both T_3 and T_4 bind to thyroid-binding proteins, primarily thyroid-binding globulin (TBG).

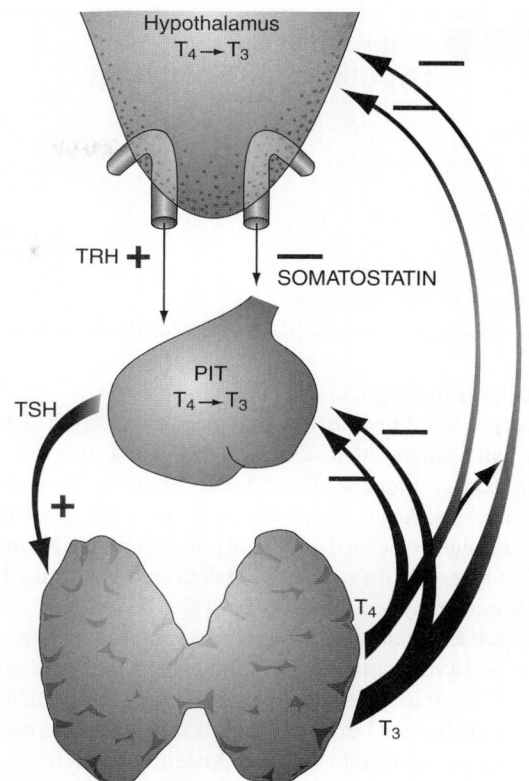

FIG. 25-2 Interrelationships of the hypothalamic–pituitary–thyroid (HPT) axis. (From Wilson JD, Foster DW, editors: *Williams textbook of endocrinology,* ed 8, Philadelphia, 1992, WB Saunders, p 169.)

The free, unbound form of T_3 and T_4 is biologically important. T_4 inhibits hypothalamic TRH and pituitary TSH secretion. Thyroid hormones influence growth and development, oxygen consumption, brain development, and metabolism of lipids, carbohydrates, and proteins.

Hypothyroidism

Description and Epidemiology. Primary hypothyroidism (hypothyroidism caused by thyroid disease) may be congenital or acquired. Congenital hypothyroidism (CH) affects 1 in 4000 infants (American Academy of Pediatrics [AAP] et al, 2006). CH is the most common cause of preventable mental retardation. Untreated hypothyroidism leads to irreversible brain damage and variable degrees of growth failure, deafness, and neurologic abnormalities.

The most common cause of acquired hypothyroidism in the U.S. is Hashimoto thyroiditis, destruction of the thyroid by the immune system (Foley, 2004). Worldwide, lack of iodine is the main cause of acquired primary hypothyroidism. Other causes are listed in Box 25-8. Hypothyroidism can also be due to a deficiency of TSH secondary to pituitary disease or tertiary to dysfunction of the hypothalamus (central hypothyroidism). TSH deficiency is usually associated with other pituitary hormone problems (especially GHF) and may be congenital or acquired (see growth section).

Acquired Primary Hypothyroidism: Etiology

- Chronic lymphocytic thyroiditis
- Goitrogens (iodide, lithium, thiouracil)
- Thyroidectomy
- I^{131} ablation
- Infiltrative disorders (Langerhans histiocytosis, cystinosis)
- Subacute thyroiditis
- Cranial/spinal radiation

Clinical Findings.

History. Slow growth, delayed puberty, delayed dentition, weight gain, fatigue, dry skin, hyperlipidemia, drop in school performance, and amenorrhea can be present in the child with hypothyroidism. A past history of risk factors for hypopituitarism (e.g., syndrome associated with hypopituitarism or CNS insult) is helpful in assessing the risk for TSH deficiency. A family history of autoimmune thyroid disease should also be sought.

Physical Examination. The clinical manifestations of primary hypothyroidism vary with the age of the child and can be very difficult to assess. There may be no overt clinical signs of CH, and the newborn may look completely normal. The most common neonatal signs are prolonged jaundice, constipation, and umbilical hernia. Infants with CH may also have a large anterior and posterior fontanelle, large tongue, and decreased muscle tone. They may have respiratory distress and poor peripheral circulation with cool, cyanotic skin in the extremities. The primary symptom in older children or those with acquired hypothyroidism may be delayed growth: small stature for their family or subnormal growth velocity. These children may be overweight for height and have delayed dentition or puberty, bradycardia, or delayed return of the deep tendon reflexes. Children with central hypothyroidism may show slow growth, increased weight for height, and features suggestive of hypopituitarism including midline facial or eye abnormalities.

Diagnostic Tests. For primary hypothyroidism:
- The diagnosis of CH usually presents in infancy, detected by newborn screening tests. Newborn screening programs test filter paper blood spots for either T_4 or TSH. When the filter paper test result is abnormal, the primary care clinician is contacted to obtain a confirmatory free T_4 and TSH serum sample. A serum sample is also indicated if clinical features of CH are detected. Retesting may be necessary and is recommended for children with Down syndrome at 6 and 12 months old and then annually (AAP, 2001).
- In older children, TSH is abnormally elevated while the free T_4 is in the normal range or low.

  For central hypothyroidism:
- Free serum T_4 is low, TSH is normal. Typically, the TSH is measurable, but there has not been enough TSH secretion to bring the free T_4 into the normal range.

  For children with TBG deficiency:
- Total T_4 will be low, but free T_4 will be normal as will TSH. This condition does not require treatment.

Management. Hypothyroidism is treated with replacement doses of levothyroxine sodium. The dose varies by age and weight (Table 25-2). The laboratory monitoring and follow-up are also age dependent. Because normal thyroid function in the first 3 years of life is crucial for normal cognitive development, more careful monitoring is necessary in that age group. In general, an elevation in TSH (in primary hypothyroidism) or depression of the free T_4 (in central hypothyroidism) indicates the need to increase the dose of medication and repeat the diagnostic test in 6 weeks to be sure the new dose is adequate.

Hyperthyroidism

Description. Hyperthyroidism occurs in childhood when the thyroid gland overproduces thyroid hormone or when a child is given too large a dose of thyroid hormone replacement.

Epidemiology. Graves disease is the most common cause of hyperthyroidism (LaFranchi & Hanna, 2005). In this condition, thyroid stimulating immunoglobulin is produced, which binds to the TSH receptor resulting in excessive thyroid hormone production. Women who have had or currently have Graves disease sometimes have babies born with neonatal Graves disease that persists until maternal antibodies dissipate at about 3 months old. Some children with Hashimoto thyroiditis will have a short (6 to 18 months) phase of hyperthyroidism. Other causes of hyperthyroidism (e.g., autonomous thyroid nodules) are less common.

Clinical Findings.

History. The history of a child with hyperthyroidism may include:
- Palpitations
- Tremor
- Increased appetite often with weight loss
- Fatigue
- Muscle weakness
- Emotional lability
- Poor concentration with decreased school performance
- Hyperdefecation

Physical Examination. Often observed findings in hyperthyroidism include:
- Goiter (almost 100%)
- Tachycardia
- Wide pulse pressure
- Underweight for height
- Eyelid lag or exophthalmus; approximately 50% of children with Graves' disease have exophthalmus

TABLE 25-2 **Thyroid Hormone Dosing**

Age	L-Thyroxine (mcg/kg)
0-3 months	12-15
3-12 months	6-10
1-5 years	4-6
6-12 years	3-5
>12 years	3-4

- A hyperfunctioning nodule in the thyroid may be present
- Warm, smooth skin
- Tremor or hyperreflexia

Diagnostic Tests. The free T_4 and total T_4 levels will be elevated and the TSH suppressed below the sensitivity of the assay. Hyperthyroidism is the one setting when measuring a T_3 level may be helpful because it may be more dramatically elevated than the T_4 and be a better marker to follow.

Management. Children with hyperthyroidism should be referred to a pediatric endocrinologist; treatment depends on the cause (LaFranchi & Hanna, 2005).

DIABETES MELLITUS

Diabetes mellitus is a group of conditions characterized by inadequate insulin secretion, insulin resistance in the tissues, or both. These dynamics lead to defective metabolism of carbohydrate, protein, and fat and subsequent hyperglycemia (Ize-Ludlow & Sperling, 2005). Diabetes is a chronic disease that affects approximately 176,500 individuals 20 years old or younger in the U.S. (National Institute of Diabetes and Digestive and Kidney Disease [NIDDK], 2005). Newly diagnosed cases appear more in the autumn and winter months (especially in adolescents) (Alemzadeh & Wyatt, 2004). In addition to the most familiar forms—type 1 (formerly called insulin-dependent diabetes mellitus [IDDM] or juvenile-onset diabetes) and type 2 (formerly called non–insulin-dependent diabetes mellitus [NIDDM] or adult-onset diabetes)—there are others (Box 25-9). Type 1 and type 2 diabetes are both on the increase in children in the U.S. and other first world countries. Table 25-3 shows the distinguishing features of type 1 and type 2 diabetes.

BOX 25-9   Types of Diabetes

Type 1
Type 2
Genetic defects in ß-cell function
- Maturity-onset diabetes of youth (MODY) syndrome
- Mitochondrial DNA mutations
- Wolfram syndrome (diabetes insipidus, diabetes mellitus, optic atrophy, deafness)
- Thiamine responsive

Drug or chemical induced
- Glucocorticoids
- L-Asparaginase
- Antirejection medications

Diseases of the exocrine pancreas
- Cystic fibrosis
- Pancreatitis
- Trauma
- Hemolytic uremic syndrome (HUS)

Infections
- Congenital rubella
- Cytomegalovirus (CMV)

Genetic syndromes with diabetes
- Prader-Willi
- Turner
- Alström
Neonatal diabetes

TABLE 25-3   Comparison of Type 1 and Type 2 Diabetes

	Type 1	Type 2
Age at onset	Two peaks: 5 years and 15 years old	Teenage year
Predominant ethnic groups affected	White	Native American Hispanic African American
Obesity	Same as general population	>90%
Hypertension	Uncommon	Common
Acanthosis nigricans	Rare	Common
Ketosis, DKA	Common	Uncommon
Islet autoimmunity	Present	Absent

DKA, Diabetic ketoacidosis.

Type 1 Diabetes

Epidemiology. Type 1 diabetes is caused by autoimmune destruction of pancreatic beta cells in the islets of Langerhans; is thought to be triggered by a preceding environmental event in genetically susceptible individuals; and results in an absolute deficiency in insulin secretion, reduced biologic effectiveness, or both. The high blood glucose is a result of the defective metabolism of carbohydrate, protein, and fats; normal metabolic function depends upon sufficient amounts of circulating insulin. The insulin deficiency results in uninhibited gluconeogenesis and a blockage in the use and storage of circulating glucose. Approximately 1 in every 400 to 600 children and adolescents in the U.S. is affected with type 1 diabetes; new cases occur at an estimated rate of 13,000 per year (NIDDK, 2005). Among children, type 1 diabetes is more common than type 2, representing 80% of all diabetes in children 9 years old and younger (0.76 cases per 1000 children), and 91% of all diabetes in non-Hispanic white youth 10 to 19 years old (2.8 cases per 1000 children). Among Hispanic youth 10 to 19 years old, 78% of diabetes is type 1; among African Americans, 69%; among Asian or Pacific Islanders, 60%; but for American Indians, only 34% of diabetes is type 1 (Liese et al, 2006).

The process of developing the disease can be gradual, but children may become ill quite suddenly once symptoms manifest. Onset of symptoms can present at any age, but there seems to be two age groups with peak incidence: at 5 to 7 years old and again at puberty (median age 7 to 15 years old). Females and males are affected in equal numbers; whites have one-third to two-thirds more disease than African-American youth (Alemzadeh & Wyatt, 2004).

Clinical Findings.

History. As diabetes develops, the symptomatology reflects the decreasing degree of β-cell mass, increasing insulinopenia and hyperglycemia, and increasing ketoacids. A provider's level of suspicion should rise when any child has inappropriate polyuria, dehydration, poor weight gain, and flulike symptoms. With type 1 diabetes, the child may have had a viral infection, cold, or flu, and parents notice increased urination and thirst during the recovery period, with additional signs and symptoms appearing over a period of days or weeks. There may be significant weight loss, fatigue, and lethargy. Twenty percent to 40% of children do not seek treatment until they are ketoacidotic (Alemzadeh & Wyatt, 2004). The following early symptoms are often reported:

- Polydipsia
- Polyphagia
- Polyuria
- Nocturia
- Blurred vision
- Weight loss
- Fatigue
- Vaginal moniliasis

As ketoacids accumulate, the following history is reported:

- Abdominal pain
- Nausea, vomiting
- Fruity-smelling breath
- Weakness (caused by dehydration)
- Mental confusion
- Coma

Physical Examination. Although children typically have polyuria, polydipsia, and weight loss, the physical examination of children with new-onset type 1 diabetes may be remarkably benign. Look for:

- Dehydration (child may not look clinically dehydrated unless actively vomiting)
- Weight loss or slow weight gain; assess height and weight over time
- Muscle wasting
- Tachycardia
- Slow, labored breathing (Kussmaul) (if ketotic)
- Flushed cheeks and face (if ketotic)
- Fruity-smelling breath (if ketotic)
- Vaginal yeast, thrush, or other infection

Diagnostic Tests. Urine testing and blood glucose measurements are generally all that are required to make the diagnosis.

- Metabolic screen for acid-base status to exclude diabetic ketoacidosis
- Blood sugar:
  - Fasting plasma glucose equal to or greater than 126 mg/dL
  - Random plasma glucose equal to or greater than 200 mg/dL
  - Postprandial (2 hours after eating) plasma glucose equal to or greater than 200 mg/dL
- Urine for glucose and ketones
- Screen for concomitant associated autoimmune conditions (primary hypothyroidism and celiac disease [if symptomatic]) (Svoren & Laffel, 2006)

Capillary blood samples, reagent sticks, and glucose meters should only be used for monitoring diabetes control.

Children older than 12 years should also be referred for an ophthalmology exam for a baseline and/or to identify and treat any diabetes-related eye complications.

Differential Diagnosis. Type 1 diabetes must be distinguished from stress-induced hyperglycemia, which in some studies occurs in up to 4% of normal children during a serious illness. Thyroiditis and celiac disease may initially present with type 1 diabetes as a symptom or may evolve afterwards.

Management. The goals of treatment of type 1 diabetes are to achieve normal growth and development, optimal glycemic control, minimal acute or chronic complications, and a positive psychosocial adjustment to diabetes. Every child is different, and treatment of new-onset type 1 diabetes must be individualized to determine the target blood sugar, diet, and insulin regimen best suited to the individual child. The American Diabetes Association periodically publishes guidelines for the management of diabetes in children (American Diabetes Association, 2006).

All children with type 1 diabetes should be started on insulin as soon as the condition is discovered. Children with ketoacidosis should be admitted to the hospital for continuous IV insulin treatment and careful monitoring to prevent cerebral edema that, although rare, can cause significant morbidity or mortality.

Most children without ketoacidosis have traditionally been hospitalized to initiate insulin therapy. However, a recent review of studies suggests that outpatient or home management at initial diagnosis of type 1 diabetes has no disadvantages as to control, complications, psychosocial factors, or total costs (Cochrane Collaboration, 2007). Some large children's diabetes centers do outpatient initial management. Whenever possible, children should be referred immediately to a children's diabetes center for initiation of insulin therapy and diabetes education. Whether followed at a diabetes center or in the primary care office, children with diabetes need ongoing access to diabetes educators, nutritionists, and psychologists and social workers when necessary.

Management of new-onset type 1 diabetes involves determining the insulin regimen and dose best suited to the individual child, target blood sugar, and a way to manage the child's diet. Children and families must learn how to inject insulin, measure blood sugar at home, quantify the amount of carbohydrate in food, prevent hypoglycemia, manage diabetes during illness, and adjust for strenuous activities. They are taught to monitor blood sugar before meals, bedtime, and sometimes in the middle of the night. Each of the components of the treatment regimen is discussed below.

Insulin. There are many potential regimens of insulin therapy. The regimen to start depends on the age of the child, the family's wishes, the family's social and educational resources and schedule, and the clinician's comfort level with the regimen. All require medical nutrition therapy that must match the insulin schedule. The available insulin preparations are listed in Table 25-4. For insulin dosing, refer to Table 25-5.

Two starting insulin strategies exist with some variations. In general, the total daily starting dose of insulin for children and teens is 1 unit/kg/day. The traditional regimen would

TABLE 25-4 Types of Insulin

Insulin	Onset (minutes)	Peak (hours)	Duration (hours)
Regular	30	2-4	4-6
Aspart (NovoLog)	5	1½	3
Lispro (Humalog)	5	1½	3
NPH	120	6-8	8-20
Detemir (Levemir)	120	Dose dependent	Dose dependent
Glargine (Lantus)	180	No peak	24

TABLE 25-5 Starting Subcutaneous Insulin Dosing (Units/Kg)

Insulin	Breakfast	Lunch	Dinner	Bedtime
Traditional Regimen				
Lispro/Aspart/ Regular	0.22	0	0.17	0
NPH	0.45	0	0	0.17
Hybrid Regimen				
Lispro/Aspart/ Regular	0.22	0	0.17	0
NPH	0.22	0	0	0
Glargine	0	0	0.31	
Basal/Bolus Regimen				
Lispro/aspart/ regular	*	*	*	*
Glargine	0	0	0	0.50†

*Bolus insulin is based on a carbohydrate-to-insulin ratio plus a high blood sugar correction:
500/wt (kg) = number of grams of carbohydrate covered by 1 unit of insulin. A 50-kg child would start with 1 unit of insulin for 10 g of carbohydrate.
1800/wt (kg) = mg/dL that 1 unit of insulin will drop an elevated blood sugar. A 50-kg child would expect 1 unit of insulin to drop the blood sugar 36 mg/dL. To start, add 1 extra unit of insulin for every 50 mg/dL the blood sugar is above 150 mg/dL.
†Give the Glargine at breakfast time for infants and toddlers, during the evening for teens.

include short-acting insulin (Lispro or Aspart) combined with intermediate-acting NPH insulin at breakfast, short-acting insulin at dinner, and NPH insulin at bedtime. This plan has the advantage that a school-age child will not need to take a shot at school, but the disadvantage that the timing of meals must stay the same each day and that the child must eat a set amount of carbohydrate at meal and snack time. Most children would have three meals and three snacks each day.

The other regimen is a basal bolus routine with Glargine insulin given at breakfast time (infants and toddlers) or bedtime (teens) to provide a steady background amount of insulin and then boluses of quick-acting insulin at meal and snack times. This allows unreliable eaters to match their carbohydrate intake with insulin; they do not need to follow a regular meal and snack schedule, but they will require more injections. Families learn to use a carbohydrate-to-insulin ratio and a high blood sugar correction to determine each quick-acting insulin dose.

A combination of the two regimens (hybrid regimen) substitutes Glargine for evening NPH, allowing only two injections per day; this is more forgiving if the family is off schedule. Although the manufacturer of Glargine did not study this insulin combined with quick-acting insulin in the same syringe, many centers are allowing children to mix the two without untoward consequences. Thus, a child could receive an injection of quick-acting insulin and NPH at breakfast and quick-acting insulin and Glargine at dinner.

The usual sites for insulin injection are the legs, arms, and upper outer quadrant of the buttocks. School-age children and adolescents can be encouraged to use their abdomen as a regular injection site. However, young children with minimal subcutaneous abdominal fat have difficulty with this site. Rotation of injection sites is necessary to prevent lipohypertrophy and poor absorption of insulin.

Insulin injection devices include regular insulin syringes, a "pen," or continuous subcutaneous insulin infusion (CSII) known as the "pump." This latter mode of delivery infuses a fast-acting insulin at an hourly rate (the basal rate) through a small, flexible, subcutaneous soft cannula. The cannula is replaced in a new site by the wearer or family every 2 or 3 days. A bolus of insulin is programmed by the user to cover the amount of carbohydrates consumed and to adjust for the level of activity. These devices are not "automatic," require more work and deeper understanding of diabetes than subcutaneous injections, and put the child at risk for ketosis if the catheter clogs up or the pump malfunctions. This method is becoming an increasingly popular way to receive insulin, requires parental supervision and glucose level testing, and may improve glycemic control in a motivated child or family.

After insulin treatment has been started, children often have a "honeymoon period" during which insulin doses decrease. Close follow up—often, daily phone calls—after beginning insulin therapy is necessary to prevent too many hypoglycemic episodes. Generally, adjustments of the insulin dose are based on the patterns of the blood glucose over several days. In general, it is wise to decrease insulin doses if there is any unexplained severe hypoglycemic event. Most often parents are given a scale or algorithm of Lispro or Aspart insulin used to correct an elevated breakfast or dinner blood sugar reading.

Parents and teens are taught to make adjustments in insulin based on patterns of blood sugar control. They analyze what time of day the blood sugar is consistently too low or high and adjust the insulin dose that caused the problem. Usually, a 10% adjustment in the problematic insulin dose can be made safely by parents. Many families with practice are able to learn to change the insulin dose independently; others may feel more comfortable conferring with their diabetes care provider.

Children taking insulin should be seen every 3 to 4 months and careful attention paid to diabetes management including:

- Home glucose monitoring results. Age-related targets for fasting and before-meal glucose are:
  - Children under 5 years old: 100 and 200 mg/dL respectively
  - 5 to 11 years old: 70 and 180 mg/dL
  - 12 years and older: 70 to 150 mg/dL
- Frequency of hypoglycemia
- Emotional adjustment to the disease
- HgbA$_{1c}$: HgbA$_{1c}$ closely correlates with average blood glucose concentrations over an 8- to 10-week time frame. Age-related targets are:
  - Children under 5 years old: less than 8.5% HgbA$_{1c}$
  - 5 to 11 years old: less than 8%
  - 12 years and older: equal to or less than 8%
- Physical activities
- Social issues, such as peer pressure
- Eating issues (young women with diabetes have an increased incidence of eating disorders) (Alemzadeh & Wyatt, 2004)
- A physical examination should focus on:
  - Growth and weight gain
  - BP
  - Stage of puberty
  - Examination of the injection sites looking for lipodystrophy
  - Clues for other autoimmune disease (thyroiditis and celiac disease affect approximately 5% of children with type 1 diabetes)

A referral for an initial dilated and comprehensive eye examination should be made 3 to 5 years after diabetes onset in children 10 years or older. The exam should be repeated yearly after that. The American Diabetes Association recommends annual testing of total urinary protein excretion in children who have had diabetes for more than 5 years (but not before puberty). Appropriate referrals for psychological counseling and nutritional review should be made as indicated.

Monitoring Blood Sugar Levels.   Children and families are taught to self-monitor blood sugar (SMBG) before meals, at bedtime, and sometimes in the middle of the night. Monitoring meters have benefited from continued advances in technology, and many different ones are on the market.

Medical Nutrition Therapy.   Nutrition is an essential component of management. Diets should be healthy and calories spread over three meals and two to three snacks daily when the child is using NPH insulin. Caloric intake is based on body size and surface area and can be calculated from a standard recommended dietary allowance (RDA) table. The division of calories is basically spread between protein (15%),

carbohydrates (55%), and fat (less than 30% with less than 7% saturated fats) and takes into consideration age, sex, activity level, and food preferences including those pertinent to culture and ethnicity. It should be the same healthy foods that clinicians recommend to all their pediatric patients. The goal is to balance food intake with insulin dose and activity so that blood glucose is kept as close as possible to the target ranges and to prevent hyperglycemia and hypoglycemia episodes.

A dietitian is essential to provide the guidance needed for the clinician, child, and family. Various approaches to nutrition therapy are being used. Counting grams of carbohydrates is one approach that allows for a total number of grams of carbohydrate for each meal and snack. Meal plans based on groups of food exchanges are also commonly used. Children with diabetes can safely eat sugary treats by including those treats in their allowed carbohydrate allotment. Low calorie (e.g., saccharin, aspartame, sucralose, acesulfame potassium) and reduced calorie (e.g., sorbitol and xylitol) sweeteners are safe in moderation. Fad diets are to be discouraged (American Diabetes Association, 2007).

Exercise.   Exercise may not improve glycemic control, but it is encouraged in all children, including children with diabetes, to promote cardiovascular fitness, control weight, and enhance social interaction and self-esteem. It improves glucose utilization, leading to an increased uptake of glucose, thereby lowering blood glucose levels. Therefore, children and families are taught how to take extra carbohydrate to compensate for exercise. Because there is commonly a prolonged hypoglycemic effect from exercise, there exists a possibility of nocturnal hypoglycemia on active days, and diet adjustments and monitoring needs to accommodate for that. All forms of exercise should be available to the diabetic child or adolescent, including competitive sports.

Complications.   Morbidity and mortality in type 1 diabetes come from metabolic derangements and from long-term complications that affect the small and large blood vessels. It has been shown that chronic high blood sugar causes the long-term complications of microvascular disease (retinopathy, nephropathy, neuropathy, depression, cognitive defects) and macrovascular disease (arterial obstruction with gangrene of extremities and ischemic heart disease). These changes can be prevented or their rate of progression slowed by intensive insulin replacement regimens consisting of multiple daily injections or CSII. After 15 years of diabetes, an individual has a 98% risk of developing diabetic retinopathy; lens opacities occur in 5% of individuals younger than 19 years old (Alemzadeh & Wyatt, 2004).

Type 2 Diabetes
Description and Epidemiology.   Type 2 diabetes begins with increased tissue resistance to insulin; as the need for insulin increases, the pancreas loses its ability to effectively secrete insulin, and there is a failure to compensate for tissue resistance. The result is hyperinsulinemia and hyperglycemia. Autoimmune destruction of pancreatic beta cells does not occur. The disease is aggravated by environmental

factors, such as obesity, sedentary lifestyles, and high-caloric lipid-rich foods. Those born to a mother with gestational diabetes, of low birth weight (sign of intrauterine undernutrition), a large increase in prepubertal body weight, and/or with a family history of type 2 diabetes are also at increased risk (Bloomgarden, 2004).

Type 2 diabetes accounts for 8% to 46% of all new total diabetes cases in the U.S. and has a stronger genetic component than type 1 diabetes (CDC, 2007; Alemzadeh & Wyatt, 2004; NIDDK, 2005). Among American Indians 10 to 19 years old, 76% of all cases of diabetes are type 2; there are 51 per 1000 cases in Pima Indians. It is least common among non-Hispanic whites (6% of all diabetes cases) (Liese et al, 2006). The prevalence of type 2 diabetes may be underdiagnosed, especially since children may have no symptoms or mild symptoms for a long period of time. Children usually are diagnosed during the teenage years, between 10 and 19 years old, and some centers have seen a greater than tenfold incidence in this age group.

Clinical Findings. The symptoms of type 2 diabetes may be absent or subtle, so children at risk should be screened. The American Diabetes Association provides guidelines for screening children at risk (ADA, 2000):

- First screen at 10 years old or at puberty, whichever comes first.
- Screen if overweight (BMI of greater than 85th percentile for age and gender), plus any two of following risk factors:
  - Family history of type 2 diabetes in first- or second-degree relative
  - Race/ethnicity (American Indian, black, Hispanic or Asian or Pacific Islander)
  - Signs of insulin resistance or condition associated with insulin resistance (e.g., acanthosis nigricans, POCS, hypertension, dyslipidemia, accelerated growth suggestive of gigantism)
- Screen if obese (BMI greater than 95th percentile) or if weight greater than 120th percentile of ideal for height without risk factors.
- Screen every 2 years.
- Use fasting plasma glucose test.
- Use clinical judgment to screen for type 2 diabetes in high-risk patients who do not meet these guidelines.

History. The history of patients with type 2 diabetes may include:

- Polydipsia
- Polyphagia
- Polyuria
- Nocturia
- Blurred vision
- Obesity, especially central
- Report of a hyperpigmented, velvetlike rash in skin folds
- Frequent or slow-healing infections
- Fatigue
- History of premature adrenarche
- Symptoms of sleep apnea
- Family history of type 2 diabetes

Physical Examination. The physical examination should include assessment of height, weight, stage of pubertal development, and blood pressure. The following findings may be present:

- Dehydration
- Overweight and obesity (BMI greater than 85th percentile for age and gender)
- Weight loss (less common)
- Acanthosis nigricans, noted in the axilla, base of the neck, groin, knuckles, and other skin folds (see Color Plates)
- Vaginal yeast, thrush, other infection
- Polycystic ovarian syndrome symptoms (e.g., acne, hirsutism)
- Hypertension

Diagnostic Tests. Screening should be conducted in high-risk children without symptoms (see earlier guidelines). An initial urine glucose screen can be done in the office. A glycosylated hemoglobin, lipid panel, TSH and free T_4, and fasting insulin level (used as a motivator rather than a true indicator of disease) should be taken. Children can have ketoacidosis if they have gone undiagnosed for a long time.

In symptomatic children, diagnosis is made if the following exist: Symptoms of diabetes plus:

- Random plasma glucose concentration equal to or greater than 200 mg/dL (11.1 mmol/L)
- Fasting plasma glucose equal to or greater than 126 mg/dL (7 mmol/L)
- Postprandial (2 hours after eating) plasma glucose equal to or greater than 200 mg/dL (11.1 mmol/L)

Depending upon the above results and differential diagnosis, further laboratory studies to evaluate thyroid dysfunction, female hyperandrogenism (serum free testosterone, 17-OHP), and sleep apnea may be indicated.

Differential Diagnosis. Some obese children get type 1 diabetes and may be misdiagnosed as type 2. The presentation of type 1 diabetes can be of slower onset in older children and adults. Maturity-onset diabetes of youth (MODY) is a group of autosomal dominant, single gene disorders that may clinically look like type 2 diabetes. Patients with MODY lack acanthosis nigricans, give a strong family history of early onset (under 25 years old) of nonautoimmune diabetes, and respond to sulfonylurea agents.

Management. As with type 1 diabetes, the treatment plan for children with type 2 diabetes must be individualized. Because the spectrum of disease is broad, ranging from apparent lack of symptoms to ketoacidosis, each case requires an individual plan of care. The goal of treatment is the normalization of blood glucose values; $HgbA_{1c}$ to less than 7%; LDL less than 110, HDL greater than 45, and triglycerides less than 125 mg/dL. Successful control of the associated complications such as hypertension and hyperlipidemia is also important. In addition to the following strategies, the child should also have an annual eye exam and urine test for albumin. $HgbA_{1c}$ should be measured every 3 to 4 months.

Lifestyle Changes: Nutrition and Exercise. When discovered early, type 2 diabetes may respond to lifestyle changes such as alterations in diet and exercise. These changes must be comprehensive. Nutritional management therapy (NMT) is an important part of the treatment plan. Referral to a registered dietitian is essential, with the goals of weight loss and regulating nutritional intake. A low-fat diet, self-monitoring of weight, eating breakfast, and being physically active are important components of NMT. Successful weight management can consist of weight maintenance rather than weight loss early on in treatment. Changes in family eating patterns can contribute to weight maintenance or loss that may normalize insulin levels. It is best to leave the weight monitoring to the adolescent and the provider and/or dietitian rather than to have the rest of the family overly vigilant. Boys have been shown to binge eat when encouraged to lose weight by their mothers (Fulkerson et al, 2002).

Sports and regular exercise are strongly encouraged in children and adolescents with diabetes. Regular vigorous exercise (30 to 60 minutes a day) helps control weight and reduce insulin resistance.

There are a number of barriers to successful weight loss in children with diabetes including accessibility of junk food at school; lack of physical exercise programs at school and home; excessive eating during holidays or festive occasions; failure of providers to offer obesity education; excessive television, videotape viewing, and videogame playing; skipping meals, heavy snacking, non-appetite-based eating and cyclic dieting; and poor family eating patterns (Alemzadeh & Wyatt, 2004). Predictors of successful weight reduction include early weight loss, male sex, younger age, greater education, social support, weight history, and behavioral and cognitive strategies (e.g., improved self-esteem, feelings of control) (Bloomgarden, 2004).

Additional lifestyle changes include tobacco cessation and breastfeeding of infants by adolescent mothers with type 2 diabetes or those who had gestational diabetes.

Pharmacotherapy. If changes in lifestyle are not successful, medication is necessary. In the U.S., one study showed that half of the children being treated with pharmacotherapy for type 2 diabetes needed oral medication and another half needed insulin (Bloomgarden, 2004). Oral medication is used to improve insulin sensitivity (Kaufman, 2005). Metformin is approved for use in children and is the drug of choice. Little research has been done on the use of other hypoglycemic agents in children. Most children are begun on metformin in doses up to 1000 mg twice a day. Metformin rarely causes hypoglycemia, so blood glucose need only be checked when fasting in the AM and two hours after dinner. Gastrointestinal side effects may often be seen with metformin use. Should the patient fail to respond to metformin, a combination of two other oral mediations is often used (Table 25-6). Lipid-reducing medications need to be used with caution in children.

When a patient with type 2 diabetes has ketonuria or is in diabetic ketoacidosis, insulin therapy will be needed initially. These patients are started on the same insulin regimen with home glucose monitoring and a precise food plan as patients with type 1 diabetes. Typically, the insulin needs are higher than in patients with type 1 diabetes. After several weeks to months of insulin therapy, it may be possible to wean the insulin and begin metformin.

TABLE 25-6 Oral Medications for Type 2 Diabetes Mellitus	
Drug	**Action/Comments**
Biguanides (Glucophage [Metformin])	Decreases the amount of sugar produced by the liver; increases insulin sensitivity of the liver and muscles. No direct effect on β-cells in pancreas. Used as first-line monotherapy.
Sulfonylureas (Amaryl [glimepiride], Diabeta, Micronase, Glynase [glyburide])	Stimulates β-cells to make more insulin; may make body tissue more sensitive to insulin. Side effects include weight gain, hypoglycemia; no effect on lipids; possible liver toxicity. Not approved for use in children. Used as second-line therapy in combination with thiazolidinediones (Bloomgarden, 2004).
Thiazolidinediones (Avandia [rosiglitazone], Actos [pioglitazone])	Increases insulin sensitivity at the cellular level; improves glucose usage. Side effects include weight gain; unknown if may cause edema and congestive heart failure in children (Bloomgarden, 2004).
Meglitinides (Prandin [repaglinide])	Stimulates β-cells; no known effect on insulin sensitivity.
Glucosidase inhibitors (Precose [acarbose], Glyset [miglitol])	Slows down the conversion of ingested carbohydrates to sugar in the intestine. Side effects primarily GI distress.

The treatment plan and child's condition should be reevaluated regularly to ensure the care given is meeting the growing child's needs. Children should be evaluated every 3 to 4 months with a history focused on lifestyle changes, nutrition management, and other complications of obesity, in addition to measures of disease control (e.g., plasma glucose levels, $HgbA_{1c}$). The child should also have an annual eye exam and urine test for albumin.

Complications. The complications are similar to those with type 1 diabetes (microvascular and macrovascular diseases). Nephropathy is a more common complication in those with type 2 than type 1 diabetes. Nonalcoholic fatty liver disease can occur and eventual dependence upon insulin for control.

Patient and Parent Education. Treatment success may be hampered by ongoing psychosocial issues and neuropsychiatric problems. Providing families and children with information that helps them gain control of a very difficult disease is crucial. Education of the child, family, and caregivers should include insulin therapy, self-monitoring of glucose, nutrition and meal planning, exercise, managing sick days, school issues, coping skills, and prevention of complications. Those with diabetes should always wear a form of medical identification. School personnel must be informed of the plan of care and must implement an individualized care plan for the child.

OBESITY

Epidemiology

Obesity is becoming increasingly common in children and adults around the world. A detailed discussion of obesity is found in Chapter 11.

In most children, overweight and obesity are thought to be due to a small imbalance between calories consumed and calories burned. Almost all children with excess caloric intake will be tall for age and/or have a normal to rapid growth velocity. Therefore, every child should have a BMI calculated and compared with normative data at each clinic visit.

From an endocrine perspective, the mechanisms of weight homeostasis are complex and involve hypothalamic hormones, hormones produced by adipocytes (e.g., leptin), and the gut (Chia & Boston, 2006). In most children, no single hormone deficiency or excess explains obesity. Recognizable syndrome and endocrine dysfunction account for, at most, 1% of children with overweight.

Several "classic" hormone situations may cause obesity, including hypothyroidism, cortisol excess, and GHD. In these conditions, the child is likely to be short or growing at a subnormal growth velocity. Several genetic conditions predispose to overweight (e.g., Prader-Willi syndrome). Developmental delay and dysmorphic features are key to identifying these conditions.

Diagnostic Tests

Children with a BMI greater than 95th percentile for age and gender should be screened for a number of conditions:

- Abnormalities in glucose tolerance with a fasting oral glucose tolerance test. This screening should be limited to children older than 10 years, or those with symptoms of hyperglycemia (e.g., polyuria and polydipsia)
- Nonalcoholic steatohepatitis with liver function tests
- Dyslipidemia with a lipid panel
- Thyroid function with a thyroid panel
- Sleep apnea by history of snoring, daytime somnolence
- Polycystic ovarian syndrome with a free and total testosterone level when there are symptoms of irregular menses, acne, or hirsutism
- Hypertension with a BP measurement
- Orthopedic issues by history
- Psychological issues by history (some children with obesity suffer from low self-esteem or behavior problems)

Management

Children with type 2 diabetes, polycystic ovarian syndrome, or other metabolic or endocrine disorders underlying their obesity should be followed in concert with a pediatric endocrinologist. Those with obesity alone are more effectively treated in the primary care office with nutritional counseling and help to achieve a more active lifestyle (Dietz & Robinson, 2005). In general, the goal is weight maintenance, not loss, in the overweight child without any of the above complications; it is expected that these children will eventually grow into their weight and achieve a BMI less than 85th percentile. For children with an overweight-related complication, weight loss of 1 pound per month would be an appropriate goal. More rapid weight loss may be associated with slowing in linear growth.

Consensus is lacking as to the most effective way to manage obesity. Goals for reducing calories consumed and increasing daily exercise must be made within the context of each family; success is more likely to be achieved if the entire family participates in lifestyle changes. Providers must work closely with families to ensure consistent follow-up, to assess the effectiveness of interventions, and to modify the treatment strategy if necessary (see Chapter 11).

POSTERIOR PITUITARY GLAND DISORDERS

Abnormal posterior pituitary function is uncommon in pediatrics. Children have inappropriately dilute urine for the clinical situation that may only become obvious when they develop hypernatremic dehydration, secondary enuresis, or polyuria. They may also be discovered in an evaluation of a child at risk for hypopituitarism. After a screening urinalysis shows low specific gravity in the absence of urinary glucose, a pediatric endocrinologist should be consulted.

◼ INTRODUCTION TO INBORN ERRORS OF METABOLISM

Inborn errors of metabolism (IEM) encompass a wide range of inherited disorders with alterations of specific biochemical reactions. The term "inborn error of metabolism" was coined by Garrod in 1908 to describe the hereditary alteration in enzyme reactions he observed in the first identified "inborn error," alkaptonuria, and use of the term has persisted (Lanpher et al, 2006; Jones & Bennett, 2002).

Although individually rare, IEM have a collective incidence of approximately 1 in 1500 live births (Raghuveer et al, 2006), and it is likely that all health care providers will encounter a child with an IEM at some point in their career. Clinical consequences for the affected individual vary from mild to severe. Early detection, accurate diagnosis, and rapid intervention are necessary to achieve favorable outcomes; prevent irreversible mental retardation, physical disability, neurologic damage, or death; and reduce long-term financial burden and human suffering. This section discusses the classification and pathophysiology of IEM; looks at newborn screening, including common clinical presentations and emergency management of conditions found in the newborn period; and presents a brief overview of the diagnosis and treatment of a few of the more common disorders.

CLASSIFICATION OF INBORN ERRORS OF METABOLISM

Classification of IEM presents a challenge because of the number and diversity of disorders. Proposed classification systems have suggested categorizing based on: affected organ (e.g., neurologic or hepatic diseases), organelle (e.g., mitochondrial or lysosomal disorders), age of presentation (e.g., neonatal or adult onset), large or small molecule diseases, or affected metabolic pathway (e.g., urea cycle defects [UCDs] or defects of amino acid metabolism). The *International Classification of Diseases ICD-9-CM* manual categorizes IEM as follows (American Medical Association [AMA], 2004):

- Disorders of carbohydrate metabolism (e.g., glycogen storage disease, galactosemia, hereditary fructose intolerance)
- Disorders of amino acid metabolism (e.g., PKU, tyrosinemia, nonketotic hyperglycinemia, maple syrup disease [MSD], homocystinuria)
- Disorders of organic acid metabolism (e.g., methylmalonic or propionic acidemia, multiple carboxylase deficiency)
- Disorders of fatty acid oxidation and mitochondrial metabolism disorders (e.g., short, medium, and very long chain acyl-CoA dehydrogenase deficiencies, CPT 1 and 2 deficiency)
- Disorders of purine and pyrimidine metabolism (e.g., Lesch-Nyhan syndrome, orotic aciduria)
- Disorders of steroid metabolism (e.g., CAH or Smith-Lemli-Opitz syndrome)
- Disorders of mitochondrial function (e.g., Kearns-Sayre syndrome, MELAS)
- Lysosomal storage disorders (e.g., Gaucher disease, mucopolysaccharidosis, Tay-Sachs, Niemann-Pick disease)

PATHOPHYSIOLOGY

IEM are caused by an inherited defect, generally of an enzyme or its cofactor, resulting in altered function of a metabolic pathway. Autosomal recessive inheritance patterns are most common.

Fig. 25-3 provides an overview of the major metabolic pathways. The majority of defects are caused by a single gene mutation encoding a specific enzyme whose function is to facilitate the conversion of various substances (substrates,

[e.g., foodstuffs]) into others (metabolic products, [e.g., urea]). The block in the pathway variably leads to: accumulation of substrate proximal to the block (e.g., lyosomal storage disorders); accumulation of toxic metabolites (e.g., galactose byproducts in galactosemia); deficiency of a product distal to the block; feedback inhibition or activation by the metabolite; or some combination thereof.

There is variability in the degree of loss of function of the enzyme, and this can alter the clinical course and response to treatment (phenotype) among persons with the same diagnosis.

ASSESSMENT OF INBORN ERRORS OF METABOLISM
Description

IEM are rare but should be included in the differential diagnosis of any critically ill neonate, as well as infants, children, adolescents, and young adults presenting with symptoms that are progressive or otherwise unexplained. The timing of symptom onset in relation to initiation of feedings can be an important clue. Babies with IEM almost always appear normal at birth with effects of the disease becoming apparent over the course of days to months. As substrates or toxic metabolites accumulate, such as in organic acidemias, nonspecific symptoms that may be indistinguishable from sepsis typically appear. Finding a cause of symptoms, however, does not necessarily rule out the possibility of an IEM (Greene et al, 2005) (e.g., electrolyte abnormalities diagnosed as renal Fanconi syndrome may be caused by underlying cystinosis).

Clinical Findings
History.   A thorough family and individual history is important to identify possibilities of IEM. Details in a family and patient history that should raise suspicion include:

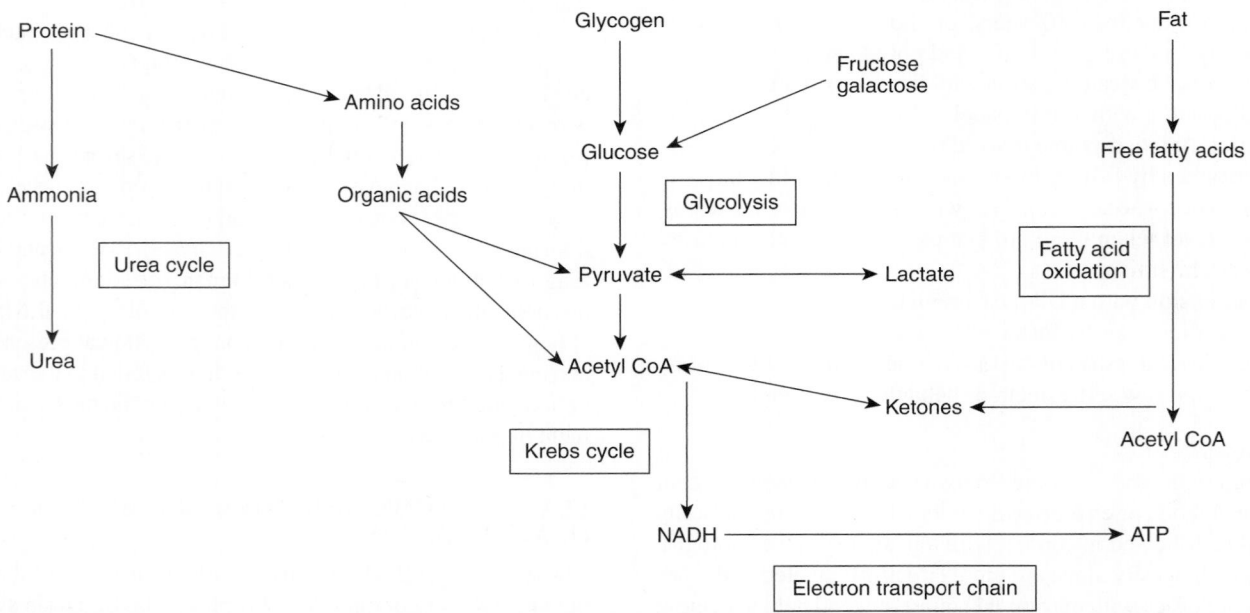

FIG. 25-3   Overview of major metabolic pathways. *Acetyl CoA,* Acetylcoenzyme A; *ATP,* adenosine triphosphate; *NADH,* nicotinamide adenine dinucleotide. (From Logan A: Metabolic disease. In Cheng A, Williams BA, Sivarajan VB, editors: *The hospital for sick children handbook of pediatrics,* ed 10, Toronto, 2004, Saunders Canada, p 474.)

- Consanguinity
- Decompensation with illness greater than anticipated for the nature of the illness (commonly seen in acidosis)
- Developmental delay, psychomotor retardation, or loss of milestones
- Failure to thrive
- Frequent infections
- Family history of IEM
- Siblings with unexplained infant or neonatal death
- Symptoms seen with a change in diet
- Unusual odor (sweat, urine, or cerumen)

Physical Examination. A complete exam is essential, with attention to dysmorphia, muscle tone, ocular symptoms, organomegaly, and respiratory function. Box 25-10 provides an overview of symptoms suspicious for an inborn error at various ages.

Diagnostic Tests. Effective intervention for IEM depends on the ability to identify the disorder before the onset of symptoms. Screening for the presence of IEM allows the provider to identify the condition before damage has occurred. The capability to screen for IEM dates to the early 1960s when an inexpensive test for PKU using a small blood sample collected on a filter paper was developed (Guthrie & Susi, 1963). Four hundred thousand newborns in 29 states were part of a pilot study that confirmed the effectiveness of this test to detect PKU. As a result, states instituted screening programs for newborn infants, and today, virtually

all of the 4 million infants born each year in the U.S. are screened.

Technologic advances have allowed for screening a wide array of disorders, and the newborn screening test encompasses much more than screening for PKU. Although every state mandates newborn screening, each state, using a developed set of criteria, independently determines which conditions will be screened (Jones & Bennett, 2002). This leads to large discrepancies between states, with screening for as few as eight to as many as forty-three disorders (National Newborn Screening & Genetics Resource Center, 2007). In 2006, only 10% of newborns in the U.S. received expanded newborn screening encompassing all test recommendations of the American College of Medical Genetics (ACMG) (Botkin et al, 2006), though this is changing rapidly.

Laboratory studies are generally necessary in the diagnosis of IEM; however, determining what studies to perform is not straightforward. Consider performing a newborn screening test on any significantly ill neonate, unless proof of prior collection is obtained. Testing for common (i.e., nonmetabolic) causes of presenting symptoms should not be sacrificed for metabolic testing, but it is not always wise to wait until all routine tests have been performed and the results known before submitting samples for metabolic disease testing. This facilitates work-up should the patient be referred to a metabolic specialist. When the ill child has signs and symptoms of what could be an IEM, the primary care provider should consult early with a metabolic specialist, rather than wait for results of tests. For chronic presentations, after common etiology are ruled out, refer to a metabolic specialist for testing beyond routine analysis.

Initial laboratory studies for the neonate with a suspected IEM includes:
- CBC with differential
- Blood gases
- Serum electrolytes with special attention to anion gap = $Na^+ - (Cl^- + HCO_3^-)$. Normal anion gap is between 8 to 12 mEq/L
- Plasma ammonia (collected free flowing [no tourniquet, no heel stick, preferably no capillary tubes] immediately placed on ice and analyzed within 45 to 60 minutes)
- Plasma lactate (collected free flowing)
- Plasma (and variably urine) quantitative amino acids; carnitine levels
- Urinalysis
- Urine reducing substances, ketones (if acidotic and hypoglycemic), organic acids, mucopolysaccharides and oligosaccharides if storage disease is suspected
- Many labs offer a metabolic screen typically on urine, but some labs prefer urine and blood. This test varies between laboratories.

Testing may also consist of biochemical or molecular (DNA) analysis obtained from blood (e.g., patients with chronic acidosis should have serum lactate and pyruvate drawn [also free flowing]), cerebral spinal fluid (glycine), or biopsy from skin, liver, or muscle (enzyme assays). Additionally, for

---

BOX 25-10 **Symptoms Suggesting an Inborn Error of Metabolism in Children by Age**

Neonates and Infants	Older Children and Adolescents (in addition to those of neonates and infants)
• Cardiomyopathy	• Ataxia
• Coarse facial features	• Dementia
• Dysmorphic features	• Dystonia or chorea
• Hyperammonemia	• Mental retardation
• Hypotonia or hypertonia	• Muscular weakness
• Jaundice	• Ophthalmoplegia
• Metabolic acidosis	• Progressive deterioration
• Neutropenia and/or thrombocytopenia	• Skeletal changes
• Ocular findings (retinitis pigmentosa, cherry red spots, cataracts or corneal clouding)	
• Organomegaly	
• Respiratory distress (apnea or tachypnea)	
• Seizures	
• Unexplained hypoglycemia	
• Vomiting	

the child with chronic encephalopathy, consider an MRI and magnetic resonance spectroscopy (MRS) for brain imaging. It is important to become familiar with the appropriate methods of specimen collection and handling (before and during shipment of the samples to the laboratory) as inappropriate practices alter the quality of the sample, potentially leading to missed cases.

Management

Management of metabolic disorders varies depending on the specific condition, its severity, and whether it is an acute or chronic presentation. Caregivers of children with a known diagnosis of inborn errors (e.g., those that cause hyperammonemia) become very astute at early recognition of symptoms in their child and should be viewed as an important part of the health care team.

Metabolic Emergencies. Emergency management of metabolic disorders requires hospital admission and specialist care. The goal of emergency management is twofold: prevent catabolism and remove toxic substrates or metabolites. Aggressive management is necessary to avert or reduce neurologic sequelae. This acute care management may require IV medications (including glucose to halt catabolism), diet restriction (e.g., no protein for 24 to 48 hours or until mental status is back to baseline), hemodialysis, or life support.

Stable Metabolic Disorders. The variability of IEM necessitates that management be tailored to the individual patient based on the specific diagnosis and phenotype. However, the following strategies provide several broad categories from which treatments are drawn.

- Control substrate accumulation:
  - Restrict dietary intake (e.g., restricting phenylalanine intake in PKU).
  - Control endogenous production of the substrate (e.g., give high-calorie, no-protein feeds during illness to prevent catabolism, which would release amino acids).
  - Accelerate removal of the substrate (e.g., administer sodium benzoate/phenylacetate in UCDs to increase elimination of waste nitrogen through an alternate pathway).
- Dietary supplementation:
  - Replace or supplement the diet with products that become deficient distal to the metabolic block or if the diet is medically restricted (e.g., arginine or citrulline in UCDs).
- Vitamin and cofactor replacement:
  - Increase the supply of certain vitamins that act as cofactors to metabolic reactions to improve function of the residual enzyme activity. Vitamin replacement is also important with severely restricted diets.
- Enzyme replacement therapy (ERT):
  - ERT (an intravenous infusion of enzyme replacement given every 1 to 4 weeks) is becoming more widely available in the clinical setting for lysosomal storage diseases (LSDs).
- Bone marrow or organ transplant:

  - Bone marrow or cord blood transplant is clinically available for some disorders, but remains controversial.
  - Organ transplant can essentially "cure" some metabolic diseases by transplanting an organ in which the mutant genes are expressed. Liver transplantation has shown success in some IEM.

Complications

Multiple complications such as renal failure, hypertension, spinal cord compression, and carpal tunnel syndrome may be seen with IEM, often necessitating a multidisciplinary management team.

SPECIFIC METABOLIC DISORDERS OF CHILDREN
Disorders of Carbohydrate Metabolism

These are a group of disorders caused by the inability to metabolize the monosaccharides glucose, galactose, and fructose and the polysaccharide glycogen. Aberrant glycogen synthesis or disorders of gluconeogenesis also contribute to faulty carbohydrate metabolism.

Glycogen Storage Diseases.

Description and Epidemiology. Glycogen is a glucose polymer stored in muscle and the liver, and deficiency of any enzyme involved in the metabolic pathway of glycogen can affect biosynthesis or degradation of glycogen in the organ in which the enzyme is expressed. This results in a variety of presentations of disease. Glucose-6-phosphatase deficiency (type 1), lysosomal acid α-glucosidase deficiency (type 2), debrancher deficiency (type 3), and liver phosphorylase kinase deficiency (type 9) are the most common early childhood presentations. Overall frequency of all forms is 1:20,000 live births (Raghuveer et al, 2006).

Clinical Findings. Signs and symptoms may include cardiomegaly, hepatosplenomegaly, hypoglycemic seizures, lactic acidosis, ketosis, hyperlipidemia, elevated transaminases, easy fatigability, hypotonia, and muscle weakness.

Diagnostic Tests. Enzyme assays and mutation analysis are available for essentially all identified forms of glycogen storage disease.

Management. Treatment varies depending on the specific defect. Types 1, 3, 4, and 9 all affect enzyme activity in the liver, which is responsible for homeostasis of plasma glucose. Treatment is aimed at maintaining normal blood glucose levels and may require continuous feedings through a gastrostomy tube, frequent feedings throughout the day, and ingestion of an uncooked cornstarch slurry at bedtime. Parents and children must be aware of symptoms of low blood sugar, and home glucose monitoring is recommended. Enzyme replacement therapy for Pompe disease (glycogen storage disease type 2) was approved by the FDA in July 2006.

Galactosemia.

Description. Galactosemia results from a disorder of galactose metabolism. The classic form of galactosemia is caused by deficient galactose-1-phosphate uridyltransferase (GALT) activity. Dietary galactose is most commonly ingested as lactose, the principle carbohydrate in human milk and commercial non-soy formulas. The metabolism of galactose undergoes many enzymatic reactions. A block at the level of the GALT enzyme results in accumulation of galactose-1-phosphate (gal-1-P) and other galactose derivatives, leading to the clinical symptoms.

Epidemiology. Incidence of the classic form is estimated at 1 in 47,000 live births (Raghuveer et al, 2006). It is an autosomal recessive trait.

Clinical Findings. Infants with classic galactosemia appear normal at birth, but demonstrate clinical manifestations after milk feeding. Although galactosemia is typically discovered on newborn screening, neonates may show clinical signs before results of the screening are known. Therefore, galactosemia should remain in the differential diagnosis of any ill neonate. Clinical manifestations of severe, untreated galactosemia include poor weight gain, lethargy, jaundice, vomiting, coagulopathies and *Escherichia coli* sepsis. Vitreous hemorrhage has been reported.

Diagnostic Tests. Urine reducing substances will be positive in recently fed infants. Serum glucose may be decreased. Measurement of GALT activity in red cells will be deficient, and liver enzymes and gal-1-P levels will be elevated.

Complications. Long-term complications of untreated galactosemia include cirrhosis, cataracts, and irreversible brain damage; death can occur. Despite treatment, most children with classic galactosemia develop speech impairment, and some develop impaired motor function. Premature ovarian failure is also common.

Management. Treatment in classic galactosemia consists of eliminating dietary galactose. There is controversy surrounding appropriate treatment of variants (e.g., Duarte) with some centers recommending dietary restriction, whereas others recommend using soy formula during the first year. Ensure that the child is receiving appropriate calcium supplementation.

Urea Cycle Disorders

Description and Epidemiology. A defect in any enzyme of the urea cycle results in hyperammonemia secondary to the body's inability to detoxify waste nitrogen through its normal conversion to urea. Ammonia is an end product of amino acid catabolism and is highly toxic to the CNS. There are five enzymes required for the conversion of ammonia to urea, and deficiency in any of these enzymes results in disease. Incidence of the disorder is approximately 1:10,000 births.

Clinical Findings. In infants, symptoms are related to the effects of hyperammonemia, start after protein ingestion, and include vomiting, lethargy, irritability, malaise, and potential seizures and coma. Older children may exhibit ataxia, confusion, agitation, irritability, and combativeness.

Diagnostic Tests. There are typically no specific findings on laboratory testing.
- Blood urea nitrogen may be low.
- Ammonia level above 100 micromoles/L (or lower in older children) evokes concern (normal values are typically less than 35 micromoles/L).
- Enzyme assays are available for diagnosis of most of the disorders.

- Genetic mutation analysis may confirm diagnosis of some of the disorders.

Complications. Despite appropriate treatment, children with UCDs are vulnerable to metabolic decompensation, mild to moderate mental retardation, and premature death.

Management. Treatment of acute hyperammonemia can be found in Box 25-11. Principles of treatment of chronic UCD are very similar, but also include limiting endogenous protein catabolism and dietary protein consumption under the supervision of a metabolic dietitian.

Amino Acid Metabolism Disorders: Aminoacidopathies and Organic Acidurias and Acidemias

There are more than 30 defects of amino acid metabolism that can be attributed to enzyme or cofactor defects. Although all of these disorders result from defects in amino acid metabolism, they are generally classified as aminoacidopathies or organic acidurias or acidemias, depending on whether amino acids or organic acids are detected in urine or plasma. The more common aminoacidopathies include: PKU, maple syrup disease (MSD), tyrosinemia types 1 and 2, and homocystinuria.

BOX 25-11 **Treatment of Acute Hyperammonemia in an Infant**

1. Provide adequate calories, fluid, and electrolytes intravenously (10% glucose and intravenous lipids 1g/kg/24 hours). Add minimal amounts of protein preferably as a mixture of essential amino acids (0.25g/kg/24 hours) during the first 24 hours of therapy.
2. Give priming doses of the following compounds:
   - To be added to 20mL/kg of 10% glucose and infused within 1-2 hours
   - Sodium benzoate 250mg/kg (5.5g/nm²)*
   - Sodium phenylacetate 250mg/kg (5.5g/nm²)*
   - Arginine hydrochloride 200-600mg/kg (4-12g/nm²) as a 10% solution
3. Continue infusion of sodium benzoate* (250-500mg/kg/24 hours), sodium phenylacetate* (250-500mg/kg/24 hours), and arginine (200-600mg/kg/24 hours†) following the above priming doses. These compounds should be added to the daily intravenous fluid.
4. Initiate peritoneal dialysis or hemodialysis if above treatment fails to produce an appreciable decrease in plasma ammonia.

*These compounds are usually prepared as a 1%-2% solution for intravenous use. Sodium from these drugs should be included as part of the daily sodium requirement.
†The higher dose is recommended in the treatment of patients with citrullinemia and argininosuccinic aciduria. Arginine is not recommended in patients with arginase deficiency and in those whose hyperammonemia is secondary to organic acidemia.
Adapted from Rezvani I: Urea cycle & hyperammonemia (Arginine, Citrulline, Ornithine). In Behrman RM, Kliegman RE, Jenson HB, editors, *Nelson textbook of pediatrics,* ed 17, Philadelphia, 2004, WB Saunders, p 426.

Phenylketonuria.

Description and Epidemiology.   Classical phenylketonuria (PKU) is the most common form of PKU and results from deficiency of the enzyme phenylalanine hydroxylase, which converts phenylalanine to tyrosine. Untreated PKU leads to elevated phenylalanine concentrations in the blood and brain and results in CNS damage with profound mental retardation. More prevalent in Caucasians, PKU is an autosomal recessive trait with an incidence of approximately 1:15,000 live births and a carrier rate estimated at 1:60 (Raghuveer et al, 2006).

Clinical Findings.   There are no clinical manifestations at birth, and the effects of high phenylalanine levels may not be apparent in the first few months, by which time, if untreated, irreversible brain damage has occurred. Children with more advanced, untreated disease tend to have lighter skin and hair than typical for their race and develop an eczematous rash and a musty or mousy odor related to phenylacetic acid.

PKU should be detected on newborn screening. Infants with PKU ingesting a normal diet will have serum phenylalanine levels greater than 20 mg/dL on confirmatory testing for PKU, whereas others with milder hyperphenylalaninemia will have intermediate levels.

Differential Diagnosis.   Biopterin is a cofactor for phenylalanine, tyrosine and tryptophan hydroxylases. Children with biopterin defects may be detected on newborn screening, but will continue to deteriorate despite usual dietary intervention for PKU. Testing blood and urine biopterins and biopterin enzymes is recommended in any child with high phenylalanine levels because treatment is different from PKU treatment.

Management.   Treatment for PKU involves limiting the dietary intake of phenylalanine, with a goal of serum phenylalanine levels below 2 to 6 mg/dL in infants and young children. Phenylalanine is an essential amino acid, so it cannot be eliminated entirely, and it is important to ensure that the infant and child are receiving enough to meet growth needs. To obtain the necessary essential amino acids, the diet is supplemented with a medically modified formula, free of phenylalanine to meet calorie and appetite needs. Over the child's first year or two of life, parents are educated on the phenylalanine content of foods; the child's phenylalanine level is frequently monitored, and a phenylalanine "allowance" is established based on the child's dietary tolerance. The current recommendation is "diet for life" to prevent long-term cognitive and neurologic sequelae. Medically modified low-phenylalanine food products are available. Pregnant teenagers with PKU must maintain strict dietary restrictions to protect the fetus. Consultation with or referral to a dietitian is essential.

Classic Homocystinuria.

Description and Epidemiology.   Homocystinuria due to cystathionine synthase deficiency is the most common form of these disorders, with a prevalence of approximately 1:100,000 to 200,000 births (Raghuveer et al, 2006). Discussion of homocystinuria caused by defects in vitamin metabolism and deficiency of methylenetetrahydrofolate reductase (MTHFR) is beyond the scope of this chapter.

Clinical Findings.   Clinical manifestations are nonspecific and include failure to thrive and developmental delay.

Diagnostic Tests.   Plasma and urine amino acid testing is done for concentrations of:
- Methionine (Elevated levels may be found on the newborn screening, but values rise slowly, and high methionine levels may not be detected on specimens obtained from affected infants in the first few days after birth; a second newborn screening is necessary.)
- Homocystine
- Total homocystine

Complications.   Treatment outcomes are variable, and these children are at high risk for metabolic stroke, though prognosis is good for those with the classical form of homocystinuria identified on newborn screening. Untreated patients develop ocular lens dislocation, progressive mental retardation, thromboembolic events, convulsions, and skeletal abnormalities resembling Marfan syndrome.

Management.   Some children respond to vitamin B_6 therapy; and plasma homocystine and methionine concentrations are monitored. If the child responds, treatment with vitamin B_6 is continued. Children who do not respond to vitamin B_6 are placed on a methionine-restricted diet with frequent monitoring of plasma amino acids and total plasma homocystine. Betaine is administered. Folate and vitamin B_{12} optimize conversion of homocystine to methionine.

Disorders of Fatty Acid Oxidation

Medium-Chain Acyl-CoA Dehydrogenase Deficiency.

Description and Epidemiology.   Fatty acids are an important energy resource for the body, used during times of fasting and stress when glycogen stores become depleted. Defects can occur at any point in fatty acid transport or the mitochondrial beta-oxidation pathway, yielding more than 20 disorders in which individuals are unable to metabolize fatty acids. The more common fatty acid oxidation disorders are: medium-chain Acyl-CoA dehydrogenase deficiency (MCAD), very long-chain Acyl-CoA dehydrogenase deficiency (VLCAD), and long-chain 3-hydroxyacyl-CoA dehydrogenase deficiency (LCHAD). The incidence of all disorders ranges from 1:8000 to 1:100,000 (Raghuveer et al, 2006). MCAD is quickly becoming one of the most common IEM identified in infants by newborn screening with an estimated incidence of 1:8500 live births (Raghuveer et al, 2006).

Clinical Findings.   Common manifestations include: hypoglycemia during fasting; cardiomyopathy; muscle weakness; and inappropriately low or absent ketone production during times of stress, fasting, and illness. Individuals with MCAD may be asymptomatic for a lifetime or have premature death. Fasting may lead to complications including hypoketotic hypoglycemia, hypotonia, lethargy and vomiting progressing to seizures, coma, encephalopathy, and death. Up to 25% of patients die during their first episode, 50% may never be symptomatic, and the overall prognosis for survivors is excellent because fasting tolerance improves with age (Venditti & Stanley, 2004).

Any increase in energy demand may tip the balance and result in a metabolic crisis as vital organs are deprived of fuel. Fatty acid oxidation disorders have been implicated as the cause of death in 5% to 8% of sudden unexpected death in infancy (Shekhawat et al, 2005).

Diagnostic Tests. Expanded newborn screening will identify the majority of fatty acid oxidation defects. Tests for MCAD include:
- Plasma acylcarnitine profile
- Enzyme assay
- Mutation analysis

Hypoglycemia or normoglycemia may be present during times of illness, and blood glucose monitoring is not a reliable measure of metabolic status in these children.

Complications. The most serious consequence of this group of disorders is the inability to use fatty acids for energy production and lack of ketone production (burned for energy) during times of fasting, which may result in death.

Management. Treatment varies and may include fasting avoidance, dietary restriction of long-chain fats, supplementing the diet with medium-chain fats, and carnitine supplementation to prevent secondary deficiency.

For individuals with MCAD, avoidance of fasting is the mainstay of treatment. Infants should not fast for longer than 4 hours for the first 4 months. For each month of age, 1 hour of fasting can be added up to a maximum of 10 to 12 hours. These guidelines do not apply during times of higher energy demand. If the child awakens during the night, this could indicate hypoglycemia and the need for a snack. Providers should maintain a low threshold for recommending intravenous glucose infusions during times of illness and fever when energy requirements increase (see Management of Metabolic Emergencies). Monitor carnitine level and supplement with oral carnitine 50 to 100 mg/kg/day in divided doses if free carnitine level is below the reference range.

Lysosomal Disorders

Lysosomal storage disorders (LSDs) are caused by an accumulation (storage) of glycoproteins, glycolipids, or glycosaminoglycans (MPS) within lysosomes and various tissues, which leads to the various clinical presentations and symptoms. Incidence for all LSD is 1:7700 live births (Raghuveer et al, 2006); the condition typically presents in later infancy to adulthood (Hoffmann & Mayatepek, 2005). Symptoms vary depending on the site of storage and the specific disorder and may include: hepatosplenomegaly, coarse facies, corneal clouding, mental retardation, thrombocytopenia, bone pain, neuralgia, abnormal liver function studies, respiratory problems, hydrocephalus, and cardiomyopathy. Enzymatic assay and/or mutation analysis are available for most disorders. Initial diagnostic testing for mucopolysaccharidosis consists of screening urinary glycosaminoglycans (urine MPS screen). Treatment varies from symptom management to ERT with varying degrees of success.

Dyslipidemia: Hypercholesterolemia and Hyperlipidemia

Description and Epidemiology. Dyslipidemias are disorders of lipoprotein metabolism, some of which lead to increased levels of total cholesterol (TC) and low-density lipoprotein cholesterol (LDL-C); a varied presentation of triglycerides (TG); and/or decreased levels of high-density lipoprotein cholesterol (HDL-C).

Dyslipidemias can be acquired (secondary) or genetic (primary). Secondary hyperlipidemias result from exogenous factors such as obesity, drugs (e.g., isotretinoin, oral contraceptives), and alcohol; endocrine or metabolic disorders (e.g., hypothyroidism, diabetes); storage disease (e.g., glycogen storage disease); obstructive liver disease (e.g., biliary atresia); and other causes such as anorexia nervosa.

Among primary dyslipidemia, familial hypercholesterolemia is most common. Familial hypercholesterolemia results from pathogenic mutation in the LDL-C receptor gene (most common) or the ApoB protein. These mutations compromise the receptor cells' ability to facilitate clearance of LDL cholesterol through the liver; as a result, LDL-C accumulates in the body. Triglycerides are usually normal. There are two types of familial hypercholesterolemia: heterozygous, which is common (1:500-1000), and homozygous, which is exceedingly rare (1:1,000,000). Homozygous hypercholesterolemia is characterized by extremely high LDL-C levels (e.g., 600 mg/dL or more) and a poor outcome without very aggressive early treatment (untreated, most individuals die by the second decade of life; even with treatment, atherosclerotic vascular disease is common by 30 years old [Tershakovec & Rader, 2004]).

Clinical Findings. Hyperlipidemia does not typically present as a clinical illness in children. There is, however, a clear relationship between high cholesterol in childhood and cardiac disease as an adult. Although not all children with dyslipidemia will have cardiovascular problems as adults, it is important to screen children at risk in order to identify those with hyperlipidemia and hypercholesterolemia and intervene in an effort to prevent problems from occurring. The Expert Panel on Blood Cholesterol Levels in Children and Adolescents of the National Cholesterol Education Program and the American Academy of Pediatrics Committee on Nutrition recommend that TC screening be done for children with parents who have a TC level greater than 240 mg/dL. Screening is recommended for children with incomplete or absent family history data and those with other risk factors related to cardiac disease (e.g., obesity, inactivity, diabetes, hypertension, cigarette smoking, low HDL-C) (Tershakovec & Rader, 2004). The National Institutes of Health (NIH) has published a childhood risk assessment and screening algorithm that includes the classification, education, and follow-up of patients based on LDL cholesterol levels (Figs. 25-4 and 25-5). A lipoprotein analysis should be done on children with a family history of premature atherosclerotic disease, and total cholesterol in others at risk or identified for screening.

History. Risk factors for hypercholesterolemia and hyperlipidemia found in the history include:
- Overweight or obesity (most predictive of dyslipidemia)
- Family history of hypercholesterolemia (e.g., parent with TC greater than 240 mg/dL)
- Family history of premature atherosclerotic disease (CHD before 55 years old in parents, grandparents, aunts, or uncles. Studies show, however, that 30% to 60% of children with elevated lipids are missed if a family history of CHD is used as the criterion for screening [Oregon Evidence-Based Practice Center, 2006]).
- Diabetes

Physical Examination. The child may have no clinical signs or symptoms or may have:
- Overweight or obesity; calculate BMI
- Hypertension
- Xanthomas (may be seen with familial hypercholesterolemia; tendon xanthomas in adolescents)

Diagnostic Tests. The clinical conditions of dyslipidemia can be determined by lipoprotein analysis (see Fig. 25-4 and Fig. 25-5). Precise genetic etiology is not needed for therapeutic decisions.

Management.

Lifestyle Changes. Dietary change has been the first step in treatment of children older than 2 years with hypercholesterolemia and, combined with other lifestyle changes, remains a mainstay of treatment—even if medications are added to the regimen. The American Heart Association revised their dietary guidelines in 2006, encouraging individuals to consider diet as only one part of a more general "lifestyle prescription for cardiovascular health," and emphasizing that a change in diet alone will not significantly change cardiovascular risks related to hypercholesterolemia (Box 25-12) (Lichtenstein et al, 2006). This approach, termed Therapeutic Lifestyle Changes (TLC), recognizes the importance of limiting total fat, saturated fatty acids, and cholesterol in the diet, but goes on to incorporate significant lifestyle changes (e.g., exercise, eliminating tobacco use, managing chronic illnesses effectively) as well.

Many issues arise with dietary changes in children (e.g., increasing dietary fiber may "fill up" the child and increase the risk of poor nutrient intake), so consultation with a pediatric dietitian is essential to ensure that children receive adequate nutrition.

Pharmacotherapy. Drug therapy should be considered in children 8 years or older who, after 6 to 12 months of diet therapy, continue to have a:
- LDL-C level greater than 190 mg/dL, OR
- LDL-C level greater than 160 mg/dL AND
  - Positive family history of premature CHD (before 55 years old) or
  - Two or more risk factors that continue despite efforts to control them (e.g., diabetes, smoking, hypertension) (Tershakovec & Rader, 2004)

First-line drugs for treatment of children with hypercholesterolemia are the bile acid sequestrants or "resins" (e.g., cholestyramine, colesevelam, colestipol). These drugs bind with bile acids, leading to increased GI excretion of bile acids. As a result, more bile acid must be synthesized. Hepatic cholesterol is used

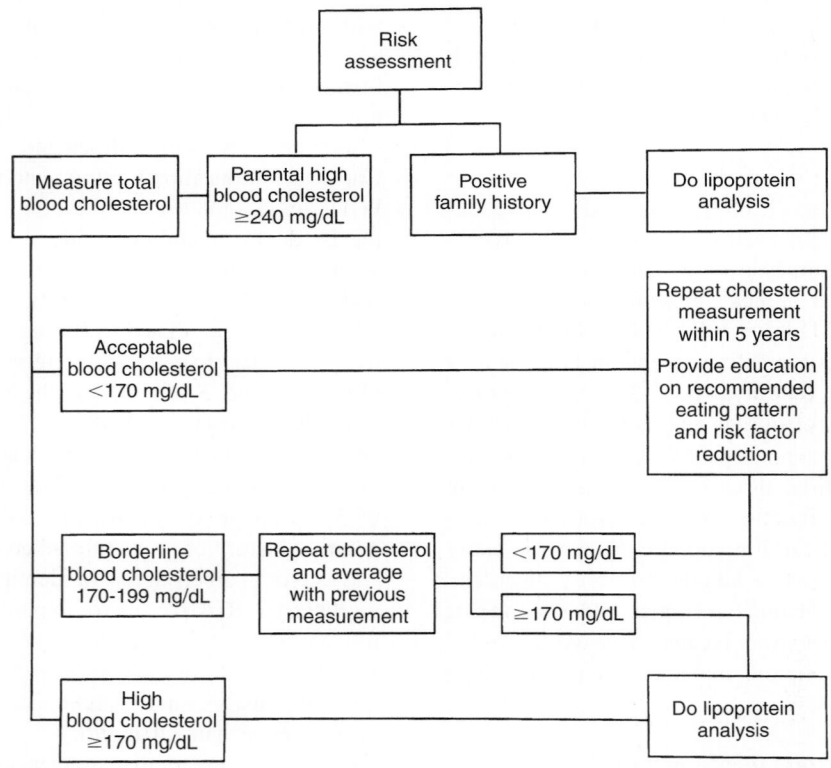

FIG. 25-4   Risk assessment of children based on high parental blood cholesterol or a positive family history of premature atherosclerotic disease. (Reprinted from National Cholesterol Education Program: *Report of the Expert Panel on Blood Cholesterol Levels in Children and Adolescents, National Heart, Lung, and Blood Institute,* US Department of Health and Human Services, PHS NIH Publication No. 91-2732, Washington, DC, 1991, US Government Printing Office.)

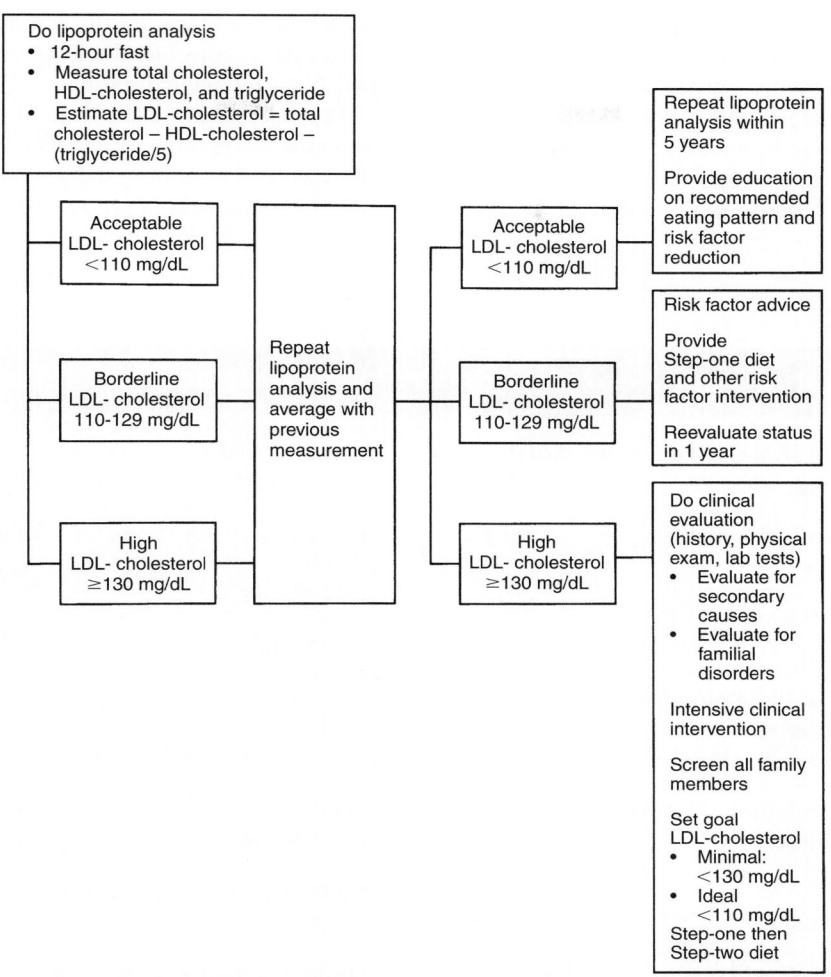

FIG. 25-5 Classification, education, and follow-up of patients based on LDL cholesterol level. (Reprinted from National Cholesterol Education Program: *Report of the Expert Panel on Blood Cholesterol Levels in Children and Adolescents, National Heart, Lung, and Blood Institute,* US Department of Health and Human Services, PHS NIH Publication No. 91-2732, Washington, DC, 1991, US Government Printing Office.)

BOX 25-12 **AHA 2006 Diet and Lifestyle Recommendations for Cardiovascular Disease Risk Reduction**

- Balance calorie intake and physical activity to achieve or maintain a healthy body weight; incorporate enough moderate physical activity to use at least 200 Kcal/day.*
- Consume a diet rich in vegetables and fruits.
- Choose whole-grain, high-fiber foods; 2 g/day of plant stanols and sterols† and 10-25 g/day soluble fiber.
- Consume fish, especially oily fish, at least twice a week.
- Limit intake of total fat to 25%-35% total calories; saturated fat to <7% of total calories, *trans* fat to <1% of total calories, and cholesterol to <200 mg/day by:
  - Choosing lean meats and vegetable alternatives
  - Selecting fat-free (skim), 1%-fat, and low-fat dairy products
  - Minimizing intake of partially hydrogenated fats (up to 10% of total calories in polyunsaturated fats; up to 20% of total calories in monounsaturated fats).
- Minimize your intake of beverages and foods with added sugars.
- Choose and prepare foods with little or no salt.
- If you consume alcohol, do so in moderation.
- When you eat food that is prepared outside of the home, follow the AHA Diet and Lifestyle Recommendations.
- Limit protein intake to approximately 15% of total calories.
- Limit carbohydrate intake to 50%-60% of total calories; mainly complex CHO.

*It is estimated that briskly walking 1 mile uses 100 Kcal of energy.
†Plant stanols and sterols occur naturally in small quantities in fruits, vegetables, nuts, seeds, cereals, legumes, and vegetable oils (particularly soybean oil); some foods (usually spreads or salad dressings) are FDA-approved fortified with stanols and sterols. To be beneficial, fortified foods must be low in saturated fat and cholesterol with no more than 13 g of total fat per serving.
From Lichtenstein AH et al: Diet and lifestyle recommendations revision 2006: a scientific statement from the American Heart Association Nutrition Committee, *Circulation* 114(1):82-96, 2006; American Heart Association: Step I, Step II, and TLC Diets. Available at *www.americanheart.org/presenter. jhtml?identifier=4764* (accessed March 23, 2007).

for this synthesis; the liver takes up circulating cholesterol for its use, and plasma LDL-C decreases. Resins are not well tolerated by many children and compliance is frequently a problem.

Use of HMG-CoA reductase inhibitors (statins) can be considered if the child has severe hypercholesterolemia or if there is a poor response to bile acid resins. The statins function by inhibiting the enzyme that synthesizes cholesterol. Recently,

as experience in children has accumulated, practitioners are often using statins initially after diet therapy has failed, skipping bile acid binding resins.

Because of the side effects of drugs and the uncertainty about their long-term use in the pediatric population, however, children who need drug therapy should be referred to a specialized pediatric lipid center for treatment.

RESOURCE BOX

National Organizations and Resources for Problems of Endocrine and Metabolic Disease

American Association of Diabetes Educators (AADE)
www.diabeteseducator.org

American College of Medical Genetics
www.acmg.net

American Dietetic Association
www.eatright.org

Barbara Davis Center for Childhood Diabetes
www.uchsc.edu/misc/diabetes
University of Colorado Health Sciences Center

Children's Diabetes Foundation at Denver
www.childrensdiabetesfdn.com

Children with Diabetes
www.childrenwithdiabetes.com

Dwarfism/Short Stature Resources
www.kumc.edu/gec/support/dwarfism.html
University of Kansas Medical Center

The Endocrine Society
www.endo-society.org

Human Growth Foundation
www.hgfound.org

Juvenile Diabetes Research Foundation International (JDRF)
www.jdrf.org

Little People of America
www.lpaonline.org

Magic Foundation
www.magicfoundation.org

MedicAlert
www.medicalert.org

Pediatric Endocrinology Nursing Society (PENS)
www.pens.org

Pituitary Network Association
www.pituitary.org

Thyroid Foundation of America
www.allthyroid.org

☑ DISCUSSION FORUM

1. The parent of a 3-week-old infant was just notified that the newborn screen on her infant was positive for hypothyroidism. She asks you, her primary care provider, why some of her baby's results were elevated (TSH) and some were low (T_3). How will you respond to her questions? What will be your management of this infant? Be sure to include pharmacologic and nonpharmacologic interventions.

2. Explain the work-up and management for a 13-year-old female with growth failure over the last 3 years accompanied by pubertal-onset delay. What are your most likely differential diagnoses? How would your answer change if the child were an 8-year-old with growth failure?

3. You do a wellness examination on an 8-year-old female who has had a growth spurt of 4 inches in the last year and who is at Tanner III breast stage and Tanner II pubic hair. Her neurologic examination is normal. How will you manage this child? Be sure to include plans for pharmacologic

management, consultation and/or referral, and anticipatory guidance.

4. You are asked by a local community group to talk about childhood diabetes. Prepare a discussion that includes the differences between type 1 and type 2 diabetes, specifically looking at pathologic conditions, epidemiology, risk factors, and clinical management.

5. You see a 2-month-old in your office for a wellness visit. Her weight gain was 7 oz/week for the first 4 weeks, but it has decreased to 4 oz/week. Her parents report she is increasingly irritable, and her suck is "not as strong as it used to be." Her bowel movements are less frequent and semiformed. Her abdominal girth has increased over her last visit. You note a high-pitched cry and generalized hypotonia and suspect galactosemia. What diagnostic testing is needed at this time? How will you manage this infant? Be sure to include anticipatory guidance, pharmacologic interventions, and guidelines for consultation and/or referral.

REFERENCES

Alemzadeh R, Wyatt DT: Diabetes mellitus in children. In Behrman RE, Kliegman RM, Jenson HB, editors: *Nelson textbook of pediatrics,* ed 17, Philadelphia, 2004, WB Saunders.

American Academy of Pediatrics (AAP) et al: Update of newborn screening and therapy for congenital hypothyroidism, *Pediatrics* 117(6):2290-2303, 2006.

American Academy of Pediatrics (AAP): Health supervision for children with Down syndrome (RE0016), *Pediatrics* 107(2):442-449, 2001.

American Diabetes Association (ADA): Nutrition recommendations and interventions for diabetes: a position statement of the American Diabetes Association, *Diabetes Care* 30:S48-S65, 2007.

American Diabetes Association (ADA): Standards of medical care in diabetes-2006, *Diabetes Care* 29(Suppl 1):S4-42, 2006.

American Diabetes Association (ADA): Type 2 diabetes in children and adolescents, *Diabetes Care* 23(3):381-389, 2000.

American Heart Association: *Step I, Step II and TLC Diets.* Available at *www.americanheart.org/presenter.jhtml?identifier=4764* (accessed Mar 23, 2007).

American Medical Association (AMA): *ICD-9-CM: International classification of diseases,* ed 6, Los Angeles, 2004, Practice Management Information Corp.

Badaru A, Wilson DM: Alternatives to growth hormone stimulation testing in children, *Trends Endocrinol Metab* 15(6):252-258, 2004.

Bloomgarden ZT: Type 2 diabetes in the young: the evolving epidemic, *Diabetes Care* 27(4):998-1010, 2004.

Botkin JR et al: Newborn screening technology: proceed with caution, *Pediatrics* 117(5):1793-1799, 2006.

Centers for Disease Control and Prevention: Diabetes projects: children and diabetes, *CDC's Diabetes Program.* Available at *www.cdc.gov/diabetes/projects/cda2.htm* (accessed Mar 17, 2007).

Chia D, Boston B: Childhood obesity and metabolic syndrome, *Adv Pediatr* 53:23-53, 2006.

Cochrane Collaboration: Home-based management of children at onset of diabetes may be as safe as hospital-based management, *The Cochrane Database of Systematic Reviews,* Issue 1, 2007, John Wiley and Sons, Ltd.

Conte FA, Grumbach MM: Diagnosis and management of ambiguous external genitalia, *The Endocrinologist* 13(3):260-268, 2003.

Cuttler L: Growth hormone treatment. In Finberg L, Kleinman RE, editors: *Saunders manual of pediatric practice,* ed 2, Philadelphia, 2002, WB Saunders.

Dietz WH, Robinson TN: Clinical practice. Overweight children and adolescents, *N Engl J Med* 352(20):2100-2109, 2005.

Foley TP: Hypothyroidism, *Pediatr Rev* 25(3):94-100, 2004.

Fulkerson JA et al: Weight-related attitudes and behaviors of adolescent boys and girls who are encouraged to diet by their mothers, *Int J Obes Relat Metab Disord* 26:1579-1587, 2002.

Greene CL, Thomas JA, Goodman SI: Inborn errors of metabolism. In Hay WH et al: *Current pediatric diagnosis & treatment,* ed 17, New York, 2005, McGraw-Hill Companies.

Greiner MV, Kerrigan JR: Puberty: timing is everything, *Pediatr Ann* 35(12):916-922, 2006.

Gunn VL, Nechyba C: *The Harriet Lane handbook: a manual for pediatric house officers,* ed 16, Baltimore, 2002, Johns Hopkins Hospital Children's Medical and Surgical Center.

Guthrie R, Susi A: A simple phenylalanine method for detecting phenylketonuria in large populations of newborn infants, *Pediatrics* 32(3):338-343, 1963.

Herman-Giddens ME et al: Secondary sexual characteristics and menses in young girls seen in office practice: a study from the Pediatric Research in Office Settings network, *Pediatrics* 99(4):505-512, 1997.

Hoffmann B, Mayatepek E: Neurological manifestations in lysosomal storage disorders—from pathology to first therapeutic possibilities, *Neuropediatrics* 36(5):285-289, 2005.

Hughes IA et al: Consensus statement on management of intersex disorders, *Arch Dis Child* 91(7):554-563, 2006.

Ize-Ludlow D, Sperling MA: The classification of diabetes mellitus: a conceptual framework, *Pediatr Clin North Am* 52(6):1533-1552, 2005.

Jones PM, Bennett MJ: The changing face of newborn screening: diagnosis of inborn errors of metabolism by tandem mass spectrometry, *Clin Chim Acta* 324(1-2):121-128, 2002.

Kaplowitz PB, Oberfield SE: Reexamination of the age limit for defining when puberty is precocious in girls in the United States: implications for evaluation and treatment. Drug and Therapeutics and Executive Committees of the Lawson Wilkins Pediatric Endocrine Society, *Pediatrics* 104(4 Pt 1):936-941, 1999.

Kaufman FR: Type 2 diabetes in children and youth, *Endocrinol Metab Clin North Am* 34(3):659-676, 2005.

LaFranchi S, Hanna CE: The thyroid gland and its disorders. In Kappy MS, Allen DB, Geffner ME, editors: *Principles and practice of pediatric endocrinology,* Springfield, IL, 2005, Charles C Thomas Ltd.

Lanpher B, Brunetti-Pierri N, Lee B: Inborn errors of metabolism: the flux from Mendelian to complex diseases, *Nat Rev Genet* 7(6):449-460, 2006.

Larsen PR et al, editors: *Williams textbook of endocrinology,* ed 10, Philadelphia, 2003, WB Saunders.

Lichtenstein AH et al: Diet and lifestyle recommendations revision 2006: a scientific statement from the American Heart Association Nutrition Committee, *Circulation* 114(1):82-96, 2006.

Liese AD et al: The burden of diabetes mellitus among US youth: prevalence estimates from the SEARCH for Diabetes in Youth Study, *Pediatrics* 118(4):1510-1518, 2006.

MacLaughlin DT, Donahoe PK: Sex determination and differentiation, *N Engl J Med* 350(4):367-378, 2004 [erratum appears in *N Engl J Med* 351(3):306, 2004].

Nathan BM, Palmert MR: Regulation and disorders of pubertal timing, *Endocrinol Metab Clin North Am* 34(3):617-641, 2005.

National Institute of Diabetes and Digestive and Kidney Diseases (NIDDK): *National diabetes fact sheet: general information and national estimates on diabetes in the United States, 2005,* National Institute of Health publication 06-3892. Available at *www.diabetes.niddk.nih.gov/dm/pubs/statistics* (accessed Mar 17, 2007).

National Newborn Screening & Genetics Resource Center: *Current newborn screening (NBS) conditions-US by state,* 2007. Available at *http://genes-r-us.uthscsa.edu* (accessed Mar 13, 2007).

Oregon Evidence-Based Practice Center: *Screening for dyslipidemia in children and adolescents: systematic evidence review for the U.S. Preventive Services Task Force,* Rockville, MD, 2006, Agency for Healthcare Research and Quality, U.S. Department of Health and Human Services.

Raghuveer TS, Garg U, Graf WD: Inborn errors of metabolism in infancy and early childhood: an update, *Am Fam Physician* 73(11):1981-1990, 2006.

Ritzen EM: Early puberty: what is normal and when is treatment indicated? *Horm Res* 60(Suppl 3):31-34, 2003.

Saenger P et al: Recommendations for the diagnosis and management of Turner syndrome, *J Clin Endocrinol Metab* 86(7):3061-3069, 2001.

Shekhawat PS, Matern D, Strauss AW: Fetal fatty acid oxidation disorders, their effect on maternal health and neonatal outcome: impact of expanded newborn screening on their diagnosis and management, *Pediatr Res* 57(5 Pt 2):78R-86R, 2005.

Stochholm K et al: Incidence of GH deficiency-a nationwide study, *Eur J Endocrinol* 155(1):61-71, 2006.

Sun SS et al: Is sexual maturity occurring earlier among U.S. children? *J Adolesc Health* 37(5):345-355, 2005.

Sun SS et al: National estimates of the timing of sexual maturation and racial differences among US children, *Pediatrics* 113(1 Pt 1):177-178, 2002.

Svoren BM, Laffel LMB: Diabetes mellitus in children and adolescents. In Burg FD et al: *Current pediatric therapy,* ed 18, Philadelphia, 2006, Saunders Elsevier.

Tershakovec AM, Rader DJ: Disorders of lipoprotein metabolism and transport. In Behrman RE, Kliegman RM, Jenson HB, editors: *Nelson textbook of pediatrics,* ed 17, Philadelphia, 2004, WB Saunders.

Venditti CP, Stanley CA: Disorders of mitochondrial fatty acid oxidation. In Behrman RE, Kliegman RM, Jenson HB, editors: *Nelson textbook of pediatrics,* ed 17, Philadelphia, 2004, WB Saunders.

Wilson TA et al: Update of guidelines for the use of growth hormone in children: the Lawson Wilkins Pediatric Endocrinology Society Drug and Therapeutics Committee, *J Pediatr* 143(4):415-421, 2003.

CHAPTER 26

Hematologic Disorders

Martha K. Swartz

Blood is a major homeostatic force of the body. Essential body functions carried out by blood include the transfer of respiratory gases, hemostasis, phagocytosis, and the provision of cellular and humoral agents to fight infection. Abnormalities of blood cells are seen in various disease states and alterations in nutrition. Therefore, diagnostic hematologic studies are essential components of pediatric practice. For the pediatric provider, the types of hematologic disorders encountered in the clinical setting range from common nutritional deficiencies in which treatment is straightforward to those rare diseases with a genetic or chronic component that necessitate extensive referral and a multidisciplinary approach. In pediatrics, particularly, early diagnosis of blood disorders is important to ensure the best possible prognosis.

■ ANATOMY AND PHYSIOLOGY

Blood is made up of a cellular component with specialized functions and a fluid component called plasma. The cellular component consists of red blood cells (RBCs), or erythrocytes; white blood cells (WBCs), or leukocytes; and platelets, or thrombocytes. Leukocytes are further differentiated into granulocytes, monocytes, and lymphocytes. Plasma is a clear yellow fluid in which proteins (primarily albumins, globulins, and fibrinogen) are the major solutes. These plasma proteins maintain intravascular volume, contribute to the coagulation of blood, and are important in acid-base balance.

Blood formation in the human embryo initially takes place in the yolk sac during the first several weeks of gestation. In the second trimester, blood is formed primarily in the liver, spleen, and lymph nodes. During the last half of gestation, hematopoiesis shifts from the fetal liver and spleen to the bone marrow where, by birth, most blood formation takes place. Bone marrow produces erythrocytes, granulocytes, monocytes, and platelets and provides lymphocytes and lymphocytic precursors to the spleen, lymph nodes, and other lymphatic tissues.

ERYTHROCYTES

Production of RBCs is regulated by the specific hormone erythropoietin, produced primarily by renal glomerular epithelial cells. In response to a decrease in the number of circulating RBCs or a decrease in the PaO_2 of arterial blood, erythropoietin stimulates the bone marrow to convert certain stem cells to proerythroblasts. Substances essential for RBC formation include iron, vitamin B_{12}, folic acid, amino acids, and other nutrients. The RBC matures through the following stages: proerythroblast, erythroblast, normoblast, reticulocyte, and erythrocyte.

As cellular differentiation occurs, the nucleus present in the early forms of the cell is extruded and replaced by hemoglobin (Hgb). The RBC assumes its characteristic nonnucleated biconcave disk shape, which is easily distorted, thereby enabling it to pass through small capillaries and sinuses without being destroyed. The large surface-to-volume ratio also facilitates rapid gas exchange.

The youngest red cells are the reticulocytes; after release from the bone marrow, they stay in circulation for about 1 day before becoming mature RBCs. The reticulocyte count is about 4% to 6% for the first 3 days of life, which reflects the relatively greater amount of erythropoiesis that occurs in the fetus. This increased reticulocyte count is followed by a sudden drop to the normal range of 0.5% to 1.5% (see Appendix C). A mature RBC lasts about 120 days before it is destroyed through phagocytosis in the spleen, liver, or bone marrow.

Hemoglobin

Hemoglobin is the oxygen-carrying protein molecule in the RBC. Each Hgb molecule is made up of two pairs of polypeptide chains (the globin portion) attached to heme groups, which are large disks containing iron and porphyrin, a nitrogen-containing organic compound. Various forms of Hgb are found in the embryo, fetus, and adult, depending on changes in globin chain synthesis. At birth, approximately 70% of Hgb is made up of fetal hemoglobin (Hgb F). By 12 months old, 95% of Hgb consists of the normal adult Hgb molecules (Hgb A), which are composed of two α- and two ß-polypeptide chains attached to four heme groups. Hgb F remains present at levels of less than 2%. Hgb A_2, another type of normal Hgb composed of two α- and two ß-globin chains, makes up about 2.5% of the total Hgb.

Each of the four iron atoms in the Hgb molecule combines reversibly with an atom of oxygen to form oxyhemoglobin. This reaction occurs when the oxygen concentration is relatively high, as in the lungs, where oxygen crosses the alveolocapillary membrane and saturates about 96% of the Hgb. This percentage is the arterial oxygen saturation (SaO_2), and it is measured through pulse oximetry or arterial blood gas determination. When the oxygen concentration is lower, as in the tissues, oxygen is released to meet cellular needs.

The level of Hgb in a newborn ranges from 15 to 22 g/dL and then drops to its lowest point at 3 to 6 months old, which is a physiologic anemia caused by the shortened survival of fetal RBCs and the rapid expansion of blood volume during this period. A decrease in Hgb can also develop secondary to a decrease in RBC production, blood loss, or increased RBC destruction. Because of these processes, transport of oxygen to the tissues is adversely affected, and the individual can become clinically anemic.

There are also altered states of Hgb, such as occurs with methemoglobin. In this condition, the ferrous form of iron is oxidized to the ferric state, and the heme moiety can not carry oxygen. If reduced Hgb levels exceed 5 g/dL, serious tissue hypoxia and cyanosis can occur. Methemoglobinemia can be congenital or caused by exposure to certain drugs and chemicals.

Antigenic Properties of Red Blood Cells

Red cells are classified into different types according to the presence of antigens on the cell membrane. The most common antigens are A, B, and Rh. A person inherits either A or B antigen (type A or B blood), both antigens (type AB blood, which is the universal recipient), or neither antigen (type O blood, which is the universal donor). Of the six types of Rh factors, the most common is D, which accounts for the Rh designation. In the U.S., 85% of whites and 95% of blacks are Rh+ (Guyton & Hall, 2006). Clinically, these distinctions become important when blood transfusions are necessary or in assessment for maternal-fetal blood incompatibilities.

LEUKOCYTES

Leukocytes, or WBCs, are larger and fewer in number than erythrocytes. Normally, about 5000 to 10,000 leukocytes are contained in a microliter of blood. The primary function of WBCs is protection of the body from invasion by foreign organisms and distribution of antibodies and other factors of the immune response.

Five distinct types of WBCs can be grouped into two broad classifications: granulocytes (also known as polymorpho-nuclear leukocytes [PMNs], or "polys") and agranulocytes (Table 26-1). Granulocytes contain large granules and horse-shoe-shaped nuclei that become segmented and are connected by thin strands (Table 26-2). With Wright stain, the cytoplasm stains blue or pink. Granulocytes are further divided into neutrophils; eosinophils, which absorb the acid dye eosin; and basophils, which absorb a basic dye. The agranulocytes include lymphocytes (also known as immunocytes) and monocytes.

Granular Leukocytes

In children, granulocytes make up 30% to 60% of all WBCs. They mature in the bone marrow through the following stages: stem cells, myeloblasts, promyelocytes, myelocytes, metamyelocytes, band forms, and mature segmented neutrophils. This maturational process takes approximately 6 to 11 days. Once a neutrophil is released into the bloodstream, it circulates for about 6 to 9 hours before entering the tissues, where the major function of PMNs is phagocytosis of harmful particles and cells, particularly bacterial organisms.

A frequency distribution of the types of WBCs is obtained by the differential count, and quantitative alterations within the categories are important diagnostically (see Table 26-1).

A relative increase in the number of circulating immature neutrophils (band forms, metamyelocytes, and myelocytes) is known as a "shift to the left," a term derived from how the differential count used to be tabulated on written forms. This phenomenon is indicative of an inflammatory process or the body's immunologic response to an acute bacterial infection.

Basophils and eosinophils are also important in the body's inflammatory and allergic responses. Basophils, which account for less than 1% of circulating leukocytes, release heparin and histamine into the bloodstream during systemic allergic reactions. They contain receptor sites for immunoglobulin E (IgE), levels of which are elevated in people with allergies; they also prevent clot formation in the microcirculation. Eosinophils are found in the mucosa of the gastrointestinal tract and in the lungs. They are weakly phagocytic. Eosinophilia is also associated with allergic reactions, in addition to parasitic infections and drug reactions.

Monocytes

Monocytes, which contain a large lobulated nucleus, are relatively immature cells that circulate for about 8 hours before migrating to tissues where they assume their mature form as macrophages. Like granulocytes, which are the first line of defense against microbe invasion, their primary function is phagocytosis of bacteria and cellular debris. Fixed and mobile macrophages are located primarily in the liver, spleen, lymph nodes, and gastrointestinal tract and make up the mononuclear phagocyte system.

Lymphocytes

Lymphocytes (or immunocytes), although not phagocytic, protect the body against specific antigens. They originate in the bone marrow, but differentiate in lymphoid tissues, such as the spleen, liver, thymus, lymph nodes, and intestines. Thymus-dependent lymphocytes, or T cells, are part of the cell-mediated immune response in which cytotoxic agents and macrophages are synthesized. B-cell lymphocytes are precursors of the humoral immune response whereby the cells are transformed into plasma cells that release immunoglobulins or antibodies into the bloodstream.

PLATELET CELLS AND COAGULATION FACTORS

The smallest cellular components in blood are the platelets, or thrombocytes, which are essential to hemostasis and clot formation. Circulating platelets are fragments of megakaryocytes, which are precursor cells that form in the bone marrow. The normal platelet count ranges from 150,000 to 300,000 cells/mm^3.

When a blood vessel is injured (or in the presence of intrinsic damage to the blood), platelets adhere to the inner surface of the vessel and form a hemostatic plug. As the platelets are degraded, a series of at least thirteen clotting factors or proteolytic enzymes are released that bring about the clotting process in a cascading sequence of successive reactions (Fig. 26-1).

The basic reactions that occur in the sequential process of blood coagulation are as follows: As factor X is activated, prothrombin (factor II) is converted to thrombin, which then

TABLE 26-1   Hematologic Values and Normal Leukocyte Differential Count During Infancy and Childhood

Hematologic Values

Age	Hemoglobin (g/dL) Mean	Range	Hematocrit (%) Mean	Range	Reticulocytes (%) Mean	MCV (fL) Lowest	Leukocytes (WBC/mm³) Mean	Range	Neutrophils (%) Mean	Range	Lymphocytes (%) Mean*	Eosinophils (%) Mean
Cord blood	16.8	13.7-20.1	55	45-65	5	110	18,000	(9000-30,000)	61	(40-80)	31	2
2 weeks	16.5	13-20	50	42-66	1		12,000	(5000-21,000)	40		63	3
3 months	12	9.5-14.5	36	31-41	1		12,000	(6000-18,000)	30		48	2
6 months-6 years	12	10.5-14	37	33-42	1	70-74	10,000	(6000-18,000)	45		48	2
7-12 years	13	11-16	38	34-40	1	76-80	8000	(4500-13,500)	55		38	2
Adult												
Female	14	12-16	42	37-47	1.6	80	7500	(5000-10,000)	55	(35-70)	35	3
Male	16	14-18	47	42-52		80						

Normal Leukocyte Differential Count

Age	Granulocytes				Agranulocytes	
	Segmented Neutrophils (%)	Band Neutrophils (%)	Eosinophils (%)	Basophils (%)	Lymphocytes (%)	Monocytes (%)
Birth	47 ± 15	14.1 ± 4	2.2	0.6	31 ± 5	5.8
6 months	23	8.8	2.5	0.4	61	4.8
12 months	23	8.1	2.6	0.4	61	4.8
2 years	25	8	2.6	0.5	59	5
4 years	34 ± 11	8 ± 3	2.8	0.6	50 ± 15	5
6 years	43	8	2.7	0.6	42	4.7
8 years	45	8	2.4	0.6	39	4.2
10 years	46 ± 15	8 ± 3	2.4	0.5	38 ± 10	4.3
12 years	47	8	2.5	0.5	38	4.4

Absolute neutrophil count (ANC) = WBC × (% seg + band)

*Relatively wide range.

FL, Femtoliters; *MCV,* mean corpuscular volume; *WBC,* white blood cell.

Data from Behrman R et al, editors: *Nelson textbook of pediatrics,* ed 17, Philadelphia, 2004, WB Saunders, p 1605 (Ch. 439: The Anemias).

Wallach J: *Interpretation of diagnostic tests,* ed 8, Philadelphia, 2006, Lippincott Williams & Wilkins.

TABLE 26-2 Overview of Leukocytes

Cell Type	Characteristics	Diagram
Granulocytes (polymorphonuclear leukocytes, polys)		
Neutrophils	Have small, fine, light pink or lilac acidophilic granules when stained and a segmented, irregularly lobed, purple nucleus.	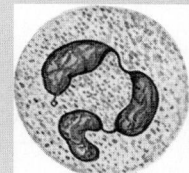
Eosinophils	Have large round granules that contain red-staining basic mucopolysaccharides and multilobed purple-blue nuclei.	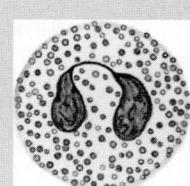
Basophils	Coarse blue granules conceal the segmented nucleus. Granules contain histamine, heparin, and acid mucopolysaccharides.	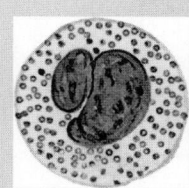
Agranulocytes		
Lymphocytes	Small cell with a large, round, deep-staining, single-lobed nucleus and very little cytoplasm. The cytoplasm is slightly basophilic and stains pale blue.	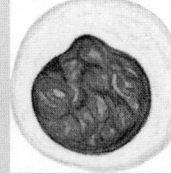
Monocytes	Large cell with a prominent, multishaped nucleus that sometimes is kidney shaped. Chromatin in the nucleus looks like lace, with small particles linked together like strands. The gray-blue cytoplasm is filled with many fine lysozymes that stain pink with Wright stain.	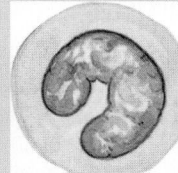

From Bullock B, Henze R: Hematology: adaptations and alterations in function. In Bullock B, editor: *Focus on pathophysiology,* Philadelphia, 2000, Lippincott Williams & Wilkins, p 359; McCance K, Huether S: *Pathophysiology: the biologic basis for disease in adults and children,* ed 5, St Louis, 2006, Mosby.

catalyzes the conversion of fibrinogen (factor I) to fibrin (Table 26-3). Fibrin provides the matrix in which blood cells aggregate to form a clot. A deficiency of any of the proteins in the pathway leads to a clotting disorder. In particular, if factor VIII is deficient (as in classic hemophilia A) or the number of platelets is inadequate (thrombocytopenia), activation of factor X is impaired.

■ PATHOPHYSIOLOGY

Hematologic problems are generally classified as disorders of RBC function, WBC function, and platelet and coagulation function. These three broad categories are further divided into disorders of blood cell production, maturation, or destruction. Knowledge of these pathophysiologic classifications gives the pediatric provider a rationale for routine screening and useful algorithms to guide further clinical investigation.

CLASSIFICATION OF THE ANEMIAS

Anemia is generally defined as a reduction in blood Hgb concentration or a decrease in red cell mass below the normal range. The reduction in the amount of circulating Hgb also causes a decrease in the oxygen-carrying potential of the RBC. Morphologically (according to RBC size, shape, and color), anemias are described as hypochromic, microcytic; as macrocytic; or as normochromic, normocytic. This approach is a useful method for ruling out particular causes of anemia when trying to determine the underlying etiology (Table 26-4). In toddlers and young children, approximately 90% of cases of anemia are accounted for by iron deficiency, lead poisoning, infections, or hemoglobinopathy.

Anemias that are caused by inadequate production include acquired and constitutional aplastic anemia, red cell aplasia, and transient erythroblastosis of childhood (TEC). Maturational anemias are caused by nutritional disturbances, such as iron deficiency, lead poisoning, and deficiencies in folic acid and vitamin B_{12}. Anemias are also a common occurrence in chronic illnesses in which either red cell survival time is decreased or the bone marrow response or transport of iron is impaired. Such conditions include chronic inflammatory illnesses, chronic infections, renal and liver disease, endocrine disorders, and malignant neoplastic diseases.

Anemias that result from increased cell destruction are hemolytic anemias and are caused by defects in the red cell membrane, hereditary hemoglobinopathies (as in sickle cell anemia), and congenital enzyme defects. These syndromes also include hereditary spherocytosis (HS) and glucose-6-phosphate dehydrogenase (G6PD) deficiency.

WHITE BLOOD CELL DYSFUNCTION

The WBC count and differential are useful diagnostic guides in the management of a variety of childhood illnesses. The normal range of granulocyte and lymphocyte counts varies throughout childhood (see Table 26-1). Leukocytosis is

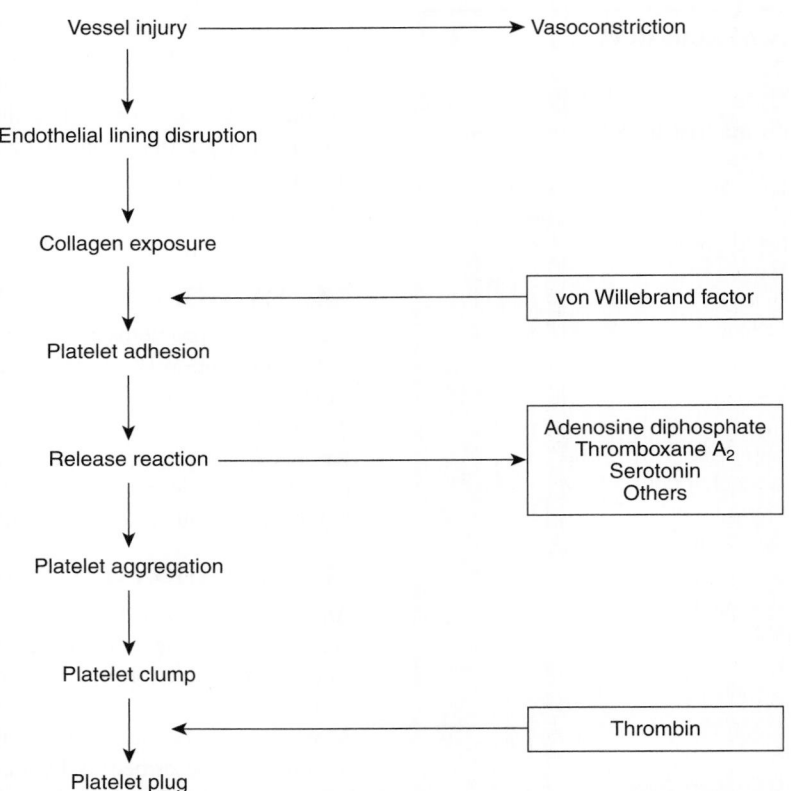

TABLE 26-3	Blood Coagulation Factors
Factor (International Nomenclature)	**Common Synonyms**
I	Fibrinogen
II	Prothrombin*
III	Tissue thromboplastin, thrombokinase
V	Proaccelerin, labile factor, accelerator globulin
VII	Proconvertin,* stable factor
VIII	Antihemophilic globulin (AHG), antihemophilic factor (AHF), antihemophilic factor A
IX	Plasma thromboplastin component (PTC), Christmas factor,* antihemophilic factor B
X	Stuart-Prower factor, Stuart factor*
XI	Plasma thromboplastin antecedent (PTA), antihemophilic factor C
XII	Hageman factor, contact factor, antihemophilic factor
XIII	Fibrin-stabilizing factor (FSF), plasma transglutaminase
Kininogen	Fitzgerald factor
Prekallikrein	Fletcher factor

*Vitamin K dependent.

an increase in the number of circulating leukocytes, with a neutrophilic response to bacterial and viral infections. A relative increase in the number of circulating immature neutrophils ("shift to the left") is a defensive mechanism in response to an inflammatory process or acute bacterial infection.

Alterations of Granulocytes

Neutropenia is defined as a decrease in the number of neutrophils and bands (the absolute neutrophil count or ANC) in the peripheral blood to less than 1500 cells/mm^3 for children older than 1 year and to below 1000 cells/mm^3 in infants older than 2 months (Sulis et al, 2006). It is classified as mild (ANC of 1000 to 1500 cells/mm^3), moderate (ANC of 500 to 1000 cells/mm^3), or severe (ANC less than 500 cells/mm^3). Neutropenia results from decreased cellular production (as in various hematologic diseases, infections, drug-induced states, and nutritional deficiencies), increased peripheral destruction (as in autoimmune disorders), or peripheral pooling (as in bacterial infections, hemodialysis, and cardiopulmonary bypass). Most cases of neutropenia are discovered during evaluation of the WBC count in a child with an acute febrile illness, and the most common infectious causes are hepatitis A and B, respiratory syncytial virus, influenza A and B, Epstein-Barr virus, and cytomegalovirus. General

TABLE 26-4   **Acute Anemia in Childhood and Adolescence**

Classification	History	Physical Findings	Screening Tests	Diagnostic Tests	Treatment
I. Microcytic					
Iron deficiency anemia	Infant and toddler Excessive cow's milk ingestion Poor solid food intake	Waxy, sallow appearance of skin	Hgb: 8-11 g/dL (moderate) <7 g/dL (severe) MCV: <60 fL Retic: ↓ to sl ↑	Serum Fe: ↓ TIBC: ↑ % Saturation: ↓	Ferrous sulfate, 4-6 mg/kg/day of elemental iron Discontinue cow's milk Limit formula to <24 oz/day and encourage solid food
Homozygous thalassemia (Cooley anemia)	Infant and toddler Growth failure Ethnic background consistent	Hepatosplenomegaly Frontal bossing	MCV: 50-60 fL	Hgb: var ↓	Hypertransfusion program; chelation therapy if iron overload, hematopoietic stem cell transplantation
II. Macrocytic					
Diamond-Blackfan anemia Megaloblastic anemia	(See III) Normocytic Variable, depending on etiology	Variable, depending on etiology	Hgb: var ↓ MCV: ↑ Retic: ↓ Platelets and WBC: ↓ Hypersegmented polys	Bone marrow: megaloblastic Vitamin B$_{12}$ level: nl to ↓ Folate Others	Variable, depending on etiology (e.g., folic acid, vitamin B$_{12}$ transfusion)
III. Normocytic **A. Production Defect**					
Diamond-Blackfan anemia	Age: 65% <6 mo old; 90% <1 yr old Insidious onset	25% with physical abnormalities	Hgb: <8 g/dL MCV: ↑ in 30% (100% after treatment) Retic: <1%	Bone marrow: erythroid hypoplasia and lymphocytosis Hgb F: ↓ RBCi antigen: ↑	Prednisone: 2-5 mg/kg/day
Transient erythroblastopenia of childhood	1 to 3 yr old Viral illness in preceding 3 mo	None	Hgb: 3-9 g/dL MCV: normal Retic: <1%	Bone marrow: erythroid hypoplasia	Supportive
Aplastic anemia	Bleeding Infection	Petechiae, purpura Infection Multiple anomalies possible with Fanconi anemia	Hgb: var ↓ MCV: ↑ in Fanconi anemia Retic: ↓ Platelets and WBC: ↓	Bone marrow: hypoplasia of all hematopoietic elements	Variable
B. Hemolytic					
Autoimmune hemolytic anemia	Jaundice Gastrointestinal symptoms Dark, red urine	Icterus Hepatosplenomegaly	Hgb: var ↓ Retic: ↑ (occ ↓) Smear: microspherocytes	Direct Coombs' test: positive	Corticosteroids: prednisone or intravenous equivalent: 2-6 mg/kg/day Transfusion indicated
Hemolytic-uremic syndrome	Infant and toddler Viral prodrome Gastrointestinal bleeding in 20% Sudden pallor, purpura CNS symptoms	Purpura Hypotension CNS abnormalities	Hgb: 7-8 g/dL Retic: ↑ Platelets: ↓ Smear: microangiopathy	None Renal tests: failure	Supportive: early dialysis ? Plasma infusion/exchange ? Antiplatelet drugs

Continued

TABLE 26-4	Acute Anemia in Childhood and Adolescence—Cont'd					
Classification	**History**	**Physical Findings**	**Screening Tests**	**Diagnostic Tests**	**Treatment**	
C. Blood loss						
Splenic sequestration crisis of sickle cell (SS) disease (internal blood loss)	SS disease: 5 mo to 2 yr old Hgb SC or S-thalassemia: all ages Sudden weakness, dyspnea, abdominal distention Shock	Hypotension Massive splenomegaly	Hgb: <4 g/dL Retic: ↑ Smear: sickle cells	None	Plasma expanders: whole or reconstituted blood	

CNS, Central nervous system; *Fe*, iron; *Hgb*, hemoglobin; *MCV*, mean corpuscular volume; *mo*, months; *nl*, normal; *occ*, occasionally; *polys*, polymorphonuclear leukocytes; *RBCi*, red blood cell i antigen; *Retic*, reticulocytes; *sl*, slightly; *TIBC*, total iron-binding capacity; *var*, variably; *WBC*, white blood cell count; *yr*, year(s).
Adapted from Burg F et al, editors: *Current pediatric therapy*, ed 18, Philadelphia, 2006, WB Saunders.

management of neutropenic patients includes careful identification and prompt treatment of any suspected or proven infections.

Neutropenia is frequently seen in preterm infants and those with intrauterine growth restriction. Because the neutrophil storage pool in newborn infants is only 20% to 30% of that of adults, it is easily depleted under stressful conditions, such as infection with resultant sepsis (Stoll, 2004). Isoimmune neonatal neutropenia is a transient process resulting from transplacental transfer of maternal antibodies to fetal neutrophil antigens (Fuleihan, 2006).

The largest group of neutropenic patients includes children who are receiving chemotherapy and are then at risk for developing severe, life-threatening bacterial infections depending on the degree and duration of neutropenia. Despite improvements in supportive care and treatment with granulocyte colony-stimulating factor (G-CSF), bacterial and fungal infections remain a major cause for morbidity and mortality in these patients (Sulis et al, 2006).

Qualitative abnormalities of granulocytes are usually related to defects of phagocytosis. Although individually rare, these defects may be genetic or acquired. Malnutrition, sepsis, diabetes, and leukemia are all acquired disorders related to defects in leukocyte function, particularly phagocytosis and microbicidal activity (Mitchell & Cotran, 2003). Granulomatous diseases are relatively rare disorders of granulocytes, particularly neutrophils, in which the enzymes necessary for bactericidal activity are lacking. Such diseases result in severe, recurrent infections of the skin, lymph nodes, lungs, liver, and bone.

Lymphocytic Disorders

Lymphocytosis is produced by viral illnesses, including mumps, measles, rubella, rubeola, varicella, and hepatitis. Pertussis and chronic lymphocytic leukemia also elevate the lymphocyte count. An increase in the number of atypical lymphocytes is evident in infectious mononucleosis, cytomegalic inclusion disease, and toxoplasmosis.

Malignant White Blood Cell Disorders

Leukemia refers to a group of malignant diseases with qualitative and quantitative changes in circulating leukocytes. Leukemia is characterized by diffuse, abnormal growth of leukocytic precursors in the bone marrow. Such an uncontrolled increase in immature WBCs suppresses normal hematopoietic stem cells and leads to anemia and thrombocytopenia. Life-threatening infections occur because of a decrease in the function of circulating WBCs. Leukemias are further classified according to the course of the illness and the types of cells and tissues involved.

Malignant lymphomas, as in Hodgkin disease, are solid neoplasms that are lymphocytic in origin. Lymphocytes are the only WBCs involved, with the malignant process occurring during their maturation or storage in bone marrow. They are associated with lymphadenopathy and tumor development in the liver, spleen, thymus, bone marrow, and submucosa of the gastrointestinal and respiratory tracts. As in leukemia, immune deficiencies develop and are followed by infection. Most lymphoid neoplasms are of B-cell origin, with T-cell tumors making up the remainder. Hodgkin lymphoma is set apart from non-Hodgkin lymphomas by the presence of Reed-Sternberg giant cells in the neoplastic tissue. Also, in Hodgkin disease, within the involved nodes the nonneoplastic inflammatory cells usually greatly outnumber the tumor cells (Aster, 2003).

PLATELET AND COAGULATION DISORDERS

In pediatrics, the most common cause of thrombocytopenia (platelet count less than 100,000/mm^3) is immune or idiopathic thrombocytopenic purpura (ITP). It is associated with destruction of circulating platelets brought about by an immune-mediated process. In approximately 70% of cases, there is a history of a viral illness approximately 1 to 4 weeks before the onset of symptoms (Briones & Abshire, 2006).

When thrombocytopenia occurs, an associated anemia, abnormalities in white blood cell numbers, or the presence of abnormal leukocytes may indicate bone marrow failure caused by aplastic anemia, leukemia, or other malignant marrow disease. If the child is febrile, meningococcemia and overwhelming sepsis should be considered. Secondary thrombocytopenia results from drug hypersensitivity, viral infections, and autoimmune conditions. Thrombocytosis, or an elevation in the platelet count, is associated with certain malignancies or with polycythemia vera.

The causes of thrombocytopenia can be grouped into the following three main categories by determining the status of the red and white blood cell lines:
- Isolated decline in platelet count with no changes in normal red and white blood cell production—caused by viral infections, immune-mediated platelet destruction, congenital diseases, gestational thrombocytopenia, splenomegaly, antiphospholipid antibody syndrome, infectious diseases of bacterial origin, and drugs
- Thrombocytopenia associated with hemolytic anemia as seen in disseminated intravascular coagulation (DIC), Evans syndrome, and thrombotic microangiopathies (hemolytic uremic syndrome and thrombotic thrombocytopenic purpura [TTP])
- Pancytopenia or thrombocytopenia associated with both anemia and white cell abnormalities—splenomegaly, aplastic anemia, myelodysplasia (primary or secondary), and myeloproliferative syndromes (Drake & Rutecki, 2006)

Disorders of coagulation can be brought about by deficiencies of any of the clotting factors. Single-coagulation-factor deficiencies are usually hereditary. The most common are deficiencies in factor VIII (classic hemophilia A), factor IX (hemophilia B), and factor XI (hemophilia C).

PANCYTOPENIA

Pancytopenia is marked by a decrease in all three formed elements of the blood—erythrocytes, leukocytes, and platelets. With this condition, a child is more likely to present with clinical findings of infection or bleeding than anemia as a result of the longer life span of RBCs compared with platelets and WBCs. Pancytopenia is caused by one of three processes (Scott, 2006):
- Failure of production (intrinsic bone marrow disease as occurs in aplastic anemia)
- Sequestration (as occurs with hypersplenism)
- Increased peripheral destruction (Scott, 2006)

The child should be referred to hematology for treatment which is focused at correcting the underlying mechanism, such as hematopoietic stem cell transplantation (failure of production), splenectomy, or other treatments aimed at reducing peripheral destruction of cells or sequestration.

■■■ ASSESSMENT
HISTORY

A comprehensive, focused history and physical assessment are important aspects of the evaluation of a child with suspected hematologic disorder. Many hematologic processes are inherited. Therefore the family history, nationality, and geographic origins are aids to diagnosis. For example, thalassemia occurs most often among patients of Mediterranean or Asian descent; G6PD deficiency is also found in these ethnic groups and is also common among blacks. The provider should obtain information about family members with a history of any of following:
- Anemia
- Jaundice
- Splenomegaly
- Gallbladder disease
- Sickle cell or thalassemia disease or trait
- Bleeding tendencies
- Drug and toxin exposure
- Bone marrow failure
- Chronic illnesses
- Lead exposure

The child's medical history and a review of systems are important, with particular attention paid to the following:
- Episodes of jaundice (including in the newborn period)
- Extremity pain
- Abdominal pain
- Blood loss (particularly from mucous membranes)
- Weight loss
- Recent infections
- Drug exposure
- Travel
- Behavioral changes
- Pallor
- Petechiae, ecchymoses
- Adenopathy
- Gastrointestinal and genitourinary disorders
- Changes in stool characteristics indicating gastrointestinal bleeding (i.e., black, tarry stools)

The nutritional history of the child (and of the breastfeeding mother) should include the following:
- Dietary intake of iron sources, vitamins, milk, and meat
- A 24-hour dietary recall
- Any history of pica (particularly when iron deficiency or plumbism is suspected)

PHYSICAL EXAMINATION

The physical examination of the child should be comprehensive, and vital signs and growth parameters should be documented. The following positive signs are particularly important to identify:
- Pallor (especially of the conjunctivae and palmar creases)
- Jaundice
- Petechiae
- Fundal hemorrhages
- Excessive bruising

- Bleeding from mucous membranes
- Lymphadenopathy
- Frontal bossing
- Joint or extremity pain
- Heart murmurs and signs of congestive heart failure
- Hepatomegaly or splenomegaly
- Congenital anomalies that are associated with hematologic disorders

SCREENING

In many states, routine screening is done on the cord blood of newborns to detect sickle cell disease, sickle cell trait, and other hemoglobinopathies. Routine Hgb screening should be done (American Academy of Pediatrics, Committee on Practice and Ambulatory Medicine, 2000; McPherson & Tender, 2006):

- at 9 to 12 months old, when fetal stores are depleted and again 6 months later
- in menstruating adolescents

Lead screening should also be an integral part of pediatric primary care (see Chapter 41). A child considered to be at risk for exposure should have blood drawn to determine the level of lead at 9 to 12 months old and again at 24 months old. Local departments of health determine the prevalence of lead poisoning in their area and issue guidelines related to blood lead level screenings for targeted children in their catchment areas (American Academy of Pediatrics, Committee on Practice and Ambulatory Medicine, 2000; Markowitz, 2004). If the initial blood lead level is 10 mcg/dL or greater, the child should be retested more frequently and needs individual case management.

Work-Up of Anemia

Anemia may be suspected on the basis of clinical judgment and the established norms of hematocrit (i.e., the percentage of blood volume occupied by RBCs) and Hgb values. The initial laboratory approach is to obtain the following:

- Complete blood count (CBC)
- Reticulocyte count
- Peripheral smear to examine the morphologic characteristics and staining properties of the RBC

In the description of the smear, *hypochromic* describes cells that are paler than usual. *Poikilocytosis* denotes a wide variation in size and shape of the RBCs and is reflected by a high RBC distribution width (RDW).

The results of the RBC indices obtained in the CBC are useful in classification of the anemia, first according to the size of the RBC and then based on the pathophysiology (see Table 26-4):

- Mean corpuscular volume (MCV) is a measure of the average volume or size of the RBC and is calculated by dividing the hematocrit by the total number of RBCs. The calculated value of the MCV is expressed in cubic micrometers. A decrease in the MCV is seen in iron deficiency or thalassemia when the RBC is microcytic or smaller than usual. The MCV is increased in the megaloblastic anemias (such as folic acid anemia or juvenile pernicious anemia) when the RBC is abnormally large.
- Mean corpuscular hemoglobin (MCH) represents the average amount of Hgb in an RBC and is computed by dividing the Hgb concentration by the number of RBCs.
- Mean corpuscular hemoglobin concentration (MCHC) is the average percentage of Hgb in an RBC and is obtained by dividing the Hgb by the hematocrit.

In addition to the above screening tests, further diagnostic studies may be indicated to identify the type of acute anemia seen in childhood. Table 26-5 presents a summary of laboratory findings in the microcytic anemias. Other laboratory tests include the following:

- Free erythrocyte protoporphyrin (FEP), which is a measure of the porphyrin precursors that have not been converted into heme.
- Serum iron (SI or Fe), which indicates iron concentration levels in plasma.
- Total iron-binding capacity (TIBC), which denotes the number of binding sites available for iron (the ratio SI/TIBC expresses the saturation).
- Serum ferritin (SF) concentration, which indicates the level of iron stores in the liver, spleen, and bone marrow. A decrease in this level is one of the earliest markers of iron deficiency.

TABLE 26-5   **Microcytic Anemias**

Diagnosis	MCV	RBC Number	RDW	Ferritin	TIBC
Iron deficiency anemia	Low or normal	Low	High (>14%)	Low	High
Thalassemia trait	Low	Normal to high	Normal (<14%)	Normal	Normal
Viral suppression or chronic depression	Normal or low	Low	Normal	High	Low
Lead poisoning	Low or normal	Low	Normal to high	Normal to high	Normal

MCV, Mean corpuscular volume, *RBC,* red blood cell; *RDW,* red (blood cell) distribution width; *TIBC,* a total iron-binding capacity.
From Burg F et al, editors: *Current pediatric therapy,* ed 18, Philadelphia, 2006, WB Saunders.

- RDW, which is the coefficient of variation of the MCV (or the standard deviation of the measured MCVs divided by their mean MCV times 100). It is a measure of variation in size of RBCs. A larger RDW indicates greater diversity in cell size. An increased RDW is seen with iron deficiency. The most common use of RDW is to differentiate thalassemia minor (in which the RDW is elevated) from iron deficiency.
- The **Mentzer index** is used to differentiate iron deficiency anemia from beta thalassemia in situations of microcytic anemias. This test has a high sensitivity but low specificity and is calculated from the results of a CBC. Divide the MCV by the RBC count (MCV/ RBC). If the quotient is less than 13, thalassemia is more likely; if greater than 14, iron deficiency anemia is more likely.
- Hgb electrophoresis, which identifies the percentages of different types of Hgb and is useful in the diagnosis of sickle cell anemia, thalassemia, and other hemoglobinopathies.
- Bone marrow aspiration, which examines for the presence of precursors of all the hematologic lines: erythroid elements, myeloid elements, and platelets/megakaryocytes. This procedure is necessary for the diagnosis of aplastic anemia (complete bone marrow failure), leukemia, and other malignancies.

White Blood Cell Count

The WBC count and differential are obtained on a smear of blood one cell layer thick, usually with a Wright stain procedure that contains both basic and acidic dyes.

The ANC is calculated from the results of the differential: if WBCs = 3600, percentage of segmented neutrophils = 20, band neutrophils = 5, lymphocytes = 60, monocytes = 10, and eosinophils = 5, then

ANC = WBC × (% Seg + Band) = 3600 × 0.25 = 900

Tests for Coagulation Disorders

- Platelet count (normal range is 150,000 to 300,000/mm^3).
- Platelet function tests, such as platelet function analyzer (PFA).
- Prothrombin time (PT) (normal range is 11.5 to 14 seconds).
- Activated partial thromboplastin time (aPTT) is the current method used to determine partial thromboplastin time (PTT) and is commonly still referred to as the PTT (normal range is 25 to 40 seconds).
- Specific coagulation factor assays determine which clotting factors are absent.

The PT and aPTT measure all of the clotting factors except factor XIII. If the platelet count is normal, the aPTT or PT is prolonged, or both, a coagulation factor deficiency is possible. The typical laboratory findings of hemophilia are normal PT and PFA and an abnormal aPTT (Hagani & Bussel, 2002).

If the PT and aPTT are elevated in association with thrombocytopenia, the probable diagnosis is DIC, which is a syndrome secondary to an underlying disorder, such as sepsis, malignancy, toxins, or liver failure. In DIC, there is a systemic activation of the coagulation process. Extensive, ongoing activation of coagulation results in the depletion of platelets and coagulation factors, which then leads to bleeding and thrombosis (Briones & Abshire, 2006).

Bone Marrow Aspiration

Bone marrow aspiration or biopsy may be necessary to evaluate the specific types of cells present, including any foreign or malignant cells and maturation of the blood cell lines. In infants, the usual sites of aspiration are the proximal end of the tibia and posterior aspect of the iliac crest. In older children, the posterior part of the iliac crest or sternum can be used.

■ MANAGEMENT STRATEGIES

The types of management strategies used to treat children with hematologic problems are as varied as the disorders themselves. Most commonly, the plan of care focuses on provision of adequate nutrition and iron supplementation. Changes may be needed in the child's environment because of lead exposure. For some problems, management centers on teaching the family ways to prevent symptom exacerbation. For other rarer disorders, the focus is on helping the child and family cope with a chronic or potentially fatal condition and on collaborating with pediatric hematologists and oncologists in the delivery of care. Effective patterns of communication and referral among all the interdisciplinary providers, including laboratory personnel, are crucial.

Improvements in technology have brought about positive changes in the clinical management of children with hematologic disorders. The recognition of blood group antigens and infectious agents makes red cell transfusion a relatively safe procedure. Advances in pediatric hematology have led to an understanding of coagulation proteins and have dramatically improved the clinical course of children with coagulopathies. Unparalleled progress in the treatment of malignant hematologic diseases is likely to continue, and future breakthroughs will be possible as a result of gene replacement therapy.

Despite these many improvements, the family coping with having a child with chronic hematologic illness may experience numerous psychological ramifications, often in the context of limited resources (Carroll & Record, 2004). In cases of sickle cell disease or bleeding disorders, the family may experience overwhelming guilt and responsibility associated with the knowledge that the disease is genetically transmitted. Families of children with leukemia may have difficulty coping with chronic uncertainty and with the needs of other siblings. Clinical issues, such as pain management and problems with venous access, may need to be addressed. Parents may be fearful that the therapeutic effects of narcotics and blood products may be outweighed by the potentially deleterious side effects. Reimbursement and financial health care coverage may become an area of real concern as children reach the maximum lifetime amount of insurance reimbursement. Families may also be hesitant to join organized support networks for fear of stigma. Health care providers need to be aware of these many issues that families of chronically ill children may face while also keeping in mind the effects of culture and ethnicity on family management styles.

Another growing field in health care involves the development and implementation of models of care for survivors of childhood cancer. With improvements in therapy for childhood cancer, such as leukemia, the expectation is that most children will survive cancer and live to adulthood. However, these survivors are at risk for long-term sequelae associated with their cancer and its treatment (Friedman et al, 2005). Programs of care are now being developed that offer childhood cancer survivors the means to monitor and manage late effects and also provide support and advocacy for psychosocial issues, health education, and assistance for financial concerns. Experts in this field have collaborated with the Children's Oncology Group to establish long-term follow-up guidelines, which may be found at *www.survivorshipguidelines.org*. Late effects of childhood cancer are discussed at the conclusion of this chapter. In addition, the Resource Box at the end of this chapter identifies other Internet sites that may be of help to families and providers caring for a child with a chronic hematologic illness.

▇ SPECIFIC HEMATOLOGIC PROBLEMS
ERYTHROCYTE DISORDERS

Anemias are classified on the basis of two overall functional disturbances: anemias caused by nutritional deficiencies or inadequate production of RBCs and anemias brought about by increased destruction (hemolysis) of RBCs. Anemias occurring in the neonatal period are generally secondary to blood loss, isoimmunization, or congenital hemolytic anemias.

Anemias Caused by Inadequate Production of Red Blood Cells
Iron Deficiency Anemia
Description. Iron deficiency anemia is a common childhood anemia that is caused by inadequate availability of iron to sustain bone marrow erythropoiesis. Anemia caused by iron deficiency is the most common hematologic disease of infancy and childhood. Mild to moderate iron deficiency anemia is characterized by Hgb levels of 8 to 11 g/dL (McPherson & Tender, 2006). Hematologic markers are important in identifying various states of iron deficiency that range from iron depletion, to iron deficiency with anemia, to iron deficiency anemia.

Epidemiology. Infants around 9 months old, toddlers, and adolescent girls are considered to be at high risk for iron deficiency anemia because of their rapid growth and inadequate iron intake and as a result of blood loss from menses in adolescent girls. Typically, the young child has a history of a diet low in iron-containing foods and a high intake of milk (more than 1 quart a day). Milk impairs iron absorption and can cause gastrointestinal irritation leading to occult blood loss, which compounds the problem. Among girls in the adolescent years after menarche, iron intake is often inadequate.

Clinical Findings
History. Clinical findings are noted as follows; however, children with mild to severe anemia may be asymptomatic:
- Irritability and restlessness are often noticed in infants and toddlers only in retrospect, after treatment, and associated with Hgb below 8 g/dL.
- Pica may be present in unusual circumstances.
- Anorexia has been reported with Hgb levels below 8 g/dL.
- Developmental delays (mental and motor areas) and behavioral disturbances that may be irreversible have been reported in infants and young children (Wu et al, 2002).

Physical Examination. In mild to moderate iron deficiency, few symptoms are seen. The child may appear normal, or pallor may be present. Rarely, in anemias that develop slowly, the physical examination may reveal tachycardia or systolic murmurs and signs of congestive heart failure.

Diagnostic Tests. The following may be seen:
- A microcytic, hypochromic anemia on CBC
- Low or normal MCV; low RBC number
- High RDW (greater than 14%)
- Low ferritin
- High TIBC
- Mentzer index greater than 14 (IDA more likely)

The two most commonly used screening tests for iron deficiency anemia are Hgb and hematocrit, with Hgb being the more direct and sensitive marker of anemia compared with hematocrit measurements (Wu et al, 2002). Iron deficiency anemia is frequently identified in routine screenings of Hgb level via finger-stick sampling. It should be noted that finger-stick technique is important to prevent inaccurate readings. Venous sampling is the most reliable indicator. If there is a low Hgb level for age (in the range of 8 to 11 g/dL), a history of low iron intake, and no concern about other possible causes for the anemia or the possibility of another hemoglobinopathy, this is suggestive of iron deficiency anemia. If the age of the child and the dietary patterns are consistent with iron deficiency anemia, many clinicians will begin a trial of iron supplementation without further diagnostic testing and then follow the child's Hgb levels. They typically see the child again in 4 weeks. If there is a response to treatment with supplemental iron, a diagnosis of iron deficiency anemia is made (Wu et al, 2002).

If there is no response to iron therapy, a more extensive work-up should include a CBC with differential, platelet count, indices, and reticulocyte count. A smear of the peripheral blood should also be examined to asses the number and morphology of RBCs, WBCs and platelets. The differential diagnosis for anemia can then be determined on the basis of whether RBC production is adequate or inadequate, and whether the cells are microcytic, normocytic, or macrocytic (Fig. 26-2). The reticulocyte production index (RPI) corrects the reticulocyte count for the degree of anemia present and indicates whether the bone marrow is responding appropriately to the anemia. The formula for calculating the RPI is (Scott, 2006):

$$RPI = \frac{\text{Reticulocyte count} \times \text{Hemoglobin}_{observed}}{\text{Hemoglobin}_{normal} \times 0.5}$$

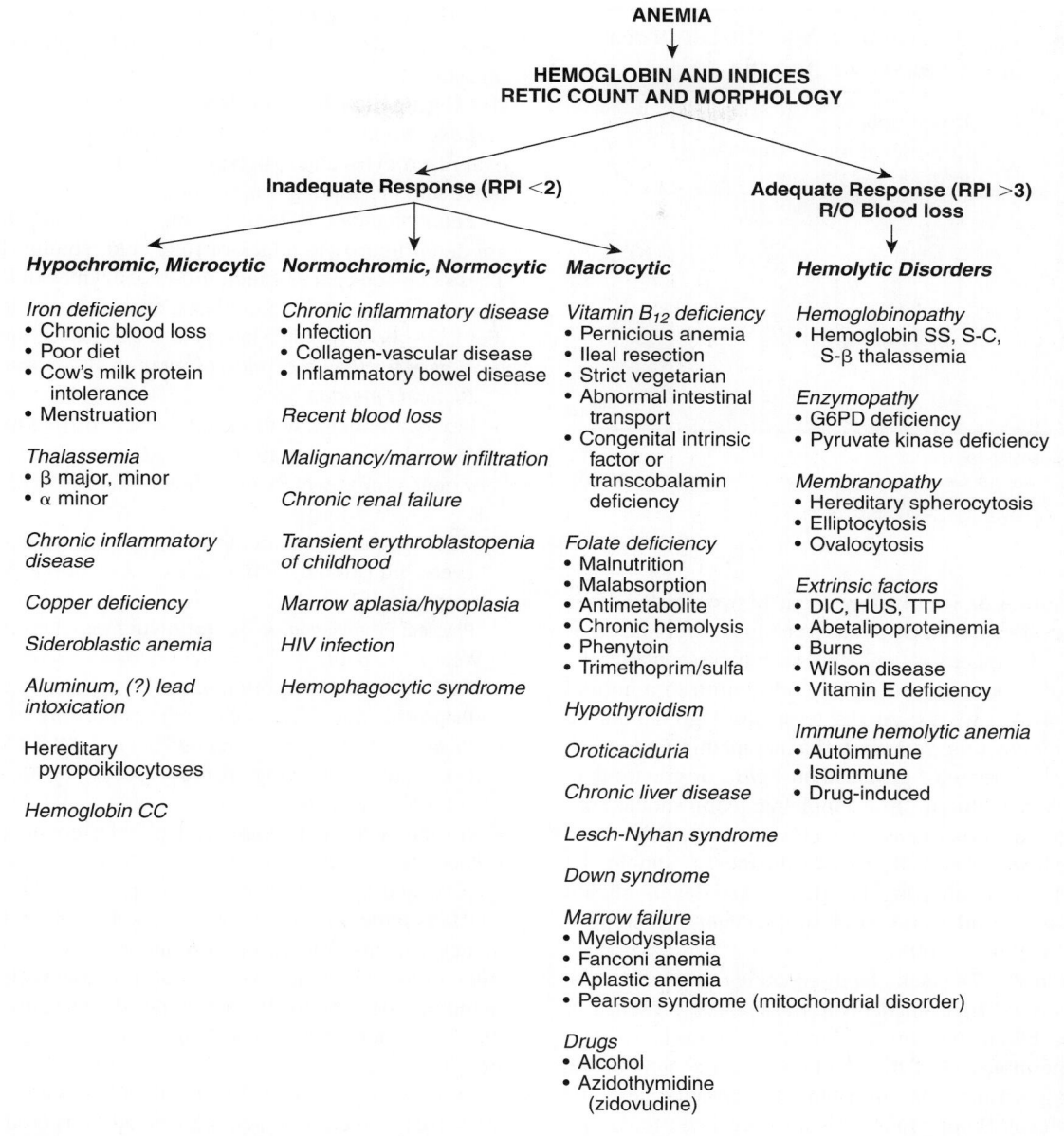

ANEMIA

↓

HEMOGLOBIN AND INDICES
RETIC COUNT AND MORPHOLOGY

Inadequate Response (RPI <2)   **Adequate Response (RPI >3)**
                                                      R/O Blood loss

Hypochromic, Microcytic   **Normochromic, Normocytic**   **Macrocytic**   **Hemolytic Disorders**

Iron deficiency
• Chronic blood loss
• Poor diet
• Cow's milk protein
  intolerance
• Menstruation

Thalassemia
• β major, minor
• α minor

*Chronic inflammatory
disease*

Copper deficiency

Sideroblastic anemia

*Aluminum, (?) lead
intoxication*

*Hereditary
  pyropoikilocytoses*

Hemoglobin CC

Chronic inflammatory disease
• Infection
• Collagen-vascular disease
• Inflammatory bowel disease

Recent blood loss

Malignancy/marrow infiltration

Chronic renal failure

*Transient erythroblastopenia
of childhood*

Marrow aplasia/hypoplasia

HIV infection

Hemophagocytic syndrome

Vitamin B$_{12}$ deficiency
• Pernicious anemia
• Ileal resection
• Strict vegetarian
• Abnormal intestinal
  transport
• Congenital intrinsic
  factor or
  transcobalamin
  deficiency

Folate deficiency
• Malnutrition
• Malabsorption
• Antimetabolite
• Chronic hemolysis
• Phenytoin
• Trimethoprim/sulfa

Hypothyroidism

Oroticaciduria

Chronic liver disease

Lesch-Nyhan syndrome

Down syndrome

Marrow failure
• Myelodysplasia
• Fanconi anemia
• Aplastic anemia
• Pearson syndrome (mitochondrial disorder)

Drugs
• Alcohol
• Azidothymidine
  (zidovudine)

Hemoglobinopathy
• Hemoglobin SS, S-C,
  S-β thalassemia

Enzymopathy
• G6PD deficiency
• Pyruvate kinase deficiency

Membranopathy
• Hereditary spherocytosis
• Elliptocytosis
• Ovalocytosis

Extrinsic factors
• DIC, HUS, TTP
• Abetalipoproteinemia
• Burns
• Wilson disease
• Vitamin E deficiency

Immune hemolytic anemia
• Autoimmune
• Isoimmune
• Drug-induced

FIG. 26-2   Use of the CBC, reticulocyte count, and blood smear in the diagnosis of anemia. *DIC,* Disseminated intravascular coagulation; *G6PD,* glucose-6-phosphate dehydrogenase; *HUS,* hemolytic uremic syndrome; *R/O,* rule out; *RPI,* reticulocyte production index; *TTP,* thrombotic thrombocytopenic purpura. (From Scott J: Hematology. In Behrman R et al, editors: *Nelson essentials of pediatrics,* ed 5, Philadelphia, 2006, WB Saunders.)

An RPI greater than 3 indicates increased production of platelets, which suggests either hemolysis or blood loss. An RPI less than 2 suggests decreased or ineffective production of reticulocytes in the marrow for the degree of anemia. Other causes of anemia, such as blood loss with occult rectal bleeding, should be considered in children with a low Hgb level on screening who eat a normal diet with adequate servings of iron-rich foods. Table 26-6 identifies age- and gender-specific laboratory cutoff values for childhood anemia.

Differential Diagnosis.   If resistant to treatment, iron deficiency should be differentiated from other microcytic, hypo-

chromic anemias, such as lead poisoning, thalassemia minor, anemia of chronic disease, and hereditary sideroblastic anemia (see Fig. 26-2). In lead poisoning, the FEP may be above 200 mcg/dL, and basophilic stippling may be seen on the RBCs in the peripheral smear. ß-Thalassemia is indicated by elevations in Hgb A$_2$.

Management.   Responses to treatment with iron supplementation are important diagnostically and therapeutically. For a child whose laboratory data reveal a microcytic, hypochromic anemia and an elevated FEP panel and whose history and physical examination are consistent with iron deficiency, a trial of iron is started (4 to 6 mg/kg/day of elemental iron in

TABLE 26-6 **Age- and Gender-Specific Laboratory Cutoff Values for Anemia**

Age (years)	Hemoglobin Concentration (g/dL)	Hematocrit (%)	MCV (fL)
1 to <2	<11	32.9	<77
2 to <5	<11.1	33	<79
5 to <8	<11.5	33.5	<80
8 to <12	<11.9	35.4	<80
12 to <15, male	<12.5	37.3	<85
15 to <18, male	<13.3	39.7	<85
12 to <15, female	<11.8	35.7	<85
15 to <18, female	<12	35.9	<85

MCV, Mean corpuscular volume.
From Burg F et al, editors: *Gellis and Kagan's current pediatric therapy*, ed 17, Philadelphia, 2002, WB Saunders.

three divided doses or 3 mg/kg/day in one to two divided doses for mild or moderate iron deficiency anemia) (McPherson & Tender, 2006). Peripheral reticulocytosis may be seen after the first 4 days of treatment, and Hgb should return to a normal level within 4 to 6 weeks. At the least, the Hgb should be rechecked 1 month after treatment. If a therapeutic response is observed (Hgb increase of greater than 1 g/dL or greater than 3% increase in hematocrit), iron supplementation should continue for 2 to 3 months to ensure adequate stores. Otherwise, compliance issues and alternative diagnoses should be explored. Dietary counseling is critical, and levels should be rechecked 6 months after iron supplements are stopped (McPherson & Tender, 2006).

Complications. The lack of a therapeutic response may be due to poor compliance, inadequate dosage, the presence of unrecognized blood loss, or an alternate diagnosis. A more extensive determination of the child's iron status is obtained by measuring serum iron, iron-binding capacity, and the venous lead level. Stool guaiac should be checked for occult blood loss.

Children with extremely low Hgb (less than 7 g/dL), hypotension, or signs of congestive heart failure should be referred and may need to be hospitalized. Laboratory results that also indicate referral are neutropenia, thrombocytopenia, nucleated RBCs, or immature myeloid elements. When disorders of erythrocytes, platelets, and leukocytes are all found, a bone marrow disorder is probable.

Education and Prevention. Parents or caretakers should be counseled about the adequacy of the child's diet. Whole cow's milk should be avoided in infants younger than 12 months old. For full-term infants, dietary iron supplementation (as in iron-enriched infant cereal) should begin at 4 to 6 months old. For preterm infants, supplementation with oral iron drops should begin as early as 2 months old. If the child is treated therapeutically with oral iron supplements, parents should be advised to avoid giving the iron with meals or milk, that vitamin C juice enhances absorption, and that the child's stools

will probably turn black. Parents should also be cautioned to keep the medication safely out of reach to prevent accidental ingestion.

Megaloblastic Anemias
Description. Megaloblastic anemias are characterized by oval macrocytes and hypersegmented PMNs in the peripheral blood and megaloblasts in the bone marrow.

Epidemiology. Relatively rare megaloblastic anemias are due primarily to a lack of folic acid, vitamin B_{12}, or both. These two substances function as coenzymes in the synthesis of nuclear protein. Megaloblastic anemias may develop if the diet lacks these two substances or if the gastric intrinsic factor necessary for the absorption of vitamin B_{12} is absent.

Clinical Findings.
History. Patients with megaloblastic anemia may include:
- Young infants who are being fed powdered milk products or goat's milk, which are deficient in folic acid and vitamin B_{12}
- Older children who are exclusively vegetarian or who have severe nutritional deficiencies, absorption problems, or tapeworm infestations

Physical Examination. The following may be seen:
- Weakness, pallor
- Beefy-red, smooth, sore tongue

Diagnostic Tests. The following results may be seen:
- Elevated MCV (greater than 95 fL) and MCHC
- Blood smear showing macroovalocytes with anisocytosis and poikilocytosis
- Normal white cell count and platelet count, but possibly decreased in more severe cases
- Large and hypersegmented neutrophils

Management. In general, management of folic acid deficiency and juvenile pernicious anemia (caused by a lack of vitamin B_{12}) is best done in consultation with a pediatric hematologist. Treatment is through dietary supplementation and correction of the underlying disorder (e.g., infection) if possible.

In folic acid deficiency confirmed by measurement of the RBC folate level, folic acid may be administered in a dose of 0.5 to 1 mg/24 hr and continued for 3 to 4 weeks. Prolonged use of folic acid should be avoided (Glader, 2004).

In vitamin B_{12} deficiency, a prompt hematologic response is usually seen after parenteral administration of vitamin B_{12}. If neurologic involvement is present, 1 mg should be given intramuscularly daily for at least 2 weeks. A maintenance dose of a 1 mg intramuscular injection of vitamin B_{12} is administered monthly throughout the patient's life (Glader, 2004).

Transient Erythroblastopenia of Childhood
Description. Idiopathic erythroblastopenia of childhood, or transient erythroblastosis of childhood (TEC), is a benign disorder of unknown cause that occurs in children during the first few years of life, usually after 1 year old. It is characterized by anemia, reticulocytopenia, and erythroid hypoplasia of the bone marrow. The cause of this acquired decrease in red cell production is not clear, although it frequently follows a viral infection (Glader, 2004; Segel et al, 2002b).

Etiology. TEC is associated with temporary failure of erythropoiesis caused by probable viral suppression or as a result of an IgG-mediated autoimmune response.

Clinical Findings

History. TEC occurs mainly in previously healthy children between 6 months and 3 years old. The child may have a history of a preceding infection.

Physical Examination. Patients have symptoms of anemia, including pallor.

Diagnostic Tests. The following are seen in TEC:

- Anemia (in which the Hgb content may be as low as 2.5 g/dL or only slightly decreased)
- Markedly low reticulocyte count
- WBC count usually normal
- Platelets normal or elevated
- High serum iron level reflecting decreased utilization
- Bone marrow aspiration results indicating erythroid hypoplasia

Differential Diagnosis. The syndrome can be differentiated from congenital hypoplastic anemia (Diamond-Blackfan syndrome) by the normal size of the RBCs (MCV less than 80 fL). Approximately 25% of children with Diamond-Blackfan syndrome have dysmorphic features (e.g., short stature, congenital heart disease, and mental retardation), whereas children with TEC have a normal physical examination (Segel et al, 2002b).

Management. TEC is self-limited, with recovery taking place 1 to 2 months after diagnosis. No specific treatment is indicated, although transfusions may be required for severe anemia. The NP should consult with a physician; a referral to a hematologist may be needed.

Hemolytic Anemias

Hemolytic anemias can be classified as either hereditary or acquired. In particular, the hereditary and congenital anemias are manifested in infancy and early childhood. They may be due to a variety of hemoglobinopathies or to defects in the red cell membrane.

Sickle Cell Anemia and Trait

Etiology. Sickle cell disease describes a group of complex, chronic disorders that are characterized by hemolysis, unpredictable acute complications that may become life threatening, and the possible development of chronic organ damage. Children who have sickle cell anemia or disease do not form the normal Hgb A molecule, but rather synthesize hemoglobin S (Hgb S), which carries the amino acid valine instead of glutamic acid. Because of this change, Hgb S tends to polymerize or come out of solution at low PaO_2, low pH, low temperature, and low osmolality. This process damages the RBC by giving it a "sickled" appearance and causes a chronic hemolytic anemia with associated ischemia and vasoocclusive problems.

Epidemiology. Sickle cell disease has an autosomal recessive inheritance pattern. It is found most often in people of African descent, but is also detected among ethnic groups from the Mediterranean, the Caribbean, and India. In the U.S., sickle cell disease occurs in about 1 of every 400 black infants

(Ambruso et al, 2005). This incidence exceeds that of most other serious genetic disorders in children, including cystic fibrosis and hemophilia.

Children with sickle cell trait who are heterozygous for the gene essentially have a benign clinical course. Their RBCs contain only 30% to 40% Hgb S, and sickling does not occur under most conditions. It is only in rare instances of hypoxia, such as in shock, while flying in unpressurized aircraft, or traveling to high elevations, that signs of vasoocclusion can occur.

Clinical Findings. Most infants with sickle cell disease born in the U.S. are now identified by routine neonatal screening. In those states that have not yet implemented universal screening, neonatal screening for sickle cell disease should be requested for those infants considered to be high risk, including those of African, Mediterranean, Middle Eastern, Indian, Caribbean, and Central and South American ancestry. A careful family medical history is also important.

Physical Examination. Symptoms begin to emerge in the second 6 months of life as the amount of Hgb S increases and Hgb F declines. Subsequently, painful, vaso-occlusive crises occur. The following may be noted:

- Pale and slightly jaundiced appearance with splenomegaly
- Painful swelling of the hands and feet (hand-foot syndrome) caused by infarction in the small bones
- Low-grade fever
- Leukocytosis
- Painful involvement of the larger bones (in older patients)
- Priapism
- Diffuse abdominal pain
- Chest pain
- Sequestration crisis, which occurs when large amounts of blood are pooled in the abdominal organs and the spleen becomes enlarged

After 5 years old, splenomegaly usually disappears because of autoinfarction. Rates of height and weight gain are usually slowed after 7 years old, and puberty may be delayed 3 to 4 years.

Diagnostic Tests. The following laboratory results are seen in sickle cell disease (Quirolo & Vichinsky, 2004; Segel et al, 2002b).

- Hematocrit of 20% to 29% with sickled cells, nucleated RBCs, and Howell-Jolly bodies on the peripheral smear
- Hgb 6 to 10 g/dL (severe sickle syndromes)
- MCV greater than 80 fL
- Reticulocyte count elevated: 5% to 15%
- Normal to increased WBC and platelet count
- Hgb electrophoresis (after infancy) showing a preponderance of Hgb S and no Hgb A
- Blood film shows irreversibly sickled cells or chronic elliptocytes

Hgb electrophoresis results in a newborn with sickle cell trait will be FAS and FS for a child with either sickle cell anemia or SB⁰-thalassemia. Normal results of Hgb electrophoresis are FA.

Differential Diagnosis. Chronic hemolytic anemia should be included in the differential diagnosis. Other syndromes characterized by hemolytic anemia and vasoocclusion are Hgb SC disease and a combination of Hgb S with α- or ß-thalassemia. These diseases may be differentiated through electrophoresis and family testing if necessary.

Management. The following measures are instituted:

- Baseline laboratory data (CBC, reticulocyte count) are monitored every few months.
- Seven-valent pneumococcal conjugate and 23-valent pneumococcal polysaccharide vaccines are administered.
- Penicillin V prophylaxis (125 mg orally, twice daily) is initiated by 2 months old. At 3 years old, the dose is increased to 250 mg orally, twice a day, and continued at least until the fifth birthday (AAP, 2002; Hilliard & Howard, 2006).
- Yearly influenza immunization is administered.
- Meningococcal vaccine is administered for children older than 2 years (Segel et al, 2002b).
- Folic acid supplementation may be indicated if the diet is low in green-leafy vegetables. Oral folic acid is administered, if needed, to prevent folic acid deficiency: 0.5 mg/day for children less than 5 years old; 1 mg/day after 5 years old (Segel et al, 2002b).
- Aggressive treatment of infections and maintenance of hydration and body temperature are used to prevent hypoxia and acidosis; volume replacement may be necessary to prevent circulatory collapse.
- Treatment of coexisting medical problems associated with lower O_2 saturations, such as asthma and obstructive sleep apnea.
- Annual stroke prevention screening of major intracranial vessels with hydroxyurea transcranial Doppler evaluation for 2- to 16-year-old children. A reading of greater than 200 cm/sec time-averaged mean maximal velocity indicates high risk for stroke (Hilliard & Howard, 2006).

Children with sickle cell disease are usually co-managed by specialists in hematology and their primary care provider. Emergency admission or referral is necessary in the presence of the following:

- Fever (to rule out sepsis) greater than 101° F (38.3° C)
- Pneumonia, chest pain, or other pulmonary symptoms (acute chest syndrome)
- Sequestration crisis (splenomegaly with decreased Hgb or hematocrit)
- Aplastic crisis (decreased hematocrit and reticulocyte count)
- Severe painful crisis
- Unusual headache, visual disturbances
- Priapism

Consultation is also necessary for the chronic sequelae of persistent bone pain or leg ulcers, in addition to issues of pregnancy and contraception. Stem cell transplantation may be a consideration in children with significant disease.

Complications. Because of functional asplenia, the greatest concern is febrile illness indicating infection and possible sepsis. In view of the serious threat of pneumococcal sepsis in children younger than 5 years old, all complaints of fever, poor feeding, lethargy, and irritability should be evaluated in the clinical setting. The consequences of hemolysis may include chronic anemia, jaundice, cholelithiasis, and delayed

growth and sexual maturation. Vaso-occlusion and tissue ischemia may result in acute and chronic injury to virtually every organ system with stroke being a major concern (AAP, 2002; Hilliard & Howard, 2006).

Patient and Family Education. The parents of children with sickle cell anemia need a great deal of support in raising a child with a genetically transmitted chronic disease. Clear patterns of communication should be established between the family and the provider. Initial education includes the genetics and pathophysiology of the disease and the importance of regular health maintenance visits. Parents should be counseled about the need for early evaluation and treatment of febrile illness, acute splenic sequestration, aplastic crisis, and acute chest syndrome. As the child grows, the family should be educated in other potential clinical complications, such as stroke, enuresis, priapism, cholelithiasis, delayed puberty, retinopathy, avascular necrosis of the hip and shoulder, and leg ulcers.

Preventive Care. Preventive measures for infants and children include the following:

- Timely administration of routine immunizations, including pneumococcal and meningococcal vaccines, and yearly influenza vaccine
- Prophylactic antibiotics
- Genetic counseling
- Support groups

Thalassemias. The thalassemias are a group of hereditary, hypochromic anemias that are associated with the absence or decreased synthesis of the normal Hgb polypeptide chains—usually the α- and ß-chains (Quirolo & Vichinsky, 2004). They occur primarily in people of Mediterranean and Southeast Asian descent.

ß-Thalassemias cover a broad clinical spectrum of disorders that are classified according to patterns of inheritance and the severity of the anemia. The heterozygous states are thalassemia minor and thalassemia minima, which are essentially silent carrier states. Homozygous forms are thalassemia intermedia and thalassemia major, or Cooley anemia.

ß-Thalassemia Minor

Description. ß-Thalassemia minor disease or trait is associated with a mild, hypochromic, microcytic anemia in which Hgb levels are 2 to 3 g/dL below normal, and the MCV averages 65 fL (Quirolo & Vichinsky, 2004). It may be confused with iron deficiency or lead poisoning and can be differentiated by measuring serum iron or lead levels, transferrin saturation, or serum ferritin levels (Table 26-7). Thus it is particularly important to avoid long-term unnecessary administration of iron supplements for a misdiagnosis that could result in iron overload. The primary diagnostic feature is increased Hgb A_2 (greater than 3.5%) on electrophoresis.

Clinical Findings. Clinically, most individuals with thalassemia trait are asymptomatic, although mild pallor and splenomegaly may be found. An Hgb of 9.5 to 11 g/dL and an MCV of less than 80 fL/cell is commonly seen in prepubertal children. The MCV/RBC count per milliliter is less than 13 (the Mentzer index). In contrast, the Mentzer index of iron

TABLE 26-7 Red Blood Cell (RBC) Disorders Associated With Anemia in Infants and Children

Disease	Clinical Presentation		Laboratory Diagnosis	Treatment
	History	Physical Findings		
Iron deficiency	Fatigue Irritability Excess milk intake	Pallor or none	RBC hypochromic, microcytic MCV ↓ Serum iron ↓ TIBC ↑ % Saturation ↓ Ferritin ↓ Blood in stool or urine Ratio of MCV/RBC >13	Correct diet Eliminate source of bleeding Ferrous SO₄ up to 6 mg/kg/ day of elemental iron
α- and β-thalassemia trait	None Pallor Family history	None Pallor	RBC hypochromic, microcytic MCV ↓↓ Basophilic stippling (β-thalassemia trait) ↑ Hgb A₂ (β-thalassemia trait) Ratio of MCV/RBC <13	None for child Test both parents Genetic counseling Avoid iron therapy

Hereditary spherocytosis	None
	Family history
	History of neonatal
	  jaundice
		Pallor, jaundice
		Splenomegaly
			Spherocytosis Coombs' test
			  negative
			Reticulocyte % ↑
			Osmotic fragility increased
			MCHC↑
				No splenectomy if Hgb
				  >10 g/dL (100 g/L) and
				  reticulocyte <10%
				Folic acid (0.5 mg daily <5
				  years old; 1 mg daily >5
				  years old)
				Splenectomy; immunizations
				  for pneumococcus,
				  Haemophilus influenzae,
				  and meningococcus;
				  penicillin prophylaxis

Chronic inflammation	Depends on the cause
	  of the inflammation
	  and the severity
	  of anemia (fatigue
	  to symptoms of
	  congestive heart
	  failure)
		Depends on the
		  cause of the
		  inflammation and
		  the severity of
		  anemia (pallor
		  to signs of
		  congestive heart
		  failure)
			Nonspecific tests: erythrocyte
			  sedimentation rate
			Acute-phase reactants:
			  C-reactive protein,
			  fibrinogen, haptoglobin
			Serum ferritin
			Serum iron and TIBC % iron
			  saturation
			Bone marrow iron stores
			Bone marrow sideroblasts
				Treat underlying disease
				  or condition
				Treat anemia

Lead intoxication	Pica—ingestion of
	  lead-containing
	  substances
	Neurobehavioral
	  problems (e.g.,
	  irritability, poor
	  appetite, inattention,
	  hyperactivity)
	Neurodevelopmental
	  delay (e.g., learning
	  problems to severe
	  cognitive dysfunction)
		Poor speech
		Visual-motor
		  integration
		  problems
		Encephalopathy,
		  neuropathy,
		  cerebral edema if
		  severe poisoning
			Basophilic stippling
			Erythrocyte protoporphyrin
			  blood lead
				Eliminate source of lead in
				  the child's environment
				Diet rich in iron and calcium
				Iron supplementation,
				  4-6 mg/kg/day to reduce
				  further absorption of lead
				Chelation therapy based
				  on lead levels and
				  symptoms (use Centers
				  for Disease Control and
				  Prevention guidelines)

MCHC, Mean corpuscular hemoglobin concentration; *MCV,* mean corpuscular volume; *RBC,* red blood cell; *TIBC,* total iron-binding capacity.
Adapted from Segel G, Hirsh M, Feig S: Managing anemia in a pediatric office practice: part 1, *Pediatr Rev* 23:75-83, 2002.

deficiency is usually greater than 13 for iron deficiency (Segel et al, 2002a). The degree of anemia may be exacerbated in concurrent illness or pregnancy.

Management. No specific treatment is known for ß-thalassemia minor. Primary emphasis should be on education of all

family members and genetic testing, and counseling should be offered.

ß-Thalassemia Major

Description. Homozygous ß-thalassemia major (or Cooley anemia) is associated with severe anemia resulting from decreased or absent production of Hgb A and hemolysis caused by the precipitation of excess α-chains in the RBCs.

Clinical Findings. Affected infants usually become symptomatic in the first year of life and have pallor, failure to thrive, hepatosplenomegaly, and a severe anemia with an average Hgb of 6 g/dL and low MCV (60 to 70 fL). RBC morphology reveals significant microcytosis, poikilocytosis, hypochromia, target cells, and nucleated RBCs. Hgb A and Hgb F levels are elevated.

Management. Proper management of the child requires collaboration with a pediatric hematologist. Exchange transfusions are usually necessary every 4 to 5 weeks with a post-transfusion level of 9.5 g/dL as the goal. Iron chelation therapy is indicated after 1 to 2 years of chronic transfusion therapy, with a serum ferritin greater than 1000 ng/dL, or hepatic iron level of 7 mg/g dry weight (Qureshi & Vichinsky, 2006). Splenectomy and bone marrow transplant may be indicated as well (Quirolo & Vichinsky, 2004).

Complications. If the condition is left untreated, the characteristic facies with frontal bossing and maxillary overgrowth will develop as a result of bone marrow expansion.

Hereditary Spherocytosis

Description. Hereditary spherocytosis (HS) is a hemolytic anemia characterized by a deficiency or abnormality of the RBC membrane protein spectrin, which reduces the RBC surface area. The RBC membranes assume a more spherical shape. Hence, RBCs are more likely to be sequestered and prematurely destroyed in the spleen (Segel et al, 2002a). The disease process of HS can range from mild chronic hemolysis to severe transfusion-dependent anemia (Berkow & Schwartz, 2006).

Incidence. HS occurs in 1 in 5000 persons of preponderantly northern European ancestry.

Clinical Findings

Physical Examination. Jaundice usually appears in the newborn period, and it may be difficult to differentiate HS from hyperbilirubinemia caused by ABO incompatibility. After 2 years old, splenomegaly is usually present. Chronic fatigue, malaise, and abdominal pain may also be noted.

Diagnostic Tests. Laboratory findings in HS include the following:

- Chronic anemia (Hgb is 6 to 10 g/dL).
- Reticulocyte count ranges from 5% to 20%.
- On peripheral smear, a small proportion of the RBCs are spherocytic and smaller than normal and lack the central pallor of the usual biconcave disk-shaped cell.
- Osmotic fragility of the cells is increased, as is the rate of autohemolysis of incubated blood.

Management. The treatment of choice for children with severe HS requiring multiple transfusions is splenectomy, which usually produces a clinical cure. It should be deferred until 5 or 6 years old because of the increased risk of infection before that age. Risks associated with splenectomy are post-splenectomy sepsis, penicillin-resistant pneumococci infection, pulmonary hypertension, and ischemic heart disease and stroke seen in HS patients (Berkow & Schwartz, 2006). Pneumococcal vaccine should be given before splenectomy.

After splenectomy, prophylactic penicillin therapy (less than 5 years old: 125 mg orally twice a day; greater than 5 years old: 250 mg orally twice a day) is recommended. Because of increased hemolysis, children with HS and active hemolysis should receive 1 mg of folic acid daily until splenectomy. There is remission of the disease after splenectomy (Segel, 2004).

Complications. Aplastic crises (which can be indicated by fever, fatigue, abdominal pain, and jaundice) associated with parvovirus and other viral infections are the most serious complications during childhood. Febrile illnesses should be vigorously treated. A splenectomized child with a temperature greater than 101.5° F (greater than 38.6° C) and without an obvious source of infection should be hospitalized and treated with intravenous antibiotics until blood cultures prove to be negative (Altman, 2002). Gall stone formation can occur as a result of chronic hemolysis, and ultrasounds should be performed every 5 years and before splenectomy (Berkow & Schwartz, 2006).

Glucose-6-Phosphate Dehydrogenase Deficiency

Description. A drug-induced hemolytic anemia can be caused by genetic deficiency of the G6PD enzyme in the RBC. Symptoms are generally associated with infections or exposure to oxidant metabolites of certain drugs that cause precipitation of Hgb, injury to the red cells, and rapid hemolysis.

Epidemiology. G6PD deficiency is transmitted as an X-linked recessive trait. In the U.S., about 10% of black males and 1% to 2% of black females are affected. It may also occur in a more severe form in Greeks, Italians, Arabs, Southeast Asians, and Chinese.

Clinical Findings

History. Patients generally have a history of recent infection (particularly hepatitis) or oxidant drug ingestion—specifically, aspirin-containing antipyretics, sulfonamides, antimalarials, antihelmintics, naphthaquinolones, and fava beans. The degree of hemolysis is dependent on the amount of the drug ingested and the extent of enzyme deficiency.

Physical Examination. The patient may have pallor and jaundice if there is chronic hemolysis, or have jaundice, pallor, lethargy, irritability, headache, and red or dark clear urine after drug ingestion.

Diagnostic Tests. Several dye reduction tests provide the diagnosis. Screening tests available to measure a deficiency of G6PD should be used in high-risk groups. These tests measure G6PD enzyme activity in the RBC. After a hemolytic crisis, however, screening may produce a false-negative result because the younger blood cells that remain after hemolysis may show normal enzymatic activity. A more representative enzyme assay can be obtained 2 to 3 months after the episode (Segel et al, 2002b).

Management. No specific treatment is available. Red cell transfusion and supportive therapy may be indicated in cases in which the anemia is severe. Keeping the child well hydrated and monitoring for renal failure are important during hemolytic crisis.

Patient and Family Education. Patients and families should be taught to avoid the offending drugs—the most common being aspirin, sulfonamide antibiotics, and antimalarials.

PLATELET AND BLOOD COAGULATION DISORDERS

Platelet disorders should be ruled out in a child before undergoing extensive surgery. Platelet disorders should also be considered in a child with petechiae, frequent nosebleeds, mucous membrane bleeding, and excessive bleeding from minor trauma. Evaluation of these complaints includes a family history of bleeding or platelet disorders and a history of drug or toxin exposure. Initial laboratory studies should include a CBC, platelet count, PT, and aPTT. Among the diagnoses that may be differentiated with these tests are ITP, hemophilia, von Willebrand disease, and leukemia.

Immune or Idiopathic Thrombocytopenic Purpura

Description.   Immune or idiopathic thrombocytopenic purpura (ITP) is the most common of the thrombocytopenic purpuras in childhood and is believed to be an autoimmune response in which circulating platelets are destroyed. It usually occurs after viral illnesses (Scott, 2006).

Epidemiology.   Most cases occur between 2 and 5 years old, and the incidence is increased in fair-skinned children.

Clinical Findings.   ITP is essentially a clinical diagnosis and does not rest on any one diagnostic test. It is characterized by the following:

- Acute onset of petechiae, purpura, and bleeding in an otherwise healthy child; the bruising or bleeding may be most prominent over the legs.
- A viral illness 1 to 4 weeks before onset in 70% of cases.
- Hemorrhage of the mucous membranes, particularly the gums and lips.
- Nosebleeds that can be severe and difficult to control.
- The liver, spleen, and lymph nodes are not generally enlarged.

Diagnostic Tests.   Laboratory findings in ITP include:

- Low platelet count (less than 150,000/mm³) with an otherwise normal CBC
- Normal PT and aPTT
- Megathrombocytes on the peripheral smear

Differential Diagnosis.   If the smear shows fragmented RBCs, blood urea nitrogen and creatinine levels should be measured to rule out hemolytic-uremic syndrome. If the PT and aPTT are elevated with thrombocytopenia, DIC is a possibility, and cultures should be taken to identify sources of infection. A prolonged PT and aPTT with a normal platelet count suggest a coagulation factor deficiency. If the syndrome is complicated by prolonged thrombocytopenia, neutropenia, anemia, bone pain, or congenital anomalies, the child should be referred to a hematologist for possible bone marrow aspiration to rule out acute lymphocytic leukemia (ALL) and other disorders. In a sick, febrile child with isolated thrombocytopenia, petechiae, or purpura, the major diagnosis to consider first is meningococcemia. Such children should also be referred, hospitalized, and treated for presumed sepsis.

Management.   The prognosis for children with ITP is excellent, with spontaneous recovery in 75% of cases in the first 3 months (Scott, 2006). Most cases of ITP can be managed on an outpatient basis without any specific therapy.

If the platelet count is greater than 50,000/mm³ and no bleeding is observed, children and parents should be taught to avoid contact sports, aspirin ingestion, and any other herbal or pharmacologic agents that interfere with platelet function and to notify the practitioner of any bleeding. Epistaxis can be treated with local measures. In severe cases (platelets less than 50,000/mm³) in which the diagnosis of leukemia is ruled out, a short course of corticosteroid therapy may reduce severity in the initial phases. Intravenous immune globulin (IVIG) is also given to children with active severe bleeding and who have contraindications for steroid use; WinRho (Anti-D) is given intravenously with dose depending on Hgb level; Rh(D) immune globulin is useful only in Rh+ individuals. Splenectomy, immunosuppressives, and anti-CD20 antibody are options for those children with refractory or chronic ITP (Briones & Abshire, 2006).

Complications.   The most serious complication is intracranial hemorrhage, which occurs in less than 1% of cases (Scott, 2006).

Hemophilia A and B and von Willebrand Disease

Description.   Inherited deficiencies are known for each of the coagulation factors, with most of them resulting in abnormal bleeding. Hemophilia refers to a deficiency of factor VIII (hemophilia A) or factor IX (hemophilia B). In hemophilia A and B, absence or deficiency of the coagulation factor results in prolonged bleeding either spontaneously from small vessels or as a result of trauma.

In plasma, factor VIII is complexed with von Willebrand factor (vWf), which is a specific circulatory protein and acts as a carrier protein. von Willebrand disease (also known as vascular hemophilia) is a heterogeneous group of hereditary bleeding disorders caused by a quantitative or qualitative abnormality of vWf protein, which also results in a bleeding disorder (Table 26-8). In type I, the protein is quantitatively reduced; in type II, it is qualitatively abnormal and is absent in type III.

Epidemiology.   Because the genes for the coagulation factors are sex linked (carried on the X chromosome) and recessive, the disease affects primarily males. Females are generally only carriers of the disorder. About 1 in 5000 males is affected with hemophilia A, which is five times more common than hemophilia B (Scott, 2006). von Willebrand disease is seen in both sexes with an incidence of 1 in 100 individuals. It is the most common inherited bleeding disorder and is associated with either a qualitative or quantitative defect in von Willebrand factor (Briones & Abshire, 2006). The primary sites of bleeding differ depending on whether the problem is hemophilia A or B or von Willebrand disease.

Clinical Findings.   The following are seen in hemophilia:

- A positive family history in the vast majority of cases
- Excessive bruising
- Prolonged bleeding from mucous membranes after minor lacerations
- Hemarthroses characterized by pain and swelling in the elbows, knees, and ankles
- A greatly prolonged aPTT

TABLE 26-8	**Comparisons of Hemophilia A, Hemophilia B, and von Willebrand Disease**		
	Hemophilia A	**Hemophilia B**	**von Willebrand Disease**
Inheritance	X-linked	X-linked	Autosomal dominant
Factor deficiency	Factor VIII	Factor IX	von Willebrand factor and VIIIC
Bleeding site(s)	Muscle, joint, surgical	Muscle, joint, surgical	Mucous membranes, skin, surgical, menstrual
PT	Normal	Normal	Normal
aPTT	Prolonged	Prolonged	Prolonged or normal
Bleeding time	Normal	Normal	Prolonged or normal
Factor VIII coagulant activity (VIIIC)	Low	Normal	Low or normal
von Willebrand factor antigen (vWF: Ag)	Normal	Normal	Low
von Willebrand factor activity (vWF: Act)	Normal	Normal	Low
Factor IX	Normal	Low	Normal
Ristocetin-induced	Normal	Normal	Normal, low, or increased at low-dose ristocetin
Platelet aggregation	Normal	Normal	Normal
Treatment	DDAVP* or recombinant VIII	Recombinant IX	DDAVP* or vWF concentrate

vWF, von Willebrand factor.
*Desmopressin (DDAVP) for mild to moderate hemophilia A or type I von Willebrand disease.
From Scott J: Hematology. In Kliegman R et al, editors: *Nelson essentials of pediatrics*, ed 5, Philadelphia, 2006, Elsevier Saunders, p 718.

A specific assay for factor VIII or IX activity confirms the diagnosis.

Clinical findings associated with von Willebrand disease include the following:

- Mucous membrane bleeding (epistaxis, menorrhagia), easy bruising, and excessive posttraumatic or postsurgical bleeding
- History of ecchymosis of trunk, upper arms, and thighs
- Factor VIII clotting activity usually decreased
- vWF antigen usually decreased
- Decreased vWF
- Normal platelet count but isolated decreased platelets associated with type IIB (Briones & Abshire, 2006)
- Bleeding time and aPTT generally prolonged, but may be normal (Montgomery & Scott, 2004)

Management. Treatment of hemophilia consists of prevention of trauma and replacement therapy to increase factor VIII or factor IX activity in plasma. Plasma-derived and recombinant factor concentrates are available for replacement with recombinant factor preferred.

Local measures include the application of cold and pressure to affected, painful joints. As with all bleeding disorders, aspirin should be avoided (Scott, 2006).

Ideally, most children with hemophilia should be enrolled in a local hemophilia treatment center to facilitate a collaborative, interdisciplinary approach to management. The primary provider should remain central to the care of the child. All immunizations should be given subcutaneously with a 26-gauge needle, followed by firm pressure at the site for several minutes. Iron replacement may also be necessary in children with severe bleeding disorders.

von Willebrand disease is treated depending on the type and severity of the bleeding. The treatment of von Willebrand disease is desmopressin (DDAVP), factor VIII-vWF concentrates, and local measures to control bleeding may be part of the treatment plan (Briones & Abshire, 2006). Adjunctive therapy (e.g., estrogen and/or aminocaproic acid) depends on the type of von Willebrand disease (Type I, IIA, IIB, IIM, IIN, or III) which is determined by the level of qualitative or quantitative factor deficiency.

A written treatment plan stating the dosage of the replacement product for the location of the bleed should be in the chart and given to the parents to carry with them. The child should wear a medical alert bracelet or necklace.

Complications. In patients with Hemophilia A and B, bleeding persists without factor replacement, particularly in closed areas, such as the joints. Brain hemorrhage can be a serious consequence of head trauma. Continued hemorrhage results in anemia and eventually hypovolemic shock.

The use of therapeutic replacement materials derived from blood carries some inherent risk. Hepatitis infection was a problem in the past. Infection with human immunodeficiency virus (HIV) unfortunately was frequently seen in patients who were exposed to multiple donors before the revision of blood donor screening tests and the use of heat-treated concentrates.

CANCER

Leukemias

Description. The leukemias represent a group of malignant hematologic diseases in which normal bone marrow elements are replaced by abnormal, poorly differentiated lymphocytes known as blast cells. Leukemias are classified according to cell type involvement (i.e., lymphocytic or non-lymphocytic) and by cellular differentiation. ALL is characterized by preponderantly undifferentiated WBCs.

Epidemiology. The leukemias are the most common form of childhood cancer and account for about one third of pediatric malignancies. ALL accounts for about 77% of cases, with a peak incidence between 2 and 6 years old. Acute myeloid leukemia (AML) accounts for about 11% of all cases. Most of the other leukemias are of the chronic myeloid form (Tubergen & Bleyer, 2004).

As with all types of malignancy, the exact cause of leukemia is unknown. Several factors associated with increased risk have been identified, including infection, radiation, chemical and drug exposure, and genetic factors.

Clinical Findings. Most of the clinical signs and symptoms of leukemia are related to leukemic replacement of the bone marrow and the absence of blood cell precursors. The child may be anemic, pale, listless, irritable, or chronically tired and have the following:
- A history of repeated infections
- Bleeding episodes characterized by epistaxis, petechiae, and hematomas
- Lymphadenopathy and hepatosplenomegaly
- Bone and joint pain

All these symptoms may be vague or nonspecific, in which case it is important for the provider to have a high index of suspicion for cancer.

Diagnostic Tests. The following are used to diagnose leukemia:
- CBC with differential WBC, platelet, and reticulocyte counts. Thrombocytopenia is present in up to 85% of cases, and anemia is also usually present. WBC count may be elevated, normal, or low with varying levels of neutropenia.
- Peripheral smear, which may demonstrate malignant cells.
- Bone marrow examination, which shows an infiltration of blast cells replacing normal elements of the marrow.

Further classification regarding cell type, morphologic characteristics, and cell surface markers is generally made at the cancer treatment center to which the child is referred.

Management. The treatment program for most types of acute leukemia involves a 28-day induction phase (usually with vincristine, prednisone, and L-asparaginase), with the goal of inducing a complete remission and restoring normal hematopoiesis. This is followed by a consolidation phase of therapy and a maintenance phase of therapy. Chemotherapy, central nervous system (CNS) therapy (cranial irradiation or intrathecal administration of chemotherapy), and systemic administration of corticosteroids are the key interventions used. The need for cranial radiation as part of therapy is decreasing. For children with ALL who relapse, the need for allogeneic stem cell transplantation is not considered until the second complete remission. However, children with the Philadelphia chromosome or those who are not in remission by the end of the first induction phases are considered high risk for relapse with the resultant need to consider transplantation sooner. For those with AML, allogeneic stem cell transplantation is considered in the first complete remission (Franklin & Steinherz, 2006). Approximately 75%

to 80% of children diagnosed with ALL are now thought to be curable. Key genetic features are now identifiable. The role of the primary care provider is crucial to facilitate proper referrals and effective interdisciplinary communication and to assist the family in their coping and adaptation processes.

Long-term sequelae of cancer therapy for ALL have been identified in research studies and include effects on cognition and neuropsychological functioning. CNS irradiation has been linked to learning disabilities and impaired IQ, especially in children younger than 5 years old who also received intrathecal therapy. As a result, cranial radiation dosages have been reduced, and earlier neuropsychological testing is recommended. Other documented potential late effects of ALL treatment include congestive heart failure, avascular necrosis, and osteoporosis (Meck et al, 2006). A discussion of late effects of the gamete of common childhood cancers is further discussed at the end of this chapter.

Risk-directed treatment based on high-risk features at diagnosis (i.e., WBC count, age, cytogenetics, response to therapy, immunophenotype, CNS status, ethnic background, and gender), response to chemotherapy, and transplantation options has drastically improved cure rates. It is hoped that the incidence and severity of late-term effects will likewise diminish (Franklin & Steinherz, 2006).

Lymphomas

Non-Hodgkin Lymphoma

Description. The non-Hodgkin lymphomas (NHLs) are a diverse group of solid tumors of the lymphatic tissues that form from malignant proliferation of T cells, B cells, or indeterminate lymphocyte cells. Different classification systems have been used. In pediatrics, the common types of NHL are small noncleaved cell lymphoma (Burkitt and non-Burkitt subtypes, B-cell origin), lymphoblastic lymphoma, and large cell lymphoma (Gilchrist, 2004).

Epidemiology. The incidence rate in children younger than 20 years old is 10.5 per 1 million white children compared with 7.3 per 1 million black children (Gilchrist, 2004). NHL occurs most frequently in children during the second decade of life and infrequently under 3 years old. It is the most frequent malignancy in children with acquired immunodeficiency syndrome (National Cancer Institute (*www.cancer.gov/cancertopics/pdq/treatment/child-non-hodgkins/healthprofessional*).

Clinical Findings. The most common site of origin is in the lymphoid structures of the intestinal tract. The most common manifestations in children are (1) acute abdomen, including abdominal pain, distention, fullness, and constipation, and (2) nontender lymph node enlargement. Histologic differences account for varying disease sites; lymphoblastic NHL often present as intrathoracic tumors; in contrast, small noncleaved cell lymphomas present in 80% of U.S. cases. Other sites include the CNS and the bone marrow (Gilchrist, 2004).

Diagnostic Tests. Diagnostic studies are ordered depending on the location of the lymphoma and symptoms. They include chest radiograph, computed tomography (CT) or magnetic resonance imaging scan or positron emission tomography of the area in question, gallium and/or bone scan, bone marrow aspirates and biopsies, lumbar puncture with CNS fluid analysis, CBC, liver function tests, lactate dehydrogenase, uric acid and electrolyte levels, and 8-hour creatinine clearance if indicated (Gilchrist, 2004).

Management. The diagnosis is confirmed by surgical biopsy, and the extent of the disease process can be determined by scans, bone marrow aspiration, and lumbar puncture. Because of rapid developments in treatment and the importance of careful histologic evaluation, these children should be referred to a major pediatric cancer center for care.

Lymphomas are sensitive to chemotherapy. Cranial irradiation or intrathecal chemotherapy is part of the treatment plan if CNS involvement is present. Maintenance therapy may be continued for 6 months to 2 years. The prognosis has improved dramatically over the past few years. For early-stage disease in which the disease is localized, 90% of patients can expect long-term disease-free survival. Patients with more extensive disease may have a 70% to 80% failure-free survival rate (Albano et al, 2005).

Hodgkin Disease

Description. Like the NHLs, Hodgkin disease is a malignancy of the lymph nodes. It usually originates in a cervical lymph node and spreads to other lymph node regions and, if left untreated, to organ systems, including liver, spleen, bone, bone marrow, and brain. Unlike in NHL, involvement of the bone marrow and CNS is rare (Gilchrist, 2004). Clinical and pathologic staging of the disease is usually done by specialists according to the Ann Arbor staging criteria.

Epidemiology. Hodgkin disease represents 50% of the lymphomas of childhood. It is rare in children younger than 5 years old. Sixty percent of children with Hodgkin disease are between 10 and 16 years old (Albano et al, 2005).

Clinical Findings. The most common manifestations of Hodgkin disease include the following:

- Painless enlargement of the lymph nodes, usually in the cervical area; the nodes may feel firm, are often matted together, and are nontender to palpation.
- Chronic cough if the trachea is compressed by a large mediastinal mass.
- Fever, decreased appetite, weight loss, and night sweats.

Diagnostic Tests. Hematologic findings are often normal, but may include the following:

- Anemia
- Elevated or depressed leukocytes or platelets
- Elevated sedimentation rate and serum copper level
- Abnormal liver function test results

Management. The diagnosis is confirmed by histologic examination of an excised lymph node, followed by bone marrow studies and gallium scans to determine the extent of the disease. The child should receive treatment at a pediatric oncology center in collaboration with the primary provider. Optimal results are obtained through irradiation and chemotherapy with numerous agents. Children with Hodgkin disease have a better response to treatment than do adults, with a 75% overall survival rate at more than 20 years follow-up (Albano et al, 2005).

LATE EFFECTS OF CHILDHOOD CANCERS

Late effects of childhood cancers can be attributed to radiation therapy, chemotherapy, or a combination of both. Common problems have been identified, and pediatric survivors of cancer need to be monitored for these issues. Problems need to be identified early and promptly addressed. They can include the following (Meck et al, 2006):

- Short stature from cranial irradiation and intensive chemotherapy.
- Avascular necrosis of the bone caused by high-dose steroid therapy—more pronounced in young children—and with local irradiation.
- Osteoporosis from cranial irradiation, glucocorticoids, and antimetabolites.
- Encephalopathy resulting from cranial irradiation, methotrexate, glucocorticoids.
- Peripheral neuropathy and hearing loss from cisplatin.
- Cognitive dysfunction, stroke, and seizures from intrathecal chemotherapy, certain systemic chemotherapy agents, and radiation.
- Vision, auditory, and skeletal changes from head and neck radiation.
- Obesity and gonadal dysfunction resulting from a neuroendocrine effect.
- Potential alterations in pubertal development and gonadal function if given high-dose alkylating agents, especially in puberty and to girls.
- Cardiomyopathy and arrhythmias if given anthracyclines. Children given these drugs are at risk for this problem. They need to be educated just before their teen years about avoiding alcohol, which increases the likelihood of cardiotoxicity, and cautioned about cigarette smoking.
- Pulmonary fibrosis from chest and thorax radiation and with such chemotherapy agents as bleomycin, carmustine.
- Malignant glioma associated with cranial irradiation and sarcomas association with musculoskeletal radiation.
- Second leukemias (usually AML) associated with therapy with alkylating agents and epipodophyllotoxins.
- Glomerular or tubular injury, renal insufficiency with heavy metals (e.g., cisplatin).
- Infertility and early menopause with alkylator therapy.
- Cystitis or bladder dysfunction with cyclophosphamide.
- Delayed recovery of normal immune function (may need readministration of immunization).
- Psychosocial effects associated with chronic illness.
- Relapse of ALL.
- Possibility of hepatitis C virus infection if the child had a blood transfusion before 1992.

All survivors of childhood cancers need regular health care supervision from a provider who is aware of their prior treatment modalities and knowledgeable of late effects, aware of their risk of occurrence, and comfortable with risk-based monitoring for such problems (Meck et al, 2006).

RESOURCE BOX

Hematologic Disorders

Cooley's Anemia Foundation
www.cooleysanemia.org

Curesearch
National Childhood Cancer Foundation
www.curesearch.org

Leukemia and Lymphoma Society
www.leukemia.org

National Hemophilia Foundation
www.hemophilia.org

Sickle Cell Disease Association of America, Inc.
www.sicklecelldisease.org

☑ DISCUSSION FORUM

1. A 15-month-old has mild pallor. A spun Hgb is 9.5. What is your approach to this child?
2. A 2-month-old is identified during newborn screening with sickle cell anemia. How would you manage this patient at 2 months, 2 years, 6 years, and at 13 years old. What are the issues for each stage in development? Where would you refer this child? How would you coordinate the care of this child?
3. A 2-week-old formula-fed African-American male has a normal direct bilirubin and liver function tests but a total bilirubin of 5. What lab tests would be diagnostic for this patient?
4. An afebrile 10-year-old has new onset of petechiae. Her labs show a normal CBC except for a platelet count of 30,000, a normal PT, and PTT. What is your next step in the management of the patient?
5. How are you going to work with a hematologist in the co-management of patient with chronic hematological problems? What is the primary care provider's role in the management of children with chronic hematologic diseases?

REFERENCES

Albano E et al: Neoplastic disease. In Hay W et al, editors: *Current pediatric diagnosis and treatment,* ed 17, New York, 2005, Lange Medical Books/McGraw-Hill.

Altman A: Hemolytic anemias. In Burg F et al, editors: *Gellis and Kagan's current pediatric therapy,* ed 17, Philadelphia, 2002, WB Saunders.

Ambruso, D et al: Hematologic disorders. In Hay W et al, editors: *Current pediatric diagnosis and treatment,* ed 17, New York, 2005, McGraw-Hill.

American Academy of Pediatrics (AAP), Committee on Genetics: Health supervision for children with sickle cell disease, *Pediatrics* 1009:526-535, 2002.

American Academy of Pediatrics (AAP), Committee on Practice and Ambulatory Medicine: Recommendations for preventative pediatric health care, *Pediatrics* 105:645, 2000.

Aster J: The hematopoietic and lymphoid systems. In Kumar V, Cotran R, Robbins S, editors: *Robbins basic pathology,* ed 6, Philadelphia, 2003, WB Saunders.

Berkow, RL, Schwartz JH: Hemolytic anemias. In Burg F et al, editors: *Current pediatric therapy,* ed 18, Philadelphia, 2006, Elsevier.

Briones M, Abshire T: Disorders of coagulation, platelet number and function. In Burg F et al, editors: *Current pediatric therapy,* ed 18, Philadelphia, 2006, Elsevier.

Carroll B, Record E: Sickle cell disease. In Jackson P, Vessey J, editors: *Primary care of the child with a chronic condition,* ed 4, St Louis, 2004, Mosby.

Drake MR, Rutecki GW: Thrombocytopenia: how best to determine the cause, *Consultant* 46(1):105-112, 2006.

Franklin A, Steinherz P: Acute leukemia. In Burg F et al, editors: *Current pediatric therapy,* ed 18, Philadelphia, 2006, Elsevier.

Friedman D, Freyer D, Levitt G: Models of care for survivors of childhood cancer, *Pediatr Blood Cancer* 46:159-168, 2005.

Fuleihan R: Immunology. In Kliegman R et al, editors: *Nelson essentials of pediatrics,* ed 5, Philadelphia, 2006, Elsevier Saunders.

Gilchrist GS: Lymphoma. In Behrman R, Kliegman R, Jenson H, editors: *Nelson textbook of pediatrics,* ed 16, Philadelphia, 2004, WB Saunders.

Glader B: Anemias of inadequate production. In Behrman R, Kliegman R, Jenson H, editors: *Nelson textbook of pediatrics,* ed 17, Philadelphia, 2004, WB Saunders.

Guyton A, Hall J: *Textbook of medical physiology,* ed 11, Philadelphia, 2006, WB Saunders.

Hagani A, Bussel J: Hemophilia. In Finberg L, Kleinman R, editors: *Saunders manual of pediatric practice,* ed 2, Philadelphia, 2002, WB Saunders.

Hilliard LM, Howard TH: Sickle cell disorders. In Burg F et al, editors: *Current pediatric therapy,* ed 18, Philadelphia, 2006, Elsevier.

Markowitz, M: Lead poisoning. In Behrman R, Kliegman R, Jenson H, editors: *Nelson textbook of pediatrics,* ed 17, Philadelphia, 2004, WB Saunders.

McPherson M, Tender J: Iron deficiency anemia. In Burg F et al, editors: *Current pediatric therapy,* ed 18, Philadelphia, 2006, Elsevier.

Meck MM, Leary M, Sills RH: Late effects in survivors of childhood cancer, *Pediatr Rev* 27:257-262, 2006.

Mitchell R, Cotran R: Acute and chronic inflammation. In Kumar V, Cotran R, Robbins S, editors: *Robbins basic pathology,* ed 6, Philadelphia, 2003, Saunders.

Montgomery RR, Scott JP: Hemorrhagic and thrombotic diseases. In Behrman R, Kliegman R, Jenson H, editors: *Nelson textbook of pediatrics,* ed 17, Philadelphia, 2004, WB Saunders.

National Cancer Institute-U.S. National Institutes of Health: *Childhood non-Hodgkin lymphoma: treatment.* Available at *www.cancer.gov/cancertopics/pdq/treatment/child-non-hodgkins/healthprofessional* (accessed Oct 24, 2007).

Quirolo K, Vichinsky E: Hemoglobin disorders. In Behrman R, Kliegman R, Jenson H, editors: *Nelson textbook of pediatrics,* ed 17, Philadelphia, 2004, WB Saunders.

Qureshi N, Vichinsky E: Thalassemia. In Burg F et al, editors: *Current pediatric therapy,* ed 18, Philadelphia, 2006, Elsevier.

Scott JP: Hematology. In Kliegman R et al, editors: *Nelson essentials of pediatrics,* ed 5, Philadelphia, 2006, Elsevier Saunders.

Segel G: Hereditary spherocytosis. In Behrman R, Kliegman R, Jenson H, editors: *Nelson textbook of pediatrics,* ed 16, Philadelphia, 2004, WB Saunders.

Segel G, Hirsh M, Feig S: Managing anemia in a pediatric office practice: part 1, *Pediatr Rev* 23:75-83, 2002a.

Segel G, Hirsh M, Feig S: Managing anemia in a pediatric office practice: part 2, *Pediatr Rev* 23:111-121, 2002b.

Stoll, BJ: Infections of the neonatal infant. In Behrman R, Kliegman R, Jenson H, editors: *Nelson textbook of pediatrics,* ed 16, Philadelphia, 2004, WB Saunders.

Sulis M, Morris E, Cairo M: Neonatal and childhood neutropenia. In Burg F et al, editors: *Current pediatric therapy,* ed 18, Philadelphia, 2006, Elsevier.

Tubergen DG, Bleyer A: The leukemias. In Behrman R, Kliegman R, Jenson H, editors: *Nelson textbook of pediatrics,* ed 17, Philadelphia, 2004, WB Saunders.

Wu A, Lesperance L, Bernstein H: Screening for iron deficiency, *Pediatr Rev* 23:171-177, 2002.

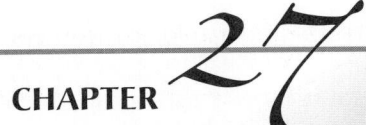
Neurologic Disorders

Catherine G. Blosser and Melissa Reider-Demer

Neurologic disorders in children are difficult for primary care providers to adequately diagnose, monitor, and medically manage. Central nervous system (CNS) problems can affect many systems and present in many ways. No other body system has as much influence on a child's development. The presenting problems may range from subtle to extreme. These CNS alterations have profound effects on the lives of children and their families. The medical care provider needs to be able to screen and identify neurologic problems; know when to appropriately refer to other health care resources; be able to monitor the general health of the patient; advocate for regional centers; serve as a case manager based upon the myriad of school and health care issues; and support families as they deal with the challenges of grief and long-term care. The coordination of resources is essential for better patient outcomes.

◼ ANATOMY AND PHYSIOLOGY

ANATOMY

An understanding of the anatomy and physiology of the brain is imperative to fully appreciate the brain's unique functional capabilities and pathway processes. The nervous system is divided into two parts: the CNS and the peripheral nervous system (PNS). The CNS consists of the brain and spinal cord. The PNS is made up of a network of afferent nerves and sense organs, which send information to the brain, and the efferent nerves, which send information out to the body for responses. Descending tracts from the brain to the gray matter of the spinal cord include the extrapyramidal tract, which conveys information from the cerebellum to the motor cells of the anterior column, and the pyramidal tract, which is the main motor pathway from the cerebral cortex to the spinal nerves and carries messages for voluntary movement. Most pyramidal tract fibers cross in the medulla, so the left half of the brain controls the right side of the body and vice versa. The anatomic units of the brain and their functions are listed in Table 27-1 and shown in Figs. 27-1 and 27-2.

AUTONOMIC NERVOUS SYSTEM

The autonomic nervous system (ANS) also involves CNS and PNS components and includes sympathetic, parasympathetic, and enteric systems. The sympathetic system begins in the thoracolumbar area of the spinal cord and extends distally; its function is often referred to as the "fight or flight" reaction. The parasympathetic system begins in the medulla and midbrain with relays to the thalamus and higher centers;

it stimulates the rest and relaxation reaction. The principal sympathetic system neurotransmitters are epinephrine and norepinephrine. The parasympathetic fibers produce acetylcholine. The two systems function in balance—one excites whereas the other inhibits (Box 27-1). The enteric system is a component of the ANS, but does not play a role specifically in neurology. This system consists of a meshwork of nerve fibers that innervate the digestive system.

PHYSIOLOGY

Nerve impulses are transmitted along a nerve fiber through changes in polarization of the membrane, during which electrical activity is produced. Certain chemicals diffuse across the synapses between nerves and end organs. The primary transmitter is acetylcholine; however, other transmitters, including norepinephrine and dopamine, are also important.

◼ PATHOPHYSIOLOGY AND DEFENSE MECHANISMS

PATHOPHYSIOLOGY

The nervous system is so intimately related to functioning of the entire body that problems in any part of the system can have neurologic implications. For example, seizures result from uncontrolled firing of cerebral neurons. Coma results from the inability of cerebral neurons to fire or the inability of the CNS to process stimuli and respond accordingly. Paralysis occurs when the peripheral nerves are unable to respond or do not receive signals through the pyramidal system of afferent and efferent nerves. Of course, more specific problems occur when special areas of the nervous system or individual nerves are damaged. Broad incapacity occurs with neurotransmitter problems.

Systemic Problems

The brain is extremely sensitive to changes in physiology anywhere in the body. Thus, any metabolic change, whether from external or internal factors, affects the CNS. Examples include delirium from toxins and diabetic coma.

Genetic Problems

All chromosomal defects are associated with some neurologic effects because they are disorders involving many genes. Some of the single-gene defects may have direct neurologic effects (such as neurofibromatosis), whereas others, typically inborn errors of metabolism, can have indirect effects via the abnormal metabolites released (e.g., phenylketonuria).

TABLE 27-1	Anatomic Units of the Nervous System and Functions
Anatomic Unit	**Functions**
I. Central nervous system	
A. Brain	
1. Forebrain—cerebrum	
a. Cortex (gray matter)	Posterior—motor skills
1) Frontal area	Anterior—decision-making, emotions, memory, judgment, ethics, abstract thinking
	Broca's area—speech
2) Parietal area	Sensory integration, language, reading, writing, pattern recognition
3) Temporal area	Memory storage, auditory processing, olfaction, limbic system in deep temporal lobe—arousal
4) Occipital area	Visual processing
b. Diencephalon	
1) Thalamus	Receives and sorts sensory input, modulates motor impulses from cortex
2) Hypothalamus	Integrates autonomic functions
2. Midbrain	Connects brain with cerebellum, pons, medulla
3. Hindbrain	
a. Pons	Bridges cerebellum, medulla, midbrain; cranial nerves V, VI, VIII arise here
b. Medulla	Proximal end of spinal cord; contains reticular system—arousal; cranial nerves IX–XII arise here
c. Cerebellum	Coordination and movement; balance; smooth movements
B. Cranial nerves	Sensory and motor components; olfaction; vision; hearing; facial, tongue, pharyngeal, eye, shoulder movements
II. Spinal cord	
A. Dorsal roots	Afferent sensory fibers
B. Ventral roots	Efferent motor fibers
III. Protective layers	
A. Meninges	Protection of delicate nervous tissues
B. Ventricles	
C. Cerebrospinal fluid	

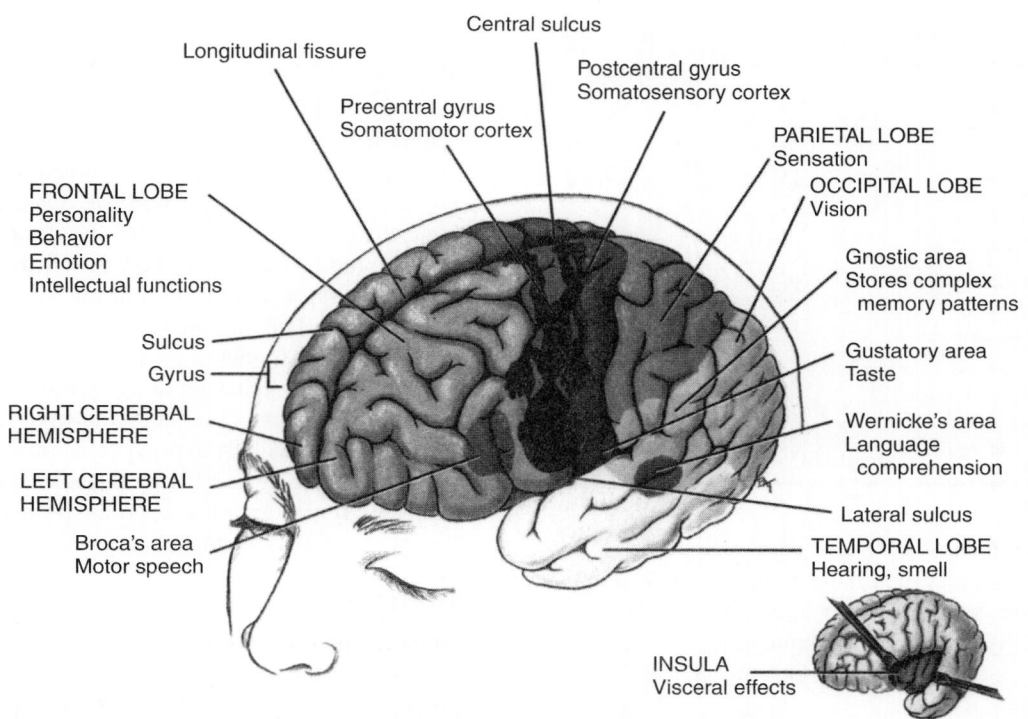

FIG. 27-1 Lobes and functional areas of the cerebrum. (From Polaski AL: *Luckmann's core principles and practice of medical-surgical nursing*, Philadelphia, 1996, WB Saunders, p. 245.)

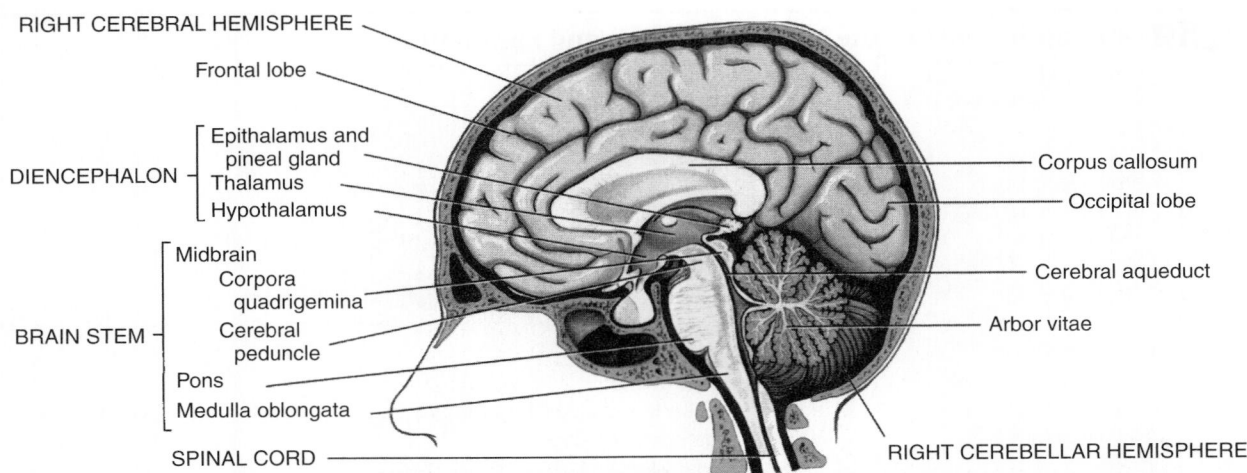

RIGHT CEREBRAL HEMISPHERE

Frontal lobe

DIENCEPHALON
- Epithalamus and pineal gland
- Thalamus
- Hypothalamus

Corpus callosum

Occipital lobe

BRAIN STEM
- Midbrain
  - Corpora quadrigemina
  - Cerebral peduncle
- Pons
- Medulla oblongata

Cerebral aqueduct

Arbor vitae

SPINAL CORD

RIGHT CEREBELLAR HEMISPHERE

FIG. 27-2 Midsagittal section of the brain showing the major portions of the diencephalon, brainstem, and cerebellum. (From Polaski AL: *Luckmann's core principles and practice of medical-surgical nursing*, Philadelphia, 1996, WB Saunders.)

BOX 27-1 **Autonomic Nervous System: Parasympathetic and Sympathetic Functions**

Parasympathetic System
Pupil constriction
Increased saliva
Lacrimal gland vasodilation
Coronary vessel vasoconstriction
Bronchial muscle constriction
Stomach peristalsis
Colon peristalsis
Genitalia vasodilation
Urinary bladder constriction
Skin vessel dilation

Sympathetic System
Pupil dilation
Decreased saliva
Coronary vessel vasodilation
Bronchial muscle relaxation
Stomach constriction
Adrenaline secretion
Colon relaxation
Sphincter relaxation
Sphincter constriction
Genitalia vasoconstriction
Urinary bladder relaxation
Skin vessel constriction

Congenital Defects

Because the CNS is structurally complex, there are many opportunities for defects to occur in utero. Examples of such defects include hydrocephaly and spina bifida.

Injuries

Head and spinal cord injuries are common and can have long-term, serious consequences for the child. Such complex

neurologic tissue does not always heal in a way that results in full recovery of function(s).

DEFENSE MECHANISMS

Peripheral nerves can regenerate somewhat if conditions are right. In the spinal cord, the axons of injured neurons cannot regrow within the cord, but they can grow in peripheral nerves outside the cord. In this case, if the cut ends are reconnected with special attention to the myelin sheath, regeneration of the injured nerve begins at the proximal end of the neuron soon after injury. The growth rate is approximately 2.5 to 3 mm per day (Menkes & Moser 2006).

■ ASSESSMENT OF THE NERVOUS SYSTEM

Assessment of the nervous system requires a careful history of the patient and family, and a detailed physical examination is essential. The examiner needs to determine (1) if a neurologic disorder exists, (2) where the disorder is located, and (3) the process that most likely produces the symptoms and affects the suspected location of the dysfunction (Menkes & Moser, 2006). For children with complex or severe neurologic problems, social, environmental, developmental, and family issues need thorough exploration. Historical information from patients more than 3 years old and from one or more family members is most likely to provide the most accurate picture of the issues. Imaging or laboratory studies may be required. See Chapter 2 for information regarding disease assessment, daily living, and developmental history.

HISTORY

Neurologic Disease History
- History of present illness:
  - Onset. When did the first symptoms appear? Was the onset insidious or sudden? Was it associated with any injury, or strain, or recent exacerbating event? If yes, describe the

trauma. Was the onset accompanied by any constitutional symptoms? How has the disorder evolved?

- Pain and/or headache. Location and character, path of radiation, severity, extent of disability produced, effect of various activities or stimuli (including light sensitivity), relief measures, changes from day to night, effects of previous treatment, presence of pain or discomfort in other parts of the body.
- Sensory deficits. Changes in hearing, vision, taste, loss of pain sensation, vertigo, dizziness.
- Injury. How, when (time and date), why, where, mechanism or manner in which the injury was produced. Immediate treatment provided.
- Reflexive responses. Vomiting, coughing, primitive reflexes, tics.
- Behavioral changes. Irritability, stupor, changes in appetite, lack of attention, random activity, emotional lability, changes in school performance.
- Motor and balance changes. Ataxia, spasticity, increased or decreased tone.
- Medical history:
  - Prenatal history: Maternal and paternal ages, alcohol, drug ingestion, radiation exposure, nutrition, prenatal care, injuries, hyperthermia, smoking, human immunodeficiency virus (HIV) exposure, maternal illness, bleeding, toxemia, diabetes, previous abortions and stillbirths.
  - Birth history and neonatal course: Complications, labor and delivery, resuscitation, trauma, congenital anomalies, feeding history (reflux, colic, frequent formula changes), jaundice, convulsions, infection, gestational age, sleep disturbances.
  - Injuries or infections. Meningitis, encephalitis, head injuries, seizures—types, frequency, medications; frequent musculoskeletal injuries (can suggest coordination or impulsive behavior).
  - Cardiovascular or respiratory disorders.
  - Environmental or drug exposure. Consider lead exposure.
  - Metabolic disorders. Diabetes mellitus, thyroid disease. Hypoglycemia causes confusion, convulsion, loss of consciousness. Hyperglycemia causes lethargy, coma. Hyperthyroidism causes tremor. Hypothyroidism causes weakness, coma.
  - Past neurologic disease and tests. Tics, hydrocephaly.
  - Psychiatric disorders. Hallucinations, delusions, and illusions.
  - Drug ingestion.
  - Urinary tract disease. Uremic syndrome manifests with confusion, convulsions, coma.
  - Physical growth.
- Family disease history:
  - Family members with similar symptoms or genetic disorders; consider obtaining a pedigree.
  - Consanguinity.
  - Migraine history.
  - Mental functioning of family members.

- Review *all* systems plus:
  - Growth pattern, including height, weight, body mass index (BMI), and head circumference.
  - Allergies, medications, immunizations, hearing, vision, dental, skin integrity, behavior, nutritional status, and eating disorders are all important areas to assess.

Developmental History

Achievement of all developmental milestones—language, gross motor, fine motor, social, and cognitive—and school performance should be reviewed. The Denver Developmental Screening Test II and WIDA-ACCESS Placement tests (W-APT) are often used to monitor these milestones. Inquire about developmental changes, loss of skills, and lack of progression.

Functional Health

Inquire about the effects of symptoms on all areas of health promotion and safety, nutrition, elimination, activity, communication, role relationships, values and beliefs, sexuality, sleep, coping (management style) and stress tolerance, temperament, and self-concept. The "management style" of family members is crucial to assess because it suggests how different family members may react over time to any chronic illness of their child (Jackson Allen & Vessey, 2004). Management styles and "chronic sorrow" are discussed more fully in Chapters 10 and 18.

Social Context

Because neurologic problems can have such profound, chronic consequences on the child and family, it is important to understand the social context of the child and family. Inquire about the family composition, home environment, stressors, strengths, resources, financial issues, identified social supports (e.g., family, friends, health professionals), and community agencies involved with the family and child (Menkes & Moser, 2006). Race and ethnicity need to be explored since they can influence family perceptions and attitudes towards social support networks (Jackson Allen & Vessey, 2004).

PHYSICAL EXAMINATION

A complete physical examination is always important. The following should be noted:

- Abnormalities of the skin (café au lait lesions, angiomas, other pigmentation changes)
- Anomalies
- Low-set ears
- Cardiovascular system (including blood pressure)
- Musculoskeletal system
- Hearing
- Vision; eye problems, including cataract, corneal clouding, cherry-red spot
- Head circumference, growth measurements
- Tanner stage
- Hepatomegaly

Neurologic Examination

The provider conducting the neurologic examination moves from the highest level of functioning to the lowest. Cerebral function is tested first; then cranial nerves, motor function, and sensory function; and finally reflexes. The neonate's neurologic functioning is largely subcortical. Therefore, the examination is more limited than in an older infant or child. In infants and children, watching them carefully while collecting the history and actively playing with them provides a great deal of neurologic information. A tennis ball, some small toys (e.g., a small car), a bell, and something that attracts attention (e.g., pinwheel) are useful throughout the examination (Menkes & Moser, 2006).

Behavior and Mental Status. Test the following cortical functions through evaluation of behavior and mental status:

- Responsiveness
- Judgment
- Language and speech (receptive, expressive, written)
- Memory
- General knowledge
- Ability to relate to others
- Mood and affect

The level of consciousness is also a CNS function and includes speech flow, voice quality, and organization of thoughts.

Cranial Nerve Function. Cranial nerves I through XII are tested. Vision (cranial nerve II) is indicated by blinking in response to a bright light. In the neonate, Cranial nerves III, IV, and VI can be tested by assessing the ability to track through the visual fields. Facial grimaces test for cranial nerves V and VII. Hearing (cranial nerve VIII) can be tested with a small bell. The gag reflex tests cranial nerves IX and X. The olfactory nerve (cranial nerve I) is not functional until 5 to 7 months old, but inhaled irritants (e.g., ammonia, vinegar) will produce a reaction in cranial nerve V in newborns (Menkes & Moser, 2006).

Motor Examination. When conducting the motor examination, look for symmetry and quality of movement. Gait, posture, coordination, balance, strength, and tone are all aspects of this examination.

- Muscle strength and size. Look at muscle size and contour. Look for symmetry. Have the child stand from a lying position. Look for Gower's sign (i.e., a child using the arms to push off from bent knees and gradually climbing the body and straightening up, which is common in children with muscular dystrophy). Ask the child to move extremities against resistance and to grip your fingers hard.
- Muscle tone. Muscle tone might be considered the resting strength of the muscle. Is the trunk or are the extremities floppy, rigid, or somewhat stiff when the child is resting? How difficult is it to move body parts passively? Tone may be increased or decreased all over or differ between the legs and the trunk and arms.
- Fine motor coordination. Fine motor coordination is tested by having the child pick up small pellets, write, stack blocks, cut with scissors, turn book pages, or do other hand activities.
- Involuntary movements. Tremors are fine involuntary movements. Chorea or choreiform movements are large, irregular

jerking and writhing movements. Athetoid movements are slow writhing movements, especially of the hands and feet. Dystonia is an uncontrolled change in tone with movement and a tendency to hyperextend the joints.

- The reflexes involve a combination of motor functioning and transmission of nerve impulses from various parts of the body to the spine and brain and back again. When a reflex is abnormal, the question is why. Did the impulse not go through, or did the child have a problem in the ability to move responsively because of either efferent signals or problems of muscle tissue contractility? The reflexes and their testing are described later.
- In an infant, assessing posture and muscle tone is fundamental. Motor testing should include observation for symmetry of movements, consistent fisting of the hands, opisthotonos, scissoring, abnormal tone, and tremors. The infant's cry can be an indicator of several diseases (e.g., it is high pitched with increased intracranial pressure, resembles mewing in cri du chat syndrome, and is hoarse with hypothyroidism).

Sensory Examination. Examine for pain sensation and stereognosis. This part of the examination is always limited in infants and young children. Use a light pinprick to check for mild pain sensation.

Reflexes. The types of reflexes tested include deep tendon, superficial, and primitive reflexes.

- Deep tendon reflexes include the biceps, brachioradialis, triceps, patellar, and Achilles.
- Superficial reflexes include the upper abdominal, lower abdominal, cremasteric, gluteal, and plantar.
- Primitive reflexes include sucking, rooting, asymmetric tonic neck, grasp, trunk incurvation, stepping, and others found in Table 27-2. These primitive reflexes can be absent or decreased in a satiated or sleepy infant. Tendon reflexes can be tested as in an older child. Babinski sign is not helpful in an infant. In older children and adults, its presence is an important sign of upper motor neuron disease.

Cranium Examination. The neurologic examination should always include measurement of head circumference and inspection of the skull for symmetry and shape. In the infant, the cranium can also be transilluminated with a flashlight outfitted with a rubber adaptor to look for structural or brain development problems (e.g., absence of cortical tissue). Auscultation over the skull or above the eyes can reveal a cranial bruit. Percussion of the skull can give a sound resembling a cracked pot when the sutures are separated, as with increased intracranial pressure. The anterior fontanelle should normally be slightly depressed with very faintly perceived pulsations.

Autonomic Nervous System. Alterations in blood pressure, sweating, or body temperature can be indicators of ANS problems.

Meningeal Signs. Evidence of meningeal irritation, such as with meningitis, include positive Kernig and Brudzinski signs. A Kernig sign is positive if resistance and head or neck pain are elicited when the patient bends over from the waist and touches fingers to toes. A positive Brudzinski is evidenced by the patient spontaneously flexing the hip and knees after the

TABLE 27-2   Primitive Reflexes

Reflex	Age Appears	Age Disappears	How to Elicit	Response	Notes
Newborn Reflexes					
Rooting	Birth	3-4 mo	Head midline, stroke perioral area	Infant opens mouth and turns head to stimulated side	Absence indicates severe CNS disease or depressed infant; sleeping infant may not respond
Sucking	Birth	3-4 mo	Place nipple or finger 3-4 cm into mouth	Suck should be strong: push finger up and back; note rate	Absence indicates CNS depression; satiated or sleeping baby may not respond well
Asymmetric tonic neck (ATNR)	Birth	4-6 mo	With baby supine, rotate head to one side; hold 15 sec	Arm and leg extend on facial side; arm and leg on other side flex	Obligatory response when child cannot get out of position is abnormal; persistence beyond 4-6 mo indicates CNS lesion (e.g., CP)
Palmar grasp	Birth	3-6 mo	Place finger into infant's palm and press against palm	Infant flexes all fingers around examiner's finger	Grasp should be strong and symmetric
Trunk incurvation (Galant)	Birth	2 mo	Suspend baby prone; stroke 2-3 cm from spine with fingernail	Baby flexes toward stimulus	Asymmetry is significant; tests for spinal cord lesions; should not persist after 6 mo
Stepping	Birth	6-8 wk	Infant is held as though weight bearing with feet on surface	Infant steps along, raising one foot at a time	Tests brainstem, spinal column; absence indicates paralysis or depressed baby
Moro	Birth	4 mo	Present loud noise or allow infant's head to drop slightly	Arms spread and fingers extend and then flex; then arms come toward each other; cry is possible	Asymmetry indicates paralysis or fractured clavicle, absence indicates brainstem problem, usually severe; persistence also abnormal
Crossed extension	0-4 mo		Passively extend one leg and press knee to table; prick sole of that foot with pin	Other leg should slightly extend and adduct	
Plantar grasp	Birth	8-10 mo	Place finger firmly against base of toes	Toes should curl down	Tests S1-S2 spinal nerves; lessens by 8 mo, suspect any asymmetry
Later Reflexes					
Landau	3 mo	15 mo-2 yr	Suspend infant prone by supporting abdomen	Infant should lift both head and legs	Abnormal if arm tone increased with internal rotation, arm held at side, or arm does not lift as noted
Neck righting	6 mo	2 yr	With infant supine, turn head to one side	Infant's trunk rotates in direction of head	Absent or decreased can indicate spasticity; can also rotate trunk and then look for head to follow; tests midbrain
Parachute	6-8 mo	Never	Suspend infant prone and lower quickly toward table	Infant should extend arms, hands, fingers	Response should be symmetric and "protective"

CNS, Central nervous system; CP, cerebral palsy; mo, month(s); yr, year(s).

examiner passively flexes the neck. In an infant, Kernig can be tested by extending the leg at the knee with the infant lying supine. A positive sign can be as subtle as facial grimacing.

DIAGNOSTIC STUDIES

- Radiographs have relatively little diagnostic value for the neurologic system since the advent of computed tomography (CT) and magnetic resonance imaging (MRI). CT scans display differences in density of the intracranial tissues and structures. An MRI can provide additional information related to aneurysms (e.g., hemorrhages, calcifications, abscesses), brain structure, and the cellular activity of various parts of the neurologic system (e.g., tumors, CNS, spinal cord, and malformations). Often times there may be a medical need to order more specific tests, such as a magnetic resonance angiogram (used to detect blood vessel stenosis and aneurysms) or functional magnetic resonance imaging (fMRI—used to detect subtle metabolic changes in the brain that indicate how certain parts of the brain are working). A neurologic consultant can advise when these would be necessary.
- Laboratory studies can provide indicators of systemic disease, infection, or inflammation. They are especially important for children receiving medication for seizures. Drug levels, liver function, and blood studies may need to be monitored routinely.
- Lumbar puncture provides a specimen of cerebrospinal fluid (CSF). The fluid provides information about metabolism, infections, and trauma within the CNS.
- The electroencephalogram (EEG) provides information about the electrical activity of the CNS, which is important in assessing function rather than structure.
- Ultrasonography can be useful in infants to evaluate brain tissue.
- Other studies can include polysomnography (helps assess narcolepsy, apnea of infancy, certain movement disorders, and nocturnal seizures); electromyography (tests muscle activity); nerve conduction studies; evoked responses (brainstem—auditory, somatosensory, and visual); electronystagmography (measures eye movements to assess vertigo and postconcussion syndrome); and cerebral arteriography (visualizes cerebral blood vessels to evaluate vascular anomalies and tumors).

■ MANAGEMENT STRATEGIES
COUNSELING

Counseling for neurologic problems involves several components. The family should understand the pathologic condition, including possible etiologies, and the treatment plan. Parents also need information about the prognosis with and without treatment and any genetic implications of the diagnosis. The latter can best be communicated through formal genetics counseling. Family members should have time to ask questions about all these issues.

Counseling also involves helping families cope with the diagnosis and its implications for the patient and family,

both short term and long term. Congenital problems are often identified at birth or shortly thereafter. Families need to receive diagnoses truthfully, compassionately, and promptly. Issues of etiology need to be addressed to relieve the guilt that some parents may feel about causing the problem. A plan of care needs to be mutually agreed on by the family and care provider before the infant or child is discharged from the hospital or clinic.

Using the sensitive, acceptable, appropriate terminology discussed below is crucial when discussing any physical limitation. Correct language can influence not only how parents relate to their child's condition but also communicate to others a more accurate reflection of the child's abilities (e.g., schools, employers).

- *Impairment:* existence of a deviation from normal movement or an inability to control an involuntary movement (one can be impaired without being disabled)
- *Disability:* a restriction in an ability to execute a normal activity of daily living that someone of similar age could execute (all people with disabilities are impaired)
- *Handicap:* existence of a disability that prevents the person from achieving a normal role in society that someone of a similar age is expected to achieve (all people with handicaps have disabilities)
- "*Extra needs*" versus "*special needs*" is a more socially acceptable and easily understood term to use when referring to a person.

ANTICIPATORY GUIDANCE
Neurologic Development

Families are sometimes concerned about problems that providers believe are within normal limits. In these situations, no neurology referral is necessary. The family needs to understand the anticipated pattern of neurologic development and be provided with time lines and markers that they can use to monitor their child's development. Misperceptions about the implications of minor variations need to be dealt with, and the family should always be given the opportunity to return for further assessment or discussion if concerns remain. The temperament of the child and the child's learned social behavior versus pathologic symptoms may need to be addressed (e.g., breath holding vs. seizures).

Educational Needs

Many neurologic problems in children affect learning, although neurologic problems are not synonymous with mental retardation. Sensory problems affect the child's ability to receive the input necessary for learning. Motor problems can affect both the child's ability to interact with the environment and the child's ability to communicate or indicate understanding. Management should always consider the educational needs of the child. Special infant or preschool early intervention educational programs can assist the child to learn by using the most appropriate learning modalities. Teachers often need assistance in understanding the limitations and strengths of the child.

Genetics Counseling

Many neurologic conditions are genetic in origin. See Chapter 40 for a discussion of genetics assessment and management, including counseling.

PHYSICAL, OCCUPATIONAL, AND SPEECH THERAPY

Physical therapy can be useful to help restore or maintain function or to teach new motor skills. The physical therapist should be accustomed to dealing with children. Physical services are often combined with occupational and speech therapy to promote maximal development. Early intervention programs offer such assistance in many states and are generally free to qualifying patients (e.g., in California there are regional centers that assist families with particular medical and physical resources). Should any services be denied, families should be advised to inquire about the appeal process for their state (e.g., in California each regional center has patient and family advocate representatives for legal counsel).

SOCIAL SERVICES

Children and families with children that experience multiple handicapping conditions frequently have ongoing issues of coping, monitoring, and management of medical and financial resources. Medical social workers and public health nurses can be a great help to these families for continuity and coordination of care.

MEDICATIONS

A variety of medications are used to control the effects of neurologic problems. These may include: antiepileptic drugs (AEDs), mood stabilizers, and antidepressants. Most require time for the effects to become apparent, need dose adjustments, and are affected by the metabolism of the individual child. Periodic measurement of blood levels is often needed. Side effects of medications need to be weighed against their beneficial effects. Many require tapering of dosages when treatment with the medication is to be discontinued. A variety of anticonvulsant medications are described later in this chapter in Table 27-5.

■ SPECIFIC NEUROLOGIC PROBLEMS OF CHILDREN

DEGENERATIVE DISORDERS

Degenerative disorders consist of a group of neurodegenerative disorders whose etiologies affect either the gray matter or white matter of the brain. Degenerative disorders are believed to be the result of biochemical or metabolic dysfunctions (in turn caused by genetic, immune-mediated demyelination or by unknown etiologies) that lead to anatomic or functional insults to major portions of the brain. These insults usually affect the basal ganglia, cerebellum, brainstem, spinal cord, peripheral and cranial nerves, or cerebrum. Such insults can also follow infections or an altered immune state.

Gray matter diseases involve neurons, and their onset is heralded by seizures, a decrease in cognitive functioning, and visual changes. Gray matter disorders include Menkes syndrome (also called kinky-hair syndrome), progressive infantile poliodystrophy, neuronal ceroid-lipofuscinoses, and Rett syndrome. White matter diseases usually lead to demyelination and are evidenced by decreasing motor skills, ataxia, and spasticity. White matter disorders include Schilder disease, acute disseminating encephalomyelitis, acute hemorrhagic leukoencephalitis, and multiple sclerosis.

The diagnosis is based on age of onset, clinical features, genetic transmission, and chemical and chromosomal studies. After identifying the major signs, symptoms, and developmental stage at which the disorder appeared, the following three steps provide a useful framework when considering etiology. The steps include: (1) determining pathogenesis (whether a genetic mechanism is involved, toxic exposure, trauma, infectious disease, or other environmental cause); (2) assessing which disease category might be involved (e.g., mitochondrial, lysozymal [lysosomal enzymes break down complex chemicals within cells; absence leads to a "storage disease" typified with developmental regression], and peroxisomal [peroxisomes are components of the cytoplasm and are indispensable for metabolism; dysfunction causes genetically heterogeneous metabolic diseases]); and (3) seeking, in the case of an inherited abnormality, a specific causative factor (e.g., an abnormal metabolite, defect with enzyme activity, mutated structural protein, gene defect, or chromosomal defect) (Brunstrom & Titan, 2005).

Only Rett syndrome and multiple sclerosis are discussed in this chapter.

Rett Syndrome

A mutation in the X-linked, methyl-CpG-binding protein 2 gene (MECP2) has been identified in 80% of females with classic Rett syndrome features (Liu & Francke, 2006). This gene contains instructions for protein synthesis of methyl cytosine–binding protein. MECP2 is abundant in the brain. When not disabled by mutation, it silences certain genes that control motion and emotion. This neurodevelopmental disorder was previously thought to affect only females and be lethal to males. However, there has been some reported variation to this X-linked Rett syndrome gene occurring in males that is not lethal and results in mental retardation and neurologic impairment (Johnston, 2004d). Defects in MECP2 have also been found in patients with autism, schizophrenia, learning disabilities, and neonatal encephalopathy (National Institute of Neurology Disorders and Stroke, 2006a).

Rather than cause brain degeneration, Rett syndrome arrests maturation of certain areas of the brain. Typically, the patient is female, with onset at 5 to 18 months old. Affected girls cease to gain developmental milestones. CNS irritability and withdrawal develop, and then these girls begin to lose skills, including speech and hand skills. Stereotypic hand movements, slowed head growth leading to microcephaly, autistic-like behavior, dementia, and disorganized breathing and apnea followed by hyperpnea occur. Seizures, scoliosis, and spastic paraparesis and quadriparesis are late developments in the syndrome.

Typically, DNA tests for presence of mutations in MECP2 are found to be about 80% accurate. This is likely attributed to the possibility that 20% to 30% of the affected patients inherit only a part of the gene that is affected, and it remains undetected with current laboratory testing.

Physical, occupational, and speech therapies and seizure management are important to preserve functional abilities. As with all neurodevelopmental problems, families need significant support and social services. Life expectancy varies (death usually occurs during adolescence or during the third decade) (Johnston, 2004d). Differential diagnoses include cerebral palsy (CP), autism, psychosis, and other neurodegenerative diseases.

Multiple Sclerosis

Description and Epidemiology. Multiple sclerosis (MS) is primarily an adult-diagnosed disease process. This disease occurs in 3% to 5% of children; it is exceptional to have symptoms occur before a child is 10 years old (0.2% to 2% of all cases). Twice as many females as males are affected. Worldwide, there are 2.5 million individuals with MS, and 400,000 cases within the U.S. It is widely believed that MS is an immune-mediated disease. Macrophages, activated T lymphocytes, and other destructive molecules are stimulated by yet not fully understood events. These inflammatory cells cause both demyelination and axon damage within the white brain matter. The biologic basis for the disease is not clear; proposals include environmental, infectious, toxic, immunologic, or genetic causes. No specific virus has been isolated. Some scientists propose that it is multifactorial. Epidemiologic data support the view that MS is caused or triggered by environmental factors in persons who are genetically sensitive (Greenburg & Kerr, 2006). The initial axonal injury in MS was not fully appreciated until newer imaging devices and staining techniques allowed closer scrutiny on the molecular level.

It is now clear that repeated attacks of cellular inflammation cause axon injury and subsequent axon loss from the brain's white matter in those with MS. Increasing axonal injury results in eventual demyelination within the CNS, including the optic nerve. The disease is typified by two phases: initial relapse and remittance and secondary progression. The episodes of focal neurologic dysfunction can last weeks or months, followed by partial or complete recovery. Repeated episodes are frequently preceded by fever, nausea and vomiting, and lethargy and may occur within months or years of each other. It is now recognized that focal inflammation of the brain is active, even during the remission phase, and there seems to be a point of no return for the brain's coping mechanism. This coping mechanism seems to allow for a degree of adaptation for different types of mechanisms of inflammation that originate from outside the CNS, from target-determined changes in immune cells and microglial activation, and from the accumulation of cortical gray matter lesions. Eventually, diffuse axonal response to the inflammation throughout the brain and meninges occurs, and the disease starts to be progressive (Perry, 2006; Arnold, 2006).

MS may be a differential diagnosis during the initial episode of a neurologic dysfunction that affects a certain region of the body and occurs over a limited period of time. The more relapses that occur earlier in the disease, the more quickly the progression to irreversible disability. Once irreversible disability begins, the rate of progression is independent of the frequency of relapses. There are no therapies to slow the disease once the progressive phase has started. Therefore, research is focused upon finding therapies to slow the early progression of the disease (Arnold, 2006).

Clinical Findings. Symptoms are the same for children as for adolescents and adults. These include (Johnston, 2004d):

- Unilateral weakness or ataxia (frequent presenting symptom).
- Headache (may be severe, prolonged, generalized).
- Vague paresthesias of lower extremities, distal portions of hands and feet, and face.
- Visual disturbance (diplopia, blurred vision, or sudden loss of vision as a result of optic neuritis).
- Concurrent optic neuritis and transverse myelitis (referred to as neuromyelitis optica or Devic disease).
- Vertigo, dysarthria, and sphincter disturbances are uncommon.

Diagnostic Studies. Neuroimaging (MRI using gadolinium enhancement to determine the number of T2 white matter lesions) early in the course of the disease can be important in predicting the clinical future. Evidence of disturbance of the blood-brain barrier is thought to be a better predictor than the number of T2 white matter lesions for developing inflammatory MS lesions and atrophy. Gray matter lesions are believed to play a role but are currently undetectable using current imaging. Later in the course of the disease, nonconventional neuroimaging techniques (magnetization transfer imaging and imaging for whole brain atrophy) are more useful than the gadolinium-enhanced MRI for tracking the progression of disability. Other studies include a lumbar puncture (may show mild pleocytosis or mild elevation in total protein during exacerbations; immunoglobulins may or may not be increased) and visual-evoked responses.

Differential Diagnoses. Brain tumor, focal encephalitis, nonviral infections with focal cerebritis or abscess formation, cerebrovascular diseases, leukodystrophies, and systemic vasculitis should be considered after initial presentation of symptoms. After a remission and exacerbation pattern is established, consider multiple cerebral emboli, systemic vasculitis, or recurrent infections in a susceptible host (Seay & DeVivo, 2003).

Management. Treatment involves exercises—resistance, aerobic, and stretching—and routines that promote agility and speed. Manage a neurogenic bladder. The use of corticosteroids during exacerbations is traditional therapy, and, in some recent studies, it was found that IV methylprednisone resulted in a faster return of visual function in adults when compared with adults receiving no medications (Galetta, 2006). This is a controversial treatment for the pediatric population. Other treatments used in adolescents and adults employ immunomodulatory therapies (high-dose, high-frequency interferon or low-frequency interferon and glatiramer acetate); both treatments reduce the frequency of contrast-enhancing lesions (Kinkel et al, 2006; Freedman, 2006). Another treatment undergoing research involves using intravenous immunoglobulins (Johnston, 2004d).

Research continues, endeavoring to target a variety of the mechanisms and processes of the disease to prevent and treat relapses, alter the progression of the disease, and discover neuroprotective factors. Treatment decisions are not solely dependent on MRI imaging alone. Tools to monitor subtle changes in abilities are often used, such as the MS Functional Composite Scale, Short Form 36, Expanded Disability Status Scale, and the MS Impact Scale (Arnold, 2006).

NONDEGENERATIVE DISORDERS

Benign Paroxysmal Vertigo

Description. Benign paroxysmal vertigo (BPV) may be incorrectly diagnosed as epilepsy. It typically develops in toddlers (median age 18 months), but rarely occurs after 3 years old. BPV is also a known precursor to the development of migraines later in life (Unger, 2006).

Clinical Findings. Features may include:

History.

- Rapid onset of attack, lasting seconds to minutes; attacks occur daily in clusters over several days then may not recur for weeks or months.
- May be a history of motion sickness.

Physical Examination. (Symptoms likely resolved by the time child is examined):

- Acute unsteadiness; child may fall or refuse to walk or sit; may grab onto a parent or object for steadiness.
- Nystagmus is common; no loss of consciousness.
- Vomiting and nausea may be present and be quite prominent.
- Appearance of child: frightened, pale.
- Child may be lethargic or drowsy; others may sleep and return to normal activities upon awakening (Johnston, 2004e).
- Neurologic exam essentially negative except for abnormal vestibular function.

Diagnostic Studies. Ice water caloric testing may be used to detect abnormal vestibular function.

Management. Clusters of attacks may be managed with diphenhydramine, 5 mg/kg/24 hours (maximum 300 mg/24 hour) PO, IM, IV, per rectum. Once diagnosis is made, parental reassurance is key.

Complications. Children may be inappropriately diagnosed as having epilepsy and put on anticonvulsants; attacks will not respond to such drugs.

Cerebral Palsy

Description. The term cerebral palsy (CP) is used to designate a mixed group of motor disorders that affect motor function and are caused by static injury to developing brains (Brunstrom & Titan, 2005). This is a chronic, nonprogressive disorder that impairs control of movement by damaging motor areas in the brain. Symptoms appear within the first few years of life. Depending on the area affected and the extent of damage, children with CP can also

have mental impairment (up to 66%); seizures (up to 50%); a lag in growth and development; neurosensory disorders affecting touch, pain, and continence; perceptual disorders; impaired vision and hearing; speech, swallowing, or chewing difficulties; and other learning or emotional difficulties. It is important to note that the degree of disability can vary from person to person and that the degree of impairment is not necessarily profound (National Institute of Neurological Disorders and Stroke [NINDS], 2006b).

There are three major types of (CP): spastic, athetoid (or dyskinetic), and ataxic. Spastic is when the muscles stiffen, causing muscle tightness. Athetoid affects the entire body. Ataxic affects balance and coordination. Children may exhibit varying degrees of involvement and severity; capabilities may improve over time depending on the degree of involvement and treatment. The health care provider is encouraged to maintain an approach that is optimistic yet realistic. Table 27-3 lists more terms that describe CP.

Epidemiology. CP was once believed to be caused only by birth complications (neonatal or perinatal asphyxia or trauma), but a recent study demonstrated that most children with CP were born at term without complicated labors and deliveries. Less than 10% of infants had evidence of intrapartum asphyxia, whereas 80% had antenatal factors that caused abnormal brain development (Johnston, 2004a). Other alternative causes being researched include prenatal factors, prematurity, or low birth weight, trauma to the brain, and congenital cerebral malformations. The condition is neither hereditary nor contagious. The etiology is unknown in a large percentage of cases. Small for gestational age, low birth weight (less than 1000 g), preterm babies (less than 37 weeks of gestation), and multiple births are at greater risk for CP. Complicated labor and delivery, breech presentation, Apgar score of less than 3 at 10 minutes or more; traumatic delivery; microcephaly; exposure to maternal infection (evidenced by chorioamnionitis, inflamed placental membranes, umbilical cord inflammation, foul-smelling amniotic fluid, maternal temperature greater than 38°C [100.4°F] during labor, or UTI); maternal vaginal bleeding (between sixth and ninth months of pregnancy); severe proteinuria late in pregnancy; maternal hyperthyroidism, mental retardation, and seizures; intracranial hemorrhage; toxemia; preeclampsia; antepartal hemorrhage; postmaturity; fetal distress; maternal stroke; coagulation in the fetus or newborn; and neonatal seizures are all considered risk factors (Menkes & Moser, 2006). Other etiologies may include intrauterine drug exposure (e.g., alcohol, cocaine, tobacco, crack), intrauterine infections (e.g., cytomegalovirus, toxoplasmosis, rubella), and congenital brain malformations. In the U.S., it is estimated that children who acquire CP postnatally account for 10% to 20% of those with the disorder. In such cases, the cause can be attributed to meningitis, encephalitis, head trauma (e.g., secondary to shaken baby syndrome or other abuse, car accidents, falls), and kernicterus (Berkowitz, 2000; Fenichel, 2001; Menkes & Moser, 2006).

The prevalence is 1 to 3 per 1000 live births across many studies. It appears that the incidence has not declined in many

TABLE 27-3 Terms Used to Describe Cerebral Palsy

Movement Type	Description	Associated Impairments
Spastic	Inability of a muscle to relax	Often evident after 4-6 months; retarded speech; convergent strabismus; toe-walking; flexed elbows; delayed walking until 18-24 months; one-third have seizures
Athetoid	Inability to control muscle movement (continuous, writhing movements)	Infant has difficult feeding as a result of tongue thrust, is initially hypotonic with head lag; increasing tone with rigidity over time; speech delay
Ataxic	Problems with balance and coordination	Tremors
Body Part Involved		
Diplegic	Affects both legs more than both arms	Most have limited use of legs; can walk often with aids; walk typically "scissor-like" with knees bent in and crisscross over each other
Hemiplegic	Affects one side of the body (upper extremity is usually affected more than the lower extremity)	Often not detected at birth; right side often more affected than left; 50% develop seizures; growth arrest on affected limb(s); individuals usually able to walk
Tetraplegia/Quadri-plegic	Affects all four extremities, trunk and head	Affects upper extremities more than lower; 50% with grand mal seizures; IQ impairment can be severe; most unable to walk or stand
Specific Problems With Movement or Function		
Dystonia	Involuntary, slow, sustained muscle contractions	Abnormal posture, writhing motion of arms, legs, trunk
Choreic	Disorganized tone	Uncontrollable jerky movements of toes and fingers
Tremor	Involuntary, rhythmic movements of opposing muscles; can affect extremities, head, face, vocal cords, trunk	
Ballismus	Violent, jerky movements; may affect only one side of body	
Rigidity	Stiffness	

years and may be slowly increasing in the very low-birth-weight population because of the higher survival rates of these infants. Children who are immobile, who are profoundly retarded, or who need special feeding have a decreased life expectancy.

Clinical Findings

History. The history should include pathologic, developmental, and functional health patterns:

Pathology

- Prenatal/natal history of risk factors as listed previously
- Seizures
- Hearing and vision or ocular problems, such as strabismus, nystagmus, optic atrophy
- Growth parameters, especially decreased head circumference
- Early head injury or meningitis
- Muscle tone (can be hypotonic before 6 months old, but then become hypertonic; unusual posture or favor one side).

Preterm infants with generalized, prolonged, and cramped synchronized movements are more often diagnosed with CP at a later time (Ferrari et al, 2002).

Development. Milestones may be delayed but should still be attained; persistent primitive reflexes are common (e.g., Moro and tonic neck). Hand preference before 1 year old is highly suspect.

Functional Health Patterns. Assess the following:

- Feeding history of regurgitating through the nose, inability to coordinate suck and swallow, inability to advance the diet to textured foods—in short, oral-motor coordination problems
- Irritability or depressed affect (including unusual sleepiness) as a neonate
- Difficulty with movement, cuddliness, grasp and release, self-feeding, and head control to look around; inability to change position per developmental level

- Persistent primitive reflexes
- Communication problems, either language or speech proficiency

Physical Examination

- Skin. Dermatologic signs of syndromes, such as neurofibromatosis, may be present.
- Orthopedic examination. Scoliosis, contractures, and dislocated hip may be present.
- Neurologic examination. The following may be seen on the neurologic examination:
  ○ Deep tendon reflexes increased
  ○ Tone increased, although occasionally decreased; hypotonia before 6 months old is common. Tone may also be mixed
  ○ Minimal muscle atrophy
  ○ No fasciculations
  ○ Persistent primitive reflexes (e.g., tonic neck and Moro after 6 months old)
  ○ Delayed reflexes (e.g., parachute reflex remains absent after 9 to 10 months old; side-protective reflexes remain absent after 5 months old)
  ○ Asymmetric movements
  ○ Preferred handedness before 1 to 2 years old
  ○ Structural defects, such as hydrocephaly or microcephaly
- Vision and hearing. Visual refractive errors occur in 50% of children, and strabismus is found in 33%. Hearing problems may have resulted from the initial brain insult.
- Development. Assessment of gross motor, fine motor, language, and personal social skills is needed. The Denver Developmental Screening Test II (Denver II) can be used for initial screening. Look also at the quality of movements (e.g., smoothness of gait, grasping, clarity of speech). In children with CP, motor milestones are commonly delayed.
- Feeding assessment. A patient with CP can have a reversed swallow wave; uncoordinated suck and swallow; decreased tone of the lips, tongue, and cheeks; increased gag reflex; involuntary tongue and lip movements; increased sensitivity to food stimuli; poor occlusion; and delayed inhibition of the suck reflex. Evaluate the diet, height, weight, and BMI for adequate nutrition.

Diagnostic Studies

- Imaging studies. A CT scan can be obtained to identify brain malformations. An MRI will aid the visualization of structures and abnormalities that are nearer to bony structures.
- Chromosomal and metabolic studies. These studies can be done to identify genetic disorders, especially single-gene defects.

Differential Diagnosis. The first and main requirement is to differentiate central from peripheral disorders. CP is always central and is characterized by brisk deep tendon reflexes. Many other conditions can have CP-motor involvement features. These conditions include sepsis from intrauterine infections, fetal alcohol syndrome, hydrocephalus, tumors, agenesis of the corpus callosum or other brain malformations, Tay-Sachs disease, phenylketonuria, Lesch-Nyhan syndrome, spinal cord injury, hypothyroidism, muscle diseases, seizures, and many genetic and metabolic disorders. Mental retardation results in

delayed milestones but should not include increased reflexes. Neuromuscular disorders are associated with signs of weakness, muscle atrophy, and decreased deep tendon reflexes. These disorders typically present with a missed milestone.

Management. The management of children with CP described here can serve as a model for the management of children with a variety of neurologic problems.

Referral of Suspected Cases. Children with CP should be evaluated and cared for at centers that provide interdisciplinary caregivers, including a developmental pediatrician, gastroenterologist, orthopedist, neurologist, nurse, speech pathologist, physical and occupational therapist, education consultant and psychologist, and social worker. The care of children with CP may also involve an ophthalmologist, feeding clinic and nutritionist services, and genetics counseling.

Family Education About the Diagnosis. Families need to understand the diagnosis and its nonprogressive but incurable characteristics. They need to understand that the extent of brain damage is not always related to the extent of disability. Thus, no one can predict what the future for a given child will be. It is known that children who receive special services, such as physical therapy, speech therapy, and other interventions, have better outcomes than do children who are left to develop on their own. United Cerebral Palsy has educational materials and a variety of services available for affected children and their families (see Resource Box at the end of the chapter).

Family Support. Generally, families grieve when given the diagnosis of CP and need support during this time. Support groups or opportunities to meet other families with affected children are often helpful. The emotional needs of siblings must not be overlooked either. The social worker can be very helpful to families trying to cope with complex health problems.

CP services are long term and expensive. Many children will be eligible for Supplemental Security Income or state program benefits for the severely handicapped. Respite care may be a benefit available to families. The Individuals with Disabilities Education Act of 1997 (IDEA) requires children with disabilities to be assessed for and instructed in the use of assistive devices along with appropriate referrals to regional centers. Again, medical social workers and public health nurses can be very helpful in connecting families to appropriate services; primary care providers can play an important role in the multidisciplinary team involved with ensuring that services are received.

Nutrition. Children with CP often have inadequate nutrition because of their problems with biting, sucking, chewing, swallowing, and self-feeding. Additionally, children with athetosis may need as much as 50% to 100% more calories to support their increased caloric needs because of their constant writhing movements. Children with spasticity, on the other hand, may need fewer calories because of their decreased movements. Occasionally, the problems are so severe that a gastrostomy is needed, sometimes with fundoplication to prevent reflux and aspiration. Special positioning, feeding therapy, and special feeding devices can help. High nutrient density is a key to providing a nutritious diet (i.e., getting more nutrients into the same volume of food; also see Chapter 11). Feeding clinics are often helpful to plan management of nutrition.

Elimination. Constipation is common because of lack of exercise, inadequate fluid and fiber intake, medications, poor positioning, low abdominal muscle tone, and other factors. Stool softeners, such as docusate sodium, may help. Laxatives, such as senna concentrate (Senokot) or milk of magnesia, may be useful but should not be used long term. The newer osmotic agents may also be used (e.g., MiraLax).

Bladder control and urinary retention are also problems for children with CP. Most achieve bladder control between 3 and 10 years old. Mental retardation makes toilet training difficult for some. Children with CP are three times more likely to suffer UTIs (Jackson Allen & Vessey, 2004).

Dentistry. Orofacial muscle tone can contribute to malocclusion, and problems with oral mobility make daily dental hygiene difficult. These children have more gum disease; the side effects of some seizure medications can include swollen gums and tooth decay. A careful dental care program is necessary.

Drooling. Inability to manage oral secretions results in drooling. Social isolation, wet clothing, skin excoriation, malodorous breath, discomfort, choking, gagging, and aspiration can make these oral secretions a serious problem. Glycopyrrolate, 0.05 to 1 mg by mouth, twice or three times daily, may help, but side effects may also be problematic (e.g., constipation, difficulty urinating, restlessness). Surgical intervention is a last resort and commonly involves removing the submandibular gland or nerves, or cutting or rerouting the salivary duct.

Pulmonary. Positioning problems, an increase in gastroesophageal reflux, and difficulty in clearing secretions place children with CP at higher risk for respiratory problems, notably pneumonias (especially from aspiration). The duration of respiratory symptoms with upper respiratory infections (URIs) is increased in these children (Jackson Allen & Vessey, 2004).

Skin. The skin in sedentary children with CP is more likely to break down and cause decubitus secondary to positioning problems. There is an increased incidence of skin latex allergies with CP (Jackson Allen & Vessey, 2004).

Movement and Mobility. Positioning and seating, standing, transportation, bathing, dressing, mobility for play and getting to school, and oral hygiene are important to assess and manage. Occupational and physical therapists are essential to these aspects of care. Families need help incorporating various strategies into their homes and lifestyles. The goals of therapy are to improve physical conditioning and gain maximal independence in mobility, fine motor activities, self-care, and communication. Therapists try to promote efficient movement patterns, inhibit primitive reflexes, and achieve isolated extremity movements. Bracing, adaptive devices, and early intervention programs beginning in infancy are important. Children need to experience different environments for developmental growth. Wheelchairs and motorized wheelchairs can be beneficial in helping children explore their environment

more efficiently. Furthermore, although the condition is not progressive in terms of the brain lesion, contractures, scoliosis, dislocated hips, and other deformities can develop if the child is allowed to maintain abnormal positions for long periods. Thus, therapy for range of motion is a long-term need for many children with CP. Orthopedic care may be necessary. Constraint-induced therapy (used in stroke patients to limit the use of the more functional side) has been demonstrated to improve mobility function and for longer periods of time than conventional physical therapy in children with CP.

Antispasmodic medications (baclofen [Lioresal], tizanidine [Zanaflex], diazepam [Valium], and dantrolene [Dantrium]) may be used to minimize contractures and spasticity.

Botulinum toxin A (Botox) injections are used to eliminate pain, minimize contractures, delay or prevent surgery, and maximize function (Pelshaw et al, 2006). Its use is dependent upon the recommendation of—and after a thorough evaluation by—a pediatric physiatrist, pediatric neurologist, or pediatric orthopedic surgeon, and after input of therapists and family. It is injected directly into muscles (sometimes guided by an electromyogram or electrical stimulation). It is common for the child to experience transient worsening of spasticity until physical and occupational therapies effectively help strengthen the antagonist and agonist muscles. The dosage administered depends upon which muscles are being selected and muscle size. Results are generally seen within 5 to 7 days and last 3 to 4 months. The toxin has been safely used in infants more than 1 month old. Resistance can occur because neutralizing antibodies can develop. Therefore, it is important that only the smallest possible effective dose be used and that at least 3 months lapse between injections. Contraindications include: diffuse hypertonia, myasthenia gravis (MG), motor-neuron disease, injection into infected muscle, caution in pregnancy (fetal complications have been seen in animal studies), and caution when it is co-administrated with aminoglycoside or another agent that interferes with neuromuscular transmission (toxin effect can be increased) (Pelshaw et al, 2006). The numerous side effects should be thoroughly understood by care providers.

Communication. With the combined problems of lack of oral-motor control and the high incidence of mental retardation, communication can be a problem for children with CP. Speech therapy is important to achieve oral speech when possible or to use augmentative devices, such as computers with voices to allow language development and communication of needs even without oral speech. Computers with specially outfitted input devices have greatly increased the ability of those with speech and movement disabilities to communicate with others. Hearing deficits need to be identified and managed by an audiologist.

Advocacy. Families often need help accessing services through schools because children with CP may have special education needs. Some insurance companies try to avoid the costs of long-term care and therapy. The primary care provider should serve as an advocate and resource for families.

Special Education. Early intervention programs and specialized educational programs through school systems are often beneficial.

Other Treatments. Drugs are sometimes used to alter muscle tone or abnormal movements. Surgery is used to release contractures or to sever overactivated nerves (called a *selective dorsal root rhizotomy*). Selective dorsal root rhizotomy (of spinal nerves) plus intrathecal baclofen decrease spasticity and increase range of motion of affected limbs. Although functional spasticity can be helped with these last two procedures, the selective motor, balance, and weakness problems are not improved. Strength training can help with balance and weakness. Functional electrical stimulation has been used to activate and strengthen muscles in the hand, shoulder, and ankle. The technique involves inserting microscopic wireless devices via a hypodermic needle into specific muscles or nerves. The devices are powered by a telemetry wand that can direct the number and strength of their pulses by remote control (NINDS, 2006b).

Complications. Approximately one third of children with CP develop seizures within the first year or two (Johnston, 2004a). Children who receive no intervention have poorer functional abilities; they make less progress developmentally and are at risk for unnecessary contractures and deformities. Box 27-2 lists associated problems seen in CP.

Prevention and Screening. The incidence of CP can be decreased to some extent through good prenatal care. Recent research is centered on several processes believed to play a causative role in CP. These research endeavors include:

BOX 27-2 **Problems Associated With Cerebral Palsy**

Cognitive
Learning disabilities
Mental retardation

Seizure Disorders
Language and Speech Disorders
Articulation
Vocal strength and quality
Language processing

Vision
Refractive errors
Strabismus
Amblyopia
Cataracts
Retinopathy of prematurity
Cortical blindness
Homonymous hemianopsia (hemiplegia)

Hearing
Conductive
Sensorineural

Other Sensory
Tactile hypersensitivity or hyposensitivity
Dyspraxia
Balance and movement problems
Proprioception difficulties
Stereognosis

Motor
Prolonged primitive reflexes
Absence of protective reflexes
Delayed motor milestones
Hip subluxation and dislocation
Scoliosis
Contractures

Feeding and Eating Problems
Chewing, sucking, and swallowing deficits
Drooling
Hypoxemia
Fatigue
Underweight and overweight
Gastroesophageal reflux
Aspiration

Bowel
Constipation
Encopresis

Urinary
Bladder control
Urinary retention
Urinary tract infections

Dental
Malocclusions
Enamel deficits and caries
Gum hyperplasia (with phenytoin)

Pulmonary
Respiratory infections
Pneumonia

Skin
Decubitus
Latex allergy

Behavioral and Emotional
Behavioral disorders
Attention-deficit disorder, with and without hyperactivity
Self-injurious behaviors
Depression
Autism
Growth failure
Other

From Jackson Allen P, Vessey J: *Primary care of the child with a chronic condition,* ed 4, St Louis, 2004, Mosby.

searching for genes associated with abnormal neuronal migration; evaluating the role that excessive amounts of glutamate in the brain play in overexcitation and death of neurons; investigating whether synthetic neuroprotective substances can be developed (neurotrophins) and given to an infant after stroke or hypoxia; and continuing to evaluate the relationship between elevations in interferons or other inflammatory cytokines that result from maternal infection and interrupt normal fetal brain development (NINDS, 2006b). Also, during pregnancy RH incompatibility may cause CP in the child if not treated (United Cerebral Palsy, 2001). During the 28th week of pregnancy, immunoglobulin (RhoGAM) can be administered to the mother to prevent CP in this situation. It is anticipated that continued research into new areas will eventually lead to further preventive interventions. Until that time, early identification and intervention can significantly improve the outlook for affected children and their families.

Bell Palsy

Description. Bell palsy is an acute unilateral paralysis or weakening of any facet of the facial nerve. The patient may initially experience localized pain or tingling in one ear and then typically be seen in the clinic with sagging on one side of the face with the eyelid completely or partially closed. When partially closed, an exposure keratitis can develop. There may be a hypersensitivity to loud noises, loss of taste on the anterior two thirds of the tongue, and changes in lacrimation and salivation on the affected side. The history usually reveals a URI within the previous two weeks or exposure to cold temperature. Onset is rapid and can progress to maximal intensity within hours. Symptoms may last for 1 to 9 weeks (average 2 to 4 weeks) with spontaneous remission and recovery. The younger the child, the more complete the remission (Legido et al, 2005).

Epidemiology. There is edema of cranial nerve VII and venous congestion in areas of the nerve canal. It is conjectured that the disease stems more from a postinfectious allergic response or immune demyelinating facial neuritis rather than from viral invasion. Implicated infectious agents include Epstein-Barr (20% of cases), mumps, herpes simplex and herpes zoster, and Lyme disease and other spirochetes. There may be a genetic predisposition that involves trigeminal and auditory nerve pathways (Legido et al, 2005).

Clinical Findings

Physical Examination. A neurologic assessment of all facial nerve functions may be difficult in children and is not critical to make an accurate diagnosis. The clinician should note the following:

- Unilateral motor changes in forehead, cheek, and perioral area; face muscles pull to the normal side when the child makes facial expressions
- Normal blood pressure
- Dribbling liquids from the weak side when offered fluids
- Eating and drinking are more difficult
- Eyelid fails to close on the affected side, and complete blinking may be absent
- Taste (50% of patients), lacrimation, and salivation may be impaired

- No limb weakness
- Any skin lesions to suggest herpes on the affected side of the face (would indicate active viral infection of the nerve or its motor neurons)

Diagnostic Studies. It is widely accepted that diagnostic testing is not indicated unless the patient fails to improve over a 6-week period or other neurologic symptoms occur.

Differential Diagnosis. Included in the differential diagnosis are Guillain-Barré syndrome (usually includes an additional symptom of absent tendon reflexes of limbs), hypertension, congenital absence of the depressor angularis oris muscle, infection, trauma (the use of forceps during delivery can cause a facial nerve compression neuropathy that spontaneously resolves within a few days to weeks), Melkersson syndrome (involves recurrent facial palsies with swollen lips, tongue, cheeks, or eyelids), Möbius syndrome, acute otitis media, polymyelitis, histiocytosis X, varicella, post-DTP (diphtheria-tetanus-pertussis) vaccine reaction, facial nerve tumors, neurofibroma, infiltration of facial nerves with leukemic cells, rhabdomyosarcoma of the middle ear, and brainstem infarcts.

Management. If lid closure is incomplete, prescribe methylcellulose eyedrops or ocular lubricant to the affected eye several times daily and patch the eye if the child plays outdoors, during active play, and when sleeping. Steroids are not indicated in children. Acyclovir is controversial in pediatric treatment. Eighty-five percent will recover fully within a few weeks; 10% may have some residual partial palsy. Of the 5% that do not recover, electrophysiologic examination of the facial nerve is indicated to discern the degree of neuropathy and regeneration. Recurrence rates are approximately 7% in children (Legido et al, 2005).

Complications. If recovery is incomplete, lack of salivation in response to food, lack of lacrimation, facial contractures, and tics may occur.

Epilepsy and Seizure Disorders

Description. Seizures are due to the misfiring of the cortical neurons of the brain. Convulsive seizures occur when misfiring causes episodes of involuntary contraction of voluntary muscles. Table 27-4 summarizes the types of seizures.

When seizures are recurrent and unrelated to fever, the disorder is called *epilepsy*. Seizures represent either brain dysfunction or significant underlying disorders. A patient may demonstrate characteristics of more than one type of seizure. Epilepsy most often has two characteristics: the seizures recur, and the seizure events are unprovoked.

Epidemiology. Different kinds of seizures arise from disorders in diverse parts of the brain. Seizures can result from a variety of genetic, symptomatic, or idiopathic conditions. More than 30,000 genes are expressed in the brain, and approximately 20% of individuals with epilepsy have a genetic etiology. Several familial epilepsies have been identified. These include benign neonatal convulsions, juvenile myoclonic epilepsy, and progressive myoclonic epilepsy (Johnston, 2004b).

TABLE 27-4 Classification of Seizures

Seizure Type	Age	Pattern	Comments
I. Partial or focal seizures			
A. Simple partial		Begin locally	Affect one hemisphere
1. With motor symptoms	Any age	Consciousness not impaired; last 10-20 seconds Any part of body; includes jacksonian seizures	From birth trauma, inflammation, stroke, tumors (individual will show progressive neurologic symptoms)
2. With sensory or somatosensory symptoms	Any age	"Pins and needles," numb; auras include lights, tastes, sounds	
3. With autonomic symptoms	Any age	Recurrent abdominal pain, headache, sweat, laugh, cry, tachycardia, dilated pupils	May have migraine quality; family history of migraine or seizures
4. Compound forms	Any age		
B. Complex partial	Any age; may be hard to recognize in young child	Consciousness impaired; clonic activity, forced head/eye deviation, focal tonic posturing, automatisms—purposeless motor activities (e.g., lip smacking, repetitious swallowing/chewing, finger/hand fidgeting, tics); lasts 1-2 minutes	
1. Impaired consciousness only		Staring spell	
2. With cognitive symptoms		May have confusion	
3. With affective symptoms		Aura of fear	
4. With "psychosensory" symptoms		May have odd smell/taste; visual or auditory hallucination	
5. With "psychomotor" symptoms		Automatisms	
6. Compound forms			
C. Partial seizures, secondary generalized		Seizure begins in one part of body but then generalizes	Aura can let person seek safe position
II. Idiopathic localization-related seizures			
A. Benign focal (or rolandic)	4-13 years		Resolve by adolescence; treatment may not be needed
1. Diurnal		Alert; unilateral twitching, drooling, paresthesia of face, gums, tongue, buccal mucosa; may progress into hemiclonic or hemitonic movements	With or without postictal weakness of affected side
2. Nocturnal		Advances to generalization	
III. Generalized seizures			
A. Absence	4-12 years	Petit mal; 5-30 seconds; lapses of consciousness (short staring "spells"); can have associated movements; no falling; no aura	Usually no aura Hyperventilation for 3-4 minutes can trigger seizure; blinking lights can also trigger
B. Myoclonic (infantile spasms)	Infancy	Head drops or sudden flexing; may suddenly cry out; older children exhibit trunk or extremity flexion	Hypsarrhythmia on EEG with no normal background activity; difficult to treat
C. Clonic		Rhythmic jerking	
D. Tonic		Intense muscle contractions	
E. Tonic-clonic	Any age; most common type of seizure	Grand mal; begins with loss of consciousness; stiffening, violent jerking; postictal phase of sleep and confusion; 15% incontinent	Aura in some; may have abdominal pain or headache; life threatening if continues, producing hypercarbia, respiratory acidosis, lactic acidosis; some occur in sleep
F. Atonic	Childhood	Similar to myoclonic; aka "drop attacks;" duration <15 minutes	Child often falls; injury protection important

aka, Also known as; *EEG,* electroencephalogram.

Clinical Findings

History. The history of a patient with seizures should include the following:

- Description of the seizure: focal or generalized, loss of consciousness, aura, length of postictal sleep or confusion, duration of the episode, and associated illness
- Any underlying medical diagnosis (e.g., diabetes, renal disease, cardiovascular disorder)
- Previous CNS infection or birth trauma
- Intrauterine infection, trauma, bleeding
- Toxic exposure or drug use
- Anticonvulsant medication stopped abruptly
- Recent head injury
- Family history of seizures
- Any noted missed milestones

Physical Examination. The following should be determined on physical examination:

- Focal abnormalities, weakness
- Presence of seizure activity during the examination
- Hypertension (for renal disease)
- Systemic disease
- Cardiovascular disorder
- Neurocutaneous disease, café au lait spots of neurofibromatosis, ash leaf spots or adenoma sebaceum of tuberous sclerosis, facial hemangioma of Sturge-Weber syndrome
- Signs of head trauma
- Transillumination of the skull in infants

Diagnostic Studies. These are typical diagnostic test recommendations. Most institutions will adopt their individual protocols:

- Complete blood count (CBC) (including platelets, liver function tests [LFTs])—useful for diagnostic purposes or as a baseline before anticonvulsant therapy is started
- Metabolic screen
- Blood glucose—standard in all patients
- Urine and serum toxicology—only if illicit drug exposure is suspected
- Lumbar puncture—only if child is younger than 6 months old; any age patient with persistent changes in mental status or failure to return to baseline functioning; patients with meningeal signs
- EEG—standard in all children after first nonfebrile seizure. An abnormal EEG supports the seizure diagnosis. However, a normal EEG when the child is not seizing does not rule out a seizure disorder
- MRI—imaging studies are not routinely indicated if the initial seizure is followed by a normal neurologic examination and return to baseline mental status. Imaging is recommended: (1) if the patient demonstrates cognitive changes after several hours and postictal focal dysfunction (signs of increased intracranial pressure, such as found with tumors, abscesses, strokes, or vascular malformations); (2) if the seizure lasted more than 15 minutes; (3) in infants younger than 6 months old; and (4) if any new onset of focal neurologic deficit has occurred. An MRI is now the preferred imaging study over CT scans because of its increased sensitivity

- CT scan—used only in cases of marked cognitive, motor, or neurologic dysfunction of unknown etiology (e.g., head injury, brain infection or tumor, abscesses); abnormal EEGs; or focal seizure symptoms that may or may not evolve into a generalized seizure
- Polysomnography (simultaneous EEG, electromyogram, electrocardiogram [ECG], and electrooculogram) can be useful to assess nocturnal seizures

Differential Diagnosis. Consider breath holding, syncope, migraine headaches, gastroesophageal reflux, night terrors, metabolic problems, tumors or other CNS problems, or a cardiovascular problem. Vertigo has been confused with epilepsy. Tics (involuntary, spasmodic, nonrhythmic, repetitive movements) are stereotypic, but not associated with impaired consciousness and at times can be suppressed by the patient.

Pseudoseizures. Pseudoseizures may be difficult to distinguish from true seizures, even after direct observation. The care provider is more likely to suspect such pseudoseizures in a patient with seizures who has gained more recent control of a seizure disorder. In such cases, the pseudoseizures serve as attention-getting behaviors for the child who misses the attention gained before control. Pseudoseizures also may be seen in adolescents, more often in girls than in boys (3:1). Incest or sexual abuse must be addressed in these girls (Fenichel, 2001). Distinguishing characteristics of pseudoseizures include the following:

- Unilaterally or bilaterally coordinated motor activity more like thrashing and jerking (scissor-like movements) rather than tonic-clonic; no aura or complaints of malaise, heart palpitations, feeling like choking before seizure onset
- Discomfort, distress expressed; sometimes ataxia, fumbling; consciousness may be impaired, but the patient is not unconscious
- No incontinence; patient does not hurt self or bite tongue
- No postictal stage
- Occur at home
- No EEG changes, even during episodes

Treatment for pseudoseizures involves developing alternative gains to seizure behavior. Most children stop after the diagnosis is made and interventions are in place. A referral for counseling may be indicated, depending on the etiology. No anticonvulsants are used in the case of children who do not have an underlying seizure disorder.

Management

Referral. A child with suspected seizures should be referred to a neurologist for diagnosis and initiation of treatment. Anticonvulsant drugs are usually prescribed, especially after a second seizure. Delaying treatment does not affect ultimate control.

Management of Stable Patients With Diagnosed Seizure Disorders. The primary care provider can monitor stable children with seizures. Monitoring activities includes prescribing anticonvulsants, monitoring drug levels, and performing case management. Approximately one third of children who have a prior history of cognitive or motor impairments will have a recurrent unprovoked seizure within 1 year.

Drug Monitoring. All providers working with patients receiving anticonvulsants should be familiar with the common drugs (Table 27-5) and their major side effects (see also Appendix A). Helping with compliance issues is also a component of the monitoring role. If possible, start with one drug with the least side effects and describe how the drug works with the child and parent, with an explanation of side effects. Key points for drug monitoring include:

- Patients can be controlled with sub-therapeutic blood levels.
- Patients can be free of side effects at levels beyond the therapeutic range.

- Phenytoin (Dilantin) saturates the enzyme system; therefore even a small increase in dosage can cause a marked increase in blood levels.
- Half-lives are longer with the introduction to a new drug; steady concentrations (and elimination) of the drug are achieved at 5 half-lives.
- Half-lives vary by patient and other drugs being taken (e.g., antibiotics, antipyretics).
- If gastrointestinal side effects occur, decreasing the dosage and increasing the frequency of administration may help; try changing to an enteric-coated pill or taking the drug after eating.

TABLE 27-5   Antiepileptic Drug Therapy for Children*

Seizure Type	Drug	Therapeutic Blood Levels (g/mL)	Laboratory Monitoring
Partial, generalized tonic-clonic in children >2 years old; contraindicated for absence and myoclonic	Carbamazepine (Tegretol)	4-12	CBC; baseline, at 6-12 wk, then annually; drug blood levels
Partial, generalized, status epilepticus	Phenytoin (Dilantin)	10-20	Drug blood levels
Simple partial, tonic-clonic	Phenobarbital (Luminal)	15-40	None
Absence	Ethosuximide (Zarontin)	40-100	None
First-line generalized seizures if >10 yr old, myoclonic, absence	Valproic acid (Depakene)	50-120	Baseline CBC with diff., LFTs, ammonia, prothrombin, partial thromboplastin; CBC with diff SGOT, drug levels especially in the first 6 months
Partial, tonic-clonic, myoclonic	Primidone (Mysoline)	5-12	None
Partial, myoclonic, infantile spasms	Vigabatrin (not approved or available in the U.S.)	1.4-14	
Partial, generalized, Lennox-Gastaut syndrome	Felbamate (Felbatol)†	Not monitored	LFTs, CBC with diff., platelets, retic ct. monthly (requires close monitoring)
Refractory partial-onset, rolandic	Gabapentin (Neurontin)—an adjunct drug with other AEDs used for partial seizures	5-15	Depends on other AED used
Partial, Lennox-Gastaut syndrome, absence, atonic, juvenile myoclonic	Lamotrigine (Lamictal)—an adjunct drug only with valproic acid	2-20	
	Topiramate (Topamax)		
Partial, generalized		2-25	None
Partial	Oxcarbazepine (Trileptal—similar to Tegretol)	5-50	None
Partial, generalized	Zonisamide (Zonegran)	10-40	None
Partial	Levetiracetam (Keppra)	20-60	None
Partial, generalized	Tiagabine (Gabitril)—adjunct drug only	5-70	None
Partial, absence, myoclonic, infantile spasms, Lennox-Gastaut, akinetic	Clonazepam (Rivotril)	>0.013	LFTs, CBC with diff

*See Appendix A for dosing information.

†Drug used only for refractory epilepsy; now approved for use in children ≥2 years old with Lennox-Gastaut; otherwise for use in children ≥ 14 years old.

AEDs, Antiepileptic drugs; *CBC,* complete blood count; *diff,* differential; *LFTs,* liver function tests; *retic ct.,* reticulocyte count; *SGOT,* serum glutamic-oxaloacetic transaminase or AST.

Data from Johnston MV: Seizures in childhood. In Behrman R, Kliegman R, Jenson J, editors: *Nelson textbook of pediatrics,* ed 16, Philadelphia, 2004, WB Saunders; Riviello JJ: General concepts in seizure management. In Burg F et al, editors: *Current pediatric therapy,* ed 18, Philadelphia, 2006, WB Saunders; Fenichel G: *Clinical pediatric neurology: a signs and symptoms approach,* ed 4, Philadelphia, 2001, WB Saunders.

- Administer drug twice daily or daily for better compliance.
- The first signs of toxicity usually include sedation, changes in behavior, and changes in cognition; other drug toxicities may cause decreases in memory and attention span or interpersonal relationship difficulties. It is important to note that some patients may exhibit these changes and have drug levels within the normal range.
- Metabolites of the drugs can cause hypersensitivity side effects.
- Do routine drug level monitoring based on the clinical picture.
- Some herbal products interfere with seizure control; Gingko and Kava are examples (Golub, 2001).

Antiepileptic Drug Withdrawal.   After 2 years or longer without seizures, most pediatric neurologists will consider gradually withdrawing anticonvulsant therapy after obtaining an EEG. Patients with histories of benign epilepsy with rolandic spikes or with idiopathic generalized seizures are more likely to be successfully withdrawn. Those with complex partial seizures and juvenile myoclonic seizures are more likely to have a recurrence once medication has been withdrawn. Drug withdrawal should span a 3- to 6-month time period because abrupt weaning can cause status epilepticus (SE) (Johnston, 2004b). Children with mental retardation, CP, focal motor deficits, age of onset younger than 2 years old, symptomatic seizures, and abnormal EEGs are not good weaning candidates. Weaning is supervised closely, with one drug removed at a time. Of children who have been seizure free for 2 years and have low risk factors, 70% to 75% remain seizure free without drugs. If seizures do recur, 50% do so within the first 6 months of weaning and 60% to 80% within 2 years. Three fourths of recurrences occur during weaning or within the first year (Bouma et al, 2002). If the onset of seizures occurred during a time of anoxia, head injury, meningitis, or encephalitis, the AED treatment can be stopped after recovery from the condition is complete. The patient can always be restarted should there be a recurrence (Camfield & Camfield, 2005).

Ketogenic Diet.   The ketogenic diet is useful in young children with all types of seizures, particularly in those with myoclonic forms, infantile spasms, atonic-kinetic types, and with the mixed seizures of Lennox-Gastaut syndrome (Fenichel, 2001). The diet is considered when the side effects of AEDs are intolerable or when allergies to AEDs preclude administration. The ideal child is between 2 and 5 years old because the desired steady state of ketosis is easier to maintain. The diet is stringent and requires utmost vigilance to the ratios of calories, protein, fat, carbohydrates, vitamins, and minerals. It is best managed under very tight control with medical and dietetic leadership. Side effects usually involve abdominal pain and diarrhea. A prescreening process, including psychological testing to determine the child's and family's emotional functioning, coping, and problem-solving abilities, is recommended. A dietitian should screen the child for nutrition and growth status. A nurse should interview the family for understanding of and education about the protocol. The diet is started while the child is admitted to the hospital, where

metabolic and neurologic states can be monitored. A recent follow-up study of children who had remained on a ketogenic diet for 3 to 6 years, demonstrated that 24% were seizure free, 51% experienced 90% seizure control, and 24% were off of all pharmacologic medications entirely (Freeman et al, 2005).

Surgery.   Surgery has been successful in helping some children with complex partial seizures. However, as with the ketogenic diet, selection of appropriate children is done with great care. Focal resection surgery is currently used only in children whose epileptic focus is localized, who have failed to respond to AEDs, and whose development has been assessed over time. Seizure-free rates after resection have been documented to reach 90%, with minimal loss of neurologic function (Finberg & Kleinman, 2002). Hemispherectomy or interhemispherectomy can be curative. Side effects of the surgery include hemiparesis, incontinence, stuttering, and poor hand coordination. Temporal lobotomies are an option for treating intractable partial complex seizures localized to the temporal area; side effects are aphasia and superior quadrant visual loss. Slightly more than 50% of candidates achieve freedom from seizures. Callosotomy and vagus nerve stimulation, as palliative surgeries, are options for children with multiple regions of hemispheric involvement that result in intractable seizures. In vagus nerve stimulation (VNS), a programmed device—"pacemaker of the brain"—is implanted in the anterior chest wall. A wire wraps around the left vagus nerve and sends regular, mild pulses of electrical energy to the brain via the nerve. A patient with an aura can stimulate the device to prevent a seizure. For those without an aura, the device is set on specific parameters given the patient's seizure pattern. With VNS, seizures and side effects can be better controlled. Both children and adults are good candidates.

Counseling.   Older children need to understand the seizures they are experiencing and their significance. They also need to know about the anticonvulsant medications they are taking. Teenagers want to drive. Laws vary from state to state, but generally a teenager who has been seizure-free for 2 years and has demonstrated good drug compliance should be allowed to drive. Parents need to understand the diagnosis, treatment, and necessary follow-up. They also need to understand the implications of seizure disorders and long-term prognoses. Negative attitudes continue to surround epilepsy and may need to be addressed. Epilepsy is not synonymous with mental retardation.

Children with epilepsy may experience social stigmas and problems with self-esteem. Other mental health problems may also occur in these children as they try to cope with a chronic disease. Parents are encouraged to treat children as normally as possible and seek appropriate support groups.

Safety.   Uncontrolled seizures can present safety hazards for an unsupervised child. The child and family need to consider the situations that the child will be in and be sure that someone knows what to do if a seizure occurs. School personnel need to be informed and prepared with appropriate guidelines. Safety helmets worn at all times are sometimes warranted if falls and head injury occur frequently. Swimming alone is never recommended, but swimming, contact sports, and climbing are to be allowed if the child is well controlled and there is constant supervision during these activities. One study revealed that fatal car crashes attributed to seizures were rare versus those caused by other medical conditions (Scherer & Krauss, 2001). Refer to Chapter 14 for a further discussion of sports and activities for those with seizure disorders.

Immunizations. The decision to give pertussis vaccine to children with neurologic seizures or other neurologic conditions needs to be made on an individual basis. Children who will be in child care centers, special clinics, or residential care centers should be immunized if possible. Progressive neurologic conditions with developmental delays are reason for deferral of pertussis vaccine. Infants and children with a personal history of seizures were noted to have a sevenfold increase in post-DPT immunization seizures. Thus, DTaP and acetaminophen at the time of administration and every 4 hours for the first 24 hours is recommended. Other neurologic conditions that predispose to seizures or neurologic deterioration or a seizure history in an infant younger than 1 year old should result in consideration of deferral of pertussis immunization (American Academy of Pediatrics Committee on Infectious Diseases, 2006).

Complications. Status epilepticus (SE) is typically defined as a prolonged single seizure lasting more than 30 minutes or recurrent seizures between which there is no recovery of consciousness (Johnston, 2004b). However, one should not determine treatment based solely upon a definition, given the dire outcomes of SE. A child who has generalized tonic-clonic seizures and who is in SE is at risk for brain damage and intellectual deficits (Wheless & Clarke, 2005). Lack of oxygenation, decreased cerebral perfusion, metabolic acidosis, hypoglycemia, hyperkalemia, lactic acidosis, increased temperature, and increased intracranial pressure can all result in significant risk of morbidity and mortality. Such an occurrence needs to be handled as a medical emergency. SE can be triggered by an acute brain infection, progressive neurologic disease, AED failure, or, rarely, a febrile seizure in an otherwise healthy child without other risk factors. However, most cases of SE occur in children with underlying neurologic deficits. It is difficult to diagnose SE in children with absence or complex partial seizures because the children may just appear confused (Fenichel, 2001). Adverse outcomes can include behavioral problems, mental retardation, and focal motor deficits. Diazepam rectal gel (Diastat) is recommended for use by health care providers, parents, and caregivers (including school personnel) in children more than 2 years old who have a seizure lasting more than 5 minutes. It is administered once and takes effect in 5 to 15 minutes. Its use has decreased emergency department visits by 67%; it is safe at higher than recommended doses; and it has less than a 1% incidence of respiratory depression. The most common side effect is somnolence. It is available in a premeasured portable packet and dosed according to age and weight (Baysun et al, 2005).

Prevention and Screening. Epilepsy cannot be prevented, but early diagnosis and intervention can often reduce the disabilities and risks associated with the condition.

Erb and Klumpke Palsies

Description. A stretch injury of the brachial plexus in neonates can occur during a difficult vaginal delivery; such injury has also been reported following cesarean births. Injury involves the upper cervical nerve roots C5 and C6 (Erb-Duchenne palsy) and the lower cervical nerve roots C7, C8, and T1 (Klumpke palsy). The injuries are attributed to traction of the involved nerves (with mild affect) to more serious complete nerve root avulsion from the spinal cord. Partial diaphragmatic paralysis can result because innervation comes from C3, C4, and C5.

Epidemiology. Neonatal risk factors for plexus injuries include high birth weight, shoulder dystocia, a lengthy labor, breech delivery, maternal gestational diabetes, and forceps or vacuum extraction. The incidence is approximately 3 per 1000 live births for Erb palsy. Klumpke palsy is rare, accounting for about 0.5% of all plexus palsies. Klumpke paralysis is believed to be caused by delivering the head before the upper arm in a breech baby whose arms are extended. Up to 81% of infants may have nerve root avulsions of the upper roots following breech delivery (Mehlman, 2003).

Clinical Findings

Physical Examination. Typically, soon after birth, the infant is found to have asymmetrical active range of motion of the arms. Upon further evaluation the following is evidenced:

- Erb palsy: "waiter's tip" positioning of the arm (shoulder adduction and internal rotation with wrist flexion); there may be some sensory impairment; ability to fist is favorable sign for a good outcome.
- Klumpke palsy: paralyzed hand and forearm with good shoulder and elbow function.
- Total plexus avulsion: completely flaccid upper extremity.
- The neonatal physical examination should include a careful evaluation of the Moro reflex (for symmetry), respiratory effort, evidence of Horner syndrome (ptosis, myosis [pupillary contraction], anhidrosis [absence of sweat]), and the neuromuscular function of the involved extremity. After the neonatal period, examine for posterior shoulder dislocation (would present as markedly limited external rotation) or bony deformity of the glenoid.

Diagnostic Studies. If nerve root avulsion is suspected, high-resolution CT myelography, fast spin-echo MRI, and electromyography and nerve conduction studies can be used to evaluate the injury.

Differential Diagnosis. Ipsilateral clavicle fracture (with resultant pain that can explain the immobility of the extremity) and Horner syndrome (also presents with ptosis, myosis, and anhidrosis in addition to avulsion of the T1 nerve root).

Management. Includes gentle range-of-motion exercises by parents and scheduled follow-up appointments to note progress by the health care provider. Surgical exploration and repair of neurolysis and nerve grafting may be undertaken in those with nerve root avulsion. However, there are no standardized outcome measurements, and comparison between studies has been inconclusive (Mehlman, 2003). Older children with permanent functional limitations may be candidates for corrective shoulder surgery (e.g., derotational humeral osteotomy).

Prognosis. The majority of brachial plexus palsies (80% to 95%) spontaneously resolve over several weeks to several months. By the third month, recovery of biceps function (active motion against gravity) is evidenced. Should wrist, thumb, and finger extension occur by this time, excellent recovery can be expected. In those with nerve root avulsions, early intervention is crucial to achieve some functional recovery.

Febrile Seizures

Description. Febrile seizures are the most common type of seizures in children. They are brief, generalized, clonic or tonic-clonic in nature, and can be either simple or complex. Fever develops in most children at the time of the attack, and temperatures can be as low as 100.1° F to 101.4° F (37.8° C to 38.5° C). Little postictal confusion is associated with febrile seizures. Simple febrile seizures last less than 15 minutes and do not recur within a 24-hour period; complex febrile seizures last longer than 30 minutes, can recur on the same day, and can have focal attributes. Most (57%) febrile seizures occur 1 to 24 hours after fever onset, and 22% occur more than 24 hours after fever onset (Wolf & Shinner, 2005).

Epidemiology. The etiology of febrile seizures is unclear and by definition excludes seizures that are caused by intracranial illness or are related to an underlying CNS problem. There is some confusion as to whether the seizures are triggered by the height of the temperature or by the action of the temperature rising. Current research slightly favors the former interpretation (Wolf & Shinner, 2005). There is believed to be a familial predisposition (24%) that inherently leaves the child with a more temperature-sensitive immature neuronal membrane (Sankar et al, 2005). Research is ongoing to identify specific genes that might play a role in this familial predisposition (e.g., mutations in GABA-A receptors).

Febrile seizures generally occur in children between 3 months and 5 years old; the median age is 18 to 22 months (93% are between 6 months and 3 years old). Boys are affected more than girls. Two percent to 4% of all children have febrile seizures. The risk for subsequent febrile seizures is 30% to 50% (Wolf & Shinner, 2005).

Clinical Findings

History. The history of a patient with a presumed febrile seizure should include the following:

- Description of seizure duration, type (generalized or focal), frequency in 24 hours
- Relationship of the seizure to a febrile episode and level of temperature
- Any abnormal neurologic findings noted before the seizure (not consistent with a febrile seizure)
- Family history of afebrile seizures
- Maternal smoking in the perinatal period
- Prematurity or neonatal hospitalizations for more than 28 days
- Parents' perception of development of child

Physical Examination. The physical examination is the same as that described earlier for seizures.

Diagnostic Studies. Diagnostic studies include the following (Johnston, 2004c):

- Lumbar puncture in infants younger than 2 months old
- Blood glucose in all children (CBC, calcium, electrolytes, urinalysis are optional but frequently included)
- EEG if neurologic signs are present or seizure was atypical
- MRI with atypical febrile seizure features

Differential Diagnosis. Consider sepsis, meningitis, metabolic or toxic encephalopathies, hypoglycemia, anoxia, trauma, tumor, and hemorrhage. Febrile delirium and febrile shivering can be confused with seizures. Breath-holding spells can mimic febrile seizures; however, the former are always related to crying or tantrums. Febrile seizures come at unpredictable times during sleep, eating, play, or other generally calm times and are related to the onset of an illness. Epileptic seizures occur without concurrent illness and at unpredictable times.

Management. The following steps should be taken in the management of a febrile seizure:

- Protect the airway, breathing, and circulation if the seizure is still occurring. Place the child in a side-lying position to prevent aspiration or airway obstruction.
- Do not put anything in the child's mouth.
- Time the duration of the seizure and observe whether it is focal or generalized.
- Reduce the fever with acetaminophen or ibuprofen, although the use of antipyretics will not necessarily prevent another febrile seizure.
- The child should be seen shortly after the seizure. Advise transport to an emergency center if the seizure lasts more than 10 minutes.
- Most medical providers agree that anticonvulsants are not recommended for febrile seizures, but they may be considered in any of the following situations:
  - The child has abnormal neurologic findings or developmental delays.
  - The initial seizure was complex febrile, *and* there is a family history of afebrile seizures.
  - The child has recurrent, prolonged simple febrile seizures.

Prophylaxis. Prolonged anticonvulsant prophylaxis is no longer recommended. Phenytoin and carbamazepine antiepileptics are not useful; sodium valproate acid can be effective, but the side effects do not justify its use (Johnston, 2004c).

If prophylaxis is indicated, diazepam by mouth 0.3 mg/kg every 8 hours (1 mg/kg/24 hours) is given during a febrile illness (usually for 2 to 3 days). Side effects of diazepam include transient ataxis, lethargy, and irritability that can be decreased by adjusting the dosage (Johnston, 2004c). An alternative to diazepam, if transient ataxis or lethargy exists, is continuous daily phenobarbital to achieve a blood level of 15 mcg/mL. Phenobarbital, however, has behavioral side effects that are often intolerable to the family.

Education. The family should receive information about febrile seizures, their risks, and their management. Education should include information explaining the febrile seizure;

reassurance that no long-term consequences are associated with febrile seizures; information that febrile seizures recur in some children and that nothing can be done to prevent the seizures; and first-aid information in case another seizure occurs at some time. The decision to use prophylaxis is up to the parents and the medical provider on a case by case basis. A follow-up phone call after the event is useful.

Complications. Death or persisting motor deficits do not occur in patients with febrile seizures. No indication has been found that intellect or learning is impaired. An affected child has an increased risk for the development of epilepsy (less than 5%) if the seizure is prolonged and focal; if the child has repeated seizures with the same febrile episode; or if the child has had a prior neurologic deficit, a family history of epilepsy, or both. Two thirds of children who have had one simple febrile seizure will not have any more. The younger the age at onset (less than 18 months old) of the first febrile seizure, the lower the temperature threshold is needed to cause the child to seize and the more likely the child is to have a recurrence.

Guillain-Barré Syndrome

Description. A paralysis that usually follows a nonspecific viral infection, Guillain-Barré syndrome is a polyneuropathy that mainly affects motor, but sometimes sensory and autonomic nerves. Most patients have a demyelinating neuropathy; axonal degeneration is another variant. A congenital form can occur. It is rare (hypotonia, weakness, areflexia); no treatment is generally required; most infants improve over the first months of life and are symptom free by 12 months old (Sarnat, 2004).

Clinical Findings

History. The following is reported:
- Nonspecific viral infection (gastrointestinal or respiratory) occurring within last 10 days
- Report of weakness beginning usually in the lower extremity and progressing up the trunk, upper limbs, and ending in the bulbar muscles (known as Landry ascending paralysis). Onset gradual, progressing over days or weeks
- Children are often irritable
- Muscle tenderness and pain may be reported in the initial stages if onset was sudden

Physical Examination
- Inability or refusal to walk to flaccid tetraplegia or quadriplegia
- Paresthesia may or may not be present
- Respiratory insufficiency
- Dysphagia, facial weakness
- Eyes: Extraocular muscle involvement rare; papilledema may be seen. Visual acuity changes not usually seen
- Miller-Fisher syndrome may be seen (acute external ophthalmoplegia, ataxia, areflexia [often early in disease])
- Signs of viral meningitis or meningoencephalitis
- Urinary retention or incontinence (20% of cases) is usually transient in nature
- Blood pressure and cardiac rate changes, including bradycardia, postural hypotension, asystole

Diagnostic Studies. The following are included in the work-up:
- CSF studies: elevated CSF protein (usually greater than twice upper limit of normal); normal glucose, no pleocytosis (less than 10 WBC/mm^3)
- Negative blood cultures; viral cultures rarely conclusive
- Normal or mildly elevated creatine kinase (CK) level; antiganglioside antibodies (against GM1, GD1) may be elevated in axonal neuropathy form of the disease
- Decreased motor nerve conduction velocities; slowed sensory nerve conduction
- Electromyogram (EMG): shows acute denervation of muscle

Differential Diagnosis. Bickerstaff brainstem encephalitis, meningitis, meningoencephalitis are included differential diagnoses.

Management. Hospitalization is paramount for observation and for handling complications of respiratory muscle paralysis. Intravenous immunoglobulin (IVIG), plasmapheresis, steroids, and/or immunosuppressive drugs may be administered. In cases unresponsive to IVIG, combination immunoglobulin and interferon can be effective. Care is supportive (respiratory, prevention of decubitus, treatment of secondary bacterial infection).

Complications. Chronic varieties of Guillain-Barré can occur, as evidenced by recurrence or lack of improvement of symptoms over months or years. Approximately 7% of children will have relapses (Sarnat, 2004). Unresolved weakness, flaccid tetraplegia or quadriplegia, bulbar and respiratory muscle compromise may linger or remain.

Headaches

Description. Headaches are common during childhood, increasing in frequency and incidence during adolescence. Headaches fall into two classifications—acute and chronic. Table 27-6 lists the more common types found in these classifications. A person may experience different types of headaches. A careful history and examination are paramount to making the diagnosis.

Epidemiology. Headaches have been reported to occur in one-third to one-half of children by 7 years old and in from 57% to 80% of those 15 years and older (Lewis, 2004). The exact physiologic mechanism for many headaches has not been determined.

Migraine headaches are common in children and often go unrecognized or are attributed to other causes. The exact etiology is still unknown; however, several theories are proposed (Miller, 2005). Pain fibers line the walls of the large intracranial blood vessels; the meninges and periosteum; the muscles around the head, neck, scalp, eyes, and jaw area; and the sinuses. The pain-sensitive blood vessels can be stimulated by inflammation and vasodilation. Intracranial pressure can cause pain as a result of traction and displacement of intracranial arteries. Low serotonin levels and temporary increases in dopamine levels are theorized as possibly contributing to the initiation of headache symptomatology (Miller, 2005).

TABLE 27-6   Most Common Types of Headaches

Characteristics	Vascular (Migraine)	Cluster	Chronic, Daily, Low Grade	Tension
Prevalence	2.5% occurrence in children <7yr old; 5% occurrence prepuberty; 5% occurrence postpuberty if male; 10% occurrence postpuberty if female Female:male = 3:2	Uncommon in children Occur mostly in females, more than 10 yr old	Most common type of chronic headaches in all ages	All ages; commonly starts during adolescence; both sexes affected
History	Positive family history (90% of patients have both parents with history); 80% have one parent with history); 50% have history of motion sickness	Family history is rare Rarely begins in childhood	Use of caffeine (including caffeinated drinks) or chronic use of nonprescription analgesics; social, psychological, emotional factors.	Positive family history with childhood onset; fatigue, stress, depression, exertion
Pattern	Recurrent pattern May be aura Transitory neurologic changes (nausea and vomiting, malaise, personality changes, photophobia, phonophobia) Appears sick Periodic "ice-pick" pain on top of head described by adolescents Resolves after sleeping Pain lasts 2-4 hr in younger children; 48-72 hr in adolescents	Unilateral headache recurring daily over 4-8 wk with 1-2 yr between occurrences Typically occurs in fall or spring Pain occurs in bursts lasting 30-90 min and repeated several times a day Hurts to lie down, pain intense (constant or throbbing); scalp tender, conjunctiva injected, tearing, nasal congestion, ptosis, eyelid edema) No nausea or vomiting	Throbbing pain, anxiety, malaise if does not take the above routinely Occurs >15 days/mo for several mo Generalized pain, low intensity, dull ache, does not interfere with most activities, but may decrease them	Bilateral, diffuse (site may shift), dull, aching pain ("tight band around head"), located in neck and back of head May appear on awakening and continue all day; does not increase with activity No nausea, vomiting, photophobia, phonophobia, or neurologic changes; negative neurologic examination Lasts 30 min, all day, or for up to 7 days Can occur at same time as more classic migraine headache
Triggers	Stress, tension, anxiety, fatigue, exercise, head trauma, menstrual cycle, sexual activity, hunger, bright lights, odors, alcohol, certain foods, noise, travel, cold weather	None	Withdrawal from caffeine or analgesics; stress or emotional upsets	May be stress, musculoskeletal dysfunction

			Tension headaches	
Differential diagnosis	Benign occipital epilepsy of childhood (same visual changes as migraine, but are followed by either unilateral or clonic-tonic; complex partial seizure pattern, then headache and nausea—occurs usually as child falls asleep)	Chronic paroxysmal one-sided head pain (hemicrania), migraines, temporal arteritis, sinusitis, glaucoma		Migraine, brain tumor, cervical, ocular and temporomandibular disorders, chronic sphenoid sinusitis
Diagnostic tests	None (EEG if: suspect benign occipital epilepsy; neurologic exam is abnormal; atypical history and pattern)	None	None	None
Treatment (see Appendix A for dosing)	Acute: See Table 27-9; Prophylaxis: See Table 27-9*; Others: biofeedback and relaxation	Suppression: prednisone 1mg/kg/day for 5 days, then taper for 2 wk; Divalproex, lithium; Acute attack: sumatriptan, oxygen, lithium. Oxygen is treatment of choice (inhale oxygen for 10min at 7-10L/min following onset [70% effective])	Acute only: acetaminophen, ibuprofen, naproxen, or other nonsteroidal antiinflammatory drugs; antidepressants	Acute: analgesics, nonsteroidal antiinflammatory drugs; amitriptyline, tizanidine; Chronic: antidepressants (treatment of choice; start with low dose and increase every 3-7 days; try for at least 1-2 mo), beta blockers, anticonvulsants; Other: massage, relaxation with techniques, cold, alternating warm compresses to occipital area

*Prophylaxis is indicated if the child has two to four severe episodes a month or cannot attend school regularly.

hr, Hour(s); min, minutes; mo, month(s); yr, year(s); wk, week(s).

Data from Fenichel GM: Clinical pediatric neurology: a signs and symptoms approach, ed 4, Philadelphia, 2001, WB Saunders, pp 77-89; Chutorian AM: Headaches. In Burg et al: Current pediatric therapy, ed 18, Philadelphia, 2006, WB Saunders; Unger J: Pediatric migraines: clinical pearls in diagnosis and therapy, Consultant Ped 5(9):545-551, 2006; Damen L, Bruijn JK, Verhagen AP: Symptomatic treatment of migraine in children: a systematic review of medication trials, Pediatrics 116(2):295-302, 2005; Silberstein SD, Young WB: Headaches and facial pain. In Goetz CG: Textbook of clinical neurology, ed 2, Philadelphia, 2003, WB Saunders.

Prevalence rates are reported to be 5% (3 to 7 years old); 4% to 11% (7 to 11 years old); 8% to 23% (11 to 15+ years old). The mean age of onset is 7.2 years for males and 10.9 years for females (Lewis et al, 2004).

Muscle contraction or *tension headaches* are common.

Traction or *inflammatory headaches* are much rarer, occurring when structural intracranial pathology (e.g., a tumor) causes traction or increases intracranial pressure on pain-sensitive structures within the brain.

Cluster headaches occur rarely in childhood; they become uncommon by the time the child reaches adolescence.

Clinical Findings. The International Headache Society provides succinct clinical criteria to help the provider evaluate and classify migraines—both with and without aura—in children less than or equal to 15 years of age (Box 27-3). Children less than 10 years of age often have a poor sense of time and may not serve as the best historians. The most important questions to ask the child and parent(s) regard frequency, location, and associated symptoms.

History. The following factors are assessed in the history of a child with headache:

• *Duration.* Recent severe onset is worrisome.
• *Frequency and triggers.* Children with recurrent, low-intensity headaches, with no neurologic changes, and who recover completely between episodes are unlikely to have serious intracranial etiology. Triggers can include ovulation or menstruation, exercise, food or odors, and stress. Other triggers can include chocolate, processed meats, aged cheeses, nuts, altered amounts of caffeine intake, diary products, shellfish and some dried fruits.
• *Location.* Occipital or consistently localized headaches can indicate underlying pathology. Facial pain might be sinusitis. Ocular motor imbalance can produce a dull periorbital discomfort, whereas temporomandibular joint pain tends to localize around the periauricular or temporal areas.
• *Quality and severity of pain.* Sharp, throbbing, or pounding pain is probably vascular (migraine). Dull and constant pain may be tension or organic. Severity can be assessed by asking about limitations to activities and missed school days. How many "different kinds of headaches" are experienced?

• *Age of onset,* progression of the headaches over time, and longest period of time without symptoms.
• *Home management* and medications used.
• *Self-coping activities.*
• *Associated symptoms* can include: nausea, vomiting, visual changes, dizziness, paresthesia, neck/shoulder pain, back pain, otalgia, abdominal pain, hypersomnia, food cravings, confusion, ataxia, pallor, photophobia, and phonophobia. Changes in gait, personality, mentation, or behavior that do not occur at the same time as the headache are worrisome and merit further evaluation with medical referral. There are some precursor symptoms and conditions that can indicate a predisposition to migraines. These include cyclic vomiting (see Chapter 32), abdominal migraine (see Chapter 32), and benign paroxysmal vertigo. Alone, they do not warrant extensive or expensive work-ups (Unger, 2006).
• *Head trauma.* If associated with headache, head trauma can represent a subdural hematoma or postconcussive syndrome.
• *Psychologic symptoms.* Evaluate for the presence of depression, school stressors, or concerns about family functioning
• *Family history.* Most children with headache, especially migraine, have a family history of headaches.

Characteristics of classic migraine include nausea; abdominal pain; vomiting; unilateral pain; pulsating pain; relief with sleep; an aura; visual changes such as dark or blind spots; and a history of a family member with migraines in 90% of cases. Dizziness and motion sickness can be described. Infants and toddlers may present with irritability, sleepiness, and pallor. In preadolescents, common migraine symptoms are more likely. Nausea and vomiting might not occur, and the pain can be more frontal. Lethargy and sleep can follow. Visual changes are rare, and the pain quality is variable. Times between headaches are pain free. Abdominal migraine is rare; symptoms include pain, nausea, and vomiting with minimal or no headache. Such symptoms can also be suggestive of complex partial seizures (Finberg & Kleinman, 2002).

There is no prodrome with muscle contraction or tension headaches. The pain is dull and bifrontal or occipital, with

---

BOX 27-3	**Classification of Pediatric and Adolescent Migraine**

With Aura
1. Meets all the criteria for migraine without aura
2. Individual has at least three of the following symptoms:
• ≥ one reversible aura symptoms
• At least one aura develops slowly over >4 hour, or two or more aura symptoms occur in succession
• Aura does not last >1 hour
• Headache follows the aura in <1 hour

Without Aura
Individual experiences ≥ five attacks
Headache episode lasts 1-72 hour
Headache has two or more of the following characteristics:
• Located bilaterally or unilaterally
• Pulsation present
• Intensity is moderate to severe
• Is aggravated by routine physical activity
Headache has one or both of the following:
• Nausea and/or vomiting
• Photophobia and/or phonophobia

Data from Headache Classification Subcommittee of the International Headache Society: International classification of headache disorders, ed 2, *Cephalalgia* 24(suppl):9-160, 2004.

nausea and vomiting occurring only rarely. Tension headaches can last for days or weeks but do not interfere with activities. In children it can be difficult to differentiate migraine and muscle contraction headaches. Psychosocial stress seems to be a major factor in tension headaches in both children and adolescents.

The key historical point for traction or inflammatory headaches is increasing pain severity, often with 88% having accompanying neurologic signs (Wilne et al, 2006). Other presenting symptoms of such headaches include:

- Headache pain that is worse in the morning on awakening and standing up
- Pain that wakens child from sleep
- Vomiting but not nausea
- Visual disturbances, diplopia, edema of the optic disk
- Increased pain with straining, sneezing, coughing, defecation, or changes in position
- Occipital region and neck pain
- Educational or behavioral alterations, irritability
- Seizures
- Unsteadiness
- Mental changes

The preceding symptoms would require prompt follow-up and referral (Box 27-4). A child with a history of a ventriculo-peritoneal shunt, meningitis, and/or hydrocephaly also needs prompt referral.

Physical Examination. The physical examination is usually normal. The following areas must be assessed:

- Blood pressure
- Neurologic examination
- Optic fundi
- Height and weight
- Head circumference (infants up to 24 months old)
- Pericranial muscles for tenderness
- Sinuses (frontal and maxillary)
- Teeth
- Temporomandibular joints (mouth and jaw)
- Thyroid gland
- Cranial bruits (over temples and orbits)

Diagnostic Studies. Imaging studies are rarely indicated unless the history suggests symptoms of increased intracranial pressure (see Box 27-4) or when a complaint of "dizziness" fits the criteria listed in Table 27-7. Parents seek medical attention for pain relief for their child, in addition to reassurance that there are no intracranial processes occurring (brain tumors). In most cases a good history and physical assessment can help the examiner distinguish the harmful from the merely painful headache. A CT scan without contrast is usually adequate to determine the presence of a brain tumor. If abnormal, an MRI should be done. An EEG should be obtained if the history and physical examination suggest a seizure process. If there was external trauma, such as from a motor vehicle accident, cervical and spinal x-rays should be ordered.

Differential Diagnosis. The differential diagnosis consists of sinusitis, an intracranial mass, pseudotumor cerebri, sleep disorder, hyperthyroidism, hypertension, cyclic vomiting, abdominal migraine, BPV, and temporomandibular joint

dysfunction. Visual acuity is rarely a cause of headaches. These and other causes of headaches in children are outlined in Table 27-8.

Management. Each child with headaches requires an individually tailored strategy that may or may not include pharmacologic and nonpharmacologic modalities. Many of the newer medications (e.g., triptans) used in adults have not been adequately tested for safety and efficacy in children and adolescents. Treatment can include general pain management, abortive therapy to interrupt migraine headaches, and prophylactic medications to prevent or reduce the frequency and severity of acute attacks.

The goals of treating acute-onset migraines include: treating the attacks quickly and consistently; restoring ability to function; minimizing back-up and rescue medications; optimizing self-care abilities of the patient and family; cost-effective treatment; and minimizing medication side effects (Lewis et al, 2004).

Prophylactic therapy is considered when headaches cause a child to miss school more than once monthly and when the child suffers severe headaches two to four times a month. The goals of preventive treatments include: reducing attack frequency, severity and duration; improving response to acute attack treatments; and restoring ability to function (Lewis et al, 2004). Anticonvulsants are also used, especially if the child has a seizure disorder. Other medications might include beta blockers, antidepressants, NSAIDs, or calcium channel

---

BOX 27-4 Signs and Symptoms Suggestive of Intracranial Structural Pathology

Infants
Full anterior fontanelle
Open metopic and coronal sutures
Poor growth
Impaired upward gaze
Abnormal head growth
Shrill cry
Lethargy
Vomiting

Children
Persistent unilateral headache
Papilledema
Abnormal eye movements (or one or both eyes suddenly turn in)
Ataxia
Hemiparesis
Abnormal deep tendon reflexes
Severe, excruciating headache of recent onset, unlike any previously experienced; no normal period of functioning between episodes of headache
Cranial bruits
Personality changes

Data from Chutorian AM: Headaches. In Burg et al: *Current pediatric therapy*, ed 18, Philadelphia, 2006, WB Saunders.

TABLE 27-7	How to Proceed When the Complaint Is "Dizziness"	

Complaint of "Dizziness"	Studies Indicated
Light-headed	None
Double vision (posterior fossa location)	MRI
Sensation of whirling motion of oneself or of room or objects (vertigo)	MRI
Confusion	MRI, EEG, comprehensive metabolic screen

EEG, Electroencephalogram; *MRI*, magnetic resonance imaging.

blockers. See Table 27-9 for treatment options compiled from sources that have reviewed random, placebo-controlled studies in the pediatric age group.

Refer all patients with organic (structural) headaches. Patients with refractory headaches (after more than three classic prophylactic regimens have failed) should be referred for adjunct counseling, relaxation, and other coping techniques (e.g., biofeedback, yoga).

Counseling. For nonorganic headaches (e.g., no tumor, aneurysm, or metabolic or structural cause), reassure the parents and patient. The patient should be taught pain and stress management techniques. There can be significant loss of school attendance as a result of headaches. School attendance should be mandatory, although a quiet rest period may be allowed at school if needed. School nurses can be helpful in developing a plan for school attendance. If the child remains home, activities should be restricted to bed and all homework completed. The child should be returned to school if the pain improves during the school day. Minimize attention to the headache. Relaxation exercises or biofeedback training can be helpful. Trigger factors should be avoided. Refer to Chapter 42 for complementary and alternative therapies.

Complications. Brain tumors, abscesses, hematomas, and arteriovenous malformations in children are generally associated with ataxia, papilledema, intellectual changes, or behavioral changes. These processes crowd out other intracranial structures, precipitating edema and interfering with the normal actions of CSF and vessels. Infants may initially accommodate well to the increase in intracranial pressure because of the ability of their cranial sutures to expand. Serious pathologic conditions are also considered when headaches interrupt sleep, increase in frequency and severity over a period of only a few weeks, occur on rising and then fade, are relieved by vomiting, are exacerbated by changes in position or with straining, are accompanied by diplopia, persist at the occiput, or are related to personality, ataxic, or behavioral changes.

TABLE 27-8	Additional Causes of Headaches in Children	

Cause	Characteristics
Drugs	
Cocaine	Migraine-like pain in patient with no history of migraine headaches
Marijuana	Frontal, mild
Analgesics and cardiovascular agents	Pain follows administration (of drug) or withdrawal (typical of analgesics)
Food additives (nitrites, monosodium glutamate common)	Pain occurs only in individual genetically sensitive; pain is diffuse, throbbing after ingestion
Physiologic	
Vasculitis	Uncommon in children; can occur as part of a collagen-vascular disease, such as systemic lupus erythematosus
Chronic hypertension	Low-grade, occipital pain on awakening or frontal during day
Eyestrain	Dull, aching pain behind eyes relieved when eyes are closed; caused by muscular fatigue during prolonged ocular convergence; not a refractive error
Temporomandibular joint syndrome (TMJ)	>8 years old; pain on one side of face and vertex of TMJ; may be a history of jaw injury
Whiplash and neck injury	Pain dull, aching in neck, shoulders, upper arms with poor neck rotation; no nausea or vomiting; caused by muscles contracted to "splint" area of dysfunction in cervical joint areas or soft tissue
Following partial or generalized seizure	Diffuse pain
Infectious illness	Uncommon
Dental disease	Uncommon
Malfunctioning shunt	History of ventriculoperitoneal, ventriculopleural, or ventriculoatrial shunt

Data from Fenichel G: *Clinical pediatric neurology: a signs and symptoms approach,* ed 4, Philadelphia, 2001, WB Saunders, pp 85-89.

TABLE 27-9	**Therapies for Pediatric Migraine**

Drug	Dosage	Notes From Studies (Unger, 2006; Lewis et al, 2004)
Acute Treatment **Nonspecific Acute Migraine Medications** (*these should be tried first in acute management*)		
• Acetaminophen*	10-15 mg/kg/dose every 4 hr up to 500 mg every 4 hr	• Acetaminophen has faster onset of action than ibuprofen
• Ibuprofen*	7.5-10 mg/kg every 4 hr up to 800 mg q 8 hrs	• Ibuprofen showed greater headache resolution than acetaminophen
• Naproxen sodium	10 mg/kg/dose every 8-12 hr up to 7 mg/kg every 8 hr	• Safe and effective
• Dimenhydrinate	5 mg/kg/24 hr in four divided doses	• Use when vomiting is a major symptom
Migraine–Specific Acute Medications* *Ergotamine preparations*		
• Ergotamine tartrate or dihydroergotamine)	1 mg PO, SQ, or per rectum suppository; may be repeated in 30 minutes	• Most effective when given early in aural stage • Consider for older children • DBCT showed no differences in effect between dihydroergotamine and placebo
5-HTI-receptor agonists (triptans):		
• Sumatriptan (Imitrex)*	Consider for children >12 yr old: Nasal spray*: 5 mg or 20 mg once as needed (may repeat once if headache unresolved after 1 hr) SQ (self-administered): 3 mg or 6 mg once (do not repeat) Tablet: 25 mg, 50 mg, 100 mg (may be repeated once after 1 hr)	Triptans are all FDA approved for those ≥18 yr old; regarded safe, and well tolerated in children ≥12 yr old; efficacy rates for the triptans (*except for sumatriptan nasal spray and oral zolmitriptan*) are essentially the same as for placebos; they may prolong an aura. If the first dose is given in the outpatient setting, the patient should be monitored for 1 hr • Side-effects: hot flushes; nausea and vomiting, chest/neck/head pressure, tingling • DBCT: when compared with placebo, nasal sumatriptan significantly reduces headache; side-effects present with sumatriptan vs placebo • Inadequate data to support use of subcutaneous sumatriptan use in children
• Zolmitriptan (Zomig)	≥18 yr. 2.5 mg PO, once prn (5 mg also available) ODT: 2.5-5 mg PO once, prn	
• Rizatriptan (Maxalt)	≥18 yr: 5-10 mg PO once, prn ODT: 5-10 mg PO once, prn	• Studies limited in children; one study found no difference in symptom relief between drug and placebo; side-effects well tolerated

Continued

TABLE 27-9 **Therapies for Pediatric Migraine—Cont'd**

Drug	Dosage	Notes From Studies (Unger, 2006; Lewis et al, 2004)
• Naratriptan (Amerge)	≥18yr: 1-2.5mg once, prn	• Do not use concurrently with an SSRI or SNRI, as serotonin syndrome can occur
• Almotriptan (Axert)	≥18yr: 6.25-12.5mg PO once, prn (start with 6.25mg)	
• Frovatriptan (Frova)	≥18yr: 2.5mg PO at onset; may use up to 3 does in 24hrs	
• Eletriptan (Relpax)	≥18yr: 20mg-40mg PO once, prn	
Prophylaxis Treatment (maintain use for at least 1yr) *Antidepressants*		
• Amitriptyline (nortriptyline and desipramine have not been studied)	Starting dosage 25-75mg at bedtime, increasing every 2weeks to maximum of 100 mg at bedtime. Maintenance dose 50-100 mg/d	• Most studies using amitriptyline in children have been open-label • Efficacy in 50%-80% of children • Adverse effects: somnolence, dry mouth, arrhythmia • Use with caution in children aged <12yr old
• Trazodone *Anticonvulsants*		• Mixed results; no appreciable side-effects
• Divalproex sodium (Depakote)	• 10-30mg/kg/day PO bid in divided doses up to 40mg/k/day	• Reduced headache frequency of 50%-70% in children aged 7-17yr old • Adverse effects: weight gain, heartburn, hair loss, dizziness • Not for use in children aged <2yr old
• Topiramate (Topamax)	5-10mg/kg/d divided bid up to maximum dose 100mg/d	• Headache frequency from one study showed reduction from 5.4 to 1.9 days per mo in children 6-15yr old: 52% attacks eliminated • Adverse effects: weight loss, episodes of paresthesia, cognitive slowing, loss of appetite, dizziness, irritability • Indicated in epilepsy for children as young as 2yr old
Antiserotonergic agents • Cyproheptadine (Periactin)	• Age <2yr: not recommended • 2-6yr: 0.25mg/kg/day PO (tablet or syrup) • Age ≥7yr: 2mg PO daily; then titrate to 3-4mg PO daily	• Used more in toddlers because weight gain and somnolence is primary adverse effect in older children • In children aged 3-12yr old, drug was effective in up to 83% of patients, per retrospective study • Do not use methysergide in children <10yr old and do not use for more than 3mo (prolonged use can cause retroperitoneal or pulmonary fibrosis)
Antihypertensives • β-blockers: Propranolol (others include atenolol, metoprolol, nadolol)†	≥7-8yr: 2-4mg/kg/day PO daily (max 4mg/kg/day); begin with lowest dose and increase gradually over 2wk until desired effect seen or max dose reached (may be divided bid or tid)	• May take up to several weeks to a month to be effective

TABLE 27-9	**Therapies for Pediatric Migraine—Cont'd**	
Drug	**Dosage**	**Notes From Studies (Unger, 2006; Lewis et al, 2004)**
• Alpha-agonist: (Clonidine)		• May lower blood pressure or cause depressive adverse effects or exercise-induced asthma • 71% of children 7-16 yr old had complete remission using 60-120 mg/day in a DBCT; other trials failed to show any improvement in headache frequency. • No significant difference in headaches between clonidine and placebo groups
• Calcium channel blockers (Nimodipine)	7-18 yr: 10-20 mg tid	• Reduces headache frequency • Adverse effect: rare mild abdominal discomfort
• Flunarizine[†]	5-13 yr: 5 mg	• Probably effective for reducing frequency • Not available in the U.S.

*Recommended as most effective treatment for acute migraine in children and adolescents (Lewis et al, 2004).

[†]Probably the most effective treatment for prophylaxis in children. Insufficient evidence for cyproheptadine, amitriptyline, divalproex sodium, topiramate, levetiracetam; conflicting evidence for propranolol and trazodone. Pizotifen, nimodipine, clonidine do not show efficacy (Lewis et al, 2004).

bid, Twice daily; *d,* day; *DBCT,* double-blind controlled trial; *hr,* hours; *max,* maximum; *mo,* month; *ODT,* orally disintegrating tablet; *PO,* by mouth; *SQ,* subcutaneous; *tid,* three times daily; *wk, weeks; yr, years.*

Data from Unger J: Pediatric migraines: clinical pearls in diagnosis and therapy, *Consultant for Pediatricians* 5(9):541-551, 2006. Other data from Haslam RH: Headaches. In Behrman RD, Kliegman RM, Jenson HB, editors, *Nelson textbook of pediatrics,* ed 17, Philadelphia, 2004, WB Saunders; Damen L, Bruijn JK, Verhagen AP, et al: Symptomatic treatment of migraine in children: a systematic review of medication trials, *Pediatrics* 116(2):295-302, 2005; Lewis D, Ashwal S, Hershey A, et al: Practice parameter: pharmacological treatment of migraine headache in children and adolescents, *Neurology* 63(12):2215-2224, 2004.

Head Injury

Description.   Head trauma involves tissue damage to the brain and its surrounding structures, and injury can range from mild to severe. Head injuries can be either open or closed. Open head trauma produces more focal injuries. Closed head trauma causes more multifocal or diffuse damage. Primary effects are from the initial injury and are related to mechanical forces that tear connections within the brain and cause contusions where the brain hits the skull surfaces (e.g., shaken baby syndrome). Axons to distant areas, fibers in the corpus callosum connecting the two hemispheres, or both can be torn. Contusions and hemorrhage can occur. Secondary effects of the trauma, such as hypoxia, ischemia, hypotension, brain swelling, hemorrhage, contusion, and SE, can affect recovery. Brain injury is the leading cause of death in those under 35 years old. Half of all deaths caused by such injuries occur in children under 15 years old, with males being victims twice as often as females.

Clinical Findings and Management.   Immediate assessment and care of a head-injured patient is outside the scope of this chapter. More information is found in Chapter 39 including the Glasgow Coma Scale (GCS), which has been traditionally used to measure the severity of head injury. The reliability of the GCS has been recently questioned as to the value of its accuracy in predicting outcome. Schaan and colleagues (2002) noted the difficulties of the requisite site-of-accident GCS score and difficulty "scaling" patients because of sedation and intubation. New scales that combine CT scans and clinical parameters (pupil dilation, hemiparesis, and brainstem signs) to predict outcome are being researched. It is acknowledged by Schaan and colleagues that predictive scales

of outcome alone should not be used to modify patient management. See Table 27-10 for a useful post-injury assessment guideline. Guidelines for sports-related injuries and when children might resume activities are found in Chapter 14.

The primary care provider is likely to encounter post-trauma patients. The duration of coma is predictive of subsequent neurologic function. A coma lasting less than 24 hours has a favorable outcome, unless there was focal brain damage. In children 10 years old or younger, normal functioning can be expected in those whose comas last less than 1.7 weeks. However, comas of less than 3 weeks can lead to borderline intelligence; comas of 8 weeks or less can result in mild retardation; and those of 11 weeks or less can lead to severe retardation (Rosman, 2006). The severity of the head injury can have significant impact on school performance and adjustment. There is a strong association between cognitive and motor development and behavioral problems before and after severe head injury. Both providers and school personnel should be alert to a lack of progress and deterioration of skills. A neuropsychological evaluation may be helpful to plan appropriate educational and behavioral management.

Children (2 to 6 years old) are usually more impaired than adolescents, secondary to immature brain development and general vulnerability. However, children and adolescents are more likely to show improvement in cognitive and social skills than adults who suffered the same degree of head trauma. Such improvement may evolve steadily over several years. Approximately 5% of hospitalized children with a head injury suffer a seizure within the first week; another 5% experience a seizure after this time (Rosman, 2006).

TABLE 27-10 **Head Injury Acuity**

Characteristics	Mild	Moderate	Severe
Length of time patient was unconscious or had posttraumatic amnesia	<1 hour	1-24 hours	>24 hours
Glasgow Coma Scale score	13-15	9-12	3-8
Symptoms	Usually alert in the emergency department with headache, lethargy, irritability, withdrawn, may or may not be labile	Occasional brain swelling and hematomas Headache, concentration, problem-solving and memory problems; symptoms can last for several months	Approximately 50% mortality rate; impaired memory, concentration, and organizational skill problems
Sequelae	Repeated "minor" damage (e.g., head trauma with sports) can result in changes in neuropsychology (attention, arousal, and information processing). ADHD, decreased attention span, emotional changes, sleep disturbances, memory problems, headache, language deficits can result	Same as for "mild"	Seizures, hemiparesis, aphasia, cognitive problems, behavior changes Anxiety, attention problems (similar to ADHD)

ADHD, Attention-deficit/hyperactivity disorder.
Data from Semrud-Clikeman M: *Traumatic brain injury in children and adolescents: assessment and intervention,* New York, 2001, Guilford Press.

The most common causes of head trauma differ according to age. Infants and toddlers are more likely to obtain head trauma from falls and physical abuse. Young children suffer head trauma from falls and pedestrian and bicycle accidents: adolescents suffer head trauma from motor vehicle accidents (Centers for Disease Control and Prevention [CDC], 2006). Concussions are commonly related to sports injuries. See Chapter 14 for information on posttrauma management of head injuries related to sports.

Prevention

- Wear helmets when using bicycles, skateboards, scooters, motorcycles, and in-line skate. The proper fitting of helmets can be found in Chapter 14.
- Protect children from falls in the home or from playground equipment.
- School-age children and adolescents should have properly fitting headgear appropriate for their sports participation.
- Use appropriate seat restraints when riding in motor vehicles.

Prevention of secondary brain trauma from hemorrhage, edema, and other factors can be maximized by the prompt management of head trauma events.

Disturbances of Head Growth

Macrocephaly. Macrocephaly is defined as a head circumference more than 2 standard deviations (SD) above the mean for age and sex or one that increases too rapidly. "Large" heads may be genetic and only of statistical significance; the provider's initial evaluation should be to measure both parents' head circumferences. Macrocephaly can also be attributed to hydrocephaly, megalencephaly (enlarged brain), subdural hematoma, tumor, thickening of the skull, or other problems. Benign familial macrocephaly occurs as or can be related to a genetic syndrome (anatomic or metabolic), such as Sotos syndrome (cerebral gigantism). Infants with anatomic megalencephaly will have macrocephaly at birth, but those with a metabolic etiology will be normocephalic at birth. In cases of excessive volumes of CSF, the fluid may be located within the brain (in the ventricular cavities) or outside the brain, in the subarachnoid spaces.

A CT scan can be diagnostic with consultation or referral if abnormal. A CT finding of "benign enlargement of the subarachnoid spaces" is transient in nature. The subarachnoid enlargement resolves by school age, though the macrocephaly will remain.

Hydrocephaly. Hydrocephaly is a condition in which an increased volume of CSF causes progressive ventricular dilation. The etiology includes a wide variety of disorders, such as infection, tumor, hemorrhage, and congenital malformation. The patient can have a large head, an excessive rate of head growth, irritability, vomiting, loss of appetite, impaired upgaze and other extraocular movements, hypertonia, and hyperreflexia. Papilledema may not be present in an infant, whereas it does appear in older children with closed cranial sutures. In a neonate, the head can sometimes be transilluminated. Prompt referral and surgical treatment are necessary.

Microcephaly. Microcephaly is defined as a head circumference two SD below the mean for age and sex or a head where the growth is increasingly slower than normal. Different ethnic groups have different standards of head circumferences. On examination, the skull will appear to be normally shaped; palpation may reveal some overlapping bones along the suture lines. This disorder can result from conditions in which the brain never formed correctly because of genetic or chromosomal abnormalities. Disease processes that interfere with normal brain growth can also be causative (these infants will have normal head circumferences at birth). Brain damage that occurs prenatally will not be evident initially, but a decreasing head circumference curve will start to occur after the infant reaches 3 to 6 months old.

Commonly, microcephalic children have delayed developmental milestones and neurologic problems. Management of microcephaly is supportive and directed toward management of the resulting deficits. Protein-calorie malnutrition, craniosynostosis, and hypopituitarism are treatable causes of microcephaly. Referral to a pediatrician or neurologist should be made for diagnosis. Development of an interdisciplinary management plan may be useful.

Craniosynostosis. The provider needs to be able to distinguish between primary and secondary skull malformations. Congenital (or "true" or "primary") craniosynostosis involves early closure or absence of one or more cranial sutures. When more than one suture is involved, there is more likely to be an associated genetic disorder; craniosynostosis can be found in more than 60 genetic syndromes (e.g., Crouzon, Apert, Carpenter, Chotzen, Pfeiffer), but all of these syndromes also have extracranial features (Consultant for Pediatricians editorial staff, 2006). Growth along the remaining open suture lines produces progressive skull deformity in one or more directions. The skull is flat over the closed suture(s). Increased intracranial pressure may result as the brain tries to grow within the confined space, but this does not always occur. Primary craniosynostosis occurs in 1 per 2000 births (Johnston & Kinsman, 2004), is ethnically neutral, and can vary in type and prominence between genders. The sagittal suture is most commonly fused (referred to as scaphocephaly or dolichocephaly) and accounts for 60% of all cases. Fig. 27-3 illustrates the different descriptions for skull deformities seen with craniosynostosis.

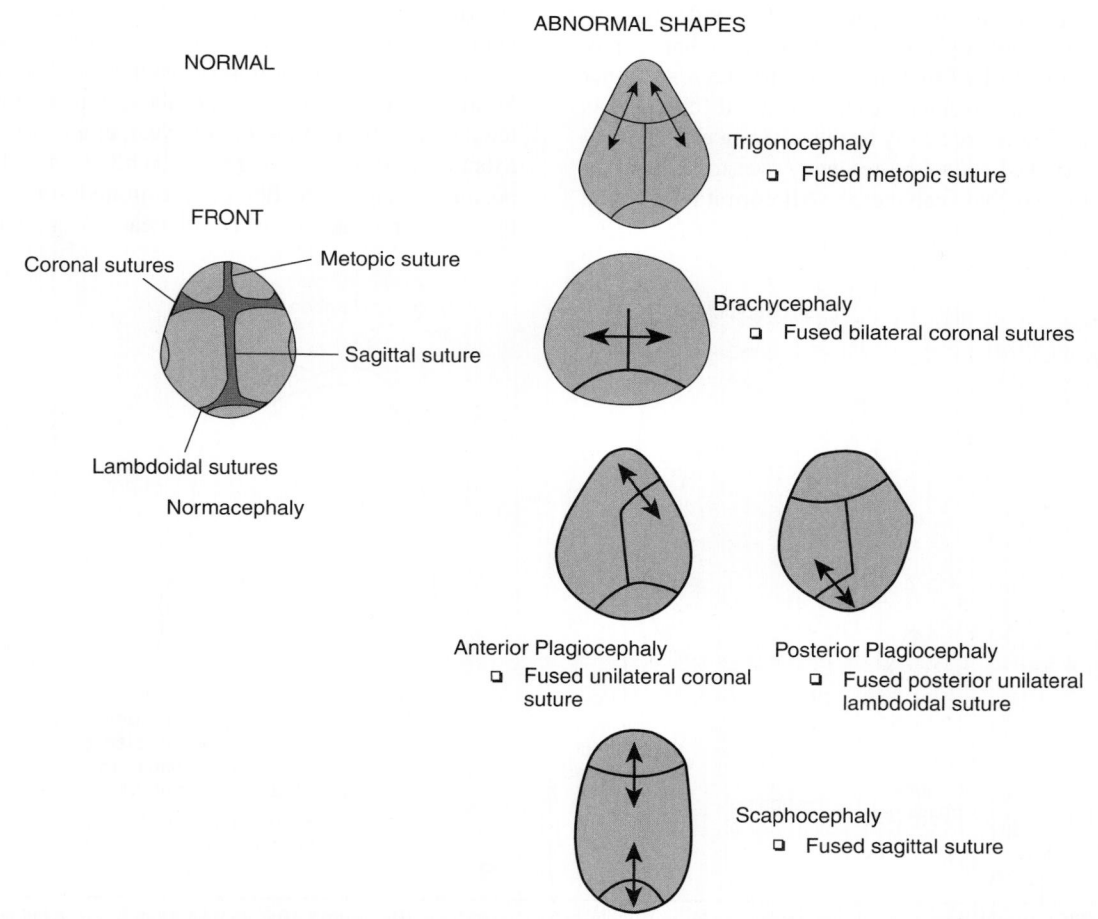

FIG. 27-3 Characteristics of skull deformities seen with craniosynostosis. (Adapted from Cohen MM: Craniosynostosis update 1987, *Am J Med Genet Suppl* 4:99-148, 1988.)

Secondary synostosis results when outside forces put pressure on the growing cranium, causing the skull to become misshapen (referred to as *deformational plagiocephaly*). Incidence is as low as 1 in 300 live births to as high as 48% depending upon the criteria used (Persing et al, 2003). Secondary synostosis is most commonly seen with premature infants (termed *deformational scaphocephaly*), after shunting an infant with hydrocephaly, in children who have microcephaly and aberrant positioning in utero, during birth, or perinatally because of torticollis or positioning traditions.

The success of the Back to Sleep campaign has resulted in an increase of infants with secondary (or pressure-related) occipital flattening. Such occipital deformity is not accompanied by compensatory suture line growth that would be seen with a primary lambdoidal synostosis, which is quite rare (0.003% of births).

Clinical Findings

Physical Examination.   Every infant's skull should be examined for cranial asymmetry up to 1 year old. This is best done by looking down at the top of the head, noting the position of the ears and cheekbones. Typically, a deformational plagiocephaly will form a parallelogram characterized by unilateral occipital flattening and contralateral occipital bossing, ipsilateral ear displacement anteriorly, and associated parietal bossing and cheekbone prominence on the side of the occipital flattening. In contrast, the deformity of lambdoidal craniosynostosis does not assume a parallelogram shape, may be present at birth, has less frontal asymmetry than positional plagiocephaly, the ear ipsilateral to the occipital flattening is posterior and displaced inferiorly to the contralateral ear, and the deformity may be become more severe over time. See Fig. 27-4 for a comparison between these two deformities (Persing et al, 2003).

Symmetry of neck rotation should also be included in the exam to rule out torticollis. Typically, infants with torticollis will have some limitation of neck rotation away from the side of their occipital flattening.

Diagnostic Testing.   An initial skull radiograph is indicated should craniosynostosis be suspected. A follow-up CT scan may be needed, as indicated by the x-ray results. Deformational plagiocephaly does not require imaging studies in most situations when the history and physical exam are diagnostic.

Differential Diagnosis.   In about 5% of young infants, the frontal metopic suture may normally be prominent. This prominence is not clinically significant, does not signify craniosynostosis, and does not require intervention (Green, 2005).

Management.   If craniosynostosis is suspected, the most expedient action for the provider to take is to refer the patient to an experienced pediatric neurosurgeon or craniofacial plastic surgeon. Treatment is often surgical, but in some cases reassurance, repositioning, exercises for any associated torticollis, and clinical follow-up is sufficient. If the condition is genetic, management will need to be planned according to the problems associated with the syndrome. Genetic counseling is important.

Health care providers can anticipate concern about deformational plagiocephaly by counseling parents at the newborn visit to: (a) lay infant down in the Back to Sleep position, alternating positions (i.e., left and right occiputs); (b) when awake and observed, place infants prone; and (c) have infants spend minimal time in car seats or other upright devices that maintain supine positioning. Improvement should occur over a 2- to 3-month period of time if the above interventions are instituted early. Throughout the first year, emphasize tummy time. Monitor head shape during all well child visits. The majority of positional plagiocephalies are self-limited; sometimes physical therapy is indicated in recalcitrant cases (e.g., with torticollis).

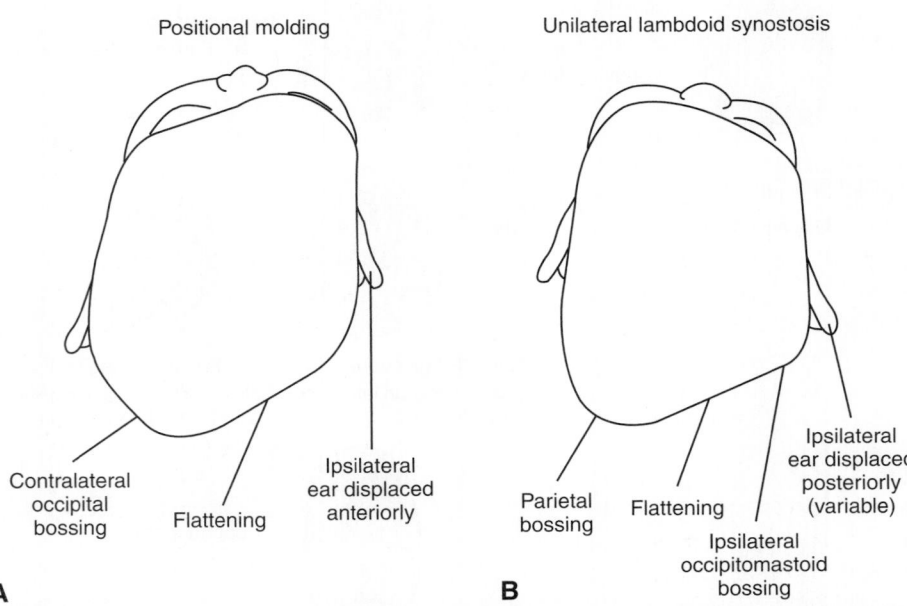

Positional molding — Unilateral lambdoid synostosis

Contralateral occipital bossing — Flattening — Ipsilateral ear displaced anteriorly

A

Parietal bossing — Flattening — Ipsilateral occipitomastoid bossing — Ipsilateral ear displaced posteriorly (variable)

B

FIG. 27-4   Differences between positional molding (**A**) and unilambdoid synostosis (**B**). (From Gruss JS, Ellenbogen RG, Whelan MF: Lambdoid synostosis and posterior plagiocephaly. In Lin KY, Ogle RC, Jane JA, editors. *Craniofacial surgery: science and surgical technique*, Philadelphia, 2002, WB Saunders.)

For positional plagiocephaly, special soft shell helmet therapy may be prescribed when repositioning and exercises are not successful. These need to be worn for 23 hours a day for 5 to 6 months, can cause skin breakdown, and are costly (Pershing et al, 2003). One study showed 36% to 54% improvement in asymmetry in those infants whose parents were most compliant in using the helmet over the 6-month study period (Bruner et al, 2004).

Central Nervous System Infections

Description.   All the infections of the CNS have similar symptoms. These infections can be manifested acutely (over 1 to 24 hours) or chronically (over 1 to 7 days or more).

Etiology.   Bacteria, viruses, fungi, spirochetes, protozoa, and parasites can all cause CNS infection. The meninges, superficial cortical structures, blood vessels, and brain parenchyma can be involved. The most common microbes are as follows (Prober, 2004):

- Newborn to 2 months old: group B and D streptococci, *Escherichia coli* and other gram-negative enterobacteria, *Listeria monocytogenes,* and occasionally *Haemophilus influenzae.*
- 2 months to 12 years old: bacterial infections most common: *H. influenzae* type B, *Neisseria meningitidis, Streptococcus pneumoniae.* In those with immune deficiencies *Pseudomonas aeruginosa, Staphylococcus aureus,* coagulase-negative staphylococci, *Salmonella* spp. and *L. monocytogenes* can be implicated.

Clinical Findings

History.   The following may be reported:

- Upper respiratory tract or gastrointestinal symptoms accompanied by fever
- Increasing lethargy and irritability
- Recent head injury or neurosurgical procedure
- Immunodeficiency diseases

Physical Examination.   Findings on physical examination include the following:

- Systemic signs, including fever; malaise; impaired heart, lung, or kidney function
- CNS signs, including headache; stiff neck and spine; nausea and vomiting; fever or hypothermia; changes in mental status, ranging from irritability to lethargy or coma; seizures; and focal or sensory deficits in cranial nerves, notably III, IV, and VI
- Presence of Kernig or Brudzinski sign of meningeal irritation (may be absent in a young infant)
- Bulging fontanelle and increasing head circumference in a young infant
- Papilledema late in the course in older children or adolescents
- Cranial nerve palsies

By age, the most common findings are as follows:

- From 0 to 3 months old: fever, hypothermia, lethargy, irritability, poor feeding, apnea, focal seizures, enteric or respiratory symptoms, nuchal rigidity, and a bulging fontanelle (infrequent)
- From 3 months to 5 years old: petechial rash, localized CNS signs as described earlier

- From 6 to 18 years old: petechial rash, cranial nerve VII palsy (Lyme disease), sinusitis symptoms, localized CNS signs

Diagnostic Studies.   Blood cultures, CBC with differential, urinalysis, chemistry panel, and lumbar puncture for CSF studies are done. Enterovirus meningitis and herpes simplex virus rapid tests are available. EEGs, CT or MRI scan, and brain biopsy may be needed.

Management and Complications.   The primary care provider needs to refer all children with potential CNS infection as rapidly as possible. Hypovolemia, hypoglycemia, hyponatremia, acidosis, septic shock, increased intracranial pressure, and other complications can occur quickly and need aggressive management. Hearing loss can occur in all forms of meningitis. Blindness, hydrocephaly, CP, seizures, and developmental delays can also occur depending on the type of organism involved. Outcomes are typically based on the following four categories:

- Type of infectious agent and severity of initial infection
- Age of patient (the younger, the worse the outcome)
- Length of symptoms before the diagnosis and initiation of treatment
- Antibiotic used and amount

The Floppy Infant

When supported with a hand under the chest, the normal infant will hold the back straight or nearly so, the arms flexed and slightly abducted at the elbows, and the head slightly up at less than 45 degrees. The "floppy" infant will droop over the hand. A floppy infant is alert but has hypotonia and depressed spontaneous movements, which should arouse suspicion. Other symptoms seen in a range of known causes include seizures, failure to react to pain, muscle wasting, absent reflexes, tongue fasciculation, and unilateral muscular movement deficits (Finberg & Kleinman, 2002). Etiologies usually focus on a metabolic or CNS dysfunction or a systemic illness. Most conditions involving the CNS are serious and lasting; others may be transitory, such as brachial plexus nerve palsy after birth or congenital myasthenia gravis (MG). Hypotonic infants can increase their tone over the first year of life and then demonstrate spastic CP. A baby can have low tone but still not lack strength when actively moving. The infant may also be weak, which means that its maximal effort lacks strength. Babies with Werdnig-Hoffmann disease (infantile spinal muscular atrophy) are weak. Floppy infants with brisk reflexes almost certainly have a CNS disorder. Acquired floppy infant syndrome has been known to occur in breastfed infants whose mothers were vegetarian; these infants were found to be deficient in cobalamin intake (Renault et al, 1999). Prenatal use of benzodiazepines has resulted in neonatal hypotonia (Gonzalez de Dios et al, 1999). All floppy babies need to be referred to specialists, including a geneticist. The diagnostic tool of choice is the MRI; sometimes muscle biopsies or various neurophysiologic studies are employed. Many conditions of floppy infant syndrome do not respond well to treatment; rehabilitation can help maximize function (Finberg & Kleinman, 2002).

Reye Syndrome

Description and Epidemiology. Reye syndrome is an encephalopathy process often associated with influenza A and B. It is a systemic disorder of mitochondrial function occurring during or after a viral infection and, more often, with the use of salicylates during such viral illnesses (Fenichel, 2001). Infrequent cases are seen with varicella or nonspecific respiratory infections, notably *H. influenzae* type B. A decline in incidence has been associated with the decreased use of salicylates in younger children.

Clinical Findings. Unless treated, the clinical course in Reye syndrome proceeds in five predictable stages after the initial prodromal symptoms of the illness. Severe vomiting progresses to irrational behavior; to stupor and coma; to apnea, fixed pupils, and decorticate posturing with increasing brain edema; and then to death.

Management. Immediate referral with admission to a hospital setting for supportive care is essential. About 70% of patients survive, some with severe neurologic sequelae. Infants are more severely affected than older children.

Tethered Cord

The spinal cord is attached to the base of the brain and free at the caudal end, allowing for freedom of movement during growth, activities, and skeletal changes (including such abnormalities as scoliotic curves). With a tethered cord, however, the caudal end is fixed by a ropelike filum terminale at or below the L2 level. This can cause abnormal stretching and damage to nerve cells, fibers, and blood vessels. Eventually, symptoms of neurologic deterioration occur. It is often associated with a congenital spinal anomaly, such as spina bifida (90%), but tethering can also result from bony protrusions, tough membranous bands, lipomas, tumors, cysts, scarring, and trauma in the caudal equina area.

Not all tethering leads to clinical symptoms. If symptoms do occur, they manifest as functional deficits to nerves that emanate from the caudal equina area. Common findings or complaints include: asymmetry of leg or foot growth and muscle wasting in an infant, leg weakness, incontinence of bladder and bowel (or worsening of such), back or leg pain (especially with flexion or extension), groin or genitorectal pain, loss of reflexes and sensation in the legs, scoliosis, or deformity of the legs or hips (Royal Australian College of General Practitioners, 2002). Symptoms are not necessarily evident in infancy but can be manifested in early childhood to adulthood (Haslam, 2004). Although not necessarily abnormal after imaging, the following skin changes are often seen in individuals later diagnosed with tethered cord or other spinal abnormalities: dimples above the gluteal cleft or within the cleft (dimples at the coccyx are generally benign), spinal hair tufts, a deviated gluteal fold, spinal fatty deposits, midline birthmarks, and sacral sinuses or tracts.

If a provider is suspicious of a tethered cord, an MRI of the spine is the gold standard for viewing the parenchymal anatomy. A referral to a pediatric neurosurgeon is also indicated.

Surgery is usually the treatment of choice and can halt and prevent further neurologic dysfunction. If a child has reached full skeletal height with minimal symptoms, monitoring is all that is often done. In children who have had surgery for tethered cord, the clinician is encouraged to be watchful for retethering, which can occur as the child gets older. A child with a history of repaired spina bifida needs to be closely monitored for early symptoms of tethered cord.

Arnold-Chiari Malformation

Arnold-Chiari malformations consist of two types of uncommon congenital spinal cord anomalies whose sequelae are usually not evident until late childhood or into adulthood. Type I malformation involves the downward elongation (herniation) of the caudal end of the cerebellar vermis through the foramen magnum. Type II malformation is present in 50% of children with lumbar meningomyelocele. The herniation can lead to brainstem and upper cervical cord compression that may ultimately cause necrosis of both structures. The etiology is believed to be secondary to embryonic segmentation disorders of the neural tube (Finberg & Kleinman, 2002).

The symptoms of a malformation may not be readily apparent. Type I malformation can cause headache, neck pain, atrophy and decreased reflexes in the lower extremities, sensory losses, and scoliosis. Any child with meningomyelocele should be suspected of having type II malformation. Type II malformation involves the same herniation as type I plus an alteration in the shape and development of the medulla. Further symptoms of type II may include hydrocephaly, respiratory distress, syncope, poor feeding, vomiting, dysphagia, tongue paralysis, and cardiopulmonary failure (Fenichel, 2001). Epilepsy is not related. Diagnosis is made by MRI and the condition may inadvertently be found at the time of an MRI for a possibly unrelated reason (e.g., headache). Management strategies are not always successful; surgery to relieve the compression or a ventriculoperitoneal shunt may be tried in symptomatic cases. Older children may benefit from a cervical laminectomy to relieve compression as the child grows.

Meningomyelocele

Description. Failure during embryogenesis of the vertebrae, skull, meninges, brain, or spinal cord to be encapsulated by the lamina of the vertebrae along the dorsal midline of the body is referred to as a *dysraphic defect*. Meningomyelocele refers to the protrusion of both the spinal cord nerve roots (myelo) and the three layers of membranes (meninges) that cover the spinal cord and brain through this spinal defect. The protruding dural sac may contain only the meninges (10% to 20% of cases) or both meninges and nerve roots (the remaining cases). The term *spina bifida cystica* is often used interchangeably with *meningomyelocele*. When the vertebral arches fail to close, but there is no subsequent herniation of cord or meninges, the term *spina bifida occulta* is used. Most cases of spina bifida cystica occur in the thoracolumbar area (90%). Meningoceles may also protrude through the skull and may or may not be covered with skin. Such a cranial meningocele consists only of a CSF-filled meningeal sac; no nerve roots are involved, and therefore no neurologic deficits exist. However, there may be brain malformation under the mass that does have neurologic consequences. Encephaloceles or cephaloceles refer to cranial lesions that contain a meningocele sac plus cerebral cortex, cerebellum, or portions of brainstem that protrude from fissures in the occipital (most common), frontal, or nasal cavity areas of the skull.

At birth a child with a meningomyelocele in the lumbosacral area would demonstrate flaccid paralysis of the legs, sensory deficits below the spinal defect, neurogenic bladder, deformities of the ankles and feet, atrophied muscles, and possibly apnea if hydrocephaly is present. Long-term dysfunction would include flaccid paraplegia, continued sensory deficits, neurogenic bladder and bowel, and recurrent UTIs.

Epidemiology. Closure of the neural tube usually occurs during the third and fourth weeks of gestation. Genetic and environmental factors are both believed to play a causative role in the failure of the closure to occur. A woman who has had a previous child born with dysraphia has about a 3% to 4% recurrence rate with future pregnancies. A lack of sufficient levels of folic acid and vitamin A increases the incidence of neural tube defects (NTDs). All women of child-bearing age are now encouraged to take 0.4 mg/day of folic acid. A woman wishing to conceive, or who has had a prior pregnancy that resulted in a neural tube defect, should take 4 mg/day for 4 weeks before conception and through the first trimester (Johnston & Kinsman, 2004). Intake of other drugs and toxins is associated with neural tube defects; such drugs and toxins include folic acid antagonists (trimethoprim, carbamazepine, phenytoin, phenobarbital, primidone), retinoic acid derivatives (e.g., vitamin A, a paradox given that insufficient levels also cause the defect), valproic acid, and alcohol. Diabetes mellitus (including gestational diabetes), maternal hyperthermia during the first month of pregnancy, trisomy 18 and 13, and Meckel syndrome are also risk factors (Johnston & Kinsman, 2004; Finberg & Kleinman, 2002).

The incidence in the U.S. is approximately 1 per 4000 live births; this rate dramatically dropped in the 1990s, but preliminary reports show rates may have leveled off by 2004. There is speculation that this leveling may be due to overall decreases in serum folate and red blood cell (RBC) folate concentrations in nonpregnant women. Such trends in serum levels were dramatically seen in nonpregnant women who participated in a National Health and Nutrition Examination Survey (NHANES) that compared data from 1999 to 2000 and 2003 to 2004 (CDC, 2007). Proposed explanations for the decline in serum folate include: increasing obesity rates (obese individuals metabolize folate differently), low carbohydrate diet trend (which requires the elimination of breads, cereals, and other products that contain the mandatory fortified folic acid-enriched flour), the popularity of whole-grain breads (which have lower natural folate levels), and the reduction in the mean folate content of certain enriched breads. Decreases in the serum folate levels spanned all races and ethnic groups (CDC, 2007).

Clinical Findings. Diagnosis is made prenatally with the use of a maternal serum test to look for an increase in the concentration of α-fetoprotein; if elevated, an ultrasound and amniocentesis are done. Alpha-fetoprotein is the primary plasma protein that exists within the fetus and amniotic fluid. The concentration of the protein is elevated if there is a defect in the skin of the fetus. If the prenatal screen indicates that the fetus has possible spina bifida cystica, a fetal ultrasound will confirm the diagnosis. Cranial ultrasounds will be done to look for hydrocephaly and cephaloceles (and in turn the Arnold-Chiari type II malformation). In the neonatal period, serial cranial ultrasounds are done to watch for the development of hydrocephaly, if this condition has not shown up prenatally. Other physical anomalies that can accompany meningomyelocele include cleft lip and palate, omphalocele, diaphragmatic hernia, tracheoesophageal fistula, congenital heart disease, bladder exstrophy, and imperforate anus. It is preferable that these infants be delivered by cesarean section.

Management and Complications. Management of a myelomeningocele entails surgical resection and closure within a week after birth of the involved neural tube structures and often shunting for hydrocephaly. If surgery is not done during that time, death may result in the first year from meningitis or sepsis. Intrauterine surgery has also been successfully done to close the defect and prevent exposure of the neural tube to amniotic fluid and possible postnatal infection. If the defect occurs in a high spinal region or there is clinical hydrocephalus at birth, survival is also compromised.

The provider's role includes delivering well child care, assessing and treating acute illnesses (especially assessing for UTIs and constipation), monitoring shunt function, and communicating and often coordinating services with the myriad of specialists that will be involved (e.g., orthopedists, ophthalmologists [strabismus is common], neurologists, nephrologists, physical therapists, social workers, geneticists).

Genitourinary management entails teaching parents (and eventually the patient) how to regularly catheterize a neurogenic bladder. Providers should also do periodic urine cultures, assess renal function (with serum electrolytes, creatinine), and, depending upon the patient's course, order appropriate imaging studies (renal scans, intravenous pyelograms [IVPs], ultrasounds). In addition, the provider needs to be alert to the onset of symptoms indicative of Arnold-Chiari type II malformation and tethered cord, watch for seizures (15% incidence), learning difficulties, and ADHD.

Prognosis. With aggressive early treatment, survival rates can be as high as 85% to 90%; deaths more commonly occur before 4 years old. Normal intelligence is seen in 70% of survivors, but they experience more learning and seizure problems. Continence can sometimes be achieved with an artificial urinary sphincter or bladder augmentation when the child is older. Bowel training can help control stool incontinence.

Functional mobility depends on the level and degree of the defect and on the intact function of the iliopsoas muscle. A child with a defect in the sacral and lumbosacral area almost certainly will be able to achieve functional ambulation. Of those with a higher defect, about half will achieve mobility using braces and canes (Johnston & Kinsman, 2004).

Myasthenia Gravis

Description. Myasthenia gravis (MG) is an autoimmune disorder that produces an immune-mediated neuromuscular blockade. It originates when circulating receptor-binding antibodies decrease the number of available acetylcholine receptors (AChR) on the postsynaptic muscle membrane or motor end plate. This leaves the motor end plate less responsive than normal (Sarnat, 2004).

MG is nonhereditary in most cases; however, three rare presynaptic congenital forms exist (believed to be due to autosomal recessive traits, not associated with plasma anti-ACh antibodies). Symptoms of congenital MG start at or close after birth and persist. Myasthenic mothers may have infants with a transient neonatal myasthenic syndrome, as a result of the transfer of placental anti-AChR antibodies. Once the infant's own receptors regenerate and reinsert into synaptic membranes, the symptoms resolve.

Children with MG can also experience other autoimmune diseases, including systemic lupus erythematosus, thyroiditis, rheumatoid arthritis, or diabetes mellitus.

Epidemiology. MG affects approximately 40 per 1 million population; about one-fifth of these develop symptoms before 20 years old. The nonhereditary form of MG can occur any time after birth, though onset before 1 year old is rare (Penn, 2003). There is no racial or geographic predilection.

Clinical Findings

Physical Examination. The key findings of this disorder include:

- Ptosis and some degree of extraocular muscle weakness (usually the first symptom). Older children may complain of double vision; younger children may endeavor to hold their eyelids open with their fingers. The ocular signs may be asymmetric.
- Dysphagia. Infants commonly have feeding problems; older children fatigue when chewing. There may be slurred speech and a snarling appearance when trying to smile.
- Muscular weakness of neck flexor muscles (infants), limb-girdle and distal muscles of the hands. Symptoms do not include muscle fasciculations, myalgias, or sensory symptoms. Ten percent of patients will have limb weakness as the initial symptom (Penn, 2003). Other times, the weakness may be so mild as to only occur after exercise.
- Rapid muscular fatigue as evidenced by:
  - Inability to hold an upward gaze for 30 to 90 seconds
  - Inability to sustain a chin to chest position, while supine
  - Inability to maintain arm abduction for more than 1 to 2 minutes
  - Inability to sustain rapid hand fisting movements for long
- Infants of myasthenia mothers: in 12%, symptoms develop within 72 hours of birth—respiratory insufficiency, dysphagia,

hypotonia, weakness, poor spontaneous motor activity, weak cry, poor sucking, choking, expressionless face, absent Moro reflex. Symptoms generally resolve within 12 weeks.
- Congenital MG: symptoms permanent, without remission, do not experience myasthenic crises.

Diagnostic Studies. The clinical test is a short-acting cholinesterase inhibitor (edrophonium chloride, or Tensilon), which should cause spontaneous improvement in the ptosis and ophthalmoplegia within seconds; other muscles should fatigue less rapidly.

An EMG is more diagnostic than a muscle biopsy. In MG an EMG will show a decremental response after repetitive nerve stimulation, then slowed muscle potentiation, then refraction. Motor nerve conduction velocity is normal. Studies can be done to determine if the transmission defect is presynaptic or postsynaptic.

Estimation of the number of AChRs per end plate and in vitro end plate function studies are also possible. An assay of plasma antibodies to AChR is often inconclusive; only one third of adolescents and an occasional prepubertal child will show these antibodies present.

Other tests can include: serologic antinuclear antibodies and immune complexes; thyroid profile; CK level (normal with MG). A chest x-ray should be done (any enlarged thymus needs to be followed up with a tomography or CT scan of the anterior mediastinum). ECG should be normal. A muscle biopsy may be done (this disorder typically demonstrates non-specific type II muscle fiber atrophy).

Differential Diagnosis. Hypothyroidism (caused by Hashimoto thyroiditis), polymyalgia rheumatica, MS, progressive external ophthalmoplegia, Guillain-Barré syndrome, Möbius syndrome, congenital ptosis, congenital myopathies, myotonic dystrophy, glycogen-storage disease.

Management. MG (including neonatal MG) is treated with anti-ChE therapy-pyridostigmine (Mestinon) because it is longer acting and produces less severe side effects that neostigmine. The initial dosage is age and weight dependent and is then titrated upwards until the patient responds, side effects are controlled, or until increases are no longer effective. Corticosteroids, cytotoxic agents (azathioprine and cyclosporine), or thymectomy may also be considered, especially if symptoms are severely debilitating (bulbar or respiratory involvement). Corticosteroids should be administered on an alternate-day regimen.

Thymectomy may relieve symptoms, but can result in possible immunodeficiency, so this requires caution. This procedure has been performed in children more than 2 years old and in adolescents with generalized MG. Remission rates of about 60% have been demonstrated (Penn, 2003).

Complications. Growth retardation from steroids; possible immunodeficiency in adulthood after thymectomy.

Tic Disorders

Tics, or habit spasms, are found in children and adults. Boys are two to three times more likely to be affected than girls. The most common time for onset is 6 to 8 years old (range is from 2 to 15 years old) (CDC, 2005). Four types of tic disorders are recognized: Tourette syndrome, transient tic disorder, chronic motor or vocal tic disorder, and unspecified type. Some tics can be suppressed with effort and are not a part of voluntary movements. Other forms of tics come and go spontaneously and tend to decrease when the child is out of school. Duration of affliction can be lifelong; half of the children with tics outgrow them in late adolescence. Others may experience this resolution only to see them recur in middle age.

Tourette syndrome is the most complex of the tic disorders. It is believed to be caused by a combination of neurobiologic, psychological, hereditary (autosomal dominant with varying levels of penetrance, which is gender related), and environmental factors. Imaging studies have demonstrated the lack of normal striatum asymmetry. The tics can vary in severity over time. Boys with Tourette syndrome frequently have concomitant ADHD, whereas girls are more likely to experience obsessive-compulsive disorder (OCD). If the onset of tics is associated with the initiation of a drug, such as one for ADHD, the relationship is generally regarded now as less causative and more an indication of a predisposition towards Tourette syndrome (Fenichel, 2001). Stopping the medication may resolve the behavior. In 50% of patients, the tic behavior does not restart after the medication is reintroduced (Boris & Dalton, 2004).

To meet the diagnostic criteria for Tourette syndrome, the tics must:
- Be a combination of motor and verbal tics
- Be repeated many times every day for more than a year with no tic-free periods of longer than 3 months
- Begin before 18 years old
- Not be related to some other medical condition (e.g., seizures, Huntington disease or postviral encephalitis), medications, or other substances (American Psychiatric Association, 2000)

Simple motor tics usually affect the head, eyes, or face (eye blinks, eyebrow raising, nose flaring, grimacing, lip smacking); head or arm jerking, kicking, toe curling, and shoulder shrugging can also occur. More complex motor tics include head shaking; touching; hitting; jumping; smelling objects; repeating movements; self-mutilating activities, such as lip biting; and other behavior. Initial vocal tics include sniffing, grunting or snorting, throat clearing, and coughing. Hissing and barking can occur, but swearing is rare in children. If swearing (or coprolalia) is repressed by the patient, it usually results in barking or coughing noises (Fenichel, 2001).

Differential Diagnosis.   Consider hyperkinesis; choreiform (harder to suppress and occurs during voluntary movements) or dystonic movements; genetic disorder, such as Huntington or Wilson disease; OCD; structural lesion in the brain; and pharmacologic side effect. Tics are not associated with degenerative diseases.

Management.   Parents should be encouraged to ignore tics, given their tendency to wax and wane. The decision to treat with medicine depends on how much the tics bother the child rather than the parents (Fenichel, 2001). Treatment should include a combination of behavioral therapy and medication. Pharmacologic management of motor or vocal tics may include haloperidol (Haldol), pimozide (Orap), fluphenazine

(Prolixin), thiothixene (Navane), clonazepam (Klonopin), and clonidine (Catapres). Fluoxetine (Prozac) and other drugs have also been used. Drugs may need to be rotated to maintain effectiveness over time. Because of the comorbidity with ADHD and OCD, management strategies must also involve the family, educational measures, and other supportive measures, including medication.

RESOURCE BOX
Neurologic Diseases

Brain Injury Association of America
www.biausa.org

International Rett Syndrome Association (IRSA)
www.rettsyndrome.org

National Headache Foundation
www.headaches.org

National Spinal Cord Injury Association
www.spinalcord.org

Spina Bifida Association
www.sbaa.org

Tourette Syndrome Association, Inc.
www.tsa-usa.org

United Cerebral Palsy
www.ucpa.org

☑ DISCUSSION FORUM

1. Are there different concerns about a new complaint of headache in a 3-year-old versus a 13-year-old? What are the similarities and differences in obtaining history, physical assessment, and differential diagnosis?
2. A 5-year-old has a tonic-clonic seizure and a temperature of 104° F (40° C)? How would your management vary if this child was 3 months old? 8 years old?
3. A 10-year-old has a chief complaint of weakness. What are key physical assessment points? What are the differential diagnoses?
4. A 17-year-old football player received a severe head injury when in a motor vehicle accident in early May. He required hospitalization and was unconscious for 30 hours. He had one seizure the week following his injury. You see him one month after his discharge. What sort of examination (including all the elements) are you going to do? What do you tell him about his returning to play on the varsity football team in late August? What sort of prediction can you make about his recovery? What sort of follow-up do you recommend?

REFERENCES

American Academy of Pediatrics Committee on Infectious Diseases: *2006 Redbook: report of the Committee on Infectious Diseases,* ed 27, Elk Grove Village, IL, 2006, American Academy of Pediatrics.

American Psychiatric Association: *Diagnostic and statistical manual of mental disorders,* ed 4, text revision, Washington, DC, 2000, American Psychiatric Association.

Arnold DL: Strategies for monitoring and assessing therapy, *Adv Stu Med* 6(7d):S701-S706, 2006.

Baysun S et al: A comparison of buccal midazolam and rectal diazepam for acute treatment of seizures, *Clin Pediatr* 44(9):771-776, 2005.

Berkowitz C: *Pediatrics: a primary care approach,* ed 2, Philadelphia, 2000, WB Saunders.

Boris NW, Dalton R: Habit disorders. In Behrman R, Kliegman R, Jenson J, editors: *Nelson textbook of pediatrics,* ed 17, Philadelphia, 2004, WB Saunders.

Bouma P, Peters A, Brouwer O: Long term course of childhood epilepsy following relapse after antiepileptic drug withdrawal, *J Neurol Neurosurg Psychiatry* 72(4):507-510, 2002.

Bruner TW et al: Objective outcome analysis of soft shell helmet therapy in the treatment of deformational plagiocephaly, *J Craniofac Surg* 15(4):643-650, 2004.

Brunstrom J, Titan A: Cerebral palsy. In Maria BL, editor: *Current management in child neurology,* ed 3, Hamilton, Ontario, 2005, BC Decker.

Camfield P, Camfield C: What is epilepsy? In Maria BL, editor: *Current management in child neurology,* ed 3, Hamilton, Ontario, 2005, BC Decker.

Centers for Disease Control and Prevention (CDC), National Center for Injury Prevention (Office of Statistics and Programming): *CDC Injury Fact Book,* 2006. Available at *www.cdc.gov/ncipc/fact_book/injuryBook 2006.pdf* (accessed Nov 10, 2007).

Centers for Disease Control and Prevention (CDC); Folate Status in women of childbearing age, by race/ethnicity—United States, 1999-2000, 2001-2002, and 2003-2004, *MMWR Morb Mortal Wkly Rep* 55(51):1377-1380, 2007.

Centers for Disease Control and Prevention (CDC): *Tourette syndrome,* Oct 5, 2005. Available at *www.cdc.gov/ncbddd/tourette/default.htm* (accessed on Jan 5, 2007).

Consultant for Pediatricians editorial staff: Scaphocephaly, *Consult Ped* 5(9):589-590, 2006.

Fenichel GM: *Clinical pediatric neurology: a signs and symptoms approach,* ed 4, Philadelphia, 2001, WB Saunders.

Ferrari F et al: Cramped synchronized general movements in preterm infants as an early marker for cerebral palsy, *Arch Pediatr Adolesc Med* 156:422-423, 2002.

Finberg L, Kleinman R: *Saunders manual of pediatric practice,* ed 2, Philadelphia, 2002, WB Saunders.

Freeman J et al: The ketogenic diet. In Maria BL, editor: *Current management in child neurology,* ed 3, Hamilton, Ontario, 2005, BC Decker.

Freedman MS: Disease-modifying drugs for multiple sclerosis: current and future aspects, *Expert Opin Pharmacother* 7(S1):S1-9, 2006.

Galetta SL: Recognizing and managing the clinically isolated syndrome, *Adv Studies Med* 6(7d):S687-693, 2006.

Green M: Structural abnormalities. In Roland LP, editor: *Merrit's neurology,* ed 11, Philadelphia, 2005, Lippincott Williams & Wilkins.

Greenburg B, Kerr D: Multiple sclerosis: 2006 update, introduction, *Adv Studies Med* 6(7d), 2006.

Golub C: Herb-medication interactions: what you don't know *can* hurt you, *Environ Nutri* 24(10):1, 2001.

Gonzalez de Dios J, Moya-Benavent M, Carratala-Marco F: "Floppy infant" syndrome in twins secondary to the use of benzodiazepines during pregnancy, *Rev Neurol* 29(2):121-123, 1999.

Haslam RH: Spinal cord disorders. In Behrman R, Kliegman R, Jenson J, editors: *Nelson textbook of pediatrics,* ed 17, Philadelphia, 2004, WB Saunders.

Jackson Allen P, Vessey J: *Primary care of the child with a chronic condition,* ed 4, St Louis, 2004, Mosby.

Johnston MV: Encephalopathies. In Behrman R, Kliegman R, Jenson J, editors: *Nelson textbook of pediatrics,* ed 17, Philadelphia, 2004a, WB Saunders.

Johnston MV: Seizures in childhood. In Behrman R, Kliegman R, Jenson J, editors: *Nelson textbook of pediatrics,* ed 17, Philadelphia, 2004b, WB Saunders.

Johnston MV: Febrile seizures. In Behrman R, Kliegman R, Jenson J, editors: *Nelson textbook of pediatrics,* ed 17, Philadelphia, 2004c, WB Saunders.

Johnston MV: Neurodegenerative disorders of childhood. In Behrman R, Kliegman R, Jenson J, editors: *Nelson textbook of pediatrics,* ed 17, Philadelphia, 2004d, WB Saunders.

Johnston MV: Conditions that mimic seizures. In Behrman R, Kliegman R, Jenson J, editors: *Nelson textbook of pediatrics,* ed 17, Philadelphia, 2004e, WB Saunders.

Johnston MV, Kinsman S: Congenital anomalies of the central nervous system. In Behrman R, Kliegman R, Jenson J, editors: *Nelson textbook of pediatrics,* ed 17, Philadelphia, 2004, WB Saunders.

Kinkel RP et al: IM interferon beta-1a delays definite multiple sclerosis 5 years after a first demyelinating event, *Neurology* 66(5):678-684, 2006.

Legido A et al: Autoimmune and postinfectious disease. In Maria BL, editor: *Current management in child neurology,* ed 3, Hamilton, Ontario, 2005, BC Decker.

Lewis DW: Headaches in children and adolescents, *Amer Fam Phy* 65(4): 625-632, 2002.

Lewis DW et al: Practice parameter: pharmacological treatment of migraine headache in children and adolescents, *Neurology* 63(12):2215-2224, 2004.

Liu J, Francke U: Identification of CIS-regulatory elements for MECP2 expression, *Hum Mol Gen* 15(11):1769-1782, 2006.

Mehlman CT: Upper extremity problems. In Rudolph CD, Rudolph AM, editors: *Rudolph's pediatrics,* ed 21, New York, 2003, McGraw-Hill.

Menkes J, Moser R: *Child neurology,* ed 7, Philadelphia, 2006, Lippincott Williams & Wilkins.

Miller V: Misunderstood and misdiagnosed: the agony of migraine headaches, *Adv Nurs Pract* 13(10):55-62, 2005.

National Institute of Neurology Disorders and Stroke (NINDS): *NINDS Rett syndrome information page.* Available at *www.ninds.nih.gov/disorders/ disorder_index.htm* (accessed Oct 23, 2006a).

National Institute of Neurological Disorders and Stroke (NINDS): *Cerebral palsy: hope through research,* NIH publication No. 06-159, Bethesda, MD, 2006b, National Institutes of Health.

Pelshaw C, Chinarian J, Dabrowski E: Botulinum toxin therapy in children: what role in managing spasticity and dystonia? *Consult Pediatr* 5(10):625-628, 2006.

Penn AS: Diseases of the neuromuscular junction. In Rudolph CD, Rudolph AM, editors: *Rudolph's pediatrics,* ed 21, New York, 2003, McGraw-Hill.

Perry VH: Mechanisms and consequences of axonal injury and degeneration in multiple sclerosis. *Adv Stud Med* 6(7D):S404-S408, 2006.

Persing J et al: Prevention and management of positional skull deformities in infants. *Pediatr* 112(1):199-202, 2003.

Prober CG: Central nervous system infections. In Behrman R, Kliegman R, Jenson J, editors: *Nelson textbook of pediatrics,* ed 16, Philadelphia, 2004, WB Saunders.

Renault F et al: Neuropathy in two cobalamin-deficient breast-fed infants of vegetarian mothers, *Muscle Nerve* 22(2):252-254, 1999.

Rosman NP: Head injury. In Burg FD et al, editors: *Current pediatric therapy,* ed 18, Philadelphia, 2006, WB Saunders.

Royal Australian College of General Practitioners: Spina bifida continence management guideline: spinal cord tethering, *Aust Fam Physician* 31(1):80-83, 2002.

Sankar R et al: Paroxysmal disorders. In Maria BL, editor: *Current management in child neurology,* ed 3, Hamilton, Ontario, 2005, BC Decker.

Sarnat HB: Neuromuscular disorders. In Behrman R, Kliegman R, Jenson J, editors: *Nelson textbook of pediatrics,* ed 16, Philadelphia, 2004, WB Saunders.

Schaan M, Jaksche H, Boszczyk B: Predictors of outcome in head injury: proposal of a new scaling system, *J Trauma* 52(4):667-674, 2002.

Scherer P, Krauss G: Seizure-related car crashes are uncommon, *Epilepsia* 42 (Suppl 7):215-216, 2001.

Seay AR, DiVivo DC: Childhood demyelinating disease. In Rudolph CD, Rudolph AM, editors: *Rudolph's pediatrics,* ed 21, New York, 2003, McGraw-Hill.

Unger J: Pediatric migraine: clinical pearls in diagnosis and therapy. *Consultant Ped* 5(9):545-551, 2006.

United Cerebral Palsy: *Cerebral palsy; what are the causes?* Oct 2001. Available at *www.ucp.org* (accessed Jan 3, 2007).

Wheless J, Clarke D: Status epilepticus. In Maria BL, editor: *Current management in child neurology,* ed 3, Hamilton, Ontario, 2005, BC Decker.

Wilne SH et al: The presenting features of brain tumors: a review of 200 cases. *Arch Dis Child* 91(6):502-506, 2006.

Wolf P, Shinner S: In Maria BL, editor: *Current management in child neurology,* ed 3. Hamilton, Ontario, 2005, BC Decker.

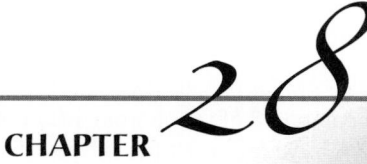

CHAPTER 28

Eye Disorders

Catherine G. Blosser

Ophthalmic diseases occur most often in the very young or elderly, with the exception of eye trauma, refractive errors, and some other disorders (e.g., retinoblastoma [RB]). Infants and children are particularly susceptible to permanent central visual loss (amblyopia), opacities (congenital cataracts), refractive errors not associated with amblyopia, strabismus (ocular misalignment), and other conditions that interfere with visual acuity (ptosis, anisometropia). With early detection and correction, these conditions will not lead to permanent loss in the mature central visual system of the older child or adult (American Academy of Ophthalmology [AAO], 2002). When caring for children with eye problems, priorities include promoting optimal growth and development of the ocular structures and maximizing visual acuity. To this end, primary care providers seek to promote good vision and health, detect abnormalities, treat those conditions that fall within their scope of practice, refer patients with conditions requiring an ophthalmologist's expertise, and provide education and reassurance to parents and children.

Care of blind or visually impaired children is discussed in Chapter 16 because of significant effects on development and learning.

▣ STANDARDS FOR VISUAL SCREENING AND CARE

The objective related to vision in the *Healthy People 2010* objectives (U.S. Department of Health and Human Services, 2000) is to:

- Increase the proportion of primary care providers who routinely refer or screen infants and children for impairments of vision, hearing, speech, and language and who assess other developmental milestones as part of well child care.

The *Guide to Clinical Preventive Services* (U.S. Preventive Services Task Force, 2004) clinical intervention states the following:

- Screening tests have reasonable accuracy in identifying strabismus, amblyopia, and refractive errors in children younger than 5 years old. Providers should be alert for signs of ocular misalignment when examining infants and children. Treating strabismus and amblyopia early greatly reduces long-term amblyopia and improves visual acuity.

The joint recommendation of the American Academy of Pediatrics (AAP), American Association of Certified Orthoptists, American Association for Pediatric Ophthalmology and Strabismus (AAPOS), and the American Academy of Ophthalmology (AAO) includes the following (AAP et al, 2003):

- All newborns and children should have the following performed at each well-child examination: an ocular history, vision assessment, external inspection of the eyes (including pupils and red light reflex), lids, and ocular mobility. This also includes an evaluation of fixation and following (binocularly and monocularly) starting at birth, with the addition of patched visual acuity screening starting at 3 years old. If the child is uncooperative, retesting should occur 6 months later. Inability to fix and follow after 3 months old warrants a referral to a pediatric ophthalmologist or an eye specialist trained to treat pediatric patients. Subsequent testing should occur at 4, 5, 10, 12, 15, and 18 years old. A subjective historical assessment should occur during visits at all other ages. Children who are difficult to screen after two attempts or who demonstrate any other eye abnormality, should undergo photoscreening techniques to detect amblyopia, media opacities, and treatable ocular disease processes. (See Tables 28-1, 28-2, and 28-3 [pp. 676-677]).

For high-risk children, the AAO (2002) recommends that asymptomatic children have a comprehensive examination by an ophthalmologist if they are at high risk because of:

- Health and developmental problems that make screening by the primary care clinician difficult or inaccurate (e.g., retinopathy of prematurity [ROP], or diagnostic evaluation of a complex disease with ophthalmologic manifestations)
- A family history of conditions that cause or are associated with eye or vision problems (e.g., RB, significant hyperopia, strabismus [particularly accommodative esotropia], amblyopia, congenital cataract, or glaucoma)
- Multiple health problems, systemic disease, or the use of medications that are known to be associated with eye disease and vision abnormalities (e.g., neurodegenerative disease, juvenile rheumatoid arthritis, systemic steroid therapy, systemic syndromes with ocular manifestations, or developmental delay with visual system manifestations)

▣ DEVELOPMENT AND PHYSIOLOGY OF THE EYE

DEVELOPMENT OF THE OCULAR STRUCTURES

At 21 days of gestation, the human embryo is one fifth of an inch in length, and the first recognizable ocular tissue is visible on each side of the head. By the end of the eighth week the eyes have moved medially toward the front of the face. The eyelids are completely formed, and the edges of the upper and lower lids fuse to seal the eye while it develops. At 16 weeks of gestation, the eyes are fully anterior, and over the ensuing weeks they continue to move closer to the bridge of the nose. By the seventh month of pregnancy, the fetus can open its eyes.

Development of the eye as a visual organ is not complete at birth, yet newborns have the ability to fix their gaze, follow an object to midline, and react to a change in the intensity of light. Over the first 2 to 3 months of extrauterine life, the ability to focus at any range develops as the eyes become coordinated horizontally and vertically. By 3 months old, infants can follow moving objects, and by 4 months old, they can indicate visual recognition of familiar objects. The shape and contour of the eyeball changes, and visual acuity and binocularity gradually increase with age. The volume of the orbits doubles by the time the child is 1 year old and almost doubles again by 6 to 8 years old. Eye growth is completed at 10 to 13 years old. The corneal dimension, however, changes minimally from full term newborn to adult.

During early childhood, the visual pathways that will ensure central vision are developing. The brain must receive equally clear, bilaterally focused images at the same time for this development to occur. The adult visual field is obtained by 10 years old. The visual pathways are amenable to the greatest corrective influences (e.g., adequate treatment of amblyopia) until 7 to 8 years old. New research has demonstrated that the visual system of teens and adults with amblyopia might still retain substantial plasticity (Scheiman et al, 2005; Zhou et al, 2006).

ANATOMY AND PHYSIOLOGY OF THE EYE

The eyeball consists of three layers of tissue: the fibrous tunic, the vascular tunic, and the inner tunic or retina. The fibrous tunic consists of the sclera and the cornea. The vascular tunic, the middle layer, is composed of the choroid, the ciliary body, and the iris (Fig. 28-1). All the structures of the eye are dedicated to accurate and efficient functioning of the innermost layer of the eyeball, the retina. The optic disc consists only of nerve fibers (no rods or cones) so no visual images are formed here. Thus, it is referred to as the blind spot.

The inside of the eyeball consists of the anterior and posterior cavities. The anterior cavity is divided into anterior and posterior chambers. The anterior chamber lies between the cornea and the iris. The posterior chamber lies between the iris and the suspensory ligament. Aqueous humor circulates throughout these chambers to maintain intraocular pressure (IOP) and link the circulatory system with the avascular lens and cornea. The other cavity within the eyeball, the posterior cavity, lies between the lens and the retina. The gelatinous vitreous humor found in this cavity contributes to the maintenance of IOP and holds the retina in place. The lens, which separates the cavities, hangs by the suspensory ligament. Six muscles guide movement of the globe. Four rectus muscles (superior, inferior, lateral, and medial) move the eyeball up, down, in, and out, respectively. Two oblique muscles (superior and inferior) rotate the eyeball on its axis. Cranial nerves III (oculomotor), IV (trochlear), and VI (abducens) innervate these muscles.

The focusing of light rays involves four basic processes: refraction of light rays, accommodation of the lens, constriction of the pupil, and convergence of the eyes. *Refraction* is the bending of light rays as they pass from one transparent medium (air) to another (cornea or lens). The lens modifies the degree of refraction to create the sharpest image on the retina. *Accommodation* is the ability of the lens to focus on close objects by increasing its curvature. The normal eye refracts

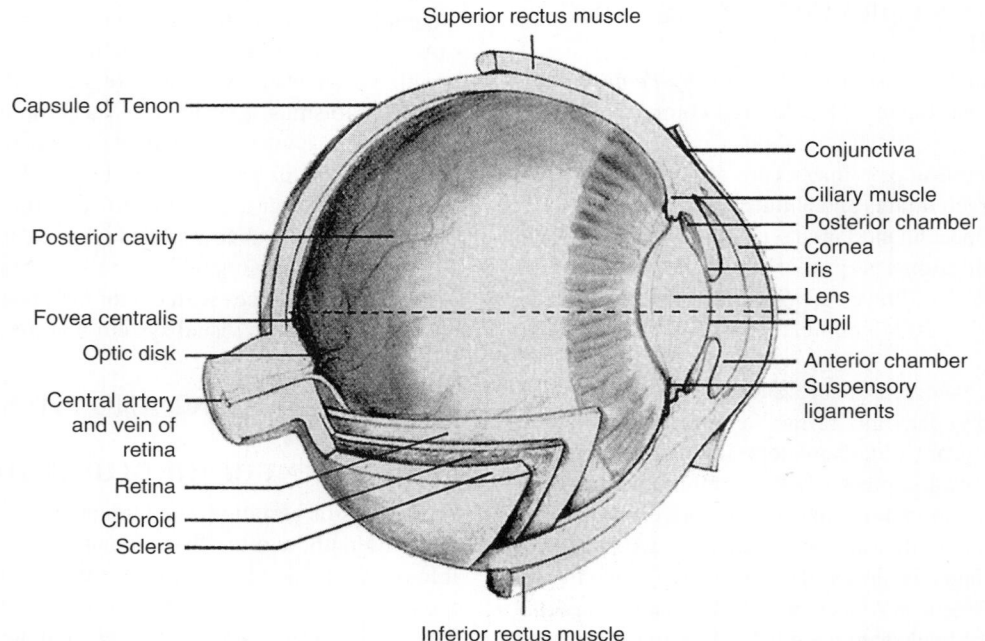

FIG. 28-1   Structure of the eye, transverse section. (From Anderson PD: *Basic human anatomy and physiology: clinical implications for the health professions,* Sudbury, MA, 1984, Jones & Bartlett. Copyright©1984, Jones & Bartlett Publishers, *www.jbpub.com*. Reprinted with permission.)

light rays from an object 20 feet away to focus a clear image onto the retina; hence the fraction 20/20 is used to denote the accepted standard of normal vision. The circular muscle fibers of the iris, which contract in response to light, cause constriction of the pupil. Regulating the light entering the eye can also facilitate production of a precise image. To maintain single binocular vision, close objects require the eyes to rotate medially so that the light rays from the object hit the same points on both retinas. This rotation is called *convergence*. A normal neonate demonstrates disconjugate fixation, but convergence and accommodation normally develop by 3 to 4 months old, with parallel alignment by 5 to 6 months old without nystagmus or strabismus. Jerky eye movements can be seen until 8 weeks after which time smooth tracking movements are expected.

After an image is formed on the retina, light impulses are converted into nerve impulses and transmitted to the visual centers located in the occipital lobes of the cerebral cortex. Lesions in various places along the neural tracts from the eye to the cortex cause different types of loss of visual fields (Fig. 28-2).

◼ PATHOPHYSIOLOGY OF THE EYES

Potential problems with the eyes or visual system can take the form of specific disorders, infections, or injuries to the eye. The most common disorders of the eye interfering with vision are refractive errors (myopia, hyperopia, astigmatism, and anisometropia). Less common disorders include strabismus, amblyopia, ptosis, nystagmus, cataracts, glaucoma, ROP, and RB. Infections and injuries may be relatively minor and superficial or be critical and involve deep tissues of the eye.

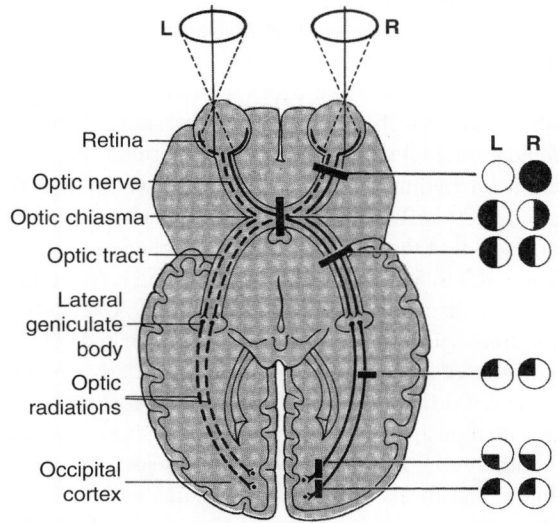

FIG. 28-2 Visual pathway. On the right are diagrams of the visual fields with areas of blindness darkened to show the effects of injuries in various locations. (From Anderson PD: *Basic human anatomy and physiology: clinical implications for the health professions*, Sudbury, MA, 1984, Jones & Bartlett. Copyright©1984, Jones & Bartlett Publishers, *www.jbpub.com*. Reprinted with permission.)

Certain systemic diseases (e.g., juvenile rheumatoid arthritis) and medications (e.g., steroids) can also affect the eyes and warrant extra assessment measures.

◼ ASSESSMENT

Assessment of the eye, as with all body systems, requires a thoughtful history, careful physical examination, and certain specialized screening tests.

HISTORY

The history should include the following:
- Medical history
- Systemic history: birth weight; pertinent prenatal, perinatal, postnatal factors (e.g., prematurity, infections); past hospitalizations and surgery; general health and development
- Ocular history, including date (and results) of the last vision screening and prior eye problems or diseases, including diagnoses and treatments
- If history of eye injury: unilateral or bilateral injury? Were there visual changes or photophobia?
- Family medical history of ocular problems (including eye surgeries), such as glaucoma, blindness, poor vision, difficulty walking in dim light, photophobia, use of thick glasses, lazy eye, strabismus, nystagmus, leukokoria, RB, congenital cataracts
- History of chronic systemic disease in patient or family (e.g., inflammatory bowel disease; connective tissue disorders; cardiac defects of Marfan syndrome; midfacial hypoplasia; abnormalities of teeth, umbilical cord, or urinary tract; neurologic or skin anomalies; developmental delay; mental retardation; diabetes; sickle cell hemoglobinopathies; Tay-Sachs disease; tuberculosis)
- Presence of allergies and to what substances
- Current medications (e.g., steroids); past or present substance abuse
- Prescription and use of eyeglasses or contact lenses (Does the child have glasses that were prescribed? Are they used? If not, why?); use of sunglasses with ultraviolet (UV) protection or protective glasses
- Present symptoms of eye dysfunction or disease
- Visual loss or change in vision, such as blurring, diplopia, spots, and halos in older children; problems with fixing or focusing (holding objects up close to see), ptosis, tracking, squinting, head tilt, eye-hand coordination, grasp, gait, balance, behavior, and changes in the ability to maintain eye contact in younger children
- Photophobia resulting in irritability and shielding or rubbing of the eyes
- Swollen eyelids, pruritus, excessive tearing or discharge, erythema, burning, eye fatigue, strabismus
- Constant blinking, chronic bulbar conjunctival injection

PHYSICAL EXAMINATION

The physical examination can be challenging, depending on the child's age. The components need to be done quickly to accommodate the child's short attention span. Knowledge of

TABLE 28-1	Normal Visual Developmental Milestones
Birth-2 weeks	Infant sees and responds to change in illumination; refuses to reopen eyes after exposure to bright light; increasing alertness to objects; fixes on contrasts (e.g., black and white); jerky movements; pupillary reflex present.
2-4 weeks	Infant fixes and follows on an object, though sporadically.
By 3-4 months	Infant recognizes parent's smile; looks from near to far and focuses close again; beginning development of depth perception; follows 180-degree arc; reaches toward toy; few exodeviations; esotropia abnormal.
By 4 months	Color vision near that of an adult; tears are present.
By 6-10 months	Infant fixes on and follows toy in all directions; movements smooth.
By 12 months	Vision is close to fully developed.

visual developmental norms is essential in assessing a child's visual capabilities (Table 28-1). The examination should include the following:

- Gross inspection should be made of the external structures with a penlight (lids, bulbar and palpebral conjunctiva, cornea, lacrimal structures, and the size, symmetry, and reactivity of the pupils), orbits, eye muscle balance, and mobility.
- The red reflex is tested in all ages. It needs to be assessed for color, intensity, and clarity (opacities or white spots).
- In children more than 5 years old, funduscopic examination allows for visualization of the retina, choroid, fovea, macula, optic disc and cup, and entry and exit of the vessels and nerves.
- Examination of the eye is sometimes facilitated by using a cotton-tipped applicator to evert the eyelid. Eyelid eversion is accomplished by having the patient look down while the examiner grasps the lashes with the thumb and index finger, places the applicator in the middle of the lid, pulls the eyelid down and out, and everts it over the applicator. Irrigation of the eye with normal saline is another technique useful in situations where removal of a foreign body or irritating substance is desired.
- Growth parameters (especially head growth and shape) and the head and neck or other structures should be examined if a systemic condition is suspected.
- A rule of thumb is that if the examiner cannot see into the eye (e.g., absent red light reflex), the patient cannot see out.

SCREENING TESTS

Conducting Screening Tests

Fatigue, hunger, anxiety, and environmental distractions can interfere with vision testing. Testing should always precede the administration of immunizations or any procedure that might cause discomfort. While testing, observe children for behavior indicating that they are having difficulty, such as straining, squinting, excessive blinking, head tilting or shaking, and thrusting of the trunk and head forward. The tendency to peek out from behind the eye shield may or may not reflect difficulty; the child may do so out of a desire to be successful and please the tester. The examiner should also resist the tendency to correct a mistake or give the child nonverbal clues that can influence the results. Three-year-old children who have difficulty performing any of the vision tests in the primary care provider's office should be tested again within 6 months; those unable to perform at older than 4 years should be retested in 1 month (AAP et al, 2003).

Red Light Reflex

Performing an adequate red light reflex test (Bruchner test) will allow the clinician to detect the presence of asymmetric refractive errors, strabismic deviations, and abnormalities in the ocular media (e.g., cataracts, corneal abnormalities, RB). Disease processes involving the cornea, lens, vitreous, or retina will block the light from entering or exiting the pupil and result in an abnormal red light reflex. The recommended technique follows:

- Darken the examination room (a lighted room will cause the pupils to constrict, causing a poor red reflex). The darker the room, the easier it is to detect more subtle asymmetries between the red reflexes.
- Stand an arms length away from the infant or child and use the ophthalmoscope light set at 0 or +1 to illuminate the face.
- Look at both pupils simultaneously and separately. Examining the red reflex slightly off axis to the center of the pupil enhances the color (ask a child to look to one side or use a distraction; infants can be approached from the side).
- The red reflexes should be symmetric; any asymmetry, dark or white spots, opacities, or leukokoria (white pupillary reflex) requires either:
  - Prompt referral to an ophthalmologist, or
  - Dilation of the pupils with 1 to 2 drops of less than 1% tropicamide ophthalmic drops to enhance the examination in questionable situations. Rare side effects to this medication include tachycardia, hypertension, urticaria, cardiac arrhythmias, or contact dermatitis (AAP, 2002).
- The red light reflex can also be documented by taking a Polaroid shot of the patient's face in a darkened room from a distance of 3 to 5 feet. Medial opacities and refractive errors can also be discerned using this technique (AAP, 2002).
- In children with fair skin pigmentation, the red reflex will be a bright red-orange color; in those with darker pigmentation, the red reflex will be a dark red-brown color.

Infants with a positive family history of RB should be referred to an ophthalmologist familiar with the disease. Eye examinations under anesthesia or dilated eye exams will be scheduled for the child on a regular basis starting at 1 to 6 weeks old, depending upon the RB disease that is present in the other family member. Infants with a history of or with a relative having congenital cataracts, congenital retinal dysplasia, or other retinal or lenticular problems should also be referred to an ophthalmologist for a dilated red reflex exam (AAP, 2002).

Some pediatric ophthalmologists are recommending routine dilation at the 2-month well-child exam. They recommend instilling 1 to 2 drops of less than 1% tropicamide drops as the infant is weighed. Adequate dilation is achieved within 15 to 30 minutes, in time for the physical exam. Such dilation would also enhance the detection of infantile cataracts (Murphee & Christensen, 2003).

Visual Acuity Testing

Visual acuity testing (Tables 28-2 and 28-3), for both near and distance vision, should be performed on all children every time they come for a routine checkup, when problems with visual acuity are suspected, and/or when eye trauma occurs. If the child wears eyeglasses or contact lenses, visual acuity measurement must be obtained with correction.

Color Vision Testing

The human retina contains 6 million red and green cones and approximately 1 million blue cones. Alterations in color vision occur when the normal photopigments in the photoreceptor cones are replaced with different ones. Color ranges are then interpreted or perceived differently.

TABLE 28-2   Visual Acuity Norms (Snellen Equivalents)

Age	Forced Choice Preferential Looking (FPL)	Visual Evoked Potential (VEP)
Birth	20/400	20/800
2 months	20/400	
4 months	20/200	20/600
6 months	20/150	20/400
12 months	20/50	20/20
18-24 months	20/25 or 20/20	
5 years	20/25 or 20/20	

VEP does not require a motor response of the primary visual cortex. FPL may involve more cortical processing, which matures more slowly than the visual cortex.
Adapted from Stout A: Pediatric eye examination. In Wright KW, Spiegel PH, editors: *Pediatric ophthalmology and strabismus*, New York, 2003, Springer. Eustis HS, Guthrie ME: Postnatal development. In Wright KW, Spiegel PH, editors: *Pediatric ophthalmology and strabismus*, New York, 2003, Springer.

TABLE 28-3   Recommended Ages and Methods for Pediatric Eye Evaluation Screening

Recommended Age	Method	Indications for Referral to an Ophthalmologist
Newborn-3 months	Red reflex	Abnormal or asymmetric
	Ocular history	
	Inspection	Structural abnormality
3-6 months (approximately)	Fix and follow	Failure to fix and follow in a cooperative infant
	Ocular history	
	Red reflex	Abnormal or asymmetric
	Inspection	Structural abnormality
6-12 months and until child is able to cooperate for verbal visual acuity	Fix and follow with each eye	Failure to fix and follow
	Alternate occlusion	Failure to object equally to covering each eye
	Ocular history	
	Corneal light reflex	Asymmetric
	Red reflex	Abnormal or asymmetric
	Inspection	Structural abnormality
≥3 years and every 1-2 years after 5 years	Visual acuity* (monocular)	3 years: 20/50 or worse; 5 years: 20/40 or worse; >5 years: 20/30 or worse, or two lines of difference between the eyes
	Ocular history	
	Corneal light reflex/cover-uncover reflex	Asymmetric/ocular refixation movements
	Red reflex	Abnormal or asymmetric
	Inspection	Structural abnormality
	Attempt ophthalmoscopy	

*Pictures (LH/LEH symbols or Allen cards for 2-4 year olds; "tumbling E" or HOTV for ≥4 year olds or vision-testing machines.
Note: These recommendations are based on panel consensus. Although the child may be retested if screening is inconclusive or unsatisfactory, undue delays should be avoided; if inconclusive on retesting, referral for comprehensive pediatric medical eye evaluation is indicated.
Use of medication for pupillary dilation facilitates evaluation of the red reflex. For infants a combined weak solution of ≤0.1% tropicamide or cyclopentolate 0.2% is associated with a quicker recovery time (within 1 day vs. 3 day with other preparations [Stout A: Pediatric eye examination. In Wright KW, Spiegel PH, editors: *Pediatric ophthalmology and strabismus,* New York, 2003, Springer]).
From American Academy of Pediatrics (AAP) Committee on Practice and Ambulatory Medicine and Section on Ophthalmology, American Association of Certified Orthoptists, American Association of Pediatric Ophthalmology and Strabismus, American Academy of Ophthalmology (AAO): Eye examination in infants, children, and young adults by pediatricians: policy statement, *Pediatrics* 111(4):902-907, 2003.

Red-green color deficiency is an X-linked inherited disorder or may indicate optic nerve disease. Inherited color deficiencies are more common in males and affect about 6% of males of European ancestry (females 0.26%); 3.1% of black, Native-American, or Hispanic males (females 0.7%); and 4.9% of Asian males (females 0.64%) (Reichel, 2000).

Color vision deficiency may also be acquired. A patient with acquired deficiency may have had normal color vision and then experienced color changes and losses. Diabetes, infections, optic neuritis, and toxins are systemic conditions that can lead to such losses. Blue-yellow deficiency is the most common type of acquired color discrepancy.

Significant color blindness can affect school performance; can have safety implications, in that the child may be unable to distinguish traffic or vehicle brake lights; and can affect career choices. Color vision is tested by using the Richmond pseudoisochromatic plates (formerly Hardy-Rand-Rittler plates) or Ishihara plates. Children 3 to 4 years old are usually able to comply with testing directions.

Peripheral Vision Testing

Examination of peripheral visual fields provides information about retinal function, the neuronal visual pathway to the brain, and the function of cranial nerve II (optic nerve). In an infant, assessment is limited to a rough estimate of peripheral visual fields by watching the child's response to a familiar object (e.g., bottle, toy) or a threatening gesture as it is brought into each of the four quadrants. In children mature enough to cooperate, peripheral visual fields can be measured by confrontation or by finger counting. Peripheral visual fields should be approximately 50 degrees upward, 70 degrees downward, 60 degrees medially (toward the nose), and 90 degrees laterally.

Testing for Ocular Mobility and Alignment

The Hirschberg test (also called the *corneal light reflex*) evaluates extraocular muscle function by projecting a small light source onto the cornea of the eye with the child looking straight ahead. A normal test reveals the reflected light as a small white dot symmetrically located in the same position of each eye (often slightly nasal of center). The cover-uncover test and the alternating cover test should be performed with the child fixating straight ahead, first on a near point and then on a far point about 20 feet away (Fig. 28-3). The process is sometimes aided by asking the child questions about the object (e.g., "How many cows do you see?"). During the alternating cover test, the examiner rapidly covers and uncovers the eye while shifting between the two eyes. Any orbital movement is an indication of misalignment.

Assessment of Visual Loss

If significant visual disturbance is suspected, the following functional vision assessments should be performed, the results documented, and the child referred immediately to an ophthalmologist:

- Shine a penlight into the eye from a lateral position and turn the light off and on several times to assess light perception. If the child can identify when the light is on or off, vision is described as "LP" (light perception).
- If hand movements can be seen 12 inches from the child's face, it is documented as "H/M at 1 ft." Indication of search and recognition should be seen as the hand is slowly moved back and forth with periodic cessation.
- Ask the child to count the number of fingers seen when one, two, or three fingers are held up 12 inches from the child's face. If the child is correct, document the vision as "C/F 1 ft."

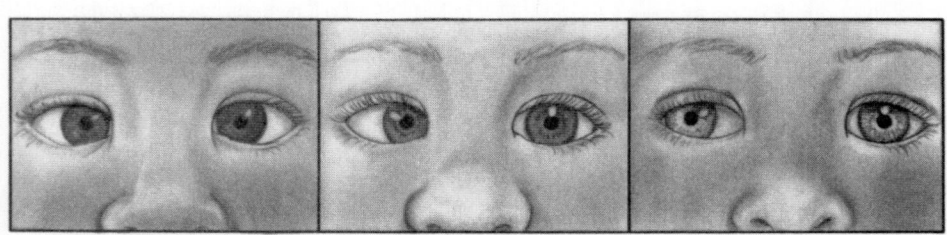

A Pseudostrabismus   **B** R Esotropia   **C** R Exotropia

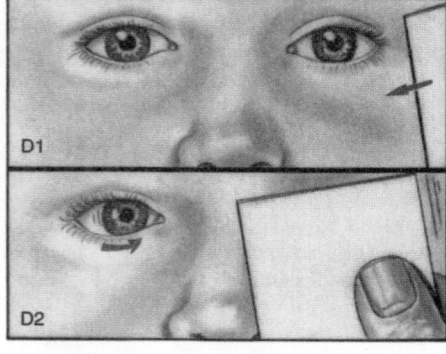

D Right, uncovered eye is weaker

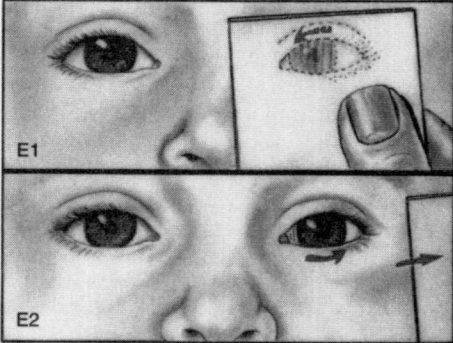

E Left, covered eye is weaker

FIG. 28-3   Extraocular muscle function testing (corneal light reflex and cover test). (From Jarvis C: *Physical examination and health assessment*, ed 2, Philadelphia, 1996, WB Saunders.)

DIAGNOSTIC STUDIES

Laboratory Studies

Cultures and Gram stain of eye discharge are done if identification of infection or particular organisms would be helpful in guiding management.

Ultrasound (not to be used in cases of a suspected ruptured globe), computed tomography (CT), or magnetic resonance imaging (MRI) are sometimes useful in determining a diagnosis of orbital cellulitis, trauma, or tumor or in substantiating a concern about the central nervous system (CNS). An MRI should not be used in the case of a suspected intraocular metal foreign body.

Fluorescein Staining

Fluorescein staining may be used to determine the extent of damage to the corneal or conjunctival epithelium as a result of trauma, infection, or exposure to a foreign body. Moisten a small strip of fluorescein tape with sterile water and place it in the lower conjunctival cul-de-sac. Allow the fluorescein to mix with tears. Examine the cornea with a cobalt blue filter light; any injury will take up the fluorescein stain and appear as a greenish area. Too much of the stain will cloud the entire cornea.

Other Visual Testing Tools

Three primary visual electrodiagnostic or electrophysiologic tests are used by ophthalmologists to provide insight into the functioning of the visual pathway. The visual evoked potentials (VEP) screening tests the optic pathway beyond the eye to the visual cortex. The electroretinogram (ERG) reflects retinal function; the electro-oculogram (EOG) indicates pigment epithelium function. These tests are often used in conjunction with other visual methods of assessment. Preferential looking, or forced choice preferential looking (FPL), testing can be done in an ambulatory care setting. This requires use of special black-and-white and gray-striped cards to provide the spatial frequencies. A Polaroid photo may be used to take images of the pupillary and red reflexes. The various visual screening procedures done in ambulatory and school settings are currently being evaluated by a three-phase Vision In Preschoolers Study (VIP) sponsored by the National Eye Institute. Results of the study will more definitively indicate which of 11 different vision screening tests are more sensitive and specific for targeting preschoolers with amblyopia, strabismus, refractive errors, and/or idiopathic decreased visual acuity. Phases I and II are complete; phase III is still recruiting Head Start preschoolers (as of May 2006) across the U.S. (National Eye Institute, 2006).

■ MANAGEMENT STRATEGIES

REFERRAL FOR OPHTHALMOLOGIC AND SPECIALTY MANAGEMENT

Many eye problems require referral to ophthalmologists or optometrists for management. See Table 28-4 for referral points. Although any child with eye pathologic conditions should be referred to an ophthalmologist, optometrists can be a valuable resource in caring for children with refractive errors or certain common eye conditions (e.g., corneal abrasions, foreign bodies). It is recommended that clinicians acquaint themselves with the statutory guidelines for scope of practice and prescription privileges as designated by the state boards of optometry within their state to optimize referral possibilities.

Ophthalmologic or optometric management of potential or present central vision deficiencies may include the following:

Occlusion

Various techniques may be employed to treat strabismus and improve or prevent amblyopia by blocking vision in the sound eye. These include occlusion (patching), occlusive contact lens (a last resort method), optical penalization (overplusses the lens on the sound eye), or pharmacologic penalization with 0.5% or 1% atropine.

Corrective Lenses

In children, eyeglasses are used to correct refractive errors. Contact lenses can be successfully worn by children older than 10 years. Keratorefractive (LASIK) surgery is undergoing worldwide research for its applicability in children as young as 2 years old with high myopia and myopic anisometropic amblyopia (Astle et al, 2002); however, its use remains controversial. The AAO discourages LASIK surgery in children under 18 years old and provides guidelines regarding suitable candidates for the procedure (AAO, 2006a).

General guidelines for glasses and contact lenses can be found in Box 28-1. Glasses must be changed frequently in children because of head growth. Because the child may be reluctant to wear eyeglasses that hurt or pinch, parents should assess the fit of the eyeglasses on a monthly basis and watch for behavior that indicates discomfort in a preverbal child (e.g., constantly removing glasses, rubbing at the frames or face).

Contact lenses (includes daily wear [hard lenses] and soft, extended and/or disposable wear lenses), in addition to the cosmetic benefit, can provide better refractive error correction than eyeglasses, thereby enhancing visual acuity and the total corrected field of vision. Eye health can be promoted by reinforcing instructions regarding proper contact lens care and reminding the patient that contact lenses should not be worn when the eye is inflamed or topical ophthalmic medications are being used.

Until recently "plano" (noncorrective, decorative or theatrical contact lenses used for cosmetic purposes) have been available for purchase from flea markets, beauty parlors, gas stations, novelty stores, and unauthorized vendors. Severe eye injuries (including blindness) resulted when people bypassed the usual regulatory safeguards (proper fit, adequate instruction on use, and hygiene). Such cases prompted AAO to sponsor legislation that required the Food and Drug Administration (FDA) to regulate the lenses as medical devices (AAO, 2005). Legislation was passed by Congress and signed into law in November 2005. The new law requires that these types of lenses be properly fitted and dispensed by prescription only from a qualified eye care professional. Another type of plano lens includes those with light-filtering tints. These are designed

TABLE 28-4	**Indications for a Comprehensive Pediatric Medical Eye Evaluation**
Indication	**Specific Examples**
Abnormalities in the screening evaluations (see Table 28-3)	Detection of a red reflex abnormality or asymmetry
	Detection of a structural eye abnormality
	Detection of an ocular alignment or motility abnormality
	Unable to perform vision screening at 3-3½ years or older
	Visual acuity 20/50 or worse, or a two-line difference in a 3-year-old
	Visual acuity 20/40 or worse, or a two-line difference in a 5-year-old
	Visual acuity 20/30 or worse, or a two-line difference in a 6-year-old or older child
Signs or symptoms of eye problems by history or observations by family members*	Defective ocular fixation or visual interactions
	Abnormal light reflex (including both the corneal light reflections and the "red" fundus reflection)
	Ocular alignment or movement abnormality
	Nystagmus (shaking of eyes)
	Persistent tearing
	Persistent ocular discharge
	Persistent redness
	Persistent light sensitivity
	Squinting
	Eye closure
	Head tilt
	Learning disabilities
Risk factors (general health problems, systemic disease, or use of medications that are known to be associated with eye disease and visual abnormalities)	Prematurity
	Perinatal complications (evaluation at birth and at 6 months old)
	Neurologic disorders or neurodevelopmental delay (on diagnosis)
	Juvenile rheumatoid arthritis (on diagnosis)
	Diabetes mellitus (twice yearly after puberty and every 1-2 months during pregnancy)†
	Systemic conditions with ocular manifestations (at 6 months old or on diagnosis)
	Chronic systemic steroid therapy or other medications (e.g., hydroxychloroquine) known to cause eye disease
A family history of conditions that cause or are associated with eye or vision problems	Retinoblastoma
	Childhood cataract
	Childhood glaucoma
	Retinal dystrophy, degeneration
	Strabismus
	Amblyopia
	Glasses in early childhood
	Sickle cell disease
	Systemic syndromes with ocular manifestations

Note: These recommendations are based on panel consensus except where noted.
*"Headache" is not included because it is rarely caused by eye problems in children. This complaint should first be evaluated by the primary care physician.
†Feist R, Blodi C, Spiegel P: Retinal vascular disorders. In Wright KW, Spiegel PH, editors: *Pediatric ophthalmology and strabismus,* New York, 2003, Springer.
From American Academy of Ophthalmology (AAO) Pediatric Ophthalmology Panel: *Pediatric eye evaluations,* San Francisco, 2002, American Academy of Ophthalmology.

to block or enhance certain colors and are designed for sports use by tennis players, golfers, baseball players, spectators, trapshooters, and skiers.

OPHTHALMIC MEDICATIONS

Caution and precision must be exercised when administering ocular medications to children because their smaller body mass and faster metabolism may potentiate the action of the drugs and result in adverse ocular and systemic side effects.

Topical ophthalmic medications, such as antibiotics, mydriatics, and corticosteroids, are frequently found in ointment or solution vehicles. These topical agents are primarily used for treating disorders affecting the anterior segment of the eye. Solubility is one of several factors that influence the absorption of topical ophthalmic medications. Those that are water soluble (e.g., anesthetics, steroids, and alkaloids) penetrate the corneal epithelium easily. Fat-soluble preparations (e.g., most antibiotics) do not penetrate the epithelium of the cornea unless it is inflamed.

Topical Antibiotics

Prescription of topical antibiotics is ideally based on empirical evidence that infection exists. The best choice of a topical

BOX 28-1   Recommendations for Use of Corrective Lenses

Eyeglasses

- Polycarbonate lenses are lightweight, strong, and shatterproof; scratch-resistant coating is recommended.
- Silicone nose pads with nonskid surfaces prevent glasses from slipping.
- Comfort cables secure frames by wrapping around the child's ears and are available for children 1 to 4 years old. Straps are recommended for infants under 1 year old and allow them to roll and lie down.
- Flexible hinges allow outward bending for easy removal by the child.
- Match the frame to the child's facial shape and features to encourage compliance; if old enough allow the child to choose the frames.
- To encourage compliance with infants and children, do not fight them when they remove glasses; be persistent, replace the glasses, and provide distraction. Parents may need to set the glasses aside for a few hours before trying again. Seek counsel from the prescribing provider for further help.
- Tinted lenses can be used for photosensitivity; UV light filters are helpful with aphakia (absence of lens), congenital absence of iris, and albinism.
- Do not place the glasses down with lenses in contact with surfaces.
- Clean glasses daily with liquid soap and a soft cloth (do not use paper products).

Contact Lenses

- Contact lenses are appropriate for children 10 to 13 years and older or in children who can demonstrate ability to manage lens hygiene, including insertion and removal.
- Contact lenses are helpful for an aphakic child who would otherwise need very thick glasses that distort images.
- Wear protective outer eyewear for sports.
- Do not wear contact lenses if one or both eyes are inflamed or when using topical ophthalmic medications. Those with recurrent conjunctival or corneal infections, inadequate tears, severe allergies, or excessive exposure to dust or smoke should not wear contact lenses.
- Extended-wear contact lenses that are usually worn overnight should be removed and not worn overnight once a week to perform lens hygiene procedures.

Adapted from American Academy of Ophthalmology (AAO): *Eyeglasses for infants and children,* Medem Medical Library website. Available at *www.medem.com* (accessed Nov 11, 2006a). Additional information from American Academy of Ophthalmology (AAO): *Extended wear of contact lenses,* Medem Medical Library website. Available at *www.medem.com* (accessed July 7, 2006c).

antibiotic is one that is not often prescribed for problems in other body systems. Topical ophthalmologic preparations, such as fluoroquinolones, sulfacetamide, and trimethoprim/polymyxin B, are effective and rarely produce a hypersensitivity reaction. Topical penicillins, on the other hand, are to be avoided. The pros and cons of these antibiotics will be addressed in later sections of this chapter. Ophthalmic ointments are generally preferred over solutions for use in children because they last longer, do not sting, do not need to be given as often, and are less likely to be absorbed into the lacrimal passage. However, they do temporarily interfere with vision because they coat the eye, and they can cause a contact dermatitis. Special care must be taken to ensure that the tip of the tube or dropper is not contaminated. Ophthalmic ointment should be transferred from the tube to moistened cotton swabs (one for each eye) and then rolled into the lower portion of each conjunctival sac (see Appendix A for ophthalmic drugs).

Ophthalmic Corticosteroids

Although ophthalmic corticosteroids are effective in the treatment of ocular inflammation and traumatic iritis (excluding ocular allergy), a patient with a condition severe enough to warrant consideration of corticosteroid use should be referred to an ophthalmologist. Steroids are associated with numerous complications, such as an increased incidence of herpes simplex keratitis and corneal ulcers, corneal perforation and intraocular sepsis, glaucoma, slowed healing of corneal abrasions and wounds, increased IOP, cataract formation, and permanent loss of sight. They should never be used for suspected eye infections, for red eye of unknown origin, in immunocompromised children, or in any eye trauma that involved plants or soils (Lichenstein, 2004; Trobe, 2001). A child receiving long-term ophthalmologic steroids should be assessed frequently for signs of adrenal suppression or other side effects. Encourage parents to keep scheduled tonometry appointments at 2- to 3-month intervals.

Other Topical Preparations

Decongestants or antihistamines or a combination of the two, mast cell stabilizers, and nonsteroidal antiinflammatory drugs are agents used in treating various ophthalmologic conditions, such as allergic conjunctivitis. Over-the-counter vasoconstrictors or vasoconstrictor-antihistamine preparations can be tried first for mild allergic conjunctivitis but are ineffective for a persistent allergic conjunctivitis (Gomi et al, 2005). Cycloplegic agents are used for iritis.

Systemic Medications

In ocular infections involving the posterior segment and the orbit, systemic antibiotic preparations are necessary. A combination of topical and systemic antibiotics can also be used. In general, these conditions warrant referral to an ophthalmologist. Systemic drugs may also cause damage to the eyes (Table 28-5).

EYE INJURY PREVENTION

Ocular trauma accounts for one third of all cases of acquired blindness in children. Male-to-female trauma incidence ratio is 4:1, with males 11 to 15 years old outnumbering all other age groups. Children under 5 years old account for 8% of all eye injuries. Most of the injuries could be prevented. The majority of the injuries are the result of sports-related accidents, toy darts, sticks, stones, fireworks, BB shot, paintball sports, other projectiles, and alpine skiing (Olitsky & Nelson, 2004). Other causes include battered child syndrome (40% have ocular

findings), birth trauma, and airbags (Wright, 2003a). Parental supervision and education of children regarding prevention of eye injury are essential to minimize these injuries. Prevention includes such fundamental concepts as the following:

- Children need to be instructed to:
  - Not run with or throw sharp objects
  - Use protective eyewear when hammering, using power tools, or participating in a sport where there is a high ocular risk (hockey, fencing, boxing, full-contact martial arts, racquetball, lacrosse, squash, basketball, baseball). Moderate-risk sports include tennis, badminton, soccer, volleyball, water polo, football, fishing, and golf. Low-risk sports include swimming, diving, skiing, noncontact martial arts, wrestling, bicycling, track and field, and gymnastics (AAO, 2006d).
  - Use orthodontic headwear that breaks away if force is applied
  - Not shine laser pointers in eyes
  - Use eye wash fountains when indicated

TABLE 28-5 Systemic Drugs, Herbs, and Nutritional Supplements That Can Cause Ocular Side Effects

Drug	Ocular Side Effects	Intervention
Corticosteroids (prednisone at dosage of 15mg/day for ≥1 year)	Cataracts	Monitor with ophthalmologic examinations.
Digoxin at moderately toxic ranges	Snowy, flickering, yellow vision	Resolves when drug is administered in correct range.
Isoniazid in greater than recommended dosages	Loss in color vision, ↓ visual acuity, and visual field changes	Effects are reversible only if discovered early. Ophthalmologic examination can be done before treatment and every 6 months; any changes warrant stopping isoniazid and referring to an ophthalmologist.
Isotretinoin	Pseudotumor cerebri (after initiating treatment) with resultant blurred vision, visual field loss, and varying visual acuity changes	Monitor for symptoms.
Minocycline hydrochloride	Pseudotumor cerebri and orthostatic blackouts, evidenced by blurred vision, visual field loss, varying visual acuity changes, diplopia; scleral pigmentation	Monitor for symptoms; scleral pigmentation may not resolve.
Phenytoin and carbamazepine	Blood levels in moderately toxic ranges can produce diplopia, blurred vision, nystagmus; sensitivity to glare	Resolves when therapeutic doses are within normal ranges.
Topiramate	Acute angle closure glaucoma; mydriasis; ocular pain; decreased visual acuity.	Onset of symptoms within 3-14 days after medication started. Stop medication. Treatment may include cycloplegics, hyperosmotic therapy, topical antiglaucoma medications.
Quetiapine (Seroquel)	Cataracts	Monitor with ophthalmologic examinations.
Herbs		
Canthaxanthine (taken to produce artificial suntan; food coloring)	Decreased visual acuity; retinopathy	
Datura (may be used by those with asthma, influenza, coughs)	Mydriasis	
Ginkgo biloba	Retrobulbar and retinal hemorrhage; hyphema	
Licorice	Decreased visual acuity	
Vitamin A	Intracranial hypertension	

Data from National Registry of Drug-Induced Ocular Side-Effects: *2006 AAO syllabus.* Available at *www.piodr.sterling.net* (accessed Jan 6, 2007). Trobe J: *The physician's guide to eye care,* San Francisco, 2001, The Foundation of the American Academy of Ophthalmology.

- Parents further need to be instructed to:
  - Store harmful chemicals and sharp objects out of the reach of small children
  - Limit and supervise the use of BB guns, air rifles, paintball devices, darts, and fireworks

Sunglasses

Ultraviolet (UV) A and UVB radiation from the sun can damage the lens and retina of the eye and cause cataracts and other conditions harmful to vision later in life. Sunglasses should be used to minimize such damage by absorbing these light wavelengths, even if wearing UV-treated contact lenses (School of Public Health, 2002). It is never too early to start wearing sunglasses. Wearing a hat with a wide (3-inch) brim cuts the radiation exposure in half.

Sunglasses that have large-framed, wraparound lenses with side shields provide the best protection. The lens and frame should be constructed of nonbreakable plastic or polycarbonate. The protection comes from the chemical coating on top of, or incorporated into, the lenses. Gray, brown, and green colors are sufficient for general purposes and lead to minimal color distortion. Darker colors or polarized lenses alone do not offer the protection that is needed. Lenses should only be purchased if they carry the American National Standards Institute (ANSI) label or American Optometry Association (AOA) notation. ANSI communicates their standards by labeling their lenses Z80.3 and "general purpose," "special purpose" (for snow and water sports), and "cosmetic use" (lowest protection). AOA sets higher UV radiation standards (School of Public Health, 2002).

Sports Protection

Eye protection is recommended for any child or adolescent participating in sports that have a high eye injury rate. Protective glasses or goggles are mandatory for all functionally one-eyed individuals (with best corrected vision worse than 20/40 in the poorer-seeing eye) or for any athlete who has had eye surgery or trauma or whose ophthalmologist recommends eye protection (AAO, 2006d). Additionally, these children or adolescents should not participate in boxing or full-contact martial arts. Caution is also recommended in these individuals if they choose to wrestle, even though there is a low rate of reported injury. Specific protective eyewear is available; however, there are no standards for eyewear in this sport. Eye protection is also recommended for pool activities, racquet sports, football, soccer, hockey, lacrosse, and squash. Eye protection also should be used in shop class or labs or when working with high-velocity projectiles (e.g., hammer on metal, power tools, or lawn mowers).

Protective eyewear should be properly fitted and selected specifically for the sport. A complete list of recommended eyewear for each sport is available on-line from the AAO website (see Resource Box at the end of the chapter). The list would serve as a useful handout for parents. A headband or wraparound earpieces should be used to secure the glasses. Parents should only buy the protective eyewear certified by American Society for Testing and Materials (ASTM), the Hockey Equipment Certification Council (HECC), Canadian Standards Association (CSA), Protective Eyewear Certification Council (PECC), or National Operating Committee on Standards for Athletic Equipment (NOCSAE) for use in the particular sport. Fashion or street-wear glasses are inadequate, as are safety eyewear that carry an ANSI Z87.1 rating.

Athletes who need prescription eyewear can either choose polycarbonate lenses in a sports frame that is ASTM F803 rated for the specific sport, wear polycarbonate contact lenses plus the appropriate protective eyewear, or wear an attached over-the-glasses eye guard that also meets specifications of ASTM F803.

Younger children who do not fit into the manufactured protective eyewear may be fitted with 3-mm polycarbonate lenses with ANSI Z87.1 rating. However, adequate protection cannot be guaranteed and perhaps another choice of sport should be discussed.

Laser Pointers

The FDA released a warning in 1997 about the misuse of laser pointers. Although harmless when used as intended by lecturers, potential injury to the retina was of concern if the pointers are used as toys. A literature review by this author found conflicting conclusions about the safety of these devices when retinas were exposed to commercially available laser pointers of 1, 2, or 5 mW for more than 10 seconds (Israeli et al, 2001; Robertson et al, 2000). It is recommended, therefore, that these devices not be made available as toys to children and adolescents.

VISION THERAPY, LENSES, AND PRISMS

Vision therapy, lenses, and prisms are controversial methods of treatment claimed by some to be effective therapy for learning disabilities and dyslexia. The joint organizational policy of the American Academy of Optometry and the American Optometric Association (1997, p. 2) states that "vision therapy does not directly treat learning disabilities or dyslexia … but is a treatment to improve visual efficacy and visual processing." These interventions consist of (1) visual training, including muscle exercises, ocular pursuit, tracking exercises, or "training" glasses (with or without bifocals or prisms); (2) neurologic organizational training (laterality training, crawling, balance board, perceptual training); and (3) wearing of colored lenses (AAP, 1998).

The AAP, AAO, and AAPOS joint statement, *Learning Disabilities, Dyslexia, and Vision: A Subject Review*, states that "vision problems are rarely responsible for learning difficulties. No scientific evidence exists for the efficacy of eye exercises ('vision therapy') or the use of special tinted lenses in the remediation of these complex pediatric developmental and neurological conditions. … Avoid remedies involving eye exercises, filters, tinted lenses, or other optical devices that have no known scientific proof of efficacy" (AAP, 1998, p. 1; AAO, 2001). Indeed current research has shown that dyslexia is a language-based disorder—not a visual-perceptual problem—caused by neurobiologic and genetic factors (International Dyslexia Association, 2007).

When counseling parents who inquire about vision therapy, the clinician should be aware of the pressure that parents may be under from optometrists advocating vision therapy for learning disabilities and the divergent opinions held by educators and the ophthalmologic community about this modality of treatment. Managing a child with academic difficulties requires a multidisciplinary approach involving education and psychological and other medical specialists. Screening for ocular defects early is a routine part of primary care practice, and defects should be referred to the appropriate specialist.

▇▇ COMMON EYE DISORDERS
VISUAL DISORDERS
Refractive Errors and Amblyopia
Description.   Alterations in the refractive power of the eye include myopia, hyperopia, astigmatism, accommodation, and anisometropia. In a normal eye, light from a distant object focuses directly on the retina. When variations in axial length of the eyeball or curvature of the cornea or lens exist, light focuses in front of or behind the retina. This abnormal focusing produces an alteration in the refractive power of the eye that results in a visual acuity deficit (Box 28-2 provides more complete definitions).

Amblyopia is usually a unilateral deficit in which there is defective development of the visual pathways needed to attain central vision. Clear focused images fail to reach the brain and result in reduced or permanent loss of vision. The condition is labeled (or typed) according to the structural or refractive problem that is causing the poor visual image to reach the brain: deprivational, or obstruction of vision (e.g., caused by ptosis, cataract, nystagmus); strabismic (caused by strabismus or lazy eye); or refractive (myopia, hyperopia, astigmatism, anisometropia).

BOX 28-2   Descriptive Terms for Refractive Errors

Myopia, or nearsightedness, exists when the axial length of the eye is increased in relation to the eye's optical power. As a result, light from a distant object is focused in front of the retina rather than directly on it. A myopic child sees close objects clearly, but distant objects are blurry.

Hyperopia, or farsightedness, exists when the visual image is focused behind the retina. As a result, distant objects are seen clearly, but close objects are blurry.

Astigmatism exists when the curvature of the cornea or the lens is uneven; thus the retina cannot appropriately focus light from an object regardless of the distance, which makes vision blurry close up and far away. Rarely, astigmatism can be caused by an alteration in the corneal sphere caused by a soft tissue mass on the inner aspect of the eyelid, such as a chalazion or hemangioma.

Anisometropia is a different refractive error in each eye. It may consist of any combination of refractive errors discussed above, or it may occur with aphakia.

Incidence.   Refractive errors are the most common visual disorder seen in children. Approximately 20% of children have significant refractive errors by their teen years. An estimated 14 million people in the U.S. older than 12 years have 20/50 or worse visual acuity that can be improved with treatment (Vitale et al, 2006). Myopia may be present at birth, but it is more likely to develop during the preteen and teen years. Mild hyperopia is normal in a young child, but should decrease rapidly between 7 and 14 years old. Amblyopia affects approximately 2% of children in the general population (Wright, 2003b).

Clinical Findings.   The following may be noted:
- Squinting
- Fatigue
- Headaches (rare)
- Pain in or around eyes
- Dizziness
- Mild nausea
- Developmental delay
- Tendency to cover or close one eye when concentrating
- Family history of refractive errors, strabismus, or amblyopia

Management.   Detection of visual problems in children at an early age is essential to prevent the development of otherwise preventable permanent visual loss. The following steps are involved:
- Refer to an ophthalmologist or optometrist for prescription corrective lenses.
- Older children should have an annual refraction and eyeglass evaluation.
- Unilateral visual occlusion may be necessary and, occasionally, surgery may be necessary.
- Extended-wear contact lenses may be prescribed in unilateral aphakia, severe anisometropia, corneal scarring with irregular astigmatism, and keratoconus.
- Support and reassurance according to the child's developmental level are needed during the period of adjustment to contact lenses or eyeglasses.
  - Infants and toddlers need distraction, with consistent replacement of glasses once removed.
  - Verbal children may be aided by the use of positive reinforcement, such as sticker charts.
  - School-age children and teenagers should participate in the selection of frames. If desired, contacts may be considered.
- Claims of certain diets or exercises as means of correcting or preventing refractive errors have not been substantiated by research efforts (see the discussion in Management Strategies earlier in this chapter).

Complications.   Untreated or insufficiently treated amblyopia in young childhood will result in irreversible and lifelong visual loss.

Strabismus
Description.   Strabismus is a defect in ocular alignment, or the position of the eyes in relation to each other; it is commonly called a "lazy eye." In strabismus, the visual

axes are not parallel because the muscles of the eyes are not coordinated; when one eye is directed straight ahead, the other deviates. As a result, one or both eyes appear crossed. In children, strabismus may be manifested as a phoria or a tropia (Box 28-3). Pseudostrabismus is present when the sclera between the cornea and the inner canthus is obscured by closely placed eyes, a flat nasal bridge, or prominent epicanthal folds (see Fig. 28-3). In children after 7 to 9 years old who have acquired tropia, double vision will occur. In those under 6 to 7 years old, cortical suppression of vision in the deviated eye will result, which stops the diplopia, but leads to amblyopia.

Variable alignment is common in the newborn. Most have straight eyes; up to 70% can exhibit transient exotropia, which should resolve by 6 months of age, and 0.5% to 2% have esotropia. Congenital esotropia is ascribed to an infant with an onset less than 6 months of age who did not have a deviation as a newborn (Wright, 2003b; Olitsky & Nelson, 2005).

Epidemiology. Strabismus affects approximately 2% to 5% of preschool children and usually develops before 5 years of age. Esodeviations are the most common type of strabismus. They account for more than 50% of deviations. Accommodative esotropia are most visible when the child is looking at a near object, occur at 2 to 3 years of age, are seen in children with a history of acquired intermittent or constant crossing, and are more likely to result in amblyopia (Olitsky & Nelson, 2005). Exodeviations occur 25% of the time, are usually intermittent, and more visible when the child is looking far away. Both types of strabismus may be hereditary or the result of various eye diseases (e.g., neuroblastoma), trauma, systemic or neurologic dysfunction that paralyzes the extraocular muscles, uncorrected hyperopia, accommodation and accommodative convergence, or diplopia after 4 to 6 years old (McManaway & Frankel, 2001; Rubin, 2001; Wright, 2003b). Esotropia can also been seen in those with a history of prematurity, cerebral palsy, hydrocephalous, and possibly maternal tobacco use and low birth weight (Olitsky & Nelson, 2005).

BOX 28-3 **Descriptive Terms for Strabismus**

A **phoria** is an intermittent deviation in ocular alignment that is held latent by sensory fusion. The child can maintain alignment on an object.

A **tropia** is a consistent or intermittent deviation in ocular alignment. A child with a tropia is unable to maintain alignment on an object of fixation.

Phorias and tropias are classified according to the pattern of deviation seen:
- **Hyper** (up) and **hypo** (down) are used to classify vertical strabismus.
- **Exo** (away from the nose) and **eso** (toward the nose) describe horizontal deviations.
- **Cyclo** describes a rotational or torsional deviation.

Clinical Findings. Clinical findings can involve the following:
- Intermittent exotropia may be seen in normal children 6 months to 4 years old who are ill or tired or when they are exposed to bright light or with sudden changes from close to distant vision. It is more often seen when the child is looking with distant fixation.
- When only one eye is affected, the child always fixates with the unaffected eye.
- When both eyes are affected, the eye that looks straight at any given time is the fixating eye.
- The angle of deviation may be inconsistent in all fields of gaze, actually changing in some forms of strabismus.
- Persistent squinting, head tilting, face turning, overpointing, awkwardness, marked decreased visual acuity in one eye, or nystagmus may be seen.
- Cataracts, RB, anisometropia, and severe refractive errors are found infrequently.

Diagnostic Testing. The corneal light reflection technique and the cover-uncover and alternating cover tests are assessments used to screen for strabismus. Asymmetry of light reflection on the cornea is indicative of a deviation in ocular alignment. The cover-uncover test is used to detect tropias, whereas the alternating cover test detects phorias (see Fig. 28-3). The photoscreener can also be used to detect strabismus.

Management. Management steps include the following:
- Any ocular misalignment seen after 4 months old is considered suspicious, and the child should be referred. Hypertropia or hypotropia, exotropia, acquired esotropia or exotropia, cyclovertical deviation, or any fixed deviation is an indication for referral as soon as it is first observed.
- The unaffected ("good") eye is occluded (patched, using an occlusive contact lens, or an overplussed lens), which forces the child to use the deviating eye. Pharmacologic penalization with the daily instillation of 0.5% to 1% atropine sulfate is also used.
- Surgical alignment of the eyes may be necessary, but this does not preclude additional amblyopia therapy.
- Orthoptic exercises as a treatment modality are indicated only in certain forms of intermittent strabismus or when the visual axes are nearly aligned.
- Corrective lenses may or may not be indicated, depending on the presence of refractive errors.
- Assessment for amblyopia should be done at every visit, even after straightening the eyes, because changes in alignment can occur through the fifth year.
- The ocular status of an affected child's siblings is monitored.
- Local botulinum toxin injection may also be used with certain deviations (Jockin, 2002).
- Age should not be used as the deciding factor for referring a child with amblyopia. A recent study showed visual improvement in previously untreated children older than 13 years (National Eye Institute, 2005).

Complications. Amblyopia (secondary visual loss) occurs in 30% to 50% of children with strabismus (Olitsky & Nelson, 2004). Uncorrected strabismus can have a negative effect on self-esteem.

Blepharoptosis

Description and Etiology. Blepharoptosis or ptosis is drooping of the upper eyelids affecting one or both eyes. It can be congenital or acquired, secondary to trauma or inflammation. Congenital ptosis is caused by striated muscle fibers of the levator muscle being replaced by fibrous tissue. It can be transmitted as an autosomal dominant trait. Other possible etiologies include trauma to cranial nerve III during the birthing process, trauma to the eyelid or neck, chronic inflammation (particularly of the anterior segment of the eye), or a neurologic disorder (myasthenia gravis, botulism, muscular dystrophy).

Parents may remark that one eye appears smaller. In severe cases, children may have a chin-up head position or adapt by raising their brow.

Management. Management involves the following steps:

- Refer to an ophthalmologist. If vision is compromised, surgery is performed in an effort to prevent amblyopia and developmental delay. The amblyopia should be addressed before surgical correction for the ptosis (Olitsky & Nelson, 2004). Surgical correction depends upon the degree of levator muscle compromise.
- Correct any underlying systemic disease.
- Evaluate for anisometropia (unequal refractive errors in each eye), anisocoria, and decrease in pupillary light reflex.

Nystagmus

Description. Nystagmus is the presence of involuntary, rhythmic movements that may be pendular oscillations or jerky drifts of one or both eyes. Movement is horizontal, vertical, rotary, or mixed.

Etiology. Nystagmus can occur in association with albinism, high refractive errors, CNS abnormalities, tumors, post-infection (e.g. Coxsackie B, cytomegalovirus [CMV], *Haemophilus influenza* meningitis), various diseases of the inner ear and the retina, middle ear trauma, visual loss before 2 years old, and pharmacologic toxicity. The child may have a birth history of prematurity, intraventricular hemorrhage, intrauterine psychogenic drug exposure, developmental delays, hydrocephaly, or be an infant of a mother with gestational diabetes.

Clinical Findings. The clinician should closely observe the nystagmus and note as much as possible about the type of movement (up, down, sideways), frequency (number of oscillations per a time unit), distance of movement, field(s) of gaze within which the nystagmus is evident (e.g., field of gaze straight ahead, left, or up), and any compensatory head or neck postures of the child. The movements may be constant or varied, depending on the direction of gaze (Strominger, 2005).

Oscillation in the newborn's eyes is common and exists for a short time during the neonatal period. Involuntary oscillation that persists or occurs beyond the initial weeks of life indicates a pathologic condition (Olitsky & Nelson, 2005).

Management. Management consists of treating any underlying systemic disorder and referring the patient to an ophthalmologist. Any acquired nystagmus is most worrisome and requires prompt evaluation.

Cataracts

Description. *Cataract,* a partial or complete opacity of the lens affecting one or both eyes, is the most common cause of an abnormal pupillary reflex. Some cataracts are considered clinically significant, others insignificant. They may exist in newborns or start in childhood.

Epidemiology. Cataracts may be congenital or a result of infection (e.g., congenital rubella, CMV, toxoplasmosis), trauma to the eye (including physical abuse, airbag deployment), metabolic disease (e.g., galactosemia, hypocalcemia), long-term use of systemic corticosteroids or ocular corticosteroid drops, prematurity, CNS anomalies (e.g., craniosynostosis, cranial defects), genetic defects (e.g., Down syndrome, albinism), and demyelinating sclerosis and ataxia-telangiectasia. They may also be seen in children who have other ocular abnormalities, such as strabismus or pendular nystagmus, and in children with diabetes mellitus, atopic dermatitis, or Marfan syndrome.

Worldwide, cataracts are responsible for visual loss in up to 10% of children. One in 250 newborns has some form of cataract (Tesser et al, 2005).

Clinical Findings. The following history and physical examination findings are present:

- A history of maternal prenatal infection, drug exposure, or hypocalcemia may be elicited.
- Cataract appears as an opacity on the lens, unilateral or bilateral.
- Visual acuity deficits may vary.
- A pale red reflex in people of color should not be confused with a cataract.

Management. Management depends upon the size, density, and location of the cataract. Often congenital or infantile cataracts can be monitored over several years for a progression that could produce amblyopia. Some types of cataracts do not progress, whereas others do (Tesser et al, 2005). Surgical removal of the lens optically clears the visual axis. The resultant aphakic refractive error is most often corrected with contact lenses. Newer research is evaluating the use of intraocular lens (IOL) implantations; some results to date show equal or better visual acuity improvement over contact lenses (Birch et al, 2005). Any sensory deprivation amblyopia is treated.

Complications. Visual delay (amblyopia), residual anisometropia, aniseikonia (unequal ocular image between eyes), intraocular competition.

Prognosis. The ultimate degree of visual function depends on the cataract type, age at time of surgery, underlying disease(s), age of onset and duration, and presence of amblyopia or other ocular abnormalities. Visual outcomes tend to be better with unilateral than bilateral cataracts. Children with histories of cataract surgery may exhibit later inflammatory sequelae, glaucoma, retinal detachment, and orbital architectural distortions (Olitsky & Nelson, 2004). Good results are more likely if cataracts are removed before 3 months old.

Glaucoma

Description.   Glaucoma is a disturbance in the circulation of aqueous fluid that results in an increase in IOP and subsequent damage to the optic nerve. It is classified according to age at the time of its appearance and other associated conditions.

Epidemiology.   Primary (infantile) glaucoma, occurs in the first 2 to 3 years of life; it occurs because of a congenital abnormality of the structures that drain the aqueous humor. Fortunately, it is rare and generally caught early. The incidence is approximately 1 in 10,000 live births and is gender and race neutral. Diagnosis is made as newborns (25% of cases), 60% before 6 months old, and 80% by 12 months old. Sixty-five to 80% occur bilaterally. It is also seen in association with other developmental anomalies, such as neurofibromatosis; diffuse facial nevus flammeus (port-wine stain); or Sturge-Weber, Marfan, Hurler, or Pierre Robin syndromes (Freedman & Walton, 2005).

Secondary or juvenile glaucoma occurs when the drainage network for aqueous humor becomes obstructed after ocular infection, trauma (airbag deployment), systemic disease, or long-term corticosteroid use.

Clinical Findings.   Parents may report that something is unusual about their child's eyes. The clinician should then note the following symptoms of infantile glaucoma:

- "Classic triad" of tearing, photophobia, and excessive blinking or blepharospasm caused by irritation (only 30% of patients manifest this triad). Infants may turn away from light (Freedman & Walton, 2005; Olitsky & Nelson, 2004).
- Hazy corneas.
- Corneal edema, corneal and ocular enlargement, bulbar conjunctival erythema, and visual impairment. If the condition is bilateral, parents may not notice any difference in the size of the corneas.

Symptoms of secondary glaucoma include the following:

- Extreme pain, vomiting
- Blurred or lost vision
- Tunnel vision
- Pupillary dilation
- Erythema (often in only one eye)
- Change in configuration of optic nerve cupping, with asymmetry between the eyes and loss of vision over time

Management.   Early diagnosis is important. The goal is normalization of IOP and prevention of optic nerve damage along with correction of associated refractive errors and prevention of amblyopia.

- Refer to an ophthalmologist. Primary treatment is surgery as early as possible (often multiple surgeries are required). Medications may be used as part of the medical management. These typically include topical β blockers, oral and topical carbonic anhydrase inhibitors (acetazolamide [Diamox], dorzolamide hydrochloride [Trusopt], brinzolamide [Azopt]), cholinergic stimulators, adrenergic agonists (epinephrine), and prostaglandins. Treatment can be difficult as a result of its prolonged nature, drug side effects, and adverse system effects.
- Parent and patient education must emphasize the importance of medication compliance and discourage excessive physical or emotional stress and straining during defecation.
- A medical identification tag is worn at all times.
- Follow-up for life, often every 3 to 6 months.
- Ophthalmoscopic examination (including tonometry) is needed for every member of the family.

Complications.   Stretching of the cornea, sclera, and permanent vision loss may occur over time despite treatment.

Retinopathy of Prematurity

Description.   Retinopathy of prematurity (ROP) is a developmental vascular disorder. It involves the abnormal growth of the retinal vessels in incompletely vascularized retinas of premature infants. Previously, ROP was called *retrolental fibroplasia.* An international classification system for ROP and the Multicenter Trial of Cryotherapy for ROP (CRYO-ROP) subclassification system provide clinicians with guidance for understanding the disease and for predicting outcome. This joint classification system describes ROP according to the distance to which the vascularization has progressed away from the optic nerve (zone I, II, or III), severity of inflammatory changes (stage), duration (clock hours), extent of disease, presence of plus disease (degree of large vessel engorgement and tortuosity), scarring patterns, prethreshold and threshold ROP (a clinical subclassification system), and presence of Rush disease (rapidly progressing ROP, especially post-retina) (Reynolds, 2005). ROP is important because of the increasing incidence, the critical window of time for treatment, and the need for monitoring for late complications.

Etiology.   ROP is a multifactorial retinal vasculopathologic disease primarily caused by early gestational age with low birth weight. It occurs primarily in premature infants born at or less than 28 weeks of gestation or weighing less than 1500 g. Infants demonstrating an unstable clinical course with weights between 1500 and 2000 g also are regarded as high risk (Olitsky & Nelson, 2004; Ober et al, 2003).

Developing retinal vessels grow outward from the optic nerve. The immature and incompletely vascularized retina is in a state of hypoxia, which stimulates the production of vascular endothelial growth factor (VEGF). Requisite levels of VEGF are needed to maintain the integrity of and stimulate retinal vessel growth. Exposure to supplemental oxygen presents an additional risk factor, although it is not totally clear what durations and concentrations of oxygen are detrimental when survival of the very smallest babies depends upon prolonged oxygen and ventilation. Higher oxygen concentrations produce lower VEGF levels and result in slowed vessel growth. Over several weeks, an avascular retina will become ischemic, and, in turn, stimulate renewed VEGF production. The increase in VEGF will stimulate vessel growth but not necessarily in an ordered manner. Other neonatal factors increase the risk of ROP (e.g., history of maternal bleeding, hydrops, anemia, intraventricular hemorrhage, sepsis, seizures, hypotension, necrotizing enterocolitis, and degree of sickness in the infant [Ober et al, 2003]). An increased incidence of the disease is noted in whites, with multiple births, and in infants with longer neonatal transport times after delivery to specialty neonatal intensive care units. There are no gender differences (Phelps, 2002).

Clinical Findings. ROP is initially diagnosed by a pediatric ophthalmologist while the infant is in the nursery, most often at 32 to 44 weeks postconception. Once the baby is discharged, the following may be seen:

- Leukokoria (white fibrovascular tissue in the retrolental space), glaucoma, cataracts
- Vitreous haziness, hemorrhage
- Retinal and iris changes
- Pallor of optic nerve
- Strabismus
- Cataracts
- Detached retinas (often with secondary glaucoma, entropion, and eye infections)

An infant (especially if full or near term) not previously diagnosed with ROP with detached retinas or leukokoria needs an ophthalmologic evaluation to rule out genetic disorders (e.g., Norrie syndrome, familial exudative vitreoretinopathy [X-linked recessive]).

Management. ROP progresses at variable rates. Initial ophthalmologic examinations should be done on all infants born at less than 28 weeks of gestation or weighing 1500 g or less or those born at 29 to 34 weeks with an unstable course during hospitalization. Examinations should occur at 4 to 6 weeks of age chronologically or 31 to 33 weeks of postconceptual or postmenstrual age; any vitreoretinal sequelae need to be followed throughout life (Ober et al, 2003). The provider's role in managing ROP is to ensure that all infants fitting these criteria (even in those whose ROP resolved or who did not have ROP) receive the initial and follow-up examinations (by 3 months after discharge). Examinations should be performed by a pediatric ophthalmologist experienced in examining preterm infants. The clinician further needs to do the following:

- Discuss with parents the implications of their child's disease.
- Monitor for late sequelae or ROP progression (e.g., strabismus, pseudostrabismus, amblyopia, myopia, anisometropia, leukokoria, cataracts).
- Assist children who have sequelae to maximize their potential by referring to early intervention services for low-vision children, to low-vision community support services, and to family support groups.
- Refer all children for yearly ophthalmologic follow-up if ROP required any treatment (even if ROP has resolved completely); less frequent follow-up is needed if no treatment was needed.

Cryosurgery or laser photocoagulation is employed to arrest the progression of abnormally growing blood vessels. Surgical reattachment of detached retinas has had disappointing results.

Complications. Complications can arise secondary to ROP or the treatment. Retinal detachment, strabismus, amblyopia, cataracts, serious myopia, astigmatism, anisometropia, uveitis, hyphema, macular burns, occlusion of the central retinal artery, glaucoma, and cicatrix (residual retinal scars) leading to later vision loss are possible. Any cicatricial formation is complete at about 8 months old. Less than 2% to 3% of infants have any visually threatening complications (Reynolds, 2005).

Prevention. Minimizing or preventing ROP can be accomplished by decreasing the occurrence of premature births and minimizing the oxygen needed. The use of vitamin E to maintain physiologic serum levels, reducing exposure to high ambient and supplemental lighting, or surfactant therapy have not been fruitful in reducing ROP (Ober et al, 2003).

Retinoblastoma

Description. Retinoblastoma is one type of intraocular tumor. It is a rare malignant tumor of the retina, but is the most common tumor in childhood. Tumors usually manifest by 2 years old, but can occur in older children (Shields & Shields, 2005). Tumors may be found in one eye or as multiple tumors in one or both eyes.

Epidemiology. Both hereditary and nonhereditary forms may occur; carrier and prenatal diagnosis is now possible. Bilateral disease and multifocal tumors are usually found in hereditary forms, whereas the nonhereditary forms are unilateral and unifocal. Unilateral disease occurs 60% of the time, is due to genetic mutation, and is commonly recognized by 25 months of age. The overall incidence is under study, but is estimated to occur once in 12,000 to 18,000 live births. New epidemiology research is showing some evidence of an increase in cases in developing countries, especially Mexico and Central America, Central Africa, and in the Indian subcontinent. A possible causal link to endemic human papillomavirus (HPV) is also under study (Murphee & Christensen, 2003).

Clinical Findings. The following may be seen:

- Positive family history
- Strabismus is often the most common finding
- Unilateral or bilateral white pupil (leukokoria), described often as an intermittent "glow, glint, gleam, or glare" by parents, usually in low-light settings (Murphee & Christensen, 2003)
- Decreased visual acuity
- Possible orbital cellulitis and photophobia (causes pain), hyphema, abnormal red reflex, nystagmus, glaucoma, hypopyon (pus in anterior chamber of eye), or signs of global rupture

Diagnosis is made via CT scan with contrast and/or echography and/or MRI. Other tests may include fundus photography, fluorescein angiography, ocular ultrasonography, or fine-needle aspiration.

Management. Refer the patient to an ophthalmologist for diagnosis and management by a multidisciplinary team. An international classification system for intraocular RB lists the criteria of tumors based upon their size, location, number, and degree of invasiveness or seeding. Depending upon the diagnosis, treatment may involve external beam radiation, cryotherapy, laser photocoagulation, episcleral plaque brachytherapy, or systemic chemotherapy. Early detection and advances in treatment have led to less enucleation and external beam radiation. In those with advanced tumors requiring enucleation, the hydroxyapatite implant provides excellent cosmetic appearance and acceptable motility of the implant

(Shields & Shields, 2005). Siblings and parents should receive a referral to an ophthalmologist for fundi examinations.

Frequent follow-up (every 3 months until 6 or 7 years old) to assess treatment and monitor for recurrence is important. An ophthalmologist, pediatric hematologist or oncologist, neurologist, pediatric surgeon, radiation oncologist, social worker, and a genetic counselor need to be involved.

Complications. Metastasis (most commonly to bone or bone marrow) is possible if the diagnosis is delayed. Those who survive are at high risk for a secondary nonocular malignancy, cataracts, vitreous hemorrhage, neovascular glaucoma, lacrimal duct or gland injury, impaired orbit bone growth, radiation retinopathy, optic neuropathy, or extraocular tumor with CNS or bone marrow suppression (Grabowski, 2006).

Prognosis. The size and extent of the tumor determine the prognosis. One third to one half of cases will develop second tumors by the time they reach 40 years old. Forty percent of those with a hereditary etiology can develop secondary, nonocular malignancies (Grabowski, 2006).

INFECTIONS
Conjunctivitis
Conjunctivitis is an inflammation of the palpebral and occasionally the bulbar conjunctiva. It is the most frequently seen ocular disorder in pediatric practice. Approximately 80% of the time, bacteria—most commonly *H. influenzae, Streptococcus pneumoniae, and Moraxella*—are responsible for the infection; both gram-negative and gram-positive organisms are implicated. *Staphylococcus aureus* is less commonly contributory, except after eye surgery or accidental eye trauma. Conjunctivitis also occurs as a viral (13%) or fungal infection or as a response to allergens (2%) or chemical irritants (Gross, 2004). Bacterial conjunctivitis is often unilateral, whereas viral conjunctivitis is most often bilateral. Unilateral disease can also suggest a toxic, chemical, mechanical, or lacrimal cause. Blockage of the tear drainage system (e.g., from meibomianitis or blepharitis), injury, foreign body, abrasion or ulcers, keratitis, iritis, herpes simplex virus (HSV), and infantile glaucoma are other known causes. A major indicator of etiology is also age of the patient (Table 28-6).

Conjunctivitis in the Newborn (Ophthalmia Neonatorum)
Description. Conjunctivitis in the newborn, also known as ophthalmia neonatorum or neonatal blennorrhea, is a form of conjunctivitis that occurs in the first month of life. In most states, conjunctivitis of the newborn is a reportable infectious disease.

Epidemiology. Conjunctivitis occurs in 0.3% to 11% of newborns. The most common cause is chemical conjunctivitis from the prophylactic instillation of silver nitrate at birth. *Chlamydia trachomatis* is the most common infectious or septic cause, and 50% of newborns with a mother positive for Chlamydia at the time of delivery will contract the disease. Various bacteria (*Staphylococcus, Streptococcus, Pseudomonas, H. influenza, Escherichia coli, Corynebacterium*

species, *Moraxella catarrhalis, Klebsiella pneumoniae, Pseudomonas aeruginosa*) plus *Neisseria gonorrhoeae* and HSV are also implicated (AAP, 2006).

Clinical Findings.
- Chemical conjunctivitis usually occurs in the first 24 to 72 hours of life.
- Septic conjunctivitis caused by:
  ○ Bacteria usually occurs from 5 to 14 days of life.
  ○ *C. trachomatis* usually begins between 5 to 14 days of life; it can also occur in newborns born via cesarean section with intact membranes.
  ○ *N. gonorrhoeae* usually appears in the first 3 to 5 days of life (up to 28 days).
  ○ HSV presents at birth or in the first four weeks of life.
  Symptoms most commonly seen include the following:
- Chemical-induced conjunctivitis frequently manifests as nonpurulent discharge and edematous bulbar and palpebral conjunctiva.
- *C. trachomatis* specifically causes moderate eyelid swelling and palpebral or bulbar conjunctival injection, moderate thick, purulent discharge.
- *N. gonorrhoeae* specifically causes acute conjunctival inflammation, lid edema, erythema, and excessive, purulent discharge.
- Bacteria presents with conjunctival erythema, purulent discharge.
- HSV specifically causes mild conjunctivitis, erythema, corneal opacity, serosanguineous discharge, and vesicular rash on eyelids and is often unilateral.

There may be a maternal history of vaginal infection during pregnancy or current sexually transmitted infection (STI).

Laboratory Studies. Swabs and scrapings must be done. Gram and Giemsa staining, direct immunofluorescent monoclonal antibody staining, cultures, enzyme-linked immunosorbent (ELISA), or polymerase chain reaction (PCR) testing can be used. Gonorrhea should be tested for in any infant younger than 2 weeks old. A culture for gonorrhea (on chocolate agar or Thayer-Martin medium) or aggressive scraping for a Gram stain are used for diagnosis (do not just sample the purulent discharge) (Schaffer, 2002). *Chlamydia* should also be tested for if gonorrhea is suspected.

Management
- Irrigate the eyes with sterile normal saline until clear of exudate.
- Gonococcal conjunctivitis: Infants should receive a 10- to 14-day course of intravenous or intramuscular ceftriaxone or cefotaxime. Ocular morbidity (corneal infection with possible scarring or perforation) can result in missed infections.
- Nongonococcal conjunctivitis: A topical ophthalmic antibiotic preparation, such as erythromycin 0.5% ointment (0.25- to 0.5-inch strip to each eye), is applied three to four times a day or moxifloxacin (four times a day for at least five days) (Rhee, 2004). The eyes should be cleansed with water or saline applied to cotton balls before instillation of the ointment into the lower conjunctival sac.

TABLE 28-6 **Types of Conjunctivitis**

Type	Incidence/Etiology	Clinical Findings	Diagnosis	Management
Ophthalmia neonatorum	Neonates: *C. trachomatis, Neisseria gonorrhoeae* (GC), herpes simplex virus (HSV). Silver nitrate reaction occurs in 10% of neonates.	Erythema, chemosis, purulent exudate with GC; clear to mucoid exudate with chlamydia	Culture (ELISA, PCR), Gram stain, R/O GC, chlamydia	Saline irrigation to eyes until exudate gone; follow with erythromycin ointment. • For GC: IM or IV ceftriaxone or cefotaxime. • For chlamydia: PO EES. • For HSV: IV or PO antivirals
Bacterial conjunctivitis	In neonates 5-14 days old; In preschoolers and sexually active teens: *H. influenzae* (nontypable), *S. pneumoniae*, GC	Erytherna, chemosis, itching, burning, mucopurulent exudate, matter in eyelashes; ↑ in winter	Cultures (optional); Gram stain (optional); Chocolate agar (for GC) R/O pharyngitis, GC, AOM, URI, seborrhea	• Neonates: Erythromycin 0.5% ophthalmic ointment. ≥1 year old: fourth-generation fluoroquinolone (e.g., moxifloxacin 0.5%) OR amoxicillin or amoxicillin/clavulanic acid oral suspension if concurrent AOM. • Warm soaks to eyes tid until clear. • No sharing towels, pillows. • No school until treatment begins.
Chronic bacterial conjunctivitis (unresponsive conjunctivitis previously treated as bacterial in etiology)	School-age children and teens: bacteria, viruses, *C. trachomatis,*	Same as above; foreign body sensation	Cultures, Gram stain; R/O dacryostenosis, blepharitis, corneal ulcers	• Depends upon prior treatment, laboratory results, and differential diagnoses. • Review compliance and prior drug choices of conjunctivitis treatment. • Consult with ophthalmologist.
Inclusion conjunctivitis	Neonates 5-14 days old, and sexually active teens: *C. trachomatis*	Erythema, chemosis, clear or mucoid exudate, palpebral follicles	Cultures (ELISA, PCR), R/O sexual activity	• Erythromycin PO for 2 week. Doxycycline, azithromycin, EES, erythromycin base PO (adolescents only).
Viral conjunctivitis	Adenovirus 3, 4, 7, HSV, herpes zoster, varicella	Erythema, chemosis, tearing (bilateral); HSV and herpes zoster: unilateral with photophobia, fever; zoster: nose lesion; ↑ spring and fall	Cultures, R/O corneal infiltration	• Refer to ophthalmologist if herpes lesions or photophobia present. • Cool compresses tid-qid.
Allergic and vernal conjunctivitis	Atopy sufferers, seasonal	Stringy, mucoid exudate, swollen eyelids and conjunctivae, itching, tearing, palpebral follicles, headache, rhinitis	Eosinophilia in conjunctival scrapings	• Vasocon 0.1%, 0.012%, 0.03% ophthalmic solution. • Refer to allergist if needed.

AOM, Acute otitis media; *ELISA,* enzyme-linked immunosorbent assay; *EES,* erythromycin ethylsuccinate; *IM,* intramuscular; *IV,* intravenous; *PCR,* polymerase chain reaction; *PO,* oral; *qid,* 4 times a day; *R/O,* rule out; *tid,* 3 times a day; *URI,* upper respiratory tract infection.

• Herpes simplex conjunctivitis: Hospitalization and topical and systemic antivirals are needed (acyclovir or vidarabine). Two thirds of infectious cases can spread to the CNS, mouth, and eyes; one third to the skin (Mills & Khazaeni, 2006).
• Chlamydia: Assess for systemic infection (pharyngitis, ear infection, pneumonia). Treatment is with oral erythromycin (50 mg/kg/day in four divided doses) for 14 days. Topical treatment is not indicated because it would not lower the risk for a subsequent pneumonia caused by Chlamydia. See Inclusion Conjunctivitis in next section.
• Chemical-induced conjunctivitis resolves spontaneously within 3 to 4 days without specific treatment.

- Mothers and their sexual partners should receive treatment if gonococcal and/or chlamydial infections occur in their newborns.

Prevention.   Prophylactic administration of silver nitrate 1% ophthalmic solution (2 drops to each eye) or an ophthalmic antibiotic ointment (or drops), such as 0.5% erythromycin (0.25- to 0.5-inch strip into each eye within 1 hour of delivery) or 1% tetracycline, is common practice for prophylaxis after birth. Povidone-iodine 2.5% solution can also be used, but such a product is not available in the U.S. Prophylaxis is required by law in most states and territories to prevent gonococcal conjunctivitis in the newborn. However, prophylaxis will not prevent neonatal chlamydial conjunctivitis or extraocular infection. It should be determined at the time of the first visit whether infants born at home have received this prophylaxis. Silver nitrate is the preferred prophylaxis in areas where there is a high incidence of penicillinase-producing *N. gonorrhoeae* (AAP, 2006).

Inclusion Conjunctivitis (Chlamydia)

Etiology.   Inclusion conjunctivitis is usually caused by one of eight known strains of *C. trachomatis* and is most often seen in a neonate or sexually active adolescent. Neonates will usually demonstrate symptoms within the first 5 to 14 days of life (to 6 weeks), whereas *N. gonorrhoeae* symptoms are usually detected earlier. Nasopharyngeal infection with *C. trachomatis* is found in 50% of those with inclusion conjunctivitis.

Clinical Findings

- Maternal history of an STI or a history of a sexual partner with an STI
- Conjunctival erythema and mild to severe mucopurulent to bloody discharge, usually bilateral
- Follicular reaction (large, round elevations) in the conjunctiva of the lower eyelids; conjunctiva may bleed if stroked
- Associated cervicitis, urethritis, or rectal infection
- Infants may have symptoms suggestive of chlamydial pneumonia at 1 to 3 months old

Laboratory Studies.   Conjunctival scrapings for Giemsa staining are indicated. A rapid screen of certain antigens can also be done using direct fluorescent antibody (MicroTrak) or electroimmunoassay (Chlamydiazyme) testing kits. A specimen should also be gathered appropriately to test for gonorrhea, because of the comorbidity of these two organisms. Ocular morbidity can result if gonorrhea is missed. Refer to Chapter 31 for guidance on pneumonia caused by *C. trachomatis*.

Management.   Treatment options have expanded from the traditional use of oral erythromycin ethylsuccinate (EES) to other macrolides, azithromycin, and clarithromycin. There is an increased incidence of idiopathic hypertrophic pyloric stenosis (IHPS) in infants less than 6 weeks old following systemic EES. However, this has not altered the recommendation of EES as the preferred treatment (AAP, 2006). The risk of using azithromycin and clarithromycin have not been fully established. Medical providers who treat newborns with EES should discuss the signs and potential risks of developing IHPS with parents.

Treatment recommendations include:

- A 14-day course of oral EES (50 mg/kg/day in four divided doses or 500 mg twice a day for 14 days). A second 14-day course is sometimes required because the failure rate with EES is 10% to 20%. Either EES is repeated, or oral azithromycin (20 mg/kg/24 hours once daily for 3 days) has been found effective (Hammerschlag, 2004). Providers are encouraged to use systemic EES with caution; if no other alternatives are viable, they need to have a high index of suspicion for the development of IHPS.
- Trimethoprim-sulfamethoxazole (0.5 ml/kg/day in two divided doses for 14 days) is an alternative systemic treatment after the neonatal period (Schaffer, 2002), and azithromycin and clarithromycin have been used, though they are not FDA approved in this age group.
- Doxycycline (200 mg twice a day for 7 days), erythromycin base (2.5 g, divided four times daily for 7 days), EES (3.2 g, divided four times daily for 7 days), azithromycin (1 g orally in a single dose), ofloxacin (600 mg divided twice daily for 7 days), or levofloxacin (500 mg daily for 7 days) can be used in young adults.
- Topical ointment (erythromycin, moxifloxacin) is sometimes recommended despite systemic drug treatment; the AAP notes that such concurrent treatment is unnecessary and ineffective (AAP, 2006).
- Mothers of infants with *C. trachomatis* conjunctivitis, partners of such mothers, and partners of sexually active adolescents also need examinations and treatment for two weeks with tetracycline or erythromycin.

Complications

Complications include chlamydial pneumonia (5% to 20% of infants will develop pneumonia if their mother had a chlamydial infection at delivery), nasopharyngeal colonization (in up to 50% of infants treated for inclusion conjunctivitis), or gastroenteritis in infants. Complications may occur 6 to 8 weeks following the conjunctivitis.

Bacterial Conjunctivitis

Description.   Acute bacterial conjunctivitis (commonly called *pinkeye*) is a contagious and easily spread disease.

Epidemiology.   Bacterial conjunctivitis is predominantly caused by nontypable *H. influenzae, S. pneumoniae,* *M. catarrhalis,* and adenovirus. It is most common in the winter and in toddlers and preschoolers (Lichtenstein, 2004). The introduction of the *S. pneumoniae* (Prevnar) vaccine in 2000 decreased the incidence of all invasive pneumococcal infections in children younger than 2 years old by 80% (AAP, 2006).

Clinical Findings.   The following may be noted:

- Erythema of one or both eyes, usually starting unilaterally and becoming bilateral (*key* finding)
- Yellow-green purulent discharge (*key* finding)
- Encrusted and matted eyelids on awakening (*key* finding)
- Burning, stinging, or itching of the eyes and a feeling of a foreign body
- Photophobia
- Petechiae on bulbar conjunctiva
- Symptoms of upper respiratory infection, otitis media, or acute pharyngitis
- Vision screen should be normal and documented in the patient's record

Laboratory Studies. Routine culture testing is *not necessary.* Gram stain and culture can be done if the conjunctivitis is chronic, recurrent, or difficult to treat.

Differential Diagnosis. Bacterial conjunctivitis requires consideration of nasolacrimal duct obstruction in infants, ear infection, Kawasaki syndrome, foreign body, corneal abrasion, uveitis, herpetic conjunctivitis, poor compliance, or wrong choice of drug. Cultures or scrapings are appropriate at that point. Leukemia can cause chronic conjunctivitis, or juvenile rheumatoid arthritis (JRA) may present with a red eye and photophobia (*Contemporary Pediatrics,* 2001; Hammerschlag, 2004).

Management. Bacterial conjunctivitis is considered a self-limited disease (unless caused by gonorrhea or chlamydia) that usually resolves within 8 to 10 days. However, because both gram-negative and gram-positive organisms have been implicated, children who receive topical antibiotics demonstrate faster clinical improvement, can return to day care or school faster, and cause less parental work loss. The common practice of prescribing antibiotics for conjunctivitis, however, has led to an increasing rate of drug resistance. It is imperative that providers make their diagnosis judiciously and then treat with an effective drug that is more likely to be tolerated and taken as directed. For this reason, older children and teens may be treated conservatively without using antibiotics. This prevents the overuse of antibiotics and takes into consideration the self-limited nature of this disease.

The provider will want to choose broad-spectrum coverage that has the lowest resistance rate, greatest compliance, and best penetration of tissues. Parents can be instructed to put pressure over the lacrimal duct when instilling the medication to prevent drainage into the nasolacrimal system. If improvement is not seen in 3 days after treatment is initiated, refer to or consult as appropriate with an ophthalmologist.

For uncomplicated bacterial conjunctivitis, the first-line drug of choice for children older than 12 months is:

- A fourth-generation fluoroquinolone because it provides excellent penetration, concentration, coverage, tolerability, compliance, and avoids the increasing levels of resistance to third-generation fluoroquinolones, such as ofloxacin. Moxifloxacin 0.5% (used tid), levofloxacin 0.5%, and gatifloxacin can be used. They are used for 5 to 7 days (Lichtenstein, 2004; Cuming et al, 2006). Insurance may not cover these drugs; if this is the case, use drugs from the following list.

Less effective but still often used drugs include:

- Third-generation fluoroquinolones, such as ofloxacin and ciprofloxacin.
- Sodium sulfacetamide 10% ophthalmic solution or ointment; poor efficacy, high resistance, stings, can cause allergic reactions (including Stevens-Johnson syndrome).
- Trimethoprim sulfate plus polymyxin B sulfate ophthalmic solution (Polytrim). There is an increasing resistance to *S. pneumoniae,* and efficacy is limited.
- Erythromycin 0.5% ophthalmic ointment is recommended for patients with sulfa allergy.

Neomycin is to be avoided because of possible sensitization. Chloramphenicol 1% can increase the chance of aplastic anemia, though rarely; the aminoglycosides (gentamycin and tobramycin) are demonstrating poor *S. pneumoniae* coverage and can cause red eye (Lichenstein, 2004).

Conjunctivitis-Otitis Syndrome. This syndrome is usually caused by *H. influenzae.* Treatment requires amoxicillin or amoxicillin with clavulanic acid (Augmentin; provides better coverage for *S. pneumoniae*) at 80 mg/kg of amoxicillin per 24 hours in children younger than 24 months old or another appropriate antibiotic for 10 days. Concurrent use of a topical antibiotic is not necessary (Giglotti, 2004).

Patient Education. If only one eye is involved, it is likely that the infection will spread within a day or two to involve both eyes. The patient (or parent) is instructed to do the following:

- Cleanse the eyelashes several times a day with a weak solution of no-tears shampoo and warm water. The importance of wiping from the inner canthus outward and using a different cloth or cotton ball for each eye should be emphasized.
- Use warm soaks three to four times a day to relieve itching and burning.
- Instill the prescribed ophthalmic solution or ointment into the lower conjunctival sac. A moistened cotton swab may be used to facilitate instillation of ointments. Dosing while the child is sleeping greatly increases compliance and, therefore, effectiveness.
- Wash hands frequently and avoid shared linens to limit spread of the infection.

Also treat seborrheic dermatitis on the scalp and face if present. Refer to Chapter 36 for treatment recommendations. Some day care centers exclude children with conjunctivitis until they have completed 1 to 2 days of treatment. Other centers allow the child to return once the treatment has started. Improvement in the child's condition should be seen within 48 hours. If medication compliance is not in question and improvement is not seen within 72 hours of administration, the parent should be instructed to return so that a smear of the exudate can be taken for culture and sensitivity testing.

Complications. If the infection proves recalcitrant to treatment, eye pain is present, vision blurred, or ophthalmoscopic examination reveals a bulging iris and a contracted, fixed pupil, suspect more serious inflammation of the uveal tract (iritis, cyclitis, or choroiditis). Refer immediately to an ophthalmologist because severe ocular morbidity can result.

Viral Conjunctivitis

Etiology. Usually caused by an adenovirus, viral conjunctivitis can also be caused by herpes simplex, herpes zoster, enterovirus, molluscum contagiosum, or varicella virus. It is more common in children older than 6 years and in the spring and fall.

Clinical Findings. The following may be noted:

- Tearing and profuse clear, watery discharge (*key* findings)
- Fever, headache, anorexia, malaise, upper respiratory symptoms (pharyngitis-conjunctivitis-fever triad with adenovirus [*key* findings])
- Pharyngitis with enlarged preauricular nodes (*key* findings)
- Itchy, red, and swollen conjunctiva
- Hyperemia and swollen eyelids
- Photophobia with measles or varicella rashes

- Herpetic vesicles on the eyelid margins and eyelashes (marginal blepharitis) or on the conjunctiva and cornea (keratoconjunctivitis)

Management

- Good hygiene is essential. Viral conjunctivitis is self-limited and should resolve in 7 to 14 days. Conjunctivitis is often difficult to distinguish from keratitis. If there is any question about diagnosis, a referral for ophthalmologic assessment is recommended.
- Warm or cold compresses and artificial tears can be used.
- Prophylaxis with antibiotics is not recommended, except in cases where keratoconjunctivitis (inflamed lesions on cornea) is suspected (Gross, 2004).
- Antihistamine or vasoconstrictive ophthalmic solutions may be used for symptomatic relief.
- With HSV infection, immediate referral to an ophthalmologist should occur because of potential complications. Vidarabine 3% or trifluridine 1% to 2% (Viroptic) or iododeoxyuridine 0.1% may be used in treatment. Topical corticosteroids should be avoided because they may worsen the course. Intravenous acyclovir (60 mg/kg/day divided into three doses for 14 days) is used in severe cases.
- Molluscum on the eyelid margins requires referral for excision.

Conjunctivitis-Pharyngitis Syndrome. This syndrome is more likely to be caused by adenovirus than by bacterium. Treat accordingly.

Complications. Involvement of deeper layers of the cornea (keratitis) can occur and must be differentiated from conjunctivitis. Scarring of the cornea resulting in blindness is a significant complication of HSV infection.

Allergic Conjunctivitis

Description. Allergic conjunctivitis usually occurs in childhood, but can occur after adolescence. Four types of allergic conjunctivitis have been identified: (1) hay fever–associated conjunctivitis is characterized by mild injection and swelling; (2) vernal conjunctivitis is more severe, is more common in 3- to 12-year-olds, and has an increased prevalence in warm weather; (3) atopic keratoconjunctivitis occurs in those with atopic dermatitis and/or asthma. It affects the lower tarsal conjunctiva, usually occurs in late adolescence, is notable for significant (beyond that seen in allergic conjunctivitis) itching, burning, and tearing that are often chronic; and (4) giant papillary conjunctivitis occurs most often in contact lens wearers allergic to the thimerosal in contact lens solutions.

Epidemiology. Seasonal allergens (notably grass pollens and ragweed) cause allergic conjunctivitis. Rhinitis, eczema, and asthma may be associated conditions. The incidence is 25% of the general population and is seen in 30% of atopic children (Boguniewicz, 2004).

Clinical Findings. The following may be noted:
- Severe itching and tearing (*key* finding)
- Family history of atopy or seasonal allergies
- Rhinitis, eczema, asthma
- Acute attacks precipitated by allergens (e.g., pollen, animals, molds, dust, dust mites, occasionally food)
- Redness and swelling of the conjunctiva or eyelid (or both)

- Follicular reaction of the conjunctiva
- Stringy, mucoid discharge
- Bilateral involvement most common
- Cobblestone papillary hypertrophy in the tarsal conjunctiva
- Vision screening should be normal; document in patient's record

Laboratory Studies. Conjunctival or nasal smears (using Wrights stain) reveal numerous eosinophils.

Management. The following steps are taken when approaching treatment:
- Prevention is best; avoid allergens.
- For mild cases, saline solution or artificial tears are administered along with cool compresses. Refrigerated eyedrops are more soothing.
- The next step is topical decongestants and oral or topical antihistamines. The decongestants will not decrease the allergic response, but they will relieve erythema, injection, and lid edema. Prescribed agents can provide quicker, more long-term relief with fewer side effects than over-the-counter agents. Vasoconstrictors (e.g., Visine) should be avoided because of rebound congestion. (Paradis & Granet, 2002).
  - Topical decongestants include: naphazoline hydrochloride (Naphcon or Vasocon) ophthalmic solution (1 to 2 drops every 3 to 4 hours).
  - A combination antihistamine-decongestant is more effective than either agent alone: Naphcon-A or Vasocon-A ophthalmic solution (1 to 2 drops four times a day) can be used sparingly to reduce ocular congestion, irritation, and itching.
- Topical mast cell stabilizers may be helpful for maintenance therapy or vernal conjunctivitis (Gomi et al, 2005).
  - Cromolyn sodium 4% (Opticrom, Crolom) 1 to 2 drops every 4 to 6 hours for children older than 4 years on a regular basis.
  - Nedocromil sodium 2% (Alocril) 1 to 2 drops twice daily.
  - Pemirolast potassium 0.1% (Alamast) or lodoxamide tromethamine 0.1% (Alomide) 1 to 2 drops four times a day for children older than 2 years.
  - Olopatadine hydrochloride 0.1% (Patanol) is a mast cell stabilizer combined with an antihistamine for children older than 3 years (1 drop 8 hours apart). Olopatadine will cover all of the symptoms of itching, redness, swelling, and discharge (Paradis & Granet, 2002).
- Nonsteroidal antiinflammatory drugs can be used for late-phase treatment of itching and burning.
  - Ketorolac tromethamine (Acular, Acular Preservative Free) 0.5%, 1 drop four times a day up to 1 week in children older than 12 years.
- Topical steroids are sometimes used in severe cases of allergy, but they must be used with caution because of possible side effects (increased IOP, potential for viral infection, contraindication with herpes, potential to cause cataracts, and poor corneal healing). An ophthalmologist should be consulted before using. At maximum they should be used for 1 week. If additional therapy is required, referral for ophthalmologic care is necessary.

- Refer to an allergist for allergen immunotherapy when rhinitis is present since therapy can lead to better control without the need for medication.
- Refer to an ophthalmologist if unresponsive to treatment or if the following is present: corneal abrasions, impaired vision, need for corticosteroids, severe keratoconjunctivitis, or atypical manifestations.
- Maintain a high threshold of suspicion for herpes-induced blepharitis or atopic keratoconjunctivitis if pain is present.

Complications. Some forms of allergic conjunctivitis (e.g., vernal conjunctivitis) can lead to cataracts, changes in the corneal curvature, and impact vision (Gross, 2004).

Blepharitis

Description. Blepharitis is an acute or chronic inflammation of the eyelash follicles or meibomian sebaceous glands of the eyelids (or both) (Table 28-7). It is usually bilateral. There may be a history of contact lens wear or physical contact with another symptomatic person.

Etiology. Blepharitis is commonly caused by contaminated makeup or contact lens solution. Poor hygiene, tear deficiency, rosacea, and seborrheic dermatitis of the scalp and face are also possible etiologic factors. The ulcerative form of blepharitis is usually caused by *S. aureus*. Nonulcerative blepharitis is occasionally seen in children with psoriasis, seborrhea, eczema, allergies, lice infestation, or in children with trisomy 21.

Clinical Findings. The following can be seen in blepharitis:

- Swelling and erythema of the eyelid margins and palpebral conjunctiva
- Flaky, scaly debris over eyelid margins on awakening; presence of lice
- Gritty, burning feeling in eyes
- Mild bulbar conjunctival injection
- Ulcerative form: hard scales at the base of the lashes (if the crust is removed, ulceration is seen at the hair follicles, the lashes fall out, and an associated conjunctivitis is present)

Differential Diagnosis. Pediculosis of the eyelashes.

Management. Explain to the patient that this may be chronic or relapsing. The patient is instructed to perform the following procedures:

- Scrub the eyelashes and eyelids with a cotton-tipped applicator containing a weak (50%) solution of no-tears shampoo to maintain proper hygiene and débride the scales.
- Use warm compresses twice daily for 5 to 10 minutes and wipe away lid debris.
- Apply antistaphylococcal antibiotic (e.g., erythromycin 0.5% ophthalmic ointment, 0.25 to 0.5 inch into each eye three to four times daily) until symptoms subside and for at least 1 week thereafter. Ointment is preferable to eyedrops because of increased duration of contact with the ocular tissue.
- Chronic staphylococcal blepharitis and meibomian keratoconjunctivitis respond to oral erythromycin (250 mg daily for maintenance). Doxycycline (50 to 100 mg twice daily), tetracycline, or minocycline can be used chronically in children older than 8 years (Ellis, 2005).

TABLE 28-7 Common Eye Infections

Condition	Clinical Findings	Management	Prevention
Blepharitis	Swelling, erythema of eyelid margins and palpebral conjunctiva, pruritus, flaking	Cleanse eyes, warm compresses, antibiotic drops or ointment	New eye makeup, clean contacts and glasses, hygiene
Hordeolum	Tender, red, swollen furuncle at eyelid margin or under eyelid	Warm compresses, remove eyelash, antibiotic drops or ointment	Hygiene
Chalazion	Initially, mild erythema and slight swelling; later, slow-growing, round painless mass	Treat cellulitis if present with oral antibiotic. Refer for evaluation to ophthalmologist.	Hygiene
Nasolacrimal duct obstruction (dacryostenosis)	Tearing or mucus, continuous or intermittent, blepharitis; express thin mucopurulent discharge from punctum	Daily massage, antibiotic ointment with inflammation or infection, normal saline for nasal congestion	Massage duct, minimize nasal congestion (see Fig. 28-4)
Nasolacrimal duct infection (dacryocystitis)	Tenderness and swelling over lacrimal duct, edema and erythema of tear sac, excoriation of skin; express purulent discharge from punctum	Warm compresses, massage, oral antibiotic	As above
Periorbital cellulitis	Acute onset, pain, swelling and erythema; temperature >102.2° F (>39° C), systemic symptoms	Outpatient systemic antibiotic therapy with close follow-up or hospitalization if moderate to severe infection, nonresponsive, poor compliance, or younger than 1 year old	HIB vaccine, hygiene, thorough cleansing of any skin disruption around eye, prompt treatment of sinusitis

HIB, Haemophilus influenzae type b.

- Treat associated seborrhea, psoriasis, eczema, or allergies as indicated.
- Remove contact lenses and wear eyeglasses for the duration of the treatment period. Sterilize or clean lenses before reinserting.
- Purchase new eye makeup.
- Use artificial tears for patients with inadequate tear pools.

Hordeolum
Description. Commonly called a stye, hordeolum is either an infection of the sebaceous glands (Zeis or Molls glands), of the eyelids (external hordeolum), or meibomian glands of the eyelid (internal hordeolum).

Etiology. The causative organism is *S. aureus* or, rarely, *P. aeruginosa*.

Clinical Findings. A tender, swollen, red furuncle is seen. In an external hordeolum, the swelling is generally smaller, superficial, and located along the lid margin. An internal hordeolum is larger and may point through the skin or conjunctival surface (Olitsky & Nelson, 2004). The patient complains of a foreign body sensation. An internal hordeolum on the palpebral conjunctiva can be inspected by rolling back the eyelid.

Differential Diagnosis. If the hordeolum does not resolve, consider cellulitis of the lid or orbit, sebaceous cell cancer, or pyogenic granuloma.

Management
- Rupture often occurs spontaneously when the furuncle becomes large and a point develops. Removal of an eyelash near the furuncle frequently promotes rupture.
- Warm, moist compresses three to four times daily, 10 to 15 minutes each time, facilitate the process of rupturing. Hygiene for the eye can be maintained by scrubbing the eyelashes and eyelids with a cotton-tipped applicator containing a weak (50%) solution of no-tears shampoo once or twice a day.
- Antistaphylococcal ointment (e.g., 0.5% erythromycin, 0.25 to 0.5 inch into each eye 3 to 4 times a day) until 2 to 3 days after resolution is effective treatment.
- Steroids are not indicated.
- Refer for incision and drainage if the hordeolum does not rupture on its own after coming to a point.
- Multiple or recurrent hordeolum: oral erythromycin 250 mg four times daily for 14 days; dicloxacillin 125 to 250 mg four times daily, or cloxacillin 500 mg four times daily for 14 days. Children older than 8 years can use prophylaxis: tetracycline 250 mg daily, doxycycline 50 to 100 mg daily, or minocycline 50 to 100 mg daily (consultation with an ophthalmologist is recommended).

Chalazion
Description. Chalazion is a chronic, sterile inflammation of the eyelid resulting from a lipogranuloma of the meibomian glands that line the posterior margins of the eyelids. It is deeper in the eyelid tissue than a hordeolum and may result from an internal hordeolum or retained lipid granular secretions.

Clinical Findings. Initially, mild erythema and slight swelling of the involved eyelid are seen. After a few days, the inflammation resolves, and a slow growing, round, nonpigmented, painless (*key* finding) mass remains. It may persist for long periods of time and is a commonly acquired lid lesion seen in children.

Management. The following steps are taken:
- Erythromycin ophthalmic ointment 0.5% (0.25 to 0.5 inch into each eye three to four times a day) or sodium sulfacetamide 10% (1 to 2 drops or 0.25 to 0.5 inch of ointment into each eye four times a day) can be used if a hordeolum is present.
- If cellulitis is present, erythromycin (30 to 50 mg/kg/24 hours in divided doses every 6 to 8 hours) or cephalexin (20 to 40 mg/kg/24 hours in divided doses every 8 hours) can be used.
- Refer to an ophthalmologist for surgical incision or topical intralesional corticosteroid injections if the condition is unresolved after medical treatment or if the lesion causes cosmetic concerns. A chalazion can distort vision by causing astigmatism as a result of pressure on the orbit.

Complications. Recurrence is common. Fragile, vascular granulation tissue called pyogenic granuloma that enlarges and bleeds rapidly can occur if a chalazion breaks through the conjunctival surface.

Nasolacrimal Duct Conditions: Dacryostenosis and Dacryocystitis
Description. Nasolacrimal duct obstruction, or dacryostenosis, is an abnormal obstruction (imperforate valve of Hasner) of the nasolacrimal duct that prevents tears from flowing into an opening in the nasal mucosa. Dacryocystitis is an inflammation of the involved nasolacrimal duct; infection can result.

Epidemiology. Nasolacrimal duct obstruction is fairly common in neonates (up to 15% of live births [Mills & Khazaeni, 2006]). It is thought to be due to a membrane at birth that covers the nasolacrimal duct, which then fails to break down quickly. It may also occur secondary to infection or trauma. Congenital failure of the duct to canalize may be unilateral or bilateral, and clinical signs appear 2 to 6 weeks after birth. When infection is present, it is most commonly caused by *S. aureus* and is often unilateral.

Clinical Findings. The following can be seen:
- Continuous or intermittent tearing, stickiness, and mucoid discharge at the inner canthus that can become purulent
- Blepharitis in lids and lashes
- Occasional nasal obstruction and drainage
- Expression of thin mucopurulent exudate from the punctum lacrimale
- Fluorescein dye, instilled bilaterally in the inferior conjunctival sac and checked in 2 and 5 minutes with a cobalt blue light source, will disappear if duct is patent.

The following additional symptoms may be noted if infection is present:
- Tenderness and swelling over the lacrimal duct
- Edema and erythema of the tear sac

- Excoriation of the surrounding skin
- Fever
- Expression of purulent material
- Mucocele of inner canthal tendon (unusual)

Laboratory Studies. A white blood cell (WBC) count (elevated) and cultures are obtained if the inflammation is severe.

Differential Diagnosis. Punctual or canalicular atresia, conjunctivitis, foreign body, congenital glaucoma, dacryocele, intraocular inflammation, and nasal mucosal edema are differential diagnoses.

Management. Treatment of dacryostenosis or chronic dacryocystitis in infancy is as follows:

- Duct blockage usually resolves spontaneously in more than 90% of infants by 12 months of age. Treatment consists of minimizing stagnation in the tear duct and preventing infection.
- Daily massage of the lacrimal sac may be performed to facilitate canalization of the duct. The technique involves placing a clean finger over the medial canthus and pressing in a posterior direction until the fingertip enters the space behind the inferior bony orbital ridge. Gentle pressure applied in a downward and medial direction transmits hydrostatic force through the nasolacrimal duct to the obstruction (Fig. 28-4). This technique should be performed about 10 times, two to three times a day.
- Topical ophthalmic ointment or ophthalmic drops (drops may penetrate more quickly), such as 0.5% erythromycin, may be prescribed (0.25 to 0.5 inch into each eye three to four times a day) for 5 days for excessive mucopurulent exudate.
- Saline drops into the nose, followed by aspiration before feeding and at bedtime, help relieve any concurrent nasal congestion.
- Refer children with persistent nasolacrimal duct obstruction to an ophthalmologist for evaluation and possible duct probing. Some ophthalmologists may probe the duct as early as 4 months old, whereas others wait until 9 to 12 months old. If probing fails to alleviate the problem (which is unusual), surgery may be required for placement of a tube stent or for a dacryocystorhinostomy (DCR).

If dacryocystitis occurs, the following actions are indicated:

- Warm compresses four times a day
- Continued lacrimal sac massage as described previously
- Topical antibiotics with the addition of an oral antistaphylococcal antibiotic that treats for ß-lactamase resistance (mild cases: amoxicillin-clavulanate potassium [Augmentin] 20 to 40 mg/kg PO three times daily for 10 days; severe cases: cefuroxime axetil [Ceftin] 50 to 100 mg/kg PO three times daily for 3 days followed by amoxicillin-clavulanate potassium PO for 7 days [Trobe, 2001])

Complications. Periorbital or orbital cellulitis is a complication of dacryocystitis.

Periorbital Cellulitis

Description. Periorbital cellulitis, or inflammation of the tissues surrounding the involved eye, is often associated with trauma or focal infection near the eye, eyelid abscess, bactere-

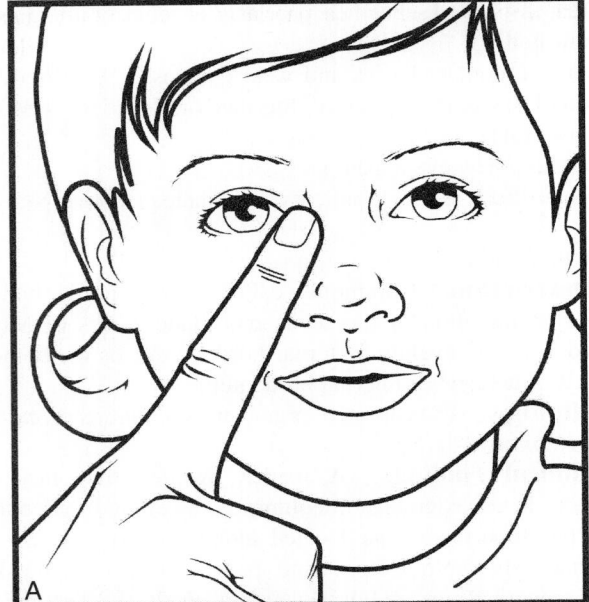

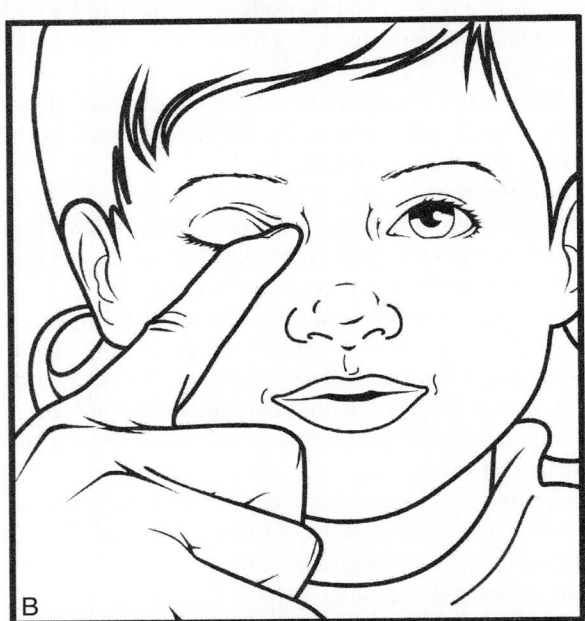

FIG. 28-4 Technique to clear nasolacrimal duct obstruction. **A,** Incorrect technique. **B,** Correct technique. The finger is pushing behind the bone, "in and up." Note that the fingertip is not visible in the proper technique.

mia, or sinusitis. It is predominantly an infection in children, spread from the upper respiratory tract or middle ear.

Etiology. Periorbital cellulitis is most commonly seen in children up to 6 years old. It can also occur with infected lacerations, abrasions, insect stings or bites, impetigo, or a foreign body where the infection is spread via venous or lymphatic channels. It may also be secondary to paranasal sinusitis (one study showed predominately ethmoid sinusitis present in 96% of children with orbital cellulitis [Ellis, 2003a]). The etiology is often unknown, but the bacteria most commonly responsible for periorbital cellulitis are streptococcal organisms, *S. aureus,* and, until the introduction of the HIB vaccine, *H. influenzae* type b. *M. catarrhalis* can also be a causative agent in children under 4 years old.

Clinical Findings. The following may be noted:

- Acute febrile illness (temperature higher than 102.2° F [39° C] if associated with bacteremia)
- Swelling and erythema of tissues surrounding the eye; upper lid affected more often than the lower lid.
- Deep red color of the eyelid (color is purple-blue with *H. influenzae* infection)
- Symptoms of bacteremia or sinusitis (headache, decreased vision)
- Orbital discomfort or pain, proptosis, or paralysis of extraocular muscles

Laboratory Studies. Depending on the severity of the cellulitis, the following can be useful:

- CBC with differential (WBC count usually greater than 15,000 if bacteremic)
- Blood cultures and culture of purulent wounds near the eye
- Lumbar puncture (infants younger than 1 year old)
- CT scan to rule out sinusitis, orbital cellulitis, or subperiosteal abscess
- Visual acuity, extraocular movement, and pupillary reaction testing

Differential Diagnosis. Conjunctivitis (bilateral conjunctival inflammation), cavernous sinus thrombosis, and orbital cellulitis (proptosis, limited extraocular movement, and reduced visual acuity) are the differential diagnoses in children; in neonates consider conjunctivitis, dacryocystitis, and ruptured dacryocystocele.

Management. The child may be managed as an outpatient if:

- The cellulitis is mild.
- The orbit is not involved (full eye movements are present, no pain with eye movement, visual changes, or ptosis).
- The child exhibits no symptoms of systemic bacterial sepsis.
- The child is older than 1 year.

Management must be made on a case-by-case basis. Consultation is needed when proptosis, ophthalmoplegia, or changes in visual acuity occur; these conditions are suggestive of orbital cellulitis.

Outpatient management consists of:

- Ceftriaxone (50 to 75 mg/kg [up to a maximum of 1 g] intramuscularly divided every 12 hours). The child is monitored daily until blood cultures are negative for 48 hours or clinical improvement is seen. Oral antibiotics may then be used to complete a 7- to 14-day course. Amoxicillin, amoxicillin with clavulanic acid, and cefixime are first-line choices for treatment (Wright, 2003c). If a rapid clinical response is not seen, further evaluation and treatment should be done. Warm soaks to the periorbital area every 2 to 4 hours for 15 minutes may provide comfort and speed healing. The parent is advised to call immediately if there is any change in condition.

Hospitalization and intravenous administration of antibiotics (usually cefuroxime) followed by a 10-day course of oral antibiotics are required for any of the following:

- Moderate to severe cases of cellulitis
- A poor response to outpatient management
- A purulent wound near the eyelid
- Children younger than 1 year old
- Children with suspected sepsis

Complications. Complications include orbital cellulitis or extension of the infection into the orbit, subperiosteal or orbital abscess, optic neuritis, retinal vein thrombosis, panophthalmitis, meningitis, epidural and subdural abscesses, and cavernous sinus thrombosis.

Keratitis and Corneal Ulcers

Description. Inflammation of the cornea (keratitis) can cause a dramatic alteration in visual acuity and can progress to corneal ulceration and blindness. A corneal ulcer begins as a well-defined infiltration at the center or edge of the cornea and subsequently suppurates and forms an ulcer that may penetrate deep into the corneal tissue or spread to involve the width of the cornea. Involvement is usually unilateral.

Etiology. Fortunately, corneal ulcers are rare in children (Wright, 2003d). Causes of keratitis include HSV-1, although other viruses and bacteria (*H. influenza, Moraxella, S. aureus, S. pneumoniae, Pseudomonas, N. gonorrhoeae*), fungi (rare), and protozoa may be responsible. Bacterial causes progress rapidly and can destroy the cornea within 24 to 48 hours. The most common risk factor for keratitis is trauma (which can also result from wearing extended-wear contact lenses). Less common causes include an allergic reaction, conjunctivitis, systemic infections, toxic chemicals, and the use of corticosteroids. The FDA has recently issued a warning against the use of improperly fitted (often purchased over-the-counter from outlets) decorative contact lenses popular with teenagers (Clinician News Staff, 2003).

Clinical Findings. Symptoms vary in intensity according to the depth and extent of ulceration. The following are reported or seen:

- Exposure to an infected individual
- History of illness, eye trauma, extended contact lens wear, foreign body, or history of recent antibiotic treatment for conjunctivitis that was unresponsive
- White lesions on cornea
- Vesicles on the skin or eyelids and herpes lesions elsewhere on the body
- Severe pain, sensation of a foreign body ("gritty"), and photophobia
- Tearing, erythema, and spasms of the eyelid
- Inflamed eye
- Blurred vision
- Occasional corneal opacification
- Area staining green with a fluorescein strip (if herpes, a dendritic ulcer is seen)

Management. When a corneal ulcer is suspected, the child should be referred immediately for a slit lamp exam. Delay can result in loss of vision in the eye. Do not attempt to treat.

- Steroids should never be used.
- Treatment with antivirals, such as trifluridine or vidarabine, may be used to speed healing in herpes simplex infections.

Complications. Corneal opacification, scarring, and loss of vision can occur if treatment is delayed.

Inflammation of the Uveal Tract

Description. Inflammation of the uveal tract (iris, ciliary body, choroids) and other ocular structures is often called *uveitis*. The inflammation may be anterior (affecting the iris, ciliary body, or both) or posterior (affecting the choroid). Adjacent ocular structures can also be involved, including the retina, vitreous, sclera, lens, and optic nerve.

Epidemiology. Many processes have been implicated. Known etiologies include viral or bacterial infections, ocular trauma, and infection elsewhere in the eye. Other causes include allergy, malignancy, and systemic diseases, such as JRA, inflammatory bowel, Kawasaki syndrome, herpes simplex, tuberculosis, Lyme disease, CMV, toxoplasmosis, syphilis, acquired immunodeficiency syndrome, ulcerative colitis, rubella retinitis, and Stevens-Johnson syndrome. The inflammation may be acute or chronic, but incidence is low in children under 16 years old (Giles et al, 2005).

Clinical Findings. The following may be noted:
- Acute onset of pain (*key* finding)
- Red eye, photophobia, and blurred or decreased vision (*key* findings)
- Excessive tearing and eyelid edema
- Conjunctival erythema
- Circumcorneal injection
- Hypopyon (pus layer in the bottom of the anterior chamber)
- Cloudy appearance of the eye with a bulging iris and a contracted, irregular, or fixed pupil
- If chronic, there may be no ocular pain, photophobia, redness, or tearing
- There may be a history of prior viral infection, joint pain, trauma, gastrointestinal problems

Differential Diagnosis. Conjunctivitis is the differential diagnosis.

Management. Evaluate and treat any underlying systemic disease. Refer the patient to an ophthalmologist. A definitive diagnosis is made by slit-lamp examination. The prognosis is improved with early treatment, and delay may result in scarring of the pupil with cataract formation or the development of glaucoma. Cycloplegics and topical or systemic corticosteroids (depending on the cause of the inflammation) are often used in treatment. Cycloplegic-mydriatics are used regularly to prevent posterior synechiae (adhesions of iris to lens and cornea). Nonsteroidal antiinflammatory agents are sometimes used as adjunct treatment.

Complications. Anterior and posterior synechiae, changes in IOP, corneal edema, various degrees of visual impairment, retinal detachment, glaucoma, enucleation, and cataracts are possible complications.

Trachoma

Description. A chronic infectious disease of the eye, trachoma is characterized by follicular keratoconjunctivitis with neovascularization of the cornea. It is the second leading cause of blindness in the world.

Epidemiology. Trachoma is a chronic keratoconjunctivitis caused by one of the two *C. trachomatis* bivars that exist in the world. It is endemic in hot, dry, dusty, poverty-stricken areas with poor personal and community hygiene. It is rare in the U.S. but is endemic among Navaho Indians in the southwestern U.S. (Hammerschlag, 2004). It is contagious, often spread from eye to eye by flies.

Clinical Findings. The following are noted:
- Inflammation
- Pain
- Photophobia
- Excessive tearing
- Granulation follicles on the upper tarsal conjunctiva, eventual inversion (entropion) of the eyelid leading to corneal trauma, scarring, and blindness

Laboratory Studies. Cultures and staining are done.

Management. Consult with an ophthalmologist because treatment is difficult and recommendations vary. The World Health Organization recommends treating with azithromycin (20 mg/kg-maximum of 1 g once per week for 3 weeks [Hammerschlag, 2004; AAP, 2006]). Other drugs used include: oral tetracycline, doxycycline (for children older than 8 years), erythromycin (rarely used), and a topical antibiotic ointment (erythromycin, tetracycline, sulfacetamide [twice daily for 2 months or intermittently over 6 months]) to rapidly reduce inflammation to prevent scar formation (AAP, 2006). Steroids are contraindicated.

Reinforce the need for frequent hand washing and careful cleansing of the eyes. Discourage sharing of towels and handkerchiefs.

▮▮▮ THE INJURED EYE
CORNEAL ABRASION

Description

Damage to or loss of the epithelial cells of the cornea in the form of a corneal abrasion or tear is relatively common (Table 28-8). Scratches from forceps delivery, paper, brushes, fingernails, contact lens overuse, improperly fitted cosmetic contact lenses, airbag deployment, plants, or a foreign body in the conjunctival sac are often responsible.

Clinical Findings

The following may be noted:
- Evidence and sensation of a foreign body
- Severe pain and photophobia
- Tearing and blepharospasm
- Decreased vision
- Conjunctival erythema
- On exam, disrupted tear film over the corneal epithelium is seen with a penlight

Other Studies. Fluorescein staining with superficial uptake is indicative of a minor corneal abrasion. If the fluorescein staining goes deep into the cornea, subepithelial corneal damage (e.g., corneal ulceration or corneal tear) is possible. Vertical striations on the cornea suggest a foreign body embedded under the eyelid.

TABLE 28-8 **Common Eye Injuries**

Injury	Clinical Findings	Treatment
Corneal injury (abrasion)	Sensation or evidence of foreign body, pain, photophobia, tearing, blepharospasm, ↓ vision, + fluorescein staining	Rest, topical antibiotics, oral analgesics, follow-up in 24 hours; refer for any severe injury.
Foreign body	Vertical striation on cornea, pain, tearing, sensation of foreign body, irregular or peaked pupil, perforating wound	Do not remove intraocular foreign body; if extraocular, irrigate eye to remove; apply topical antibiotic and patch; follow-up in 24 hours.
Burns Chemical Thermal UV radiation	Pale, necrotic appearance to skin and eyelids, opaque cornea, visual impairment, photophobia, tearing, pain with UV injury only	Chemical and thermal: emergency; continuous irrigation for 20-30 minutes; to ophthalmologist with ongoing irrigation. UV: topical antibiotic, patch, analgesics, heals in 1-2 days.
Hyphema	Pain, tearing, photophobia; blood in anterior chamber, hazy iris, or inability to detect red reflex, change in visual acuity	Refer to ophthalmologist; restrict intake, place eye shield; increased risk if child has sickle cell trait or disease or other hematologic disorder.
Lacerations	Irregular pupil, poor RLR, pain, visual disturbance, uveal prolapse, black tissue or fluid under conjunctiva	Apply eye shield and refer immediately to ophthalmologist.
Retinal detachment	Visual field impairment, "flashing light" sensation	Refer immediately to ophthalmologist.
Hematoma/ contusion of orbit	Visual field impairment, "flashing light" sensation	Refer immediately to ophthalmologist.
Orbital fracture	Pain, diplopia, numbness below orbit, facial bruising, globe displacement, swelling, corneal laceration, irregular pupil, hyphema or absent red light reflex	Plain film radiography, CT scan; refer immediately to an ophthalmologist; may need surgery.

↓, Decrease; +, positive; *CT*, computed tomography; *MRI*, magnetic resonance imaging; *RLR*, red light reflex; *UV*, ultraviolet.

Management

The following steps are taken:

- Refer severe corneal injuries or possible subepithelial damage to an ophthalmologist. Refer those who wear contact lenses with an abrasion to an ophthalmologist to rule out bacterial corneal infection.
- If no symptoms of corneal infection, use topical antibiotics (0.5% erythromycin or Polysporin drops or ointment) four times daily and apply a pressure patch (patching is inconsistently recommended in the literature; if used apply a 1-inch tape across the lid margin or tape obliquely in parallel strips from forehead to cheek [Wright 2003a; Catalano, 2005]). An abrasion generally heals in 24 to 48 hours.
- Advise the patient to return daily for follow-up evaluation or refer for slit-lamp examination within 24 to 36 hours. If responding continue the ointment for 2 to 3 days after removal of the patch. If no improvement is seen after 24 to 48 hours or if symptoms worsen, refer to an ophthalmologist.
- Use elbow restraints for the infant to ensure that the eye is not rubbed or further irritated.
- Do not use topical anesthetics because they are toxic to the epithelium. Oral analgesics or ophthalmologic nonsteroid antiinflammatory agents (0.5% Acular, Acular Preservative Free) may be used to ease the discomfort.

FOREIGN BODY

Description

A superficial foreign body in the eye is usually lodged on the surface of the eye or superficially in the cornea. It rarely results in serious trauma. Foreign objects may penetrate the globe (intraocular) with more serious consequences.

Etiology. Foreign bodies commonly occur in younger children during play and in older children during sports. Foreign bodies can include dirt, dust, metallic particles, or alkaline products from the deployment of an airbag.

Clinical Findings. The following may be noted:
- Pain and foreign body sensation
- Foreign body in conjunctival sac
- Tearing
- Inflammation
- Irregular or peaked pupil
- Photophobia
- Opaque lens
- Perforating wound to the cornea or iris

Other Studies. Fluorescein staining may be useful if no foreign body is visualized. Ultrasonography or CT scan may be needed, depending on the foreign body and its location. An MRI is contraindicated. Refer any suspected intraocular penetration by a metal object or fragment (ask if patient had been engaged in a metal-on-metal activity).

Management.   Recommendations include the following:

- Never remove an intraocular foreign body and never remove a foreign body if the history indicates that a projectile object was possibly involved in the injury. Refer immediately to an ophthalmologist.
- View the upper bulbar conjunctiva by having the patient look down while the upper lid is pulled away from the globe and the upper recess illuminated. Evert the eyelid to visualize the superior tarsal conjunctiva.
- Use of a topical anesthetic (proparacaine 0.5% or tetracaine 0.5%, 1 drop—may repeat at 3- to 5-minute intervals) facilitates patient cooperation.
- If not visualized but suspected, remove an extraocular foreign body via irrigation with sterile saline or Dacriose.
- If the object is visualized, a moistened cotton swab may be used. Cautiously and gently roll it across the cornea to remove the extraocular foreign body, but only in cooperative patients because this maneuver might cause considerable additional damage to the epithelial surface (Eisenbaum, 2003; Trobe, 2001).
- If any difficulty is encountered, stop all efforts, patch the eye, and refer the patient immediately to an ophthalmologist.
- After removing any extraocular object, instill fluorescein stain and inspect the cornea with cobalt-blue light to look for green staining or lines. Instill an ophthalmic antibiotic drop or ointment, patch the eye, and follow guidelines for managing a corneal abrasion.
- Reschedule the patient in 24 hours or refer to an ophthalmologist for follow-up.
- In the case of an airbag deployment, irrigate the eyes with a balanced salt solution (e.g., sterile saline or Dacriose [Wright, 2003a]).

Complications.   Sympathetic ophthalmia, chronic siderosis, or a uveitis of the injured eye can occur any time from 10 days to many years after a penetrating injury of the globe.

BURNS
Etiology
Burns to the eyes and surrounding tissues can be thermal (caused by exposure to steam, flame, intense heat, cinders, or cigarettes), chemical (e.g., cleaning agents, fertilizers, pesticides, battery fluid, or laboratory products), or induced by UV light (e.g., from bright snow, laser pointers, or a sunlamp). The amount of damage to the eye is directly related to the length of exposure and the nature of the source of the burn. Chemical burns are true emergencies because of the progressive damage that can occur. Alkaline solutions are especially damaging. Burns on the eyelids are classified and treated the same as burns elsewhere on the body.

Clinical Findings
The following may be noted:
- Pale or necrosed appearance of the surrounding skin and eyelids
- Opacity of corneal tissue
- Visual impairment (decreased acuity)

- Initial exquisite pain or delayed complaints of pain (e.g., in UV burns, pain emerges about 6 hours after exposure)
- Photophobia
- Tearing within 12 hours of exposure
- Swollen corneas
- Fluorescein stain revealing pinpoint uptake

Management
The following steps are taken:
- Instill a topical anesthetic if available.
- Chemical burns require immediate, ongoing irrigation. With the eyelids held apart, instill a steady, gentle solution of tepid water, saline, or Ringer irrigation for 20 to 30 minutes or until the pH of the tear film is 7.3 to 7.7. Refer to an ophthalmologist after irrigation to determine the extent of the damage. Do not patch the eye; allow tearing to continue to cleanse the eye. Cool compresses applied to the surrounding skin may be comforting. Hospitalization may be needed for sedation and analgesia.
- Thermal burns may be treated the same way as acid or alkaline chemical burns, (Wander, 2000).
- UV burns are treated by using topical antibiotic prophylaxis, patches, and analgesics. Healing should occur in 1 to 2 days.

LACERATIONS OF THE ORBIT
Description
Lacerations from injuries cause perforation of the cornea and lead to uveal prolapse. They are described as to whether they are of the anterior segment (cornea, anterior chamber, iris, lens) or posterior segment (sclera, retina, vitreous).

Clinical findings
The clinical findings (only a few of the more obvious are mentioned here) depend upon which segment is involved (Wright, 2003a).

Anterior segment:
- Irregular pupil (retracted or peaked)
- Iris prolapse

Posterior segment:
- Poor red light reflex
- Decreased vision
- Black tissue or fluid seen under the conjunctiva

Management
Apply an eye shield to protect the eye. Refer the patient immediately to an ophthalmologist to rule out damage to the globe and surrounding structures.

TRAUMATIC HYPHEMA
Description
A hyphema is an accumulation of visible blood or blood products in the anterior chamber of the eye.

Epidemiology
A hyphema is the result of blunt trauma to the globe without penetration or perforation. This condition is most often caused by balls, fists or fingers, elbows, rocks, exploding airbags, and

sticks. It may also occur in infants with birth trauma or in patients with RB, abnormal iris vessels (rubeosis), leukemia, juvenile xanthogranuloma of the iris, or abnormal hematologic profiles, such as sickle cell trait or disease (Wright, 2003a). Hyphema is the most common contusion injury to the eye seen in children and occurs in approximately 2 per 10,000 children per year. It is responsible for more hospitalizations than any other ophthalmologic condition.

Clinical Findings

Vision, pupil motility, the lids and adnexa, the cornea and anterior segment, and the red reflex should all be assessed. The following may be noted:

- History of traumatic eye injury
- Somnolence (often associated with intracranial trauma)
- Blood appearing as a dark red fluid level between the cornea and iris on gross examination or as a hazy-appearing iris
- Inability to detect a bilateral red light reflex
- Pain, photophobia, and tearing
- Visual acuity changes and impaired vision (light perception and hand motion perception)
- Abnormal pupillary reflex

Management

The goals of treatment include resolving the hyphema, making the patient comfortable, and preventing complications; however, no consensus has been reached on how to best accomplish such treatment (e.g., hospitalization or not, systemic medication or not, which medications). There is a risk of recurrent bleeding. However, the following steps should be taken:

- Refer the patient immediately to an ophthalmologist. A slit-lamp examination is indicated.
- Restrict oral intake until the child has been seen by an ophthalmologist.
- Place a perforated eye shield (not a patch) over the eye—avoid pressure to prevent reinjury.
- If a hematologic disorder is detected, ensure quick intervention and close follow-up.

The following steps are commonly recognized for treatment of traumatic hyphemas:

- Outpatient management is acceptable for those with small hyphemas (grade I): Elevate the head of the bed to 30 degrees. Child should wear a Fox shield; maintain bed rest with bathroom privileges for 5 days; participate in no strenuous activites for 10 days; have daily eye exams to check for blood staining and IOP. Cycloplegic agents may be used (Wright, 2003a).
- Children should be hospitalized with a hyphema of grade II or III, those with sickle cell, if there is an increase in IOP, or if there is a question about compliance with outpatient treatment.
- Atropine drops, antibiotics, tonometry, topical anesthetics, antiglaucoma agents, steroids, systemic antifibrinolytic agents (in sickle cell cases), or topical dilating agents are usually not indicated or their efficacy has not been proven (Wright, 2003a).

- Acetaminophen is the analgesic of choice; avoid aspirin and nonsteroidal antiinflammatory agents because they may add to the risk of a rebleed. Sedatives may be necessary in pediatric patients.
- Surgery may be necessary to remove the trapped blood from the chamber if: it is causing an increase in IOP; in sickle cell patients; to prevent corneal blood staining; if the hyphema remains without some clearing in the first four days; or a clot is pressing against the corneal epithelium (Wright, 2003a).
- Hospital discharge is usually after a week. The child should be followed closely by an ophthalmologist because long-term monitoring is necessary to detect possible traumatic cataract, retinal detachment, or glaucoma. Systemic corticosteroids may be used to reduce rebleeds (Wright, 2003a).

Complications

A second hemorrhage can occur within 3 to 5 days of the first, leading to glaucoma, amblyopia, or corneal blood staining that can result in permanent visual loss. The larger the hyphema, the more likely the child is to rebleed (up to 60% versus 15% for small, grade I hyphemas). Patients with abnormal hematologic profiles (e.g., sickle cell hemoglobinopathies) are more likely to have visual loss because of optic atrophy (Wright, 2003a).

RETINAL DETACHMENT

Description and Etiology

Retinal detachment is detachment of the neurosensory retina from its retinal pigment epithelium base within the globe. It is rare in children, so suspicion should be high for traumatic causes (e.g., child abuse), a congenital abnormality or syndrome (aphakia, cataracts, Ehlers-Danlos, Stickler, Marfan, Norrie), or specific disease (ROP, viral retinitis, RB, or various retinopathies). Some detachments may not be diagnosed for months or years after a blunt trauma injury (Weichel et al, 2005). There may be concurrent ocular disease or a family history of retinal detachment.

Clinical Findings

The following may be noted:

- Blurry vision that becomes progressively worse
- Dark cloud in one visual field, flashing lights, or a "shower of floaters"
- Darkening of retinal vessels on funduscopic examination
- Gray elevation at the site of detachment

Management

Instruct the patient not to eat and refer to an ophthalmologist for evaluation.

ORBITAL HEMATOMA/CONTUSION OF THE GLOBE

Etiology

This condition is usually the result of a blow to the globe. The degree of damage depends on the energy of the object hitting the globe. Such injuries commonly occur as a result of sports activities, motor vehicle accidents, assault, BB gun accidents, or airbag deployment.

Clinical Findings

The following may be seen:

- Milky white appearance of the retina
- Visual acuity changes
- Severe bruising of the eyelids and periorbital tissues
- Lens dislocation
- Retinal detachment or edema
- Vitreous, retinal, or choroid hemorrhage
- Rupture of the eyeball

Management

Refer the patient immediately to an ophthalmologist. A closed head injury, damage to the skull, and facial bone fractures will need to be ruled out via CT scan, MRI, or ultrasound radiography. Occasionally, cryopexy or laser photocoagulation surgery is needed for contusions of the globe.

Complications

Possible complications include permanent visual loss, retinal necrosis, subretinal hemorrhage, and retinal or macular holes.

ORBITAL FRACTURES
Description and Etiology

An orbital fracture is a fracture of the walls of the orbit secondary to blunt trauma to the orbital rim or eye(s). The orbital floor is thin and subject to fracture. The inferior rectus muscle may become caught in the fracture site.

The usual cause of an orbital fracture is a blow or blunt trauma to the orbit (e.g., ball, fist, motor vehicle accident [hitting the dashboard], fall).

Clinical Findings

The following may be noted:

- Pain, diplopia
- Numbness below orbit
- Ecchymosis of the lids, nosebleed, trouble chewing
- Limited ocular movement (especially upward) and weakness in downward movement
- Globe displacement with a sunken-eye appearance or a protruding eye
- Bony discontinuity or "step-off"
- Subcutaneous emphysema in surrounding tissues and edema
- Enophthalmos
- Corneal laceration
- Irregular pupil
- Hyphema or absent red light reflex

  Diagnostic Studies. Plain film radiography and CT scan are the best imaging modalities.

Management

- An orbital fracture is an ophthalmologic emergency requiring immediate intervention and referral. Diagnostic studies are performed to rule out injury to the skull and cranial contents. Open reduction may be necessary if any of the orbital bones are displaced or to rule out displacement of the globe or enophthalmos.

- Icing the injury for 24 hours, followed by heat for 2 to 3 days, allows the swelling to subside before surgical repair. Surgery is often best done within 2 to 7 days up to 2 to 4 weeks, depending upon the injury (Wright, 2003a).
- Antibiotics and nasal decongestant may also be used.

PTERYGIUM

A pterygium is a fibrovascular mass of thickened bulbar conjunctiva that extends beyond the limbus onto the cornea. Elastic and hyaline degenerative changes occur. The lesion is usually triangular and more commonly found on the nasal side of the orbit. It is caused by irritation of the bulbar conjunctiva from sunlight, wind, dust, fumes, or airborne allergens; it can also be hereditary. Growth rates of the lesions vary. A pinguecula may precede the pterygium, which will occur as a yellow-white, slightly raised mass on the bulbar conjunctiva. The lesion is usually painless, may itch, and may be accompanied by occasional complaints of blurred vision if the lesion enlarges.

Because a pterygium is uncommon in children, the clinician needs to consider other causes: papillomas, dermoids, keratoacanthomas, an epithelial inclusion or a dermoid cyst, or a rare malignancy (Wilson et al, 2003). Treatment involves protecting against irritants (use of goggles or sunglasses, or topical lubricants, such as artificial tears) and using mild vasoconstrictors or short-term steroids for inflammation. Surgical removal may be needed if the pterygium impedes vision. Recurrence after surgical removal, restricted ocular mobility (especially with abduction), and diplopia may be complications.

SUBCONJUNCTIVAL HEMORRHAGE

Subconjunctival hemorrhage is splotchy bulbar conjunctival redness that spontaneously occurs or is secondary to increased intrathoracic pressure (from coughing, sneezing, straining, or trauma) that results in the bursting of conjunctival vessels. It is commonly found in neonates as a benign occurrence to a vaginal delivery. The hemorrhages usually spontaneously resolve within 1 to 2 weeks. No treatment is indicated. Spontaneous hemorrhages can (rarely) occur with HTN, diabetes mellitus, a bleeding tendency, or be a sign of a ruptured globe if there is a history of trauma (Wright, 2003a).

■ DEFORMITIES OF THE EYELIDS
ENTROPION

Entropion is a condition in which the eyelids invert so that the cilia or epithelium rubs against the corneal surface, causing abrasion or irritation. Both the upper and lower eyelids may be involved. There is a rare congenital form. On examination, there is evidence of lid laxity. Pain or irritation and photophobia are typical symptoms. Complications include corneal scarring and corneal infections. Management involves surgical intervention.

ECTROPION

Ectropion is a rare condition in which the eyelid margins evert. It may be congenital, seen after infection, or secondary to scarring after trauma, radiation, or prior surgery. It can be confused with an euryblepharon. Management involves lubrication for mild cases; surgery is indicated for chronic or symptomatic cases.

EURYBLEPHARON

An euryblepharon appears as a wide palpebral fissure with the appearance of a sagging half of the lower eyelid (temporal side) or a pulling away of the lid from the orbit. It can have a genetic etiology (e.g., Down syndrome), be associated with other ocular anomalies (e.g., congenital cleft lip, strabismus, congenital ptosis), or be seen in association with other anomalies (e.g., hypospadia, inguinal hernias, dental anomalies). It is often confused with ectropion. It is usually a mild cosmetic condition, and the child may outgrow it. No treatment is indicated unless chronic tearing and inflammation occur (Ellis, 2003b).

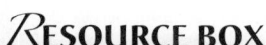

RESOURCE BOX

Eye Problems

Blind Childrens Center
www.blindchildrenscenter.org

National Federation of the Blind: National Organization of Parents of Blind Children
www.nfb.org/nfb/Parents_and_Teachers.asp

Prevent Blindness America
www.preventblindness.org

Vision World Wide
www.visionww.org

American Academy of Ophthalmology
www.aao.org

☑ DISCUSSION FORUM

1. You are vision screening a 4-year-old. The exam is 20/70 right eye and 20/30 left eye. Cover-uncover testing is normal, and the extraocular movements are intact. What is your next step in this child? What is the risk of an untreated refractive error? If you get the same results in a 13-year-old, would it have the same significance?
2. A 13-year-old comes in during late April with bilateral red eyes without discharge and no history of trauma. What do you need to document on your note? What is the differential diagnoses? What would be included in your management plan?
3. How do resistance rates affect what drugs you prescribe for conjunctivitis? How are your prescribing practices affected by the pharmaceutical industries? Insurance companies?

REFERENCES

American Academy of Ophthalmology (AAO), Pediatric Ophthalmology Panel: *Preferred practice guidelines: pediatric eye evaluations,* San Francisco, 2002, American Academy of Ophthalmology.

American Academy of Ophthalmology (AAO): *Summary recommendations for LASIK,* revised 2006a. Available at *www.aao.org/education/statements/recommendations/lasik.cfm* (accessed July 5, 2006).

American Academy of Ophthalmology (AAO): *Academy applauds second study on unregulated plano contact lenses confirming need for legislation,* 9/26/2005. Available at *www.aao.org/newsroom/release20050926.cfm* (accessed July 7, 2006).

American Academy of Ophthalmology (AAO): *Protective eyewear for young athletes: joint policy statement* revised 2003. Available at *www.aao.org/about/policy/upload/Protective-Eyewear-for-young athletes.pdf* (accessed on July 7, 2006).

American Academy of Ophthalmology (AAO) Complementary Therapy Task Force: *Complementary therapy assessment: vision therapy for learning disabilities, 2001.* Available at *www.aao.org/education/guidelines/cta/loader.cfm?url=/commonspot/security/getfile.cfm&page10=1224* (accessed on July 7, 2006).

American Academy of Optometry, American Optometric Association: Vision, learning and dyslexia, *J Am Optom Assoc* 68:284-286, 1997.

American Academy of Pediatrics (AAP) Committee on Practice and Ambulatory Medicine and Section on Ophthalmology, American Association of Certified Orthoptists, American Association of Pediatric Ophthalmology and Strabismus, American Academy of Ophthalmology (AAO): Eye examination in infants, children, and young adults by pediatricians: policy statement, *Pediatrics* 111(4):902-907, 2003.

American Academy of Pediatrics (AAP): Policy statement: red reflex examination in infants, *Pediatrics* 109(5):980-981, 2002.

American Academy of Pediatrics (AAP): Learning disabilities, dyslexia, and vision: a subject review, *Pediatrics* 102:1217-1219, 1998.

American Academy of Pediatrics (AAP): R*ed book: 2006 report of the Committee on Infectious Diseases,* ed 27, Elk Grove Village, IL 2006, American Academy of Pediatrics.

Astle WF, Huang PT, Ells AL et al: Photorefractive keratectomy in children, *J Cataract Refract Surgery* 28(6):932-41, 2002.

Birch EE, Cheng C, Stager DR Jr et al: Visual acuity development after the implantation of unilateral intraocular lenses in infants and young children, *J AAPOS* 9(6):527-32, 2005.

Boguniewicz M: Ocular allergies. In Behrman RE, Kliegman R, Jenson H, editors: *Nelson textbook of pediatrics,* ed 17, Philadelphia, 2004, WB Saunders.

Catalano RA: Ocular trauma and its prevention. In Nelson LB, Olitsky SE, editors: *Harley's pediatric ophthalmology,* ed 5, Philadelphia, 2005, Lippincott, Williams & Wilkins.

Clinician News staff: Improper use of cosmetic lenses a disturbing national trend, *Clinician News* 7(2), Mar 2003.

Contemporary Pediatrics editorial staff: Management of conjunctivitis: mimics and non-bacterial disease, *Contemp Pediatr* Suppl 2001.

Cuming GS, Dorfman MS, Murphey DK: Bacterial conjunctivitis in children: containing the infection, *Inf Dis Child* monograph, Jan 2006.

Eisenbaum A: Eye. In Hay WW et al, editors: *Current pediatric diagnosis and treatment,* ed 16, New York, 2003, McGraw-Hill.

Ellis FD: Pediatric eyelid disorders. In Nelson LB, Olitsky SE, editors: *Harley's pediatric ophthalmology,* Philadelphia, 2005, Lippincott, Williams & Wilkins.

Ellis FD: Proptosis and orbital diseases. In Wright KW, Spiegel PH, editors: *Pediatric ophthalmology and strabismus,* New York, 2003a, Springer.

Ellis FD: Lid malformations, malpositions, and lesions. In Wright KW, Spiegel PH, editors: *Pediatric ophthalmology and strabismus,* New York, 2003b, Springer.

Freedman SF, Walton DS: Glaucoma in infants and children. In Nelson LB, Olitsky SE, editors: *Harley's pediatric ophthalmology,* Philadelphia, 2005, Lippincott, Williams & Wilkins.

Giglotti F: Co-infections of conjunctivitis. Infections Diseases in Children Editorial Staff: Ocular infections in children: best practices in diagnosis and treatment, *Inf Dis Child* CME ed, Mar 2004.

Giles CL, Capone A, Joshi MM: Uveitis in children. In Nelson LB, Olitsky SE, editors: *Harley's pediatric ophthalmology,* Philadelphia, 2005, Lippincott, Williams & Wilkins.

Gomi CF, Robbins SL, Heichel CW et al: Conjunctival diseases. In Nelson LB, Olitsky SE, editors: *Harley's pediatric ophthalmology,* Philadelphia, 2005, Lippincott, Williams & Wilkins.

Grabowski E: Intraocular and extraocular retinoblastoma. In Burg FD, Ingelfinger JR, Polin RA et al, editors: *Current pediatric therapy,* ed 18, Philadelphia, 2006, Saunders/Elsevier.

Gross RD: Differential diagnosis of conjunctivitis. Infectious Diseases in Children Editorial Staff; Ocular infections in children: best practices in diagnosis and treatment, *Inf Dis Child* CME ed, Mar 2004.

Hammerschlag M: Chlamydial infections. In Behrman RE, Kliegman R, Jenson H, editors: *Nelson textbook of pediatrics,* ed 17, Philadelphia, 2004, WB Saunders.

International Dyslexia Association: Website. *Dyslexia basics,* 2007. Available at *www.interdys.org/ewebedit pro5/upload/Dyslexia_Basics_FS_-_final-81407.pdf* (accessed Nov 9, 2007).

Israeli D, Hod Y, Geyer O: Retinal injury induced by laser pointers, *Harefuah* 140(1):28-9, 86, 2001.

Jockin Y: Strabismus and amblyopia. In Burg F et al, editors: *Gellis and Kagan's current pediatric therapy,* ed 17, Philadelphia, 2002, WB Saunders.

Lichtenstein S: Treatment options for pediatric conjunctivitis. Infectious Diseases in Children Editorial Staff: Ocular Infections in Children: best practices in diagnosis and treatment, *Inf Dis Child* CME ed, Mar 2004.

McManaway J, Frankel C: Strabismus. In Hoekelman R, editor: *Primary pediatric care,* ed 4, St Louis, 2001, Mosby.

Mills M, Khazaeni L: Red eye. In Burg FD, Ingelfinger JR, Polin RA et al, editors: *Current pediatric therapy,* ed 18, Philadelphia, 2006, Saunders/Elsevier.

Murphee AL, Christensen LE: Retinoblastoma and other malignant intraocular tumors. In Wright LB, Spiegel SE, editors: *Pediatric ophthalmology and strabismus,* New York, 2003, Springer.

National Eye Institute: *Vision in Preschool Study (VIP Study).* Available at *www.clinicaltrials.gov* (accessed July 5, 2006).

National Eye Institute: *Older children can benefit from treatment for childhood's most common eye disorder, 2005.* Available at *www.nei.nih. gov* (accessed on July 7, 2006).

Ober RA, Palmer EA, Drack AV et al: Retinopathy of prematurity. In Wright KW, Spiegel PH, editors: *Pediatric ophthalmology and strabismus,* New York, 2003, Springer.

Olitsky S, Nelson LB: Disorders of the eye. In Behrman R, Kliegman R, Jenson H, editors. *Nelson textbook of pediatrics,* ed 17, Philadelphia, 2004, WB Saunders.

Olitsky S, Nelson LB: Strabismus disorders. In Nelson LB, Olitsky SE, editors: *Harley's pediatric ophthalmology,* ed 5, Philadelphia, 2005, Lippincott, Williams & Wilkins.

Paradis A, Granet D: Don't let children rub their eyes! *Infect Dis Child* 15(5):66-67, 2002.

Phelps DL: Retinopathy of prematurity. In Fanaroff A, Martin F, editors: *Neonatal-perinatal medicine,* vol 2, *Diseases of the fetus and infant,* ed 7, St Louis, 2002, Mosby.

Reichel E: Hereditary gene dysfunction syndromes. In Albert D et al, editors: *Principles and practice of ophthalmology,* ed 2, Philadelphia, 2000, WB Saunders.

Reynolds JD: Retinopathy of prematurity. In Nelson LB, Olitsky SE, editors: *Harley's pediatric ophthalmology,* ed 5, Philadelphia, 2005, Lippincott, Williams & Wilkins.

Rhee R: Question and answer session. In Alcon Laboratories: Advances in the treatment of ocular infections in children, *Inf Dis Child* symposium coverage issue, 2004.

Robertson DM, Lim TH, Salomao DR et al: Laser pointers and the human eye: a clinicopathologic study, *Arch Ophthalmol* 118:1686-1691, 2000.

Rubin S: Management of strabismus in the first year of life, *Pediatr Ann* 30(8):474-480, 2001.

Schaffer D: Conjunctiva. In Burg F et al, editors: *Gellis and Kagan's current pediatric therapy,* ed 17, Philadelphia, 2002, WB Saunders.

Scheiman MM, Hertle RW, Beck RW et al. Randomized trial of treatment of amblyopia in children aged 7 to 17 years, *Arch Ophthalmol* 123(4):437-447, 2005.

Shields JA, Shields CL: Ocular tumors of childhood. In Nelson LB, Olitsky SE, editors: *Harley's pediatric ophthalmology,* ed 5, Philadelphia, 2005, Lippincott, Williams & Wilkins.

School of Public Health, University of California-Berkeley: The best pair of shades, *Wellness Letter* 18(10):4, 2002.

Strominger MB: Nystagmus. In Nelson LB, Olitsky SE, editors: *Harley's pediatric ophthalmology,* ed 5, Philadelphia, 2005, Lippincott, Williams & Wilkins.

Tesser RA, Hess DB, Buckley EG: Pediatric cataracts and lens anomalies. In Nelson LB, Olitsky SE, editors: *Harley's pediatric ophthalmology,* ed 5, Philadelphia, 2005, Lippincott, Williams & Wilkins.

Trobe J: *The physician's guide to eye care,* San Francisco, 2001, Foundation of the American Academy of Ophthalmology.

US Department of Health and Human Services: *Healthy people 2010,* vol 1, *Child and adolescent focused objectives,* Washington, DC, 2000, US Department of Health and Human Services.

US Preventive Services Task Force: Screening for visual impairment in children younger than age 5 years: recommendation statement. In *Guide to clinical preventive services,* ed 3: periodic updates. Agency for Healthcare Research and Quality, Rockville, MD, May 2004. Available at: *www.ahrq. gov/clinic/3rduspstf/visionscr/vischrs.htm* (accessed May 12, 2006).

Vitale S, Cotch MF, Sperduto RD: Prevalence of visual impairment in the United States, *JAMA* 295:2158-2163, 2006.

Wander A: Thermal burns. In Fraunfelder F, Roy F, editors: *Current ocular therapy,* ed 5, Philadelphia, 2000, WB Saunders.

Weichel ED, Vander JF, Tasman W et al: Diseases of the retina and vitreous. In Nelson LB, Olitsky SE, editors: *Harley's pediatric ophthalmology,* ed 5, Philadelphia, 2005, Lippincott, Williams & Wilkins.

Wilson MW, Haik BG, Karcioglu ZA et al: Pediatric conjunctival tumors. In Wright KW, Spiegel PH, editors: *Pediatric ophthalmology and strabismus,* Philadelphia, 2003, Lippincott, Williams & Wilkins.

Wright KW: Pediatric ocular trauma. In Wright KW, Spiegel PH, editors: *Pediatric ophthalmology and strabismus,* New York, 2003a, Springer.

Wright KW: Binocular vision and introduction to strabismus. In Wright KW, Spiegel PH, editors: *Pediatric ophthalmology and strabismus,* New York, 2003b, Springer.

Wright KW: Eyelid and orbital masses. In American Academy of Pediatrics (AAP): *Pediatric ophthalmology for primary care,* ed 2, Elk Grove Village, IL, 2003c, American Academy of Pediatrics.

Wright KW: Corneal abnormalities. In American Academy of Pediatrics (AAP): *Pediatric ophthalmology for primary care,* ed 2, Elk Grove Village, IL, 2003d, American Academy of Pediatrics.

Zhou Y, Huang C, Xu P et al: Perceptual learning improves contract sensitivity and visual acuity in adults with anisometropic amblyopia, *Vis Res* 46(5):739-50, 2006.

CHAPTER 29

Ear Disorders

Ann M. Petersen-Smith and Shirley Becton McKenzie

The ear provides the body with the ability to hear and maintain equilibrium. Appropriate functioning of the ear is essential for hearing, acquisition of speech, and the ability to maintain an upright position. The ear extends from the external to the inner ear structures. Malfunction of any of the structures of the ear can have an impact on both the ear and surrounding tissue. Additionally, ear dysfunction can cause systemic problems that can have a lifelong impact. Adequate hearing is important for learning, socialization, and language development. Caring for children with ear problems is an important role of pediatric primary care providers; understanding ear anatomy, physiology, and disorders requires a thoughtful assessment of the system and its functions.

STANDARDS FOR HEARING SCREENING

Universal detection of hearing loss before 3 months old is advocated by the Joint Committee on Infant Hearing (2000a, 2000b), the *Healthy Hearing 2010* initiative (U.S. Department of Health and Human Services, 2000), and the National Institutes of Health (NIH) (1993). These bodies also recommend follow-up by 3 months old and appropriate family-centered intervention by 6 months old. Screening of newborns or infants can be done by using evoked otoacoustical emission testing or the auditory brainstem response. Currently, 38 states, the District of Columbia, and various places in Canada and Europe have mandated newborn hearing screening programs (Jacobson & Jacobson, 2004). In 2001 the U.S. Preventive Services Task Force (USPSTF) stated that there is insufficient evidence to recommend for or against routine screening of asymptomatic newborns; this recommendation is currently under review (USPSTF, 2007). The USPSTF does agree with the need for predischarge screening of newborns with one or more neonatal risk factors and screening for hearing loss in children 1 month to 3 years old with certain risk factors.

During childhood, routine screening of asymptomatic children older than 3 years is debated. The USPSTF (2001) does not recommend screening beyond 3 years old or in adolescence. However, the Joint Committee on Infant Hearing, the American Academy of Pediatrics (AAP), and Bright Futures Guidelines all recommend pure-tone audiometry at 3, 4, 5, 10, 12, 15, and 18 years old, with subjective assessment at other ages. In 1997, the American Speech-Language-Hearing Association recommended annual pure-tone audiometry from 3 years old to third grade (U.S. Public Health Service, 1997); this recommendation remains unchanged. Screening of high-risk children, including those with frequently recurring otitis media (OM), middle ear effusion (MEE), or both, or those with chronic exposure to loud noises, should include annual audiologic screening and monitoring the development of communication skills.

DEVELOPMENT, ANATOMY, AND PHYSIOLOGY

DEVELOPMENT

Development of the ear begins during the third week of gestation and is complete by the third month of embryonic life. Insult to the fetus during this time can cause irreparable damage to the ear. Ear development occurs at the same time as kidney development, so malformation or dysfunction in one system should alert the health care provider to problems in the other.

ANATOMY AND PHYSIOLOGY

The external ear is responsible for transmission of sound waves from outside the ear to the middle ear and for clearance of debris. The canal contains glands that secrete sweat, sebum, and cerumen, which help lubricate the hair follicles and aid in the removal of debris. Patency of the ear canal is imperative for proper functioning.

The tympanic cavity constitutes the middle ear. The tympanic membrane (TM) is at the proximal end of the external auditory canal (EAC) and separates the external ear from the middle ear. The middle ear is a small chamber in the temporal bone that contains the ossicles—the malleus, incus, and stapes—which function to transmit sound waves from the EAC to the inner ear. The malleus lies against the TM, which vibrates when sound waves hit it. The stapes rests against the oval window, and its vibration causes the oval window to stimulate the fluids of the inner ear.

The eustachian tube has three physiologic functions with respect to the middle ear: (1) ventilation of the middle ear to equalize air pressure in the middle ear with atmospheric pressure and to replace oxygen that has been absorbed; (2) protection from nasopharyngeal sound, pressure, and secretions; and (3) drainage of secretions from the middle ear into the nasopharynx.

The inner ear functions to transmit sound and aid in balance. Vibrations of the TM, ossicles, and oval window set the inner ear fluids in motion. The fluid sound waves reach the cochlea, wherein lies the organ of Corti, which contains the hearing receptor hair cells. The hair cells transmit impulses to the

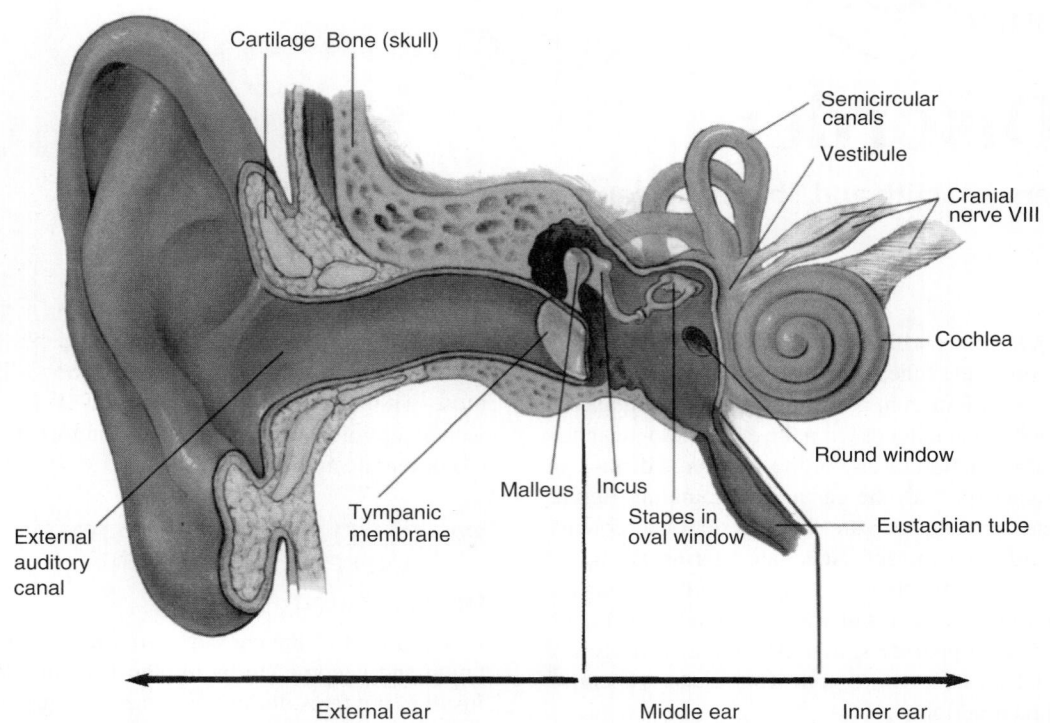

Cartilage Bone (skull)

Semicircular canals

Vestibule

Cranial nerve VIII

Cochlea

Round window

Eustachian tube

Stapes in oval window

Incus

Malleus

Tympanic membrane

External auditory canal

External ear

Middle ear

Inner ear

FIG. 29-1 Anatomy of the ear. (From Jarvis C: *Physical examination and health assessment*, ed 2, Philadelphia, 1996, WB Saunders, p. 365.)

auditory nerve (cranial nerve VIII), which transmits stimuli to the auditory cortex of the temporal lobe in the brain. The equilibrium receptors lie in the semicircular canals and vestibule of the inner ear. The semicircular canals respond to changes in direction of movement. The vestibule contains receptors essential to the maintenance of equilibrium (Fig. 29-1).

PATHOPHYSIOLOGY AND DEFENSE MECHANISMS
PATHOPHYSIOLOGY

The processes that negatively affect the ear are usually localized; however, pathologic ear conditions can be related to systemic dysfunction or disorders. Common localized pathologic conditions include disruption of defense mechanisms; viral, bacterial, or fungal infections in the inner, middle, and outer ear; foreign bodies in the ear; and trauma. Neurologic dysfunction, poor immunologic competence, and congenital anomalies are common disorders that can affect the ear and its functions. External influences, such as excessive noise in the environment, can cause irreparable damage to the ear's hearing function.

DEFENSE MECHANISMS

Debris formed by keratinizing cells in the ear is lubricated and extruded by the cilia in the EAC. Maintenance of an acidic pH in the ear canal prevents the growth of pathogenic bacteria. Additionally, the surface lining of the external ear is water resistant and has ample blood and lymph supply. These characteristics and the antibacterial properties of cerumen help protect against invading microorganisms. In comparison with the distal end of the EAC, the proximal end has fewer hair fibers, a thinner epithelial layer, and more nerve fibers that cause great discomfort when touched. This sensitivity to pain serves a protective function by deterring the insertion of foreign bodies into the ear, thus preventing damage to the middle ear.

The inner ear is also well protected inasmuch as the structures for both hearing and equilibrium are set deep within the skull.

ASSESSMENT
HISTORY

The history of a patient with an ear disorder should include the following:
- Previous medical history significant for craniofacial abnormalities (e.g., cleft lip or palate) or syndromes associated with craniofacial anomalies (Down syndrome, Treacher Collins syndrome)
- Prematurity
- Past medical history pertinent to ear conditions (e.g., infections, trauma, etc.)
- Pain (onset, location, quality, duration, alleviating or aggravating factors)
- Associated symptoms, such as fever, vomiting and diarrhea, nasal congestion, or other symptoms of upper respiratory infection
- Itching or discharge
- Tinnitus or hearing loss
- Exposure to risk factors: environmental tobacco smoke (ETS), bottle propping, pacifier use, day care, noise, swimming
- Diabetes mellitus
- Family history of ear dysfunction
- Family history of or presence of kidney malformation

PHYSICAL EXAMINATION

The physical examination includes the following:

* Inspection of the external structures of the ear for symmetry, skin abnormalities, discharge, or lesions.
  * The inner and outer canthi of the eye should form a straight line with the superior portion of the pinna. If the pinna inserts below this line, the ear is considered low set, which can be associated with a number of genetic and congenital syndromes.
* Assessment of developmental milestones related to hearing and speech development (Box 29-1).
* Palpation and rotation of the external ear for tenderness and inflammation; push on the tragus and apply pressure to the mastoid process.
* Otoscopic examination, which is best accomplished in a young child at the end of the physical examination with the child on an examining table or seated on the parent's lap. Pulling the ear downward, outward, and backward can enhance visualization of the EAC in infants and small children. In older children and adolescents, the EAC is lifted upward and backward, slightly away from the head.
* Decreased TM mobility secondary to effusion is noted through pneumatic otoscopy, tympanometry, or acoustic reflectometry.

BOX 29-1   **Developmental Milestones Used to Assess Hearing**

Birth to 3 Months
Startles (Moro reflex) to loud noise
Awakens to sounds
Blinks or widens eyes to noises

3 to 6 Months
Quiets to parent's voice
Stops activity to listen to new sound
Looks for source of sound
Reciprocates vocally and initiates sounds

6 to 12 Months
Coos and gurgles with inflection
Responds to simple phrases
Turns to localize sound in any plane
Responds to own name

12 to 18 Months
Points to unexpected sound or familiar objects when asked
Follows simple direction without cues
Imitates some sounds, first words by 12 to 15 months old

18 to 24 Months
Points to body parts when asked
Has expressive vocabulary of 20 to 50 words
50% of speech intelligible to strangers

Data from Northern J, Downs M: *Hearing in children,* ed 4, Baltimore, 1991, Williams & Wilkins.

---

* Examine the canal for redness, edema, or discharge. Assess all 360 degrees of the TM, the bony processes, and the cone of light (see Color Plate). Look for air-fluid level or bubbles behind the TM. Note any retraction or perforation.

COMMON DIAGNOSTIC STUDIES

* *Evoked otoacoustic emission testing* (EOAE) is the method of hearing screening being used for universal newborn screening. Dr. Kemp first described the phenomenon of otoacoustic emissions in 1978. He found that the normal-hearing ear emits detectable 20 decibels (dB) sounds called *spontaneous otoacoustic emissions*. The normal ear also emits these sounds when given a stimulus and provides evidence that the outer hair cells of the cochlea are functioning appropriately and hearing is likely to be intact. EOAE is efficient, highly sensitive, and easy to perform in a quiet, cooperative child, which makes it conducive for use in newborns. However, the EOAE does not quantify hearing deficit and may not identify auditory nerve dysfunction; ambient room noise and an uncooperative child may interfere with the test and provide unreliable results (DiMichelle & Ruth, 2005; Gregg et al, 2004; Jacobson & Jacobson, 2004). Improvements in EOAE and auditory brainstem response (ABR) technology have resulted in highly acceptable levels of hearing sensitivity and specificity at relatively low cost (Kenna, 2003).
* *Auditory brainstem response* measures the initiation of sound-induced electrical signals in the cochlea. The ABR measures the functioning of the peripheral auditory system and neurologic pathways related to hearing. Although it is not a direct measure of hearing, ABR allows for inferences to be made about hearing thresholds (Gregg et al, 2004; DiMichelle & Ruth, 2005). The ABR is useful in identifying hearing loss in a young infant or in children unable to cooperate with EOAE or audiometry. Occasionally, sedation is required. Neurologic abnormalities may make interpretation of an ABR impossible. Automated ABR is now available as a screening device.
* *Audiometry,* useful in assessing hearing loss in children, measures hearing threshold via bone or air conduction, or both, in decibels at varying frequencies (Tables 29-1 and 29-2). Twenty dB is about as loud as a whisper, 90 dB produces pain, and 40 dB is normal speaking loudness. The frequencies of normal speaking range from 250 to 4000 Hz. Hearing loss, especially in the higher frequencies (2000 to 6000 Hz), can cause significant problems in understanding speech. A screening audiogram that tests each ear at 20 dB and frequencies of 500, 1000, 2000, and 4000 Hz is a useful assessment tool in office pediatrics. If a more detailed audiogram is needed, a qualified audiologist should perform it. Box 29-2 lists the various types of audiometry.
* *Pneumatic otoscopy* helps assess TM mobility. A good seal with the speculum and otoscope is required before insufflation of air into the ear canal. Brisk movement of the membrane should be seen; altered mobility suggests MEE or possible perforation.

TABLE 29-1 **Audiologic Tests for Infants and Young Children**

Test	Characteristics	Age Range	Advantages	Disadvantages
Behavioral observation audiometry (BOA)	Behavioral test: responses to noisemakers or calibrated sounds are observed	0-5 mo	Low cost	Insensitive to unilateral or less than severe hearing loss; highly subject to observer bias; child tires rapidly when subjected to repeated stimuli
Visual reinforced audiometry (VRA)	Behavioral test: child is given an animated toy for turning to sounds	5-24 mo	Low cost; child responds at softer levels and for longer periods compared with BOA	Insensitive to unilateral loss (unless earphones used); need two examiners to reduce bias
Play audiometry	Behavioral test: child is trained to respond to tones by playing game	2-5 yr	Low cost; can detect unilateral and mild hearing loss	Requires cooperation of child
Screening audiometry	Behavioral test: child raises hand or responds verbally to tones at fixed levels (20-25 dB)	4 yr and older	Can be performed by trained paraprofessional in most children 4 yr and older; can detect unilateral and mild hearing loss	Further tests required if failed
Otoacoustic emissions (OAE)	Physiologic test: response of inner ear to brief clicks or tones is measured with specialized instrument	Any	Child's response not needed; takes fewer than 2 min if child is quiet; can be performed by a trained paraprofessional; low cost; can detect unilateral and mild hearing loss	Cannot tell type or degree of loss; further tests required if failed
Auditory brainstem response (ABR) audiometry	Physiologic test: averaged number of responses of brainstem to brief tones or clicks	Any	Child's response not needed; can detect unilateral and mild loss; can determine degree and slope of loss (with tone bursts and bone conduction testing)	Requires audiologist and equipment to administer and interpret; expensive; requires sedation beyond about 6 mo old

dB, Decibels; *min*, minutes; *mo*, months; *yr*, years.
From Daly KA, Hunter LL, Giebink GS: Chronic otitis media with effusion, *Pediatr Rev* 20(3):85-93, 1999.

TABLE 29-2 **Evaluation of Audiometric Results**

Average Threshold at 500-2000 Hz (decibels)	Description	Significance
−10 to +15	Normal	
16-25	Slight loss	Difficulty hearing faint speech, slight verbal deficit
26-40	Mild loss	Auditory learning dysfunction, language, or speech problems
41-55	Moderate loss	Trouble hearing conversational speech, may miss 50% of class discussion
56-70	Moderately severe loss	
71-90	Severe loss	Educational retardation, learning disability, limited vocabulary
90	Profound loss	

- *Tympanometry* evaluates the function of the middle ear by assessing the movement of the TM by applying from -400 to $+100$ mm H_2O pressure to the ear canal. Movement of the TM is translated into a graph called a *tympanogram* (Fig. 29-2).

BOX 29-2   Types of Audiometry

- Behavioral Observational Audiometry (BOA) is used for young infants, birth to 6 months old. The BOA involves observation of any behavioral responses of an infant to sound stimulation under structured conditions. Limitations of the BOA include the need for high-intensity stimuli and examiner bias; consequently there are a high number of false-positive and false-negative test results (Jacobson & Jacobson, 2004).

- Visual Reinforcement Audiometry (VRA) is the most appropriate test for children older than 12 months but less than 3 to 4 years old. Sounds are presented into the examination room and when the child responds to the sound a visual reinforcement is given in the form of a lighted toy. Because VRA is not ear specific, a unilateral hearing loss may be missed (Gregg et al, 2004).

- Play audiometry is for children 2 years and older and involves the child responding to hearing a sound that is emitted from a speaker or through a set of headphones by performing a task. Pure-tone audiometry is intended for older children and adolescents and can measure both air conduction (AC) and/or bone conduction (BC). AC helps to establish the well-being of the entire auditory pathway. BC helps to differentiate conductive hearing loss from sensorineural hearing loss (SNHL). In pure-tone audiometry, children respond to signals generated by an audiometer.

The type A tympanogram has a compliance peak between ±100 mm H_2O and reflects a normal TM. The type B tympanogram generally has no peak or a flattened wave and suggests effusion, perforation, or the presence of a pressure-equalizing tube. The type C tympanogram has a sharp peak between -100 and -200 mm H_2O and reflects negative ear pressure (see Fig. 29-3 for types of tympanograms). Tympanograms are helpful when OM with effusion is persistent or a question remains regarding the results of physical examination of the eardrum. Tympanograms are of little use in children younger than 7 months old because their ear canals are hypercompliant in response to pressure from the tympanometer.

- *Acoustic reflectometry* is used to detect a MEE by directing a sound of varying frequency toward the TM and measuring the intensity of reflected sound. The reflectometer directs sounds of varying frequency toward the TM and measures the intensity of the reflected sound. The fluid-filled middle ear space restricts vibration of the eardrum, so sound is intensified when returning to the device. Unfortunately, the reflectometer cannot distinguish if a MEE is serous or suppurative. Acoustic reflectometry is less accurate than pneumatic otoscopy; however, it has a sensitivity of 80% to 87% and a specificity of 54% to 70%.

- *Tympanocentesis* with aspiration of middle ear fluid is helpful for the relief of pain and identification of persistent infecting organisms. It is rarely used in clinical pediatrics and is generally considered outside the scope of practice of the primary care provider.

- Laboratory tests of blood and urine are rarely indicated unless questions remain regarding perinatal infection, systemic illness, or concomitant kidney dysfunction.

A normal tympanogram is depicted below. Four features of the tympanogram can be used to evaluate the ear under test:

❶ Static admittance (Peak Ya) is a measure of the height of the tympanometric peak. Given appropriate norms, static admittance is a useful indicator of middle ear disease.

❷ Equivalent ear canal volume (+200 Vea) is the admittance value determined with an ear canal air pressure of +200 daPa (dekapascals). An abnormally high equivalent ear canal volume suggests the presence of a tympanic membrane perforation, or a patent tympanostomy tube.

❸ Tympanometric peak pressure (TPP) is the position of the tympanometric peak on the pressure axis. TPP is an imprecise measure of the middle ear pressure. By itself, TPP is not an accurate indicator of middle ear disease.

❹ Tympanometric gradient (GR) or tympanometric width is a measure of the width of the tympanometric peak. Defined as the pressure interval required for a 50% reduction of peak eardrum admittance, tympanometric width is a good indicator of the presence of **middle ear effusion**.

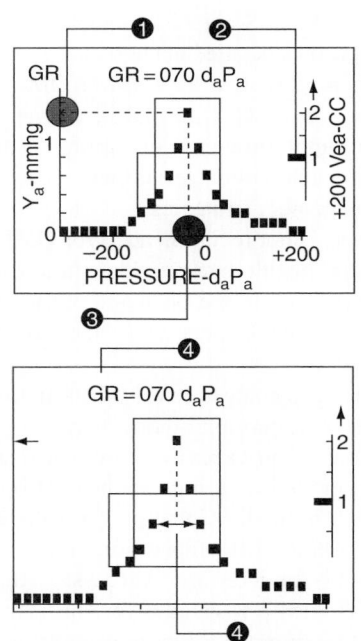

FIG. 29-2   A normal tympanogram. (From WelchAllyn: *MicroTymp Portable Tympanometric Instrument operating instructions*. Available at *www.welchallyn.com*, Skaneateles Falls, NY.)

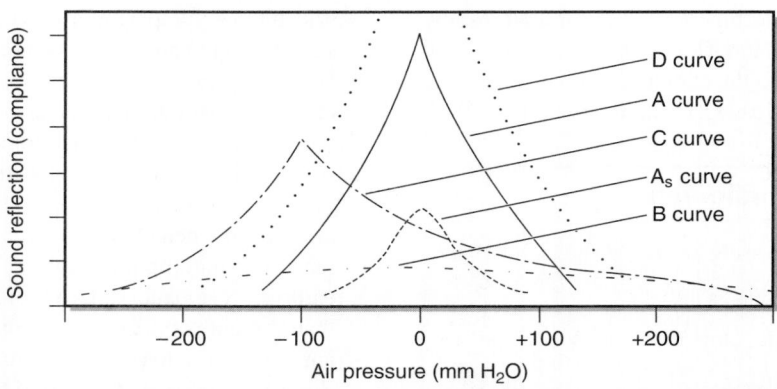

FIG. 29-3 Tympanogram. Five types of tympanogram curves. Generally, an *A* curve indicates a normal TM, a *B* curve is abnormal, a *C* curve may be abnormal, and a *D* curve indicates hypermobility. An A_s curve may be normal in infants. (From Harrison CJ, Belhorn TH: Acute otitis media: Management and prophylaxis, *Clin Rev Apr* 1992, p. 55.)

- Genetic testing can be used to evaluate deaf and hard-of-hearing persons to provide a diagnosis, plan treatment and interventions, and to determine whether the hearing loss may be genetically inherited. Approximately 80% of sensorineural hearing loss (SNHL) is recessive (Smith, 2003).

■ MANAGEMENT STRATEGIES
MEDICATIONS

The AAP and the American Academy of Family Physicians (AAFP) in 1998 published principles for the judicious use of antibiotics to treat infections including OM (Dowell et al, 1998). The same concepts were endorsed by the Centers for Disease Control and Prevention. In 2004 AAP and AAFP further defined treatment for both acute otitis media (AOM) and otitis media with effusion (OME). Some of the chief concepts are bulleted below, with specifics detailed in the sections on these topics.
- OM should be classified as AOM or OME. Correct differentiation between AOM and OME is one of the essential principles of appropriate use of antibiotics in children.
- Pain management, antibacterial therapy, and watchful waiting are management strategies.
- Antibiotic use is not recommended for OME.

The pediatric health care provider should be familiar with these recommendations and be aware of their role in the prevention of superinfections caused by the indiscriminate use of antibiotics.

Antipyretics and analgesics are useful in treating fever and discomfort. Use of ceruminolytics or removal of the impaction is essential when excessive cerumen impedes examination of the ear or alters hearing. Acidic eardrops help maintain an environment in the EAC that prevents the growth of fungi and bacteria. Ototopical preparations must be administered appropriately to help ensure successful treatment. These medications should be warmed before instilling the drops, the tragus should be pumped a few times after instillation of the drops, and the affected ear should remain up for at least 2 to 3 minutes after the procedure is complete.

EDUCATION AND COUNSELING

Education and counseling of the patient and family regarding the watchful waiting concept, the prevention of additional problems, and the treatment course are key counseling points in the treatment of ear problems. Areas of particular importance include avoiding passive smoke exposure, avoiding bottle propping, minimizing exposure to other children with minor acute illnesses, decreasing exposure to loud noises, receiving an annual influenza vaccine for all children 6 months or older, completing the pneumococcal conjugate vaccination series for children under 2 years old, and breastfeeding during the first 6 months of life.

PREVENTION OF NOISE-INDUCED HEARING LOSS

Noise is a common cause of SNHL in children, and the pattern of damage depends on the frequency, intensity, and duration of the noise (Kenna, 2003). According to the U.S. Department of Labor, 85 dB is the boundary between acceptable and damaging noise, whether the noise is continuous or intermittent. Any structure in the ear can be permanently damaged by noise greater than or equal to 140 dB. Firearms, fireworks, loud music, recreational vehicles, and power tools can all contribute to SNHL. The health care provider should actively educate patients and parents to avoid damaging sources of sound and use protective devices. Three types of protective devices are readily available at pharmacies or hardware stores: earmuffs, form-fitting foam earplugs, and premolded earplugs. Maintaining an awareness of risk factors should lead the provider to early detection of cochlear damage and hearing loss. The decibel levels of common noises are listed in Table 29-3.

REMOVAL OF CERUMEN

Cerumen in the ear canal can be removed mechanically, with the use of a ceruminolytic/softening agent, by gently irrigating the ear, or by a combination of these techniques (Dimmitt, 2005). Before irrigation 2 to 3 drops of docusate sodium (Colace), triethanolamine (Cerumenex), mineral oil, or other

TABLE 29-3	How Loud is Safe?
Decibels	**Sounds**
20	Watch ticking
30	Whispering, quiet library
40	Leaves rustling, refrigerator humming, quiet street noises
50	Neighborhood street, average home
60	Dishwasher, normal conversation
70	Car, alarm clock, city traffic
80	Garbage disposal, noisy restaurant, vacuum cleaner, outboard motor, hair drying
90	Factory, screaming child, portable stereo at high volume, motorcycle
100	Power lawn mower, highway driving in a convertible
110	Diesel truck, subway train (outside, not as a passenger), chain saw, snowmobile
120	Rock concert, propeller plane, portable stereos on max volume, screaming baby, car horn
130	Jet plane (100 feet away), air-raid siren
140	Fireworks, shotgun blast, explosion

Modified from sound of 80 decibels (dB) or less are believed to be safe for nearly all healthy adults, no matter how long you hear them. Sounds of 85 dB should be limited to no more than 8 hours a day, and 91 dB to 2 hours for a healthy adult. Limit the 100 dB sounds to 15 minutes and 120 dB sounds to about 9 seconds. Sounds in the 125-140 dB range are loud enough to cause pain unless you protect your ears with earplugs. The long-term effects of high noise levels for children are unknown; therefore, the thresholds cited here may be too high for them.
Hearing loss: a guide to prevention and treatment—a special health report from Harvard Medical School, copyright 2006 by the President and Fellows of Harvard College; American Academy of Otolaryngology—Head and Neck Surgery (AAO-HNSF): *Noise and hearing protection.* Available at *www.entnet.org/health.info/hearing/noise_hearing.cfm* (accessed Feb 2007); Ohio State University: *A fact sheet on noise.* Available at *www.ohioline.ag.ohio-state.edu/cd-fact/0190* (accessed Jan 2007).

warm oil may be instilled to help soften the obstructive wax. Baking soda mixed with water is also effective. Mix one-half of a teaspoon of baking soda with 2 oz of water and instill a few drops in the affected ear two times daily for 1 week. After 1 week the solution should be discarded. Tap water irrigation alone is also as effective as using a softener before irrigation. For dry, hardened wax, softeners may decrease the amount of irrigant required. Irrigation is then accomplished by using a bulb syringe or "water pick" (on low setting). The irrigation solution can be warm water or hydrogen peroxide diluted 1:1 with warm water. Irrigation should not be attempted if the TM is possibly perforated or tympanostomy tubes are in place.

Mechanical cerumen removal (curettage) requires skill and the use of a cerumen spoon. This method is not as messy and may be as effective as irrigation. Blunt plastic ear curettes may be less traumatic than the metal variety. Always carefully explain the procedure to parents and inform them that the ear canal is extremely sensitive and fragile and bleeds easily when touched. This may prevent an adverse parent reaction when there is blood on the curette or in the ear canal.

FOLLOW-UP AND REFERRAL

Follow-up of ear signs and symptoms and assessment for hearing loss are necessary to detect changes in hearing and monitor recurrence of illness. This is especially true with the watchful waiting option in OM. A follow-up ear exam is recommended in 3 to 4 weeks after a confirmed AOM. An otolaryngology referral is indicated for unusual ear conditions, congenital malformation of the head and neck structures, craniofacial anomalies, sensory dysfunction involving hearing or speech, when appropriate therapy for OM has failed, or if ongoing effusion or infection persists (American Academy of Pediatrics Policy Statement, 2004). Myringotomy or placement of pressure-equalization tubes (PETs) can help relieve discomfort and decrease the likelihood of further infection. Audiologic referral is necessary if the ear pathology is prolonged or when the child's ability to hear is questioned. Speech and language evaluations are imperative to resolve questions about whether the child's verbal development is delayed because of persistent or recurring ear problems. Chapter 31 addresses criteria for tonsillectomy and adenoidectomy.

Pressure-Equalizing Tubes

Indications for tympanostomy and the insertion of PETs are listed in Box 29-3. Every child with recurrent or persistent AOM or chronic OME must be considered on an individual basis for the placement of PETs. Baseline hearing status should be established in any child having PETs inserted. Otolaryngologists may wait until the fall or winter months to insert PETs because the tubes require more care during the summer, and most ear disease wanes in the summer months.

Paradise and colleagues (2005) reported that the immediate placement of PETs in children less than 3 years old with persistent OME did not have a significant improvement in developmental outcomes, including speech and language acquisition. The authors concluded that waiting to insert PETs (6 months for bilateral effusion and 9 months for unilateral effusion) had no detrimental effect on development and resulted in fewer procedures with equal outcomes.

Insertion of PETs in a child with recurrent OM or prolonged MEE results in less discomfort with AOM, appropriate ventilation of the middle ear space, and improved hearing and necessitates only having to prescribe antibiotic otic drops when treating ear infections while the PETs are patent. Additionally, the use of PETs may decrease the incidence of AOM in some children. The effectiveness of the PETs is dependent on their insertion in the correct place and being functional. The procedure takes less than 15 minutes and is usually done using general anesthesia. The child is usually discharged after about an hour and is treated with otic drops for several days. The average life span for PETs is 14 months (Paradise & Bluestone, 2005). Children with persistent hearing loss after PETs are placed should be further evaluated (AAP Section on Otolaryngology and Bronchoesophagology, 2002).

The examiner can establish that the tube is functioning properly if the tube spans the eardrum, the lumen is unobstructed, and no MEE is present. If appropriate functioning of

---

BOX 29-3 **Indications for Tympanostomy and the Insertion of Pressure-Equalizing Tubes**

- Sustained hearing loss that is moderate (31 to 60 dB HL) or severe (61 to 90 dB HL)
  - Questionable or disturbed speech or language development, with hearing loss that is at least moderate
  - History of frequent or severe episodes of AOM
  - History of adverse reaction to multiple antibiotics
  - Regular exposure to large numbers of other children
  - Children between 1 and 4 years old, children with craniofacial anomalies or syndromes (e.g., cleft palate), and other children at high risk for acute and recurrent AOM benefit
  - At-risk children (sensory, physical, cognitive, or behavioral developmental delays) (e.g., hearing loss independent of OME, speech and language delay, pervasive developmental delay, blindness)
  - Documented OME lasting more than 4 months or recurrent OME regardless of hearing
  - Structural damage to TM or middle ear: severe retraction pocket, ossicular erosion, areas of atelectasis or atrophy
  - Severe ETD (persistent ear popping, pain, vertigo, tinnitus, or fluctuating hearing loss)
  - Complications of OM present or suspected (mastoiditis, facial nerve paralysis, brain abscess, labyrinthitis)

AOM, Acute otitis media; *ETD,* eustachian tube dysfunction; *OME,* otis media with effusion; *TM,* tympanic membrane.
Data from Paradise JL, Bluestone CD: Tympanostomy tubes: a contemporary guide to judicious use, *Pediatr Rev* 26(2):60–65, 2005.
DeRosa J, Grundfast KM: Surgical management of otitis media, *Pediatr Ann* 31(12):814-820, 2002.

the tube cannot be established, pneumatic otoscopy or tympanometry may be useful. A flat (type B) tympanogram with large volume measurements confirms appropriate function of the PET. A normal (type A) tympanogram suggests a clogged or extruded tube.

The use of ototopical drops for 5 to 7 days can occasionally clear clogged PETs. Otic suspensions that are mildly acidic should be used because they are less irritating to middle ear mucosa. Water and ceruminolytics are contraindicated. If the child can taste the drops or complains of stinging, the drops are most likely reaching the middle ear space and indicate a functioning tube.

Generalized water precautions for children with PETs are controversial. Water does not enter the middle ear space via the PET during bathing, showering, or surface swimming. Diving and head dunking may allow water into the middle ear space; however, chlorinated pools have few bacteria, and earplugs are probably unnecessary. However, lakes, ponds, rivers, and bath water may have increased bacterial counts, so earplugs are recommended if head dunking may occur.

Viral myringitis or early AOM without otorrhea in a child with PETs will most likely resolve spontaneously because of

increased middle ear ventilation. Antibiotics (oral or ototopical) are not indicated. Tympanostomy tube otorrhea (TTO) occurs usually when a child with PETs has an upper respiratory infection and has drainage coming from the tubes. TTO occurs in about 20% of all children with PETs, most of which are self-limited episodes (Rosenfeld, 2004b). TTO usually involves the same bacterial pathogens seen in AOM. Ototopical antibiotics are recommended because of their ability to concentrate the medication in the ear. Eardrops containing fluoroquinolone with or without a corticosteroid additive are the preferred treatment for TTO (Dohar et al, 2006; Leibovitz, 2006; Myer, 2004; Roland, 2004; Rosenfeld, 2004b). Ototopical medications are listed in Table 29-4. If the otorrhea has not improved after 5 to 7 days of topical therapy, treatment with oral antibiotics is appropriate. If the otorrhea is resistant to oral and ototopical agents, referral to an otolaryngologist is recommended.

Many PETs fall out well before their usefulness has been expended; some children will require a second set. Once the PET has been extruded from the TM, follow-up every 6 to 12 months is suggested until the tube falls out of the external canal. For the rare set of PETs that remain in situ, surgical removal is suggested after 2 years (AAP Section on Otolaryngology and Bronchoesophagology, 2002). Complications of PETs include otorrhea, otitis externa (OE), granuloma, cholesteatoma, PET obstruction, persistent TM perforation, and tympanosclerosis.

■ SPECIFIC EAR PROBLEMS IN CHILDREN
OTITIS EXTERNA
Description
Otitis externa (OE), commonly called "swimmer's ear," is an inflammatory reaction of the EAC, which may also involve the pinna or TM. Inflammation is evidenced as (1) simple infection with edema, discharge, and erythema; (2) furuncles or small abscesses that form in hair follicles; or (3) impetigo or infection of the superficial layers of the epidermis. OE can also be classified as mycotic OE, caused by fungus, or as chronic external otitis, a diffuse low-grade infection of the EAC. Severe infection or systemic infection can be seen in children who have diabetes, who are immunocompromised, or who have received head and neck irradiation.

Epidemiology
OE results when the protective barriers in the EAC are damaged by mechanical or chemical mechanisms (Schroeder, 2004). OE is most frequently caused by retained moisture in the external ear canal, which changes the acidic environment of the external ear canal to a neutral or basic environment, thereby promoting bacterial or fungal growth. Chlorine in swimming pools adds to the problem because it kills the normal ear flora and allows the growth of pathogens. The most common pathogens in "swimmer's ear" are *Pseudomonas aeruginosa* and *Staphylococcus aureus*. *Pseudomonas* is also associated with the use of hearing aids or protectors, drainage from AOM, and ear trauma (Schroeder, 2004).

TABLE 29-4 Commonly Used Topical Preparations for Ear Disease

Product Name (Manufacturer)	Antibiotic	Antiinflammatory	Acid	Comments
Auralgan (Wyeth-Ayerst)	None	None	None	Benzocaine in a glycerin and propylene base; used for anesthesia in cases of severe AOM; **do NOT use in presence of TM perforation**
Cipro HC Otic (Alcon Labs)	Ciprofloxacin	Hydrocortisone	Glacial acetic acid	Use ≥1 year old
CiproDex (Alcon)	Ciprofloxacin	Dexamethasone		Use ≥6 months old
Ciloxan Ophthalmic (Alcon Labs)	Ciprofloxacin	None	Acetic	Sterile ophthalmic preparation demonstrated safety and efficacy for use with open TM
Cortisporin Otic Solution (Monarch Pharmaceuticals)	Polymyxin B and neomycin	Hydrocortisone	Hydrochloric	May be painful on instillation; demonstrated to be ototoxic in animal models; human studies have demonstrated no ototoxicity in children or adults
Cortisporin Otic Suspension	Polymyxin B and neomycin	Hydrocortisone	None	May be used when solution is poorly tolerated
Cortisporin Ophthalmic	Polymyxin B and neomycin	Hydrocortisone	Sulfuric	May be used when this combination is desired and both otic solution and suspension are poorly tolerated
Debrox Otic Solution (SmithKline Beecham)	None	None	Citric	Excellent choice for cleansing of the EAC; also contains carbamide peroxide as an added ceruminolytic
Domeboro Otic (Bayer Pharmaceutical Division)	None	None	Acetic and boric	Excellent antimicrobial and antifungal activity; may be used in conjunction with other topicals
Floxin Otic (Daiichi Pharmaceuticals)	Ofloxacin	None	Hydrochloric	Use ≥6 months old
Gentamicin Ophthalmic	Gentamicin	None	Hydrochloric	May be used by some otolaryngologists as a first-line agent in patients with a sulfa allergy; demonstrated ototoxicity in animal models
Inflamase Mild (1/8%), Inflamase Foret (1%) (Ciba Vision Ophthalmics)	None	Prednisolone	None	Excellent choice for inflammatory conditions, such as granular myringitis
Pediotic (King Pharmaceuticals)	Polymyxin B and neomycin	Hydrocortisone	None	Usage has declined dramatically with introduction of Floxin
TobraDex Ophthalmic (Alcon Labs)	Tobramycin	Dexamethasone	Sulfuric	No documented ototoxicity with either agent; excellent broad-spectrum coverage
Vasocidin Ophthalmic (Ciba Vision Ophthalmics)	Sulfacetamide	Prednisolone	Hydrochloric	Used by some otolaryngologists as a first-line agent and as a prophylactic
Vigamox Ophthalmic (Alcon Labs)	Moxifloxacin	None	Hydrochloric	Use ≥1 year old

AOM, Acute otitis media; *EAC,* external auditory canal; *FDA,* food and drug administration; *TM,* tympanic membrane.

Many cases of acute OE are polymicrobial with aerobic and anaerobic bacteria (Sifuentes, 2005). Other pathogens commonly associated with acute OE include *S. epidermidis,* and *Streptococcus pyogenes.* Furunculosis of the external canal is generally caused by *S. aureus* and *S. pyogenes* carried by dirty fingers. Otomycosis is usually caused by *Aspergillus* or *Candida* and is caused by recent use of systemic or topical antibiotics or steroids. Otomycosis is also more common in children with diabetes or immune dysfunction, accounts for 10% of OE, and is most commonly caused by *A. niger. Escherichia coli, Klebsiella pneumoniae,* and group B streptococci are more common in neonates (Sifuentes, 2005).

Long standing ear drainage may suggest a foreign body, chronic middle ear problem, such as a cholesteatoma, or granulomatous tissue. Bloody drainage may indicate trauma, severe OM, or granulation tissue. Chronic or recurrent OE may result from eczema, seborrhea, or psoriasis. Eczematous dermatitis, moist vesicles, and pustules are seen in acute infection, and crusting is more consistent with chronic infection (Schroeder, 2004).

Clinical Findings

History. The following can be found:
- Itching and irritation progressing to severe pain
- Pressure and fullness in ear and occasionally hearing loss that can be conductive or sensorineural
- Rare systemic complaints and symptoms
- Rare hearing loss and otorrhea
- Sagging of the superior canal, periauricular edema, and preauricular and postauricular lymphadenopathy with more severe disease. Extension to the surrounding soft tissue results in the obstruction of the canal with or without cellulitis (Sifuentes, 2005).

Physical Examination. Findings on physical examination can include the following:
- Pain, often quite severe, with movement of the tragus or on attempts to examine the ear with an otoscope
- Swollen EAC with debris, making visualization of the TM difficult or impossible
- Rare otorrhea
- Occasional regional lymphadenopathy
- Tragal tenderness with a red, raised area of induration that can be deep and diffuse or superficial and pointing, which is characteristic of furunculosis
- Red, crusty or pustular spreading lesions
- Black spots over the TM, indicative of mycotic infection
- Dry-appearing canal with some atrophy or thinning of the canal and virtually no cerumen visible with chronic OE
- Presence of PET or perforation of TM (avoid use of ototoxic drops)

Diagnostic Studies. Culturing the discharge from the ear is not customary, but may be indicated if: clinical improvement is not seen during or after treatment; there is severe pain; the child is immunocompromised; in neonates; chronic OE is suspected (Lye, 2004). Culturing requires a swab premoistened with sterile nonbacteriostatic saline or water.

Differential Diagnosis

AOM with perforation, TTO, chronic suppurative otitis media (CSOM), necrotizing OE, cholesteatoma, mastoiditis, posterior auricular lymphadenopathy, dental infection, and eczema are all in the differential diagnoses.

Management

Box 29-4 outlines the management of OE. Additional steps listed below:
- Debridement with a cotton-tipped applicator, self-made cotton wick, or calcium alginate swabs is the most critical step (Shroeder, 2004).
- Burow's solution is soothing, decreases edema, and kills *Pseudomonas*.

BOX 29-4 **Management of Otitis Externa**

Treatment Guidelines
- Administer analgesics as needed
- Remove any foreign body
- Lance any furuncles
- Irrigate and débride with saline or Burow's solution or 2.5% acetic acid solution if no perforation
- Instill antibiotic drops; insert wick if significant swelling
- If impetigo: cleanse, rinse, and apply antibiotic ointment
- If mycotic: cleanse with 5% boric acid in ethanol solution, followed by antifungal solution

Prevention
- Avoid water in ears
- Use acidic eardrops in ear after swimming
- Avoid scratching, cleaning, and prolonged use of ceruminolytics
- Use blow dryer to dry the external auditory canal

- Eardrops (antiseptic, nonquinolone antibiotic, quinolone antibiotic or steroid-antibiotic) are the mainstay of therapy for OE (see Table 29-4). Sixty-five percent to 90% of children with OE improve within 7 to 10 days regardless of type of therapy (AAO-HNSF, 2006). Antibiotic choice should be chosen based on efficacy, low incidence of adverse effects, cost, and likelihood of compliance.
  - Steroid combined with antimicrobial provide better cure rates than steroid drops alone (AAO-HNSF, 2006) and may help to control the development of granulation tissue involving the TM and middle ear space (Shroeder, 2004).
  - Topical antibiotics preparations free of potential ototoxic agents (quinolones), though they are quite costly, are preferred when the child has tympanostomy tubes or a perforated TM.
  - The quinolone products are effective against *Pseudomonas, S. aureus,* and *S. pneumoniae,* which may be a factor if the OE is a complication of AOM.
  - Neomycin is effective against *S. aureus,* but has no activity against *Pseudomonas* (Capoot et al, 2002); additionally, neomycin has been reported to cause an allergic contact dermatitis in some recipients. Polymyxin, which is often found in combination with neomycin, also has good *S. aureus* and *Pseudomonas* coverage.
- It is important to apply tragal pressure after each drop of medication to ensure that the medication gets to the middle ear space.
- If significant swelling is present, insert a wick soaked with the antibiotic eardrop solution (Schroeder, 2004). A foam (Pope™), cotton, hydrogel polymer (Merocel XL™) or gauze (0.25 inch) wick usually works well. The tip of the wick is lubricated with water-based lubricant just before insertion into the ear. Once in place, the wick should be impregnated

with antiobiotic for as long as it remains in the auditory canal. (This may require reapplication of drops every 2 to 3 hours). Wicks are usually removed after several days if they have not fallen out on their own. The wick falls out when the swelling has subsided, and treatment with direct application of drops to the ear canal should continue for the entire course.

- If the child is not improved within 72 hours (relief of otalgia, itching, and fullness), recheck to confirm diagnosis. Lack of improvement may be due to obstructed ear canal, poor adherence, or contact sensitivity among other things.
- Oral or parenteral antibiotics are generally not needed except for systemic illness or failed topical treatment.
- Avoid cleaning, manipulating, and getting water into the ear. Swimming is prohibited during acute infection.
- Administer analgesics for pain, as needed. Narcotic analgesics may be necessary for severe pain and are indicated for short-term use.
- Lance a furuncle that is superficial and pointed with a 14-gauge needle. If it is deep and diffuse, a heating pad or warm oil-based drops can speed resolution.
- If impetigo is present, clear the canal by using half-strength hydrogen peroxide or other antiseptic solutions, followed by a warm-water rinse. Apply an antibiotic ointment (mupirocin) once or twice a day for 5 to 7 days. The child should avoid touching the ear. Fingernails should be short and hands cleansed with antibacterial soap. Systemic antibiotics are generally unnecessary.
- Mycotic OE is treated with a solution of 5% boric acid in ethanol, which is antiseptic and promotes drying. Clotrimazole-miconazole solution can be used alone or with a topical antibiotic corticosteroid solution for 5 to 7 days.
- A follow-up visit may be necessary after 1 to 2 weeks for reevaluation of the OE and removal of debris.
- A dermatology consultation is indicated if no improvement is seen within 1 week.

Complications

Infection of surrounding tissues with impetigo, irritated furunculosis, and malignant OE with progression and necrosis caused by *Pseudomonas* infection are possible complications. Involvement of the parotid gland, mastoid bone, and infratemporal fossa are rare complications (Sifuentes, 2005).

Prevention

The patient should be instructed to do the following:

- Avoid water in the ear canals.
- Use well-fitting earplugs for swimming especially in "dirty water."
- Use acidic drops (diluted vinegar or diluted alcohol) three to five drops daily, especially after swimming, to prevent the recurrence of OE. Over-the-counter drugs, such as VoSol Otic™ eardrops can be used (5 drops in each ear after swimming).
- Use a blow dryer on warm setting to dry the EAC (Sifuentes, 2005).
- Avoid persistent scratching or cleaning of the external canal.
- Avoid prolonged use of ceruminolytic agents.

FOREIGN BODY IN THE EAR CANAL

Description

A foreign body in the external ear canal is a problem frequently seen in pediatric patients.

Epidemiology

Foreign bodies are usually placed or thrown in the ear canal by the child or other children. Insects can also be found in the canal.

Clinical Findings

History.   The history can include the following:

- Child reports putting something into the ear or having something thrown at them
- Complaints of buzzing, fullness, or an object in the ear
- Persistent cough or hiccups (Engstrom, 2005; Kadish, 2005)
- Unilateral otalgia and otorrhea.

Physical Examination.   A foreign body is visible with the naked eye or by otoscopic examination.

Management

Foreign bodies in the lateral one-third of the ear canal are the easiest to remove. Foreign bodies in the medial two-thirds of the ear canal are more difficult to remove because the canal is narrower; it is lined with bone, is quite vascular, and exquisitely sensitive. The TM lies at the most medial part of the EAC. Otolaryngologists have a greater success rate removing objects in this area (Kadish, 2005). Spherical objects are the most difficult to remove and should be referred to otolaryngology. If available suctioning with a Schuknecht foreign body catheter with umbrella may work well.

- Straighten the ear canal by pulling on the pinna and gently shake the patient's head; occasionally the foreign body will fall out.
- Soft, irregularly shaped objects are generally graspable with a Bayonet forceps or curved hook.
- If the object is made of iron, nickel, or cobalt, try using a magnet to retrieve it.
- Kill insects in the ear canal before flushing. Ethanol, isopropyl alcohol, vinegar, 1% or 4% lidocaine, or lidocaine with epinephrine and water may be used to kill the insects (Anderson, 2005).
- Irrigation, if appropriate, should be done using a commercial irrigator or 60-mL syringe with an angiocatheter on the end. Irrigation may only serve to push the object further into the ear canal (Shroeder, 2004).
  - Do not irrigate if the object is a disk battery or vegetable matter or if the TM is not intact (Anderson, 2005; Kadish, 2005).
- Refer the patient to an otolaryngologist if you are unable to extract the object on the first attempt, cannot remove the object without causing further damage or worse pain, the child is unable to cooperate, or the foreign body has a higher likelihood of failure (in the medial third of the ear canal, spherical shape, etc.) (Kadish, 2005).

- Ear blocks (regional anesthesia) are not recommended.
- Consider conscious sedation if the clinical setting is appropriate (Brown, 2004).
- Topical antibiotic drops with steroid are recommended for any drainage and to decrease inflammation.

Complications

Infection, perforation of the TM, and damage to the ossicles are possible if the object is not removed.

Prevention

Educate children and their parents not to put objects in the ear.

ACUTE OTITIS MEDIA

Description

AOM is an acute infection of the middle ear (see Color Plate). The AAP and AAFP Clinical Practice Guidelines (2004a) require the presence of the following three components to diagnose AOM:

- Recent, abrupt onset of signs and symptoms of middle ear inflammation and effusion (ear pain, irritability, otorrhea and/or fever)
- MEE as confirmed by bulging TM; limited or absent mobility by pneumatic otoscopy; air-fluid level behind TM; otorrhea
- Signs and symptoms of middle ear inflammation as confirmed by distinct erythema of the TM or distinct otalgia interfering with normal sleep or activity

Characteristics of different types of AOM are defined in Table 29-5.

Epidemiology

AOM often follows eustachian tube dysfunction (ETD). Young children have shorter, more horizontal, and more flaccid eustachian tubes that are easily disrupted by viruses, which predisposes them to AOM. Day care attendance is also a significant risk factor. Other risk factors include being white, a male, and having a history of ear infections in

TABLE 29-5	**Types of Acute Otitis Media**
Type	**Characteristics**
AOM	Suppurative effusion of the middle ear
Bullous myringitis	AOM in which bullae form between the inner and middle layers of the TM and bulge outward
Persistent AOM	AOM that has not resolved when antibiotic therapy has been completed or AOM recurs within days of treatment
Recurrent AOM	Three separate bouts of AOM within a 6-month period or four within a 12-month period; often a positive family history of OM and other ENT disease in family

AOM, Acute otitis media; *ENT,* ear, nose, throat; *TM,* tympanic membrane.

parents or siblings. Predisposing factors include upper respiratory infection, bottle propping during feedings, ETS, asthma and allergies, cleft palate, and Down syndrome. ETS leads to functional eustachian tube obstruction and decreases the protective ciliary action in the eustachian tube. When the eustachian tube is obstructed, negative pressure develops as air is absorbed in the middle ear (see Color Plate). The negative pressure pulls fluid from the mucosal lining and causes an accumulation of sterile fluid. Bacteria pulled in from the eustachian tube lead to the accumulation of purulent fluid.

S. pneumoniae, Haemophilus influenzae, and *M. catarrhalis* are the most common infecting organisms (Pelton, 2005). In the past, the distribution of these organisms was *S. pneumoniae* (30% to 50%), *H. influenzae* (15% to 30%) and *M. catarrhalis* (10% to 15%). With the introduction of the heptavalent pneumococcal conjugate vaccine (PCV7 or Prevnar) in 2000, the incidence of AOM caused by *S. pneumoniae* has decreased by 80% for children under 2 years old; it has also decreased infections in older children. In some areas, however, there has been an increase in AOM caused by other serotypes of *S. pneumoniae* that are not contained in the PCV7. There has also been up to a twofold increase in nontypable *H Influenza,* especially B-lactamase positive strains (Block & Correa, 2006; Block et al, 2004; Casey & Pichichero, 2004; Revai et al, 2006). Respiratory syncytial virus and influenza are two of the viruses most responsible for the increase in the incidence of AOM seen from January to April.

Although immunization with pneumococcal vaccine has affected the types of pathogens causing AOM, the change may also be attributed to the recommendations made in the 1990s: curtailing the use of prophylactic chemoprophylaxis; reducing the use of antibiotics in OME; and observing AOM with pain treatment before initiating antibiotics (Harrison, 2005).

Children with recurrent AOM are more likely to have a family history of AOM and have other ear, nose, and throat (ENT) diseases. Most episodes of AOM occur in the first 24 months of life, with almost 50% of infants in the U.S. having their first AOM before 6 months old. Sixty-five percent to 90% of children will suffer at least one episode by 2 years old (Siegel & Bien, 2004). AOM is the most common indication for antibiotic prescriptions in the U.S. (Friedman et al, 2006).

Clinical Findings

History. Rapid onset of signs and symptoms:

- Ear pain with possible ear pulling in the infant; may interfere with activity and/or sleep
- Irritability in an infant or toddler
- Otorrhea
- Fever

Other key factors or symptoms:

- Prematurity or craniofacial anomalies or congenital syndromes associated with craniofacial anomalies
- Exposure to risk factors (ETD, bottle propping, ETS, and day care)
- Disrupted sleep or inability to sleep
- Lethargy, dizziness, tinnitus, and unsteady gait
- Diarrhea and vomiting

- Sudden hearing loss
- Stuffy nose, rhinorrhea, and sneezing
- Rare facial palsy and ataxia

Physical Examination

- Presence of MEE, confirmed by pneumatic otoscopy, tympanometry or acoustic reflectometry, as evidenced by:
  - Bulging TM (see Color Plate)
  - Absent or decreased mobility of the TM (see Color Plate)
  - Air-fluid level behind the TM
  - Otorrhea
- Signs and symptoms of middle ear inflammation indicated by either:
  - Erythema of the TM *or*
  - Distinct otalgia that interferes with normal activity or sleep

  In addition, the following TM findings may be present:
- Increased vascularity and obscured or absent landmarks (see Color Fig. 4).
- Red, yellow, or purple color (redness alone should not be used to diagnose AOM, especially in a crying child)
- Thin-walled, sagging bullae filled with straw-colored fluid seen with bullous myringitis

Diagnostic Studies.   Tympanometry reflects effusion (type B pattern). Tympanocentesis to identify the infecting organism is helpful in the treatment of infants younger than 2 months old. In older infants and children, tympanocentesis is rarely done and is useful only if the patient is in a toxic state or immunocompromised or in the presence of resistant infection or acute pain from bullous myringitis (Bluestone & Klein, 2004). If a tympanocentesis is warranted, refer the patient to an otolaryngologist for this procedure.

Differential Diagnosis

OME, mastoiditis, dental abscess, sinusitis, lymphadenitis, parotitis, peritonsillar abscess, trauma, ETD, impacted teeth, temporomandibular joint dysfunction, and immune deficiency are differential diagnoses. Any infant 2 months old or younger with an AOM should be evaluated for fever without focus and not just treated for an ear infection.

Management

Over the last decade, changes have been made in the treatment of OM primarily because of the increasing rate of antibiotic-resistant bacteria related to the injudicious use of antibiotics. Ample evidence has been presented that symptom management is all that is required because many cases of AOM, usually those caused by *H. influenzae* or *M. catarrhalis*, resolve without antibiotics (Friedman et al, 2006; Siegel & Bien, 2004). Treatment options are decided based on the child's age, the illness severity, and the certainty of diagnosis (Fig. 29-4).

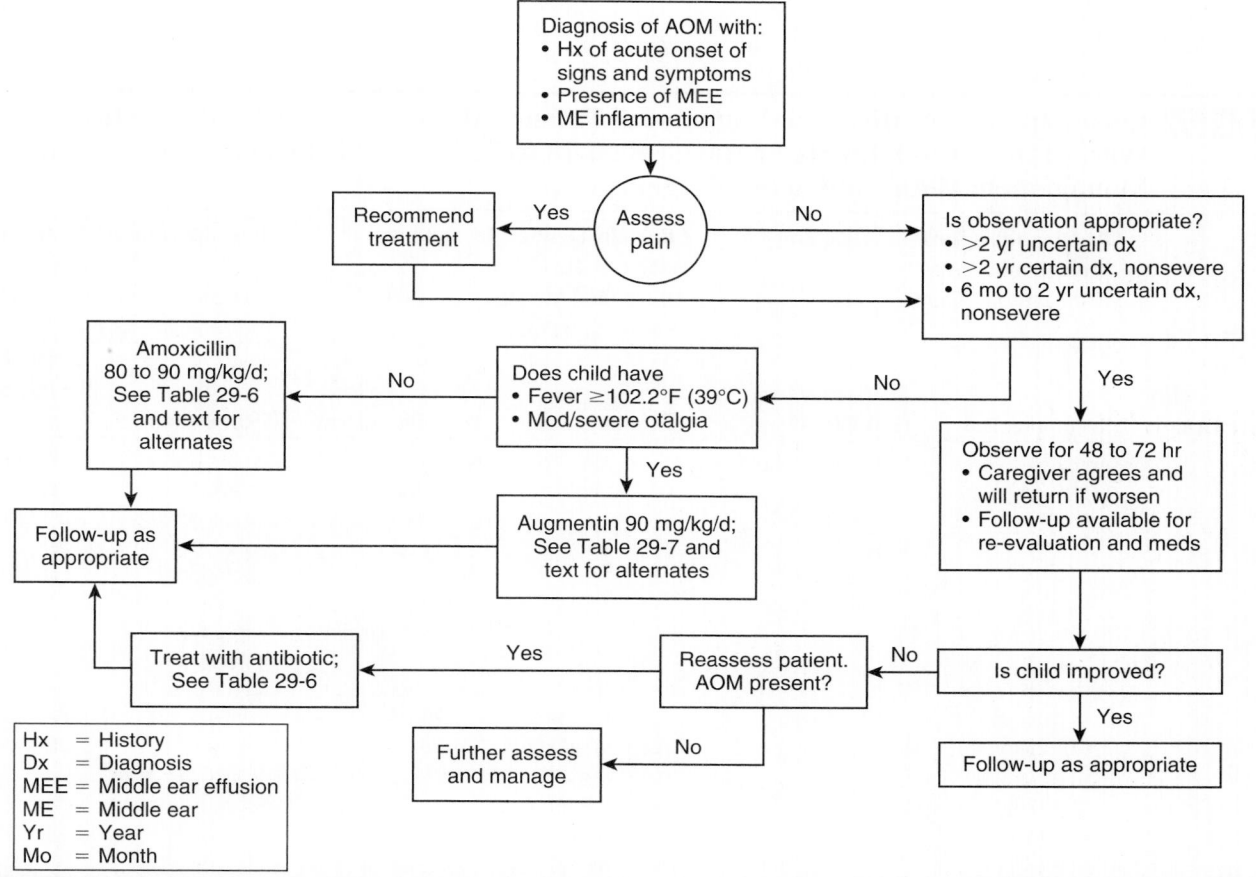

FIG. 29-4   Management of AOM. (Also see Tables 29-4, 29-5, 29-6, and 29-7.) (Data from American Academy of Pediatrics (AAP) and American Academy of Family Physicians: Clinical practice guideline: diagnosis and management of acute otitis media, *Pediatrics* 113[5], 2004.)

1. Pain management is the first principle of treatment.
   - Acetaminophen or ibuprofen should be given as needed for pain or fever management.
   - Topical analgesic agents, such as benzocaine or antipyrine/benzocaine otic preparations (Auralgan), for pain relief in children older than 5 years in the absence of perforation or PETs; naturopathic agents have comparable relief.
   - Distraction, oil application, or external use of heat or cold may be of some use.
2. Observation or "watchful waiting" for 48 to 72 hours allows the patient to improve without antibacterial treatment. Pain relief should be provided, and a means of follow-up must be in place; options for follow-up include:
   - Parent-initiated visit or phone call for worsening or no improvement.
   - Scheduled follow-up appointment.
   - Routine follow-up phone call.
   - Antibiotic prescription to fill if child is not improved.
   - Communication with the parent, reevaluation, and the ability to obtain medication must be in place.
   - Watchful waiting option can be used for children as outlined in Table 29-6.
   - After 48 to 72 hours, if a child has not showed improvement in ear symptomatology, the presence of AOM should be confirmed or excluded, and antibacterial therapy should be started (Table 29-7).

TABLE 29-6 Criteria for Antibacterial Agent Treatment or Observation in Children With Acute Otitis Media

Age	Certain Diagnosis	Uncertain Diagnosis
<6 months	Antibacterial therapy	Antibacterial therapy
6 months to 2 years	Antibacterial therapy	Antibacterial therapy if severe illness; observation option* if nonsevere illness
≥2 years	Antibacterial therapy if severe illness; observation option* if nonsevere illness	Observation option*

*Observation option discussed in text; see details.
From American Academy of Pediatrics (AAP) and American Academy of Family Physicians: Clinical practice guideline: diagnosis and management of acute otitis media, *Pediatrics* 113(5), 2004, p 1454.

TABLE 29-7 Recommended Antibacterial Agents for Patients Who Are Being Treated Initially With Antibacterial Agents or Have Failed 48 to 72 Hours of Observation or Initial Management With Antibacterial Agents

Temperature 102.2° F (≥39° C) and/or Severe Otalgia	At Diagnosis for Patients Being Treated Initially With Antibacterial Agents		Clinically Defined Treatment Failure at 48–72 Hours After Initial Management With Observation Option		Clinically Defined Treatment Failure at 48–72 Hours After Initial Management With Antibacterial Agents	
	Recommended	Alternative for Penicillin Allergy	Recommended	Alternative for Penicillin Allergy	Recommended	Alternative for Penicillin Allergy
No	Amoxicillin, 80-90mg/kg/day	Non-type I: cefdinir, cefuroxime, cefpodoxime; Type I:* azithromycin, clarithromycin	Amoxicillin, 80-90mg/kg/day	Non-type I: cefdinir, cefuroxime, cefpodoxime; Type I:* azithromycin, clarithromycin	Amoxicillin-clavulanate, 90mg/kg/day of amoxicillin component, with 6.4 mg/kg/day of clavulanate	Non-type I ceftriaxone, 3 days, Type I: * clindamycin
Yes	Amoxicillin-clavulanate, 90mg/kg/day of amoxicillin, with 6.4mg/kg/day of clavulanate	Ceftriaxone, 1 or 3 days	Amoxicillin-clavulanate, 90 mg/kg/day of amoxicillin, with 6.4mg/kg/day of clavulanate	Ceftriaxone, 1 or 3 days	Ceftriaxone, 3 days	Tympano-centesis, clindamycin

*Type I allergic reaction is an anaphylactic reaction.
From American Academy of Pediatrics (AAP) and American Academy of Family Physicians: Clinical practice guideline: diagnosis and management of acute otitis media, *Pediatrics* 113(5), 2004, p 1454.

- Watchful waiting studies in children 6 months to 12 years old with nonsevere AOM have demonstrated the safety, effectiveness, and decreased antibiotic use when parents share in the decision-making and there is close follow-up (Finkelstein et al, 2005; McCormick et al, 2005; Merenstein et al, 2005). Likewise, watchful waiting, provided there is close follow-up, does not increase the incidence of mastoiditis (Little, 2006; Marcy et al, 2001).

3. Antibacterial therapy should be instituted for: all children under 6 months old with a diagnosis of AOM; for those 6 months to 2 years old with a definitive diagnosis; and for children older than 2 years with severe illness. See Table 29-6.
   - Amoxicillin remains the first-line antibiotic for AOM with a dosage of 80 to 90 mg/kg/day divided in two doses.
   - With severe illness (fever greater than 102.2° F[39° C] or moderate to severe otalgia) or suspected B-lactamase bacteria, amoxicillin-clavulanate should be started at 90 mg/kg/day of amoxicillin component, with 6.4 mg/kg/day of clavulanate divided in two doses.

   If there is a documented hypersensitivity reaction to amoxicillin, the following antibiotics are acceptable:
   - Nontype I hypersensitivity reaction
     - Cefdinir 14 mg/kg/day in one or two doses
     - Cefpodoxime 10 mg/kg/day once daily
     - Cefuroxime 30 mg/kg/day in two divided doses
   - Type 1 hypersensitivity reaction, macrolides can be used, though they provide poor coverage for *H. influenzae*:
     - Azithromycin (10 mg/kg on day 1 and 5 mg/kg on days 2 to 5)
     - Clarithromycin (15 mg/kg/day in two divided doses)
   - Other possibilities include:
     - Erythromycin-sulfisoxazole (50 mg/kg/day of erythromycin)—not an option for treatment failure.
     - Clindamycin 30 to 40 mg/kg/day in three divided doses (may be considered for ceftriaxone failure).
     - Ceftriaxone 50 mg/kg given parenterally daily in one to three doses is effective for the vomiting child, the child unable to tolerate oral medications, or the child who has failed amoxicillin-clavulanate (3 days of treatment is felt to be superior, AAP, 2004b).
   - A listing of medications that are acceptable to treat OM is found in Table 29-8.

4. Recommendations for follow-up include:
   - After 48 to 72 hours, if a child has not showed improvement in ear symptomatology, the child should be seen to confirm or exclude the presence of AOM. If the initial management option was an antibacterial agent, the agent should be changed.
   - If the child shows clinical improvement, follow-up in 3 to 4 weeks is recommended.

5. Optimal treatment duration for AOM is uncertain. Most studies support the 10-day therapy course for children younger than 6 years old and for children with severe disease. A shorter course (5 to 7 days) is acceptable for treating uncomplicated AOM in children older than 6 years.

6. Persistent and recurrent AOM
   - Persistent AOM occurs when antibiotic therapy has been completed and evidence of AOM is still present, or AOM recurs within days of treatment. Retreatment with a broader-spectrum antibiotic is suggested.
   - Persistent MEE is common after resolution of acute symptoms and should not be seen as a need for continuing antibiotics (see section on OME).
   - Recurrent AOM is present when more than three distinct and well-documented bouts of AOM have occurred in 6 months or four or more episodes in 12 months.

7. An otolaryngology referral is indicated when appropriate therapy for OM has failed. Myringotomy or placement of PETs can help relieve discomfort and decrease the likelihood of further infection. Indications for tympanostomy and the insertion of PETs are listed in Box 29-3 and discussed in an earlier section. Every child with recurrent or persistent AOM must be considered on an individual basis for the placement of PETs.

8. The pediatric provider is encouraged to keep current on updated recommendations for the treatment of AOM because of the rapid changes in resistance patterns and newly developed treatments.

9. Other issues in treating AOM
   - Decongestants and antihistamines are not helpful in the treatment of AOM.
   - Antimicrobial ototopical drops (ofloxacin, ciprofloxacin, or Cortisporin) or ophthalmic drops (tobramycin or gentamicin) are indicated if the TM is perforated, the child has otorrhea, or has patent, draining PETs. Oral antibiotics are not needed in the case of functioning PETs.
   - Xylitol, a sugar found in fruits and the bark of birch trees, has bacteriostatic effects against S. pneumoniae and interferes with bacterial adhesion to mucous membranes. It appears to have some suppressive effects in preventing ear infections. Having the child chew at least three to five sticks a day of xylitol chewing gum may reduce the recurrence rate. However, there are conflicting data about its ability to decrease the number of episodes of AOM; side effects can include excessive gas and diarrhea (Tonnaer et al, 2006).
   - There is no safe or effective herbal treatment for the treatment of AOM or OME; however, there was one study showing that homeopathy resulted in fewer symptoms and treatment failures than with placebo. Homeopathy may be an adjunct for those wishing to hold off on using antibiotics for their child (Kemper, 2002).

Complications

Persistent AOM, persistent OME, TM perforation (see Color Plate), OE, mastoiditis, cholesteatoma, tympanosclerosis (see Color Plate), hearing loss of 25 to 30 dB for several months, ossicle necrosis, pseudotumor cerebri, cerebral thrombophlebitis, and facial paralysis are possible complications.

Prevention and Education

The following interventions, shown to be helpful in preventing AOM, should be encouraged:
- PCV7 is recommended because it has decreased the incidence of pneumococcal AOM (Pelton, 2005; Block, 2005; Block et al, 2004).

TABLE 29-8	Medications Used to Treat Acute Otitis Media	
Drug	**Dose**	**Comments**
Amoxicillin	40-90 mg/kg/day every 12 hr	First choice unless contraindicated
Amoxicillin-clavulanate (Augmentin)	40-90 mg/kg/day every 12 hr with clavulanate <10 mg/kg/day	Good β-lactamase coverage; costly and more likely to cause diarrhea
Amoxicillin-clavulanate (Augmentin 600 ES)	90/6.4 mg/kg/day every 12 hr	Higher amoxicillin per tsp than Augmentin; less diarrhea than with Augmentin
Azithromycin (Zithromax)	10 mg/kg/day on day 1 (max dose 500 mg/day) then 5 mg/kg/day on days 2-5 given daily (max dose 250 mg/day)	Children older than 6 mo, 5-day treatment course; macrolide; primarily used with penicillin allergy
Cefdinir (Omnicef)	14 mg/kg/day every 12 hr or daily	Broad-spectrum third-generation cephalosporin
Cefixime (Suprax)	8 mg/kg every 12 hr or daily	Broad-spectrum third-generation cephalosporin; reduced efficacy against *S. pneumonia*
Cefpodoxime (Vantin)	10 mg/kg/day daily	Broad-spectrum of coverage, costly; third-generation cephalosporin
Cefprozil (Cefzil)	30 mg/kg/day every 12 hr	Broad-spectrum of coverage, cost similar to other cephalosporins; intermediate potency second-generation cephalosporin; moderate taste
Ceftibuten (Cedax)	9 mg/kg/day given daily	Children older than 6 mo; third-generation cephalosporin; active against β-lactamase; reduced efficacy against *S. pneumonia*
Ceftriaxone (Rocephin)	50 mg/kg/day IM in 1-3 doses over 3 days	Costly; third-generation cephalosporin
Cefuroxime (Ceftin)	30 mg/kg/day every 12 hr	Broad-spectrum of coverage, costly; most potent second-generation cephalosporin; poor taste
	125 mg every 12 hr if younger than 2 yr old 250 mg every 12 hr if 2-12 yr old 250-500 mg every 12 hr if older than 12 yr	
Clarithromycin (Biaxin)	15 mg/kg/day every 12 hr	Children older than 6 mo; macrolide; primarily used with penicillin allergy
Clindamycin	30-40 mg/kg/day given every 8 hr	

hr, Hours; *IM,* intramuscularly; *IV,* intravenously; *max,* maximum; *mo,* months; *yr,* years.
From American Academy of Pediatrics (AAP) and American Academy of Family Physicians: Clinical practice guideline: diagnosis and management of acute otitis media, *Pediatrics* 113(5), 2004, p 1454.

- Annual influenza vaccine may help prevent OM, especially in high-risk children who attend day care centers (Ozgur et al, 2006). Early treatment of influenza with the antiviral oseltamivir can also help reduce OM (Meissner, 2005).
  - *H. influenzae* type b vaccine, although recommended, is not helpful in the prevention of AOM because the *H. influenzae* responsible for AOM is usually nontypable.
- Xylitol chewing gum, as discussed previously.
  The following issues should be addressed:
- Exclusive breastfeeding until at least 6 months old is protective against single and recurrent episodes of AOM (Chantry et al, 2006).
- If the child is in day care, a less populated child care environment may need to be considered.
- Avoid bottle propping, feeding infants lying down, and passive smoke exposure.
- Avoid the use of pacifiers. Although the relationship cannot be fully explained, multiple studies have shown that pacifier use increases the incidence of AOM (Siegel & Bien, 2004).

- Educate regarding the problem of drug-resistant bacteria and the need to avoid the use of antibiotics unless absolutely necessary; if antibiotics are used, the child needs to complete the entire course of the prescription and keep the follow-up appointment.

OTITIS MEDIA WITH EFFUSION

Description

The diagnosis of OME is made when there is evidence of MEE or fluid without signs or symptoms of acute ear infection (see Color Plate). MEE decreases the mobility of the TM and interferes with sound conduction.

Epidemiology

OME can occur spontaneously with ETD caused by an inflammatory process after AOM, viral illness, anatomic abnormalities, barotrauma, allergies, or a combination of these conditions. ETD changes the middle ear mucosa in the following sequence: (1) the mucosa becomes secretory with increased mucus production; (2) the mucus becomes viscous as the mucosa absorbs water; and (3) fluid becomes stuck behind the TM. Bacterial biofilms may explain the persistence of OME; biofilms are mixed microorganisms enclosed in a polymeric matrix that adhere to surfaces, such as the middle ear mucosa (Hall-Stoodley et al, 2006; Tonnaer et al, 2006).

In another process, ETD causes OME, which then becomes AOM. OME is a natural consequence of both treated and untreated AOM. Approximately 90% of children will have OME at some time before school age, with an increased frequency between 6 months and 4 years old. Most episodes of OME resolve within 3 months, but 30% to 40% will have recurrent OME (AAP, 2004b). Renko et al (2006) found that almost 70% were effusion free within 2 weeks of diagnosis, with a median of 50 days.

Risk factors for chronic OME are listed in Box 29-5.

Clinical Findings

History.   The following features may be noted in the affected child:

- Often asymptomatic, afebrile, with mild, intermittent or no complaints of ear pain
- Fullness in the ear, "popping" or the feeling of "talking in a barrel"
- Complaint of hearing loss in older children
- Dizziness or impaired balance
- Chronic vomiting with failure to thrive, which can be related to chronic OME

Physical Examination.   Pneumatic otoscopy reveals decreased TM mobility and is the primary tool used to diagnose OME. An abnormal-appearing TM, often described as dull, varying from bulging and opaque with no visible landmarks to retracted and translucent with visible landmarks and an air-fluid level or bubble, may be seen (see Color plate). Head and neck structures should be examined for abnormalities.

Diagnostic Studies.   The tympanogram is flat-type B. The audiogram can show hearing loss of 15 to 31 dB.

Differential Diagnosis

Differential diagnoses include AOM; all causes of hearing loss and anatomic abnormalities; unilateral OME can indicate nasopharyngeal carcinoma.

Management

Recommendations in the 2004 OME guidelines (AAP, 2004b) pertaining to children 2 months to 12 years old include:

- Documenting in the medical record at each visit the presence and duration of effusion, whether it is unilateral or bilateral, and any associated symptoms
- Identifying children at risk for speech, language, or learning problems
- Using watchful waiting in those children who are not at risk because of the likelihood of spontaneous resolution of OME

1. At-risk children are defined as having developmental delays because of sensory, physical, cognitive, or behavioral factors (e.g., hearing loss independent of OME, speech or language delays, pervasive or other developmental disorders, syndromes or craniofacial disorders, blindness, cleft palate). These children should be promptly referred for hearing, speech, and language evaluation.

2. Children considered not at risk should be watched for 3 months from the onset of effusion or diagnosis because 75% to 90% of effusion resulting from AOM resolves within 3 months.
   - Follow-up during the 3 months with pneumatic otoscopy and/or tympanogram is at the clinician's discretion.
   - Reexamination is recommended at 3- to 6-month intervals until the effusion dissipates, significant hearing loss is identified, or structural abnormalities of the TM or middle ear are suspected (retraction pockets, ossicular erosion, areas of atelectasis or atrophy)
   - Hearing and language testing is recommended if OME lasts for 3 months or longer or at any point if language delay, learning problems, or significant hearing loss is suspected. Box 29-6 lists risk factors for hearing loss.

3. Referral rationale, expectations, and decision-making process should be communicated to the parent when referral to an otolaryngologist is made. Duration of effusion, reason for referral, and any relevant information should be communicated to the otolaryngologist.

Bilateral myringotomy with insertion of tympanostomy tubes is recommended in children with:

- Documented bilateral effusion that persists 4 months or longer
- An identified persistent hearing loss
- Sensory, physical, cognitive, or behavior factors that make a child more susceptible for developmental delay or disorder

---

BOX 29-5   Risk Factors for Chronic OME or Longer Duration of OME

Environmental
- Group child care
- Number of hours in child care
- Exposure to children at home or in child care
- Number of smokers and cigarettes smoked in household
- Feeding in supine position
- Shorter duration of breastfeeding
- Autumn season

Characteristics of Child or Specific Disease History
- Early onset of OM
- Several prior episodes
- Bilateral OME
- Male gender
- Lower socioeconomic status
- Having a sibling with a history of OM

AOM, Acute otitis meida; *OM,* otitis media; *OME,* otitis media with effusion.
NOTE: Many of these are also implicated in the increased risk of AOM and recurrent OM.

BOX 29-6   Risk Factors for Hearing Loss Caused by OME*

- Bilateral OME for 4 months or longer
- If two or more present:
  - OME present for longer than 8 weeks
  - Speech development slower than peers
  - Speech less clear than previously
  - Child decreases amount of talking
  - Child less responsive to name and other familiar sounds
  - Child says "Huh?" or "What?" frequently
  - Child sits close to TV or wants volume louder
  - Child has difficulty learning (reading, spelling)
  - Child is hyperactive or overly inattentive

*Child should be tested audiologically if one or two of the above are present.
OME, Otitis media with effusion.
Modified from Daly KA, Hunter LL, Giebink GS: Chronic otitis media with effusion, *Pediatr Rev* 20(3):89, 1999.

- Recurrent or persistent OME regardless of his or her hearing status
- Structural damage to the TM or middle ear
4. Other recommendations:
   - There is insufficient evidence of therapeutic efficacy for either antihistamines or decongestants and the adverse effects of these agents are well known. Limited studies suggest OME associated with allergies may be helped by antihistamine (Nowak-Wegrzyn, 2005).
   - Antimicrobial therapy and corticosteroids do not have long-term efficacy and are not recommended for routine management of OME.
   - Tonsillectomy or adenoidectomy alone should not be used to treat OME.
   - The use of complementary and alternative medicine as a treatment for OME lacks scientific evidence documenting efficacy and the uncertain balance of harm and benefit.

Complications

Complications include recurrent AOM and hearing loss that may be temporary conductive or, over time, permanent high-frequency SNHL. It is debated how much of an effect chronic OME has on cognitive ability, language, and learning, including attention and behavior.

Prevention and Education

- Stress the importance of follow-up until the TM and hearing are normal. Advise parents of the length of time (weeks to months) required for resolution of OME.
- Remind parents of their important role in language development of their child. Conversation and parent interaction through reading and play, along with affirmative sounds and gestures, are the most important factors in language development and school readiness.

- Strategies for maximizing hearing for the child:
  - Face the child and get within 3 feet before speaking.
  - Enunciate clearly, speak slower and louder.
  - Use visual clues and repeat as necessary.
  - Turn off competing background noise (music, radio, television).
  - Request preferential seating in the classroom.

CHOLESTEATOMA

Description

Cholesteatoma is an epidermal inclusion cyst of the middle ear or mastoid consisting of desquamated debris from the keratinizing, squamous epithelial lining of the middle ear (see Color Plate).

Epidemiology

Cholesteatomas can be congenital or acquired. Varied theories explaining their formation include the following: an inflammatory process, perforation of the TM, and failure of desquamated tissue to clear from the middle ear. The incidence rate is unknown.

Clinical Findings

History.   The history can include:
- Chronic OM with malodorous purulent otorrhea
- Vertigo and hearing loss

Physical Examination.   A pearly white lesion is present on or behind the TM. Aural polyps are considered cholesteatomas unless proven otherwise. Congenital cholesteatomas are often in the most anterior, inferior position of the TM.

Differential Diagnosis

Tympanosclerosis, debris from chronic OME, malignant rhabdomyosarcoma, and aural polyps are some of the differential diagnoses.

Management

Accurate diagnosis and immediate otolaryngologic referral for surgical excision are needed.

Complications

Complications include irreversible structural damage, permanent bone damage, facial nerve palsy, hearing loss, and intracranial infection, especially in untreated cases.

MASTOIDITIS

Description

Mastoiditis is a suppurative infection of the mastoid cells.

Epidemiology

Mastoiditis may accompany OM. The mucoperiosteal lining of the mastoid air cells becomes inflamed, with subsequent progressive swelling and obstruction of drainage from the mastoid. Common organisms identified include *S. pneumoniae, H. influenzae, M. catarrhalis, S. aureus, S. pyogenes,* and *Mycobacterium tuberculosis* (rare). Gram-negative organisms, such as *E. coli, Proteus,* or *Pseudomonas* are more common in chronic mastoiditis, in more virulent infections, and in young infants. Antibiotic treatment for AOM does not safeguard against and may actually mask mastoiditis with a normal TM. Intracranial complications of mastoiditis are not rare and may develop despite treatment.

The exact incidence is unknown; however, it is described as low since the introduction of antibiotics. It is most common between 2 months to 18 years old, with a peak between 6 to 13 months old; gender distribution is equal. Although uncommon, it is potentially life threatening. Watchful waiting with AOM or OME has not increased the incidence of acute mastoiditis (Rosenfeld, 2004b).

Clinical Findings

History and Physical Examination.
- Concurrent or recurrent AOM
- Fever and otalgia
- Persistent OM unresponsive to antibiotic therapy
- Postauricular swelling

Infants may have swelling above the ear, displacing the pinna inferiorly or laterally. In older children, the swelling pushes the earlobe superiorly and laterally.

Diagnostic Studies.   Radiography may show coalescence of mastoid air cells and loss of bony trabeculation, though this may lag behind clinical findings.
- CT can provide definitive anatomic information.
- Tympanocentesis with culture and Gram stain help identify offending organism.

Management

Urgent ENT referral is imperative. Hospitalization, intravenous antibiotics, and mastoidectomy are usually required.

Prevention

The pneumococcal conjugate vaccine may reduce the incidence of mastoiditis caused by *S. pneumoniae*.

SENSORINEURAL AND CONDUCTIVE HEARING LOSS

Description

Hearing loss is defined as bilateral pure-tone hearing loss of 40 dB or more at frequencies of 500, 1000, and 2000 Hz in the better ear. Three types of hearing loss are recognized—sensorineural, conductive, central—although there may also be a combined type. Either or both ears may be involved. Before the institution of universal newborn hearing screening, many children with profound hearing loss were not identified until 18 to 36 months old, and many children with mild hearing loss were not identified until 4 years old (Gregg, 2004; Jacobson & Jacobson, 2004).

Sensorineural hearing loss (SNHL) is most commonly associated with dysfunction of or damage to the cochlea (inner ear) and less often associated with damage to the auditory nerve (eighth cranial nerve) (Gregg et al, 2004). SNHL that is related to the auditory nerve is usually labeled auditory neuropathy or auditory dyssynchrony, neither of which are amenable to treatment with hearing aids, but may respond to cochlear implants. SNHL can be congenital or acquired, be mild or severe, and is permanent.

Conductive hearing loss, either congenital or acquired, results from blocked transmission of sound waves from the EAC to the inner ear (e.g., AOM, OME). The cochlea functions normally. Bone conduction is usually normal with decreased air conduction. Conductive hearing loss is usually in the range of 20 to 60 dB (Gregg, 2004). MEEs result in an average hearing loss of 27 to 31 dB.

Mixed hearing loss occurs when there are abnormalities identified in outer, middle, and inner ear spaces. Central hearing loss occurs when the nerves or nuclei of the central nervous system, either in the pathways to the brain or the brain itself, are damaged or impaired (Kenna, 2004).

Epidemiology

SNHL and conductive hearing loss can be associated with craniofacial anomalies (e.g., aural atresia, cleft lip or cleft palate, external ear deformity without atresia, dysmorphic facies without external ear deformity), genetic aberrations or congenital deformities (e.g., white forelock, café au lait spots, family history of SNHL, metabolic abnormalities), or environmental exposure (e.g., ototoxic drugs, bacterial or viral meningitis, other infectious diseases, loud noises, head trauma) (Kenna, 2004).

SNHL can occur when hair cells in the cochlea are injured by exposure to excessive noise over a variable period. SNHL can also come from prenatal and perinatal exposure (e.g., intrauterine infections, toxic chemicals, erythroblastosis fetalis). It is estimated that 80% of congenital SNHL is due to recessive inheritance (Nance, 2003). Recently, multiple genes associated with various types of SNHL have been identified.

Conductive hearing loss can also be congenital or acquired. Congenital causes include aural stenosis or atresia and ossicle malformations. Acquired conductive hearing loss can be caused by AOM, OME, foreign bodies in the ear canal, cerumen impaction, TM perforation, cholesteatoma, ossicular discontinuity, collapsing ear canals, otosclerosis, and tympanosclerosis (Gregg et al, 2004).

The overall prevalence of congenital deafness is estimated to be 1 in 1000 births. The incidence for varying degrees of hearing loss in healthy infants is 3 in 1000 and increases to 6 in 1000 when well and at-risk infants are pooled together (Gregg et al, 2004). The incidence of bilateral mild (20 to 40 dB) to moderately severe hearing (60 to 70 dB) SNHL for children is 2 to 4 per 1000, and for children with significant unilateral hearing loss the incidence is 10 per 1000 (Nozza, 2002).

Clinical Findings

History.   Hearing loss is often a "silent disease." Careful consideration and attention to identified risk factors are essential in identifying hearing loss in children.

The risk factors for SNHL in newborns include the following (Joint Committee on Infant Hearing, 2000a, 2000b; Kenna, 2004):
- Birth weight less than 1500 g
- Severe depression at birth (e.g., Apgar score of 0 to 3 at 5 minutes, failure to initiate a response by 10 minutes, or hypotonia at up to 2 hours old)
- Neonatal intensive care unit admission for 2 days or longer

- Prolonged mechanical ventilation for greater than 10 days
- Persistent pulmonary hypertension
- Long Q-T syndrome (usually profound hearing loss)
- Congenital infections, such as toxoplasmosis, bacterial meningitis, syphilis, rubella, cytomegalovirus, and herpes
- Metabolic disorders, such as PKU and galactosemia
- Endocrine disorders, such as adrenal hyperplasia and hypothyroidism
- Craniofacial anomalies, including morphologic abnormalities of the pinna and ear canal
- Genetic syndromes, such as sickle cell disease, Usher syndrome, neurofibromatosis, Waardenburg syndrome, osteopetrosis, or findings associated with other genetic syndromes known to include hearing loss
- Hyperbilirubinemia requiring exchange transfusion or causing kernicterus
- Family history of hereditary childhood SNHL
- Ototoxic drug exposure

The risk factors for hearing loss in children 1 month to 3 years old include the following (Joint Committee on Infant Hearing, 2000a, 2000b; Kenna, 2004):

- Parental or caregiver concern regarding hearing, speech, language, or developmental delay; parents tend to be about 12 months ahead of care providers in identifying hearing loss in children (Bachman & Arvedson, 1998)
- Kidney malformation
- Family history of permanent childhood hearing loss
- Stigmata or other findings associated with a syndrome known to include SNHL, conductive hearing loss, or ETD
- Syndromes associated with progressive hearing loss, such as neurofibromatosis and osteopetrosis
- Neurodegenerative disorders, such as Hunter syndrome, or sensorimotor neuropathies, such as Friedreich ataxia and Charcot-Marie-Tooth disease
- Head trauma with loss of consciousness or skull fracture
- Bacterial meningitis
- Ototoxic medication exposure
- Diabetes mellitus
- Recurrent or persistent OME for at least 3 months

Other risk factors or indicators for hearing loss include the following:

- Failure to learn to speak at the appropriate age or failure to respond to auditory stimuli; speech that sounds like baby talk or is monotone and difficult to understand; avoidance of speaking
- Failed school screening audiogram; decreased note taking; seeming to misunderstand, ignore, confuse, or miss what is being said
- Aggression, increased physical complaints, difficulty in school and social situations
- Environmental exposure to firecrackers, toy cap pistols, firearms, loud music, loud television, squeaking toys, and machines (e.g., snowmobiles, farm equipment, lawn mowers)
- History of head or neck irradiation

Physical Examination. The following may be found in children with SNHL and conductive hearing loss:

- Abnormal hearing screening during routine well child care visits or other office visits. For children younger than 6 months old, an ABR test is recommended. Behavioral testing using a conditioned response or an ABR is appropriate for children older than 6 months.
- A complete physical examination with special attention to the eyes, skin, and skeletal and nervous systems is needed.
- Ears—preauricular pits, auricular malformation or appendage, abnormal TM integrity, or impaired mobility with pneumatic otoscopy.
- Eyes—cataracts, corneal opacities, coloboma, blindness, nystagmus, exophthalmos, night blindness, heterochromia iridis, or blue sclerae (associated with genetic disorders that can cause SNHL).
- Craniofacial anomalies or genetic stigmata associated with SNHL (see Epidemiology).

Diagnostic Studies. EOAE or ABR are the diagnostic tests used for newborn hearing screening. After that period of time, audiometry is the preferred hearing testing of choice. If the cause of the hearing impairment is evident (cholesteatoma, ossicle malformation, OM) then the diagnostic work-up is limited. If the cause of the hearing loss is not readily apparent, then consider the following diagnostic tests (Kenna, 2004):

- Urinalysis, serum blood urea nitrogen, and creatinine to rule out renal disease
- Complete blood count, thyroid function tests, sickle cell screen
- TORCH (toxoplasmosis, other agents, rubella, cytomegalovirus, herpes simplex) screen in newborns
- Genetic testing
- ECG (Long Q-T syndrome)
- Ophthalmologic examination (TORCH, retinitis pigmentosa associated with Usher Syndrome)
- CT as indicated to rule out inner ear malformation

Differential Diagnosis
Mixed SNHL with conductive hearing loss and central hearing loss are included in the differential diagnosis.

Management
The following should occur for any child with suspected hearing loss:

- Refer any child with suspected hearing loss to an audiologist and otolaryngologist for full evaluation as soon as possible. In the referral, include information about the patient's symptoms, history or physical findings, and any known diagnosis associated with hearing loss.
- Refer for surgical intervention as indicated.
- Treat known medically related conditions (diabetes, hypothyroidism).
- Genetic counseling.
- Encourage the use of amplification devices as appropriate. They may be personal (e.g., hearing aids) or group (e.g., teacher microphone).
- Cochlear implants with an external speech processor are sometimes used for profound SNHL. If implants are in place, assume proper immunizations are given.

- Recommend special school and teaching strategies, such as front-of-room placement and facing the child when speaking.
- Evaluate and treat AOM and OME if present (see the AOM and OME sections).
- Screen for hearing loss if bilateral MEE is present for 3 months or longer.
- Ensure a family-centered approach in making decisions regarding interventions for the child (e.g., Individuals with Disabilities Education Act [IDEA]).
- Refer to Chapter 16 for discussion of children who are deaf.

Complications

Significant hearing loss impedes speech, language, cognitive development, and social interaction skills.

Prevention

- Good prenatal care.
- Provide $Rh_o(D)$ immune globulin to prevent erythroblastosis fetalis in susceptible women.
- Treat prenatal and perinatal infections promptly.
- Avoid ototoxic drug use.
- Immunize against mumps, rubella, varicella, *H. influenzae* type b, *S. pneumoniae,* influenza, and other diseases that can cause SNHL through central nervous system damage.
- Recommend avoidance of environmental factors associated with hearing loss.

✓ DISCUSSION FORUM

1. The treatments of relatively well children with OM have changed to a watch and see approach. How would you handle a resistant parent who wants to dictate how you prescribe?
2. The insurance company will not cover a fluoroquinolone-based otic preparation for an 8-year-old with an external otitis following swimming in his pool for a week. What is your next step and why?
3. A 3-year-old has a foreign body in the ear canal. It turns out the foreign object is a roach. How do you inform the parent? What factors need to be considered?
4. A mother reports that her febrile sick-appearing 18-month-old with AOM is allergic to a variety of antibiotics. On careful questioning, the child gets diarrhea when these antibiotics are taken, but has no other side effects. Discuss this scenario.

RESOURCE BOX
Eye Problems

AHQR National Guideline Clearinghouse
www.guideline.gov

American Academy of Audiology
www.audiology.org

American Academy of Family Physicians
www.aafp.org

American Academy of Pediatrics Virtual Classroom
www.aap.org/otitismedia
Online case studies and pneumatic otoscopy course

Centers for Disease Control and Prevention
www.cdc.gov

Intermountain Ear, Nose, and Throat Online Center http//:intermountainhealthcare.org/xp/public/managehealth/patiented/otitismedia

Johns Hopkins University School of Medicine
A View Through the Otoscope:
Distinguishing Acute Otitis Media with Effusion

University of Michigan Health Topics Index
www.med.umich.edu/1libr/topics

University of Iowa Virtual Hospital Education Materials
www.uihealthcare.com/topics/medicaldepartments/otolaryngology/index.html

REFERENCES

American Academy of Otolaryngology-Head and Neck Surgery (AAO-HNS): Clinical practice guideline: acute otitis externa, *Otolaryngol Head Neck Surg* 134 2006, 54-523.
American Academy of Otolaryngology-Head and Neck Surgery (AAO-HNS): Noise and hearing protection. Available at www.entnet.org/healthinfo/hearing/noise_hearing.cfm (accessed February 2007).
American Academy of Pediatrics (AAP), American Academy of Family Physicians: Clinical practice guideline: diagnosis and management of acute otitis media, *Pediatrics* 113(5):1451-1465, 2004a.
American Academy of Pediatrics (AAP): Clinical practice guideline: Otitis media with effusion, *Pediatrics* 113(5):1213-1429, 2004b.
American Academy of Pediatrics (AAP) Section on Otolaryngology and Bronchoesophagology: Follow-up management of children with tympanostomy tubes, *Pediatrics* 109(2):328-329, 2002.
Anderson A: Removing foreign bodies with magnets and butter, *Pediatric News* 39(11), 2005.
Block S: Diagnosing acute otitis media: It's what you see, not what you hear, *Contemp Pediatr* 22(suppl. 12):3-8, 2005.
Block SL, Correa AG: Update on the management of pediatric acute otitis media and acute bacterial sinusitis, *Contemp Pediatr* 23(suppl. 12):1-10, 2006.
Block SL, Hedrick J, Harrison CJ, et al: Community-wide vaccination with the heptavalent pneumococcal conjugate significantly alters the microbiology of acute otitis media, *Pediatric Infect Dis J* 23(9):829-833, 2004.
Bluestone CD, Klein JO: Surgical and mechanical management. In *Otitis media in infants and children: management update,* Philadelphia, 2004, Elsevier.
Brown L, Denmark T, Wittlake W et al: Procedural sedation use in the ED: management of pediatric ear and nose foreign bodies, *Am J Emerg Med* 22:310-314, 2004.
Capoot GD et al: The child with otitis externa: current and comprehensive management, *Contemp Pediatr* (suppl.):4-18, 2002.
Casey JR: Treatment of acute otitis media post PCV &: judicious antibiotic therapy, *Contemp Pediatr* 23 (suppl. 12):16-23, 2006.
Casey JR, Pichichero ME: Changes in frequency and pathogens causing acute otitis media in 1995-2003, *Pediatric Infect Dis J* 23(9):824-828, 2004.

Chantry CJ, Howard CR, Auinger P: Full breastfeeding during and associated decrease in respiratory tract infection in US children, *Pediatrics* 117(2): 425-432, 2006.

DeMichelle A, Ruth R: *Newborn hearing screening for deafness.* Available at *www.emedicine.com/ent/topics576.htm,* 2005.

Dimmitt P: Cerumen removal products, *J Pediatr Health Care* 19(5):332-336, 2005.

Dohar J, Giles W, Roland P: Topical ciprofloxacin/dexamethasone superior to oral amoxicillin/clavulanic acid in acute otitis media with otorrhea through tympanostomy tubes, *Pediatrics* 118(3):e1-e9, 2006.

Dowell SF et al: Otitis media-principles of judicious use of antimicrobial agents, *Pediatrics* 101:165-171, 1998.

Engstrom, Removing foreign bodies with magnets and butter. *Clin Rounds* 39(11), 2005.

Finkelstein JA, Stille CJ, Rifas-Shiman et al: Watchful waiting for acute otitis media: are parents and physicians ready? *Pediatrics* 115(6):1466-1473, 2005.

Friedman NR, McCormick DP, Pittman C et al: Development of a practical tool for assessing the severity of acute otitis media, *Pediatric Infect Dis J* 25(2):101-107, 2006.

Gregg R, AuD L, Wiorek M et al: Pediatric audiology: a review, *Pediatr Rev* 25(7):224-233, 2004.

Hall-Stoodley L, Hu FZ, Gieseke A et al: Direct detection of bacterial biofilms on the middle-ear mucosa of children with chronic otitis media, *JAMA* 296(2):202-211, 2006.

Harrison CF: The microbiology of acute otitis media: past, present, and future, *Contemp Pediatr* 22(suppl. 12):8-16, 2005.

Jacobson J, Jacobson C: Evaluation of hearing loss in infants and young children, *Pediatric Annals* 33(12):811-822, 2004.

Joint Committee on Infant Hearing: Joint Committee on Infant Hearing 2000 position statement, *Pediatrics* 106:798-817, 2000a.

Joint Committee on Infant Hearing: Joint Committee on Infant Hearing 2000 position statement: principles and guidelines for early hearing detection and intervention programs, *Am J Audiol* 9:9-29, 2000b.

Kadish H: Ear and nose foreign bodies: it is all about the tools, *Clin Pediatr* 44:665-670, 2005.

Kemper K: Otitis media: when parents don't want antibiotics or tubes, *Contemp Pediatr* 19:47-58, 2002.

Kenna M: Neonatal hearing screening, *Pediatric Clin North Am* 50:301-313, 2003.

Leibovitz E: The use of fluoroquinolones in children, *Curr Opinions Pediatr* 18(1):64-70, 2006.

Little P: Delayed prescribing-a sensible approach to the management of acute otitis media, *JAMA* 296 (10):1290-1291, 2006.

Lye P: Earache. In Kliegman R, Greenbaum L, Lye P, editors: *Practical strategies in pediatric diagnosis and therapy,* Philadelphia: Elsevier, 2004.

Marcy M, Takata G, Shekelle P et al: Management of acute otitis media, *Evidence Rep/Tech Assess* No 15, Rockville, MD, Agency for Healthcare Research and Quality, 2001.

McCormick DP, Chonmaitree T, Pittman C et al: Nonsevere acute otitis media: a clinical trial comparing outcomes of watchful waiting versus immediate antibiotic treatment, *Pediatrics* 115(6):1455-1465, 2005.

Meissner HC: Reducing the impact of viral respiratory tract infections in children, *Pediatric Clin North Am* 52(3):695-710, 2005.

Merenstein D, Diener-West, Krist A et al: An assessment of the shared-decision model in parents of children with acute otitis media, *Pediatrics* 116(6):1267-1275, 2005.

Myer CM: The evolution of ototopical therapy: from cumin to quinolones, *Ear Nose Throat J* 83(1 suppl.):9-11, 2004.

Nance W: The genetics of deafness, *Ment Retardation Developmental Disability Res* Rev 9(2):109-119, 2003.

National Institutes of Health: Early identification of hearing impairment in infants and young children, *NIH Consensus Statement* 11(1):1-24, 1993.

Nowak-Wegrzyn A: Similar allergic inflammation in the middle ear and the upper airway: evidence linking otitis media with effusion to the united airways concept, *Pediatrics* 116(Suppl. 1):552-553, 2005.

Nozza R: The assessment of hearing and middle ear function in children. In Bluestone C, Stool S, editors: *Pediatric otolaryngology,* ed 4, Philadelphia, 2002, WB Saunders.

Ozgur SK, Beyazova U, Kemaloglu YK et al: Effectiveness of inactivated influenza vaccine for prevention of otitis media in children, *Pediatric Infect Dis J* 25(5):401-405, 2006.

Paradise JL, Bluestone CD: Tympanostomy tubes: a contemporary guide to judicious use, *Pediatr Rev* 26(2):60-65, 2005.

Paradise JL, Campbell TF, Dollaghan CA et al: Developmental outcomes after early or delayed insertion of tympanostomy tubes, *N Engl J Med* 353(6):576-586, 2005.

Pelton SI: Otitis media: re-evaluation of diagnosis and treatment in the era of antimicrobial resistance, pneumococcal conjugate vaccine, and evolving morbidity, *Pediatric Clin North Am* 52:711-728, 2005.

Renko M, Kontiokari T, Jounio-Ervasti K et al: Disappearance of middle ear effusion in acute otitis media monitored daily with tympanometry, *Acta Paediatrica* 95(3):359-363, 2006.

Revai K, McCormick DP, Patel J et al: Effect of pneumococcal conjugate vaccine on nasopharyngeal bacterial colonization during acute otitis media, *Pediatrics* 117(5):1823-1829, 2006.

Roland PS: Contemporary management of childhood ear infection, *Patient Care Nurse Practitioner* 1(2):1-8, 2004.

Rosenfeld RM: Otitis, antibiotics, and the greater good, *Pediatrics* 114(5):1333-1335, 2004a.

Rosenfeld RM: Antibiotic use for otitis media: oral, topical, or none? *Pediatric Annals* 33(12):833-842, 2004b.

Schroeder A, Darrow D: Management of the draining ear in children, *Pediatric Annals* 33(12):843-852, 2004.

Siegel RM, Bien JP: Acute otitis media in children: a continuing story, *Pediatr Rev* 25(6):187-192, 2004.

Sifuentes M: Disorders of the ear. In Osborn L, Dewitt T, First L et al, editors: *Pediatrics,* Philadelphia, 2005, Elsevier.

Smith R, Hone S: Genetic screening for deafness, *Pediatric Clin North Am* 50:315-329, 2003.

Tonnaer ELGM, Graamans K, Sanders EAM et al: Advances in understanding the pathogenesis of pneumococcal otitis media, *Pediatric Infect Dis J* 25(6):546-552, 2006.

US Department of Health and Human Services: *Healthy people 2010. Objectives: draft for public comment: child and adolescent focused objectives, 2000.* Available at *http://web.health.gov/healthypeople* (accessed Oct 21, 2002).

US Preventive Services Task Force (USPSTF): *Recommendations and rationale for newborn hearing screening, 2001.* Available at *www.ncbi.nlm. nih.gov/books/bv.fcgi?highlight-screening.recommendations.rationale. newborn.hearing/rid-hstat3.chapter.458* (accessed Feb 24, 2007).

US Public Health Service: *Put prevention into practice: the clinician's handbook of preventive services,* ed 2, Germantown, MD, 1997, International Medical Publishing.

CHAPTER 30

Cardiovascular Disorders

Julie Martchenke and Catherine G. Blosser

Most cardiovascular problems in the pediatric population are due to congenital heart disease (CHD), which occurs in 0.5% to 0.9% of all live births, 3% to 4% of stillborns, 10% to 25% of abortuses, and 2% of premature infants (patent ductus arteriosus (PDA) excluded) (Bernstein, 2004). Incidence rates vary depending on diagnostic techniques used and the inclusion and exclusion criteria of studies. By 1 week of age, 40% to 50% of infants with CHD have been detected (Bernstein, 2004). Some defects, such as small ventricular septal defects (VSDs) or a bicuspid aortic valve, may cause no disability to a child; however, they pose a risk for bacterial endocarditis and may cause great concern for parents and caregivers.

Pediatric cardiologists can accurately diagnose CHD through noninvasive procedures in almost every instance. Fetal echocardiographers now diagnose CHD as early as 16 to 18 weeks of gestation in many cases and as early as 10 weeks of gestation with the newer high-frequency transvaginal echocardiography. In addition to cardiac malformations, fetal echocardiography is used to diagnose arrhythmias and hemodynamic changes (Allen et al, 2001). Fetal detection of CHD may decrease the morbidity and mortality rates associated with undiagnosed heart problems and give parents time to emotionally prepare for their child.

Gender affects the incidence of various types of CHD. Transposition of the great vessels and aortic stenosis (AS) are more common in males; atrial septal defects (ASDs), VSDs, and PDAs occur more in females.

The primary care provider (PCP) must maintain a high index of suspicion regarding any signs or symptoms of cardiovascular disease. This facilitates early identification and referral of infants and children with potential cardiovascular problems. PCPs also assist in the management of patients with CHD before and after heart surgery or procedures. Providers need to be attentive to the needs of the whole child because the focus of subspecialists and the family is on the heart disease. They also support families and children once a diagnosis is made and educate families about prevention of acquired heart disease.

■ ANATOMY AND PHYSIOLOGY
FETAL CIRCULATION

Knowledge of the fetal circulation is essential for understanding the circulatory changes that occur in the newborn at delivery (Fig. 30-1). Fetal circulation has four unique features that differ from postnatal circulation:

- Oxygenation of the blood occurs in the placenta, not the lungs.
- Fetal pulmonary vascular resistance is high, and systemic vascular resistance is low (high pressure on the right side of the heart, low pressure on the left side).
- The foramen ovale, the opening in the septum between the two atria, permits a portion of the blood to flow from the right atrium directly to the left atrium.
- A PDA provides a connection between the pulmonary artery and the aorta that allows blood to flow from the pulmonary artery to the aorta and bypass the fetal lungs.

Oxygen is diffused into the fetal circulation from the maternal uterine arteries in the placenta. From the placenta, oxygenated blood flows through the umbilical vein and is diverted through the liver to the inferior vena cava (IVC) by the ductus venosus. When this well-oxygenated blood reaches the right atrium, it flows preferentially toward the atrial septum, through the foramen ovate, and into the left atrium. Oxygenated blood then flows into the left ventricle and out the aorta. Approximately two thirds of the blood from the aorta flows toward the head and neck to ensure that the fetal brain constantly receives well-oxygenated blood.

Venous blood returns from the head and upper extremities through the superior vena cava (SVC) to the right atrium. This blood preferentially flows toward the tricuspid valve into the right ventricle. From the right ventricle, the blood enters the pulmonary artery. Because pulmonary vascular resistance is high and systemic resistance is low, most blood in the pulmonary artery flows through the ductus arteriosus into the descending aorta to supply oxygen and nutrients to the trunk and lower extremities. Only a small amount of blood flows into the pulmonary circuit to perfuse the lungs.

The fetal circulation is best described as two parallel circuits, with the left ventricle supplying blood to the upper extremities and the right ventricle serving the lower extremities and the placenta. At the time of transition to extrauterine life, these separate blood flows become a serial circuit.

NEONATAL CIRCULATION

A number of complex events occur at birth that rapidly shift the fetal circulation toward a neonatal circulation. Clamping the umbilical cord with subsequent removal of the placenta as the oxygenating organ causes an immediate circulatory change in which the lungs become the new source of oxygenation. This change causes an increase in systemic vascular resistance (systemic BP). With the first breath, mechanical inflation of

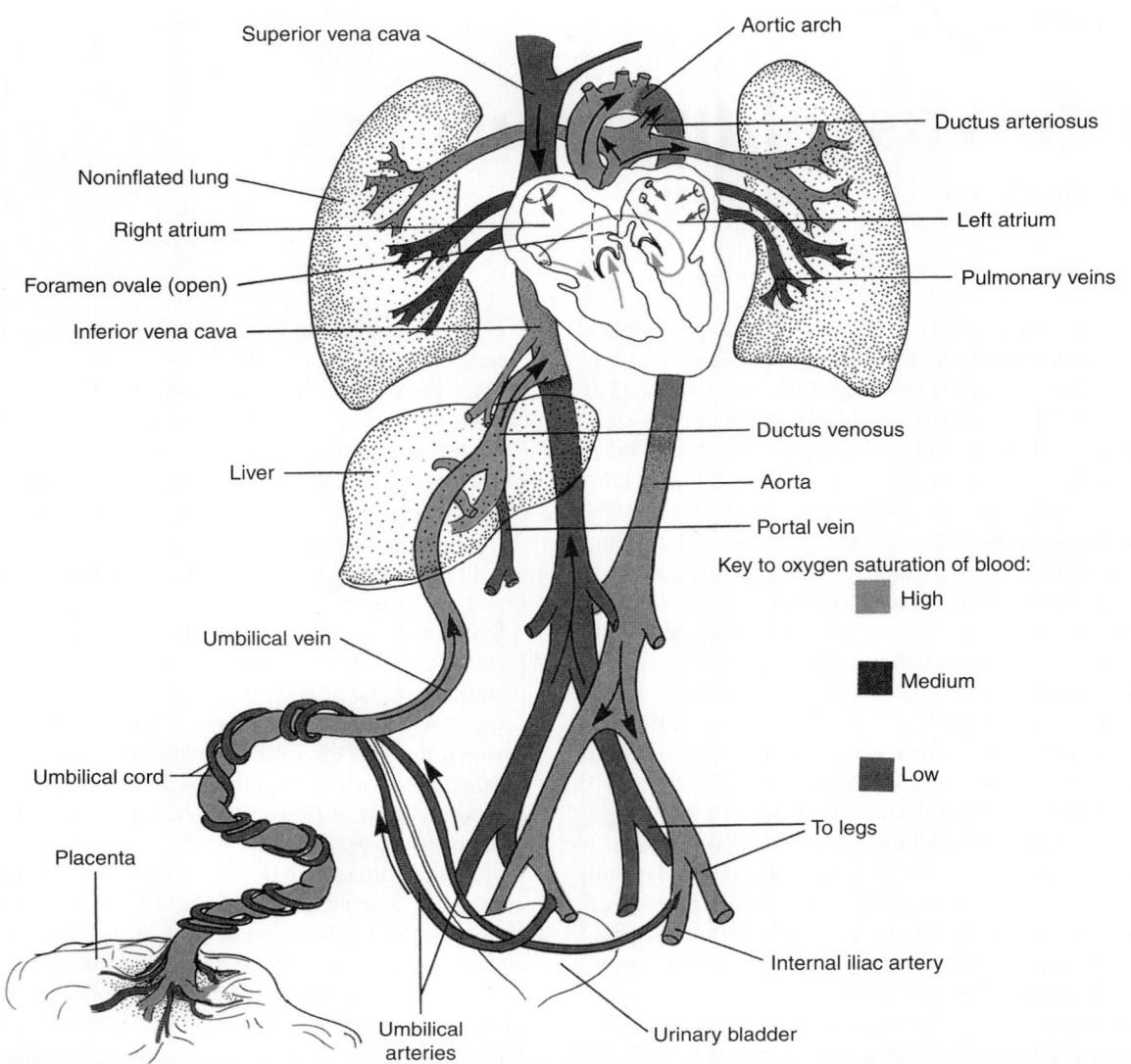

FIG. 30-1 Fetal circulation. (From Gorrie TM, McKinney ES, Murray SS: *Foundations of maternal-newborn nursing,* Philadelphia, 1994, WB Saunders.)

the lungs and an increase in oxygen saturation bring about a dramatic fall in pulmonary vascular resistance and, consequently, increased pulmonary blood flow. This activity leads to beginning constriction of the ductus arteriosus. As the pressures within the heart become relatively higher on the left side and lower on the right, the foramen ovale closes. Functional closure of the ductus arteriosus and foramen ovale usually occurs within the first hours to days of life, and a serial circuit forms out of the once-parallel pulmonary and systemic circulation.

The transition toward complete anatomic closure, or obliteration of fetal structures by tissue growth or constriction, is more gradual. Pulmonary vascular resistance drops gradually over the first 6 to 8 weeks of life, which may protect the pulmonary circulation against volume overload in some congenital heart anomalies. Shunt murmurs or symptoms of congestive heart failure (CHF) gradually become apparent as the infant approaches 8 weeks of age. At this time, resistance to flow is less, and shunting to the pulmonary bed increases.

Conditions that cause persistence of fetal shunts, thus allowing unoxygenated blood to flow from the right side of the heart to the left, may cause cyanosis. Any murmur or cyanosis in a newborn should be carefully monitored and evaluated to detect cardiac abnormalities.

NORMAL CARDIAC STRUCTURE AND FUNCTION

The heart is a muscular, four-chambered organ located in the mediastinum, the space in the chest between the lungs. The four chambers are divided into two larger muscular pumping chambers, the ventricles, and two smaller receiving chambers, the atria. Desaturated systemic blood returns to the right atrium by way of the inferior and superior venae cavae. The blood passes from the right atrium through the tricuspid valve to the right ventricle. The right ventricle pumps the blood through the pulmonic valve into the pulmonary artery and the lungs, where it is oxygenated. Blood returning from the lungs enters the left atrium by way of the pulmonary veins and then passes through the mitral valve into the left ventricle.

The left ventricle pumps the blood through the aortic valve into the aorta to provide oxygenated blood for the systemic circulation.

The heart valves are one-way valves that open and close because of pressure changes within the heart, controlling the flow of blood from chamber to chamber. The tricuspid valve has three cusps held in place by the chordae tendineae. The pulmonary valve directs blood flow from the right ventricle into the pulmonary artery, which bifurcates into right and left arteries to allow flow into both lungs. The pulmonary veins entering the left atrium contain no valves, so blood can flow freely from the lungs into the atrium. The mitral valve controls flow from the left atrium into the left ventricle. The aortic valve controls flow from the high-pressure left ventricle out to the body.

CONDUCTION SYSTEM

Myocardial contraction is stimulated by electrical depolarization along the conduction tract within the heart. Depolarization begins at the sinoatrial node, which is high in the wall of the atrium. This node acts as the pacemaker of the heart by regularly beginning the depolarizing impulses of each heartbeat. The wave of depolarization travels from the sinoatrial node throughout the atria and produces contraction of the atrial muscle. The impulses reach the atrioventricular (AV) node, which is located in the lower portion of the right atrium at the junction of the atrium and ventricle. From the AV node, the depolarization wave passes through the bundle of His, the fibers extending from the AV node along the intraventricular septum. Depolarization spreads through the left and right branches of the bundle of His and through the Purkinje fibers extending into the ventricular muscle. Impulses then spread throughout the ventricles and cause contraction. The electrocardiogram (ECG) can demonstrate this pattern of changing electrical impulses.

HEART SOUNDS

At the time of ventricular contraction, the beginning of systole, the mitral and tricuspid valves close and produce the first heart sound (S_1). S_1 is the "lubb" of lubb-dupp. Although the left side of the heart reacts slightly before the right side, closure of the mitral and tricuspid valves occurs so closely together that S_1 appears as a single sound. S_1 is best heard at the apex of the heart and is synchronous with the apical and carotid pulses.

After the blood has been ejected, the heart relaxes, the mitral and tricuspid valves open, and the aortic and pulmonary valves close to keep the blood from rushing back into the ventricles. This closure results in the second heart sound (S_2). S_2 is normally split with inspiration in children. S_2 reflects the onset of diastole and is the "dupp" of lubb-dupp. The intensity and splitting of S_2 is one of the most important parts of the pediatric cardiac examination.

◼ PATHOPHYSIOLOGY

The term *congenital heart disease* implies only that a cardiovascular malformation is present at birth. It does not indicate the etiology or the cause of the malformation. When CHD is diagnosed in an infant or child, parents may incorrectly assume that they are somehow responsible for the child's defect. Health care professionals must be clear about what is and what is not known about CHD to spare parents needless worry and guilt.

Most CHD is due to a complex interaction of genetic and environmental or intrauterine factors, a pattern called *multifactorial inheritance*. The heart is essentially formed by 6 weeks of fetal life, a time when the fetus is most susceptible to infectious or teratogenic exposure or to predisposing genetic or chromosomal factors. Up to 25% of children with CHD also have noncardiac abnormalities (Stevenson, 2006).

Our understanding about the genetic involvement in CHD is evolving rapidly. Table 30-1 lists the most common known chromosomal abnormalities associated with heart disease. Providers can access *http://genetests.org* (funded by the National Institutes of Health [NIH]) for specific information about ordering genetic tests and resources for families. The Online Mendelian Inheritance in Man (OMIN) website at *www.ncbi.nlm.nih.gov* has more in-depth information about specific genetic defects or syndromes. Children who have multiple congenital anomalies, dysmorphic features, or neurocognitive deficits, in addition to CHD, should be referred to a clinical geneticist (Goldmuntz, 2004).

Two percent to 4% of CHD is caused by well-documented teratogens and maternal conditions or environmental influences. Teratogens known to affect the heart include maternal thalidomide, cocaine, lithium, fluconazole, phenothiazine, alcohol, anticonvulsants, and retinoic acid. Maternal exposure to pesticides and solvents has also been associated with CHD. Infection, especially cytomegalovirus, mumps, or rubella, contracted in the first 8 weeks of gestation can cause CHD. Infants born to mothers with insulin-dependent diabetes, lupus erythematosus, and phenylketonuria also have increased risk for various cardiac defects (Lin et al, 2006). See Box 30-1 and Table 30-1.

◼ ASSESSMENT OF THE CARDIOVASCULAR SYSTEM

Cardiac assessment includes a comprehensive history, a thorough physical assessment, and a variety of diagnostic tests.

HISTORY

Cardiac evaluation includes review of the family, maternal, fetal, neonatal, and infant medical history, in addition to growth and development (see Box 30-1 for risk factors).

PHYSICAL EXAMINATION

Physical assessment in a child with suspected CHD should be adapted to the age of the child (Box 30-2). It is not always possible to follow the same pattern of assessment with each child. Be flexible, yet thorough, in any evaluation and include all aspects of the physical examination in an order that best suits the comfort and needs of the infant or child.

TABLE 30-1	Congenital Malformation Syndromes Associated With Selected Congenital Heart Disease

Syndrome With Chromosomal/Gene Disorders	Resultant Heart Defect(s)/Occurrence
Trisomy 21 (Down syndrome)	Atrioventricular septal defect, VSD, ASD, PDA, TOF (50%)
Trisomy 18 (Edwards syndrome)	VSD, ASD, PDA, COA, bicuspid aortic or pulmonary valve (99%)
Trisomy 13 (Patau syndrome)	VSD, PDA, dextrocardia (90%)
Turner syndrome (XO)	Bicuspid aortic valve, COA (35%)
Marfan syndrome (FBN1 gene)	Mitral valve prolapse, aortic root dilation
DiGeorge, Velocardial Facial, Takeo, Catch 22 syndromes (22q11.2 deletion)	Interrupted aortic arch, truncus arteriosus, TOF, perimembranous VSD, aortic arch anomalies
Klinefelter variant (XXXXY)	PDA, ASD (15%)
Noonan syndrome (PTPN11)	Valvar pulmonic stenosis, hypertrophic cardiomyopathy
CHARGE (gene CHD7)	Truncus arteriosus, interrupted aortic arch type B
Jacobsen (11q23 deletion)	Hypoplastic left heart syndrome, COA
Long QT syndrome	Palpitations, syncope, sudden death
Cri du chat syndrome (5p)	VSD, PDA, ASD (25%)
Neurofibromatosis	PS
Nonhereditary Syndromes	
Fetal alcohol syndrome	VSD, PDA, ASD, TOF (25%-30%)
Fetal hydantoin syndrome	PS, AS, COA, PDA, VSD, ASD (<5%)
Fetal trimethadione syndrome	TGA, VSD, TOF (15%-30% incidence)
Infant of diabetic mother	TGA, VSD, COA (3%-5%); cardiomyopathy (10%-20%)
Pierre Robin syndrome	VSD, PDA (29%); ASD, COA, TOF (less commonly)
VATER association	VSD, other defects (>50%)
Congenital diaphragmatic hernia	VSD, TOF (25%)
Cornelia de Lange (de Lange) syndrome	VSD, (30%)
Other System Malformations	
Hydrocephalus	VSD, ECD, TOF (6%)
Dandy-Walker syndrome	VSD (3%)
TE fistula and/or esophageal atresia	VSD, ASD, TOF (21%)
Imperforate anus	TOF, VSD (12%)

AS, Aortic stenosis; *ASD,* atrial septal defect; *COA,* coarctation of the aorta; *ECD,* endocardial cushion defect; *PDA,* patent ductus arteriosus; *PS,* pulmonary stenosis; *TGA,* transposition of the great arteries; *TOF,* tetralogy of Fallot; *VSD,* ventricular septal defect.
Data from Goldmuntz E: The genetic contribution to congenital heart disease, *Pediatr Clin of North Am* 51:1721-1737, 2004. Lin A, Belmont J, Malik S: Heart. In Stevenson R, Hall J: *Human malformations and related anomalies,* ed 2, Oxford, 2006, Oxford University Press; Park MK, Troxler RG: *Pediatric cardiology for practitioners,* ed 4, St Louis, 2002, Mosby.

Vital Signs

Heart rate, respiratory rate, and BP vary considerably throughout childhood. Measurements of vital signs must be obtained on each visit with the child at rest because crying and exercise affect results. Refer to charts for normal ranges for various age groups, gender, and height for comparison.

- *Heart rate* (see Table 30-2). Heart rates should always be obtained by auscultation of the heart in children younger than 10 years old. Assessment should include rate and rhythm variations. An increased heart rate can be caused by excitement, anxiety, hyperthyroidism, heart disease, anemia, or fever. Assess the rhythm for regularity.

- *Pulses.* Pulses should be checked in the upper and lower extremities and evaluated for character (strength) and variation between the different sites. A bounding pulse may indicate a PDA or aortic insufficiency. Weak or "thready" pulses may indicate CHF or an obstructive lesion, such as severe AS. Good brachial pulses in conjunction with weak or absent femoral pulses indicate coarctation of the aorta (COA).

- *Blood pressure (BP).* The National Institutes of Health National High Blood Pressure Education Program (NIH-NHBPEP) on BP control in children and adolescents recommends measuring BP annually beginning at 3 years old (2004). Providers should auscultate BP on children 3 years or older. In selected cases, providers should check BPs in younger children. It is important to always use a BP cuff that is appropriate for the child's size. For arm pressure, the width of the cuff should be two thirds the length of the upper arm measured from the axilla to the antecubital space. A cuff that is too narrow or does not fit around a chubby arm may cause an erroneously high reading. Initial evaluation should compare the pressure in all four extremities. Pressure in all extremities should be equal, with pressure in the legs being slightly higher (10 to 20 mm Hg) in a child who walks. The NIH publishes norms for BP by gender, age, and height periodically and are found in Tables 30-3 and 30-4 (NIH-NHBPEP, 2004).

| BOX 30-1 | **Risk Factors Suggestive of Congenital Heart Disease** |

Perinatal Risk Factors

Maternal infections and exposures (CMV, rubella, other viral syndromes)

Maternal use of tobacco, alcohol, street drugs, retinoic acid, hydantoins, lithium, valproates

Maternal chronic disease (CHD, lupus, insulin-dependent diabetes, phenylketonuria)

Maternal age at child's birth (increase in chromosomal abnormalities after 40 years old)

Maternal pregnancy history (excessive weight gain, gestational diabetes)

Neonatal Risk Factors

Fetal or newborn distress (aspiration, hypoxia, cyanosis)

Prematurity (increased incidence of CHD in premature infants)

Presence of associated anomalies (genetic or chromosomal abnormalities or syndromes)

Neonatal infections (GABHS)

Birth weight (term infants, <2500 g; SGA, <2 standard deviations from the mean for gestational age)

Newborn Risk Factors

Murmur at birth or early infancy

Hypertension (at birth or beyond)

Feeding difficulty (SOB, easily fatigued, diaphoresis, poor intake)

Cyanosis (increase with crying, feeding, exertion)

Tachypnea (persistent, with crying, feeding)

Toddler, School-Age, and Teenage Risk Factors

Deviation from normal growth and development (normal milestone development, following own growth curve)

Deviation from activity level appropriate for chronologic age (unable to keep up with peers; unable to run or ride bike)

Frequent respiratory tract infections (pneumonia, URIs that last longer than normal)

Prior murmurs, blue spells

Documented GABHS infection

Hypertension (documented on a minimum of three separate visits)

Chest pain with exertion

SOB with exertion (beyond normal peers)

Syncope or dizziness (especially associated with noted heart rate change)

Tachycardia or bradycardia (fluttering in chest, racing heart)

Family History Risk Factors

CHD (especially siblings, parents, first-degree relatives)

Sudden death or premature myocardial infarction (before 50 years old)

Hypertension

Rheumatic fever

Genetic syndromes

Hypercholesterolemia

CHD, Congenital heart disease; *CMV,* cytomegalovirus; *GABHS,* group A β-hemolytic streptococcus; *SGA,* small for gestational age; *SOB,* shortness of breath; *URIs,* upper respiratory infections.

○ The pulse pressure (difference between systolic and diastolic pressure) is normally 20 to 50 mm Hg throughout childhood. A wide pulse pressure caused by an abnormally low diastolic pressure may be an indication of PDA, aortic regurgitation, or other cardiac pathologic conditions.

- *Respiratory rate.* Evaluation of the respiratory system includes the respiratory rate, assessment of effort, and breath sounds in all five lobes of the lungs. It is important to evaluate the respiratory rate in a quiet infant or child. A respiratory rate above 40 in a young child or 60 in a newborn who is quiet, resting, and afebrile warrants further evaluation. An infant with CHD may be happily tachypneic and not show significant signs of grunting, intercostal retractions, nasal flaring, or tracheal pulling.

- *Oxygen saturation.* Oxygen saturation is now considered to be an essential vital sign in many settings. It is important to establish oxygen saturations in new babies or new patients because cyanosis is often subtle and not always readily perceptible to all examiners. Pulse oximetry is a sensitive screening tool in detecting cyanotic heart disease in asymptomatic newborns (Koppel et al, 2003).

General Appearance

- The provider should observe an infant while obtaining a history and before performing any other part of the physical examination. General nutritional state, respiratory effort, color, physical abnormalities, and distress or discomfort level should be observed.

- During this observation period, one should also note the presence of unusual facial characteristics (e.g., malformed ears, wide-spaced eyes, noticeable anomalies) or extracardiac anomalies (e.g., cleft lip or palate, polydactyly, microcephaly) that may be associated with a syndrome or chromosomal abnormalities. Children may have obvious stigmata, such as those seen with Down syndrome, Marfan syndrome (unusually tall with an arm span wider than the head-to-toe height), Turner syndrome (webbed neck, prominent ears), or fetal alcohol syndrome (microcephaly and pinched facies), all of which are associated with CHD.

- Overall skin color should be assessed for signs of mottling or central cyanosis while the infant is at rest. Cyanosis caused by heart disease is recognized as a pale blue or ruddy red color of the mucous membranes (lips, tongue, nail beds). The tongue is the best indicator because it lacks pigmentation and is abundantly served by the vascular system. Peripheral cyanosis or acrocyanosis, a blueness or pallor noted around the mouth and on the hands or feet, can be a normal variant, especially if it intensifies when the child is cold or crying. Clubbing of the fingers and toes may be seen in children with long-standing cyanosis.

BOX 30-2   Developmental Approach to Cardiac Assessment

Infants
Complete the assessment with the infant in the parent's arms to keep the infant quiet and cooperative.
Perform uncomfortable aspects of the examination after auscultation to ensure a quiet listen.
Keep the infant covered and warm to minimize discomfort and physiologic changes associated with chilling.
Observe color, respiratory effort, and general effort level while the baby is quiet.

Toddlers
Approach the child quietly, calmly, and slowly. A loud, boisterous greeting may frighten the toddler.
Complete the assessment wherever the child is most comfortable—sitting on the floor, in the parent's lap, on the examination table.
Allow the child to handle a stethoscope while the history is being taken.
Have a toy or distraction item available during the examination.
Consider "listening" to the parent first to improve comfort with the examination.

School Age
Clearly explain the plan and expectations before the examination.
Answer the child's questions honestly.
Talk about topics of interest (school, sports) during the examination.
School-age children may be modest and prefer to keep a gown on during most of the examination.
School-age children may be helpful in discussion of symptoms and events surrounding current concerns.

Adolescents
Questions should be directed at the adolescent and parent.
Communicate in a manner that conveys honesty, professionalism, and interest in their concerns.
Ensure privacy related to both the physical examination and information sharing.
Provide a choice of having a parent present for any or all aspects of the history and examination.
Adolescents are very "body aware" and need reassurance that their concerns are valid, even when the symptom is within normal limits.

TABLE 30-2   Normal Heart Rates (Beats per Minute) in Infants and Children

Age	Resting (Awake)	Resting (Asleep)	Exercise/ Fever
Newborn	100-180	80-160	Up to 220
1 week-3 months	100-220	80-200	Up to 220
3 months-2 years	80-150	70-120	Up to 220
2-10 years	70-100	60-90	195-215
10-20 years	55-90	50-90	195-215

- Note any wheezing, nasal flaring, retractions, prominent neck veins, or head bobbing with respirations.
- Note also signs of peripheral or periorbital edema. Edema or puffiness around the eyes may be evident in an infant with CHF even in the absence of peripheral edema of the hands or feet. True pitting edema of the feet is an unusual finding in an infant with CHF.
- Measure and plot height and weight on standardized charts, including Down and Turner syndrome charts, at each assessment. Although many children with CHD fall within the normal ranges of height, weight, and development, a large number of infants and children with heart disease experience poor weight gain, less than normal linear growth, and delays in achieving developmental milestones.

Palpation
- Palpate all five areas of the chest: the aortic, pulmonic, tricuspid, and mitral areas and Erb's point (Fig. 30-2). Chest palpation is best accomplished by using the open palm of the hand near the base of the fingers. The hand should be gently moved across the chest to assess abnormal precordial activity, including pulsations, lifts, heaves, or thrills, and to determine the location of the apical impulse. The apical impulse is used to determine the size of the heart and is the most lateral point at which cardiac activity can be palpated. In infants and children, the impulse is normally palpated at the apex of the heart in the fourth intercostal space just to the left of the midclavicular line. At approximately 7 years old, the point shifts to the fifth intercostal space. In the presence of cardiomegaly, the apical impulse is shifted laterally or downward.
- Thrills are a palpable vibration caused by turbulent blood flow through abnormal structures or defects in the heart. The turbulent flow may be due to valvular narrowing or stenosis or defects, such as VSD.

TABLE 30-3   **Blood Pressure Levels in the 90th and 95th Percentiles for Girls 1 to 17 Years Old by Percentiles of Height**

	Height Percentiles*	Systolic BP (mm Hg)							Diastolic BP (mm Hg)						
Age	BP†	5%	10%	25%	50%	75%	90%	95%	5%	10%	25%	50%	75%	90%	95%
1	90th	97	97	98	100	101	102	103	52	53	53	54	55	55	56
	95th	100	101	103	104	105	106	107	56	57	57	58	59	59	60
2	90th	98	99	100	101	103	104	105	57	58	58	59	60	61	61
	95th	102	103	104	105	107	108	109	61	62	62	63	63	65	65
3	90th	100	100	102	103	104	106	106	61	62	62	63	64	64	65
	95th	104	104	105	107	108	109	110	65	66	66	67	68	68	69
4	90th	101	102	103	104	106	107	108	64	64	65	66	67	67	68
	95th	105	106	107	108	110	111	112	68	68	69	70	71	71	72
5	90th	103	103	105	106	107	109	109	66	67	67	68	69	69	70
	95th	107	107	108	110	111	112	113	70	71	71	72	73	73	74
6	90th	104	105	106	108	109	110	111	68	68	69	70	70	71	72
	95th	108	109	110	111	113	114	115	72	72	73	74	74	75	76
7	90th	106	107	108	109	111	112	113	69	70	70	71	72	72	73
	95th	110	111	112	113	115	116	116	73	74	74	75	76	76	77
8	90th	108	109	110	111	113	114	114	71	71	71	72	73	74	74
	95th	112	112	114	115	116	118	118	75	75	75	76	77	78	78
9	90th	110	110	112	113	114	116	116	71	72	72	73	74	75	75
	95th	114	114	115	117	118	119	120	76	76	76	77	78	79	79
10	90th	112	112	114	115	116	118	118	73	73	73	74	75	76	76
	95th	116	116	117	119	120	121	122	77	77	77	78	79	80	80
11	90th	114	114	116	117	118	119	120	74	74	74	75	76	77	77
	95th	118	118	119	121	122	123	124	78	78	78	79	80	81	81
12	90th	116	116	117	119	120	121	122	75	75	75	76	77	78	78
	95th	119	120	121	123	124	125	126	79	79	79	80	81	82	82
13	90th	117	118	119	121	122	123	124	76	76	76	77	78	79	79
	95th	121	122	123	124	126	127	128	80	80	80	81	82	83	83
14	90th	119	120	121	122	124	125	125	77	77	77	78	79	80	80
	95th	123	123	125	126	127	129	129	81	81	81	82	83	84	84
15	90th	120	121	122	123	125	126	127	78	78	79	79	80	81	81
	95th	124	125	126	127	129	130	131	82	82	82	83	84	85	85
16	90th	121	122	123	124	126	127	128	78	78	79	80	81	81	82
	95th	125	126	127	128	130	131	132	82	82	83	84	85	85	86
17	90th	122	122	123	125	126	127	128	78	79	79	80	81	81	82
	95th	125	126	127	129	130	131	132	82	83	83	84	85	85	86

*Height percentile determined by standard growth curves.
†BP percentile determined by a single measurement.
From National Institutes of Health, National High Blood Pressure Education Program Working Group on High Blood Pressure in Children and Adolescents (NIH-NHBPEP): The fourth report on the diagnosis, evaluation, and treatment of high blood pressure in children and adolescents, *Pediatrics* 114:555-576, 2004. Available at *www.nhlbi.nih.gov/guidelines/hypertension/child_tbl.pdf.* (accessed December 14, 2007).

- Assess peripheral pulses (radial, brachial, carotid, dorsalis pedis, and posterior tibial) for amplitude and intensity. In COA, the examiner will note decreased or absent femoral pulses and impulse lag if the radial pulse is palpated simultaneously. A fast pulse rate may indicate arrhythmia or CHF.
- The liver and spleen should be assessed for enlargement. A liver more than 1 cm below the right costal margin may indicate hepatomegaly and is an important finding. Infants may have a palpable liver edge as a normal finding.

- The back should be examined for scoliosis, a finding associated with enlarged hearts.

Auscultation of Heart Sounds
- The examiner should approach auscultation of the heart in the same manner for every child either beginning at the base or apex of the heart. Ideally, assess heart sounds in a quiet environment when the child is cooperative.
- Evaluate heart sounds and listen for murmurs in each of five previously noted areas of the heart (see Fig. 30-2).

TABLE 30-4 **Blood Pressure Levels in the 90th and 95th Percentiles for Boys 1 to 17 Years Old by Percentiles of Height**

Age	Height Percentiles* BP†	Systolic BP (mm Hg)							Diastolic BP (mm Hg)						
		→ 5%	10%	25%	50%	75%	90%	95%	5%	10%	25%	50%	75%	90%	95%
1	90th	94	95	97	99	100	102	103	49	50	51	52	53	53	54
	95th	98	99	101	103	104	106	106	54	54	55	56	57	58	58
2	90th	97	99	100	102	104	105	106	54	55	56	57	58	58	59
	95th	101	102	104	106	108	109	110	59	59	60	61	62	63	63
3	90th	100	101	103	105	107	108	109	59	59	60	61	62	63	63
	95th	104	105	107	109	110	112	113	63	63	64	65	66	67	67
4	90th	102	103	105	107	109	110	111	62	63	64	65	66	66	67
	95th	106	107	109	111	112	114	115	66	67	68	69	70	71	71
5	90th	104	105	106	108	110	111	112	65	66	67	68	69	69	70
	95th	108	109	110	112	114	115	116	69	70	71	72	73	74	74
6	90th	105	106	108	110	111	113	113	68	68	69	70	71	72	72
	95th	109	110	112	114	115	117	117	72	72	73	74	75	76	76
7	90th	106	107	109	111	113	114	115	70	70	71	72	73	74	74
	95th	110	111	113	115	117	118	119	74	74	75	76	77	78	78
8	90th	107	109	110	112	114	115	116	71	72	72	73	74	75	76
	95th	111	112	114	116	118	119	120	75	76	77	78	79	79	80
9	90th	109	110	112	114	115	117	118	72	73	74	75	76	76	77
	95th	113	114	116	118	119	121	121	76	77	78	79	80	81	81
10	90th	111	112	114	115	117	119	119	73	73	74	75	76	77	78
	95th	115	116	117	119	121	122	123	77	78	79	80	81	81	82
11	90th	113	114	115	117	119	120	121	74	74	75	76	77	78	78
	95th	117	118	119	121	123	124	125	78	78	79	80	81	82	82
12	90th	115	116	118	120	121	123	123	74	75	75	76	77	78	79
	95th	119	120	122	123	125	127	127	78	79	80	81	82	82	83
13	90th	117	118	120	122	124	125	126	75	75	76	77	78	79	79
	95th	121	122	124	126	128	129	130	79	79	80	81	82	83	83
14	90th	120	121	123	125	126	128	128	75	76	77	78	79	79	80
	95th	124	125	127	128	130	132	132	80	80	81	82	83	84	84
15	90th	122	124	125	127	129	130	131	76	77	78	79	80	80	81
	95th	126	128	129	131	133	134	135	81	81	82	83	84	85	85
16	90th	125	126	128	130	131	133	134	78	78	79	80	81	82	82
	95th	129	130	132	134	135	137	137	82	83	83	84	85	86	87
17	90th	127	128	130	132	134	135	136	80	80	81	82	83	84	84
	95th	131	132	134	136	138	139	140	84	85	86	87	87	88	89

*Height percentile determined by standard growth curves.
†BP percentile determined by a single measurement.
From National Institutes of Health, National High Blood Pressure Education Program Working Group on High Blood Pressure in Children and Adolescents (NIH-NHBPEP): The fourth report on the diagnosis, evaluation, and treatment of high blood pressure in children and adolescents, *Pediatrics* 114:555-576, 2004. Available at *www.nhlbi.nih.gov/guidelines/hypertension/child_tbl.pdf.* (accessed December 14, 2007).

- Four individual heart sounds can be heard: S_1, S_2, S_3, and S_4. S_1 and S_2 represent normal heart sounds, whereas the presence of S_3 or S_4 may indicate cardiac enlargement or volume overload. At each area of examination, the provider should accurately identify the first (S_1) and second (S_2) heart sounds.
- S_1 has the following characteristics:
  - It is heard in the beginning of systole and indicates closure of AV valves (mitral and tricuspid).
  - It may be differentiated from early systolic clicks by the low frequency of the sound (clicks have a higher frequency). It is best heard with the diaphragm of the stethoscope.
  - It is usually loudest at apex.
- S_2 has the following characteristics:
  - It is composed of the aortic (A_2) and pulmonic (P_2) components and marks the end of systole.
  - S_2 is normally split with inspiration because pulmonic valve closure lags behind aortic valve closure. S_2 becomes single with expiration.
  - S_2 is best assessed at the upper left sternal border in the pulmonic area.
  - Pulmonary hypertension causes early closure of P_2 and accentuation of S_2, which may sound like a loud, single second heart sound.

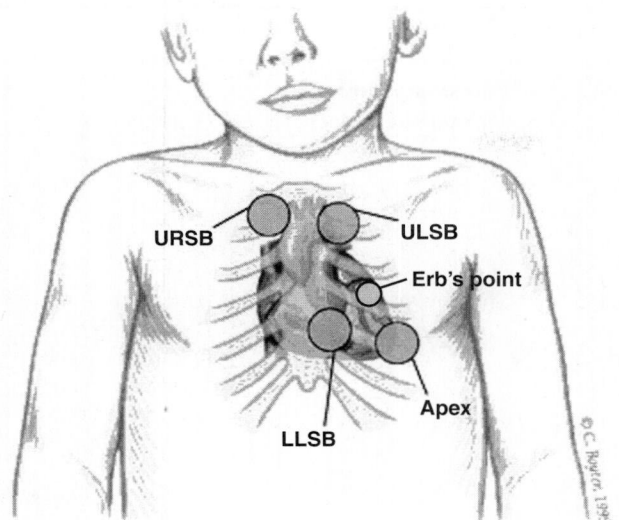

Upper right sternal border (URSB; aortic listening area)
• Aortic valve clicks of aortic stenosis, venous hum

Upper left sternal border (ULSB; pulmonic listening area)
• Pulmonary valve clicks of pulmonary stenosis, pulmonary flow murmurs, atrial septal defect, PDA, venous hum

Lower left sternal border (LLSB; tricuspid area)
• Ventricular septal defects, Still's murmur, tricuspid value regurgitation, hypertrophic cardiomyopathy, subaortic stenosis

Apex (mitral area)
• Aortioc or mitral valve clicks, mitral valve regurgitation

Erb's point
• Aortic ejection click of aortic stenosis, or dilated aortic root

FIG. 30-2 Traditional auscultatory areas for clicks and murmurs. (Adapted from McConnell M, Adkins S, Hannon D: Heart murmurs in pediatric patients: when do you refer? *Am Fam Pract* 60[2]:558–565, 1999. © C Boyter, 1999.)

° Absence of one of the semilunar valves (as in pulmonary atresia) causes single S_2.
° Wide splitting of S_2 without becoming a single sound on expiration may indicate increased pulmonary flow (typical of atrial septal defect [ASD]).
• S_3 and S_4 have the following characteristics:
° S_3 is associated with rapid ventricular filling; it may be heard in a quiet infant or child with a rapid heart rate.
° S_3 "gallop" is best heard at the apex with the bell of the stethoscope during early diastole. When combined with S_1 and S_2, it gives an impression of the word "Kentucky." S_3 is easier to appreciate when the child is in the left lateral decubitus position.
° S_4 is always pathologic; it represents increased force of atrial contraction and ventricular distention.
° S_4 "gallop" sounds like the word "Tennessee." It is best heard in late diastole just before S_1.
° S_4 is low pitched and is best heard at the apex with the bell of the stethoscope.
• Clicks: Ejection clicks are heard early in systole, immediately after S_1, and may sound like a split first heart sound. Pulmonic ejection clicks are high in frequency, vary with

respiration, and disappear with inspiration. An aortic ejection click, heard best at Erb's point, is constant in intensity with a sound of a "snap" or a "click." Nonejection clicks are heard best in midsystole, or midway between S_1 and S_2 in the cardiac cycle at the apex. These clicks are best heard in patients who are leaning forward or standing, may disappear with inspiration, and are due to mitral valve prolapse (Park & Troxler, 2002). See Fig. 30-2 for a description of cardiac conditions associated with each of these clicks.

Murmurs

Up to 80% of children may have a murmur, especially beginning at 3 to 4 years old (Park & Troxler, 2002). It may be caused by normal blood flow through normal cardiac structures (innocent or physiologic murmur) or by turbulent blood flow caused by a defect or abnormal cardiac structures. Murmurs may be intensified by anything that increases cardiac output (e.g., anemia, fever, exercise).

Innocent or Functional Murmurs. Functional or innocent cardiac murmurs are common in children and can be evident in newborns. Table 30-5 describes common types of innocent murmurs; Box 30-3 describes the characteristics of an innocent murmur. Families and older children with innocent murmurs should be reassured that nothing is wrong with the heart. They should be informed that this murmur may come and go and may be louder at times of fever, anxiety, pain, or exercise, but in no way represents cardiac pathology. Families should be reminded that activities do not need to be limited or any special precautions taken.

Criteria for Describing a Heart Murmur. Every murmur is assessed according to the criteria listed in Table 30-6. These are further illustrated and discussed in Fig. 30-3. Characteristics of pathologic murmurs needing referral are listed in Box 30-3. It is important to note that the presence of a murmur causes great anxiety for a family awaiting a diagnosis.

All murmurs should have a second opinion from a pediatric colleague or pediatric cardiologist if the diagnosis is uncertain or there is a suspicion of heart disease (Driscoll, 2006).

Common Diagnostic Studies. If the provider intends to refer for a cardiology consult, performing any of the following routine diagnostic studies is not cost-effective. The cardiology consultant will be able to determine with greater discrimination which, if any, tests should be ordered (Driscoll, 2006).

• *Chest radiograph.* Radiography provides the following information: cardiac size and size of specific chambers and great vessels, cardiac contour, status of pulmonary blood flow, and status of the lungs and other surrounding tissue (Fig. 30-4).
• *ECG.* ECG monitors the electrical activity of the heart from different locations and in different planes of the body. The ECG gives information about forces of ventricular contraction, hypertrophy, chamber dilation, and rhythm.
• *Echocardiogram.* Echocardiography uses reflected sound waves to identify intracardiac structures and their motion. The types of recordings include two-dimensional, M-mode, contrast, Doppler, and Tissue Doppler studies (Fig. 30-5).

TABLE 30-5 **Common Innocent Murmurs**

	Stills	Pulmonary Flow Murmur of Childhood	Pulmonary Flow Murmur of Infancy	Venous Hum
Other names	Innocent Vibratory Functional Physiologic "Head Start" murmur	Flow murmur	Peripheral pulmonary stenosis	
Description	Midsystolic, louder in supine position or with inspiration	Early systolic to midsystolic; decreases or disappears with standing; increases with cardiac output or in supine position	Short, midsystolic ejection murmur	Constant swishing sound, disappears with head turning, compression of jugular vein(s), or supine position; varies with respirations
Age	Any age, but most common between 2-6 years	Any age, but more commonly heard in thin-chested adolescents between 8-14 years	Common during newborn period, especially in preterm infants	Any
Best heard	Midpoint, left midsternal border to apex	Pulmonary outflow area; radiates to lung fields	Murmur radiates from left upper sternal border to both axilla and back, usually gone by 6 months	In upright position, left and right upper chest
Quality	Short, vibratory, musical, "twangy string"	Soft, blowing with normally split S_2; no click or thrill	Soft with middle to high pitch	Soft, high pitch; does not radiate
Intensity	Grade II-III	Grade I-III	Grade I-II	Grade II-III
Differential diagnosis	Small VSD, IHSS	ASD, PS	Supravalvular PS or AS	PDA

NOTE: Innocent murmurs typically increase with cardiac output (excitement, fever, anemia).
AS, Aortic stenosis; *ASD,* atrial septal defect; *IHSS,* idiopathic hypertrophic subaortic stenosis; *PDA,* patent ductus arteriosus; *PS,* pulmonic stenosis; *VSD,* ventricular septal defect.
Adapted from Allen H, Phillips J, Chan D: History and physical examination. In Allen H et al: *Moss and Adams' heart disease in infants, children, and adolescents: including the fetus and young adult,* ed 6, Philadelphia, 2001, Lippincott Williams & Wilkins; Asprey D: Innocent heart murmur. In Burg F et al: *Gellis and Kagan's current pediatric therapy,* Philadelphia, 2002, WB Saunders.

BOX 30-3 **Auscultatory Findings—the Innocent Versus Pathologic Murmur**

The Innocent Murmur
- Usually grade I-II/VI in intensity and localized
- Changes with position (sitting to lying)
- May vary in loudness or presence from visit to visit
- May increase in loudness (intensity) with fever, anemia, exercise, or anxiety
- Musical or vibratory in quality
- Systolic in timing except for venous hum, which is continuous
- Duration is short
- Best heard in LLSB or pulmonic area (except for venous hum)
- Rarely transmitted
- May disappear with Valsalva maneuver, position, or gentle jugular pressure
- Vital signs: normal
- ECG: normal
- General health status: good

Possible Pathologic Murmur: *Refer these*
- A murmur in a patient with a syndrome known to have a high incidence of CHD (e.g., trisomy 21)
- Any diastolic murmur
- Any systolic murmur that is associated with a thrill
- Pansystolic murmurs
- Continuous murmurs that cannot be suppressed
- Systolic clicks
- Opening snaps
- Fixed splitting of the second heart sound not associated with bundle branch block
- An accentuated S_2
- S_4 gallops
- Not positional
- Grade $\geq$ III/VI
- Harsh quality

ECG, Electrocardiogram; *LLSB,* left lower sternal border.
Data from Lucas JF, Saul JP: Innocent murmurs. In Burg FD, Ingelfinger JF, Polin RA et al: *Current pediatric therapy,* ed 18, Philadelphia, 2006, WB Saunders.

TABLE 30-6	DESCRIBING A HEART MURMUR
Grade or Intensity: • Does not necessarily indicate severity of the problem • May be altered with positional change from supine to sitting	Grade I: Barely audible; heard faintly after a period of attentive listening Grade II: Soft but easily audible Grade III: Moderately loud, no thrill Grade IV: Loud, present Grade V: Loud, audible with stethoscope barely on the chest Grade VI: Heard without stethoscope (rare)
Timing with cardiac cycle	Systolic Diastolic Continuous
Location on chest where murmur is loudest	Aortic Pulmonic
Radiations or transmission to other locations	To back To apex To carotids
Quality	Musical Harsh blowing
Duration	Point of onset and length of time systole and diastole murmurs last (e.g., "early systole, heard throughout cardiac cycle")
Pitch	Low Middle High

• *Complete blood count (CBC)*. CBC rules out severe anemia or polycythemia as a cause of a murmur.
  Other diagnostic tests may include the following:
• *Cardiac catheterization*. An opaque catheter is introduced into the heart chambers via the large peripheral vessels. The cardiologist measures pressures and saturation in chambers and vessels and uses dye to outline anatomy. This provides information about cardiac output, vascular resistance, and the response of the heart to exercise and medications.
• *Hyperoxia test*. Supplementation of 100% oxygen results in "pinking" and increased arterial oxygen saturation when the disease is primarily pulmonary; minimal or no color improvement indicates that the disease is cardiac. More commonly, simple pulse oximetry saturations are used to evaluate for cyanosis.
• *Magnetic resonance imaging*. This technique uses a strong magnetic field to cause movement of nuclei to yield an image of the heart structures and information about chamber volumes and function.
• *Exercise testing*. A graded treadmill or bicycle ergometer is used to determine cardiac output (myocardial blood flow and rhythm) response to exercise for endurance and capacity measurement.

■ MANAGEMENT STRATEGIES
REFERRAL

If a provider suspects cardiac disease or is unsure about findings, it is best to refer to a pediatric cardiologist if available. These specialists can best determine the extent of work-up necessary to confirm or eliminate a diagnosis (Bernstein, 2004). Findings suggestive of cardiac disease are the presence of cyanosis, symptoms of CHF, a pathologic murmur, or a murmur

SYSTOLIC MURMURS

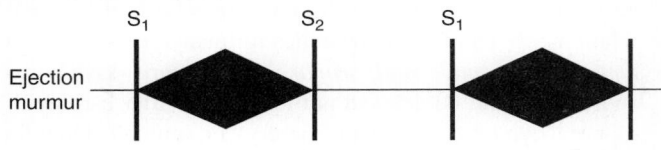

Ejection murmur

• Comprise most murmurs heard and occur between S1 and S2.
• Are either regurgitation murmurs (e.g., the holosystolic murmur of a VSD that begins with S1 and continues throughout systole) or ejection murmur caused by flow of blood through narrowed or stenotic areas (e.g., AS).
• Best heard at second left or right intercostal space (ICS)
• Begin after S1 and end before S2.
• Include all innocent and physiologic murmurs

DIASTOLIC MURMURS

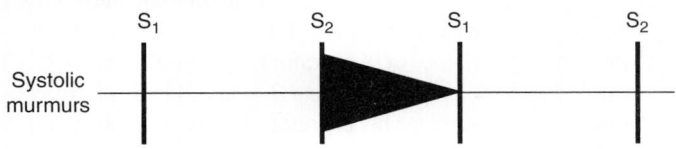

Systolic murmurs

• Occur between S2 and the return to S2.
• Always indicate cardiac pathology.
• Murmur that starts with S2 and has a decrescendo quality is most commonly due to aortic or pulmonic regurgitation.
• Mid-diastolic "rumble," a short low-pitched rumble heard best at the apex, is commonly due to atrioventricular valve stenosis or increased flow across a nonstenotic valve, such as seen with a large VSD or PDA.

CONTINUOUS MURMURS

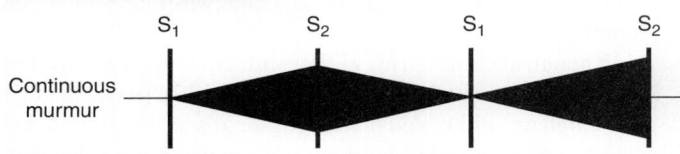

Continuous murmur

• Start at S1 and go completely through systole and diastole.
• Most common cause is PDA.
• These murmurs need to be differentiated from the coexistence of separate systolic and diastolic murmurs and venous humns.

FIG. 30-3 Types of heart murmurs. (Adapted from Allen H et al: *Moss and Adams' heart disease in infants, children, and adolescents, including the fetus and young adult*, ed 6, Philadelphia, 2001, Lippincott Williams & Wilkins, p 150.)

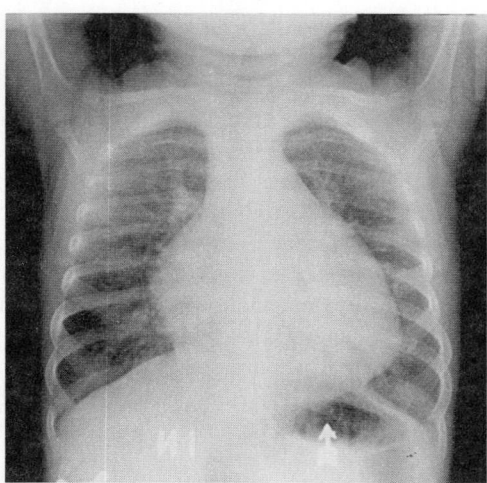

FIG. 30-4 Chest radiogram of a 3-month-old with VSD and CHF. Cardiomegaly with increased pulmonary vascular markings from pulmonary venous congestion is visible.

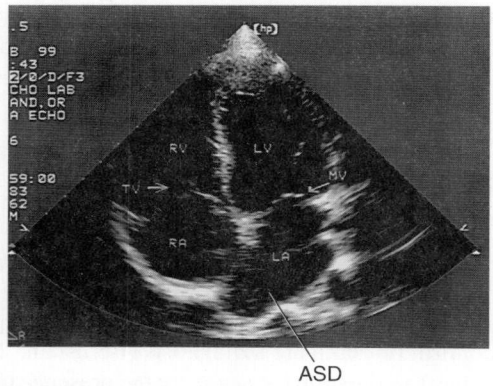

ASD

FIG. 30-5 Echocardiogram of a 2-year-old with an ASD.

that is difficult to differentiate in the presence of poor growth and development. A murmur alone in a child who is otherwise doing well should be referred to a pediatric cardiologist for further evaluation in a timely but not urgent time frame (2 to 4 weeks). An infant with suspected disease who has a murmur, symptoms of CHF, cyanosis, or poor feeding should be evaluated as soon as possible by a pediatric cardiologist. Newborns should be evaluated within 1 or 2 days of noticeable signs. An older child with dizziness, chest pain with exertion, dysrhythmia, dyspnea, syncope, signs of CHF, or abnormal vital signs should also be referred as soon as possible.

FAMILY SUPPORT

Families with infants or children in whom a cardiac problem has been diagnosed may feel fearful, confused, and even guilty. Families need the support of their PCP to help them understand the diagnosis, to cope with the short- and long-term consequences, and to advocate for them within the referral system, which may be an overwhelming experience. Because of the stress involved in initial diagnosis, many parents do not absorb all information presented and may need multiple opportunities to ask questions and learn about the diagnosis.

Parents and their designated support people should clearly understand the diagnosis and have diagrams of the defect and general information to take away with them for future reference. Should medication be necessary, parents should understand the reason for the treatment and the regimen for administration and side effects. They should have a good understanding of the signs and symptoms of deterioration (e.g., CHF) and clear information regarding how to proceed should symptoms develop. Infant and child cardiopulmonary resuscitation certification is critical for anyone caring for a child with a heart condition.

PRIMARY HEALTH CARE FOR CHILDREN WITH CARDIOVASCULAR DISEASES

The goals of primary health care for a child with cardiovascular disease include the following:

• *Adequate nutritional intake and optimal growth.* Depending on the child's condition, the family may need help in modifying the diet to provide maximum calories or limit various types of foods. The young infant with CHF may need 24, 27, or 30 kilocalories per ounce of formula or breast milk. The child may further need a nasogastric or gastric tube to obtain adequate calories because they are unable to suck adequately. Children with cyanotic conditions may initially have adequate weight gain. The provider should refer to a nutritionist if available for assistance with complex diets (see Chapter 11 for more detailed information).

• *Optimal psychosocial development and functioning.* Discuss with the family the need to treat the child as normally as possible. Encourage the family members to contact health care providers when they have questions or need reassurance. Direct parents to support groups that provide informational and emotional support for families. See Resource Box for some internet support groups. Provide support to siblings of the affected child as well. Poor sibling bonding and unexpressed fears and anger in young siblings toward an infant with a severe or chronic disease can affect their relationships and family dynamics for many years.

• *Optimal preventive and primary health care.* Live virus vaccines should be delayed until 6 months after cardiopulmonary bypass (open heart surgery) or immune globulin exposure. (American Academy of Pediatrics [AAP], 2006). This most often affects 1-year-old infants who are due for varicella and measles, mumps, and rubella vaccines. Other vaccines can be given on a regular schedule. The AAP recommends provision of respiratory syncytial virus (RSV) prophylaxis for infants less than 2 years old who have cyanotic or severe CHD. This currently involves monthly injections of palivizumab (Synagis) from November through May each year (AAP, 2006).

• *Prevention of avoidable complications.* Prevention of respiratory infections through good hand washing should be emphasized.

Although uncommon in children, infective endocarditis (IE) (also called subacute bacterial endocarditis [SBE]) is associated with a high morbidity and mortality rate (discussed later in this chapter) and warrants primary prevention whenever indicated. New standards for prophylaxis against SBE were published in

2007 by the American Heart Association (Box 30-4, and Tables 30-7 and 30-8) (Wilson et al, 2007). A high index of suspicion for IE should be maintained if any unusual clinical findings (e.g., petechiae, fever) are present after any procedure. Children with CHD appear to have more severe gingival inflammatory conditions, with concomitant increase in *Haemophilus* species, *Actinobacillus actinomycetemcomitans, Cardiobacterium hominis, Eikenella corrodens,* and *Kingella* species (HACEK) and other microbes known to cause endocarditis compared with other children (Steelman et al, 2003). The reason for this is not clear. Good dental hygiene is extremely important for these patients.

- *Optimal fitness.* Reassure the parents that the child generally "self-limits" activity according to ability. Exercise tolerance studies should be completed before entrance into sports or any activities that require strenuous physical exertion. Parameters for sports participation for children with carditis, hypertension, CHD, dysrhythmias, mitral valve prolapse, and heart murmurs are available from the American College of Cardiology Bethesda conference (Maron et al, 2005). Also see Chapter 14, Table 14-2.
- *Optimal neurodevelopmental adaption to school and life tasks.* Several recent studies have shown relatively high incidences of neurodevelopmental impairments in school-age children who had open heart surgery in infancy. (Bellinger et al, 2003; Hövels-Gürich et al, 2006). Although mean

---

BOX 30-4 **Cardiac Conditions Associated With the Highest Risk of Endocarditis: Prophylaxis Recommended**

Prophylaxis is recommended for those individuals who had:
- Prior procedures that involved the application of prosthetic valves
- Prior procedures that involved the use of prosthetic material to repair cardiac valves
- A history of infective endocarditis
- Unrepaired cyanotic congenital heart disease, including palliative shunts and conduits
- Completely repaired congenital heart defect with prosthetic material or device(s) whether done via surgery or catheterization*
- Repaired congenital heart disease with residual defects (e.g., residual ventricular septal defect) at the site of or adjacent to an area of a prosthetic patch or prosthetic device*
- A cardiac transplant who develop cardiac valvulopathy

*For the first 6 months after the procedure due to the endothelialization of prosthetic material within that period of time.
Data from Wilson W, Taubert KA, Gerwitz M et al: Prevention of infective endocarditis. Guidelines from the American Heart Association. A guideline from the American Heart Association Rheumatic Fever, Endocarditis, Kawasaki Disease Committee, Council on Cardiovascular Disease in the Young, and the Council on Clinical Cardiology, Council on Cardiovascular Surgery and Anesthesia, and the Quality of Care and Outcomes Research Interdisciplinary Working Group, *Circulation* 116:1736-1754, 2007.

---

intelligence scores are generally within the average range, many of these children have difficulties with visual-spacial tasks, fine motor functions, and attention. They may be impaired in their ability to coordinate lower-order skills to perform higher-order tasks. In one study, 37% of children required remedial services in school (Bellinger et al, 2003). PCPs can assist parents in observing for and assessing these difficulties and obtaining appropriate services early.

Specific developmental areas that may require additional attention at various ages are listed in Box 30-5.

■ CONGENITAL HEART DISEASES
CONGESTIVE HEART FAILURE

CHF is the most common symptom complex in children with heart disease. It is the major reason, other than elective procedures, for hospitalization of these children. Those under 6 months old usually have an underlying intracardiac left-to-right shunt (e.g., VSD), whereas those older than 4 years succumb to CHF from acquired heart diseases or as a consequence of CHD (Allen et al, 2001).

CHF refers to a set of clinical signs and symptoms that indicate myocardial dysfunction. This dysfunction results in cardiac output that is inadequate to provide blood and oxygen to body tissues. Compensatory mechanics in the body respond by affecting fluid homeostasis. Electrolyte and hormonal imbalances and water retention result, further complicating pulmonary and peripheral congestion (Anderson et al, 2002). VSD and PDA are examples of conditions that lead to increased myocardial workload caused by excessive volume secondary to shunting of blood. Structural or valvular abnormalities (e.g., coarctation and AS) impede the normal flow of blood through cardiac structures and thereby increase the pressure load on the heart. Any condition that decreases the effectiveness of myocardial function (e.g., myocarditis, anemia, dysrhythmia) can also result in failure of the heart to maintain adequate cardiac output (Table 30-9).

Alterations in cardiac function occur because the cardiac muscle is overtaxed and compensation mechanisms are activated in an attempt to maintain adequate cardiac output. Ventricular dilation and hypertrophy are early indicators of the heart's reaction to increased workload. Tachycardia is an adaptive mechanism to increase cardiac output and promote delivery of oxygen to the heart and body. If demands on the heart are increased past the point of maximal effectiveness, the result is decreased cardiac output, pulmonary and systemic congestion, and associated clinical symptoms (Box 30-6).

ACYANOTIC CONGENITAL HEART DISEASE (LEFT-TO-RIGHT SHUNTS)

Acyanotic lesions have a communication between the two sides of the heart through which extra blood shunts from the high-pressure, oxygenated, left side of the heart to the low-pressure, deoxygenated, right side of the heart. The result is an increase in pulmonary blood flow (Fig. 30-6).

TABLE 30-7 Procedures for Which Endocarditis Prophylaxis Is or Is Not Recommended in High-Risk Individuals

	Prophylaxis Recommended	Prophylaxis NOT Recommended
Dental	Dental extractions Periodontal procedures Dental implant placement and reimplantation of avulsed teeth Root canal instrumentation Initial placement of orthodontic braces but not brackets Teeth or implant cleaning where bleeding is expected	Restorative dentistry Routine anesthetic injections through noninfected tissue Intracanal endodontic treatment; postplacement and buildup Rubber dam placement Postoperative suture removal Placement of removable prosthodontic or orthodontic appliances Bleeding from trauma of lips or oral mucosa Taking oral impressions Fluoride treatments Taking oral radiographs Orthodontic appliance adjustment or placement of brackets Shedding of primary teeth
Respiratory tract	Tonsillectomy or adenoidectomy Surgery involving respiratory mucosa	Endotracheal intubation Flexible bronchoscopy without biopsy Pressure tympanostomy tube insertion/removal Rigid bronchoscopy
Skin	Procedures involving infected skin or skin structures	Uncomplicated skin biopsy Tattooing (but this is highly discouraged in high risk individuals)
Musculoskeletal tissue	Procedures involving infected musculoskeletal tissue	
Genitourinary tract	Cystoscopy or urinary tract manipulation in patients with entococcal infection	Vaginal delivery Cesarean section Urethral catheterization without infection Therapeutic abortion Circumcision Hysterectomy
Gastrointestinal tract		Any GI tract procedures including esophagogastroduodenoscopy or colonoscopy
Other procedures		Cardiac catheterization, including device placement and pacemakers

Data from Helpin ML & Berg JH: Dental problems. In Burg F et al, editors: *Gellis and Kagan's current pediatric therapy*, ed 18, Philadelphia, 2006, WB Saunders; Wilson W, Taubert KA, Gerwitz M et al: Prevention of infective endocarditis. Guidelines from the American Heart Association. A guideline from the American Heart Association Rheumatic Fever, Endocarditis, Kawasaki Disease Committee, Council on Cardiovascular Disease in the Young, and the Council on Clinical Cardiology, Council on Cardiovascular Surgery and Anesthesia, and the Quality of Care and Outcomes Research Interdisciplinary Working Group, *Circulation* 116:1736-1754, 2007.

Atrial Septal Defect

Description. An atrial septal defect is a defect or hole in the atrial septum. Of the four types of ASD, the most common involves the midseptum in the area of the foramen ovale and is called an ostium secundum–type defect (Fig. 30-7). Defects of the sinus venosus type are high in the atrial septum, near the entry of the superior vena cava (SVC), and are frequently associated with anomalous pulmonary venous return. A primum ASD is in the lower portion of the septum and is most often seen in children with Down syndrome. The rarest form of ASD is an unroofed coronary sinus (Driscoll, 2006).

Incidence. ASD of the ostium secundum variety is twice as common in females and accounts for 7% to 10% of CHD (Driscoll, 2006).

Clinical Findings

History
- Often completely asymptomatic
- May fatigue easily or have exertional dyspnea
- May be somewhat thin
- May have a history of frequent upper respiratory tract infections or pneumonia

Physical Examination
- Typically a murmur may not be noticed until the child is 2 to 3 years old, when examination of a quiet child can be performed.
- Mild left precordial bulge or palpable lift at the left sternal border may be seen.
- S_1 is normal or split, with accentuation of the tricuspid valve closure sound.

TABLE 30-8   Prophylactic Regimens for Dental Procedures*

Route	Agent	Regimen†
Able to take oral medication	Amoxicillin	Adults: 2g PO; children: 50mg/kg PO (max 2g)
Unable to take oral medication	Ampicillin	Adults: 2g IM or IV; children: 50mg/kg IM or IV (max 2g)
	or‡	
	Cefazolin or ceftriaxone	Adults: 1g IM or IV; children: 50mg/kg IM or IV (max 1g)
If Penicillin allergic, oral	Clindamycin	Adults: 600mg PO; children: 20mg/kg PO (max 600mg)
	or‡	
	Cephalexin or cefadroxil	Adults: 2g PO; children: 50mg/kg PO (max 2g)
	or‡	
	Azithromycin or clarithromycin	Adults: 500mg PO; children: 15mg/kg PO (max 500mg)
Penicillin allergic and unable to take oral medication	Clindamycin	Adults: 600mg IM or IV; children: 20mg/kg IM or IV (max 600mg)
	or‡	
	Cefazolin or ceftriaxone	Adults: 1g IM or IV; children: 50mg/kg IM or IV (max 1g)

IM, Intramuscularly; *IV*, intravenously; *max*, maximum, *PO*, orally.
* Antibiotic regimens are procedure specific; refer to the American Heart Association reference for nondental prophylaxis recommendations.
† Take 30-60 minutes prior to the procedure.
‡ Or other first- or second-generation oral cephalosporin in equivalent adult or pediatric dosage. Cephalosporins should not be used if there is a history of anaphylaxis, angioedema, or urticaria with penicillins.
Wilson W, Taubert KA, Gerwitz M et al: Prevention of infective endocarditis. Guidelines from the American Heart Association. A guideline from the American Heart Association Rheumatic Fever, Endocarditis, Kawasaki Disease Committee, Council on Cardiovascular Disease in the Young, and the Council on Clinical Cardiology, Council on Cardiovascular Surgery and Anesthesia, and the Quality of Care and Outcomes Research Interdisciplinary Working Group, *Circulation* 116:1736-1754, 2007.

BOX 30-5   Key Areas of Primary Health Care for Children With Cardiovascular Disease

Infancy (Birth to 2 Years)
Growth and development
Nutrition
Immunizations
Attention to siblings

Preschool Years
Development
Discipline
Dental care
Endocarditis prophylaxis

School Age (6 to 12 Years)
School program
Activity recommendations and sports
Endocarditis prophylaxis

Adolescence
Sexuality concerns, contraception, and pregnancy
Delayed puberty
Genetic counseling
Athletic exercise
Vocational counseling
Endocarditis counseling

TABLE 30-9   Conditions That Can Lead to Congestive Heart Failure in Children

Age	Condition
Premature infant	Patent ductus arteriosus
Birth-1 week	Hypoplastic left heart syndrome
	Coarctation of the aorta
	Critical aortic stenosis
	Interrupted aortic arch
	Arteriovenous malformations
	Tachycardia
	Cardiomyopathy
1 week-3 months	Ventricular septal defect
	Truncus arteriosus
	Atrioventricular canal (endocardial cushion defect)
	Total anomalous pulmonary venous return
	Coarctation
	Tachycardia
	Patent ductus arteriosus
	Aortic stenosis
	Tricuspid atresia
Older than 1 year	Bacterial endocarditis
	Rheumatic fever
	Myocarditis

BOX 30-6	**Signs and Symptoms of Congestive Heart Failure**

Infants
Tachypnea
Tachycardia
Rales or wheezing
Cardiomegaly and hepatomegaly
Periorbital edema
Poor feeding
Poor weight gain
Diaphoresis

Children
Tachypnea
Tachycardia
Rales or wheezing
Cardiomegaly and hepatomegaly
Orthopnea
Shortness of breath or dyspnea with exertion
Peripheral edema
Poor growth and development

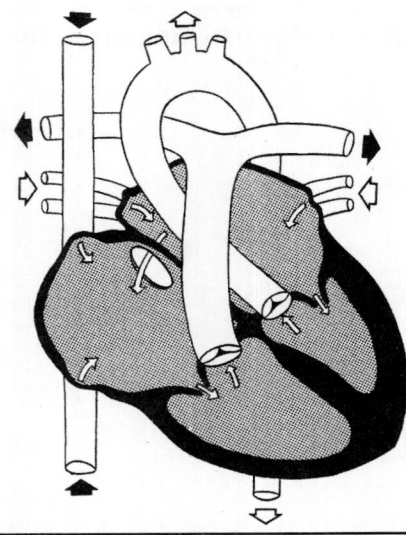

FIG. 30-7 Atrial septal defect. (Used with permission of Ross Products Division, Abbott Laboratories, Columbus, OH 43216. From *Clinical education aid no 7.* Copyright 1970 Ross Products Division, Abbott Laboratories.)

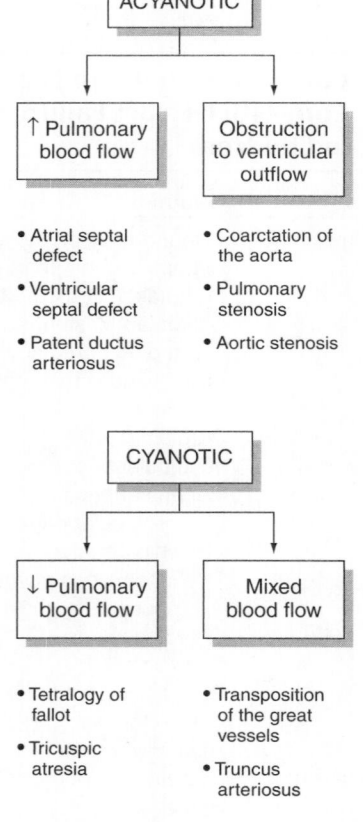

FIG. 30-6 Classification of CHD.

- S_2 is split widely and is relatively fixed in relation to respiration in patients with normal pulmonary pressure.
- A grade I to III/VI, widely radiating, medium-pitched, not harsh systolic ejection murmur is heard best at the pulmonic area. If the shunt is large, increased blood flow across the tricuspid valve is responsible for a middiastolic, rumbling murmur at the left lower sternal border (LLSB).
- In older patients (teenage or older), pulmonic and tricuspid murmurs decrease in intensity, and the second heart sound may be single and accentuated. A diastolic murmur of pulmonic incompetence can appear.

Diagnostic Studies

- Chest radiography may reveal cardiac enlargement. The main pulmonary artery may be dilated and the pulmonary vascular markings increased.
- The ECG shows right axis deviation with right atrial enlargement. Lead V1 usually shows a right bundle branch block with a rsR' pattern. However, the ECG can be normal in small left-to-right defects.
- The echocardiogram identifies the specific location of the defect in the atrial septum and shows chamber enlargement.
- Cardiac catheterization is rarely necessary unless the diagnosis is in doubt, shunt size is indeterminable, or pulmonary vascular disease is suspected (Bernstein, 2004).

Management. Management of ASD includes the following:

- Small defects found in infancy may close on their own.
- Larger defects require intervention, usually after 1 year and before school entry or when the defect is identified in an older child. Interventional cardiologists can now close most ASDs in the cardiac catheterization lab with a closure device. If the defect is quite large or unfavorable to device closure, cardiac surgeons can patch the defect. Surgical mortality rate is less than 1%.

- No SBE prophylaxis precautions are necessary if the defect is small and isolated (see Box 30-4 and Table 30-7).
- Long-term outcome is excellent for patients after ASD repair.

Ventricular Septal Defect

Description. A VSD is a hole or defect in one of the areas of the ventricular septum. There are four types of VSDs: perimembranous, supracristal is, inlet/inflow, and muscular (Driscoll, 2006). The most common type is the perimembranous VSD (Fig. 30-8).

Incidence. VSD is the most common childhood cardiac defect, accounting for 25% of diagnosed CHD. It is associated with Down syndrome, but 95% of all VSD cases have no chromosomal anomaly. Approximately 30% to 50% of these defects are small; the vast majority of these close by 4 years old.

Clinical Findings

History

- A murmur is often not heard immediately after birth. When pulmonary vascular resistance falls (normally at 2 to 8 weeks old), more blood is shunted across the VSD from left ventricle to right ventricle and hence to the pulmonary circulation. This causes a classic loud murmur and possibly heralds the beginning of CHF symptoms.
- Parents may note signs and symptoms of CHF, such as pale skin color, poor weight gain, feeding difficulty, increased respiratory rate and effort, and diaphoresis with crying or feeding.
- Small defects may be completely asymptomatic.

Physical Examination

- Small VSD
  - Harsh, high-pitched, grade II to IV/VI holosystolic murmur at LLSB
  - All other findings within normal limits
- Large VSD
  - Low-pitched, grade II to V/VI holosystolic murmur at LLSB
  - VSD murmur that becomes higher pitched over time indicates that the defect is becoming smaller

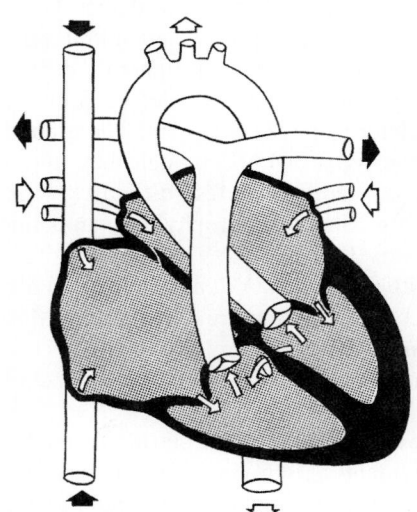

FIG. 30-8 Ventricular septal defect. (Used with permission of Ross Products Division, Abbott Laboratories, Columbus, OH 43216. From *Clinical education aid no 7.* Copyright 1970 Ross Products Division, Abbott Laboratories.)

- Diastolic rumble at the apex
- "Thrill" along the left sternal border
- Signs of progressing CHF (e.g., hepatomegaly, rales, fatigability, tachypnea, failure to thrive) after the first weeks of life
- S_3 or S_4 gallop if CHF is present (Driscoll, 2006)

Diagnostic Studies

- Chest radiography findings vary depending on the size of the shunt. Children with small shunts have normal heart size and pulmonary vascular markings that are just beyond the upper limits of normal. Patients with large shunts have cardiac enlargement involving both the left and right ventricles and left atrium, as well as pulmonary vascular markings that are significantly increased (see Fig. 30-4).
- The ECG is normal for patients with small defects and may show left ventricular hypertrophy (LVH) or biventricular hypertrophy (BVH) with large shunts.
- Echocardiography provides visualization of defects and pinpoints the exact anatomic location. In "pinhole" VSDs, a murmur may be present; however, a defect may not be visualized on the echocardiogram.
- Cardiac catheterization is rarely necessary except when there is a question of elevated pulmonary vascular resistance (Driscoll, 2006).

Management

- Infants with small defects and no symptoms of CHF are monitored every 3 to 6 months throughout the first year of life and then biannually to assess for closure of the defect. Some defects may never close and cause no difficulty. See SBE prophylaxis guidelines in Table 30-7 and Box 30-4.
- Larger defects with signs of CHF are managed as follows:
  - Lanoxin, diuretics, ACE inhibitors, and beta-blocker dosages are prescribed, as needed, by a cardiologist.
  - The provider must monitor nutritional intake and weight gain in these infants and children. It is also important to teach families to fortify infant's calories to 24, 27, or even 30 kcal/oz, as needed, and arrange enteric nutritional support via nasogastric tube in young infants struggling to meet their caloric needs.
  - Families must be taught the signs and symptoms of developing or progressing CHF.
- The pediatric cardiologist will arrange surgery or device closure in the cardiac catheterization lab if no improvement is seen over weeks or months.
  - Surgical repair consists of closure of the defect with a Gortex patch.
  - SBE prophylaxis precautions are necessary for 6 months after surgery.

Long-term outcome is excellent after VSD repair (Driscoll, 2006).

Atrioventricular Septal Defect (AV Canal Defect or Endocardial Cushion Defect)

Description. The endocardial cushion is a central cardiac structure that includes the septal portions of the mitral and tricuspid valves and lower portion of the atrial septum and upper portion of the ventricular septum. In AV septal defects, variable portions of the endocardial cushion are absent. Complete AV septal defect implies the absence of this cushion, leading to a primum ASD, a single AV valve (composed of leaflets of the intended mitral and tricuspid valves), and an inlet VSD. There may also be partial and intermediate defects with less profound abnormalities and usually less severe symptoms (Fig. 30-9).

Incidence. Two percent of congenital heart defects are complete endocardial cushion defects, and 1% to 2% have partial or intermediate AV canal defect. Forty percent of patients with complete AV canal defect have Down syndrome (Driscoll, 2006).

Clinical Findings
History
- Children with only a primum ASD (partial AV canal) may not manifest symptoms.
- In infants with complete AV canal defects, parents may note signs and symptoms of CHF, such as pale skin color, poor weight gain, feeding difficulty, increased respiratory rate and effort, and diaphoresis with crying or feeding. These children may experience increased respiratory distress of CHF with common respiratory infections as well.

Physical Examination
- Partial AV canal (primum ASD) findings are the same as those with secundum ASD. There may also be a soft blowing murmur of mitral regurgitation in the apex and or infrascapular area.
- Complete AV canal defect
  - Low-pitched, grade II to V/VI holosystolic murmur at LLSB. A murmur may not be evident at birth. When pulmonary vascular resistance falls (normally at 2 to 8 weeks old), more blood is shunted across the VSD and ASD from the left ventricle to right ventricle and hence to the pulmonary circulation. This causes a classic loud murmur and the beginning of CHF symptoms.
  - Diastolic rumble at the apex.

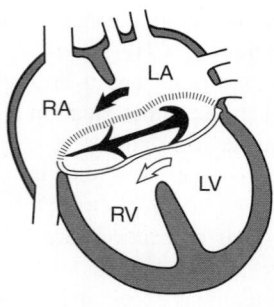

Complete

FIG. 30-9   Complete atrioventricular canal defect (also known as a complete endocardial cushion defect). An ostium primum atrial septal defect (*solid arrow*) and an inlet VSD (*open arrow*) are present. *LA*, left atrium; *LV*, left ventricle; *RA*, right atrium; *RV*, right ventricle. (Used with permission of Park MK, Troxler RG: *Pediatric cardiology for practitioners*, ed 4, St Louis, 2002, Mosby.)

- "Thrill" along the left sternal border.
- Signs of progressing CHF (e.g., hepatomegaly, rales, fatigability, tachypnea, diaphoresis, failure to thrive) after the first weeks of life.
- S_3 or S_4 gallop if CHF is present.
- Some infants maintain neonatal high pulmonary vascular resistance and do not show signs of CHF. Instead they may manifest signs of pulmonary hypertension with loud single S_2, precordial heave, minimal murmur, and perhaps desaturation with agitation or effort (Driscoll, 2006).

Diagnostic Studies
- Chest radiography findings vary depending on the size of the shunt. Children with small shunts have normal heart size and pulmonary vascular markings that are just beyond the upper limits of normal. Patients with large shunts (complete AV canal defect) have cardiac enlargement involving both the left and right ventricles and left atrium, as well as increased pulmonary vascular markings that are significantly increased (see Fig. 30-4).
- The ECG usually shows superior axis between −40 and −160 degrees. Right ventricular hypertrophy (RVH) is usually present, and LVH or BVH in large shunts may be present. In 50% of children, the PR interval is prolonged.
- Echocardiography (two-dimensional, Doppler, or transesophageal) provides visualization of the size of ASD and VSD defects and the size and other characteristics of the AV valve(s). Echocardiography can also evaluate the relative sizes of the RV and LV. This is important to discern because some children have right or left ventricles that are too small for a two-ventricle repair.
- Cardiac catheterization is rarely necessary except when there is a question of elevated pulmonary vascular resistance (Driscoll, 2006).

Management
- Children with a partial AV canal defect that consists of a primum ASD and possibly a cleft mitral valve are monitored every 3 to 6 months throughout the first year of life and then biannually until the defect is closed surgically during toddler or preschool years. These children usually do not have signs of CHF, though they may gain weight slowly. They rarely manifest difficulty with pulmonary hypertension. See SBE prophylaxis guidelines in Table 30-7 and Box 30-4.
- Infants with a complete AV canal defect usually need surgical correction in the first 6 months of life. Most need CHF medical management before surgery:
  - Digoxin, diuretics, ACE inhibitors, and beta-blockers are used.
  - The provider must monitor nutritional intake and weight in these infants and children. Families need to be taught to fortify an infant formula or breast milk to 24, 27, or even 30 kcal/oz. Enteric nutritional support via nasogastric tube can be arranged in young infants struggling to meet their caloric needs.

- ° Families must be taught the signs and symptoms of developing or progressing CHF.
- ° Surgical repair consists of closure of the defect with a Gortex patch and reconstruction of the common AV valve into separate tricuspid and mitral valves. Residual mitral and/or tricuspid insufficiency is common after surgery.
- ° After this repair, SBE prophylaxis precautions are necessary for 6 months.

Patent Ductus Arteriosus

Description. In the normal newborn, functional closure of the ductus arteriosus occurs in the first 12 to 72 hours. Permanent sealing of the ductus arteriosus occurs in 2 to 3 weeks (Driscoll, 2006). The ductus arteriosus may remain patent in some infants and leave a connection between the aorta and the pulmonary artery. As pulmonary vascular resistance falls, aortic blood is shunted into the pulmonary artery and recirculates through the lungs (Fig. 30-10).

Incidence. PDA accounts for 9% to 12% of all cases of CHD. The incidence in females outnumbers that in males 2:1. The frequency of PDAs increases with decreasing gestational age in premature infants; it is as high as 45% to 80% in very young infants less than 1750 g (Driscoll, 2006).

Clinical Findings

History

- The infant or child may be asymptomatic if the PDA is small.
- Increasing signs of CHF may appear in the first weeks of life in larger PDAs.

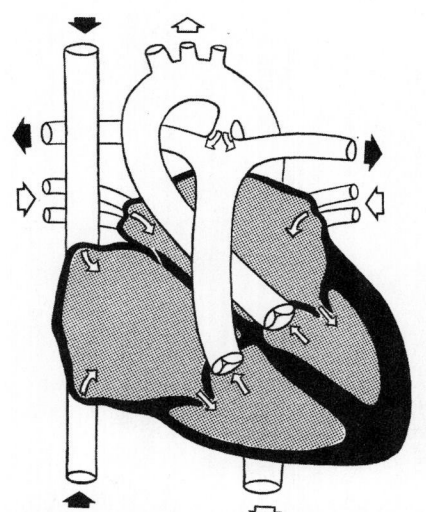

FIG. 30-10 Patent ductus arteriosus. (Used with permission of Ross Products Division, Abbott Laboratories, Columbus, OH 43216. From *Clinical education aid no 7.* Copyright 1970 Ross Products Division, Abbott Laboratories.)

Physical Examination

- In the immediate postnatal period, the murmur is soft, systolic, and heard along the left sternal border, under the left clavicle, and in the back.
- After the first weeks of life, a typical grade II to V/VI, harsh, rumbling, continuous "machinery murmur" is heard in the left infraclavicular fossa and pulmonic area with a thrill at the base.
- Physical findings of CHF (e.g., hepatomegaly, rales, fatigability, tachypnea, failure to thrive) may be present with a large shunt.

Diagnostic Studies

- Chest radiographic findings include the following:
  - ° With a small to moderate shunt, the heart is not enlarged.
  - ° If the shunt is large, evidence of both left atrial and ventricular enlargement is apparent. Pulmonary vascular markings may be increased.
- ECG reveals LVH with large shunts. QRS axis will be normal or rightward.
- An echocardiogram demonstrates the patent ductus and usually shows enlargement of the left atrium (Driscoll, 2006).

Differential Diagnosis. See Table 30-10.

Management

- Indomethacin, a prostaglandin inhibitor that constricts and closes the ductus, may be given to preterm infants to effect closure when there is significant left-to-right shunt.
- An asymptomatic infant with a small left-to-right shunt from a PDA is followed for spontaneous closure for approximately 2 years. Patients with large shunts or infants with pulmonary hypertension should have their PDA surgically closed within the first few months of life to prevent the development of progressive pulmonary vascular obstruction. Surgical ligation of the ductus is a low-risk procedure because cardiopulmonary bypass is not necessary.
- Interventional cardiologists now close many PDAs in children older than 1 year by inserting coils into the shunt in the cardiac catheterization laboratory.
- Families should be reassured that their child will live an active, normal life.
- SBE prophylaxis precautions are recommended until 6 months after the repair.

CYANOTIC CONGENITAL HEART DISEASE (RIGHT-TO-LEFT SHUNTS)

Cyanotic CHD (see Fig. 30-6) represents 10% to 18% of all congenital heart lesions (Lin et al, 2006). Cardiac cyanosis is due to obstruction of pulmonary blood flow or mixing of oxygenated and unoxygenated blood. Visible cyanosis occurs when greater than 3 to 5 g/dL of desaturated hemoglobin is present in arterial blood. Cyanosis is more readily apparent with polycythemia and less readily apparent with anemia or the presence of fetal hemoglobin. Polycythemia is a compensatory mechanism to increase the oxygen-carrying capacity in cyanotic patients; however, it increases the risk for cerebral

TABLE 30-10 Congenital Heart Disease: Differential Diagnosis of Cardiac Defects

Feature	Atrial Septal Defect	Ventricular Septal Defect	Patent Ductus Arteriosus	Transposition of the Great Vessels	Tetralogy of Fallot	Tricuspid Atresia	Aortic Stenosis	Pulmonic Stenosis	Coarctation of the Aorta
Incidence of total CHD	10%, 2:1 female to male	20%	10%	5%, 3:1 male to female	8%	2%	5%, 4:1 male to female	8%	5%
Age at initial presentation	Variable; may be asymptomatic into adulthood	Variable depending on size; large by 4-8 wk old; small by 6 mo old	Neonate to 3 mo old	Immediately at birth	Usually by 6 mo old	Usually newborn	Depends on severity; critical in newborn	Depends on severity; newborn to school-age children	First wk of life or 3-5 yr old
Clinical findings	Murmur on preschool examination	CHF or murmur	CHF or murmur	Cyanosis	Cyanosis	Cyanosis	Murmur, CHF; older child, chest pain	Cyanosis or murmur	CHF in newborn; hypertension in preschooler
Auscultation	Midsystolic murmur at ULSB with wide-split second heart sound	Holosystolic murmur at LLSB	Continuous murmur under left clavicle, referred to back	Usually no murmur	Early systolic ejection murmur at second left intercostal space; holosystolic murmur at LLSB	ASD murmur, may be associated with PDA	Systolic ejection murmur at URSB, constant systolic click apex with bicuspid valve	Late systolic ejection murmur at ULSB, intermittent systolic to back ejection click	Systolic ejection murmur in left intraclavicular region with transmission

Radiologic findings	May have mild cardiomegaly	Normal or cardiomegaly	Cardiomegaly	Egg-shaped heart	Boot-shaped heart	Cardiomegaly	Normal	Normal	Rib notching
Pulmonary vasculature	Normal to slightly increased	Normal or increased	Increased markings	May have increased markings or be normal	Decreased pulmonary vascularity	Decreased pulmonary markings	Normal	Decreased in severity	Normal
ECG	May have RsRi in V1, right atrial enlargement	Combined ventricular hypertrophy	Combined ventricular hypertrophy	RV hypertrophy	RV hypertrophy	Right atrial enlargement, absent RV voltage	LVH	RV hypertrophy	RV hypertrophy
Associations	Holt-Oram syndrome, Down syndrome in PAPVR, mitral valve prolapse	Associated with many defects	Associated with many defects	VSD, PDA, coronary artery anomalies	Down syndrome	VSD, PDA, ASD	Marfan syndrome, Turner syndrome, Williams syndrome	Turner syndrome, Williams syndrome, neurofibromatosis	Turner syndrome, neurofibromatosis PDA
Treatments	Surgical closure	Observation, digoxin and/or diuretics; if large, surgical closure	Surgical closure if large	Newborn PGE, septostomy, arterial switch (Jatene)	Tetralogy repair, BT shunt	Shunt and surgical repair	Catheter valvulotomy or surgical repair	Catheter valvuloplasty or surgery	Surgical repair or balloon dilation

ASD, Atrial septal defect; BT, blalock-taussig; CHF, congenital heart failure; ECG, electrocardiogram; LLSB, left lower sternal border; LVH, left ventricular hypertrophy; mo, month(s); PAPVR, partial anomalous pulmonary venous return; PDA, patent ductus arteriosus; PGE, prostaglandin E; RV, right ventricular; ULSB, upper left sternal border; URSB, upper right sternal border; wk, week(s); VSD, ventricular septal defect; yr, year(s).

thromboses (Bernstein, 2004). Common heart conditions causing cyanosis in the immediate newborn period include transposition of the great arteries (TGA), tetralogy of Fallot (TOF), truncus arteriosus, and tricuspid atresia.

Transposition of the Great Arteries

Description. TGA results from incomplete septation and migration of the truncus arteriosus during fetal development. In TGA, the aorta arises from the right ventricle and the pulmonary artery arises from the left ventricle. The aorta receives the deoxygenated systemic venous blood and returns it to the systemic arteries. The pulmonary artery receives oxygenated pulmonary venous blood and returns it to the pulmonary circulation (Fig. 30-11). There may be a number of other heart malformations, most commonly a(n) VSD and ASD.

Incidence. TGA accounts for 2% to 5% of all cases of CHD and occurs 60% to 70% more frequently in males (Lin et al, 2006). Without treatment, there is a 50% mortality rate in the first month of life and 90% by the first year. With surgery, 90% to 98% survive.

Clinical Findings

History

- Cyanosis is immediately evident by 1 hour of birth (52%) or within the first day after birth (92%). Because TGA and VSD allow mixing of oxygenated and unoxygenated blood, occasionally children with these defects who are less cyanotic present as late as 3 months old.
- CHF symptoms may be present.
- Affected infants are often large for gestational age with retardation of growth and development after the neonatal period.

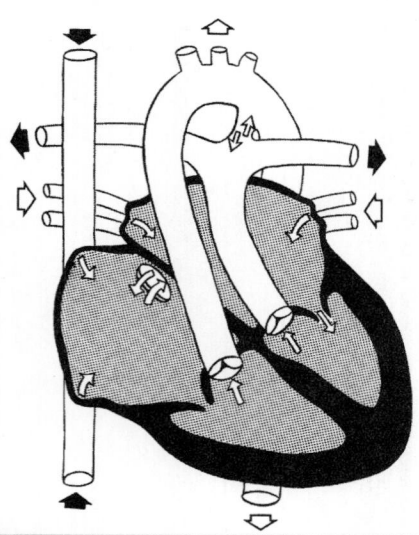

FIG. 30-11 Complete transposition of the great vessels. (Used with permission of Ross Products Division, Abbott Laboratories, Columbus, OH 43216. From *Clinical education aid no 7.* Copyright 1970 Ross Products Division, Abbott Laboratories.)

Physical Examination

- Infants may have no murmur at birth or may have a murmur characteristic of associated lesions, such as VSD, ASD, or PDA.
- S_2 is loud and single because of the anatomic placement of the great arteries in TGA.

Diagnostic Studies

- Chest radiography and ECG findings may be normal in the early newborn period, or the heart may appear egg shaped.
- ECG findings show right axis deviation and RVH.
- Echocardiography shows the pulmonary artery arising from the left ventricle and the aorta arising from the right (Driscoll, 2006).

Management

- Immediate referral and transfer if necessary to a pediatric cardiac center are necessary. Correction of electrolyte and acid-base imbalance may be necessary.
- Give intravenous prostaglandin E_1 (PGE_1) to delay closure or reopen the ductus arteriosus.
- A balloon atrial septostomy may be performed in the catheterization laboratory to promote mixing of oxygenated and unoxygenated blood in the atria.
- The arterial switch (Jatene procedure) is usually performed in the first few days of life.
- These patients are monitored closely throughout life with annual echocardiogram follow-up.
- SBE prophylaxis precautions are indicated.

Prognosis. Operative mortality is from 5% to 17% with excellent long-term results (Driscoll, 2006). However, long-term patency and growth of the coronary arteries warrant close monitoring. Neopulmonic stenosis and neoaortic regurgitation may occur after the arterial switch. The PCP should refer any patient with history of arterial or atrial switch to a pediatric cardiologist, especially with a history of palpitations, syncope, and/or shortness of breath with exertion.

Tetralogy of Fallot

Description. The tetralogy of Fallot (TOF), also referred to as TET, is a combination of four anatomic cardiac defects resulting in right ventricular outflow tract obstruction: (1) pulmonary valve stenosis, (2) RVH, (3) VSD, and (4) an aorta that overrides the ventricular septum (Fig. 30-12). There is a spectrum of severity in TOF. In the most severe forms, the pulmonary valve and artery are atretic (not patent). This is referred to as TOF pulmonary atresia, and these infants are quite cyanotic as newborns. In the mildest form, "pink TETs," the infant may not display signs of cyanosis because the valvular stenosis is mild, and their symptoms may be similar to a large VSD. In most cases of TOF, however, right-to-left shunting across the VSD and cyanosis increases over the first months of life as a result of increasing obstruction in the right ventricular outflow tract (Driscoll, 2006).

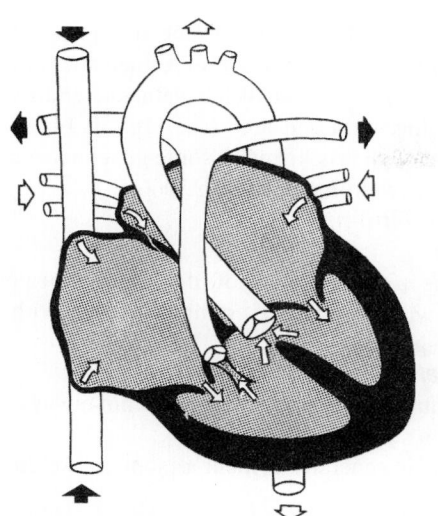

FIG. 30-12 TOF. (Used with permission of Ross Products Division, Abbott Laboratories, Columbus, OH 43216. From *Clinical education aid no 7*. Copyright 1970 Ross Products Division, Abbott Laboratories.)

Epidemiology. TOF, the most common cyanotic lesion, accounts for 3.5% to 9% of all cases of CHD. There is no racial bias; the defect occurs up to 56.4% more frequently in males (Lin et al, 2006). Approximately 16% of children with TOF have a chromosome 22q11 deletion. This is usually a spontaneous mutation and not present in the parents (Goldmuntz, 2005).

Clinical Findings

History

- Cyanosis
  - Cyanosis (in cases with mild right ventricular outflow obstruction) may be so slight that it is not initially evident, or it may be present at birth (with severe obstruction).
  - Cyanosis (including hypercyanotic episodes, or TET spells) and dyspnea increase by 2 to 4 months old, especially with crying, feeding, and/or defecation. The infant may have a history of poor weight gain.

Physical Examination.
The severity of symptoms depends on the degree of right ventricular outflow obstruction. The following examination findings may be evident:

- Cyanosis of the mucous membranes and dyspnea.
- A grade III to V/VI, harsh systolic ejection murmur is heard at the left mid to upper sternal border (VSD murmur and symptoms of a large VSD). There may be palpable thrill and a holosystolic murmur at the LLSB.
- A sternal lift secondary to right ventricular hypertrophy.

Diagnostic Studies

- Chest radiography may show a boot-shaped heart with decreased pulmonary vascular markings.
- ECG shows RVH, right axis deviation and may show a conduction delay in V_1.
- An echocardiogram shows the extent of the pulmonary obstruction and demonstrates the anatomy of the overriding aorta and VSD.

- Pulse oximetry values decrease over time, with resultant increase in hemoglobin and hematocrit values.
- Cardiac catheterization is done before surgery in the most severe forms to delineate pulmonary artery anatomy.

Management

- In neonates with severe pulmonary obstruction, the ductus arteriosus is maintained or reopened with PGE_1 until more definitive repair or palliation is possible.
- For hypercyanotic episodes, or TET spells, the child should be cradled in a knee-chest position, soothed, and given oxygen and perhaps morphine sulfate subcutaneously until the spell subsides. The knee-chest maneuver increases systemic resistance, decreases right-to-left shunting, and increases pulmonary blood flow, perhaps alleviating symptoms. Immediate intervention is required for infants who are "spelling," especially if the above maneuvers do not end the spell. Children have died from TET spells that were not adequately addressed. Most children are surgically repaired before hypercyanotic spells begin (Driscoll, 2006).
- Complete repair with open-heart surgery is usually performed in infancy (Driscoll, 2006).
- These children need lifelong cardiology follow-up for pulmonic regurgitation or late arrhythmias. Recent studies indicate that progressive right ventricular dilation leads to increasing QRS duration on ECG. (Gatzoulis, 2003). Children and young adults with QRS duration greater than 160 milliseconds have increased risk of sudden death (presumably from atrial or ventricular arrhythmia). Sports participation is usually unrestricted if there are no residual defects after surgery. The provider should seek a cardiology consult before clearing for sports participation (Maron et al, 2005).
- SBE prophylaxis precautions are indicated prior to surgery and generally 6 months after repair.

Tricuspid Atresia, Hypoplastic Left Heart Syndrome, and Other Single Ventricle Defects

Description and Epidemiology. Hypoplastic left and right heart and single ventricle defects are a heterogenous group of heart problems that together comprise perhaps 5% to 6% of congenital defects. In most cases there is functionally one ventricle involving either right or left morphology that must do the work of pumping blood to both the systemic and pulmonary circulations (Figs. 30-13, 30-14, and 30-15). Oxygenated and deoxygenated blood mix in this ventricle, and the child is cyanotic. Most of these children will require palliative cardiac procedures.

Tricuspid atresia results in the absence of communication between the right atrium and the right ventricle (see Fig. 30-13). TGA also occurs in 50% of these patients. The right ventricle is usually hypoplastic. Less than 3% of all children with CHD have tricuspid atresia. Up to 20% have multiple cardiac abnormalities. The etiology of this condition is unknown (Driscoll, 2006).

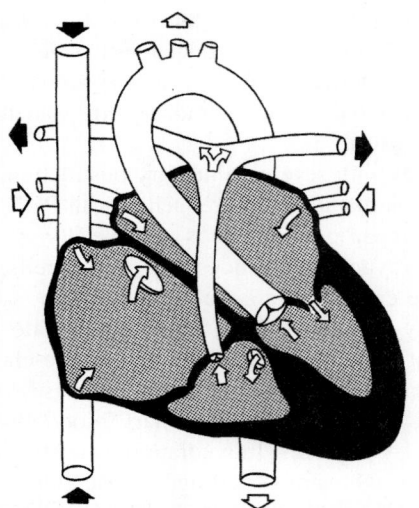

FIG. 30-13 Tricuspid atresia. (Used with permission of Ross Products Division, Abbott Laboratories, Columbus, OH 43216. From *Clinical education aid no 7.* Copyright 1970 Ross Products Division, Abbott Laboratories.)

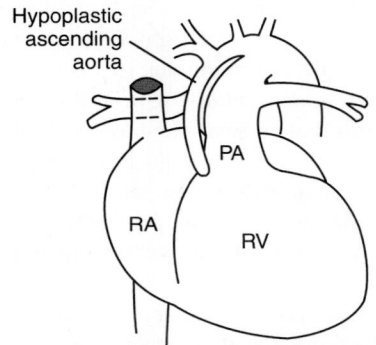

FIG. 30-14 Hypoplastic left heart syndrome. (Adapted from Park MK, Troxler RG: *Pediatric cardiology for practitioners,* ed 4, St. Louis, 2002, Mosby.)

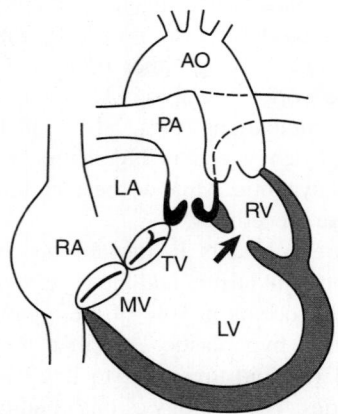

FIG. 30-15 Single ventricle defect. (Used with permission of Park MK, Troxler RG: *Pediatric cardiology for practitioners,* ed 4, St. Louis, 2002, Mosby.)

Hypoplastic left heart syndrome occurs in 2.5% of heart defects. Intrauterine stenosis of either the mitral or aortic valves results in a small left ventricle and hypoplasia of the ascending aorta and arch (see Fig. 30-14). The cause is unknown though it is linked to some genetic syndromes, such as Jacobsen syndrome (Driscoll, 2006).

Clinical Findings
History
- Cyanosis in the first week of life with dyspnea on exertion
- Fatigue with the effort of crying or feeding with subsequent poor weight gain.

Physical Examination
- A murmur may be present although not always.
- Usually a single S_2 is heard.
- Cyanosis is generally evident as soon as the ductus arteriosus closes.
- Hepatomegaly (may or may not be present).

Diagnostic Studies
- Chest radiography is generally normal initially, with changes occurring as the degree of cardiomegaly and obstruction of the pulmonary blood flow progresses.
- ECG findings depend on type of single ventricle disease, but are always abnormal for age.
- Two-dimensional echocardiography is diagnostic and shows the specifics of the anatomy (Driscoll, 2006).

Management
- Intravenous PGE_1 may be indicated in newborns. Most children are palliated with aortopulmonary shunts or Norwood procedures depending on their anatomy. At 6 months of age, palliation is continued with a Glenn anastomosis of the SVC to the pulmonary artery. The third stage of palliation is the Fontan procedure which occurs at 2 to 4 years old. In this procedure, the IVC is connected to the pulmonary artery. Some children are considered for cardiac transplantation early in life if their anatomy is not amenable to the Fontan pathway (Driscoll, 2006).
- Families require support throughout the child's life. Frequent surgeries and hospitalizations can interfere with normal social development. Early recognition and intervention for developmental delays are important to the child's future.
- SBE prophylaxis is no longer considered necessary except in 6 month post-operative period or if prosthetic material was used (Box 30-4).

Complications. Complications include development of collateral arterial and venous vessels, protein-losing, enteropathy, and many others. A decrease in exercise tolerance throughout life can be expected, in addition to left or right ventricular dysfunction. There may be less complications with surgical palliation at earlier ages. For patients with severe long-term complications, heart transplantation can be an option (Driscoll, 2006).

OBSTRUCTIVE CARDIAC LESIONS
Aortic Stenosis and Insufficiency
Description. Aortic stenosis (AS) or narrowing may occur at the aortic valvular, subvalvular, or supravalvular level. Valvular stenosis is the most common form (Fig. 30-16). The

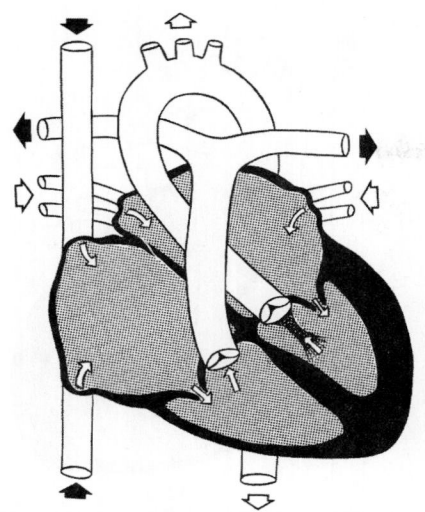

FIG. 30-16 Subaortic stenosis. (Used with permission of Ross Products Division, Abbott Laboratories, Columbus, OH 43216. From *Clinical education aid no 7.* Copyright 1970 Ross Products Division, Abbott Laboratories.)

stenotic AV is usually bicuspid rather than tricuspid. Stenosis causes increased pressure load on the left ventricle leading to LVH and, ultimately, ventricular failure. Obstruction of the AV may decrease coronary artery blood flow leading to the risk of fatal ventricular arrhythmias. The bicuspid AV generally becomes more stenotic and often regurgitant (insufficient) over time. However, some infants are born with critical AS and require urgent intervention.

Incidence. AS accounts for 5% of all cases of CHD and is four times more common in males. Twenty percent of patients with AS have associated cardiac abnormalities, such as COA and VSDs (Driscoll, 2006).

Clinical Findings
History

- The patient may be asymptomatic, depending on the severity of the defect.
- Growth and development may be normal.
- Activity intolerance, fatigue, chest pain (angina pectoris), or syncope can develop or increase with age.
- CHF, low cardiac output, and shock may be evident in newborns with severe AS (Driscoll, 2006).

Physical Examination

- BP may reveal a narrow pulse pressure. The apical impulse may be pronounced with moderate to severe stenosis.
- A grade III to IV/VI, loud, harsh systolic ejection murmur is best heard at the upper right sternal border with radiation to the neck, LLSB, and apex.
- With a valvular lesion, a faint, early systolic click at the LLSB may be heard.
- With aortic insufficiency, an early diastolic blowing murmur is heard at the LLSB to apex.
- In the most severe lesions, S_2 is single or closely split.
- S_3 or S_4 heart sounds may also be heard.
- A thrill may be present at the suprasternal notch (Driscoll, 2006).

Diagnostic Studies

- Chest radiographs are usually normal or may show LVH.
- ECG can be normal or reveal LVH and inverted T-waves.
- Echocardiograms are the diagnostic examinations of choice (Driscoll, 2006).

Management

- The timing of treatment depends on the severity of the obstruction. Treatment is usually not necessary unless the stenosis is moderate to severe.
- Balloon valvuloplasty of the stenotic valve is the initial palliative treatment of AS in the newborn. However, the AV will generally have to be surgically addressed later (Driscoll, 2006).
- In older children, AV replacement is necessary for severe AS and/or insufficiency. Unfortunately, none of the current AV options (mechanical, heterograph [pig- or cow-engineered valves]), homograft (human cadaver) or autograft (the Ross procedure—moves the pulmonic valve to the aortic position), are ideal or enduring options for children. Mechanical valves are prothrombotic and require anticoagulation with warfarin. Heterograph and homograft valves have limited durability in the aortic position, and the Ross procedure requires placement of the homograft in the pulmonic position, leading to future replacements of that valve as it stenoses. (Tchervenkov et al, 2003).
- Patients with mild AS can participate in all sports, but should have annual cardiac examinations. Patients with moderate AS should chose low-intensity sports, such as golf, bowling, table tennis, or softball, as guided by their cardiologist. Patients with severe AS or moderate AS with symptoms should avoid competitive or intensive sports. (Maron et al, 2005).
- SBE prophylaxis is always necessary (Driscoll, 2006).

Pulmonic Stenosis

Description. Normally, the pulmonary valve opens to allow the flow of blood from the right ventricle into the pulmonary artery. In pulmonic stenosis, there is narrowing at the subpulmonic, valvar, or supravalvar area. Right-sided pressure is increased as the ventricle pumps against the obstruction. RVH occurs as a result of this increased load. Pulmonary stenosis can also occur in the main and/or branch pulmonary arterial system. Mild pulmonic stenosis is usually identified on routine examination.

Incidence. Isolated pulmonic stenosis makes up approximately 6% to 8% of all cases of CHD. Approximately 1% to 2% may have other cardiac defects (Lin et al, 2006).

Clinical Findings
History

- The patient is usually asymptomatic, with a murmur noted on routine physical examination.
- Exertional dyspnea and fatigue are noticeable as stenosis progresses.
- Cyanosis from right-to-left shunting over the foramen ovale may be evident with severe pulmonic stenosis in the newborn.
- Growth and development are usually normal except in cases of Noonan syndrome where short stature is common.

Physical Examination

- A grade II to IV/VI, harsh, mid-to-late systolic ejection murmur is heard at the upper left sternal border over the pulmonic region with transmission along the left sternal border, neck and back, and into both lung fields.
- An intermittent systolic ejection click may be evident in the pulmonic area that decreases with inspiration and increases with expiration.
- Cyanosis and symptoms of right-sided CHF can occur in severe pulmonic stenosis in the newborn.

Diagnostic Studies

- Chest radiographs may be within normal limits in infants or show prominent main pulmonary artery segments in 80% to 90% of cases. Right-sided cardiac enlargement and decreased peripheral pulmonary vascular markings may be evident if heart failure develops.
- ECG may be normal with mild stenosis. In moderate to severe pulmonic stenosis, the ECG will show right axis deviation and RVH.
- Echocardiograms confirm the diagnosis, identifying the gradient, and monitoring progression of the stenosis.
- Cardiac catheterization may be used to delineate location of the main and branch pulmonary artery stenoses before intervention with balloon or stenting devices or surgical repair.

Management

- Interventional cardiologists will perform balloon valvuloplasty in neonates and older children with stenosis greater than 50 mm Hg. If unsuccessful, surgical valvuloplasty or replacement may be indicated. Interventional catheterization with stents and balloons is also used for branch stenosis.
- With mild stenosis, families need to be encouraged to treat their children normally and not limit their activity. In those with moderate stenosis, the stenosis can progress to severe narrowing during periods of rapid growth, such as during infancy or adolescence.
- SBE prophylaxis is no longer considered necessary except in the 6 month post-operative period or if prosthetic material was used (Box 30-4).

Coarctation of the Aorta

Description.   Coarctation of the aorta is a narrowing of a small or long segment of the aorta (Fig. 30-17). Coarctation may occur as a single defect caused by a disturbance in the development of the aorta or may be secondary to constriction of the ductus arteriosus. The severity of the coarctation, its location, and the degree of obstruction determine the effect of the coarctation. Systolic and diastolic hypertension exists in vessels proximal to the narrowing. Hypotension is present in vessels below the area of narrowing.

Incidence.   Coarctation accounts for 5% of CHD with the prevalence in 1.4 cases per 100,000 live births. Patients with Turner syndrome have close to a 35% incidence of coarctation (Lin et al, 2006).

Clinical Findings

History.   In older children, coarctation may go unnoticed until the BP is checked and mild hypertension is noted in the upper extremities or a murmur is detected. Retrospectively,

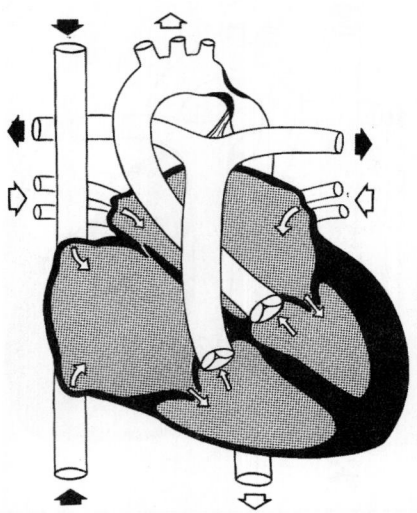

FIG. 30-17   COA. (Used with permission of Ross Products Division, Abbott Laboratories, Columbus, OH 43216. From *Clinical education aid no 7*. Copyright 1970 Ross Products Division, Abbott Laboratories.)

children with coarctation may have had complaints of leg pain with exercise or headaches. Severe neonatal coarctation will present early in life with tachypnea, poor feeding, and possibly cool lower extremities. COA in newborns is not always apparent until the ductus closes and decreases blood flow to the lower body.

Physical Examination

- Upper extremity hypertension with lower extremity hypotension is present, although milder cases may cause only a minimal discrepancy between upper and lower extremity BPs. In severe cases, poor lower extremity perfusion may be noticed with lower body mottling or pallor.
- Delayed timing and absent or weak arterial femoral and other distal pulses may occur.
- Bounding brachial, radial, and carotid pulses may occur.
- Signs of CHF may be evident.
- A systolic ejection murmur may be detected in the left infraclavicular region with transmission to the back.
- A ventricular heave at the apex can be palpated.
- Gallup rhythm may occur in infants with CHF.

Diagnostic Studies

- Chest radiography may reveal a normal or slightly enlarged heart and increased pulmonary vascular markings.
- ECG findings depend on the severity of the lesion and the age of the patient. In infants, RVH may be seen; in older children, LVH develops secondary to hypertension.
- Echocardiography is helpful in confirming the diagnosis and locating the constricted aortic segment. It may also show associated cardiac abnormalities.
- Magnetic resonance imaging (MRI) can define the location, severity, and anatomy of the aortic arch.

Management

- In critical neonatal coarctation, PGE_1 is used to maintain or reopen the ductus.
- Surgeons resect the constricted area and anastomose the upper and lower portions of the aorta if possible. Restenosis

is more likely to occur if repair was done before 1 year old (Driscoll, 2006). Cardiologists may dilate or stent the coarcted area in recoarctation or mild coarctation. Other procedures, including bypass grafting, may be necessary with unusually long coarcted segments. Surgical mortality is rare (Backer & Mavroudis, 2003).

- In older children with long-standing hypertension, antihypertensive medication may be required for several months after repair. Long-term prognosis is excellent unless there are associated intracardiac defects. PCPs should monitor BP postoperatively for recoarctation.
- Patients with previous coarctation repairs may participate in any competitive sport if residual BP gradient between arm and legs is less than 20 mm Hg and peak systolic BP is normal at rest and with exercise. However, during the first year after surgery, high-intensity static exercises, such as weight lifting and wrestling, should be avoided (Maron et al, 2005).
- SBE prophylaxis is no longer considered necessary except in the 6 month post-operative period or if prosthetic material was used (Box 30-4).

LONG-TERM PROGNOSIS FOR CHILDREN AND YOUNG ADULTS WITH CONGENITAL HEART DISEASE
Description

Because of the success of pediatric cardiac surgery, 85% of children born with CHD live to adulthood. As more and more of these children survive into adulthood, they require close supervision to assess their cardiac function and may need further interventions as appropriate. Some studies estimate there are now more adults with CHD than children with the same problems. Surgeries performed on these adults during their childhood were not corrective, but palliative to different degrees. The severity of residual problems varies depending upon the defect, type of surgical correction, and individual patient. However, very few of these individuals born with CHD would have made it to adulthood without some residual cardiac problem. To assist these patients, regional centers for the care of adults with CHD are developing (Gatzoulis & Webb, 2003).

Management

Adolescent patients should be referred to adult congenital heart specialists for follow-up of moderate to complex lesions, for determining when future surgeries (cardiac and noncardiac) may be best performed, and for risk assessment for pregnancy. Details about residual problems for each cardiac defect are beyond the scope of this text. However, key points in the evaluation of an older child or young adult with CHD are presented:

Chronic Cyanosis. Chronic cyanosis leads to difficulty with homeostasis and polycythemia. Clotting properties of platelets are often adversely affected, and friable collateral vessels develop in the pulmonary circulation. Conversely, polycythemia and dehydration can predispose these patients to thromboemboli. Cyanotic older children and young adults often have limited cardiac reserve and a tendency for renal dysfunction associated with surgery, anesthesia, or physiologically stressful events.

Cardiac Chamber Dilation (Atrial or Ventricular). Many older CHD patients have insufficiency in one or more valves, often as a residual effect of previous surgery. Over long periods this leads to chamber dilation in the chamber receiving backflow. This dilation is well tolerated for many years but will eventually affect function, lead to arrhythmias initiated in the dilated tissues, and dilation of other valves. Because the process is gradual, patients are often not cognizant of a change in function and may wait until the process is quite advanced before seeking care.

Arrhythmias and Heart Blocks. Rhythm disturbances can occur as a result of long-standing cyanosis, the above mentioned chamber dilation, and fibrotic suture lines. Often episodes of palpitations bring older congenital heart patients to care (Shore, 2003).

Ventricular Hypertrophy. Ventricular hypertrophy caused by stenotic outflow vessels or valves can, over time, predispose patients to myocardial ischemia, poor ventricular compliance, and serious ventricular arrhythmias (Gatzoulis & Webb, 2003).

▮▮ ACQUIRED HEART DISEASE
CHEST PAIN
Description

Chest pain in the pediatric population is a common complaint and does not usually represent a serious cardiovascular problem. However, chest pain of any kind can cause great anxiety for children, adolescents, and their parents. It is important to thoroughly evaluate this complaint with a careful history (especially a family history of sudden death or early cardiac disease) and a thorough physical examination. ECG and other laboratory tests may be indicated if findings are present. Reassurance is of utmost importance.

Epidemiology

The most frequent cause of chest pain is musculoskeletal, originating in the chest wall or chest cage. Costochondritis, Tietze syndrome, idiopathic chest pain, precordial catch syndrome, slipping-rib syndrome, hypersensitive xiphoid syndrome, trauma, and muscle strain are diagnoses assigned to specific types of chest pain; all are of musculoskeletal origin, benign, and rarely require any treatment. The pain is often related to sports or casual athletic activity. Chest pain secondary to a pulmonary problem (asthma, pneumonia, embolism, pneumothorax) or gastrointestinal problem (reflux esophagitis, esophageal foreign body), herpes zoster, or sickle cell disease should be included in the differential diagnosis. Chest wall pain, particularly with exercise, may indicate exercise-induced asthma, but rarely indicates cardiac disease. Chronic chest pain that is vague and occurs over many months in a variety of circumstances, particularly around stressful events, may be psychogenic (anxiety or hyperventilation). Pain associated with syncope, exertional dyspnea, or irregularities in heart rhythm needs careful evaluation for a cardiac cause. Usually, children or adolescents who have pain of cardiac origin describe a specific history with details that are consistent from event to event. Most pediatric patients with chest pain do not have cardiac pathologic conditions.

The incidence of chest pain is approximately 0.288%, and it occurs slightly more often in males. The mean age at initial evaluation is 12 to 14 years old. Most cases resolve spontaneously (Driscoll, 2006).

Clinical Findings

History. To determine the etiology of the chest pain, the provider should inquire about the following:

- Past medical history or family history for sudden death, heart disease or condition, asthma, eczema, Marfan syndrome, sickle cell disease
- Past sports activities, including friendly wrestling at the home
- Previous trauma or muscle strains
- Characteristics of the chest pain
  - Relationship of pain to exercise; any syncope or exertional dyspnea
  - Any burning, substernal pain that worsens with reclining or with spicy foods (gastrointestinal etiology)
  - Pain that is sharp or stabbing, lasting several seconds to minutes, located over the midsternum or infranipple area, and occurring with nonexertion or deep inspirations (more likely musculoskeletal in origin)
  - Pain that awakens the patient (more likely organic)
- Any other associated symptoms, such as fever, nausea, vomiting, headaches, choking episodes
- Any recent, major stressful events
- Medication, tobacco, or other drug use, including oral contraceptives (embolism)

Physical Examination. A complete chest (lungs and heart) and abdominal examination should be performed. Key findings to focus on include the presence of the following:

- Cardiac murmur, rubs, or clicks
- Point tenderness of one or more costochondral joints exaggerated with physical activity or deep inspirations (costochondritis or Tietze syndrome [if associated with warmth, swelling, or tenderness over costochondral junction])
- Irregular heart rhythm (cardiac disease)
- Shortness of breath, coughing, wheezing, chest pain with exercise
- Rales, wheezing, tachypnea, decreased breath sounds (pulmonary disease)

Diagnostic Studies. In most cases, only the history and physical are necessary to make the diagnosis; other tests are not indicated unless the following problems are suspected:

- Febrile, cardiac, or pulmonary condition: chest radiograph
- Exercise-induced asthma: pulmonary function testing with exercise
- Rhythm disturbance: 24-hour Holter monitor or stress test (or both)
- Signs of CHD, pericarditis, or myocarditis: ECG

Musculoskeletal, respiratory, psychogenic, and gastrointestinal disorders, as discussed earlier, as well as miscellaneous entities, such as sickle cell crisis, aortic abdominal aneurysm (Marfan syndrome), pleural effusion (collagen-vascular disorders), and shingles, are in the differential diagnosis.

Management

- When chest pain has no clear-cut etiology, the child appears well, and all aspects of the evaluation are normal, reassurance may be the most important treatment. Frequently, when reassured that the pain has no organic cause, the pain subsides or becomes less of an issue for the child.
  - Costochondritis and Tietze syndrome are usually responsive to nonsteroidal antiinflammatory treatment and rest.
  - Antacids may be tried if esophagitis is suspected; see Chapter 32.
  - See management of esophageal foreign body ingestion in Chapter 32.
  - See Chapters 14 and 32 for management of asthma and respiratory diseases.
- In cases in which pulmonary, gastrointestinal, or cardiac disease is a concern, treatment, referral, or evaluation is necessary. Chest pain associated with exercise should be referred to a cardiologist.
- Follow-up is indicated to ensure that no new findings have emerged and the child is participating in normal activities and to monitor for potential psychoemotional problems.

HYPERTENSION

Definition

Hypertension is defined as a systolic or diastolic (or both) BP in the 95th or higher percentile for age, sex, and height on at least three consecutive occasions. High-normal or prehypertensive BP is defined as average systolic or diastolic BP in the 90th percentile or higher, but less than the 95th percentile. Normal BP is defined as systolic and diastolic BP below the 90th percentile for age, sex, and height. Stage 1 hypertension is BP that ranges from the 95th percentile for age, sex, and height to 5 mm Hg above the 99th percentile. Stage 2 hypertension is BP greater than 5 mm Hg above the 99th percentile (NIH-NHBEP, 2004).

Epidemiology

Hypertension is a significant problem in children and young adults and results from the interaction of genetic and environmental factors. Increasingly, children are found to have high BP associated with obesity, sedentary lifestyles, and stress. The etiology is genetic in 60% of cases. Secondary hypertension is more commonly seen in children under 6 years old with significant or severe hypertension (NIH-NHBEP, 2004). The primary cause of secondary, severe hypertension is renovascular or parenchymal renal diseases. Other causes include cardiovascular, endocrine, metabolic and drug-induced, and central nervous system conditions (NIH-NHBEP, 2004). The onset of primary hypertension is more likely to occur after

10 years old. Neonates with hypertension are severely ill with neurologic and cardiac symptoms.

Clinical Findings

The goal of the clinical history and physical examination is to look for causes of secondary hypertension, comorbidities of primary hypertension, and signs of end-organ damage of prolonged hypertension of either type.

History

- Neonatal history of prolonged mechanical ventilation, umbilical catheterization
- Diet, activities, and other habits (e.g., smoking, drinking)
- Sleep history, particularly symptoms of sleep apnea (Enright et al, 2003)
- Medications taken, including oral contraceptives, cold medications, steroids, and diet aids
- Chronic illness, especially renal disease, past history of urinary tract infections, diabetes, or seizures
- Headache, chest pain, dyspnea, muscle weakness, palpitations, abdominal pain, facial palsy, decreased vision, excessive sweating
- Family history of a first-degree relative with myocardial infarction (especially before 50 years old), stroke, hypertension, diabetes, hyperlipidemia, sudden cardiac death, polycystic kidney disease, neurofibromatosis, pheochromocytoma, or obesity

Physical Examination

- Body habitus, especially overweight (per body mass index); poor growth (height, weight); signs of metabolic syndrome
- Dysmorphic features
- Edema, pallor, flushing, skin lesions (suggestive of tuberous sclerosis or systemic lupus erythematosus [SLE])
- Absent, diminished, or pounding pulses in all extremities
- Fundi, thyroid gland, abdominal mass, flank bruit; decreased visual acuity, facial palsy
- Elevated BP

Accurate BP measurement is essential. An appropriately sized cuff must be used with the cubital fossa supported at the heart level. The right arm is preferred for comparison with normative charts, but right thigh measurement is also recommended if elevated pressure is suspected. The child or adolescent should be seated and have been resting in that position for 3 to 5 minutes. Deflation should be controlled at 2 to 3 mm Hg per second. Systolic pressure is recorded at the onset of tapping sounds; diastolic pressure is recorded at the disappearance (not the muffling) of sounds. Some authorities recommend recording the pressure twice on each occasion and using an average of each to record. BP elevation must be confirmed on three separate occasions.

Management

See Fig. 30-18 for an algorithm to manage children with high BP.

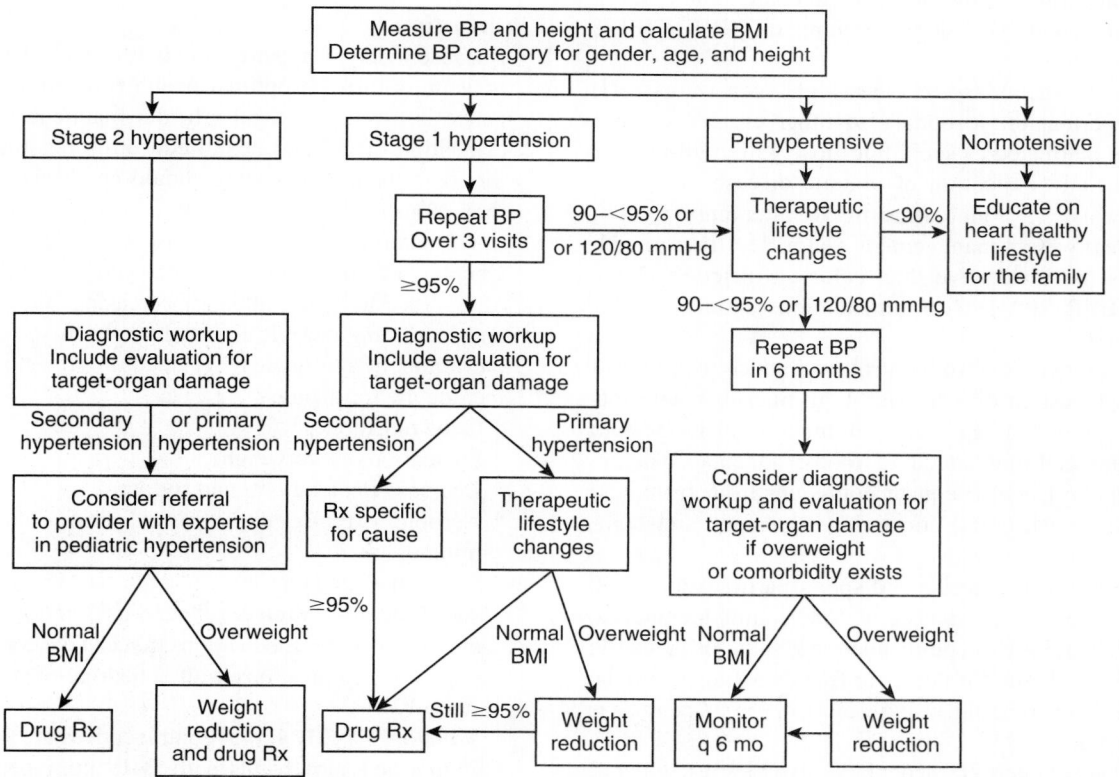

FIG. 30-18 Hypertension management algorithm. *BMI,* Body mass index; *BP,* blood pressure; *q,* every; *Rx,* prescription. (Used with permission of the National Institutes of Health, National High Blood Pressure Education Program Working Group on High Blood Pressure in Children and Adolescents (NIH–NHBPEP): The Fourth Report on the Diagnosis, Evaluation, and Treatment of High Blood Pressure in Children and Adolescents, *Pediatrics* 114[Suppl]: 555–576, 2004, p. 571.)

- BP measurements should be done annually on all children 3 years and older, with baseline and serial measurements documented carefully in the child's record. Standardized measurements are available (see Tables 30-3 and 30-4).
- Prehypertension: At least two follow-up BP measurements should be taken within 1 to 2 months of the initial reading to determine whether this high reading is a single, isolated event. If subsequent readings fall below the 95th percentile, the child should continue with routine BP checks during annual visits.
- Stage 1 or 2 hypertension: Laboratory evaluation should focus on searching for causes of secondary hypertension, comorbidities of primary hypertension, and target organ damage of either primary or secondary hypertension. The search for secondary causes of hypertension needs to be individualized. Children under 10 years old with stage 2 hypertension require more aggressive laboratory evaluation compared with older children with stage 1 hypertension and obesity. History and physical exam may focus suspicion. CBC, erythrocyte sedimentation rate (ESR), urinalysis and culture, electrolytes, blood urea nitrogen, creatinine, and plasma renin levels, renal nuclear medicine scans, and renal ultrasound are screening studies for the most common secondary causes of hypertension. If renal vascular disease is suspected, the work-up is best managed by a nephrologist because newer technologies, such as MRI and spiral CT, are replacing angiography. Additional organ assessments would include echocardiography for LVH and coarctation of aorta and a thorough ophthalmologic examination (NIH-NHBEP, 2004).
- Hypertension, secondary to overweight, can be as serious as hypertension secondary to other organic disease and should be treated as such. For those with high-normal BP without any indication of organic disease, treatment should consist of nonpharmacologic intervention: diet, exercise, and weight management. Caloric restriction with exercise is more effective than caloric restriction alone. (NIH NHBEP, 2004). Recommendations should include the following:
  - Dietary intervention to control or reduce overweight includes ingestion of a low-fat, high-fiber diet with lots of fresh fruits and vegetables; elimination of foods high in sodium and salt added to foods; adequate calcium (1200 mg/day); and adequate potassium from fruits and beans. Eliminate sugar-containing beverages and high-energy snacks.
  - Increase physical exercise and sports participation to 30 to 60 minutes a day balanced with relaxation techniques. Aerobic exercise is recommended, not static or isometric exercise. It is helpful if family or friends participate in the exercise regimen; maintaining a diary or log of exercise is encouraged.
  - Concurrently, decrease sedentary activities to under 2 hours/day, including television viewing, computer, and video games.
  - Avoid smoking, caffeine, alcoholic beverages, and illicit drug consumption.

- Patients with secondary hypertension, primary hypertension with symptoms, LVH, or insufficient change in hypertensive status after 6 to 12 months of diet and exercise therapy should start medications (NIH-NHBEP, 2004). The provider should refer the patient to a specialist who has experience using antihypertensive agents in children. The goal is to reduce systolic or diastolic BP below the 95th percentile. If a concurrent condition(s) exist, the goal becomes reducing BP to the 90th percentile. The most recent medication recommendations, based on available studies and expert opinion from the National High Blood Pressure Education Program Working Group on High Blood Pressure in Children and Adolescents, are found in Table 30-11. A single drug, usually an ACE inhibitor, angiotension-receptor blocker (ARB), beta blocker, calcium channel blocker, or diuretic should be started at the lowest recommended dose and advanced until the desired BP is reached. If maximum dose or adverse side effects are reached, a second medication should be added. Step-down therapy may be possible for overweight children who lose weight and achieve BP goals.

Complications

Long-term BP elevation leads to an increase in left ventricular mass, increased carotid intimal medial thickness, and coronary artery calcification, especially if combined with overweight, lipid and lipoprotein abnormalities, and tobacco use. Yearly echocardiograms may be recommended to evaluate LVH.

Prevention

- Because much of hypertension is lifestyle-related in origin, prevention through optimal health promotion and maintenance is essential. Regular health maintenance, including evaluation of BP and health education regarding risk factors, is critical. Counseling should emphasize both behavioral modification and parental involvement. It is especially important for fathers to exercise with their children (see Chapter 14 for further information) (American College of Sports Medicine, 2003). Decreasing body mass index and increasing aerobic fitness have been shown to reduce elevations in age-related BP. Specific preventive measures include the following:
  - Good nutrition
  - Prevention of overweight
  - Decrease in dietary fat and sodium
  - Aerobic exercise daily for a period of at least 30 minutes
  - Stress management
  - Avoidance of caffeine, tobacco use, and prescription or over-the-counter medications that can exacerbate high BP (e.g., cold medications with ephedrine or phenylephrine, steroids)
  - Monitoring of BP if oral contraceptives are used
- Children and adolescents with systemic hypertension may have significant rise in their BP during exercise. Athletes with significant hypertension should have their BP measured regularly (every 2 months) to monitor the impact of exercise on BP. Patients with stage 1 hypertension in the absence

TABLE 30-11   Antihypertensive Medications for Children

Class	Drugs	Dose and Dosing Interval	Comments
ACE inhibitors	Captopril	Initial 0.3-0.5 mg/kg/dose: max dose: 6 mg/kg/day. tid dosing.	• ACE inhibitors are contraindicated in pregnancy.
	Enalapril	Initial dose: 0.08 mg/kg/day up to 5 mg/day; max dose: 0.6 mg/kg/day up to 40 mg. Daily to bid dosing.	• Check serum potassium and creatinine periodically.
	Lisinopril	Initial 0.07 mg/kg/day up to 5 mg/day: max dose: 0.6 mg/kg/day up to 40 mg/day. Daily dosing.	• All can be compounded into a suspension.
Alpha and beta blocker	Labetalol	Initial dose: 1-3 mg/kg/day: max dose: 10-12 mg/kg/day up to 1200 mg/day. bid dosing.	
Beta-adrenergic antagonist	Propranolol	Initial dose: 1 mg/kg/day divided bid; usual dose 2-4 mg/kg/day; max dose: 16 mg/kg/day.	• Asthma, heart failure, and insulin-dependent diabetes are contraindications.
	Metoprolol	Initial 1-2 mg/kg/day: max dose: 6 mg/kg/day up to 200 mg/day. bid dosing.	• Monitor heart rate for excessive bradycardia.
	Atenolol	Initial 0.5-1 mg/kg/day: max dose: 2 mg/kg/day up to 100 mg/day. Daily to bid dosing.	• Athletic performance may be impaired.
Angiotensin-receptor blocker	Irbesartan	6-12 yr: 75-150 mg/day. >13 yr: 150-300 mg/day.	• ARB inhibitors are contraindicated in pregnancy.
	Losartan	Daily dosing. Initial 0.7 mg/kg/day up to 50 mg/day: max dose: 1.4 mg/kg/day up to 100 mg/day. Daily dosing.	• Check serum potassium and creatinine periodically. • Losartan can be compounded into a suspension.
Calcium channel blocker	Amlodipine	Children 6-17 yr: 2.5-5 mg once daily.	• Amlodipine and isradipine can be compounded into a suspension.
	Isradipine	Initial 0.15-2 mg/kg/day: max dose: 0.8 mg/kg/day up to 20 mg/day. tid-qid dosing.	• May cause tachycardia.
	Extended-release nifedipine	Initial 0.25-0.5 mg/kg/day up to 5 mg/day: max dose: 3 mg/kg/day up to 120 mg/day. Daily to bid dosing.	
Central-adrenergic agonists	Clonidine	Children 12 yr: initial dose: 0.2 mg/day, divided bid; max dose: 2.4 mg/day.	• May cause dry mouth or sedation. • Sudden cessation can cause rebound.
Peripheral alpha agonist	Prazosin	Initial dose: 0.05-0.1 mg/kg/day; max: 0.5 mg/kg/day up to 50 mg/day once. tid dosing.	May cause hypotension and syncope.
Direct vasodilators	Hydralazine	Initial dose: 0.75 mg/kg/day; max dose 7.5 mg/kg/day up to 200 mg/day divided. Dosed qid.	• Fluid retention and tachycardia commonly occur.
	Minoxidil	Initial dose: 0.2 mg/kg/dose once daily; up to 50 mg/day. Daily to tid dosing.	• Hydralazine can cause lupus-like syndrome in some patients. • Minoxidil can cause hypertrichosis.
Diuretics	Chlorthalidone	Initial dose: 0.3 mg/kg/dose once daily; max 2 mg/kg/day up to 50 mg/day. Daily dosing.	• Patients on diuretics should have electrolytes monitored.
	Furosemide	0.5-2 mg/kg/day per dose; max 6 mg/kg/day; dosed daily to bid.	• Potassium-sparing diuretics (spironolactone, triamterene, amiloride) can cause hyperkalemia especially when give with ACE inhibitor or ARB.
	Hydrochlorothiazide	1 mg/kg/day, max 3 mg/kg/day up to 50 mg/day; dosed daily.	• Chlorthalidone may cause azotemia in patients with renal disease.
	Spironolactone	1.5 mg/kg/day, max 3.3 mg/kg/day; dosed daily or bid.	

ACE, Angiotensin-converting enzyme; *ARB,* angiotensin-receptor blocker; *bid,* twice daily; *max,* maximum; *tid,* three times daily dosing; *qid,* four times a day dosing; *yr,* year(s).
Adapted from National High Blood Pressure Education Program Working Group on High Blood Pressure in Children and Adolescents: The Fourth report on the diagnosis, evaluation, and treatment of high blood pressure in children and adolescents, *Pediatrics* 114:555-576, 2004.

of LVH or concomitant heart disease are eligible for any competitive sport. Athletic participation in individuals with stage 2 hypertension should be restricted, especially high static sports, until hypertension can be controlled (Maron et al, 2005).

KAWASAKI DISEASE

Description

Kawasaki disease (KD) (also known as mucocutaneous lymph node syndrome or infantile polyarteritis) is characterized by an acute generalized systemic vasculitis occurring throughout the body. During the initial stage (acute phase), inflammation of the arterioles, venules, and capillaries of the heart occurs and can later progress to coronary artery aneurysm in 15% to 25% of untreated children. KD is self-limited and is the most common cause of acquired heart disease in children in Japan and the U.S. (Newburger et al, 2004).

Epidemiology

Although the etiology of KD remains unknown, clinical evidence supports an infectious cause. It exhibits geographic and seasonal outbreaks, in the late winter and early spring. Person-to-person spread is low, but it occurs with greater frequency in siblings (1%). Genetic susceptibility is probably an important contributor, as evidenced by the differential racial incidence and higher rates of occurrence among siblings. Between 9.1 and 32.5 per 100,000 children (depending on race) contract KD each year in the U.S. (Newburger et al, 2004). Although children of all racial groups are susceptible, the incidence is highest in Asian-American children, followed by African Americans, Hispanics, and lowest in white children. There is a 1.5:1 male-to-female ratio. More than 85% of cases occur in children younger than 5 years old (Newburger et al, 2004).

Clinical Findings

The classic diagnostic criteria are listed in Box 30-7. However, children can have atypical or incomplete KD with coronary anomalies shown by echocardiogram. Children younger than 6 to 12 months old may have more atypical findings. See Fig. 30-19 for a decision-making algorithm for suspected atypical or incomplete KD. There are four stages in which changes in cardiovascular pathology occur, depending on the length of time since the onset of symptoms.

Stage 1. The acute phase (days 0 to 14) begins with an abrupt onset of high fever (greater than 102.2° F [39° C]) that is unresponsive to antipyretics or antibiotics. Typically, significant irritability, bilateral nonpurulent conjunctival injection, erythema of the oropharynx, dryness and fissuring of the lips, "strawberry tongue," cervical lymphadenopathy, a polymorphous rash, erythema of the urethral meatus, tachycardia, and edema of the extremities are noted. During the acute phase, there may be pericardial, myocardial, endocardial, and coronary artery inflammation. The child typically is tachycardic and has a hyperdynamic precordium with a gallop rhythm and a flow murmur. Rarely, children have low cardiac output syndrome from poor myocardial function.

BOX 30-7 **Diagnostic Criteria for Kawasaki Disease**

The child must exhibit fever for 5 days plus four of the other five criteria *or,* if fewer than four criteria, coronary vessel involvement:

1. Bilateral conjunctival injection without exudate
2. Polymorphous rash that may be urticarial or pruritic
3. Inflammatory changes in the lips and oral cavity
4. Changes in the extremities, such as peripheral edema, erythema of the palms and soles, or desquamation of the hands and feet (convalescent period)
5. Cervical lymphadenopathy that is often unilateral, anterior cervical

Data from Newburger J, Takahasi M, Gerber M et al: Diagnosis, treatment and long-term management of Kawasaki diseases: a statement for health professionals from the Committee on Rheumatic Fever, Endocarditis, and Kawasaki Disease, Council on Cardiovascular Disease in the Young, American Heart Association, *Pediatrics* 114:1708-1733, 2004.

- Laboratory findings: an elevated ESR and platelet count (as high as 700,000/mm^3), positive C-reactive protein (CRP), leukocytosis with left shift, slight decreases in red blood cells and hemoglobin, hypoalbuminemia, increased a^2-globulin, and sterile pyuria. It is important to note that the platelet count may be initially normal, with gradual increase after the seventh day of fever.

Stage 2. The subacute phase (2 to 4 weeks after illness onset) begins with resolution of the fever and lasts until all other clinical signs have disappeared.

- Irritability may be prolonged throughout this phase.
- Desquamation of the fingers (at the junction of nail tip and digit) occurs first, followed by the toes.
- Transient jaundice, abnormal liver function tests, arthralgia or arthritis, transient diarrhea, orchitis, facial palsy, and sensorineural hearing loss may occur.
- Coronary artery aneurysms appear during this period in 15% to 25% of untreated children and less than 5% of treated children. Common sites for aneurysm, in order of frequency, are the proximal left anterior descending coronary, proximal right coronary, left main coronary, left circumflex, and distal right coronary artery.
- Deaths from KD occur from cardiac sequelae 15 to 45 days after onset of fever (Newburger et al, 2004).

Stage 3. During the convalescent phase, all clinical signs of KD have resolved, but laboratory values may not have returned to normal. This phase is complete when all blood values are normal (6 to 8 weeks from onset).

Stage 4. The chronic phase is from 40 days to years after illness onset. Coronary complications, if present, can persist into adulthood. Children with coronary dilation or aneurysms (especially those greater than 4 mm) may have long-term coronary endothelial changes, which place the child at risk for early ischemic disease (Iemura et al, 2000). Children with KD may also develop dyslipidemias (Newburger et al, 2004).

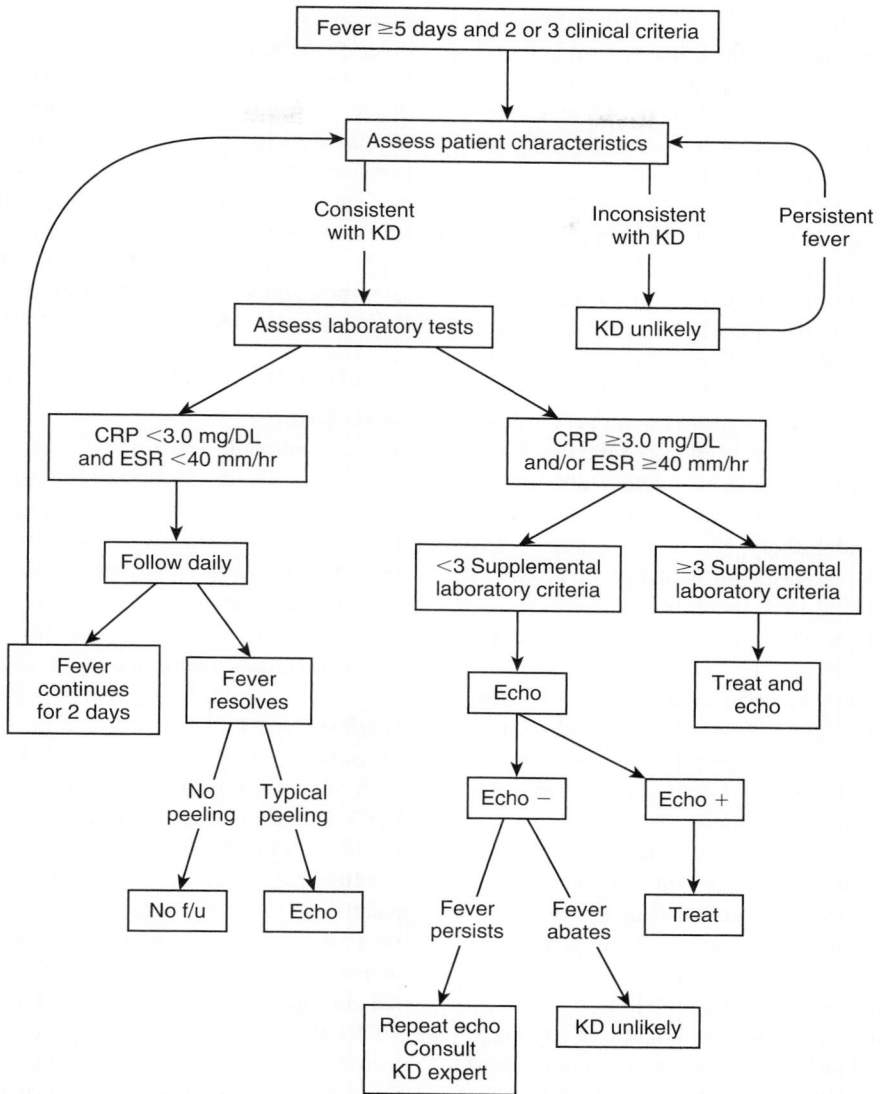

FIG. 30-19 Algorithm for evaluation of suspected incomplete KD. (Redrawn from Newburger J, Takahashi M, Gerber M et al: Diagnosis, treatment and long-term management of Kawasaki diseases: a statement for health professionals from the Committee on Rheumatic Fever, Endocarditis, and Kawasaki Disease, Council on Cardiovascular Disease in the Young, American Heart Association, *Pediatrics* 114[6]:1708-1733, 2004, p. 1709.

Diagnostic Studies

- CBC with differential, ESR, platelet count, CRP, liver transaminases, γ-glutamyltransferase (GGT), and urinalysis are done. Occasionally, the ESR is normal, but there is an elevated CRP.
- Blood, urine, cerebrospinal fluid, and group A ß-hemolytic streptococcus (GABHS) pharyngeal cultures may be indicated given the patient's symptomatology (to rule out other sources of fever).
- Echocardiograms are performed to evaluate for coronary, myocardial, and pericardial inflammation. Angiography, MRI, and or cardiac stress testing may be considered.

Differential Diagnosis

Measles, adenovirus, scarlet fever, drug reactions, Stevens-Johnson syndrome, erythema multiforme, mononucleosis,

juvenile arthritis, leptospirosis, inflammatory bowel disease, sarcoidosis, SLE, rickettsial infection, and toxic shock are differential diagnoses for the triad of red eyes, prolonged fever, and rash (Newburger et al, 2004).

Management

Early diagnosis is essential to prevent aneurysms in the coronary arteries and extraparenchymal muscular arteries. Goals of treatment include: (1) evoking a rapid antiinflammatory response, (2) preventing coronary thrombosis by inhibiting platelet aggregation, and (3) minimizing long-term coronary risk factors by exercise, diet, and smoking prevention.

- Treatment includes the following (Newburger et al, 2004):
  - Intravenous gamma globulin therapy (a single dose of 2 g/kg over a period of 10 to 12 hours, ideally in the first 10 days of the illness) reduces the incidence of coronary

artery abnormalities. The use of immunoglobulin after the tenth day must be individualized. If a patient is found to have an abnormal echocardiogram, fever, tachycardia, or other signs of inflammation beyond the tenth day, then gamma globulin is still indicated. Retreatment with immunoglobulin may be useful for persistent or recurrent fevers

○ High-dose aspirin is given for its antiinflammatory properties (80 to 100 mg/kg/day in four divided doses every 6 hours initially). After the fourteenth day of illness and once the child has been afebrile for 48 hours, aspirin is continued at an antiplatelet dose (3 to 5 mg/kg once daily) in patients without echocardiographic evidence of coronary artery changes. Low-dose aspirin continues until the ESR and platelet count have returned to normal (typically 6 to 8 weeks). If significant coronary artery abnormalities develop and do not resolve, aspirin or other antiplatelet therapy is used indefinitely. Warfarin (Coumadin) is sometimes added in patients with evidence of turbulent flow through the affected vessel sections.

Additional management strategies include (Newburger et al, 2004):

• An echocardiogram should be obtained as soon as the diagnosis is established as a baseline study, with subsequent studies done at 2 weeks and 6 to 8 weeks after onset of illness. If a child is found to have abnormalities, then more frequent evaluations may be indicated.

• All patients on chronic aspirin therapy should receive influenza vaccination. If varicella or influenza develops, aspirin treatment should be stopped for 6 weeks and another antiplatelet drug substituted to minimize the risk of Reye syndrome.

• Live-virus vaccines should be delayed until 11 months after administration of intravenous gamma globulin.

• Patients without coronary or cardiac changes at any stage on echocardiography should be followed by a cardiologist throughout the first year. Afterwards, the PCP may follow the patient; no activity restrictions are imposed at that point.

• Patients with any range of transient coronary artery dilation (including giant aneurysms) should be followed by a cardiologist for years. Physical activity limitations depend on degree of cardiac abnormality and whether warfarin therapy is used.

Complications

The acute disease is self-limited; however, if left untreated, significant cardiac sequelae will develop in 15% to 25% of cases (Newburger et al, 2004). The process of aneurysm formation and subsequent thrombosis or scarring of the coronary artery may occur as late as 6 months after the initial illness. Possible complications include recurrence (less than 2%); coronary aneurysm (less than 25%); CHF or massive myocardial infarction myocarditis or pericarditis, or both (30%); and pericardial effusion, mitral valve insufficiency, and coronary vessel stenosis.

Prognosis

There is a 1.25% mortality rate. The risk of coronary aneurysm is reduced to 3% in patients older than 1 year if intrave-

nous immunoglobulin is given within 10 days of the illness. Aneurysm regression occurs in half of all patients who develop them, commonly by 1 year after the illness (80% resolve within 5 years), but vessels do not dilate normally in response to increased oxygen demand by the myocardium. Patients with coronary artery abnormalities are at risk for myocardial infarction, sudden death, and myocardial ischemia for years after the illness. Prompt treatment of chest pain, dyspnea, extreme lethargy, or syncope is always warranted. Surgical revascularization and transcatheter revascularization are used for some coronary sequelae of KD (Newburger et al, 2004).

ACUTE RHEUMATIC FEVER

Description

Acute rheumatic fever (ARF) is an exaggerated autoimmune response in a susceptible host to group A streptococcus. Epitopes on certain subspecies of group A streptococcus are similar to human myosin and tissue of the mitral annulus and chordae. Antistreptococcal immunoglobulins, stimulated by repeated streptococcal infections, attack the patient's own heart and joints, CNS, and cutaneous tissue. Repeated episodes lead to rheumatic heart disease (RHD) (Carapetis et al, 2005).

Epidemiology

Conservatively, worldwide 500,000 children acquire ARF each year with 15.6 million people carrying the burden of RHD. However, the prevalence varies dramatically around the world with an incidence of 0.5 per 1000 in most developed countries; it occurs at a much higher rate in less developed countries where poverty is greater. In sub-Saharan Africa, the prevalence is 5.7 per 1000 children. ARF is also endemic in Pacific Islander peoples, Southeast Asia, and in aboriginal communities around the world. During the late 1960s and 1970s, the disease almost disappeared in the U.S. and Western Europe only to resurge in the mid-1980s in the intermountain states. It is the leading cause of acquired heart disease in children worldwide. It occurs most commonly in school-age children 5 to 15 years old (Carapetis et al, 2005).

Fig. 30-20 shows the pathogenic pathway of ARF and RHD. In developed countries, the strains of streptococci that induce ARF are rare and usually cause throat infection; they do not cause skin infections, such as impetigo. However, this is not always true in developing countries or subpopulations with high ARF prevalence (such as aboriginal Australians). In these populations, impetigo streptococcal infections do precede ARF (Carapetis et al, 2005). Some children are also more susceptible to the ARF immune response based on their human leukocyte antigen (HLA) class.

Repeated streptococcal infections appear to prime the immune response in the child before the first episode of ARF. Once the immune system is primed to the pathogen and triggered by repeated exposures, CD4 cells attack cardiac myosin and laminin (in valve membranes) because these proteins appear similar to the M protein on the streptococci. This classically occurs during a latent period of 10 to 20 days following streptococcal infection. First episodes of ARF usually occur before adolescence, and any cardiac

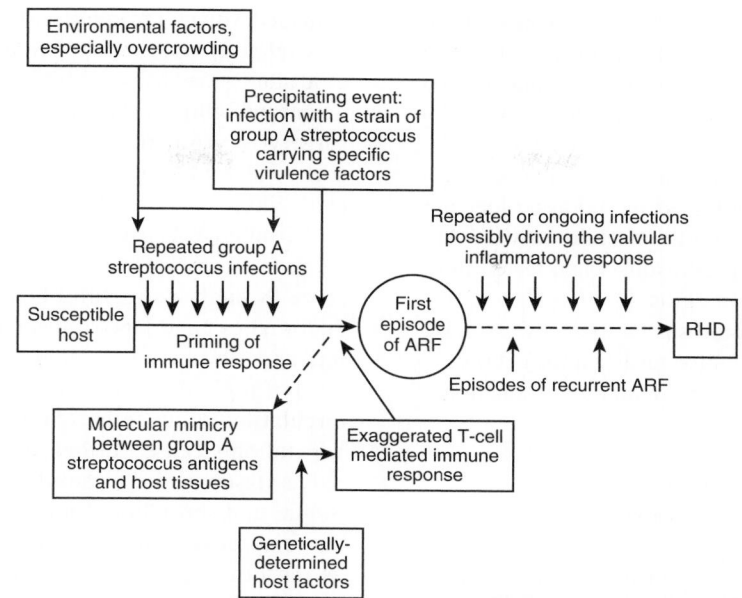

FIG. 30-20 Pathogenetic pathway for ARF and RHD. (Used with permission of Carapetis J, McDonald M, Wilson N: Acute rheumatic fever, *Lancet* 366:155-168, 2005, p 157.)

BOX 30-8 Jones Criteria for Rheumatic Fever*

Evidence of Preceding GABHS Infection
- Positive throat culture or rapid streptococcal antigen test result
- Elevated or rising streptococcal antibody titer

Minor Manifestations
- Arthralgia
- Fever
- Elevated acute-phase reactants
- Elevated erythrocyte sedimentation rate
- Elevated C-reactive protein

Major Manifestations
- Carditis
  - Tachycardia out of proportion to degree of fever
  - Cardiomegaly
  - New murmurs or change in preexisting murmurs
    Muffled heart sounds
    Precordial friction rub
    Precordial pain
    Changes in electrocardiogram (especially prolonged PR interval)

- Polyarthritis
  Swollen, hot, red, painful joint(s)
  After 1 to 2 days, affects different joints (migratory)
  Favors large joints—knees, elbows, hips, shoulders, wrists
- Erythema marginatum
  Erythematous macules with clear center and wavy, well-demarcated border
  Transitory
  Nonpruritic
  Primarily affects trunk and extremities (inner surfaces)
- Chorea
  Sudden, aimless, irregular movements of extremities
  Involuntary facial grimaces
  Speech disturbances or emotional lability
  Muscle weakness (can be profound)
  Muscle movements exaggerated by anxiety and attempt at fine motor activity; relieved by rest
- Subcutaneous nodes
  Nontender swelling
  Located over bony prominence
  May persist for some time and then gradually resolve

*The presence of two major or one major and two or more minor criteria with evidence of preceding GABHS infection indicates a high probability of rheumatic fever.
From Dajani AS et al: Guidelines for the diagnosis of rheumatic fever: Jones criteria, updated 1992, *Circulation* 87:302-307,]1993. Ferrieri P, for the Jones Criteria Working Group: Proceedings of the Jones criteria workshop, *Circulation* 106(19):2521, 2002. Reviewed and reaffirmed the prior updated 1992 Jones criteria.

---

damage may resolve if no further episodes occur (through prevention by antibiotic prophylaxis). However, in the developing world or in high prevalence communities, reexposure without prophylaxis is common, inducing worsening RHD with each new episode.

Clinical Findings

The diagnosis of ARF is based on a set of guidelines known as the Jones criteria (Dajani et al, 1993; Ferrieri, 2002) (Box 30-8). The presence of two major or one major and two minor criteria with evidence of a preceding GABHS infection indicates a high probability of ARF. Children with fewer manifestations can also have ARF. Arthritis of large joints occurs in 65% of cases, carditis in 50%, chorea in 15% to 30%, cutaneous nodules in 5%, and subcutaneous nodules in less than 7%.

Diagnostic Studies

- Rapid streptococcal antigen screening or streptococcal culture is done during the acute illness in children older than 2 years. However, up to two-thirds of children with ARF may have negative streptococcal results when tested in the latency period after acute pharyngitis.
- Other tests include antistreptolysin O titer (ASO), CBC, ESR, and CRP (see Chapter 24 for further information).
- Echocardiograms to evaluate valve damage and function.

Management

See Chapter 24 for further discussion of ARF.

- Treatment and prevention of GABHS infection are essential.
- Use antiinflammatory agents to control clinical manifestations of the disease because 50% of patients with ARF have carditis to a greater or milder extent. The more severe carditis may require steroids; the lesser cases are given salicylates (Carapetis et al, 2005).
- Supportive therapy as appropriate for CHF and choreiform movements.
- Prevention of recurrence can be achieved with prompt identification and treatment of future GABHS infections. In approximately 70% to 80% of patients, valvar disease will resolve if they are compliant in taking antibiotic prophylaxis after the first episode of RHD. This will require either a monthly penicillin injection or daily oral antibiotics (Carapetis et al, 2005).

INFECTIVE ENDOCARDITIS

Description

Infective endocarditis, formerly referred to as subacute bacterial endocarditis (SBE), is a condition in which a bacterial or fungal infection invades traumatized endocardial surfaces of the heart, most commonly the cardiac valves. IE usually occurs in children or adults with underlying structural cardiac abnormalities (CHD, ARF), but it does rarely occur in those without structural heart disease. IE also occurs in children or adults with indwelling catheters and devices that are commonly used in oncology or neonatal patients. The incidence of IE has increased as more children with CHD are surviving because of aggressive treatments. Half of the cases occur in children older than 10 years, but infection can occur in any age group. Infection carries high morbidity and mortality rates and can lead to destruction of heart valves or disseminated sepsis. The importance of prevention in patients who are at risk and the importance of early diagnosis and treatment cannot be overemphasized.

Epidemiology

In developing counties where there is a high prevalence of RHD, there is a concurrent increase in IE since RHD damaged valves are quite vulnerable to IE. Endocarditis is now relatively rare in the U.S. It accounts for 1 in 1280 pediatric admissions per year, 92% of these admissions have CHD or an indwelling catheter. Patients who have had palliative surgery for cyanotic heart disease and those with prosthetic aortic valve replacements are at highest risk for IE (Ferrieri et al, 2002).

Turbulence caused by stenotic valves, previous surgical repairs, or high-velocity jets (from blood flowing under force through a structural heart defect) traumatize cardiac endothelium and lead to thrombogenesis. Clumps of platelets and fibrin provide a nidus for circulating bacteria or rarely fungi. The bacteria or fungi multiply, shielded from circulating white cells by the platelet-fibrin matrix. These vegetations cause further damage by destroying nearby valve tissue and extending to surrounding endothelium. Septic and thrombotic emboli from these vegetations can cause abscesses and ischemic damage to distant areas, such as the brain, abdominal viscera, and extremities (Ferrieri et al, 2002).

Gram-positive cocci cause most cases of IE in children. *S. viridans* is the most common causative organism, followed by *S. aureus*. Together, these two groups account for 80% of IE cases. HACEK organisms are less commonly implicated (Ferrieri et al, 2002). Children with CHD appear to have more severe gingival inflammatory conditions, increased plaque accumulation, and more HACEK microbes, which lead to endocarditis (Steelman et al, 2003).

Clinical Findings

History and Physical Examination

- Exposure within 2 weeks before onset of symptoms
- Acute manifestations: short duration of illness, high fever (greater than 102.2° F [39° C]), myalgias, night sweats, arthralgias, headache, general malaise, decreased appetite, increase in intensity of preexisting murmur or new onset of murmur
- Embolization symptoms: hematuria, acute onset of respiratory distress, splenomegaly, neurologic changes (stroke, brain abscesses, hemorrhage, meningitis), petechiae (in conjunctiva, buccal mucosa, palatal area, nail beds, palms, and soles)

Diagnostic Studies

- The diagnosis is based on clinical findings and results of blood cultures. A persistent low-grade fever in a patient with known cardiac abnormalities should be evaluated immediately with three sets of blood cultures over 24 hours from different sites before the administration of empirical antibiotic therapy. This will detect 97% of cases of IE. When three cultures are positive for the same organism, IE must be considered and treatment instituted.
- The ESR, CRP, and WBC count are elevated in the acute stage; anemia may be evidenced.
- Two-dimensional echocardiography is helpful in detecting vegetation, new valvular insufficiency, or obvious damage to a valve (Ferrieri et al, 2002).

Management

- Treatment should begin as soon as IE is suspected in order to decrease the subsequent morbidity and mortality associated with untreated bacteremia.
- High doses of appropriate antibiotics are given intravenously for 4 to 6 weeks.

Prevention

For children with high-risk cardiac conditions (previous endocarditis; unrepaired or palliated cyanotic CHD; prosthetic or bioprosthetic valve, shunt or conduit; repaired CHD with residual defects adjacent to site of prosthetic patch or device; and heart transplant recipients) prophylactic antibiotic therapy is given before all dental procedures involving manipulation of gingival tissue. Antibiotics are also recommended for procedures on respiratory tract or infected skin in the above listed patients (see Tables 30-7 and 30-8). (Wilson et al, 2007).

MYOCARDITIS

Myocarditis is a rare inflammatory illness of the muscular walls of the heart. It may go unrecognized in children whose inflammatory process resolved spontaneously, or it may progress to fulminant disease resulting in chronic cardiomyopathy or even death. Myocarditis is often caused by viral infections, most commonly enteroviruses, coxsackievirus A and B, echoviruses, and poliovirus. Influenza, cytomegalovirus (CMV), varicella, mumps, human immunodeficiency virus, RSV, and rubella are other viral causes. Nonviral infections (fungal, bacterial, protozoan, rickettsial), various medications, autoimmune or inflammatory disorders (e.g., ARF, SLE), toxic reactions to infectious agents, or other disorders (e.g., KD) may also be etiologic agents; however, the etiology is often unknown. Myocarditis may occur in epidemics, usually in infants in association with coxsackievirus B (Colan, 2006).

Clinical Findings

History. Symptoms of myocarditis, which are secondary to reduced myocardial function, are caused by interstitial inflammation or damage. As a result, muscle function decreases and causes enlargement of the heart with decreased contractility. As this process progresses, cardiac function decreases and symptoms of CHF become evident. The following history is characteristic:

- Infants:
  - Fever, irritability or listlessness, episodes of pallor, diaphoresis
  - Tachypnea or respiratory distress
  - Poor appetite and vomiting
- Children and adolescents:
  - Recent flulike or gastrointestinal viral illness (10 to 14 days previously)
  - Lethargy, low-grade fever, pallor
  - Decreased appetite and abdominal pain
  - Exercise intolerance, malaise, rashes, palpitations, respiratory distress (late finding), decreased pulse oximetry reading

Physical Examination

- Pallor, mild cyanosis, skin cool and mottled with poor perfusion (in infants)
- Rapid laborious respirations, grunting, decreased pulse oximetry reading
- Tachycardia, gallop rhythm, muffled heart sounds, apical systolic murmur, weak pulses
- Hepatomegaly

Diagnostic Studies. The PCP should refer patients with symptoms suggestive of myocarditis to a pediatric cardiologist. Diagnostic testing will usually involve chest radiography, ECG, two-dimensional echocardiography, CBC, ESR, CRP, cardiac and liver enzymes, viral titers, blood cultures, metabolic studies (e.g., thyroid and carnitine), and viral cultures from the myocardium.

Differential Diagnosis

Sepsis, asthma, recurrent vomiting, and chronic viral illness are in the differential.

Management

Treatment is supportive with bed rest and medications, such as digitalis, diuretics, ACE blockers, and beta-blockers. Occasionally, cardiologists may use anticoagulation and antiarrhythmia medications. Many experimental therapies are under study, including the use of intravenous gamma globulin and vaccines for enteroviruses (Colan, 2006). Severe cases may require hospitalization for mechanical ventilation and inotropic support. Recovery often takes 2 to 3 months; follow-up is indefinite. Pericardial effusion and pericarditis can occur concurrently. Scarring of the myocardium may occur and cause persistent heart failure and ventricular arrhythmias.

Prognosis

Cardiac transplantation may be necessary in some patients with myocarditis or cardiomyopathy. In a recent review of patients with myocarditis, 66% of children made a complete recovery, 10% had partial recovery, and 24% required transplant or died (English et al, 2004).

PERICARDITIS

Pericarditis refers to an inflammation or other abnormality of the pericardium, the sac that surrounds the heart. Excess fluid accumulates in the pericardial space and causes the normally compliant pericardium to distend. As intrapericardial pressure increases, the heart becomes compressed and its ability to fill is limited. Pericarditis may be seen in individuals without a prior history of cardiac disease. Viral infection (usually coxsackievirus or adenovirus) is the most common cause of pericarditis in children (40% to 75% of cases). Other etiologic agents include infections (tuberculosis, other bacteria), trauma, hypersensitivity to medication (INH, hydralazine), collagen-vascular and connective tissue diseases (ARF, juvenile rheumatoid arthritis, SLE), KD, postsurgical complications, and complications of systemic infection. Pericarditis is most common in children younger than 2 years old and demonstrates equal sex distribution (Nowlen & Bricker, 2000). It is a serious illness that may have rapidly fatal consequences if not diagnosed and treated in a timely manner. The following findings should alert the provider to refer the patient to a pediatric cardiologist:

- History of precordial or substernal chest pain altered by respiration, coughing, or position (may not be found in small children); lethargy, loss of appetite, abdominal pain; fever, irritability; tachycardia; viral illness 10 to 14 days before onset of symptoms
- Physical examination findings: distended neck veins; tachycardia, pericardial friction rub (an early sign heard best along the left sternal border with the patient leaning forward) or muffled heart sounds (if the effusion is large); Kussmaul sign (slow, deep respirations); pulsus paradoxus, a decrease in BP of greater than 10 mm Hg during inspiration with patient in a supine position; hepatomegaly

Myocarditis is the main differential diagnosis. Management consists of pericardiocentesis if tamponade becomes evident, nonsteroidal antiinflammatory and analgesic medications, or, rarely, sternotomy or thoracotomy to control any intrapericardial bleeding. Cardiac tamponade can occur with large or rapid effusions. There is a relapse rate of 15% if the causative agent was viral. Most children recover fully within a 3- to 4-week period.

◼ HEART CONDUCTION DISTURBANCES
CARDIAC ARRHYTHMIAS
Epidemiology
Approximately 14 per 100,000 pediatric emergency department (ED) visits are for cardiac arrhythmias or dysrhythmias. Children tend to come to EDs either in early infancy or adolescence with dysrhythmias. The most common dysrhythmias are sinus tachycardia (most prevalent), supraventricular tachycardia (SVT), bradycardia, and atrial fibrillation (Doniger & Sharieff, 2006). There are genetic defects that cause some arrhythmias, most notably long QT syndrome and familial ASD or conduction abnormality defect (Goldmuntz, 2004). Most abnormal heart rhythms in children with structurally normal hearts are benign, but an arrhythmia in a child with a cardiac abnormality can be lethal. Any patient who has an arrhythmia or syncope with exertion requires an evaluation for underlying cardiac disease.

Types of Dysrhythmia
Dysrhythmias can manifest as a primary disorder or as a consequence of cardiac or other systemic disorders. The PCP should be familiar with the following dysrhythmias (see Table 30-3 for normal heart rates):
- Sinus arrhythmia—variable heart rate that increases with inspiration and decreases with expiration. This is a normal finding in children.
- Bradycardia or slow heart rate for age.
  - Sinus bradycardia is the most common cause of bradycardia in children and may be due to hypoxia, acidosis, increased intracranial pressure, abdominal distention, hypothermia, or hypoglycemia. It may also be caused by drugs, such as beta-blockers or digoxin. Mild slowing may be due to increased vagal tone or cardiac conditioning (e.g., athletes) (Doniger & Sharieff, 2006).

  - Complete AV block can either be congenital, as seen in infants of mothers with an autoimmune disease, such as SLE, or may be acquired after cardiac surgery. Certain rare cardiac defects, such as L-transposition of great arteries and heterotaxy, are also associated with complete heart block. The hemodynamic effect of a slow heart rate depends on how slow it is (Doniger & Sharieff, 2006).
- Tachycardias
  - Sinus tachycardia is caused by predisposing factors that increase cardiac output, including fever, anxiety, infection, drug exposure, dehydration, pain, hyperthyroidism, or anemia among many others. Treatment is directed at the underlying disorder (Doniger & Sharieff, 2006).

SVTs are the most common pathologic tachycardias in children:
- AV reentrant tachycardia is the most common SVT. In AV reentrant tachycardia, there is an additional pathway for impulse transmission from atria to ventricles besides the normal AV node. Conduction occurs more rapidly down the accessory pathway, setting up a cyclical rhythm that is faster than the rhythm generated by the sinus node. A subgroup of these children have Wolff-Parkinson-White syndrome (WPW), which has classic findings on the ECG (once the SVT rhythm has been broken) of short PR interval and delta wave (a positive inflection in upstroke of QRS). AV reentrant tachycardias often first present in infants younger than 4 months old and again in young adolescents (Doniger & Sharieff, 2006).
- Less common SVT is AV nodal tachycardia, which is also a reentrant tachycardia caused by dual AV node pathways.
- The rarest type of SVT is ectopic atrial tachycardia caused by an ectopic focus in the atrium. There are usually different p-wave morphologies on ECG (Doniger & Sharieff, 2006). This SVT is much more difficult to diagnose and treat.
- Long QT syndrome-induced ventricular tachycardia. Patients with a prolonged QT interval may have episodes of torsades de pointes (a type of ventricular tachycardia that is often fatal). The QT interval on the ECG is a measure of repolarization of the ventricles. This interval is longer than normal in some people as a result of a congenital abnormality or exposure to certain drugs and toxins (a list of such substances are available at www.qtdrugs.org). A QT interval corrected for the heart rate (QTc) of greater than 0.45 seconds is worthy of investigation (Walsh et al, 2006).

  Researchers have linked the congenital form of long QT syndrome to seven gene defects. If the provider suspects long QT syndrome based on ECG and concerning symptoms (dizziness, palpitations, syncope) or family history, refer to a pediatric cardiologist. All family members need screening if an index case is identified. Treatment includes beta-blocker medications, activity restrictions, and implantable defibrillators (Walsh et al, 2006).
- Premature atrial contractions. Depolarization may or may not be conducted through the AV node. Premature contractions can be seen in an infant or child with an

otherwise normal heart. It is not unusual to see multiple premature atrial contractions on the ECG of a newborn.

- Premature ventricular contractions—premature QRS complex with a prolonged duration or morphologic difference from the preceding QRS. Occasional premature ventricular contractions are also seen in otherwise normal infants. Premature ventricular contractions that are uniform in appearance, which means that they have the same QRS complex appearance every time, are usually of no consequence.

Clinical Findings
History

- Bradycardia with a sudden decrease in heart rate can cause syncope or severe dizziness.
- SVT can be of sudden onset and variable duration.
  - Infants tolerate several hours of SVT with rates up to 250 beats per minute before demonstrating evidence of poor feeding, irritability, or pallor that can eventually lead to CHF if not converted.
  - Older children may feel quite ill after a few minutes and have complaints of "butterflies" in the chest, dizziness, palpitations, pain in the neck, abdominal pain with nausea and vomiting, and syncope

Physical Examination

- Slow or fast heart rate; rhythm—regular, irregular, or regularly irregular

Diagnostic Studies.   Tests include ECG (the basic screening tool) and 24-hour Holter monitor or event monitor if symptoms are sporadic and the ECG is normal.

Differential Diagnosis

The differential diagnosis includes any condition that may elevate or slow heart rate.

Management

Identification of an arrhythmia can be challenging. A sinus arrhythmia requires no treatment. Refer all other rhythm abnormalities to a pediatric cardiologist for evaluation. Other findings that require a referral include the following:

- Abnormal ECG
- History of unusual heart rhythm
- History of syncope or dizziness on exertion with palpitations
- History of cardiac abnormality, heart surgery, or Wolff-Parkinson-White syndrome

Complications

Death can occur with some arrhythmias if untreated.

Education and Prognosis

- Recurrent SVT—the child or parent may be taught to monitor the heart rate and use vagal maneuvers to break the spell.

RESOURCE BOX
Cardiovascular Disorders

AMERICAN HEART ASSOCIATION
www.amhrt.org

PARENT AND PATIENT SUPPORT
Mended Hearts, Inc.
www.mendedhearts.org

Congenital Heart Information Network
www.tchin.org
   An international organization that offers information, support, and resources to parents of children and adults with congenital and acquired heart disease

PediHeart
www.pediheart.org
   Provides information and support for children and their parents with heart disease

National Center for Biotechnology Information
www.ncbi.nlm.nih.gov

✓ DISCUSSION FORUM

1. How is the assessment and evaluation of a 10-day-old infant with a new-onset systolic ejection murmur different from that of a 2-year-old? How are they the same? Be sure to cover physical and developmental differences.
2. You see a 2-year-old with Down syndrome in your outpatient clinic. He has a large VSD and is scheduled for surgical repair in 2 months. He is on digoxin at 7.5 mcg/g/day for control of his CHF. Create a plan of care to coordinate this child's care through surgery making sure you include interventions for this child's physical, developmental, and family needs.
3. How would you explain the need for SBE prophylaxis to the mother of an infant with a PDA? Would it be different if the child had a COA or an AV canal?
4. You see a 3-year-old with hypertension (documented on three different visits) in your outpatient clinic. Describe the work-up, differential diagnoses, assessment, and management. Be sure to include pharmacologic and nonpharmacologic interventions. How would your plan of care be different if the child were 10 years old?

REFERENCES

Allen H, Phillips J, Chan D: History and physical examination. In Allen H et al: *Moss and Adams' heart disease in infants, children, and adolescents, including the fetus and young adult,* ed 6, Philadelphia, 2001, Lippincott Williams & Wilkins.

American Academy of Pediatrics (AAP): *2006 Red book: report of the Committee on Infectious Diseases,* ed 27, Elk Grove Village, IL, 2006, American Academy of Pediatrics.

American College of Sports Medicine: Girls more likely to be active when parents participate, *News Release,* Sept 4, 2003. Available at *www.acsm.org* (accessed July 29, 2006).

Anderson R et al: *Paediatric cardiology,* ed 2, New York, 2002, Churchill Livingstone.

Backer C, Mavroudis C: Coarctation of the aorta. In Mavroudis C, Backer C: *Pediatric cardiac surgery,* ed 3, Philadelphia, 2003, Mosby.

Bellinger D, Wypij D, duPlessis A et al: Neurodevelopmental status at eight years in children with dextrotransposition of the great arteries: the Boston Circulatory Arrest Trial, *J Thor Card Surg* 126:1385-1396, 2003.

Bernstein D: The cardiovascular system. In Behrman RE, Kliegman RM, editors: *Nelson essentials of pediatrics,* ed 17, Philadelphia, 2004, WB Saunders.

Carapetis J, McDonald M, Wilson N: Acute rheumatic fever, *Lancet* 366:155-168, 2005.

Colan S: Cardiomyopathies. In Keane J, Lock J, Fyler D: *Nadas' pediatric cardiology,* ed 2, Philadelphia, 2006, Saunders Elsevier.

Dajani AS et al: Guidelines for the diagnosis of rheumatic fever: Jones criteria, updated 1992, *Circulation* 87:302-307, 1993.

Doniger SJ, Sharieff GO: Pediatric dysrhythmias, *Ped Clin North Am* 53(1):85-105, 2006.

Driscoll D: *Fundamentals of pediatric cardiology,* Philadelphia, 2006, Lippincott Williams & Wilkins.

English R, Janosky J, Ettedgui J et al: Outcomes for children with acute myocarditis, *Cardio Young* 14:488-493, 2004.

Enright P, Goodwin J, Sherrill D et al: Blood pressure elevation associated with sleep-related breathing disorder in a community sample of white and Hispanic children, *Arch Pediatric Adolesc Med* 157:901-904, 2003.

Ferrieri P, for the Jones Criteria Working Group: Proceedings of the Jones criteria workshop, *Circulation* 106(19):2521, 2002.

Ferrieri P, Gewitz M, Gerber M et al: Unique features of infective endocarditis in childhood, *Circulation* 105:2115, 2002.

Gatzoulis M: Tetralogy of Fallot. In Gatzoulis M, Webb G, Daubeney P: *Diagnosis and management of adult congenital heart disease,* Edinburgh, 2003, Churchill Livingstone.

Gatzoulis M, Webb G: Adults with congenital heart disease: a growing population. In Gatzoulis M, Webb G, Daubeney P: *Diagnosis and management of adult congenital heart disease,* Edinburgh, 2003, Churchill Livingstone.

Goldmuntz E: The genetic contribution to congenital heart disease, *Pediatr Clin North Am* 51:1721-1737, 2004.

Goldmuntz E: DiGeorge syndrome: new insights. *Clin Perinat* 43(6):519-522, 2005.

Hövels-Gürich H, Konrad K, Skorzenski D et al: Long-term neurodevelopment outcome and exercise capacity after corrective surgery for tetralogy of Fallot or ventricular septal defect in infancy, *Ann Thor Surg* 81(3):958-966, 2006.

Iemura M. Ishii M, Sugimura T et al: Long term consequences of regressed coronary aneurysms after Kawasaki disease: vascular wall morphology and function, *Heart* 83(3):307-11, 2000.

Koppel RI, Druschel CM, Carter T et al: Effectiveness of pulse oximetry screening for congenital heart disease in asymptomatic newborns, *Pediatrics* 111(3):451-455, 2003.

Lin A, Belmont J, Malik S: Heart. In Stevenson R, Hall J: *Human malformations and related anomalies,* ed 2, Oxford, 2006, Oxford University Press.

Maron B, Zipes D, Ackerman M et al: 36th Bethesda conference: eligibility recommendations for competitive athletes with cardiovascular abnormalities, *J Am Coll Card* 45(8):1313-1377, 2005.

National Institutes of Health, National High Blood Pressure Education Program Working Group on High Blood Pressure in Children and Adolescents (NIH-NHBPEP): The Fourth Report on the Diagnosis, Evaluation, and Treatment of High Blood Pressure in Children and Adolescents, *Pediatrics* 114:555-576, 2004.

Newburger J, Takahashi M, Gerber M et al: Diagnosis, treatment and long-term management of Kawasaki diseases: a statement for health professionals from the committee on Rheumatic Fever, Endocarditis, and Kawasaki Disease, Council on Cardiovascular Disease in the Young, American Heart Association, *Pediatrics* 114:1708-1733, 2004.

Nowlen T, Bricker J: Pericardial diseases. In Moller J, Hoffman J: *Pediatric cardiovascular medicine,* New York, 2000, Churchill Livingstone.

Park MK, Troxler RG: *Pediatric cardiology for practitioners,* ed 4, St Louis, 2002, Mosby.

Shore D: Late repair and reoperations in adults with congenital heart disease. In Gatzoulis M, Webb G, Daubeney P: *Diagnosis and management of adult congenital heart disease,* Edinburgh, 2003, Churchill Livingstone.

Steelman R, Rosen DA, Nelson ER et al: Gingival colonization with selective HACEK microbes in children with congenital heart disease *Clin Oral Invest* 7(1):38-40, 2003.

Stevenson R: Human malformations and related anomalies. In Stevenson R, Hall J: *Human malformations and related anomalies,* ed 2, Oxford, 2006, Oxford University Press.

Tchervenkov C, Chu V, Shum-Tim D: Left ventricular outflow tract obstruction. In Mavroudis C, Becher C: *Pediatric cardiac surgery,* ed 3, Philadelphia, 2003, Mosby.

Walsh E, Berul C, Treidman J: Cardiac arrhythmias. In Keane J, Lock J, Fyler D: *Nadas' pediatric cardiology,* ed 2, Philadelphia, 2006, WB Saunders Elsevier.

Wilson W, Taubert KA, Gerwitz et al: Prevention of bacterial endocarditis: Recommendations by the American Heart Association, *JAMA* 277: 1794-1801, 1997.

CHAPTER 37

Respiratory Disorders

Margaret A. Brady

Respiratory problems are a leading cause of illness in children and a major reason for health care visits. Viral upper respiratory tract infections (URIs) and otitis media are common diagnoses seen every day by practitioners. Guiding parents in the appropriate management of upper respiratory disorders is often a challenge for health care providers seeking to treat such problems as the common cold, otitis media, rhinitis, tonsillopharyngitis, and sinusitis. Parents seeking to relieve their child's upper respiratory tract symptoms are often tempted to use a variety of over-the-counter medications readily available to them or to pressure the primary care provider to prescribe needless antibiotics. In contrast, a child with a lower respiratory tract disorder such as asthma or bacterial pneumonia can experience a potentially life-threatening illness that demands prompt attention. Providers who ask key questions about the history of the respiratory symptoms; do a systematic and complete examination of the upper and lower airways, including the sinuses; and, if indicated, order specific laboratory tests and radiographic examinations can determine an accurate diagnosis and develop a successful treatment plan in most cases. When children have complicated problems, they can be referred with baseline information to the appropriate medical specialist for additional studies and treatment.

■ ANATOMY AND PHYSIOLOGY
UPPER RESPIRATORY TRACT

The upper respiratory tract includes the nostrils, nasopharynx, larynx, upper part of the trachea, eustachian tubes, and sinuses. Air is warmed and humidified as it travels through the nasal passages, and particles are filtered out by coarse nasal hairs. A blanket of mucus covers the surface epithelium of the nasal mucosa. Nasal secretions contain lysozymes and secretory immunoglobulin A (IgA) to defend against microbial invasion. Similarly, the paranasal sinuses are lined with ciliated, mucus-secreting epithelium, and the mucociliary action of the paranasal epithelium moves secretions from the sinuses to the nasal cavity and then to the pharynx. The maxillary and ethmoid sinuses are the earliest sinuses to develop and can be visualized on plain radiographs when the child is 1 to 2 years old. The sphenoid and frontal sinuses become visible on radiographs at approximately 5 to 6 years old. The sinuses become clinically significant sites of infection as follows:
- Maxillary and ethmoid sinuses as early as infancy
- Sphenoid sinuses around the third and fourth year of life
- Frontal sinuses around the sixth to tenth year of life

The sinuses continue to grow through adolescence.

The epiglottis deflects swallowed material toward the esophagus to protect the larynx. The vocal cords form a V-shaped opening known as the glottis. The subglottic space is beneath the vocal cords, and its walls converge toward the cricoid ring, a complete ring of cartilage. In children less than 2 to 3 years old, the cricoid ring is the narrowest part of the airway; in older children and adults, the glottis is narrowest. The rings of cartilage support the trachea and the main stem bronchi.

LOWER RESPIRATORY TRACT

The right lung has three lobes, upper, middle, and lower, with the upper and middle being separated by a minor fissure. The left lung has two lobes, upper and lower, separated by a major fissure. The upper left lobe has an area called the *lingula* that corresponds to the right middle lobe. The right main stem bronchus is shorter and wider than the left bronchus. It forms a smaller angle away from the trachea than the left bronchus does. This anatomic variation explains why foreign bodies (FBs) usually end in the right main stem bronchus. Although the body surface and the number of respiratory airways and alveoli increase tenfold from birth to adult life, the tissue available for gas exchange increases approximately twentyfold. The newborn's chest is cylindrically shaped and has relatively horizontal ribs, which limits the infant's ability to expand his or her chest. The shape of the chest changes during the first few years of life because of greater transverse growth in the lower part of the chest wall. This differential growth results in the ribs being positioned lower anteriorly than posteriorly. The change in positioning of the ribs adds rigidity to the thorax of older children.

The diaphragm is the main muscle of respiration, and the intercostal, sternocleidomastoid, spinal, neck, and abdominal muscles are accessory muscles that can be used to increase effort. Normal exhalation occurs from elastic recoil of the lung.

Primitive airways appear at approximately the fourth week of gestation. At about the sixteenth week of gestation, the number of bronchial branches equals that in adults. Subsequent growth continues by increasing the length of the respiratory tract. During the sixteenth to twenty-sixth weeks of gestation, vascularization of the future respiratory portion of the lung occurs. Cartilage, glands, and muscles of the airways and type II alveolar cells are formed by the twenty-eighth week. Type II cells allow the fetus to produce surfactant. The airways continue to grow, and terminal sac formation occurs.

At approximately the thirty-sixth week, the terminal sacs divide, and alveoli are formed. Approximately 50 million primitive alveoli are present at birth.

After birth, the alveolar ducts branch off the third respiratory bronchioles. Alveoli continue to form and number 100 to 200 million in older children and 200 to 600 million in adolescents. The alveolar sacs continue to increase in size. The adult lung contains approximately 300 million alveoli.

Other structures important for gas exchange and pulmonary function are present at birth and include cartilage, mucous glands, goblet cells, and ciliated cells of the conducting airways. Smooth muscle is also present; therefore even very young infants can have bronchospasm.

Airway resistance is higher in newborns and young children than in adults. The airways of young infants and children are easily obstructed by inflammation, FBs, or mucous secretion. The maximal inspiratory pressure generated by an infant is equal to that of an adult. However, the chest wall and supporting structures are softer and more flexible, so chest wall retraction is greatest in young infants. The chest wall of a newborn is highly compliant (Behrman et al, 2004; Marshall & Debley, 2006).

■ PATHOPHYSIOLOGY INVOLVED IN AIRWAY DISEASE

All lung disorders eventually result in some form of airway obstruction. Narrowing of the lumen of the airway results from one or more of the following:
- Presence of intraluminal material (e.g., secretions, tumors, or foreign matter)
- Mural thickening (e.g., edema or hypertrophy of the glands or mucosa)
- Contraction of smooth muscle (e.g., spasm)
- Extrinsic compression

These factors rarely occur in isolation. They cause pulmonary malfunction by impairing tracheobronchial hygiene and impeding normal airflow. Severe airway obstruction can result from very small blockages because of the proportional size of an infant's or young child's airway.

The two major types of airway obstruction are complete and partial. In complete obstruction, neither airflow nor drainage of secretions occurs. Such occlusion leads to lobar atelectasis after the residual gas diffuses into the pulmonary circulation. In partial obstruction, flow of air and drainage of secretions occur but are impaired. Partial obstruction can be further divided into the following two separate classifications.

The first consists of a bypass valve obstruction caused by narrowing of the lumen; a wheeze may be produced. Although resistance to flow is increased, air can still flow in during inspiration and out during expiration. The second is a check-valve or ball-valve obstruction; air entry is possible, but during expiration the lumen is completely occluded so that escape of air is impossible. Bronchial FBs and emphysema are associated with bypass, check-valve, or ball-valve obstructions that result in overinflation of lung airways.

High airway obstruction occurs above the level of the secondary bronchi and generally interferes more with inspiration than expiration. If the obstruction is complete and above the bifurcation of the trachea, asphyxia and death can result. Partial obstruction may result in severe dyspnea, stridor (a harsh, high-pitched inspiratory sound), and subcostal retractions. Coughing is the mechanism to remove nonfixed, high airway obstruction. Poor inspiratory airflow limits the effectiveness of coughing. The sound produced by coughing can help detect the level of obstruction and assists in making a diagnosis. Obstructions next to the larynx produce a cough that sounds croupy or barking; obstructions in the trachea or major bronchi produce a brassy sound.

Lower airway obstructions are caused by peripheral lesions that are usually diffuse in location and involve bronchioles smaller than 3 mm. The usual mechanism of narrowing is spasm, accumulation of secretions, edema of the mucous membrane, extrinsic compression, or any combination of these factors.

Complete obstruction causes atelectasis. A large percentage of the lung volume needs to be involved before symptoms become apparent; small atelectatic changes do not produce obvious clinical manifestations.

The primary clinical manifestation of lower airway obstruction is expiratory-phase symptoms. Wheezing is the principal sound patients make if the obstruction allows enough air to pass through the narrowed lumen. Chest excursion is diminished, and the expiratory phase is prolonged. Increased airway resistance during exhalation results in overinflation of the lungs, which in turn eventually increases the anteroposterior diameter of the chest. Chronic overinflation results in the "barrel chest" typical of a patient with chronic lung disease such as cystic fibrosis (CF) or emphysema. The accumulation of fluids and inflammation in the lower airways usually result in a repetitive hacking, ineffectual cough. On physical examination, percussing an overinflated chest elicits hyperresonance.

The more marked the obstruction, the more symptoms induced. The body attempts to compensate by using accessory muscles to assist in breathing. Dyspnea can result, often in association with orthopnea and exercise intolerance. Cyanosis is an ominous sign that can suggest impending death. Mild obstruction is marked by reduced respiratory rate and increased tidal volume; severe obstruction is characterized by increased respiratory rate, increased retractions with the use of accessory muscles, anxiety, and cyanosis.

Fine crackles or rales also indicate pathologic respiratory conditions and are short, crackling sounds heard during inspiration. These sounds are not cleared by coughing and are caused by airways suddenly opening after having been previously closed. The gas pressure between the compartments equalizes and creates the crackling sound.

Airway obstruction is the underlying etiology for the most common forms of pediatric lung diseases. Restrictive disease is less common in pediatric patients and is characterized by decreased lung compliance with relatively normal flow rates. Examples of causative factors include neuromuscular weakness, lobar pneumonia, pleural effusion or masses, severe pectus excavatum, or abdominal distention. Key findings of restrictive lung disease are rapid respiratory rate and decreased tidal volume (Marshall & Debley, 2006).

■ DEFENSE SYSTEMS

The respiratory defense system includes both mechanical and biologic processes. Mechanical defenses include:

- Filtering of particles
- Warming and humidifying of inspired air
- Clearing of airway through mucociliary and coughing actions
- Spasm and breathing changes

Approximately 75% of inspired air is warmed as it passes through the nose, paranasal sinuses, pharynx, larynx, and upper portion of the trachea. Final warming and humidifying of the airstream take place in the trachea and large bronchi. Heat and moisture are removed during the expiratory phase of respiration. The nose has a large surface area on which particles larger than 5 mm are impacted and filtered to prevent them from entering the lower airways. The trachea and bronchioles are lined with various defensive cells and mucous glands. Goblet cells secrete the mucous layer that lies on the tip of cilia. Particles entering the conducting airway are quickly cleared by the mucociliary defenses. Coughing is a reflex mechanism. Through forceful expiration, FBs and other materials can be removed from the airways. Coughing can propel particles, but in young infants and children, coughing is often unproductive in expectorating mucus. Instead, infants and young children swallow rather than expectorate secretions. Loss of the cough reflex can lead to aspiration and pneumonia.

The temporary cessation of breathing, reflex shallow breathing, laryngospasm, and even bronchospasm are compensatory efforts aimed at stopping foreign matter from further entry into the lower respiratory tract. However, these respiratory efforts offer limited protection and have significant drawbacks.

Biologic processes that protect the respiratory system include:

- Phagocytosis
- Absorption of noxious gases in the vasculature of the upper airway
- Absorption of particles by the lymph system

Phagocytosis, aided by the secretory immunoglobulins IgA plus interferon, lysozyme, and lactoferrin, is the principal antimicrobial defense. Particles reaching the alveoli can be phagocytized by alveolar macrophages and polymorphonuclear cells, cleared from the lung by the mucociliary system, or carried by lymphocytes into regional nodes or the blood. These particles can take days to months to clear.

The respiratory defense system is at risk for compromise from numerous environmental factors. Damage to epithelial cells is caused by a variety of substances and gases such as sulfur, nitrogen dioxide, ozone, chlorine, ammonia, and cigarette smoke. Hypothermia, hyperthermia, morphine, codeine, and hypothyroidism can adversely alter mucociliary defenses. Dry air from mouth breathing during periods of nasal obstruction, tracheostomy placement, or inadequately humidified oxygen therapy results in dryness of the mucous membrane and slowing of the cilia beat. Cold air is also irritating to the lower airways.

Phagocytic ability is also reduced by many substances, including ethanol ingestion and cigarette smoke. Hypoxemia, starvation, chilling, corticosteroids, increased oxygen, narcotics, and some anesthetic gases also impair phagocytosis. Recent acute viral infections can reduce antibacterial killing capacity. Damage from infection and chemical irritants may or may not be reversible (Behrman et al, 2004; Marshall & Debley, 2006).

■ ASSESSMENT OF THE RESPIRATORY SYSTEM

HISTORY

- History of the present illness:
  - *Onset.* Was the onset acute or insidious or preceded by the common cold?
  - *Key signs and symptoms.* Has the child had symptoms or signs of a daytime or nighttime cough, fever, vomiting, malaise, rhinorrhea, sore throat, lesions in the mouth, retractions, cyanosis, dyspnea, or increased respiratory effort? See Table 31-1 for key characteristics and causes of cough.
  - *Progression.* Are the respiratory signs or symptoms increasing in severity, lessening, or about the same? Is the child easily fatigued, less active, having trouble sleeping, or working harder to breathe?
  - *Associated symptoms.* Has there been a decrease in appetite or feeding or are breathing problems impacting the child's ability to sleep and eat? Any rashes, headache, or abdominal pain?
  - *Contacts.* Are any family members or close contacts (day care, school) ill with similar signs and symptoms?
  - Similar illnesses in the past. Does the child have a history of respiratory tract infections, allergies, or asthma? How many similar past infections has the child had (e.g., croup, pneumonia, sinusitis, streptococcal tonsillopharyngitis, frequent colds)?
  - *Treatment.* Have any over-the-counter or prescription drugs been used? Have any other treatment modalities been used, including folk cures, complementary therapies, or home remedies?
- Family history:
  - Do others in the family have a history of allergies or asthma? Is there any family history of ear-nose-throat or respiratory problems that could be familial or genetic diseases such as CF?
- Review of systems:
  - Note any infections, constitutional diseases, or congenital problems that might have a respiratory component.
- Environment:
  - Does anyone in the family or in the day care setting smoke? Does the child live or attend school in an urban or industrial area subject to air pollution (e.g., near a major highway or industrial plant)?

TABLE 31-1 **Key Characteristics of Cough, Common Causes, and Questions to Ask in a Pediatric History**

Purpose	A cough is a protective reflex to ensure airway patency.
Characteristics	
Age factor	Infants have a weak, nonproductive cough.
Quality	Staccato-like, brassy, barking (LTB), whooping in young infants (pertussis), weak, honky (psychogenic).
Duration	Acute (most causes are infectious), recurrent (associated with allergies and asthma), or chronic (e.g., CF); continuous or intermittent; a *chronic cough* is defined as coughing that lasts more than 2 to 4 weeks.
Productivity	Mucus producing or nonproductive.
Timing	During the day, night (associated with asthma), or both.
Associated symptoms	Fever—may indicate bacterial infection (pneumonia).
	Rhinorrhea, sneezing, wheezing, atopic dermatitis—associated with asthma and allergic rhinitis.
	Malaise, sneezing, watery nasal discharge, mild sore throat, no or low fever, not ill appearing—typical of URI.
	Tachypnea—pneumonia or bronchiolitis in infants (infants may not have a cough).
Causes	
Congenital anomalies	Tracheoesophageal fistula, laryngeal cleft, vocal cord paralysis, pulmonary malformations, tracheobronchomalacia, congenital heart disease, congestive heart failure.
Infectious agents	Viral (RSV, adenovirus, parainfluenza), bacterial (tuberculosis, pertussis, *S. pneumoniae*), fungal, and others (*Chlamydia* and *Mycoplasma*).
Allergic conditions	Allergic rhinitis, asthma.
Other	FB aspiration, gastroesophageal reflux, psychogenic cough, environmental triggers (air pollution, tobacco smoke, wood smoke, glue sniffing, volatile chemicals), CF, drug induced, HIV, tumor.

CF, Cystic fibrosis; *FB,* foreign body; *HIV,* human immunodeficiency virus; *LTB,* laryngotracheobronchitis; *RSV,* respiratory syncytial virus; *URI,* upper respiratory infection.
Adapted from Noble JE: Cough. In Berkowitz C, editor: *Pediatrics: a primary care approach,* ed 2, Philadelphia, 2000, WB Saunders, pp 271–274; McNamara M: Cough. In Schwartz MW, editor: *The 5-minute pediatric consult,* ed 2, Philadelphia, 2000, Lippincott Williams & Wilkins, pp 20–21.

PHYSICAL EXAMINATION

Chapter 2 covers physical examination of the respiratory system. Additional information pertinent to the physical examination of a child with suspected respiratory disease includes the following:

- Measurement of vital signs and observation of general appearance:
  - A normal respiratory rate is age dependent and, if elevated, is a key indicator of lower respiratory involvement.
  - The level of anxiety, nasal flaring, and position of comfort are useful indicators of respiratory distress. Changes in skin color may be subtle or obvious depending on the level of deoxygenation.
- Inspection of:
  - The nose for rhinorrhea—clear, mucoid, mucopurulent; FBs, erosion, polyps, lesions, bleeding; and color of the mucous membrane.
  - The throat, pharynx, and tonsillar areas for lesions, vesicles, exudate, enlargement of any structure, or other abnormalities. If epiglottitis is a consideration, do not inspect the mouth.
  - The chest for the depth, ease, symmetry, and rhythm of respiration. These elements are key indicators of lower respiratory tract involvement. The use of accessory muscles and the presence of retractions should be noted. A prolonged expiratory phase is associated with respiratory obstruction in the lower airways.
- Palpation or percussion (or both) of:
  - The paranasal and frontal areas to check for signs of sinus tenderness.
  - The chest for signs of dullness or hyperresonance caused by consolidation, fluid, or air trapping.
- Auscultation of the chest:
  - Upper tract involvement frequently causes rhonchi or referred breath sounds.
  - Lower tract involvement is suggested by fine crackles or rales (interrupted abnormal breath sounds) or by wheezing.
- Determination of respiratory distress is based on physical findings—consider the anxiety level, respiratory rate and rhythm, use of accessory muscles, color, breath sounds, and pulse oximetry.

DIAGNOSTIC TESTS

Diagnostic procedures used to evaluate respiratory illness in children managed as outpatients include the following:

- Monitoring oxygenation by pulse oximetry and blood gases:
  - Pulse oximetry can be used to continuously measure pulse rate and peripheral oxygen saturation in arterial blood. The oxyhemoglobin saturation percentage (SpO_2) is digitally displayed. Results generally correlate well with simultaneous arterial saturation (SaO_2). The equation to determine the partial pressure of O_2 (PaO_2) is $PaO_2 = FiO_2 (Ba - PH_2O) - 1.2\ PaCO_2$. FiO_2 is the fractional oxygen concentration (FiO_2) of the inspired gas. The partial pressure of H_2O is constant at 47 and that of CO_2 is usually 45. This dependence on barometric pressure (Ba) is the limiting factor: the higher the altitude at which one lives, the more hypoxic one becomes (e.g., the PaO_2 of room air at sea level $= 0.21\ [760 - 47] - 1.2 \times 45 = 95.73$). If Ba falls 50 mm Hg, the resultant PaO_2 of room air changes drastically (e.g., $PaO_2 = 0.21[710 - 47] - 1.2 \times 45 = 85$). People living in higher altitudes suffer from chronic hypoxia. When first arriving at a high elevation, many individuals experience a transient mountain sickness with symptoms that include headache, insomnia, irritability, breathlessness, nausea, and vomiting. This phenomenon can last approximately 1 week before acclimatization begins to occur. The affected person begins to increase production of red blood cells. Changes in hemoglobin result in decreased O_2 affinity, which makes more O_2 available to the cells. Finally, a functional nonpathologic right ventricular hypertrophy takes place. These effects last as long as the person remains at high altitude. Severe altitude sickness can lead to cerebral and pulmonary edema and be life threatening.
- Blood gas studies can help the provider in assessing possible respiratory collapse. A rising $PaCO_2$ is an ominous sign. Box 31-1 lists normal values for blood gases at sea level.
- Radiographic imaging, including radiographs, ultrasonography, magnetic resonance imaging (MRI), and computed tomography (CT) of the sinuses, soft tissues of the neck, and chest. Chest radiographs should be done in both posteroanterior and lateral positions because lesions may only be seen in one of the two views. Fluoroscopy is useful in the evaluation of stridor and abnormal movement of the diaphragm. Contrast studies (e.g., barium esophagogram) are useful for patients with recurrent pneumonia, persistent cough, or suspected fistulas.
- Pulmonary function tests are discussed in Chapter 24 in the section on asthma.
- Other specialized tests, including cultures and blood work, are addressed under the specific illness.
- Other imaging studies that might be needed to assess these children include bronchograms (useful in delineating the smaller airways), pulmonary arteriograms (evaluation of the pulmonary vasculature), and radionuclide studies (evaluation of the pulmonary capillary bed). Endoscopy (bronchoscopy and laryngoscopy), bronchoalveolar lavage, percutaneous tap, lung biopsy, sweat testing, and microbiology studies are other helpful diagnostic procedures if used appropriately. Children who are significantly ill or have unusual signs and symptoms that require such procedures should be referred to medical specialists.

BASIC RESPIRATORY MANAGEMENT STRATEGIES

GENERAL MEASURES

General management measures include the following:

- *Fluid.* Hydration is important to keep mucous membranes and secretions moist. Intake of fluids should be encouraged and parents of young children given guidelines regarding the amount of fluids that their child should take and the frequency of feedings.
- *Oxygen administration.* The use of supplemental oxygen is important to help relieve hypoxemia in most children who have acute respiratory distress. Depression of the respiratory drive is possible with supplemental oxygen administration if the central nervous system chemoreceptors are blunted by hypercapnia. However, children at risk for blunting are those with issues related to chronic hypercapnia and are generally easily recognized because they tend to have chronic severe respiratory diseases such as CF and bronchopulmonary dysplasia. In acute situations, administer oxygen using an appropriately sized mask or a high-flow O_2 source held near the child's face if a mask frightens the child. The safe, acceptable range of O_2 saturation is 92% to 95%; higher levels may lead to oxygen toxicity (Marshall & Debley, 2006).
- *Humidification.* For a child with laryngotracheobronchitis (LTB), taking the child out into the cold night air, opening a freezer door, or turning on the shower to create a hot steamy room at home is often beneficial. A cold-mist vaporizer helps provide moisture to the nares and oropharynx; the vaporizer must be cleaned daily so that it will not become a source of infection.
- *Bulb syringe.* Because infants are obligate nose breathers, parents should be instructed in use of the bulb syringe to relieve obstruction of the infant's nares with mucus. Use the bulb syringe gently and intermittently because improper use

---

BOX 31-1 **Normal Blood Gas Values at Sea Level**

- Normal PaO_2: 90 to 100 mm Hg
- Normal $PaCO_2$: 38 to 42 mm Hg
- Capillary PO_2: roughly one-half arterial PO_2
- Capillary PCO_2: same as arterial PCO_2
- Hypoventilation: $PaCO_2$ greater than 45 mm Hg; as $PaCO_2$ rises, the risk of respiratory failure increases
- Hyperventilation: $PaCO_2$ less than 35 mm Hg (usually need a respiratory rate greater than 60 breaths/minute)

can cause irritation, inflammation, and respiratory obstruction from tissue damage. Providing parents with written instruction on suctioning the infant's nose with a bulb syringe is advantageous. Cincinnati Children's Hospital Medical Center has home instructions for this technique available on its website (*www.cincinnatichildrens.org/health/info/newborn/home/suction.htm*).

- *Normal saline nose drops or spray.* Use before feedings and when mucus is thick or crusted. Follow by suctioning the nares with a bulb syringe.
- *Children who are significantly ill or have unusual manifestations need referral* to or consultation with a pediatrician or pediatric subspecialist.

MEDICATIONS

The following pharmacologic agents may be needed to treat various respiratory illnesses:

- *Antibiotics.* Specific agents are discussed in the section on individual illnesses. If an antibiotic is prescribed, the drug should be taken until completed.
- *Analgesics and antipyretics.* Acetaminophen and ibuprofen may be prescribed for relief of pain or fever.
- *Decongestants and antihistamines.* The use of decongestants and antihistamines is controversial. They do not shorten the course of a disease, but can provide relief of nasal symptoms. Use these agents with caution, in children older than 2 years. Their use in children under the age of 2 years is contraindicated. A Federal Drug Administration public health advisory about the use of nonprescription cold and cough medicine in children under 2 years old was issued in 2007.
- *Expectorants.* Water is one of the most effective expectorants. Over-the-counter agents provide some symptomatic relief, but do not shorten the course of respiratory illnesses. Do not use in children under 2 years old.
- *Cough medication.* Cough suppressant medications should be prescribed judiciously because coughing is a protective mechanism to clear secretions. Prescribing a cough suppressant at bedtime can help the child and parent sleep. Do not use in children under 2 years old.

The American Academy of Pediatrics (AAP) has guidelines for the judicious use of antimicrobial agents in pediatric patients with common respiratory illnesses, such as otitis media, pharyngitis, sinusitis, and cough or bronchitis. These guidelines can be accessed online at *www.aap.org*. Pediatric providers should be familiar with these recommendations. All health care providers must be cognizant of their role in the prevention of superinfections caused by the indiscriminate use of antibiotics.

PATIENT AND PARENT EDUCATION

Parents should be educated about assessment and management of changes in the child's condition. Significant educational issues are identified in Box 31-2.

▬ INDICATIONS FOR TONSILLECTOMY AND ADENOIDECTOMY

In considering the need to refer a child for tonsillectomy, adenoidectomy, or both, the following guidelines are used

---

BOX 31-2   Parental Education for At-Home Care of the Child With a Respiratory Tract Infection

Infection: Issues to Discuss

Fluid: Give guidelines on amount and frequency of fluids child should take.

Humidification: For laryngotracheobronchitis, take the child out into the cold night air, open a freezer door, or turn on the shower at home. In dry climates, humidifiers help in respiratory illnesses; instruct about cleaning of nebulizers and humidifiers (see below).

Bulb syringe: Instruct to use the bulb syringe gently and intermittently for suctioning the nares.

Normal saline nose drops or spray: Use before feedings and when mucus is thick or crusted. Follow by suctioning nares with bulb syringe.

Other educational issues to cover:

- Indications for immediate reevaluation of child:
- Signs and symptoms of respiratory distress
- Other indicators of worsening of illness (e.g., toxic appearance, malaise, feeding difficulty)
- Information on when to expect improvement in the child's symptoms and, if symptoms do not improve as expected, what to do next
- Clear instructions about medications—how much to give, when to give, side effects to watch for, how long to give, and the necessity of completing the course of antibiotics
- Infection control information if needed—hand washing and disposal of infected secretions
- Care of nebulizers and humidifiers—to prevent the growth of organisms, nebulizers and humidifiers should 1be cleaned first with soapy water, rinsed thoroughly, soaked for one half hour in a solution of one part vinegar to two or three parts distilled water, and then air-dried. Control 3™ is a commercial product that can be substituted for vinegar. However, it is expensive.
- Instructions on next return visit

(Hiltzik & de Serres, 2006). *Absolute* indications for tonsillectomy include:

- More than seven documented (streptococcal) recurrent pharyngotonsillitis per year for 2 years or five infections per year for 2 years or three infections per year for 3 years
- Obstructive symptoms (nighttime awakenings or "hot potato" voice)
- Recurrent peritonsillar abscess

Relative indications for tonsillectomy include chronic tonsillitis unresponsive to medical treatment, tonsillolithiasis, halitosis, and acute peritonsillar abscess.

Absolute indications for adenoidectomy include:

- Massive adenotonsillar hypertrophy causing extreme breathing difficulties and dysphagia
- Clinically evident obstructive sleep apnea

Adenoidectomy can also be considered if appropriate medical treatment fails to correct any of the following: obstructive adenoidal hypertrophy, recurrent or chronic otitis media (after tympanostomy tube placement has been tried), and chronic, unresponsive sinusitis. Adenoidectomy may also be the treatment of choice for other medical reasons such as decreased olfaction, dental-facial abnormalities, and attention-deficit/hyperactivity disorder (ADHD) (10% of children have obstructive sleep apnea as the cause of their ADHD).

For any relative indication for tonsillectomy, the risk-benefit ratio of the procedure must be weighed. Significant morbidity and mortality rates are associated with tonsillectomy including complications such as anesthesia problems, hemorrhage, and infection. The morbidity and mortality rates connected with adenoidectomy are not as high as with tonsillectomy. This procedure may often be accompanied by tonsillectomy (Hiltzik & de Serres, 2006; Wetmore, 2004).

■ UPPER RESPIRATORY TRACT DISORDERS

NASOPHARYNGITIS (COMMON COLD OR UPPER RESPIRATORY TRACT INFECTION) AND TONSILLOPHARYNGITIS

Description

Nasopharyngitis and tonsillopharyngitis are frequent problems seen in pediatric practice. Young children have, on average, six to ten URIs, or colds, per year. (Table 31-2 includes a differential diagnosis of URI from sinusitis and purulent rhinitis.) When tonsillar involvement is significant, the term *tonsillopharyngitis* or *tonsillitis* is used; when tonsillar involvement is minor, the term *nasopharyngitis* is used. Nasopharyngitis is most often caused by a viral agent (Turner & Hayden, 2004).

Management

Only supportive care is needed for a viral URI as addressed in the sections entitled General Measures and Patient Education under Basic Respiratory Management Strategies. Antibiotics are not appropriate treatment. The use of antipyretics, analgesics, decongestants, antihistamines, and cough medication is controversial but can help alleviate the distress caused by URI symptoms if used cautiously. The use of nonprescription cough and cold medication in children under 2 years old is contraindicated.

Acute Viral Pharyngitis and Tonsillitis

Epidemiology. Viral infection is the leading cause of nasopharyngitis and tonsillopharyngitis. Adenovirus is the most common cause of viral pharyngitis and tonsillitis. Adenoviruses are more likely to cause pharyngitis as a prominent symptom. Other viruses (e.g., rhinovirus) are associated with pharyngitis as a minor symptom and rhinorrhea or cough as predominant features. The enteroviruses (coxsackievirus, echovirus), herpesvirus, and Epstein-Barr virus are also common. Although not a virus, *Mycoplasma pneumoniae* is a frequent cause of pharyngitis and tonsillitis in school-age children. Viral infections occur year-round, but peak during winter and spring, and it is helpful to know what agents are currently infecting children in the community. It can be difficult to differentiate viral from bacterial infections because of overlapping symptoms. However, hoarseness, cough, coryza, conjunctivitis, diarrhea, and characteristic enanthems and exanthems are classic features of a viral infection, which is often

spread to siblings and classmates via close contact (Gerber, 2006; Marshall & Debley, 2006).

Clinical Findings

History. The following may be reported:
- Gradual onset
- Prominent nasal symptoms of rhinorrhea (key finding)
- Sore throat and dysphagia
- Mild cough
- Low-grade fever

Physical Examination. Virus-specific findings include the following:
- Epstein-Barr virus can produce exudate on the tonsils, soft palate petechiae, and diffuse adenopathy.
- Adenovirus can produce exudate on the tonsils and cervical adenopathy.
- Enteroviruses can produce vesicles or ulcers on the tonsillar pillars and posterior fauces; coryza, vomiting, or diarrhea may be present.
- Herpesvirus produces ulcers anteriorly and marked adenopathy.

Diagnostic Tests. If a diagnosis of viral infection is in doubt, a culture should be done. Cultures are useful in differentiating viral infection from group A β-hemolytic streptococci (GABHS) infection. If infectious mononucleosis is suspected, a heterophil antibody test and complete blood count (CBC) can be helpful in confirming the diagnosis.

Management. For viral infection, only supportive care is needed, including fever and sore throat pain relief with acetaminophen or ibuprofen. Fluid intake should be encouraged.

Acute Bacterial Pharyngitis and Tonsillitis

Epidemiology. The three most common bacterial causes of pharyngitis and tonsillitis in children and adolescents are GABHS, *Neisseria gonorrhoeae,* and *Corynebacterium diphtheriae.* GABHS accounts for about 15% to 30% of infections in children with acute sore throat and fever. *N. gonorrhoeae* pharyngitis is a sexually transmitted disease that can mimic GABHS pharyngitis or can run a subclinical course. *C. diphtheriae* causes diphtheria and is discussed later in this chapter. The latter two organisms are rare causes of tonsillopharyngitis.

Clinical Findings

History. The following characterize GABHS infection:
- Less commonly seen in children younger than 2 years old; most commonly found in 5- to 15-year-old children
- Abrupt onset without nasal symptoms
- Moderate to high fever, malaise, prominent sore throat, dysphagia
- Nausea, abdominal discomfort, vomiting, headache
- Presentation in winter or early spring

Physical Examination. The following may be seen:
- Petechiae on soft palate and pharynx, swollen beefy-red uvula, red enlarged tonsillopharyngeal tissue
- Tonsillopharyngeal exudate that is yellow, blood-tinged (frequently)
- Tender and enlarged anterior cervical lymph nodes
- Stigmata of scarlet fever may be seen—scarlatiniform rash, strawberry tongue, circumoral pallor

TABLE 31-2 **Differentiation of Common Upper Respiratory Infections in Children**

Site of Infection	Symptoms	Duration of Symptoms (days)	Etiologic Agent	Management	Duration of Treatment	Comments
The common cold (viral URI)	Malaise, sneezing, watery nasal discharge, mild sore throat, may have a fever, not ill appearing	0-10	Adenovirus, rhinovirus, RSV, parainfluenza, enterovirus	No antibiotics: Symptomatic Rx, e.g., saline nose drops, increased fluids; for infants, bulb-syringe the nose before meals and bedtime; for older children, cough suppression at night if unable to sleep; humidifier		If lasts longer than 10-14 days, consider other diagnosis (e.g., sinusitis).
Acute purulent rhinorrhea	Thick, yellow nasal discharge (often associated with URI)	>3	Part of the natural history of URI; superinfection by S. pneumoniae, H. influenzae, β-hemolytic streptococci	Symptomatic care; a wait-and-see approach for antibiotics: if >10- to 14-day duration, reconsider diagnosis as may be sinusitis	Best approach, wait and see	Avoid indiscriminate and frequent use of antibiotics (development of antibiotic resistance)
Acute sinusitis	Persistent nasal symptoms for more than 10 days with URI, nasal drainage—purulent or discolored, cough, recalcitrant asthma	10-30	S. pneumoniae, M. catarrhalis, nontypable H. influenzae	Amoxicillin, erythromycin; sulfamethoxazole-trimethoprim, or amoxicillin-clavulanate	10-14 days	By 7 days should be asymptomatic; change antibiotics 48-72 hours after start of treatment if no response
Subacute sinusitis	Same as above but persistent for at least 30 days	30-84	Same as above; may be β-lactamase producing	Amoxicillin-clavulanate		Initial acute infection did not clear, need to switch antibiotics
Chronic/recurrent sinusitis	Malaise, easy fatigability, unilateral or bilateral nasal discharge, postnasal discharge, nasal obstruction if middle turbinate significantly obstructed	Recurrent >10 to <28 but symptom free for at least 10 days in between bouts; Chronic >84	Same as above plus α-hemolytic streptococci and S. aureus	Amoxicillin-clavulanate, azithromycin, staph coverage	3-6 weeks	May need endoscopic sinus surgery if chronic sinusitis does not respond to prolonged medical management; investigate differential diagnoses or underlying issues (e.g., allergic rhinitis)

RSV, Respiratory syncytial virus; *Rx*, medication; *URI*, upper respiratory infection.

- Variable presentation; may have mild pharyngeal erythema without tonsillar exudate or cervical adenopathy

Diagnostic Tests. A positive throat culture confirms the diagnosis and is still the test of choice; however, a positive culture can also identify a carrier state. Some rapid streptococcal identification tests are not as sensitive as culture in detecting GABHS; therefore a negative rapid test result must be followed by culture. The specificity of the rapid streptococcal test is very good (95%); therefore if the rapid test result is positive, the diagnosis of GABHS is confirmed. Documentation of past GABHS infection is obtained by antibody titer to various streptococcal enzymes such as antistreptolysin O (ASO).

Management. The goal of antibiotic therapy is to prevent the development of rheumatic fever (the incubation period is 1 to 3 weeks), the spread of illness to others, and the development of suppurative complications. Antibiotics also shorten the course of the illness and the severity of symptoms. If the rapid strep test result is positive, antibiotics should be started immediately. The drug of choice for the treatment of GABHS is penicillin for children not allergic to it because of its cost, narrow spectrum of antimicrobial activity, and infrequent adverse drug reactions (Gerber, 2006). The management plan includes the following:

- Antimicrobial therapy (based on clinical need)—one of the following (Jenson & Baltimore, 2006; Young & Strong, 2006):
  - Benzathine penicillin G intramuscularly (600,000 units if less than 60 lb; 1.2 million units for larger children and adults).
  - Phenoxymethyl penicillin (penicillin V potassium) orally for 10 days: for children, 40 mg/kg divided 3 times; adult dose is 500 mg two to three times a day for 10 days. Alternative dosage is 250 mg/dose bid to tid for children and 500 mg/dose bid to tid for adults with a 10-day course of therapy.
  - Amoxicillin suspension is often used with young children because it is more palatable (efficacy seems equal to penicillin). It too must be taken for 10 days. A recent study has demonstrated that once daily administration of amoxicillin is as effective as twice daily administration for the treatment of GABHS. The dosage was 750 mg once daily for children less than 40 kg and 1000 mg once daily for children more than 40 kg. The duration of therapy was 10 days (Clegg et al, 2006).
  - If allergic to ß-lactams:
    - For smaller children: Erythromycin estolate (20 to 40 mg/kg/day in 2 to 4 divided doses for 10 days) or erythromycin ethylsuccinate (40 to 50 mg/kg/day in 2 to 4 divided doses).
    - For larger children and adults: Erythromycin 1 g/day in 2 to 4 divided doses for 10 days.
  - A 10-day course of a narrow-spectrum (first-generation), orally administered cephalosporin is now acceptable, particularly if the child is allergic to penicillin. However, a substantial number of patients allergic to penicillin also are allergic to the cephalosporins.
  - If evidence of penicillin resistance is present, a β-lactamase-resistant antibiotic can be used, such as amoxicillin-clavulanate or dicloxacillin.
- Results from preliminary studies indicate a once-daily amoxicillin therapy is an effective therapy (Gerber, 2006).

- Supportive care—antipyretics, fluids, rest.
- Reculture is not generally needed except in situations in which it is necessary to ensure eradication of the organism.
- If the child continues to have symptoms of streptococcal pharyngitis and a positive culture for streptococcus, this child may represent an actual treatment failure or have a new infection with a different serologic type of streptococcus.
- Noncompliance with pharmacologic therapy can explain treatment failure, and in these instances, an injection of benzathine penicillin is recommended.
- For a compliant patient with recurrence soon after completion of antimicrobial therapy, treat with any of the following drugs: the same antimicrobial agent, amoxicillin-clavulanate, clindamycin, narrow-spectrum cephalosporin, erythromycin, or another macrolide (Jenson & Baltimore, 2006).
- If clinical relapse occurs, a second course of antibiotic is indicated, as discussed earlier. If recurrent infection is a problem, culturing of the family for the chronic carrier state is advised. Toothbrushes or orthodontic devices may harbor GABHS and should be cleaned or discarded.
- Children can return to school when they are afebrile and have been taking antibiotics for at least 24 hours.

Complications. Major late complications caused by GABHS are rheumatic fever and acute glomerulonephritis. Suppurative complications include cervical adenitis, sinusitis, otitis media, pneumonia, mastoiditis, and retropharyngeal or peritonsillar abscess. Recurrent GABHS tonsillopharyngitis can also be a problem. Sydenham chorea is linked to GABHS infection. In addition, the onset or worsening of other neuropsychiatric disorders (e.g., obsessive-compulsive disorder, Tourette syndrome, or tic disorder) has been associated with streptococcal infection. The acronym used to describe this phenomenon is PANDAS (pediatric autoimmune neuropsychiatric disorders) (Morer et al, 2006).

ACUTE PURULENT RHINITIS

Description

Acute purulent rhinitis often represents a superinfection of a common cold or purulent sinusitis. Remember that thick, yellow discharge is a common sequela of an uncomplicated URI.

Etiology

Likely organisms involved in the superinfection are pneumococci, *H. influenzae,* β-hemolytic streptococci, and *Staphylococcus aureus.*

Clinical Findings

History. Complaints of URI with characteristic symptoms and a profuse and continuous, purulent, yellow- to-green nasal discharge for more than 3 days are reported.

Physical Examination. A yellow-to-green nasal discharge is seen.

Differential Diagnosis

A nasal FB and sinusitis are the differential diagnoses. The mucopurulent discharge associated with the common cold (acute viral rhinitis) is intermittent and worse in the early morning on awakening. Allergic rhinitis is discussed in Chapter 24.

Management

Controversy surrounds the appropriateness of early intervention with antibiotic therapy if the only major symptom is a purulent nasal discharge. Overuse of antibiotics to treat "purulent" rhinorrhea has lead to resistant strains of bacteria. The following approaches should be considered:

- *Take a wait-and-see plan.* Advise symptomatic treatment because the discharge may be only a symptom of an uncomplicated URI.
- *Remove purulent material.* May need to instill saline into the nares and use a bulb syringe or do saline washes.
- *Family education.* Tell to return should symptoms persist for more than 10 to 14 days or if worsening.

SINUSITIS

Description

Inflammation and secondary infection of the paranasal sinuses can be either an acute or a chronic problem. Sinusitis often complicates the common URI and allergic rhinitis in children. Persistence of URI symptoms for longer than 10 days without improvement separates a simple URI from sinusitis. The maxillary and anterior ethmoid sinuses are most frequently involved in children because they are present at birth, but only the ethmoidal sinuses are pneumatized. The frontal sinuses begin their development at 7 years old with complete development at adolescence. Inflammation and edema of the mucous membranes lining the sinuses cause obstruction and set up an ideal situation for bacteria to invade the sinus cavities. Certain conditions predispose children to chronic sinus infections, including allergies, nasal deformities, CF, nasal polyps, and human immunodeficiency virus (HIV) infection.

Differentiation of acute from subacute, recurrent, chronic and acute-on-chronic sinusitis is based on the duration of respiratory symptoms. In acute sinusitis, respiratory symptoms last more than 10 days but less than 30 days. When respiratory symptoms persist more than 30 days (4 weeks) to 12 weeks and do not improve, a diagnosis of subacute sinusitis is made. Recurrent sinusitis is defined as episodes of acute sinusitis (each lasting less than 4 weeks), but separated by symptom-free intervals of at least 10 days. If symptoms last more than 12 weeks, a diagnosis of chronic sinusitis is appropriate. If patients with chronic sinusitis develop new symptoms of sinusitis, this is referred to as acute-on-chronic sinusitis. Remember that sinus inflammation is part of the natural history of a cold or allergic rhinitis. Thick, yellow discharge is a common and normal finding with a URI. Therefore the pediatric provider must be cautious to not overdiagnose sinusitis and subsequently indiscriminately use antibiotics (Shrime & Keller, 2006).

Epidemiology

The common bacterial organisms responsible for superinfections are *S. pneumoniae,* nontypable *H. influenzae, Moraxella catarrhalis,* and less often *S. aureus,* other streptococci, and anaerobes. The presence of antibiotic-resistant organisms is associated with prior antibiotic therapy. The role of viruses in sinusitis is not clear. Anaerobic and staphylococcal agents are implicated in chronic sinusitis. The various sinuses develop, aerate, and become clinically important at different times during childhood. Ethmoiditis can occur after 6 months old, in contrast to frontal sinusitis, which is first seen around 10 years old. Cases of recurrent and chronic sinusitis are often caused by recurrent viral URIs associated with day care attendance, smoking in the home, older siblings at home who reinfect the child, or certain predisposing conditions, such as allergies, nasal polyps, immunodeficiency disorders, or CF—the latter two conditions predispose to infections with *Aspergillus* and *Zygomycetes.*

Clinical Findings in Acute Sinusitis

The time frame of symptoms determines the classification of sinusitis as described above. To make a diagnosis of acute sinusitis, the following set of clinical findings must be present. The child must have **two major** criteria or **one major** and **two minor** criteria as listed below (Gerber, 2006).

   Major Criteria
- Facial congestion and/or fullness
- Fever (acute sinusitis only)
- Purulent rhinorrhea and/or discolored nasal discharge or postnasal drip on nasal examination
- Facial pain and/or pressure
- Nasal obstruction
- Hyposmia or anosmia
   Minor Criteria
- Headache
- Halitosis
- Fatigue
- Dental pain
- Cough
- Otalgia and/or aural fullness

   Diagnostic Tests. If the clinical findings suggest sinusitis, radiographs are not needed. Facial swelling, acute sinusitis unresponsive to 48 hours of antibiotics, a child with a toxic appearance, chronic or recurrent sinusitis, and chronic asthma are indications for imaging studies, including either sinus radiographs, ultrasonograms, or CT scanning. CT is now the accepted imaging study for acute or chronic sinusitis. However, because it has only a 40% to 85% predictive value in children with clinical sinusitis, the AAP recommends its use only as an adjunct in children older than 6 years or for those children undergoing operative procedures. A Waters' view is usually sufficient to demonstrate sinusitis on a radiograph. Nasal cultures are not useful, and transillumination is difficult to perform in children.

Differential Diagnosis

Viral upper respiratory tract illness, allergic rhinitis, and other causes of headache are the differential diagnoses. Remember that sinusitis may exacerbate asthma.

Management

Although 60% to 80% of acute sinusitis episodes resolve without antibiotics in about 4 weeks, antimicrobial therapy increases the speed of resolution and reduces the amount of mucosal damage. Antibiotics should be prescribed for a course of at least 10 to 14 days in sinusitis or, if the child is responding slowly but not symptom-free, an additional 7 days. Most children show dramatic improvement in 3 to 4 days (fever and nasal discharge abating). Failure to improve in 48 hours suggests a resistant organism or complications. The course of therapy may be up to 21 days in acute sinusitis and up to 6 weeks in chronic sinusitis.

In uncomplicated acute sinusitis in children, treatment can include (Gerber, 2006; Jenson & Baltimore, 2006):

- Amoxicillin (80 to 90 mg/kg/day), amoxicillin-clavulanate, cefpodoxime, proxetil, or cefuroxime axetil as initial therapy if the child has NOT taken antibiotics in the past 4 to 6 weeks. The AAP has also recommended amoxicillin 40 to 45 mg/kg/day, but this treatment should not be given if there are high rates of resistance (Shrime & Keller, 2006).
  - If allergic to amoxicillin—azithromycin, clarithromycin, erythromycin, or sulfamethoxazole/trimethoprim (SMT) (failure rates are up to 38% with SMT).
- Children at risk for resistant bacterial infections (antibiotic therapy within prior 1 to 3 months, day care attendance, less than 2 years old, failure to respond within 72 hours) should be given high-dose amoxicillin-clavulanate (80 to 90 mg/kg/day amoxicillin and 6.4 mg/kg/day of clavulanate).

The management of chronic sinusitis is more complicated because bacteria are generally only one of other contributing factors. Referral to an otolaryngologist is often needed.

Additional management considerations include the following:

- The use of decongestants, antihistamines, or both, and nasal saline irrigations. The use of intranasal steroids in the treatment of acute or chronic sinusitis is controversial and has not proved effective. Antihistamines and intranasal steroids may have a role in recurrent or chronic sinusitis if allergic manifestations are present (see the management section for allergic rhinitis). See Chapter 24 for information on the use of decongestants and antihistamines.
- Children with complications or signs of invasive infection should be referred to the appropriate medical specialist. Surgical drainage by an otolaryngologist, treatment of allergies and control of allergic rhinitis by an allergist, or both may be necessary.
- Comfort measures include the use of acetaminophen, ibuprofen, or codeine for severe pain. A humidifier helps relieve the drying of mucous membranes associated with mouth breathing. Increase oral fluid intake. Saline irrigation of the nostrils is recommended by some allergists.
- Diving is contraindicated with sinusitis.

Complications

Chronic or recurrent sinusitis can become a problem often requiring referral to an otolaryngologist or allergist. Orbital cellulitis secondary to ethmoiditis, manifested by swelling and erythema of the eyelids, proptosis, decreased extraocular movements, and altered vision, is a serious, life-threatening complication that is a medical emergency. Intracranial complications, such as cavernous sinus thrombosis, subdural empyema, and brain abscess, can also occur. Chronic sinusitis is also associated with intractable wheezing in children with asthma (Behrman et al, 2004; Gerber, 2006).

DIPHTHERIA

Description

Diphtheria occurs as an acute infection of the upper respiratory tract, the trachea, or both. Diphtheria can cause membranous obstruction of the upper airway. It also produces a neurotoxin. Although only about five cases of diphtheria are reported annually in the U.S., it remains an important and dangerous disease.

Epidemiology

C. diphtheriae is a gram-positive rod with three strains that can be either toxigenic or nontoxigenic. Diphtheria is caused by the toxigenic strain of C. diphtheriae or, less commonly, C. ulcerans. Transmission results from intimate contact with an infected person or carrier. Discharge from the nose, throat, eye, and skin lesions can produce infection. Although rare, fomites can act as a vehicle of transmission, and food-borne outbreaks have been reported. Asymptomatic carriers can transmit the organism. The incubation period averages from 2 to 5 days; communicability lasts for 2 weeks or less in untreated cases. Chronic carriage can occur even with antimicrobial therapy.

Clinical Findings

Disease may be mild or asymptomatic in partially or fully immunized individuals and severe if unimmunized. Characteristic signs and symptoms follow.

Primary Infection.   Low-grade fever
- Grayish, adherent pseudomembrane found in either the nasopharynx, pharynx, or trachea
- Sore throat, serosanguineous or seropurulent nasal discharge, hoarseness, cough
- Cutaneous lesions (nonhealing ulcers with dirty gray membrane or colonization of preexisting dermatoses) infected with diphtheria (seen less often)

Toxin Production.   The ability of a strain of C. diphtheriae to produce toxin is related to bacteriophage infection of the bacterium, not to colony type.
- Toxin production is more lethal than the primary infection and can induce the following:
  - Myocarditis and electrocardiographic changes
  - Respiratory compromise
  - Cranial nerve and local neuropathies
  - Peripheral neuritis

Diagnostic Tests.   A confirmatory diagnosis is based on a positive culture of C. diphtheriae. Specimens should be obtained from the nose, throat, any skin lesions, and either beneath the membrane or from a portion of the membrane. A special culture medium is needed, and toxigenicity tests are performed if *C. diphtheriae* is confirmed. Culture results take 8 to 48 hours; however, treatment begins when diphtheria is suspected. Do not wait for laboratory confirmation. Results of the CBC may be normal or show a slight leukocytosis and thrombocytopenia.

Differential Diagnosis

Acute streptococcal pharyngitis and infectious mononucleosis are included in the differential diagnosis of pharyngeal diphtheria. A nasal FB or purulent sinusitis can resemble nasal diphtheria; epiglottitis and viral croup can also cause obstruction, as does laryngeal diphtheria.

Management

Children with diphtheria require hospitalization. Treatment consists of the following:

- Antitoxin administration (hyperimmune equine antiserum) and antimicrobial therapy with erythromycin or penicillin (either aqueous, procaine, or penicillin G)
- Supportive care for respiratory, cardiac, and neurologic complications as appropriate
- Standard and droplet precautions until two cultures are negative
- Immunization of the child after recovery because disease does not necessarily confer immunity
- Monitoring and antimicrobial prophylaxis of contacts regardless of immunization status
- Care for respiratory, cardiac, and neurologic complications as appropriate

Prevention

Universal immunization against diphtheria with regular booster injections is the only effective method of control. Infection can occur in immunized or partially immunized children, but the severity of the disease is greatly diminished. Disease generally occurs in nonimmunized children; the frequency of severe life-threatening complications in this group is high. Care of a child exposed to diphtheria is individualized and based on immunization status, likelihood of follow-up, and compliance with antimicrobial therapy. The AAP Committee on Infectious Diseases *Red Book* lists specific guidelines that should be followed for the care of exposed children.

PERTUSSIS

Description

Pertussis is commonly known as whooping cough because of the high-pitched inspiratory whoop that is characteristic of this illness in young children. The cough is an attempt to dislodge plugs of necrotic bronchial epithelial tissue and thick mucus. It is an acute, highly contagious infection that produces a toxin responsible for the severe symptoms associated with pertussis. If this disease occurs in unvaccinated infants younger than 1 year old, it is often associated with pneumonia, seizures, and encephalopathy. Pertussis in older children

and vaccinated children produces a milder respiratory illness (Behrman et al, 2004). Outbreaks of pertussis still occur despite the availability of an effective vaccine. Older children and adults can be the vector of pertussis because their symptoms are not severe.

Epidemiology

Classic pertussis is caused by *Bordetella pertussis,* either as a primary disease or reinfection. Similar disease (pertussis syndrome) can be caused by related species, such as *Bordetella parapertussis, Bordetella holmesii,* and *Bordetella bronchiseptica;* they cause milder illness and are not affected by *B. pertussis* vaccination. Transmission of these gram-negative pleomorphic bacilli is via aerosol droplet spread by coughing from close contact with infected individuals, who generally have mild or atypical illness that is not recognized as pertussis. The incubation period is between 6 and 21 days; the period of communicability is greatest during the catarrhal stage until before or during the early paroxysmal stage of coughing. Cases of pertussis occur in adults, who constitute a reservoir for the disease. Thus, the usual source of *B. pertussis* infection in infants is an adult family member with a cough caused by *B. pertussis* that was not recognized as such. The highest incidence of mortality occurs under 1 month old (Cherry & Harrison, 2006; Jenson & Baltimore, 2006).

Clinical Findings

Manifestations of this disease vary by age group, stage of disease, and whether the child has received any immunization against pertussis.

Characteristics of the disease in infants and young children include the following:

- Catarrhal stage—1 to 2 weeks
  - Mild cough, coryza, sneezing, and low-grade fever (to 101° F [38.3° C])
- Paroxysmal stage—2 to 4 weeks
  - Persistent staccato, paroxysmal cough ending with an inspiratory whoop
  - Vomiting at the end of paroxysmal coughing and whoop
  - Cyanosis, sweating, prostration, and exhaustion after coughing
- Convalescent stage—2 to 3 weeks
  - Waning of paroxysmal coughing episodes

Specific findings in infants younger than 6 months old are generally severe, particularly in neonates, and include:

- Apnea (common) often with seizures caused by hypoxemia
- No inspiratory whoop
- Severe pneumonia and pulmonary hypertension is common
  Findings in older children include:
- Persistent irritating cough but no inspiratory whoop (resembles a prolonged bronchitic illness)
- Low-grade fever

Diagnostic Tests. Culturing for *B. pertussis* requires special media and takes 7 days for incubation. It is the gold standard for the diagnosis of pertussis. Nasopharyngeal aspiration or collection of the specimen using a calcium alginate fiber tip swab is necessary. The organism is found most frequently during the catarrhal or early paroxysmal stage. A positive culture from the nasopharynx aspiration is diagnostic; however, false-negative results do occur. Leukocytosis (20,000 to 50,000/mm³) with 70% to 80% lymphocytes (lymphocytosis) is a common finding in young children (but rare in young infants) and appears around the end of the catarrhal stage. Polymerase chain reaction (PCR) is useful. Direct fluorescent antibody (DFA) staining has low specificity and sensitivity and is technologically difficult.

Diagnostic Criteria. Criteria used to make the diagnosis of pertussis include (Cherry & Harrison, 2006):
- Paroxysmal cough
- Illness more than 2 weeks duration with no or minimal fever
- Leukocytosis (greater than 11,100/mm³) with absolute lymphocytosis (greater than 6300/mm³)
- Positive culture or PCR (nasopharyngeal specimen)
- Positive DFA (nasopharyngeal specimen)
- ELISA demonstration of high single-IgG antibody titer to pertussis between an acute-phase and convalescent-phase serum specimen or in adolescents and children who have not received a pertussis immunization within the previous year.

Management
The following steps are involved (Cherry & Harrison, 2006):
- Young infants and children with severe respiratory symptoms require hospitalization for management of respiratory symptoms and hydration and nutrition needs.
- Erythromycin (40 to 50 mg/kg/day [maximum, 2 g/day] in four divided doses for 14 days) can improve symptoms if given in the catarrhal stage. If given to neonates younger than 4 weeks old, it has a rare association with pyloric stenosis.
- Other antimicrobial agents that can be used in lieu of erythromycin:
  - Azithromycin (5-day treatment: a single dose of 10 mg/kg/day [maximum of 500 mg] on day one; then a single dose of 5 mg/kg/day [maximum of 250 mg] on days 2 to 5).
  - Clarithromycin (15 to 20 mg/kg in 2 divided doses for 7 days with a maximum dose of 1 g/day).
  - Trimethoprim-sulfamethoxazole: 8 to 12 mg/kg trimethoprim, 40 to 60 mg/kg sulfamethoxazole/day in 2 doses for 14 days (maximum 320 mg trimethoprim). This drug is not recommended as a first-line therapy; use if there is demonstrated pertussis resistance to erythromycin.
- Antimicrobial therapy given in the paroxysmal stage does not alter the course of pertussis per se, but administration of erythromycin limits spreading of the organism (eradicates nasopharyngeal carriage within 3 to 4 days).
- Corticosteroids should not be used. Albuterol nebulization may modestly reduce symptoms, but the associated fussing from the treatment may trigger paroxysms (Behrman et al, 2004; Cherry & Harrison, 2006).

Care of Exposed Children. Recommendations regarding the need for isolation and prophylactic measures for exposed children and adults include the following (Cherry & Harrison, 2006):

- Immunization coverage with diphtheria-tetanus-acellular pertussis (DTaP).
- Chemoprophylaxis with erythromycin (40 to 50 mg/kg/day [maximum, 2 g/day] orally in four divided doses for 14 days) for all household and close contacts, including children in day care and playmates, irrespective of their immunization status; azithromycin or clarithromycin are better tolerated by adolescents. Start as soon after exposure as possible. An alternate approach that can be used with only adults is to follow closely and treat with macrolides with the first appearance of respiratory signs or symptoms.
- Close monitoring of respiratory symptoms for 20 days after last contact with an infected individual.

Complications
Secondary bacterial pneumonia, seizures, epistaxis, subconjunctival hemorrhage, encephalopathy, and death can occur. Activation of tuberculosis is associated with pertussis infection.

Prevention
Immunity following either natural pertussis infection or illness or vaccination is **not** long lasting. Reinfections are mild and may not be noticed. Young infants are at greatest risk for pertussis. The recommended guidelines for giving the initial series of DTaP vaccines and booster doses should be followed. Remember that just one DTaP immunization can reduce the severity of symptoms in an infant infected with pertussis. Universal immunization of children younger than 7 years old is crucial to control this disease.

Only children with valid contraindications to receiving pertussis vaccine, as identified in Chapter 23, should be excluded from receiving the vaccine. Immunity from pertussis immunization wanes over time, and the vaccine does not confer active immunity. Pertussis in older children, adolescents, and adults is a mild, often unrecognized disease that, if transmitted to an unimmunized infant, can result in life-threatening illness.

RECURRENT EPISTAXIS
Epidemiology
Recurrent epistaxis is commonly seen in children living in dry climates or during the winter months when artificial heating is used. The cause is often benign and typically related to mechanical trauma to the area (e.g., nose picking), and, thus, it is generally self-limiting. Other factors that can cause mucosal irritation that results in bleeding include allergies, neoplasms (e.g., polyps, hemangiomas), chronic rhinitis, URI, FB, chronic use of nasal sprays or drying agents, such as decongestants, and viral or bacterial infections of nasal tissue. In adolescents, the use of recreational drugs such as cocaine causes local mucosal irritation. The anterior portion of the nasal septum, Kiesselbach area, has a rich vascular supply and is the usual site of involvement (Lavelle, 2006). Hypertension is a rare cause of acute or recurrent epistaxis in children; a coagulopathy, generally von Willebrand disease or platelet aggregation disorders, can manifest as recurrent epistaxis.

Clinical Findings

History. The following may be reported:

- Frequent nosebleeds
- Recent URI
- Allergic rhinitis
- Tarry stools as a result of swallowing of blood (occasionally noted)

Physical Examination. Bleeding from the nares can often be seen, and the anterior aspect of the nares is red and raw with or without fresh clots or old crusts. The nasal mucosa on the medial surface of the anterior septum of one naris may be dry, cracked, or excoriated, and scabbing may be seen. The presence of blood in both nares or in the oropharynx or bleeding that is hard to control suggests posterior bleeding.

Diagnostic Tests. A baseline hematocrit may be indicated in severe or chronic epistaxis. It can reveal iron deficiency anemia secondary to the bleeding. In the vast majority of causes, hemoglobin, platelets, and clotting times need not be ordered.

Differential Diagnosis

A bleeding disorder or nasal tumor is characterized by epistaxis that is severe, prolonged, and recurrent. Be suspicious of epistaxis in a child younger than 2 years old, evidence of bleeding at other sites, and bleeding that lasts longer than 20 minutes. If these abnormalities occur and a coagulopathy is suspected, order a CBC, platelet count, prothrombin time (PT), activated partial thromboplastin time (PTT), and ristocetin cofactor. If epistaxis is associated with a traumatic injury, evaluate for the presence of a nasal fracture and/or septal hematoma.

Management

The following steps are taken:

- Have the child sit upright and lean forward to prevent swallowing the blood.
- Apply pressure to the nose (pinch the nares together at the bony structure) for 10 minutes.
- Packing and topical vasoconstrictor drugs are occasionally needed.
- Use a bedside humidifier to moisten the air in dry climates or in winter with forced air heating.
- Apply petroleum jelly or topical antibiotic to the site of the septal scab for 5 to 7 days to keep moist, reduce itching, and assist healing.
- Silver nitrate sticks can be used to cauterize exposed vessels if bleeding persists; however, the site must be easily accessible, visible, and not bleeding briskly. It has a high failure rate and has been associated with atrophy of the nasal septum.
- Nasal packing with absorbable oxycellulose material if bleeding continues or the site cannot be localized; if packing is used, prescribe oral antibiotics to reduce the risk of secondary sinusitis and toxic shock syndrome.
- Treat the underlying cause of the problem (e.g., tumor, polyp).

Prevention

Use of a vaporizer and normal saline nose drops and application of petroleum jelly (e.g., Vaseline) to the inside of the nares are preventive measures.

NASAL FOREIGN BODY

Description

It is not uncommon for young children to insert all types of FBs into any body orifice. Nasal FBs can be noted immediately by the parent or lie undetected until classic symptoms appear.

Clinical Findings

History. A persistent or recurrent unilateral purulent nasal discharge is reported.

Physical Examination. FB is typically associated with purulent, foul-smelling nasal discharge.

Differential Diagnosis

Nasal polyps, purulent rhinitis, adenoiditis, sinusitis, and nasal tumors are conditions that are also associated with either bilateral or unilateral discharge.

Management

Management involves the following (Tom & Shah, 2006):

- Detection of a foreign body (FB) in the nasal cavity, which secures the diagnosis
- Removal of the nasal FB, depending on its location, its composition, and the skill of the practitioner
- Good lighting (use a headlight) is essential, as is immobilization of the young child via papoose board
- Elevation of the child's head and suctioning of blood and secretions
- Use of alligator forceps, suction with narrow tips, cotton-tipped applicators with collodion, and topical vasoconstrictor drugs (to reduce swelling) if needed to remove the object, depending on its size and consistency; can also consider using a hook or curette to roll the object out
- Referral to an otolaryngologist for young children who cannot cooperate or when the FB is extremely difficult or dangerous to remove, such as paper clips or staples

■ EXTRATHORACIC AIRWAY DISORDERS

LARYNGOTRACHEOBRONCHITIS—INFECTIOUS CROUP

Description

Laryngotracheobronchitis (LTB) is an inflammatory process involving the upper trachea and larynx. It results in rapid, acute, upper airway obstruction of varying degrees at the larynx characterized by a harsh, barking cough and inspiratory stridor.

Epidemiology

Viral agents are responsible for most cases of croup, with the parainfluenza viruses (types 1, 2, and 3) being the leading viral organisms, followed by respiratory syncytial virus (RSV). Adenoviruses and influenza are less common agents

(Jacobs, 2006; Jenson & Baltimore, 2006). Viral croup is most common in children between 6 and 36 months old (60% younger than 24 months old) and occurs most often in the cold season of the year. Males are affected more often than females. Recurrent croup and recurrent laryngitis can develop in children until 6 years old. A positive family history has been noted in a small percentage of children in whom croup develops. Croup lasts approximately 5 days. With growth, the child's laryngeal tracheal airway is less vulnerable to the effects of viral infections and less susceptible to obstruction.

Clinical Findings

Clinical manifestations depend on the type of infectious agent responsible for the croup and the area of the upper airway affected.

History. The history includes the following:
- Prodrome of URI symptoms (rhinorrhea, conjunctivitis, or both) is sometimes present before stridor.
- Intermittent stridor—mild to moderate.
- Gradual onset of symptoms (2 to 3 days).
- Symptoms worse at night.
- May or may not have sore throat.
- Most children with viral croup improve within a few days.

Physical Examination. The following can be seen:
- Slight dyspnea, tachypnea, and retractions
- Mild, brassy, or barking cough (harsh sounding)
- Stridor—a high-pitched, harsh sound from turbulent airflow that is generally inspiratory, but may be biphasic
- Temperature typically low grade, but may be elevated to 104° F (40° C)
- Decreased breath sounds bilaterally with rhonchi
- Wheezing and rales may be heard if there is additional lower airway involvement

Diagnostic Tests. Usually the diagnosis is evident clinically. Radiography of the soft tissues of the neck and chest displays a classic pattern of subglottic narrowing ("steeple sign"), but is usually not done unless there is a question about the diagnosis. Microbiology cultures can be helpful in selected cases that have atypical presentations.

Differential Diagnosis

The differential diagnoses include acute epiglottitis; acute spasmodic croup (no signs of infection); aspiration of a FB; retropharyngeal abscess; extrinsic compression from tumors, trauma, or congenital malformations; angioedema (anaphylaxis) or early asthmatic attack; bacterial tracheitis, infectious mononucleosis; and psychogenic stridor.

Table 31-3 differentiates acute infectious LTB from other common causes of stridor.

Management

Therapy depends on the cause, severity, and location of the disease. The aim of therapy is to provide adequate respiratory exchange.
- Symptomatic relief of mild croup can be provided with the judicious use of steam from a hot shower or bath or "cold"

steam from a humidifier. These measures usually end the laryngeal spasm. Often a ride in a car at night with the windows down accomplishes the same result. Occasionally, vomiting also relieves the spasm.
- Cough and cold medicines sometimes help, especially if the child has URI symptoms.
- If bronchospasm is also suspected, the use of bronchodilators in the usual doses prescribed for relief of asthma as discussed in Chapter 24 may be advantageous.
- Corticosteroids as part of the management of LTB are beneficial in decreasing the edema of the laryngeal mucosa. Corticosteroids (oral prednisone at 1 to 2 mg/kg/day or dexamethasone either oral or IM for outpatients with mild or moderate croup) reduce inflammatory edema and prevent destruction of ciliated epithelium (Behrman et al, 2004; Jenson & Baltimore, 2006). A one-time dose of dexamethasone (0.6 mg/kg) can be given as part of outpatient management. Antibiotics are not indicated.

Indications for Hospitalization. Children in distress with respiratory rates between 70 and 90 breaths per minute or exhibiting stridor at rest should be hospitalized. A child with a temperature higher than 102.2° F (39° C) should be carefully evaluated; hospitalization may be necessary if other worrisome symptoms are present. Racemic epinephrine by aerosol may help, but typically leads to rebound swelling several hours later. Corticosteroids are used (dexamethasone 0.5 to 2 mg/kg/dose every 8 hours IV), and intravenous hydration may be necessary (Jacobs, 2006; Jenson & Baltimore, 2006).

Complications

Increasing obstruction of the airways causes continuous stridor, nasal flaring, and suprasternal, infrasternal, and intercostal retractions. With further obstruction, air hunger and restlessness occur and are quickly followed by hypoxia, weakness, decreased air exchange, decreased stridor, increased pulse rate, and eventual death from hypoventilation. Anything that taxes the child's respiratory efforts, such as crying or feeding, causes more respiratory distress. Examination of the nasopharynx with a tongue depressor may result in sudden respiratory compromise. Severely ill children should be evaluated for acute epiglottitis. Viral pneumonia complicates about 1% to 2% of croup cases.

ACUTE SPASMODIC CROUP

Description

Some children are prone to recurrent episodes of acute LTB, which may be related to airway hypersensitivity or allergy. The term *acute spasmodic croup* is used to describe this condition. In spasmodic croup, symptoms come on suddenly and without the typical URI prodrome. The episode is usually milder and of short duration, but symptoms may be severe and recurrent. The treatment plan is the same as indicated for acute LTB. Spasmodic croup tends to respond well to exposure to cool or humidified air. The causes of spasmodic croup cannot be differentiated from the usual causes of croup; most likely a viral agent triggers the airway reaction.

TABLE 31-3 | **Differentiating Common Respiratory Diseases That Can Cause Stridor or Similar Signs**

Characteristic	LTB	Epiglottitis	Bacterial Tracheitis	Diphtheria	Foreign Body
Peak age	3-36 months old	1-5 years old	3-10 years old	Any age/ unimmunized	Toddlers
Onset	Gradual, acute onset at night	Rapid	Acute	Gradual onset	Acute symptoms or gradual onset
Common findings	URI, seal-bark cough, mild-moderate dyspnea, symptoms worse at night	Sore throat, drooling, aphonia, looks toxic, dysphagia, tripod position	URI, may have cough, looks toxic, purulent sputum	Pharyngeal membrane, sore throat, nasal discharge, hoarseness	Coughing and/or choking episode, dyspnea, wheezing, cyanosis, signs and symptoms of secondary infection
Respiratory efforts	Rate generally <50	Marked distress	Marked distress	Minor to significant signs and symptoms of obstruction	Minor to significant distress
Fever	Common—low grade	High (102.2° F [39° C])	High (102.2° F [39° C])	Low grade	Normal to low grade
CBC	Generally normal	High, left shift	High, left shift	Normal to slight leukocytosis, decreased thrombocyte count	Normal unless secondary infection
Organism(s)	Usually viral: parainfluenza, adenovirus, RSV	Usually *H. influenzae* type b (HIB)	Usually *S. aureus*	*C. diphtheriae*	
Specific laboratory tests	None	None	None	Positive culture	None
Radiographic view/findings	Lateral or AP of neck/subglottic narrowing	Lateral of neck/ thumb sign	Lateral of neck/ subglottic narrowing	Signs of obstruction in severe cases	May see localized hyperinflation, mediastinal shift, atelectasis
Treatment	Humidification, corticosteroids in selected cases	Hospitalization, cephalosporin, corticosteroids	Hospitalization, staphylococcus coverage	Hospitalization, erythromycin/ penicillin, antitoxin	Removal of FB, treatment of secondary infection or bronchospasm
Intubation	Rare	Usually necessary	Frequently necessary	May be necessary	Endoscopy to remove FB
Prevention	None	Immunization—HIB	None	Immunization—DTaP	Education on child proofing home and monitoring child

AP, Anteroposterior; *CBC,* complete blood count; *FB,* foreign body; *LTB,* laryngotracheobronchitis; *RSV,* respiratory syncytial virus; *URI,* upper respiratory tract infection.

EPIGLOTTITIS
Epidemiology
Epiglottitis, an acute inflammation of the epiglottis and the supraglottic larynx, occurs in children generally between 1 and 5 years old with 25% of cases in children younger than 2 years old. *H. influenzae* type b is usually the cause of this illness. However, the use of *H. influenzae* type b vaccine beginning at 2 months old has resulted in a drastic decline in the number of children with invasive infections caused by this organism; fortunately, epiglottitis is now a rare event. Group A streptococcus is a rare cause of epiglottitis (Jacobs, 2006; Jenson & Baltimore, 2006).

Clinical Findings
History. An affected child has a sudden escalating course of fever, sore throat, and dyspnea and looks sick.

Physical Examination. Findings include the following:
- Inspiratory and sometimes expiratory stridor
- Drooling, aphonia (muffled voice), and high fever
- Rapidly progressive respiratory obstruction and prostration
- Flaring of the ala nasi and retraction of the supraclavicular, intercostal, and subcostal spaces
- Child assuming a position of hyperextension of the neck
- In older children, one may find:
  ○ Complaints of sore throat and dysphagia

- Stridor, irritability, restlessness, and brassy cough (uncommon)
- Child assuming a "tripod" position with head held forward, jaw thrust forward, mouth open and tongue hanging out

A rare, unusual finding is that of just a hoarse cough and a cherry-red epiglottis. No attempt should be made to examine the posterior pharynx because stimulation of the area can induce spasm and obstruction of the epiglottis and lead to respiratory arrest.

Diagnostic Tests. Blood cultures should be ordered. If the possibility of epiglottitis is thought to be remote in a patient with croup, a lateral neck radiograph may be obtained before the physical examination is undertaken. Absence of the "thumb" sign on the radiograph rules out the condition. A health care professional capable of supporting the airway and skilled in intubation must accompany the child to the radiology department and back.

Management

The time from the onset of symptoms until death may be only a matter of hours. Acute epiglottitis is a pediatric emergency because of the risk of sudden airway obstruction! If epiglottitis is suspected, do not examine the throat. The child should not be placed in the supine position and should be immediately transported to the hospital. The child should be examined in the operating room by someone who can do an emergency tracheostomy. An airway must be established, either a nasotracheal airway or a tracheostomy. The diagnosis is confirmed in the operating room by depressing the tongue to view the swollen cherry-red epiglottis. Such children have a risk of reflex laryngospasm and acute and complete airway obstruction.

Begin the following treatments:

- Administer intravenous broad spectrum antibiotics to cover *H. influenzae.*
- Administer oxygen and respiratory support.

The acute infection rarely lasts more than 48 to 72 hours. As improvement occurs, the child can be extubated, but antibiotic therapy should be continued for 10 days. Patients heal completely. Untreated or undertreated patients have a significant mortality rate. Remember that the time from the onset of symptoms to death can be a matter of hours. If *H. influenzae* is identified as the causative agent, rifampin prophylaxis (20 mg/kg in a single dose [maximum, 600 mg] for 4 days) should be given to all family contacts with children younger than 4 years old and all child contacts younger than 4 years old.

Prevention

Routine immunization against *H. influenzae* type b, the leading cause of epiglottitis, is the primary means of prevention.

BACTERIAL TRACHEITIS (MEMBRANOUS CROUP)

Epidemiology

Bacterial tracheitis, also known as membranous croup, is an acute, potentially dangerous bacterial infection of the upper airway that does not involve the epiglottis. This condition can occur at any age, but typically is seen in the 3- to 10-year-old child. Bacterial tracheitis usually follows a viral respiratory infection (generally parainfluenza virus type 1). The child typically has had a prior croup episode or influenza virus and then becomes secondarily infected with *S. aureus,* the most common organism cultured, *H. influenzae, or M. catarrhalis.* No gender differentiation has been noted in the incidence or severity of symptoms (Behrman et al, 2004; Jenson & Baltimore, 2006).

Clinical Findings

History. A brassy cough as part of a "typical viral LTB or URI" and a high fever (greater than 102° F [38.9° C]) may be reported. A normal or hoarse voice is reported, and the illness is typically biphasic with rapid deterioration.

Physical Examination. Copious purulent sputum is seen in older children. Inspiratory stridor develops, and the child begins to look "toxic."

Diagnostic Tests. The diagnosis is based on confirming a bacterial upper airway infection. The white blood cell (WBC) count will be elevated. Bacterial tracheitis can be differentiated from epiglottitis by its slower clinical course and a normal-appearing epiglottis on examination. The "classic" features of acute epiglottitis are absent (e.g., no thumb sign on a lateral neck film). Leukocytosis with a left shift is noted.

Management

Management includes the following:

- The usual treatments for croup are ineffective, and hospitalization is necessary.
- Intubation or tracheostomy is usually necessary to bypass the swelling that develops at the level of the cricoid cartilage and to manage the copious purulent secretions.
- Antibiotics that cover staphylococcus are administered.
- Oxygen and airway support are necessary.
- Most patients become afebrile in 48 to 72 hours; the child is weaned from the artificial airway and usually does well.

■ INTRATHORACIC AIRWAY DISORDERS
FOREIGN BODY ASPIRATION

Description

The symptoms and physical findings associated with aspiration of a FB depend on the nature of the material aspirated plus the location and degree of the obstruction. The cough reflex protects the lower airways, and most aspirated material is immediately expelled with coughing. Onset of a sudden episode of coughing without a prodrome or signs of respiratory infection should make the provider suspicious of FB aspiration.

Epidemiology

Objects that are either too large to be eliminated by the mucociliary system or cannot be expelled by coughing eventually lead to some form of respiratory symptomatology. Obviously, a large FB occluding the upper airway can cause suffocation.

A small object in the lower respiratory tree may not produce symptoms for days to weeks. Obstruction results from either the FB itself or edema associated with its presence. Hot dogs are one of the most common causes of fatal aspiration. Toddlers are the group of children who most commonly aspirate an FB; however, FB aspiration does occur in children of all ages.

Laryngeal Foreign Body
Clinical Findings
History.   A rapid onset of hoarseness and the development of a chronic croupy cough with aphonia are reported. Be suspicious of a prior FB aspiration in children with cough, unilateral wheezing, and recurrent pneumonia.

Physical Examination.   The child can also have hemoptysis, dyspnea, wheezing, and cyanosis.

Diagnostic Tests.   Because most FBs are not radiopaque, radiographs may not be useful in the diagnosis. However, if a chest radiograph does not reveal a FB but shows local emphysema—an area that does not inflate or deflate—suspect FB aspiration (Jenson & Baltimore, 2006; Kinane & Scirica, 2006). If the history suggests FB aspiration, bronchoscopy must be undertaken. Direct laryngoscopy might reveal the presence of foreign matter.

Tracheal Foreign Body
Clinically, the child has a history of a brassy cough, hoarseness, dyspnea, and possibly cyanosis. The most characteristic signs of tracheal FB aspiration are the asthmatic wheeze and the audible slap and palpable thud sound produced by the momentary expiratory impact of the FB at the subglottic level.

Bronchial Foreign Body
The initial clinical findings are similar to those seen in either tracheal or laryngeal FB aspiration. Blood-streaked sputum may be expectorated. Children aspirating a metallic object often complain of a "metallic taste" in their mouths. If the object is nonobstructive and nonirritating, few or no initial symptoms may be seen. A small object can act as a bypass valve, and wheezes can be heard; emphysema or atelectasis can develop as the result of a large obstruction caused by a bronchial FB. The child may have limited chest expansion, decreased vocal fremitus, atelectasis, or emphysema-like changes with resulting hyporesonance or hyperresonance. Diminished breath sounds are often found. Crackles, rhonchi, and wheezes can be present if air movement is adequate. Most objects are aspirated into the right lung. A careful medical history may reveal a forgotten episode of choking.

Clinical Findings
History.   An initial episode of coughing, gagging, and choking is described. Some objects are inhaled with no choking (e.g., a spear of grass). Hemoptysis rarely occurs as an early symptom but, on rare occasions, does occur as an initial symptom months or years after the aspiration event took place.

Physical Examination.   If the acute episode is missed or not appreciated, a latent period of mild "wheezing" or cough may be seen. Lobar pneumonia, intractable wheezing, and status asthmaticus can develop.

Diagnostic Tests.   Clinical suspicion is the clue to this diagnosis. Inspiratory and forced expiratory chest radiographs and chest fluoroscopy are useful in identifying radiolucent FBs (Fig. 31-1).

Management.   If the object is removed via bronchoscopy before permanent damage occurs, recovery is usually complete. Secondary lung infections and bronchospasms should be treated as suggested in the section on management of pneumonia and asthma.

Complications.   If the FB is vegetable matter, vegetal or arachidic bronchitis can occur. This severe condition can be characterized by sepsis-like fever, dyspnea, and cough. If the material has been there for a long time, suppuration can occur.

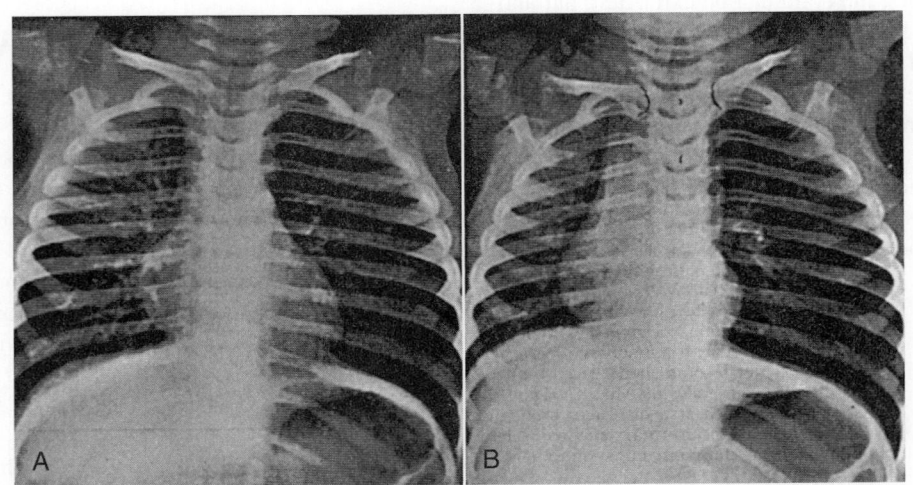

FIG. 31-1   Obstructive overinflation caused by a peanut fragment in the left main stem bronchus. **A,** Inspiration. **B,** Expiration. (From Orenstein D: Foreign bodies in the larynx, trachea, and bronchi. In Behrman RE, Kliegman RM, Jenson HB, editors: *Nelson textbook of pediatrics,* ed 16, Philadelphia, 2000, WB Saunders, p 1281.)

BRONCHITIS

Description

The diagnosis of bronchitis is often made by health care providers and can be classified as acute or chronic. Acute bronchitis is usually caused by a viral agent resulting in inflammation of the tracheal and major bronchial mucosa. Chronic bronchitis, which is characterized by a productive cough lasting for more than 3 months, is usually a symptom of another chronic disorder (e.g., allergies, asthma, CF, cigarette smoking). Bronchitis involves fully cartilaginized conducting airways. As such, it probably does not exist as a single pathologic entity in children (Allen, 2006).

Epidemiology

This condition is usually preceded by a viral URI. Although a virus is the most common cause of true bronchitis, weakened tissue can succumb to a secondary bacterial infection. The common viral agents implicated in bronchitis are rhinovirus, RSV, and parainfluenza. *S. pneumoniae, B. pertussis,* and *H. influenzae* are the most commonly cultured bacterial organisms. *M. pneumoniae* and *C. pneumoniae* are also causative agents. *Pseudomonas aeruginosa* is the common agent in children with CF.

Clinical Findings

History. The following are reported:

- A dry, hacking, unproductive cough begins a few days after the onset of rhinitis.
- The patient complains of low substernal discomfort or burning chest pain aggravated by coughing.
- The cough becomes productive after a few days, and shortness of breath can occur.

Physical Examination. Findings can vary and include the following:

- Low-grade or no fever
- Signs of nasopharyngeal infection, conjunctivitis, and rhinitis (common)
- Coarse breath sounds and coarse to fine moist rales
- The presence of rhonchi, which can be high pitched and resemble wheezes

Differential Diagnosis

Children with recurrent acute bronchitis must be evaluated for underlying pathologic conditions. Respiratory tract anomalies, FB aspiration, bronchiectasis, immunodeficiency, allergy, sinusitis, tonsillitis, exposure to air pollutants, adenoiditis, and CF must be considered in the differential diagnosis. Check for tobacco or marijuana use in teenagers.

Management

No specific therapy is known, and most patients require none. Care is primarily supportive. Postural drainage and the use of a humidifier can be helpful. Cough suppressants should be prescribed judiciously and only for children over 2 years old. Antihistamines should not be used because of their excessive drying effect; these drugs tend to prolong the symptoms. If evidence of a bacterial infection such as high fever and crackles is observed, antibiotics may be considered. Mucus generally thins in 5 to 10 days, and the cough decreases.

Complications

In normal, healthy children, the condition is not serious; however, malaise continues for another week or so after the cough lessens. In undernourished or chronically ill children, otitis, sinusitis, and pneumonia are common.

BRONCHIOLITIS

Description

Bronchiolitis is a common acute disease of the lower respiratory tract that causes inflammation leading to obstruction of the small respiratory airways as a result of swelling of the small bronchioles with resultant inadequate expiratory flow. In addition, infection of bronchiolar epithelial cells causes necrosis and sloughing of cells into the airways. In mild cases, symptoms can last for 1 to 3 days. In severe cases, cyanosis, air hunger, retractions, and nasal flaring with symptoms of severe respiratory distress within a few hours may be seen. Bronchiolitis is the term used for an infant seen with wheezing for the very first time and is the leading cause of hospitalizations for infants.

Epidemiology

Bronchiolitis is a viral illness with RSV responsible for more than 50% of cases. Human metapneumovirus, parainfluenza virus (type 3), influenza virus, adenovirus, rhinovirus, or *M. pneumoniae* (in older children) generally cause the remainder of cases. Adenovirus and RSV can cause long-term complications. The incubation period for RSV is 4 to 6 days and typically occurs late fall through early spring. Bronchiolitis commonly occurs in young children from infancy to 2 years old, is very contagious, and spread by close contact with infected respiratory secretions or fomites. The most frequent mode of transmission is hand carriage of contaminated secretion. Viral shedding in nonimmunocompromised patients can be up to 21 days (Allen, 2006). The source of infection is an older family member with a "mild" URI. Older children and adults have larger airways and tolerate the swelling associated with this infection better than infants do. Most cases of bronchiolitis resolve completely, but recurrence of infection is common, and symptoms tend to be mild.

Traditional risk factors for severe RSV disease are premature birth, chronic lung disease, and immunodeficiency. However, the vast majority of infants admitted to hospitals for bronchiolitis were previously healthy. An interesting study by Aurivillius and colleagues (2005) reported a potential genetic link with susceptibility to severe RSV infection in previously healthy infants (Jenson & Baltimore, 2006).

Clinical Findings

History. The following are reported:

- Initial presentation of URI symptoms (cough, coryza, and rhinorrhea) lasting for 3 to 7 days
- Gradual development of respiratory distress marked by noisy, raspy breathing with audible wheezing
- Low-grade to moderate fever up to 102° F (38.9° C)

- Decrease in appetite
- No prodrome in some infants; rather they have apnea as the initial symptom

Physical Examination.   Findings include the following:

- Paroxysmal wheezing
- Crackles may be heard throughout the breathing cycle
- High respiratory rate (approximately 60 to 80 breaths per minute)
- Varying signs of respiratory distress and pulmonary involvement (e.g., nasal flaring, grunting, retractions, cyanosis, prolonged expiration)
- Palpable liver and spleen because of their being pushed down by hyperinflated lungs

Diagnostic Tests.   A chest radiograph displays air trapping with hyperinflation of the lungs and increased anterior-posterior diameter. The routine use of chest radiographs in previously healthy infants with mild to moderate RSV bronchiolitis is currently being debated as to their benefit in determining the management plan versus the radiation exposure to the infant. Some infants may have scattered areas of consolidation caused by atelectasis or inflammation of the alveoli. Early bacterial pneumonia can be difficult to detect and cannot be ruled out by radiographs. Immunofluorescence analysis of nasal washings is helpful to confirm RSV, parainfluenza viruses, influenza viruses, and adenoviruses. PCR is helpful in deciding about isolation of cohorts with the same infection in the hospital setting. A mild leukocytosis may be seen with 12,000 to 16, 000/microliter. Routine laboratory tests are usually not required to confirm the diagnosis because they lack specificity.

Differential Diagnosis

Making the diagnosis is not usually a problem. In mild afebrile cases, bronchial asthma can be confused with bronchiolitis. A successful challenge with bronchodilators favors the diagnosis of asthma. Less than 5% of cases of recurrent bronchiolitis have a virus as their cause. Other, rarer conditions to be ruled out include congestive heart failure, tracheal FB aspiration, organophosphate poisoning, CF, and bronchopneumonia with generalized obstructive emphysema.

Management

Most infants with mild signs of respiratory distress can be treated as outpatients.

- Supportive care consists of adequate hydration and use of antipyretics.
- Careful instructions must be given to parents regarding the following:
  - Management of rhinitis (use of saline drops)
  - Signs of increasing respiratory distress or dehydration that call for hospitalization
  - Indications for the use of antipyretics
  - Guidelines for feeding an infant with signs of mild respiratory distress (amount of fluid needed per 24 hours; smaller, more frequent feedings; monitoring of the respiratory rate; and guarding against vomiting)

Infants younger than 2 months old and older infants with signs of severe respiratory distress should be hospitalized.

Signs that suggest increasing respiratory distress include the following (Jenson & Baltimore, 2006):

- Progressive stridor or stridor at rest
- Apnea
- Increasing respiratory rate (sleeping rate of greater than 50 to 60 breaths per minute)
- Restlessness, pallor, or cyanosis
- Hypoxia recorded by either blood gas (Po_2 less than 60 mm Hg) or pulse oximetry (less than 92% on room air)
- Rising PCO_2 (recorded by blood gas)
- Inability to tolerate oral feedings
- Depressed sensorium
- Presence of chronic cardiovascular or immunodeficiency disease
- Parent unable to manage at home for any reason

In-hospital management focuses on supportive care and includes suctioning of upper airways, which is critical, humidified supplemental oxygen, and elevation of the child to a sitting position at a 30- to 40-degree angle. The infant's neck should be extended to 30 to 40 degrees. Intravenous fluids are frequently needed because respiratory distress interferes with nursing or bottle feeding. Monitoring oxygenation levels using pulse oximetry is helpful. The use of ribavirin, epinephrine, ipratropium bromide, ß₂-agonist bronchodilators, inhaled and oral corticosteroids, and antibiotics have demonstrated no convincing evidence of effectiveness. There are subsets of infants with bronchiolitis who demonstrate significant bronchodilator responsiveness. Therefore, all infants (especially those with a family history of asthma or atopy) with significant wheezing should be given a one-time trial of an aerosolized ß₂-adrenergic treatment. If after an initial one-time trial there is no improvement, additional use of bronchodilators should be abandoned (Allen, 2006).

Occasionally, a hospitalized child is not able to be quickly weaned back to room air. Home management of these patients requiring oxygen is extremely difficult and should be undertaken only by someone with excellent pulmonary skills and in consultation with a pediatrician or pediatric pulmonologist. The child should have an O_2 saturation study before discharge to help determine the O_2 requirements at rest, feeding, play, and sleep. A pneumogram to rule out apnea may also be indicated. Strict outpatient follow-up is mandatory for as long as the child is receiving home O_2.

Complications

The first 48 to 72 hours after the onset of cough is the most critical. Apneic spells are common in an infant. The child can be desperately ill, but gradually improves. The fatality rate associated with bronchiolitis is about 1% to 2%. Prolonged apnea, uncompensated respiratory acidosis, and profound dehydration secondary to loss of water from tachypnea and an inability to drink are the factors leading to death in young infants with bronchiolitis. In some children, bronchiolitis can cause minor pulmonary function problems and a tendency for bronchial hyperreactivity that lasts for years. RSV bronchiolitis has been associated with the development of asthma, but its role in the causality of asthma is still debated (Allen, 2006).

Prevention

Palivizumab (Synagis) is an RSV-specific monoclonal antibody used to provide some protection from severe RSV infection for high-risk infants (see Chapter 23). Educate caregivers about decreasing exposure to and transmission of RSV especially to families with high-risk infants. Advice should include limiting exposure to child care centers, if possible; hand washing; avoiding tobacco smoke exposure; and scheduling RSV prophylaxis vaccination.

PNEUMONIA

Pneumonia is a lower respiratory tract infection with consolidation of the alveolar spaces involving the airways and parenchyma of the lung. Pneumonitis is a general term used to describe lung inflammation that may or may not be associated with consolidation. Several subclassifications of pneumonia are recognized: bacterial, viral, other infectious agents, mycotic, aspiration, and a few other rare syndromes. It can also be characterized as lobar, interstitial, or bronchopneumonia. Lobar pneumonia involves depositions in the alveolar space that result in consolidation; it is described as "typical" pneumonia. Atypical pneumonia describes patterns of consolidation that are not localized. In interstitial pneumonia, cellular infiltrates attack the interstitium, which makes up the walls of the alveoli, the alveolar sacs and ducts, and the bronchioles; this type of pneumonia is typical of acute viral infections, but may be a chronic process. In bronchopneumonia, the inflammation is centered in the bronchioles and is characterized by the production of mucopurulent exudate, which obstructs small airways resulting in patchy consolidation of adjacent lobules.

Lobar and interstitial pneumonia and bronchiolar and bronchial inflammation can coexist in a child (Foca, 2006; Jenson & Baltimore, 2006). Table 31-4 differentiates the various forms of pneumonia commonly found in infants, children, and adolescents. Of note, clinical diagnosis of pneumonia may be required in very young infants and children when physical examination is less revealing. Treatment is often empirical and varies with age.

Description

Primary bacterial pneumonia is less common in childhood than secondary bacterial infection after a viral infection. Viral pneumonia often involves both the conducting airways and the alveoli. This type of pneumonia is a common problem in young children and can result in serious illness in a young infant. Viral infection affects the lung defenses by altering normal secretions, inhibiting phagocytosis, modifying the normal bacterial flora, and disrupting the epithelial layer. Thus, the many childhood viruses set the stage for secondary bacterial infection. Children with immunologic problems or chronic illnesses are prone to primary bacterial pneumonia and experience recurrent pneumonias or fail to clear the initial infection completely. Differentiating bacterial from viral pneumonia is particularly important in infants younger than 6 months old.

TABLE 31-4   Differentiating Various Forms of Pneumonia in Infants, Young Children, and Adolescents

Characteristic	Bacterial	Viral	Mycoplasmal	Chlamydial
Common age	All ages	All ages	>5 years old	2-19 weeks old (typically 1-3 months old)
Onset	Acute; gradual	Acute; gradual	Slow	Gradual
Clinical findings	Depend on age; starts with URI, cough, dyspnea, tachypnea, rales, decreased breath sounds, grunting, retractions, toxic look; potential progression to severe respiratory distress	Depend on age; cough, coryza, hoarseness, crackles, wheezing, stridor	Persistent cough, malaise, headache	Tachypnea, staccato cough, crackles, wheezing rare, 50% have signs or history of conjunctivitis
Fever	Acute onset of fever (≥102.2° F [≥ 39° C])	Present	>102.2° F (>39° C)	Afebrile
CBC	WBCs often elevated >15,000/microliter	Normal or slight elevation of WBCs	Normal	Eosinophilia in 75% of cases
Organism(s)	90% caused by *S. pneumoniae*	RSV, parainfluenza, influenza (types A and B)	*M. pneumoniae*	*C. trachomatis*
Radiographic findings	Lobar consolidation	Transient lobar infiltrates	Varies, interstitial infiltrates	Hyperinflation, infiltrates
Treatment	Depends on bacteria; penicillin, methicillin, cefuroxime, gentamicin, vancomycin	Supportive care	Erythromycin/ clarithromycin	Erythromycin

CBC, Complete blood count; *RSV,* respiratory syncytial virus; *URI,* upper respiratory infection; *WBCs,* white blood cells.

Mycoplasmal pneumonia, or primary atypical pneumonia, is the most common cause of pneumonia in children older than 5 years through the young adult years. This disease is usually mild and self-limited. Chlamydial pneumonia is a characteristic pneumonia resulting from the transmission of *C. trachomatis* from the infected genital tract of the mother to the infant. It does not become apparent until the infant is 2 to 19 weeks old.

Epidemiology

Infecting organisms associated with pneumonia vary by age (Box 31-3). The usual cause of bacterial pneumonia is *S. pneumoniae*. It causes more than 90% of cases of childhood bacterial pneumonia. Pneumococcal pneumonia occurs most commonly in the late winter and early spring, after the cycle of viral URIs. Asymptomatic carriers play a more important role in dissemination of disease than do sick contacts. Children younger than 4 years old suffer the highest attack rate. Pneumonia caused by community-acquired methicillin-resistant *Staphylococcus aureus* (MRSA) has become a worrisome occurrence.

Viruses commonly causing pneumonia in children of all ages are identified in Box 31-3. *M. pneumoniae*, an organism without a cell wall, is responsible for mycoplasmal pneumonia. It is transmitted from one symptomatic patient to another by droplet spread. The incubation period is 2 to 3 weeks, and asymptomatic carriage after infection can last for weeks. *C. trachomatis* is an organism that has many subtypes within the species. Approximately 50% of infants born to infected mothers acquire this infection, but only 5% to 20% of these infants develop chlamydial trachomatis pneumonia with a typical onset between 1 to 3 months old.

Clinical Findings in Infants and Young Children

Age influences the clinical manifestations of pneumonia. Depending upon the type of pneumonia, it may also have characteristic findings. However, the difference in presentation of viral or bacterial pneumonia is not always clear or easy to differentiate. Remember that neonates may have respiratory manifestations without a fever, or fever only with subtle or no physical findings suggestive of pneumonia.

History. The following may be reported (Jenson & Baltimore, 2006):
- Initial history of a mild URI for a few days—similar for both bacterial and viral.
- Abrupt high fever with temperatures above 103.3° F (39.6° C), chills, cough, and dyspnea suggest bacterial pneumonia.
- Slower onset of respiratory symptoms, cough, wheezing, or stridor with less prominent fever suggest viral pneumonia.
- Other manifestations include restlessness, shaking chills, apprehension, shortness of breath, malaise, and pleuritic chest pain.
- With *C. trachomatis*, infant is typically afebrile; prior, concurrent, or no history of inclusion conjunctivitis reported.

Physical Examination. Findings include the following:
- Nasal flaring, grunting, retractions
- Tachypnea generally if greater than 60 breaths per minute in infants less than 2 months old, greater than 50 breaths per minute in children 2 to 11 months old, or greater than 40 breaths per minute at rest in children 1 to 5 years old (may be the only clue), tachycardia, air hunger, cyanosis are significant findings
- Fine crackles, dullness, diminished breath sounds
- Other findings can include:
  ○ Presence of a pleural effusion and signs of congestive heart failure
  ○ Abdominal distention, downward displacement of the liver or spleen
  ○ Nuchal rigidity without meningeal infection from involvement of the right upper lobe
  ○ Decreased peripheral perfusion and capillary refill; lethargy
- May have signs specific to the individual viral organism
- *C. trachomatis* pneumonia characterized by repetitive, staccato cough with tachypnea, cervical adenopathy, crackles, tachypnea, rarely wheezing

Clinical Findings in Children and Adolescents

History. The patient can have:
- Initial history of URI
- Sudden onset of shaking chills, followed by a high fever, cough, chest pain (more suggestive of bacterial pneumonia)
- Intermittent periods of drowsiness, restlessness, rapid respiration
- Dry, hacking, productive cough (with rust-colored or bloody sputum if expectorated)
- With mycoplasma—URI symptoms, low-grade fever (temperature greater than 39° C), dry cough with scant sputum; often associated with a prodrome of chills, headache, sore throat, gastrointestinal symptoms, and malaise; rhinorrhea not commonly reported

Physical Examination. The following may be seen:
- Retractions, tachypnea, decreased tactile and vocal fremitus, diminished breath sounds.
- Dullness plus fine and crackling rales on the affected side.

BOX 31-3   Pneumonia—Frequently Associated Pathogens by Pediatric Age Group

- RSV, influenza, cytomegalovirus, parainfluenza, adenoviruses, human metapneumovirus, and rhinovirus—ALL ages
- Group B β-*hemolytic streptococcus*, gram-negative organisms, and *Listeria monocytogenes*—neonates
- *S. aureus*, (a very serious infection) *C. trachomatis*, *S. pneumoniae*—infants 1 to 3 months old
- *S. pneumoniae*, nontypable *H. influe zae*, and *M. pneumoniae*—4 months to 5 year olds
- *M. pneumoniae*, *C. pneumoniae*, and *S. pneumoniae*—5 years and older

Data from Foca MD: Pneumonia. In Burg FD WB et al, editors: *Current pediatric therapy*, ed 18, Philadelphia, 2006, WB Saunders Elsevier.

- Splinting of the affected side to minimize pleuritic pain or lying on the side in a fetal position—helps compensate for decreased air exchange and improves ventilation.
- Progression to delirium, circumoral cyanosis, and posturing.
- Mycoplasmal pneumonia—typically see minimal changes or harsh breath sounds and rhonchi heard on auscultation.

Diagnostic Tests.   DFA testing of nasopharyngeal washings may be helpful in determining the viral agent, but are generally reserved for children needing hospital admission. The typical radiograph in viral pneumonia shows patchy bronchopneumonia (diffuse infiltrates). Hyperinflation (hyperexpansion of the lungs) is a common radiographic finding (Fig. 31-2). The WBC count is normal or mildly elevated with a predominance of lymphocytes. Usual findings in a bacterial infection include the following:

- The WBC count is elevated (greater than 20,000/mm³) with neutrophils predominant.
- Arterial blood gases are consistent with hypoxia.
- The organism may be found by culture of nasopharyngeal scrapings (not always accurate), tracheal aspirates, blood (10% to 20% of cases are positive; however, if positive, confirms the causative pathogen), or lung tap fluid.
- Counterimmunoelectrophoresis results are positive.
- Radiographs are consistent with lobar or segmental consolidation or a round pneumonia with pleural effusion in up to 30% of children. Frontal and lateral films are needed for adequate visualization. Staphylococcal pneumonia involves the right lobe 65% of the time. Pneumatoceles are common in staphylococcal pneumonia (Behrman et al, 2004; Jenson & Baltimore, 2006).
- Blood, urine, and cerebrospinal fluid cultures should also be obtained in infants younger than 3 months old as part of a septic work-up.

Mycoplasmal pneumonia is suspected if cold agglutinins are present in peripheral blood samples and is confirmed by mycoplasma IgM or PCR testing. Chest radiograph findings are nonspecific and reveal bronchovascular markings or bronchopneumonia with areas of atelectasis. Remember that chest radiographs may be read as normal in early pneumonia and then reveal infiltrates later during treatment when there is more fluid from edema.

C. trachomatis pneumonia has chest radiographic findings of hyperinflation and bilateral diffuse infiltrates. Mild eosinophilia is characteristic (greater than 400 cells/mm³), and elevated serum IgG and IgM concentrations are indirect evidence of infection. An elevated serum titer of chlamydia-specific IgM is diagnostic of the disease, but this test is not available in all laboratories. The organism may be cultured. Hyperinflation with minimal interstitial or alveolar infiltrates is a consistent finding on chest radiograph (Behrman et al, 2004).

Differential Diagnosis

The age of the child and characteristic signs and symptoms as identified above help distinguish viral from bacterial pneumonia. Other disease entities and conditions to consider in the differential diagnosis are bronchiolitis, congestive heart failure, acute bronchiectasis, aspiration of a FB, pulmonary abscess, parasitic pneumonia, and endotracheal tuberculosis. Also, right lower lobe pneumonia can be confused with appendicitis. Right upper lobe pneumonia can often closely resemble meningitis.

Management

Most healthy older children can be managed as outpatients. Neonates must always be admitted to the hospital if diagnosed with pneumonia regardless of infecting pathogen. Young infants up to 4 months old may also need hospitalization unless chlamydia is suspected (Box 31-4). The healthy older infant or child with a viral pneumonia generally only needs supportive care (antipyretics, hydration, rest); however, if secondary bacterial infection is suspected, antibiotic therapy is appropriate. Management of bacterial pneumonia consists of appropriate antibiotic coverage, adequate fluid intake, and respiratory therapy (humidified oxygen, pulmonary therapy, intubation) if needed. Older children with pneumococcal pneumonia can usually be treated safely at home if not in severe respiratory distress. Most children who are moderately ill and can be treated at home will respond to amoxicillin. Pharmacologic therapy is based on age and the common organisms that are found in a particular age group.

Guidelines for outpatient and inpatient treatment of pneumonia by age and certain specific pathogens are as follows (Foca, 2006; Jenson & Baltimore, 2006):

Outpatient antibiotic treatment (7 to 10 days duration of therapy):

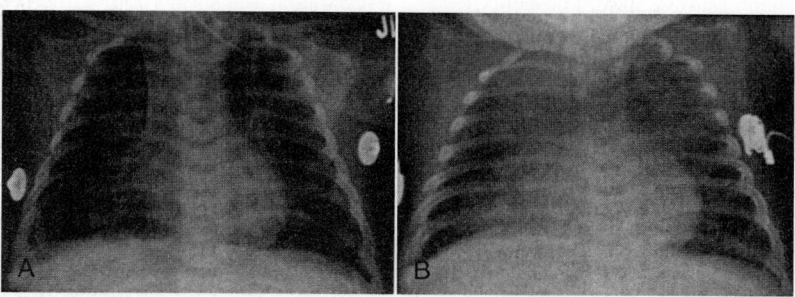

FIG. 31-2   Six-month-old infant with rapid respirations and fever. An anteroposterior radiograph of the chest shows hyperexpansion of the lungs with bilateral fine air space disease and streaks of density, indicating the presence of both pneumonia and atelectasis. (From Prober CG: Pneumonia. In Behrman RE, Kliegman RM, Jenson HB, editors: *Nelson textbook of pediatrics*, ed 16, Philadelphia, 2000, WB Saunders, p 761.)

BOX 31-4 **Criteria for Hospital Admission**

- Tachypnea: >60 breaths/minute in infants <2 months; >50 breaths/minute in children 2 to 11 months old; or >40 breaths/minute at rest in children 1 to 5 years old
- Grunting, severe respiratory distress
- Decreased oxygen saturations (pulse oximetry reading or arterial blood gas) with need for supplemental oxygen
- Toxic appearance
- Failure to respond to appropriate oral antibiotic
- Neonate; consider for young infants 1 to 6 months old
- Feeding issues, vomiting, or dehydration
- Pulmonary complications noted on radiographs—abscess, empyema, pneumatocele
- Social issues at home that indicate parent or caretaker cannot appropriately monitor and/or care for the child

---

- *One month to 4 months old:* May need to admit unless chlamydia suspected: Treat chlamydia with erythromycin 20 to 50 mg/kg/day, divided every 6 hours.
- *Four months to 5 years old:* Amoxicillin 80 to 100 mg/kg/day, divided bid or tid.
- *Five years and older:* Azithromycin 12 mg/kg/day daily (maximum dose 500 mg) or amoxicillin 80 to 100 mg/kg/day divided bid or tid.
- Erythromycin, azithromycin, or clarithromycin is the recommended treatment if *M. pneumoniae* suspected.

  Inpatient treatment: testing to identify the pathogen is important for selection of appropriate antimicrobial therapy:
- *Neonate must be admitted:* Ampicillin and cefotaxime or ceftriaxone or gentamicin.
- *One month to 5 years old:* Cefuroxime and add vancomycin if rapid progression of illness.
- *Five years and older:* Cefotaxime and azithromycin and add vancomycin if rapid progression of illness.
- The recommended treatment for *S. aureus* pneumonia is nafcillin or oxacillin with vancomycin as an alternative.

Prognosis

By the second to third day, auscultation reveals a change in respiratory sounds as the infection begins to consolidate. Increased fremitus, tubular breath sounds, and the disappearance of crackles may be noted. As resolution occurs around the seventh day, which is typically the day when children and adolescents who are untreated may become quite sick, crackles can recur. Most children have an uneventful recovery, but it is important to inform parents that their child's cough can last for several weeks. It may take 6 to 8 weeks before radiographic findings are normal. If pneumonia recurs or persists for longer than one month, the child needs further evaluation for underlying disease.

Complications

Empyema is common in staphylococcal and GABHS infections. Scarring of the airways and lung tissue can cause dilated bronchi, which results in bronchiectasis. Lung abscess can result if the pneumonia causes necrosis of the lung tissue.

M. pneumoniae can spread to the blood, central nervous system, heart, skin, or joints. A child with sickle cell disease and mycoplasmal pneumonia has more severe pulmonary disease than the average child does.

Prevention

Identify and treat pregnant women with *C. trachomatis*. The need for influenza and pneumococcal immunization and monthly injections of humanized monoclonal RSV antibody for high-risk neonates is essential (see Chapter 23).

Guidelines for Radiographic Follow-up After Pneumonia

A follow-up chest radiograph should be obtained if there is no trend toward improvement; if there is persistent cough, dyspnea, or other physical findings; or if there is a worsening or recurrence of symptoms or physical findings. Patients who have had lobar pneumonia, mycoplasmal pneumonia, or *C. pneumoniae* tend to have a cough for weeks and moderate dyspnea on exertion for 2 to 3 months as part of a normal course in recovery. Children with recurrent pneumonias should be referred for further pulmonary evaluation.

TUBERCULOSIS

Tuberculosis is discussed in Chapter 23.

CYSTIC FIBROSIS

Description

CF is a multisystem genetic disorder manifested by chronic obstructive pulmonary disease (COPD), gastrointestinal disturbances, and exocrine dysfunction.

Epidemiology

CF is an autosomal recessive genetic disorder involving mutation of the CF transmembrane conductance regulator gene on chromosome 7. It occurs in approximately 1 in 2500 white births. Although not common, it does occur in 1 in 17,000 African-American, 1 in 9000 Hispanic and 1 in 90,000 Asian births. The basic insult is an inability to clear mucoid secretions and inadequate salt and water secretion on the cellular level. This occurs because of problems in regulation of the chloride ion channel and other proteins that conduct ions across the epithelial cell membranes in the airways, biliary tree, pancreas, intestines, vas deferens, and sweat glands. The end result of this dysfunctional epithelial transport (both in its secretory and absorptive function) is inadequate hydration and obstruction of the target organ ducts. The endobronchial spaces are not cleared of their mucoid secretions, which leads to colonization by bacteria with resulting chronic inflammation and infection. Inadequate water secretion also causes desiccation of mucoid and proteinaceous secretions and, consequently, pulmonary and exocrine duct obstruction and tissue damage (Behrman et al, 2004; Dovey, 2006).

Clinical Findings

CF is a multisystem, progressive illness with varying levels of severity. Clinical manifestations may include the following (Behrman et al, 2004; Dovey, 2006; Marshall & Debley, 2006):

- *Pulmonary*. CF is a major cause of severe chronic lung disease in children. The respiratory epithelium exhibits marked impermeability to chloride and excessive reabsorption of sodium. Mucus is viscous, and dehydration of the airway secretions occurs leading to dysfunctional mucociliary transport and airway obstruction and chronic infections. The pulmonary system manifestations run the clinical spectrum from chronic, dry, frequent cough and sputum production to respiratory failure. Bronchitis, bronchiolitis, bronchiolectasis, and pneumonia are frequent. Bronchospasm resembling acute or chronic asthma may be present. The airways become colonized with *S. aureus, H. influenzae,* and, finally, *P. aeruginosa. Burkholderia cepacia* is a slower-growing organism found in children with CF. Pulmonary disease usually becomes progressive and leads to cor pulmonale, respiratory failure, and death. Other respiratory problems associated with CF include recurrent acute sinusitis, nasal polyps, and allergic bronchopulmonary aspergillosis. Digital clubbing is common.
- *Gastrointestinal tract and nutrition*. Meconium ileus develops in up to 15% of newborns born with CF. A meconium ileus syndrome equivalent can also develop in older patients, with desiccated fecal material causing gastrointestinal obstruction. Eighty-five percent of affected children have failure to thrive because of pancreatic enzyme insufficiency. Edema-hypoproteinemia may also be present. These children have thick, fat-laden stools (steatorrhea), poor muscle mass, and delayed maturation. Infants with CF who are fed soy-based formulas do very poorly, and severe hypoproteinemia and anasarca quickly result. Other gastrointestinal problems associated with CF include intussusception, volvulus, duodenal inflammation, gastroesophageal reflux, bile reflux, fibrosing colonopathy, rectal prolapse, and vitamin A, K, E, and D deficiencies with resulting bleeding diathesis or bleeding disorders.
- *Hepatobiliary tract*. Biliary cirrhosis occurs in 2% to 3% of children with CF and is characterized by jaundice, ascites, hematemesis from esophageal varices, and splenomegaly. Hepatic steatosis is also a known complication of CF. Adolescent patients experience biliary colic and cholelithiasis.
- *Pancreas*. Recurrent acute pancreatitis is not uncommon. Diabetes mellitus with relative insulin deficiency develops in 8% of such patients, usually in the second decade of life.
- *Genitourinary tract*. Affected children have delayed sexual development. Males are almost always azoospermic as a result of atrophy or absence of the vas deferens. The incidence of inguinal hernia, hydrocele, and undescended testes is higher. Females experience secondary amenorrhea, cervicitis, and decreased fertility. A pregnancy is usually carried to term if pulmonary function is not severely compromised.
- *Sweat glands*. Excessive salt loss can lead to hypochloremic alkalosis, especially in warm weather or after gastroenteritis. Children with CF often taste salty because of elevated amounts of NaCl lost in endogenous sweat. Dehydration and heat exhaustion are concerns.

Diagnostic Tests. The diagnosis of CF is based on an abnormal sweat analysis. Sweat tests should be done at a laboratory that regularly deals with children and routinely does these tests. At least 75 mg of sweat should be collected to ensure accuracy and precision of the sweat test. A result of greater than 60 mEq/L of chloride on two specimens is considered diagnostic of CF. Forty to 60 mEq/L is borderline, and less than 40 mEq/L is negative. Children with hypoproteinemia may elicit false-negative sweat test results.

Pancreatic function tests include 3-day stool collection to measure fat balance (a cumbersome test) and quantification of trypsin and chymotrypsin activity in a fresh stool sample (patients with CF have decreased stool trypsin and chymotrypsin activity). Glycosylated hemoglobin levels may be elevated in older children because of impaired pancreatic functioning (Behrman et al, 2004). Pulmonary function tests are used to follow the clinical course.

Prenatal diagnosis has a greater than 90% sensitivity for detecting a CF gene mutation on the long arm of chromosome 7. Genotyping identifies 95% of all alleles associated with CF; however, a child may have CF without an identified allele carrying the mutation. To establish a diagnosis of CF, the following criteria are required:

- Positive result from a newborn screening test or sibling with CF
- Two or more positive sweat test results
- One or more typical CF features (chronic sinopulmonary disease, characteristic gastrointestinal and nutritional abnormalities, salt-loss syndromes, obstructive azoospermia)
- Identified characteristic abnormality in ion transport across the membranes of epithelial cells
- Identification of two mutations known to cause CF

Treatment

Children with CF have complicated treatment regimens and should be monitored by a multidisciplinary team at a CF accredited center. Pulmonary, nutritional, physical, and pharmacologic (antibiotic and antiinflammatory) therapy and psychological counseling must be individualized for each child at each stage of the illness. Home-based maintenance therapy for pulmonary and nutritional interventions is critical. With pulmonary exacerbations, children with CF generally have hospital stays for at least 2 weeks for aggressive pulmonary and antibiotic therapy.

■ SYNCOPE

Syncope is a transient loss of consciousness and muscle tone. A child with a syncopal episode requires a thoughtful approach. Many possible etiologies can produce syncopal episodes. Neurocardiogenic syncope (NCS), resulting in fainting, is common and needs to be differentiated from cardiac syncope, which is rare and potentially life threatening. Additional causes of syncope that should be considered include neurologic (headache, seizure, transient ischemic attack), psychiatric (depression, panic attack, conversion reaction), and systemic or metabolic (drugs, carbon monoxide, electrolyte imbalance/problems) (Alexander, 2006).

The initial approach to the assessment and management of syncope includes a thorough history and analysis of the symptom, a careful physical examination, and selected screening tests if indicated. NCS is typically benign and involves the voluntary and involuntary nervous system controlling heart rate, blood pressure, and related blood flow to the heart. Cardiogenic syncope is due to hemodynamic collapse from pathologic arrhythmias and/or mechanical obstruction or myopathy. It often comes without prodromal symptoms or may be associated with palpitation or chest pain (Alexander, 2006).

HISTORY

Important information to obtain about the syncopal incident includes whether the child had:

- A triggering factor, such as exercise, pain, or an emotional event
- A prior incident or incidents of syncope or fainting
- An associated injury, clonic-tonic movements, or vertigo
- Associated chest pain or palpitations
- A family history of sudden death
- The possibility of pregnancy or the use of drugs
- A history of exercise-induced asthma or respiratory distress
- A known psychological stress or stressors at home or school or in social environments

NCS generally has a history of a prodrome characterized by dizziness, warmth, and visual changes (visual spots or dimming) before the loss of consciousness. It is commonly associated with marked pallor and may be caused by standing or a clear trigger. School-age children and adolescents are prone to orthostatic intolerance. Recovery is quick (duration less than 1 minute) and is associated with residual complaints of headache, fatigue, and nausea. Cyclonic jerks, abrupt collapse, or urinary or fecal incontinence are not characteristic of NCS. About 25% of the population has a history of fainting, with the peak incident occurring in adolescent girls.

Cardiac syncope is considered a potentially life-threatening event that may herald the potential for sudden death. Syncope triggered by exercise or associated with injury or incontinence, a family history of sudden death (less than 40 years old) or cardiomyopathy, long QT syndrome, past history of heart disease, or history of an abnormal electrocardiogram (ECG) or cardiac exam suggest cardiac syncope (Alexander, 2006).

PHYSICAL EXAMINATION

A detailed neurologic examination is needed if the syncopal episode suggests a seizure disorder. Careful evaluation of the head, eyes, ears, nose, and throat is done if vestibular disease is likely. A cardiovascular examination is always important.

DIAGNOSTIC TESTS

For possible cardiac causes of syncope, a 12-lead ECG is performed and a 24-hour ambulatory monitor is used if there is concern about intermittent cardiac arrhythmia. Check orthostatic heart rate and blood pressure readings. If a seizure disorder is suspected, appropriate neurologic evaluation is done as outlined in Chapter 27. Note that a CBC, random glucose test, and glucose tolerance test have low yields and are not recommended as routine tests for a syncopal episode. Tilt-testing is expensive and is rarely needed to diagnosis NCS (Steinberg & Knilands, 2005).

MANAGEMENT

If cardiac syncope is suspected, a cardiac referral is needed. Restrict the child from sports participation until seen by a pediatric cardiologist. NCS is best treated by education, prevention (avoid long periods of standing in one place), and fluids. Having the child rest for 5 to 10 minutes either supine or legs up after a fainting episode is important because quick restanding may trigger repeated syncope.

Appropriate referral to pediatric specialists for further evaluation and diagnostic testing is suggested for children whose history, physical examination, or diagnostic tests suggest a potential pathologic problem that is outside the range of practice for the primary care provider. See Chapter 30 for discussion about cardiac etiologies.

▆ PECTUS DEFORMITY

DESCRIPTION

Pectus excavatum, or funnel chest, is an abnormality of the skeleton and chest wall resulting in sternal concavity. Midline narrowing of the thoracic cavity and restriction in chest wall movement are characteristic. Pectus carinatum describes a chest wall where the sternum bows out, commonly called "pigeon breast." Although this shape may be cosmetically unattractive, it does not cause problems with ventilation.

EPIDEMIOLOGY

Children with upper airway obstruction have a higher incidence of pectus excavatum, but many children with this defect are identified at birth or within the first year of life and have no underlying pulmonary problem. The cause of pectus excavatum in these instances is often unknown. About 79% of cases occur in males, and a positive family history of chest wall deformity is found in about 37% of cases. In pectus carinatum, underlying pulmonary problems may contribute to this deformity, but again it can be found in healthy children (Marshall & Debley, 2006).

CLINICAL FINDINGS

History

The parent may note a depression (excavatum) or bowing out (carinatum) of the sternum.

Physical Examination

Findings include posterior depression of the sternum and costal cartilage (in cases of excavatum) and anterior bowing of the sternum (carinatum).

Diagnostic Tests

Diagnostic tests include:

- Chest radiography
- Exercise testing if substantial pectus excavatum deformity is present

- Other cardiac (echocardiogram) and pulmonary function studies as suggested by the degree of excavatum deformity and symptomatology

MANAGEMENT

If the excavatum deformity is the result of a pulmonary disease, early treatment of the underlying pulmonary problem occasionally resolves the skeletal deformity. Surgical repair depends on the severity of the defect, demonstration of a decrease in pulmonary function, progression of the defect on serial radiographs, or sometimes the patient's and parents' wish for cosmetic repair. If the patient is male with an associated scoliosis or has a severe pectus carinatum or excavatum, evaluate for Marfan syndrome. Surgery for children with pectus carinatum, if done, is usually for cosmetic purposes.

COMPLICATIONS

Pectus excavatum can also affect cardiac and pulmonary function.

☑ DISCUSSION FORUM

1. A 3-year-old child has a 4-day history of temperature to 100.5° F (38.1° C) maximum, cough mostly at night, and thick, yellow-green nasal discharge. Previous medical history is negative for allergies or any chronic disease. Mom reports that his appetite and activity levels are normal and states, "I'm sure he has a sinus infection since his drainage is yellow." Physical exam reveals a nontoxic-appearing child, lungs clear to auscultation, no cervical lymphadenitis, moderate nasal congestion, and copious clear postnasal drainage. What is your management plan for this child? What education regarding sinus infections will you provide?

2. A mother calls because her 11-year-old daughter baby-sat an ill 4-month-old infant 10 days ago who has just been diagnosed with pertussis. Her daughter's last pertussis vaccine was at 4 years old (DTaP), and she is currently showing signs of URI. What is your response to the parent?

3. A 14-month-old previously healthy child has acute-onset expiratory wheezing, fine rales in the lung bases, and copious thick, clear rhinorrhea. The child's respiratory rate is 52, pulse is 134, and O_2 saturations in room air are 96%. She had a 3-day history of temperature to 101.5° F (38.7° C), nasal congestion, and cough, which has worsened considerably in the last 24 hours. The child is eating and drinking less than normal and had a wet diaper approximately 2 hours ago. Family history is positive for asthma in an older sibling. Social history is positive for day care attendance. What additional testing with rationale (if any) do you need to establish your diagnosis? What is your management of this child? Be sure to include physical, educational, and follow-up needs.

4. Compare and contrast the outpatient management of a 5-year-old and a 15-year-old with acute bacterial pneumonia. Be sure to consider physical and epidemiologic differences between the age groups.

5. Develop a phone protocol for a 2-year-old with acute LTB that incorporates (1) essential management components, (2) signs that require further evaluation, (3) patient educational guidance, and (4) follow-up plan.

REFERENCES

Alexander ME: Syncope. In Burg FD et al, editors: *Current pediatric therapy*, ed 18, Philadelphia, 2006, WB Saunders Elsevier.

Allen JL: Bronchitis and bronchiolitis. In Burg FD et al, editors: *Current pediatric therapy*, ed 18, Philadelphia, 2006, WB Saunders Elsevier.

Aurivillius M et al: Is susceptibility to severe respiratory syncytial virus (RSV) infection genetically determined? *Acta Paediatr* 94:414-418, 2005.

Behrman RE, Kliegman RM, Jenson HB, editors: *Nelson textbook of pediatrics*, ed 16, Philadelphia, 2000, WB Saunders,

Behrman RE, Kliegman RM, Jenson HB, editors: *Nelson textbook of pediatrics*, ed 17, Philadelphia, 2004, WB Saunders.

Cherry JD, Harrison RE: *Bordetella* pertussis (whooping cough). In Burg FD et al, editors: *Current pediatric therapy*, ed 18, Philadelphia, 2006, WB Saunders Elsevier.

Clegg HW et al: Treatment of streptococcal pharyngitis with once-daily compared with twice-daily amoxicillin: a noninferiority trial, *Pediatr Infect Dis J* 25:761-767, 2006.

Dovey ME: Cystic fibrosis. In Burg FD et al, editors: *Current pediatric therapy*, ed 18, Philadelphia, 2006, WB Saunders Elsevier.

Foca MD: Pneumonia. In Burg FD et al, editors: *Current pediatric therapy*, ed 18, Philadelphia, 2006, WB Saunders Elsevier.

Gerber MA: Group A streptococcal infections. In Burg FD et al, editors: *Current pediatric therapy*, ed 18, Philadelphia, 2006, WB Saunders Elsevier.

Hiltzik DH, de Serres LM: Tonsillectomy and adenoidectomy. In Burg FD et al, editors: *Current pediatric therapy*, ed 18, Philadelphia, 2006, WB Saunders Elsevier.

Jacobs IN: Croup and epiglottitis. In Burg FD et al, editors: *Current pediatric therapy*, ed 18, Philadelphia, 2006, WB Saunders Elsevier.

Jenson HB, Baltimore RS: Infectious diseases. In Kleigman RE et al, editors: *Nelson essentials of pediatrics*, ed 5, Philadelphia, 2006, WB Saunders Elsevier.

Kinane TB, Scirica CV: Asthma. In Burg FD et al, editors: *Current pediatric therapy*, ed 18, Philadelphia, 2006, WB Saunders Elsevier.

Lavelle JM: Epistaxis and nasal trauma. In Burg FD et al, editors: *Current pediatric therapy*, ed 18, Philadelphia, 2006, WB Saunders Elsevier.

Marshall SG, Debley JS: The respiratory system. In Kliegman RE et al, editors: *Nelson essentials of pediatrics*, ed 5, Philadelphia, 2006, WB Saunders Elsevier.

Morer A et al: Antineuronal antibodies in a group of children with obsessive-compulsive disorder and Tourette syndrome, *J Psychiatr Res* 42(1):64-68, 2006.

Shrime MG, Keller JL: Pediatric rhinitis and acute and chronic sinusitis. In Burg FD et al, editors: *Current pediatric therapy*, ed 18, Philadelphia, 2006, WB Saunders Elsevier.

Steinberg LA, Knilands TK: Diagnostic tests to investigate children with syncope… high cost, low yield, *Pediatrics* 146:355-358, 2005.

Tom LW, Shah UK: Foreign bodies in the ears, nose, and pharynx. In Burg FD et al, editors: *Current pediatric therapy*, ed 18, Philadelphia, 2006, WB Saunders Elsevier.

Turner RB, Hayden GF: The common cold. In Behrman J, Kliegman RM, Jenson HB, editors: *Nelson textbook of pediatrics,* ed 17, Philadelphia, 2004, WB Saunders.

Wetmore RF: Tonsils and adenoids. In Behrman J, Kliegman RM, Jenson HB, editors: *Nelson textbook of pediatrics,* ed 17, Philadelphia, 2004, WB Saunders.

Young TH, Strong WB: Acute rheumatic fever. In Burg FD et al, editors: *Current pediatric therapy,* ed 18, Philadelphia, 2006, WB Saunders Elsevier.

CHAPTER 32

Gastrointestinal Disorders

Ann M. Petersen–Smith and Shirley Becton McKenzie

The gastrointestinal (GI) system functions to ingest and absorb nutrients and discard waste products. Appropriate functioning of the system is essential for normal growth and development and maintenance of other organ systems.

The pediatric primary care provider plays an integral role in the care of children with GI dysfunction. A thorough understanding of the anatomy, physiology, and common disorders of the GI system is needed to appropriately assess and treat pediatric GI problems. This chapter focuses on GI disorders that involve organic pathologic conditions. Functional problems of the GI system, such as obesity, anorexia, bulimia, encopresis, and constipation, are discussed in Chapters 11 and 13.

ANATOMY AND PHYSIOLOGY

The GI system begins to develop during the third week of gestation. The primitive gut is initially formed and then divides into the foregut, midgut, and hindgut. The structures further develop in an intricate and complex fashion to become the digestive tract and accessory organs.

The GI tract extends from the mouth to the anus. It includes the organs of digestion and accessory organs, such as the liver, pancreas, and gallbladder. The system provides the following functions:

- Ingestion of food
- Movement of food from the mouth toward the rectum
- Mechanical dissolution of food
- Chemical dissolution of food
- Absorption of nutrients
- Expulsion of waste products

The mouth serves as the site for ingestion, chewing, and mixing of food with saliva. The tongue senses the texture and taste of foods, which initiates salivation and release of gastric juices in the stomach. The esophagus transports food from the mouth to the stomach by *peristalsis*, the sequential contraction and relaxation of the musculature in the esophagus. The upper esophageal sphincter prevents air from being swallowed while breathing. The lower esophageal sphincter (LES) prevents food from being regurgitated from the stomach, which is important because intraabdominal pressure exceeds intrathoracic and atmospheric pressures. The stomach serves as a reservoir for ingested foods. It secretes digestive juices, mixes food with the gastric fluids, and propels the liquid material into the small intestine. The small intestine's primary function is absorption of nutrients (carbohydrates, fats, proteins, minerals, and vitamins) into the systemic circulation. Absorption occurs through villi, which cover the mucosal folds and serve

as the functional unit of the intestine. Each villus contains an artery, a vein, and a lymph vessel, which serve to transport nutrients from the intestine into the systemic circulation. The villi are covered with enterocytes, whose major role is the digestion of carbohydrates and proteins. Enterocytes secrete proteins and enzymes known as brush border enzymes, which assist in digestion.

Carbohydrates must be converted to monosaccharides before their absorption is possible. This process begins in the mouth, where the salivary enzyme amylase breaks down complex starches into disaccharides. The brush border enzymes in the small intestine convert disaccharides into monosaccharides (sucrose to glucose and fructose, lactose to glucose and galactose, and maltose to glucose). When this process is hindered, disaccharides remain osmotically active and can cause diarrhea.

Fat absorption, which occurs mainly in the jejunum, is accomplished through the addition of lipases secreted by the pancreas. Lipases break down fats into particles that are easily absorbed by the villi. Fats then rely on the lymphatic system for absorption.

Proteins are converted to amino acids by pancreatic enzymes. The resulting amino acids are further divided into smaller amino acid particles that are absorbed via the brush border into the systemic circulation. After appropriate absorption of nutrients, the small intestine is left with the initial fecal liquid. This liquid is then propelled by peristalsis into the large intestine. The large intestine removes water from the fecal liquid and allows for short-term storage. The fecal mass, which consists of waste products, bacteria, intestinal secretions, and shed cells, is pushed into the sigmoid colon.

Entry of feces into the rectum stimulates the defecation reflex. This reflex stretches the rectal wall, relaxes the internal anal sphincter, and thereby creates the need to defecate. If this urge is ignored, further fluid resorption occurs as the stool is retained, increases in mass, and becomes very dry. Excessive stretching of the colon from the hard, dry stool bolus can lead to decreased peristalsis, further complicating the retention of stool.

PATHOPHYSIOLOGY

The GI tract can be affected by illness, injury, or generalized problems that prevent it from functioning normally. Dysfunction can be localized or systemic. Categories of dysfunction include the following:

- Disorders of motility
- Infection
- Malabsorption syndromes

- Impairment of digestion, absorption, and nutrition
- Congenital malformations
- Genetic syndromes
- Metabolic disorders
- Behavioral problems
- Injuries and trauma

■ ASSESSMENT

HISTORY

The history assesses the following:

- Family history of gallbladder disease, ulcers, or allergy to any food product
- Past medical history related to the GI system (e.g., illnesses, surgeries, anatomic problems, such as cleft lip or palate, esophageal atresia)
- Presence of pain (onset, location, type, quality, and aggravating and alleviating factors)
- Bowel habits (frequency, times per week, consistency, associated pain, the need for aids, such as medications or enemas)
- Constipation and diarrhea (patient's definition of each, how often they occur, treatment tried thus far)
- Changes in appetite
- Thirst level (increased or decreased)
- Food intolerance or allergy (what foods, symptoms, treatment)
- Belching and flatulence
- Vomiting
- Heartburn
- Feeding habits and nutrition history or current diet (what, when, how often, what tolerated)
- Other signs or symptoms, such as apnea or asthma, may be caused by gastroesophageal reflux (GER)

PHYSICAL EXAMINATION

When assessing a suspected GI problem, a head-to-toe physical examination is frequently indicated.

- Plot growth parameters, including weight for height, to establish proportionality of the patient and exclude certain growth aberrations from the diagnosis.
- Determine body mass index (BMI). The BMI is one of the first indicators used to assess body fat and is a common method of tracking weight problems and obesity in children 2 years and older (see Chapter 11 for more details).
- Determine hydration status (skin turgor, mucous membranes, peripheral pulses, tears).
- Inspect the abdomen for visible peristalsis, rashes, lesions, asymmetry, masses, enlarged organs, and pulsations.
- Auscultate for frequency of bowel sounds (normal is 5 to 20 per minute).
- Percuss for density and to measure organs.
- Palpate both lightly and deeply.
- Assess peritoneal irritation:
  ○ Have the patient walk standing straight up or cough.
  ○ Have the patient stand on tiptoes and fall onto the heels or jump once.
  ○ Palpate for rebound tenderness.
  ○ Check for the obturator sign: A supine patient flexes the right thigh at the hip with the knee bent and internally rotates the hip. The sign is positive when it induces abdominal pain.
  ○ Check for the psoas sign: The patient lies on the left side and extends and then flexes the right leg at the hip. A positive sign is one that induces abdominal pain.
- Perform a rectal examination when intraabdominal, pelvic, or perirectal disease is suspected. This examination includes external inspection and internal palpation for masses, stool, or irregularities. The index finger is typically used because of its increased sensitivity; however, in infants and young children, use the fifth finger. Insert a gloved, lubricated finger into the rectum. Place the other hand on the abdomen for a bimanual examination. Young pediatric patients should be supine with their feet held together and knees and hips flexed, putting their legs over their abdomen. Adolescent males can be lying on their side or standing with the hips flexed and the upper part of the body on the examination table. Adolescent females can be lying on their side or, if a concurrent pelvic examination is to be done, in the lithotomy position.
- Perform a gynecologic examination if a pathologic pelvic condition is suspected (see Chapter 35).

COMMON DIAGNOSTIC STUDIES

Laboratory tests are performed as indicated by the history, initial symptoms, and physical examination and include the following:

- Urinalysis (UA) and urine culture
- Complete blood count (CBC) with differential
- Serum chemistry screen, liver profile, lipid profile, erythrocyte sedimentation rate (ESR), C-reactive protein (CRP), thyroid function
- Stool examination for ova and parasites (O&P), culture, blood, white blood cells, pH, Clinitest for reducing substances
- Fecal fat collection for 72 hours to rule out fat malabsorption
- Radiologic examination, including abdominal radiographs, computerized axial tomography scan, abdominal and pelvic ultrasonography (US), chest radiographs (there can be referred abdominal pain with pneumonia), upper and lower GI series, and radionuclide studies with scintiscan, depending on the suspected pathologic condition
- Bone age to assess suspected growth abnormalities
- Pregnancy test
- Urine tests for gonorrhea or chlamydia, Papanicolaou smear and vaginal cultures and/or smears if pelvic or gynecologic pathologic condition is suspected

Additional, more specialized tests can be ordered after consultation with a physician:

- Duodenal aspirate to identify existing infection
- Esophageal pH probe to establish GER, with a pH of less than 4 representing a reflux episode
- Capsule endoscopy
- Breath hydrogen test if lactose intolerance is suspected
- Sweat chloride test if cystic fibrosis (CF) is suspected (see Chapter 31).

MANAGEMENT STRATEGIES
MEDICATIONS

Many common medications are used to treat various GI disorders:

- Antibiotics or antifungals may be necessary for bacterial or fungal infection.
- Antiemetics can be used to treat nausea or vomiting.
- Antidiarrheals are occasionally appropriate for persistent diarrhea or diarrhea associated with chronic disease, but they are never appropriate with acute diarrheal diseases because toxins need to be excreted from the body.
- Stool softeners, laxatives, and cathartics are useful in the acute treatment and long-term management of constipation and encopresis.
- Medications that alter GI motility or tone can be used to treat GER.
- Oral steroids, parenteral steroids, and other immunosuppressants may be indicated in the treatment of inflammatory bowel disease.
- Pain medication and antispasmodics may occasionally be used in selected acute and chronic GI conditions.
- Medications that alter gastric acidity can be used to treat GER and ulcer disease.
- Iron supplementation may be needed as supportive therapy for chronic disease.

Probiotics

Probiotics can be used as dietary supplements. Probiotics are live microorganisms that, when ingested and colonized in the bowel, can have a therapeutic or preventive health benefit. Their effects have been most extensively studied in diarrheal disease and inflammatory bowel disease. Probiotics may be antagonistic to *Helicobacter pylori*, reduce symptoms of atopic disease, and be helpful in infant immunity (Markowitz & Bengmark, 2002; Vanderhoof & Young, 2002; Weng & Walker, 2006). Huebner and Surawicz (2006) found there may be a role for probiotics in traveler's diarrhea, antibiotic-associated diarrhea, and recurrent *Clostridium difficile*–associated disease. See Chapter 42 for further information.

NUTRITION

Normal nutrition that meets the recommended daily needs should be encouraged to promote normal GI function, growth, and development. Intake of fluids to ensure hydration is equally important. Dysfunction of the GI tract can be either short term or long term and can require alterations in dietary intake. Consultation with a registered dietitian is important in designing an adequate diet for a child with a long-term GI problem. See Chapter 11 for more detail.

ACTIVITY

Age-appropriate activity should be encouraged on a regular basis to help maintain normal GI function. Some GI maladies require short-term rest, but generally the system functions better when activity is regular and consistent.

COUNSELING AND EDUCATION

It is important to spend time assessing and planning for the unique needs of a child with GI dysfunction. Helping the family understand the disease or disorder and its course, prognosis, and management is essential. Planning for specific needs related to medication, diet, and activity assists the family to normalize life for the child.

UPPER GASTROINTESTINAL TRACT DISORDERS
DYSPHAGIA
Description

The pathophysiology of feeding and swallowing is complex. There are three phases of feeding and swallowing known as oral, pharyngeal, and esophageal (Miller & Willging, 2003). The oral phase refers to ingestion, mastication, and the propulsion of food to the back of the mouth. Problems with the oral phase are generally sensory and/or oral motor dysfunction. The pharyngeal phase includes the swallowing and transfer of food from the pharynx to the esophagus. Airway closure is critical during the pharyngeal phase, and the child needs to have intact motor and sensory pharyngeal protective mechanisms to prevent aspiration. The esophageal phase allows for food to pass into the stomach. Problems in this phase are most commonly associated anatomic, functional, and inflammatory esophageal disorders.

In dysphagia, younger children are unable to swallow, and older children can have awareness that something is wrong with their swallowing ability. The number of children with swallowing difficulties has escalated in the last 20 years because the advances in technology have increased the survival of children with special health care needs (Miller & Willging, 2003).

Epidemiology

As many as 50% of children with feeding difficulties have a mixed etiology for their feeding disorder, and there is often an interplay of environmental and biologic factors (Rommel et al, 2003; Rudolph et al, 2002). Miller and Willging (2003) described a classification system for pediatric dysphagia including structural abnormalities, neurologic conditions, cardiorespiratory issues, metabolic dysfunction, oral-sensory and behavioral issues, or a dysfunctional feeding relationship between child and feeder. Pharyngeal, laryngeal, and esophageal lesions, foreign bodies, and tumors can also be responsible for symptoms.

Clinical Findings

History.   The following may be reported:

- Progressive dysfunction
- Persistent drooling or cough
- Symptoms, such as discomfort with swallowing or a sense of food getting stuck
- Picky eating (e.g., a child who prefers liquids to solids) or food refusal

Physical Examination

- Observe the infant or child feeding paying special attention to the adequacy of the child's oral motor skills and safety of swallowing.
- Perform a complete physical examination paying particular attention to mouth, throat, and neck.

Diagnostic Studies. Diagnostic tests may include:
- Lateral neck films
- Barium swallow
- Videofluoroscopy is the gold standard
- Fiberoptic endoscopic evaluation of swallowing
- Endoscopy and manometry
- Functional magnetic resonance imaging
- Electromyography

Differential Diagnosis

Obstructive and compressive lesions usually cause trouble only with solids. Physiologic dysfunction is usually associated with systemic disease, and the patient has trouble with both liquids and solids. Cricopharyngeal dysphagia involves nasopharyngeal regurgitation and aspiration and is associated with Chiari I malformation (Ruark et al, 2002). Eosinophilic esophagitis causes feeding difficulty or refusal, pain, vomiting, or food impactions (Khan, 2003).

Management

A multidisciplinary approach is recommended including health professionals from the following specialty areas: otolaryngology, gastroenterology, nutrition, occupational therapy, psychology, and speech-language pathology. This approach provides a comprehensive, cost-effective evaluation and promotes consistent care for the child and family.

VOMITING AND DEHYDRATION

Description

Vomiting is the forceful emptying of gastric contents. Nonbilious vomit is generally caused by infection, inflammation, metabolic, neurologic, or psychological problems. An obstructive lesion generally causes bilious vomiting. Bloody vomit accompanies active bleeding in the GI tract.

Dehydration is the loss of water and extracellular fluid. In 2003 the Centers for Disease Control and Prevention (CDC) recommended there be only two classifications of dehydration: mild to moderate (3% to 9%) and severe (greater than 9%) because the treatment for mild and moderate is essentially the same (Bender et al, 2005). Depending on the cause of dehydration, water and salts (primarily sodium chloride) may be lost in physiologic proportion or lost disparately, producing one of three types of dehydration: isonatremic (isotonic), hypernatremic (hypertonic), and hyponatremic (hypotonic). When dehydration is caused by simple diarrhea, homeostatic mechanisms can usually maintain sodium concentrations in the serum, resulting in isonatremia. When vomiting occurs with diarrhea and water intake is less, there is greater water loss than salt loss, potentially resulting in hypernatremic dehydration. When there is massive stool loss of water and salt and only water is ingested, there is a large salt loss, potentially resulting in hyponatremia.

Epidemiology

Vomiting is one of the most common symptoms in childhood. Following is a list of potential causes of vomiting by site of origin:

- Oropharynx: cleft palate and laryngopharyngeal cleft
- Upper GI: congenital stricture, foreign body, gastritis and/or esophagitis, gastric web pyloric stenosis, tracheoesophageal fistula, vascular ring, peptic ulcer disease (PUD)
- Small intestine: annular pancreas, choledochal cyst, intestinal atresias and stenoses, intestinal malrotation with volvulus, intestinal pseudoobstruction
- Colon: Hirschsprung disease, intussusception, meconium ileus, necrotizing enterocolitis, fecal impaction
- Hepatobiliary or pancreatic dysfunction
- Infections: bacterial enteritis, otitis media, sepsis, urinary tract infection (UTI), viral gastroenteritis (VGE), hepatitis
- Neurologic: congenital anatomic malformation, gray and white matter degenerative disorders, hydrocephalus, kernicterus, brain tumors, migraine headache, head trauma
- Other: cow's milk protein allergy, inborn errors of metabolism, maternal drug exposure and/or withdrawal, toxic ingestions, appendicitis, cyclic vomiting, pneumonia, drug or alcohol ingestion, eating disorders, pregnancy

Clinical Findings

History. The history should assess the following:
- Parent concern regarding decreased tearing or depressed fontanelle in infants (this concern has been found to be directly associated with more severe dehydration and metabolic acidosis (Porter et al, 2003)
- Past history of illnesses, surgeries, or hospitalizations
- Medications currently being taken (including over-the-counter, herbal, cultural, and homeopathic remedies)
- Recent exposure to illness, injury, or stress
- Possibility of poisoning
- Family history of GI disease or fetal or neonatal deaths (metabolic syndrome, congenital anomaly)
- Onset and duration of vomiting, quality and quantity, presence of blood or bile, odor, precipitating event
- Relationship of vomiting to meals, time of day, or activities
- Vomiting early in the morning
- Presence of associated symptoms: diarrhea, fever, ear pain, UTI symptoms, vision changes, cough, headache, seizures, high-pitched cry, polydipsia, polyuria, polyphagia, anorexia
- Symptoms of dehydration (Table 32-1)

Physical Examination. The following are needed:
- Assessment of dehydration (see Table 32-1). One of the most useful clinical signs of hydration is capillary refill time (CRT). Normal CRT is less than 2 seconds. Steiner and colleagues (2004) found that CRT, skin turgor, and tachypnea, when considered together, were the most helpful in the determination of dehydration.
- Growth parameters and vital signs.
- Neurologic examination: nuchal rigidity, decreased level of consciousness, and behavioral changes, which can include irritability or lethargy. Sensorium remains intact until there is greater than 6% of weight loss as a result of dehydration. Hypotension is a late manifestation of dehydration.
- Abdominal examination: Inspect for distention, abdominal scars from previous surgery (may be associated with obstruction and/or adhesions), or visible peristaltic waves. Auscultate

TABLE 32-1 **Estimation of Dehydration**

Characteristic	Extent of Dehydration			
	Mild	**Moderate**	**Severe**	**Shock**
Weight loss—infants (%)	3-5	5-10	10-15	>15
Weight loss—children (%)	3-4	6-8	10	
Pulse	Normal	Slightly increased	Very increased	Rapid and weak
Blood pressure	Normal	Normal to orthostatic, >10 mm Hg change	Orthostatic to shock	
Behavior	Normal	Irritable, more thirsty	Hyperirritable to lethargic	Difficult to awaken or unresponsive; too weak to stand; very dizzy
Thirst	Slight	Moderate	Intense	
Mucous membranes*	Normal	Dry	Parched	
Tears	Present	Decreased	Absent; sunken eyes	
Anterior fontanelle	Normal	Normal to sunken	Sunken	
External jugular vein	Visible when supine	Not visible except with supraclavicular pressure	Not visible even with supraclavicular pressure	
Skin* (signs and symptoms less useful in children >2 yr old)	Capillary refill >2 sec	Slowed capillary refill, 2-4 sec (decreased turgor)	Very delayed capillary refill (>4 sec) and tenting; skin cool, acrocyanotic, or mottled*	CRT >4 sec; cold and/or acrocyanotic
Urine production	Slight decrease	Infants: no urine for >8 hr; children: no urine for >12 hr	Very decreased or absent	Anuria
Urine specific gravity	>1.020	>1.020; oliguria	Oliguria or anuria	

*These signs are less prominent in patients who have hypernatremia.
CRT, Capillary refill time; *hr*, hour(s); *sec*, seconds; *yr*, years.

bowel sounds (i.e., increased with gastroenteritis, decreased with obstruction, absent with ileus or peritonitis). Palpate the abdomen for pain. Assess abdominal organs (liver and spleen size, masses). Perform a rectal examination as indicated.
- Respiratory examination: tachypnea, decreased oxygen saturation.
- Perform a pelvic examination as indicated.

   Diagnostic Studies.   Diagnostic studies are performed as indicated by the probable diagnosis:
- CBC with differential, blood culture.
- Electrolytes, glucose, and liver function tests. Steiner and colleagues (2004) found that serum bicarbonate below 15 to 17 mEq/L was the most valuable laboratory test to make the diagnosis of dehydration.
- CRP and ESR.
- Blood and urine tests for metabolic disorders may only be abnormal during episodes of vomiting, and measurements of serum lactate, serum and urine carnitine, and urine for δ-aminolevulinic acid and porphobilinogen may be helpful (Orenstein & Peters, 2004).
- UA and urine culture.
- Toxicology screen.
- Stool for culture and occult blood, leukocytes, parasites, fat, pH as indicated.
- Rapid strep test and/or throat culture.

- Pregnancy test.
- Abdominal radiographs (suspected obstruction or foreign body ingestion, organomegaly, or a palpable mass).
- Chest radiograph (suspected pneumonia).
- US (abscesses, masses, stenoses, cysts, appendicitis, pyloric stenosis).
- Barium swallow or enema (malrotation, pyloric stenosis, GER, masses).
- Endoscopy (obstruction, hemorrhage, infection; collect biopsies).
- Esophageal pH probe analysis.
- Computed tomography (CT) scan or magnetic resonance imaging (MRI) to diagnose masses, inflammation, herniations, perforations, and obstructions.
- Electroencephalogram (EEG).

Differential Diagnosis

The age of the child may help to formulate an appropriate list of potential diagnoses (Orenstein & Peters, 2004). For the newborn, vomiting may be a symptom of a congenital obstructive malformation, such as an atresia or web, meconium ileus, or Hirschsprung disease. Infants may be overfed, have gastroenteritis, UTI, a mild obstructive lesion, pyloric stenosis, malrotation, or volvulus. Vomiting in infants may also be due to intussusception, a metabolic disorder or an inborn error of metabolism, nutrient intolerance, GER, or a psychosocial disorder, such as rumination associated with emotional maltreatment. A child of any age may have gastroenteritis, PUD, GER, UTI, pyelonephritis, hepatic disease, small bowel obstruction, cholecystitis, appendicitis, pneumonia, rheumatologic disorders, increased intracranial pressure, migraine headache, poisoning, or many other conditions. In addition, vomiting in later childhood and adolescence may signal pregnancy, pelvic inflammatory disease (PID), alcohol or drug ingestion, or an eating disorder.

Management

The following steps are taken:
- Determine the degree of dehydration and treat the cause.
- Use antiemetics as indicated. A single dose of an oral disintegrating tablet of ondansetron (2 mg for children 8 to 15 kg, 4 mg for children 15 to 30 kg, and 8 mg for greater than 30 kg) reduces vomiting, which decreases the chance of dehydration, increases the success of oral hydration, decreases the need for intravenous hydration, and decreases time at the hospital (Freedman et al, 2006; Roslund et al, 2006; Stork et al, 2005).
- Rehydrate (Table 32-2). A period of gut rest is not recommended (King et al, 2003). Introduce an appropriate rehydration solution. Avoid plain water, apple juice, soda, milk, and sports drinks because none of these liquids provides appropriate replacement of sugars and electrolytes (Table 32-3).

Begin with small amounts (as little as 5 to 10 ml) of clear liquids every 5 to 10 minutes. Breastfed infants should continue to breastfeed more frequently for shorter periods of time.
- ○ Oral rehydration should be attempted with every patient, if possible, because it can be instituted more quickly and less time is spent in the emergency department compared with intravenous rehydration management (Spandorfer et al, 2005).
- ○ Oral rehydration is not indicated in cases of hemodynamic shock, abdominal ileus, or suspected bowel obstruction (King et al, 2003).
- Resume maintenance fluid levels (see Table 32-2).
- Refeeding should resume as quickly as possible because the gut needs nutrition to facilitate mucosal repair following injury. Breastfed infants should continue breastfeeding during an episode of vomiting if possible. Formula-fed infants should resume full strength formula as quickly as possible. There is no benefit in giving a child diluted formula. Children should return to a regular diet as soon as possible, eating smaller amounts of bland solids more often. Bland solids might include complex carbohydrates, bananas, applesauce, pretzels, and rice or rice cereal.
- Monitor urine output.
- Treat fever.
- Refer if the child has a toxic appearance or moderate to severe dehydration, projectile vomiting, abnormal examination, vomiting for greater than 12 hours, or vomiting of blood, bile, or fecal matter.

TABLE 32-2	Treatment of Dehydration

Rehydration (With Increased Sodium Concentration)		
Mild	ORS	40-50 mL/kg over 4 hr (10 mL/kg/hr)
Moderate	ORS	60-100 mL/kg over 4-6 hr (20 mL/kg/hr)
Severe	IV fluids	Ringer's lactate or normal saline, 20-mL/kg bolus over 1 hr; may repeat bolus if needed (until pulse, perfusion, mental status are normal)
		Follow with 5% dextrose with NaCl and KCl added (once the child has voided) for maintenance fluids and abnormal loss replacement (see later); if severe dehydration, give one half amount over 8 hr, the other one half over the next 16 hr; include bolus amounts in the 24-hr total
		Begin ORS as soon as possible
Maintenance		
Total water volume	0-10 kg	100 mL/kg/24 hr
	10-20 kg	1000 mL + 50 mL/kg for each kg over 10 kg/24 hr
	>20 kg	1500 mL + 20 mL/kg for each kg over 20 kg/24 hr
Replacement of fluid losses (if continued, heavy losses)		
10 mL/kg or 4-8 oz of ORS for each diarrhea stool (1 to 1.5 times the amount of stool)		
Refeeding		
Reintroduce age-appropriate diet as quickly as possible. Avoid fatty foods and foods high in simple sugars.		
Encourage complex carbohydrates, lean meats, yogurt, bananas, and applesauce.		
Formula-fed infants should have full-strength formula. If that is not tolerated, use lactose-free or soy formula.		
Breastfeeding infants should continue to breastfeed with shorter duration and more frequent feedings.		
For children quickly return to regular milk in smaller amounts more often. May give up to 150 mL/kg in first 24 hr.		

hr, Hours; *IV,* intravenous; *ORS,* oral rehydration solution.

TABLE 32-3   **Rehydration Solutions**

Stool	Sodium*	Chlorine*	Potassium*	Base Type	Base Concentration*	Carbohydrate Type	Carbohydrate Concentration (g/L)	Osmolality
Pediatric diarrheal stool	50-100	75-90	25-35	HCO_3	25-40	—	—	250-300
Oral Rehydration Solutions								
Recommended:								
WHO ORS[‖]	90	80	20	Citrate	30	Glucose	20	<300
WHO recommendations for ORS solutions	60-90	50-80	20-30	Citrate	20	Glucose	25-35	<300
Pedialyte (Ross)	45	35	20	Citrate	30	Glucose	25	<264
Rehydralyte (Ross)	75	65	20	Citrate	30	Glucose	25	<327
Cereal-based ORS	60-90	—[†]	—[†]	—[†]	—[†]	Starch[‡]	50	200-225
Infalyte (Mead-Johnson)	50	45	25	Citrate	34	Rice syrup solids	30	
Home sugar-salt solution	30-60	30-60	—	—	—	Sucrose	40	170-230
Other solutions:								
Soft drinks, cola, etc.	2	(—)[§]	0.1	HCO_3	13	F/G	50-150	<550
Apple juice	3	(—)[§]	32	—	0	F/G/S	63	<700
Chicken broth	250	(—)[§]	5	—	0	—	0	<450
Gatorade	20	(—)[§]	3	HCO_3	3	G/others	45	<330
Intravenous Solutions								
Recommended:								
Ringer's lactate	135	90	4	Lactate	49	—	—	<278
Normal saline	135	135	0	—	0	—	—	<270
5% dextrose in saline	135	135	0	—	0	Glucose	50	<545
Not recommended:								
5% dextrose in water	0	0	0	—	0	Glucose	50	<275

*In millimoles or milliequivalents per liter.
[†]Variable.
[‡]From various cereals: rice, wheat, sorghum, etc.
[§]Value not reported.
[‖]Not available in the U.S., but used worldwide.
F, Fructose; *G*, glucose; *ORS*, oral rehydration solution; *S*, sucrose; *WHO*, World Health Organization.
From Northrup RS, Flanigan TP: Gastroenteritis, *Pediatr Rev* 15(12):461-472, 1994.

CYCLIC VOMITING SYNDROME

Description

Cyclic vomiting syndrome (CVS), first described by Samuel Gee in 1882, is characterized by at least three episodes of recurrent, intense nausea and unremitting vomiting between which the child is completely well. The periods of vomiting may last hours or even days, and the symptom-free periods may last for weeks or even months. There is no evidence of metabolic, GI, central nervous system, or biochemical disease (Lindley & Andrews, 2005). CVS is sometimes referred to as abdominal migraine. Cyclic vomiting may occur any time between infancy and adulthood; however, it is most commonly diagnosed between 3 and 7 years old (Bullard & Page, 2005).

Although the typical child with CVS is healthy up to 90% of the time, there is substantial morbidity and medical costs when episodes occur because of missed days of school per child (average 20), high rate of intravenous rehydration, and the cost of laboratory and imaging studies, endoscopic procedures, emergency department visits, and missed work by parent.

Epidemiology

There is strong evidence that CVS has a maternal inheritance pattern. Affected individuals tend to have mothers and maternal grandmothers who have a higher incidence of migraine headaches, depression, anxiety, irritable bowel syndrome (IBS), and hypothyroidism (Boles et al, 2005). Most children appear to outgrow CVS before or during the preteen years; however, approximately 28% of children with CVS suffer migraine headaches as adolescents and adults (Li & Balint, 2000).

Clinical Findings

History

- Very careful listening is important! This diagnosis is made primarily on history.
- Three questions are essential to make the diagnosis of CVS (Li & Howard, 2002):
  - Has the child had at least three episodes? (100% respond, "Yes.")
  - Is the child completely asymptomatic between episodes? (100% respond, "Yes.")
  - Are the episodes stereotypical? (98% respond, "Yes.")
- Recurrent episodes tend to be stereotypic for the child. Episodes usually last 24 to 48 hours; they occur at regular intervals, usually every 2 to 4 weeks, although many children have unpredictable episodes.
- The child may have a prodromal period (some combination of pallor, anorexia, nausea, abdominal pain, or lethargy) or a recovery period (from ill to playing again) that is brief.
- Episodes more likely to occur at night (2:00 to 4:00 AM) or early in the morning (6:00 to 7:00 AM).
- Episodes generally begin and end abruptly.
- There is an identifiable trigger in 80% of children—infection, psychological stress, food products (e.g., chocolate, cheese, monosodium glutamate), physical exhaustion or lack of sleep, atopic events, motion sickness, and menstruation (Lindley & Andrews, 2005).
- There is intense nausea not relieved by vomiting.
- Vomiting may occur as frequently as every 5 to 10 minutes, unmatched in any other disorder.
- Abdominal pain, retching, diarrhea, and fever may occur.
- Headache, motion sickness, photophobia, phonophobia, or vertigo may occur.
- Family history positive for migraine headache is common.

  Physical Examination. Children with CVS appear substantially more ill than children with VGE.

- There may be abnormal posturing (parkinsonian or fetal), social withdrawal, lethargy that may be profound (unable to walk or talk, may look semicomatose), pallor, and excessive salivation (Lindley & Andrews, 2005).
- Other symptoms of autonomic dysregulation (hyperpyrexia, skin blotching, headache, abdominal pain, hypertension, tachycardia, and leukocytosis).

  Diagnostic Studies. Laboratory testing during a vomiting episode is needed to exclude other diagnoses:

- Electrolytes, serum pH, glucose, lactate, ammonia, amino acids, carnitine species, and amylase
- UA, urinary ketones and organic acids, urine microscopy, and urine culture
- Upper GI contrast studies
- Abdominal and renal US
- Intestinal biopsy
- MRI or CT of head or sinuses

Differential Diagnosis

CVS is a diagnosis of exclusion. Less than four bouts of emesis per hour or more that two episodes per week is more likely to be chronic vomiting and suggests other pathologic conditions. "Red flags" to be aware of and to guide further evaluation include severe GI symptoms (bilious vomiting, abdominal tenderness, and/or severe abdominal pain) that could indicate hydronephrosis, cholelithiasis, pancreatic disease, or ureteropelvic junction obstruction (Schulte-Bockholt et al, 2002; Weinstein, 2005). CVS precipitated by concurrent illness, fasting, or high-protein meals could indicate a metabolic disorder. An abnormal neurologic exam (e.g., altered mental status, abnormal eye movements, or gait abnormalities) is suggestive of increased intracranial pressure. Approximately 12% of children with CVS-like history have a specific underlying disorder and may require referral to a gastroenterologist (Li & Howard, 2002; Lindley & Andrews, 2005).

Management

Treatment and supportive measures include the following (Bullard & Page, 2005; Cyclic Vomiting Syndrome Association, 2005; Khasawinah et al, 2003; Lindley & Andrews, 2005):

- Identify and treat and avoid precipitating factors.
- Medications to treat the episode once it has started (ondansetron, granisetron, sumatriptan, ketorolac, diphenhydramine, lorazepam). Early pharmacotherapy is essential. May need to consider sublingual, rectal, and intravenous routes of administration.
- Prokinetics (e.g., erythromycin)
- Prophylactic medication to prevent episodes:
  - Antimigraine medications: cyproheptadine, amitriptyline, propranolol
  - Anticonvulsants: phenobarbital, carbamazepine
  - Antidepressants: amitriptyline, nortriptyline
  - Contraceptives for episodes associated with menstruation
- Sedation to reduce nausea and induce sleep (lorazepam or chlorpromazine given with diphenhydramine)
- Analgesics as needed (ketorolac, ibuprofen)
- Intravenous fluids to replace losses and prevent dehydration
- H_2 receptor antagonists to prevent peptic esophagitis (cimetidine, famotidine, and ranitidine)
- Quiet, dark room
- Alternative modalities (e.g., biofeedback, massage, and/or imagery)
- Family support

  Referral to a gastroenterologist is recommended when further testing is needed (endoscopy), when atypical or "red flag" symptoms occur (see Box 32-3, p. 820), or if the child fails to respond to treatment.

GASTROESOPHAGEAL REFLUX

Description

GER refers to the passage of gastric contents into the esophagus from the stomach through the LES. Three classifications of GER are recognized:

- *Physiologic:* Infrequent, episodic vomiting. Suwandhi and colleagues (2006) suggest that physiologic GER is a normal phenomenon that usually resolves by 1 year old, but can last up to 18 months old. After 18 months, an increase in frequency or duration of reflux episodes or impaired esophageal acid clearance indicates a pathologic process.

- ○ *Functional:* Painless, effortless vomiting with no physical sequelae.
- ○ *Pathologic:* Frequent vomiting with alteration in physical functioning (e.g., esophagitis, failure to thrive [FTT], and aspiration pneumonia). This combination of symptoms is labeled gastroesophageal reflux disease (GERD). Older children are likely to have GERD similar to adults.

Epidemiology

The etiology is unclear and probably multifactorial. Inappropriate relaxation of the LES is the likely cause of most GER with failure to prevent gastric acid reflux into the esophagus, prolonged esophageal clearance of the gastric refluxate, and impaired esophageal mucosal barrier function (Suwandhi et al, 2006). The LES usually is influenced by intraabdominal pressure, hormones, neurologic control, and age. LES tone is normal in infants and children with GER. Young infants have increased intraabdominal pressure because of their inability to sit upright.

Alterations in swallowing, pharyngeal coordination, and esophageal motility and delayed gastric emptying are also potential factors related to GER. Children with neurodevelopmental disability commonly have GER. Increased muscle tone, chronic supine positioning, and altered GI motility exacerbate GER.

Up to 70% of infants less than 1700g have pathologic GER. Forty percent have symptomatic improvement by 4 months old, and 85% are symptom free by 12 months old (Sondheimer, 2005).

Clinical Findings

History. Important historical information to elicit includes the following:

- Careful birth, medical, and social history
- Concerns about feeding difficulty, pulling from the bottle or breast, refusing to eat, crying, choking, coughing, wheezing, apnea, weight loss, irritability, continuous unexplained crying, recurrent respiratory infections, pneumonia, and bloody emesis in younger children
- FTT
- Acute life-threatening event (ALTE)
- Sandifer syndrome (abnormal behavior and posturing with tilting of the head to one side and bizarre contortions of the trunk) generally considered to be the result of a protective reflex to prevent refluxate from reaching the upper esophagus (Cavataio & Guandalini, 2005; Rudolph, 2003)
- Heartburn, painful belching, headache, dyspnea, abdominal pain, stool pattern changes, dental caries, or recurrent pneumonia
- A 24-hour diet history and discussion of feeding circumstances

Physical Examination. Findings can include the following:

- Signs of FTT
- Torticollis
- Hoarseness
- Anemia

- Tooth erosion resulting from destruction of enamel by gastric acids caused by frequent vomiting
- Rash, recurrent diarrhea, persistent vomiting, or early-morning vomiting (symptoms of other primary disease with GER as a secondary problem)

Diagnostic Studies. In most infants with vomiting and in older children with regurgitation and heartburn, a history and physical examination are sufficient to reliably diagnose GER, recognize complications, and initiate treatment. The following tests may be obtained. Special studies should be ordered as indicated following consultation with a physician or a pediatric gastroenterologist.

- Esophageal pH monitoring is the gold standard to diagnose (Suwandhi et al, 2006). The test is a reliable way to diagnose GER, with a pH lower than 4 indicating reflux; however, esophageal pH may be normal in some patients with GER, especially those with respiratory complications (Cavataio & Guandalini, 2005; NASPGN, 2001, Rudolph et al, 2001).
- Upper GI series (test is neither sensitive nor specific for the diagnosis of GER, but is useful for the evaluation of anatomic abnormalities, such as pyloric stenosis or malrotation) (Cavataio & Guandalini, 2005; Rudolph, 2003).
- Endoscopy to obtain a biopsy, rule out esophagitis and other pathologic conditions if deemed necessary.
- Intraluminal esophageal impedance that measures episodes of GER independent of the pH of the fluid is especially useful for making a diagnosis in children with respiratory events related to GER because it can measure multiple indices, such as heart rate, oxygenation, sleep state, and apnea episodes. Unfortunately, this study lacks validation and established normal values in the pediatric population (Suwandhi et al, 2006).
- Radionucleotide scan with scintiscan can help to establish whether or not aspiration is caused by GER.
- Abdominal US to rule out pyloric stenosis if age-appropriate.
  Nonradiologic diagnostic tests as indicated:
- CBC with differential to rule out anemia and infection
- UA and urine culture
- Stool for occult blood
- Testing for *H. pylori*

Differential Diagnosis

Included in the differential diagnosis are anatomic obstruction, antral or esophageal webs, masses, malrotation, *H. pylori* infection, otitis media, UTI, gastroenteritis, formula intolerance, inborn errors of metabolism, brain tumors, increased intracranial pressure, Reye syndrome, obstructive uropathy, pancreatitis, and hepatobiliary problems.

Management

- See Figs. 32-1 and 32-2.
- A period of empiric therapy may be useful in determining if GER is causing a specific symptom. Treat first and refer for endoscopy later (Fox & Forgacs, 2006).
- Breastfed infants should continue to breastfeed.
- Formula-fed infants: There is evidence that a 1- to 2-week trial of a hypoallergenic formula in formula-fed infants

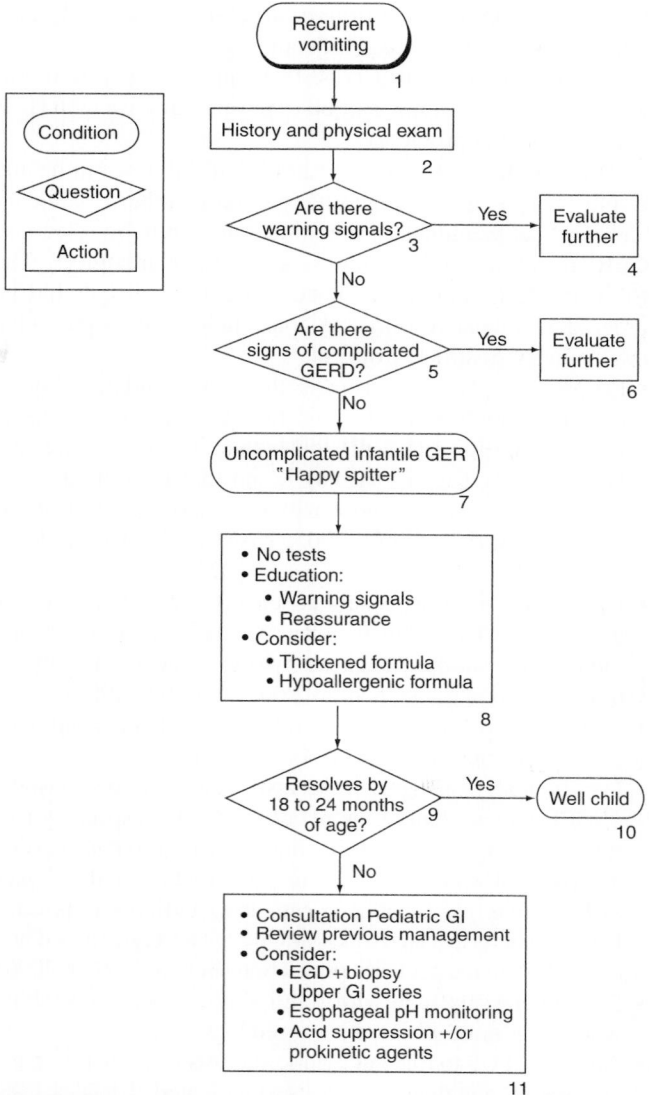

FIG. 32-1 Management of an infant with uncomplicated GERD (the "happy spitter"). *EGD*, esophagogastroduodenoscopy; *GI*, gastrointestinal. (From Mazur LJ, Smith HD: Gastroesophageal reflux. In Burg FD, Ingelfinger JR, Polin RA, et al: *Current pediatric therapy*, ed 18, Philadelphia, 2006, WB Saunders, p 533.)

is helpful. Use smaller, more frequent feedings and frequent burping during feedings. Milk-thickening agents or prethickened formulas may decrease the number of episodes of regurgitation, decrease the amount regurgitated per event, and decrease choke-gag-cough response to GER episode. However, it may not change the pH probe monitoring results, decrease the amount of crying, or increase the amount of time spent sleeping (Rudolph et al, 2001; Vanderhoof et al, 2003).

- Prone positioning is the most beneficial for infants with GER; however, the risk of sudden infant death syndrome (SIDS) outweighs the benefits associated with lying prone. The supine position is preferred in all infants, including

those with GER. In children older than 1 year, there is benefit to left-side positioning during sleep with the head of the bed elevated (McGuirt, 2003). Car seats should be avoided after meals.

- For older children, avoid chocolate, caffeine, high-fat foods, spicy foods, alcohol, and bedtime snacks. For children who are obese, weight loss is recommended.
- See Table 11-10 for feeding strategies in patients with GER.
- Medications can be helpful when the aforementioned measures have failed to give relief (Table 32-4). Lansoprazole is effective in healing erosive esophagitis and relieving GER symptoms. Children with asthma who had abnormal 24-hour pH studies, with and without GER, had clinical improvement of their asthma when treated medically for GERD (McQuirt, 2003; Rudolph, 2003).
  - Antacids short term may relieve symptoms by buffering acidic stomach acids; antacids containing aluminum should be used with caution.
  - H_2PAs provide healing of esophagitis.
  - PPIs maintain higher gastric pH and are indicated when H_2PA treatment fails.
  - Prokinetic agents theoretically should increase sphincter tone and help with delayed gastric emptying; potential severe side effects make their use controversial.
- Close follow-up of growth parameters to ensure adequate weight gain is important.
- Refer for Nissen fundoplication or similar surgical procedures if the GER is severe, not well managed medically, or causing significant secondary morbidity.

Complications

Complications include chronic cough, FTT, irritability, and malnutrition. Esophageal injury secondary to GER results in bleeding, stricture formation, and Barrett's esophagus (Suwandhi et al., 2006). GER and GERD are circumstantially associated with significant asthma, pneumonia, or laryngeal disorders; however, there may be clinical improvement of these conditions with treatment strategies for GER and GERD (Chang et al, 2006; McGuirt, 2003; Rudolph, 2003). GER may have a role in the initiation of otitis media with effusion (Tasker et al, 2002). The role of GER in infant apnea has been looked at; there is evidence, however, that only 12% of reflux events in infants are acidic, and there is no temporal relationship between non-acidic reflux and apnea in preterm infants. In fact, there is evidence that the apnea occurring with a GER episode may be protective in nature and prevents aspiration (Rudolph, 2003).

Patient Education

- Assure parents of infants that GER is usually self-limited and symptoms improve as the child grows.
- Remind parents that GER may temporarily worsen during illness.
- Review medication information, including dosages and side effects.

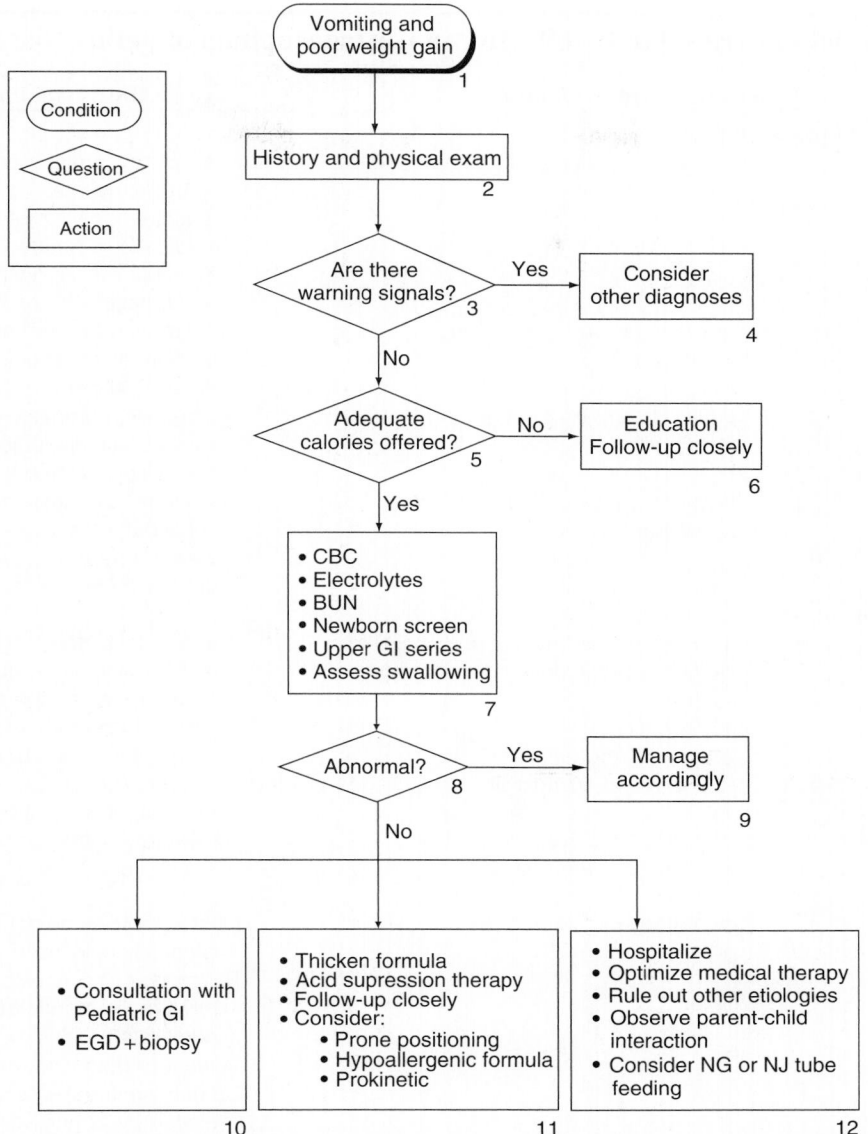

FIG. 32-2   Management of an infant with vomiting and poor weight gain. *BUN,* Blood urea nitrogen; *CBC,* complete blood count; *EGD,* esophago-gastroduodenoscopy; *GI,* gastrointestinal, *NG,* nasogastric; *NJ,* nasojejunal. (From Mazur LJ, Smith HD: Gastroesophageal reflux. In Burg FD, Ingelfinger JR, Polin RA, et al: *Current pediatric therapy,* ed 18, Philadelphia, 2006, WB Saunders, p 534.)

PEPTIC ULCER DISEASE (PUD)

Description

PUD consists of a group of gastric and duodenal disorders. With duodenal ulcers (DU), mucosal defects penetrate the duodenal mucosa and submucosa. Gastric ulcers (GU) result from mucosal defects that penetrate the gastric mucosa and submucosa.

Epidemiology

Most primary ulcers are duodenal, have no underlying cause, and tend to be chronic with resulting granulation tissue and fibrosis (Hassall, 2001). Secondary ulcers are more often gastric, generally more acute, and associated with known ulcerogenic events (Sondheimer, 2005). Ulceration in children is commonly associated with stressful situations, medications, and critical illness. A strong familial predisposition for PUD has been noted. There is no evidence that diet plays a role in the formation of ulcers. Chronic aspirin therapy and nonsteroidal antiinflammatory drugs (NSAIDs) cause gastric mucosal damage but are not associated with ulcer formation. Smoking can cause DUs and slow the rate of healing.

Primary GUs are about seven times less likely than DUs to occur in children. *Cytomegalovirus* (CMV) and *H. pylori* are associated with PUD in children. The incidence of *H. pylori* infection is 10% in children with PUD. Colonization rates have been suggested to be 8% to 63%. Colonization with *H. pylori* likely occurs early in life, but the infection often

TABLE 32-4   Drugs Demonstrated to Be Effective in Gastroesophageal Reflux Disease

Type of Medication	Recommended Oral Dosage	Adverse Effects and Precautions
Histamine₂-Receptor Antagonists		
Cimetidine (Tagamet)	40 mg/kg/day divided tid (adult dose: 400 qid-800 bid)	Rash, bradycardia, dizziness, nausea, vomiting, hypotension, gynecomastia, reduces hepatic metabolism of other medications, neutropenia, thrombocytopenia, agranulocytosis, doses should be decreased with renal insufficiency
Famotidine (Pepcid)	1 mg/kg/day divided bid (adult dose: 20-40 mg bid)	Headache, dizziness, constipation, diarrhea, nausea, doses should be decreased with renal insufficiency
Nizatidine (Axid)	7-8 mg/kg/day divided bid or tid (adult dose: 150 mg bid)	Headaches, dizziness, constipation, diarrhea, nausea, anemia, urticaria, doses should be decreased with renal insufficiency
Ranitidine (Zantac)	7-8 mg/kg/day divided bid or tid (adult dose: 150 mg bid)	Headache, dizziness, fatigue, irritability, rash, constipation, diarrhea, thrombocytopenia, elevated transaminases, doses should be decreased with renal insufficiency
Proton Pump Inhibitors		
Omeprazole (Prilosec)	1 mg/kg/day divided daily or bid; if ≥20 kg give 20 mg (adult dose: 20 mg daily)	Headache, diarrhea, abdominal pain, nausea, rash, constipation, vitamin B₁₂ deficiency Approved 2 years and older
Lansoprazole (Prevacid)	1-2 mg/kg/day daily or bid; 15 mg daily if <30 kg or 30 mg daily if >30 kg (adult dose 15-30 mg daily)	Headache, diarrhea, abdominal pain, nausea, elevated transaminases, proteinuria, angina, hypotension Approved 1 year and older
Rabeprazole (Aciphex)	No pediatric dose available (adult dose: 20 mg daily)	Headache, diarrhea, abdominal pain, nausea
Prokinetic		
Cisapride	0.8 mg/kg/day divided qid (adult dose: 10-20 mg qid)	Most authorities do not recommend, though it is occasionally used with GI consultation Rare cases of serious cardiac arrhythmia (FDA recommends ECG before administration) Beware of drug interactions Do not use in patients with liver, cardiac, or electrolyte abnormalities (FDA recommends checking K⁺, Ca⁺⁺, Mg⁺⁺, and creatinine before administration)

bid, Twice a day; *ECG*, electrocardiogram; *FDA*, Food and Drug Administration; *hs*, at bedtime; *qid*, four times daily; *tid*, three times daily.

remains asymptomatic with low-grade inflammation or no mucosal changes at all (Kato et al, 2004; Rothenbacher et al, 2004). *H. pylori* is transmitted person to person or by contaminated water sources (fecal-oral or oral-oral transmission). It induces a chronic inflammation in the stomach and duodenal mucosa that destroys the protective mucosal layer. No correlation between *H. pylori* infection and recurrent abdominal pain (RAP) has been found in children.

Most children with DUs have a positive family medical history, a key finding. PUD is rare in children under 10 years old and usually related to secondary causes. It is most common between 12 and 18 years old, with boys being affected more frequently. The male-to-female ratio is about 2:1 to 3:1.

It is more common among children of low socioeconomic status; African Americans and Hispanics; and children living in crowded, unsanitary conditions who share a bed (Bechtel, 2002). Approximately 10% of children in the U.S. will be positive for *H. pylori* by 10 years old (Manfredi & Israel, 2006).

Clinical Findings
History
- Box 32-1 delineates major and minor criteria for the diagnosis of peptic disease.
- Asymptomatic or symptoms can wax and wane.
- Pain (onset, location, duration, severity) with eating, dyspepsia, awakens from sleep (key finding).

> **BOX 32-1** **Major and Minor Criteria for the Diagnosis of Peptic Disease**
>
> **Major Criteria**
> Epigastric abdominal pain; periumbilical pain in young children
> Recurrent vomiting (at least three times per month)
> **Minor Criteria**
> Hematemesis
> Pain awakening the child at night
> Heartburn, oral regurgitation
> Anorexia, early satiety, chronic nausea; irritability with eating in young children
> Excessive belching and/or hiccupping, oral regurgitation
> Family history of PUD, dyspepsia, or IBS
> Anemia
> Guaiac positive or melena stools

IBS, Irritable bowel syndrome; *PUD,* peptic ulcer disease.
Data from Manfredi MA, Israel EJ: Gastritis and peptic ulcer disease. In Burg FD, Ingelfinger JR, Polin RA et al: *Current pediatric therapy,* ed 18, Philadelphia, 2006, WB Saunders, p 532-540; Chelimsky G, Czinn S: Peptic ulcer disease in children, *Pediatr Rev* 22(10):349-355, 2001.

- Infants: poor feeding, GI bleeding, vomiting, intestinal perforation.
- Toddlers and preschoolers: poorly localized abdominal pain, vomiting, GI bleeding.
- School-age children and adolescents: poorly localized epigastric or right lower quadrant (RLQ) pain. Pain may be relieved by food, milk, and antacids and may be referred to the back.
- Predisposing factors: alcohol, smoking, aspirin, NSAIDs, or corticosteroids.

    Physical Examination.   A careful physical examination should be performed; however, there may be no physical findings. The physical examination should include the following:
- Height, weight, head circumference, BMI, and percentiles
- Funduscopic examination
- Careful mouth inspection looking for ulcers (associated with Crohn disease) and dental enamel erosion (associated with GER)
- Lung examination for wheezing (associated with GER)
- Abdominal examination for tenderness and hepatosplenomegaly
- Rectal examination to assess perirectal disease

    Diagnostic Studies
- CBC: Anemia is associated with chronic infection with *H. pylori* (Kato et al, 2004); albumin (low) and ESR (high) are red flags for systemic disease.
- Endoscopy is the diagnostic test of choice with mucosal biopsy.
- Evaluation for *H. pylori* in children is controversial and should only be done when: there is suspicion of organic disease or endoscopic evidence of a duodenal or gastric ulcer; the child has mucosa-associated lymphoid tissue (MALT) lymphoma; occasionally to determine if the infection has been eradicated.

- Tests to detect *H. pylori* (Amieva, 2005; Manfredi & Israel, 2006; Stockman, 2004):
  - Histologic exam and culture of biopsies obtained via endoscopy is the gold standard; sensitivities to antibiotics should be done concurrently.
  - Urea breath test: sensitive in children older than 2 years, but requires special equipment.
  - Stool monoclonal antibody test is sensitive and specific; useful to monitor after eradication.
  - Serum IgG antibody titer for *H. pylori* (level greater than 500 units [normal 0 to 200]) in children older than 12 years; if positive only means exposure to disease. This test should not be the sole basis for starting therapy nor should it be used to test for eradication.

Differential Diagnosis
All other causes of abdominal pain (see Table 32-7, p. 810), GERD, IBS, GI bleeding, cholelithiasis, cholecystitis, pancreatitis, lactose intolerance, hyperkalemia, and hypercalcemia are included in the differential diagnosis.

Management
- A 2- to 4-week trial of the following may be helpful:
  - Antacids: any liquid preparation, 0.5 mL/kg, given between 1 and 3 hours after eating and before bed.
  - H_2 antagonist or PPI (Table 32-5).
- Referral to a gastroenterologist should occur if:
  - Lack of improvement.
  - Inability to wean off meds.
  - History of hematemesis, melena, occult blood in stools, anemia, and/or weight loss.
- Eradication therapy for *H pylori* is indicated for children with a duodenal or gastric ulcer identified by endoscopy and histopathology; children diagnosed with MALT lymphoma; and children with atrophic gastritis and proven metaplasia; iron deficiency anemia unexplained by other causes
  - Empirical therapy for suspected *H. pylori* is not recommended. There is increasing antibiotic resistance to *H. pylori* (Stockman, 2004). Therapy is not indicated for gastritis without PUD, RAP, nor children with asymptomatic PUD or family member with PUD.
  - See Table 32-6 for treatment guidelines. Compliance with the treatment regimen is the single most important determinant of eradication.
  - Follow-up noninvasive studies (urea breath or stool antigen) 8 weeks after treatment may be done (Amieva, 2005).

Complications
Recurrence (*H. pylori* treatment failure rate of 25%), hemorrhage, perforation, gastric outlet obstruction, gastric adenocarcinoma, and gastric lymphoma are possible complications.

Patient Education/Prevention/Prognosis
Treatment success depends on the child completing the drug regimen. PUD in children is being actively studied; pediatric primary care providers must be aware of ongoing changes in recommendations for therapy.

TABLE 32-5 **Medications Used in the Treatment of Acid-Peptic Disease**

Medication	Pediatric Dose	How Supplied
Histamine$_2$-Receptor Antagonists		
Cimetidine (Tagamet)	20-40 mg/kg/day up to 400 mg divided bid; infants 1-2 mg/kg/day every 6 hr	Syrup: 60 mg/mL; tabs: 100, 200, 300, 400, and 800 mg
Famotidine (Pepcid)	1-2 mg/kg/day up to 20 mg every 8-12 hr; 40 mg/day daily for young adults	Syrup: 40 mg/5 mL; tabs: 20 and 40 mg
Nizatidine (Axid)	>6 mo old: 5-10 mg/kg/day divided bid	Solution: 15 mg/mL; capsule: 150 and 300 mg; tab: 75 mg
Ranitidine (Zantac)	2-6 mg/kg/day up to 150 mg divided bid	Syrup: 15 mg/mL; tabs: 150 and 300 mg
Proton Pump Inhibitors		
Lansoprazole (Prevacid)	1-2 mg/kg/day daily or bid; start at 1 mg/kg/day	Oral suspension: 15 mg and 30 mg per packet; solutab: 15 and 30 mg; capsules: 15 and 30 mg
Omeprazole (Prilosec)	0.5-1.5 mg/kg/day daily or bid; start at 1 mg/kg/day; dose range 0.3-3.3 mg/kg/day has been reported; 20 mg/day daily for young adults	Capsules: 10, 20, and 40 mg
Cytoprotective Agents		
Sucralfate	40-80 mg/kg/day up to 1 g qid; 1 g qid for young adults	Suspension: 1 g/5 mL; tabs: 1 g

hr, Hours; *mo*, months; *qid*, four times daily.

TABLE 32-6 **Recommended Eradication Therapies for *H. pylori* Disease in Children**

Medications	Dosage
First-Line Options	
1. Amoxicillin	50 mg/kg/day up to 1 g bid
Clarithromycin	15 mg/kg/day up to 500 mg bid
Omeprazole (or comparable acid inhibitory doses of another PPI)	1 mg/kg/day up to 20 mg bid
2. Clarithromycin	15 mg/kg/day up to 500 mg bid
Metronidazole	20 mg/kg/day up to 500 mg bid
Omeprazole (or comparable acid inhibitory doses of another PPI)	1 mg/kg/day up to 20 mg bid
Second-Line Option	
3. Bismuth subsalicylate	1 tablet (262 mg) qid *or* 15 mL (17.6 mg/mL qid)
Metronidazole	20 mg/kg/day up to 500 mg bid
PPI or H$_2$ blocker	1 mg/kg/day up to 20 mg bid
Tetracycline*	50 mg/kg/day up to 1 g bid

*Only for children 8 years or older. Initial treatment should be provided in a twice-daily regimen (to enhance compliance) for 7 to 14 days.
bid, Twice daily; *PPI*, proton pump inhibitor; *qid*, four times daily.
Data from AAP, Committee on Infectious Diseases: Report of the Committee on Infectious Diseases, ed 27, Elk Grove Village, IL, 2006, American Academy of Pediatrics.

■ LOWER GASTROINTESTINAL TRACT DISORDERS

INFANTILE COLIC

Description

Infantile colic is characterized by persistent crying in infants younger than 3 months old. The average infant cries for 2 to 3 hours per day. In contrast, an infant with colic usually cries for more than 4 hours per day. One definition of colic is the rule of threes: a healthy infant who cries for more than 3 hours per day, more than 3 days per week, for more than 3 weeks (Goldstein et al, 2003). The crying is unpredictable and spontaneous, and the child cannot be comforted (Roberts et al, 2004). Illingsworth (1954) described colicky infants as having attacks of screaming in the evening with classic motor features that included flushed face, furrowed brow, and clenched fists, with legs drawn up and a piercing, high-pitched scream.

Epidemiology

No specific cause of colic has been identified, although both physical and psychosocial factors may play a role. Organic causes account for less than 5% of infants with excessive crying. Certain physical factors have been implicated and include sensitivity to diet (e.g., cow's milk), excessive gas, and swallowed air during feeding, inadequate burping, hypermotile bowel, and cigarette smoke in the infant's environment. Smoking is linked to increased plasma and intestinal motilin levels, and higher than average levels of motilin are linked to elevated risk of colic (Shenassa & Brown, 2004). Psychosocial factors can include the perception of a stressful pregnancy, negative childbirth experience, unsatisfying interactions among family members, and overstimulation. However, there is no evidence that parental personality or anxiety causes colic (Barr, 2002). The parents' inability to accurately interpret and respond to the infant's cries may contribute to colic. The infant may become overstimulated, underfed, or overfed. The stress created by a crying baby contributes to ineffective parental communication and interventions, family dysfunction, parental anxiety and fatigue, and can exacerbate the problem. Carey's classic study on colic (1972) revealed that colicky babies have a low sensory threshold. More recent studies do not support the notion that colic is a manifestation of a child with "difficult temperament," but more likely just a manifestation of typical behavioral development (Barr, 2002; Keefe et al, 2006a; Keefe et al, 2006b; Roberts et al, 2004; White et al, 2000). The fact that colic tends to go completely away by 4 months old may support this notion.

The incidence of colic varies greatly depending on the definition used. Various studies using the Wessel definition find the incidence to be about 20% of infants (Clifford et al, 2002) to 30% to 40% of infants with 15% to 40% continuing with colic symptoms past 3 months of life (Goldstein et al, 2003; Weisbluth, 2006).

Clinical Findings

History.   Parents or caregivers report that the infant is less than 3 months old and cries 3 hours or more a day for 3 days or more per week (Goldstein et al, 2003). Additional findings include the following:

- Demands frequent feeding and is often fussy while feeding
- Has excessive gas
- Is inconsolable or is comforted for short periods only
- Is "tense" or "tight" and keeps legs stiff and fists clenched tightly
- Red flags in the history indicating a potential organic cause for crying:
  - Apnea, cyanosis, struggling to breathe
  - Excessive spitting or vomiting

Physical Examination.   If possible see the family during a crying time. A thorough examination must be completed to rule out other pathologic conditions and should include the following:

- Body temperature
- Evaluation of growth parameters
- Full body exam to look for signs of trauma or abuse
- Abdominal examination for masses, tenderness, and bowel sounds
- Stool for blood or mucus

Diagnostic Studies.   If the child is gaining weight and has a normal examination, no other laboratory tests are indicated.

Differential Diagnosis

All other causes of abdominal pain are in the differential diagnosis (Table 32-7), in addition to undetected corneal abrasion, UTI, other infection, or traumatic injury. Persistent mother-infant distress syndrome (increased crying and colicky behaviors that persist beyond 3 months old) and latent distress (no colicky behavior at 6 weeks old, but present at 3 months old) are newer subcategories of colic being researched.

Management

- No cure is known for infantile colic. The goal of treatment is to manage the situation until the colic resolves itself. Parents and providers who are flexible, creative, and persistent in seeking solutions are most likely to be successful. See Box 32-2 for management strategies.
- There may be benefit from eliminating milk products, eggs, peanuts, tree nuts, wheat, soy, and fish from the diet of breastfeeding mothers (Cirgin-Ellet, 2003; Hill et al, 2006).
- Altering the infant's diet may improve colic:
  - Removing cow's milk protein (CMP) and soy from the infant or breastfeeding mother's diet improved colic in 10% to 34% of infants with colic (Brown, 2002).
- Herbal teas (chamomile, vervain, licorice, fennel, and lemon balm) used three times a day decrease crying in colicky infants.
- Gripe Water (mixture of herbs and herb oils) is touted to provide relief from flatulence and indigestion, but is not entirely without risk. Parents need to avoid products made with sugar or alcohol and to use products made in the U.S. (Roberts et al, 2004).
- Medications (e.g., simethicone) are not useful in treating colic. The use of medications may give the parents "something to do," but can actually potentiate the myth of a physical cause.
- A 4-week nurse home visit program with inquiries about the parent and baby, limiting overstimulation and sensory overload, and promoting regularity and predictability of feeding and sleeping were beneficial in decreasing crying time (Keefe et al, 2006b).
- Kangaroo care (skin to skin) contact may be beneficial.
- Dr. Brown's Natural Flow Bottle decreased fussing and crying in babies with colic (Cirgin-Ellett et al, 2006).
- Car ride simulators, crib vibrators, infant massage, and increased holding during noncrying times are generally not helpful, but do calm some children and give parent's a sense of "doing something."
- Rao and colleagues (2004) found that infants who had excessive uncontrolled crying that persisted beyond 3 months old, without other neurologic deficits, were more likely to have cognitive deficits in childhood. These infants should be followed closely.

Text continued on p. 815

TABLE 32-7 Differential Diagnosis of Gastrointestinal Causes of Abdominal Pain in Children

Disease	Major Symptoms	Signs	Excreta	Tests	Age of Onset
Abdominal migraine	Paroxysmal episodes of intense; acute periumbilical pain. Intervening periods of usual health	Abdominal pain associated with at least two of the following: anorexia, nausea, vomiting, headache, photophobia, or pallor	Normal	None	Mean onset at 7 yr old with peak between 10 and 12 yr old.
Anal fissure	Constipation, crying with defecation, bright red blood on stool or in diaper	Small tears in anal mucosa	Constipation with bloody streaks	Stool occult blood	Any
Appendicitis	Fever, anorexia, vomiting; process evolves over 12 hr	Diffuse, then localized to right-sided (RLQ) tenderness, guarding, maximal pain over McBurney point + Rovsing sign	Constipation or diarrhea, rare blood and pus	CBC: increased neutrophils UA: pyuria Abdominal radiograph: may show fecalith US: may be abnormal CT with contrast test of choice	Frequency increases with age, peaking between 15-30 yr old
Cholelithiasis	Episodic and colicky pain that may radiate to the scapula, back, or other parts of the abdomen. Uncommon in children, but is associated with hemolytic anemias, cholestatic diseases, prematurity, and medications	Pain and vomiting Diaphoresis, pallor, tachycardia, weakness, nausea, and lightheadedness There may be a pear-shaped palpable mass in the RUQ Pain can be diurnal, but is generally worse at night Acute cholecystitis: fever, mild jaundice, severe abdominal pain, emesis, nausea and leukocytosis Biliary obstruction: sudden onset of severe, sharp tight upper quadrant pain, localized deep tenderness in the RUQ			Any depending on the cause
Colic	Persistent crying in infant	Duration of crying >3hr/day for 3 or more days/wk	Normal	Stool: r/o blood, mucus	<3mo old

Constipation	Poor appetite, soiling, straining with stools	Possible tenderness over colon and small bowel, rectal fissures, encopresis, fewer than 3 stools/wk	Hard or soft, may have blood on outer surface of stool	Abdominal radiograph Barium enema if unresponsive to intervention	Peaks between 2-4yr old
Foreign body	Children may be asymptomatic or have coughing, choking, gagging, pain in throat or chest, anorexia, pain with swallowing	May have increased salivation, refusal to swallow, respiratory symptoms Normal abdominal examination	May see passage of FB	Chest radiograph if respiratory symptoms Abdominal radiograph if FB not seen to pass in stool or signs of abdominal pain and/or obstruction present	Highest incidence between 14mo-6yr old
Gastroenteritis, viral or bacterial	Vomiting, diarrhea	General abdominal tenderness	Watery, bilious (green) vomitus, may or may not have blood in stool	Stool: may show bacteria, WBCs, blood, mucus	Any
Gastroesophageal reflux	Regurgitation, vomiting, irritability, recurrent pain after bedtime	Infants: gastric distention, effortless regurgitation during or after feedings; FTT, stridor, apnea, recurrent pneumonia, bronchospasm Older children: vomiting, sour taste in mouth, abdominal pain, burning sensation in substernal area; chronic nocturnal cough, wheezing, pneumonia; dysphagia, nausea, FTT	Rare hematemesis Never bilious	24-hr esophageal pH probe study Barium swallow with fluoroscopy; Esophageal manometry Endoscopy for esophageal biopsy	Commonly 0-24mo old with 60%-80% spontaneous resolution; can occur in specific disease disorders and in premies, older children and adolescents
Hepatitis	Nausea, anorexia	Tender liver with or without splenomegaly, jaundice	Pale stools, diarrhea	Elevated ALT and AST Mild elevations of LDH and alkaline phosphatase Elevated bilirubin (direct and indirect) May have mild lymphocytosis Hepatitis panel may show active or carrier status	Any—dependent on type of hepatitis

Continued

TABLE 32-7 Differential Diagnosis of Gastrointestinal Causes of Abdominal Pain in Children—Cont'd

Disease	Major Symptoms	Signs	Excreta	Tests	Age of Onset
Hernia (strangulated)	Vomiting, crying	Distention, bulge in inguinal area	Fecal vomitus	None—refer for immediate surgical evaluation	70% occur in first yr
Hirschsprung disease	Failure to pass stool within 24hr in an infant or rectal stimulation required to pass stools; history of constipation since infancy in children	FTT, abdominal distention, palpable stool throughout abdomen, but empty rectal ampulla	May have diarrhea, bilious (green) vomiting	Abdominal radiograph Barium enema Rectal examination: absence of stool in rectal ampulla Electrolytes, CBC	Infancy to adult
Inflammatory Bowel Diseases Crohn disease	Umbilical or RLQ pain, diarrhea, weight loss, anorexia	Short stature, tender abdominal mass, fever, arthralgias or arthritis, perianal lesions	Loose and usually nonbloody stools unless anal fissures present	CBC, total protein, albumin, ESR, CRP Stool for blood and WBCs Bone age Refer for endoscopy	Childhood and adolescence with peak at 20-30yr old
Ulcerative colitis	Weight loss, abdominal pain	Tender colon	Bloody stools	Same as above	Peak incidence at 16-20yr old
Intestinal obstruction	Vomiting, abdominal distention; failure to pass feces in newborn after 24hr; acute or gradual onset of periumbilical or lower abdominal pain	Alternating crampy and quiescent periods of periumbilical to lower abdominal pain, increased bowel sounds, obstipation	Bilious (green) emesis	Abdominal radiograph (flat, upright views)	Neonates; if occurs after 2mo old, usually as a result of intussusception or other causes
Intussusception	Episodic, cyclic abdominal pain with vomiting alternating with calm periods	Tender, sausage-shaped mass in RUQ, distention, legs drawn up at time of pain followed by periods of lethargy, absence of bowel sound in RLQ; these "classic" symptoms occur in <50% of cases	Blood-tinged mucus ("currant jelly" stool); this occurs as a late sign	Abdominal US 100% reliable (abdominal radiography misses diagnosis in 33%-55% of cases) Barium enema	70% <2yr old with peak incidence at 5mo and 3yr old; as age of onset increases, further pathologic conditions are often present

Condition	Clinical Findings		Diagnostic Studies	Comments
Irritable bowel syndrome	Recurrent, intermittent, dull, crampy abdominal pain, diarrhea, or constipation	Intense thirst, fluctuating abdominal distention, increased bowel sounds; history of others in family with RAP especially with social stimulation, travel, holidays, trauma; healthy appearance; borborygmus and flatus in school-age and older children; vague tenderness in RLQ, LLQ, and epigastrium; pain usually not related to eating or defecation; occasional pallor and nausea	Watery, malodorous stools; first stool of day may be formed, followed by 3 or more watery stools through the day	CBC, ESR, UA, stools for O&P and occult blood; Abdominal US; Upper GI series with small bowel follow-through	5-15yr old
Lactose intolerance	Bloating, gaseousness, crampy abdominal pain	Pain and diarrhea within hours of lactose ingestion; may have history of recent severe VGE. In infants: vomiting, distention, abdominal pain after lactose-containing formula or bovine milk ingestion by breastfeeding mother	Acidic diarrhea	Breath hydrogen test after lactose challenge; Reducing substances in stool; Lack of normal increase in blood glucose after ingestion of lactose	5-15yr old rare in infancy; prominent in some ethnic groups
Mesenteric lymphadenitis	Fever, vomiting	Right-sided (RLQ often) or diffuse tenderness		Abdominal US may show mesenteric adenitis	
Meckel diverticulum	Painless rectal bleeding	Anemia, periumbilical or lower abdominal pain may be manifested similar to appendicitis or volvulus	Bloody stools	CBC; Stools for occult blood; Refer for surgical consultation	65% incidence in children <5yr old with peak at 2yr old
Necrotizing enterocolitis	Feeding intolerance; abdomen distended, tense, and tender	Possible palpable abdominal mass and cellulitis of abdominal wall, GI bleeding, shock		CBC, chemistry panel; Abdominal radiograph/US	Premature and term infants

Continued

TABLE 32-7 Differential Diagnosis of Gastrointestinal Causes of Abdominal Pain in Children—Cont'd

Disease	Major Symptoms	Signs	Excreta	Tests	Age of Onset
Pancreatitis	Intense epigastric pain that is steady, ache-like, worse in the recumbent position, and may radiate to the back	Protracted, occasionally bilious emesis Low-grade fever Hunched-over or knee-to-chest position Dehydration or shock Pain may last 7-10 days		Serum amylase/lipase CBC US CT	Supportive care NG decompression IV fluids Pain medications Endoscopic sphincterotomy Enteral alimentation to prevent an ileus
Parasites	Parasite dependent: possibly diarrhea, bloating, distention, flatulence	Parasite dependent: rectal itching, weight loss, malaise, cough, hepatomegaly, vague abdominal pain, anemia	May or may not have diarrhea, which may be bloody, greasy, or foul smelling; visible worms in stool or vomitus	Stools for O&P CBC: may show increased eosinophils	Any
Peptic ulcer disease	Poor appetite, weakness, epigastric pain with or without nausea	Vague abdominal pain or RLQ localization; epigastric tenderness, which can occur at night; vomiting	Black stools or coffee-ground vomitus	Endoscopy and biopsy PCR of tissue for *H. pylori* Serum IgG antibody titer for *H. pylori* Urea breath testing	Any, usually above 8yr old
Recurrent abdominal pain	At least 3 episodes of abdominal pain over 3-mo period	Periumbilical to generalized abdominal pain, sometimes sharp or dull and lasting 1-3hr; occasional nausea and vomiting	Normal	CBC, ESR, chemistry screen UA and urine culture Stool O&P, culture, pH, reducing substances	Usually between 6 and 19yr old with peak at 9yr old
Volvulus or malrotation	Bilious (green) vomiting	Abdominal distention, GI bleeding, palpable epigastric mass, dehydration, lethargy, shock	May be bloody	CBC Abdominal radiograph Barium enema Upper GI series Refer immediately for surgical consultation	First mo of life

ALT, Alanine aminotransferase; *AST*, aspartate aminotransferase; *CBC*, complete blood count; *CRP*, C-reactive protein; *CT*, computerized tomography; *ESR*, erythrocyte sedimentation rate; *FB*, foreign body; *FTT*, failure to thrive; *GI*, gastrointestinal; *hr*, hour(s); *LDH*, lactate dehydrogenase; *LLQ*, left lower quadrant; *mo*, months; *NG*, nasogastric; *O&P*, ova and parasites; *RLQ*, right lower quadrant; *r/o*, rule out; *RUQ*, right upper quadrant; *UA*, urinalysis; *US*, ultrasound; *WBCs*, white blood cells; *wk*, week(s); *yr*, year(s).

Management Strategies for Infantile Colic

- Affirm the baby's good health and reinforce the parents efforts to comfort their infant.
- Acknowledge the importance of the concern.
- Help parents distinguish infant cries and understand infant state.
- Encourage parents to take time off by seeking help from family or friends.
- Remind parents that colic is temporary.
- Allow parents to express feelings of anger, guilt, and frustration.
- Repeat information because parents are often sleep deprived and anxious.
- Encourage sucking at breast, fist, fingers, or pacifier.
- Provide rhythmic activities: rock, swing, jogger, bouncing, walking, dancing, car ride.
- Swaddle, massage or snuggle in front carrier.
- Provide "white" noise: lullabies, shushing, nature-recorded sounds, heartbeat or womb-recorded sounds, hair dryer or vacuum cleaner sounds.
- Meet the infant's needs: feed, sleep, hold, suck, stimulate.
- Ensure proper feedings (correct latch-on, frequent burping, avoidance of early addition of solids, change in diet if lactose intolerance or milk allergy is a problem).
- Reduce stimulation (quiet, dark, motionless).
- Avoid the overtired state (nap within 1 to 2 hour of wakefulness).
  ○ Keep a diary of baby's fussing, crying, and sleeping; analyze to develop a clear daily routine and identify patterns that may be addressed by behavioral intervention (e.g., attunement, self-soothing).

Complications

Stress created by a crying baby can contribute to parental feelings of hostility, anger, and guilt, ultimately leading to poor parent-child interaction. Parents may respond by unintentionally physically or emotionally abusing their infant.

Patient Education/Prevention/Prognosis

Given the risk for child abuse, the National Center for Shaken Baby Syndrome "Period of PURPLE Crying" campaign has materials to educate parents about the characteristics of early (first 3 months of life) crying. *P* stands for peak, *U* for unpredictability of crying bouts, *R* for resistance to soothing, *P* for painlike expression, *L* for long crying bouts, and *E* for evening clustering. See the Resource Box at the end of this chapter for contact information.

ACUTE ABDOMINAL PAIN

Description

The location and character of abdominal pain can be helpful in identifying the disease process. Visceral pain is generally dull and diffuse. Visceral pain fibers are located in the muscular wall of hollow viscera and the capsule of solid viscera. Visceral nerves are stimulated by tension and stretching. Parietal pain is usually sharp, localized, and stimulated by inflammation in the parietal peritoneum. The shared innervation of many abdominal organs leads to poor localization of pain.

- *Epigastric* pain usually indicates pain from the liver, pancreas, biliary tree, stomach, and upper part of the small bowel.
- *Periumbilical* pain is generated from the distal end of the small intestine, cecum, appendix, and ascending colon.
- *Suprapubic* discomfort indicates distal intestine, urinary tract, and pelvic organ dysfunction.
- *Referred* pain is usually sharp, localized pain felt in remote areas innervated by the same nerves as the affected organ. When visceral pain is overwhelming, referred pain occurs.
- *Acute* continuous pain is more indicative of an acute process.

Epidemiology

Primary GI causes of abdominal pain in children include appendicitis, viral and bacterial enteritis, inflammatory bowel disease, PUD, intussusception, pancreatitis, cholecystitis, and liver dysfunction.

Primary GI causes of abdominal pain that do not originate in the GI tract include ovarian cyst, salpingitis, sexually transmitted diseases, otitis media, pneumonia, pharyngitis, UTI, Henoch-Schönlein purpura, rheumatic fever, sickle cell disease, pleurisy, kidney pain, rectal or uterine disease, and hernia. Referred pain in the shoulder can be generated from pneumonia, subphrenic abscess, pleurisy, pancreatitis, and the spleen, gallbladder, and liver. Testicular pain occurs with kidney disease and appendicitis. Back pain can also accompany retroperitoneal hematoma, pancreatitis, and rectal or uterine disease.

Clinical Findings

History.   The history should assess the following:
- Family history of gallbladder disease, hernia, kidney or liver disease, and other incidences of abdominal pain
- Past medical history of illnesses or surgeries
- History of trauma or abuse
- Pain: onset, location, duration, distribution, quality, radiation, changes in location, awakens child from sleep
- Activity level
- Appetite and food intake
- History of recent infection
- Fever (high fever is usually not associated with acute abdomen)
- Nausea, vomiting, diarrhea, or constipation
- Aggravating and alleviating factors
- Hematuria, dysuria, frequency, incontinence
- Menstrual history and last period, vaginal discharge, sexual activity, birth control, and penile discharge

Physical Examination.   Adolescents should be examined with parents out of the room (for privacy and to elicit a complete history). The following are needed for all children:
- Determine the level of pain by using a reliable pain tool
- Complete physical examination
- Weight, BMI, and vital signs (temperature, heart rate, respiratory rate, and blood pressure)
- Abdominal examination, including rectal examination, psoas and obturator signs, rebound tenderness, decreased bowel sounds

- Pelvic examination as indicated
- Repeated examinations as necessary to observe for changes
  See Differential Diagnosis for specific findings; also see sections on appendicitis and intussusception.

Diagnostic Studies. The following are performed as indicated:

- CBC with differential, serum electrolytes, ESR, amylase, pregnancy test (as indicated by the history and examination)
- UA and urine culture
- Stool for occult blood
- Pelvic examination—gonococcal or chlamydial culture (or both), Papanicolaou smear, vaginal smears
- Abdominal radiographs with or without contrast
- Chest radiograph (anteroposterior and lateral as indicated) to rule out pneumonia
- Abdominal or pelvic (or both) ultrasound
- CT

Differential Diagnosis
See Table 32-5 and Fig. 32-3.

Management
Treatment involves the following:

- Consultation and referral, including surgery as indicated
- No sedatives or pain medication until the diagnosis is made
- Intravenous rehydration and gastric decompression as necessary
- Treatment of the cause

Complications
Complications include ruptured viscera, intraabdominal bleeding, strangulation leading to ischemia of the gut, and shock leading to death.

APPENDICITIS
Description
Appendicitis is inflammation of the appendix. Although a classic presentation is easy to discern, appendicitis can mimic many other intraabdominal conditions, making diagnosis tricky.

Epidemiology
Following obstruction of the appendiceal lumen by a fecalith, lymphoid tissue, tumor, parasite, foreign body, or inspissated CF secretions, the appendix becomes distended and subject to ischemia and necrosis. Peritoneal inflammation around the infected appendix causes the characteristic symptoms. There is about a 36- to 48-hour window from the onset of pain to the rupture of the appendix at which the child may have signs of peritonitis including "high fever, abdominal pain and tenderness, a rigid board-like abdomen, leukocytosis, and right lower quadrant mass" (Kliegman, 2004).

Appendicitis is the source of abdominal pain most commonly treated with surgery, and it affects four of every 1000 children (McCollough & Sharieff, 2006). Frequency increases with age, but the average age of appendicitis in children is 10 years old, with boys and girls equally affected. Perforation is most common under 5 years old (Nance et al, 2000).

Clinical Findings
- The most reliable information is gained from the sequence of symptoms.
  - Periumbilical pain is felt (earliest sign).
  - Child awakens with pain that peaks in 4 hours, then subsides and migrates to RLQ (classic sign).
  - After a few hours, vomiting may occur (this follows periumbilical pain; in gastroenteritis, vomiting precedes the pain).
  - Anorexia occurs (although up to 50% of children state that they are hungry).
  - Stool is low volume with mucus (gastroenteritis has high-volume, watery stools).
  - Fever is neither sensitive nor specific for appendicitis (Cardall et al, 2004).
- A scoring system may be helpful (Kharbanda et al, 2006). A score of 5 or less was highly sensitive in the exclusion of the diagnosis of appendicitis.
  - Nausea (2 points)
  - Focal RLQ pain (2 points)
  - Migration of pain (1 point)
  - Difficulty walking (1 point)
  - Rebound tenderness and/or pain with percussion (2 points)
  - Absolute neutrophil count less than 6.75×10^3/microliter (6 points)
- The process evolves over 12 hours, with the potential for infants and young children to become sick much more quickly.
- Following perforation, symptoms lessen, with less vomiting, fever greater than 101° F (38.3° C), and the most comfortable position being on the side with the legs flexed.
- Infants demonstrate irritability, pain with movement, and flexed hips.
- The child may become quiet because crying and movement hurt.

Physical Examination. A complete physical examination is necessary. Reexamination may be needed in 4 to 6 hours. The following can be found:

- Presence of involuntary guarding, RLQ rebound tenderness, maximal pain over McBurney's point (1.5 to 2 inches in from the right anterior superior iliac crest on a line toward the umbilicus) on abdominal examination (most reliable finding); percussion is best method for eliciting rebound tenderness.
- Heel-drop jarring test (on toes for 15 seconds, drops on heels); inability to stand straight or climb stairs; winces when getting off examination table or riding in a car over bumps.
- Positive psoas sign or obturator sign (or both).
- Rovsing sign (pressure deep in left lower quadrant with sudden release elicits RLQ pain). A positive Rovsing sign and rebound tenderness have high sensitivity and specificity in children (McCollough & Sharieff, 2006).
- Tenderness and possibly a mass on the right side on rectal examination.
- Scoring systems are available and can help focus attention on signs and symptoms necessary for the diagnosis.

Differential Diagnosis

Accidental injury	Ectopic pregnancy	Pneumonia
Accidental ingestion	Food intolerance	Renal stones
Anaphylactoid purpura	Gastroenteritis	Sickle cell anemia
Appendicitis	Hemolytic uremic syndrome	Tortion of ovary or testicle
Child abuse	Mechanical obstruction	Trauma
Constipation	Mononucleosis	Urinary tract infection
		Viral syndrome

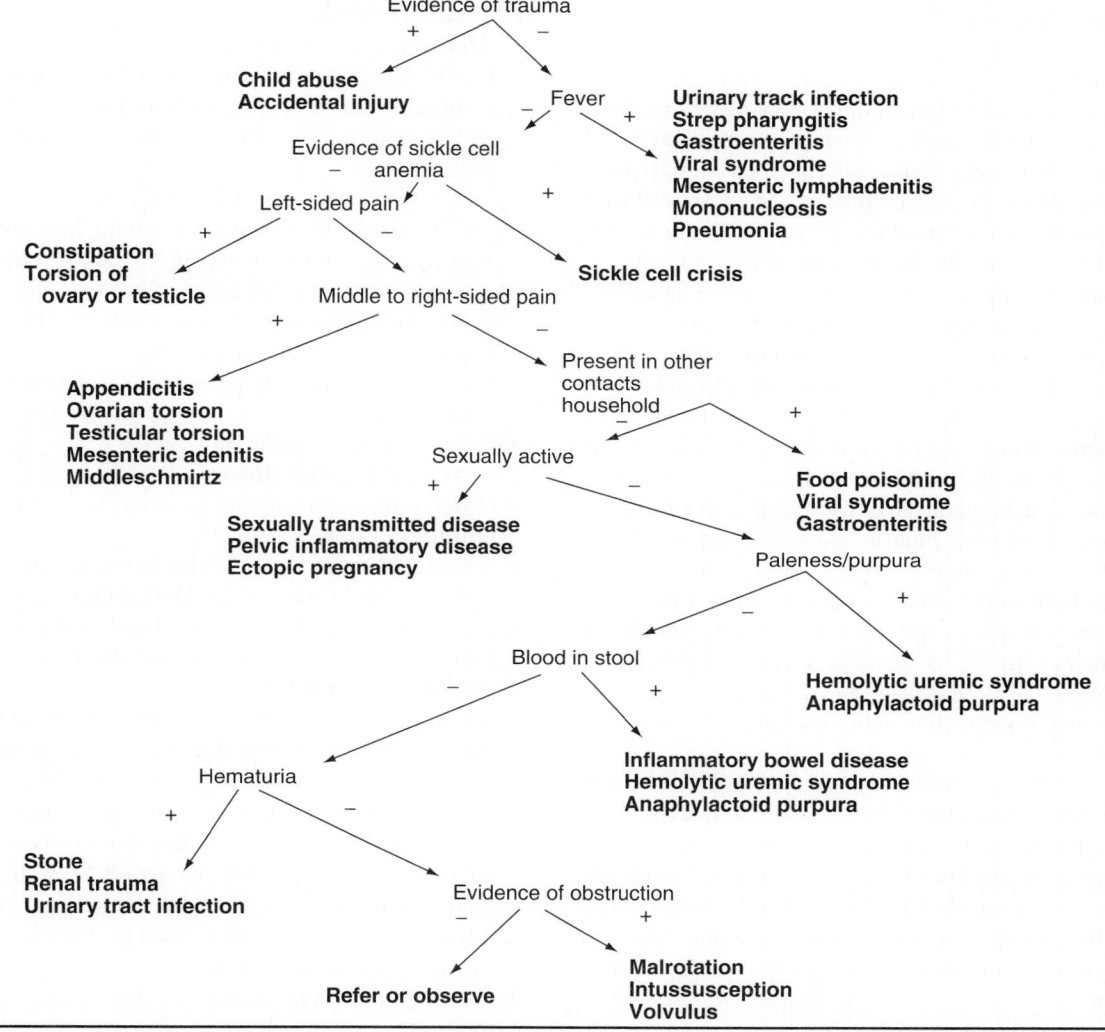

FIG. 32-3   Decision tree for differential diagnosis of acute abdominal pain. (From Schwartz MW et al, editors: *Pediatric primary care: a problem-oriented approach*, ed 3, St Louis, 1997, Mosby.)

Diagnostic Studies.   The following may be noted with appendicitis:

- CBC with differential may show an increased white blood cell (WBC) count (greater than 10,000) with an increased neutrophil count (greater than 75%). However, an elevated WBC count may be neither sensitive nor specific in the clinical diagnosis of appendicitis (Cardall et al, 2004).
- CRP may be elevated if symptoms have been present for longer than 12 hours (greater than 1.5 mg/dL on first day after the onset of symptoms, greater than 4 mg/dL on the second day, and greater than 10.5 mg/dL on the third day) (Wu et al, 2005).
- UA can show pyuria.

- Examination of stool may demonstrate blood and pus (rare finding).
- Abdominal radiographs can show a fecalith, especially if rupture has occurred.
- US demonstrates thickened, noncompressible, larger than 6 mm mass (not as helpful if appendix is perforated). US has excellent specificity, but only fair sensitivity and is operator dependent (Morrow & Newman, 2007).
- CT with contrast has highest accuracy, especially in adolescents. CT compared with US has higher sensitivity and specificity, is not operator dependent, and may be more cost effective in preventing an unnecessary appendectomy (Terasawa et al, 2004).

Differential Diagnosis

The differential diagnosis includes vomiting and gastroenteritis (fever and crampy abdominal pain with vomiting, diarrhea, or both), constipation, UTI (fever, chills, and urinary symptoms), PID or organ pathologic condition, pneumonia, duoderal ulcer (gnawing and burning pain), intestinal obstruction (crampy pain), peritonitis (worse pain when jumping or coughing), and intussusception (child younger than 2 years old with a right upper quadrant [RUQ] mass).

Management

- A surgical consultation for an appendectomy is needed. Administering opioid narcotics for pain before surgical consultation effectively reduces acute abdominal pain, does not impede the diagnostic process, and does not lead to an inappropriate increased use of CT scanning preoperatively (Green et al, 2005; Neighbor et al, 2005).
- Open appendectomy (OA) or laparoscopic appendectomy (LA) is indicated in nonperforated appendicitis. LA is marginally more expensive than OA; however, LA allows for earlier return to normal activities (Lintula et al, 2004).
- Urgent appendectomy may not be indicated in cases of perforated appendicitis. If the clinical course is less than 4 to 5 days in duration, surgeons may choose to perform appendectomy once fluid resuscitation and antibiotics have been administered. Some surgeons will choose a nonoperative approach as long as the child's clinical condition improves with antibiotic treatment and may or may not perform an appendectomy 8 to 12 weeks after recovery (Morrow & Newman, 2007).
- Intravenous and preoperative antibiotics are given if perforation is suspected.
- Patients should be seen in follow-up 2 to 4 weeks after surgery. If appetite, bowel function, energy, and activity level are normal; no pain or fever is present; findings on physical examination are normal; and the wound is well healed, the child can resume unrestricted activity. If at the 2- to 4-week follow-up the child has signs of delayed infection, abnormal bowel function, or unexplained weight loss, refer back to the surgeon.

Complications

Perforation, peritonitis, pelvic abscess, ileus, obstruction, sepsis, shock, and death can occur.

INTUSSUSCEPTION

Description

The invagination of bowel begins proximal to the ileocecal valve and is usually ileocolic, but it can be ileoileal or colocolic.

Epidemiology

The cause is not generally apparent. Polyps, Meckel's diverticulum, Henoch-Schönlein purpura, constipation, lymphomas, lipomas, parasites, rotavirus, adenovirus, and foreign bodies can be predisposing factors. Intussusception may be a complication of CF. Intussusception is most common between 3 months and 5 years old with a peak incidence between 6 and 11 months old (McCullough & Sharieff, 2006). In younger infants, intussusception is generally idiopathic. Children older than 5 years are more likely to have a lead point caused by polyps, lymphoma, Meckel's diverticulum, or Henoch-Schönlein purpura; therefore, a cause must be investigated (McCullough & Sharieff, 2006).

Clinical Findings

History. The following can be reported:
- The classic triad for intussusception, intermittent colicky abdominal pain, vomiting, and bloody mucous stools, are present in only 20% to 24% of cases (McCullough & Sharieff, 2006):
  - Paroxysmal, episodic abdominal pain with vomiting every 5 to 30 minutes. Some children will not have any pain at all.
  - Screaming with drawing up of the legs with periods of calm, sleeping, or lethargy between episodes.
  - Stool, possibly diarrhea in nature, with blood ("currant jelly").
- Fever may or may not be present.
- May follow an uncomplicated gastroenteritis or upper respiratory infection.
- Possible severe prostration.

Physical Examination
- Observe the baby's appearance and behavior over a period of time.
- A sausagelike mass may be felt in the RUQ of the abdomen with emptiness in the RLQ (Dance sign).
- The abdomen is often distended and tender to palpation.
- Grossly bloody or guaiac-positive stools.

Diagnostic Studies
- An abdominal flat-plate radiograph can appear normal, especially early in the course (Fig. 32-4). A plain radiograph may show sparse or no intestinal gas or stool in the ascending colon. "A 'target sign' on plain film consists of concentric circles of fat density, similar in appearance to a doughnut, visualized to the right of the spine" (McCullough & Sharieff, 2006).
- Abdominal US shows the same "target sign" and the "pseudokidney" sign. Can also be used to evaluate resolution following air or barium enema.
- An air or barium enema is diagnostic and frequently therapeutic.

Differential Diagnosis

The differential diagnosis includes incarcerated hernia, testicular torsion, acute gastroenteritis, appendicitis, colic, and intestinal obstruction.

Management

The following steps are taken:
- Emergency management and consultation with a pediatric radiologist and a pediatric surgeon.
- Rehydration and stabilization of fluid status.
- Radiologic reduction using an air or barium enema under fluoroscopy is the gold standard.
- Surgery if perforation, peritonitis, or hypovolemic shock is suspected or radiologic reduction fails.

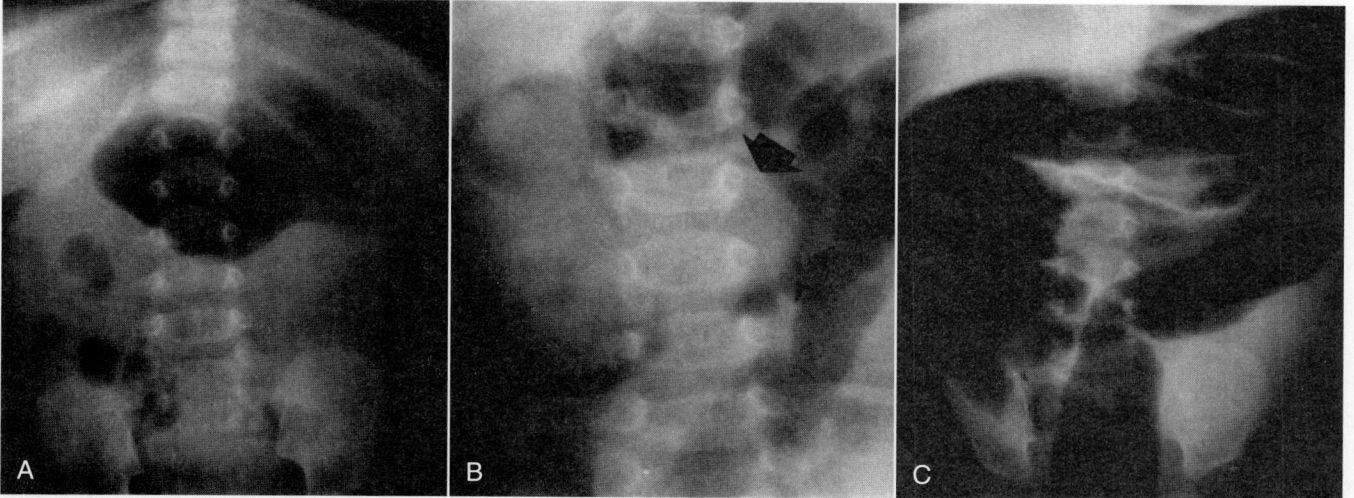

FIG. 32-4 Intussusception. **A,** Plain abdominal radiograph demonstrating a gas-filled stomach and relatively little gas in the distal end of the bowel. This baby had typical clinical features of intussusception and a palpable upper abdominal mass. Therefore an enema with air was performed. **B,** The intussusception *(arrows)* is outlined by air. **C,** Reduction is proved by air refluxing into loops of small bowel. (From Burg FD et al, editors: *Gellis and Kagan's current pediatric therapy*, ed 15, Philadelphia, 1999, WB Saunders.)

- Intravenous antibiotics are often administered to cover potential intestinal perforation.
- A period of observation following radiologic reduction is recommended; clear discharge instructions to return with any recurrence of symptoms are required, and close phone follow-up for up to 72 hours is prudent.

Complications
Swelling, hemorrhage, incarceration, and necrosis of the bowel requiring bowel resection may occur. Perforation, sepsis, shock, and reintussusception (5% to 10%, usually within 24 hours of radiologic reduction) can all occur.

FUNCTIONAL ABDOMINAL PAIN (FAP) AND FUNCTIONAL ABDOMINAL PAIN SYNDROME (FAPS)
Description
Diagnostic criteria (also known as Rome III criteria) for functional abdominal pain (FAP) (Rasquin et al, 2006), also known as recurrent abdominal pain (RAP) include:
- Episodic or continuous abdominal pain
- Insufficient criteria for other functional GI disorders
- No evidence of an inflammatory, anatomic, metabolic, or neoplastic process to explain symptoms

These criteria must be fulfilled at least once per week for at least 2 months before diagnosis.

Diagnostic criteria for FAPS must include childhood FAP at least 25% of the time and one or more of the following (Rasquin et al, 2006):
- Some loss of daily functioning
- Additional somatic symptoms, such as headache, limb pain, or difficulty sleeping

These criteria must be fulfilled at least once per week for at least 2 months before diagnosis.

Epidemiology
The cause of the pain remains unclear, but the pain is genuine. There is no evidence of visceral hypersensitivity in the rectum (Rasquin et al, 2006). Affected children have an involuntary predisposition for the development of physiologic pain (e.g., a family history of FAP). Temperament and personality can make the child more vulnerable to environmental stressors (often minor) that precipitate the sensation of pain. Children who are perfectionists, are dependent, or have low self-esteem may be more likely to experience FAP. Maternal anxiety and depression, overprotectiveness, and poor conflict resolution in the household are also contributing factors. However, some studies have shown that children with FAP have similar scores on measures of psychological distress as children with an organic cause for their pain (Thiessen, 2002). Occasionally a precipitating event occurs, but commonly none is found. Daily stress and negative life events can be related to increased frequency of episodes and the persistence of chronic abdominal pain. Positive and negative reinforcement can modify the pain.

Approximately 10% to 15% of children with FAP have an organic etiology (Thiessen, 2002). The prevalence of FAP ranges from 0.3% to 19%. It is more common in females and has the highest prevalence between 4 and 6 years old and in early adolescence (Chitkara et al, 2005). Males and females are affected equally until 9 years old; between 9 and 12 years old, the female-to-male ratio is 1.5:1. FAPS prevalence is approximately 0.5% to 2% with a peak in the fourth decade of life (Clouse et al, 2006).

Clinical Findings
History
- A complete review of systems and a careful psychosocial history (home, school, parents, friends); note any parental history of FAP

- Associated symptoms, such as headache, joint pain, anorexia, vomiting, nausea, excessive gas, and altered bowel pattern
- Anxiety and/or depression (in children or adults), behavioral problems, a negative life event
- Alarm symptoms (Box 32-3); there is an association between the presence of alarm symptoms and an organic cause to the chronic pain (AAP & NASPGHAN, 2005).
- Rome criteria for FAP or FAPS (see description)
- Pain often accompanied by a dramatic reaction (clutching abdomen, doubling over, or throwing self to ground)
- School avoidance
- Pain medications do not alleviate pain
- Illicit drug use
- Sexual activity or abuse and possibility of pregnancy

Physical Examination. Following initial examination, reexamination should be done during an acute episode and with each subsequent visit. The physical examination is usually normal, but should include the following:

- Weight, height, and BMI plotted on growth curves
- Vital signs (temperature, heart rate, respiratory rate, blood pressure)
- Abdominal examination: presence of pain, rebound tenderness, masses
- Perianal and rectal examination
- Complete neurologic examination
- Pelvic examination as indicated
- Examination of skin and joints
- Alarm symptoms (see Box 32-3); there is an association between the presence of alarm symptoms and an organic cause to the chronic pain (AAP & NASPGHAN, 2005).

BOX 32-3 **Alarm Symptoms for Functional Abdominal Pain**

Red Flags on History
Localization of the pain away from the umbilicus, especially right or left upper
Pain associated with a change in bowel habits, particularly chronic, severe diarrhea; constipation; or nocturnal bowel movements
Pain associated with night wakening
Repetitive, significant emesis, especially if bilious
Constitutional symptoms, such as recurrent fever, loss of appetite or energy
Recurrent abdominal pain occurring in a child younger than 4 years old

Red Flags on Physical Examination
Unexplained fever
Unintentional loss of weight or decline in height velocity
Organomegaly
Localized abdominal tenderness, particularly removed from the umbilicus
Perirectal abnormalities (e.g., fissures, ulceration, or skin tags)
Joint swelling, redness, heat, or discoloration
Ventral hernias of the abdominal wall

Diagnostic Studies. Any testing should be reserved for the presence of alarm symptoms or specific symptoms of organic disease.

- CBC, ESR, CRP, UA, and urine culture if FAPS is suspected. If indicated, a biochemical profile (liver and kidney function); stool for ova, parasites and culture; and breath hydrogen testing may be useful
- US, endoscopy with or without biopsy, and esophageal pH monitoring as indicated with alarm symptoms

Differential Diagnosis

There is no evidence that the presence of the associated symptoms, a negative life event, or the presence of anxiety or depression can help distinguish between organic and FAP (AAP & NASPGHAN, 2005). Fig. 32-5 outlines a decision tree for differential diagnosis of chronic abdominal pain. The following are included in the differential diagnosis:

- All organic causes of abdominal pain, including urinary tract, GI tract, and extraabdominal causes
- Malabsorption syndromes (usually with diarrhea, belching, flatulence, and bloating)
- Abdominal pain associated with depression (usually includes social isolation, decreased activity and attention span, difficulty sleeping, and irritability)
- School avoidance (usually associated with severe pain and anxiety on weekday mornings only)

Management

- Establish a therapeutic parent-child-practitioner relationship to improve patient satisfaction, adherence to treatment, symptom reduction, and other outcomes (Drossman, 2006). Explain the brain-gut interaction.
- Use medications judiciously (Rudolph & Miranda, 2004). H_2 blockers should not be used unless dyspepsia is present. Citalopram is in clinical trials with promising results.
- Discuss the possibility with the child and parent that the pain can be functional (inorganic) early in the visit. Assure them that the symptoms are real and will be addressed.
- Encourage return to school and normalization of lifestyle. Limit attention given for pain episodes.
- Consider the use of complementary and alternative (CAM) medical approaches (see Chapter 43). If certain dietary practices seem to cause pain, a more bland diet may be helpful (e.g., a lactose-fee diet with documented lactose intolerance). Avoiding sorbitol and fructose may be useful if malabsorption is considered a contributing factor. A mind-body approach is often useful, combining relaxation, behavioral management, stress coping training, meditation, and biofeedback. Acupuncture, massage, and hypnosis have also been shown to help with chronic abdominal pain. (Rudolph & Miranda, 2004; Scharff & Kemper, 2003).
- Explore psychological triggers and use management strategies for the pain:
  ○ Discuss how stressful events and emotional issues might affect the pain.
  ○ Distraction to shift attention from abdominal pain to other activities; attending school is a good distraction.

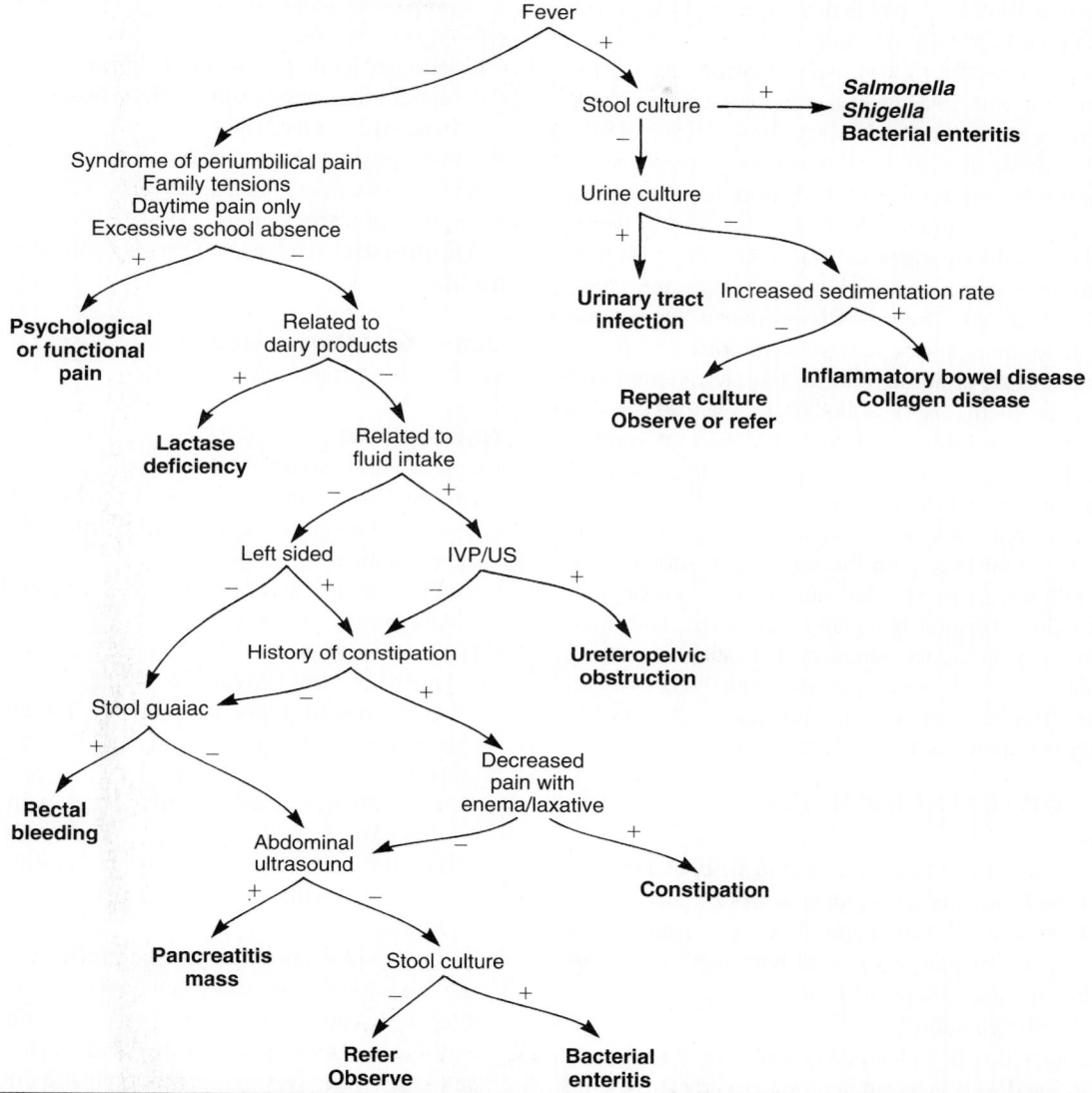

Differential Diagnosis

Bacterial enteritis	Functional	Tumor
Collagen vascular disease	Inflammatory bowel disease	Ureteropelvic obstruction
Constipation	Lactase deficiency	Urinary tract infection
Enteritis	Pancreatitis	

FIG. 32-5   Decision tree for the differential diagnosis of chronic abdominal pain. (From Schwartz MW et al, editors: *Pediatric primary care: a problem-oriented approach*, ed 3, St Louis, 1997, Mosby.)

- Biofeedback to provide evidence to the child that he or she can change muscle tension, skin temperature, and relaxation.
- Relaxation and guided imagery decrease abdominal pain (Ball et al, 2003).
- Identify, treat, and refer for any significant psychological issues.
  - Psychotherapy and family therapy may be of some benefit.
  - Cognitive behavioral therapy has also been helpful for all forms of FAP.

- Using a biopsychosocial approach is especially helpful for FAPS.
- Refer for psychological dysfunction (maladaptive behavior, conversion reaction, depression, anxiety).
- Discuss alarm symptoms (see Box 32-3) so that the parents and child can identify changes in status and illness.
- Establish regular follow-up.

Prognosis/Complications

RAP can be a lifelong and chronic condition, though one third of cases resolve within 2 months of diagnosis, one third have a long-term disorder with similar complaints in adulthood, and the final third have chronic complaints of pain (often headache) instead of abdominal pain (Kohli & Li, 2004). Male gender, onset of FAP before 6 years old, a delay in diagnosis greater than 6 months, and a family history of somatic pain, as first reported in 1958 by Apley and Naisch, are factors still predictive of a poor long-term prognosis.

Youssef and colleagues (2006) found that quality of life scores for children with FAP were lower than healthy peers and the same as peers with inflammatory bowel disease (IBD) and GERD. They also showed that the parents' perceptions of quality of life for their children with FAP were lower than the children's perceptions. Parents tend to feel helpless in being able to help their children with FAP and worry about finding the underlying etiology and receiving appropriate treatment (vanTilburg et al, 2005). There is also evidence that people with chronic abdominal pain have more symptoms of anxiety and depression and are at higher risk for long-term emotional and psychiatric problems (AAP & NASPGHAN, 2005).

Pain-associated disability syndrome (PADS) is described by Hyams (2005a) and Hyman and Elder Danda (2004) as 2 months of continuous or RAP that disrupts daily life. There is impairment in normal functioning (cannot eat or go to school) that the patient attributes to pain. Strategies that should have otherwise ameliorated the pain fail, and there is no organic cause of the pain. The pain is usually functional, and there is a comorbid psychological stressor. Persistent searching for an organic cause only serves to make the PADS worse. Collaborative effort between patient, clinician, mental health, and the family is imperative for successful treatment.

IRRITABLE BOWEL SYNDROME (IBS)
Description
The criteria for IBS (also known as Rome III criteria) must include *all* of the following (Rasquin et al, 2006):
- Abdominal discomfort (an uncomfortable sensation not described as pain) or pain associated with two *or more* of the following at least 25% of the time:
  - Improved with defecation
  - Onset associated with a change in frequency of stool
  - Onset associated with a change in form (appearance) of stool
- No evidence of an inflammatory, anatomic, metabolic, or neoplastic process that explains the subject's symptoms

Epidemiology
Visceral hypersensitivity related to infection, inflammation, intestinal trauma, or allergy has been documented. Disordered gut motility may be associated with IBS, as may be genetic predisposition, early stressful events, and ineffective coping mechanisms. Psychological comorbidity (somatic symptoms, anxiety, and depression) has also been reported. Diagnosis of IBS in primary care has been cited as 0.2% with a mean age of 52 months; however, it is as high as 22% to 45% in tertiary care (Rasquin et al, 2006).

Clinical Findings
History. The following symptoms *may* be present (Hyman & Elder Danda, 2004; Rasquin et al, 2006):

- Rome criteria for IBS (see description)
- Abnormal stool frequency (four or more stools per day and two or less stools per week)
- Abnormal stool form (lumpy/hard or loose/watery)
- Abnormal stool passage (straining, urgency, or feeling incomplete evacuation)
- Passage of mucus
- Bloating or feeling of abdominal distention
- Potential triggering events and psychosocial factors

Physical Examination
- Normal physical examination
- Normal growth curves and BMI
- Absence of alarm signals

Diagnostic Studies. There are no laboratory markers for IBS.

Differential Diagnosis
See FAP for differential diagnosis.

Management
- Confirm and explain diagnosis.
- The goal is to modify severity of symptoms. Identify and develop strategies to deal with triggering events and psychosocial factors.
- Antidepressants and serotoninergic agents have not been widely used in children.
- Treatment options for IBS include:
  - Antispasmodics (Poynard et al, 2001).
  - Enteric-coated peppermint oil for 2 weeks, which may decrease the severity of the abdominal pain (Kemper, 2003).
  - Anticholinergics, useful only if the pain is predictable (after a meal).
  - Tricyclic antidepressants may be helpful (more so with adults); use with care and obtain an ECG before initiation of therapy.
- Dietary modifications may be helpful with IBS. Avoid trigger foods known to exacerbate pain episodes (caffeine, sorbitol, fatty food, large meals, gas-producing foods, such as carbonated beverages, lactose (with lactose intolerance), and cruciferous vegetables (Rudolph & Miranda, 2004).

ABDOMINAL MIGRAINE
Description
Abdominal migraine is thought to be part of a continuum with cyclic vomiting and migraine headache. Affected individuals often progress from one disorder to another. The diagnostic criteria for abdominal migraine (also known as Rome III criteria) must include *all* of the following (Rasquin et al, 2006):
- Paroxysmal episodes of intense, acute periumbilical pain that lasts for an hour or more
- Intervening periods of usual health lasting weeks to months
- Pain that interferes with normal activities
- Pain that is associated with two or more of the following:
  - Anorexia, nausea, vomiting, headache, photophobia, pallor
- No evidence of an inflammatory, anatomic, metabolic, or neoplastic process that explains the symptoms

These criteria need to be present two or more times in the preceding 12 months.

Epidemiology

Abnormal visual-evoked responses, hypothalamic-pituitary-adrenal axis abnormalities, and autonomic dysfunction are possible mechanisms. Abdominal migraine affects 1% to 4% of children and tends to be more common in girls than boys (3:2), with a mean onset at 7 years old and a peak at 10 to 12 years old (Rasquin et al, 2006).

Clinical Findings

History
- Rome criteria for abdominal migraine (see description)
- Family history of migrane
- History of motion sickness
- Most episodes last hours to days

Physical Examination
- Normal physical examination
- Normal growth curves and BMI
- Absence of alarm signals

Diagnostic Studies.   There are no laboratory markers for abdominal migraine.

Differential Diagnosis

Obstructive GI and renal processes, biliary tract disease, recurrent pancreatitis, familial Mediterranean fever, and metabolic disorders, such as porphyria, should be ruled out.

Management
- Identify and avoid triggers: caffeine, nitrates, and amine-containing foods; excessive emotional stress; travel; prolonged fasting; altered sleep; flickering or glaring lights
- Abdominal migraine should respond to migraine prophylactic therapy (pizotifen, propranolol, cyproheptadine, or sumatriptan). A positive response helps confirm diagnosis.

MALABSORPTION SYNDROMES

Description

Malabsorption syndromes can be caused by many different genetic, congenital, and acquired conditions. Malabsorption syndromes usually cause an initial decrease in weight followed by a deceleration in height velocity. A complete listing of the causes of malabsorption is beyond the scope of this chapter. Celiac disease (CD), lactose intolerance, and cow's milk protein intolerance (CMPI) will be discussed here. Otherwise, this section offers a general approach to all malabsorption syndromes.

Epidemiology

Celiac disease (CD) is thought to be the most common genetically predetermined condition to affect mankind today. CD is not well understood. However, there is strong evidence of an association of human leukocyte antigen (HLA) with immune response. Once the inflammatory reaction is activated by gluten, intestinal damage occurs (Gelfond & Fasano, 2006). There may also be an association between repeated rotavirus infections and increased risk of CD (Stene et al, 2006). CD can be associated with autoimmune diseases including type I diabetes, thyroid disease, and Sjögren syndrome and with nonautoimmune diseases, such as Down syndrome, IgA deficiency, Williams syndrome, and Turner syndrome. CD has a worldwide distribution. The incidence of CD is estimated to be 1 in 250 people. The most typical presentation is between 6 months and 2 years old. Hoffenberg and colleagues (2003) found that CD affects 0.9% of children in Denver by 5 years old and that girls are at increased risk for disease.

Lactose intolerance is a clinical syndrome that causes abdominal pain, diarrhea, nausea, flatulence, and bloating after the ingestion of foods containing lactose. *Lactose malabsorption* causes lactose intolerance and is caused by the imbalance of the amount of lactose ingested and the capacity for lactase to hydrolyze lactose (Heyman & the Committee, 2006). Lactose is a disaccharide that consists of glucose and galactose, and it is found exclusively in mammalian milk. It requires the enzyme lactase, which is found on the small intestinal brush border, to hydrolyze the two monosaccharides apart and make them fit for absorption into the gut. Lactose that cannot be absorbed creates an osmotic load in the gut and draws fluid and electrolytes into the intestine thereby causing loose stool or diarrhea. The unabsorbed lactose is metabolized by intestinal bacteria creating gases (methane, carbon dioxide, and hydrogen) that then cause bloating and flatulence. Lactose intolerance causes symptoms related to lactose ingestion; it does not cause any intestinal damage.

Primary lactase deficiency, also known as lactase non-persistence or hereditary lactase deficiency, is the most common cause of lactose intolerance and occurs when there is an absence of lactase. It usually develops in childhood, at varying ages, and is more common in various ethnic groups. *Secondary lactase deficiency* results from small bowel injury (e.g., gastroenteritis, chemotherapy, chronic diarrhea) and is more common in infancy. *Congenital lactase deficiency* is a congenital absence of lactase, is extremely rare, and if left untreated, can be fatal in early infancy. *Developmental lactase deficiency* describes the lactase deficiency that occurs in preterm infants born before 34 weeks because of the immaturity of the intestinal tract (Heyman, 2006). The incidence of primary lactase deficiency has been estimated to be 70%. It is more common in Hispanic, Black, Ashkenazi Jewish, Asian, and American-Indian populations.

Cow's milk protein intolerance (CMPI) and *cow's milk allergy* (CMA) have a similar clinical picture; however, the body's immune response is much different in each of these conditions. Both CMPI and CMA are caused by the body's inability to digest CMP and can result in bloody diarrhea, anemia, dehydration, poor growth, and FTT. CMPI is non-IgE mediated, may cause elevated T-cell levels, and does not have the same long-term adverse effects of CMA (Ewing & Jackson-Allen, 2005). CMPI occurs when large molecules, such as CMP, pass through the infant's permeable GI tract and are absorbed rather than broken down (Cirgin-Ellet, 2003; Ewing & Jackson-Allen, 2005). CMA is IgE mediated and causes antibody production that has been associated with other atopic illnesses. Heine and colleagues (2002) described three stages of CMPI. They include, *immediate*, which is IgE mediated, occurring within 30 minutes and having signs of hives, angioedema, and anaphylaxis; *intermediate*, which is not IgE mediated, resulting in GI symptoms within hours of ingestion of CMP; and *late*, which causes GI symptoms days after consumption. GER, infantile proctocolitis, esophagitis, atopic dermatitis, constipation, and enterocolitis are all manifestations of intermediate and late reactions (Dupont & de Boissieu, 2003).

Clinical Findings

History. Careful past medical and family medical histories are very important in the evaluation of malabsorption syndrome and are often the key to the diagnosis. In addition, a complete dietary history is needed to distinguish between undernutrition and malabsorption. Important historical findings include the following:

- Past surgical and trauma history is needed.
- Growth failure (a common symptom of nutritional deficiency and malabsorption).
- Delayed puberty can coexist with malabsorption.
- A voracious appetite or particular food avoidance may be present in small children with malabsorption syndromes.
- Chronic diarrhea with frequent, large, foul-smelling, pale stools.
- Excessive flatus with abdominal distention.
- Pallor, fatigue, hair and dermatologic abnormalities, digital clubbing, dizziness, cheilosis, glossitis, peripheral neuropathy (symptoms of vitamin deficiency seen with malabsorption).

Disease Specific Findings

Celiac Disease

- Impaired growth, chronic diarrhea, frank steatorrhea, abdominal distention, muscle wasting with hypotonia, poor appetite, and lack of energy (Gelfond & Fasano, 2006).
- May have no symptoms at all despite having evidence of small bowel changes or may have isolated short stature, delayed puberty, anemia, dermatitis herpeticus, and symmetrical dental enamel hypoplasia in all four quadrants of the mouth involving the second dentition (Hill & Hill, 2005).
- Children with chronic diarrhea should be screened for CD (Imanzadeh et al, 2005).

Lactose intolerance

- Symptoms are often related to the amount of lactose ingested and include abdominal pain, diarrhea, nausea, flatulence, and bloating.

CMPI and CMA

- Family history of allergy and/or atopy
- May have only GI symptoms or only cutaneous symptoms or only respiratory symptoms or only anaphylaxis or with any combination of the above (Ewing & Jackson-Allen, 2005).
- Symptoms start early in infancy: there is less CMP in breast milk; therefore breastfed infants are generally more sensitized to CMP, more likely to have CMA, and may have long-term sequelae (Brown, 2002).
- Most common GI symptoms are bloody stools, diarrhea, vomiting, food refusal.

- Skin manifestations include eczema, atopic dermatitis, itching, hives, and angioedema.
- Cough and wheeze associated with ingestion of CMP.
- Anaphylaxis is rare.
- Food refusal and FTT.

Physical Examination. The following should be included:

- Growth parameters and percentiles (weight, height, BMI, head circumference)
- Skinfold thickness and lean body mass
- Tanner stage
- Examination for delayed growth and puberty

Diagnostic Studies. The following are ordered as indicated:

- Stool assessment for occult blood, O&P, WBCs, and culture; liquid stool for pH and reducing substances; 72-hour fecal fat collection or Sudan stain for stool fat.
- Spot stool testing for α_1-antitrypsin level to establish the diagnosis of protein-losing enteropathy.
- In the presence of steatorrhea, a sweat chloride test for CF is necessary.
- Stool culture and O&P. Giardiasis is a common intestinal infection causing malabsorption.
- CBC with differential, red cell concentration, iron, folic acid, and ferritin.
- Serum calcium, phosphorus, magnesium, alkaline phosphatase, serum protein, liver function tests, vitamin D and its metabolites, vitamins A, B_{12}, E, and K.
- HIV testing because FTT and chronic diarrhea may be presenting symptoms.
- Small bowel biopsy will help to identify diseases of the small bowel mucosa and to obtain material for culture and sensitivities.
- Plain abdominal radiographs and barium contrast studies as indicated.
- Abdominal US can detect masses and stones in the hepatobiliary system.
- Retrograde studies of the pancreas and biliary tree if indicated.
- Bone age.

Specific Tests for CD

- Endoscopy and biopsy needed for definitive diagnosis of CD.
- Test for CD if there is any clinical suspicion of disease; child has associated disorder, or there is a first-degree relative with CD.
- Multiple serologic tests are recommended because single serologic tests have a higher false-positive rate especially if there are GI symptoms. Tests include:
  - Elisa of IgA and IgG anti-TTG (antitissue transglutaminase antibodies) for detection and follow-up of CD (Baudon et al, 2004). This test has a higher correlation to intestinal biopsy-proven CD (Hill & Hill, 2005).
  - Children with CD who are ingesting a gluten-containing diet have increased levels of antigliadin antibodies (AGA) of IgA and IgG classes and antiendomysium antibodies (EMA). EMA is more expensive and less accurate in children under 2 years old (Gelfond & Fasano, 2006).
- Monitoring of CD should include careful follow-up of growth parameters, TTG testing after 6 months of gluten-free diet (GFD), and then yearly (NASPGHN, 2005).
- Bone density testing (bone problems may be first symptom of CD).

Specific Tests for Lactose Intolerance

- Trial of a lactose-free diet for 2 weeks, being aware of hidden sources of lactose. Symptoms should disappear with the diet and reappear when lactose reintroduced.
- Lactose and sucrose breath hydrogen testing for carbohydrate intolerance. Children should not be taking antibiotics at the time of the study (Ulshen, 2004).
- Stool for Clinitest and reducing substances.
- Bone density (lactose is necessary for calcium absorption into bone, and lactose-free diets may predispose to osteoporosis).
- If secondary cause of lactose intolerance suspected, continue work-up for all other causes of malabsorption.

CMP I and CMA

- Allergy testing often delayed until 1 year old.
- Test of choice is double-blind placebo controlled food challenge done in an allergist's office over a few hours time.
- Screening tests for infants and children may include serum allergy testing.
- Diagnosis is made when there is clinical improvement on CMP-free diet.
- Endoscopy and/or colonoscopy.

Differential Diagnosis

Organic and inorganic FTT, colic, short stature, chronic diarrhea, CF, immune deficiency, cholestatic liver disease, GER, and IBD are included in the differential diagnosis.

Management
Celiac Disease

- CD is treated by instituting a strictly gluten-free diet (GFD) for life. The standard for being gluten free is a limit of 20 ppm of gluten (NASPGHN, 2005). The ingestion of pure oats does not cause symptoms nor prevent mucosal healing in CD (Hogberg et al, 2004). Unfortunately, oats are often contaminated with gluten during manufacturing.
- A lactose-free diet for young children may be necessary. This is generally not the case in adolescence and adults unless they are lactose intolerant (NASPGHN, 2005).

Lactose Intolerance

- Avoid lactose-containing milk and other dairy products (including goat's milk); however, remain cognizant of the child's need for calcium and vitamin D.
- Use lactose-free dairy products.
- Use alternate milk sources (soy, rice, etc.).
- Many people with lactose intolerance can tolerate small amounts of lactose.
- Oral lactase supplements.

CMPI and CMA

- Restrict milk and milk products from the diet of infant or breastfeeding mother.
- Switch infant to soy formula or hydrolyzed formula or amino-acid formula.
- Avoid milk, eggs, fish, shellfish, peanuts, and tree nuts for breastfeeding mothers and infants for the first 2 years of life.
- Have EpiPen if anaphylaxis is a concern.
- Monitor growth and development carefully.

- Refer to an allergist or gastroenterology if symptoms are severe.

Complications and Prognosis
Celiac Disease

- Growth failure.
- Osteoporosis with reduced bone mineral density with delayed diagnosis and inadequate treatment (Kavak et al, 2003). Can be reversible with GFD (Gelfond & Fasano, 2006).
- Idiopathic cerebellar ataxia (prolonged GFD relieves the ataxia somewhat) (Sander et al, 2003).
- Associated with chronic headache, developmental delays, hypotonia, learning disorders, and attention-deficit/hyperactivity disorder (ADHD) (Castano et al, 2004).
- Increased risk for intestinal adenocarcinoma, esophageal cancer, melanoma, and non-Hodgkins lymphoma.
- Tuberculosis (Ludvigsson et al, 2006).
- Untreated CD can lead to infertility, endocrine disturbances, pathologic bone conditions, and dilated cardiomyopathy.
- Celiac crisis consisting of abdominal distention, explosive watery diarrhea, dehydration with electrolyte imbalance, hypotensive shock, and lethargy (Gelfond & Fasano, 2006).
- Prognosis is improved with lifelong GFD.

CMPI and CMA

- CMPI usually resolves by 1 to 3 years old.
- When there are only GI symptoms, CMPI resolves completely (Dupont & de Boissieu, 2003).
- There is no reversal of the sensitization that occurs in CMA, and there is a high likelihood of other food allergies.

POLYPS
Description

The hallmark of intestinal polyps is painless, bright red rectal bleeding often without changes in stooling pattern (Attard &Young, 2006). There are a number of other polyposis syndromes that are diagnosed based on biopsy.

Sporadic juvenile polyps are the most common and are generally isolated, colorectal juvenile (hamartomatous) polyps (Attard &Young, 2006). Gupta and colleagues (2001) described that sporadic juvenile polyps are up to 3 cm long and have no known association with colorectal cancer. There are typically only one or two polyps usually on the left side of the colon; up to one-third are located proximal to the splenic flexure (Attard & Young, 2006).

Juvenile polyposis coli (JP) occurs when there are five or more colorectal polyps or in the proximal GI tract, the child has any number of juvenile polyps, and a family history of JP (Jass et al, 1998). There are multiple hamartomatous polyps. There is no absolute histologic difference between sporadic and syndromic polyps (Attard & Young, 2006).

Familial adenomatous polyposis involves hundreds to thousands of polyps in the colon and rectum and may include colorectal and duodenal adenomas. If left untreated, there is nearly a 100% risk of colorectal cancer and very high risk for other types of cancer.

Peutz-Jeghers syndrome (PJS) is characterized by hamartomatous polyps that can involve the jejunum and other parts of the GI tract. PJS often presents as a bowel obstruction or hemorrhage (Attard & Young, 2006). There may also be melanin spots on the buccal mucosa, labia, and digits. There is an increased risk of colorectal cancer and a variety of other cancers, including testicular cancer that may present as gynecomastia.

Gastric polyps are usually an incidental finding on endoscopy, but can be associated with other polyposis syndromes. If they occur with familial adenomatous polyposis, there is a high likelihood of malignancy.

Epidemiology

Sporadic juvenile polyps affect approximately 2% of children and present between 5 and 6 years old (Attard & Young, 2006). JP is thought to be caused by genetic mutation (Howe et al, 2001). Familial adenomatous polyposis is an autosomal dominant inherited form of colorectal cancer, and it occurs in 1:8000 to 10,000 people. PJS is an "autosomal dominant trait of intermediate frequency" (Attard & Young, 2006). Gastric polyps are more common in caucasians than blacks with equal distribution between men and women.

Clinical Findings
History

- Painless, bright red rectal bleeding. Usually the blood coats or is mixed in with the stool. Bleeding can be daily, intermittent, or infrequent. Large volume blood loss is extremely rare.
- Duodenal polyps may cause vomiting and abdominal pain.
- Gastric polyps may cause abdominal pain, nausea, vomiting, and/ or GI hemorrhage.
- A careful family history is imperative.

Physical Examination. A thorough physical examination is needed with special attention to the following:

- Anorectal examination to find polyp or other source of rectal bleeding.
- Pallor and edema caused by anemia and hypoproteinemia from GI hemorrhage and protein-losing enteropathy (indicate a heavy polyp burden) (Attard & Young, 2006).
- Macrocephaly, digital clubbing, and skin and nail pigmented macules are associated with PJS.
- Characteristic ophthalmologic findings: dental anomalies (supernumerary or unerupted teeth): skull, jaw, and extremity osteomas: and multiple lipomas are associated with familial adenomatous polyposis.

Diagnostic Studies

- Fecal occult blood test, even if blood appears to be present.
- Stool culture for bacterial pathogens and parasites.
- CBC with differential and ESR, prothrombin time, and partial thromboplastin time.
- Complete colonoscopy to the terminal ileum with biopsy evaluation is the diagnostic test of choice.
- An upper endoscopy may be warranted if there is concern for gastric or duodenal polyps. Capsule endoscopy may be an alternative, but lacks the ability to procure a biopsy.

- A barium swallow with small bowel follow-through is less invasive, but also less sensitive in diagnosing polyps in the small intestine.
- Abdominal CT with oral and intravenous contrast can also be used to identify larger polyps.

Management

- Referral to gastroenterologist.
- Sporadic juvenile polyps require colonoscopy and biopsy. Children with one to four juvenile polyps at diagnosis usually need no further follow-up unless there are recurrent symptoms.
- If there are five or more juvenile polyps or there is a family history of colon polyps or the biopsied polyps are unusual, follow-up is recommended in 6 to 12 months.
- In JP all of the polyps must be removed and close follow-up maintained. Follow-up includes a colonoscopy 1 year after initial diagnosis and then, if no new polyps are noted, every 2 to 3 years.
- Familial adenomatous polyposis and other polyposis syndromes require careful follow-up by a specialist.
- Ophthalmologic evaluation.
- Genetic counseling.

ANAL FISSURE
Description
Anal fissures are small tears in the anal mucosa.

Epidemiology
The usual cause of an anal fissure is passage of frequent or hard stools. Anal stenosis and other trauma can also be causative factors. Anal fissures are the most common cause of rectal bleeding in all pediatric groups.

Clinical Findings
History. The following can be reported:
- Crying with bowel movement
- Bright red streaks of blood in the stool or diaper
- Withholding of stool

Physical Examination. With the patient in the knee-chest position and the anus slightly everted, small tears in the anal mucosa can be visible. An otoscope with a large speculum is needed if the external fissures are not readily visible. A digital anal examination with the fifth finger rules out anal stenosis.

Differential Diagnosis
Other sources of lower intestinal hemorrhage, such as infection, formula intolerance, necrotizing enterocolitis, intussusception, juvenile polyps, hemolytic-uremic syndrome, Henoch-Schönlein purpura, irritable bowel disease, and vascular lesions are included in the differential diagnosis. Sexual abuse should be considered in children with large, irregular, or multiple fissures.

Management
- Treat the cause (see Constipation in Chapter 13).
- Local wound care should include sitz baths twice a day and application of 0.5% hydrocortisone cream or K-Y jelly to the anus.

Complications

Recurrence of fissures is common (e.g., constipation causes a fissure, which leads to a retention-constipation cycle).

Prevention

Preventive measures include the following:
- Prevent constipation.
- Encourage regular toileting habits.
- Avoid the use of laxative medications and enemas.

■ INFLAMMATORY BOWEL DISEASE

Inflammatory bowel disease (IBD) is thought to be due to inappropriate and ongoing activation of the mucosal immune system with likely defects in both the barrier function of the intestinal epithelium and the mucosal immune system (Podolsky, 2002). IBD involves a genetic predisposition and environmental factors that serve to exacerbate the immune system response (Innis et al, 2006). Children with IBD are usually diagnosed before 20 years old, with about one third having at least one extraintestinal manifestation. See Table 32-8 for features of Crohn disease in contrast to ulcerative colitis (UC). Age of diagnosis of a chronic illness, such as IBD, can have differing impact on psychosocial functioning. According to Mackner & Crandall (2006) and Szigethy and colleagues (2006), adolescents may be at higher risk for social functioning difficulties, anxiety, or depression than a childhood diagnosis. Family dynamics have been reported as similar between healthy adolescents and those with IBD. Professionals working with adolescents with IBD should encourage participation in social activities, such as support groups and IBD camps. Palsson & Drossman (2005) identified depression, anxiety, and somatization disorders as the most frequent psychiatric disorders seen in clinical IBD patients. Incorporating psychosocial interviewing, development of a therapeutic relationship, and appropriate utilization of medications is key to achieving a satisfactory clinical outcome.

CROHN DISEASE

Description

Crohn disease is a chronic inflammatory disease with exacerbations and remissions involving any portion of the intestinal tract. Areas of intestine that are unaffected are called skip areas.

Epidemiology

The cause is largely unknown, though it is most likely a genetically determined response that is immunologically mediated. Crohn disease has a multifactorial basis (heredity, diet, immunologic aberrations, and ineffective mucosal integrity) that is probably influenced by environmental factors. The disease occurs in 400 of every 100,000 individuals, affects males and females equally, and is more common in white people. Twenty-five percent to 40% of cases are diagnosed in childhood and adolescence. Siblings are more likely to get Crohn disease than is the general population (Kugathasan & Amre, 2006; Loftus, 2006).

Clinical Findings

History. The following can be reported:
- Fever, usually low grade, of unknown etiology
- Weight loss (average of 5 to 7 kg)
- Delayed growth velocity, short stature, delayed bone age (Kim & Ferry, 2004)
- Arthralgias and/or arthritis in large joints, occasional joint destruction
- Obstructive symptoms associated with meals, bloating, early satiety
- Pain in the umbilical region and RLQ; may awaken at night
- Anorexia
- Malabsorption and lactose intolerance
- Diarrhea (with or without blood or mucus) and pain with stooling
- Jaundice
- Mouth sores, especially during exacerbations of the illness
- Use of NSAIDs, use of tobacco (Loftus, 2006; Podolsky, 2002)
- Positive family history

Physical Examination
- A complete physical examination is required.
- Carefully measure growth parameters (height, weight, and BMI).
- An abdominal examination is performed while observing for RLQ tenderness and a mass.
- Perianal skin tags, deep anal fissures, and perianal fistulas strongly suggest Crohn disease.
- Clubbing of digits may be present.
- Erythema nodosum is common.

Diagnostic Studies. The following are ordered as needed:
- Inflammatory markers: ESR, CRP
- Nutritional labs: albumin, total protein, (consider iron panel, calcium, zinc, alkaline phosphatase, folate, vitamin B_{12})
- Other blood tests: CBC with differential (consider liver enzymes—AST, ALT, total bilirubin, GGT; amylase; lipase)
- Stool: routine culture, O&P, C. difficile (with recent antibiotic use), blood, WBCs, and fecal α_1-antitrypsin
- Radiologic studies: bone age (usually delayed by 2 years), abdominal plain films, Upper GI series with small bowel follow-through, abdominal CT with contrast (or consider DEXA scan or endoscopic studies)

Differential Diagnosis

Rheumatoid arthritis, systemic lupus erythematosus, hypopituitarism, acute appendicitis, peptic ulcer, intestinal obstruction, intestinal lymphoma, anorexia, and growth failure are included in the differential diagnosis (Sondheimer, 2005).

Management

The goals of therapy are to (1) control the disease and induce a lasting remission; (2) prevent relapses; and (3) achieve normal nutrition, growth, and lifestyle. Treatment is pharmacologic, nutritional, surgical, and psychosocial. The following management steps are taken:
- Refer for endoscopy, definitive diagnosis, consultation, and follow-up care.

TABLE 32-8   Features of Crohn Disease and Ulcerative Colitis

Feature	Crohn Disease	Ulcerative Colitis
Age at onset	10-20 years old	10-20 years old
Area of bowel affected	Oropharynx, esophagus, and stomach, rare; small bowel only, 25%-30%; colon and anus only, 25%; ileocolitis, 40%; diffuse disease, 5%	Total colon, 90%; proctitis, 10%
Distribution	Segmental; disease-free skip areas common	Continuous distal to proximal
Pathologic conditions	Full-thickness, acute, and chronic inflammation; noncaseating granulomas (50%), extraintestinal fistulas, abscesses, stricture, and fibrosis may be present	Superficial, acute inflammation of mucosa with microscopic crypt abscess
X-ray findings	Segmental lesions; thickened, circular folds, cobblestone appearance of bowel wall secondary to longitudinal ulcers and transverse fissures; fixation and separation of loops; narrowed lumen, "string sign"; fistulas	Superficial colitis; loss of haustra; shortened colon and pseudopolyps (islands of normal tissue surrounded by denuded mucosa) are late findings
Intestinal symptoms	Abdominal pain, diarrhea (usually loose with blood if colon involved), perianal disease, enteroenteric or enterocutaneous fistula, abscess, anorexia	Abdominal pain, bloody diarrhea, urgency, and tenesmus
Extraintestinal symptoms		
Arthritis/arthralgia	15%	9%
Fever	40%-50%	40%-50%
Stomatitis	9%	2%
Weight loss	90% (mean 5.7 kg)	68% (mean 4.1 kg)
Delayed growth and sexual development	30%	5%-10%
Uveitis, conjunctivitis	15% (in Crohn colitis)	4%
Sclerosing cholangitis	—	4%
Renal stones	6% (oxalate)	6% (urate)
Pyoderma gangrenosum	1%-3%	5%
Erythema nodosum	8%-15%	4%
Laboratory findings	High ESR; microcytic anemia, low serum iron and total iron-binding capacity; increased fecal protein loss; low serum albumin; antineutrophil cytoplasmic antibodies present in 10%-20%; *Saccharomyces cerevisiae* antibodies positive in 60%	High ESR, microcytic anemia; high WBC count with left shift; antineutrophil cytoplasmic antibodies present in 80%

ESR, Erythrocyte sedimentation rate; *WBC*, white blood cell.
From Kirschner BS: Inflammatory bowel disease in children, *Pediatr Clin North Am* 35:189, 1989. Cited in Sundheimer J: Gastrointestinal tract. In Hay WW et al, editors: *Current pediatric diagnosis and treatment*, ed 16, New York, 2003, Lange Medical Books.

- Medications:
  - Antidiarrheals will not help inflammation, but will help make the symptoms manageable.
  - Corticosteroids (e.g., prednisone, budesonide) are used orally, rectally, or intravenously for acute exacerbations for mild to moderate disease. They are not intended for use in remission.
  - Aminosalicylates (sulfasalazine, olsalazine, and mesalamine) are given topically (enema) or orally for mild disease.
  - Immunomodulator agents may be used (azathioprine, 6-mercaptopurine, methotrexate, and cyclosporine) for severe small or large bowel disease, steroid-dependent or refractory disease, severe fistula, growth failure.

○ Antibiotics are used for acute exacerbation (ampicillin, gentamicin, clindamycin, ciprofloxacin, or metronidazole) with perirectal fistula, or abscess in bowel.

○ Adjunctive therapy, administration of healthy bacteria (probiotics [e.g., *Lactobacillus GG, Saccharomyces boulardii*]).

○ Biologic agents (e.g., infliximab, a chimeric, antitumor necrosis factor alpha-antibody) for steroid-dependent or refractory disease, perirectal fistula, maintenance of remission (Hyams, 2005).

• Severe disease can require hospitalization, total parenteral nutrition, a nasogastric tube for decompression, and surgery. Seventy percent of patients eventually (10 to 20 years following diagnosis) require surgery (Sondheimer, 2005).

• Monitor growth.

• If the small bowel is involved, an ophthalmologic examination is needed to rule out underlying ophthalmologic manifestations of the disease.

• Refer for nutritional therapy to help induce remission, prevent or correct malnutrition, and maintain and promote growth. See Box 11-9 for specific nutritional recommendations.

• Refer for psychosocial therapy as indicated. Depressive disorders are common.

Complications

Growth failure, fistula and abscess formation, intestinal obstruction, vitamin D deficiency, and malnutrition can occur. Perforation and hemorrhage are rare. Cholelithiasis, nephrolithiasis, pancreatitis, pericarditis, arthritis, and peripheral neuropathy are other complications of Crohn disease (Papa et al, 2006; Sawczenko et al, 2006; Sondheimer, 2005). There is also an increased risk of colon cancer (Friedman, 2006).

Prevention and Prognosis

Follow recommended therapy to prevent sequelae. Crohn disease is usually progressive. More than 50% experience symptoms affecting quality of life, 20% have severe disability, and 20% describe themselves as healthy (Sondheimer, 2003). Approximately 99% have more than one relapse after diagnosis and therapy (Hyams, 2005b).

ULCERATIVE COLITIS

Description

Ulcerative colitis is characterized by recurring bloody diarrhea with acute and chronic inflammation limited to the colon. Patients with UC have significant weight loss secondary to chronic caloric insufficiency.

Epidemiology

The cause is largely unknown, but is probably a genetically determined response that is immunologically mediated. It is thought to be an altered immunologic response in the intestinal mucosa. The disease has a multifactorial basis (heredity, diet, immunologic aberrations, and ineffective mucosal integrity) influenced by environmental factors (Moreels & Pelckmans, 2005). The overall incidence is two to six cases per 100,000, with the peak onset occurring among 16- to 20-year-olds. Approximately 20% occur in children younger than 20 years old (Snyder, 2002).

Clinical Findings

History.   The following can be reported:
• Fever
• Weight loss (average of 4 kg)
• Delayed growth and sexual maturation
• Arthritis and/or arthralgias of the large joints
• Anorexia
• Diarrhea
• Lower abdominal cramping, left lower quadrant pain
• Pain increased before stooling and passing flatus
• Stool with bright red blood and mucus
• Oral ulcers possible with active disease
• Skin lesions (erythema nodosum, pyoderma gangrenosum, and diffuse papulonecrotic eruptions)

Physical Examination
• Perform a complete physical examination.
• Carefully measure growth parameters (weight, height, and BMI).
• Abdominal examination can reveal rebound tenderness if the disease is severe.

Diagnostic Studies.   The following are ordered as needed:
• CBC with differential, iron-binding capacity, total protein, albumin, ESR, CRP, platelet count
• Stool for WBCs, blood, and culture
• Bone age (usually delayed up to 2 years)
• Colonoscopy
• Positive perinuclear neutrophil cytoplasmic antigen in 60% to 70%
• High fecal calprotectin in active disease

Differential Diagnosis

Shigella, Salmonella, Yersinia, Campylobacter, E. coli, C. difficile, IBS, and Crohn disease are the differential diagnoses (Sondheimer, 2005).

Management

The goals of therapy are to (1) control the disease and induce a lasting remission; (2) prevent relapses; and (3) achieve normal nutrition, growth, and lifestyle. Treatment is pharmacologic, nutritional, surgical, and psychosocial. Management involves the following:
• Refer for endoscopy, definitive diagnosis, consultation, and close follow-up care.
• Medications:
  ○ Aminosalicylates (sulfasalazine, mesalamine) orally or rectally
  ○ Parenteral or oral steroids for moderate to severe disease, tapered doses for remission.
  ○ Immunomodulatory agents (azathioprine or 6-mercaptopurine) to wean off steroids
  ○ Hydrocortisone rectal preparation for tenesmus
  ○ Antispasmodics before meals
  ○ Iron supplementation to correct anemia

- Nutrition (see Box 11-9 for nutritional recommendations):
  - Diet: high in protein and carbohydrate, normal amount of fat, and decreased roughage.
  - Lactose is poorly tolerated (Sondheimer, 2005).
  - Vitamin and iron supplementation is recommended.
  - Parenteral or enteral nutritional supplements (60 to 70 cal/kg/day) may be used.
  - Refer for nutritional therapy to prevent or correct malnutrition and maintain and promote growth.
- Monitor growth.
- Refer for surgery as indicated (can be curative).
- Refer for ophthalmologic examination to rule out ophthalmologic manifestations of the disease.
- Refer for psychosocial therapy as indicated. Depressive disorders are common.

Complications

Complications can include growth failure, toxic megacolon, intestinal perforation, liver disease, sepsis, colitis (children with pancolitis experience a much more severe course), cancer of the colon (can be a long-term sequela—1% to 2% per year after 10 years of disease), arthritis, uveitis, malnutrition, and behavioral and emotional problems (Sondheimer, 2005).

Prevention and Prognosis

Follow the recommended therapy to prevent complications. Prognosis is good. Seventy percent will go into remission within 3 months of diagnosis, following initiation of therapy. Fifty percent will remain in remission. Up to 26% with severe disease require colectomy, whereas only 10% with mild disease do (Hyams, 2005b).

FOREIGN BODIES IN THE GASTROINTESTINAL TRACT

Description

Most swallowed foreign bodies pass through the GI tract without difficulty. Some objects get lodged at points of narrowing (e.g., cricopharyngeal muscle, the carina, Schatzki ring, cardioesophageal junction, pylorus, ligament of Treitz). Anything 3 to 5 cm or larger might have trouble passing the ligament of Treitz. In 10% to 20% of the cases, a nonoperative intervention, such as endoscopy, balloon-tipped catheter, or esophageal bougienage dilation technique, will be required (Uyemura, 2005; Waltzman et al, 2005). The need for surgical intervention for a GI foreign body is about 1% or less (Li et al, 2006).

Epidemiology

The cause is a swallowed foreign body, with the highest incidence occurring between 6 months and 3 years old (Uyemura, 2005). Foreign body ingestion occurs equally in boys and girls, with developmentally delayed children at higher risk. Common items include coins (most commonly pennies), food, toys, marbles, buttons, safety pins, bottle tops, and batteries. Bezoars are foreign bodies that have accumulated over time in the alimentary tract (Wyllie, 2004). They are most often caused by plant or vegetable matter (phytobezoar), hair (trichobezoar), and persimmons (disopyrobezoar). Bezoars eventually cause obstructive symptoms because of increasing size.

Clinical Findings
History

- Often there is no history of swallowing a foreign body.
- Initially the child might have experienced a coughing, choking, or gagging episode, even though the parents may not have observed the episode. Persistent wheezing that is unresponsive to bronchodilators may indicate a foreign body in the esophagus or lung.
- Subsequent symptoms can include discomfort in the throat or chest, refusal to eat, increased salivation, vomiting, pain with swallowing, and respiratory difficulty (Little et al, 2006; Uyemura, 2005).

Physical Examination

- Most children are asymptomatic.
- GI examination is normal.
- Respiratory symptoms may be found if the foreign body is lodged in the esophagus and pressing on the trachea.

Diagnostic Studies

- If symptoms of obstruction persist, radiographic studies are ordered to rule out a foreign body. A dime is 17 mm, a penny 18 mm, a nickel 20 mm, and a quarter 23 mm in size. The radiographic studies should include the neck, the chest, and the upper abdomen (Uyemura, 2005). Abdominal radiographs can be ordered if an object has not been seen in the stool and symptoms of distress or obstruction are present. Most ingested foreign bodies are radiopaque; however, wooden, plastic, and glass objects and fish and chicken bones may not be seen on radiographs.
- A contrast study (barium esophagogram), forced expiratory film, CT scan, US, or MRI may be needed if a foreign body is suspected but is not radiopaque.
- An alternative to radiography is a hand-held metal detector.

Management

If asymptomatic or if the foreign body is in the stomach or intestine, no intervention is necessary, and the family can be reassured. Smooth objects, buttons, and most coins can remain in the intestines for months without symptoms. The exception is new, mostly zinc pennies, which can cause a chemical reaction and poisoning. Watch for fecal passage and report any new associated symptoms. Follow-up radiography is indicated after 2 weeks if a coin has not been identified in stool. Emergent endoscopic removal of all batteries should be done because burns and injury can occur within 4 hours of ingestion.

If symptomatic or if the object is sharp or very large, give the child nothing by mouth until a decision is made. Consult with a physician and pediatric surgeon. Generally, foreign bodies that remain in the esophagus longer than 3 hours or in the small intestine longer than 5 days need to be removed. Removal is often accomplished via a Foley catheter technique or by gastroesophagoscopy. Sharp objects (e.g., open safety pins, wooden toothpicks, and fish bones) and small batteries also need to be removed; this is generally accomplished by endoscopy (Little et al, 2006; Uyemura, 2005). When it is unclear how long a foreign body has been in the esophagus or if it has been there more than 48 hours, it should be retrieved with an endoscope. Foreign bodies can erode into esophageal tissue and ultimately cause catastrophic perforation (Little et al, 2006).

Complications

Perforation or stricture formation can occur in up to 10% of children. With esophageal foreign bodies that have been present for an extended period of time, FTT or recurrent aspiration pneumonia may be seen (Uyemura, 2005).

Prevention

Parent education, anticipatory counseling, and careful supervision of children are needed. Avoid ear piercing in children younger than 2 years old because earrings are easily ingested. Keep toys with small parts that might come off and any small objects (especially sharp ones and batteries) out of the reach of children.

■ FAILURE TO THRIVE (ORGANIC)

DESCRIPTION

Failure to thrive (FTT), also called growth deficiency (Brayden et al, 2003), is described as inadequate weight gain as determined by standardized growth charts. The diagnosis is based on a child's weight being below the 3rd to 5th percentile or falling more than two major percentile groups or becoming flat (Block & Krebs, 2005). Weight falls before height and head circumference do. Organic FTT is also referred to as undernutrition or inadequate growth caused by major organ system disease (Brayden et al, 2003; Gahagan, 2006). The conceptualization of FTT as either organic or nonorganic has changed. FTT is now understood to be the product of interaction between the environment and the individual's health, development, and behavior (Gahagan, 2006).

EPIDEMIOLOGY

FTT can be unintentional (difficulties with breastfeeding, formula preparation errors, inappropriate food selection with poor transition in the 6- to 12-month-old age group, excess juice consumption), associated with multiple medical conditions (Table 32-9), or psychological factors (see Chapter 18). The purpose of this section is to discuss the assessment, laboratory findings, and differential diagnosis related to medical or organic causes of FTT; however, it is necessary to consider all physical and psychological factors concurrently when evaluating FTT. Eight percent to 10% of children seen for primary care have signs of growth failure, with the number rising to 15% to 30% in inner-city emergency departments (Brayden et al, 2003). Poverty is the primary risk factor for FTT worldwide, including the U.S. (Block et al, 2005).

CLINICAL FINDINGS

A thoughtful approach to the history, physical examination, and laboratory evaluation of children with FTT includes the following (Block et al, 2005; Brayden et al, 2003; Gahagan, 2006):

History

- Three-day diet history (72 hours)
- Careful family history of weight, height, BMI, growth patterns, and chronic health conditions
- Prenatal factors: drug, alcohol, and tobacco exposure; length of gestation; illnesses; weight gain; nutrition; TORCH (toxoplasmosis, other agents, rubella, cytomegalovirus, herpes simplex); and human immunodeficiency virus (HIV) exposure
- Perinatal factors: birth weight, Apgar scores, complications, length of stay in the hospital, congenital anomalies, neurologic insults, newborn screening results
- Collection and interpretation of growth data for the child's measurements, percentiles, BMI, height for weight over time
- General parental concerns about the child's weight and growth

---

TABLE 32-9   **Major Organic Causes of Failure to Thrive**

System	Cause
Gastrointestinal	GER, CD, pyloric stenosis, cleft palate or cleft lip, lactose intolerance, Hirschsprung disease, milk protein intolerance, hepatitis, cirrhosis, pancreatic insufficiency, biliary disease, IBD, malabsorption, food alkalines
Renal	UTI, renal tubular acidosis, diabetes insipidus, chronic renal insufficiency
Cardiopulmonary	Cardiac diseases leading to congestive heart failure, asthma, bronchopulmonary dysplasia, CF, anatomic abnormalities of the upper airway; obstructive sleep apnea (snoring)
Endocrine	Hypothyroidism, diabetes mellitus, adrenal insufficiency or excess, parathyroid disorders, pituitary disorders, growth hormone deficiency
Neurologic	Mental retardation, cerebral hemorrhage, degenerative disorders
Infectious	Parasitic or bacterial infections of the GI tract, tuberculosis, HIV disease
Metabolic	Inborn errors of metabolism
Congenital	Chromosomal abnormalities, congenital syndromes (e.g., fetal alcohol syndrome), perinatal infections
Miscellaneous	Lead poisoning, malignancy, collagen-vascular disease, recurrently infected adenoids and tonsils

CD, Celiac disease; *CF*, cystic fibrosis; *GER*, gastroesophageal reflux; *GI*, gastrointestinal; *HIV*, human immunodeficiency virus; *IBD*, inflammatory bowel disease; *UTI*, urinary tract infection.

From Bauchner H: Failure to thrive. In Behrman RE, Kliegman R, Jenson HR, editors: *Nelson textbook of pediatrics*, ed 17, Philadelphia, 2004, WB Saunders, p 134.

- General health history: hospitalizations, medications, surgeries, accidents, illnesses
- Developmental history
- Nutrition history: caloric intake; feeding behavior; feeding cues; cues to hunger and satiety; ability to suck, swallow, chew; progression to solids; frequency of feedings; amount taken per feeding; preparation of formula (overdilution), family eating patterns (meals and child feeding)
- Stooling and voiding history: diarrhea, constipation, vomiting, poor urine stream
- Social and family factors: family composition, caregiving environment, day care, family support, finances, parent-child relationship, parenting attitudes, typical day
- Careful review of systems

Physical Examination

- Weight, height, BMI, and head circumference (in those younger than 2 years old) plotted on standardized growth curves and percentiles, including weight-for-height graphs (include past and present growth parameters)
- Skinfold measurements
- Vital signs (temperature, pulse, respiratory rate, blood pressure)
- Evidence of abuse or neglect
- Presence of dysmorphic features
- Upper and lower segment measurements (Fig. 32-6) to rule out dwarfism
- Skin, hair, nails, and mucous membranes
  - Scaling skin seen with zinc deficiency
  - Rough or hard skin with hypothyroidism
  - Edema with protein deficiency
  - Alopecia with hypervitaminosis or syphilis
  - Spoon-shaped nails with iron deficiency or GI diseases
  - Cyanosis with heart disease
  - Labial fissures with vitamin deficiency
- Oral findings: dental caries, tonsillar hypertrophy, submucous cleft palate, or tongue enlargement
- Lymphadenopathy and splenomegaly with malignancy and immune deficiency
- Endocrine: thyroid enlargement, precocious or ambiguous sexual development
- Neuromuscular tone and strength
- Disproportionate somatic growth (dwarfism)

Diagnostic Studies

Appropriate use of laboratory tests as indicated by the history and physical examination:

- Review of newborn metabolic screening tests
- UA and urine culture
- CBC, differential and platelets, ESR
- Serum electrolytes (make sure to get total CO_2 to rule out renal tubular acidosis)
- Lead level
- Purified protein derivative (PPD) with *Candida* control
- HIV screening

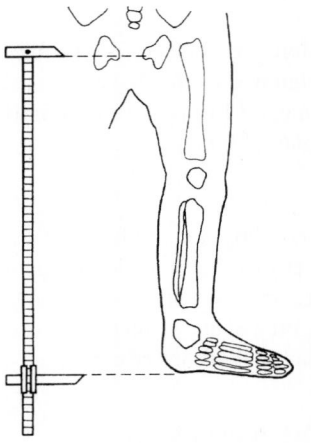

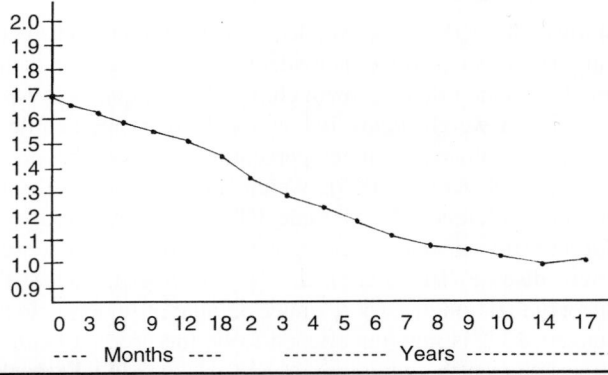

FIG. 32-6   Upper:lower (U:L) segment ratios. **A,** To calculate U:L segment ratios use the following formula: (height − lower segment)/lower segment. **B,** Normal U:L segment ratios. 1.7 at birth, 1.3 at 3 years old, 1 at 14 years old. High U:L ratios are characteristic of short limb dwarfism or bone disorders, such as rickets. (From Siberry GK, Iannone R, editors: *The Harriet Lane handbook*, ed 15, St Louis, 2000, Mosby, p 278.)

- Serum protein, albumin, alkaline phosphatase, blood urea nitrogen (BUN), and creatinine
- Thyroid function and growth hormone (expensive, often done later in work-up)
- Stool studies for fat, reducing substances, O&P, and culture
- Sweat test
- Bone age
- Chest radiograph
- Renal US and voiding cystourethrography
- Developmental testing

DIFFERENTIAL DIAGNOSIS

See Table 32-7.

MANAGEMENT

- Manage treatable causes with prompt attention to urgent, life-threatening medical conditions.
- Provide nutritional support: vitamin supplementation with iron, zinc, and minerals; calorically enriched formula and foods (up to 150 cal/kg/day). See Box 11-4 for further information related to FTT.

- Provide parent education and support.
- Make referrals as needed.
- Provide close follow-up, initially every 1 to 2 weeks. Day care may provide structure for eating and other activities.
- Normal weight gain by age (Brayden et al, 2003; Gahagan, 2006):
  - Birth to 3 months old: 20 to 30 g/day
  - Three to 6 months old: 15 to 20 g/day
  - Six to 9 months old 10 to 15 g/day
  - Nine to 12 months old: 6 to 12 g/day
  - Twelve to 18 months old: 5 to 8 g/day
  - Eighteen to 24 months old: 3 to 7 g/day

■ LOWER GASTROINTESTINAL TRACT INFECTIONS

ACUTE DIARRHEA

Description

Acute diarrhea involves an excessive loss of fluid and electrolytes in the stool. Children of different ages normally have differing volumes, numbers, and frequency of stools. According to Limbos (2005) diarrhea is, therefore, defined as either an increase in stool frequency or decrease in stool consistency.

Epidemiology and Incidence

Four types of diarrhea are recognized (Limbos, 2005):

1. Osmotic diarrhea results when osmotically active particles in the intestine draw excess fluid into the stool; this condition occurs with dumping syndrome, lactase deficiency, overfeeding, malabsorption syndromes, and excess ingestion of hypertonic juices.
2. Secretory diarrhea occurs because there is active secretion of water and electrolytes from mucosal crypt cells in the small intestine into the bowel lumen. There tends to be large volumes of watery diarrhea even if the child is not being fed. Causes include endotoxin production from bacteria, congenital disorders, mucosal disorders, and tumors.
3. Motility disorders cause diarrhea but not malabsorption. Bile salt and pancreatic enzyme deficiency can cause diarrhea by deletion or inhibition of the normal absorption process. Toddler's diarrhea is thought to be caused by an alteration in intestinal motility.
4. Inflammatory processes, such as bacterial invasion, celiac sprue, and IBS, or surgical procedures can change the anatomy and functional ability of the intestine. Abnormal peristalsis for any reason can result in acute diarrhea.

Acute diarrhea can be caused by various viruses, bacteria, and parasites (Table 32-10). Viruses injure the absorptive surface of mature villous cells, which reduces the amount of fluid absorbed and causes a disaccharide deficiency. Bacterial agents cause damage to the intestinal mucosa by direct invasion and through the release of endotoxins (Berman, 2003).

Viral causes of acute diarrhea include:

- *Rotavirus* affects children 4 to 24 months old, causes half of all cases of acute gastroenteritis, occurs mostly in the cooler months, and can cause significant dehydration. Virtually all children are infected by 3 years old (Dennehy, 2005). It is spread via fecal-oral route, though the virus can be found on toys and hard surfaces. Rotavirus tends to have an acute onset with fever, vomiting, and diarrhea.
- *Adenoviruses* are the second most common type of viral diarrhea. This illness does not generally include the high fever or respiratory symptoms associated with nonenteric adenovirus (Dennehy, 2005). Transmission is via fecal-oral route.
- *Noroviruses* cause most of the diarrhea in industrialized countries (Dennehy, 2005). Fifty percent of food-borne outbreaks of diarrhea are caused by *noroviruses* (Fankhauser et al, 2002). These viruses are spread via fecal-oral route either in contaminated water or person to person. *Norovirus* infection usually starts with nausea, vomiting, watery, nonbloody diarrhea, and abdominal cramping and lasts about 24 to 60 hours.

Bacterial diarrhea, which is much less common, can be caused by:

- *Campylobacter jejuni* is a gram-negative rod found mostly in raw or undercooked poultry or meat. It is transferred person to person by the fecal-oral route and has a low infective dose (one drop of raw chicken juice) (Dinolfo, 2005). Shedding of the bacteria can persist for 2 to 3 weeks. It is most common in the summer months. Symptoms include diarrhea, abdominal pain, malaise, and fever. In neonates bloody diarrhea may be the only symptom (Dennehy, 2005).
- *Salmonella* is a gram-negative rod found in contaminated, improperly cooked poultry, eggs, dairy products, and sausage. It is spread by human-to-human contact. *Salmonella* is most common in children younger than 4 years old. The peak incidence is in the first months of life (AAP, 2003). Invasive disease is more common in children with underlying chronic illness or who are immunocompromised.
- *Shigella* is a gram-negative rod found in contaminated food and water. Humans are the host and reservoir, and the organism is spread by the fecal-oral route. The organism multiplies and releases cytotoxin, which causes epithelial damage and ulceration. There is usually a high spiking fever and bloody diarrhea. *Shigella* is most common in children 6 months to 3 years old.
- Enteroadherent and enterotoxigenic strains of *E. coli* usually cause mild traveler's diarrhea.
- Enterohemorrhagic *E. coli* (O157:H7) can be associated with a mild, self-limited diarrhea that causes bloody stool and abdominal cramping, hemorrhagic colitis, hemolytic-uremic syndrome, and postdiarrheal idiopathic thrombocytopenic purpura. *E. coli* O157:H7 is the prototype and can cause mild to severe, profuse, and bloody diarrhea. Incubation is from 10 hours to 6 days; *E. coli* O157:H7 infection usually lasts 3 to 4 days and can be fatal. The bacteria are shed in cow feces and can be found in undercooked ground beef, contaminated water, raw fruits and vegetables, and unpasteurized milk and can be transmitted from infected persons. Outbreaks are linked to unpasteurized fruit juice, ground beef, petting zoos, salami, yogurt, spinach, lettuce and contaminated drinking water.

TABLE 32-10 **Infectious Diarrhea: Signs, Symptoms, Treatment, and Complications**

Cause	Diarrhea	Blood in Stool	Abdominal Pain	Vomiting	Fever	Treatment	Potential Complications
C. jejuni	+++ Foul smelling		+	+	+	Erythromycin, 40mg/kg/day in 3 divided doses for 5-7 days decreases fecal excretion in 24-48hr; illness lasts 7-12 days, or Azithromycin 10mg/kg/day the first day of treatment then 5mg/kg/day daily for 4 days.	Hemorrhagic necrosis of the jejunum, reactive arthritis, seizures, pseudotumor in the mesenteric lymph nodes, and hemolytic anemia
C. difficile	++	+	+		–	Discontinue offending antibiotic (see text). Metronidazole, 30mg/kg/day in 4 divided doses for 7-10 days *or* Vancomycin, 40mg/kg/ day in 4 divided doses for 7-10 days. Cholestyramine helps bind the toxin and decrease diarrhea.	Pseudomembranous colitis, toxic megacolon, colonic perforation, relapse, intractable proctitis, and death in debilitated children
Y. enterocolitica	+ Green, malodorous	+	+ RLQ pain		+	Usually resolves spontaneously in 3-4 days; if septic, TMP-SMZ, 8mg TMP/kg/day in 2 divided doses for 7-10 days, or Chloramphenicol, 50-75mg/kg/day in 4 divided doses for 7-10 days, or Tetracycline, 25-50mg/kg/day in 4 divided doses for 7-10 days (older teens only).	Septicemia and acute ileitis syndrome
Salmonella	++	+	+ Rebound tenderness	+	+	No treatment if uncomplicated. Usually resolves spontaneously. Antibiotics can prolong the carrier state. Antibiotics indicated for children younger than 1yr old who are at risk for bacteremia and for patients who are immunosuppressed or have cardiac or valvular disease, lymphoproliferative diseases, sickle cell disease, or hemolytic anemias.	Bacteremia, focal infection, and carrier state

					Treatment	Complications
					If indicated use Amoxicillin, 40mg/kg/day in 3 divided doses for 7-10 days or TMP-SMZ, 8mg TMP/kg/day for 7-10 days in 2 divided doses. Steroids and prostaglandins may be necessary for severe illness.	
Shigella	+++(initially + (after 1-3 days)	+		+	Need susceptibility information. Resistance is common. TMP-SMZ, 8mg TMP/kg/day in 2 divided doses for 5 days or If resistant to TMP-SMZ or if susceptibility is unknown then ceftriaxone, fluoroquinolones, or azithromycin may be indicated.	Toxic megacolon, cholestatic hepatitis, hemolytic-uremic syndrome, Reiter syndrome, and bacteremia
E. coli	++	+ Cramps and abdominal pain	−/+	+	No treatment is indicated for inflammatory or bloody diarrhea. Antibiotic resistance is common. If diarrhea is severe then consider: TMP-SMZ, 8mg TMP/kg/day in 2 divided doses for 7-10 days if diarrhea is moderate to severe or Azithromycin 10mg/kg/day the first day of treatment then 5mg/kg/day daily for 4 days or Ciprofloxacin 20-30mg/kg/day divided bid. Do CBC, platelets, and kidney function tests.	Hemolytic-uremic syndrome
Virus	+++ Watery	+ Cramps		+	Symptomatic treatment and maintenance of fluids.	

hr, Hours; *yr*, years; +, small amount; ++, moderate amount; +++, large amount; ± may or may not; −, not a clinical finding.

- *Yersinia enterocolitica* is a gram-negative rod found in contaminated food (e.g., uncooked pork and unpasteurized milk) and water. It produces an enterotoxin that causes secretion of fluid and electrolytes into the bowel. *Y. enterocolitica* causes diarrhea in children of all ages.
- *C. difficile* is a gram-positive anaerobic bacillus. Asymptomatic carriers of *C. difficile* who take antibiotics (usually ampicillin, clindamycin, and cephalosporins) experience increased growth of the organism. *C. difficile* intestinal colonization rates in healthy neonates and young infants can be as high as 50%, but are usually less than 5% in children older than 2 years and adults (AAP, 2006). Illness caused by *C. difficile* is generally mild, but can be severe and cause death, especially with an emerging more virulent strain (McDonald et al, 2005).

There are nongastrointestinal, referred to as parenteral, causes of acute diarrhea in children including other infectious processes (e.g., otitis media, UTI, pneumonia, and meningitis), endocrinopathies, neoplasms, antibiotic use, and allergic disorders (e.g., milk, soy, foods).

Acute diarrhea accounts for approximately 20% of acute care visits in children younger than 2 years old. It is the cause of 8 in 1000 hospitalizations in children younger than 1 year old and is the reason for 10% of preventable deaths in the U.S. Acute diarrhea is responsible for 500 deaths per year in the U.S. among children 1 to 4 years old. Poor access to care and poverty are correlated with increased mortality rates from diarrhea.

Clinical Findings

History.   The following should be included (see Table 32-10):

- Pattern of diarrhea: when diarrhea began, number of stools, frequency, quality of stools
- Signs and symptoms associated with infectious diarrhea: bloody stool, abdominal pain, vomiting, or fever
- Number of wet diapers in the past 24 hours and approximate time of last void
- Dietary record, changes in diet that might correlate with increased stooling
- Family members with similar illness or other GI diseases
- Day care or school illness patterns and contacts
- Travel history
- Most recent weight and previous growth pattern.

Physical Examination.   Assess the following (see Table 32-10):

- Complete physical examination including vital signs, assessment of behavior, and evaluation of anterior fontanelle, if it is still open.
- Assessment of dehydration (see Table 32-1). Steiner and colleagues (2004), found that CRT, skin turgor, and tachypnea, when considered together, were the most helpful in the determination of dehydration. Normal CRT is less than 2 seconds. Research has shown that a CRT of 2 to 2.9 seconds corresponds to a 50- to 90-ml/kg loss, 3 to 3.5 seconds corresponds to a 90- to 110-ml/kg loss, 3.5

to 3.9 corresponds to a 110- to 120-ml/kg loss, and more than 4 seconds corresponds to a 150-ml/kg loss (Finberg, 2002).

Diagnostic Studies.   Most diarrheal illness does not require any lab testing. The following are ordered as indicated:

- Stool examination (color, consistency, blood, mucus, pus, odor, volume).
- Stool pH, Clinitest, and heme test.
- Stool cultures should be considered for bloody or prolonged diarrhea, suspected food poisoning, or recent travel abroad (Banks, 2004).
- Specific laboratory findings (Table 32-11).
- *Rotavirus* is diagnosed using enzyme immunoassay and latex agglutination for group A rotavirus antigen in the stool, electron microscopy, and reverse transcriptase PCR (Dennehy, 2005).
- *Adenoviruses* are diagnosed by antigen detection by immunoassay.
- *Noroviruses* are diagnosed via reverse transcriptase PCR.
- *Campylobacter* is diagnosed by stool culture.
- *E. Coli O157:H7* is diagnosed using MacConkey agar base with sorbitol.
- The following are criteria to culture stool for *C. difficile*:
  - Test patients who are older than 1 year. *C. difficile* is commonly found in asymptomatic children less than 1 year old.
  - Severe diarrhea lasting at least 2 days.
  - The presence of other GI symptoms (cramping, abdominal pain).
- If intravenous fluids are necessary, serum bicarbonate will help establish the severity of the dehydration. Other serum electrolytes and glucose may help to evaluate complicated diarrhea (Banks, 2004).

Differential Diagnosis

Numerous causes, including infection (bacterial or viral), medication ingestion, parasitic infestations, anatomic abnormalities, dietary intolerances, and appendicitis, may be responsible for acute diarrhea.

Management

The following steps are taken:

- Restore and maintain hydration. Oral rehydration with an oral electrolyte solution should be attempted. Appropriate rehydration solutions include Pedialyte and Infalyte. It is inappropriate to use fruit juices, Kool-Aid, sports drinks, or soda. If the child is not vomiting, oral rehydration can be accomplished quickly (less than 4 hours) (see Tables 32-2 and 32-3). For formula-fed infants, returning to full-strength formula as quickly as possible is recommended. If the child is unable to tolerate full-strength formula, a diluted formula (one fourth to half strength) can be used for a short time (4 to 6 hours) as tolerated. The child's regular formula can be used initially as long as it is tolerated. If not tolerated, use soy or hydrolysate formula. Breastfed infants should continue to breastfeed more frequently for shorter periods.

TABLE 32-11 **Laboratory Findings Associated With Infectious Diarrhea**

Cause	Bloody Stool	WBCs in Stool	Stool Culture	CBC	Other
C. jejuni	+ Gross	+	+	↑ WBCs	Darting and motility on microscopy
C. difficile	+ Gross	+	+ for toxin	Slightly ↑ WBCs, ESR nl	
Y. enterocolitica	+ Gross or occult	+	+		
Salmonella	+ Gross	+	+	↓, nl, or slightly ↑ WBCs with left shift	
Shigella	+ Gross	+	+	nl or slightly ↑ WBCs with left shift	
E. coli	+ Gross	—	+		Hemolytic-uremic syndrome as a complication
Virus	—	—	±*		

*If virus is suspected, consider studying stool for reducing substances, Clinitest, heme test, and pH. Can test stool using ELISA and latex agglutination assay for rotavirus.

CBC, Complete blood count; *ESR*, erythrocyte sedimentation rate; *nl*, normal; *WBCs*, white blood cells; *+*, present; *−*, not a clinical finding ±, may or may not be present; ↑, increased; ↓, decreased.

- Resume early refeeding because contents of the bowel stimulate the growth of enterocytes and help to facilitate mucosal repair following injury. The resumption of a regular diet once rehydration has been accomplished or continuing with a regular diet despite the diarrhea has been shown to shorten the duration of the disease. There is no additional benefit to the BRAT diet; a diet tolerated by the child is recommended.
- Administer parenteral hydration if necessary for the following:
  ○ Impaired circulation and possible shock
  ○ Weight less than 4 to 5 kg or a child younger than 3 months old
  ○ Intractable diarrhea, lethargy, anatomic anomalies
  ○ Failure to gain weight or continued weight loss despite oral fluids
- Prescribe medications as indicated (see Table 32-10)
- Antidiarrheals are not generally recommended because the offending organism must be excreted. Most over-the-counter products intended for diarrhea now contain salicylates, and there is concern for Reye syndrome. If diarrhea persists beyond the initial infection, cautious use of those agents without salicylates in older children is acceptable.
- *Lactobacillus* given early in a viral diarrheal illness or antibiotic-associated diarrhea can shorten the duration of the diarrhea and lessen the number of stools per day (Banks, 2004; Szajewska et al, 2006). *Lactobacillus* is most effective if a dose above threshold (10 billion colony-forming units) is given during the first 24 to 48 hours of diarrhea.
- Dioctahedral smectite, an adsorbent clay, has been found to protect the intestinal mucosa by absorbing viruses, bacteria, and bacterial toxins with few side effects. Studies have shown that smectite can reduce the duration of diarrhea by 20% to 50% (Szajewska et al, 2006; Yen & Lai, 2006).
- Peppermint oil and capsules can be used for diarrhea, cramping, and bloating. Peppermint can produce smooth muscle relaxation and slow food transit through the intestines (Goerg & Spilker, 2003).
- Studies looking at the efficacy of zinc given to children with acute diarrhea show a decrease in the duration of illness (King et al, 2003).
- Enteroadherent and enterotoxigenic *E. coli* may respond to trimethoprim-sulfamethoxazole and bismuth subsalicylate; however, treatment should be started when the diarrheal illness starts. Prophylaxis for travel is not recommended because of the potential severe medication side effects.

Complications

Acute diarrhea can cause dehydration, metabolic acidosis, cardiovascular collapse, and possible death.

- Rotavirus has been linked to bacteremia in children with recurrent fever or new onset of fever in children who had no fever associated with the initial diarrheal illness (Lowenthal et al, 2006).
- See Table 32-10 for complications associated with bacterial diarrhea.

Prevention

Preventive measures include the following:

- Good hand washing by the child and care providers. Liquid soap and paper towels are recommended at day care centers.

- Good sanitation and appropriate removal of soiled clothing and diapers. The diapering area should be cleaned after changing each baby at day care centers.
- Avoiding contaminated sources; meat should be properly cooked.
- With *Shigella*, culture all symptomatic contacts and treat those with positive stool cultures.
- Avoid unnecessary antibiotic usage.

CHRONIC DIARRHEA
Description
Chronic (persistent) diarrhea is defined as the passage of three or more watery stools per day for more than 2 weeks in a child who either fails to gain or loses weight (Bhutta et al, 2004).

Epidemiology
Infants
- The most common cause of chronic diarrhea in infants is CMPI. Symptoms start between 2 weeks to 2 months of age and include poor feeding, vomiting, diarrhea, and occasionally bloody stools (Limbos, 2005). There may also be recurrent respiratory infections, coughing, wheezing, and eczema. The stool may contain leukocytes and reducing substances.
- Hirschsprung disease
- Other neonatal or infant enteropathies (rare):
  ○ *Microvillus inclusion disease* causes chronic diarrhea that can begin on the first day of life; stool can be so watery it looks like urine, can cause severe dehydration, shock, and death (Sherman et al, 2004). Continuous intravenous total parenteral nutrition or intestinal transplant is the only treatment. There is often a prenatal history of polyhydramnios.
  ○ *Tufting enteropathy* presents in the first few months of life with chronic diarrhea and growth failure. Children with tufting enteropathy tend to have dysmorphic features (Sherman et al, 2004). Total parenteral nutrition is needed for optimal growth.
  ○ Autoimmune enteropathy causes chronic diarrhea in the first year of life; often there are other symptoms of autoimmunity.
  ○ IPEX syndrome, which is X-linked, and involves immune dysregulation, polyendocrinopathy, and enteropathy.
- Munchausen by proxy occurs when caregivers give laxatives that cause chronic diarrhea.

Toddlers
- Toddler diarrhea is a chronic diarrhea with no definitive cause in an otherwise healthy child 6 to 24 months old who is growing normally.
- Diarrhea caused by vomiting and gastroenteritis can become protracted when treated with a high-carbohydrate, low-fat, and low-protein diet, which causes an osmotic diarrhea and results in mucosal injury and persistent enteritis (Limbos, 2005).
- Celiac disease addressed elsewhere in this chapter.

School Age and Adolescent
- Acquired lactase deficiency in older children primarily of African, Asian, or Middle Eastern descent (Keating, 2005)
- Short-bowel syndrome, IBS, Crohn disease, UC, intestinal lymphangiectasia, secretory tumors

- Perforated appendix
- Constipation with encopresis is often interpreted by caregivers as chronic diarrhea
  #### Any Age
- Viral or bacterial enteritis
- Immunodeficiency syndromes
- Radiation therapy

Clinical Findings
History. The following should be assessed:
- Occurrence of three or more watery stools per day for more than 2 weeks
- Red flags (Keating, 2005)
  ○ Hematochezia or melena
  ○ Persistent fever
  ○ Weight loss or growth arrest
  ○ Anemia
- Dietary history (including amount of fruit juices ingested per day)
- Stool consistency, blood, mucus, pus, particles of food
- Stool incontinence
- Day care exposure and other ill exposures
- Contact with pets or other animals
- Teething
- Treatment by parents (any dietary manipulation, drug, or home treatments)
- Recent travel

Physical Examination. Look for physical findings associated with the underlying pathologic condition (see Differential Diagnosis). The complete physical examination includes
- Assessment of hydration status
- Weight and height measurements
- Skin and hair condition, color of skin and conjunctivae
- Vital signs (heart rate and blood pressure)
- Palpation of the thyroid
- Abdominal examination
- Rectal exam (skin tags, impaction, tenderness)

Diagnostic Studies. The following are ordered as indicated:
- Stool for culture, O&P, pH, Clinitest (for reducing substances), heme test, leukocytes, fat stain
- CBC with differential, ESR, CRP, and serum electrolytes and albumin
- Hormonal studies to assess for secretory tumors (VIP, gastrin, secretin, urine assay for 5-HT)
- Breath hydrogen test for lactose or sucrose intolerance
- Viral serologies, such as HIV or CMV
- UA and urine culture
- Sweat chloride test
- Endoscopy

Differential Diagnosis
The differential diagnosis includes allergy (the patient usually has other systemic symptoms), hyperthyroidism (enlarged thyroid, increased heart rate), malabsorption (weight loss and growth retardation), CF (clubbing, respiratory symptoms), celiac disease, Crohn disease, and nonacute UTI.

Management

The following steps are taken:
- Treat the underlying cause.
- Provide enteral or parenteral support if the patient is unable to maintain adequate intake orally.
- Treat toddler's diarrhea (chronic nonspecific diarrhea) as follows:
  - Normalize the diet.
  - Remove offending foods and fluids.
  - Eliminate sorbitol-containing fluids.
  - Give half of fluid as milk (whole or 2%).
  - Increase fat in the diet to a total of 4 g/kg/day.
  - Increase fiber.
- Refer the following patients to a gastroenterologist:
  - Newborns with diarrhea in first hours of life
  - Patients with abnormal growth delay or failure or abnormal physical findings (anorexia, abdominal pain, chronic bloating, vomiting, or weakness)
  - Those with severe illness

Complications

Malnutrition and growth failure can occur.

INTESTINAL PARASITES

Description

Multiple organisms cause parasitic infestation in the GI tract. *Giardia lamblia, Enterobius vermicularis* (pinworm), *Ascaris lumbricoides* (roundworm), and *Taenia* (tapeworm) are some of the most common intestinal parasites that affect pediatric patients.

Epidemiology

Giardia lamblia. *G. lamblia* is a flagellate protozoan generally found in contaminated mountain water sources, municipal water supplies, and food. It has a worldwide distribution. Humans are the principal reservoir, but Giardia can also infect dogs, cats, beavers, and other animals (Hvlavsa et al, 2005). Person-to-person spread is via the fecal-oral route from an infected person or via contaminated water. Epidemics are seen in child care settings and institutions for people with developmental disabilities (AAP, 2006). The organism resides in the small intestine and the biliary tract. Encystation occurs as feces dehydrate in transit. Cysts can be excreted for months or years. Many infected individuals remain asymptomatic.

Enterobius vermicularis. Pinworms are nematodes or roundworms that usually occur in family clusters, but are also found worldwide (AAP, 2006). They are 1 cm long, white, and threadlike and live in the colon and rectum. The female lays eggs in the perianal area and dies. The eggs come from contaminated fomites and the anus, fingers, and mouth. They can survive in bedding, clothing, and house dust for 2 weeks. The eggs are ingested, hatch, and become larvae in the small intestine; once mature, they migrate to the rectum. Eggs are easily transmitted within families, day care settings, and institutions. Humans are the only natural source.

Ascaris lumbricoides. Roundworms come from fecal contamination of soil and contaminated vegetables. Ingested eggs hatch, and the larvae penetrate the wall of the small intestine and enter the pulmonary system via the circulatory and portal systems. They break out of blood vessels into the lungs, are coughed up and swallowed, then become adult worms in the small intestine. The process takes 2 months. The worms can grow to 30 cm in length and can live, if untreated, for 12 to 18 months, surviving cold, drying, and chemicals. They can penetrate the liver or perforate the intestine. Found in the rural southern part of the U.S., they are most common in children younger than 10 years old. *A. lumbricoides* is the most widespread of all human roundworms (AAP, 2006).

Taenia. Tapeworm, also known as "beef" or "pork" tapeworm, comes from the consumption of raw or undercooked beef or pork with encysted parasites. The larval form of pork tapeworm causes cysticercosis, with space-occupying lesions in the viscera, brain, and muscle. The incidence is unknown; however, there is a worldwide distribution.

Clinical Findings

See Tables 32-12 and 32-13.

Differential Diagnosis

The differential diagnosis includes all other causes of infectious and noninfectious diarrhea; pinworms, in particular, can be associated with "pinworm neurosis" after successful therapy or as a fantasy infestation in unaffected contacts.

Management

See Table 32-12.

Complications

See Table 32-12.

Prevention

Most parasitic infestations can be prevented by good hand washing and good sanitation. The following parasites can be avoided or eliminated:

- *G. lamblia*: Encourage good hand hygiene. Prevent contamination of water sources. Treat questionable water with iodine, boiling for 20 minutes, or commercial filters that are available to filter contaminated water. Exclude symptomatic children and staff from school and child care until asymptomatic.
- *E. vermicularis*: Avoid scratching. Wash sheets and clothing in hot water and detergent.
- *A. lumbricoides*: Appropriate food preparation is necessary to prevent infection.
- *Taenia*: Avoid raw or undercooked beef or pork.

TABLE 32-12 **Intestinal Parasite Infection: Signs, Symptoms, Treatment and Complications**

Parasite	Gastrointestinal Symptoms	Diarrhea	Weight Loss	Treatment	Possible Complications
G. Lamblia	+ Abdominal cramps, flatulence, bloating, anorexia, weight loss, FTT; may be intermittent, protracted, or debilitating disease. Asymptomatic infection is common	++ Rarely bloody, watery, greasy, foul smelling	+	Treat all positive stool cultures with the following: Top 3 choices: Metronidazole, 15 mg/kg/day in 3 divided doses for 5 days *or* Nitazoxanide, children 1-4 yr old 100 mg bid for 3 days; children 5-11 yr old 200 mg bid for 3 days *or* Tinidazole 50 mg/kg/dose single dose (max 2 g) Alternatives: Paromomycin 25-35 mg/kg/day in 3 divided doses for 7 days *or* Furazolidone, 6 mg/kg/day in 4 divided doses for 7-10 days (liquid formulation) *or* Quinacrine 2 mg/kg/dose tid for 5 days (max 300 mg/day) Can repeat if treatment fails	Debilitating disease, leading to malabsorption. Anorexia, weight loss, and FTT
E. vermicularis (pinworms)	—	—	—	Mebendazole, 100 mg tab for 1 dose, then repeat in 2 wk, *or* Pyrantel pamoate, 11 mg/kg (max 1 g) for 1 dose, then repeat in 2 wk *or* Albendazole 400 mg po as single dose Vaginitis is self-limiting Simultaneously treat family members	Perirectal/vaginal itching Urethritis, vaginitis, salpingitis, and pelvic peritonitis have been reported
A. lumbricoides (roundworm)	Worms in stool or vomit Bowel or biliary obstruction Peritonitis Common bile duct obstruction: biliary colic, cholangitis, or pancreatitis Most infections are asymptomatic	—	+ Malnutrition	Reinfection is common Albendazole 400 mg single dose *or* Mebendazole, 100 mg tab bid for 3 days or 500 mg once *or* Ivermectin 150-200 mcg/kg as a single dose Surgical intervention may be necessary	Löffler syndrome (fever, respiratory symptoms, pulmonary infiltrates, excessive serum eosinophilia) caused by an allergic response as the larvae migrate to the lungs Systemic cysticercosis
Taenia (tapeworm)	Worms in stool, abdominal pain, nausea, diarrhea, excessive appetite Infection often asymptomatic	+	—	Praziquantel 5-10 mg/kg once *or* Niclosamide 50 mg/kg once *or* Nitazoxanide children 1-3 yr old: 100 mg bid for 3 days; children 4-11 yr old: 200 mg bid for 3 days	

bid, Twice daily; *FTT,* failure to thrive; *max,* maximum; *tab,* tablet; *tid,* three times daily; *wk, week(s); yr,* year(s); *+,* present; *++,* significantly present; *−,* not present.

TABLE 32-13 Laboratory Findings Associated With Intestinal Parasite Infestation

Parasite	Stool Findings	Stool for Ova and Parasites	Stool Culture	CBC	Duodenal Aspirate	Other
G. lamblia		±	+ Three cultures over 1 week		Rarely duodenal biopsy is needed	EIA for Giardia
E. vermicularis (pinworm)						Transparent tape test during night (2-3 hours after child goes to sleep Three consecutive specimens
A. lumbricoides (roundworm)	Worms in stool May also pass worms through the nose and mouth	+	—	Marked eosinophilia		
Taenia (tapeworm)		+ Ova in stool or in perianal region				

CBC, Complete blood count; EIA, enzyme immunoassay; +, present; —, negative; ±, may or may not be present.

RESOURCE BOX

Gastrointestinal Disorders

Children's Digestive Health & Nutrition Foundation
www.cdhnf.org

Crohn's and Colitis Foundation of America (CCFA)
www.ccfa.org
   Newsletter, informational materials (including Spanish), referrals to local resources, local chapters, advocacy, fund research

Cyclic Vomiting Syndrome Association
www.cvsaonline.org
   Empiric guidelines available, newsletter, informational materials, networking, referrals to local resources, local chapters, fund research, maintain research registry

International Foundation for Functional Gastrointestinal Disorders (IFFGD)
http://www.iffgd.org/
   Newsletter, informational materials, referrals to local resources, advocacy

National Digestive Diseases Information Clearinghouse
www.digestive.niddk.nih.gov

National Institute of Diabetes and Digestive and Kidney Diseases
www.niddk.nih.gov

National Center on Shaken Baby Syndrome
www.dontshake.com
   Materials for the prevention of shaking in relation to crying and colic

North American Society for Pediatric Gastroenterology, Hepatology, and Nutrition
www.naspgn.org

Rome Foundation: Functional Gastrointestinal Disorders
www.romecriteria.org

☑DISCUSSION FORUM

1. You are caring for a 6-year-old whose mother tells you she was just diagnosed with FAP. What clinical findings in the child would be associated with FAP? What is your role in caring for this child?
2. An 18-month-old who attends daycare and has been camping over the weekend presents with acute diarrhea. Outline the components of your assessment. Develop a management plan including both traditional and complementary modalities.
3. You suspect that a 9-year-old has CD. What tests do you order? What is your plan of care? What are some of the issues that can arise during adolescence? What techniques may be helpful in caring for a noncompliant adolescent?

REFERENCES

American Academy of Pediatrics (AAP) Committee on Infectious Diseases: *Report of the committee on infectious diseases*, ed 27, Elk Grove Village, IL, 2006, American Academy of Pediatrics.

American Academy of Pediatrics (AAP) and North American Society for Pediatric Gastroenterology, Hepatology, and Nutrition (NASPGHAN) Committee on Chronic Abdominal Pain: Chronic Abdominal Pain in Children: a technical report of the American Academy of Pediatrics and the North American Society for Pediatric Gastroenterology, Hepatology, and Nutrition, Journal of Pediatric Gastroenterology and Nutrition, *Pediatrics* 40:249-261, 2005.

Amieva MR: Important bacterial gastrointestinal pathogens in children: a pathogenesis perspective, *Pediatr Clin North Am* 52(3):749-777, 2005.

Apley J, Naish N: Recurrent abdominal pains: a field survey of 1000 school children, *Arch Dis Child* 168:165-170, 1958.

Attard T, Young R: Diagnosis and management of gastrointestinal polyps, *Gastroenterology Nurs* 29(1):16-22, 2006.

Ball T, Shapiro D, Monheim C et al: A pilot study of the use of guided imagery for the treatment of recurrent abdominal pain in children, *Clin Pediatr* 42:527-532, 2003.

Banks J, Sullo E: What is the best way to evaluate and manage diarrhea in the febrile infant? *J Fam Pract* 53(12):996-998, 2004.

Barr RG: Changing our understanding of infant colic, *Arch Pediatr Adolesc Med* 156:1172-1174, 2002.

Baudon J, Johanet C, Absalon Y, et al: Diagnosing celiac disease: a comparison of human tissue transglutaminase antibodies with antigliaden and antiendomysium antibodies, *Arch Pediatr Adolesc Med* 158:584-588, 2004.

Bechtel B: Treating *H. pylori* in childhood may stave off cancer in adulthood, *Inf Dis Child* 15:59, 2002.

Bender B, Skae C, Ozuah P: Oral rehydration therapy: the clear solution to fluid loss, *Contemp Pediatr* 22(4) 72-76, 2005.

Berman J: Heading off the dangers of acute gastroenteritis. *Cont Peds* 2003.

Bhutta Z, Grishan F, Lindley K, et al: Persistent and chronic diarrhea and malabsorption: working group report of the second world congress of pediatric gastroenterology, hepatology, and nutrition, *JPGN* 39: 5711-5716, 2004.

Block RW, Krebs NF, Committee on Child Abuse and Neglect and the Committee on Nutrition: Failure to thrive as a manifestation of child neglect, *Pediatrics* 116(5):1234-1237, 2005.

Boles R, Adams K, Li B: Maternal inheritance in cyclic vomiting syndrome, *Am J Med Genetics* 133:71-77, 2005.

Brayden RM, Daley MF, Brown JM: Growth deficiency. In Hay WW et al, editors: *Current pediatric diagnosis and treatment*, ed 16, New York, 2003, Lange Medical Books.

Brown H: The spectrum of milk intolerance syndromes, *J Nutr Environ Med* 12(3):153-175, 2002.

Bullard J, Page N: Cyclic vomiting syndrome: a disease in disguise, *Pediatr Nurs* 31(1):27-30, 2005.

Cardall T, Glasser J, Guss D: Clinical value of the total white blood cell and temperature in the evaluation of patients with suspected appendicitis, *Acad Emerg Med* 11(10):1021-1027, 2004.

Carey WB: Clinical applications of infant temperament measurements, *J Pediatr* 81:823-828, 1972 (Classic).

Castano L, Blarduni E, Ortiz L et al: Prospective population screening for celiac disease: high prevalence in the first three years of life, *JPGN* 37:80-84, 2004.

Cavataio F, Guandalini S: Gastroesophageal reflux. In Guandalini S, editor: *Essential pediatric gastroenterology and nutrition*, New York, McGraw Hill, 2005.

Chang A, Lasserson T, Kiljander T et al. Systematic review and meta-analysis of randomized controlled trials of gastro-esophageal reflux interventions for chronic cough associated with gastro-esophageal reflux, *Br Med J* 332:11-17, 2006.

Chitkara D, Rawat D, Talley N: The epidemiology of childhood recurrent abdominal pain in western countries: a systematic review, *Am J Gastroenterol* 100:868-1875, 2005.

Cirgin-Ellet M: What is known about infant colic? *Gastroenterol Nurs* 26(2):60-65, 2003.

Cirgin-Ellett M, Perkind S: Examination of the effect of Dr. Brown's Natural Flow Baby Bottles on infant colic, *Gastroenterol Nurs* 29(3):226-231, 2006.

Clifford TJ, Campbell MK, Speechley KN: Sequelae of infant colic: evidence of transient infant distress and absence of lasting effects on maternal mental health, *Arch Pediatr Adolesc Med* 156:1183-1188, 2002.

Clouse R, Mayher E, Aziz Q et al: Functional abdominal pain syndrome, *Gastroenterology* 130:1492-1497, 2006.

Cyclic Vomiting Syndrome Association: *Empiric guidelines for the management of cyclic vomiting syndrome*. Available at *www.cvsaonline.org* (accessed December 16, 2007).

Dennehy P: Acute diarrheal disease in children: epidemiology, prevention, and treatment, *Infect Dis Clin* 19:585-602, 2005.

Dinolfo E: *Campylobacter* infection, *Peds Rev* 26(9):339-340, 2005.

Drossman D: The functional gastrointestinal disorders and the Rome III process, *Gastroenterology* 130(5):377-1390, 2006.

Dupont C, de Boissieu D: Formula feeding during cow's milk allergy, *Minerva Pediatrica* 53(3):209-216, 2003.

Ewing W, Jackson-Allen P: The diagnosis and management of cow milk protein intolerance in the primary care setting, *Pediatr Nurs* 31(6): 486-493, 2005.

Fankhauser R, Monroe S, Noel J et al: Epidemiologic and molecular trends of Norwalk-like viruses associated with outbreaks of gastroenteritis in the US, *J Infect Dis* 186:1-7, 2002.

Finberg L, Kleinman RE: *Saunders manual of pediatric practice*, ed 2, Philadelphia, 2002, WB Saunders.

Fox M, Forgacs I: Gastro-esophageal reflux disease, *Br Med J* 332:88-93, 2006.

Freedman S, Adler M, Seshadri R et al: Oral ondansetron for gastroenteritis in a pediatric emergency department, *N Engl J Med* 354:1698-1705, 2006.

Friedman S: Cancer in Crohn's disease, *Gastroenterol Clin North Am* 35(3):621-639, 2006.

Gahagan S: Failure to thrive: a consequence of undernutrition, *Pediatr Rev* 27(1):e1-e11, 2006.

Gelfond D, Fasano A: Celiac disease in the pediatric population, *Pediatr Ann* 35(4):275-279, 2006.

Goerg K, Spilker T: Effect of peppermint oil and caraway oil on gastrointestinal motility in healthy volunteers: a pharmacodynamic study using simultaneous determination of gastric and gallbladder emptying and oral ceocal transit time, *Ailment Pharmacol Ther* 17(2):445-451, 2003.

Goldstein E, Hagerman R, Reynolds A: Child development and behavior. In Hay WW et al, editors: Current pediatric diagnosis and treatment ed 16, New York, 2003, Lange Medical Books.

Green R, Bulloch B, Kabani A et al: Early analgesia for children with acute abdominal pain, *Pediatrics* 116(4):978-983, 2005.

Gupta S, Fitzgerald J, Croffie J et al: Experience with juvenile polyps in North American children: the need for pancolonoscopy, *Am J Gastroenterol* 96(6):1695-1697, 2001.

Hassall E: Peptic ulcer disease and current approaches to *H. pylori*, *J Pediatr* 138:462-468, 2001.

Heine R, Elsayed S, Hoskings C et al: Cow's milk allergy in infancy, *Curr Opinion Allergy Clinic Immunol* 2:217-225, 2002.

Heyman M, The Committee on Nutrition: Lactose intolerance in infants, children, and adolescents, *Pediatrics* 118:1279-1286, 2006.

Hill D, Toy N, Heine R et al: Effect of low-allergen maternal diet on colic among breastfed infants: a randomized controlled trial, *Pediatrics* 116(5):709-715, 2006.

Hill K, Hill I: Celiac disease: fundamentals for pediatricians, *Contemp Pediatr* 22(10):65-78, 2005.

Hoffenberg E, et al: A prospective study of the incidence of childhood celiac disease, *J Pediatr* 143:308-314, 2003.

Hogberg L, Faith-Magusson K, Grant C: Oats to children with newly diagnosed celiac disease: a randomized double-blinded study, *Gut* 53:645-654, 2004.

Howe J, Bair J, Sged M et al: Germline mutations of the gene encoding bone morphogenetic protein receptor 1A in juvenile polyposis, *Nat Genetics* 28(2):184-187, 2001.

Huebner ES, Surawicz CM: Probiotics in prevention and treatment of gastrointestinal infections, *Gastroenterol Clin* 35(2):355-365, 2006.

Hvlavsa M, Watson J, Beach M: Giardiasis surveillance: United States, 1998-2002, *MMWR* 54(SSO1):9-16, 2005.

Hyams J: Treatment of functional gastrointestinal disorders associated with abdominal pain, *J Pediatr Gastroenterol Nutr* 41:S47-S48, 2005a.

Hyams J: Inflammatory bowel disease, *Pediatr Rev* 26(9):314-320, 2005b.

Hyman P, Elder Danda C: Understanding and treating childhood bellyaches, *Pediatr Ann* 33(2):98-104, 2004.

Illingsworth R: Three-months' colic, *Arch Dis Child* 29:165-174, 1954 (Classic).

Imanzadeh F, Sayyari A, Yagboodi M et al: Celiac disease in children with diarrhea is more frequent than previously suspected, *JPGN* 40:309-311, 2005.

Innis SM, Pinsk V, Jacobson K: Dietary lipids and intestinal inflammatory disease, *J Pediatr* 149(5):S89-S96, 2006.

Jass J, Williams C, Bussey H et al: Juvenile polyposis—A precancerous condition, *Histopathology* 13(6):619-630, 1998.

Kahn S, Orenstein S, DiLorenzo C et al: Eosinophilic esophagitis: strictures, impaction, dysphagia, *Dig Dis Digest* 48:22-29, 2003.

Kato S, Nishino Y, Ozawa K et al: The prevalence of Helicobacter pylori in Japanese children with gastritis, or peptic ulcer disease, *J Gastroenterol* 39:734-738, 2004.

Kavak U, et al: Bone mineral density in children with untreated and treated celiac disease, *JPGN* 39:80-84, 2003.

Keating J: Chronic diarrhea, *Pediatr Rev* 26(1):5-13, 2005.

Keefe M, Karlson K, Dudley W et al: Reducing parenting stress in families with irritable infants, *Nurs Res* 55(3):198-205, 2006a.

Keefe M, Lobo M, Froese-Fretz A et al: Effectiveness of an intervention for colic, *Clin Pediatr* 45:123-13, 2006b.

Kharbanda A, Taylor G, Fishman S et al: A clinical decision rule to identify children at low risk for appendicitis, *Pediatrics* 116(3):709-716, 2005.

Khasawinah I, Ramirez A, et al: Preliminary experience with dexmedetomidine in the treatment of cyclicvomiting syndrome. *Am J Ther* 10, 303-307, 2003.

Kim SC, Ferry GD: Inflammatory bowel diseases in pediatric and adolescent patients: clinical, therapeutic, and psychosocial considerations, *Gastroenterology* 126(6):1550-1560, 2004.

King C, Glass R, Breese J et al: Managing acute gastroenteritis among children: oral rehydration, maintenance, and nutritional therapy, *MMWR* 52(RR-16):1-16, 2003.

Kliegman R: Acute and chronic abdominal pain. In Kliegman R, Greenbaum L, Lye P, editors: *Practical strategies in pediatric diagnosis and therapy*, Philadelphia, 2004, Elsevier.

Kohli R, Li B: Differential diagnosis of recurrent abdominal pain: new considerations, *Pediatr Ann* 33(2):113-122, 2004.

Kugathasan S, Amre D: Inflammatory bowel disease-environmental modification and genetic determinants, *Pediatr Clin North Am* 53(4):727-749, 2006.

Li BU, Balint J: Cyclic vomiting syndrome: evolution in our understanding of a brain-gut disorder, *Adv Pediatr* 47:117-161, 2000.

Li BU, Howard J: New hope for children with cyclic vomiting syndrome, *Contemp Pediatr* 19:121-130, 2002.

Li Z-S, Sun Z-X, Zou D-W et al: Endoscopic management of foreign bodies in the upper-GI tract: experience with 1088 cases in China, *Gastrointest Endosc* 64(4):485-492, 2006.

Limbos A: Approach to the child with diarrhea. In Osborn L, DeWitt T, First L, editors: *Pediatrics*, Philadelphia, 2005, Mosby.

Lindley K, Andrews P: Pathogenesis and treatment of cyclical vomiting, *JPGN* 41:S38-S4, 2005.

Lintula H, Kokki H, Vanamo K et al: The costs of laparoscopic appendectomy in children, *Arch Pediatr Adolesc Med* 158:34-37, 2004.

Little DC, Shah SR, St Peter SD et al: Esophageal foreign bodies in the pediatric population: our first 500 cases, *J Pediatr Surg* 41(5):914-918, 2006.

Loftus EV: The new epidemiology of IBD: a unique phenomenon or part of a global trend? *Inflammatory Bowel Dis* 12(10):S1-S2, 2006.

Lowenthal A, Livni G, Amr J et al: Secondary bacteremia after rotavirus gastroenteritis in infancy, *Pediatrics* 117(1):224-226, 2006.

Ludvigsson J, Wahlstrom J, Grunewald J et al: Celiac disease and risk of tuberculosis: a population based cohort study, *Thorax* 62(1):23-28, 2006.

Mackner LM, Crandall WV: Brief report: psychosocial adjustment in adolescents with inflammatory bowel disease, *J Pediatr Psychol* 31(3): 281-285, 2006.

Manfredi MA, Israel EJ: Gastritis and peptic ulcer disease. In Burg FD, Ingelfinger JR, Polin RA et al: *Current pediatric therapy*, ed 18, Philadelphia, 2006, Saunders.

Markowitz JE, Bengmark S: Probiotics in health and disease in the pediatric patient, *Pediatr Clin North Am* 49(1):127-141, 2002.

McCullough M, Sharieff G: Abdominal pain, *Pediatr Clin North Am* 53: 107-137, 2006.

McDonald L, Kilgore G, Thompson A et al: An epidemic, toxic gene variant strain of clostridium difficile, *N Engl J Med* 353(23):2433-2441, 2005.

McGuirt W: Gastroesophageal reflux and the upper airway, *Pediatr Clin North Am* 50(2):487-502, 2003.

Miller C, Willging J: Advances in the evaluation and management of pediatric dysphagia, *Curr Opinion Otolaryngol Head Neck Surg* 11:4432-446, 2003.

Moreels TG, Pelckmans PA: Gastrointestinal parasites—Potential therapy for refractory inflammatory bowel diseases, *Inflammatory Bowel Dis* 11(2):178-184, 2005.

Morrow S, Newman K: Current management of appendicitis, *Semin Pediatr Surg* 16:34-40, 2007.

Nance M, Adamson W, Hedrick H: Appendicitis in the young child: a continuing diagnostic challenge, *Pediatr Emerg Care* 16:160-162, 2000.

Neighbor M, Baird C, Kohn M: Changing opioid use for the right lower quadrant abdominal pain in the ED, *Acad Emerg Med* 12:1216-1220, 2005.

North American Society for Pediatric Gastroenterology and Nutrition: Pediatric GE reflux guidelines, *J Pediatr Gastroenterol Nutr* 32:S1-S31, 2001.

North American Society for Pediatric Gastroenterology and Nutrition: Guideline for the diagnosis and treatment of celiac disease in children, *JPGN* 40:1-19, 2005.

Orenstein S, Peters J: Vomiting and regurgitation. In Kliegman R, Greenbaum L, Lye P, editors: *Practical strategies in pediatric diagnosis and therapy*, Philadelphia, 2004, Elsevier.

Palsson OS, Drossman DA: Psychiatric and psychological dysfunction in irritable bowel syndrome and the role of psychological treatments, *Gastroenterol Clin* 34(20):281-303, 2005.

Papa HM, Gordon CM, Saslowsky TM et al: Vitamin D status in children and young adults with inflammatory bowel disease, *Pediatrics* 118(5): 1950-1961, 2006.

Podolsky D: Inflammatory bowel disease, *N Engl J Med* 347:417-429, 2002.

Porter S, Fleisher G, Kohane I et al: The value of parental report for diagnosis and management of dehydration in the emergency department, *Ann Emerg Med* 41(2):196-205, 2003.

Poynard T, Regimbeau C, Benhamou Y: Meta-analysis of smooth muscle relaxants in the treatment of irritable bowel syndrome, *Ailment Pharmacol Ther* 15:355-361, 2001.

Rao M, Brenner R, Schisterman T et al: Long term cognitive development in children with prolonged crying, *Arch Dis Child* 89:989-992, 2004.

Rasquin A, DiLorenzo C, Forbes D et al: Childhood functional gastrointestinal disorders: child/adolescent, *Gastroenterology* 130:1527-1537, 2006.

Roberts D, Ostapchuk M, O'Brien J: Infantile colic, *Am Fam Physician* 70(4):735-740, 2004.

Rommel N et al: The complexity of feeding problems in 700 infants presenting to a tertiary care institution, *J Pediatr Gastroenterol Nutr* 37:75-84, 2003.

Roslund G, Hepps T, McQuillen K: The ED role of ondansetron in oral rehydration of children in with gastroenteritis related vomiting, *Acad Emerg Med* 13(5):5147-5153, 2006.

Rotenbacher D, Inceogln J, Brenner H et al: Acquisition of Heliobader pylori infection in a high-risk population occurs within first 2 years of life. *J Peds,* 136(6):744-748, June 2000.

Ruark J, McCullough G, Peters R et al: Bolus consistency and swallowing in children and adults, *Dysphagia* 17:24-33, 2002.

Rudolph C, Link D: Guidelines for evaluation and treatment of gastroesophageal reflux in infants and children: recommendations of the North American Society for Pediatric Gastroenterology and Nutrition, *J Pediatr Gastroenterol Nutr* 32(suppl 2):S14, 2001.

Rudolph C: Gastroesophageal reflux. In Lifschitz, editor: *Pediatric gastroenterology and nutrition in clinical practice,* New York, 2003, Marcel Dekker.

Rudolph C, Link D: Feeding disorders in infants and children, *Pediatr Clin North Am* 49:97-112, 2002.

Rudolph C, Miranda A: Treatment options for functional abdominal pain, *Pediatr Ann* 33(2):105-112, 2004.

Sander H, Magda P, Chin R et al: Cerebellar ataxia and celiac disease, *Lancet* 362:1548-1555, 2003.

Sawczenko A, Ballinger AB, Savage MO et al: Clinical features affecting final adult height in patients with pediatric onset Crohn's disease, *Pediatrics* 118(1):124-129, 2006.

Scharff L, Kemper K: For chronic pain, complementary and alternative medical approaches, *Contemp Pediatr* 20(10):117-141, 2003.

Schulte-Bockhold A, Kugathasan S, Mesrobian H et al: Ureteropelvic junction obstruction: an overlooked cause of cyclic vomiting, *Am J Gastroenterol* 97(4):1043-1045, 2002.

Shenassa E, Brown M: Maternal smoking and infantile gastrointestinal dysregulation: the case of colic, *Pediatrics* 114:497-505, 2004.

Sherman P, Mitchell D, Cutz E: Neonatal enteropathies: defining the causes of protracted diarrhea in infancy, *JPGN* 38:16-26, 2004.

Snyder JP: Inflammatory bowel disease: ulcerative colitis and Crohn disease. In Finberg L, Kleinman RE, editors: *Saunders manual of pediatric practice,* ed 2, Philadelphia, 2002, WB Saunders.

Sondheimer JM: Gastrointestinal tract. In Hay WW et al, editors: *Current pediatric diagnosis and treatment,* ed 17, New York, 2005, Lange Medical Books.

Spandorfer P, Alessandrini E, Joeefe M et al: Oral versus intravenous rehydration of moderately dehydrated children: a randomized, controlled trial, *Pediatrics* 115(2):259-301, 2005.

Steiner M, DeWalt D, Byerly J: Is this child dehydrated? *JAMA* 291(22):2746-2754, 2004.

Stene L, Honeyman M, Hoffenber E et al: Rotavirus infection frequency and risk of celiac disease autoimmunity in early childhood: a longitudinal study, *Am J Gastroenterol* 101:2333-2340, 2006.

Stockman J: Gastroenterology, year book in pediatrics, St. Louis, 2004, Elsevier.

Stork C, Reily T, Brown K et al: Dexamethasone vs. ondansetron in children with refractory vomiting from acute vial gastritis, *J Acad Emerg Med* 12(5)Suppl 1:19-20, 2005.

Suwandhi E, Ton M, Schwarz S: GER in infancy and childhood, *Pediatrics Ann* 35(4):259-266, 2006.

Szajewski H, Setty M, Mrukowic J et al: Probiotics in gastrointestinal disease in children: hard and not so hard evidence of efficacy, *JPGN* 42:454-475, 2006.

Szigethy E, Carpenter J, Baum E et al: Case study: longitudinal treatment of adolescents with depression and inflammatory bowel disease, *J Am Acad Child Adolesc Psychiatry* 45(4):396-400, 2006.

Tasker A, DEttmar P, Panetti M et al: Is gastric reflux a cause of otitis media with effusion in children, *Laryngoscope* 112:1930-1934, 2002.

Terasawa T, Blackmore C, Bent S et al: Systematic review: computed tomography and ultrasonography to detect acute appendicitis in adults and adolescents, *Ann Intern Med,* 141(7):537-546, 2004.

Thiessen P: Recurrent abdominal pain, *Pediatr Rev* 23:39-46, 2002.

Ulshen M: Malabsorptive disorders. In Behrman R, Kliegman R, Jenson H, editors: *Nelson textbook of pediatrics,* ed 17, Philadelphia, 2004, WB Saunders.

Uyemura MC: Foreign body ingestion in children, *Am Fam Physician* 72(2):287-291, 2005.

Vanderhoof JA, Young RJ: Probiotics in pediatrics, *Pediatrics* 109(5):956-957, 2002.

Vanderhoof J, Moran J, Harris C et al: Efficacy of a pr-thickened infant formula: a multicenter, double-blind, randomized, placebo-controlled parallel group trial in 104 infants with symptomatic gastroesophageal reflux, *Clin Pediatr* 42:483-495, 2003.

vanTilburg M, Venepalli N, Ulshen M et al: Parent's worries about recurrent abdominal pain in children, *Gastroenterol Nurse* 29(1):50-55, 2005.

Waltzman ML, Baskin M, Wypij D et al: A randomized clinical trial of the management of esophageal coins in children, *Pediatrics* 116(3):614-619, 2005.

Weinstein M: Underlying disorders in cyclic vomiting syndrome, *Clin Pediatr* 44:805-807, 2005.

Weissbluth M: Colic. In Burg FD, Ingelfinger JR, Polin RA et al: *Current pediatric therapy,* ed 18, Philadelphia, 2006, Saunders.

Weng M, Walker WA: Bacterial colonization, probiotics, and clinical disease, *J Pediatr* 149(5):S107-S114, 2006.

White B, et al: Behavioral and physiological responsivity, sleep, and patterns of daily cortisol production in infants with and without colic, *Child Dev* 71:862-877, 2000.

Wu H, Lin C, Chang C et al: Predictive value of C-reactive protein at different cutoff levels in acute appendicitis, *Am J Emerg Med* 23:449-453, 2005.

Wyllie R: Foreign bodies and bezoars. In Behrman RE, editor: *Nelson textbook of pediatrics,* ed 17, Philadelphia, 2004, WB Saunders.

Yen. Z, Lai M: Best evidence topic report: smectite for acute diarrhea in children, *Emerg Med J* 23(1):65-66, 2006.

Youseff N, Murphy T, Langseder A et al: Quality of life for children with functional abdominal pain: a comparison study of patients' and parents' perceptions, *Pediatrics* 117:54-59, 2006.

CHAPTER 33

Dental and Oral Disorders

Peter Milgrom, Ohnmar K. Tut, Donald L. Chi, Mary Ann Draye, and Michele E. Acker

The mouth serves many functions, including speech, and is richly endowed with special systems that serve complex needs. For this reason, good oral health is essential for normal growth and development.

The mouth has been increasingly recognized as a barometer of health and well-being throughout life. In fact, in many cases, saliva is replacing serum and blood as the vehicle for noninvasive diagnostic tests for systemic diseases. Many of these tests are already on the market.

In children, microbial infections caused by bacteria, viruses, and fungi cause tooth decay (dental caries), periodontal or gum diseases, herpes labialis, and candidiasis. Moreover, inherited and congenital conditions result in impairments and cosmetic defects that have serious impacts on children as they grow and develop. Lifestyle choices, such as tobacco and drug use, body art, and piercing, create challenges for maintaining oral health (U.S. Department of Health and Human Services, 2000).

Dental problems, particularly tooth decay, are much more common than asthma and can restrict normal daily activity. Visits to the dentist for treatment and prevention result in lost time from school and work (Gift et al, 1992). Thus, a primary care provider is in a unique position to play an essential role in the prevention of oral disease, identifying and minimizing the impact of disease, and providing guidance to parents and children about mouth care.

To develop this chapter, we interviewed and surveyed pediatric and family nurse practitioners to identify the oral health problems they face in daily practice and to clarify which areas should be covered. Those surveyed practiced in varied settings. The typical provider reported being asked to provide guidance or treatment for an oral health problem at least once per week. One fifth of those responding faced such questions nearly every day. In response, this chapter offers information and practical answers for providers in everyday practice.

NORMAL GROWTH AND DEVELOPMENT

ANATOMY OF THE MOUTH

The structures of the mouth include the mucosa (buccal and gingival), palate, salivary glands, frenula, tongue, and teeth.

The Teeth

Anatomy of a Tooth. Primary and permanent teeth have similar anatomy, differing primarily in the size and external shape of each tooth. Fig. 33-1 shows a cross section of the typical tooth including the crown (white part) and root (encased in bone).

Pattern of Tooth Eruption. The first primary tooth (also called baby tooth or deciduous tooth) may be present at birth. Normally the eruption of primary teeth begins with the anterior primary teeth, occurs during the first 6 to 8 months of life, and ends at about 30 to 36 months old with the maxillary second molars. The sequence of eruption and the timing of eruption for each tooth are similar for both sexes. Variability in the age of children at emergence of the individual teeth is small, with a standard deviation of 2 to 3 months. In most children, the 20 primary teeth (10 per arch) erupt in a period spanning about 2 years.

The permanent teeth begin erupting as children reach school age (about 6 years old), and the jaws grow. The eruption of permanent dentition begins with eruption of the mandibular central incisors and ends with the eruption of the maxillary third molars. The primary teeth are shed as the permanent ones erupt. The permanent molars erupt behind the primary molars. The shedding and replacement of the primary molars by permanent premolars is usually complete around the fifth grade or by 12 years of age. This period, when both primary and permanent teeth are present, is called the transitional dentition. In most children, the total period of eruption of permanent teeth (except for the third molars) spans about 6 years.

In general, the variability in eruption times for the permanent dentition is much greater than the variability observed in the primary dentition, with standard deviation of 8 to 18 months (about five times greater than in the primary dentition). The sequence of permanent tooth eruption is almost identical for both sexes. However, all teeth erupt earlier in girls than in boys. The gender difference in eruption times averages approximately 6 months. The tooth eruption pattern for both the primary and permanent dentitions is listed in Table 33-1.

Managing Teething. Often, teeth pierce the gums without causing any symptoms. However, some children will show local symptoms, such as redness and swelling in the oral mucosa overlying the erupting tooth. These symptoms appear a few days before clinical eruption. The child may also show signs of irritation, drooling, and sometimes, slight fever.

Recommended treatments for teething discomfort include topical treatments, such as chewing on a cold teething ring, pacifier, or even ice (McIntyre & McIntyre, 2002). Massaging the gums with a wet finger or a cold spoon may also be helpful. Topical analgesics containing benzocaine gel are marketed for

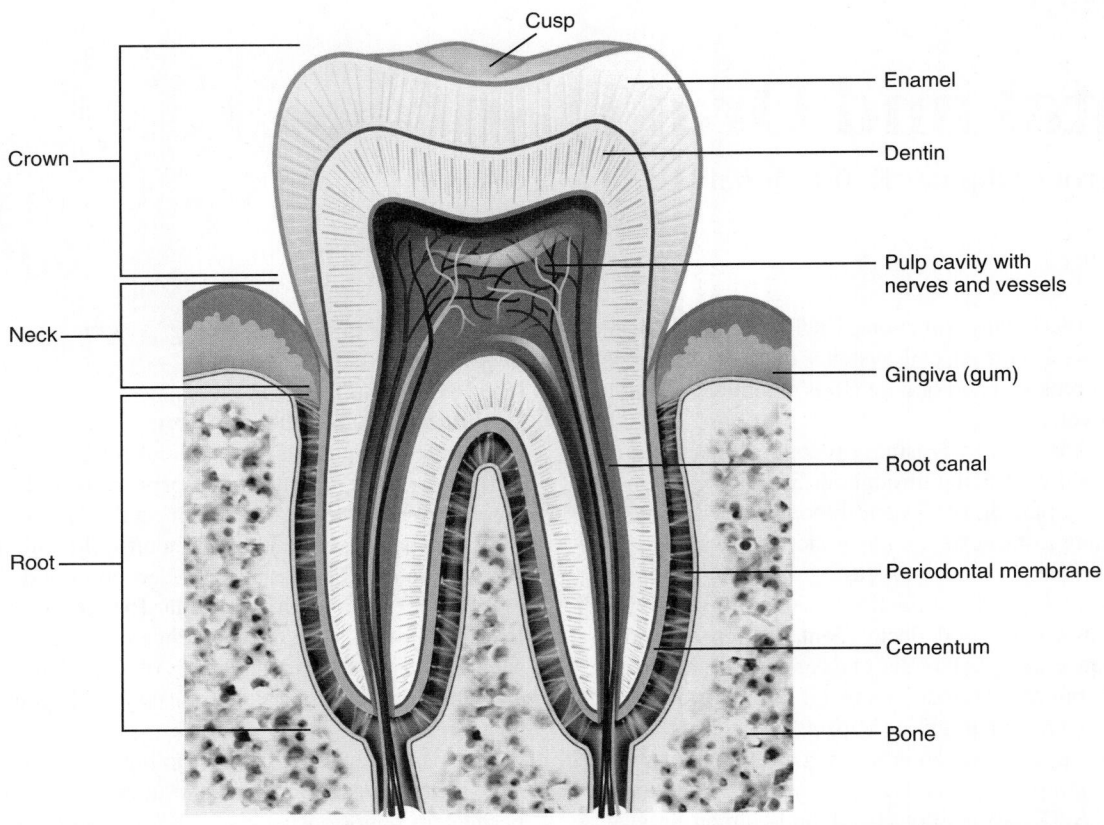

Cusp

Crown

Neck

Root

Enamel

Dentin

Pulp cavity with
nerves and vessels

Gingiva (gum)

Root canal

Periodontal membrane

Cementum

Bone

FIG. 33-1 Anatomy of a tooth. (From Thibodeau GA, Patton KT: *Structure and function of the body*, ed 12, 2004, Mosby, p 396.)

this purpose and may be recommended. Exercise caution regarding topical benzocaine because of potential sensitivity. At least one case of methemoglobinemia has been reported. Similarly, there are topical salicylates available, but overuse of these can cause burns. Oral acetaminophen is an effective remedy. All such remedies should be stored carefully out of the reach of children.

A great number of folk remedies are used, especially in communities without good access to medical care (Smitherman et al, 2005). Among those practices not recommended are rubbing whiskey on the gums or tying a penny on a string around the child's neck (creates a potential risk of strangulation). In addition, parents should be cautioned against honey-coated pacifiers that might cause tooth decay in already erupted teeth or introduce botulism.

■ THE ORAL EXAMINATION
PERFORMING AN INFANT OR CHILD ORAL EXAM

Trying to examine the mouth and teeth with the child sitting in the parent's lap is not recommended because the provider has to bend over to see the upper teeth, and the crying and movement of the child makes visibility very poor.

An infant's teeth and oral tissues are examined most easily by placing the child on his or her back on an examining table

with the head toward the end of the table. Have the parent restrain the legs and hands. Standing at the head of the table, use a tongue blade or toothbrush as a mouth prop. Use a penlight and intraoral mirror for optimal visualization. Tip the head back to see the upper teeth. The exam table approach is also useful for looking at the teeth of older children.

An alternative for examining a small child is the knee-to-knee approach favored by many dentists. In this approach, the provider and parent sit knee to knee. The parent holds the child facing him or her and then lowers the head into the provider's lap. The child's legs are wrapped around the parent's waist. Again the parent restrains the hands. Small children will cry during the exam, but the crying will stop as soon as the exam is completed.

CLINICAL FINDINGS

An oral and dental exam should be systematic. During the exam, take the opportunity to point out abnormalities (e.g., tooth decay) to the parent.

The Oral Mucosa

The soft mucosal tissues are examined before the teeth. This part of the examination should also include an assessment of the tonsils for size and the presence of inflammation or exudate.

TABLE 33-1   Calcification, Crown Completion, and Eruption

Tooth	Age of Eruption
Primary Dentition	
Maxillary	
Central incisor	7½ months
Lateral incisor	8 months
Canine	16-20 months
First molar	12-16 months
Second molar	20-30 months
Mandibular	
Central incisor	6½ months
Lateral incisor	7 months
Canine	16-20 months
First molar	12-16 months
Second molar	20-30 months
Permanent Dentition	
Maxillary	
Central incisor	7-8 years
Lateral incisor	8-9 years
Canine	11-12 years
First premolar	10-11 years
Second premolar	10-12 years
First molar	6-7 years
Second molar	12-13 years
Third molar	17-21 years
Mandibular	
Central incisor	6-7 years
Lateral incisor	7-8 years
Canine	9-10 years
First premolar	10-12 years
Second premolar	11-12 years
First molar	6-7 years
Second molar	11-13 years
Third molar	17-21 years

Adapted from Logan WHG, Kronfeld R: Development of the human jaws and surrounding structures from birth to age fifteen years, *J Am Dent Assoc* 20:379, 1993.

Start the exam with the inside of the lips and continue to the mucosa on the inside of the cheeks, including the mucosal surfaces that connect and surround each tooth. Inspect the palate directly by tipping the child's head backward. Use a mirror to help direct light to the soft palate. Examine the dorsal and ventral mucosal surfaces of the tongue and floor of the mouth by retracting the tongue with a tongue blade, a dental mirror, or by holding the tongue with cotton gauze. Ulcerations, changes in color and surface texture, swellings, or fistulae of any of these tissues should be noted.

When examining the gums, give special attention to any swelling or retraction of the gingiva where the gums meet the tooth surface. Such symptoms can be a notable sign of tooth or gingival abnormality typical of periodontal disease in peripubertal children and adolescents. Note the presence and attachment of frenula, with special emphasis on the possible complicating effects of high insertion of such frenula on the periodontal tissues.

The Saliva

Salivary flow does not appreciably change over the life span. Note the quantity and quality of the saliva; thick or ropy saliva or a dry mouth may be abnormal. Decreased salivary flow and changes in sensation in the area of the facial nerve can result from infection or tumor in the parotid space or facial musculature, or it can be a side effect of dehydration or medications.

The Teeth

Examine the teeth systematically by beginning with the upper right buccal or facial surfaces and moving around to the left. Then go from left to right, examining the lingual surfaces of the upper teeth. Then examine the biting surfaces in the same systematic manner. After this, move to the lower jaw. The number and types of teeth erupted, color changes, irregularities, and asymmetries should be noted.

Variations in number, morphology, color, and surface structure should then be observed under good light after drying the teeth with cotton gauze. Primary teeth may be malformed or have incompletely formed or chalky or pitted enamel comorbidly with other systematic conditions, such as ectodermal dysplasia. In the case of traumatically injured teeth, the color and translucency of the injured tooth or teeth should be evaluated. Slight color changes are often found as one of the first signs of intrapulpal damage after trauma and may lead to an abscessed tooth.

Early tooth decay can be detected most effectively by cleaning the teeth with a toothbrush and then drying them with gauze. Note any surface roughness or loss of surface continuity.

ABERRATIONS IN PRIMARY TOOTH ERUPTION

NATAL AND NEONATAL TEETH

The prevalence of natal or neonatal teeth is estimated at 1 case per 2000 to 3000 births and is equally common in boys and girls. The teeth usually erupt in pairs. Natal and neonatal teeth have been shown to occur in about 50 different syndromes, of which about 10 are associated with chromosomal aberrations. More than 90% of these prematurely erupting teeth are mandibular central incisors belonging to the normal dentition, and they have a normal shape and color. Supernumerary teeth may be abnormal in shape and color and only loosely attached to the gingiva. Natal or neonatal teeth can lead to gingivitis, self mutilation of the tongue, and trauma to the mother's breast. However, they should be extracted only if they are loose enough to involve risk of aspiration or if feeding is severely disturbed. Most will develop normally with normal root structure (Leung & Robson, 2006).

DELAYED TOOTH ERUPTION

In general, children with chronic diseases who show delay in both physical and dental development will experience delayed but otherwise normal tooth eruption. Parents may need reassurance if there is some delay. Once the child is old enough to tolerate dental x-rays, typically no earlier than 4 years old and often later, diagnostic films can be taken to provide a better assessment of the developing dentition.

OTHER GUM EVENTS

Preeruption Cysts

When a tooth starts erupting through the gingival tissue, a blood-filled cyst may precede it. Alarmed parents may report a purple, reddish, black, or blue bump or bruise in their child's mouth. If the enlargement is on the alveolar ridge, reassurance is all that is required. The symptom will resolve as the tooth erupts (Fig. 33-2).

Congenital Epulis

Congenital epulis is a fibrous, pedunculated, soft tissue enlargement that occurs on the maxillary alveolar ridge at birth. This condition is more common in female babies. It typically regresses with time, but large lesions should be excised.

Bohns Nodules

Bohns nodules are present at birth and appear as firm, non-painful nodules on the buccal surface of the alveolar ridge. They are remnants of dental lamina connecting the developing tooth bud to the epithelium of the oral cavity. No treatment is required because they will resolve spontaneously. If they appear in the midline of the palate, they are referred to as Epstein pearls.

▇▇ PROFESSIONAL DENTAL CARE
FEAR OF THE DENTIST

As many as one in five adults in North America are fearful of the dentist (Smith & Heaton, 2003). Many of the parents of children with whom primary care providers interact may have this fear and consequently avoid dental visits

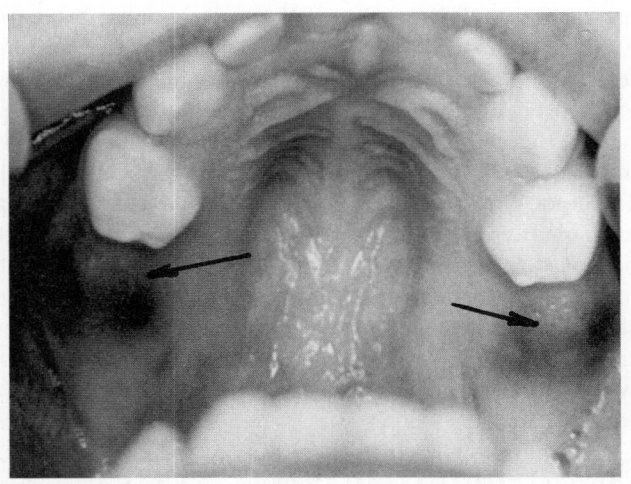

FIG. 33-2 Preeruption cyst. Eruption hematomas (*arrows*) have developed before the eruption of the second primary molars. (From McDonald RE, Avery DR, Dean JA: *Dentistry for the child and adolescent,* ed 8, 2004, Mosby, p 182.)

themselves. Among poorer and ethnic and racial minority families, episodic care and racial discrimination may have led to a cycle of emergency care with poor treatment, pain, and then more symptomatic care. Many low-income parents have little experience with preventive care for themselves or their children. In contrast to its progress in improving access to medical care, Medicaid has largely failed to reduce the inequalities in dental access associated with poverty (Bloom et al, 2006).

The best preventive measure for the development of fear and avoidance is early and consistent primary prevention (Milgrom & Weinstein, 2001; Weinstein & Milgrom, 2006). Allowing tooth decay to go untreated until a child is school age results in extensive restorative intervention—a traumatic experience for any child. Dental restorative care is the only area of medicine in which children are expected to endure extensive surgery while they are awake. Hospitalizing children and performing reparative services under general anesthesia is an option, but a scarce, expensive, and risky procedure. Moreover, the majority of children experience recurrence of disease within 6 months because the surgical treatment does not address the underlying disease.

If access to a dentist is limited, then primary care providers become primary dental hygiene educators and diagnosticians with the following goals:

- Reducing the burden of disease in preschool children by educating parents on diet and oral hygiene
- Prescribing appropriate fluorides and other preventive agents (e.g., applying fluoride varnish, which will be discussed later)
- Promptly detecting early signs of tooth decay so that an intensive secondary prevention program can be instituted. This effort should not be just for preschool children because many children in the U.S. experience preventable tooth decay in 6-year molars.

CHOOSING A DENTIST

For children who have had poor previous experiences, the choice of a dentist is critical. Many general dentists are skilled at working with children, so the absence of a pediatric specialist is not a huge barrier. A dentist new to the child should be told about any prior dental experiences.

Parents of dentally naïve children should be counseled to choose a dentist known to like and work well with children in order to provide the best chance at having a successful visit and outcome. Even within a dental clinic, there are differences in provider skills. Parents should be encouraged to ensure that their child has had a good night's sleep and is fed before a visit. The child's teeth should be brushed before any visit to the dentist. A parent or caretaker who is comfortable with the dentist should accompany the child into the treatment room; avoid dentists who do not allow this.

Counsel parents to avoid dentists that rely only on pharmacologic types of behavior management, such as nitrous oxide, oral antihistamines, or narcotics. The most effective strategies are behavioral. Combinations of behavioral and pharmacologic methods—such as distraction and nitrous oxide—can be effective, whereas the drug alone may not be.

Dentists and parents who rely solely on authoritarian approaches or who are permissive are likely to fail with a fearful child. Preparation should focus on helping the child develop coping skills and ways to gain control. Children gain control when the dentist briefly explains procedures and allows them to signal any discomfort. An example of a coping skill is relaxation breathing. Finding a dentist who tells stories and riddles, sings to the children, or otherwise distracts them is particularly effective. Directed guidance strategies—specific kinds of direction followed by praise—are also very effective in managing children's behaviors. For fearful children, practitioners can be successful by using structured rehearsals, in which procedures are broken into small steps, and teaching coping strategies. (Weinstein & Milgrom, 2006).

Older children do better when the dentist treats them more like adults and encourages coping. Many are afraid of getting hurt, and poor pain control can be a problem. The key is to teach older children good coping skills, including how to signal and communicate with the dentist. Dentists who explain things well, structure rest breaks, and provide opportunities for feedback do best with older children. Providing distractions—video, music, and games—are useful strategies.

Parents should be cautious about dentists with laser-based diagnostic devices. These devices are often marketed to dentists as being capable of detecting "invisible" cavities. They are being misused to justify unnecessary fillings, often called "preventive resins." The standard method of examination of the teeth is visual, using strong light and transillumination (shining light through the tooth) without using sharp probes. Research has shown that the sharp probes, especially when used in the grooves of teeth, cause damage. The probes also transfer potential pathogenic bacteria from one groove or surface to another. Most tooth decay in permanent teeth in children occurs on the biting surface, and x-rays are of limited diagnostic value in such cases. Parents should be urged to seek second opinions whenever a lot of fillings are recommended.

■ DENTAL HEALTH EDUCATION

Dental health education is a common, long-standing, and crucial preventive strategy. Tailoring health education messages and instruction to an individual's capacity to "obtain, process, and understand" reflects a health literacy approach to oral health education. Low parental health literacy is most often associated with early childhood caries (tooth decay), low income, and inadequate maternal education. This problem of low reading literacy combined with low health literacy is of particular concern given the dual role a parent plays as decision-maker for self and child. The potential negative consequences for health and safety escalate.

Health information that is accessible to individuals with limited literacy is now just beginning to influence dentistry. A review of dental education materials for parents found many required reading skills above the seventh to ninth grade. Additionally, many materials included dental jargon and unnecessarily difficult words. The same study found that more than 80% of secondary school children (spanning a reading level equivalent to that of adults) were unsure of many dental terms, such as "fluoride tablets" and "gum disease" (Alexander, 2000). The advice given in published materials often was inconsistent.

A good source of reference material on the web is *www.medlineplus.gov*, the consumer side of PubMed from the National Library of Medicine. Access is free, and materials are often in multiple languages. The site includes brochures that can be freely downloaded and copied.

REDUCING DISPARITIES THROUGH PREVENTIVE INTERVENTION

Weinstein et al have shown that parents of young children are willing and able to change home preventive oral health practices. Weinstein's intervention approach uses the transtheoretical "stages of change" model of Prochaska and Norcross. Applying the model, individuals overcome self-identified barriers to change by setting goals that are perceived to be attainable and of personal value (Weinstein et al, 2004; Weinstein & Milgrom, 2006).

Demonstrations by staff and parental practice of toothbrushing in the primary care clinic, preschool, Head Start, or WIC can be powerful reinforcing strategies to improve parents' toothbrushing skills and oral hygiene education. Studies of young primary school children tested the additive effects of home- and school-based intervention on oral hygiene and gingivitis. Researchers found that oral hygiene and gingivitis scores improved in children when instructions about oral health were reinforced both in the home and at school (Rayner, 1992; Kwan et al, 2005). Davies and colleagues (2005) reported positive benefits of a series of "gifts" by mail to parents of infants 8 through 32 months old. The gifts included written educational pamphlets, a trainer cup, toothpaste, and a toothbrush. Parents who received the repeated mailings versus those who did not, were more likely to report favorable feeding behaviors, initiation of toothbrushing before 12 months old, and twice daily toothbrushing.

■ BACTERIAL DISEASES OF THE MOUTH
TOOTH DECAY (CAVITIES, DENTAL CARIES)
Description and Epidemiology

Tooth decay is a bacterial disease resulting in irreversible damage and potential loss of teeth. The decay is caused by lactic acid demineralization of the teeth. The acid is produced by an alpha hemolytic streptococcus (*Mutans streptococci*, in older literature referred to as *S. mutans*). Active cavities are also frequently infected with lactobacilli. The bacterial species are part of the biofilm adherent to the teeth. The bacteria are usually transmitted to the child by oral contact with the mother or female caretaker. Infection and colonization peak around the time of the eruption of the primary teeth, but may occur before. There is also child-to-child transmission. These bacteria metabolize carbohydrates in the diet, producing acid and demineralization of the tooth subsurface enamel. Unless neutralized and buffered by saliva (remineralized), the demineralization process will lead to cavitation.

In infants, the carbohydrates may be present in the form of prolonged exposure to formula or breast milk, especially if the infant is allowed to sleep with the nipple in his or her mouth (van Palenstein Helderman et al, 2006; Azevedo et al, 2005). Before and after weaning, carbohydrates may also come from milk sweetened with honey or sugar or from juices in baby bottles or training cups, especially when given at bed, naptime, or when a child is allowed to take swigs of the fluid throughout the day. In older children, the source of the carbohydrates may be Tang, Kool-Aid, sports drinks, and/or soda. This frequent carbohydrate exposure keeps the pH of mouth fluid near the tooth surface below 5 and results in an environment conducive to demineralization. The neutralization process does not have enough time to increase the mouth pH to a level that would allow remineralization. In patients undergoing chemotherapy or radiation to the head and neck and in patients who are immunocompromised, normal salivary flow and salivary buffering of acids is disrupted. Cavities result.

State surveys suggest that 50% to 60% of third graders have had at least one cavity; a minimum of 25% of third graders has untreated decay. In some states, the rate approaches four in ten children with untreated tooth decay (CDC, 2006).

Clinical Findings

Clinical findings can include the following:
- Early caries lesions. These appear as whitish or brown opaque changes in the tooth enamel near the gumline on either the tongue or lip side of the front teeth in populations using baby bottles because the cavity-causing fluids pool in these areas of the mouth. In cultures where bottle use especially at night or naptime is less common, the damage may occur in back teeth first as a function of other dietary patterns. When white lesions occur, the dentin is initially damaged. Then, as the lesion progresses, the hard enamel breaks and a clinical cavity is evident (see Color Plate).
- Advanced tooth decay. This appears as cavitations in the teeth. Nearly all cavities in permanent teeth in children in the U.S. begin on the biting surface of the molars. The initial lesion appears as a pinhole surrounded by a white, opaque halo. As the lesion enlarges, greater damage to the enamel becomes apparent. Lesions typically appear about 1 year after the eruption of the tooth and frequently begin while the tooth is still erupting. A gumboil may form if the tooth becomes abscessed (Fig. 33-3).
- Sensitivity. Cavities can be hot and cold and sweet sensitive.
- Localized pain. Lesions that progress can begin to hurt all the time, disrupting normal activity, sleeping, and eating.
- Inflammation and abscesses. Bacterial invasion of the pulpal tissue in the tooth causes inflammation and necrosis. In severely decayed primary teeth, a gumboil or draining fistula will form on the gum tissue above the root end of the tooth. This also occurs in permanent teeth, but is a late stage (see Fig. 33-3).
- Facial pain
- Gingival swelling, erythema
- Possible lymphadenopathy
- Possible fever

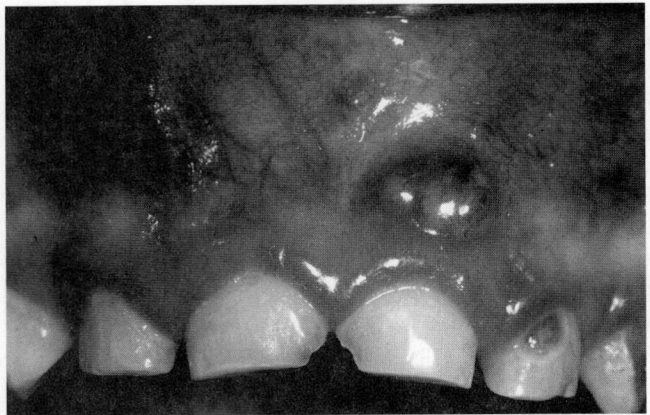

FIG. 33-3 Advanced tooth decay with gumboil. (Courtesy John Davis, DDS MSD, Professor Emeritus, University of Washington, Seattle, Department of Pediatric Dentistry.)

- In the mouths of methamphetamine users ("meth mouth"), accelerated tooth decay on the facial surfaces of the teeth and between the teeth is typically seen. In later stages, the teeth are blackened, stained, and appear to be crumbling. There may be signs of severe grinding and dry mouth (Klasser & Epstein, 2005).
- Cavities may spontaneously arrest. This is thought to occur, for example, when cavities are exposed to saliva high in fluoride or when the diet changes (such as after weaning). Children from outside the U.S. may have open cavities that are black or dark brown in color and arrested. If the child has such open cavities, is asymptomatic, the teeth are primaries, and access to dental care is problematic, they can be left alone and allowed to shed normally. Ideally, these children should receive dental care, but many of these arrested cavities in primary teeth will not need treatment. The discoloration also may be the result of topical treatment with diamine silver fluoride or silver nitrate.

Management and Prevention Strategies for the Primary Care Provider

Primary care providers are often the first to detect tooth decay, whether it comes in the form of subtle white spots on the upper central incisors near the gumline, extensive cavitations, or complaints of toothache. Many interventions are available. The following treatments should be in every provider's oral health toolbox.

Fluoride varnish. Early white spot lesions in primary and permanent teeth can be remineralized using topical fluoride varnish. In many states, primary care providers and nurses are permitted to apply fluorides (Fig. 33-4). Marketed fluoride varnish preparations contain from 1000 ppm (Fluor Protector, 0.1% silane fluoride) to 22,600 ppm (CavityShield, Duraflor, and Duraphat, sodium fluoride, 5%). Typically the 5% varnish preparations are used for children. All of the 5% varnishes for sale in the U.S. are essentially similar, varying in flavor or color. Twice-yearly applications have been shown to reduce tooth decay by about one-third. Frequent

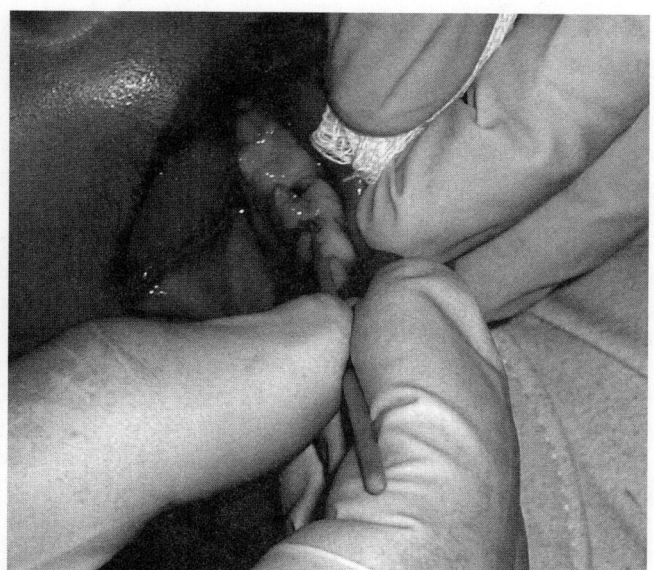

FIG. 33-4 Applying fluoride varnish. (Courtesy Peter Milgrom, DDS.)

application of fluoridated toothpaste will also promote repair (Helfenstein & Steiner, 1994). See the Resources Box to find sources for ordering fluoride varnish. The low plasma fluoride levels following applications of varnish are not associated with toxicity or fluorosis. Fluoride varnish is the agent of choice for young children and has been shown to be more effective than the fluoride gels that are still widely used in the U.S. Fluoride gels are dangerous and difficult to apply in preschool children and are not recommended because of the risk of acute toxicity.

Fluoride therapy.   The most effective preventive measure against dental caries is optimizing the fluoride content of communal water supplies to 1 ppm. However, only about 50% of children in the U.S. drink fluoridated water. Children who consume fluoride-deficient water supplies and who are at risk for caries will benefit from dietary fluoride supplementation (CDC, 2001). The fluoride level of public water supplies can usually be ascertained by calling the local health department. If the patient uses a private water supply, the fluoride level should be tested before prescribing fluoride supplements. To prevent potential overdoses, no fluoride prescription should be written for more than a total of 120 mg of fluoride. See Table 33-2 for adjusting the dose of fluoride supplements in relationship to that found in the community water supply. Box 33-1 lists the usual doses of fluoride supplementation for those without a source of fluoridated water.

Bottled water.   Many children drink bottled water. Although some bottled waters marketed in the U.S. contain an optimal concentration of fluoride (approximately 1 ppm), most contain less than 0.3 ppm fluoride. Thus, a person substituting bottled water with a low fluoride concentration for fluoridated community water might not receive the full benefits of community water fluoridation. For water bottled in the U.S., current FDA regulations require that fluoride be listed on the label only if the bottler adds fluoride during processing. The overall concentration of fluoride is regulated, but does not have to be stated on the label.

Toothbrushing techniques.   Parents should be taught to clean a child's teeth with a brush or washcloth as soon as they erupt using the "lift the lip" method. Simple flip charts are available to teach parents how to do this; a demonstration by the provider during a well-child visit is ideal. Essentially, the technique involves having a parent lift the child's upper lip monthly to check closely for horizontal white or brown lines or spots along the upper central gumline or gingival margin. If a parent detects a problem, early intervention can prevent demineralization progression. Parents often have difficulty brushing an infant's teeth. As the infant is repeatedly exposed, the behavioral aspects get easier. Toothbrushing does not hurt. It may be easier to brush a child's teeth on the floor or on a couch with the child's head in the parent's lap. A second adult can help by holding the hands and feet if necessary. Brushing in the bathroom standing up is more difficult.

TABLE 33-2   **Fluoride Supplementation Based Upon Drinking Water Fluoride Concentration**

	Fluoride Ion Level in Drinking Water (ppm)*		
Age	**Less Than 0.3 ppm**	**0.3–0.6 ppm**	**Greater Than 0.6 ppm**
Birth-6 months	None	None	None
6 months-3 years	0.25 mg/day[†]	None	None
3-6 years	0.50 mg/day	0.25 mg/day	None
6-16 years	1 mg/day	0.50 mg/day	None

*1 part per million (ppm) = 1 milligram/liter (mg/L)
[†]2.2 mg sodium fluoride contains 1 mg fluoride ion.
Only children living in nonfluoridated areas should receive supplements between the 6 months and 16 years old. If the fluoride level is not known, it should be tested first. State and local health departments can provide information on testing drinking water for fluoride levels.
From Centers for Disease Control and Prevention (CDC): *Dietary fluoride supplement schedule*, 2002. Available at *www.cdc.gov/oralhealth/factsheets* (accessed Mar 14, 2007). Approved by the American Dental Association, the American Academy of Pediatrics, and the American Academy of Pediatric Dentistry (AADP).

BOX 33-1 **Dosage of Fluoride Supplementation for Children Without a Source of Fluoridated Water**

6 months-3 years old: Fluoride drops 0.25 mg/0.6 mL. Administer 0.6 mL daily. Give directly by mouth; may be mixed with water or juice **but not** with milk products.

3-6 years old: Fluoride tablets 0.5 mg. Dispense 100 tablets, refill prn. Administer one tablet daily. Chew slowly or dissolve in mouth.

6-16 year old: Fluoride tablets 1 mg. Dispense 100 tablets, refill prn. Administer one tablet daily. Chew slowly or dissolve in mouth.

---

prn, As needed.

The type of toothbrush, manual or electric, is not clinically relevant. The effectiveness of tooth cleaning is primarily a function of the person doing the cleaning. Most children and adults are not systematic and do not spend enough time cleaning to be effective. The toothbrush songs and timers are helpful in teaching children and parents how long to brush. Very small children can have their teeth cleaned with a washcloth or special finger brushes made for parents to use. Small soft brushes are widely available for children, and large handled brushes are available for children with physical disabilities that make holding a regular brush difficult.

Toothpaste. Fluoridated toothpaste works by creating a reservoir of fluoride in the fluid layer of the plaque and in the saliva that is available to remineralize or repair teeth that are being damaged by bacterial acids. A small amount of toothpaste (about the size of a pea) should be used. The amount should be controlled by an adult because children swallow a large amount of what is brushed on. Longer supervised toothbrushing results in more effective prevention of childhood cavities.

Diet. Dietary advice is essential to parents. Bottles should only be filled with formula or water and the child weaned at 12 months old. Bottles should never be propped during naps or sleep. Training cups should be started at 4 to 6 months old for water and juices for both breastfed and bottle-fed infants. Some WIC centers in the U.S. distribute training cups to promote appropriate eating behaviors and prevent tooth decay caused by inappropriate bottle use. However, personnel may not be aware of the potential danger of the cups themselves if sugary drinks or juice are available *ad lib*. Nursing mothers should not allow their infants to sleep attached to the nipple.

Xylitol gum and syrup. Xylitol, a naturally occurring sugar, has been demonstrated to prevent and control tooth decay when used at least three times per day with a minimum dose of about 6 g. Xylitol is FDA approved and works by reducing the adhesiveness of oral bacteria in the dental plaque and reducing the overall numbers of virulent organisms. The effect is topical not systemic.

Chewing gum and mints are the most frequent source of xylitol. Products should contain at least 50% xylitol, and xylitol should be the first ingredient listed on the label. The gum should be chewed for about 5 minutes or until the sweetness disappears. Chewing gum is not appropriate for preschoolers because of the risk of choking. In the dosage range used for tooth decay prevention, side effects are rare and are limited to abdominal cramping (Ly et al, 2006). More severe abdominal pain and diarrhea may occur in children who consume sorbitol in excess from other products.

Xylitol syrups have been shown experimentally to help reduce the number of episodes of acute otitis media, but the syrups are not as yet available commercially. Children of mothers who use xylitol chewing gum at least three times per day for 2 years after the baby is born will have less tooth decay because of reduced or postponed bacterial colonization. (Isokangas et al, 2000).

"Meth mouth." Methamphetamine users should be encouraged to seek drug treatment. Any dental intervention will fail without control of the underlying condition. Encourage the patient to drink lots of water and switch to artificially sweetened drinks. Over-the-counter fluoride mouth rinse, remineralizing solutions or xylitol chewing gum, and prescription chlorhexidine gluconate mouth rinse may be recommended. Instructions for the chlorhexidine gluconate mouth rinse are: half a capful swished in the mouth for 30 seconds twice daily and then spit out. Individuals should not rinse the mouth afterwards or eat for 30 minutes. It is necessary to use it at least 60% of the time to have any clinical effect.

Toothache. If tooth decay has resulted in a toothache and draining tract, analgesics, warm water or saline rinses, and a bland diet are recommended. In the presence of cellulitis and fever, antibiotic therapy is appropriate, and follow-up dental treatment is needed. Penicillin is the drug of choice; in the case of allergy, clindamycin or erythromycin are alternatives (Schneider et al, 2007). The child needs an emergency dental visit (not an emergency department visit) after several days if not responding to antibiotic treatment.

Management and Prevention Role of the Dentist

The American Academy of Pediatrics and the American Academy of Pediatric Dentistry (AAPD) both recommend that children be examined by a dentist by 12 months old or within 6 months of the eruption of the first tooth. The AAPD has a useful website (see Resource Box at the end of the chapter) containing guidance on the prevention and treatment of dental disease in children. Box 33-2 defines some common dentistry terms that will be discussed throughout the rest of this chapter.

Larger cavities in primary teeth can be repaired with plastic fillings or with steel or plastic crowns. Deep cavities involving the pulp tissue in primary teeth require a form of therapy called a pulpotomy, removing the inflamed or necrotic pulp tissue, followed by the placement of a stainless steel crown. Teeth with deep cavities and draining gumboil are generally extracted. Thus, a decision to repair teeth or remove them depends on the extent of damage and the length of time until the tooth would be normally exfoliated. Retention of primary molars is important because they hold space to allow the normal eruption of permanent successors. However, many times the correct treatment for a badly decayed primary tooth is

BOX 33-2 Glossary of Terms Used in Dentistry

Amalgam filling: Metal filling material used to replace tooth structure affected by decay in permanent teeth. Contains silver, mercury, copper, and other metals. Usually referred to generically as amalgam. Not commonly used in primary teeth now.

Composite filling: Tooth colored acrylic filling material used to replace tooth structure affected by decay. Also used to as an aesthetic material for replacement of discolored tooth structure. Main filling material used in children's teeth.

Crossbite: Type of malocclusion in which one or more upper teeth are located behind the opposing teeth. Usually caused by premature tooth loss.

Erythroplakia: Matted red plaques located on the soft tissues of the oral cavity in smokers and those using smokeless tobacco, which can be a sign of oral cancer.

Extrusion: Condition in which a tooth is loosened from its normal tooth position in the direction of tooth eruption.

Glass ionomer: Tooth-colored filling material often used in atraumatic restorative procedures in young children.

Gumboil: Fistula associated with an abscessed tooth draining through the gums.

Intrusion: Condition in which a tooth is loosened from it normal position in the opposite direction of tooth eruption.

Leukoplakia: Matted white plaques located on the soft tissues of the oral cavity that can be a sign of oral cancer.

Luxation: Condition in which a tooth is loosened from its normal tooth position.

Malocclusion: A term to describe abnormalities in the way maxillary and mandibular teeth articulate. Includes crossbites, open bites, and abnormal spacing. May or may not have functional significance. Can usually be corrected by a dentist or orthodontist.

Nitrous oxide: Laughing gas. Commonly used as a relaxing agent mixed with oxygen for mildly anxious or nervous patients during conscious sedation. Usually used at less than 50% in an open anesthesia system.

Open bite: Type of malocclusion in which the front teeth do not touch together when the back teeth are biting.

Periapical pathosis: Tooth infection that often presents as a radiolucency on a dental radiograph.

Pericoronitis: Inflammation around the crown of an unerupted tooth.

Pulp: Part of the tooth anatomy containing the nerves and blood vessels. When invaded by bacteria in tooth decay, it swells and necroses, resulting in gumboils and pain and the need for pulpotomy or root canal treatment.

Root canal: Space that houses a tooth's neurovascular bundle. Root canal treatment involves removing the infected neurovascular bundle and replacing it with an inert filling material.

Sealants: Plastic coatings placed on the chewing surfaces of permanent molars at about 6 to 7 years and again at about 13 to 14 years old, when the tooth is fully erupted. Also called pit and fissure sealants or occlusal sealants.

Xerostomia: Dry mouth that results from reduced salivary flow or production. May be secondary to medications.

---

extraction. Young children may need to be sedated or receive treatment under a general anesthetic to cope with the treatment.

Cavities in permanent teeth are repaired with either silver amalgam or plastic composite fillings. Mercury-containing silver amalgam fillings are safe (DeRouen et al, 2006). The longevity of plastic fillings is very much shorter than silver fillings except when small and not involved with the bite. There are no dependable alternatives to the mercury-containing amalgams. Severe cavities resulting in abscess formation in permanent teeth are treated with root canal therapy. Permanent molars either need to be capped (crown) after root canal therapy or treated with large silver fillings. If the family cannot afford a gold or tooth-colored crown, a prefabricated stainless steel crown can be substituted for several years.

Pit and fissure (occlusal) sealants are recommended for children at moderate or high risk for tooth decay. These are children who have experienced a lot of tooth decay in their primary teeth, have poor oral hygiene, or diets with lots of refined carbohydrates and pop. Sealants are plastic coatings placed on the biting surfaces of permanent molars at about 6 to 7 years old and 13 to 14 years old, depending on tooth eruption. Sealants are very effective in preventing decay and do not involve drilling. The treatment involves cleaning and conditioning the surface and then placing a light polymerizing resin in the grooves on the biting surface where decay is most likely to occur (Fig. 33-5). Sealants are underused in the U.S. for children at high or moderate risk. A child at low risk for tooth decay does not need sealants.

Complications

A complication of too much systemic fluoride exposure is fluorosis. About 22% of children in the U.S. have some level of fluorosis, but most is very mild and not clinically significant. About 1% have moderate fluorosis. Very few children have fluorosis that is cosmetically unacceptable (CDC, 2001). This occurs primarily in children who drink naturally fluoridated water with high levels of fluoride or in children who receive systemic supplements (fluoride tablets or drops) and who also use fluoridated toothpaste before 3 years old. The advisability of introducing toothpaste for very young children should always depend on the risk of tooth decay. When risk is high (e.g., if the mother and siblings have tooth decay, poor hygiene and diet) the benefit outweighs the minimal consequences of fluorosis. Nevertheless, toothpaste should always be metered by parents.

Some teeth abscess after fillings are placed in them. Permanent teeth may be sensitive to hot and cold for many weeks after fillings are placed. Untreated abscesses may

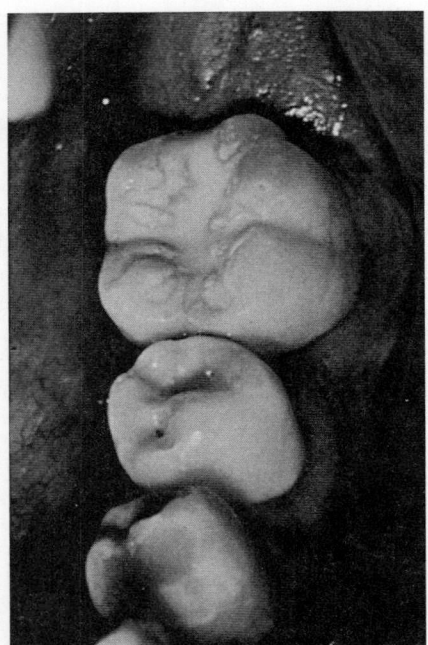

FIG. 33-5   Sealant. (From Pinkham JR: *Pediatric dentistry: Infancy through adolescence*, ed 4, St. Louis, 2005, Elsevier WB Saunders, p. 537.)

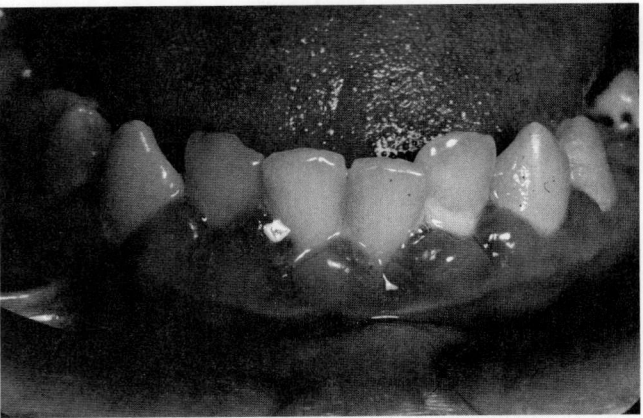

FIG. 33-6   Periodontitis (gross gingivitis). (From Davis J, Peterson D: *Atlas of pediatric dentistry*, Seattle, 2004, University of Washington.)

develop into life-threatening facial space infections, requiring surgical drainage and parenteral antibiotic treatment.

AGGRESSIVE PERIODONTITIS

Description and Epidemiology

Periodontitis is an aggressive bacterial infection that results in loss of periodontal attachment and supporting bone around teeth. This is a bacterial infection of the gums and bone with phagocyte abnormalities and hyperresponsive macrophages. The primary infection is by *Actinobacillus* and *Bacteroides* species in younger children and by *Treponema* species and other gram-negative rods in older children. There is a localized and more generalized form of the disease as defined by the location of the loss of attachment and which teeth are affected.

The incidence is about 0.2% to 0.5% in children and adolescents, especially those 12 years and older; African-American children are at slightly more risk. Age of onset is typically circumpubertal, with a familial aggregation of cases (American Academy of Pediatric Dentistry [AAPD], 2005-2006a).

Clinical Findings

This condition can be localized (around the primary incisors and molars) or more generalized (all teeth affected). The teeth may become loose, but in the localized form there is generally no inflammatory response, suppuration, or fever. This localized disease is not oral hygiene related, and the damage happens within months.

Individuals with the generalized form of gum disease often have poor oral hygiene. This condition is more common in patients with special health care needs brought about by such systemic diseases as Papillon-Levre disease, Down syndrome,

and cyclic neutropenia. A history of periodontal disease in parents may be found. Fig. 33-6 illustrates this condition.

Management

If gum disease is caught early, local debridement of the teeth and systemic antibiotics are used. Management with tetracyclines or metronidazole in combination with amoxicillin is appropriate. Tetracyclines should not be prescribed while the crowns of the permanent teeth are still unerupted and developing in the jaws. Individual circumstances may vary, but typically the tetracyclines would be safe for children 8 years and older.

Complication

The major complication of gum disease is loss of teeth.

Education and Prevention

For patients with a familial history of gum disease, frequent dental examinations and radiographs during the peripubertal period are essential to identify the condition early. Patients should be counseled to avoid tobacco products since they increase the risk of all periodontal diseases; damage to dentition is permanent.

NECROTIZING PERIODONTAL DISEASE

Description and Epidemiology

This is an aggressive bacterial disease resulting in damage to the gum tissue between the teeth. The gum tissues harbor high levels of spirochetes, and invasion of the tissues has been demonstrated. Predisposing factors are viral infections (including HIV and other systemic diseases), malnutrition, emotional stress, and lack of sleep. The incidence in North America is fewer than 1% of children and adolescents; the prevalence is 2% to 5% in those age groups from Africa, Asia, or South America (AAPD, 2005-6a).

Clinical Findings

Children have severe gingival pain and fever. The triangular area of gums between the teeth is ulcerated and necrotic and covered with a gray film. There may be a fetid mouth odor.

Management

If the provider notes this condition and the patient is febrile, metronidazole and penicillin should be started and a dental referral made. Careful oral hygiene and a bland diet are recommended. Dental treatment involves a thorough cleaning of the teeth and mechanical debridement under local anesthesia. Address the predisposing conditions.

Complications

The major complication of this disease is loss of teeth.

Education and Prevention

Early treatment is needed to prevent disfigurement of the gums with chronic infection.

■ OTHER DENTAL CONDITIONS
PYOGENIC GRANULOMA

Pyogenic granuloma is an inflammatory hyperplasia that is usually caused by low-grade localized infection, trauma, or hormonal factors. It is usually a small exophytic (outward growing) lesion that is smooth or lobulated and sometimes hemorrhagic. The surface color ranges from pink to red to deep purple, depending on how long the lesion has been present in the oral cavity. A pyogenic granuloma most commonly occurs in pregnant females. Possible treatments include improved oral hygiene, chlorhexidine rinses (previously described), surgical excision, cryosurgery, or intralesional injections of corticosteroids. If hygiene or chlorhexidine does not resolve the problem, then the patient should be referred.

SOURCES OF DAMAGE TO THE TEETH
Bruxism/Grinding

Description and Epidemiology. Bruxism is a condition of excessive grinding of the teeth. Studies of the prevalence of bruxism or excessive tooth grinding are limited to clinical populations and plagued by poor design and measurement. A study by Cheifetz and colleagues (2005) stands out as being well designed. However, the conclusions should be viewed cautiously. A group of predominantly Caucasian, well-educated parents estimated the prevalence of bruxism in their 8-year-old children at 38%. Almost all the grinding was at night, and no facial pain or other symptoms were associated with the grinding. Many of the children who ground their teeth had a familial history of bruxism or had undefined "psychological disorders." This study suggests that underlying stressors may be a cause, and as such, may provide an opportunity for intervention and education.

Clinical Findings. Primary teeth show marked wear, and parents report that their child grinds his or her teeth during sleep. Children with excess wear in the permanent teeth usually have an orthodontic problem that needs attention. Some adolescents may experience facial muscle pain and develop temporomandibular joint disorder (discussed later).

Management. No treatment is required for most grinding and tooth wear. The use of plastic night guards for children or adolescents rarely eliminates grinding. Behavioral methods, such as relaxation training and other self-management skills including control of gum chewing, have been shown to be effective in helping to manage facial muscle pain and headache. Clicking of the jaw on opening or closing is not a pathologic condition, and is seen mostly in adults.

Complications. Children or adolescents who have either limited mouth opening, pain on opening or closing, or deviation of the jaw to one side during opening may have a jaw fracture or another serious problem, such as a tumor or infection.

Education and Prevention. Parents should be told that tooth grinding is normal in young children and that no intervention is needed. It is not associated with any damage to permanent dentition. Teens may experience headache or facial muscle pain, particularly at stressful times. Stress management guidance may be offered. Parents should be counseled to avoid dentists who routinely prescribe expensive plastic mouth guards or similar appliances for this complaint.

Dental Erosion

Description and Epidemiology. Dental erosion is a chemical process that leads to irreversible acid demineralization of tooth structure. Acids that cause dental erosion can be classified as intrinsic or extrinsic. Intrinsic acids include stomach acid introduced into the oral cavity by diagnosed or silent gastroesophageal reflux disorder (GERD), bulimia nervosa, and vomiting. Extrinsic acids include acidic beverages, methamphetamines, citrus fruits (e.g., sucking on lemons), and medications (e.g., chewable vitamin C tablets or HCl supplements). Factors that can aggravate dental erosion include xerostomia (dry mouth) secondary to decreased salivary flow; medications that interfere with saliva composition or production (e.g., clonidine); dental attrition; and dental abrasion. Asthmatic children have greater amounts of dental erosion than other children, but no association has been found with specific medications (Al-Dlaigan et al, 2002). One of the latest studies demonstrated an erosion prevalence rate of 41% to the upper permanent incisors in children 11 to 13 years old in the U.S. (37% in the United Kingdom) (Deery et al, 2000).

Clinical Findings. Clinical manifestations of dental erosion include smooth, cupped-out teeth on chewing surfaces; fillings that are raised above the normal level of the tooth; overly shiny silver fillings; enamel cuffing along the gums; and tooth hypersensitivity. Bulimic patients usually have very smooth lingual surfaces of the permanent teeth (Fig. 33-7).

Differential Diagnosis. Consider abrasion caused by gritty substances, such as coarse toothpaste or hard toothbrushes, and attrition caused by mechanical forces, such as tooth grinding (bruxism). Also consider tooth decay.

Management. Early detection, diagnosis, and treatment of dental erosion are critical. Hot and cold sensitivity can be managed by the use of "sensitive teeth" fluoridated toothpastes or topical treatments applied by the dentist. Referral to medical professionals, such as gastroenterologists or psychiatrists, is warranted in suspected cases of GERD or bulimia. Dietary counseling may be appropriate. Unless the erosion is deep, fillings are not required. Deep groves in teeth can be repaired by the dentist using atraumatic techniques and materials.

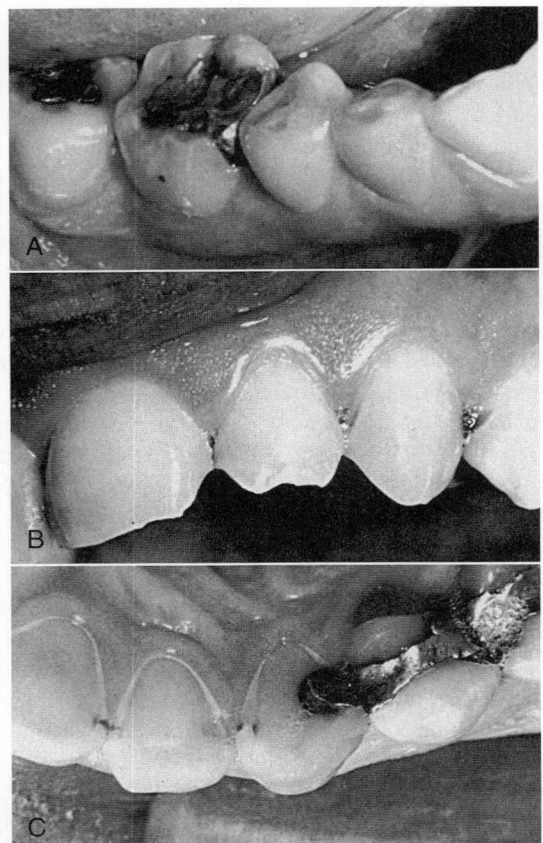

FIG. 33-7 Dental erosion from bulimia. **A,** Loss of occlusal enamel with exposure of dentin. **B,** Ragged incisal edges. **C,** Lingual exposure of dentin highlighted by outlines of remaining enamel and exposed surfaces of restorations. (From Casamassimo P, Castaldi C: Considerations in the dental management of the adolescent, *Pediatr Clin North Am* 29:648, 1982.)

Complications. Patients with mild to moderate dental erosion may report tooth hypersensitivity. Severe dental erosion can lead to dental nerve (pulp) exposures, which can necessitate root canal treatment.

Education and Prevention. Typically the problem can be managed by identifying and eliminating the etiologic agent. Over-the-counter products, such as soft toothbrushes, low-abrasive fluoridated toothpaste, and fluoride rinses, are helpful. Patients with bulimia should be referred for behavioral therapy.

PERICORONITIS ASSOCIATED WITH PARTIALLY ERUPTED WISDOM TEETH

Description and Etiology
This condition is due to a partially erupted lower wisdom tooth with a tissue flap covering part of the crown. A foreign body, such as a piece of food, is forced under the flap, causing a localized infection. In some cases, upper wisdom teeth will erupt with the crown rubbing against the buccal mucosa and cause pain. The problem is common in college-age students.

Clinical Findings
The gum tissue partially covering the tooth is inflamed and painful. The patient may be febrile. The tissue flap may be traumatized by biting. Partially erupted wisdom teeth can create an environment in which the distal surface of the second molar becomes decayed because it cannot be cleaned.

Differential Diagnosis
Aggressive periodontal diseases and severe tooth decay may have similar clinical presentations.

Management
Primary care providers may recommend irrigation of the area with sterile water or saline, prescribe analgesics, and start amoxicillin if the patient is febrile. If the tooth is impacted, it should be surgically removed. Upper teeth that are erupted toward the buccal mucosa should be removed. Not all patients having third molar extractions require general anesthesia, although this is commonplace in the U.S. It may be possible to operate on only one side at a single session. Oral benzodiazepines and nitrous oxide sedation may help young patients successfully cope with the surgery.

Complications
Removal of wisdom teeth always requires a risk-benefit calculation because there is significant morbidity associated with the surgery (Friedman, 2007). Temporary or permanent nerve damage is possible. A common complication of wisdom tooth surgery is alveolar osteitis or dry socket. This painful condition is associated with the loss of the normal clot in the healing socket. The cause of the pain is exposed bone. Smoking and the use of oral contraceptives are risk factors. Pretreatment rinsing with 0.12% chlorhexidine gluconate mouth rinse reduces the risk of complications. Treatment at the time of surgery with a nonsteroidal antiinflammatory may reduce the extent of swelling postoperatively. Pain and foul taste in the mouth are the main symptoms, beginning 4 to 5 days after surgery. The patient should be referred back to his or her dentist. The treatment is symptomatic with analgesics because the problem is self-limiting.

Education and Prevention
Not all wisdom teeth need to be removed. Wisdom teeth do not cause other teeth to become crooked. Teeth fully covered in bone do not need to be removed and carry no significant risk. Similarly, if there is space for the erupting teeth, there is no reason to remove them. Partially erupted teeth are the source of most problems.

It is appropriate to wait for the teeth to fully erupt as much as they can. Studies show they may still erupt at 23 or 24 years old. Waiting maximizes the chance they will not need to be removed and minimizes the morbidity associated with the surgery.

TRAUMATIC INJURIES TO ORAL STRUCTURES

Description
Injuries to the face usually result in trauma to the teeth or jaws. Such trauma is one of the most common presentations of young children to dentists. Dental injuries occur secondary to falls, motor vehicle accidents, violence, abuse, and

sporting activities. Fewer traumas are presently seen from supervised, organized sports because most children wear mouth guards; nevertheless, a disproportionate amount of trauma results from leisure activities, such as skateboarding, swimming, and other noncontact sports. Upper incisors are particularly vulnerable to dental injuries.

Epidemiology

Age is a significant consideration in trauma to teeth, with most injuries occurring between 7 and 12 years of age. Luxation (loosening) injuries to upper anterior teeth predominate in toddlers because of their frequent falls during attempts at walking. Studies show that boys have dental injuries more frequently than girls. Other risk factors for trauma-related dental injuries include participation in sports, cerebral palsy, and misaligned bites. Between 25% and 50% of all accidents in children up to 14 years of age involve the head. Sports-related injuries can result from falls, collisions, and direct contact with balls or other hard surfaces. Children 6 to 15 years old are most likely to come to the emergency department with a sports-related tooth injury. (AAPD, 2005-6b).

It is important to rule out caregiver abuse. The orofacial region is commonly traumatized during episodes of child abuse. Injuries that do not match the given history, bruising of soft tissue not overlying bony prominences, an injury that takes the shape of a recognizable object, or multiple injuries at different ages may be indications of nonaccidental trauma.

Clinical Findings

History. Because a dental injury may become the subject of litigation, a thorough history and examination is mandatory. When possible, an injury should be photographed. The provider should ask the following questions:

- When and how did the trauma occur?
- Were there any other injuries?
- Have there been any injuries in the past?
- Is there any concern for the safety of this child and family?
- Is there any history of abuse, drug or alcohol use in family?
- Are any problems occurring as a result of the trauma?
- Is tetanus immunization current (within the last 5 years)? This question is especially important with dirty wounds or with complete displacement of a tooth from its socket (Jasper et al, 2007).

Physical Examination. The examination should include:

- Soft tissue. Palpate the jaws and the rest of the facial skeleton to determine if a fracture is possible.
- Skin. Look for extraoral lacerations and facial wounds.
- Intraoral mucosa. Look for wounds, swelling, and bruising of the oral mucosa, gingiva, tongue, cheeks, and/or palate.
- Teeth. Look for:
  - Displacement: a tooth forced from its normal socket position (intrusion, extrusion)
  - Luxation: loosened, mobile tooth
  - Avulsion: tooth knocked out
  - Tooth fractures: classified as complicated (those involving nerve exposure) and uncomplicated (those involving enamel or dentin)
  - Root fracture: caused by injury to the tooth root
  - Bite problems: check for abnormalities in occlusion
  - Pulp exposure: bleeding from the broken stump of the tooth itself
  - Color change: the whole tooth turning dark from internal bleeding when the tooth is intact
  - Jaw movement: deviation to one side or pain and limitation on opening

Management

Blunt trauma tends to cause greater damage to soft tissues and supporting structures, whereas high velocity or sharp injuries cause luxation and fractures of the teeth. Children with sports-related injuries can have teeth that are avulsed, fractured, luxated, intruded, or extruded.

Most minor injuries to the intraoral mucosa do not require suturing unless bleeding is a problem. Wound care should consist of irrigating the area with sterile saline and prescribing water-based 0.12% chlorhexidine gluconate mouth rinse. Avoid the alcohol-based rinse because its use maybe painful.

Children with avulsed and fractured teeth, those unable to bite normally, and those with jaw injuries should be referred promptly. Left untreated, dental injuries secondary to trauma can lead to tooth abscesses, dental pain, and problems with the eruption of permanent teeth.

- Tooth avulsion. Primary teeth cannot be replanted. If permanent teeth are knocked out, timing is important, and management information can be given over the telephone (Koch & Poulsen, 2001). Replant an avulsed clean tooth immediately or within 5 minutes. If the tooth is dirty, rinse it gently in cold milk, saline, or room temperature water and then replant it. Do not rub the root surface. If the tooth can be replanted, have the child bite gently on a handkerchief or clean cloth to keep the tooth in place, and seek immediate dental treatment in order to be sure the tooth is in the right position and stabilized. Prescribe amoxicillin (loading dose 1000 mg followed by 500 mg three times per day for seven days). In the case of a penicillin allergy consider clindamycin (Lin et al, 2007). If unable to replant the tooth, it may be kept several hours in cold milk, saline, or room temperature tap water and wrapped in plastic wrap to prevent dehydration. The tooth can also be kept in the child's mouth next to the cheek, being careful that the child does not swallow it. If available, the best transport media are Viaspan or Hanks Balanced Salt Solution. The prognosis for successful reimplantation decreases with time. A tooth that is allowed to dehydrate will not be viable after 1 hour. The dentist should also x-ray to rule out an alveolar fracture and for placement of a flexible plastic splint to maintain proper tooth position.
- Tooth fracture. If possible, have the patient keep the pieces of permanent incisors and place them in saline or water to prevent drying. Sometimes the dentist can temporarily repair the tooth if the fragment is large enough. Tooth fractures with bleeding from the stump are emergencies. Simple fractures not involving the pulp or nerve tissue are not emergencies, but still may be repaired.

The provider should be alert to the possibility of a closed head injury if severe trauma is reported. See Chapter 14 for a discussion of head injuries after sports participation and return-to-play policies. See Chapter 27 for further discussion of head injuries.

Complications

Trauma not only compromises a previously healthy dentition but also may affect self-esteem and quality of life. In some cases, the traumatized tooth may be asymptomatic and appear to be clinically normal. This tooth can subsequently become darker, which is an important indication that the tooth needs assessment by a dental professional. The tooth can also become spontaneously symptomatic, with the patient reporting cold sensitivity, pain on chewing, or unprovoked pain.

Education and Prevention

It is important to identify and educate children who are at high risk for dental trauma-related injuries. Children and teenagers who participate in sports should be encouraged to wear mouth guards and helmets. Parents and coaches should also encourage youths to remove all intraoral piercings (e.g., tongue and lip rings or studs) while engaging in sports.

Parents, coaches, and physical education teachers should also be alerted to the importance of making saline part of first-aid kits to treat tooth avulsions. Parents and caregivers with children who are learning to walk should be instructed on how to childproof their homes. To prevent dental trauma in motor vehicle accidents, it is important to ensure that caregivers know how to select an appropriate-sized car seat for younger children. (The top of the child's head should not be above the back of the car seat.)

TEMPOROMANDIBULAR JOINT DISORDER

Description and Incidence

Temporomandibular joint disorder (TMD) includes chronic facial pain and mandibular dysfunction. In the past, this disorder was evaluated strictly based on the physical state of the jaws or bite. This led to a great many inappropriate, ineffective, and even dangerous treatments. Today the significance of the condition is evaluated within the context of a biopsychosocial model. This model is based on the premise that physical changes alter physiologic processes. These processes then stimulate nociceptive pathways that come to the consciousness of an individual in the form of perceived discomfort or pain. The individual then adapts behaviorally to that pain by being anxious, depressed, avoiding social interaction, developing other physical symptoms, or by seeking treatment or pharmacologic relief (Dworkin & Drangsholt, 2003).

Patients who do not respond to the basic recommendations in this chapter need referral to specialized centers where teams of dentists and psychologists work together. Diagnosis involves assessment of physical findings and both Axis I and II dimensions of the mental state.

Onset of most TMD is in adolescence. A well-designed Swedish study of 28,899 youths 12 to 19 years old found a prevalence of 4.2% with a rate of 6% in girls and 2.7% in boys (Nilsson et al, 2005). Similar rates have been found in American children. The diagnosis includes both pain and other functional and psychological components (Leresche et al, 2006).

Clinical Findings

Two clinical symptoms are predictive of TMD: (a) self-reported facial pain once or more per week associated with a limitation in normal ability to open the mouth wide and (b) pain once a week or more in the temples, face, or jaws (Nilsson et al, 2006). Facial muscles are tender to palpation, often unilaterally, but there is usually no swelling or skin bruising. The individual will be afebrile. Tooth pain, if present, is non-specific. There may be a deviation to the painful side when the mouth is opened.

Differential Diagnosis

Consider infection of the face or teeth, traumatic injury (fracture of the jaw), myositis, dislocation of the jaw, neoplasm, arthritis, collagen diseases (systemic lupus erythematosus [SLE]), congenital and developmental anomalies of the joint (rare), and capsulitis.

Management

This disorder should be conceived of as a biopsychosocial problem for which surgical interventions, particularly changes to the teeth, are inappropriate. Current treatment recommendations include a soft diet, muscle relaxation and stretching exercises, analgesics, and antiinflammatory medication. Previously, expensive plastic guards or splints and similar appliances to reposition the bite were used to treat this problem. However, the current treatment recommendations were found to be less expensive and as efficient (Truelove et al, 2006). A clinician's guide to self-help treatment is available from NIH at no cost and can be downloaded from the Internet (see reference citation for Dworkin & Drangsholt, 2003).

Complications

Chronic headaches, otalgia, tinnitus, and lost time from work, school, or activities may result.

GINGIVAL HYPERPLASIA

Description and Etiology

Gingival hyperplasia is a fibrous enlargement of gingival tissue around the teeth. The enlargement is typically caused by drugs (phenytoin, cyclosporine, nifedipine), hormones, chronic inflammation, leukemia, or heredity. It can be idiopathic.

Clinical Findings

The gingival tissue can be normal or red-blue in color or lighter than the surrounding tissue. It may be spongy or firm and dense. The tissue is generally not inflamed, and patients are asymptomatic.

Management

Treatment consists of improved oral hygiene and chlorhexidine mouth rinses. In cases where the overgrowth interferes with chewing, gingivectomy is required.

RANULA

A ranula is a cyst filled with saliva products. It is associated with a major salivary gland in the sublingual area and is caused by lip or cheek biting. A common clinical problem occurring

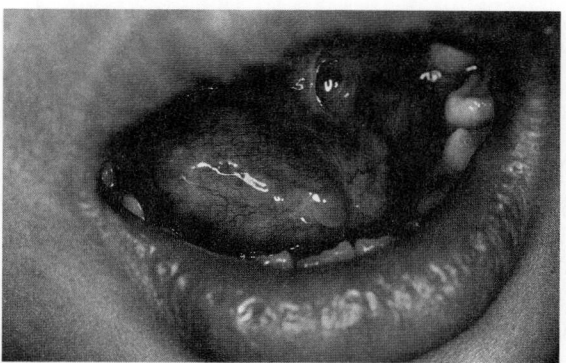

FIG. 33-8   Ranula of the floor of the mouth. (From Pinkham JR: *Pediatric dentistry: infany through adolescence*, ed 4, St. Louis, 2005, Elsevier/WB Saunders, p 44.)

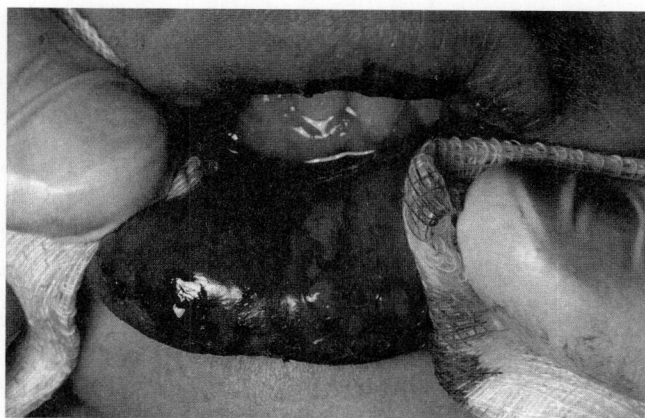

FIG. 33-9   Herpes stomatitis in an infant. (From Davis J, Peterson D: *Atlas of pediatric dentistry*, Seattle, 2004, University of Washington.)

at any age, including infancy, a ranula is evidenced by a large, soft, mucus-containing swelling in the floor of the mouth. The cyst should be excised by an oral surgeon (Fig. 33-8).

MUCOCELE

A mucocele is a salivary gland lesion caused by a blockage of a salivary gland duct. It is most common on the lower lip and has the appearance of a fluid-filled vesicle or a fluctuant nodule with the overlying mucosa normal in color. The patient should be referred to an oral surgeon for surgical excision of the involved tiny accessory salivary gland.

▨ VIRAL DISEASES OF THE MOUTH
HERPETIC HERPES STOMATITIS
Description and Epidemiology

Herpetic herpes stomatitis is a viral disease that results in oral and circumoral ulcers. It is caused by herpes simplex virus (HSV-1). Asymptomatic herpetic stomatitis occurs in the majority of children, but up to 5% under 5 years old will experience symptomatic disease (Annunziato, 2004). Approximately 80% of the adult population in North America is seropositive to herpes simplex virus, and 45% experience recurrent herpes labialis (Gordon & Ganatra, 2006; Dock & Creedon, 2003).

Clinical Findings

The following clinical findings are typical (Fig. 33-9):

- Oral or perioral vesicles. Abrupt history of onset, with pain in the mouth, excess salivation, bad breath, refusal to eat, and fever as high as 40° C (104° F). Fever and irritability may precede the oral lesions by several days. Lip lesions, which are initially papular, progress to being ulcerative and eventually crust over.
- Gingivostomatitis, as evidenced by yellow- or white-filled vesicles that rupture and form painful, erythematous ulcers on the mucosal surfaces of the mouth. Gums bleed easily.

Differential Diagnosis

Herpes stomatitis/labialis may be confused with aphthous ulcers (canker sores), ulcerative gingivitis, hand-foot-and-mouth disease, trauma, herpangina, or chemical burns. Rare conditions that may also cause lesions are neutrophil defects, systemic lupus, Behçet syndrome, and Crohn disease.

Management

Lesions heal without treatment in 7 to 10 days. Supportive therapy is appropriate, such as cold liquids and analgesics. Topical treatment with an equal mixture of diphenhydramine and Maalox may provide symptomatic relief. Antimicrobials are not appropriate. Exclude the child from day care or school during the drooling phase of the illness. Encourage parents to clean the teeth with a soft toothbrush or cloth.

For children under 12 years old, oral acyclovir (20mg/kg) every 8 hours for 5 days has been recommended (Bentley et al, 2003). Single-dose oral famciclovir is effective in reducing the healing period of initial or recurrent labial lesions by about 1 day over no treatment (Hull et al, 2006). The adult dose—typically given to children—is 1500 mg, taken as a single dose as early in the episode as possible. However, the efficacy and safety of famciclovir for children under 18 years old has not been fully established.

Complications

Children are at risk for dehydration. Parents should be instructed to watch for such signs and symptoms and seek medical care in such an event. Careful hand washing should be recommended to the child and the caregivers to prevent autoinoculation or transmission of infection to the eyes.

Education and Prevention

Reactivation of the virus resulting in recurrent lip lesions is thought to be the result of exposure to ultraviolet light, tissue trauma, stress, or fevers. Use of Vaseline-based lip products to protect the lips during cold weather, sports, or direct sun may be helpful. Over-the-counter topical agents for the treatment of erupted lip lesions are largely unproven, and some topical treatments that deaden lesions may prolong healing.

▨ FUNGAL DISEASES OF THE MOUTH
CANDIDIASIS/THRUSH
Description and Epidemiology

Thrush is a fungal disease caused by an overgrowth of *Candida albicans*, a normal part of the oral flora in nearly half the population. Overgrowth occurs when host resistance is lowered, after exposure to broad-spectrum antibiotics, or in association with immunosuppression or systemic disease. The disease may be acquired by neonates from mothers with a vaginal infection. Infants may acquire it from sucking fingers, from the breast or bottle nipples, or after receiving antibiotics. Patients using inhaled corticosteroids for asthma or rhinitis are also subject to oral candidiasis. Fig. 33-10 illustrates this overgrowth. The presence of thrush/candida in an adolescent should prompt investigation of his or her immune status because it can be a symptom of underlying immunosuppression (e.g., HIV).

Clinical Findings
White, patchy, raised, adherent, furry, or curdled milk-like lesions are typically located on the buccal mucosa, pharyngeal surfaces (often seen in infants), gums, and tongue. The lesions may bleed if scraped with a tongue blade. Neonates may experience oropharyngeal involvment (Kaufmann & Campbell, 2007). Young children often have white lesions only, whereas adolescents may have areas of bleeding. However, many children are asymptomatic. There may be mild lymphadenopathy. Infants may be totally asymptomatic or may refuse to eat as a result of discomfort from the infection. Individuals with oropharyngeal candidiasis may report a cottony feeling in the mouth, loss of taste, and sometimes pain on eating and swallowing. The diagnosis can be confirmed by direct microscopic examination on potassium hydroxide smears and culture of scrapings from the lesions.

Management
Oropharyngeal infections in the healthy newborn are usually self-limiting in 3 to 8 weeks. Treatment with nystatin will hasten

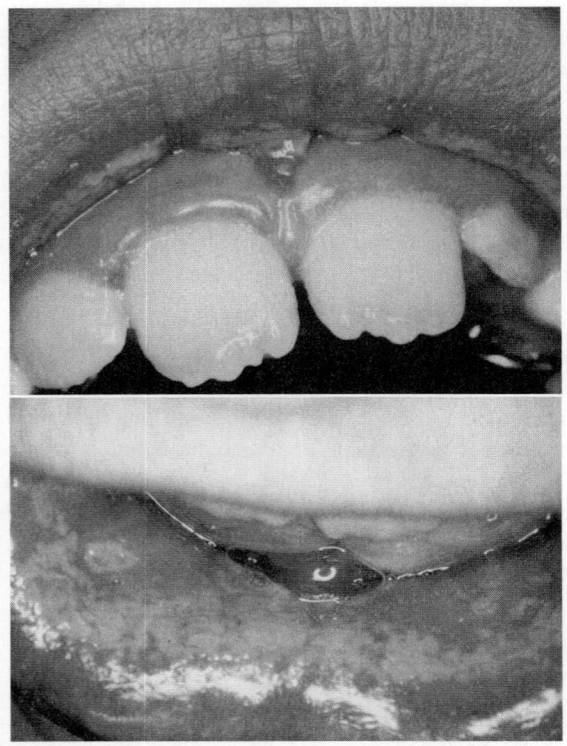

FIG. 33-10 Acute candidiasis on the upper and lower lips of a young patient. (From McDonald RE, Avery DR, Dean JA: *Dentistry for the child and adolescent*, ed 8, 2004, Mosby, p 423)

recovery and reduce the risk of spread. Typical dosages for the oral suspension are: infants, 200,000 units four times per day and children, 400,000 to 600,000 units four to five times per day. The medication should be used until at least 48 hours after the disappearance of the perioral symptoms. Treatment with oral troches or pastilles should be 200,000 to 400,000 units four to five times per day. Persistent infections should be treated with fluconazole. The typical pediatric dose is 6 mg/kg on day 1 followed by 3 mg/kg once daily for 2 weeks.

If infection is caused by the use of oral corticosteroids for asthma, the patient should be instructed to rinse his or her mouth after using the inhaler.

Complications
If the disease is recurrent, look for underlying causes. Many organ systems may be affected in advanced cases. For example, candida endocarditis is seen in children with congenital heart disease or a history of surgery.

Education and Prevention
Educate children and their parents about the importance of rinsing the mouth after using inhaled steroids.

◼️ IDIOPATHIC ORAL CONDITIONS
APHTHOUS ULCERS
Description and Epidemiology
This is a condition of recurrent oral ulcers. The etiology is not well understood. Infectious agents, such as *H. pylori*, HSV-1, or even measles have been implicated in the etiology. Alterations of cell-mediated immunity may be associated with the disease. Emotional and physical stress, hormonal factors, and food hypersensitivity have been implicated. Sodium lauryl sulfate in toothpaste has been associated with recurrent ulcers. Vitamin and mineral deficiencies also can cause recurrent oral aphthae, particularly deficiencies in several B vitamins (1, 2, 6, and 12), iron, folic acid, and zinc. Aphthous ulcers are reported to develop in 20% of the population and are most common in childhood and adolescence.

Clinical Findings
Single or multiple small mucosal lesions are present on alveolar or buccal mucosa, tongue, soft palate, or the floor of the mouth. The ulcers are surrounded with an erythematous halo and a pale center.

Differential Diagnosis
Consider HSV-1 infection.

Management
Lesions generally last 10 to 14 days and heal without treatment and without scarring (Goldstein & Goldstein, 2006). A bland diet and oral analgesics may be appropriate. Vitamin or mineral replacement may prevent recurrence. Over-the-counter treatments, such as triamcinolone hexacetonide in Orabase, fluocinonide gel covered by Orabase, or amlexanox 5% oral paste (Aphthasol), may be applied four times per day

for 3 to 4 days. Early treatment leads to a quicker recovery (Murray et al, 2005). There are homeopathic and complementary remedies as well (see Chapter 42). Maintaining good oral hygiene is essential.

BENIGN MIGRATORY GLOSSITIS (BMG)

Also known as geographic tongue, BMG usually presents as asymptomatic, circular lesions that appear on the anterior two-thirds of the dorsum of the tongue. The lesions may heal and reappear on other areas of the tongue. The etiology is unknown. Proposed risk factors for BMG include hormonal changes, use of oral contraceptives, diabetes mellitus, and stress. Patients can be reassured that the lesions are benign and do not require treatment.

HALITOSIS

Description

Halitosis is oral malodor or bad breath. It is primarily associated with poor oral hygiene. It is more common in individuals who are mouth breathers, who suffer from postnasal drip, or who use tobacco products.

Management

Encourage proper oral hygiene, including regular brushing, flossing, and dental visits. Provide reassurance and encourage patients to avoid breath mints and other sugar-containing candies that might cause tooth decay or erosion. Sugarless gum or mints may be helpful. Patients who have not had their teeth cleaned or an oral examination within the last 6 months should be referred to a dentist.

The provider should evaluate the patient for systemic disease, sleep apnea, and other airway-related conditions.

OCCLUSAL AND TOOTH SPACING IRREGULARITIES

Malocclusion

Description. Dental occlusion is the way the maxillary and the mandibular teeth articulate. From birth to adulthood and beyond, dental occlusion undergoes significant changes. To be able to diagnose any abnormal development, it is important to understand and recognize the scope of the changes that are normally occurring in the dentition.

Epidemiology. Malocclusions have their basis in hereditary or genetic and/or environmental factors. Prevention of genetic causes for malocclusion is not possible at this time, but the prevention of environmental factors holds much promise. An estimated 57% to 59% of U.S. children under 18 years of old need orthodontic treatment for malocclusions. Severe problems related to occlusion and crowding occur in 15% to 20% of children (Proffit et al, 1998). Ethnic minorities and the uninsured and underinsured have higher levels of need.

Clinical Findings. The most common malocclusions that may require early diagnosis and interception include an anterior or posterior crossbite or an open bite. Retention of a primary tooth beyond the normal period can deflect the eruption of the permanent successor and lead to a crossbite. Crossbites are classified as follows:

- Anterior crossbite. The most common cause is crowding where one or two teeth are either behind or in front of the teeth in the opposing jaw while the others are in good alignment.
- Posterior crossbite. In the posterior jaw, one or more of the upper teeth is inside the opposing lower tooth. In the upper jaw, the premature loss of a second primary molar in a crowded mouth may result in forward movement of the first permanent molar, forcing the second premolar to erupt palatally.
- Anterior open bite. In the anterior jaw, the front teeth do not touch together when the back teeth are biting. Children with this problem may have a habit of passing their tongues through the space and can have problems speaking or chewing.

In early stages of the mixed dentition period when both primary and permanent teeth are present, a child may have a temporary open bite, usually either a result of the still incomplete eruption of the incisors or a result of mechanical interference from a persistent finger habit. Sucking habits are normal in infancy, and pacifiers do not normally cause lasting effects. Thumb and finger sucking or long-term use of a pacifier that is not discontinued by the time the permanent teeth erupt may result in an anterior open bite. The upper front teeth will tip and push out. Tongue habits described above exacerbate the open bite.

Management. Control of habits and the prevention of premature loss of primary teeth are examples of effective preventive measures. Dental health education and improved caries prevention have lowered the number of children who develop malocclusion because of premature loss of primary teeth. However, this premature loss is still one of the most common controllable causes of malocclusion.

The recognition and referral of a malocclusion or a condition that could lead to a malocclusion is the most important orthodontic service a primary care provider can offer his or her patients. Malocclusion has an important effect on the function and aesthetics of the entire dentition, and can have a lifelong impact on the self-esteem of a child or an adolescent. Most crossbites in the permanent dentition are readily treated by a dentist or orthodontist. A persistent open bite in a school-aged or older child is difficult to correct and requires referral to an orthodontic specialist.

Diastema

Spacing issues also affect the dentition. A space between any neighboring two teeth is referred to as a *diastema*. During the mixed dentition stage, when both primary and permanent teeth are present, a midline space between the upper front teeth is normal. If the teeth are not otherwise crowded or malaligned, these spaces usually close by the time the permanent maxillary canines fully erupt, and referral is not needed. Diastemas caused by missing incisors or midline supernumerary tooth or teeth will persist in the permanent dentition stage and require referral.

Another cause of a diastema is a prominent labial frenum, which is the tissue connecting the upper lip to the area of the gums between the front upper teeth. Sometimes the frenum is large and appears to be causing space between the front teeth. Generally the space closes as the jaws grow, and referral is not needed. Unnecessary or premature excision can result in scarring. A prominent labial frenum attachment that persists in the permanent dentition stage may require excision.

ANKYLOGLOSSIA ("TONGUE-TIE")

Ankyloglossia or "tongue-tie" is caused by a short lingual frenum that hinders tongue movement. The frenum may lengthen as the child gets older. Usually no treatment is needed. If the extent of the ankyloglossia is severe, speech may be affected and referral for a surgical correction indicated. In the absence of speech effects, referral can result in unnecessary excision and damage to the gums around the lower teeth.

◼ LIFESTYLE CHOICES THAT IMPACT DENTAL HEALTH
SMOKELESS TOBACCO: GUM DISEASE AND CANCER
Description

Smokeless tobacco is a highly addictive substance that is held in the oral cavity, allowing nicotine to enter the bloodstream.

Epidemiology

Smokeless tobacco is commonly used by individuals who think chewing tobacco is a healthier alternative to smoking cigarettes. Smokeless tobacco may also be associated with weight-loss attempts. About 8% of all teens nationwide report using smokeless tobacco (Marshall et al, 2006). Popular cultural events (e.g., baseball) and heroes (e.g., rodeo riders and baseball players) make the habit "look cool."

Clinical Findings

Examine the posterior buccal vestibule of the lower jaw and the anterior buccal vestibule of the upper jaw. These are the areas where smokeless tobacco is commonly held in the mouth. The intraoral findings of smokeless tobacco users include:

- Oral leukoplakia (white changes and scarring)
- Erythroplakia (red changes)
- Gingivitis and gum recession (particularly in the lower jaw)
- Periodontitis
- Stained teeth
- Halitosis
- Tooth decay, which may be associated with tobacco products that have added sweeteners.

Management

Although tobacco use is associated with a variety of health problems, three main factors make it difficult to quit: its association with pleasurable activities, social factors (peer pressure), environmental cues (media bombardment), and nicotine addiction.

Patients who use tobacco products should be assessed for willingness to undergo tobacco cessation treatments. Recent research suggests ways to apply cessation principles in the pediatric patient population (see Weinstein & Milgrom, 2006). See Chapter 10 for a discussion of an effective strategy to use with adolescents.

Complications

Complications include lip and oral cancer, gingivitis, gum recession, periodontitis, and stained teeth.

Education and Prevention

It is important for the family to be actively involved in the lives of their children to prevent the start of smokeless tobacco. In addition, direct patient education parlayed by a caring health professional can help. Likewise, behavior modeling, whereby caregivers indirectly teach a child by avoiding tobacco themselves, is effective. If young patients have relatives who use tobacco products, the primary care provider may need to focus tobacco-cessation efforts on these family members.

ORAL BODY ART
Piercing and Intraoral Tattoos

Description. Studs and other body ornaments pierce the tongue and lower lip. Some patients may also have tattoos on the buccal mucosa of the lips.

Clinical Findings. Tissue around tongue studs may be infected as evidenced by inflammation, swelling, and pain. Some individuals may exhibit inflammation and pain as an allergic response to the metals in the studs or piercings, particularly to nickel. There also may be fractures of the lower anterior teeth from metal studs that habitually click against the teeth or gum recession.

Management. Tongues, especially just after stud insertion, are swollen. The mouth heals quickly, and the inflammatory response should be resolved within 8 to 10 days without treatment. Swelling beyond this period suggests infection or an allergic response. Infection should be treated with chlorhexidine gluconate mouthwash twice per day for at least 1 week and a broad-spectrum systemic antibiotic, such as penicillin or clindamycin (Jasper et al, 2006). If mouth tissue is infected, the ornament should be removed at least temporarily. If an allergic reaction to nickel is suspected, have the patient change to gold or silver. Devices that cause chronic allergic reactions should be removed permanently. The patient's immune status to tetanus and hepatitis B should be ensured.

Complications. Deep neck infection, airway obstruction, bleeding, nerve damage, tooth fracture, and hepatitis have been noted. Systemic infections also have been reported.

Education and Prevention. Adolescents contemplating or who have oral piercings should be counseled about:

- The potential for acquiring an infectious disease
- Using only regulated practitioners
- Ensuring that only sterile equipment and noble metals are used
- Completing a hepatitis B vaccination series before seeking piercing
- The potential damage to the teeth and gums
- Removing studs and piercings during sports

TOOTH WHITENING (BLEACHING)
Description

Patient requests for "whiter and brighter" smiles have resulted in increased demands for tooth whitening. The procedure may be indicated for permanent teeth stained by trauma, fluorosis, tetracycline consumed during tooth development, or colored foods and beverages.

Tooth whitening can involve the use of over-the-counter kits, in-office treatment, or take-home bleaching trays that are customized for each patient. The in-office tooth whitening process involves repeated short-term exposure of teeth to carbamide peroxide (typically in the range of 10% to 38%) until desired results are achieved. Over-the-counter kits include lower concentration carbamide peroxide in trays or hydrogen peroxide in strips. Most are used for 2-week periods. There are also numerous gels, rinses, gums, toothpastes, and paint-on films. Most have been inadequately studied. Higher concentrations of hydrogen peroxide are more effective than lower concentrations.

In all cases, the effect of the treatment is temporary, and the teeth will eventually return to their normal coloring. As far as we know, repeated treatments do not carry great risk for complications, but published aftermarket studies are limited and potentially biased (Hasson et al, 2006).

Clinical Findings

The most common clinical evidence of tooth bleaching in children and adolescents is a complaint of hypersensitive teeth and gum irritation. In some studies, one-third to one-half of subjects experienced tooth sensitivity or gingival inflammation or both. There are no studies of these products in children.

Management

In most cases, teeth will return to their normal sensation, gum status, and color if treatments are not repeated.

Education and Prevention

Health providers can remind parents and caregivers that permanent teeth are naturally darker than primary teeth and in most cases do not need whitening. Unless there are major aesthetic concerns that could affect a child's psychosocial development, tooth whitening should not be undertaken until all permanent teeth have fully erupted. This measure will also prevent shade mismatching that can occur when teeth are whitened during the mixed dentition stage (when both permanent and primary teeth are in the mouth). The potential side effects should be mentioned. The patient or parent should consult with a dental professional.

▪ DENTAL CARE OF CHILDREN WITH SPECIAL NEEDS

Children with chronic disease or with congenital or acquired physical and/or mental disabilities require extra preventive strategies and individualized dental appointments based upon their particular needs and conditions (Koch & Poulsen, 2001). Success in treating children with disabilities can be enhanced by knowledge of a particular child's disabilities and by knowledge of the dental, educational, social, and psychological skills needed to successfully treat the individual.

At-risk children include those with neuropsychological disabilities (mental retardation, autism spectrum); sensory disabilities (blindness, visual impairment, deafness and hearing impairments); muscular difficulties (osteogenesis imperfecta, cerebral palsy, spina bifida, paralysis); and chronic diseases (asthma, cardiovascular disorders, chronic renal failure, diabetes mellitus, bleeding disorders, malignant disease, and epilepsy). Some individuals have a higher incidence of oral disease either because of the systemic problem itself or because of the secondary effects on diet, medications, or the inability of caretakers to clean or maintain the teeth. These include the following:

- Diet. A number of conditions, such as congenital heart disease, facial clefts, esophageal defects, generalized hypotonia, muscular dysfunction, or mental retardation involve feeding problems. A child's sucking or chewing problems may lead to meals lasting for an hour or more. Liquid—or soft and often high, cavity-causing sugar foods—are common. Food is often retained in the mouth for a long time before it is swallowed.
- Elimination. Many children with disabilities experience chronic constipation or diarrhea. Sweet remedies, such as dried fruits or sodas and juices, are often used to cure such conditions. Frequent intake of beverages is often recommended for children on medication to prevent kidney failure. To increase hydration, parents often resort to sugar-containing drinks.
- Medications. Long-term use of sweetened medicines or syrups can also present a hazard to dental health. Various drugs, such as the antihistamines, may also reduce salivation and thereby increase susceptibility to caries. Phenytoin commonly causes gingival hyperplasia.
- Cognition. In some children, problems may relate to an inability to understand the meaning behind oral hygiene procedures.
- Muscular function. Hypotonia may influence salivation and cause drooling or chewing problems. Impaired manual dexterity may make it difficult for children to perform preventive oral hygiene routines. Hyperfunction may result in extensive tooth wear as a result of grinding of teeth. This is also seen in some children with mental retardation. Children with feeding tubes face many difficulties.

MANAGEMENT STRATEGIES

The ability of parents to follow recommendations for preventive dental care will vary with the difficulties presented by the child's condition. In addition, the ability of parents to take full responsibility over time for the preventive dental care of a child may vary. Therefore, recommendations for professional checkups and preventive services, such as fluoride treatments, should be individualized. If hygiene is poor, preventive treatments need to be provided more often. Counseling parents to maintain good communication involving both medical and dental providers is essential.

The primary care provider is advised to frequently ask about the status of dental visits and whether routine oral hygiene is taught and practiced in the school the child attends. Specific areas to cover include:

Diet

For children with reduced salivary secretion or impaired self-cleaning mechanisms of the oral cavity, parents or caretakers must be especially attentive to the diet. Restrictions in cavity-causing foods are necessary to prevent rampant tooth decay. Chronic use of sweetened medicinal syrups can cause severe decay. If sweetened medicines cannot be replaced by sugar-free alternatives, medicines should be taken at mealtime. Water or sugar-free beverages should be recommended for drinks between meals.

Topical Fluorides

A child with reduced salivary secretion, impaired muscular function, or with a cavity-causing diet may need an intense fluoride program in addition to careful oral hygiene. Primary care professionals can apply 5% sodium fluoride topical varnish or prescribe a fluoride rinse, gel, or high-fluoride toothpaste for home use. Primary care practitioners should carefully monitor the teeth of these patients and make prompt referrals when problems are noted.

Topical Iodine

The teeth and gums can be painted with topical Betadine once every 4 to 6 months. There is evidence that topical 10% povidone iodine suppresses tooth decay–causing flora without major changes in the overall flora (Zhan et al, 2006). Children who have had major dental treatment under general anesthesia because of extensive dental caries are obvious candidates for repeated iodine treatments. Iodine can be painted on the teeth at the same visit in which fluoride varnish is applied with the iodine wiped off with gauze before applying the varish. The primary care provider can do this treatment if dental services are lacking.

Chemical Plaque Control

Chemical plaque control with a 0.12% chlorhexidine gluconate mouth rinse is recommended in cases where oral hygiene is difficult to perform (Milgrom & Weinstein, 2001). Gels and toothpastes with chlorhexidine are available outside the U.S. However, compounding pharmacists can be asked to create a facsimile. Chlorhexidine rinses can be used daily during periods of certain medical treatment procedures 7 to 10 days before dental treatment to minimize bleeding or bacteremia in children with hemophilia, cardiac disease, or immunodeficiency.

☑ DISCUSSION QUESTIONS

1. What is the level of fluoride in the water within the communities that you live? What information do you need before you prescribe fluoride? What are other sources of fluoride that children have access to?
2. An adolescent has multiple carious teeth. What are your differential diagnoses? How would the differential vary if this were a 2-year-old or an 8-year-old?
3. A 16-year-old admits to the use of smokeless tobacco. How does the use of the transtheoretical model of change help you in caring for this client?
4. Why do children and adolescents with special health care needs have an increased risk for oral problems? How can you help coordinate care for these children and their families?
5. A child with multiple carious teeth has no dental insurance. What options are there for this family? Which groups of children need prophylactic antibiotics before dental care?
6. Research your state's practice requirements for ordering, and learning how to apply, fluoride varnish as part of your practice. How would you incorporate its use in your practice?

*R*ESOURCE BOX

Dental and Oral Disorders

Parent handouts and similar information are widely available. Here are some key sources:

American Academy of Pediatric Dentistry
www.aapd.org

American Dental Association
www.ada.org

Medline Plus (in Spanish and English)
www.medlineplus.gov

National Maternal and Child Oral Health Resource Center
www.mchoralhealth.org

SUGGESTED REFERENCES OR USEFUL MATERIALS

Dental Behavioral Publications:
Milgrom P, Weinstein P: Early childhood caries and Weinstein P, Milgrom P: Oral self care: strategies for preventive dentistry. Available from www.dentalbehavioralresources.com
Lift the Lip Video and flip charts (in multiple languages) available at www.dental.washington.edu/conted/store/documents/lift the lipappl.pdf

FLUORIDE VARNISH AND OTHER DENTAL PRODUCTS RESOURCES

Sources for fluoride varnish:

Colgate Duraphat Varnish
www.colgateprofessional.com

Omnii Cavity Shield or White Varnish
www.omniipharma.com

Duraflor fluoride varnish
www.medicom.com

MPL VarnishAmerica
www.medicalproductslaboratories.com/public-health/ varnishamerica.html

WHERE TO BUY MOUTH MIRRORS

Disposable or autoclavable dental mouth mirrors are widely available from dental supply companies. Examples are *www. practicewares.com* or *www.henryschein.com*.

FREE OR DISCOUNTED TOOTHPASTE AND TOOTHBRUSHES

See website *www.dentalcare.com* for information on Crest courtesy pricing for kits. Check with local pediatric dentists for information about how to reach a Procter and Gamble representative to request donations. The similar Colgate website is *www.colgateprofessional.com*. Both companies have free downloadable educational materials on their websites.

REFERENCES

Al-Dlaigan YH, Shaw L, Smith AJ: Is there a relationship between asthma and dental erosion? A case control study, *Int J Paediatr Dent* 12 (3):189, 2002.

Alexander RE: Readability of published dental educational materials, *J Am Dent Assoc* 131(7):937, 2000.

American Academy of Pediatric Dentistry (AAPD): *Reference manual 2005-6a: periodontal diseases of children and adolescents*. Available from *www.aapd.org/media/PoliciesGuidelines* (accessed Nov 3, 2006).

American Academy of Pediatric Dentistry(AAPD): *Reference manual 2005-6b: policy on prevention of sports-related orofacial injuries*. Available from *www.aapd.org/media/PoliciesGuidelines* (accessed Feb 2, 2007).

Annunziato PW: Herpes simplex virus infection. In Gershon AA, Hotez PJ, Katz SL, editors: *Krugman's infectious diseases of children*, ed 11, St Louis, 2004, Mosby.

Azevedo TD, Bezerra AC, de Toledo OA: Feeding habits and severe early childhood caries in Brazilian preschool children, *Pediatr Dent* 27(1):28, 2005.

Bentley JM, Barankin B, Guenther LC: A review of common pediatric lip lesions: herpes simplex/recurrent herpes labialis, impetigo, mucoceles, and hemangiomas, *Clin Pediatr* 6:475, 2003.

Bloom B, Dey AN, Freeman G: Summary health statistics for U.S. children: National Health Interview Survey, 2005, *Vital Health Stat 10* 231:1, 2006.

Centers for Disease Control Prevention (CDC): Recommendations for using fluoride to prevent and control dental caries in the United States, *Morb Mortal Wkly Rep* 50(RR14):1-42, 2001.

Centers for Disease Control Prevention (CDC): *National Oral Health Surveillance System. Caries experience: percentage of 3rd grade students with caries experience (treated or untreated tooth decay), 2006*. Available from *www.apps.cdc.gov/nohss/Indicators.asp?indicator-2* (accessed Nov 3, 2006).

Cheifetz AT, Osganian SK, Allred EN et al;: Prevalence of bruxism and associated correlates as reported by parents, *J Dent Child* 72:67, 2005.

Davies GM, Duxbury JT, Boothman NJ et al: A staged intervention dental health programme to reduce early childhood caries, *Community Dent Health* 22(2):118, 2005.

Deery C, Wagner ML, Longbottom C et al: The prevalence of dental erosion in a United States and a United Kingdom sample of adolescents, *Pediatr Dent* 22:505-510, 2000.

DeRouen TA, Martin MD, Leroux B et al: Neurobehavioral effects of dental amalgam in children: a randomized clinical trial, *JAMA* 19:295(15):1784-1792, 2006.

Dock M, Creedon RL: The teeth and oral cavity. In Rudolph CD, Rudolph AM, editors: *Rudolph's pediatrics*, ed 21, NY, 2003, McGraw-Hill.

Dworkin SF, Drangsholt M: Clinical trials in temporomandibular disorders. In Max MJ, Lynn J: *Interactive textbook of clinical symptom research*, 2003. Available from *www.symptomresearch.nih.gov/chapter_22* (accessed Feb 8, 2007).

Friedman JW: The prophylactic extraction of third molars: A public health hazard. *Am J Pub Health* 97(9):1554-1559, 2007.

Gift HC, Reisine ST, Larach DC: The social impact of dental problems and visits, *Am J Public Health* 82(12):1663-1668, 1992.

Goldstein BG, Goldstein AO: Oral lesions. *Up To Date*, 15.3. Available at *www.uptodateonline.com* (accessed December 20, 2007)/electronic text book.

Gordon SC, Ganatra S: Viral infections of the mouth. Emedicine. Updated January 4, 2007. www.emedicine.com/derm/topic765.htm. (accessed December 20, 2007).

Hasson H, Ismail AI, Neiva G: Home-based chemically-induced whitening of teeth in adults, *Cochrane Database of Systematic Rev* 4(CD006202), 2006.

Helfenstein U, Steiner M: Fluoride varnishes (Duraphat): a meta-analysis, *Community Dent Oral Epidemiol* 22(1):1, 1994.

Hull C, Spruance S, Tyring S et al: Single-dose famciclovir for the treatment of herpes labialis, *Curr Med Res Opin* 9:1699, 2006.

Isokangas P, Soderling E, Pienihakkinen K et al: Occurrence of dental decay in children after maternal consumption of xylitol chewing gum: a follow-up from 0 to 5 years of age, *J Dent Res* 79:1885, 2000.

Jasper J, Losh G, Endom EE: Evaluation and repair of tongue lacerations. *Up to Date Online* 15.3. Available at *www.uptodateonline.com.* (accessed December 20, 2007) electronic textbook.

Kauffman CA, Campbell JR: Clinical manifestations of *Candida* infection in children. *Up To Date* Online 15.3. Available at *www.uptodateonline.com.* (accessed December 20, 2007).

Klasser GD, Epstein J: Methamphetamine and its impact on dental care, *J Can Dent Assoc* 71:759, 2005.

Koch G, Poulsen S: *Pediatric dentistry: a clinical approach*, Copenhagen, 2001, Munksgaard.

Kwan SY, Peterson PE, Pine CM et al: Health-promoting schools: an opportunity for oral health promotion, *Bull World Health Organ* 83(9):677, 2005.

LeResche L, Mancl LA, Drangsholt MT et al: Predictors of onset of facial pain and temporomandibular disorders in early adolescence, *Pain*, 129(3): 269-278, 2007.

Leung AK, Robson WL: Natal teeth: a review, *J Natl Med Assoc* 98(2):226, 2006.

Lin S, Zuckerman O, Fuss Z et al: New emphasis in the treatment of dental trauma: Avulsion and luxation, *Dent Traumatol* 23(5),297-303, 2007.

Ly KA, Milgrom P, Rothen M: Xylitol, sweeteners and dental caries, *Pediatr Dent* 28(2):154, 2006.

Marshall L, Schooley M, Ryan H et al: Centers for Disease Control and prevention. Youth tobacco surveillance—United States, 2001-2002, Morb Mortal Wkly Rep 55(SS03):1-56 2006.

McIntyre GT, McIntyre GM: Teeth troubles? *Brit Dent J* 192:251, 2002.

Milgrom P, Weinstein P: *Early childhood caries*, Seattle, 2001, Behavioral Dental Publications. Available from *www.Dentalbehavioralresources. com*. (Accessed Dec 20, 2007).

Murray B, McGuinness N, Biagioni P, et al: A comparative study of the efficacy of Aphtheal in the management of recurrent minor aphthous ulceration, *J Oral Pathol Med* 7:413, 2005.

Nilsson IM, List T, Drangsholt M: Prevalence of temporomandibular pain and subsequent dental treatment in Swedish adolescents, *J Orofac Pain* 19(2):144,2005.

Nilsson IM, List T, Drangsholt M: The reliability and validity of self-reported temporomandibular disorder pain in adolescents, *J Orofac Pain* 20(2):138, 2006.

Proffit WR, Fields HW Jr, Moray LJ: Prevalence of malocclusion and orthodontic treatment need in the United States: estimates from the NHANES III survey, *Int J Adult Orthodon Orthognath Surg* 13:97,1998.

Rayner JA: A dental health education programme, including home visits, for nursery school children, *Br Dent J* 172(2):57-62, 1992.

Schneider K, Segal G: Dental abscess. Emedicine. Updated Oct. 12, 2007. www.emedicine.com/ped/topic2675.htm (accessed December 21, 2007).

Smith TA, Heaton LJ: Fear of dental care: are we making any progress? *J Am Dent Assoc* 134(8):1101-1108, 2003.

Smitheman LC, Janisse J, Mathur A: The use of folk remedies among children in an urban black community: remedies for fever, colic, and teething, *Pediatrics* 3:e297-304, 2005.

Truelove E, Huggins KH, Mancl L et al: The efficacy of traditional, low-cost and nonsplint therapies for temporomandibular disorder: a randomized controlled trial, *J Am Dent Assoc* 8:1099, 2006.

US Department of Health and Human Services: *Oral Health in America: a report of the surgeon general–executive summary*, Rockville, MD, 2000, US Department of Health and Human Services, National Institute of Dental and Craniofacial Research, National Institutes of Health.

van Palenstein Helderman WH, Soe W, van 't Hof MA: Risk factors of early childhood caries in a Southeast Asian population, *J Dent Res* 85(1):85-88, 2006.

Weinstein P, Harrison R, Benton T: Motivating parents to prevent caries in their young children: one-year findings, *J Am Dent Assoc* 135(6):731-8, 2004.

Weinstein P, Milgrom P: *Oral self care: strategies for preventive dentistry*, ed 4, Seattle, 2006, Behavioral Dental Publications. Available from www. *Dentalbehavioralresources.com* (accessed December 20, 2007).

Zhan L, Featherstone JD, Gansky SA et al: Antibacterial treatment needed for severe early childhood caries, *J Public Health Dent* 3:174, 2006.

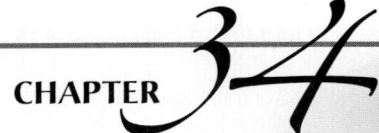
Genitourinary Disorders

Nan M. Gaylord and Nancy Barber Starr

The genitourinary system is responsible for maintaining an optimal environment for metabolism, including regulation of water and electrolytes (sodium, potassium, chloride, calcium, phosphate, and magnesium), excretion of waste products (urea, creatinine, poisons, and drugs), acid-base regulation, and hormonal secretion (vitamin D, renin, erythropoietin, and prostaglandins). The male system has both reproductive and excretory functions. Genitourinary problems in children and adolescents range from commonly occurring easily treated diseases to significant congenital or acquired conditions. Pediatric primary care providers play a significant role in working with children, adolescents, and families to identify problems, manage disorders, maintain optimal function, and provide education and support related to genitourinary function. First-line assessment and management, provision of continuity of care, and referral to and collaboration with pediatric urologists and nephrologists are important components of patient management.

Discussion of related functional health problems—enuresis and dysfunctional voiding—is included in Chapter 13.

■ STANDARDS OF CARE

The *Pocket Guide to Clinical Preventive Services* (U.S. Preventive Health Services Task Force, 2005) does not recommend any urine screening for asymptomatic bacteriuria in any child of any age. The *Preventive Services for Children and Adolescents Guideline* (Institute for Clinical Systems Improvement [ICSI] AHRQ, 2005) concurs with this recommendation as does the American Academy of Pediatrics (AAP), Committee on Practice and Ambulatory Care (2007), Also, dipstick leukocyte esterase testing is recommended yearly by all of the aforementioned authorities, the Centers for Disease Control and Prevention (2006), and *Bright Futures* (2007) to screen for sexually transmitted infections (STIs) in sexually active adolescents.

Hypertension is frequently renal in origin in children. Blood pressure (BP) screening is recommended by the AAP, Committee on Practice and Ambulatory Care (2007), and *Bright Futures* (Hagan, 2002) at every recommended preventive health care visit beginning at 3 years old. The other authorities previously listed suggest BP screening for children periodically, but no specific times are suggested. The management and treatment of hypertension is discussed in Chapter 30.

■ ANATOMY AND PHYSIOLOGY

The renal system is composed of two kidneys, two ureters, a bladder, and a urethra. The kidneys are positioned posteriorly on the abdominal wall. The main features of the kidney are the cortex, the medulla, and the collecting system. The renal medulla and nephrons are present at birth, but the peripheral tubules are small and immature. By adolescence, the kidneys are of adult size and weight. The ureters are muscular tubes that convey urine from the kidneys to the bladder by peristaltic contractions. The bladder is a muscular reservoir to collect the urine. It lies close to the anterior abdominal wall in early childhood. With growth, it descends into the pelvis and changes shape from cylindrical to pyramidal. As the bladder nears its capacity, nerve signals are transmitted to the brain to indicate that urination is required. When urination occurs, the sphincter between the bladder and urethra opens and contractions of the bladder create pressure that forces the urine out the urinary meatus. The male urethra is significantly longer than the female's as it leaves the bladder in the lower pelvis, passes through the prostate with openings for the release of bulbourethral gland fluids and semen with sexual activity, and extends the full length of the penile shaft. The urethral meatus is normally located on the tip of the glans in the male. In the female, the urethra descends from the bladder and exits the body inside the labia minora, midline, just posterior to the clitoris.

Physiologically, the kidneys serve to filter, clear, reabsorb, and secrete substances essential to the body's metabolism. The urinary system begins forming and excreting urine at 3 months of gestational age. Glomerular filtration and renal blood flow begin to increase at birth and become stable by 1 to 2 years old. In infants, total extracellular fluid volume is significantly greater than that of adults, and fluid composition tends to have a lower bicarbonate concentration. Normal urine excretion is 1.5 to 3 mL/kg/hour. The kidneys are still maturing throughout infancy, although all measurable variables of kidney function approach adult values between 6 and 12 months of life.

■ PATHOPHYSIOLOGY AND DEFENSE MECHANISMS
PATHOPHYSIOLOGY

Problems in the urinary system can occur at any point in the system from the kidneys to the urethral meatus. If the kidneys and ureters are involved, the disease is considered to be in the upper tract; if the problem is in the bladder, urethra, or meatus, it is considered a disease of the lower urinary tract. These differentiations can be difficult because frequently disease in one part of the system affects the entire system. Additionally, disease can be relatively silent in clinical presentation or noticeably problematic at any age. The main mechanisms of disorders can be classified as follows:

- Infection
- Inflammatory response
- Congenital malformation or condition
- Abnormalities acquired from injury, infection, or malfunction within the system

DEFENSE MECHANISMS

The urinary tract is normally a sterile system. The mucosal lining of the bladder serves as the first line of defense and provides inhibition of bacterial growth and adherence. The acid pH of the urine also protects the urinary system by inhibiting bacterial growth. Finally, actual flow of urine out of the bladder provides mechanical defense by its flushing action. If these defenses are compromised, the body initiates an inflammatory response within the urinary system.

▇▇▇ ASSESSMENT OF THE GENITOURINARY SYSTEM

HISTORY

The following information should be obtained:
- History of the present illness
  - Onset and pattern of symptoms
  - Fever, abdominal pain, or both
  - Preceding injury or illness, especially streptococcal infection
  - Vomiting
  - Voiding pattern-stream force and direction, any dribbling or discharge
  - Color, odor, frequency, and volume of urine, dysuria, urgency; enuresis, or incontinence
  - Diarrhea or chronic constipation
  - Sexual activity or abuse
- Family history
  - Any familial history of renal disease, deafness, high BP, structural abnormalities, or syndromes involving the genitourinary system
- Past history of urinary tract infection (UTI), hematuria, proteinuria, or any other related finding

PHYSICAL EXAMINATION

Pertinent findings to assess:
- Growth parameters—failure to thrive (FTT) can be associated with UTI in infants; increased weight can be associated with nephrotic syndrome
- BP—often elevated with nephritis and nephrotic syndrome
- Edema, pallor, dehydration
- Ear position and formation—if low set or abnormal, may have concurrent renal involvement

- Abdominal masses, ascites, flank or suprapubic tenderness
- Costovertebral tenderness
- External genitalia abnormalities

DIAGNOSTIC STUDIES

Diagnostic studies are ordered as indicated. The proper collection, transport, and storage of urine are essential to obtain accurate results. Most tests on urine, unless otherwise indicated, are best done on a first morning void. A second morning void, collected before the ingestion of large amounts of fluid, is recommended for microscopic examination. This second void collects fresh urine and increases the likelihood of seeing cellular casts, which can dissolve within 10 to 30 minutes. Urine should be evaluated within 30 minutes and, if stored, kept below 39.2° F (4° C), but not overnight unless in a special preservative (e.g., boric acid). The efficacy and cost efficiency of routine UA is much debated.

The following should be noted on UA:
- Physical characteristics. Color, clarity, odor, specific gravity, and osmolality are noted.
- Chemical characteristics. Urine dipsticks are available, are among the waived tests by the Clinical Laboratory Improvement Amendment (CLIA), and widely used to determine pH, specific gravity, glucose, ketones, protein, bile pigments, hemoglobin, nitrites, and leukocyte esterase. For correct results, strips must remain in their original containers and not be exposed to moisture, light, cold, or heat until used. Urine must be fresh, warmed if refrigerated, and read at correct time intervals for each test strip (Table 34-1).
  - Urine pH can vary from 4.6 to 8 and is reflective of the body's ability to maintain acid-base balance. Specific gravity is a measure of hydration and renal concentration ability and varies from 1.003 to 1.030. A random first-voided urine specimen specific gravity of 1.023 or more indicates intact renal concentrating ability. Urine with a specific gravity greater than 1.020 is considered concentrated (Wallace & Sadovsky, 2005).
  - A dipstick positive for blood indicates the presence of hemoglobin. Intact erythrocytes cause spotty changes on the dipstick, whereas free hemoglobin or myoglobin causes uniform changes of color.
  - The nitrite test is an indirect measure of bacteria in the urine. Common urinary pathogens contain enzymes that reduce nitrate in urine to nitrite. However, the urine should have been in the bladder at least 4 hours to show accurate results. Urine culture should be done on any urine sample positive for nitrites for confirmation of infection.
- Microscopic examination of urine. Urine can be spun by centrifuge and the sediment examined, or it can be examined unspun. When evaluating results, consideration must be given to which method was used, and repeated examination is recommended. Urine should be examined under the microscope for red blood cells (RBCs), white blood cells

TABLE 34-1	**Chemical Characteristics of Urine**		
Constituent	**Positives Indicate**	**False Positives Caused By**	**False Negatives Caused By**
Glucose	Metabolic problem (e.g., diabetes), recent high glucose intake, galactosemia	Antibiotics, delay in reading, myoglobin, oxidizing contaminants	Ascorbic acid intake, ketones, high specific gravity
Ketones	Dehydration, starvation, strenuous exercise, stress, fever, metabolic problems (e.g., diabetes)		If urine left standing, acetone evaporates
Protein	Renal disease, orthostatic proteinuria	Exercise, fever, dehydration, alkaline or concentrated urine (specific gravity >1.020), semisynthetic penicillin, oxidizing, cleansing agents	Dilute or acidic urine
Blood (hemoglobin)	If concurrent microscopic examination is negative for RBCs: • Free hemoglobin secondary to chemicals, illness, or drugs; myoglobin secondary to burns, muscle trauma, physical child abuse, myositis, strenuous exercise • If concurrent microscopic examination is positive for RBCs: renal problems	Menses, oxidizing cleansing agents, dilute urine	Ascorbic acid
Nitrite	Bacteria causing UTI	Rare	Common; urine should be in bladder at least 4 hours
Leukocyte esterase	Pyuria (WBCs in urine); inflammation from irritation or infection of vulva, vagina, or urethra; inflammation of bladder or kidneys with or without infection	Oxidizing agents	Immunocompromised
Urobilinogen	Hemolytic disease; hepatic disease	Rare	Rare
Bilirubin	Hepatic disease; biliary obstruction	Rare	Rare

RBCs, Red blood cells; *UTI,* urinary tract infection; *WBCs,* white blood cells.

(WBCs), bacteria, casts, and crystals. Microscopic examination of a fresh specimen is essential if blood or protein is found on the dipstick or urinary tract symptoms are present (see earlier comments).

- RBCs—The number of RBCs per high-power field (hpf) that are thought to be abnormal varies; in general more than 2 to 5/hpf (×40) in unspun urine or more than 2 to 10/hpf in spun urine is thought to be abnormal (Finberg & Kleinman, 2002; Patel, 2006) (Fig. 34-1). If cells are dysmorphic, the origin of the blood is most likely the kidney.
- WBCs—Fewer than 2 WBCs/hpf should be seen. More than 10 WBCs often indicates a symptomatic infection. If between 2 and 10 WBCs/hpf are seen, urine culture or other work-up should be performed (Patel, 2006) (Fig. 34-2).

- Bacteria and leukocytes seen in an unspun sample are associated with colony counts on culture of 100,000 (Fig. 34-3).
- Casts—RBC, hyaline, waxy, epithelial, leukocyte, or fatty casts are seen in various disease states (Fig. 34-4).
- Crystals, if amorphous, are not unusual. Calcium oxalate, cystine, tyrosine, leucine, cholesterol, or sulfa crystals are abnormal.

Depending on the results of the UA and/or clinical symptoms, other tests may be indicated, including:

- Gram stain. A Gram stain of the urine can be helpful in identifying organisms when examining urine under the microscope.
- Urine culture and sensitivities. The method of collection of urine is an important factor to note when interpreting culture results. Bag collection is considered reliable only if the

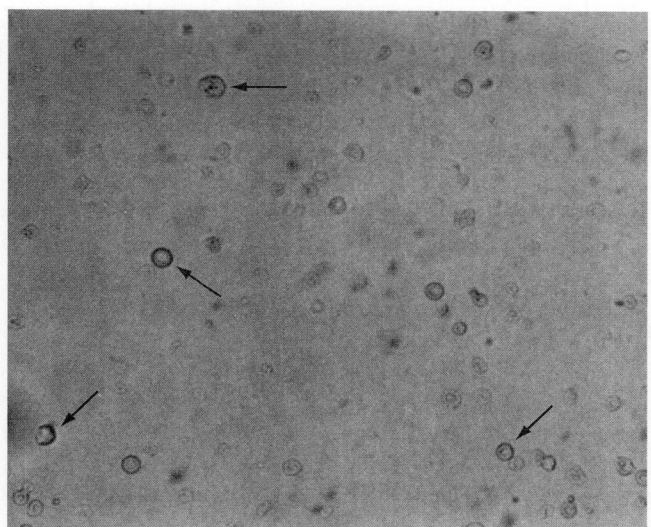

FIG. 34-1 RBCs may originate from any part of the renal system. The presence of large numbers of RBCs suggests a pathologic condition. (From Graff SL: *A handbook of routine urinalysis*, Philadelphia, 1983, JB Lippincott.)

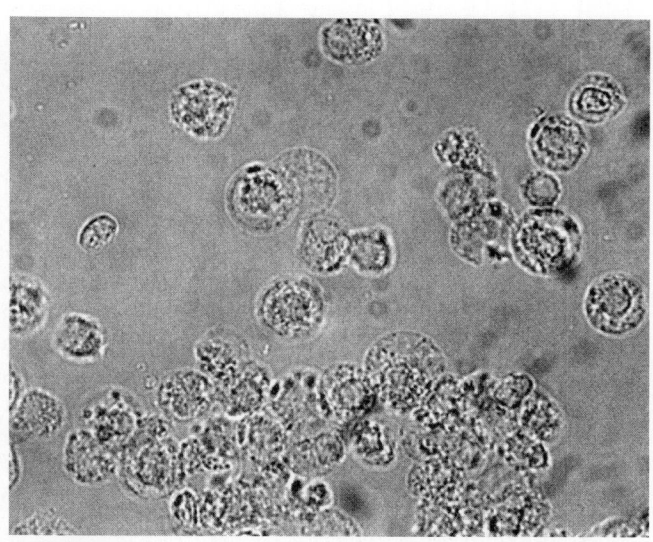

FIG. 34-2 WBCs in the urine (pyuria) may originate from any part of the renal system. The presence of more than 5 WBCs per hpf suggests a pathologic condition. (From Graff SL: *A handbook of routine urinalysis*, Philadelphia, 1983, JB Lippincott.)

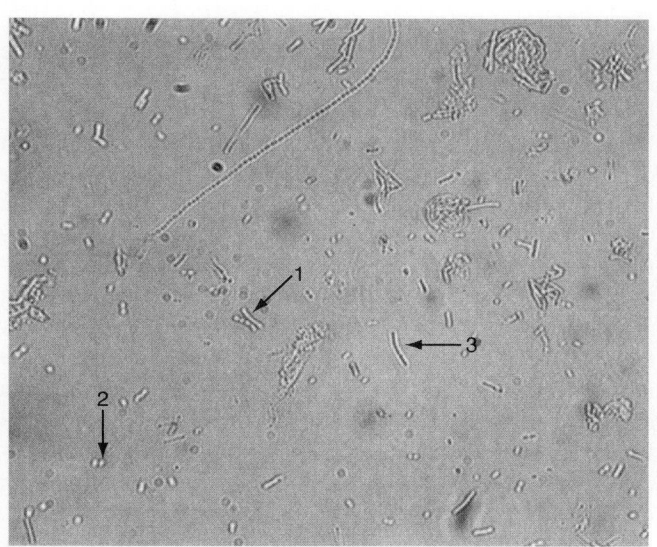

FIG. 34-3 Bacteria (rods *[1]*, cocci *[2]*, and chains *[3]*) (500×). (From Graff SL: *A handbook of routine urinalysis*, Philadelphia, 1983, JB Lippincott.)

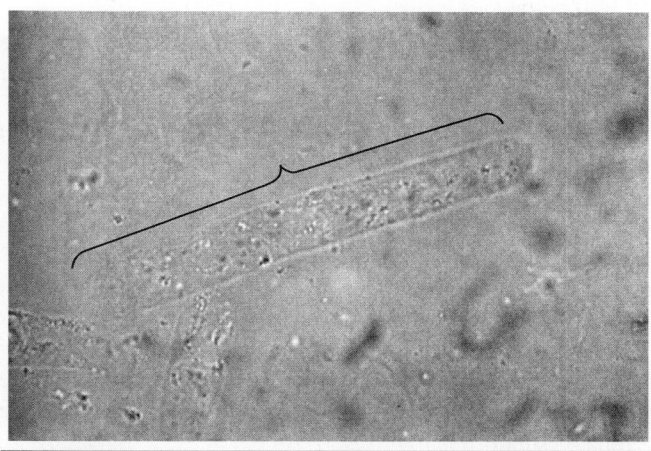

FIG. 34-4 Hyaline casts. Viewed with an 80A filter (400×). (From Graff SL: *A handbook of routine urinalysis*, Philadelphia, 1983, JB Lippincott.)

results are negative because there are more false positives in bagged urine (rate of 85% or higher) than catheterized specimens (Chang & Shortliffe, 2006). Sterile catheterization or suprapubic bladder tap is recommended if a culture is indicated on children less than 24 months old and for those unable to provide a midstream clean-catch urine. Although these standard collection recommendations have been questioned (Schroeder et al, 2005), researchers concluded that the choice of the collection method depends upon the patient's age, the need for immediate diagnosis and treatment, and plans for future imaging studies (Raszka & Khan, 2005; Schroeder et al, 2005).

○ Urine culture is easily done by standard culture methods or with a dipslide incubated overnight at room temperature. Urine should be cultured immediately, but may be refrigerated for up to 24 hours before plating. Urine specimens unrefrigerated for 2 hours or more are subject to bacterial overgrowth, change in pH, and dissolution of RBC and WBC casts (Wallace & Sadovsky, 2005). Bacterial identification and sensitivities need only be performed in complicated or nonresponsive cases.

- Urethral swabs. Either urethral swabs (insertion of the specified sterile swab 1 to 2 cm into the urethral opening with a slow gentle twisting action on removal) or vaginal swabs are accurate methods of culture acquisition for diagnosis of *Neisseria gonorrhoeae* and *Chlamydia trachomatis* and are the only diagnostic methods available in some areas of practice. The culture media are specific for each of those organisms. This method of specimen collection for culture, however, is being replaced with screening tests using a urine nucleic acid amplification test (NAAT) for detection of these organisms (CDC, 2006). If the urine test for these organisms is available, the specimen should only be between 10 and 20 mL of the first-catch urine with no cleansing of the perineum or penis.
- A 24-hour urine collection. Collecting a 24-hour sample of urine is done to determine calcium excretion, the calcium-creatinine ratio, and quantification of protein.
- Blood work.
  - Serum or blood urea nitrogen (BUN) estimates the urea concentration in serum or blood and is a measure of toxic metabolites that can cause uremic syndrome.
  - Serum creatinine in combination with creatinine clearance is used to estimate the glomerular filtration rate (GFR) or kidney function.
  - Serum electrolytes and acid-base status can detect renal tubular abnormalities.
- Ultrasonography. Ultrasonography of the renal system provides noninvasive structural information and is useful as a first-line evaluation of the renal system.
- Voiding cystourethrogram (VCUG). A VCUG is the most accurate test to evaluate reflux of urine from the bladder back into the ureters and kidneys.
- Intravenous pyelogram (IVP). IVPs are readily available and provide structural and functional information about the renal system.
- Nuclear imaging scans. These scans provide less structural and functional detail than an IVP, but involve less radiation exposure. Nuclear scans are especially helpful in the early identification of pyelonephritis and parenchymal scarring and in monitoring reflux.

■ MANAGEMENT STRATEGIES
EDUCATION AND COUNSELING

Education and counseling are essential components in the management of genitourinary tract disorders. Parents and children must be informed about the pathologic condition, etiology, treatment, and prognosis with and without treatment. A plan of care that the family and care provider is comfortable with must be decided on and initiated. Urinary problems can occur as early as the newborn period or anytime throughout childhood or adolescence. They vary in severity and chronicity.

The nurse practitioner (NP) must modify appropriate strategies for each individual situation.

MEDICATION, DIET, AND ACTIVITY

Depending on the diagnosis, medications can include antibiotics and steroids. Diet and activity may need to be modified in some chronic renal conditions. These modifications are usually carried out in consultation with appropriate specialists.

REFERRAL

Referral to a pediatric urologist, nephrologist, or surgeon may be required. When a referral is made, the primary care provider retains the essential role of serving as case manager for the child and providing continuity of care over time. The primary care provider is often the one whom the family best knows and is most comfortable with in discussing concerns, potential plans, and long-term management.

■ GENITOURINARY TRACT DISORDERS
URINARY TRACT INFECTION AND PYELONEPHRITIS
Description

UTIs are frequently seen in primary care, and are also the most commonly seen serious bacterial infection in young febrile children without an obvious source of infection. Because young children have limited symptoms, a high degree of suspicion must be maintained to diagnose UTI. Inflammation and infection can occur at any point in the urinary tract, so a UTI must be identified according to location. Bacteriuria is bacteria in the urine without other symptoms and is notable as a marker for possible underlying anatomic abnormality. Cystitis is infection of the bladder that produces lower tract symptoms. Pyelonephritis is the most severe type of UTI involving the renal parenchyma or kidneys and must be identified because of its potential for causing renal damage. Clinical signs thought to indicate pyelonephritis are a febrile infant with no other sign of infection or an older child with significant bacteriuria, systemic symptoms, or renal tenderness. UTIs may also be differentiated according to the type of infection. A UTI may be symptomatic or asymptomatic. It may also be complicated or uncomplicated. A *complicated UTI* is defined as a UTI with fever, toxicity, and dehydration or occurring in a child younger than 3 to 6 months old. It is also defined as a UTI associated with a structural or functional abnormality, such as vesicoureteral reflux (VUR), obstruction, voiding dysfunction, instrumentation, or pregnancy (Raszka & Khan, 2005). Additionally, a UTI must be identified as a first occurrence, recurrent (within 2 weeks with the same organism or any reinfection with a different organism), or chronic (ongoing, unresolved, often caused by an abnormality or resistant organism). Finally, age at the time of occurrence and gender of the child are important factors in determining the course of treatment.

Epidemiology

The organism most commonly associated with UTI is *Escherichia coli* (75% to 95%), although other organisms, such as *Enterobacter, Klebsiella, Pseudomonas*, and *Proteus* can be found. UTI secondary to group B *streptococci* is more common in neonates than older populations (Chang & Shortliffe, 2006). Several factors are believed to contribute to the etiology of UTIs. Most UTIs are thought to be ascending (i.e., the infection begins with colonization of the urethral area and ascends the urinary tract). If the infection progresses to the kidney, intrarenal reflux deep into the kidneys can lead to scarring. However, the most important risk factor for the development of pyelonephritis in children is VUR and is detected in 10% to 45% of young children who have symptomatic UTIs. Furthermore reflux of infected urine from the bladder increases the risk of pyelonephritis (Raszka & Khan, 2005). This damage to the kidney occurs in the composite papillae, which have wide and gaping openings allowing intrarenal reflux. Simple papillae have angled, slitlike openings that resist intrarenal reflux (Fig. 34-5). The composite papillae are located in the upper and lower poles of the kidney, which is the usual site of scarring.

Host resistance factors and bacterial virulence factors are also important in the etiology of UTIs. Host resistance factors include the presence of a structural abnormality or dysplasia (such as VUR, obstruction, or any other anatomic defect) or the presence of functional abnormalities (such as

dysfunctional voiding or constipation). Other factors affecting resistance include female gender (having a short urethra), poor hygiene, irritation, sexual activity or sexual abuse, and pinworms.

Several bacterial factors are known, but the two most important ones are adherence and virulence of the bacteria. Bacteria that have fimbriae or pili are able to anchor or adhere to the surface of the bladder mucosa. This adherence allows the bacteria to resist the bladder's defensive cleansing flow of urine and causes tissue inflammation and cell damage. Adherence may also play a role in bacteria ascending the urinary tract. Virulence refers to the toxicity of substances released by bacteria. The greater the virulence, the greater the damage to the urinary tract. Both of these factors enhance colonization of the urinary tract and aid in the persistence and impact of the bacteria.

The incidence of UTI in newborns is 1% to 1.4%, with a greater frequency in premature and low-birth-weight infants and a slightly greater frequency in uncircumcised males. One study showed a UTI incidence of 1:47 in uncircumcised males during the first year of life, compared with 1:445 in circumcised males and 1:49 in females (Schöen et al, 2000). After the first year of life, it is also more common to find a UTI in females than in males (1:10). The overall incidence is 3% to 5% in girls and 1% in boys (Elder, 2004). Symptomatic UTI is found in 3% to 8% of females and 1% to 2% of males of all ages. By 11 years old, 3% of girls and 1% of boys will have had a UTI (Alon, 2006; Larcombe, 2002). The incidence of UTI is often increased in adolescent girls as they become sexually active with an incidence of 10.8% in females 18 to 24 years old (Chang & Shortliffe, 2006). Recurrence is common, often within the first year after the initial infection.

Clinical Findings

History. The following information should be obtained:
- Previous infection? Request records from the evaluation of past infections and diagnostic studies performed.
- Hygiene habits
- Voiding and bowel patterns: frequency, completeness, dribbling, daytime enuresis, and weak stream
- Irritants, such as nylon underwear, or clothing (spandex, tight pants or shorts that rub)
- Masturbation, sexual activity, or sexual abuse
- Family history of VUR, recurrent UTI, or kidney problems
- Other infection: pinworms, diaper rash

Physical Examination
- See Table 34-2 for age-related symptoms.
- BP, temperature, and general appearance (toxic appearing?)
- Growth parameters—growth may be decreased with chronic UTI or renal insufficiency, especially in infants
- Flank pain or tenderness in the costovertebral angle
- Abdominal examination—suprapubic tenderness, bladder distention or a flank mass (obstructive signs), mass from fecal impaction

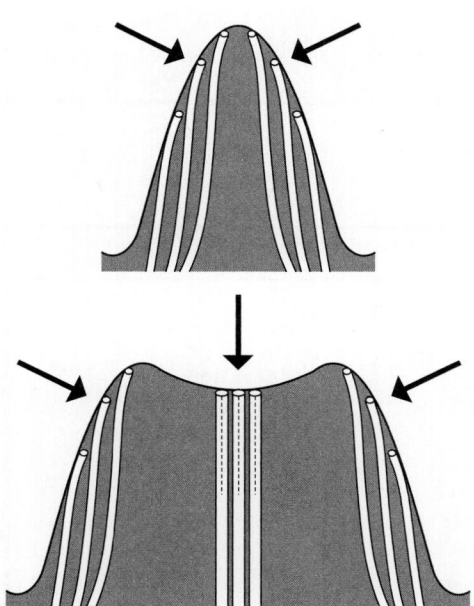

FIG. 34-5 Most renal papillae are conical, with papillary ducts that open obliquely into the renal pelvis *(top)*. These do not allow intrarenal reflux. But some kidneys have compound papillae, formed by the fusion of conical papillae *(bottom)*. These have papillary ducts with gaping openings at right angles to urine flow and do permit intrarenal reflux. (From Ransley PG: Intrarenal reflux: anatomical, dynamic and radiological studies–part I, *Urol Res* 5:61-69, 1977.)

- Genitalia—vaginal erythema, edema, irritation, or discharge; labial adhesions; uncircumcised male, urethral ballooning; weak, dribbling, threadlike stream
- Neurologic examination (if voiding is dysfunction)—perineal sensation, lower extremity reflexes, sacral dimpling, or cutaneous abnormality

Diagnostic Studies. The method used to collect urine has an impact on the interpretation of results. Urine collected in a bag, because of the high degree of contaminants, is accurate only if negative. Voided midstream, clean-catch specimens are somewhat more accurate, especially if collected as a first morning specimen and kept refrigerated (less than 24 hours) until it can be cultured. Having the female child sit backward on the toilet separates the labia and decreases contamination. In assessing for infection, suprapubic bladder aspiration is the most accurate method (99%), but sterile catheterization is 95% sensitive (Table 34-3). Either aspiration or catheterization, one of these collection methods, should be used in very ill children and infants. See the diagnostic studies section in the first part of this chapter for other pertinent information.

- UA has limited value in diagnosing UTI because it can have negative results even with a positive culture. It should be used only to raise or lower suspicion. Suspicious findings include foul odor, cloudiness, nitrites and/or leukocytes, alkaline pH, proteinuria, hematuria, pyuria, and bacteriuria.
  - Nitrite chemical tests are reliable on urine specimens collected after sleeping all night, when gram-negative bacteria are present, and when the urine has been in the bladder for 4 hours or longer. False-positive results are rare, whereas false-negative results are common.
  - Leukocyte esterase chemical tests detect pyuria, but pyuria may arise from causes other than UTI.
- Microscopic evaluation of uncentrifuged urine is helpful if bacteria are seen.
- Urine culture by standard culture methods or by dipslide is essential to confirm the diagnosis. See Table 34-3 for evalu-

---

TABLE 34-2 | **Clinical Findings of Urinary Tract Infection in Children of Various Ages**

Neonates	Infants	Toddlers and Preschoolers	School-Age Children and Adolescents
Jaundice	Malaise	Altered voiding pattern	"Classic dysuria" with frequency, urgency, and discomfort
Hypothermia	Irritability	Malodor	
Failure to thrive	Difficulty feeding	Abdominal/flank pain*	Malodor
Sepsis	Poor weight gain	Enuresis	Enuresis
Vomiting or diarrhea	Fever*	Vomiting or diarrhea*	Abdominal/flank pain*
Cyanosis	Vomiting or diarrhea	Malaise	Fever/chills*
Abdominal distention	Malodor	Fever*	Vomiting or diarrhea*
Lethargy	Dribbling	Diaper rash	Malaise
	Abdominal pain/colic		

*Findings especially likely with pyelonephritis.

TABLE 34-3 | **Criteria for Diagnosis of Urinary Tract Infections**

Method of Collection	Colony Count (Pure Culture)	Probability of Infection (%)
Suprapubic aspiration	Any organism	>99
Catheterization	>10^5	95
	≥10^4-10^5	Infection likely, especially if obstruction or if frequent voider
	10^3-<10^4 single organism	Suspicious, repeat
	<10^3	Infection unlikely
Clean voided		
Boy	>10^4, single organism	Infection likely
Girl	Three specimens, >10^5	95
	Two specimens, >10^6	90-95
	One specimen, >10^6	80-90
	5×10^4-10^5	Suspicious, infection possible, repeat
	10^4-5×10^4	Suspicious, if symptomatic, repeat
	10^4-5×10^4	Infection unlikely if asymptomatic
	<10^4	Infection unlikely

From Omokaro S: Nephrology. In Robertson J, Shilkofski N, editors: *Johns Hopkins Hospital: the Harriet Lane handbook,* ed 17, St Louis, 2005, Mosby.

ation of culture results. If culture growth is 10,000, repeat the culture unless the sample was collected by suprapubic aspiration or catheterization. Gram stain is helpful if bacteria are identified.

- Bacterial identification and determination of sensitivities are necessary in patients who appear toxic or could have pyelonephritis, have relapses or recurrent UTI, or are nonresponsive to medication.
- CBC (elevated WBC count), erythrocyte sedimentation rate (ESR), C-reactive protein, BUN, and creatinine should be done if the child appears ill, is less than 1 year old, or pyelonephritis is suspected.
- Blood culture should be done if sepsis is suspected or in infants younger than 1 year old (see Chapter 23, Fever without a Focus).

Differential Diagnosis

The differential diagnosis includes a foreign body, urethritis, vaginitis, viral cystitis, sexual abuse, dysfunctional voiding, dysuria-pyuria syndrome, appendicitis, pelvic abscess, and pelvic inflammatory disease. Any child who has fever without focus, a fever of unexplained origin, FTT, chronic diarrhea, or recurrent abdominal pain should be evaluated for UTI.

Management

1. Goals of treatment are to quickly identify the extent and level of infection; to treat appropriately to eradicate infection; to provide symptomatic relief; to find and correct anatomic or functional abnormalities; and to prevent recurrence and new or progressive renal damage. When deciding on a treatment plan, the child's age, sex, and symptoms and the suspected location of the UTI must be kept in mind.
2. Bacteriuria. Whether asymptomatic bacteriuria should be treated is controversial. Those who advocate treatment do so with the intent of preventing further infection or sequelae and identifying any underlying abnormalities.
3. Afebrile UTI (Fig. 34-6):
   a. Antibiotic treatment for 10 days (Alon, 2006; Chang & Shortliffe, 2006; Tran et al, 2001). First-line drugs as recommended by the AAP practice parameter on UTIs (AAP, 2002) are as follows:
      - Trimethoprim-sulfamethoxazole (6 to 12 mg/kg trimethoprim plus 30 to 60 mg/kg/day sulfamethoxazole) in two divided doses if older than 2 months.
      - Amoxicillin (40 mg/kg/day) in two or three divided doses if no resistance is found in the community.

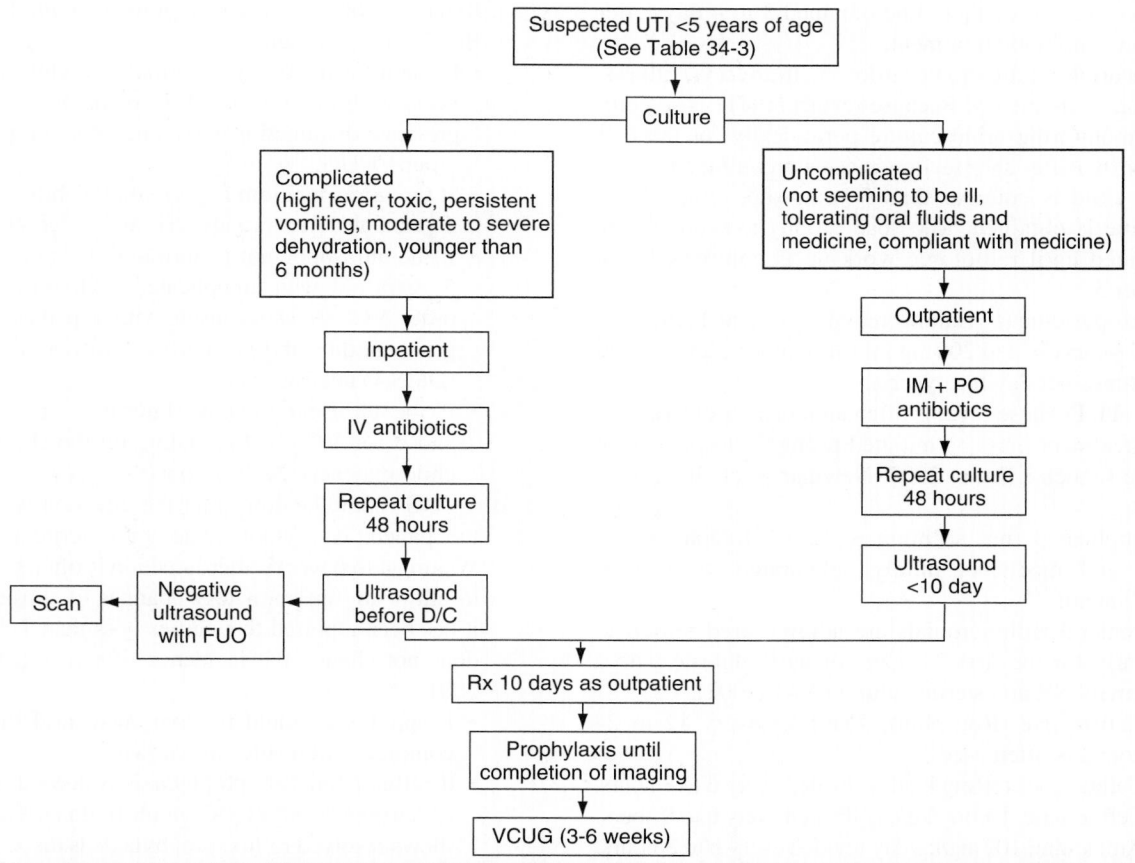

FIG. 34-6 Evaluation of UTI in a child less than 5 yr old. *D/C*, Discharge; *FUO*, fever of unknown origin; *IM*, intramuscular; *IV*, intravenous; *PO*, oral; *Rx*, prescribe; *VCUG*, voiding cystourethrogram; *VUR*, vesicoureteral reflux.

Also recommended are the following:

- Augmentin (20 to 40 mg/kg/day) in three divided doses.
- Sulfisoxazole (120 to 150 mg/kg/day) in three or four divided doses if older than 2 months
- Nitrofurantoin (5 to 7 mg/kg/day) three or four times a day if older than 1 month

  If allergic to the drugs just mentioned or a broader spectrum antibiotic is needed:
- Cefixime (8 mg/kg/day) in one or two doses
- Cephalexin (25 to 50 mg/kg/day) in three or four divided doses
- Cefprozil (30 mg/kg/day) in two divided doses
- Cefpodoxime (10 mg/kg/day) in two divided doses
- Loracarbef (15 to 30 mg/kg/day) in two divided doses

b. Follow-up urine culture should be done 48 to 72 hours after initiating treatment, especially if symptoms persist or organism resistance is found in the community.
  - If the culture is sterile, continue antibiotic therapy.
  - If the culture is not sterile or if no clinical improvement is seen, urine should be sent for bacterial identification and sensitivity studies, and an alternative broad-spectrum antibiotic should be used pending those results. Culture should again be repeated after 48 to 72 hours and, if sterile, antibiotic therapy continued.

c. Follow-up cultures should be obtained 3 to 4 days after finishing antibiotic treatment.

d. Repeat urine culture should be done with any fever, illness, dysuria, or frequency. Because recurrent UTI is so common, monitoring urine culture periodically for the first year or two after an infection is often recommended.

e. If the child is younger than 5 years old, once a sterile urine is obtained, low-dose prophylaxis should be continued until radiologic work-up is completed (see number 5).

f. Phenazopyridine (Pyridium) may be given at 100 mg for 6 to 12 years old and 200 mg for those older than 12 years three times per day for dysuria.

4. Febrile UTI. Because fever is often an indicator of pyelonephritis, treatment must be initiated promptly to prevent or minimize sequelae (Lum, 2007; Newman et al, 2002) (see Fig. 34-6).

a. Uncomplicated (not seeming to be ill, tolerating oral fluids and medicine, mildly dehydrated, with good compliance):
  - Parenteral antimicrobials are administered intramuscularly for the first 24 hours or until afebrile with a normal ESR and sterile culture (AAP, 2002).
    - Ceftriaxone (Rocephin), 75 mg/kg every 12 to 24 hours, is often used.
    - Cefotaxime, 150 mg/kg/day divided every 6 to 8 hours.
    - Ceftazidime, 150 mg/kg/day divided every 6 to 8 hours.
    - Ampicillin, 100 mg/kg/day divided every 6 to 8 hours.
    - Gentamicin, 5 mg/kg/day divided every 8 to 12 hours.
  - Oral antibiotics (see the section on cystitis) are administered following intramuscular therapy for a total of 10 to 14 days, followed by prophylaxis until the radiologic work-up is complete; if pyelonephritis is the final diagnosis, continue prophylactic antibiotics for at least 6 months.
  - Repeat urine culture after 48 hours of antibiotic therapy and periodically for the first year or two after an infection.
  - Ultrasonography should be performed as soon as convenient, VCUG within 6 weeks.

b. Complicated (high fever, toxic, persistent vomiting, moderate to severe dehydration, poor compliance, younger than 3 to 6 months old):
  - Inpatient treatment with intravenous antibiotics (see intramuscular antibiotics earlier) until afebrile for 24 to 36 hours with a normal ESR and sterile culture.
  - The remainder of treatment is as presented earlier.

5. Radiologic work-up:

a. Box 34-1 lists the suggested criteria for the radiologic work-up of children with UTI; Table 34-4 details radiologic studies that can be done.

b. In a child older than 10 years with a first uncomplicated UTI and no voiding dysfunction before the UTI, no further work-up is needed.

c. Renal and bladder ultrasonography should be done. See Box 34-1 for guidelines.
  - If the ultrasonogram is normal in a child older than 5 years with complicated UTI or involves a child with previous dysfunctional voiding, start prophylaxis and order VCUG.
  - If the ultrasonogram is normal in a child younger than 5 years old, start prophylaxis and order VCUG.
  - If the ultrasonogram is normal in a child younger than 5 years old with complicated UTI, start prophylaxis, order VCUG, and consult with a pediatric nephrologist regarding the need for a dimercaptosuccinic acid (DMSA) nuclear scan.
  - If the ultrasonogram is abnormal, start prophylaxis, and order VCUG. Depending on the abnormality, the child may need referral to a urologist.

d. VCUG should be done after the infection is treated, once the patient is asymptomatic with sterile urine culture. Waiting 4 to 6 weeks after infection is often recommended to allow any inflammatory changes to subside, although it has been reported that earlier (less than 7 days) VCUG does not change the incidence of reflux (Mahant et al, 2001).
  - Prophylaxis should be continued until the VCUG is complete and results are known.
  - If reflux is present, prophylaxis is needed for 1 year, at which time repeat VCUG should be done. If repeat VCUG shows resolved reflux, prophylaxis is discontinued.

BOX 34-1   Radiologic Work-up and Prophylaxis for Urinary Tract Infections

Why Do a Radiologic Work-up?
- To identify any structural or functional abnormality of the urinary tract
- To identify any renal scarring or damage

Who Requires a Work-up?
Recommendations vary among experts. Those who recommend the most aggressive work-up do so to identify scarring early and prevent further damage.
- All children with the first infection (Chang & Shortliffe, 2006; Lum, 2007)
- Infants or any child younger than 4-5 years old (Alon, 2006; Elder, 2004)
- All children younger than 6 years old (Elenberg & Travis, 2002)
- Any child with pyelonephritis
- Any child younger than 8 years old with acute symptoms, especially fever or toxicity (at least 50% have reflux or obstructive lesions)
- All children younger than 10 years old and all children 10 years and older with signs and symptoms of pyelonephritis who respond slowly to therapy and are prepubertal (Friedman, 2004)
- Males with a first infection; females after a second infection if no other criteria are met
- Any child with suspicious factors (e.g., HTN, abnormal urine stream, poor growth) or with a positive family history of UTI or abnormal voiding patterns
- Adolescents with pyelonephritis or after a second UTI with documented culture and no history of recent sexual activity

What Should Be Done?
- Renal and bladder ultrasound: done initially in all children. May be deferred if prenatal ultrasound normal. (Alon, 2006)
- VCUG: done if ultrasound is abnormal, if child is younger than 5 years old, or if voiding dysfunction was present before UTI, febrile UTI, or complicated UTI
- Nuclear imaging scan: done to detect renal scars or parenchymal inflammation
- IVP: done if further definition of structure or function of the kidney is needed

When Should It Be Done?
- Ultrasonography: during hospitalization or within 10 days in any child younger than 5 years old or with complicated UTI
- VCUG: before discharge from the hospital if inpatient, some authorities recommend 2 to 6 weeks after the diagnosis of UTI for the urine to become sterile and the patient asymptomatic (Elder, 2004)
- VCUG: recommended follow-up for the diagnosis of vesicoureteral reflux

When Should Prophylaxis Be Used?
- After resolution of UTI and before VCUG or IVP
- To suppress recurrent UTI after VCUG or IVP

What Should Be Used for Prophylaxis?
- Approximately one third to one half of the treatment dosage of antibiotic should be given at bedtime. Although prophylaxis is generally recommended, well-designed, randomized, placebo-controlled trials are still required to determine if long-term, low-dose antibiotic administration prevents UTI in children (AAP, 2002; Elder 2004, Wald, 2006).
- Nitrofurantoin 1 to 2 mg/kg daily if older than 2 months; max dose 50 mg; expensive
- TMP 1-2 mg/kg and SMX 5-10 mg/kg daily if older than 2 months; TMP 5 mg/kg and SMX 25 mg/kg bid twice per week (max dose 40 mg); a yearly CBC should be done to monitor for neutropenia
- TMP 1-2 mg/kg, max dose 50 mg at bedtime if older than 3 months
- Cephalexin 15 mg/kg divided every 12 hours
- Sulfisoxazole 10-20 mg/kg divided every 12 hour if older than 2 months
- Penicillin or ampicillin can be used for a newborn or premature infant
- Nalidixic acid 30 mg/kg divided every 12 hours
- Methenamine mandelate 75 mg/kg divided every 12 hours

bid, Twice daily; *CBC*, complete blood count; *HTN*, hypertension; *IVP*, intravenous pyelogram; *SMX*, sulfamethoxazole; *TMP*, trimethoprim; *US*, ultrasound; *UTI*, urinary tract infection; *VCUG*, voiding cystourethrography.

TABLE 34-4   Radiologic Studies Done for Evaluation of Urinary Tract Infection

Study	Cost	Advantages	Disadvantages	Use
Ultrasound	Least expensive	Shows structure, shape, and growth Detects structural abnormality, obstruction, pyelonephritis, large scars Painless, low risk, no radiation, noninvasive, available	Does not detect small scars of VUR Poor visualization of ureters Does not measure renal function or transient injury to kidney	Initial evaluation and follow-up
VCUG (radiographic)	Least expensive	Detects and grades VUR—if high or low pressure, high or low bladder volumes, during voiding, during early or late bladder filling Visualize bladder and urethra (especially in males) and diverticula	Does not detect obstruction, pyelonephritis, scars Risk of urethral trauma from catheterization Greater radiation than with scan	Initial evaluation In infants and children younger than 5 year old with abnormal ultrasound or dysfunctional voiding
VCUG (nuclear)	More expensive	Visualize bladder and reflux Constantly monitors for transient reflux Less radiation	Discomfort of catheterization No urethral visualization Unable to grade reflux	Follow-up of VUR To evaluate siblings of child with VUR Follow-up of surgery
IVP	Less expensive	Detects obstruction, pyelonephritis, large scars, stones, nephrocalcinosis Details pelvicaliceal system, shows ureters Estimates renal function Readily available	Does not detect small scars or VUR Risk of allergic reaction, acute renal failure, pain of injection, radiation Requires good renal function Only identifies structural damage	Better defines level of obstruction Not used very often
Nuclear scans	Most expensive	Detects acute inflammation, scars, and obstruction	Does not detect VUR or measure renal function	Follow-up
• DMSA		Earlier detection of parenchymal damage—large or small scars, permanent or focal—than with IVP (1-3 year old) Good in neonates	Does not evaluate calyces, ureters, bladder, or urethra	Fever of unknown origin and negative ultrasound in neonates To diagnose APN To detect renal scars
• Tc-DTPA		Shows renal outline, estimates renal and tubular function, measures changes Less radiation		
CT scan (contrast)	Expensive	Detects obstruction, pyelonephritis, large scars	Does not detect small scars or VUR Risk of allergic reaction, acute renal failure	Trauma

APN, Acute pyelonephritis; *CT*, computed tomography; *DMSA*, dimercaptosuccinic acid; *IVP*, intravenous pyelography; *Tc-DTPA*, technetium-labeled diethylenetriamine pentaacetic acid; *VCUG*, voiding cystourethrography; *VUR*, vesicoureteral reflux.

e. Nuclear scans (DMSA or technetium-labeled diethylene-triamine pentaacetic acid [Tc-DTPA]) can be performed to diagnose acute pyelonephritis and to evaluate for scarring. These tests are especially helpful in neonates and in children with fever of unknown origin. However, they are the most expensive tests available and should be ordered only as indicated and after consultation with a pediatric nephrologist.

  • Any evidence of acquired kidney damage requires antibiotic suppression therapy.

6. Recurrent infection (two or more in 1 year):
  a. Initial treatment is as for UTI.
  b. Perform a radiologic work-up if not previously done.
  c. Once urine is sterile, administer prophylactic antibiotics and monitor urine cultures for 6 to 12 months (see Fig. 34-6 and Box 34-1).

Patient Education, Prevention, and Prognosis

The following should be discussed with parents and/or patients:

• Clear explanation of the cause, potential complications, and overall treatment plan, including both short- and long-term plans.

• Frequent and complete voiding and increased quantities of fluids, especially water. Sometimes scheduled voiding times or double voiding (voiding and then immediately attempting to void again) can be helpful.

• Proper hygiene and avoidance of irritants, such as bubble baths and perfumed soaps. Avoidance of tight pants, especially spandex pants, is recommended along with cotton underwear. Treat perineal inflammation to help prevent UTI.

• Sexually active females should be encouraged to drink water before intercourse and void immediately afterward.

• Home monitoring of urine with nitrite sticks on first morning urine is helpful. If positive result or questionable or the child is symptomatic, a culture must follow.

• Decrease intake of bladder irritants, such as the "four *Cs*" (caffeine, carbonated beverages, chocolate, citrus), aspartame (NutraSweet), alcohol, and spicy foods.

• Prevent constipation. Stool softeners and timed defecation may be helpful.

• Three-day rule. To prevent delay in treatment, no infant or young child with unexplained fever should go longer than 3 days without examination of urine.

• Cranberry juice is considered helpful in preventing the adherence of *E. coli* in the urethra (see Chapter 42).

Recurrent infection, chronic UTI, FTT, and irreversible renal scarring (the most significant complication) can occur. Major risk factors for renal damage include delay in treatment of pyelonephritis, younger than 1 year old, anatomic or neurogenic obstruction, severe reflux, dysplasia, and multiple infections. The same acute inflammatory process responsible for eradication of bacteria is also responsible for damage to renal tissue and subsequent scarring.

VESICOURETERAL REFLUX

Description

Regurgitation of urine from the bladder up the ureter to the kidney is called vesicoureteral reflux (VUR). Primary VUR is the most common type and is typified by a congenital, abnormally short ureter and ineffective valve. Secondary VUR is due to bladder outlet obstruction and can be functional or structural. It is graded according to an international classification (Fig. 34-7). Grade I does not reach the renal pelvis; grade II extends up to the renal pelvis without dilation; grade III describes reflux to the renal pelvis with mild to moderate dilation of the ureter and the renal pelvis; grades IV and V (high grade) include definite distention of the ureters and renal pelvis and can include hydronephrosis or reflux into the intrarenal collecting system (American Urological

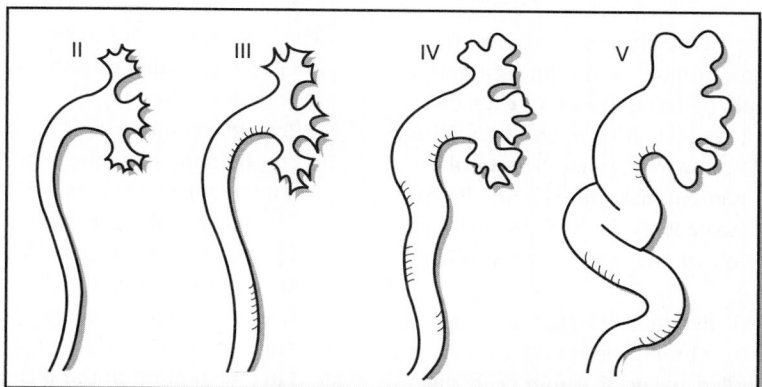

FIG. 34-7 International reflux grading. Grade I: ureter only. Grade II: ureter, pelvis, and calyces; no dilation, normal calyceal fornices. Grade III: mild or moderate dilation or tortuosity (or both) of ureter, and mild or moderate dilation of renal pelvis but no or slight blunting of the fornices. Grade IV: moderate dilation or tortuosity (or both) of ureter and moderate dilation of renal pelvis and calyces. Complete obliteration of sharp angles of fornices but maintenance of papillary impressions in majority of calyces. Grade V: gross dilation and tortuosity of ureter; gross dilation of renal pelvis and calyces; papillary impressions are no longer visible in majority of calyces. (From Lebowitz RL et al: International system of radiographic grading of vesicoureteral reflux, International Reflux Study in Children, *Pediatr Radiol* 15[2]:105, 1985.)

Association [AUA] Practice Parameters, Guidelines and Standards Committee, 1997; Greenbaum & Mesrobian, 2006; Elder, 2004).

Epidemiology

Reflux occurs because of congenital abnormalities and can persist with recurrent infection. Reflux provides a route for bacteria to ascend to the kidney and cause pyelonephritis. VUR is the most common anatomic abnormality found in children with UTI, with an incidence of 20% to 50% when studied after the first UTI (Chang & Shortliffe, 2006; Decter, 2001). Approximately 30% to 40% of siblings of children with reflux also have reflux, and 50% of children whose mothers have reflux also have reflux (Elder, 2004).

Clinical Findings

History. The history may be positive for a previous UTI, abnormal voiding pattern or dysfunction, unexplained febrile illness, or UTI symptoms.

Diagnostic Studies. The following are ordered, as indicated, to identify obstructive uropathy and dysplasia:

- Ultrasonography (may be normal even in the presence of reflux)
- VCUG—establishes the presence of reflux, determines the grade, and gives high detail
- Nuclear scan—uses less radiation to identify VUR, but gives less detail (no grading) and requires someone skilled in interpretation; most helpful in long-term follow-up and with neonates
- IVP—may be done if the VCUG is positive because it gives more defined structural and functional information

Management

The goal of treatment is the prevention of infection and subsequent scarring. Early identification and appropriate treatment of infection achieve this goal.

Management involves the following (Tables 34-5 and 34-6):

- Grades I, II, and III reflux. Most children outgrow their reflux probably secondary to an increase in the intramural length of the ureter and should be left to do so. Grades I and II VUR resolve spontaneously in up to 85% of children, 50% in grade III, 30% in grade IV; however, grade V is unlikely to resolve spontaneously (Greenbaum & Mesrobian, 2006). Primary VUR resolves spontaneously in 85%; secondary VUR resolves with correction of the underlying problem (Arant, 2002).
  - Prophylactic antibiotics to prevent UTI (see Box 34-1) should be continued until the child has been infection free for 12 months as documented by urine cultures. If antibiotics are not taken or the child has recurrent infection, surgery may be needed. A recent study (Garin et al, 2006) questions the need for antibiotic therapy for grades I, II, or III reflux; additional studies will assist in clarifying this issue.
  - Interval urine cultures are performed with symptoms of unexplained illness (see Fig. 34-6).
  - Repeat the VCUG once after the diagnosis of reflux at 12 to 18 months to monitor reflux and scarring. Routine follow-up studies are recommended every 2 to 3 years, depending on the reflux grade, sex, and whether both or only one kidney is affected (Alon, 2006).
  - CBC, BUN, and creatinine annually to monitor renal function.
  - Circumcision may be recommended for the male infant (Cascio et al, 2001).
  - In children with reflux who are toilet trained, regular, low-volitional, low-pressure voiding with complete bladder emptying should be encouraged. If uninhibited bladder contractions are suspected, anticholinergic therapy may be helpful (AUA Practice Parameters, Guidelines and Standards Committee, 1997).
- Grades IV and V reflux are managed medically or surgically by a pediatric urologist and pediatric nephrologist.
- Adolescents may need surgery because reflux in this age group is rarely outgrown.
- Surgery is indicated for progressive renal injury and breakthrough infection (especially acute pyelonephritis) or with associated anatomic abnormalities.
- Nephrology consultation is indicated in the presence of notable scarring, a solitary or atrophic kidney, hypertension, elevated creatinine, or evidence of abnormal kidney function with any grade of reflux.

Patient Education, Prevention, and Prognosis

- VUR does not cause scarring, infection does—but VUR is a risk factor for pyelonephritis and subsequent scarring.
- Screening ultrasonography should be done on an infant born to parents with VUR, on any young siblings of a child with VUR, and on any older siblings with any history of UTI.
- Management, prevention of UTIs, and compliance must be understood by families. The necessity of urine culture with any suspicious symptoms should also be emphasized. The potential for untreated, chronic UTI leading to chronic renal disease must be explained. Other points to emphasize include the following:
  - Prompt treatment of UTI should be instituted.
  - Prophylactic medicines are best given at night because of urinary stasis while asleep.
  - BP and growth should be monitored.
  - The guidelines discussed in the Patient Education and Prevention section of UTIs should be reviewed.

Preexisting renal damage may be present, and new renal scarring can occur. Children with grades I and II reflux usually have resolution of the reflux if infections are thwarted or treated early. Children with grades III or IV reflux have up to 50% reported incidence of scarring at the time of diagnosis (Decter, 2001). These complications can lead to ongoing renal disease, atrophy, growth failure, elevated BP, and decreased renal functioning.

TABLE 34-5 Treatment Recommendations for Children Without Scarring at Diagnosis

Recommendations were derived from a survey of preferred treatment options for 36 clinical categories of children with reflux.
The recommendations are classified as follows:
Guidelines = treatments selected by 8 or 9 of 9 panel members, given the strongest recommendation language.
Preferred options = treatments selected by 5-7 of 9 panel members.
Reasonable alternatives = treatments selected by 3-4 of 9 panel members.
No consensus = treatments selected by no more than 2 of 9 panel members.
The treatment recommendations apply to both boys and girls with primary VUR.

Clinical Presentation (Age at Presentation)		Treatment				
		Initial (Antibiotic Prophylaxis or Open Surgical Repair)		Follow-up* (Continued Antibiotic Prophylaxis, Cystography, or Open Surgical Repair)		
VUR Grade Laterality	Age (Years)	Preferred Option — Guideline	Reasonable Alternative	Guideline	Preferred Option	No consensus†
I-II unilateral or bilateral	<1	Antibiotic prophylaxis				Boys and girls
	1-5	Antibiotic prophylaxis				Boys and girls
	6-10	Antibiotic prophylaxis				Boys and girls
III-IV unilateral or bilateral	<1	Antibiotic prophylaxis				
	1-5	Unilateral: antibiotic prophylaxis	Bilateral: antibiotic prophylaxis	Bilateral: surgery if persistent‡	Unilateral: surgery if persistent‡	
	6-10	Unilateral: antibiotic prophylaxis Bilateral: surgery	Bilateral: antibiotic prophylaxis		Surgery if persistent‡	
V unilateral or bilateral	<1	Antibiotic prophylaxis		Surgery if persistent‡		
	1-5	Bilateral: surgery Unilateral: antibiotic prophylaxis	Bilateral: antibiotic prophylaxis Unilateral: surgery	Surgery if persistent‡	Surgery if persistent‡	
	6-10	Surgery				

*For patients with persistent uncomplicated reflux after extended treatment with continuous antibiotic therapy.
†No consensus was reached regarding the role of continued antibiotic prophylaxis, cystography, or surgery.
‡The duration of reflux regarding the length of time that clinicians should wait before recommending surgery is dependent on the child's age, whether the disease is unilateral or bilateral, the grade of the reflux at diagnosis, and the percent chance of reflux resolution from diagnosis to 5 years (AUA, 1997, p. 23, Table 2).
From American Urological Association (AUA) Pediatric Vesicoureteral Reflux Clinical Guidelines Panel: *The management of primary vesicoureteral reflux in children: clinical practice guidelines,* Baltimore, 1997, The Association, p 52.

TABLE 34-6 **Treatment Recommendations for Children With Scarring at Diagnosis**

Recommendations were derived from a survey of preferred treatment options for 36 clinical categories of children with reflux.
The recommendations are classified as follows.
Guidelines = treatments selected by 8 or 9 of 9 panel members, given the strongest recommendation language.
Preferred options = treatments selected by 5-7 of 9 panel members.
Reasonable alternatives = treatments selected by 3-4 of 9 panel members.
No consensus = treatments selected by no more than 2 of 9 panel members.
The treatment recommendations apply to both boys and girls with primary VUR.

Clinical Presentation (Age at Presentation)		Treatment					
		Initial (Antibiotic Prophylaxis or Open Surgical Repair)			Follow-up* (Continued Antibiotic Prophylaxis, Cystography, or Open Surgical Repair)		
VUR Grade Laterality	Age (Years)	Guideline	Preferred Option	Reasonable Alternative	Preferred Guideline	Option	No consensus†
I-II unilateral or bilateral	<1	Antibiotic prophylaxis					Boys and girls
	1-5	Antibiotic prophylaxis					Boys and girls
	6-10	Antibiotic prophylaxis					Boys and girls
III-IV unilateral	<1	Antibiotic prophylaxis			Girls: surgery if persistent‡	Boys: surgery if persistent‡	
	1-5	Antibiotic prophylaxis			Girls: surgery if persistent‡	Boys: surgery if persistent‡	
	6-10		Antibiotic prophylaxis		Girls: surgery if persistent‡		
II-IV bilateral	<1	Antibiotic prophylaxis			Girls: surgery if persistent‡		
	1-5		Antibiotic prophylaxis	Surgery	Girls: surgery if persistent‡		
	6-10		Surgery		Girls: surgery if persistent‡		
V unilateral or bilateral	<1		Antibiotic prophylaxis	Surgery	Girls: surgery if persistent‡		
	1-5	Bilateral: surgery	Unilateral: surgery			Surgery if persistent‡	
	6-10	Surgery					

*For patients with persistent uncomplicated reflux after extended treatment with continuous antibiotic therapy.
†No consensus was reached regarding the role of continued antibiotic prophylaxis, cystography, or surgery.
‡The duration of reflux regarding the length of time that clinicians should wait before recommending surgery is dependent on the child's age, whether the disease is unilateral or bilateral, the grade of the reflux at diagnosis, and the percent chance of reflux resolution from diagnosis to 5 years (AUA, 1997, p. 23, Table 2).

From American Urological Association (AUA) Pediatric Vesicoureteral Reflux Clinical Guidelines Panel: *The management of primary vesicoureteral reflux in children: clinical practice guidelines*, Baltimore, 1997, The Association, p. 52.

HEMATURIA

Description

Hematuria refers to blood in the urine that may be persistent, recurrent, or transient. It is detected by dipstick, by microscopic examination, or with the naked eye (macroscopic) and can arise from any point in the urinary system. Hematuria is a symptom of disease or injury to the urinary system, although a few RBCs can be normal in a pediatric patient. The number of RBCs/hpf considered to be abnormal varies and ranges from any to more than 5 RBCs/hpf in unspun urine to more than 5 to 10 RBCs/hpf in spun urine (Friedman, 2004; Patel, 2001; Patel 2006). For management purposes, *hematuria* in this text is defined as more than 2/hpf in unspun or 5/hpf in spun urine.

Epidemiology

Factors causing hematuria can arise from anywhere in the urinary system from the urinary meatus to the kidneys. The term *gross hematuria* is related to the concentration of RBCs rather than to the location or significance of the disorder. The causes of macroscopic hematuria are as follows: hypercalciuria (23%), immunoglobulin A (IgA) nephropathy (16%) glomerulonephritis (GN) 9%, and no cause 38%. UTI, hydronephrosis, tumor, cystitis cystica, polyps, or epididymitis are characterized by macrohematuria less than 1% of the time (Bergstein et al, 2005; Halverson & Alper, 2006). However, according to Bloom & Kolon (2005) 50% of children with gross hematuria have UTIs. Brownish, tea-colored urine with casts or protein is usually glomerular in origin; clots and red to pink urine with isomorphic RBCs but no protein usually originate from the lower tract. The incidence of hematuria is 0.5% to 2% when confirmed with repeat UA (VanDeVoorde & Bissler, 2006).

Clinical Findings

History. The following information is obtained:
- Previous medical history of cystic kidney disease, sickle cell, SLE, malignancy
- Family or previous history of hematuria, nephrolithiasis, cystic kidney, hemoglobinopathy, sickle cell disease or trait, systemic lupus erythematosus (SLE), hypertension, congestive heart disease, malignancy, deafness, renal failure
- Preceding illness—viral or streptococcal pharyngitis or impetigo
- Onset, duration, pattern, and timing of hematuria
- Color of urine
- Dysuria, urgency, or frequency
- Presence of pain—back, abdominal, or flank, with voiding
- Straining or squatting with urination (tumor)
- Strenuous exercise or trauma (including bladder catheterization)
- Enuresis
- Trauma, foreign body, or sexual activity or abuse
- Current menstruation or medication
- Edema, rash, pallor, or arthralgias

- Drug ingestion, especially nonsteroidal antiinflammatory drugs (NSAIDs), aspirin, or antibiotics
- Symptoms related to chronic renal disease (Box 34-2)

Physical Examination. Findings include:
- FTT or falling growth curves (chronic renal insufficiency or long-standing acidosis)
- Malformed ears (congenital renal disease)
- Oliguria or anuria, edema, hypertension, and proteinuria, which are suggestive of glomerular disease
- Flank pain, which is suggestive of a lower tract disorder
- Abdominal or flank mass, which suggests an obstruction, such as Wilms' tumor, cystic disease, or posterior valves
- External genitalia—excoriation, bleeding, foreign body, abuse

Diagnostic Studies. The following studies are essential:
- UA (dipstick):
  - Color—a tea or smoky color indicates a nephrologic disorder; red indicates a urologic disorder.
  - If greater than 1+ hematuria by dipstick (which equals 3 RBCs/hpf or 0.02 mg/dL hemoglobin) for blood, microscopic examination for RBCs is needed to differentiate hemoglobin or myoglobin from RBCs.
  - If protein is present, refer to the section on proteinuria and nephritis for further work-up. *Note: The most significant differentiating factor is the presence of proteinuria. If present, rapid evaluation and early referral to a nephrologist are essential.*
- Microscopic examination for RBCs, including size and shape, casts, crystals, and WBCs:
  - A few RBCs/hpf can be normal in a pediatric patient (see description of hematuria).
  - Distorted, misshapen RBCs of different size suggest glomerular disease.
  - A negative microscopic examination occurs in dilute urine because RBCs undergo lysis as a result of the hypotonicity of urine.
- Urine culture
- For persistent hematuria:

| BOX 34-2 | Seven "Red Flags" for Chronic Renal Failure |

1. Failure to thrive (poor growth, fatigue, anorexia, nausea, gastroesophageal reflux, vomiting)
2. Chronic anemia (normochromic, normocytic, nonresponsive to medication)
3. Complicated enuresis (daytime frequency, urgency, incontinence, chronic constipation, encopresis, infrequent voiding, straining to void, recurrent UTI)
4. Prolonged, unexplained vomiting or nausea (especially in the morning), anorexia, weight loss without diarrhea
5. Hypotension
6. Unusual bone disease (rickets, valgus deformity, fracture with minor trauma)
7. Poor school performance (headache, fatigue, inattention, withdrawal from family activity)

○ UA on first-degree relatives.
○ Consider a CBC with platelets, electrolytes, BUN, creatinine, sickle cell screen, tuberculin purified protein derivative (PPD), complement components C3 and C4, antinuclear antibody (ANA), antistreptolysin O (ASO) titers, immunoglobulins, hepatitis serologies, and human immunodeficiency virus (HIV) (Omokaro, 2005).
○ Renal ultrasonography is performed if any concerns remain along with other indicated radiologic studies.
• If the diagnosis is isolated, transient hematuria, monitor every year with UA, growth performance, and BP.

Differential Diagnosis

Five patterns of hematuria have been identified and may be helpful when considering the differential diagnosis of hematuria (Boineau & Lewy, 1989):
Type 1—microscopic and persistent
Type 2—microscopic and intermittent
Type 3—persistent macroscopic
Type 4—intermittent or recurrent macroscopic
Type 5—intermittent or recurrent macroscopic with persistent microscopic

Types 1 and 2 account for most cases of hematuria in pediatrics. Type 3 is common in urologic and nephrologic disorders, such as UTI, GN, hemoglobinopathies, renal stones, and trauma. Types 4 and 5 occur with IgA nephropathy, hypercalciuria, and benign recurrent hematuria.

Other differential diagnoses to consider include the following:
• *Pseudohematuria* occurs when a false-positive dipstick reading is noted, but no RBCs are found on the microscopic examination. The two most common causes are myoglobinuria and hemoglobinuria (see Table 34-1).
• *Extrarenal hematuria* is common with systemic bleeding disorders and is evidenced by macroscopic and microscopic hematuria.
• The presence of RBC casts, proteinuria, or both is a manifestation of *glomerular hematuria*, such as acute or chronic GN.
• *Idiopathic hypercalciuria* is an inherited tubulointerstitial disorder with excessive urinary calcium excretion in the presence of macroscopic and microscopic hematuria. It is the most common cause of isolated cases of hematuria in children and occurs more frequently in children living in the southern U.S. and southern Canada. This metabolic disease is characterized by excessive calcium excretion in the urine in the absence of hypercalcemia or other known causes of hypercalciuria. The diagnosis is made by laboratory examination of urine. The spot calcium-creatinine ratio done on the first morning specimen is elevated (greater than 0.21 mg/dL). Elevated 24-hour calcium excretion (greater than 4 mg/kg/24 hours) confirms the diagnosis. Idiopathic hypercalciuria is responsible for 22% of asymptomatic hematuria in children (Bergstein et al, 2005; Pan, 2006).

• Although rare, *renal stones (nephrolithiasis)* or *calcification (nephrocalcinosis)* can occur. If suspected, a renal ultrasonogram can be included as part of the work-up.
• *Exercise-induced hematuria* occurs when hematuria is present after vigorous exercise, but not at other times.
• Although rare in children, a UTI, viral illness with adenovirus (hemorrhagic cystitis), renal tuberculosis, and parasites are known to cause hematuria and may need to be considered in the work-up for hematuria (Pan, 2006).
• Hematuria caused by external irritation of the urinary meatus will resolve with healing and removal of the offending irritant (e.g., soaps, bubble bath, lotions) or avoidance of the offending behavior (e.g., scratching, masturbation, sexual activity).

Management

A progressive approach to evaluating hematuria should be undertaken with the goal of not overlooking serious, treatable, progressive conditions while at the same time avoiding unnecessary studies. Guidelines for specific clinical presentations include:
1. Macroscopic hematuria without proteinuria or casts (Fig. 34-8).
   • Urine culture is done initially to rule out UTI.
   • Ultrasonography may be done to evaluate for renal stones, an obstructive lesion, or tumor; as indicated by clinical symptoms. IVP or VCUG is performed as indicated.
   • Type 4 or 5 hematuria may need an immunologic work-up—ASO, C3, ANA, anti-DNA, BUN, creatinine.
   • Consultation or referral to a nephrologist or urologist may be necessary, depending on the findings.
2. Microscopic hematuria. Initially, three first morning urine samples should be examined within 7 to 14 days to confirm persistent hematuria (Fig. 34-9).
   • If exercise-induced hematuria is suspected, recheck the urine after refraining from exercise for 72 hours.
   • If repeated urine specimens are negative, recheck the urine in 1 month and again in 6 months.
   • If protein or casts are found in the urine (a red flag), suspect glomerular hematuria and see the section on nephritis.
   • If urine culture is positive, see the section on UTI.
   • If the calcium-creatinine ratio is greater than 0.21, suspect idiopathic hypercalciuria:
     ○ Increase fluid to dilute the calcium concentration.
     ○ Refer to a nephrologist.
     ○ Perform ultrasonography if nephrolithiasis is suspected.
     ○ Monitor BP.
   • If asymptomatic microscopic hematuria is suspected:
     ○ Perform microscopic examination of family members' urine.
     ○ Consult with or referral to a nephrologist may be warranted.
   • Monitor UA, BP, and growth every 6 to 12 months.
3. Refer to a nephrologist for persistent microhematuria, recurrent gross hematuria, proteinuria, RBC or other casts detected by UA, family history of kidney disorders, or any signs of renal failure.

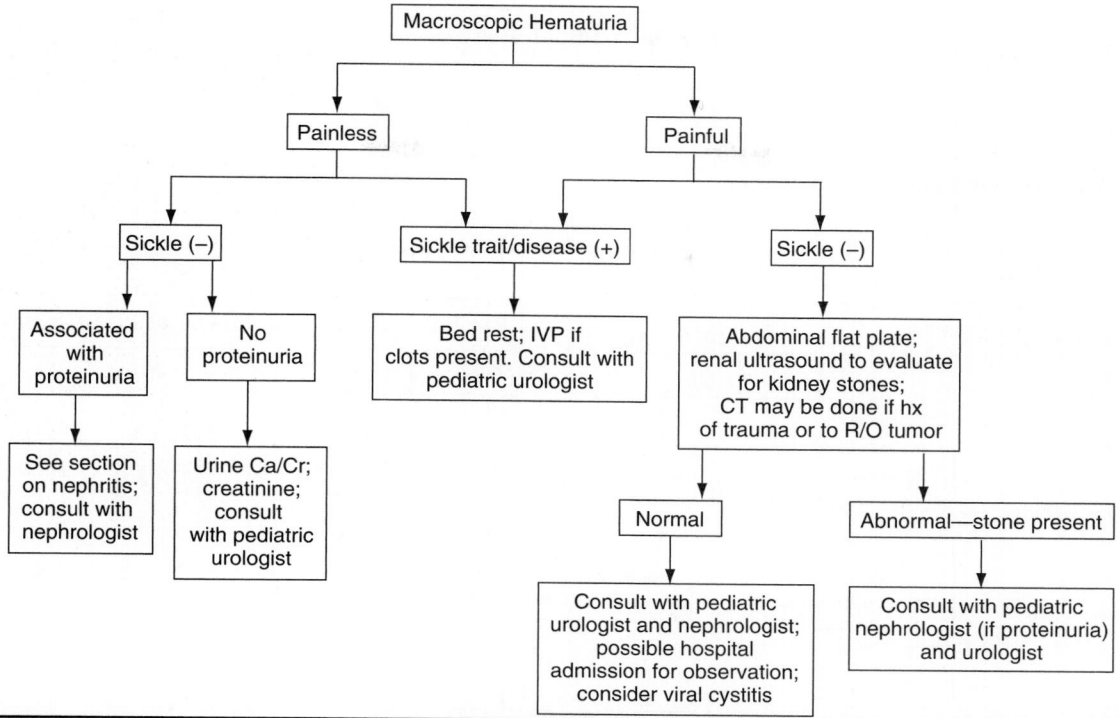

FIG. 34-8   Management of macroscopic hematuria. *Ca/Cr*, calcium/creatinine ratio; *CT*, computed tomography; *hx*, history; *IVP*, intravenous pyelogram; *R/O*, rule out. (Adapted from Dershewitz RA, editor: *Ambulatory pediatric care*, ed 3, Philadelphia, 1999, JB Lippincott-Raven.)

Patient Education, Prevention, and Prognosis

Patient education should stress the importance of follow-up for the evaluation of the hematuria. Microscopic hematuria is a transient benign finding in the vast majority of patients, and the finding is rarely a sign of renal disease, but deserves follow-up. Gross hematuria requires a thorough diagnostic evaluation. Prognosis depends upon the cause of the hematuria. A definitive cause is found in only 17% of cases of microscopic hematuria (16% are due to hypercalciuria), but in 62% of children with gross hematuria, 22% are due to hypercalciuria. The risk of developing kidney stones is not known, but may be increased in patients with gross hematuria or microscopic hematuria with hypercalciuria. Of note, there are no long-term studies validating that early detection is beneficial in preventing kidney stones (Bergstein et al, 2005; Lum, 2007; Pan, 2006).

PROTEINURIA

Description

Protein in the urine is commonly detected by dipstick tests. It may be transient, recurrent, or fixed. Proteinuria can be a symptom of disease, or it can reflect a benign, self-limited condition. The quantity of protein and the timing of its presence determine its significance. Qualitative protein in urine, as tested by dipstick, is considered a positive result if it registers 1+ (30 mg/dL) or more in urine with a specific gravity of less than 1.015. Quantitative protein is tested by measuring a volume of urine over a set period of time. A level of less than $4 \, mg/m^2$/hour is considered normal, 4 to $40 \, mg/m^2$/hour is abnormal, and greater than $40 \, mg/m^2$/hour indicates nephritic disease.

Four groups of proteinuria exist: isolated, transient or functional, glomerular, and tubulointerstitial.

- Orthostatic proteinuria and persistent asymptomatic proteinuria, which are members of the first group, termed *isolated proteinuria*, are the most common.
  - *Orthostatic proteinuria* accounts for up to 60% (75% in adolescents) of cases of proteinuria (Finberg & Kleinman, 2002; Vogt & Avner, 2004). In this condition, the child excretes abnormal amounts of protein when upright but normal amounts when lying down. Orthostatic proteinuria is demonstrated by collecting urine as described under diagnostic studies.
  - *Persistent asymptomatic proteinuria* is a common, transient phenomenon in which an otherwise healthy child, with normal clinical and laboratory work-up, has an abnormally high level of protein in the urine.
- The second group of proteinuria is *transient or functional proteinuria* and is caused by some type of stress.
  - *Exercised-induced proteinuria* is documented by collecting a urine sample, having the patient exercise vigorously for several minutes, and then collecting another sample. The post-exercise sample is usually strongly positive.
  - *Fever-induced proteinuria* can accompany any febrile state and usually subsides with resolution of the fever. Other stress-related causes include cold exposure, infection, congestive heart failure, and seizures. This type

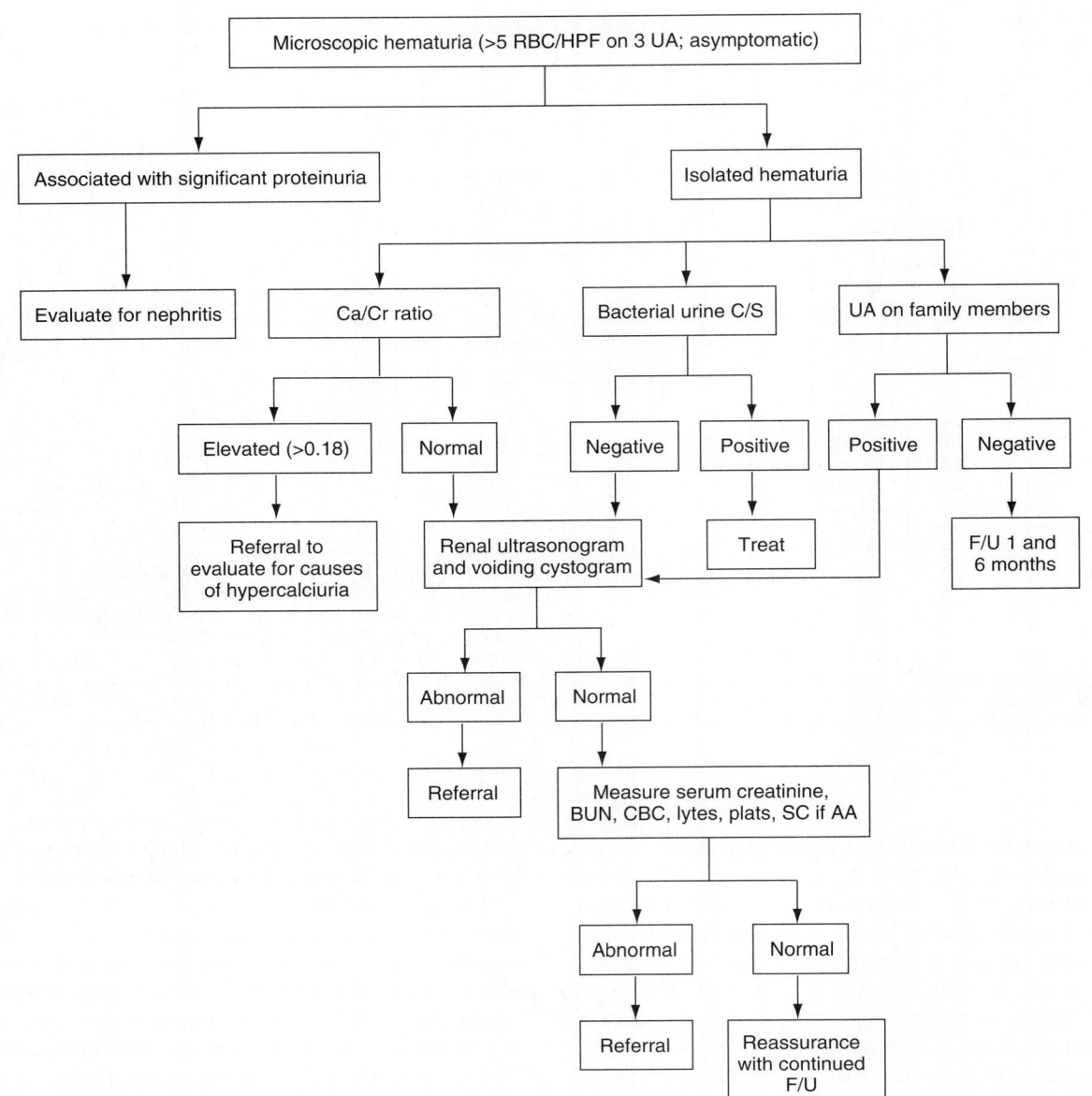

FIG. 34-9 Management of asymptomatic microscopic hematuria. *AA,* African American; *BUN,* blood urea nitrogen; *CBC,* complete blood count; *Ca/Cr,* calcium/creatinine ratio; *C/S,* culture/sensitivity; *F/U,* follow-up; lytes, electrolytes; plats, platelets; *RBC/HPF,* red blood cells per high-power field; *SC,* sickle cell; *UA,* urinalysis. (Adapted from Dershewitz RA, editor: Ambulatory pediatric care, ed 3, Philadelphia, 1999, JB Lippincott-Raven.)

of proteinuria usually resolves in 1 to 2 weeks, and if resolution has been verified, no further work-up is required.

- The third and fourth groups, *glomerular proteinuria,* which is typified by GN, and *tubulointerstitial proteinuria,* are least common and are characterized by high levels of proteinuria. Some authorities believe that children with persistent proteinuria, even at low levels, should be followed with a high index of suspicion for an underlying, progressive renal disorder.

Epidemiology

Proteinuria originates from problems with glomerular filtration, tubular reabsorption or secretion, or both. The child is often asymptomatic. If proteinuria is significant enough to cause hypoproteinemia, edema is present.

The incidence of proteinuria is cited at 5% to 15% in school-age children. It drops to 2% if a criterion of 1+ protein is used and to 0.1% if greater than 2+ is used. It persists, however, in only 1% of children when four consecutive urine specimens are tested. (Finberg & Kleinman, 2002; Vogt & Avner, 2004).

Clinical Findings

History.   The following may be reported:
- Family history of deafness, visual problems, and renal disease
- Recent strenuous exercise or febrile illness
- Polydipsia or polyuria
- Vague symptoms, such as malaise, fatigue, or pallor
- Symptoms related to chronic renal disease (see Box 34-2)

Physical Examination
- BP (hypertension), pulse, respiratory rate
- Growth and development parameters (poor weight gain or FTT with chronic disease; weight gain with nephrotic syndrome)
- Edema, especially periorbital edema, or symptoms of fluid retention
- Abdominal examination for a mass, enlarged kidney, fluid, tenderness

Diagnostic Studies.   The following are done as indicated:
- UA (repeated three times over 1 to 2 weeks), preferably done on a first-voided specimen:
  - 1+ protein (30 mg) is significant if the specific gravity is less than 1.015; 2+ protein (100 mg) is significant if the specific gravity is greater than 1.015.
  - False-positive results occur in highly concentrated or alkaline (pH greater than 5.5) urine. False-negative results occur in dilute or acidic urine.
  - At least 75% of asymptomatic patients with proteinuria in a single urine specimen have normal urine on repeated testing.
- A urine sample collected immediately after arising in the morning can be compared with a specimen collected after several hours of activity to rule out orthostatic etiology. The child must have voided before sleep to obtain accurate results. A typical result yields negative to trace amounts on the first morning specimen, but 1+ or greater on the second specimen. If the result is equivocal, back-to-back urine samples (from arising to bedtime and bedtime to arising) can be evaluated for quantitative protein.
- Microscopic urine:
  - RBCs or WBCs (or both), casts, bacteria, oval fat bodies, or other abnormalities are present in most pathologic conditions.
- The protein-to-creatinine ratio on a random daytime urine sample is elevated. Normal values are less than 0.5 mg/dL in children younger than 2 years old and less than 0.2 mg/dL in children older than 2 years; greater than 2 mg/dL is considered nephritic (Lum, 2007).
- A 12- or 24-hour timed urine collection for creatinine (normal, 14 to 20 mg/kg/24 hours) and protein excretion (normal less than 4 mg/m^2/hour) is elevated (Lum, 2007). A back-to-back collection (e.g., bedtime to arising, arising to bedtime) is done to compare active or upright and resting levels.
- If protein in urine is greater than 4 mg/m^2/hour, check the CBC, electrolytes, BUN, creatinine, albumin/total protein, C3, C4, cholesterol, liver function tests, and urine culture. Perform an ultrasonogram, VCUG, and radionuclide scans as indicated. Evaluate for systemic disease as indicated (e.g., ANA, ASO, streptozyme, hepatitis B, HIV, tuberculosis).

Differential Diagnosis

Pseudoproteinuria can be caused by semisynthetic penicillins or benzalkonium chloride.

Management

The persistence, quantity, and presence of other abnormalities (e.g., hematuria) are key to evaluating proteinuria.
1. If protein by dipstick is trace or 1+ and specific gravity is greater than 1.015:
   - Offer reassurance.
   - Do monthly recheck of urine for 4 to 6 months.
   - If protein is persistent, refer the patient to a nephrologist.
2. If protein by dipstick is greater than 1+, see Fig. 34-10. Evaluate the child for orthostatic proteinuria.
3. If morning's urine protein is 1+ or 2+, perform either:
   - A quantitative 12- to 24-hour urine protein excretion test:
     - If less than 4 mg/m^2/hour, reassure.
     - If greater than 4 mg/m^2/hour, proceed as in Fig. 34-7.
   - A random urine total protein-creatinine ratio and UA with microscopic:
     - If UA is normal and there is less than 0.2 mg of protein/mg of creatinine, reassure as normal.
     - If protein/creatinine ratio is greater than 0.2 mg of protein/mg of creatinine, proceed as in Fig. 34-10.
4. If protein by dipstick is greater than 2+, evaluate for nephrotic syndrome (see later section).
5. If hematuria is present, evaluate for nephritis (see later section).
6. Follow-up is important to monitor for any change in status.
7. Refer the following to a nephrologist: persistent unexplained nonorthostatic proteinuria, any hematuria or RBC or WBC casts, polyuria or oliguria, nephrotic levels of protein, elevated BUN or creatinine, elevated BP, systemic complaints (joint pain, rashes, or arthralgias), or a child with a family history of renal failure, GN, sensorineural hearing loss, or kidney transplantation.

Patient Education, Prevention, and Prognosis

Patient education should stress the importance of follow-up to evaluate the cause of proteinuria. Orthostatic proteinuria with a 10-year follow-up showed resolution in 50% and the remainder with a normal GFR.

NEPHROTIC SYNDROME

Description

Nephrotic syndrome is due to excessive excretion of protein in urine. The classic definition of nephrotic syndrome is massive proteinuria (greater than 40 mg/m^2/hour and a protein-creatinine ratio on spot urine of greater than 1), hypoalbuminemia (less than 2.5 g/dL), edema, and hyperlipidemia. The latter two findings may not be present in all cases or at all times. The main mechanism of the massive protein loss is increased

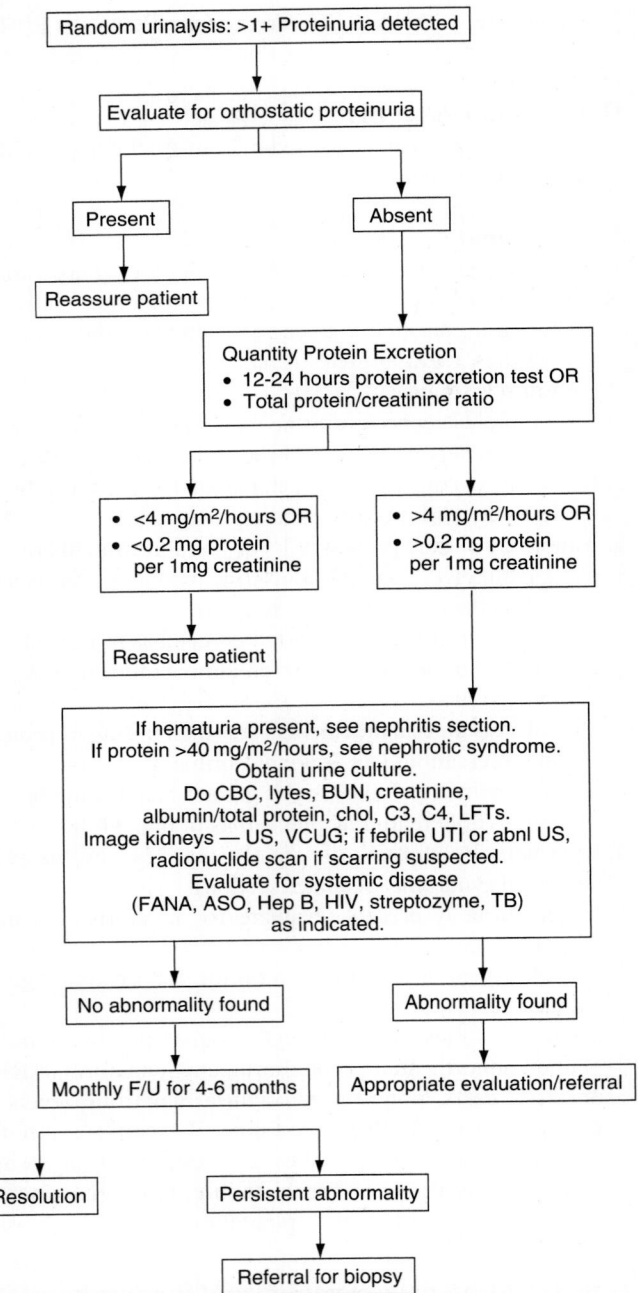

FIG. 34-10 Evaluation of proteinuria. *abnl,* Abnormal; *alb/TP,* albumin/total protein; *ANA,* antinuclear antibody; *ASO,* antistreptolysin O; *BUN,* blood urea nitrogen; *C3,* complement 3; *C4,* complement 4; *CBC,* complete blood count; *chol,* cholesterol; *Cr,* creatinine; *FANA,* fluorescent antinuclear antibody; *F/U,* follow-up; *Hep B,* hepatitis B; *HIV,* human immunodeficiency virus; *LFTs,* liver function tests; *lytes,* electrolytes; *US,* ultrasound; *VCUG,* voiding cystourethrogram. (Adapted from Dershewitz RA, editor: *Ambulatory pediatric care,* ed 3, Philadelphia, 1999, JB Lippincott-Raven.)

glomerular permeability. The loss can be selective (albumin only) or nonselective (including most serum proteins), and such selectivity is an important distinction in diagnosis. With protein loss, the liver increases its synthesis of protein and thereby causes concurrent hyperlipidemia and lipiduria.

The classification of nephrotic syndrome as described by the International Collaborative Study of Kidney Diseases in Children (Warshaw, 1994) is as follows:

- Primary nephrotic syndrome, unrelated to systemic disease, is also called minimal change nephrotic syndrome (MCNS) or idiopathic nephrotic syndrome, lipoid nephrosis, or nil disease. Minimal change disease is characterized by the child's age (1 to 7 years old), normal vascular volume despite edema (normal BP and normal heart size), absence of gross hematuria or urinary casts, and absent or transient microhematuria with normal serum creatinine, complement components, and ANA. Histopathologic examination shows glomerular lesions without inflammation and mild to no morphologic abnormality. This type occurs in 80% to 90% of cases and is usually characterized by resolution of symptoms in response to steroids.
- Secondary nephrotic syndrome occurs in association with or secondary to systemic disorders (e.g., SLE, Henoch-Schönlein purpura [HSP]), infectious processes (e.g., syphilis, hepatitis B, HIV, or malaria), drug toxicities (e.g., NSAIDs, mephenytoin), allergens, or other renal disorders (e.g., IgA or congenital nephritis). Histopathologic examination shows moderate to severe morphologic abnormality. This type occurs in 10% of cases.

Nephrotic syndrome is a chronic disease characterized by periods of remission (when both the urinary protein excretion and serum albumin normalize) and relapses (recurrence of proteinuria and hypoalbuminemia after complete remission). Most children are steroid responders, with remission subsequent to treatment with steroids. Of the remainder, most are steroid resistant and show no response to steroids. A small number of cases are either partial responders with minimal response to steroids or are steroid dependent and require high doses of prednisone with frequent relapses.

Epidemiology

Nephrotic syndrome occurs as a result of immune, systemic, nephrotoxic, allergic, infectious, malignant, vascular, or idiopathic processes. The actual mechanism of nephrotic syndrome has been extensively studied, and the understanding of its histopathology is better than the understanding of its pathogenesis. The primary mechanism is believed to be immunologic rather than renal (Lum, 2007).

The incidence of nephrotic syndrome is 2 to 3 per 100,000, with a fifteen times greater incidence in children than in adults. Ninety percent of children with nephrotic syndrome have a form of idiopathic nephrotic syndrome with a peak incidence at 2 to 6 years old. Eighty-five percent of patients are steroid responders. In early childhood, the male-to-female ratio is 2:1; however, by midadolescence the rate of occurrence is equal (Vogt & Avner, 2004).

Clinical Findings

History. The following may be reported:

- Edema, which is a cardinal clinical feature, especially periorbital edema, in dependent areas (tight shoes or underwear) and lax tissues (puffy eyes)
- Low urine production
- Gastrointestinal symptoms: anorexia, paleness, listlessness, diarrhea, vomiting, abdominal pain (right upper quadrant)
- Recent prodromal infection
- Respiratory difficulties secondary to ascites, effusion, pneumonia, if advanced disease

Physical Examination. Findings include:

- Edema—periorbital in the morning, dependent in the evening
- Hypertension, normal BP if hypovolemic
- Chronically ill appearing
- Muscle wasting, malnourishment, growth failure if prolonged
- If the disease is progressive, hydrothorax with respiratory difficulty or ascites with labial edema

Diagnostic Studies. The following are ordered as indicated:

- UA and microscopic examination (protein of 2+ or greater, hyaline and fine granular casts, microhematuria (in 33%), elevated specific gravity, fat bodies, and casts in urine)
- Quantitative urine protein excretion (24-hour collection or protein-creatinine ratio on a random first morning urine)
- CBC; electrolytes, BUN, creatinine (normal); calcium; serum albumin (less than 2 g/dL), total protein; liver enzymes; triglycerides, lipoproteins, cholesterol (elevated); C3 and C4 (normal); ANA
- Consideration of Venereal Disease Research Laboratories (VDRL), hepatitis B surface antigen, HIV, malaria, PPD as indicated by history
- Kidney biopsy is recommended in the following circumstances:
  - If criteria for MCNS are not met
  - If systemic disease is present
  - In the presence of hypertension and hematuria
  - With hypocomplementemia or nonselective proteinemia
  - If the patient is older than 7 years or an adolescent
  - If the patient is nonresponsive to steroids
  - If relapses are frequent

Differential Diagnosis

Infants (newborn to 1 year old) usually have congenital renal problems, children 7 years and older are likely to have focal glomerulosclerosis or mesangial proliferative GN, and teens have membranous nephropathy. The differential diagnosis includes hypoproteinemia from starvation, liver disease, and protein-losing enteropathy; none of these conditions has associated proteinuria. GN should also be considered in the differential diagnosis.

Management

Nephrotic syndrome is a complex, often chronic disorder that responds to careful management with a gratifying long-term outcome. The diagnosis is made with 95% certainty on clinical impressions. A major goal is to control edema while awaiting definitive remission. Management involves the following:

- Consultation with and/or referral to a nephrologist is important because of the constantly changing strategies for managing these children.
- Hospitalization may be necessary initially if disease is severe.
- Prednisone (2 mg/kg/day; maximum, 60 mg) to induce remission, which can occur as early as 14 days as evidenced by diuresis. Steroids are continued for at least 4 to 6 weeks. A crushed or quartered pill is economical and often easier to give than liquid. Once remission occurs, steroid therapy is tapered and weaned over several months. Relapses are treated with a short course of steroids and the patient weaned as soon as the proteinuria resolves.
- Activity and diet recommendations. No limitation is placed on activity. During active disease, salt may be restricted. At other times, a diet appropriate for age is recommended. A high-protein, low-salt or no-salt diet with less than 35% fat and less than 300 mg of cholesterol per day is sometimes recommended.
- Diuretics and albumin replacement are sometimes used in the acute phase. Monitoring of BP at home is sometimes recommended.
- Proteinuria testing at home is recommended to monitor the child and identify exacerbations as soon as possible. Relapses begin with persistent proteinuria of greater than 2+ every day for 3 days.
- Routine immunizations, especially live vaccines and including varicella vaccine, should be given during remissions and at least 3 months after immunosuppressive drugs. Pneumococcal and influenza vaccines are recommended for these children.
- Monitoring and prompt treatment of infection are essential. Exposure to varicella zoster requires that varicella zoster immune globulin be given within 72 hours of exposure. Sepsis work-up should be done with any fever and broad-spectrum antibiotics given until the organism is identified (Lum, 2007).

Patient Education, Prevention, and Prognosis

Children with nephrotic syndrome are susceptible to pneumococcal, *E. coli, Pseudomonas,* and *Haemophilus influenzae* infection because of stasis of fluid; such infection is seen as peritonitis, pneumonia, cellulitis, or septicemia. Hypertension or hypotension is a possibility. Because the child is in a hypercoagulable state, thromboembolism is possible. Protein losses and compromising edema are also potential complications.

Patient education should stress the importance of continued, regular care to monitor renal function and the early treatment of the disease or concurrent infections. Families must know that relapses are the rule. An understanding of the disease process, side effects of steroids, recognition of infection, and the importance of monitoring proteinuria for relapses is crucial. If chronic steroid treatment is needed, the child and family must understand the side effects of the medication. The prognosis is good in steroid responders, with relapses that decrease in frequency as the child grows older without any residual renal dysfunction (Chan & Foreman, 2006; Vogt & Avner, 2004).

NEPHRITIS OR GLOMERULONEPHRITIS

Description

Nephritis is a noninfectious, inflammatory response of the kidneys characterized by varied degrees of hypertension, edema, proteinuria, and hematuria that can be either microscopic or macroscopic with dysmorphic RBCs and casts. Nephritis is classified as acute, intermittent, or chronic. Primary GN occurs when the original and predominant structure impaired is the glomerulus. Secondary GN occurs when renal involvement is secondary to systemic disease (e.g., SLE, HSP, primary vasculitis, Goodpasture syndrome, or drug hypersensitivity reactions). Involvement can be in the glomerulus or the interstitium and either localized in one part of the kidney or generalized throughout. GN refers to inflammation primarily in the glomeruli; interstitial nephritis refers to inflammation in the interstitium primarily caused by drug reactions. Poststreptococcal GN (PSGN) is the classic form of GN.

Acute nephritis most commonly occurs as PSGN, which is characterized by a history of streptococcal infection within the prior 2 weeks and an acute onset of edema, oliguria, hypertension, and gross hematuria. Consider an alternative diagnosis if the following findings are present:

- Nephrotic levels of protein
- Lack of evidence for a postinfection mechanism
- Rapidly deteriorating renal function
- Clinical or laboratory findings suggesting other forms of GN (e.g., rash, positive ANA)

Intermittent gross hematuria and proteinuria syndromes include the following:

- *IgA nephropathy,* or *Berger disease,* is the most common chronic GN in children of European-Asian descent and is uncommon in blacks; it has a 2:1 male preponderance. It is an immunologic entity causing recurrent gross and microscopic hematuria and often proteinuria. It is present in about one third of persons biopsied for persistent microscopic hematuria. It is often precipitated by viral infections or strenuous exercise, and each episode lasts less than 72 hours. BP is normal; no edema is present, and C3 is normal. Definitive diagnosis is made by biopsy. The prognosis is good in the absence of elevated serum creatinine or nephrotic-range proteinuria, although progression to chronic renal insufficiency can occur in 10% to 30%. Berger disease and idiopathic hypercalciuria (see the section on hematuria) are responsible for 50% or more cases of isolated hematuria in children (Blowey, 2002).
- *Hereditary* or *familial nephritis* involves many disorders, but the best known is Alport syndrome. More common and

severe in males, with onset before 15 years old in 75% of children, this condition is inherited as an X-linked dominant trait. The initial manifestation is isolated, persistent microscopic hematuria with intermittent macrohematuria and variable proteinuria occurring with an upper respiratory infection or exercise. Laboratory abnormalities are variable; biopsy verifies the diagnosis. Extrarenal abnormalities, including neurogenic deafness (hearing loss in 50% with females often spared), ocular abnormalities (30%), and macrothrombocytopenia, are often found (Elias et al, 2006). Vision and hearing screening is essential with referral for any abnormalities. Severe forms of the disease can lead to end-stage renal disease, which is often heralded by hypotension.

- *Familial* or *benign recurrent nephritis,* also known as thin-basement-membrane disease, is a disorder inherited as an autosomal dominant trait with unknown etiology. Macroscopic and microscopic hematuria and mild proteinuria, often precipitated by upper respiratory tract infection, characterize episodes. Laboratory values other than UA are normal. The diagnosis is confirmed by biopsy, which may not be needed if the disease is mild and confirmed in relatives. In the absence of notable proteinuria, deafness, ocular defects, renal failure, and with normal biopsy findings, the prognosis is excellent.

- Chronic nephritis is most commonly known as *membranoproliferative GN* (MPGN) and is distinguished by four types based on biopsy. Chronic nephritis can be found after acute nephritis or when investigating nonspecific complaints, such as anorexia, intermittent vomiting, and malaise. It is manifested by diminished renal function that ultimately has detrimental effects on other organ systems. Types I and II may respond to steroids, but the overall prognosis is guarded.

Pyelonephritis, discussed earlier in the UTI section, is inflammation of the renal parenchyma, calyces, and pelvis caused by bacteria.

Epidemiology

The inflammatory response of the kidneys results from various causes, such as infection, an immunologic response, a drug or toxin, and vascular or systemic disorders. PSGN is an immune response by the host to a Group A ß-hemolytic streptococcal infection, whereas acute postinfectious GN (APGN) can be caused by bacterial, fungal, viral, parasitic, or rickettsial agents.

PSGN is the most common form of nephritis in childhood, occurs most often between 5 and 12 years old, more often in males (2:1), and is unusual in children younger than 3 years old. The incidence of APGN is difficult to determine because of the large number of patients with subclinical cases, most younger than 5 to 10 years old (Davis & Avner, 2004; Blowey, 2002).

Clinical Findings

History. The following may be reported:

- Streptococcal skin (more likely) or pharyngeal infection within the past 2 to 3 weeks (PSGN). Classically, a latent period of 7 to 10 days elapses between infection and the onset of symptoms; if less than 5 days or more than 14 days, consider other causes.

- Abrupt onset of gross hematuria
- Reduced urine output
- Lethargy, anorexia, nausea, vomiting, abdominal pain
- Chills, fever, backache (pyelonephritis)
- Medication for any infection taken in the last few weeks

Physical Examination. Findings may include:

- Hypertension that is transient and resolves in 1 to 2 weeks
- Edema, especially periorbital edema, of abrupt onset with weight gain
- Ear malformations
- Flank or abdominal pain or a mass (in polycystic kidney or malignancy [e.g., Wilms' tumor])
- Costovertebral angle tenderness (in pyelonephritis)
- Circulatory congestion—dyspnea, cough, pallor, pulmonary edema if severe
- Oliguria, with diuresis in 5 to 7 days
- Rashes or arthralgias (with SLE, HSP, or impetigo)
- Evidence of trauma or abuse

Diagnostic Studies. The following are done as indicated:

- UA with microscopic examination—tea color, elevated specific gravity, macrohematuria and microhematuria, proteinuria not exceeding the amount of hematuria, pyuria in PSGN; granular, hyaline, WBC, or RBC casts and dysmorphic RBCs

- Serum C3/C4 (low early in disease, returning to normal in 6 to 8 weeks), total protein and albumin (elevated)
- CBC, ESR, ASO titer (elevated), Streptozyme test (positive), anti-DNA antibody titer
- Electrolytes, BUN, creatinine, and cholesterol
- Fluorescent antinuclear antibody (SLE), hepatitis titers, sickle cell or hemoglobin electrophoresis, tuberculin PPD, and fluorescent treponemal antibody absorption (syphilis)

Differential Diagnosis

Acute nephritis also occurs as part of systemic illnesses, such as SLE, HSP, hemolytic-uremic syndrome, vasculitis, or as a reaction to drugs or irradiation.

Management

See Fig. 34-11. Consultation with a nephrologist is recommended in all cases.

- PSGN treatment is supportive because resolution occurs spontaneously 90% of the time within 6 to 24 months. The course does not seem to be affected by corticosteroids, immunosuppression, or other treatment modalities. During the peak of oliguria and hypertension in the first few days of illness, hospitalization may be required with fluid and sodium limitation and diuretic, antihypertensive, and antibiotic treatment if cultures are positive. Resolution occurs once diuresis begins. Gross hematuria persists for 1 to 2

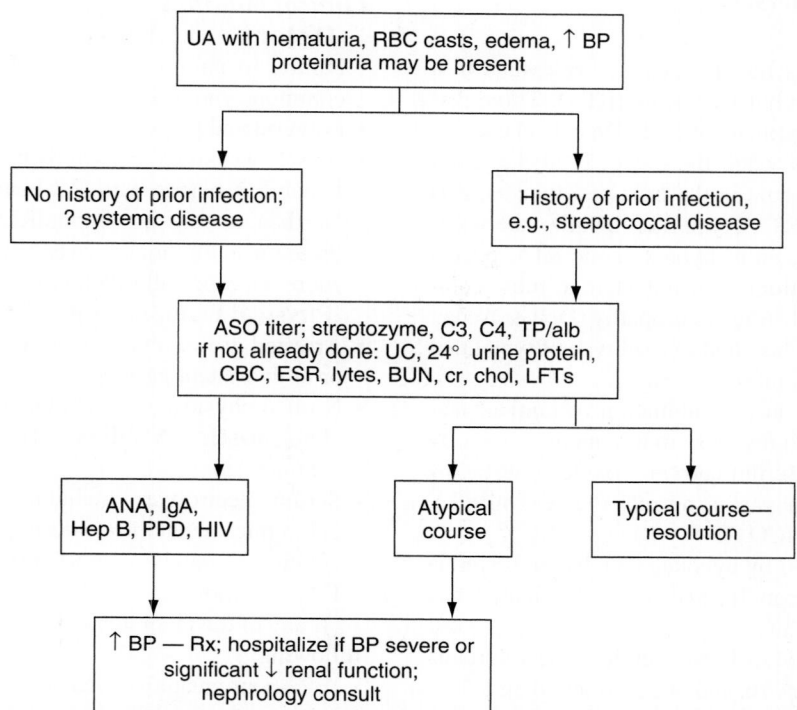

FIG. 34-11   Evaluation of nephritis. *alb*, albumin; *ANA*, antinuclear antibody; *ASO*, antistreptolysin O; *BP*, blood pressure; *BUN*, blood urea nitrogen; *C3*, complement 3; *C4*, complement 4; *CBC*, complete blood count; *chol*, cholesterol; *cr*, creatinine; *ESR*, erythrocyte sedimentation rate; *Hep B*, hepatitis B; *HIV*, human immunodeficiency virus; *IgA*, immunoglobulin A; *LFT*, liver function test; *PPD*, purified protein derivative; *RBC*, red blood cell; *Rx*, prescribe; *TP*, total protein; *UA*, urinalysis.

weeks, urine can be abnormal for 6 to 12 weeks, and microscopic hematuria can persist for up to 2 years. Complement levels return to normal in 3 to 6 weeks.

- Acute nephritis—possible hospitalization with treatment, as just described.
- IgA nephropathy—annual follow-up with BP, UA, and determination of renal function.
- Benign familial or hereditary nephritis—perform audiometry and review family medical history. Hereditary markers are being developed for this disease.
- Benign recurrent nephritis—monitor UA and renal function every 1 to 2 years.
- Chronic nephritis—a team approach is required to adequately provide care.

Patient Education, Prevention, and Prognosis

Prolonged oliguria and renal failure can occur if acute nephritis progresses. Hypertensive encephalopathy or congestive heart failure can occur secondary to PSGN. Irreversible parenchymal damage causes hypertension and renal insufficiency.

Patients with PSGN may have macrohematuria or microhematuria for up to 6 to 12 months, but the long-range outcome is excellent. Thin-basement-membrane disease has a good outcome. IgA nephropathy with severe histologic findings has a poor outcome, especially if the child is black. Patient education should stress the importance of continued, regular care to monitor renal function.

RENAL TUBULAR ACIDOSIS

Description

Dysfunction of renal tubule transport capability results in a condition known as renal tubular acidosis (RTA). Three distinct types of RTA have been identified. Type I, classic or distal RTA (dRTA), occurs when the defect is in the distal tubule. When the defect occurs in the proximal tubules, it is known as proximal RTA (pRTA), type II, or bicarbonate-wasting RTA. Type IV, also known as hyperkalemic RTA, occurs with problems in the functioning of aldosterone most commonly following relief of obstructive uropathy (Dell & Avner, 2004). Type III has been reclassified as a subtype of type I that occurs primarily in preterm infants.

The diagnosis depends on a combination of clinical features, laboratory values, and response to treatment.

RTA is suggested by a serum carbon dioxide level below 20, especially if the anion gap is normal ($12 \pm 4\,mEq/L$). Anion gap = $Na^+ - (Cl^- + HCO_3^-)$.

- dRTA (type I) is suggested by hypokalemia, hyperchloremia with a serum CO_2 less than 16, and urine pH greater than 5.5.
- pRTA (type II) is suggested by hypokalemia, hyperchloremia with a serum CO_2 less than 16, and urine pH less than 5.5.
- Type IV is suggested by hyperkalemia.

Fanconi syndrome is an uncommon and more complex form of pRTA (type II) with associated glycosuria, phosphaturia, aminoaciduria, and a defect in vitamin D metabolism manifested as nausea, anorexia, intermittent vomiting, and possibly rickets.

Epidemiology

The dysfunction in the transport capability of the renal tubules affects either the reabsorption of filtered bicarbonate, excretion of hydrogen ion, or both and results in a metabolic acidosis. RTA is often an isolated and primary problem with unknown cause, but diseases or intoxication can cause it. It is seen most typically in children evaluated for growth failure and is often revealed when illness, dehydration, or starvation stresses a child. RTA is more common in males than females, with pRTA being the most common form seen in children.

The proximal tubule, which normally absorbs 85% of bicarbonate, is able to reabsorb only 60% of bicarbonate from filtered urine in patients with pRTA. The distal tubule continues to function and reabsorbs approximately 15% of the bicarbonate, and the urine is acidified (pH less than 5.5). However, a large amount of bicarbonate is wasted. As the body adapts, a new threshold for serum bicarbonate is set, usually around 14 to 16 mEq (Dell & Avner, 2004).

A defect in the ability of the distal renal tubule to excrete hydrogen is the cause of dRTA. This defect causes complete loss of reabsorption of the final 15% of bicarbonate and an inability to acidify urine (pH greater than 5.5). Type IV RTA is characterized by a deficiency in the production or responsiveness of aldosterone and impaired ammonia production. Type IV RTA is often associated with an obstructive uropathy or other transient phenomenon in infancy (Alon, 2002; Friedman, 2004).

Clinical Findings

History. The following is often reported:
- Failure to gain weight (especially) and height—the most common symptoms
- Polyuria and polydipsia
- Muscle weakness (caused by hypokalemia)
- Irritability before eating, satiation after eating, vomiting, diarrhea, or constipation in dRTA
- Preference for liquids over solid foods, poor appetite, or anorexia, especially with type IV

Physical Examination. Findings can include:
- Arrested growth curve toward the end of the first year with prior consistent growth
- Normal physical examination and development

Diagnostic Studies. The following studies are recommended:
- Serum electrolytes, including CO_2 (hypokalemia, hyperchloremic metabolic acidosis), renal function tests (BUN, creatinine), calcium, phosphorus, alkaline phosphatase, and UA (first morning void) to test for glucose and pH

If any of the laboratory findings are abnormal, consider the following:
- A 24-hour creatinine clearance to establish the normal GFR, calcium (normal less than 4 mg/kg/24 hours), calcium-to-creatinine ratio (normal less than 0.21 mg/dL for children older than 6 years, less than 0.42 for children 19 months to 6 years old, less than 0.6 for children 7 to 18 months old, and

less than 0.86 for children younger than 7 months old), citrate, potassium oxalate (Chan et al, 2001; Omokara, 2005)
- Renal ultrasonography to determine the anatomy and rule out nephrocalcinosis, nephrolithiasis, hydronephrosis, obstructive uropathy, and parenchymal damage

Differential Diagnosis

Primary RTA must be differentiated from secondary RTA, which can be due to many disease states or conditions, such as other causes of growth failure (FTT), hypothyroidism, and systemic acidosis.

Management

Goals of management include correcting the acidosis and maintaining normal bicarbonate (greater than 20 mEq/L), thereby restoring growth and minimizing complications.

- Oral alkalizing medications given to achieve these goals include the following:
  - Bicitra (sodium citrate and citric acid or Shohl solution), which equals 1 mEq bicarbonate/mL and is relatively pleasant tasting.
  - Polycitra (sodium and potassium citrate and citric acid), which equals 2 mEq bicarbonate/mL and is less palatable. Giving it in juice, water, or formula may ease its administration. Polycitra is especially useful if the child is hypokalemic or requires an excess quantity or if compliance is an issue.
  - $NaHCO_3$ tablets are available in 325 mg strength (4 mEq bicarbonate) and 650 mg strength (8 mEq bicarbonate).
  - Eight oz of baking soda mixed with 2.65 L of distilled water equals 1 mEq/mL of bicarbonate.
  - Dosing is determined by the type of RTA. dRTA requires low doses, often between 2 and 5 mEq/kg/day. pRTA requires high doses, often between 5 and 15 mEq/kg/day and sometimes as high as 20 mEq/kg/day. The dose must be titrated to the child's response as determined by weight and laboratory results (CO_2 and electrolytes). Initiate medication at 3 mEq/kg/day and check laboratory results in a few days. Titrate the dose until a serum bicarbonate level of 20 to 22 mEq/L is achieved (Dell & Avner, 2004).
- To maintain as normal a bicarbonate level as possible, doses should be given frequently throughout the day (with meals) and as late as possible at night (at bedtime). A larger dose at bedtime has been advocated to coincide with growth hormone secretion at night to maximize growth (Chan et al, 2001).
- The response to medication helps confirm the diagnosis and type of RTA. dRTA has a rapid response to treatment, and normal bicarbonate levels are maintained with little difficulty. pRTA requires higher doses to normalize bicarbonate and is less easily maintained. Type IV RTA requires mineralocorticoid treatment if aldosterone is deficient.
- Maximizing caloric intake to enhance growth can be accomplished as follows:
  - Solid foods should be emphasized for all meals and snacks and water and noncaloric foods avoided.
  - Provide nutritional supplements.

- Meticulous follow-up is imperative.
  - Weight and laboratory results should be monitored biweekly to monthly until weight gain is established and CO_2 is stabilized. Weighing on the same scale and by the same person is essential.
- Pseudoephedrine should be avoided because it is minimally excreted in alkalinized urine and associated with a risk of intoxication.
- Referral to a pediatric nephrologist is necessary for any child whose laboratory values are not normalizing and who is not growing well with treatment, has unusual laboratory results, has type IV RTA, or has any complication of RTA.

Patient Education, Prevention, and Prognosis

It is rare to have complications with pRTA. Hypercalciuria leading to nephrocalcinosis, nephrolithiasis, renal parenchymal destruction, and occasionally renal failure can occur with dRTA. Rickets are sometimes found in type IV RTA.

Isolated pRTA responds quickly to treatment, with children showing catch-up growth and obtaining normal maximum height. pRTA resolves spontaneously without recurrence of symptoms, often within 1 to 2 years but at worst over the first decade of life (Constantinescu 2006; Dell & Avner, 2004). dRTA usually lasts a lifetime; type IV resolves with correction of the underlying problem. Patient education should stress the importance of continued, regular care to monitor renal function and growth.

NEPHROLITHIASIS AND UROLITHIASIS

Description

Urinary stones can be found anywhere in the urinary tract system. In North America, most children with stones have stones that are found in the kidneys; bladder stones occur in less than 10% of the pediatric cases and are most often related to urologic abnormalities. Bladder stones are endemic to other parts of the world and seem related to diet (Nicoletta & Lande, 2006).

Epidemiology

The prevalence of urinary stones varies by region, with a higher incidence in the Southeast U.S. and in Caucasians, with a slightly higher incidence in males than in females. Seventy-five percent of children who have nephrolithiasis have an identifiable predisposition to stone formation. Metabolic risk factors account for more than 50% of cases, structural abnormalities account for 32%, and infection account for 4%. Hypercalciuria is the most common metabolic cause (accounts for 30% to 50%) of urinary calculi and is a condition with many causes including renal tubular dysfunction, endocrine disturbances, bone metabolic disorders, UTI, familial idiopathic hypercalcemia, and medications (Gillespie & Stapleton, 2004). Hyperoxaluria is found in up to 20% of children with nephrolithiasis. Hyperuricosuria has been documented in 2% to 10% of children with stone formation. Cystine stones account for less than 1% of urinary stones.

Clinical Findings

History

- Family history of nephrolithiasis, arthritis, gout or renal disease
- Stones or fragments passed in urine
- Dietary history high in protein, sodium, calcium, and oxalate intake.
- Colic in an infant
- History or symptoms suggestive of a UTI in a preschooler

Physical Examination

- Abdominal, flank, or pelvic pain (occurs at all ages, but present in 94% of adolescents)

Diagnostic Studies

- Urine UA and culture
  - Gross or microscopic hematuria in 33% to 90% of children
  - Stone or stone fragments with chemical analysis
- Abdominal radiography
- Abdominal ultrasound
- Computed tomography (CT)
- If stone or fragments are passed or seen in the urinary system on imaging studies, refer to urology and initiate complete metabolic evaluation.
  - Serum levels of uric acid, electrolytes, creatinine, calcium, phosphorus, bicarbonate, parathyroid hormone level, and alkaline phosphatase.
  - Random urine sample for offending constituents with 24-hour collection for abnormal values (Gillespie & Stapleton, 2004; Omokaro, 2005).
- Calcium/Creatinine
  - <0.8 mg/mg (0 to 6 months old)
  - <0.6 mg/mg (7 to 12 months old)
  - <0.21 mg/mg (>2 years old)
- Oxalate/Creatinine
  - <0.3 mg/mg (0 to 6 months old)
  - <0.15 mg/mg (6 months to 4 years old)
  - <0.1 mg/mg (4 years old to adult)
- Cystine/Creatinine <0.02 mg/mg (all ages)
- Citrate/Creatinine <0.51 mg/mg (all ages)
- Uric Acid/GFR <0.56 mg uric acid/dL of GFR (GFR = urine uric acid × serum creatinine)

Differential Diagnosis

Other diagnoses causing flank pain should be considered especially (e.g., UTI or pyelonephritis and trauma) in adolescents but also with younger children. Other afebrile illnesses including gastrointestinal viral syndromes, early appendicitis, chronic recurrent abdominal pain of no known cause, and emotional stress should be considered in the preschool child because just more than half of those with nephrolithiasis have flank pain.

Management

Increased fluid intake is the first line of therapy for all stone types regardless of the cause. In adolescents, a goal of 2 liters of urine output per day would be helpful. (Nicoletta & Lande, 2006). Stone removal may be required if the stone is not passed and severe symptoms continue for a significant amount of time. Extracorporeal shock wave lithotripsy (ESWL) is safe in children, as long-term kidney damage has not been validated in follow-up studies. Skin bruising and hematuria are almost universal side effects of ESWL. Stones may also be removed by using rigid or flexible endoscopes passed through the urethra into the bladder or ureter. Renal calculi may also be removed percutaneously, and open surgical lithotomy is still an option if other techniques fail (Gillespie & Stapleton, 2004). Dietary restrictions control stone formation and renal injury in most metabolic disorders contributing to stone formation. Referral to a dietary expert for nutritional advice is advantageous.

Patient Education, Prevention, and Prognosis

Recurrence rates are high if left untreated, and patients with hyperuricosuria may continue to have symptomatic or asymptomatic calculi. Despite an excellent response to therapy, children with nephrolithiasis require long-term follow-up with a nephrologist because the potential for renal insufficiency and end-stage renal disease is significantly increased in these children (Nicoletta & Lande, 2006).

WILMS' TUMOR

Description

Wilms' tumor, the most common malignancy of the genitourinary tract, is typically recognized as a firm, smooth mass in the abdomen or flank. It is staged according to the National Wilms' Tumor Study as follows:

- Stage I is limited to the kidney and can be completely excised with the capsular surface intact (35%).
- Stage II extends beyond the kidney but can still be completely excised (30%).
- Stage III has postsurgical residual nonhematogenous extension confined to the abdomen (20%).
- Stage IV has hematogenous metastasis, most frequently to the lung (12%).
- Stage V is bilateral kidney involvement (3% to 5%) (Nachman & Abelson, 2004; Steinhurz, 2002).

Epidemiology

This malignancy is manifested as a solitary growth in any part of either or both kidneys. Two forms are recognized: heritable (less than 1%) and nonheritable. An important feature of Wilms' tumor is the occurrence of associated congenital anomalies in 15% of children, including renal abnormalities, such as cryptorchidism, hypospadias, duplication of the collecting system, ambiguous genitalia (4.4%), hemihypertrophy (2.9%), aniridia (1.1%), cardiac abnormalities, and Beckwith-Wiedemann, Drash, and Perlman syndromes. Wilms' tumor will develop in 15% to 20% of children with neurofibromatosis. It occurs with equal frequency in both sexes and has a 3:1 black-to-white incidence. Fifty-five percent occur on the left side. The incidence of Wilms' tumor is 1 per 10,000/year in children younger than 15 years old, or about 400 to 500 cases annually, with 80% being diagnosed before 5 years old.

The peak incidence and median age at diagnosis is 3 years old (Ferguson, 2006; Jaffe & Huff, 2004; Nachman & Abelson, 2004).

Clinical Findings

History

- The most frequent finding is increasing abdominal size or an actual palpable mass.
- Pain is reported if the mass has undergone rapid growth or hemorrhage (25% to 50%).
- Fever, dyspnea, diarrhea, vomiting, weight loss, or malaise may be reported.

Physical Examination

- A firm, smooth abdominal or flank mass that does not cross the midline may be noted.
- BP is elevated if renal ischemia is present (rare).
- A left varicocele is found in males if the spermatic vein is obstructed.
- A careful examination is needed to rule out congenital anomalies.

Diagnostic Studies

- Chest and abdominal radiography is performed to differentiate neuroblastoma, which is usually calcified.
- Abdominal ultrasonography is used to differentiate a solid from a cystic mass or hydronephrosis and multicystic kidney.
- UA demonstrates hematuria in 25% to 33% of children.
- A CBC, reticulocyte count, and liver and renal chemistry studies are performed.
- A CT scan of the chest, abdomen, and pelvis to stage the disease and bone marrow is done by the oncology team.

Differential Diagnosis

Neuroblastoma is the main differential diagnosis (the mass often crosses the midline). Multicystic kidney, hydronephrosis, renal cyst, or other renal malignancies are additional conditions to consider.

Management

Diagnostic work-up is the initial urgent priority, with concurrent referral to a pediatric cancer center for treatment. Surgery is scheduled to remove the affected kidney and possibly the ureter and adrenal gland; combined chemotherapy and radiotherapy are instituted if the disease is advanced or histologic findings are unfavorable. Close follow-up after the initial treatment should be coordinated with the cancer team.

Patient Education, Prevention, and Prognosis

The lungs and liver are the most common sites of metastasis. High BP is possible because of renal ischemia and will occasionally lead to cardiac failure. Scoliosis resulting from radiation therapy is uncommon because radiation exposure is carefully controlled.

The prognosis is determined by the histology of the neoplasm, by the patient's age (the younger the better), the size of the tumor, positive nodes, and, most significantly, the extent or stage of the disease. If the child has favorable histologic parameters, the 4-year survival rate is as follows: 97% if stage I, 92% if stage II, 87% if stage III, and 73% if stage IV. Forty-five percent of relapses occur within 6 months, 28% more within 12 months (Nachman & Abelson, 2004).

Children with one kidney should not participate in contact sports, although there are kidney protectors available that one may consider. New information on the long-term sequelae for the treatment of Wilms' tumors and the present trials and treatment recommendations can be accessed at The National Wilms' Tumor Study (see Resource Box at the end of the chapter).

■ COMMON GENITOURINARY CONDITIONS IN MALES

HYPOSPADIAS

Description

Hypospadias is a common congenital abnormality in which the urethral meatus is located anywhere from the proximal glans to the perineum on the ventral surface (underside) of the penis. Chordee, a ventral bowing of the penis, occurs when a tight band of fibrous tissue pulls on the penis. Torsion refers to rotation of the penis to the right or left.

Epidemiology

The etiology of hypospadias is unclear. It is believed that the endocrine system probably has an important role, but what that role is remains unclear. The primitive gonad in the eighth week of embryonic development differentiates into male or female. As the genital tubercle enlarges, developmental arrest occurs along the line of urethral fusion and causes hypospadias.

Hypospadias occurs in 1 in 250 male infants (Elder, 2004). There was a major increase in incidence in the 1990s, especially in low-birth-weight babies and babies whose mothers had taken fertility drugs or undergone in vitro fertilization. The cause of this may be due to genetic factors (e.g., endocrine abnormalities) or environmental factors (e.g., androgen blockers and estrogen or endocrine disruptors), and it probably occurs early in gestation. Risk is increased if family members have hypospadias: 8% if the father, 14% if a sibling, and 21% if two family members. Hypospadias occurs more commonly in whites, in Italians and Jews, and in winter conceptions. Nine percent of boys with hypospadias also have undescended testicles, inguinal hernia, or hydrocele (Hussain et al, 2002; Kurzrock, 2004.)

Clinical Findings

History

- A family history of a male relative with genitourinary problems is reported.
- The child sits to void, urinates on the floor in front of the toilet unless he holds his penis to direct the stream.

Physical Examination.   In a newborn, the classic finding is a dorsally hooded foreskin. It is essential to visualize the urethral meatus. Pulling the ventral shaft skin in a downward

and outward direction facilitates visualization. Anatomic classification is made by location:
- Anterior (70%), glanular, coronal, or anterior penile
- Middle (10%)
- Posterior (20%), scrotal, penoscrotal, or posterior penile
  Other findings include:
- Urinary stream that aims downward rather than straight
- Inguinal hernia or undescended testicles (9%)
- Chordee

Differential Diagnosis
The differential diagnosis includes intersex abnormalities.

Management
The goal of surgical repair is to have a functional penis that appears normal. Circumcision must not be done because the foreskin may be used in the surgical repair. Referral should be made to a urologist at birth for evaluation. Surgery to correct hypospadias is best done at around 6 to 18 months old. Considerations in scheduling surgery at this age include the following: it is psychologically less damaging; a caudal block is easily performed; the wound heals more rapidly; and there is more time to repair complications before toilet training begins. Surgery scheduled after 18 months old minimizes anesthesia risk, the larger anatomy makes surgery easier, and the patient can participate in the decision-making process. Repair is usually accomplished in a one-stage outpatient procedure unless it is a complex defect. Generally, fewer than 8% of patients experience complications (Snodgrass, 2004).

Patient Education, Prevention, and Prognosis
With unrepaired hypospadias, peer taunting of boys and problems with erections are possible complications. Intersex abnormalities are possible if associated with cryptorchidism.

Hypospadias is usually an isolated anomaly, but it does require further work-up to assess the anatomy of the urinary system for other anomalies. Education and reassurance regarding cause, repair, and outcome should be provided. Careful assessment of the newborn should be done when hypospadias is reported in a male family member.

CRYPTORCHIDISM (UNDESCENDED TESTES)
Description
Cryptorchidism describes a testis that does not reside in and cannot be manipulated into the scrotum. A retractile testis is out of the scrotum, but can be brought into the scrotum and remains there. A gliding testis can be brought into the scrotum, but returns to a high position in the scrotum once released. An ectopic testis lies outside the normal path of descent. An ascended testis is one that has fully descended, but has spontaneously reascended and lies outside the scrotum. A trapped testis is one dislocated after herniorrhaphy. Any testis that is not in the scrotum is subject to progressive deterioration. Undescended testes are a common disorder that often causes great anxiety for parents.

Epidemiology
Testes develop in the abdomen and descend in the seventh fetal month to the upper part of the groin, subsequently progressing through the inguinal canal into the scrotum. Failure of the testes to descend can be caused by mechanical lesions or can be secondary to hormonal, chromosomal, enzymatic, or anatomic disorders.

Undescended testis is the most common genitourinary disorder in boys. It is more common in preterm, low-birth-weight, and twin infants. The incidence of cryptorchidism is 0.2% to 1.8% in young adults, 0.5% to 0.8% in 1-year-olds, 2.5% to 4% in term infants, 20% to 30% in premature infants, more than 60% if infant birth weight is under 1500 g, and nearly 100% in 900-g neonates (Elder, 2004; Reiter & Saenger, 2002). A great majority of undescended testes descend spontaneously by 6 months old. After 6 months old, it is rare for them to descend. The best time for repair is under discussion. One belief is that the optimal timing for repair is 6 months old because the critical time for maturation and transformation of gonocytes to adult dark spermatogonia is before 6 months old. However, others believe that surgical management within the first 2 years of life improves future fertility (MacLellan & Diamond, 2006). The frequency of bilateral occurrence is 10% to 25%; unilateral involvement (55% to 66%) is more likely to be right sided. Retractile testes are bilateral and most common in boys 5 to 6 years old.

Clinical Findings
History. The history can include the following:
- Family history of undescended testes or testicular malignancy
- Testes not consistently descended during the infant's bath
- Associated urinary problems
- Prematurity
- Risk factors (Callaghan, 2000; MacLellan & Diamond, 2006): first born, cesarean section, toxemia, hypospadias, congenital subluxation of the hip, low birth weight, winter conception, Down syndrome, maternal age less than 20 and more than 35 years old
- Other congenital, endocrine, chromosomal, or intersex disorders

Physical Examination. Having the child sit cross-legged or frog legged, squat, or stand can facilitate testicle descent and palpation. Findings include the following:
- Scrotal rugae less full
- Bilateral or unilateral absence of a testicle
- Retractile testes, which move between the scrotum and external ring, but can be manipulated to the lower part of the scrotum and remain there; retraction especially common with tactile stimulation of the area or cold between 3 months and 7 years old
- Gliding testes that lie between the scrotum and external ring and can be manipulated to the lower part of the scrotum, but return to the high position
- Location:
  - Prescrotal (at the external inguinal ring), 25%

- Canalicular, high or low (between the external and internal rings), the most common type, 40%
- Ectopic (superficial inguinal, femoral, or perineal), 25%
- Intraabdominal (above the internal inguinal ring), not palpable, occurring in less than 15% of males with undescended testes
- Indirect inguinal hernia, 90%

Diagnostic Studies. None are indicated except in newborns with potential sex abnormalities, hypopituitarism, Down syndrome, or congenital adrenal hyperplasia. The risk of intersex abnormality is 27% if hypospadias and unilateral or bilateral cryptorchidism are present.

Differential Diagnosis

Retractile testes, anorchism, and chromosomal abnormalities are the differential diagnoses.

Management

The goals of treating undescended testes are to improve fertility outcome, decrease malignancy potential, and minimize the psychological stress associated with an empty scrotum. Management has come full circle from an initial recommendation for surgery, to treatment with hormonal therapy, and back to early surgical intervention. Both forms of treatment are still options.

- If the testes are undescended by 6 months old with the peak of postnatal testosterone, they are unlikely to descend spontaneously. The AAP, Action Committee of the Urology Section (1996), issued a statement recommending orchiopexy by 1 year old if performed by a skilled pediatric urologist or surgeon with an attendant, skilled pediatric anesthesiologist. Laparoscopy is the surgical procedure of choice, although repair can be done by inguinal incision or the intraabdominal route, depending on placement of the testes (MacLellan & Diamond, 2006).
- Hormonal therapy can be used to differentiate a retractile testis from a true cryptorchid one. Human chorionic gonadotropin (hCG) by the intramuscular route is the only approved method in the U.S., although intranasal gonadotropin-releasing hormone (GnRH) is used in some countries.
- In a child younger than 1 year old, regular examination to assess the position of the testes should be performed at every well child care visit. If the testes remain undescended, referral to a pediatric urologist or surgeon should occur by 1 year old. Referral should also occur if a retractile testis does not retain scrotal residence.
- If undescended testes are found after 1 year old, the child should be immediately referred to a pediatric urologist or surgeon for treatment.

Patient Education, Prevention, and Prognosis

Poor development, infertility, malignancy, vulnerability to trauma, testicular torsion, and inguinal hernia are possible complications of undescended testicles.

Families and patients should be informed of the following:

- Histologic changes have been shown in an undescended testis as early as 6 months old, with irreversible changes shown by 2 years old contributing to infertility and associated with malignancy (Ferrer & McKenna, 2000).
- Infertility as a complication of cryptorchidism has been reported in as many as 32% to 40% of men with unilateral undescended testes and in 59% to 70% if bilateral (Ferrer & McKenna, 2000).
- There is a 50% occurrence of torsion in nonfixed testes.
- Testicular malignancy in males with cryptorchidism is reported to have an incidence 4 to 10 times higher than the general population. Correction of undescended testes does not diminish the incidence of testicular cancer (Reiter & Saenger, 2002). Malignancy is more common with an intraabdominal testis. A progressive increase in the incidence of testicular tumor as the age at orchiopexy increases has been observed. A testicular neoplasm in one child mandates examination of his male siblings. Testicular self-examination should be taught to all adolescents but especially to these young men (Fig. 34-12). The website for the Testicular Cancer Awareness Week (see Resource Box at the end of the chapter) has a patient handout sheet on testicular self-examination and also provides the opportunity to sign up to receive monthly reminders to perform testicular self-examination.
- No evidence has indicated that undescended testes resolve with puberty; retractile testes generally settle into the scrotum by puberty.
- Open discussion of the problem, management, and potential complications is essential both initially and over time.
- Participation in contact sports is discouraged because of the risk of losing the one viable testicle to trauma.

HYDROCELE

Description

A common cause of painless scrotal swelling is a *hydrocele*, a collection of serous fluid in the scrotal sac. A *noncommunicating hydrocele* has a collection of fluid only in the scrotum. If the processus vaginalis remains patent so that fluid moves from the abdomen to the scrotum, it is called a *communicating hydrocele* and is more likely to be associated with a hernia (Fig. 34-13).

Epidemiology

Incomplete closure of the processus vaginalis through which the testes descend into the scrotum allows a hydrocele to develop. Incidence is 0.5% to 2% of males, appearing primarily under 1 year old (Kaplan, 2000; Schnitzer, 2006).

Clinical Findings

Hydroceles that persist beyond 1 year old are assumed to be in conjunction with a hernia. In older children, hydroceles appear after trauma or with inflammatory illness or neoplasm.

History. The history includes the following:

- Intermittent or constant bulge or lump in the scrotum, often more distally placed. Scrotal size increases with activity and decreases with rest.

In the realm of "if it ain't broke, don't fix it," there has been a substantial increase in information about prostate cancer. However, testicular cancer is the most common cancer in men 15 to 35 yr old, an age when we do not want to admit the possibility of illness. If detected early, it is among the easiest to cure. For men in this age group, a once-a-month simple self-examination is suggested. This can help catch this cancer at an early stage.

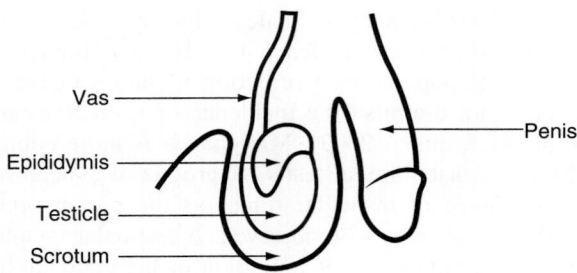

The most convenient time to examine yourself is while taking a shower or bath. The warm water causes the skin to relax, making the examination of the underlying tissues easier.

First:

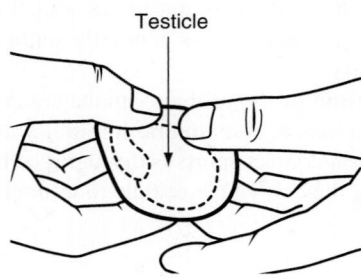

Examine your testicles. Slowly roll each testicle between thumb and forefingers. Try to find any hard, nonsensitive bumps.

Second:

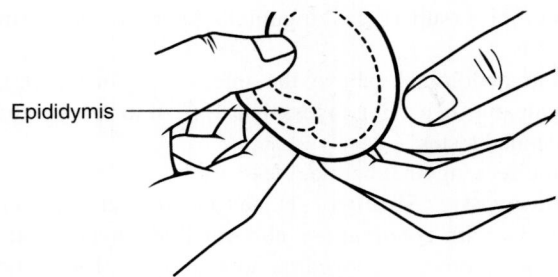

Examine the epididymis for lumps. This crescent-shaped cord is behind each testicle. This area is tender so do not be alarmed.

Third:

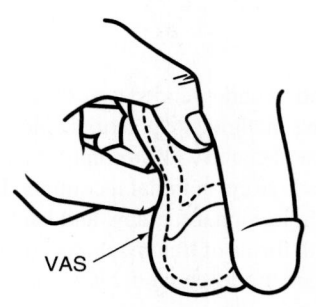

Examine the vas deferens, the sperm carrying tube that extends from the epididymis of each testicle.

Symptoms:

In early stages, testicular cancer may be symptomless. When symptoms do occur, they include:
* Lump on testicle, epididymis, or vas deferens
* Enlargement of a testicle
* Heavy sensation in groin area or testicles
* Dull ache in groin or abdomen area

If you find a lump or have any of the above symptoms, see your physician or NP immediately for an accurate diagnosis.

FIG. 34-12 Self-examination for testicular cancer. (From National Men's Resource Center: *Self exam for testicular cancer: "in the shower" guide,* San Anselmo, CA, 1994, The Center.)

* Overlying skin may be tense.
* No distress or vomiting.

Physical Examination. Findings include the following (Table 34-7):
* Asymmetry or a scrotal mass present; if swelling is present in the inguinal area, a hernia is probable
* Testes descended
* Usually unilateral swelling
* Translucent on transillumination (pink or red glow)
* Noncommunicating hydrocele—scrotal sac tense, slightly blue tinged, fluctuant, and does not reduce; no swelling in the inguinal region

* Communicating hydrocele—fluid in the scrotal sac comes and goes (probably flat in the morning, swollen later in the day)

Differential Diagnosis
Hernia, undescended testicle, retractile testicle, and inguinal lymphadenopathy are the differential diagnoses.

Management
The following steps are taken:
* Noncommunicating hydrocele—fluid is generally absorbed spontaneously; no treatment is indicated unless the hydrocele is so large that it is uncomfortable or persists longer than 1 year.

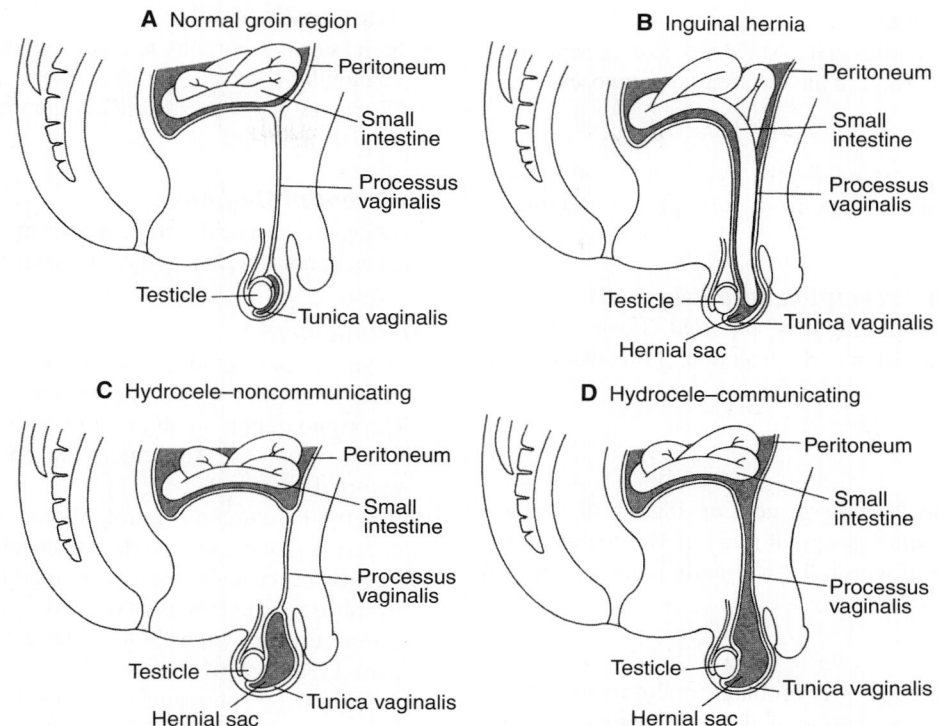

FIG. 34-13 Hydroceles and hernias. **A,** Groin region of the normal male infant. **B,** An inguinal hernia is the protrusion of bowel into the groin region. **C,** A hydrocele is a collection of fluid within the processus vaginalis. In a noncommunicating hydrocele, the scrotal swelling does not change in size or shape because there is no connection with the abdominal cavity. **D,** In a communicating hydrocele, the processus vaginalis remains open from the scrotum to the abdominal cavity, and scrotal swelling may vary in size during the course of an infant's day. (From Betz CL, Hunsberger M, Wright S: *Family-centered nursing care of infants,* ed 2, Philadelphia, 1994, WB Saunders.)

TABLE 34-7	**Physical Findings in Scrotal Swellings**				
			Cremasteric		Transillu-
Condition	**Tender**	**Red**	**Blue**	**Reflex**	**mination**
Chronic					
Hydrocele	–	–	+	+	+
Tumor	–	–	–	+	–
Varicocele	–	–	–	+	–
Acute					
Torsion					
Newborn	–	–	+	–	–
Other	+	+	–	–	–
Torsion of appendage	+	+	–	+	–
Epididymitis	+	+	–	+	–
Trauma	+	–	+	±	–

From Kaplan GN: Scrotal swelling in children, *Pediatr Rev* 21(9):312, 2000.

- Communicating hydrocele—can resolve, but more likely to develop a true hernia requiring surgical repair. Refer if persistent after 1 year old; surgical intervention is generally recommended.
- Surgery is usually done on an outpatient basis.

Patient Education, Prevention, and Prognosis

Reassure that the increased size of the scrotal sac will resolve, usually by 1 year old and involves no danger. Signs of hernia must be explained, and parents must be alerted to observe and report any abnormal findings.

SPERMATOCELE

Description

A benign, painless scrotal mass or cyst on the head of the epididymis or testicular adnexa containing sperm is called a *spermatocele.*

Epidemiology

A spermatocele is an uncommon finding (less than 1%), but when found is usually in the neonatal period, late childhood, or early adolescence with a peak at 14 years old (Leslie & Cain, 2006).

Clinical Findings
   History
- Scrotal swelling but asymptomatic otherwise
   Physical Examination
- Painless, mobile cystic nodule usually less than 1 cm in size, superior and posterior to the testicle that transilluminates
- No change in size with the Valsalva maneuver

Differential Diagnosis

A varicocele and an epididymal cyst (identical in appearance, but not containing sperm) are the differential diagnoses.

Management

No treatment is required unless the cyst is large and painful. Refer for ultrasound or to a urologist if diagnosis suspected.

Patient Education, Prevention, and Prognosis

Any pain or discomfort should be reported. Testicular self-examination would assist in early detection of this disorder in later adolescence.

VARICOCELE

Description

A varicocele is a benign enlargement or dilation of testicular veins causing a painless scrotal mass of varying size that may feel like a "bag of worms." It is usually found on the left side.

Epidemiology

The etiology of varicoceles is probably multifactorial, with the physiologic changes associated with puberty playing some role. A varicocele is caused by valvular incompetence of the spermatic vein resulting in dilated or varicose veins. Varicoceles are rare before 10 years old and may be indicative of malignancy. They occur in 5% of adolescent males and 15% of adult males (Elder, 2004). In males 10 to 25 years old, the average incidence is 16% (Adelman & Joffe, 2000) and as high as 20% of adolescents and young adults (Kaplan, 2000). Up to 85% to 95% arise on the left side because the left spermatic vein drains into the left renal vein and arterial compression of the renal vein obstructs blood flow from the vein. In contrast, the right spermatic vein drains into the vena cava (Ogunfiditimi, 2005). However, 22% of varicoceles occur bilaterally.

Clinical Findings

History

- Usually a painless swelling is noted in the left side of the scrotum, occasionally a "dull ache" or "heavy" feeling if large.
- Pain can occur with strenuous physical activity.
- Scrotal swelling with prolonged standing causes pain; swelling and pain resolve on reclining.

Physical Examination

- In the standing position, a "bag of worms" can be felt posterior and superior to the testis that collapses on lying and enlarges with the Valsalva maneuver.
- Measure and compare the size of both testes (length, width, and depth) using a standard orchidometer.
- Grade 3 varicoceles, the classic "bag of worms," are larger than 2 cm and easily visualized; grade 2 varicoceles are 1 to 2 cm in diameter and are easily palpable when the adolescent is standing, but not visualized; grade 1 varicoceles are the most common, very small, and difficult to palpate (the Valsalva maneuver may help).

Diagnostic Studies

- Serial ultrasonography to measure testicular size every 6 to 12 months
- Ultrasonography to rule out malignancy in children younger than 10 years old

Differential Diagnosis

Varicoceles must be differentiated from other testicular masses, such as lipoma, hernia, hydrocele, spermatocele, and tumors.

Management

- Asymptomatic grade 1 varicoceles with normal testicular volumes usually do not require intervention in adolescence. Ultrasonographic monitoring of testicular size can be done every 6 months. Any change in comfort level should be reported.
- Referral to a surgeon or urologist should be made if the varicocele is grade 2 or 3, if the varicocele is painful, if the difference in testicular volume is marked (greater than 2 mm by ultrasound), if the varicocele is right sided or bilateral, or if testicular growth becomes retarded over a 6- to 12-month period (Kass, 2001).
- Treatment by spermatic vein embolization or ligation may be attempted in adolescents. Ligation is the usual procedure, completed on an outpatient basis and has few complications.

Patient Education, Prevention, and Prognosis

Atrophy or testicular growth arrest, as noted by a discrepancy in testicular size, can occur. Lower fertility rates with decreased sperm concentration and motility have been noted and are factors in an aggressive surgical approach for the adolescent male with grade 2 or 3 varicocele. Hydrocele may be an insignificant, self-limiting complication following surgery.

A varicocele is the most common cause of infertility. Because of this, early identification is essential. All patients should be counseled about the long-term risks to fertility. Correction of testicular atrophy and an improved sperm count and fertility have been noted in 80% to 90% of those undergoing surgery early in adolescence. Testicular self-examination assists in early detection of this disorder.

INGUINAL HERNIA

Description

A scrotal or inguinal swelling (or both) that includes abdominal contents is an inguinal hernia (see Fig. 34-12). In females, inguinal hernias cause swelling in the inguinal area and labia majora.

Epidemiology

Incomplete closure of the processus vaginalis through which the testes descend into the scrotum allows the presence of abdominal contents in the inguinal canal or scrotum (labia majora in females) and thus the development of a hernia. Males who are obese or weight lifters or have a family history of undescended testes are at high risk for hernias (Sheldon, 2001).

Inguinal hernias are much more common in males than in females (8 to 10:1), occurring in 1% to 5% of boys. Premature infants are at increased risk (7% to 30% of males, 2% of females), with an additional 60% risk of incarceration (Schnitzer, 2006). More than 50% of hernias are diagnosed during the first year of life, with the peak incidence in the first 3 months of life. Bilateral hernias are common (10% to 20%). Unilateral hernias are more likely to occur on the right side (50% to 60%) than the left (30%) (Aiken, 2004; Ingelfinger, 2002). Indirect hernias are a congenital condition and are the most common type in children younger than 3 years old. Direct hernias increase in incidence after 3 years old and are usually acquired.

Clinical Findings
History
- Family history of undescended testes
- Swelling in the inguinal area, scrotum, or both that comes and goes and increases with crying or straining
- Weight lifting or obesity
- Prematurity
Physical Examination.   Findings include the following:
- Swelling is found in the inguinal area, scrotal area (labia majora in females), or both.
- The hernia is reducible with pressure on the distal end.
- Transillumination does not occur unless the bowel is filled with fluid.
- Direct hernias push outward through the weakest point in the abdominal wall.
- Indirect hernias push downward at an angle into the inguinal canal.
- The child is fussy and has a distended abdomen if the hernia is incarcerated.
- Silk glove sign—a sensation of two surfaces rubbing against each other while one palpates the spermatic cord as it crosses the pubic tubercle.
Diagnostic Studies.   An abdominal radiograph can be helpful if air is present below the inguinal ligament. Ultrasonography can differentiate a hernia from a hydrocele and is especially helpful if an incarcerated hernia is suspected.

Differential Diagnosis
Hydrocele, undescended testes (coexist in 15%), and inguinal lymphadenopathy are included in the differential diagnosis.

Management
If a child is seen with a hernia, an attempt should be made to reduce it, and the child should be referred to a surgeon or urologist for repair within 1 to 2 weeks. Even if no swelling is seen at the visit but is elicited by the history, the child should be referred to a surgeon or urologist. Inguinal hernias do not resolve spontaneously. Premature infants can be deferred until 42 weeks of gestation if the hernia is reducible. If the hernia is not easily reduced, if it is painful, or if a hard, tender, or red mass is present, refer immediately. If reduction has been difficult and ischemia is ongoing, hospitalization and surgical repair within 24 to 48 hours are indicated.

Patient Education, Prevention, and Prognosis
Incarceration and strangulation of a hernia cause pain, irritability, erythema, vomiting, and abdominal distention. The risk of incarceration is greater than 60% in premature infants, so repair is recommended before discharge (Schnitzer, 2006). The overall incidence of incarceration is 12% to 17%, and two thirds of incarcerated hernias occur during the first year of life (Aiken, 2004). Either of these conditions should be treated as a surgical emergency. Bowel ischemia is of immediate concern, and testicular injury can occur from torsion as a result of the direct pressure of the incarcerated hernia or as a result of ischemia from cord compression (Leslie & Cain, 2006).

Because of the 40% to 60% contralateral occurrence of hernias in children, bilateral exploration is usually done at the time of surgery in infants younger than 1 year old. If surgery is deferred, parents must be aware of the signs and symptoms of incarceration (tenderness, redness, crying, nausea, vomiting, abdominal distention) and be cautioned to seek immediate evaluation by a medical provider should they occur.

TESTICULAR MASSES
Description
A mass located on the testicle is most often a malignancy.

Epidemiology
Testicular tumors are most common between 15 and 35 years old, but can be found anytime after 14 years old. Three percent of all cancer deaths in this age group are due to testicular cancer, affecting 1 in 10,000 teens. Bilateral tumors occur in 2% to 4% of patients; however, one third of all tumors are benign (Adelman & Joffe, 2005; Kaplan, 2000).

Clinical Findings
History
- Family history of testicular cancer
- Sensation of fullness or heaviness
- Possibly no complaints because testicular masses cause little or no pain and are often small
- Cryptorchidism, trauma, and atrophy
Physical Examination
- A hard, painless lump the size of a pea is palpated on the testis. Note the character and extension of the mass.
- The mass does not transilluminate.
- A hydrocele is present in 10% of malignancies; swelling in up to 73% of malignancies (Adelman & Joffe, 2005).
- The abdomen and supraclavicular areas should be assessed for any palpable nodes.
Diagnostic Studies
- Scrotal sonography to establish the exact location of the mass and differentiate a cystic from a solid mass
- CT scan to evaluate for metastasis

- Once a tumor is suspected levels of α-fetoprotein, ß-unit of hCG, and lactate dehydrogenase are indicated

Differential Diagnosis

Intratesticular masses, which are almost always malignant, must be differentiated from extratesticular masses, such as hernia, varicocele, hydrocele, or spermatocele.

Management

Any child or adolescent with a testicular mass must be referred immediately for further evaluation. Treatment is dependent on the stage and type of tumor and can include orchiectomy, irradiation, and chemotherapy.

Patient Education, Prevention, and Prognosis

Metastasis may have occurred before the initial tumor is noticed. Pay attention to complaints about back or abdominal pain, unexplained weight loss, dyspnea (pulmonary metastases), gynecomastia, supraclavicular adenopathy, urinary obstruction, or a "heavy" or "dragging" sensation (Adelman & Joffe, 2005).

Early detection and therapeutic intervention can lead to a 90% survival rate. Ninety percent of relapses occur in the first 12 months after treatment. Testicular examination must not only be routinely done during physical examinations but must also be taught to adolescent males (see Fig. 34-12).

PHIMOSIS AND PARAPHIMOSIS

Description

Phimosis refers to a foreskin that is too tight to be retracted over the glans penis. Physiologic or primary phimosis occurs over the first 6 years of life when the glans has not completely separated from the epithelium. Pathologic or secondary phimosis occurs when the foreskin cannot be retracted after previously being retracted or after puberty. Paraphimosis is the opposite, a retracted foreskin that cannot be reduced to the normal position.

Etiology and Incidence

Phimosis can be congenital or acquired from infection and inflammation under the foreskin. Paraphimosis causes constriction of the penis and results in edema of the glans, pain, and possible necrosis. Paraphimosis is most common in adolescents and can follow masturbation, sexual abuse, or forceful retraction.

Clinical Findings
History
- May be a history of infection or inflammation of the penis
- Retraction of the foreskin with an inability to reduce it (paraphimosis)
- Pain and dysuria
- Signs of urinary obstruction
  - Ballooning of the foreskin with urination
  - Abnormal intermittent urinary stream
Physical Examination
- Phimosis—a tight, pinpoint opening of the foreskin with minimal ability to retract the foreskin; foreskin flat and effaced
- Pathologic phimosis—thickened rolled foreskin

- Paraphimosis—edema and bluish discoloration of the glans and foreskin

Management
Management includes the following:
- Phimosis:
  - Normal cleansing with gentle stretching of the foreskin until resistance. Most foreskins are retractable by 5 or 6 years old. Never forcefully retract the foreskin.
  - Circumcision is indicated if urinary obstruction or infection is present.
  - Persistent phimosis can be treated with a 0.05% or 0.1% betamethasone cream for 2 to 6 weeks. This frequently allows successful retraction of the foreskin and promotes awareness of improved hygiene (Leslie & Cain, 2006).
- Paraphimosis:
  - A trial of ice may be done to reduce the swelling and allow reduction of the foreskin. Reduction may be accomplished by using the index and third fingers to hold the penis with gauze proximal to the foreskin and by pushing the glans penis back with the thumbs. If this technique is not successful, surgical release of the constricting band must be done to prevent necrosis of the glans.
  - Severe paraphimosis is a surgical emergency.
  - Investigation of events leading to the paraphimosis is needed to rule out sexual abuse.

Patient Education, Prevention, and Prognosis
Infection, urinary obstruction, and reflux can occur with phimosis; however, a tight foreskin in uncircumcised males is normal and usually resolves by 6 years old. It is not an indication for circumcision. Necrosis of the penis is possible with paraphimosis. The foreskin of infants and children should never be forced back.

BALANITIS AND BALANOPOSTHITIS

Description
Balanitis is an inflammation of the glans; balanoposthitis is an inflammation of the foreskin and glans penis occurring in males with phimosis or in uncircumcised males.

Epidemiology
Accumulation of debris under the foreskin, probably resulting from poor hygiene, irritates the foreskin and glans and leads to infection. If purulent discharge with fiery-red erythema and moist translucent exudates is present, streptococcal etiology should be considered. Skin flora are the usual causes of infection, but gram-negative bacteria can be involved. If a urethral discharge is present, an STI must be considered (Leslie & Cain, 2006). Occasionally, trauma or allergy can be the cause.

Clinical Findings
History
- A fussy infant
- Pain and dysuria in an older child
Physical Examination
- Edema and inflammation are noted on the foreskin and glans.

Diagnostic Studies
- Cultures

Management
Antibiotics, both topically and orally, as directed by the cultures, along with warm soaks in the bathtub are prescribed. Depending on the swelling, topical steroids might also be prescribed (Leslie & Cain, 2006).

Patient Education, Prevention, and Prognosis
Paraphimosis can occur with severe infections; however, forcible retraction of the foreskin is to be avoided. A review of proper hygiene and the removal of irritants are needed. Occurrence is not an indication for circumcision.

SCROTAL TRAUMA
Description
Trauma to the scrotum most often occurs as a result of sports participation or play.

Epidemiology
Direct blows to the scrotum and straddle injuries are the most common causes of trauma. In a prepubertal child, the testicle is often spared damage because of the small size and mobility of the testes. Damage can occur when the testicle is forcibly compressed against the pubic bones. Significant symptoms (swelling, discoloration, and tenderness) from minor trauma suggest an underlying tumor.

Clinical Findings
History
- Pain after some type of injury; older children and adolescents usually report a specific mechanism of injury, time, and place (Leslie & Cain, 2006).
Physical Examination
- Swelling, discoloration, ecchymosis, and tenderness of the scrotum.
- Clear transillumination is compromised if a hematoma is present.

Diagnostic Studies. Ultrasound is useful to differentiate the degree and type of injury and assess for testicular rupture (Leslie & Cain, 2006).

Differential Diagnosis
Urethritis, epididymitis, orchitis, and prostatitis should all be included in the differential diagnosis. Degrees of injury include the following:
- Traumatic epididymitis—inflammation, but no infection. Pain and tenderness with scrotal erythema and edema and a tender indurated epididymis develop within a few days after injury. UA and Doppler ultrasonographic findings are normal. The course is usually acute, but short lived.
- Intratesticular hematoma.
- Hematocele with contusion and ecchymosis of the scrotal wall with severe scrotal injury.
- Testicular torsion.

Management
- NSAIDs, cool compresses, scrotal support or elevation, and bed rest are modalities used to help relieve pain.
- An enlarging scrotum merits immediate surgical exploration, as does hematocele.

Patient Education, Prevention, and Prognosis
On rare occasion, testicular rupture can occur and be manifested by massive swelling and ecchymosis. An athletic cup should be worn when participating in any sport in which injury could occur. A testicular mass should be considered cancer until proved otherwise.

TESTICULAR TORSION
Description
Testicular torsion, a severely painful condition of acute onset in which interruption of the blood supply to the testis causes subsequent ischemic injury, results in an emergency surgical situation.

Epidemiology
Normal fixation of the testis is absent, so the testis can rotate and block lymphatic and then blood flow. Torsion can occur after physical exertion, trauma, or on arising.

Torsion occurs at any age, but most commonly in adolescence, with a peak at 15 to 16 years old (1 in 4000 males younger than 25 years old and a cluster in infancy) (Adleman & Joffe, 2000; Leslie & Cain, 2006). The left side is twice as likely to be involved because of the longer spermatic cord.

Clinical Findings
History. The following may be reported:
- Unilateral pain that starts acutely and gradually and progressively worsens (the cardinal symptom); it can be scrotal or testicular and may worsen if elevated.
- Minor trauma, physical exertion, or onset of acute pain on arising is possible.
- Prior episodes of transient pain are reported in about half of the patients.
- Nausea, vomiting, or anorexia may occur.
- May be described as abdominal or inguinal pain by the embarrassed child.
- Fever is minimal or absent.

Physical Examination. Findings include the following:
- Ill-appearing and anxious male resisting movement.
- Gradual, progressive swelling of involved scrotum with redness, warmth, and tenderness.
- The ipsilateral scrotum can be edematous, erythematous, and warm.
- Testis swollen larger than opposite side, elevated, lying transversely, exquisitely painful.
- Spermatic cord thickened, twisted, and tender.
- Slight elevation of the testis increases pain (in epididymitis it relieves pain).
- Transillumination can reveal a solid mass.
- The cremasteric reflex is absent on the side with torsion.

- Neonate—hard, painless, nontransilluminating mass with edema or discolored scrotal skin.

Diagnostic Studies. Potential studies to consider include:

- Doppler ultrasound
- CBC (possible elevated WBC count); probably not useful
- UA (usually normal)
- Radiographic imaging (color ultrasonography or nuclear scintigraphy) to measure intratesticular blood flow if the diagnosis is in question (Bennett et al, 2002)

Differential Diagnosis

Torsion of the testicular or epididymal appendage, acute epididymitis (mild to moderate pain of gradual onset), orchitis, trauma (pain is better within an hour), hernia, hydrocele, and varicocele are included in the differential diagnosis.

Management

Testicular torsion is a surgical emergency, and identification with prompt surgical referral must occur immediately. If surgery is performed within 3 hours, the testicle salvage rate is 100%; the rate drops to 92% by 6 hours, 62% between 6 and 12 hours, and 38% at 12 to 24 hours. Intervention beyond 48 hours rarely results in salvage (Leslie & Cain, 2006). Occasionally, manual reduction can be performed, but surgery should follow within 6 to 12 hours to prevent retorsion, preserve fertility, and prevent abscess and atrophy. Contralateral orchiopexy may be done because of a 50% occurrence of torsion in nonfixed testes. Rest and scrotal support do not provide relief.

Patient Education, Prevention, and Prognosis

Testicular atrophy, abscess, or decreased fertility and loss of the testis as a result of necrosis can occur if the torsion persists more than 24 hours.

EPIDIDYMITIS

Description

Epididymitis is an inflammation of the epididymis that is painful and acute.

Epidemiology

Epididymitis is commonly caused by *N. gonorrhoeae* or *C. trachomatis* in the sexually active adolescent, with infection initially present in the urethra or bladder. However, it can also be caused by a viral, coliform bacterial, or tubercular infection; by chemical irritation; by anomalies of the genitourinary tract; or by dysfunctional voiding. It is rare before puberty, but does occur in children younger than 2 years old with genitourinary tract abnormalities (Ogunfiditimi, 2005).

Clinical Findings

History. The following may be reported:

- Sexual encounters within 45 days
- Painful scrotal swelling, usually gradual but can be acute in onset
- Dysuria and frequency or obstructive voiding
- Trauma (less than 50%)
- Fever, nausea, vomiting (less than 50%)

Physical Examination. Findings include the following:

- Scrotal edema and erythema are noted.
- The epididymis is hard, indurated, enlarged, and tender; the spermatic cord is tender.
- The testis has normal position and consistency.
- The cremasteric reflex is normal (not present in older adolescents).
- Prehn's sign—elevation of testis relieves pain (in torsion it increases pain)—can be elicited.
- Hydrocele may be present as a reaction to inflammation.
- Urethral discharge may be present, purulent in gonorrhea, and scant and watery in chlamydial infection if associated with urethritis.
- Rectal examination reveals prostate tenderness and can produce a urethral discharge.

Diagnostic Studies. The following are done as indicated:

- UA (pyuria and occasional bacteria may be present)
- CBC (elevated WBC count)
- Urethral culture and Gram stain (urine nucleic acid amplification tests may be done for gonococci and chlamydia)
- Testing for other STIs if there is a history of sexual activity
- Doppler ultrasonography or radionuclide imaging to differentiate torsion of the testis
- Follow-up VCUG, ultrasonography, or both in prepubertal children and in those who deny sexual activity, to rule out urogenital problems

Differential Diagnosis

The differential diagnosis includes testicular torsion of the spermatic cord or appendix testis, hernia, hydrocele, varicocele, spermatocele, trauma, tumor, or concomitant urethritis. Testicular cancer has been confused with epididymitis.

Management

Management is directed toward symptom relief and treatment of a causative organism if found. The following steps are taken:

- Bed rest, scrotal support, and elevation; apply ice packs as tolerated.
- Sitz baths and analgesics or NSAIDs are administered to relieve pain.
- Antibiotic treatment (CDC, 2006):
  - First line: ceftriaxone (250 mg intramuscularly one time) plus doxycycline (100 mg twice a day for 10 days)
  - Alternative treatments: ofloxacin (300 mg twice a day for 10 days) or levofloxacin (500 mg once a day for 10 days)
- Referral to a urologist is indicated if a solitary testicle is involved, if a prompt response to treatment does not occur, or if a question about the diagnosis remains.
- Treatment of sexual partner(s) from the last 60 days is indicated if caused by an STI. Intercourse should be avoided until cured.

- Follow-up is needed within 3 days if no improvement is seen or if symptoms recur after treatment. Follow-up after antibiotics is recommended to ensure that no palpable mass remains.

Patient Education

Infertility, abscess formation, testicular infarction, and late atrophy are possible but rare complications of epididymitis.

Because epididymitis is usually caused by an STI, partners must be evaluated and treated. Patients must understand the sexually transmitted etiology of this disease. Pain and edema usually resolve within 1 week.

RESOURCE BOX

American Association of Kidney Patients
www.aakp.org
Newsletter, informational materials, networking, advocacy, maintain research registry

American Foundation for Urologic Disease
www.auafoundation.org
Organization that helps the prevention and cure of urologic diseases with its research, advocacy, and education of health care professionals and the public

IgA Nephropathy Support Network
www.igansupport.org

National Cancer Institute: Wilms Tumor Information
www.cancer.gov/CancerInformation/CancerType/wilms-tumor

National Institute of Diabetes and Digestive and Kidney Disease
www.niddk.nih.gov

National Kidney and Urologic Diseases Information Clearinghouse
www.kidney.niddk.nih.gov/index.htm
Newsletter, informational materials, networking, referrals to local resources, maintain research registry

National Kidney Foundation
www.kidney.org
Newsletter, informational materials, referrals to local resources, local chapters, fund research

National Wilms Tumor Study
www.nwtsg.org

Testicular Cancer Awareness Week
www.tcaw.org
Patient handout sheet on testicular self-examination and the opportunity to sign up to receive monthly reminders to perform testicular self-examination

✓ DISCUSSION FORUM

1. How does your follow-up vary in a 3-month-old with a UTI, 8-year-old female, and a 16-year-old female? What things are you concerned about in each age group?
2. A 4-year-old male has a chief complaint of "his foreskin will not retract." The exam is otherwise normal. What do you want to advise the parent? How would this vary if the child was a 13-year-old male, Tanner IV?
3. What would you do if a 15-year-old refused a genitalia exam during a well visit?
4. What are the recommendations for a screening UA from the AAP, *Bright Futures*, and U.S. Preventive Health Task Force for an 8-year-old? What are the recommendations for an adolescent? Why do the recommendations vary? Why do they vary by age?

REFERENCES

Adelman WP, Joffe A: Testicular masses/cancer, *Pediatr Rev* 26(9):335-337, 2005.
Adelman WP, Joffe A: The adolescent with a painful scrotum, *Contemp Pediatr* 17(3):111-128, 2000.

Agency for Healthcare Research and Quality (AHRQ): *Pocket guide to clinical preventive services, 2005*. Available from www.ahrq.gov/clinic/ppipx (accessed September 24, 2006).
Aiken, JJ: Inguinal hernias. In Behrman RE, Kliegman RM, Jensen HB, editors: *Nelson textbook of pediatrics*, ed 17, Philadelphia, 2004, WB Saunders.
Alon US: Renal tubular acidosis. In Finburg L, Kleinman RE, editors: *Saunders manual of pediatric practice*, ed 2, Philadelphia, 2002, WB Saunders.
Alon US: Urinary tract infection and perinephric/intranephric abscess. In Burg FD et al, editors: *Current pediatric therapy*, ed 18, Philadelphia, 2006, WB Saunders.
American Academy of Pediatrics (AAP): The diagnosis, treatment, and evaluation of the initial urinary tract infection in febrile infants and young children. In *Pediatric clinical practice guidelines and policies: a compendium of evidence-based research for pediatric practice*, ed 7, Elk Grove Village, IL, 2007, American Academy of Pediatrics.
American Academy of Pediatrics (AAP), Action Committee of the Urology Section: Timing of elective surgery of the genitalia of children with particular reference to the risks, benefits and psychological effects of surgery and anesthesia, *Pediatrics* 97:590-594, 1996.
American Academy of Pediatrics (AAP), Committee on Practice and Ambulatory Care: Recommendations for preventive pediatric health care, *Pediatrics* 105(3):645-646, 2000.
American Urological Association (AUA) Practice Parameters, Guidelines and Standards Committee: *Report on the Management of Primary Vesicoureteral Reflux in Children*, Baltimore, 1997, American Urological Association (a classic study).

Arant BS: Vesicoureteral reflux and evidence-based management, *J Pediatr* 139(5):620-621, 2002.

Bennett S et al: *Ultrasound findings as predictors of clinical outcomes in the acute scrotum (abstract 427).* Program and Abstracts of the American Urological Association 97th Annual Meeting in Orlando, FL, May 25-30, 2002.

Bergstein J, Leiser J, Andreoli S: The clinical significance of asymptomatic gross and microscopic hematuria in children, *Arch Pediatr Adolesc Med* 159:353-355, 2005.

Bloom TL, Kolon TF: Gross hematuria in a healthy adolescent, *Clinical Advisor* 8:99-100, 2005.

Blowey DL: Acute glomerulonephritis. In Finburg L, Kleinman RE, editors: *Saunders manual of pediatric practice,* ed 2, Philadelphia, 2002, WB Saunders.

Boineau FG, Lewy JE: Evaluation of hematuria in children and adolescents, *Pediatr Rev* 11(4):101-107, 1989.

Bright Futures: guidelines for health supervision of infants, children and adolescents, ed 2, revised, Arlington, VA, 2000-2002, National Center for Education in Maternal and Child Health.

Callaghan P: Undescended testis, *Pediatr Rev* 21(11):395, 2000.

Cascio S, Colhoun E, Puri P: Bacterial colonization of the prepuce in boys with vesicoureteral reflux who receive antibiotic prophylaxis, *J Pediatr* 139(1):160-162, 2001.

Centers for Disease Control and Prevention (CDC): *Sexually transmitted diseases: 2006 treatment guidelines.* Available from *www.cdc.gov/std/treatment/default.htm* (accessed Sept 24, 2006).

Centers for Disease Control and Prevention (CDC): Screening tests to detect *Chlamydia trachomatis* and *Neisseria gonorrhoeae* infections—2002, *MMWR* 2002:51(No. RR-15). Available from *www.cdc.gov/STD/labguidelines/* (accessed Sept 24, 2006).

Chan JC, Foreman JW: The nephrotic syndrome. In Burg FD et al, editors: *Current pediatric therapy,* ed 18, Philadelphia, 2006, WB Saunders.

Chan KM, Scheinman JI, Roth KS: Renal tubular acidosis, *Pediatr Rev* 22(8):277-286, 2001.

Chang SL, Shortliffe LD: Pediatric urinary tract infections, *Pediatr Clin North Am* 53(3):379-400, 2006.

Constantinescu AR: Renal tubulopathies. In Burg FD et al, editors: *Current pediatric therapy,* ed 18, Philadelphia, 2006, WB Saunders.

Davis ID, Avner ED: Conditions particularly associated with hematuria. In Behrman RE, Kliegman RM, Jensen HB, editors: *Nelson textbook of pediatrics,* ed 17, Philadelphia, 2004, WB Saunders.

Decter RM: Vesicoureteral reflux, *Pediatr Rev* 22(6):205-209, 2001.

Dell KM, Avner ED: Tubular disorders. In Behrman RE, Kliegman RM, Jensen HB, editors: *Nelson textbook of pediatrics,* ed 17, Philadelphia, 2004, WB Saunders.

Elder JS: Urologic disorders in infants and children. In Behrman RE, Kliegman RM, Jensen HB, editors: *Nelson textbook of pediatrics,* ed 17, Philadelphia, 2004, WB Saunders.

Elias ER, Tsai AC, Manchester DK: Genetics and dysmorphology. In Hay WW et al: *Current pediatric diagnosis and treatment,* ed 18, New York, 2006, McGraw Hill.

Ferguson WS: Visceral tumors. In Burg FD et al, editors: *Current pediatric therapy,* ed 18, Philadelphia, 2006, WB Saunders.

Ferrer FA, McKenna PH: Current approaches to the undescended testicle, *Contemp Pediatr* 17(1):106-111, 2000.

Finberg L. & Kleinman R: *Saunders manual of pediatric practice,* ed 2, Philadelphia, 2002, WB Saunders 2002.

Friedman AL: Nephrology: fluids and electrolytes. In Behrman RE, Kliegman RM, editors: *Nelson essentials of pediatrics,* ed 17, Philadelphia, 2004, WB Saunders.

Garin EH et al: Clinical significance of primary vesicoureteral reflux and urinary antibiotic prophylaxis after acute pyelonephritis: a multicenter, randomized controlled study, *Pediatrics* 117:626-632, 2006.

Gillespie RS, Stapleton FB: Nephrolithiasis in children, *Pediatr Rev* 25:131-11138, 2004.

Greenbaum LA, Mesrobian HO: Vesicoureteral reflux, *Pediatr Clin North Am* 53(3):413-428, 2006.

Halverson L, Alper BS: Hematuria, *Clin Advisor* 9(3):93-94, 2006.

Hussain N et al: Hypospadias and early gestation growth restriction in infants, *Pediatrics* 109(3):473-478, 2002.

Ingelfinger JR: Disorders of the bladder and urethra, ureter and collecting system. In Burg FD et al, editors: *Gellis and Kagan's current pediatric therapy,* ed 17, Philadelphia, 2002, WB Saunders.

Institute for Clinical Systems Improvement [ICSI]: *Healthcare guideline: preventive services for children and adolescents,* Bloomington, MN, 2005, National Guideline Clearinghouse at Agency for Healthcare Research and Quality (AHRQ). Available from *www.guideline.gov* (accessed Sept 24, 2006).

Jaffe N, Huff V: Neoplasms of the kidney. In Behrman RE, Kliegman RM, editors: *Nelson essentials of pediatrics,* ed 17, Philadelphia, 2004, WB Saunders.

Kaplan GW: Scrotal swelling in children, *Pediatr Rev* 21(9):311-314, 2000.

Kass EJ: Adolescent varicocele, *Pediatr Clin North Am* 48(6):1559-1570, 2001.

Kurzrock EA: Hypospadias. In Behrman RE, Kliegman RM, editors: *Nelson essentials of pediatrics,* ed 17, Philadelphia, 2004, WB Saunders.

Larcombe J: Urinary tract infection, *Clin Evidence,* June 2002, pp 65-67.

Leslie JA, Cain MP: Pediatric emergencies and urgencies, *Pediatr Clin North Am* 53(3):513-528, 2006.

Lum GM: Kidney and urinary tract. In Hay WW et al, editors: *Current pediatric diagnosis and treatment,* ed 18, New York, 2007, McGraw-Hill.

MacLellan DL, Diamond DA: Recent advances in external genitalia, *Pediatr Clin North Am* 53(3):449-464, 2006.

Mahant S, To T, Friedman J: Timing of voiding cystourethrogram in the investigation of urinary tract infections in children, *Pediatrics* 139(4):568-571, 2001.

Nachman JB, Abelson HT: Wilms tumor. In Behrman RE, Kliegman RM, editors: *Nelson essentials of pediatrics,* ed 17, Philadelphia, 2004, WB Saunders.

The National Wilms Tumor Study. Available from *http://nwtsg.org* (accessed Oct 20, 2006).

Newman TB et al: Urine testing and urinary tract infections in febrile infants seen in office settings, *Arch Pediatr Adolesc Med* 156(1):44-54, 2002.

Nicoletta JA, Lande MB: Medical evaluation and treatment of urolithiasis, *Pediatr Clin North Am* 53(3):479-492, 2006.

Ogunfiditimi F: Testicular disorders: What you should know, *Clin Advisor* 8(9):31-36, 2005.

Omokaro S: Nephrology. In Robertson, Shilkofski, editors: *Johns Hopkins Hospital: the Harriet Lane handbook,* ed 17, St Louis, 2005, Mosby.

Pan CG: Evaluation of gross hematuria, *Pediatr Clin North Am* 53(3):401-412, 2006.

Patel HP: The abnormal urinalysis, *Pediatr Clin North Am* 53(3):325-338, 2006.

Patel HP, Bissler JJ: Hematuria in children, *Pediatr Clin North Am* 48(6):1519-1538, 2001.

Raszka WV, Khan O: Pyelonephritis, *Pediatr Rev* 26:358-363, 2005.

Reiter EO, Saenger PH: Undescended testes. In Finberg L, Kleinman RE: *Saunders manual of pediatric practice,* ed 2, Philadelphia, 2002, WB Saunders.

Schnitzer JJ: Hernias and hydroceles. In Burg FD et al, editors: *Current pediatric therapy,* ed 18, Philadelphia, 2006, WB Saunders.

Schöen EJ, Colby CJ, Ray GT: Newborn circumcision decreases incidence and costs of urinary tract infection during the first year of life, *Pediatrics* 105(4):789-793, 2000.

Schroeder AR et al: Choice of urine collection methods for diagnosis of urinary tract infection in young, febrile infants, *Arch Ped Adol Med* 159:915-922, 2005.

Sheldon CA: The pediatric genitourinary examination: inguinal, urethral and genital diseases, *Pediatr Clin North Am* 48(6):1339-1380, 2001.

Snodgrass WT: Hypospadias, *Pediatr Rev* 25:62-66, 2004.

Steinhurz PG: Wilms tumor. In Finburg L, Kleinman RE, editors: *Saunders manual of pediatric practice,* ed 2, Philadelphia, 2002, WB Saunders.

Tran D, Muchant DG, Aronoff SC: Short-course versus conventional length antimicrobial therapy for uncomplicated lower urinary tract infections in children: a meta-analysis of 1279 patients, *J Pediatr* 139(1):93-99, 2001.

US Preventive Health Services Task Force: *Pocket guide to clinical preventive services, 2005.* Available from *www.ahrq.gov/clinic/pocketgd05* (accessed Sept 24, 2006).

VanDeVoorde RG, Bissler JJ: Hematuria and proteinuria. In Burg FD et al, editors: *Current pediatric therapy*, ed 18, Philadelphia, 2006, Elsevier.

Vogt BA, Avner, ED: Conditions particularly associated with proteinuria. In Behrman RE, Kliegman RM, editors: *Nelson essentials of pediatrics*, ed 17, Philadelphia, 2004, WB Saunders.

Wald ER: Vesicoureteral reflux: the role of antibiotic prophylaxis, *Pediatrics* 117:919-922, 2006.

Wallace M, Sadovsky R: What clinicians should know about urinalysis, *Clin Advisor* 4:39-47, 2005.

Warshaw BL: Nephrotic syndrome in children, *Pediatr Ann* 23(9):495-504, 1994 (a classic study).

CHAPTER 35

Gynecologic Conditions

Teral Gerlt and Nancy Barber Starr

Pediatric gynecology can provide the health care provider with varied and interesting challenges. Knowledge, sensitivity, and comfort with gynecology will aid the pediatric provider in working with the child or adolescent and the parent. Educating children and adolescents about their bodies as they mature is essential. Approaching issues that may be considered personal or embarrassing, openly and directly allows more comprehensive care and an opportunity for anticipatory guidance. Establishing and maintaining a good relationship with both parents and adolescents helps ease the transition during which adolescents take an increasingly larger role in determining their own care.

Gynecologic (GYN) issues range from normal transitions that may be perceived as abnormal to serious systemic diseases or abnormalities. The provider should have an elevated index of suspicion in all cases so as to not overlook significant signs and symptoms. At the same time, most conditions are normal and can be easily addressed, reassuring the child, adolescent, and/or parent that all is well and that her body is developing normally.

■ STANDARDS OF CARE

Healthy People 2010 (U.S. Department of Health and Human Services, 2000) has multiple objectives that are applicable to children and adolescents. Those that fall into pediatric gynecology are to promote responsible sexual behaviors, and reduce teen pregnancies, sexually transmitted infections (STIs), and human immunodeficiency virus (HIV) infections in adolescents.

The American Medical Association (AMA) *Guidelines for Adolescent Preventive Services (GAPS)* (AMA, 1997) recommends as a routine part of annual health supervision asking all adolescents about sexual health behaviors that place them at risk for pregnancy, STIs, and HIV. Further, they should receive counseling about responsible sexual behavior, including abstinence and the use of contraception and condoms to prevent pregnancy and infection with STIs and HIV. All sexually active adolescents should be screened for STIs (gonorrhea [GC], chlamydia, and syphilis if living in an endemic area) and HIV infection. The *Guide to Clinical Preventive Services* (U.S. Preventive Services Task Force, 2005) also recommends screening all sexually active women 25 years old and younger for chlamydia.

■ ANATOMY AND PHYSIOLOGY

For the first 6 to 7 weeks of gestation, male and female fetuses are sexually undifferentiated, both having two bipotential gonads and bilateral paramesonephric (müllerian) and mesonephric (wolffian) ducts. At this point, testicular differentiation begins at the direction

of the testes-determining factor on the Y chromosome. In the male gonad, the Sertoli cells produce antimüllerian hormone (AMH) which inhibits müllerian duct development, and the Leydig cells produce testosterone, which maintains wolffian duct development and causes them to differentiate into the epididymis, vas deferens, and the seminal vesicles.

Without the influence of the Y chromosome, the female gonads develop into ovaries by about 8 weeks gestation, and by 20 weeks the fetal ovary reaches mature compartmentalization. The müllerian ducts become the uterus and fallopian tubes, and the wolffian ducts regress. By week 22 of gestation, canalization to create the uterine cavity, cervical canal, and the vagina is complete.

The external genitalia are neutral primordial and able to develop into either male or female structures. The presence of testosterone from the testes will masculinize the external genitalia, whereas the lack of androgens allows female genitalia to form.

In utero, maternal estrogen thickens and enlarges the female genital structures. After birth, maternal hormones are withdrawn resulting in the desquamation of the hypertrophic walls of the uterus. The mucus from the cervix results in the physiologic leukorrhea of the newborn period. As the hormonal influences continue to decrease, the endometrial shedding may be accompanied by bleeding.

Between 8 weeks and 7 years of age, without maternal or endogenous estrogens, the labia majora are flat, the labia minora are thin, and neither offer protection to the genitalia. The absence of fat pads results in an open labia whenever the child is in the squatting position. In addition, this thin atrophic genital epithelium is readily traumatized.

The function of the reproductive system is controlled by the hypothalamic-pituitary-ovarian (HPO) axis. This complex process begins in the neurologic system (the hypothalamus), involves the endocrine system (the anterior pituitary), and completes its cycle with the gonads (ovaries). Initially, this cycle causes sexual maturation, and, once that is completed, the ongoing release of hormones controls the menstrual cycle, pregnancy, and lactation.

■ ASSESSMENT OF THE GYNECOLOGIC SYSTEM
HEALTH SUPERVISION VISITS FOR FEMALE ADOLESCENTS

The American College of Obstetricians and Gynecologists (ACOG) now recommends that young female adolescents have an initial reproductive health visit between 13 and 15 years old to provide preventive care, anticipatory guidance, and screening (ACOG, 2006b). This visit would include discussions of sexual development and reproductive issues rather than problem-focused care (Holland-Hall et al, 2005). Counseling and education about normal menses and patterns, pregnancy prevention, STIs, and HIV are essential; a pelvic exam would only be performed if indicated.

This visit is the perfect opportunity to discuss confidentiality with the patient and her parents. All need to understand the importance of confidentiality in the health care provider-patient relationship and the limits to confidentiality imposed by state and local statutes and/or medical necessity. A relationship of trust and mutual respect is extremely important to establish so that the adolescent to be willing to discuss intimate matters.

History

The history taken will depend on the age of the child and chief complaint. Histories for specific conditions are included later in this chapter. An in-depth sexual history for the adolescent can be found in Chapter 19. The sexual history should be completed with the parent out of the room.

The general history includes the following:
- Family history
  ◦ Maternal age at menarche and any problems encountered
  ◦ Dysmenorrhea, dysfunctional uterine bleeding (DUB), or endometriosis
  ◦ Diabetes mellitus
  ◦ Thyroid disease
  ◦ Bleeding or clotting disorders
  ◦ Cancer of the female reproductive system
  ◦ Genetic disorders
- Pubertal development
  ◦ Knowledge of pubertal development
  ◦ Age at breast and pubic hair development
  ◦ Age at menarche
  ◦ Length of cycles, longest and shortest interval between menses, duration of flow, estimated blood loss
  ◦ Last normal menstrual period (LNMP)
  ◦ Dysmenorrhea
- Sexual history
  ◦ Knowledge about sexuality and discussions with parent or guardian (see Chapter 19)
  ◦ Age at first intercourse (voluntary or forced)
  ◦ Current sexual activity
  ◦ Type of activity (oral, vaginal, anal)
  ◦ Partners of opposite sex, the same sex, or both
  ◦ Number of sexual partners in previous 60 days, 12 months, lifetime
  ◦ Previous vaginal infections or STIs
  ◦ Current exposures to STIs
  ◦ Last Pap test
  ◦ History of abnormal Pap test
- Contraceptive history
  ◦ Current method—type, duration, frequency of use, problems and satisfaction
  ◦ Past methods—type, duration, frequency of use, problems and satisfaction
  ◦ Obstetric history, as appropriate
  ◦ Review of systems: urinary, gastrointestinal, endocrine, dermatologic, general health, growth, stressors, medications, allergies, and substance use.

Physical Examination

A girl's first gynecologic examination can influence her attitude toward future gynecologic care. When a gynecologic examination is performed, the child or adolescent should maintain a feeling of being in control. It is important that the provider take the time to establish rapport, preserve modesty, give choices, and obtain consent to examine. It is also important that the parent understands what the exam entails and why it is necessary.

The adolescent should be given as many choices as possible; would she like someone else in the room with her; the position of the table; use of a hand mirror to observe; and when possible, the timing of the examination. This requires flexibility and time from the care provider, but demonstrates respect for the adolescent.

Prepubertal Child.   There are a variety of positions in which to examine the vulva, vestibule, and lower vagina of a prepubescent girl. Lying on a table, supine, with feet together and knees out ("frog legged") is generally the most comfortable for patients and provides ease of examination and obtaining of cultures if necessary. Another alternative is sitting up in the parent's lap with feet and knees frog legged. Putting the parent on the examination table with feet in the stirrups and the child on his or her lap with feet to the outside of the parent's legs is another alternative. If examination of the entire vagina is necessary, putting the child in knee-chest position on the examination table is the best position for noninvasive, internal examination of the vulva and vagina.

Examine or note the following:
- Breasts, abdomen, and inguinal area
- Presence and distribution of pubic hair
- Presence and distribution of body hair: face, chest, back, abdomen, legs, arms
- Skin lesions
- State of hygiene
- Anus for cleanliness, excoriation, or erythema
- Sexual maturity rating (SMR) or Tanner staging (see Chapter 8 and Figs. 8-3 and 8-4)
- Genital exam with gentle traction on the labia majora
  ◦ Size of clitoris (approximately 3×3 mm prepubertal)
  ◦ Signs of estrogenization (prepubertal vaginal mucosa—moist, thin, and red; postpubertal vaginal mucosa—moist and dull pink)
  ◦ The hymen is normally smooth and continuous
    - Described as crescent shaped, annular, or redundant (Fig. 35-1)
    - Presence of notches or tags—normal variation (Sugar & Graham, 2006)
    - Presence of hymenal ridge—usually without sequela (Sugar & Graham, 2006)
    - Imperforate hymen
  ◦ Periurethral bands

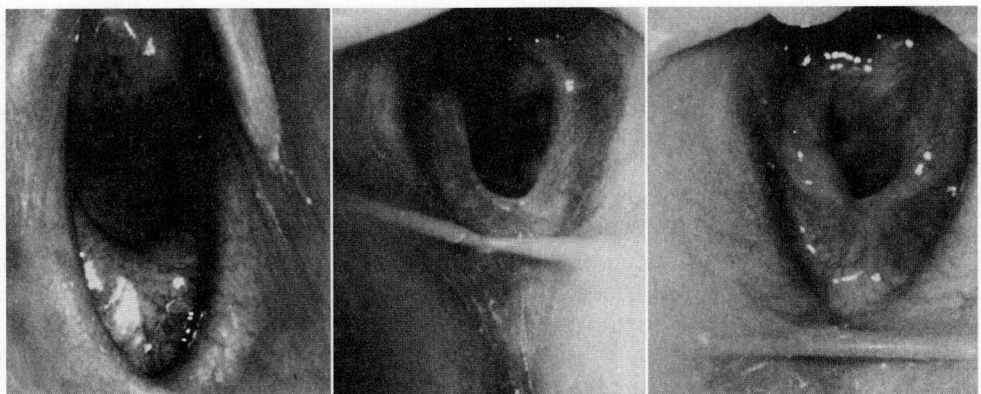

FIG. 35-1 Types of hymens, photographed through a colposcope. **A,** Crescentic hymen. **B,** Annular hymen. **C,** Redundant hymen with crescent appearance after retraction. (From Emans SJ: Vulvovaginal problems in the prepubertal child. In Emans SJ, Laufer MR, Goldstein DP, editors: *Pediatric and adolescent gynecology*, ed 5, Philadelphia, 2005, Lippincott Williams & Wilkins.)

The significance of the diameter of the hymenal opening as a diagnostic finding is debated. Both transverse and anterior-posterior diameters are dependent on age, relaxation, method of examination, and type of hymen. In general, the older and more relaxed the child, the larger the opening. It is also larger with retraction and in the knee-chest position. In the 3- to 6-year-old, a range of normal findings for the transverse diameter is 1 to 6 mm and for the anterior-posterior diameter, 1 to 7 mm. Obesity in young children is associated with hymenal openings larger than average for age (e.g., a 2-year-old with a 4-mm opening when average is 2 mm).

Adolescent

- Inspect the skin for acne.
- Examine the breasts; note Tanner stage.
- Palpate the thyroid.
- Inspect hair distribution on face, chest, back, arms, legs, and abdomen.
- Inspect the external genitalia and determine Tanner stage.
- Vaginal examination alone may be adequate to assess for irregular bleeding, severe dysmenorrhea, vaginal discharge, and amenorrhea. However, a speculum and a bimanual examination may be necessary based on symptoms and history.

Diagnostic Studies

The routine care of the child and adolescent without gynecologic complaints will not require diagnostic studies.

The following studies can be helpful as diagnostic tools. Specific studies and techniques are discussed with each diagnosis. Collection of specimens must be done with care. Techniques that are helpful include using a small amount of saline as a vaginal wash, using a soft plastic eyedropper or feeding tube, or using a moistened cotton swab.

- Wet mounts of vaginal secretions
  - Saline for microscopic examination to look for white blood cells (WBCs), clue cells, trichomonads, and bacteria
  - 10% KOH for whiff test and microscopic examination to look for yeast (branching hyphae and spores) (Fig. 35-2)
- pH of vaginal mucus (neutral in prepubescent; less than 4.5 once pubertal)

- Urine-based nucleic acid amplification test (NAAT), cultures, and/or serologic blood tests for STIs
- Other tests as indicated including pregnancy test by urine or serum, Biggy agar culture (suspected yeast infection), or ultrasound

Cervical Cancer Screening. The American Cancer Society recommends that cervical cancer screening with Pap testing should begin approximately 3 years after a young woman has initiated vaginal intercourse and no later than 21 years old (Saslow et al, 2002). After the initiation of cervical screening, the young women should have annual Pap testing with conventional cytology or every 2 years with liquid-based cytology.

The rationale for this recommendation is the increasing understanding of the natural history of human papillomavirus (HPV) infections, the causative agent of most cervical cancer. It is estimated that between 32% and 50% of sexually active young

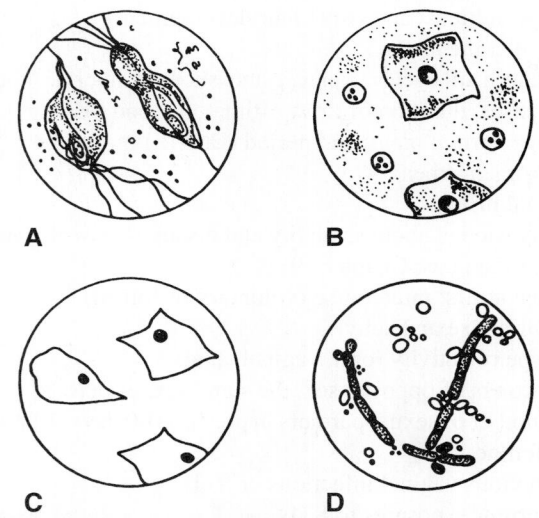

FIG. 35-2 Drawings of vaginal smears showing **A,** *Trichomonas*; **B,** clue cells of bacterial vaginosis; **C,** leukorrhea; **D,** *Candida*. **A, B,** and **C** are saline preparations; **D** is a potassium hydroxide (KOH) preparation. (From Emans SJ: Vulvovaginal problems in the prepubertal child. In Emans SJ, Laufer MR, Goldstein DP, editors: *Pediatric and adolescent gynecology*, ed 5, Philadelphia, 2005, Lippincott Williams & Wilkins.)

women have HPV (Kahn & Hillard, 2004). There is evidence that the majority of low grade HPV lesions will regress spontaneously. Therefore, Pap testing prior to recommended 3 years post-initiation of vaginal intercourse, was leading to overdiagnosis of cervical pathologic conditions and unnecessary interventions.

The health care provider's judgment should still play a role as to when to initiate Pap testing. It is important to get a thorough and accurate sexual history to assess for risk factors that could place the adolescent at increased risk of a high-grade cervical lesion. The ACOG (2004) recommends the following factors be considered:

- Early age of first vaginal intercourse
- Multiple sexual partners
- Male partner with multiple partners
- History of other STIs
- Immunocompromised status
- Risk of loss to follow-up

The ACOG Committee on Adolescent Health Care published a statement on the evaluation and management of cervical cytology in the adolescent (see ACOG, 2006a for complete recommendations). For an initial Pap test result of atypical squamous cells of undetermined significance (ASC-US) or low-grade squamous intraepithelial lesions (LSIL) the recommendation is to repeat the Pap in 6 and 12 months or do HPV-DNA testing at 12 months. Figure 35-3 includes a complete algorithm.

Hopefully, in the future, fewer young women will need colposcopy and cervical therapy with the advent of HPV vaccine and the change in management guidelines related to cervical cytology.

MANAGEMENT STRATEGIES
ANTICIPATORY GUIDANCE

Anticipatory guidance related to gynecologic issues is important to both the child or adolescent and parents. Attention to appropriate genital hygiene can help prevent some potential childhood problems. The transition to puberty and establishment of menses will be eased with appropriate education and counseling beforehand. With the advent of puberty and the increasing interest in sexuality, a great deal of guidance is needed to help the adolescent and her parents through these transitions. See Chapters 8 and 19 for further discussion of these topics.

COUNSELING AND EDUCATION

Counseling and education related to normal gynecologic conditions and disorders of the gynecologic system need to be tailored to the child or adolescent and the parents. Confidentiality is a matter to be established with both the parents and the adolescent. Some states have specific laws that allow providers to treat adolescents for obstetric and family planning conditions without parental knowledge or consent.

NORMAL GYNECOLOGIC SYSTEM AND COMMON VARIATIONS
PUBERTY

Puberty is the "coming together of multiple systems and influences, including genetic, metabolic, and hormonal factors" (Speroff & Fritz, 2005, p. 178). It is a process usually starting

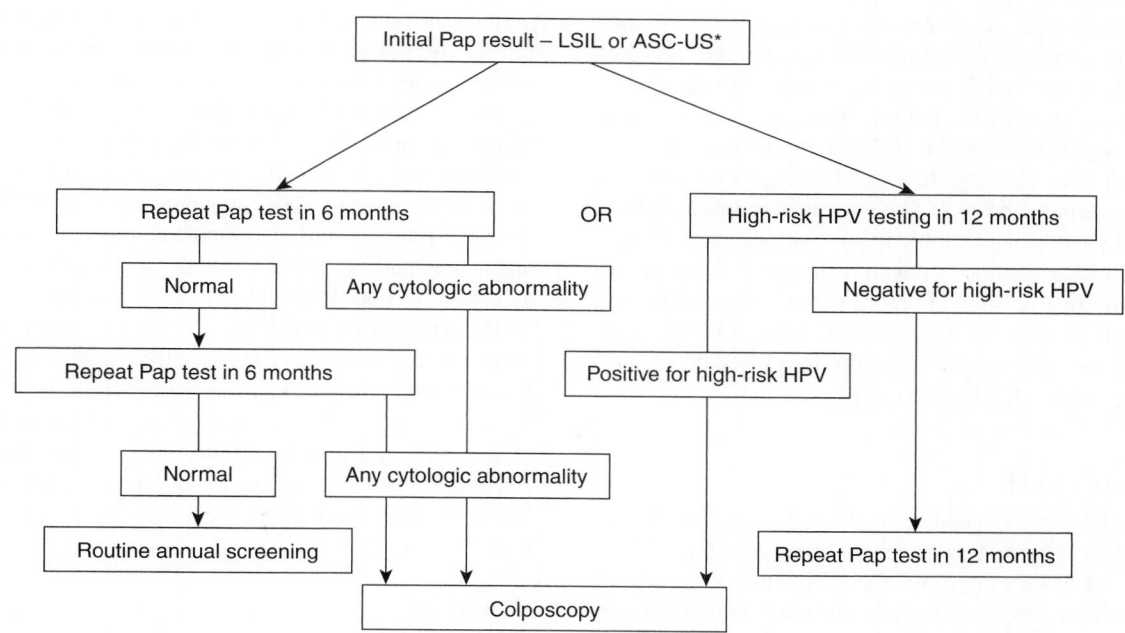

*Immediate colposcopy is an acceptable alternative for adolescents with LSIL or ASC-US

FIG. 35-3 *HPV*, Human papillomavirus. Management of low-grade squamous intraepithelial lesions (LSIL) or atypical squamous cells of undetermined significance (ASC-US) in the adolescent patient. (From American College of Obstetricians and Gynecologists: Committee opinion: evaluation and management of abnormal cervical typology and histology in the adolescent, *Obstet Gynecol* 107:966, 2006.)

with early breast development (thelarche), then growth of pubic and axillary hair (pubarche), and finally the first menses (menarche).

What sets this all in play is the reactivation of the HPO axis that has been suppressed since shortly after birth. The catalyst for this is unknown; however, there is a reduction of gonadotropin-releasing hormone (GnRH) suppression and decreased sensitivity of the negative feedback to estrogen, which leads to increasing GnRH pulsations to the anterior pituitary. This stimulates the anterior pituitary to release the gonadotropins; follicle-stimulating hormone (FSH) and luteinizing hormone (LH). These, in turn, stimulate the ovaries to synthesize estrogen (gonadarche). Increasing estrogen stimulates breast development, vaginal and uterine growth, skeletal growth, and female fat distribution. Independent of the HPO axis, increasing levels of adrenal androgens (adrenarche) lead to the growth of pubic and axillary hair. Finally, by midpuberty there is enough estrogen to cause endometrial proliferation, and the first menses occurs (menarche). Because early cycles are anovulatory 50% to 80% of the time in the first 2 to 3 years after menarche, menstrual irregularities and 21- to 45-day cycle lengths are common. Anovulatory cycles may continue 10% to 20% of the time up to 5 years after menarche (Harel, 2005).

On average, it takes approximately 4.5 years to traverse all the pubertal stages. The mean age of menarche in white American girls is between 12 and 13 years old and slightly earlier for African-American girls. This age has remained unchanged for more than 50 years. If a girl has not started breast development by 13 years old or had menarche by 16 years old, she is experiencing delayed puberty and should be evaluated for medical or genetic conditions. Likewise, precocious puberty, the early development of secondary sex characteristics, needs further evaluation. However, the age a further work-up is recommended varies by source. Traditionally, the definition of precocious puberty is breast or pubic hair development under 8 years old. In 1999, the Lawson Wilkins Pediatric Endocrine Society developed revised guidelines in response to research findings. Their recommendation, which remains unchanged since 1999, is to evaluate only if secondary sexual characteristics develop before 7 years old in Caucasian-American girls and before 6 years old in African-American girls (Kaplowitz & Oberfield, 1999). Others argue that lowering the age of work-up will miss girls with significant pathology (Mansfield, 2005).

MENSTRUAL CYCLE

The menstrual cycle is controlled by the HPO axis. It is essential that pediatric providers have an understanding of this complicated feedback system for the evaluation of menstrual disorders. GnRH from the hypothalamus plays both a permissive and supportive role. It has only positive actions on the anterior pituitary and causes syntheses, storage, activation, and secretion of gonadotropins. The GnRH secretion must be within a critical range of both frequency and concentration for the anterior pituitary to respond and secrete the FSH and LH

in a pulsatile fashion. The gonadotropin levels are then controlled by ovarian steroid feedback to the anterior pituitary.

Low levels of estrogen enhance FSH and LH synthesis and storage and inhibit FSH secretion but have little effect on LH secretion. High levels of estrogen induce the midcycle LH surge, and high steady levels lead to sustained elevated LH secretion. Low levels of progesterone act on the pituitary to enhance the LH response to GnRH and are responsible for the FSH surge at midcycle. High levels of progesterone antagonize pituitary response to GnRH with estrogen action and inhibit GnRH pulses at the hypothalamus. This results in inhibited pituitary secretion of gonadotropins.

The average adult menstrual cycle is 28 days with a range of 21 to 34 days. Fig. 35-4 illustrates the female reproductive cycle. The four phases of the cycle are:
- Menses—4 days plus or minus 2 days
- Follicular—10 to 14 days
- Ovulation—10 to 12 hours after LH surge
- Luteal—consistently close to 14 days plus or minus 3 days

The Follicular Phase

Initial follicular development occurs without hormonal influence. However, it is the stimulation by FSH that moves the follicles to the preantral stage.

Antral Follicle. The dominant follicle is established during cycle days 5 to 7, leading to increased levels of estradiol by day 7 (Figs. 35-4 and 35-5). The increasing estradiol suppresses FSH and leads to LH secretion. Estrogen also modifies the gonadotropin molecule, increasing the quality and the quantity of FSH and LH midcycle. LH levels rise steadily during the late follicular phase, stimulating the theca in the production of androgen. The action of FSH in the granulosa permits the dominant follicle to use androgen to make estrogen, further increasing estrogen production. FSH also stimulates LH receptors to form on the granulosa cells.

It is not the gonadotropins alone acting on the follicle; growth factors and autocrine and paracrine peptides also influence the feedback loop. Inhibin B, which is secreted by the granulosa cells in response to FSH, suppresses pituitary FSH. Activin, from the pituitary and the granulosa, augments FSH secretion and action, and insulin-like growth factor (IGF) acts to enhance all actions of both FSH and LH (Speroff & Fritz, 2005).

Preovulatory Follicle. When the estrogen levels are sufficient to induce the LH surge, the increasing LH initiates luteinization and progesterone production in the granulosa. This rise in progesterone assists the positive feedback action of estrogen and may be needed to stimulate the FSH peak midcycle. An increase in local and peripheral androgens also occurs midcycle from the thecal tissue of lesser follicles (Fig. 35-6).

Ovulation

The LH surge stimulates continuation of miosis in the oocyte, luteinization of the granulosa, and production of progesterone and prostaglandins within the follicle. Progesterone augments the activity of the proteolytic enzymes that, together with prostaglandins, are responsible for the digestion and rupture of the

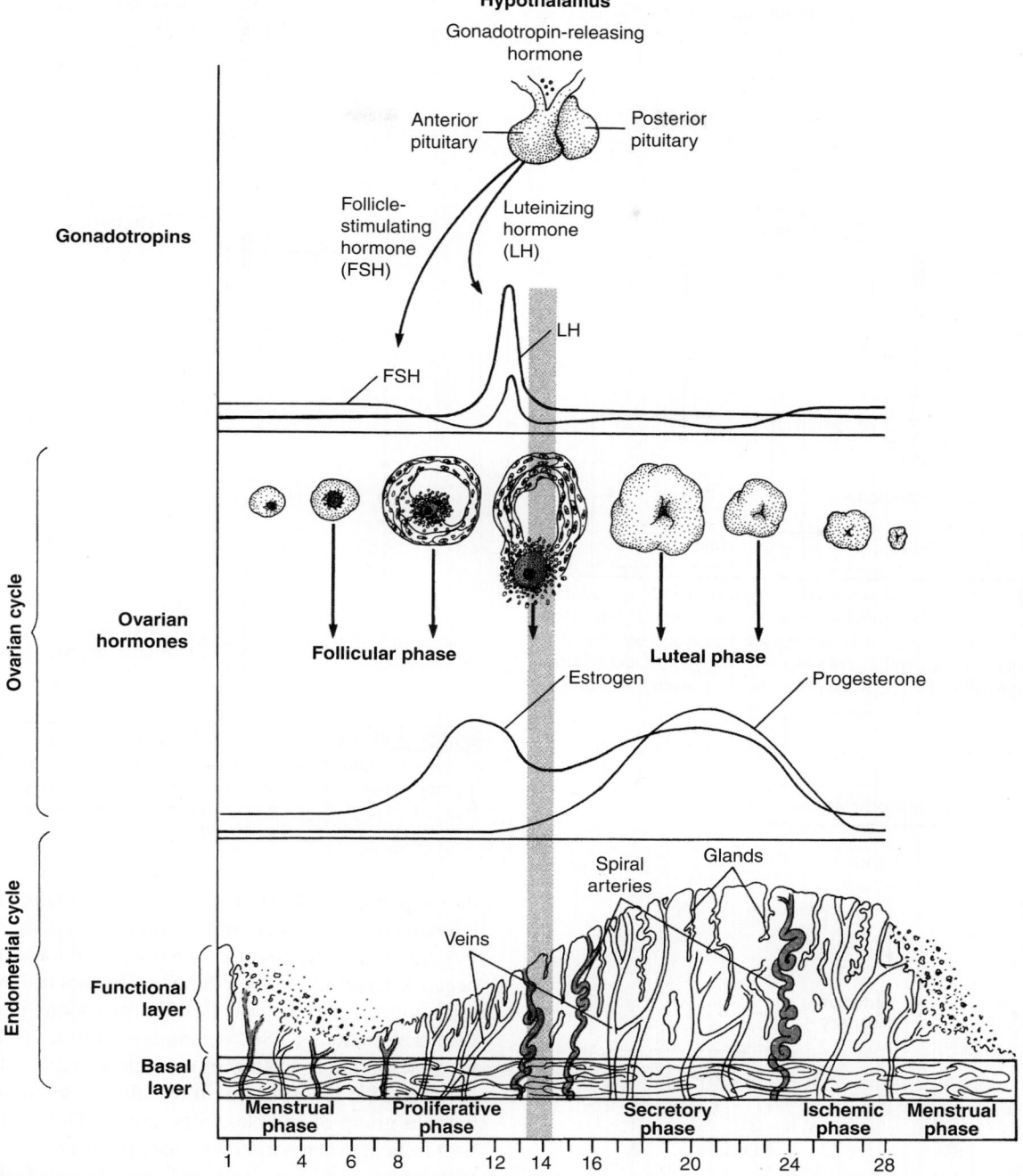

FIG. 35-4   Female reproductive cycle showing changes in hormone secretion and in the ovary and the uterine endometrium. (From Gorrie T, McKinney E, Murray S: *Foundations of maternal newborn nursing*, ed 2, Philadelphia, 1998, WB Saunders.)

follicular wall. The progesterone-influenced midcycle rise in FSH assists to free the oocyte from follicular attachments, to convert plasminogen to the proteolytic enzyme, plasmin, and to guarantee that adequate LH receptors are present to allow a normal luteal phase.

The Luteal Phase
A normal luteal phase requires both consummate preovulatory follicular development and the continued support of LH.

Centrally, progesterone, estrogen, and inhibin-A suppress new follicular growth. The regression of the corpus luteum may involve the luteolytic action of estrogen produced by the corpus luteum itself and is interceded by a modification in local prostaglandin and endothelin-1 concentrations (Fig. 35-7).

Luteal-Follicular Transition.   The loss of the corpus luteum causes a fall in circulating levels of estradiol, progesterone, and inhibin-A. The decreasing inhibin-A eliminates

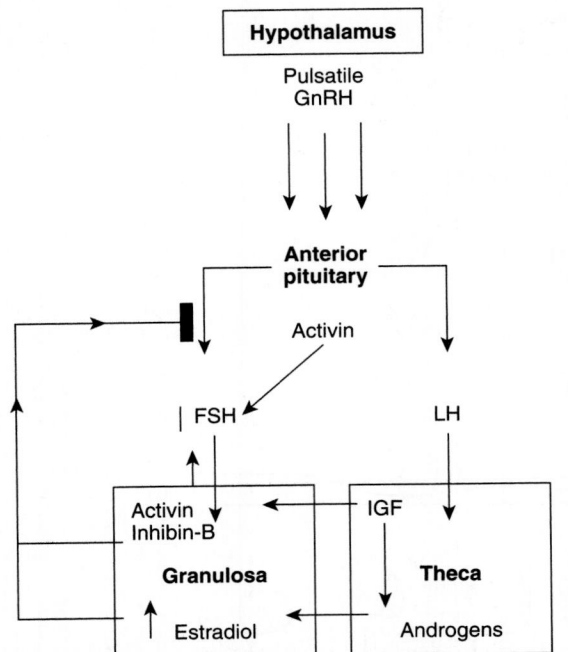

FIG. 35-5 Early follicular to midfollicular phase. *GnRH,* gonadotropin-releasing hormone; *FSH,* follicle-stimulating hormone; *LH,* luteinizing hormone; *IGF,* insulin-like growth factor; dark box represents negative feedback. (Data from Speroff L, Fritz MA: *Clinical gynecologic endocrinology and infertility,* ed 7, Philadelphia, 2005, Lippincott, Williams & Wilkins.)

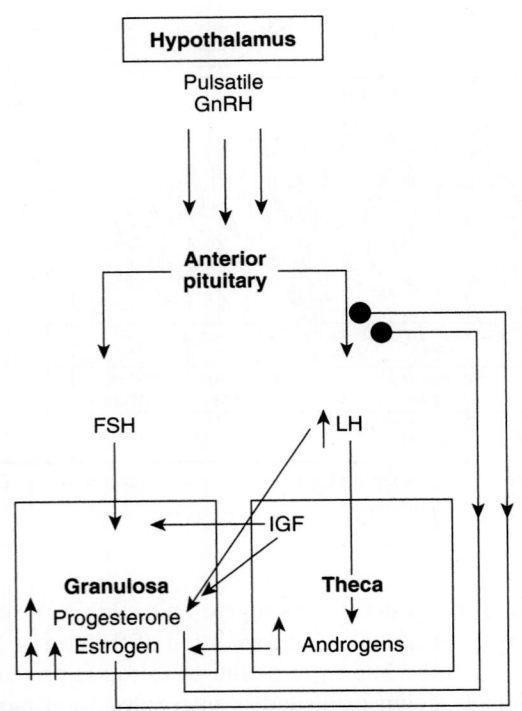

FIG. 35-6 Late follicular phase to ovulation. *GnRH,* Gonadotropin-releasing hormone; *FSH,* follicle-stimulating hormone; *LH,* luteinizing hormone; *IGF,* insulin-like growth factor; dark circle represents positive feedback. (Data from Speroff L, Fritz MA: *Clinical gynecologic endocrinology and infertility,* ed 7, Philadelphia, 2005, Lippincott, Williams & Wilkins.)

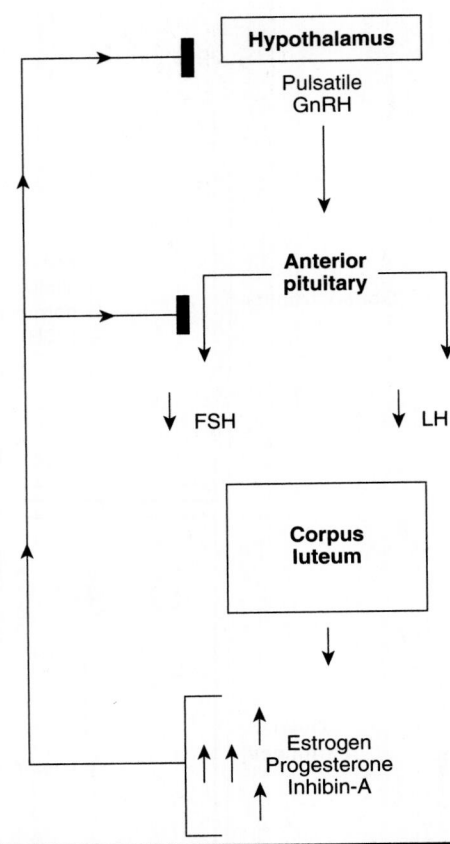

FIG. 35-7 Early luteal to midluteal phase. *GnRH,* Gonadotropin-releasing hormone; *FSH,* follicle-stimulating hormone; *LH,* luteinizing hormone; dark "boxes" represents negative feedback. (Data from Speroff L, Fritz MA: *Clinical gynecologic endocrinology and infertility,* ed 7, Philadelphia, 2005, Lippincott, Williams & Wilkins.)

the suppression of FSH secretion in the pituitary. The decrease in estradiol and progesterone permits a rapid increase in the frequency of GnRH pulsatile secretion and the elimination of negative feedback on the pituitary. The loss of inhibin-A and estradiol and the increasing GnRH pulsations join to permit greater secretion of FSH as compared with LH, which in turn increases in the frequency of episodic secretion of FSH. This increase FSH is influential in rescuing an approximately 70-day-old group of follicles from atresia. This allows a dominant follicle to begin its emergence, and the cycle begins again (Fig. 35-8).

MITTELSCHMERZ

Description
Pelvic pain that occurs at the time of ovulation, midway between menstrual periods, is referred to as *mittelschmerz* (middle pain).

Epidemiology
The etiology is unclear, but pain is probably caused by follicular rupture and the irritation of the peritoneum from the follicular fluid. The incidence is unknown, although some ultrasonographic studies have detected follicular fluid midcycle in 40% of women with normal cycles (Laufer & Goldstein, 2005).

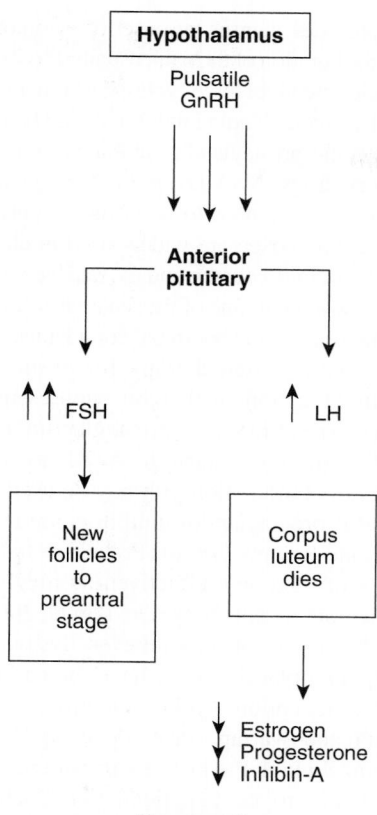

FIG. 35-8   Luteal-follicular transition. *GnRH*, Gonadotropin-releasing hormone; *FSH*, follicle-stimulating hormone; *LH*, luteinizing hormone. (Data from Speroff L, Fritz MA: *Clinical gynecologic endocrinology and infertility*, ed 7, Philadelphia, 2005, Lippincott, Williams & Wilkins.)

Clinical Findings

History.

- Pain occurs midway between cycles, although not with irregular cycles
- Dull, achy pain in lower abdomen lasting a few minutes to several hours
- Recurrent discomfort at same time in each cycle
- Pain occasionally severe and crampy, persisting up to 3 days

Physical Examination.   Pain on palpation in either or both sides of lower abdomen overlying ovaries may be present.

Differential Diagnosis

Included in the differential diagnosis is appendicitis, torsion or rupture of an ovarian cyst, and ectopic pregnancy.

Management

The etiology and benign nature of the pain should be explained to the adolescent and parent.

A heating pad may provide some relief, and analgesics, especially prostaglandin inhibitors (ibuprofen, naproxen), may be used. Box 35-1 lists the dosages. Rarely, oral contraceptives (OCs) may be prescribed to suppress ovulation.

BOX 35-1   Common Prostaglandin Inhibitors Used to Treat Adolescent Menstrual Disorders

- Ibuprofen (Advil, Motrin): 400-800 mg three times a day with a loading dose of 800 mg and a maximum dose of 2400 mg/24 hours
- Naproxen: 500 mg at onset followed by 250-500 mg every 6-12 hour, maximum dose of 1250 mg/24 hours
- Naproxen sodium (Aleve, Anaprox): 550 mg at onset followed by 275 mg every 6-12 hours; maximum dose of 1375 mg/24 hours
- Mefenamic acid: 500 mg at onset followed by 250 mg every 6 hours
- Meclofenamate: 100 mg initially; 50-100 mg every 6 hours

Patient Education

Provide reassurance and comfort measures as outlined in the management section. The adolescent should be encouraged to return if the pain worsens or changes or if she is concerned.

DYSMENORRHEA

Description

Painful menstruation with cramping in the lower abdomen or pelvis is the most common gynecologic problem seen in adolescence. Primary dysmenorrhea has no pelvic pathologic condition identified, whereas secondary dysmenorrhea is due to a pelvic pathologic condition.

Epidemiology

Primary dysmenorrhea is painful menses caused by an exaggerated production of prostaglandins, primarily prostaglandin F_{2a}, in the secretory endometrium. This causes uterine contractions and vasoconstriction leading to ischemia and pain. The elevation of prostaglandins is brought about by falling progesterone levels during the luteal phase of ovulatory cycles.

Secondary dysmenorrhea may be prompted by endometriosis; complications of pregnancy; outflow obstruction; ovarian cysts, fibroids, or other uterine abnormalities; or infection. Dysmenorrhea is present in more than 50% of adolescents and has been reported in up to 90%. It is the leading cause (greater than 10%) of absenteeism from school or work, with increasing incidence in those who describe the pain as severe (Laufer & Goldstein, 2005; Proctor & Farquhar, 2004).

Clinical Findings

History.   The history should assess the following:

- Primary dysmenorrhea
  - Menstrual history
  - Attitudes and beliefs about menstruation
  - Onset—usually 6 to 24 months after menarche
  - Location—lower midabdominal area radiating to back, thighs

- Duration and timing of pain—usually begins with menses and lasts less than 2 days
- Character—mild to severe cramping
- Associated symptoms—nausea, vomiting, diarrhea, headache, fatigue, nervousness, dizziness, urinary frequency, lower back or thigh pain
- Ameliorating or aggravating factors
- Treatments or medications tried, including complementary and alternative medicine (CAM)
- Sexual activity
- Number of days of school or activities missed
- Cigarette smoking
- Family history of dysmenorrhea
- Secondary dysmenorrhea (add the following history)
  - Onset (with menarche or 2 to 3 years postmenarche)
  - Pelvic pain at times other than menstruation (worsens over time)
  - Character of pelvic pain (dull and constant rather than crampy)
  - History of infection, menorrhagia, intermenstrual bleeding, or abnormal vaginal discharge
  - Dyspareunia
  - History of sexual abuse
- Family history of endometriosis

Physical Examination. A complete physical examination is recommended and required for secondary dysmenorrhea. A speculum and bimanual examination may be deferred if the adolescent is not sexually active, if the dysmenorrhea is mild, does not interfere with daily activities, or if the dysmenorrhea is responding to treatment and without suspicion of pathologic condition (Durain, 2004). However, the external genitalia should be examined and a cotton swab inserted in the vagina to rule out hymenal abnormalities and/or a vaginal septum. A rectoabdominal examination will also help rule out adnexal tenderness and masses (Laufer & Goldstein, 2005).

Diagnostic Studies. The following are ordered only if indicated:

- NAATs or cervical cultures for GC and chlamydia
- Complete blood count (CBC) with sedimentation rate if pelvic inflammatory disease (PID) is suspected
- Pregnancy test
- Pelvic ultrasound if abnormalities are suspected

Differential Diagnosis

Endometriosis, PID, chronic pelvic pain, obstructive malformations and/or other pathologic conditions of the reproductive tract are included in the differential diagnosis. Nongynecologic causes of pelvic pain, such as Crohn disease and irritable bowel syndrome, should be considered.

Management

The following steps are recommended:

- Primary dysmenorrhea:
  - Prostaglandin synthetase inhibitors provide relief in 70% to 80% of patients (Laufer & Goldstein, 2005; Speroff & Fritz, 2005). They should be administered at onset of menses or, if

cramping precedes menses, at onset of symptoms. Treat the patient for the duration of the pain, usually 1 to 2 days. The trial period should extend for three cycles; if no relief is experienced, an alternative prostaglandin inhibitor should be tried. See Box 35-1 for specific prostaglandin inhibitors. Nonsteroidal anti-inflammatory drugs (NSAIDs) are advantageous as first-line therapy because they need to be taken for only 2 to 3 days. Ibuprofen and naproxen are widely used in clinical practice, are available over the counter, and are relatively inexpensive. If ineffective, move on to one of the fenamates. Taking NSAIDs with food helps prevent abdominal complaints.

- OCs are a widely used therapy for dysmenorrhea. The mechanism of action is that by suppressing ovulation, total progesterone-induced prostaglandin production is decreased in the endometrium. A 30- to 35-mcg estrogen-progestin combination pill may be used for a 3- to 6-month trial if prostaglandin inhibitors are not successful. The Cochrane Review Group (Proctor & Farquhar, 2004) found OCs of unknown effectiveness for dysmenorrhea; however, a more recent study (Davis et al, 2005) found that low-dose birth control pills relieved dysmenorrhea more effectively than placebo. OCs have the additional advantages of contraception, cycle regulation, protection from endometrial and ovarian cancer, decreased iron deficiency anemia, and slowing the progression of endometriosis.
- CAM is likely to be beneficial per Cochrane Review Group (Proctor & Farquhar, 2004) (see Chapter 42, Table 42-5 for further CAM therapies)
  - Application of topical heat
  - Thiamine 100 mg/day
  - Toki-shakuyaku-san (herbal remedy) 2.5 g three times daily
  - High-frequency transcutaneous electrical nerve stimulation (TENS)
  - Vitamin E 500 units/day
- Follow up by telephone or visit to adjust dose or change medication as needed; the adolescent should be seen again in 3 to 4 months. If there is failure to respond after 6 months of treatment or if pain worsens over time, a further work-up is warranted.
- Secondary dysmenorrhea:
  - Would require a full diagnostic work-up and usually requires referral for gynecologic care.

Patient Education and Prevention

- Encourage exercise and stress reduction, which may help to decrease pain.
- A well-balanced diet with ample amounts of fiber and water, in addition to decreasing caffeine, chocolate, and salt intake, may be useful to control dysmenorrhea (Durain, 2004).
- Smoking cessation may help decrease dysmenorrhea. A longitudinal study of women found that 41% of smokers compared with 26% of nonsmokers experienced moderate or severe dysmenorrhea (Chen et al, 2000).

ADOLESCENT PREGNANCY PREVENTION

There are several common goals in adolescent pregnancy prevention. These goals can be achieved by supporting a positive or protective environment, connecting the adolescent to an intervention program, and providing appropriate health care services.

Prevention goals include the following:

- Maintain sexual health.
- Promote sexual responsibility.
- Assist adolescents to make informed choices, recognizing educational, social, and economic impact of choices.
- Encourage abstinence.
- Delay onset of intercourse.
- Provide contraceptive counseling and selection of a contraceptive device for any adolescent who has recently experienced a spontaneous abortion, as part of third-trimester health teaching before delivery, or at the time of an elective termination of pregnancy.

Dryfoos (1998) identified common components of successful intervention programs; they include:

- Intensive individualized attention
- Early identification of at-risk children
- Early intervention to prevent high-risk behavior
- Youth empowerment
- Social skills training
- Parental involvement and training in parenting
- Community-wide multiagency collaborative approaches

A home environment that protects against pregnancy was outlined by The National Campaign to Prevent Teen Pregnancy in Parent Power (2003):

- Close relationship with parents
- Clear and honest discussions about sexuality, love, and relationships
- Clear messages about the value of abstinence and/or use of protection
- Parental supervision
- Valuing education and goals for the future

Appropriate health care services are also important and include the following:

- Confidential services with minimal or no financial barriers
- Easy availability (e.g., timed for easy access, on site at school, or easy transportation to site)
- A full range of contraceptive services for male and female adolescents (see section on contraception for specific methods)

CONTRACEPTION

Contraceptive Counseling and Education

Significant and specific knowledge is required for pediatric providers to offer reproductive health and contraceptive services to adolescents. An in-depth discussion is beyond the scope of this text; however, excellent management references are available. The authors would recommend *Contraceptive Technology* by Hatcher et al, 2004 and *A Clinical Guide for Contraception* by Speroff & Darney, 2005 (see Chapter 19 for more information on sexuality counseling).

Contraceptive counseling needs to be individualized and at the adolescent's developmental level. It is also important not to overwhelm the patient with too much information at one time. Ascertain what methods she knows about or is thinking about

using. Frequently, the provider needs to dispel misconceptions about risks related to various methods and educate on the menstrual and health benefits. It may take more than one visit to find a compatible contraceptive method. However, the adolescent should not leave the office without understanding the risk of pregnancy and STIs and HIV with unprotected sex. She should have education about and a prescription for emergency contraception (ECs) and know that condoms are a must for safer sex.

A number of factors have been identified as predictors of failure or success with contraception. These include the following:

- Age. Adolescents 15 years old and younger are at highest risk for pregnancy because 35% report using no method of contraception at their first episode of intercourse. In comparison, only 17% of females 19 years or older report using no method (Abma et al, 2004).
- Noncompliance with the first method chosen (previous method failure).
- Not acquiring a method of contraception at the first reproductive health visit.
- Frequency of family planning visits in the preceding 12 months. Increased compliance with clinic attendance appears to correlate with effective contraceptive use by client.
- Coital frequency. Adolescent females who have sexual intercourse more than six times per month are at greater risk of becoming pregnant.
- Length of time between first coitus and initiation of birth control use. The longer adolescents delay seeking services for contraception, the less likely they are to use a highly reliable method consistently and correctly.

Antecedent risk factors to unintentional pregnancy include the following:

- Early onset of sexual activity, especially before 15 years old
- Early onset of substance use, including cigarettes, alcohol, and illicit drugs
- Lesbian or bisexual; these females are as likely to have sex with males as heterosexuals, but their pregnancy rate is more than doubled (Meininger et al, 2002)
- Low educational expectation
- Low perception of life options
- Poor grades and academic achievement
- Behavior problems, including truancy and delinquency
- Negative peer influence
- Poor contraceptive compliance or failure with a contraceptive device
- Nonintact families (those without both biologic mother and father present)
- Depression
- Cultural values that favor adolescent pregnancy
- Prior history of sexual or physical abuse or violence at home (Neinstein & Farmer, 2002)

Initial Screening to Assess for Appropriate Contraception

History. For the most part, adolescent women are healthy with no contraindications for hormonal contraceptive methods.

However, it is important to get a personal history related to cardiovascular and peripheral vascular disease, diabetes, headaches, liver and gallbladder disease, and current medications (including prescription, OTC, herbal, and dietary supplements). The World Health Organization (WHO), using evidence-based methodology, has developed medical eligibility criteria for starting contraceptive methods (2004). The authors would recommend using the WHO website to access the most recent criteria updates (see Resource Box).

Physical Examination.
- Height and weight; body mass index (BMI)
- Blood pressure
- Thyroid examination
- Breast examination, including Tanner staging
- Auscultation of heart and lungs
- Abdominal examination
- Pelvic examination (not a requirement to start oral contraceptive pills [OPCs])

Diagnostic Studies.
- Pap smear if indicated by current guidelines
- NAAT on urine or cultures for GC and chlamydia
- Wet mounts when indicated by presence of abnormal vaginal discharge
- CBC or hemoglobin or hematocrit and rubella titer as indicated
- Syphilis serology with known STI, particularly condylomas or genital ulcers and if residing in endemic areas
- HIV

HORMONAL METHODS OF CONTRACEPTION (COITUS-INDEPENDENT METHODS)

Protocol for Initial Use of Oral Contraceptive Pills
The initial use of an oral contraceptive pill (OCP) requires special attention to dosing, preparation, timing, patient education, and follow-up.

Dosing. Initial dosing for a combination OCP should be at 30 to 35 mcg estrogen, with low progestin potency per tablet. Most providers have one to two OPCs that are favorites for first-time use in women without special conditions. There are 20-mcg combination OCPs available, should an ultra-low dose estrogen formulation be desired. The selection of an OCP can also be individualized based on menstrual characteristics or patient sensitivity. For example, a client with a history of cystic acne can be tried on an OCP where the progestins are desogestrel or norgestrel, or on Ortho Tri-Cyclen or Estrostep, the only OCs with Food and Drug Administration (FDA) approval for use in acne. For clients with hirsutism or polycystic ovarian syndrome (PCOS), a low androgenic potency pill is used, such as Ortho-Cyclen, Desogen, or Ovcon-35. For clients who miss pills, using a monophasic 30- to 35-mcg pill provide more protection against escape ovulation than a 20-mcg estrogen, progestin only, or triphasic pill. Adolescents who demonstrate estrogen sensitivity can be tried on a more androgenic pill, such as Lo/Ovral, Nordette, or Loestrin or a 20-mcg preparation, such as Alesse.

Preparation. Given the vast selection of products available to the health care provider, Hatcher and colleagues (2004) developed a flow chart to assist clinicians in choosing a combined OC with low-dosage estrogen. The selection process contains four steps:

1. Does the adolescent have a contraindication to estrogen use?
2. If yes, consider the use of a progestin-only formulation.
3. If the client can use estrogen, the provider can select between numerous products, considering the following:
   - The number of micrograms of estrogen in the preparation
   - Availability of the pill on formulary
   - Ease of understanding the packaging of the pill
   - Price of the pill to the adolescent and possibly the clinic
   - Previous adverse event or experience the adolescent may have had with a specific preparation
4. Consider other clinical factors, such as acne, nausea or vomiting, spotting or breakthrough bleeding, and absence of withdrawal bleeding.

Timing. Ideally, OCs should not be started until the adolescent has had three to six regular periods after menarche, but sexually active or other high-risk teens can be put on OCPs even before menarche. OCs can be started 3 to 4 weeks postpartum (if breastfeeding, use progestin-only pill [POP]) or after a first-trimester therapeutic abortion (Hatcher et al, 2005; Nelson & Neinstein, 2002a).

There are several ways in which OCPs can be initiated:
- Quick start—same day start in certain circumstances
  - If within 72 hours of unprotected sex, use ECs now and start OCPs the next day
  - If pregnancy can be ruled out or there was no unprotected sex since the last menses, may start same day and use backup (condoms) for 7 days or until menses starts. This is a preferable method for adolescents because it is less complicated and has a higher rate of continuation
- Start first day of menses
- Start within 5 days after menses and use backup (condoms) for 7 days
- First Sunday after menses started and use backup (condoms) for 7 days

Another timing issue is the pattern of combination OC (COC) use. The majority of pill packs come with 28-day cycling: 21 days of active tablets and 7 days of placebo tablets, with the woman having a monthly withdrawal bleed during the placebo week. For years, providers have recommended various patterns of monophasic COC use to prevent withdrawal bleeds. Women can skip the placebo week of their pill packs for one, two, or three cycles to decrease the number of withdrawal bleeds per year. This is particularly helpful in women with endometriosis, menorrhagia, severe dysmenorrhea, and menstrual migraines. In 2003, Seasonale came on the market and is packaged with eighty-four active pills and seven inactive pills, giving women only four withdrawal bleeds per year.

Patient Education.
- Provide clear instructions on how to start OCPs
- Emphasize correct and consistent use of the OCP

○ Take the pill every day in the order presented in the pill pack—no matter what your body is doing or what your friends say
- How to make up missed or forgotten pills and the use of a backup method
  ○ One missed pill—take ASAP and take next pill as usual
  ○ Two missed pills—take one pill ASAP and one pill in 12 hours. Then continue with the remainder of the pack and use backup for 7 days. Additionally, offer EC if pills missed in first week of pack
  ○ If more than two pills are missed—take EC and restart OPCs the next day and use backup for the next 7 days. If declines EC, skip missed pills and continue the rest of the pack and use backup until next menses (Hatcher et al, 2005)
- Explain common side effects and the need to call if questions or concerns arise
- Stress the importance of duel methods for protection from STIs and HIV
  ○ All adolescents should use condoms along with any other method used for contraception
- All adolescents should have a prescription for ECs and understand how to use them

Follow-up Management. Provide an emergency follow-up number and instruct the client on indications for calling. Schedule a return appointment. The return visit gives the health care provider an opportunity to assess the physiologic effects of the OCP and the adolescent's acceptance and use of this particular contraceptive method.

Adolescents tend to be acutely aware of and sensitive to body changes and processes. As a result, they may incorrectly interpret physical signs, exaggerate the effects of OCs on their bodies, and discontinue the OCP use without consulting their health care provider. At the follow-up visit, the provider should reemphasize the noncontraceptive benefits of the OCP, have the client discuss concerns about the OCPs, discuss the lower risks of OCPs compared with those of pregnancy, and review and reclarify directions and side effects.

The use of the acronym ACHES can help guide assessment questions, but should be used carefully to help the teenager understand more clearly the advantages and risks of OCPs without unduly concerning her:

- **A**bdominal pain. Have you experienced abdominal pain (severe)?
- **C**hest pain. Have you noticed chest pain (severe), cough, or shortness of breath?
- **H**eadaches. Do you have headaches (severe), dizziness, weakness, or numbness?
- **E**ye problems. Have you had a change in vision (loss or blurring) or other eye problems or speech problems?
- **S**evere leg pain. Have you had any severe leg pain, especially in the calf or thigh?

Also interview the client for STI exposure, compliance, satisfaction with medication, and perceived side effects. Physical examination parameters during the return visit include weight and blood pressure measurements and any laboratory follow-up.

Preparations of Oral Contraceptive Pills

Types of Preparations. Two basic preparations are available: a combination formulation (COC) that contains estrogen (less than 50 mcg) and progestin in a low dose and a progestin-only minipill. Most women in the U.S. use the combination formulation, in either monophasic or triphasic formats. Progestin-only pills (POP) are prescribed for women in whom estrogens are contraindicated (e.g., lactating women or women with medical contraindications to estrogen). Generally, they are not the first choice for nonlactating adolescents because of irregular bleeding and higher failure rates.

Mechanisms of Action.
- Suppression of ovulation (90% to 95% with COC and 50% with POP)
- Thickening of cervical mucus, blocking penetration of sperm
- Alteration of endometrial lining
- Alteration of tubal motility

Theoretic and Use Effectiveness.
- Perfect use failure rate is 0.3%
- Typical first-year failure rate in all women is 8%

Benefits.
- High rate of effectiveness
- Simple method to use
- Ease of discontinuing use
- Rapid reversal of effects after discontinuing medication
- Beneficial effects on the menstrual cycle
  ○ Reduction of premenstrual symptoms
  ○ Decreased dysmenorrhea
  ○ Decreased flow

Medical Benefits. For women younger than 20 years old, the estimated death rate while on an OCP is 0.3 per 100,000 nonsmoking users (2.2 per 100,000 smoking users), as compared with that of childbirth, for which the estimated maternal death rate is 7 per 100,000 live births (Emans, 2005b).

Other health benefits:
- Reduction of anemia
- Decreased incidence of gonorrheal PID, which results in less morbidity in the areas of chronic pelvic pain, decreased incidence of ectopic pregnancies, and less infertility
- Protection against formation of ovarian cysts (COCs)
- Reduction of ovarian and endometrial cancer (COCs)
- Ortho Tri-Cyclen and Estrostep are approved by FDA for treatment of acne

Disadvantages.
- No protection from STIs—need to use condoms
- Daily use difficult for some women

Disadvantages of Triphasic OCP.
- Confusion about color of package
- Less flexibility of use by the prescribing person (e.g., difficult to use for periods greater than 21 days or for management of ovarian cysts, endometrial bleeding, or DUB)
- Some adolescents find the triphasic preparation confusing, especially if they forget to take a pill

Disadvantages of Progestin-Only OCP.
- Irregular bleeding
- Effectiveness decreases dramatically if even one pill is missed; manufacturer recommends that POPs be taken at

the same time every day and that a backup method of birth control be used if even one pill is missed or taken more than 3 hours late (Hatcher et al, 2004).

- May increase acne
- No protection from STIs—need to use condoms

Side Effects.

- Nausea and vomiting
- Breakthrough bleeding (spotting)
- Breast tenderness
- Headaches
- Mood changes

Failure/Lack of Efficacy. Reasons for failure of OCPs include the following:

- Method failure or method ineffectiveness
- Patient failure/user effectiveness—68% of women still use OCPs 1 year after initiation; most discontinuance is for non-medical reasons
- Concurrent drug interaction, such as with anticonvulsants, tetracycline, St. John's wort (see Chapter 42, Table 42-2 for a more complete list), and possibly oral antifungals
- OCPs can increase the action of diazepam, Librium, tricyclics, and theophylline.

Evra Contraceptive Patch

The Evra patch is a 20-cm^2 transdermal adhesive patch consisting of progestin (17-deacetylnorgestimate) and ethinyl estradiol. It is placed on the trunk, buttock, or arm once a week for 3 weeks and removed for 1 week to allow for a withdrawal bleed. The advantage of the patch is that it does not require the user to remember a daily OCP. Disadvantages include the visibility of the patch, which precludes privacy of method, and the need to remember to replace the patch when indicated. The patch also has decreased efficacy in women who weigh more than 90 kg. It costs about the same as OCPs (except for generic forms) and has the same precautions and side effects as OCPs. There is currently some evidence that the Evra patch may have an increased risk of nonfatal venous thromboembolism (VTE) over OCPs in some women. Careful screening of VTE risk is recommended.

Nuva Ring

The Nuva Ring is a self-administered contraceptive, consisting of a soft, flexible, 2-inch transparent plastic ring with a hole in the middle. It is 0.125 inch thick and is impregnated with both estrogen and progestin. It is inserted vaginally once a month on or before the fifth day of menses, left in place for 3 weeks, removed for 1 week to allow for a withdrawal bleed, and then a new ring inserted. Placement over the cervix is not necessary. As long as it is in contact with the vagina, it is working. The failure rate is the same as OCPs: typical use 8%, and perfect use 0.3%. Advantages include: is coitus independent, does not involve the use of messy creams or gels, and is only dealt with once a month. It does not provide protection against STIs; there is some initial breakthrough bleeding, and the user must be comfortable inserting and removing the device and be able to adhere to the usage schedule.

Subdermal Implant Contraception

Implanon is the new, and currently only, implanted form of progestin-only contraception on the market in the U.S. Implanon is a one-rod, 3-year subdermal implant that has a newer form of progestin (etonogestrel). The method of action is the same as other progestin-only methods. The advantage of an implant is that it provides long-acting contraception. Disadvantages include surgical insertion and removal procedures and side effects, such as irregular bleeding, weight gain, and acne. It is a more successful method for mature adolescents committed to long-term contraception.

Injectable Contraception

Medroxyprogesterone Acetate (Depo-Provera).

Protocol for Initial Use. Always evaluate for pregnancy before giving the initial dose. A single 150-mg injection inhibits ovulation for 13 weeks. Dosage adjustment for body weight is not necessary. It is preferable to deliver the initial injection before day 5 of the menstrual cycle to minimize pregnancy potential. Injections are usually given at 12-week intervals. If more than 13 weeks have transpired between injections, evaluate for pregnancy before giving the injection.

Mechanism of Action.

- Inhibits ovulation by inhibiting LH surge (normal ovulation occurs within 6 months after the last injection in approximately 50% of women; however, 25% will take up to 1 year to return to a normal menstrual pattern) (Speroff & Darney, 2005)
- Creates shallow, atrophic endometrium, unsuitable for implantation
- Increases thickening of cervical mucus, decreasing sperm penetration

Theoretic and Use Effectiveness. The lowest expected pregnancy rate is 0.3 per 100 women-years with the typical failure rate of 3%.

Benefits.

- One-time dosing every 3 months
- Good method for adolescents who want to keep their contraception private from family and friends
- Gynecologic benefits (e.g., decreases in PID, ectopic pregnancy, and endometriosis)

Disadvantages.

- Menstrual irregularities
- Amenorrhea or decreased menstrual flow
- Weight gain
- Headache
- Breast tenderness
- Acne
- Hirsutism
- Psychological effects, such as moodiness, depression, change in libido
- Evidence of bone density loss in adolescents; osteopenia
- Intramuscular injection
- Need to use condoms to prevent STIs
- Increased risk for low birth weight in infants exposed in utero

Patients Appropriate for Depo-Provera. Depo-Provera is a contraceptive method of choice for patients with the following characteristics:

- Seeking a long-term, reversible, highly reliable, private method of contraception
- Those for whom use of estrogen is contraindicated (e.g., patients with a previous thromboembolic episode, lupus, sickle cell anemia)
- Those with seizure disorders—improves control (Speroff & Darney, 2005)
- Those with poor compliance using other contraceptive methods
- Those with menstrual hygiene issues, such as individuals who are mentally retarded, because Depo-Provera often causes amenorrhea after two injections

Postcoital Hormonal Contraception or Emergency Contraception

Preparation. Emergency contraception (EC) is designed to be used after unprotected intercourse to prevent an unwanted pregnancy. Plan B is the only FDA-approved oral emergency contraceptive (EC) marketed in the U.S. and is now approved for purchase without a prescription for women older than 18 years. Plan B is a two-tablet progestin-only method that should be taken within 72 hours of unprotected intercourse for the highest efficacy. The dosage is either one tablet taken immediately with the second tablet taken in 12 hours or both tablets taken at one time. Regular OCPs (combination) may also be used at recommended dosages; this regimen is referred to as the Yuzpe method. Progestin-only OCPs are another alternative (see Hatcher et al, 2004 for specifics).

Clinical Management. All adolescents should have a prescription, in advance, for self-administration as needed. The prescription is intended for such times as when a condom breaks or there has been a lapse in birth control method. EC is more effective the earlier it is taken after unprotected intercourse. Studies have shown that when readily available, the use of EC does not increase unprotected sex (Speroff & Darney, 2005).

If a client has a need for EC within 72 hours after unprotected intercourse:

- Assess for pregnancy using a rapid high-sensitivity urine pregnancy test. If LNMP has been within 1 month, a pregnancy test is not necessary
- Instruct patient to return for a pregnancy test if no menses occurs within 3 weeks
- Instruct patient to abstain from intercourse until the start of her next cycle or use condoms 100% of the time
- Discuss a long-term birth control method; review current method and effectiveness for client
- Schedule return visit in 3 to 4 weeks

Mechanism of Action.
- Inhibits ovulation
- May affect tubal transport

Side Effects.
- Side effects include nausea, vomiting, breast tenderness, headache, and dizziness
- The progestin-only methods have fewer side effects (Speroff & Darney, 2005)

Contraindications to Emergency Contraception.
- None for progestin-only formulations

Effectiveness.
- Plan B has a 1% failure rate
- 2% to 3% failure rate with COCs by Yuzpe method

BARRIER METHODS OF CONTRACEPTION (COITUS-DEPENDENT METHODS)

Condoms

Condoms are the most common barrier method of contraception. Used effectively, they can prevent pregnancy and decrease STI transmission. In the Centers for Disease Control and Prevention's (CDC's) 2005 Youth Risk Behavior Surveillance data, 63% of high school students stated they used condoms for their last act of sexual intercourse (CDC, 2006d). This is up 5% from the 58% reporting condom use in the 2001 survey.

More than 100 brands of condoms are available in an array of sizes (most are 170 by 50 mm), textures, lubricants, colors, and scents. Ninety-nine percent use latex condoms, and less than 1% use either natural skin or the newer polyurethane condoms. The polyurethane condoms are not subject to breakdown by petroleum-based lubricants, are latex free, and have an improved taste over latex. However, they are less elastic, which increases slippage and breakage. They should be reserved for those with latex allergies.

Protocol for Use.
- Use every time!
- Apply correctly, allowing for 0.5-inch tip at end and removing any trapped air
- Remove correctly after intercourse. Hold onto the condom while withdrawing the penis from the vagina to prevent the condom from coming off in the vagina. Replace if used for oral or anal sex before intravaginal intercourse
- Avoid use of petroleum-based lubricants, such as petroleum jelly, shortening, and oil-based vaginal therapeutics, such as Monistat or Femstat
- Check expiration date on the package and make sure package is intact
- Use only once and discard
- Keep a prescription for EC handy

Mechanism of Action.
- Prevent sperm from entering vagina

Theoretic and Use Effectiveness.
- First-year failure rate among typical users is 15%
- First-year failure rate among perfect users is 2%
- Concomitant, perfect use of condoms with a spermicide has an estimated probability of contraceptive failure of 0.3%. This is equivalent to perfect-use failure rate with an OCP

Benefits.
- Encourages male participation
- Appeals to those who have episodic intercourse and for sexual debuts (Nelson & Neinstein, 2002b)
- Is inexpensive and accessible
- Use of lubricated condoms reduces mechanical friction and vaginal or penile irritation
- Decreases the risk of transmitting STIs
- Eliminates postcoital vaginal discharge
- Helps maintain erection for some men
- Has few contraindications

Disadvantages.

- Condom breakage or slippage approximately 2% to 6% of condoms fail as a result of breakage or slippage
- Natural-skin condoms are contraindicated if there is a risk of infection by sexually transmitted viruses (e.g., hepatitis B virus, HPV, herpes simplex virus [HSV], and HIV)
- Either partner may be allergic to latex
- Male partner may fail to accept responsibility for use
- Some men cannot maintain an erection when a condom is used

Diaphragm

Available for more than 100 years, there are currently three types of diaphragms in sizes from 50 to 105 mm, available by prescription only. For most adolescents, the 65 to 75 mm sizes are commonly prescribed. These are:

- Arching spring (Koroflex, Allflex, Ramses Bendex)
- Coil-spring rim (Koromex, Ortho, Ramses)
- Wide-seal rim (Milex) available only from the manufacturer

The diaphragm can be placed in the vagina over the cervix up to 1 hour before intercourse and can be left in place for 24 hours, but it must be left a minimum of 6 to 8 hours. Reapplication of spermicide is required with subsequent intercourse.

Cervical Cap

The Prentif Cavity Rim Cervical Cap is the only type of cervical cap approved by the FDA for use in the U.S. It comes in four sizes that properly fit 80% of women's cervices. The cap can be left in place for 48 hours, and subsequent intercourse within 6 hours or more requires additional intravaginal spermicide. The cervical cap should probably be reserved for those adolescents who are older, more motivated to comply with contraception, and able to place and remove the device (Speroff & Darney, 2005). The association of abnormal Pap smear results with the use of the cervical cap is unresolved. FDA protocol recommends obtaining a Pap smear at the time of fitting, then 3 months after onset of use and annually thereafter.

Female Condom

The female condom is a device with an inner ring or dome that fits next to the cervix. An outer ring fits around the external opening to the vagina. The single-use condom acts as a barrier to prevent sperm from entering the vagina and may reduce the risk of STIs.

Today Sponge

The sponge is made of soft, disposable polyurethane foam and contains the spermicide nonoxynol-9. After it is moistened with water and inserted into the vagina, it becomes effective immediately and protects against pregnancy for the next 24 hours without the need to add spermicidal cream or jelly—even with repeated acts of intercourse.

Protocols for Using Other Barrier Methods. These vary depending on the barrier method; however, **use every time** is applicable to all!

Theoretic and Use Effectiveness. Effectiveness of any of these methods is influenced by the patient's ability to use the method consistently and correctly, along with her own personal fertility characteristics. Patients who are younger than 30 years old and have intercourse four or more times a week experience higher failure rates.

- Diaphragm failure rate is 16% in typical users
- Cervical cap failure rate averages 16% to 32%
- Female condom pregnancy rates are reported to be 21%
- *Today* Sponge failure rate with typical use is 14% to18%

Benefits.

- Diaphragms and female condoms help prevent transmission of STIs and decrease risk of PID, bacterial and viral infection, and cervical neoplasia
- Female condoms and the *Today* Sponge are accessible over the counter

Disadvantages.

- Barrier methods are contraindicated if there is a history of toxic shock syndrome
- Female condoms cost $3.00 versus $1.00 for male condoms and have a visible outer ring
- The *Today* Sponge costs about $3.00 per sponge
- Caps are contraindicated if there has been a full-term delivery within the last 6 weeks, if there has been a recent spontaneous or induced abortion, or if there is vaginal bleeding from any cause, including menstrual flow
- Allergic reaction may occur in those sensitive to spermicide, rubber, latex, or polyurethane
- Abnormalities in vaginal anatomy can interfere with satisfactory fit or placement of any of the devices
- Diaphragm can cause recurrent urinary tract infections
- For diaphragms and caps, trained personnel may not be available to fit device or lack the time to instruct patient adequately on use of method
- Patient must be able to learn correct insertion and extraction techniques
- Patient may not feel comfortable touching self or may find procedure messy and unpleasant

Spermicides

Protocol for Use.

- Use every time!
- Keep adequate supply and store properly
- Be alert to timing of product placement before intercourse. Place in vagina at appropriate time
- Insert new application of product before every episode of repeated intercourse

Mechanism of Action. Spermicides are a combination of an inert base or carrier (foam, cream, jelly, suppository, or tablet) with active spermicidal agent nonoxynol-9 or octoxynol, which kills sperm by permeating the cell membrane. Spermicides are marketed in various formats:

- Foams, creams, or jellies that can be used alone or in combination with a condom or diaphragm
- Spermicidal suppositories that are intended for use alone or with a condom; require a 10- to 15-minute wait before intercourse to allow the product to effervesce
- Vaginal contraceptive film that can be used alone or with a condom or diaphragm; film contains 72 mg of nonoxynol-9 in a thin sheet that is placed next to the cervix 15 minutes before intercourse

Theoretic and Use Effectiveness.
- Estimated 15% failure rate among perfect first-year users
- Among typical users, failure is about 29%

Benefits.
- Medically safe, with same efficacy as barrier methods or condoms
- Available over the counter without a prescription; no need to access medical system
- No need for partner involvement with decision-making or implementation
- Used as backup option while waiting to start OCPs, for missed OCPs, or between relationships

Disadvantages.
- Can cause allergic reaction in those sensitive to spermicidal agent or base
- Can be difficult for some people to learn correct insertion technique
- Abnormalities in vaginal anatomy can prevent correct placement or product retention (e.g., septum, prolapse, double cervix)

LESS USEFUL CONTRACEPTIVE METHODS FOR ADOLESCENTS

Most methods may be considered for use in the mature and motivated adolescent. However, the following methods are usually not recommended for use with sexually active adolescents because of higher failure rates, the need for more maturity, and proven and committed use of contraceptives:
- Periodic abstinence
- Fertility awareness or rhythm method because of the more irregular cycles of adolescents
- Implanted contraception, as a result of intolerance of side effects and costs associated with early removal
- POPs, unless indicated
- Intrauterine devices, as a result of increased risk of STIs and irregular bleeding

ADOLESCENT PREGNANCY

Description

Adolescent pregnancy occurs in girls or young women between 13 and 19 years old, although pregnancy is possible for any girl who has ovulatory cycles. Pregnancy has been seen in girls before their first menstrual cycle and in those as young as 10 or 11 years old.

Epidemiology

There has been a steady decrease in teen pregnancy over the last decade and a half. This is regarded as evidence of more effective contraceptive practices, delayed sexual debuts, and a decrease in sexual activity. Of teen pregnancies, approximately 51% end in live births, 14% in miscarriage or stillbirth, and 35% in therapeutic abortions (Klein, 2005).

Social factors that correlate with adolescent pregnancy are poverty (83% of adolescents giving birth and 61% of those having abortions are from low-income households); being the product of an adolescent pregnancy themselves (one third of cases); history of childhood physical or sexual abuse (as many as 50%

to 60% of early adolescent or midadolescent girls who become pregnant); and having a child already (25% of teen births are to adolescents who have had another child.) (Klein, 2005). Having a sibling who is a teen parent, decreased parental monitoring of the adolescent, academic underachievement, poor sense of personal efficacy, depression, and substance abuse have all been associated with teen pregnancy (Nicoletti, 2005).

Assessment

History. The history should include the following:
- Menstrual history
  - Menarche
  - Cycle regularity—normally how many days apart, how many days of flow
  - LNMP and/or last bleed
  - Contraceptive use—method, consistency of use. If on a hormonal method—any missed pills, late patch or ring replacement, late Depo, etc.
- Sexual history (see Boxes 19-2 and 19-3)
- Associated symptoms: breast sensitivity, nipple tenderness (1 to 2 weeks after conception), fatigue, nausea, urinary frequency (2 weeks after conception)
- Patients often have vague complaints (e.g., headache, abdominal discomfort, dizziness, and vaginal and urinary symptoms)

Physical Examination. There are three classic signs of pregnancy, each of which may be observed during the pelvic examination:
1. Hegar sign—softening of the isthmus of the uterus (the area between the cervix and the uterine body). This may be observed before there is uterine enlargement.
2. Chadwick sign—dark-bluish or purplish discoloration of the vaginal and cervical epithelium, the result of increased blood supply to the pelvis. This is usually observed before uterine growth.
3. Uterine enlargement—occurs at 5 to 6 weeks and initially is due to changes in the uterine muscle rather than growing gestation. Uterine sizing is traditionally done by bimanual examination and recorded in weeks of estimated gestation.

Fetal heart tones may be auscultated by Doppler at 10 to 12 weeks gestation.

Diagnostic Studies. The following laboratory studies are done in cases of suspected pregnancy:
- Pregnancy testing—Urine testing is the chosen test for the ambulatory setting because results can be obtained rapidly, and the test is accurate and inexpensive.

The current urine tests can detect human chorionic gonadotropin (hCG) in the urine down to 25 international units/L. Normal serum levels at the time of the first missed menses are between 50 to 100 international units/L.

Serum testing is of two types; a qualitative test can detect hCG down to 5 international units/L, but will not measure the exact amount. A quantitative ß-hCG can measure the exact amount of ß-hCG in the serum and is indicated for serial measurements to evaluate for ectopic pregnancy, molar pregnancy, or to rule out gestational trophoblastic neoplasia (GTN) following a molar pregnancy.

- If the pregnancy test result is positive, routine laboratory diagnostics include the following:
  - Cervical cultures for GC and chlamydia
  - Cervical cytology
  - Vaginal pH with saline and KOH wet mounts
  - Urinalysis and culture
- Routine prenatal blood work includes: blood type and Rh, syphilis serology, rubella titer, CBC with differential, and screening for hepatitis B and HIV. Another test to consider is an abnormal hemoglobin screen in women of African-American, Asian, and Mediterranean descent for sickle cell trait and thalassemias. Women of Ashkenazi Jewish, French-Canadian, and Cajun descent should be referred for testing for Tay-Sachs.
- Possibly, vaginal and/or pelvic ultrasonography to determine gestation accurately

Differential Diagnosis

The differential diagnoses for pregnancy are as follows:
- Amenorrhea from another etiology
- Nonviable intrauterine pregnancy
- Ectopic pregnancy
- Molar pregnancy

Management and Education

Prompt diagnosis assists with pregnancy planning, early onset of prenatal precautions (e.g., avoidance of OTC medications and herbal preparations without provider approval; the dangers of alcohol, smoking, and illicit drug use), and prenatal care. Early care also allows women considering an abortion ample time for counseling, decision-making, and obtaining an abortion in the first trimester, when the procedure is safest.

The health visit should include a pregnancy test, physical examination, and health counseling. If the pregnancy test result is negative, the provider should talk with the adolescent about her situation. Is she in a steady relationship, was this date rape, were drugs and alcohol involved, was this forced or consensual sex, how old is the partner, etc? The counseling should be tailored to her individual needs, in addition to general education regarding the risk of unprotected intercourse, the potential for pregnancy and STIs and HIV, and reliable methods to protect her in the future.

If the pregnancy test result is positive, the visit should include the following:
- Dating parameters and pelvic examination to determine gestational age
- Counseling for pregnancy options, including continuing pregnancy and retaining custody of child, continuing pregnancy and placing child for adoption, or termination
- Assessment of the involvement of her social support system including family, partner, and any significant others. The provider should encourage parental involvement in the decision-making and may need to role-play and/or serve as mediator for the teenager in informing others. Some states have parental notification laws in place around the issue of abortion, and in most, health care providers are mandatory

reporters of statutory rape. Providers must be aware of laws of the state in which they practice
- Initiation of referrals as appropriate for the decision made:
  - If the choice is continuing the pregnancy and prenatal care is not part of the provider's practice, the adolescent should be referred to another provider or, if available in the community, a comprehensive adolescent pregnancy program to initiate medical, nutritional, psychosocial, and educational services
  - If adoption is the option of choice, refer to the appropriate legal or social service agency, or both. Look for agencies in the community that offer comprehensive preadoption and postadoption counseling
  - If the choice is terminating pregnancy, refer to an appropriate resource for abortion counseling and the procedure
- Make additional referrals as indicated:
  - Women, Infants, and Children (WIC) program
  - Medicaid coverage
  - Community health nurse

Public health–based research indicates that there is a significant positive effect on pregnancy, parenting, and child-rearing outcomes if home visits are made by public health nurses. It is recommended that all pregnant teens be referred to such a service (Koniak-Griffin et al, 2002).

Complications

Young age in a pregnant woman is an inherent risk factor, even with good prenatal care. Adverse outcomes are common in pregnant teenagers and include the following:
- Maternal
  - Anemia
  - Preeclampsia
  - Excessive weight gain or poor weight gain
  - Puerperal complications
  - Potential social consequences (e.g., educational, economic, and occupational delay)
- Fetal and neonatal
  - Low birth weight
  - Intrauterine growth retardation
  - Prematurity
  - Minor acute infections

◼ PATHOPHYSIOLOGY AND DEFENSE MECHANISMS OF THE GYN SYSTEM

PATHOPHYSIOLOGY

The primary disorders of the gynecologic system can be classified as menstrual cycle disorders, inflammatory reactions, infection, and reproductive problems.

Menstrual Cycle Disorders

Pubertal development is a complex but normal process. Adolescents may be seen with common menstrual problems, such as mittelschmerz or dysmenorrhea. Abnormal uterine bleeding, endometriosis, and amenorrhea are three less common disorders that require the provider to differentiate normal growth and developmental variations from systemic disorders or disease (especially neurologic, endocrine, and reproductive problems). The female athlete is especially prone to exercise-related menstrual problems.

Inflammatory Reactions

An inflammatory response can occur in either the external or internal genitalia. Local reactions involve the external genitalia and can be caused by dermatologic disorders or skin irritation from such factors as normal leukorrhea, chemical or allergic reactions, or nonspecific causes. Internal inflammation caused by infection is not always obvious.

Infections

The warm, moist environment of the reproductive tract provides an ideal place for infection. Viral pathogens, such as HSV and HPV, or fungal infection can manifest as a vulvitis or vaginal infection. *Trichomonas*, a protozoan infection, colonizes the vaginal vault. By contrast, bacterial infections caused by chlamydia and GC can ascend into the upper genital tract where PID can cause tubal damage.

Reproductive Problems

Reproductive problems occur as a result of structural, hormonal, or endocrine disorders or as sequelae of infection. Refer to a gynecologic or endocrine text for further information.

DEFENSE MECHANISMS

The gynecologic system has both anatomic and physiologic defense mechanisms. The labia majora and the pubic hair provide a barrier that serves as the first line of defense. The vagina, serving as an exit for mucosal secretion, menstrual fluids, and products of conception, also provides a means of defense with its natural downward and outward flow of secretions.

Additionally, with increasing estrogen exposure, the vaginal epithelial tissue thickens and an acid pH develops, discouraging infection. The small external cervical os, a thick mucous plug, and the downward flow of cervical secretions provide barriers to entry to the uterus. A chemical barrier is also established by the cervical enzymes and antibodies.

▊ SPECIFIC GYNECOLOGIC PROBLEMS OF CHILDREN

LABIAL ADHESIONS

Description

The fusion of tissue between the labia minora that appears to cover the vaginal opening is a common, benign condition in infants and prepubertal girls. It is also called agglutination, synechia vulvae, or vulvar adhesion if only the lower half of the labia minora is involved (Fig. 35-9).

Epidemiology

Before puberty, the vaginal tissues are in a hypoestrogenized state and are prone to inflammation and denudation. As the tissues heal, adhesion of the labia can occur. Mechanisms

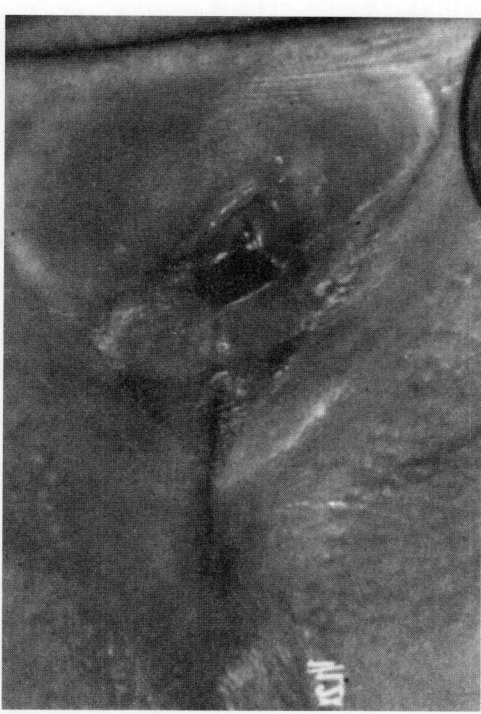

FIG. 35-9 Labial adhesions that are thinned and almost translucent inferiorly following topical estrogen therapy. (From Craighill MC: Pediatric and adolescent gynecology for primary care pediatricians, *Pediatr Clin North Am* 45:1668, 1998.)

for the initial insult are irritation, infection, and trauma. The most common precipitant is an asymptomatic, nonspecific vulvovaginitis caused by poor hygiene. There is debate about whether lack of hygiene, masturbation, fondling, and subsequent irritation from sexual abuse are potential causes in older females. Labial adhesions occur primarily in girls 3 months to 6 years old, but can persist until puberty (Emans, 2005d).

Clinical Findings

History. The history can include the following:
- Concern about rash in genital area
- Parental concern about vaginal opening
- Dysuria, difficulty voiding, or local discomfort

Physical Examination. Physical examination reveals a thin, flat membrane of varying length from the posterior fourchette to the clitoris. The degree of opening near the clitoris varies. The vulva appears flat with a central line of fusion. The urethra may or may not be visualized, and there may be urinary dribbling.

Differential Diagnosis

Scarring, imperforate hymen, clitoral hypertrophy, and intersex problems are the differential diagnoses.

Management

The treatment of labial adhesions is somewhat controversial; Table 35-1 outlines steps that are generally accepted. In asymptomatic labial adhesions, observation is often the best

TABLE 35-1 Treatment of Labial Adhesions

Degree of Involvement	Treatment	Prognosis
No urinary tract infection, no obstruction, no parental concern.	No treatment. Reassure and observe.	Resolution with puberty and estrogenization of tissue.
Opening ensures urinary and vaginal drainage, but treatment desired.	Apply ointment (e.g., A & D or Vaseline) nightly with cotton-tipped swab with gentle pressure. Following separation, maintain good hygiene and mild ointment (e.g., Vaseline) nightly for 6-12 mo.	Separation within 8 wk. If not, double check technique to ensure gentle pressure is being applied. If persists, see use of estrogen cream below.
Urinary and vaginal drainage impaired.	Apply estrogen-containing 1% cream (e.g., Premarin) bid for 3 wk with cotton-tipped swab then at hs for another 2-3 wk. Use gentle pressure until separation occurs. Following separation, use Vaseline nightly as outlined above.	Separation occurs approximately 50% of the time within 2-3 wk. If not, check technique to ensure pressure is being applied and continue for another 3 wk. If unresponsive, may anesthetize with 5% lidocaine ointment or EMLA cream then gently tease the adhesions with a Calgiswab (Emans, 2005d). Always avoid forceful separation.

hs, At bedtime; mo, months; wk, weeks.

treatment. If treatment is desired, applying A & D ointment or Vaseline at bedtime may be helpful. The presence of symptoms of urinary tract infection, pain with activity, and change in behavior dictates treatment (Bacon, 2002). Forceful separation is always contraindicated because it may result in both trauma to the child and recurrence of adhesions. The use of Premarin cream is discussed in Table 35-1.

Complications
Urinary tract infections and readhesion following mechanical lysis can occur.

Patient Education
Premarin cream can cause breast tenderness, transient enlargement, and vulvar pigmentation or erythema, which resolves with discontinuation of the cream. The incidence of recurrence can be decreased with careful attention to perineal hygiene and the daily application of A & D ointment until puberty.

VULVOVAGINITIS
Description
Vulvovaginitis refers to inflammation, often with discharge, from infection or irritation. Vulvitis refers to inflammation of the vulva alone, whereas, vaginitis refers to vaginal discharge, often with pruritus and irritation that may be secondary to the vulvitis. (Hamel-Teillac, 2004)

Epidemiology
Age is important in differentiating the etiology of vulvovaginitis. In prepubescent children, several factors make vulvovaginitis a common problem. The lack of estrogen stimulation leaves the vulvar skin thin and the vaginal mucosa atrophic and contributes to minimal vaginal secretions with neutral pH. The lack of pubic hair and labial fat pads diminishes barrier protection, and the proximity of the vaginal opening to the anus predisposes prepubertal females to irritation and infection of the vulva and vagina. Poor hygiene, including wiping technique and lack of hand washing, irritants such as bubble bath, harsh soaps, sand from playtime, or tight-fitting clothing provide additional insults. Being overweight is also a risk factor. Prepubescent vulvovaginitis most commonly is nonspecific (up to 80%). Other causes include foreign bodies (most often toilet paper), bacterial infection (often group A ß-hemolytic streptococci), or pinworms (Emans, 2005d).

Clinical Findings
The clinical findings pertaining to vulvovaginitis are found in Table 35-2.

History. The history for the prepubertal child includes the following:
- Onset—less than 1 month usually associated with specific diagnosis, whereas a longer period of time more likely nonspecific (Emans, 2005d)
- Characteristics:
  ○ Genital irritation, itching, pain, inflammation
  ○ Vaginal discharge—note onset, quantity, color, type (bloody, mucoid), odor, consistency, and duration
  ○ Nighttime perianal itching
  ○ Urinary complaints, including dysuria and enuresis
- Recent medications, especially antibiotics

TABLE 35-2   Evaluation and Treatment of Vulvovaginitis

	Signs and Symptoms	Vaginal Discharge	Etiology	Laboratory Data	Treatment
Nonspecific vaginitis	Itching, burning; dysuria; varied vulvitis	Scant to copious; brown to green; mucoid; foul smelling	Irritation from contact with various substances; poor hygiene	pH variable; no odor on whiff test; micro: leukocytes, bacteria, debris; normal UA	Refractory cases may need topical estrogen or antibiotics
Physiologic leukorrhea	None or minimal itch or burn; minimal vulvitis; 6-12 mo before menarche; possible mild erythema	Scant to moderate; clear to white; odorless; nonirritating	Endogenous hormones 6-12 mo before menarche	pH <4.5; no odor on whiff test; micro: epithelial cells, lactobacilli; normal UA	No treatment needed; explain and reassure
Chemical or mechanical	Itch, erythema, vulvar inflammation, dysuria	Scant amount; yellow to white	Bubble bath, perfumed soap, lotion; tight-fitting clothes, sand or dirt from playground, overweight	pH <4.5; no odor on whiff test; micro: leukocytes, epithelial cells	Remove irritant; topical steroids
Foreign body	Dysuria, discomfort, bleeding, minimal vulvar excoriation; history of foreign body in other orifices	Purulent, persistent, dark brown, foul smelling (18%), bloody (82%)	Toilet paper (prepubescent); tampons (adolescent); condoms or object used for masturbation	pH >4.5; odd odor on whiff test; micro: WBCs, epithelial cells with bacteria and debris; UA normal	Remove foreign body with forceps or by irrigating with saline and small feeding tube; knee-chest position may work best
Bacterial	Acute respiratory, enteric, or skin infection	Green color, foul, copious with possible bleeding	*Streptococcus* (most common), *Escherichia coli*, *Enterococcus*, *Shigella*, *Staphylococcus*, or other bacteria	Strep test positive; culture positive	Penicillin, erythromycin, amoxicillin, broad-spectrum cephalosporin or other antibiotic as indicated
Candidiasis	Itching, burning, vulvar inflammation, external dysuria, dyspareunia	Thick, white, curdy cottage cheese, adherent, odorless; vulva red, edematous with satellite lesions	*Candida albicans*; recent antibiotic or steroid use; diabetes or immunodeficiency; pregnancy	pH <4.5; no odor on whiff test; micro: fungal hyphae and buds or spores, culture positive for *Candida* (see Fig. 35-2)	Azole cream topically or intravaginally; or Fluconazole 150-mg oral tab—single dose
Pinworms	Recent exposure to pinworms; perineal itching, especially at night; anal excoriation, erythema, and lesions from scratching	No discharge	*Enterobius vermicularis* spread from anus	Normal UA; tape test reveals eggs	Mebendazole 100 mg once; repeated in 2 wk; treat family members
Bacterial vaginosis	Foul odor, especially after menses or intercourse; often asymptomatic; no inflammation; abdominal pain or irregular prolonged bleeding	Homogeneous, thin milky white discharge adherent* to vaginal walls and pools in posterior fornix; increased amount	*Gardnerella vaginalis*, mycoplasmas, and anaerobic bacteria; caused by replacement of normal vaginal flora; may or may not be sexually transmitted	pH >4.5*; fishy odor on whiff test*; micro: clue cells,* few lactobacilli, gram-negative rods, no WBCs	Treat if symptomatic with metronidazole 500 mg orally twice a day for 7 days or metronidazole gel 0.75% 5 g intravaginally at hs for 5 days or clindamycin cream 2% 5 g intravaginally at hs for 7 days

Continued

TABLE 35-2 **Evaluation and Treatment of Vulvovaginitis—Cont'd**

	Signs and Symptoms	Vaginal Discharge	Etiology	Laboratory Data	Treatment
Trichomoniasis	Lower abdominal discomfort, dysuria, symptoms worse before and after menses; history of sexual contact; vulvar itching and erythema	White to yellow-grey, frothy, foul odor, profuse, purulent, slightly watery; vaginal mucosa erythematous, cervix friable with petechiae	*Trichomonas vaginalis*, flagellated protozoa, primarily sexually transmitted	pH >4.5, frequently has fishy odor on whiff test; micro: motile, flagellated organisms, WBC >10/hpf on UA	Prepubertal: Metronidazole 15mg/kg in 3 divided doses for 7-10 days; or 40mg/kg in single dose Postpubertal: 2g in single dose

*Need three of these findings to diagnose bacterial vaginosis.
hpf, High-power field; *hs*, at bedtime; *micro*, microscopic examination; *mo*, months; *UA*, urinalysis; *WBC*, white blood cell; *wk*, weeks.

- Possible trauma, foreign body, pinworm infestation, or sexual abuse
- Previous occurrences and treatment used
- Underlying illnesses (e.g., streptococcus infection, dermatosis, diabetes, immunosuppression)
- Perineal hygiene
- Use of harsh soaps and bubble bath
- Tight-fitting or nylon underwear or clothing
- Superabsorbent diapers

Physical Examination. A good light and magnifying glass may aid in the physical examination. Prepubertal examination includes inspection, possible vaginal otoscopy in frog-leg or knee-chest position, and rectal examination.

Diagnostic Studies. The following should be considered:
- pH of vaginal secretions
- Wet mounts of vaginal secretions
  ○ Saline for microscopic examination to look for WBCs, clue cells, trichomonads, and bacteria
  ○ 10% KOH for whiff test and microscopic examination to look for yeast (branching hyphae and spores) (see Fig. 35-2)
- Bacterial culture of vaginal secretions
- Slide with 20% KOH of skin scraping for yeast
- Pinworm eggs visualized on tape slide under microscope
- Cultures for GC and chlamydia if suspected sexual abuse

Differential Diagnosis

Atopic dermatitis, psoriasis, seborrhea, lichen sclerosus, or other dermatosis; labial adhesions; polyps or tumors; systemic diseases, such as Kawasaki or Crohn; STIs; and sexual abuse are included in the differential diagnosis.

Management

General treatment measures for any type of vulvovaginitis are listed in Box 35-2.

Specific recommendations include the following (see also Table 35-2):
- Prepubertal nonspecific etiology:

BOX 35-2 **General Treatment Measures for Vulvovaginitis**

1. Hygiene
   - Wash hands frequently
   - Wipe front to back
   - Change underwear every day
   - Blow dry perineal area with cool to warm air (especially if overweight)
2. Clothing
   - Wear absorbent white underwear, changing once or twice daily; do not wear underwear at night
   - Wear loose clothing—no pantyhose or tight clothes
   - Avoid spandex and sleeper pajamas
   - Change out of swimsuit after swimming
3. Comfort and healing measures
   - Take sitz bath with thorough drying
   - Blow dry for 10-15 minutes once or twice daily with cool to warm air or pat dry with towel
   - Apply hydrocortisone cream 1% once or twice daily for itching
   - Use oral diphenhydramine or hydroxyzine if itching is severe
4. Protective measures
   - Avoid bubble baths and perfumed lotions or powder
   - Use mild soap (e.g., Dove, Basis, Neutrogena)
   - Avoid shampoo in bath water
   - Use protective ointment twice a day (e.g., Vaseline, A & D, Aquaphor)
   - Avoid bleach or fabric softener in wash, double rinse
   - Urinate with knees spread apart to minimize urinary reflux

  ○ If persistent, prescribe antibacterial cream at night (e.g., Bactroban, Sultrin, or clindamycin) for 2 weeks
  ○ If persistent after 3 weeks, prescribe a trial of amoxicillin, Augmentin, or one of the cephalosporins
  ○ If symptoms still persist, use estrogen cream at bedtime for 2 to 3 weeks, then every other night at bedtime for 2 weeks to thicken vulvar epithelium

○ If recurrent vulvovaginitis, a 1- to 2-month course of low-dose cephalexin or trimethoprim-sulfamethoxazole (TMP-SMX) at bedtime should be tried

○ If a specific infection is found, treat as outlined herein or refer to appropriate section

○ If therapy fails, refer to a pediatric gynecologist

○ If an STI is found in a child, a complete work-up for sexual abuse is indicated

• Contact dermatitis:
  ○ Steroids and hormonal cream can be used to thicken vaginal skin and minimize irritation

• Foreign body:
  ○ Prepubertal: Irrigate with warm normal saline with a small feeding tube at the hymenal opening with the child in the frog-leg position. If foreign body remains after irrigation, refer to a pediatric gynecologist
  ○ A broad-spectrum antibiotic, such as amoxicillin or a cephalosporin, may be indicated if infection is apparent

• Bacterial infection:
  ○ Obtain cultures and prescribe appropriate treatment; penicillin or erythromycin is usually used

• Candida infection:
  ○ Topical antifungal creams are usually successful
  ○ Treatment failure or recurrence may indicate a resistant organism
  ○ If appropriate, evaluate for STIs
  ○ Complicated candidal infections (severe local, recurrent in an immunocompromised host) require documentation by culture, work-up for predisposing conditions, longer duration of treatment

• Pinworms:
  ○ Mebendazole (one chewable 100-mg tablet, repeated in 2 weeks)
  ○ Hand washing is important to minimize the spread of infection
  ○ See Chapter 32 for further discussion

• GC, chlamydia, or trichomoniasis in prepubescent children needs to be treated and evaluated as suspected child abuse. See the section on STIs in this chapter and 2006 CDC guidelines for treatment of STIs (CDC, 2006a) for more details

Complications
Labial adhesions can occur.

Patient Education, Prognosis, and Prevention
• Follow up in 5 days if there is no improvement
• Recurrence is common, especially with poor hygiene, in overweight girls, and during upper respiratory infection

▮▮ SPECIFIC GYNECOLOGIC PROBLEMS OF ADOLESCENTS

AMENORRHEA

Description
Amenorrhea is lack of menstruation and is described as either primary or secondary. *Primary amenorrhea* is defined as one of the following (Emans, 2005a; Speroff & Fritz, 2005; Wilson et al, 2005).

• Absence of menarche by 16 years old with normal pubertal growth and development
• Absence of menarche by 14 years old in the absence of secondary sexual characteristics

Secondary amenorrhea is defined as the absence of menstruation for at least three cycles or more than 6 months in females who have an established menstrual pattern.

Epidemiology
There are multiple etiologies for primary and secondary amenorrhea. When evaluating a young woman for amenorrhea, pregnancy should be ruled out first, regardless of sexual history given. Amenorrhea is usually categorized by clinical findings and laboratory results into broad areas of causation. Speroff and colleagues (Speroff et al, 1973) devised a compartmental system to categorize amenorrhea that is still in use today (Speroff & Fritz, 2005). He distinguishes between: compartment 1, disorders of the outflow tract or uterine target organ; compartment 2, disorders of the ovary; compartment 3, disorders of the anterior pituitary; and compartment 4, disorders of the CNS (hypothalamic). Emans (2005a) uses the organs in the HPO axis to categorize etiology. Others (Wilson et al, 2005), using the lab results of the gonadotropins and prolactin, categorize etiology into: hypogonadotropic, hypergonadotropic, normogonadotropic, hyperprolactinemic, and anatomic. Grouping in some manner assists the provider to delineate the origin of an individual adolescent's amenorrhea (see Table 35-3).

Clinical Findings
History. The history should assess the following:
• Maternal and sibling age of menarche
• Family history of menstrual irregularities
• Family history of eating disorders, diabetes, thyroid disease, or genetic disorders
• Any prenatal exposure to hormones
• Detailed history of growth and pubertal development (sequence and tempo)
• Menstrual calendar (last menses, number and pattern of cycles, age at menarche)
• Chronic systemic disease or illness or previous surgery, radiation, or chemotherapy
• Nutrition, including eating habits, dieting, weight fluctuations
• Exercise patterns, including amount and intensity, level of participation, weigh ins, or standards for weight that must be kept
• History of stress fractures
• Bowel patterns or abdominal pain
• Headache or visual change
• Galactorrhea, hirsutism, acne
• Medication use (contraceptives, phenothiazines, antihypertensives)
• Sexual activity, contraceptive use
• Stress, recent change in environment, or depression
• Substance use

TABLE 35-3 **Differential Diagnosis of Amenorrhea**

	Primary	Secondary
Hypogonadotropic		
Compartment IV	Delayed puberty	Psychological disorder
Hypothalamic	Chronic illness	Depression
	Eating disorders	Eating disorders
	Excessive exercise	Excessive exercise
	Kallmann syndrome	
Compartment III	Pituitary disease	Pituitary disease
Pituitary	Hyperprolactinemia	Hyperprolactinemia
		Sheehan syndrome
Thyroid		Hypothyroid
Hypergonadotropic		
Compartment II	Premature ovarian failure	Premature ovarian failure
Ovaries	Gonadal dysgenesis	PCOS
	PCOS	
Adrenals	Adrenal hyperplasia	Adrenal hyperplasia
Anatomic	Müllerian agenesis	Asherman syndrome
Compartment I	Androgen insensitivity	
Outflow	Imperforate hymen	
	Vaginal septum	
Hyperprolactinemia		
Compartment III	Medication/drugs	Medication/drugs
Pituitary	Macroadenoma	Macroadenoma
	Tumor	Tumor
		Lactation

PCOS, Polycystic ovarian syndrome.
Data from Emans SJ: Amenorrhea in the adolescent. In Emans SJ, Laufer MR, Goldstein DP, editors: *Pediatric and adolescent gynecology*, ed. 5, Philadelphia, 2005a, Lippincott Williams & Wilkins; Speroff L, Fritz MA: *Clinical gynecologic endocrinology and infertility*, ed 7, Philadelphia, 2005, Lippincott Williams & Wilkins; Wilson GR, Haddad JE, Haddad CJ: Amenorrhea: common causes and evaluation, *Comp Ther* 31:270-278, 2005.

Physical Examination. The physical examination should include the following:
- Height, weight, BMI, nutritional status, blood pressure, pulse
- Sexual maturation rating
- Complete neurologic examination, including cranial nerves, funduscopic examination, and visual fields
- Midline facial defects or other congenital anomalies or stigmata of Turner syndrome
- Palpation of thyroid
- Breast examination with gentle compression to identify galactorrhea
- Palpation of abdomen and groin for masses, tenderness
- Examination of skin, hair distribution, and genitalia for signs of virilization
- External genital examination for estrogenization of vaginal mucosa (indicates ovarian function), vaginal and hymenal patency, and clitoromegaly (androgen excess)
- Digital vaginal examination and speculum examination if any abnormality is suspected
- Bimanual examination

Diagnostic Studies
- Initial laboratory studies with an essentially normal exam include:
  - Pregnancy test regardless of sexual history
  - TSH
  - FSH
  - Prolactin
- Follow the algorithm (Fig. 35-10) for complete evaluation.

Differential Diagnosis

The differential diagnoses for primary amenorrhea and secondary amenorrhea have considerable overlap (see Table 35-3). The exceptions are a few genetic conditions that cause primary amenorrhea (e.g., Turner syndrome). The most common causation of amenorrhea in the adolescent falls within the hypogonadotropic-hypothalamic category. An important marker of hypogonadotropic hypogonadism is the female athlete triad of amenorrhea, eating disorder, and osteoporosis (Emans, 2005a; Greydanus & Patel, 2002), especially common in gymnasts, figure skaters, ballet dancers, and long-distance runners at elite or highly competitive levels. The pressure for the ideal body for the sport and the intense exercise required may lead to this triad (also see Chapter 14 for a discussion of this triad).

Management

The treatment of amenorrhea obviously depends on its cause. Restoration of ovulatory cycles leads to the best long-term prognosis, and this is often accomplished through estrogen-progestin therapy. The primary care pediatric provider may

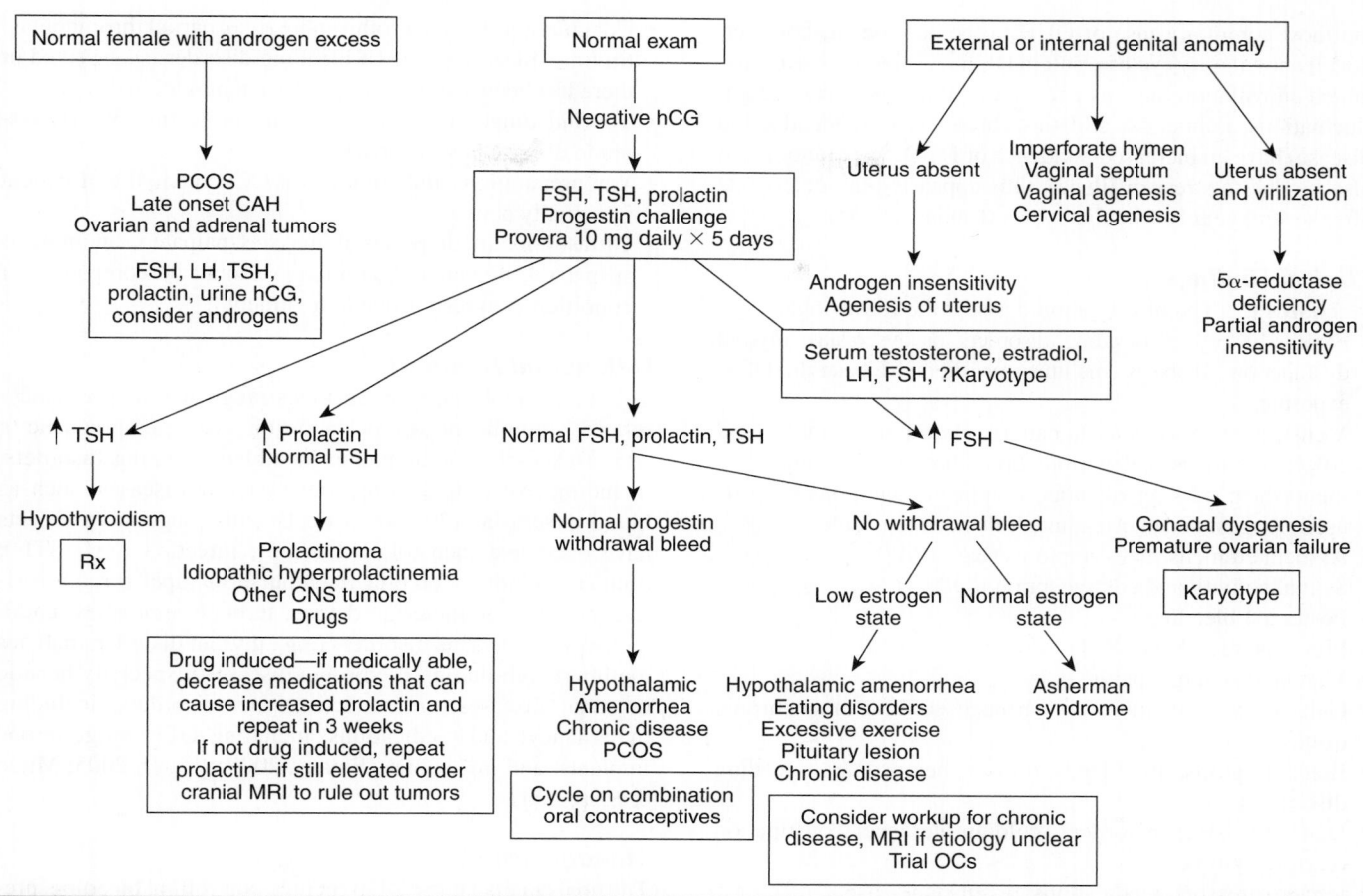

FIG. 35-10 Evaluation and management of amenorrhea. *CAH*, Congenital adrenal hyperplasia; *CNS*, central nervous system; *FSH*, follicle-stimulating hormone; *hCG*, human chorionic gonadotropin; *LH*, luteinizing hormone; *MRI*, magnetic resonance imaging; *OC*, oral contraceptive; *PCOS*, polycystic ovarian syndrome; *Rx*, medication; *TSH*, thyroid-stimulating hormone. (Adapted from Emans SJ: Amenorrhea in the adolescent. In Emans SJ, Laufer MR, Goldstein DP, editors: *Pediatric and adolescent gynecology*, ed 5, Philadelphia, 2005, Lippincott, Williams & Wilkins.)

need to consult and/or refer to a pediatric gynecologist or endocrinologist depending on the etiology. Anxiety about amenorrhea is common, and frequent reassurance is necessary. Young women should be made aware of the long-term skeletal effects of amenorrhea and instructed on adequate diet, reasonable exercise, and calcium supplementation to prevent osteoporosis.

DYSFUNCTIONAL UTERINE BLEEDING

Description
Dysfunctional uterine bleeding (DUB) refers to abnormal uterine bleeding that is excessive, prolonged, or unpatterned. It can be described as follows:

- *Polymenorrhea*: less than 21 days between menses
- *Menorrhagia*: normal intervals with excessive flow or duration of menses
- *Metrorrhagia*: irregular frequency of cycles with bleeding between cycles
- *Menometrorrhagia*: excessive amount of bleeding with irregular frequency of cycles

DUB is a diagnosis of exclusion, so any other causes of pathologic conditions must first be ruled out. DUB can be

classified as mild, moderate, or severe based on hemoglobin level, duration of cycle, and quantity of bleeding.

Epidemiology
The mechanism of DUB appears to be a delay in the maturation of the negative feedback cycle and is not related to structural pathologic conditions or medical illness (Emans, 2005c). Estrogen production continues without the balancing decrease in FSH, which would suppress estrogen. This results in abnormal endometrial thickening. The abnormal endometrium then sheds in a disorderly manner manifested by heavy, irregular, or prolonged bleeding. There is great variation in what is considered to be a normal menstrual cycle, especially in adolescents. Normal can range from 21 to 45 days between periods, with duration of flow from 3 to 7 days and 30 to 40 mL of blood loss (10 to 15 soaked tampons or pads) per cycle. Periods that last longer than 8 to 10 days and blood loss in excess of 80 ml are considered excessive (Emans, 2005c).

Abnormal uterine bleeding is frequently seen in adolescents (Emans, 2005c; Matytsina, 2006; Harel, 2005). Anovulation is the most common cause of DUB in the adolescent; however, not all anovulatory cycles result in DUB. Adolescents with sustained anovulation (e.g., as a result of eating disorders, weight fluctuations, competitive athletics, chronic illness, or endocrine disease) have an increased incidence of DUB. Anovulation can also be due to stress or illness, thus appearing in adolescents after several years of regular cycles (Emans, 2005c).

Clinical Findings

History. The history should assess the following:

- Family history of bleeding disorders or dyscrasias, thyroid dysfunction, diabetes mellitus, or diethylstilbestrol (DES) exposure
- Menstrual history: onset, pattern, duration, quantity, and color; last menstrual period; breakthrough bleeding; dysmenorrhea; passing of clots, number of tampons or pads used; longest and shortest intervals between cycles
- Associated menstrual symptoms (e.g., PMS)
- Sexual activity and contraception used
- Postcoital bleeding
- Previous infection or STIs
- Vaginal discharge, pelvic pain
- Galactorrhea, hirsutism (endocrine disease), or other chronic disease
- Bleeding gums, nosebleeds, bruises, hemorrhage (bleeding disorders)
- Hair loss, sleep disorders, cold intolerance, constipation (thyroid symptoms)
- Recent stressors, medications, or substance use
- Exercise and eating patterns, weight, weight fluctuations, laxative use, body image
- Genital trauma, sexual abuse
- Impact of bleeding on lifestyle

Physical Examination. The physical examination should include the following:

- Height, weight, BMI, body type, and fat distribution
- Vital signs (temperature, pulse, respiratory rate), orthostatic blood pressures
- Observation for acne, hirsutism, clitoromegaly (evidence of androgen excess)
- Breast examination for galactorrhea
- Thyroid palpation
- Observation for petechiae, bruising, pale color
- Abdominal examination for mass or tenderness
- Pelvic examination, including digital and speculum examination for foreign bodies, cervical lesions. In young, nonsexually active girls, the speculum exam may not be necessary per provider discretion.
- Tanner staging
- Bimanual and rectoabdominal examination

Diagnostic Studies. The following are ordered as indicated:

- Pregnancy test regardless of sexual history
- CBC with differential, platelet count, reticulocyte count
- Sedimentation rate or CRP (if infection or inflammation is suspected)
- Coagulation studies: prothrombin time, partial thromboplastin time, bleeding time (if bleeding disorder is suspected or there has been a significant drop in hemoglobin)
- Thyroid function test, blood sugar, prolactin level (if systemic disease is suspected)
- Wet preparations and cultures for GC, chlamydia, if patient is sexually active
- Ultrasonogram of pelvis if mass is palpated, anomaly is suspected, bimanual examination cannot be completed, or condition is unresponsive to treatment

Differential Diagnosis

The differential diagnosis includes pregnancy or pregnancy-related complications (postabortion, ectopic pregnancy); stress; excessive participation in athletics; eating disorders, including overweight; drug use; systemic diseases, such as blood dyscrasias (20% of patients with coagulation defects have excessive menstrual bleeding); infection (e.g., STIs); trauma, including forceful intercourse or rape; foreign bodies, including intrauterine device; tumors; anomalies; endometriosis; endocrine disorders (e.g., thyroid disorder, diabetes mellitus); debilitating or chronic diseases (especially hepatic or renal diseases); reproductive tract disorders, including malignancy; and medications, including OCs, progesterone implants, and injectables (Emans, 2005c; Harel, 2005; Mitan & Slap, 2002).

Management

The goals in managing DUB include controlling bleeding, preventing endometrial hyperplasia, preventing and treating anemia, restoring quality of life, and preventing recurrence. The following will enable the provider to manage DUB (Emans, 2005b; Mitan & Slap, 2002; Levine, 2006).

- Mild DUB: a shortened cycle or menses longer than normal with flow slightly to moderately increased or unpredictable; hemoglobin greater than 12 g/dL:
  - Observe and reassure.
  - Have patient start and maintain a menstrual calendar
  - Prescribe iron supplementation and dietary interventions to prevent anemia
  - Use prostaglandin inhibitors to reduce heavy bleeding (see Box 35-1)
  - Consider OCs for 3 to 4 months to decrease menorrhagia and stabilize menses
  - Reevaluate in 3 months
- Moderate DUB: shortened (1 to 3 weeks), irregular cycle with moderate to heavy bleeding, hemoglobin between 10 and 12 g/dL:
  - Prescribe 35 mcg monophasic combination OCs
    - If not currently bleeding, use same day start (see contraception section)
    - If currently bleeding, start with one OC bid for 3 to 4 days until bleeding stops. Then continue with one daily until finished with that pack, skip the placebo week, and start another pack without a withdrawal bleed. If bleeding resumes when OCs are decreased to one per day, again take one bid until

first pack is completed and start a second pack, taking one OC daily without a withdrawal bleed. Occasionally, the bid dose will not stop the bleeding. Add one OC every 3 to 4 days up to four OCs per day. After the bleeding stops, decrease the dose by one pill every 3 to 4 days until down to one per day. Continue OCs without a withdrawal bleed until the patient is completing a regular pill pack at one pill per day. If unable to control bleeding with four OCs per day, consult and/or referral is necessary
  - Add antiemetic to control the nausea of higher doses of estrogen
  - Usual length of treatment with OCs is 6 months
  ○ Alternatively, prescribe a progestin, such as medroxyprogesterone acetate (5 to 10 mg every day for 10 to 14 days started on the fourteenth day of cycle for 1 to 2 months). OCs are more effective at stopping active bleeding
  ○ Have patient start and maintain a menstrual calendar
  ○ Prescribe iron supplementation plus 1 mg folic acid per day
  ○ Reevaluate at least monthly until condition is stable
  ○ Reassess after 6 months
- Severe DUB: irregular, prolonged, heavy bleeding; hemoglobin less than 10 g/dL:
  ○ Refer to GYN and hospitalize if actively bleeding heavily and hemodynamically symptomatic; treatment may include transfusion, intravenous hormonal therapy, and dilation and curettage
  ○ Manage as moderate DUB if not actively bleeding

Complications

Anemia, profuse bleeding, shock, and side effects of OCs can occur. A long history of anovulation and DUB increases the risk of infertility and endometrial carcinoma.

Patient Education and Prognosis

- Encourage individual to keep a calendar of bleeding days and amounts. This includes keeping track of the number of pads or tampons used to increase accuracy
- Educate the patient and her parents about the use of OCs as a medication in the treatment of DUB. It is important, as with any medication, that it be taken as directed. Suddenly stopping it midcycle will result in resumed bleeding
- Prognosis is excellent if DUB is due to anovulation and immaturity of the HPO axis; these adolescents respond well to treatment, and most will develop regular menstrual patterns within 4 years of menarche (Matytsina, 2006)

ENDOMETRIOSIS

Description

Endometriosis is the proliferation of ectopic endometrial tissue outside the pelvic cavity. It is primarily manifested by dysmenorrhea that progressively worsens. Other symptoms include acyclic pelvic pain, gastrointestinal complaints, and dyspareunia. Adolescents usually experience pain, and as many as 62% of adolescents with endometriosis have both cyclic and acyclic pain.

Epidemiology

The cause of endometriosis is unknown. A risk factor is early menarche. Several theories have been developed to explain the possible cause of endometriosis, including retrograde menstruation; embryonic müllerian remnants, coelomic metaplasia; lymphatic, vascular, and iatrogenic dissemination; genetic factors; and immunologic or hormonal problems or defects.

The incidence rate in adolescents is difficult to obtain because endometriosis has only recently been studied in this age group. Estimates of 7% in the population with a first-degree relative with endometriosis, and 1% otherwise, are reported. Between 50% and 70% of adolescents with untreatable dysmenorrhea or pelvic pain are found to have a diagnosis of endometriosis on laparoscopy. This incidence of endometriosis on laparoscopy in adolescents increases with age, from 12% among 11- to 13-year-olds to 54% among 20- to 21-year-olds (Laufer & Goldstein, 2005).

Clinical Findings

History. The history can include the following:
- First-degree relative with endometriosis
- Deep unilateral or bilateral pain described as sharp or dull
- Chronic pelvic pain that is cyclic and/or acyclic and mildly to severely disabling, disrupting routine and causing missed school days or emergency department visits without definitive diagnosis
- Bladder and bowel dysfunction; rectal pain
- Dyspareunia
- Cyclic leg pain

Physical Examination. The following may be seen:
- Tender, enlarged, or fixed ovaries
- Adnexal masses, thickening, or tenderness
- The pelvic examination is most often unremarkable, with mild to moderate pelvic tenderness on palpation

Diagnostic Studies. The following are ordered as indicated:
- CBC, urine testing, or cervical cultures for GC and chlamydia to rule out infectious cause
- Ultrasound (helpful to evaluate anatomic structures; however, nonspecific for diagnosing endometriosis)

Differential Diagnosis

Primary dysmenorrhea, PID, appendicitis, ovarian cysts, müllerian anomalies, eating disorders, lactose intolerance, irritable bowel syndrome, chronic constipation, and depression are included in the differential diagnosis.

Management

- Have adolescent keep pain diary
- Trial of cyclic OCs and NSAIDs
- If unresponsive and the patient is under 18 years old, refer for a laparoscopic evaluation. If older than 18 years, may try empiric trial of GnRH agonist. If pain improves, a diagnosis of endometriosis can be made (ACOG, 2005)
- Supportive phone follow-up for side effects of medications and painful flare-ups is essential

- See at 1- to 3-month intervals to provide support and reevaluate
- Diet and exercise are important aspects in coping with chronic pain
- Stress reduction techniques and support groups may also be helpful
- A website specific to adolescent endometriosis is available (see Resource Box at the end of the chapter).

Complications

Miscarriage and infertility can occur. Endometriomas are rare in the adolescent age group. Gastritis, that may be treated with histamine-2 blockers, is seen frequently.

Prognosis and Prevention

Endometriosis is a chronic disease, and remission and exacerbation are to be expected. Stressful events often cause exacerbation. The goals of treatment are to control pain and prevent infertility.

VAGINITIS AND VAGINAL DISCHARGE

Description

Vaginitis refers to an inflammation or infection of the vulva and vaginal wall with or without discharge from the vagina.

Epidemiology

At puberty, the pH changes from 7 to 4.5, vaginal mucosa thickens, acidogenic bacteria predominate, and lactobacillus stabilizes the environment, all offering protection from infection. Adolescent vaginitis is most often due to a specific cause, often secondary to sexual contact. Normal physiologic leukorrhea occurs 6 to 12 months before puberty. Yeast, group A ß-hemolytic streptococci or other infections, foreign bodies (toilet paper fragments, tampon), and pinworms are possible causes. Bacterial vaginosis (BV), *Trichomonas*, or other STIs (discussed later in this chapter) must also be considered. Up to one half of female gynecologic complaints are related to vaginitis. *C. vaginitis*, BV, and *Trichomonas* infections are the most common infecting agents (Syed & Braverman, 2004).

Clinical Findings

The clinical findings pertaining to vaginitis are found in Table 35-2.

History. The history should include the following:
- Onset—How long have the symptoms been present?
- Location—vulva, vagina, perineum, and/or anus
- Characteristics:
  - Genital irritation, itching, pain, and inflammation
  - Vaginal discharge—note onset, quantity, color, type (bloody, mucoid), odor, consistency, and duration
  - Urinary complaints, including dysuria
  - Pelvic pain
  - Dyspareunia
- Ameliorating or aggravating factors
- Treatments or medications tried including CAM
- Previous occurrences and treatment used

- Recent medications, especially antibiotics
- Use of contraception
- Possible trauma, foreign body, or sexual abuse
- History of sexual activity or menstrual irregularities
- History of or recent exposures to STIs
- Perineal hygiene
  - Use of harsh or perfumed soaps and bubble bath
  - Use of tampons or pads, with deodorant
  - Douching, personal sprays
  - Any other hygiene measures
- Underlying illnesses (e.g., streptococcus infection, dermatosis, diabetes, immunosuppression)

Physical Examination. The examination of the adolescent would include the careful inspection of the perianal area and a speculum exam to visualize the cervix and vaginal walls. If the adolescent has not initiated vaginal intercourse, vaginal secretions can be collected with a saline moistened cotton swab. See Table 35-2 for physical examination findings.

Diagnostic Studies. The following should be considered:
- pH of vaginal secretions
- Wet mounts of vaginal secretions
  - Saline for microscopic examination to look for WBCs, clue cells, trichomonads, and bacteria
  - 10% KOH for whiff test and microscopic examination to look for yeast (branching hyphae and spores) (see Fig. 35-2)
- NAATs on urine or cultures for GC and chlamydia if suspected
- Urinalysis and culture if UTI suspected

Differential Diagnosis

The differential includes normal physiologic discharge, yeast vaginitis, BV, trichomoniasis and other STIs, foreign body, and contact or allergic dermatitis.

Management

See Table 35-2 for treatment.
- CAM recommendations:
  - For yeast: decrease foods high in simple carbohydrates; avoid foods with yeast or mold; increase fiber, garlic, ginger, cinnamon; live lactobacillus (1 to 2 billion live organisms per day) and acidophilus in diet
  - For BV: lactobacillus in the diet, and vaginal boric acid capsules

Complications

BV can contribute to PID, endometritis, postsurgical infection (abortion), and adverse pregnancy outcomes, such as preterm labor and birth, premature rupture of the membranes, and chorioamnionitis. Trichomoniasis has been linked with premature rupture of membranes and preterm delivery.

Patient Education, Prognosis, and Prevention

- Follow up in 5 days if there is no improvement
- For the sexually active adolescent, recommend not using diaphragm or condom until 3 days after treatment with topical vaginal cream or tablet
- Recommend frequent changes of tampons and use of a pad, especially at night, or ceasing the use of tampons

SEXUALLY TRANSMITTED DISEASES

Description

Multiple organisms are responsible for STIs in adolescents and children. GC, chlamydia, syphilis, HSV, and HPV are the most common STIs affecting the lower female reproductive tract. *Trichomonas* (discussed in previous section), hepatitis B, and HIV infections also are recognized as STIs. See Chapter 23 for discussion of hepatitis B and HIV (systemic STIs). The term sexually transmitted infection (STI) is often used instead of sexually transmitted diseases (STDs). Diagnosis can also be made in terms of the location of the infection (e.g., vaginitis, cervicitis, or urethritis) if causal organism is unknown.

STIs are a significant public health problem, placing a heavy financial health burden on society, having a tremendous impact on individuals' lives, and playing an important role in the transmission of HIV. The past 40 years have brought progress in treating STIs, with historic low incidence rates for GC and syphilis. However, the highest STI rates in the industrial world still occur in the U.S.

Epidemiology

Considered an epidemic, STIs have the highest rates in adolescents. The CDC reports that of the 19 million new STIs per year almost half occur in adolescents and young adults 15 to 24 years old. Furthermore, young women between 15 to 19 years old have the highest rates of *Neisseria gonorrhoeae* and *Chlamydia trachomatis* (CDC, 2005). Adolescents at highest risk for acquiring STIs include youth in detention facilities, male homosexuals, and injection drug users. Minorities, especially African Americans, are disproportionally affected.

Factors contributing to this epidemic are the increasingly early age and frequency of sexual activity, inconsistent use of contraceptive and protective devices, physiologic characteristics that predispose adolescents to infection, adolescents' lack of access to and use of health care, and societal influences (Box 35-3). Another factor that may contribute to higher reported numbers of STIs is the increased use and availability of accurate screening tests for diseases, especially chlamydia.

Most STIs must be reported, and the provider must be aware of each state's specific rules. All fifty states allow adolescents to be evaluated and to receive treatment for STIs confidentially. Management of children younger than 13 years old with STIs requires a coordinated effort between the pediatric provider and child protective authorities.

GC, caused by *N. gonorrhoeae*, a nonmotile, gram-negative diplococcus, is often found in carriage with chlamydia or other STIs. The GC rate for 2005 was 115.6 cases per 100,000, which is down 11% from 2002, but still far exceeds the 19 cases per 100,000 *Healthy People 2010* objective (CDC, 2006c). The highest rate for adolescents occurs in the 15- to 19-year-old group. There are more reported cases of GC in African Americans than Caucasians (18:1). The infection is often asymptomatic, with as many as 80% of young women infected with GC reporting no symptoms

---

| BOX 35-3 | **Risk Factors for Sexually Transmitted Diseases** |

- Adolescent younger than 15 years old
- Sexually active adolescent, especially with 2 or more partners in 6 months, high frequency of intercourse, or high rate of new partners
- Use of drugs or alcohol or other high-risk behaviors
- Pregnancy or abortion
- Homosexual
- Victim of abuse, rape, or incest
- Incarcerated, runaway, homeless, in group shelter or detention home
- Clients in STI clinics or with any other STI or previous history of STI
- Lack of family availability; low level of parental support and monitoring
- Beliefs about normative behaviors among peers
- Inappropriate health care behaviors (e.g., not seeking medical care, not adhering to treatment regimen, failure to recognize symptoms, delay in notifying partners, nonuse of barrier contraceptive)

Data from Biro FM, Rosenthal SL: Adolescent STDs: diagnosis, developmental issues, and prevention, *J Pediatr Health Care* 9:256-262, 1995; Bonny AE, Biro FM: Recognizing and treating STDs in adolescent girls, *Contemp Pediatr* 15:119-143, 1998; Shrier LA: Bacterial sexually transmitted infections: gonorrhea, chlamydia, pelvic inflammatory disease, and syphilis. In Emans SJ, Laufer MR, Goldstein DP, editors: *Pediatric and adolescent gynecology*, ed 5, Philadelphia, 2005, Lippincott Williams & Wilkins.

(Stamm & McGregor, 2001). Untreated GC can progress to PID.

C. trachomatis infection is the most frequently reported bacterial STI, with a rate of 332.5 cases per 100,000 reported in 2005, up 5.1% from 2004 (CDC, 2006c). Adolescent females have the highest percentage of these cases. Young women 15 to 19 years old account for 37% of the chlamydial infections, whereas 20- to 24-year-olds represent 36%. All sexually active young women in this age group should be screened at least annually because chlamydia is frequently asymptomatic. Untreated chlamydia can progress to PID; as many as 40% of the women with untreated infections develop PID, and 20% of those may loose their fertility (CDC, 2005).

Syphilis, caused by *Treponema pallidum*, is a motile spirochete with a rate of 3 cases per 100,000 in 2005, an increase of 11% from 2004. The majority of this increase (8.5%) was in males and primarily in men having sex with men (MSM) (CDC, 2006c). The MSM population had 64% of the new cases in 2004 (CDC, 2005). The rate for women increased for the first time in more than a decade (from 0.8 per 100,000 to 0.9 in 2005) with the rate of congenital syphilis down 12% from 2004 to 2005 at 8 per 100,000 live births (CDC, 2006c).

There are two identified serotypes of HSV: HSV-1 and HSV-2. Although either type may infect any part of the body, most recurrent genital herpes is a result of HSV-2. Asymptomatic HSV infections are responsible for the transmission of most cases of genital herpes. Type 2 in prepubescent children is reportable in some states.

HPV is a small DNA virus. More than thirty types of HPV can infect the genital tract. Visible warts are usually caused by HPV types 6 or 11. A person may be infected with multiple types of HPV. Types 16, 18, 31, 33, and 35 have been strongly associated with cervical cancer and vulvar, penile, and anal squamous intraepithelial neoplasia (CDC, 2006a).

Clinical Findings

History. Many patients are asymptomatic. The history should assess the following:
- Type of sexual activity (including oral, vaginal, anal sex/intercourse) and contraceptive use
- Number of sexual partners over 60 days, 12 months, and lifetime; heterosexual or homosexual (or both) activity
- Known exposure or previous STIs
- Use of drugs or alcohol
- Vaginal discharge (amount, color, odor), pruritus, irregular or painful bleeding, dysmenorrhea, dyspareunia
- Dysuria, urinary urgency or frequency
- Abdominal or pelvic pain
- Skin rashes or lesions, ulcers, warts
- Systemic symptoms, such as fever, malaise, headache
- See Box 35-3 for risk factors for STIs; Box 35-4 for CDC's five Ps; and Table 35-4 for history specific to each STI
- See Chapter 19 for further details on obtaining history

Physical Examination

The physical examination should include the following:
- General examination—skin rashes and lesions, lymphadenopathy
- Abdominal examination—hepatic or splenic enlargement or tenderness in right upper quadrant
- Pelvic examination—inspection of external genitalia and vaginal mucosa, vaginal pH and discharge, cervical erythema, friability and mucopus, bimanual examination for cervical motion tenderness, uterine size, adnexal tenderness
- Rectal examination
- See Table 35-4 for physical findings specific to each STI

Diagnostic Studies. In deciding which studies to order, the provider needs to know the difference in and accuracy of tests. Methods that are sufficiently accurate for adolescents (presumptive tests) are not adequate for children who are being evaluated for possible abuse.
- GC. Culture on selective media with determination of penicillin resistance is the definitive test for GC in women. Nucleic acid hybridization tests (DNA probes) and NAAT are also available for GC testing (Spigarelli & Biro, 2004). NAATs are more reliable when done by cervical swab testing than with urine testing for GC (Shrier, 2005). Gram stains of vaginal discharge or cervical secretions are not recommended (CDC, 2006a)
- *Chlamydia*. Culture is the only acceptable method to diagnose possible sexual abuse cases; many family planning clinics use direct immunofluorescent smears; however, DNA probes and NAATs are acceptable in adolescents,

---

| BOX 35-4 | CDC's The Five Ps |

PARTNERS, PREVENTION OF PREGNANCY, PROTECTION FROM STIs, PRACTICES, PAST HISTORY OF STIs

1. Partners
   - "Do you have sex with men, women, or both?"
   - "In the past 2 months, how many partners have you had sex with?"
   - "In the past 12 months, how many partners have you had sex with?"
2. Prevention of pregnancy
   - "Are you or your partner trying to get pregnant?" If no, "What are you doing to prevent pregnancy?"
3. Protection from STIs
   - "What do you do to protect yourself from STIs and HIV?"
4. Practices
   - "To understand your risks for STIs, I need to understand the kind of sex you have had recently."
   - "Have you had vaginal sex, meaning 'penis in vagina sex'"?
   - If yes, "Do you use condoms: never, sometimes, or always?"
   - "Have you had anal sex, meaning 'penis in rectum/anus sex'?"
   - If yes, "Do you use condoms: never, sometimes, or always?"
   - "Have you had oral sex, meaning 'mouth on penis/vagina'?"

   For condom answers:
   - If "never:" "Why don't you use condoms?"
   - If "sometimes": "In what situations or with whom, do you not use condoms?"
5. Past history of STIs
   - "Have you ever had an STI?"
   - "Have any of your partners had an STI?"

   Additional questions to identify HIV and hepatitis risk:
   - "Have you or any of your partners ever injected drugs?"
   - "Have any of your partners exchanged money or drugs for sex?"
   - "Is there anything else about your sexual practices that I need to know about?"

From Centers for Disease Control and Prevention (CDC): *Sexually transmitted diseases: treatment guidelines, clinical prevention guidance*, Atlanta, 2006, U.S. Department of Health and Human Services. Available from *www.cdc.gov/std/treatment/2006/clinical.htm* (accessed Jan 8, 2007).

---

especially in high-prevalence populations. Only NAATs can be done on either a cervical swab or urine and are therefore preferable for adolescents
- Syphilis. Direct visualization with dark-field microscopy or direct immunofluorescent antibody (DFA) test is definitive. Serologic nontreponemal tests (Venereal Disease Research Laboratories [VDRL], rapid plasma reagin [RPR], or automated reagin test) correlate with disease activity, decline after treatment, and are used to monitor disease progress. Treponemal tests (fluorescent treponemal antibody absorption [FTA-ABS] or microhemagglutination test for *T. pallidum*

TABLE 35-5   Sexually Transmitted Disease: History, Physical Examination, and Initial Treatment

	History	Physical Examination	Treatment
Gonorrhea (GC) N. gonorrhoeae	Often asymptomatic (33%); dysuria; vaginal discharge or bleeding; dyspareunia	Profuse, thick, green discharge, urethritis, cervicitis; Skene's or Bartholin gland abscess; exudative pharyngitis	Ceftriaxone 125 mg IM 1 time *or* Cefixime 400 mg PO 1 time *or* Ciprofloxacin 500 mg 1 time* *or* Levofloxacin 250 mg 1 time* *or* Ofloxacin 400 mg PO 1 time* *If chlamydial infection not ruled out also give* Azithromycin 1 g PO in a single dose *or* Doxycycline 100 mg PO bid for 7 days[†] Report to state health department Do culture and sensitivity 2 wk after treatment if symptoms persist
Chlamydia C. trachomatis	Often asymptomatic (30%-70%); spotting, vaginal discharge; dysuria, pyuria; mild abdominal pain or foreign body sensation in eyes possible	Clear to white or yellow discharge, mucopurulent cervicitis with edema, erythema, hypertrophy; Fitz-Hugh–Curtis syndrome (right upper quadrant pain); conjunctivitis	Azithromycin 1 g PO in a single dose *or* Doxycycline 100 mg PO bid for 7 days[†] Alternative medications: Erythromycin base 500 mg PO qid for 7 days *or* Erythromycin ethylsuccinate 800 mg PO qid for 7 days *or* Ofloxacin 300 mg PO bid for 7 days* *or* Levofloxacin 500 mg PO for 7 days* Report to state health department Test of cure not recommended unless pregnant or compliance questioned
Syphilis T. pallidum	*Primary:* vaginal, anal, or oral chancre *Secondary:* copper-penny rash especially on palms and soles, lymphadenopathy, mucocutaneous lesions	Single painless papule with serous discharge, smooth base, raised edges; painless regional lymphadenopathy	Benzathine penicillin G 2.4 million units IM *or* If penicillin allergy and not pregnant: Doxycycline 100 mg PO bid for 14 days[†] *or* Tetracycline 500 mg PO qid for 14 days[†] Test for GC, chlamydia, and HIV at time of infection and in 3 mo Follow with RPR or VDRL titers at 6 and 12 mo; should have fourfold decline by 6 mo Report to state health department
Herpes simplex virus (HSV)	Painful rash, blisters and ulcers; burning and irritation 24 hr before outbreak; dysuria; other systemic complaints	Clear to white to yellow discharge; vesicles on erythematous base that become ulcers in 1-3 days; extragenital lesions; lymphadenopathy	Primary—Acyclovir 400 mg tid for 7-10 days (*or* 200 mg 5 times a day for 7-10 days) *or* Famciclovir 250 mg tid for 7-10 days *or* Valacyclovir 1 g bid for 7-10 days Recurrent—Acyclovir 400 mg tid for 5 days *or* Acyclovir 800 mg bid for 5 days *or* Acyclovir 800 mg tid for 2 days *or* Famciclovir 125 mg bid for 5 days *or* Famciclovir 1 g bid for 1 day Comfort measures—sitz bath, dry heat, lidocaine jelly 2%
Human papillomavirus (HPV)	Asymptomatic or subclinical unrecognized; can be painful	Warts, friable or pruritic (or both); moist, cauliflower-like anogenital and inguinal 4-6 wk after exposure	*Patient applied treatment* (see text): Podofilox or imiquimod *Provider applied treatment* (see text): Cryotherapy, podophyllin resin, trichloroacetic acid or bichloroacetic acid, or surgical removal

*Contraindicated under 18 yr old, in pregnancy, or during lactation. Quinolones should not be used in persons with a history of recent foreign travel or partner's travel, infections acquired in California or Hawaii, or infections acquired in other areas with increased quinolone-resistant *N. gonorrhoeae* prevalence.
[†]Contraindicated under 8 yr old.
bid, Twice a day; *HIV,* human immunodeficiency virus; *hr,* hours; *IM,* intramuscular; *mo,* months; *PO,* by mouth; *qid,* 4 times daily; *RPR,* rapid plasma reagin; *tid,* three times daily; *VDRL,* Venereal Disease Research Laboratories; *wk,* weeks.
Data from Centers for Disease Control and Prevention (CDC): Sexually transmitted diseases: treatment guidelines, *MMWR Morb Mortal Wkly Rep* 55(RR-11): 1-100, 2006.

[MHA-TP]) are confirmatory, but once positive they usually remain so for years

- Herpes. Culture of scraped vesicle or ulcer is most accurate. Tzanck stain, DFA, and enzyme immunoassay (EIA) are quicker but less sensitive. Blood tests are being studied, but are not routinely used because they are not readily available and are expensive
- HPV. ViraPap is the specific test. Pap testing that shows koilocytosis, dysplasia, atypia, or cervical intraepithelial neoplasia is suspicious. The use of HPV nucleic acid tests for typing visible genital warts is not recommended. Biopsy for histologic and cytologic microscopic evaluation and typing by DNA hybridization are more specific but rarely needed

Differential Diagnosis

Chancroid, lymphogranuloma venereum, cytomegalovirus, hepatitis, granuloma inguinale, and molluscum are included in the differential diagnosis.

Management

The guidelines identified in this section are those recommended by the CDC (2006a) for uncomplicated, initial treatment of STIs. Other recommendations and options for children weighing less than 45 kg and for recurrent and complex cases are also found in that CDC resource or in adolescent gynecology or child abuse literature.

The goals of treatment include making a prompt diagnosis, determining the mode of acquisition, instituting appropriate treatment, preventing complications, contacting appropriate authorities, ensuring appropriate follow-up, and educating the adolescent and partner about risk reduction. All adolescents in the U.S. can consent to confidential diagnosis and treatment of STIs.

Several options for treatment are given for each disease (see Table 35-4). When determining appropriate treatment, consideration should be given to the site of infection, the resistance patterns in the community, concurrent infections, side effects of the medication, and cost. See Box 35-5 for general treatment measures for STIs.

1. GC (uncomplicated, patient weighing more than 45 kg):
   - See Table 35-4
   - Cefixime 400 mg orally in a single dose is recommended as the single-dose treatment
   - Fluoroquinolones should not be used for treatment of GC if the infection was acquired in Asia, the Pacific Islands (including Hawaii), or California because the prevalence of fluoroquinolone-resistant *N. gonorrhoeae* is high in those areas
   - Evaluate and treat all partners exposed in the previous 30 to 60 days and treat last sexual partner if more than 60 days since last intercourse
2. Chlamydia (uncomplicated genital infection):
   - See Table 35-4
   - Treat last partner and any partner exposed within the 60 days before the onset of symptoms
   - Rescreen 3 to 4 months after positive test result because a high prevalence of *C. trachomatis* infection is found in women with a chlamydial infection in the preceding several months. Reinfection is usually the cause of infection and elevates the risk for PID

BOX 35-5 **General Treatment Measures for Sexually Transmitted Infections**

1. Have patient abstain from sexual intercourse until patient and partner are cured (treatment complete and symptoms resolved). Consequences of untreated STIs should be explained.
2. Test for other STIs, including hepatitis B, HIV, BV, and *Trichomonas*.
3. Notify, examine, and treat all partners of patient for any STI identified or suspected.
4. Report STIs to state health department. Reporting to appropriate authorities is important to identify those at risk, recognize new strains, and assess extent of infection in community and the effect of prevention efforts.
5. Provide regular sex health assessment including Papanicolaou testing, vaginal examination, and testing for STIs.
6. Give hepatitis B, HPV vaccines if not done already.
7. Discuss safer sex practices, including abstinence and use of condoms.
8. Educate and counsel about complications and transmission of STIs and perinatal consequences.

---

3. Syphilis (primary or secondary):
   - See Table 35-4
   - The same laboratory tests (RPR or VDRL) should be used for follow-up and should decrease fourfold by 6 months and become nonreactive 1 year after treatment in primary cases. If still reactive after 12 months, retreat and reevaluate for HIV
   - Treat all partners exposed during symptomatic period and for the 3 months before onset of infection
   - An acute febrile reaction (Jarisch-Herxheimer reaction) with myalgia, headache, and other symptoms can occur within 24 hours after treatment
   - Refer if symptoms of secondary or tertiary syphilis are present
4. Genital herpes. No treatment will eradicate the disease. Treatment or prevention of acute outbreaks is the goal of therapy:
   - See Table 35-4
   - Use daily suppressive treatment if episodes occur six times or more in a year. This reduces the frequency of episodes by more than 70% to 80%
     ○ Acyclovir 400 mg orally twice a day or
     ○ Famciclovir 250 mg orally twice a day or
     ○ Valacyclovir 500 mg once a day or 1000 mg once a day
   - Test for other STIs as indicated
   - Counsel to abstain from sexual activity when active lesions are present and inform sexual partners
   - Inform that transmission of HSV can occur during asymptomatic periods
   - Stress the risk of perinatal infection and follow pregnancies closely
   - Educate regarding course of disease, self-inoculation, transmission, and asymptomatic viral shedding

- Suggest dietary modifications including increased intake of vitamin C, B-complex and B$_6$ vitamins, zinc, and calcium to boost the immune system. A diet high in lysine and low in arginine (e.g., eating fish, chicken, cheese, and most fruits and vegetables and avoiding chocolate, peanuts, and white and wheat flour) may be helpful

5. HPV. No treatment will eradicate this disease. The goal should be to remove visible warts and reduce symptoms. The benefit of identification and treatment of subclinical infections has not been established. Patient preference and treatment availability should guide treatment course; spontaneous resolution will occur in most cases. Warts on moist surfaces respond better to topical treatment than do warts on drier surfaces:

- Patient-applied treatment: treat with (1) podofilox 0.5% solution or gel twice a day for 3 days, no treatment for 4 days, for a total of four cycles (safety in pregnancy has not been established) or (2) imiquimod 5% cream applied with finger at bedtime three times a week for up to 16 weeks. Wash treated area with mild soap and water 6 to 10 hours after application. Warts should clear after 8 to 10 weeks. Safety in pregnancy is not determined
- Provider-applied treatment: treat external visible warts with (1) cryotherapy with liquid nitrogen or cryoprobe every 1 to 2 weeks or (2) 10% to 25% podophyllin resin in benzoin washed off in 1 to 4 hours to decrease local irritation, repeated weekly (safety in pregnancy not established), or (3) trichloroacetic acid (TCA) or bichloroacetic acid (BCA) applied in small amounts, dried to frosting consistency, followed by baking powder or baking soda to remove unreacted acid, repeated weekly, or (4) surgical removal with scissors, shave, curette, or electrosurgery
- Change treatment if there is no response after three patient-applied treatments or six provider-applied treatments
- Use only one treatment modality at a time to prevent increased complications
- Advise patient that an inflammatory reaction is common before resolution
- After cryotherapy, pain, necrosis, and blistering are common
- Refer patients with cervical warts, suspected abuse, or extensive lesions in difficult areas for gynecologic treatment. Intralesional interferon or laser surgery may be necessary in severe cases
- No change in the schedule for Pap testing is necessary with clinical warts
- Advise patient that recurrence is common, most often in the first 3 months following treatment

Complications

In general, perinatal transmission, disseminated infection, and increased risk for chronic hepatitis are possible. PID, ectopic pregnancy, and infertility are possible sequelae to GC and chlamydia. Tertiary disease is a risk with syphilis. An increased risk of HIV transmission has been found with other STIs. HPV infection is linked with cervical dysplasia and cancer.

Patient Education and Prevention

- Prevention occurs at a variety of levels and in a variety of ways. The following approaches are recommended (Bonny & Biro, 1998; Stevens-Simon, 1998):
  - Primary prevention seeks to reduce the number of new cases of STIs. This best occurs before sexual debut, focusing on delaying initiation of sexual intercourse, encouraging noncoital sexual behavior, promoting condom negotiating skills, and avoiding exposure to STIs if the intent is to become sexually active. These topics must be addressed specifically, using knowledge, attitudes, and behaviors to guide education. Developmental needs, cultural values, misperceptions, and social skills are areas to be addressed. Peer facilitators are often useful. Hepatitis B, HPV, and possibly hepatitis A immunizations are recommended
  - Secondary prevention seeks to reduce the numbers of existing cases by early detection and treatment through well-woman care, annual Pap testing, and STI screening (recommended every 6 months for those at risk). Access to health care for treatment and follow-up, monitoring for sequelae, partner notification, and evaluating risk behaviors are important aspects to successful secondary prevention
  - Tertiary prevention seeks to minimize the psychological and biologic sequelae of STIs. This includes minimizing perinatal complications and infant morbidity and mortality rates and reducing the frequency of PID and its complications. Identifying coping strategies and means of increasing self-esteem are also important aspects
- Treatment of any STI in a child should be coordinated with the laboratory, child protective services, and the state authorities
- Important family factors that reduce risk behaviors include the following:
  - Perceived parental support
  - Degree of family closeness
  - Communication among family members
  - Parenting style
  - Parental supervision and monitoring

PELVIC INFLAMMATORY DISEASE

Description
Considered an ascending infection, PID refers to infection and inflammation involving the upper genital tract (uterus, fallopian tubes, ovaries, or peritoneal tissue). PID is either acute (less than 3 weeks duration) or chronic. The classic picture is acute salpingitis that causes lower abdominal pain, vaginal discharge, and fever with an onset after menses. However, PID is difficult to diagnose because symptoms are widely varied (CDC, 2006a).

Epidemiology
PID is often a polymicrobial infection, with GC and chlamydia being the two most common STIs causing PID. Vaginal flora, other aerobic and anaerobic organisms, group B streptococcus, genital mycoplasma, and gram-negative bacteria also are implicated. There are one million new cases of PID every year, with approximately 20% occurring in adolescents (Banikarim & Chacko, 2004).

The two risk factors considered to be most significant among teenagers are multiple sexual partners and the high prevalence of STIs in this age group. Other risk factors include increased susceptibility of adolescents to infection, cervical ectopy and thinner cervical mucus, recent instrumentation or intrauterine device use, previous PID, history of lower genital tract infection (including GC, chlamydia, trichomoniasis, and BV), and nonuse of contraceptives of any type.

Clinical Findings

PID in adolescents is often subtle and can go undiagnosed, contributing to the inflammatory sequelae. Criteria for diagnosis of PID have been identified, including a set of minimal, low-threshold criteria prompting early intervention (Box 35-6).

History
- Sexual history, including number of partners and type of activity
- Last menstrual period, contraceptive use, and previous STI or PID
- Lower abdominal pain or tenderness (acute onset with GC, subtle with chlamydia)
- Intermenstrual bleeding
- Malaise, dysuria, nausea, vomiting, chills, dyspareunia

Physical Examination
- Abdominal examination—bilateral lower quadrant tenderness (most common initial symptom) and possibly right upper quadrant pain (Fitz-Hugh–Curtis syndrome: inflammation of liver capsule); occasional peritoneal signs
- Speculum examination—cervical or vaginal mucopurulent discharge

---

BOX 35-6   **Criteria for Diagnosing Pelvic Inflammatory Disease (PID)**

Minimum criteria for treating PID in sexually active adolescents with no other cause for illness identified:
Cervical motion tenderness **OR** Uterine tenderness **OR** Adnexal tenderness
Additional criteria that support a diagnosis of PID:
  Oral temperature >101° F (>38.3° C)
  Abnormal mucopurulent cervical or vaginal discharge
  Presence of abundant WBCs in saline microscopy of vaginal secretions
  Elevated erythrocyte sedimentation rate
  Elevated C-reactive protein
  Laboratory documentation of cervical infection with GC or chlamydia
Most specific criteria for diagnosing PID, warranted in selected cases:
  Endometrial biopsy with histopathologic evidence of endometritis
  Transvaginal sonography or magnetic resonance imaging showing thickened fluid-filled tubes with or without free pelvic fluid or tuboovarian complex
  Laparoscopic abnormalities consistent with PID

Data from Centers for Disease Control and Prevention (CDC): Sexually transmitted diseases: treatment guidelines, *MMWR Morb Mortal Wkly Rep* 55(RR-11):i-100, 2006.

- Bimanual examination—cervical motion tenderness, uterine or adnexal tenderness (may be unilateral)

Diagnostic Studies
- CBC (WBCs greater than 10,000), erythrocyte sedimentation rate (greater than 15 mm/hour), C-reactive protein (elevated)
- Microscopic examination of cervical discharge
- NAATs or culture for GC and chlamydia
- Serologic test (syphilis)
- Pregnancy test (ectopic)
- Urinalysis and culture if symptoms of pyelonephritis or cystitis
- Pelvic ultrasound (if adnexal enlargement or tuboovarian abscess suspected)
- Culdocentesis (pus)

Differential Diagnosis

Acute appendicitis, ectopic pregnancy, torsion of an ovarian cyst, ruptured corpus luteal cyst, salpingitis, tuboovarian abscess, endometritis, acute pyelonephritis, gastroenteritis, vaginitis, and functional pain are included in the differential diagnosis.

Management

- Goals of treatment include the relief of acute discomfort and prevention of infertility and other sequelae. More than one diagnosis is possible. Empiric treatment should be initiated in sexually active young women if the minimal criteria are met. Treatment should be initiated as soon as possible with broad-spectrum coverage to minimize long-term sequelae
- Hospitalization is recommended in the following situations: surgical emergency cannot be excluded; pregnancy; lack of response to oral antibiotics; inability to tolerate oral antibiotics; severe illness with nausea, vomiting, or high temperature; or tuboovarian abscess (CDC, 2006a)
- Outpatient treatment regimens are delineated in Table 35-5
- Follow up within 72 hours. Patients should demonstrate clinical improvement as evidenced by defervescence, decreased abdominal tenderness, and decreased uterine, adnexal, and cervical motion tenderness. If no clinical improvement, the patient will need hospitalization
- Treatment of any sexual partners exposed within 60 days of onset of symptoms is imperative. No intercourse until partners have been treated
- Follow up 7 to 10 days after treatment
- Rescreen for chlamydia and GC 4 to 6 weeks after treatment in documented cases
- HIV screening should be offered
- PID is a reportable STI in some states

Complications

Infertility (8% to 50% attributable to PID, a higher percentage with subsequent episodes); tuboovarian abscess; ectopic pregnancy (threefold to tenfold increased risk); perihepatitis (Fitz-Hugh-Curtis syndrome); chronic pelvic pain; dyspareunia; repeated PID (Banikarim & Chacko, 2004).

Prevention

Decrease prevalence and transmission of STIs by promoting abstinence and barrier methods (condoms, diaphragms, cervical caps, and spermicidal foams). Screen sexually active adolescents for GC and chlamydia every 6 months.

TABLE 35-5 **Outpatient Treatment Regimens for Pelvic Inflammatory Disease**

	Regimen A	Regimen B
Oral	Levofloxacin 500 mg orally once daily for 14 days* **OR** Ofloxacin 400 mg orally twice daily for 14 days* **With or Without** Metronidazole 500 mg twice daily for 14 days	Ceftriaxone 250 mg IM in a single dose **Plus** Doxycycline 100 mg orally twice a day for 14 days **With or Without** Metronidazole 500 mg twice daily for 14 days **OR** Cefoxitin 2 g IM in a single dose and Probenecid 1 g orally administered concurrently in a single dose **Plus** Doxycycline 100 mg orally twice a day for 14 days **With or Without** Metronidazole 500 mg twice daily for 14 days

*Contraindicated under 18 yr old, in pregnancy, or during lactation. Quinolones should not be used in persons with a history of recent foreign travel or partners' travel, infections acquired in California or Hawaii, or infections acquired in other areas with increased quinolone-resistant *N. gonorrhoeae* prevalence.
IM, Intramuscular.
Data from Centers for Disease Control and Prevention (CDC): Sexually transmitted diseases: treatment guidelines, *MMWR Morb Mortal Wkly Rep* 55(RR-11): 1-100, 2006a.

RESOURCE BOX

National Resources for Pediatric and Adolescent Gynecology

Abstinence Clearinghouse
www.abstinence.net

American College of Obstetricians and Gynecologists (ACOG) (pamphlets)
www.acog.com
Pamphlets available

American Social Health Association
www.ashastd.org

Association of Reproductive Health Professionals
www.arhp.org
Pamphlets available

Centers for Disease Control and Prevention (CDC) STD information
www.cdc.gov/std
Hotline: 1-800-227-8922

Center for Young Women's Health, Children's Hospital Boston
www.youngwomenshealth.org

Education Training Resource Associates
www.etr.org
Pamphlets available

Medical Institute for Sexual Health
www.medinstitute.org

The National Campaign to Prevent Teen and Unplanned Pregnancy
www.teenpregnancy.org

National Herpes Hotline
1-800-227-8922

National STD Hotline
1-800-227-8922

North American Society for Pediatric and Adolescent Gynecology (NASPAG)
www.naspag.org

Planned Parenthood Federation of America, Inc.
www.plannedparenthood.org

ReproLine
www.reproline.jhu.edu

Sexuality Information and Education Council of the United States (SIECUS)
www.siecus.org

Society for Adolescent Medicine
www.adolescenthealth.org

World Health Organization—Medical Eligibility Criteria for Contraceptive Use
www.who.int/reproductive-health/publications/mec

☑ DISCUSSION FORUM

1. As a provider you may have religious beliefs that are against abortion and birth control. In addition, you may work with providers with similar beliefs. How can you work with sexually active adolescents or adolescents who are pregnant and may want an abortion?

2. A sexually active 13-year-old is not using any contraceptive method. She does not want her parents to know that she is sexually active. How would you approach this child? How would you counsel her about contraceptive use? What methods might be more suitable? What other things do you want to include in your discussion?

3. A 12 ½-year-old female has had secondary amenorrhea for 3 months. She started her menses at 9 years old and had a 28-day cycle for the past 2 years. What do you want to do and why? How would your approach vary if the patient were 10 years old and had her menses for only 6 months?

4. A 6-year-old has a yellow discharge. The exam is otherwise normal. What are key points in the history and physical exam? How would your approach differ if the patient was a sexually active 16-year-old? What are similarities and differences in the approach?

REFERENCES

Abma JC et al: Teenagers in the U.S.: sexual activity, contraceptive use, and childbearing, 2002. National Center for Health Statistics, *Vital Health Stat* 23(24):2004. Available from *www.cdc.gov/nchs/data/series/sr_23/sr23_024.pdf* (accessed Jan 7, 2007).

American College of Obstetricians and Gynecologists (ACOG): Committee opinion, cervical cancer screening in adolescents, *Obstet Gynecol* 104:885-889, 2004.

American College of Obstetricians and Gynecologists (ACOG): Committee opinion, endometriosis in adolescents, *Obstet Gynecol* 105:921-927, 2005.

American College of Obstetricians and Gynecologists (ACOG): Committee opinion, evaluation and management of abnormal cervical cytology and histology in the adolescent, *Obstet Gynecol* 107:963-968, 2006a.

American College of Obstetricians and Gynecologists (ACOG): Committee opinion, the initial reproductive health visit, *Obstet Gynecol* 107:1215-1219, 2006b.

American Medical Association (AMA): *Guidelines for adolescent preventive services (GAPS): recommendations monograph*, Chicago, 1997 American Medical Association.

Bacon JL: Prepubertal labial adhesions: evaluation of a referral population, *Am J Obstet Gynecol* 187:327-332, 2002.

Banikarim C, Chacko M: Pelvic inflammatory disease in adolescents, *Adolesc Med Clin* 15:273-285, 2004.

Bonny AE, Biro FM: Recognizing and treating STDs in adolescent girls, *Contemp Pediatr* 15:119-143, 1998.

Centers for Disease Control and Prevention (CDC): Sexually transmitted diseases: treatment guidelines, *MMWR Morb Mortal Wkly Rep* 55(RR-11):i-100, 2006a.

Centers for Disease Control and Prevention (CDC): *Sexually transmitted diseases: treatment guidelines, clinical prevention guidance*, Atlanta, 2006b, U.S. Department of Health and Human Services. Available from *www.cdc.gov/std/treatment/2006/clinical.htm#clinical2* (accessed Jan 8, 2007).

Centers for Disease Control and Prevention (CDC): *Trends in reportable sexually transmitted diseases in the United States, 2005*, Atlanta, 2006c, U.S. Department of Health and Human Services. Available from *www.cdc.gov/std/stats/05pdf/trends-2005.pdf* (accessed Jan 7, 2007).

Centers for Disease Control and Prevention (CDC): Youth risk behavior surveillance—United States, 2005, *MMWR Morb Mortal Wkly Rep* 55(SS-5):i-110, 2006d.

Centers for Disease Control and Prevention (CDC): *Trends in reportable sexually transmitted diseases in the United States, 2004*, Atlanta, U.S. Department of Health and Human Services 2005. Available from *www.cdc.gov/std/stats/trends2004.htm* (accessed Sept 15, 2006).

Chen C et al: Prospective study of exposure to environmental tobacco smoke and dysmenorrhea, *Environ Health Perspect* 108:1019-1022, 2000.

Davis AR et al: Oral contraceptives for dysmenorrhea in adolescent girls: a randomized trial, *Obstet Gynecol* 106:97-104, 2005.

Dryfoos JG: Thirty years in pursuit of the magic bullet, *J Adolesc Health* 23:338-343, 1998.

Durain D: Primary dysmenorrhea: assessment and management update, *J Midwifery Womens Health* 49:520-528, 2004.

Emans SJ: Amenorrhea in the adolescent. In Emans SJ, Laufer MR, Goldstein DP, editors: *Pediatric and adolescent gynecology*, ed 5, Philadelphia, 2005a, Lippincott Williams & Wilkins.

Emans SJ: Contraception. In Emans SJ, Laufer MR, Goldstein DP, editors: *Pediatric and adolescent gynecology*, ed 5, Philadelphia, 2005b, Lippincott Williams & Wilkins.

Emans SJ: Dysfunctional uterine bleeding. In Emans SJ, Laufer MR, Goldstein DP, editors: *Pediatric and adolescent gynecology*, ed 5, Philadelphia, 2005c, Lippincott Williams & Wilkins.

Emans SJ: Vulvovaginal problems in the prepubertal child. In Emans SJ, Laufer MR, Goldstein DP, editors: *Pediatric and adolescent gynecology*, ed 5, Philadelphia, 2005d, Lippincott Williams & Wilkins.

Greydanus DE, Patel DR: The female athlete: before and beyond puberty, *Pediatr Clin North Am* 49:829-855, 2002.

Hamel-Teillac D: Vulvo-vaginal disorders. Pediatric and adolescent gynecology. evidence-based clinical practice, *Endocr Dev* 7:39-56, 2004.

Harel Z: In training, approach to the adolescent girl as she transits from irregular to regular menstrual cycles, *J Pediatr Adolesc Gynecol* 18:193-200, 2005.

Hatcher RA et al: *Contraceptive technology*, ed 18, New York, 2004, Ardent.

Hatcher RA et al: *A pocket guide to managing contraception*, ed 8, Tiger, GA, 2005, Bridging the Gap Foundation.

Holland-Hall C, Hewill G, Breech L: Tips for clinicians, the 'well girl' exam, *J Pediatr Adolesc Gynecol* 18:289-291, 2005.

Kahn JA, Hillard PA: Human papillomavirus and cervical cytology in adolescents. *Adolesc Med Clin* 15(2):301-321, 2004.

Kaplowitz PB, Oberfield SE: Reexamination of the age limit for defining when puberty is precocious in girls in the United States: implications for evaluation and treatment, *Pediatrics* 104:936-941, 1999.

Klein JD: Adolescent pregnancy: current trends and issues, *Pediatrics* 116:281-286, 2005.

Koniak-Griffin D et al: Public health nursing care for adolescent mothers: impact on infant health and selected maternal outcomes at 1 year postbirth, *J Adolesc Health* 30:44-54, 2002.

Levine SB: In training, dysfunctional uterine bleeding in adolescents, *J Pediatr Adolesc Gynecol* 19:49-51, 2006.

Laufer MR, Goldstein DP: Gynecologic pain: dysmenorrhea, acute and chronic pelvic pain, endometriosis, and premenstrual syndrome. In Emans SJ, Laufer MR, Goldstein DP, editors: *Pediatric and adolescent gynecology*, ed 5, Philadelphia, 2005, Lippincott Williams & Wilkins.

Mansfield J: Precocious puberty. In Emans SJ, Laufer MR, Goldstein DP, editors: *Pediatric and adolescent gynecology*, ed 5, Philadelphia, 2005, Lippincott Williams & Wilkins.

Matytsina LA et al: Dysfunctional uterine bleeding in adolescents: concepts of pathophysiology and management, *Prim Care* 33:503-515, 2006.

Meininger E et al: Gay, lesbian, and bisexual adolescents. In Neinstein LS, editor: *Adolescent health care, a practical guide*, ed 4, Philadelphia, 2002, Lippincott Williams & Wilkins.

Mitan LA, Slap GB: Dysfunctional uterine bleeding. In Neinstein LS, editor: *Adolescent health care, a practical guide*, ed 4, Philadelphia, 2002, Lippincott Williams & Wilkins.

Neinstein LS, Farmer MY: Teenage pregnancy. In Neinstein LS, editor: *Adolescent health care, a practical guide*, ed 4, Philadelphia, 2002, Lippincott Williams & Wilkins.

Nelson AL, Neinstein LS: Combination hormonal contraceptives. In Neinstein LS, editor: *Adolescent health care, a practical guide*, ed 4, Philadelphia, 2002a, Lippincott Williams & Wilkins.

Nelson AL, Neinstein LS: Barrier contraceptives. In Neinstein LS, editor: *Adolescent health care, a practical guide*, ed 4, Philadelphia, 2002b, Lippincott Williams & Wilkins.

Nicoletti AM: Teen pregnancy. In Emans SJ, Laufer MR, Goldstein DP, editors: *Pediatric and adolescent gynecology*, ed 5, Philadelphia, 2005, Lippincott Williams & Wilkins.

Proctor ML, Farquhar CM: Dysmenorrhoea, *Clin Evid* 12:2524-2547, 2004.

Saslow D et al: American Cancer Society guideline for the early detection of cervical neoplasia and cancer, *CA Cancer J Clin* 52:342-362, 2002.

Shrier LA: Bacterial sexually transmitted infections: gonorrhea, chlamydia, pelvic inflammatory disease, and syphilis. In Emans SJ, Laufer MR, Goldstein DP, editors: *Pediatric and adolescent gynecology*, ed 5, Philadelphia, 2005, Lippincott Williams & Wilkins.

Speroff L, Darney PD: *A clinical guide for contraception*, ed 4, Philadelphia, 2005, Lippincott Williams & Wilkins.

Speroff L, Fritz MA: *Clinical gynecologic endocrinology and infertility*, ed 7, Philadelphia, 2005, Lippincott Williams & Wilkins.

Speroff L, Glass RH, Kase NG: *Clinical gynecologic endocrinology and infertility*, Baltimore, 1973, Williams & Wilkins.

Spigarelli MG, Biro FM: Sexually transmitted disease testing: evaluation of diagnostic tests and methods, *Adolesc Med Clin* 15:287-299, 2004.

Stamm CA, McGregor JA: Diagnosing and treating STDs in young women, *Contemp Pediatr* 18:53-67, 2001.

Stevens-Simon C: Providing effective reproductive health care and prescribing contraceptives for adolescents, *Pediatr Rev* 19(12):409-417, 1998.

Sugar NF, Graham EA: Common gynecologic problems in prepubertal girls, *Pediatr Rev* 27:213-222, 2006.

Syed TS, Braverman PK: Vaginitis in adolescents, *Adolesc Med Clin* 15: 235-251, 2004.

The National Campaign to Prevent Teen Pregnancy: *Parent power: what parents need to know and do to help prevent teen pregnancy*, 2003. Available from *www.teenpregnancy.org/resources/reading/parentpower/ default.asp* (accessed Sept 7, 2006).

US Department of Health and Human Services: *Healthy people 2010: understanding and improving health*, ed 2, 2000. Available from *www. healthypeople.gov/Document/tableofcontents.htm#topofpage* (accessed Aug 19, 2006).

US Preventive Services Task Force: *Guide to clinical preventive services*, 2005. Available from *www.ahrq.gov/clinic/pocketgd.htm* (accessed July 8, 2006).

Wilson GR, Haddad JE, Haddad CJ: Amenorrhea: common causes and evaluation, *Comp Ther* 31:270-278, 2005.

World Health Organization, Reproductive Health and Research: *Medical eligibility criteria for contraceptive use*, ed 3, Geneva, 2004. Available from *www.who. int/reproductive-health/publications/mec/mec.pdf* (accessed Jan 9, 2007).

CHAPTER 36

Dermatologic Diseases

Peggy Vernon, Margaret A. Brady, and Nancy Barber Starr

The skin is the body's largest organ and one of its most important. The condition of the skin reflects physical and emotional health, plays a major role in defining identity and supporting survival, and often gives clues to underlying conditions. Skin functions are multiple. Beauty is often defined by the appearance of the skin. Emotions are expressed by blushing and sweating. Skin conveys many impressions through its sensory functions, including reaction to touch, heat, cold, pressure, and pain. Additionally, the skin provides a protective physiologic covering, the first line of defense against injury from chemical, physical, and microorganic invaders. Homeostasis is maintained through fluid regulation and thermoregulation.

Disruptions in the skin account for a significant percentage of all pediatric office visits. The primary care provider plays an essential role in maintaining skin integrity, identifying and minimizing skin disruptions, maximizing healing, and educating parents and children about skin care.

SKIN DEVELOPMENT

Skin development is constant from embryogenesis throughout life. During the embryonic period (the first 2 months of gestation), the skin differentiates into several layers. During the fetal period, appendages (hair, nails, and sebaceous, apocrine, and eccrine glands) develop, and all skin layers continue to mature. Neonatal skin continues to change and develop throughout childhood and adolescence, achieving adult skin thickness and characteristics in the late teenage years. Melanin in the skin reaches adult levels by 1 year old. Vascularization is well developed by the end of the second year of life. Cutaneous nerves develop until puberty and beyond. Sebaceous glands cease production between 6 and 12 months old, but become active again at around 7 years old. Eccrine sweat function begins between 2 and 18 days old, although full function is not in place until 2 or 3 years old. The apocrine glands become active at puberty. Hair goes through three stages: growth (anagen), rest (telogen), and regression (catagen), with approximately 1 cm of growth per month. Nails, formed in the fifth fetal month, are spoon shaped and thin from infancy until 2 to 3 years old.

ANATOMY AND PHYSIOLOGY

The skin is composed of three layers: the epidermis, the dermis, and the subcutaneous layer (Fig. 36-1). Skin thickness, including its epidermis and dermis, varies from 1.5 mm to 4 mm thick (Weston et al, 2007).

The epidermis, the thinner outer layer, functions as a protective barrier between the body and the environment. It comprises five layers of stratified squamous epithelium. The majority of epidermal cells are keratinocytes, and the replication and maturation of the keratinocytes is called keratinization. New keratinocytes of the basal layer mature and shed approximately every 28 days (Cohen, 2005). The outer horny layer, the stratum corneum, is responsible for much of the barrier protection against microorganisms and irritating chemicals. It also impedes the exchange of fluids and electrolytes with the environment and provides strength of the skin. Melanin serves to protect DNA from damage by ultraviolet (UV) light irradiation. It is produced in the basal layer of the epidermis and contributes to the color of the skin, eyes, and hair. The water content of the environment influences the epidermal barrier, with either excess or inadequate amounts contributing to microscopic and macroscopic breaks.

The thicker middle layer, the dermis, contributes strength, support, and elasticity to the skin. It is a tough, leathery mechanical barrier that also regulates heat loss, provides host defenses of the skin, and aids in nutrition and other regulatory functions. The dermis is primarily composed of fibrous connective tissue (made up of fibroblasts and collagen), with some elastic fibers and a mucopolysaccharide gel. It includes mast cells, inflammatory cells, and blood and lymph vessels, in addition to cutaneous nerves that elicit sensations (touch, pain, pressure, itch, warmth, and cold). These specialized receptors serve as a defense mechanism to protect the skin surface from environmental trauma.

Underlying the dermis is subcutaneous tissue primarily composed of adipose tissue. Networks of arteries lie here and branch into the dermis as small arterioles; these arteries assist in the thermoregulation of the skin. The subcutaneous tissue is an insulator, a cushion against trauma, and a source of energy and hormone metabolism (see Fig. 36-1).

Skin appendages include the hair, nails, sweat glands, and sebaceous glands. Hair follicles are found over the entire body except for the palms, soles, knuckles, distal and interdigital spaces, lips, glans and prepuce of the penis, and areolae and nipples. Two types of hair can be found on the body. Terminal hair is thick and visible and found on the scalp, axillae, and pubis. Very fine vellus hair is found over the remainder of the body. The visible portion of the hair is the shaft. The root of the hair is embedded in the dermis as a pilosebaceous unit, consisting of a hair follicle and a sebaceous gland. The hair shaft may be straight, wavy, helical, or spiral. Following an acute febrile illness

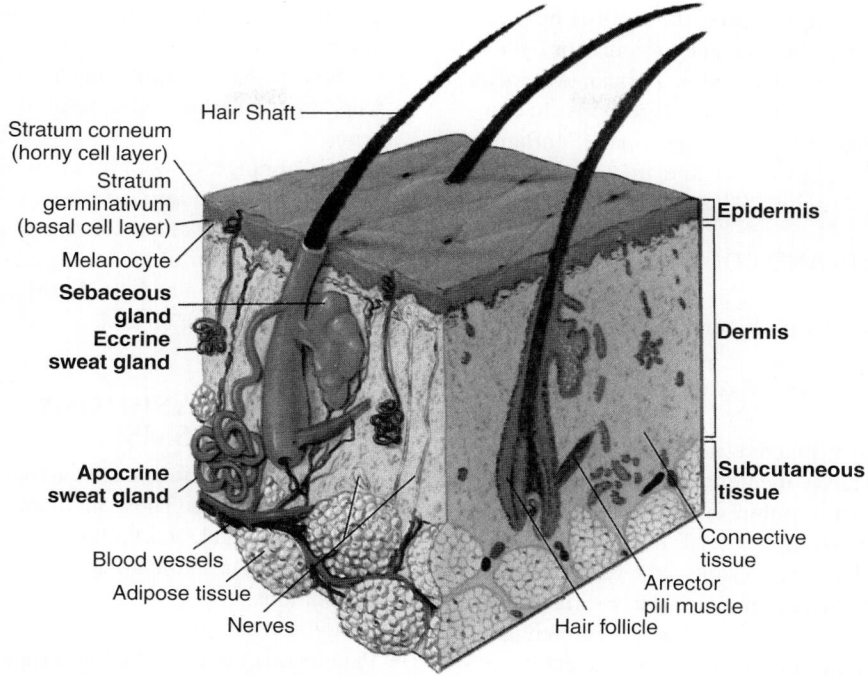

Stratum corneum
(horny cell layer)
Stratum
germinativum
(basal cell layer)
Melanocyte
**Sebaceous
gland
Eccrine
sweat gland**

Hair Shaft

Epidermis

Dermis

**Apocrine
sweat gland**

Blood vessels
Adipose tissue
Nerves

**Subcutaneous
tissue**

Connective
tissue
Arrector
pili muscle
Hair follicle

FIG. 36-1   Structure of the skin. (From Jarvis C: *Physical examination and assessment*, ed 2, Philadelphia, 1996, WB Saunders.)

or stress, many hairs convert from anagen to telogen stage, resulting in a noticeably thinned amount of hair for several months.

Nails are epidermal cells converted to keratin that grow continually. The body of the nail (or nail plate) is visible. The nail bed, underneath the nail plate, is composed of layers of epidermis and dermis, which serve as structural support. The root of the nail lies just under the epidermis.

Sweat glands can be grouped into three categories: eccrine, ceruminous, and apocrine. Eccrine glands are numerous and are distributed over the entire body. The coiled bodies of the eccrine glands lie in the dermis and empty onto the surface of the skin, helping maintain fluid and electrolyte balance and body temperature, in addition to providing some excretory function. Ceruminous glands, thought to be modified sweat glands, are located in the external ear canal and secrete a waxy pigmented substance, cerumen. Apocrine glands, located primarily in the axillary, genital, and periumbilical areas, are larger coils than eccrine glands. They open into hair follicles, require androgens to stimulate their secretions, and are thought to be responsible for body odor.

Sebaceous glands, found in conjunction with hair follicles, are distributed over the entire body except the soles, palms, and dorsa of the feet and contribute to the protection of the epidermis. These glands secrete sebum (oil) when stimulated by androgen and function to prevent excessive water evaporation, minimize heat loss, and lubricate the skin and hair.

SPECIAL DERMATOLOGIC CONSIDERATIONS IN CHILDREN WITH DARK SKIN OR FROM DIVERSE CULTURAL OR ETHNIC GROUPS

Knowledge of the normal variations in children both with different levels of pigmentation of the skin and from diverse ethnic or cultural groups is important for assessing and treating dermatologic conditions. Skin reactions to injury, inflammation, common skin conditions, and cultural practices are varied. A wise pediatric health care provider listens to parents because they are often the first to detect subtle changes in color or texture of the skin.

CUTANEOUS REACTION PATTERNS

Three identified patterns of cutaneous reactions are pigment lability, follicular response, and mesenchymal response Pigment lability manifested as postinflammatory hypopigmentation or hyperpigmentation is common and tends to be more obvious in dark-skinned individuals regardless of race. If superficial, with changes in the epidermis only, normal pigmentation returns in about 6 months (e.g., in diaper rash, seborrhea, tinea, pityriasis alba). If dermal changes occur, dermal tattooing may occur, causing long-term or permanent changes (e.g., excoriated acne, impetigo, varicella, contact dermatitis). The exaggerated follicular response can be seen in prominent papules and follicles, especially with atopic dermatitis, pityriasis rosea (PR), syphilis, or tinea versicolor. The mesenchymal response causes hypertrophic scars and keloids (which extend beyond the edge of the scar), often following varicella, ear piercing, burns, or any surgical procedure. Other exaggerated responses include lichenification and vesicular or bullous reaction to bites or staphylococcal infection. African-American children may have an exaggerated cutaneous response to common disorders of the skin. Of note, erythema of inflamed black skin may be difficult to detect and may appear as a purplish tinge (Paller & Mancini, 2006).

NORMAL VARIATIONS AND COMMON PROBLEMS

The following are normal variations or common problems in children with darker skin:

- Variation in color and texture of skin from one part of the body to another
- Pigmentation of gingiva, mucous membrane, sclerae, and nails correlates with degree of cutaneous pigmentation
- Increased areas of melanin in thicker-skinned areas (elbow, knee)
- The term, *Futcher's* or *Ito's line*, describes the vertical line that separates the hyperpigmented dorsal and extensor surfaces from less pigmented ventral surfaces. This line of differentiation follows Voigt's lines and is most noticeable on the extremities
- Mongolian spots and increased numbers of café au lait spots (see discussion later in chapter)
- Normal exfoliation produces a fine layer of gray scales
- Color alterations (jaundice, anemia, cyanosis)—difficult to assess
- Kinky, wooly, tightly curled hair with closely knit growth that tangles when dry and mats when wet
- Tinea versicolor (see section on fungal disorders), initially papular with hypopigmentation or hyperpigmentation, occurring only on the face
- Atopic dermatitis (see Chapter 24) with prominent follicular pattern with pityriasis alba and postinflammatory hypopigmentation
- PR (see section on papulosquamous disorders) often confused with tinea, primarily follicular, inverse distribution (face, neck, extremities, and torso)

Conditions occurring more commonly in African-American children include tinea capitis, tinea versicolor, papular urticaria, infantile acropustulosis, dermatosis papulosa nigra, lichen nitidus, lichen spinulosus, lichen planus, pseudofolliculitis barbae, transient neonatal pustular melanosis, keloids, dermatosis papulosa (appearing during adolescence, especially in females) and acanthosis nigricans (AN). Lichen planus is more severe, and keloids are more frequent. Pediculosis capitis is less common in African-American children.

CULTURAL OR ETHNIC PRACTICES WITH SKIN SEQUELAE

Grooming, cosmetic, or healing practices of cultural or ethnic groups contribute to various conditions that may be seen. These include the following:

- Hair pomade—acne
- Bleaching creams—discoloration and erythematous nodules
- Chemical or thermal hair straighteners—alopecia, fragile hair shaft, scalp contact dermatitis

- Coining—petechiae and ecchymoses, especially on chest and back
- Cornrowed hair or tight ponytails—traction alopecia
- Cupping—circular ecchymoses on neck, chest, back, and arms
- Henna—orange discoloration of skin, increased bilirubin levels in infants if applied topically
- Scars or tattoos from decorative practices
- Healing practices used during significant illness that produce burns—circular 1- to 2-cm scars on chest, periumbilicus, wrists, ankles, or back

PATHOPHYSIOLOGY AND DEFENSE MECHANISMS

Disruption of the skin and subcutaneous tissue occurs through a variety of assaults. These include:

- Bacterial, fungal, and viral infections
- Allergic and inflammatory reactions
- Infestations
- Vascular reactions
- Papulosquamous and bullous eruptions
- Congenital lesions
- Hair and nail disorders

The skin's outer layers provide the body's first line of defense from chemical, physical, and microorganic injury. The epidermis provides a functional barrier, the dermis provides strength and protection through the cutaneous nerves, and the subcutaneous tissue ensures insulation, cushion from injury, energy source, and hormonal metabolism. These layers, in turn, protect the other body systems. The water content of the skin enhances the protective barrier of the skin. If the skin becomes too dry or too wet, breaks in the barrier occur that elicit an inflammatory response. As a continuously growing system, the skin not only heals itself but controls growth or colonization of microorganisms by continual shedding.

ASSESSMENT OF THE SKIN AND SUBCUTANEOUS TISSUE
HISTORY

The history should assess the following (Lembo, 2006; Weston et al, 2007):

- History of present illness
  - Onset and length of present or recent illness (e.g., respiratory or gastrointestinal)
  - Most common concerns: pruritus, scaling, and alterations in cosmetic appearance
  - Symptom analysis—Questions to ask about an eruption or lesions include: What did the rash or lesion(s) originally look like, and how has it changed in appearance? Where did the eruption first begin, and has it spread to other locations (pattern of spread)? How long has the rash or lesion been present? Is the way it looks today typical of its appearance? Does the rash come and go? Has the lesion blistered, bled, or had discharge? Does it itch? What have you used to treat it and what was the effect? What parts of

the body are not affected by the rash or lesions (e.g., face, soles, or palm)?

- ○ Associated systemic symptoms: fever, malaise, pain associated with lesion or eruption
- ○ Factors that alleviate or worsen skin symptoms or seem to trigger them
- ○ Exposures or allergies: medication, foods, animals, plants? Known allergens? New substances? Persons with similar symptoms or illness? What soaps, hair products (shampoos, gels, pomade, etc), lotions, and detergents are used?
- ○ All medication (prescription and over-the-counter) taken over the last few days, including creams, ointments, powders, or lotions (it is often helpful to have patients bring medications they have used to the appointment)
- ○ Prior incidents of similar rash
- ○ Recent travel
- Family history
  - ○ Similar symptoms
  - ○ Skin disorders or history of atopy disorders (asthma, seasonal or drug allergies or atopic dermatitis)
- Review of systems and past medical history
  - ○ Usual state of health and recent illnesses
  - ○ Skin, hair, and nails: skin type (dry or oily), recent and long-term changes, previous incidence of skin disease
  - ○ Eyes, ears, nose, and throat: swelling, itching, crusting, discharge or circles around eyes, nasal mucus discharge, patency or irritation, dry mouth, lesions, or pain
  - ○ Chest: wheezing, coughing, or respiratory difficulty

PHYSICAL EXAMINATION

A key question is, "Does the patient appear ill?" This clinical impression is important to differentiate the few serious illnesses from the majority of dermatologic conditions. The entire body needs to be examined, not just exposed skin. Attention should be given to the eyes, nose, mouth (mucous membranes, teeth), lymph nodes, and lungs because a skin disorder may be a cutaneous manifestation of other disease. The dermatologic examination includes a thorough look at the skin, scalp, hair, palms and soles, nails, and anogenital region.

Special techniques for examination of the skin may be required. Good light (daylight is best) is essential to a good examination. A source of direct light, such as a gooseneck lamp, is the best alternative. Other helpful tools include a magnifying glass, a ruler, a glass slide, and a Wood's lamp (UV light). A glass slide gently pressed on the skin (diascopy) allows viewing of the skin with and without capillary filling. A Wood's lamp is used to examine fluorescent-positive fungal infections and depigmenting skin disorders, such as vitiligo.

Identification of the type of lesion and correct use of terminology are essential to good dermatologic care. Essential documentation includes the following:

- Location and type of lesion
- Color, color changes, size, and shape
- Arrangement (e.g., isolated, grouped, linear, annular, zosteriform)
- Pattern (e.g., sun-exposed area, symmetry)
- Distribution of lesion (e.g., regional, generalized, crops)

- Border (e.g., indistinct, well circumscribed)
- Consistency (e.g., firm, soft, mobile)

Primary skin lesions (Box 36-1) include changes that arise from previously normal skin. These descriptions should be memorized and used. *Secondary* skin lesions (Box 36-2) result from changes in primary lesions. *Vascular* skin lesions (Box 36-3) involve the blood supply. Other useful descriptive terms are listed in Box 36-4. The presence of vesicles, pustules, scaling, and color changes should be noted when considering differential diagnoses.

DIAGNOSTIC STUDIES

A few simple laboratory tests are helpful in identifying or excluding dermatologic disorders. Proper procurement of the

---

BOX 36-1 Primary Skin Changes to Lesions

Macule—flat, nonpalpable, discolored lesion, 1 cm or smaller
Patch—macule, larger than 1 cm
Papule—solid, raised lesion of varied color with distinct borders, 1 cm or smaller
Plaque—solid, raised, flat-topped lesion with distinct borders, larger than 1 cm
Nodule—raised, firm, movable lesion with indistinct borders and deep palpable portion, 2 cm or smaller
Tumor—large nodule, may be firm or soft
Wheal—fleeting, irregularly shaped, elevated, itchy lesion of varied size, pale at center, slightly red at borders
Vesicle—blister filled with clear fluid
Bulla—vesicle larger than 1 cm
Cyst—palpable lesion with definite borders filled with liquid or semisolid material
Pustule—raised lesion filled with pus, often in hair follicle or sweat pore
Comedo—plugged, dilated pore; open (blackhead), closed (whitehead)

BOX 36-2 Secondary Skin Changes to Lesions

Crusts—dried exudate or scab of varied color
Scales—thin, flaking layers of epidermis
Desquamation—peeling sheets of scale
Lichenification—thickening of skin with deep visible furrows
Excoriation—abrasion or removal of epidermis; scratch
Fissure—linear, wedge-shaped cracks extending into dermis
Erosion—oozing or moist, depressed area with loss of superficial epidermis
Ulcer—deeper than erosion; open lesion extending into dermis
Atrophy—thinning skin, may appear translucent
Scar—healed lesion of connective tissue
Keloid—healed lesion of hypertrophied connective tissue
Striae—fine pink or silver lines in areas where skin has been stretched

BOX 36-3   Vascular Skin Lesions

Angioma or hemangioma—papule made of blood vessels

Ecchymosis—bruise, purple to brown in color, macular or papular, varied in size

Hematoma—collection of blood from ruptured blood vessel, larger than 1 cm

Petechiae—pinpoint, pink to purple macular lesions that do not blanch, 1 to 3 mm

Purpura—purple macular lesion, larger than 1 cm

Telangiectasia—collection of macular or raised, dilated capillaries

BOX 36-4   Descriptive Terms for Dermatologic Lesions

Acral—involving extremities (hands, feet, ears, etc.)

Annular—ring-shaped

Arcuate—arc-shaped

Circinate—circular

Confluent—running together

Contiguous—touching or adjacent

Discrete—distinct and separate

Diffuse or generalized—scattered, widely distributed

Eczematous—referring to vesicles with oozing crust

Grouped—arranged in sets

Guttate—small, droplike

Herpetiform—referring to grouped vesicles resembling those of herpes

Iris—arranged in concentric circles, one inside the other

Linear—arranged in a line

Localized—in a limited area

Nummular—coin-shaped

Pedunculated—having a stalk

Polycyclic—oval with more than 1 ring

Reticular—netlike

Serpiginous—snakelike, creeping

Symmetric—balanced on both sides

Target lesion—(iris or targetoid) erythematous papule or plaque characterized by a red-to-violet dusky center surrounded by a raised, edematous pale ring and red periphery

Telangiectatic—referring to dilated terminal vessels

Umbilicated—depressed or shaped like a navel

Verrucous—wartlike

Zosteriform—resembling shingles, following a nerve root or dermatome

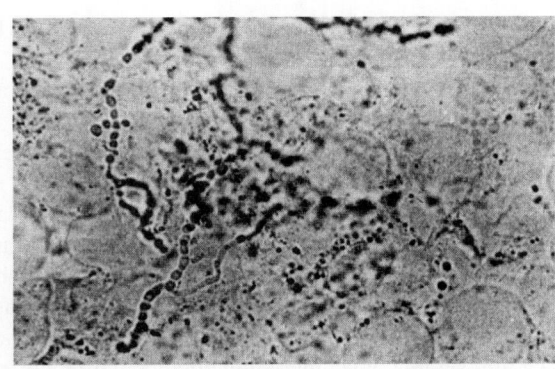

FIG. 36-2   Fungal elements (hyphae) as seen on microscopic examination of a potassium hydroxide preparation. (From Hurwitz S: *Clinical pediatric dermatology*, ed 2, Philadelphia, 1993, WB Saunders, p 374.)

- Microscopic examination of skin scrapings:
  - Potassium hydroxide (KOH) can be used to examine for fungal disorders (hyphae or spores; Fig. 36-2). Scrape fine scales from the edge of the lesion onto a glass slide. Add a drop of KOH 20% to dissolve debris and cover with a coverslip. Let sit for 20 to 30 minutes or heat gently (do not boil). Use × 10 magnification to examine.
  - Wright, Giemsa, or Gram stains are used to examine for bacteria or herpes simplex or herpes zoster (HZ) giant cells. Allow scrapings to air-dry, then stain with Wright or Giemsa stain. Use × 40 magnification to examine for bacteria.
- Tzanck smear for herpes, varicella, or zoster.
- Microbial culture of lesions for bacteria, viruses, or fungi. Simple, inexpensive culture methods for fungal organisms (Dermatophyte Test Medium or InTray CCD [includes *Candida*]—see Resource Box at the end of the chapter) can be done at room temperature. Skin or nail scrapings or hairs, including the root, are applied so that they break the agar surface. A color change is noted in 1 to 5 days.
- Patch or skin testing for allergic or contact reactions is usually done by dermatologists or allergists.
- Skin biopsy following local anesthesia may be done by punch or shave method for any tumor, palpable purpura, persistent dermatitis, or blister that is not otherwise definitively diagnosed. Such procedures often require referral to a dermatologist.
- Complete blood count (CBC) and erythrocyte sedimentation rate (ESR) may be done to evaluate infection or inflammation.

■ MANAGEMENT STRATEGIES
HYDRATION AND LUBRICATION

Maintenance of skin hydration is essential to prevent and treat skin conditions. If the skin is overhydrated, the bonds between cells at the stratum corneum loosen and the barrier is broken. If the skin is too dry, it cracks, again breaking the barrier.

Bathing

Although less frequent, bathing is often recommended, especially with dry skin or in dry climates. Proper bathing and lubrication

sample is important. Scraping of lesions can be done with a No. 15 blade or a toothbrush and scales or debris placed on a glass microscope slide or in culture material. The No. 15 blade is also useful for exfoliating a blister. It is important to scrape under any scabs to get a sample of the organisms. Moistening the lesion may facilitate this. Scrapings can be obtained from the edges of skin lesions; from plucked hair (getting the root is essential); from the nail plate; or from subungual debris. Laboratory tests that can be used include the following:

will enhance addition and retention of water in the skin. Lukewarm, not hot, water should be used. The bath should not last long enough for skin to become supersaturated. In general, soap substitutes or mild soaps, such as Dove, Neutrogena, Aveeno, or Purpose should be used. Soap substitutes include Cetaphil and Purpose Gentle Cleansing Wash. Bubble-bath solutions are especially irritating and should be avoided. Soaping and shampooing should be done at the end of the bath followed by thorough rinsing. The skin should be gently dried and a lubricating agent applied immediately. See Chapter 24 for further information on lubricating baths. Baths including baking soda or Aveeno colloidal ointment may be helpful to relieve pruritus. Tar baths can be used for psoriasis (e.g., Zetar, Polytar, or Balnetar). It is worth noting that bathing and other heat exposures can make a rash seem worse temporarily.

Environmental Considerations

Because water is essential to skin integrity, environmental humidity also plays a role. Excessive humidity (greater than 90%) or deficient humidity (less than 10%) can cause disruption of the skin. Macerated skin, for example, benefits from less humidity (e.g., wet dressings enhance evaporation and relieve symptoms). Itching from excessively dry skin is often relieved by increased humidity provided by humidified heating in winter or by using a vaporizer or humidifier. In hot temperatures, itching can be alleviated by cool air conditioning. Water consumption also plays a role in maintaining proper skin hydration, and children should be encouraged to drink plenty of water.

Skin Care Agents

Soaps, Oils, and Colloids.   Mild soaps include Dove, Aveeno, Neutrogena, Basis, Alpha Keri, Oilatum, and Lubriderm. Cetaphil lotion and Purpose Gentle Cleansing Wash are soap substitutes. Bath oils include Alpha Keri and Domol. Colloids include Aveeno.

Moisturizers and Lubricants. Moisturizers and lubricants treat chronic dryness and inflammation of the skin by retaining water in the skin. Composed of petrolatum or a mixture of petrolatum and lanolin, moisturizers and lubricants are most effective when applied to damp skin. Petrolatum-based lubricants include Moisturel, Purpose, Dermasil cream, Vaseline Pure Petrolatum Jelly, and Vaseline Dermatology Formula Lotion. Petrolatum and lanolin combinations include Aquaphor ointment, Eucerin cream and lotion, Lubriderm lotion, and Keri Creme. Glycerin preparations without lanolin or petrolatum include Corn Huskers Lotion, Cetaphil, Keri Light, and Neutrogena.

Sunscreens and Sunblocks. Sunscreens and sunblocks protect the skin from UV light and are graded by their ability to provide sun protection. Daily application of a fragrance-free sunscreen with a minimum sun protection factor (SPF) of 15 is recommended. Children who are extremely photosensitive should use sunscreen with levels of SPF 30 or higher. Sunscreens that act by absorbing UV light in the B range include para-aminobenzoic acid (PABA) or PABA esters, cinnamates, salicylates, benzophenones, and anthranilates. Only benzophenones protect from UV rays in the longer UVA range. Sunblocks, including titanium dioxide, zinc oxide, and talc, scatter light and act as protective barriers. They are especially useful on the nose, ears, and lips (see Box 36-10 on p. 980).

Chemical-containing sunscreens ideally should be applied 30 minutes before exposure to the sun to allow binding of the agents to the stratum corneum. Sunblocks can be applied immediately before sun exposure. Reapply sunscreens after swimming, excessive periods of perspiration, or after washing or showering. Sunscreen is never a substitute for sensible sun protection, which always includes limiting exposure to intense sun rays. Other protective strategies include protective clothing, wearing of hats with visors, and sunglasses with UV protection.

Wet Dressings

When skin is in an acute stage of oozing, crusting, or itching, wet dressings are useful to help dry the skin, decrease itching, and remove crusts. Thin cloths, such as diapers, handkerchiefs, or strips of sheets, make the best wet dressings. Dressings should be moderately wet, but not dripping, with lukewarm water and applied for 10 to 20 minutes four to six times daily for 48 to 72 hours. During the treatment, dressings must be kept wet either by removing and rewetting or by applying water. Alternative solutions include saline (1 tsp salt with 1 pint of water) or Burow's solution (one Domeboro [aluminum acetate; calcium acetate] Tablet with one pint of cool or tepid water). Creams or ointments applied following wet dressings enhance absorption of the medication in the cream. A slightly more intense technique includes applying a steroid ointment or cream to the skin, covered with a wet dressing and then a dry dressing (e.g., a sleeper, pajamas, or long johns are wetted and put on, and covered with a dry sleeper or long johns) (Paller & Mancini, 2006; Weston et al, 2007). The dressing is changed every 6 hours for 24 to 72 hours or is used overnight for five to ten nights. Care must be taken to prevent excessive steroidal absorption using this technique by applying steroid only to areas needing it, especially in infants and young children.

Occlusive Dressings

Occlusive dressings decrease evaporation of water from the skin and enhance hydration and absorption of topical medications. Plastic wrap is placed over the affected area after hydrating the skin and applying cream or ointment; these dressings should not be left on longer than 8 hours. Ointments, oils, urea compounds, and propylene glycol used alone are occlusive. Skin folds serve as naturally occurring occlusive areas. Lichen simplex chronicus, dyshidrotic eczema, and psoriasis are skin conditions that benefit from occlusion.

Other Considerations

- Irritants and sensitizing agents, such as wool, sweat, and saliva, should be avoided.
- Allergens and foods that most commonly cause skin reactions include milk, eggs, wheat, tomato, citrus, chocolate, fish, and nuts.

MEDICATIONS

Topical therapeutics are most commonly used for dermatologic conditions. Topical therapy can achieve the following goals:

- Restore hydration
- Alleviate symptoms
- Reduce inflammation
- Protect the skin
- Reduce scale and debris
- Cleanse and débride
- Eradicate causative organisms

Thought must be given not only to the medication used in treating skin conditions but also to its preparation (Box 36-5)

BOX 36-5 Preparations of Topical Medications

Shampoos—liquid soaps or detergents for cleaning the hair (e.g., tar for psoriasis or seborrhea)

Powders—absorb moisture and reduce friction, provide cooling, decrease itching, increase evaporation

Pastes—made of a combination of powder and oil, which makes them somewhat difficult to apply and remove, but effective in providing dryness and protection for skin

Lotions—mixtures of powder and water, useful for drying, cooling, and soothing actions; *emulsion lotions* contain some oil, so are not as drying as lotions; lotions come in suspension or solution

Gels—alcohol based, provide good penetration of skin, but can burn on application; primarily used for acne and in hairy areas

Creams—contain more water than oil and therefore are less occlusive; better used with less dry skin, in high-humidity areas, in summertime, and on parts of body that naturally cause occlusion (body folds); often accepted better by patient, but must be applied every 2-3 hours

Ointments—best used with dry skin; composed primarily of oil with little or no water; provide most potent concentration of medication because of their occlusive action on skin; generally need to be used only every 12 hours; tend to leave a greasy feeling and can cause heat retention from decreased evaporation; come as water in oil, absorbent, or water repellent

Oils—fluid fats that hold medication to the skin as barriers or occlusive agents

---

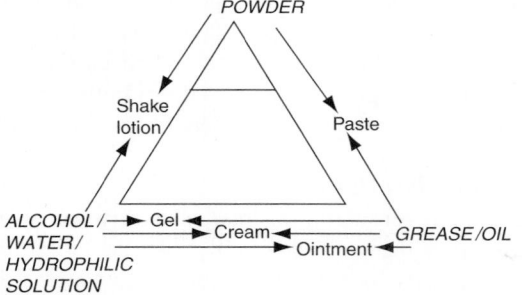

FIG. 36-3 Vehicles for dermatologic therapy. See Box 36-5 for description.

and vehicle (Fig. 36-3), including stabilizers, preservatives, and perfumes. Sensitization, and thus aggravation rather than relief of symptoms, is occasionally caused by the medication vehicle or its preparation. Common agents causing sensitization include ethylenediamine, lanolin, parabens, thimerosal, diphenhydramine, "caines," and neomycin. The following guidelines for use of preparations may be helpful:

- Acute inflammation—wet dressings, powders, suspension lotions, alcohol- or water-based lotions, or aerosols
- Chronic inflammation—creams, oil-based lotions or gels, ointments
- Patient's tolerance for and willingness to use certain vehicles
- Patient's environment (dry or humid)

All preparations of topical medication except powders have enhanced absorption if applied to skin immediately after it has been saturated with water. Absorption is also enhanced by occlusion (skin folds or plastic wraps; see previous discussion). Application of the topical medication is best done in one direction, preferably along the hair follicles, without rubbing, applied with a single motion. Use an adequate but not excessive amount.

Antibacterial Agents

Topical antiseptics, soap, and antibacterial soap reduce the number of bacteria on the skin and provide thorough cleansing. Examples of antiseptics include povidone-iodine (Betadine), chlorhexidine gluconate (Hibiclens), and pHisoderm. Topical antibiotics, such as mupirocin (Bactroban), applied directly to the skin, are used to treat minor skin infections. Neomycin should be avoided because of the high incidence of contact sensitization. Oral antibiotics used to treat more significant bacterial infections include penicillins, erythromycin, cephalosporins, and tetracycline.

Antifungal Agents

Antifungal agents are used to treat *Candida, Malassezia (Pityrosporum)*, and dermatophyte infections. Many topical antifungals are over-the-counter medications. Oral antifungals are used for hair and nail infections or refractory skin infections. They are used with caution in children, not only because of the side effects but also because the newer agents are not Food and Drug Administration (FDA)-approved for children, or clinical experience with children is minimal. The traditional drugs are usually the first line of treatment. Antifungal agents are listed in Table 36-4 in the section on fungal infections on p. 956.

Antiviral Agents

Topical antivirals are used to control cutaneous herpes infections. Oral antivirals, such as acyclovir for herpes infections, are reserved for more complicated or extensive cases.

Wart therapy agents destroy keratinocytes. These include salicylic acid and lactic acid collodion, salicylic plaster, salicylic solution, liquid nitrogen, cantharidin, podophyllum, and trichloroacetic acid.

Antiacne Agents

Topical keratolytics are used in acne to relieve follicular obstruction by inhibiting bacteria and promoting peeling of

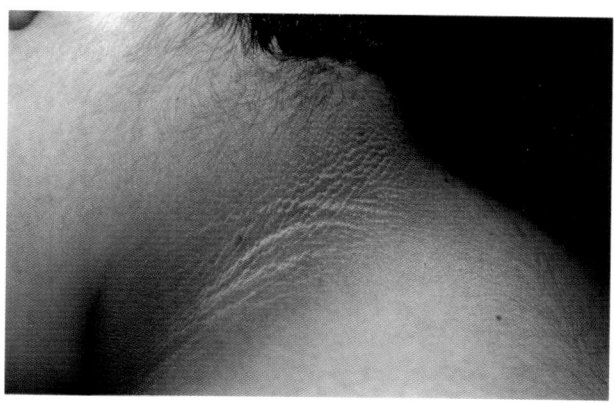

Acanthosis nigricans of a child's neck. (From Weston WL, Lane AT, Morelli JG: *Color textbook of pediatric dermatology*, ed 4, St Louis, 2007, Mosby, p 331.)

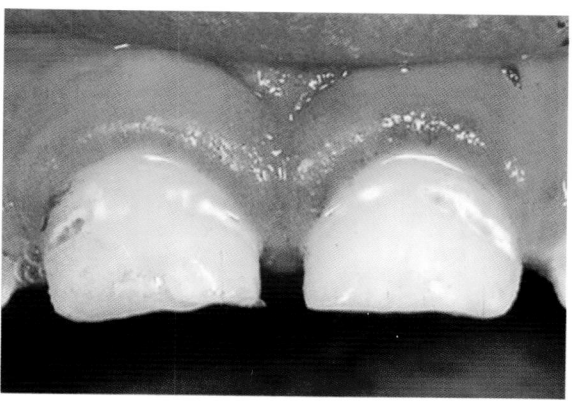

Early childhood caries. Upper incisor white spots. (Courtesy John Davis, DDS MSD, Professor Emeritus, University of Washington, Seattle, Department of Pediatric Dentistry.)

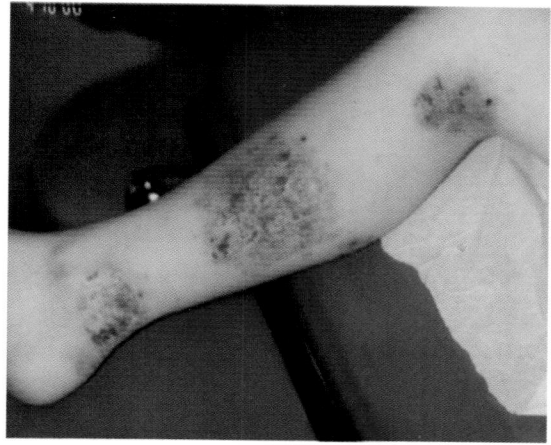

Acute atopic dermatitis. (Photograph courtesy Peggy Vernon, RN, MA, CPNP, Aurora/Parker Skin Care Center, CO.)

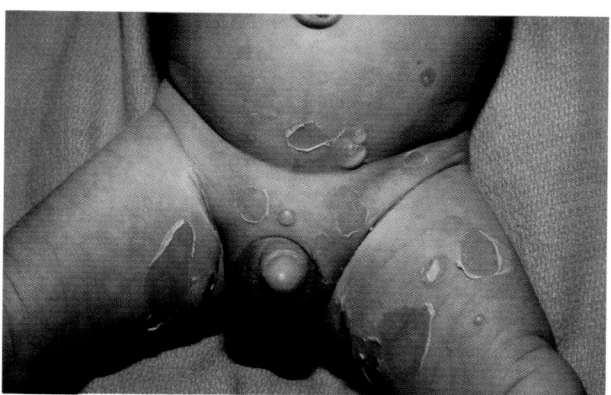

Bullous impetigo in a newborn. Multiple areas of flaccid blisters and shallow erosions on a red base. (From Weston WL, Lane AT, Morelli JG: *Color textbook of pediatric dermatology*, ed 4, St Louis, 2007, Mosby, p 62.)

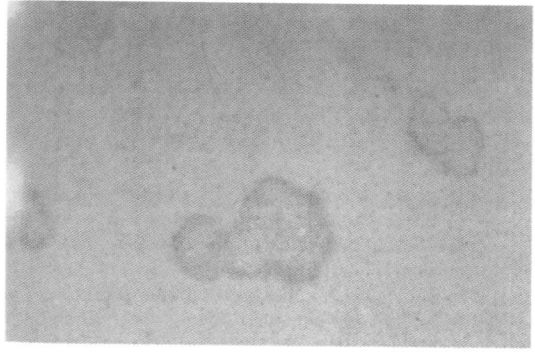

Tinea corporis. Lesions are annular with a raised inflammatory edge and central clearing. (From Aly R, Maibach H: *Atlas of infections of the skin*, Philadelphia, 1999, WB Saunders, p 23.)

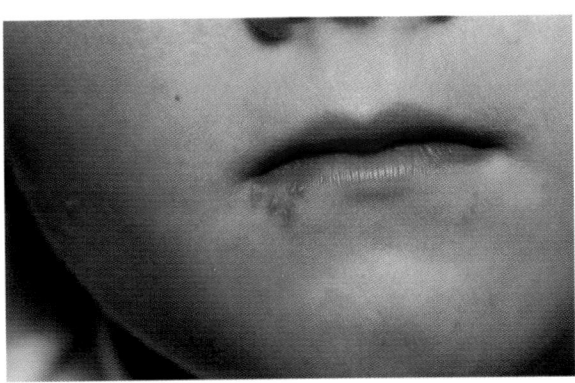

Recurrent herpes labialis of the lower lip and adjacent skin in a child. (From Weston WL, Lane AT, Morelli JG: *Color textbook of pediatric dermatology*, ed 4, St Louis, 2007, Mosby, p 128.)

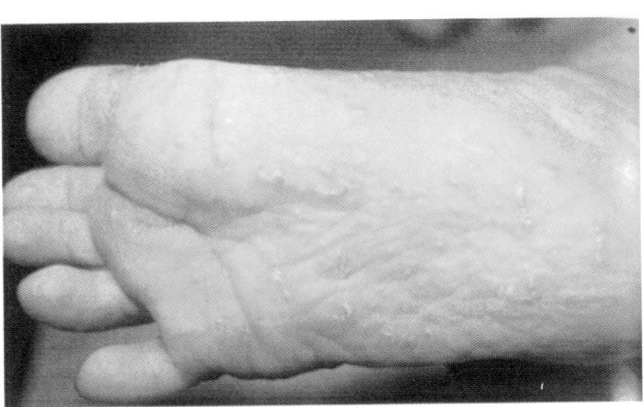

Scabies in an infant with multiple burrows and pustules on soles. (From Aly R, Maibach H: *Atlas of infections of the skin*, Philadelphia, 1999, WB Saunders, p 176.)

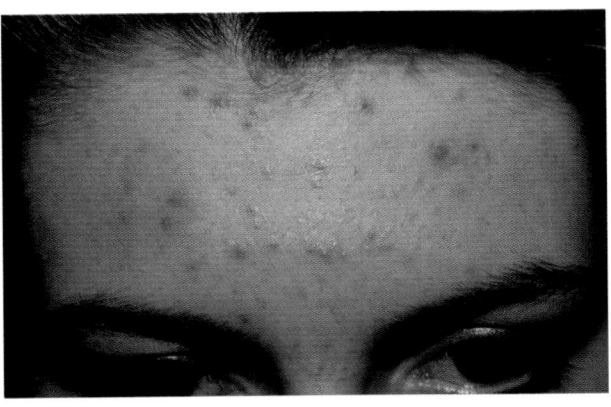

Mild inflammatory acne. Several inflammatory papules. (From Weston WL, Lane AT, Morelli JG: *Color textbook of pediatric dermatology*, ed 4, St Louis, 2007, Mosby, p 27.)

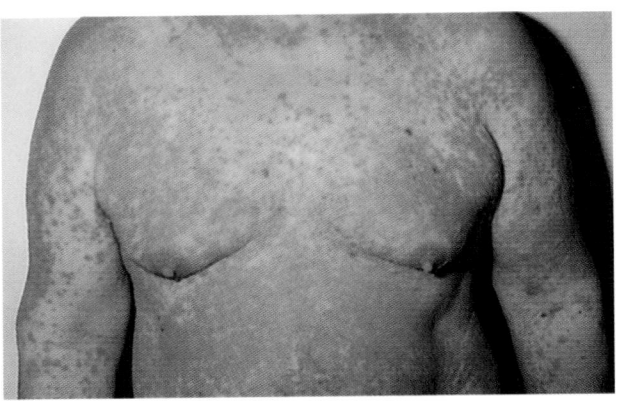

Allergic drug eruption in an erythematous and symmetric rash, usually generalized. (From Lookingbill DP, Marks JG: *Principles of dermatology*, ed 2, Philadelphia, 1993, WB Saunders, p 218.)

Urticaria. (From Weston WL, Lane AT, Morelli JG: *Color textbook of pediatric dermatology*, ed 4, St Louis, 2007, Mosby, p 259.)

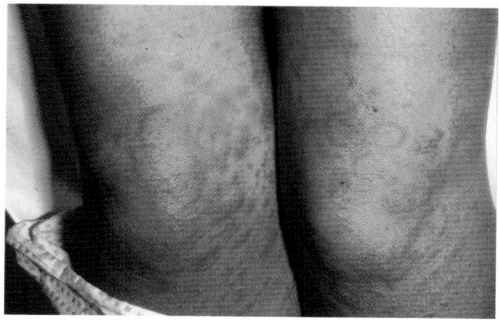

Erythema multiforme secondary to herpes simplex. (From Arndt KA et al: *Primary care dermatology*, Philadelphia, 1997, WB Saunders.)

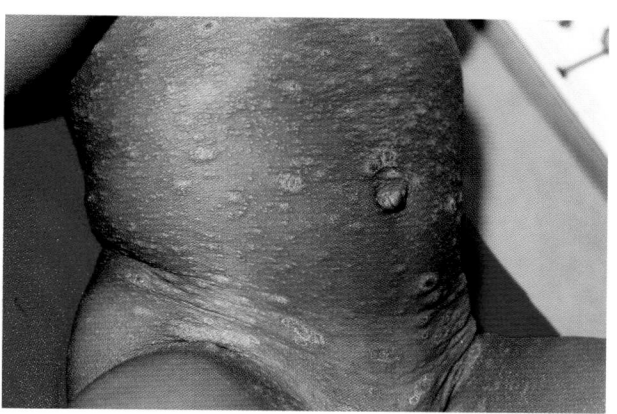

Pityriasis rosea. Truncal involvement with larger plaques and predominantly round papular lesions, most commonly seen in young children and African-Americans. Note the peripheral scale and distribution along skin lines. (From Paller AS, Mancini AJ: *Hurwitz clinical pediatric dermatology: a textbook of skin disorders of childhood and adolescence*, ed 3, Philadelphia, 2006, WB Saunders, p 101.)

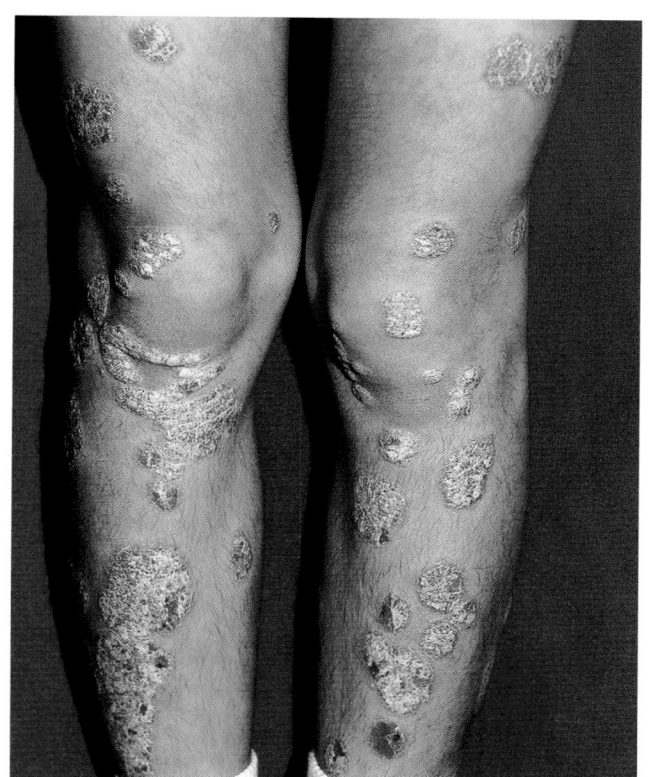

Psoriasis. Typical plaques of psoriasis with thick, micaceous scale overlying erythema. (From Paller AS, Mancini AJ: *Hurwitz Clinical pediatric dermatology: a textbook of skin disorders of childhood and adolescence*, ed 3, Philadelphia, 2006, WB Saunders, p 86.)

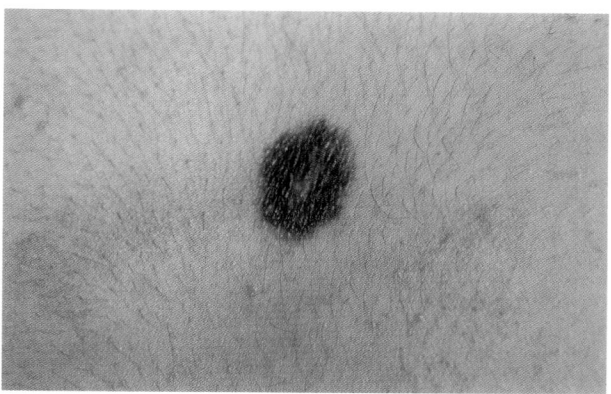

Halo nevus. Loss of pigment around regressing central intradermal nevus. (From Weston WL, Lane AT, Morelli JG: *Color textbook of pediatric dermatology*, ed 4, St Louis, 2007, Mosby, p 329.)

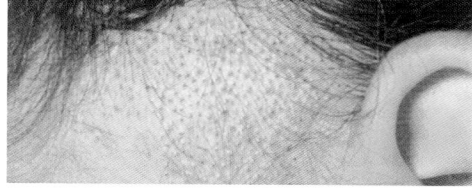

Tinea capitis showing a black dot variety with minimal inflammation. (From Aly R, Maibach H: *Atlas of infections of the skin*, Philadelphia, 1999, WB Saunders, p 20.)

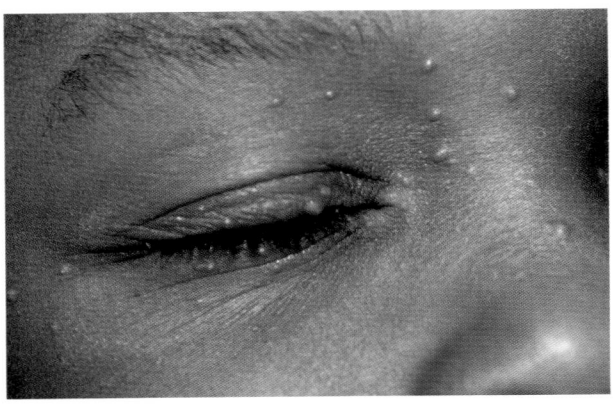

Multiple molluscum papules on an infant's face. (From Weston WL, Lane AT, Morelli JG: *Color textbook of pediatric dermatology*, ed 4, St Louis, 2007, Mosby, p 144.)

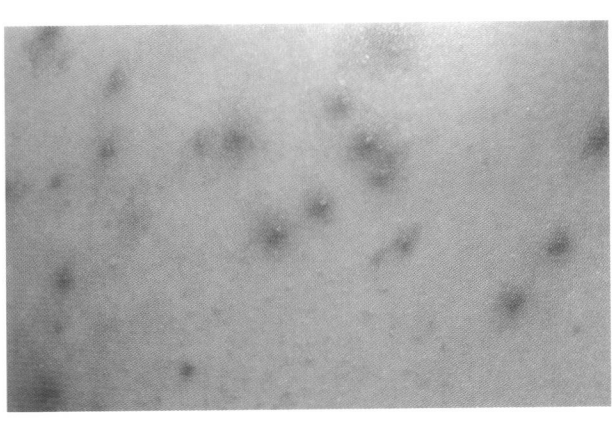

Staphylococcal superficial folliculitis. Multiple pustules on a red base. (From Weston WL, Lane AT, Morelli JG: *Color textbook of pediatric dermatology*, ed 4, St Louis, 2007, Mosby, p 69.)

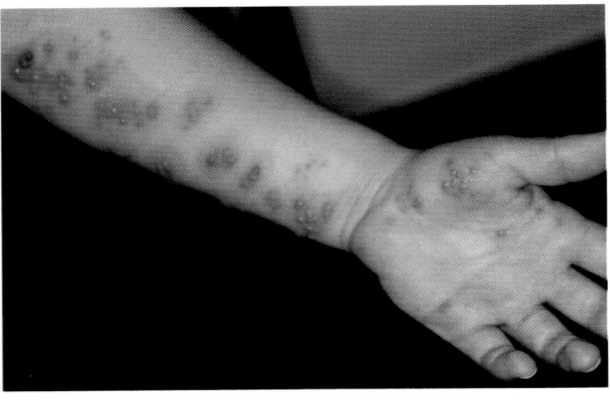

Many groups of blisters occurring over the arm in a child with herpes zoster. (From Weston WL, Lane AT, Morelli JG: *Color textbook of pediatric dermatology*, ed 4, St Louis, 2007, Mosby, p 134.)

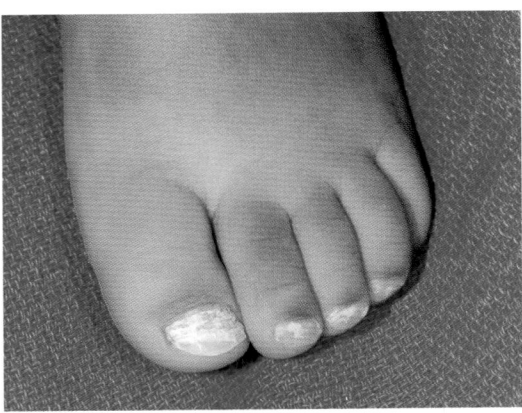

Onychomycosis, proximal subungual type. White discoloration of the nail plate, with the process originating in the proximal nail fold regions. (From Paller AS, Mancini AJ: *Hurwitz clinical pediatric dermatology: a textbook of skin disorders of childhood and adolescence*, ed 3, Philadelphia, 2006, WB Saunders, p 461.)

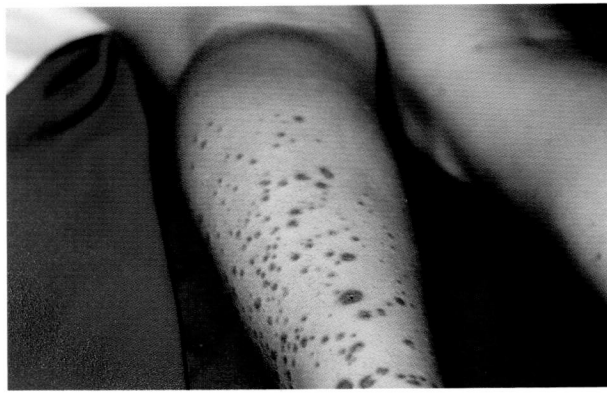

Heinlich-Schönlein purpura. (From Paller AS, Mancini AJ: *Hurwitz clinical pediatric dermatology: a textbook of skin disorders of childhood and adolescence*, ed 3, Philadelphia, 2006, WB Saunders, p 558.)

the skin. Benzoyl peroxide and retinoic acid are two main agents. They are the first line of treatment for mild acne and used in combination with other agents for moderate or severe acne. Topical antibiotics have few side effects and are most effective in maintaining control of acne. Common ones used include clindamycin, erythromycin, and sulfacetamide (Paller & Mancini, 2006). Systemic antibiotics are effective in inflammatory acne. Tetracycline and erythromycin are the most commonly used. Antibiotics exert their effect by decreasing the population of *Propionibacterium acnes*. Oral retinoid (isotretinoin), effective in nodulocystic acne not responding to other treatment, is contraindicated in pregnancy because of its teratogenic effects, and prescription of this agent is tightly controlled (see Table 36-8 and acne discussion later in the chapter).

Antiinflammatory Agents

Topical glucocorticoids are frequently used to reduce inflammation, to decrease itching, and for vasoconstriction without having the widespread systemic effects of oral steroids. They are subdivided into three categories: low-potency, moderate-potency, and high-potency agents (Table 36-1).

TABLE 36-1   Topical Corticosteroids

Class	Generic name	Trade name	Potency
1	Betamethasone dipropionate, augmented 0.05%	Diprolene 0.05% Diproline AF 0.05%	High potency
	Clobestasol propionate 0.05%	Temovate 0.05% Dermovate 0.05% Embelline (US) Cormax (US)	
	Diflorasone diacetate 0.05%	Psorcan 0.05%	
	Halobetasol propiate	Ultravate 0.05%	
	Diflucortolone valerate	Nerisone forte 0.3% (UK)	↑↑↑↑
2	Amcinonide	Cyclocort ointment 0.1%	
	Betamethasone dipropionate	Diprosone ointment 0.05%	
	Diflorasone diacetate	Florane ointment 0.05% Maxiflor ointment 0.05%	
	Halcinonide	Halog cream 0.1% Halciderm 0.1%	
	Fluocinonide	Lidex cream 0.05% Metosyn 0.05% Lidex ointment 0.05%	
	Desoximetasone	Topicort cream 0.25%	
	Mometasone furoate	Elocon ointment 0.1%	
	Desoximetasone	Topicort cream 0.25% Stiedex 0.05% cream (UK)	
	Beclometasone dipropionate	Propaderm cream/ointment 0.25% (UK)	↑↑↑
3	Betamethasone dipropionate	Diprosone cream 0.05%	
	Betamethasone benzoate	Benisone gel 0.025%	
	Betamethasone valerate	Valisone ointment 0.1% Betacap 0.1%	
	Fluticosone propionate	Cutivate ointment 0.05%	
	Clobetasone butyrate 0.05%	Eumovate (UK)	↑↑
4	Triamcinolone acetonide	Aristocort ointment 0.1% Kenalog ointment 0.1% Adocortyl 0.1%	
	Fluradrenolide	Cordran ointment 0.05%	
	Fluocinolone acetonide	Synalar cream 0.025%	↑
5	Desonide	Tridesilon ointment 0.05%	↓
	Triamcinolone acetonide	Aristocort cream 0.1%	
	Fluradrenolide	Cordan SP cream 0.05%	
	Fluocinolone acetonide	Fluonid cream 0.01% Synalar 0.025% Synalar cream 0.01%	
	Triamcinolone acetonide	Kenalog cream 0.1%	
	Betamethasone valerate	Valisone cream 0.1%	
	Hydrocortisone valerate	Westcort cream 0.2%	
	Hydrocortisone butyrate	Locoid cream 0.1%	
	Prednicarbate 0.1%	Dermatop cream/ointment	

Continued

TABLE 36-1	Topical Corticosteroids—Cont'd		
6	Hydrocortisone 1%, urea 10%	Alphaderm cream 1%	↓↓
	Flumetasone pivalate	Locorten cream 0.03%	
	Desonide 0.05%	Tridesilon cream 0.05%	
		DesOwen cream	
	Alclometasone dipropionate	Aclorate cream 0.05%	
		Modrasone 0.05%	
		Desonide 0.05%	
7	Hydrocortisone 1%	Hytone cream 1% Cobadex 1%	↓↓↓
		Dioderm 0.1% Mildison 1%	
		Hydrocortisyl 1%	
		Hytone ointment 1%	
	Dexamethasone	Hexadrol cream 0.04%	
	Methylprednisolone acetate	Medrol ointment 0.25%	
	Prednisolone	Meti-derm cream 0.5%	
8	Hydrocortisone 0.5%	Cortoid cream	Low potency

From Cohen BA: *Pediatric dermatology,* ed 3, Philadelphia, 2005, Mosby, p 11.

High-potency steroids should not be used in children. Only low-potency agents should be used on the face, in the diaper area, and in young children and only for short periods of time. Steroids are also classified as fluorinated or nonfluorinated. Nonfluorinated steroids are less potent and have fewer side effects; fluorinated steroids are rarely used in pediatrics.

Oral glucocorticoids (prednisone) are used only in acute situations and are limited to short courses. Intralesional steroid injections may be used by the dermatologist to control localized eczema, lichen planus, or psoriasis.

A key to using steroids is to be familiar with a few low-, medium-, and high-level steroids and use them consistently. Use the lowest possible potency that has the desired effect and with the least possible frequency. Brand name preparations often have a more consistent base and potency. Only low-potency or medium- to low-potency steroids (in severe cases) should be used on the face, groin, and axillae. Remember that ointments are more potent than creams, and lotions are better in hairy areas. Absorption is enhanced in areas that are traumatized or denuded. Side effects are possible when using topical steroids, especially with prolonged use or more potent preparations. Common side effects with long-term use include skin atrophy, striae, increased fragility of the skin, hypopigmentation, secondary infection, acneiform eruption, folliculitis, miliaria, hypertrichosis, telangiectasia, and purpura. Apply only a thin coat of these agents to the affected area.

Antipruritic Agents

Antihistamines are used both for sedation and to relieve itching. The most commonly used antihistamines are hydroxyzine and diphenhydramine. Topical antihistamines, especially diphenhydramine HCl (Benadryl) and "caine" medications, should be avoided because of the possibility of contact sensitization. Menthol and pramoxine are topical anesthetics that do not cause sensitization (Paller, 1999). Nonsteroidal antiinflammatory drugs (NSAIDs) are used for relief of pain and in the treatment of sunburn. Ibuprofen and indomethacin are the two mainstays.

Topical Calcineurin Inhibitors

This relatively new class of nonsteroidal antiinflammatory topical medication is used for short-term or intermittent long-term treatment of atopic dermatitis when conventional therapy is inadvisable, ineffective, or not tolerated. Immunomodulators are expensive and cannot be used in children under 2 years old. See Chapter 24 for more information.

Scabicides and Pediculicides

These agents are toxic to mites and lice. Crotamiton (Eurax), permethrin (Elimite, Nix), and pyrethrin plus piperonyl butoxide are used in children and should be used sparingly. Lindane (Kwell) is no longer recommended for use in children.

Hair and Scalp Preparations

Antimicrobial, tar, keratolytic, and detergent shampoos are agents used on the hair and scalp.

Herbal Remedies

Herbal or natural health practices are often used to treat acne, minor wounds, eczema, yeast and fungal infections, herpes simple virus, and poison ivy. See Chapter 42 for more information.

Other Medications and Treatments

Other medications and treatments used in dermatologic care include retinoids, topical tars, anthralin, calcipotriene (a vitamin D analogue), masking preparations, agents to relieve excessive sweating (aluminum chloride or chlorohydrate), cytotoxic and immunosuppressive agents, and phototherapy.

COUNSELING AND ANTICIPATORY GUIDANCE

Spending adequate time with the patient and parents to discuss the child's skin condition and the family's concerns and needs is essential to the successful management of skin and subcutaneous disorders. Education regarding the disease, plan of treatment, and potential risks and benefits should be provided.

Because disorders of the skin are so visible, time must be spent discussing the short- and long-term prognoses and potential plans to prevent complications, recurrence, and spread.

Ideas for preventive care for the dark-skinned patient should be implemented in routine care. The following are initial areas to include:

- Prevent acne or contact dermatitis.
- Avoid pomades.
- Prevent traction alopecia.
- Immunize for varicella to prevent scarring.
- Use insect repellents to minimize insect bite reactions.
- Treat early signs and symptoms of pruritic or inflammatory conditions (acne, eczema) and infections.
- Use moisturizing agents and eliminate soaps for dry, itchy skin.
- Use oral antipruritics for dry, itchy skin.
- Caution about the use of topical medications, especially high-potency steroids, benzoyl peroxide, and isotretinoin.
- Avoid trauma and any procedures that can induce keloids.

■ BACTERIAL INFECTIONS OF THE SKIN AND SUBCUTANEOUS TISSUE

Diagnosis and treatment of common bacterial infections are listed in Table 36-2.

IMPETIGO

Description

Impetigo is a common contagious bacterial infection of the superficial layers of the skin. Nonbullous impetigo usually follows some type of skin trauma (e.g., bites, abrasions, varicella) or other skin disease (most commonly atopic dermatitis). Bullous impetigo develops on intact skin and is caused by *Staphylococcus aureus* toxin production (see Color Plate).

Epidemiology

Impetigo is the primary bacterial infection of the skin in children. Nonbullous impetigo (sometimes referred to as crusted impetigo) accounts for more than 70% of cases with *S. aureus* as the usual pathogen; group A β streptococcus and anaerobic organisms play a lesser role as causative agents. Bullous impetigo occurs sporadically and is more common in infants and young children. Certain epidermal toxin-producing types of *S. aureus* are the primary pathogens responsible for bullous impetigo. In impetigo the organism usually spreads from autoinoculation via hands, towels, clothing, or nasal discharge or via droplets. *Streptococcus pyogenes*, responsible for 30% to 40% of cases, is found most commonly in preschool children and is uncommon on open skin in children under 2 years old. Both organisms may be found in an impetiginous lesion. Impetigo occurs more frequently with poor hygiene; during the summer months; in warm, humid climates; and in lower socioeconomic groups (Darmstadt & Sidbury, 2004; Paller & Mancini, 2006). Streptococcal types that cause pharyngitis rarely cause impetigo and vice versa.

Clinical Findings

History

- Pruritus, spread of the lesion to surrounding skin, and earlier skin disruption at the site
- Weakness, fever, diarrhea may accompany bullous impetigo

Physical Examination.   The following can be found:

- Nonbullous, classic, or common impetigo—begins as 1- to 2-mm erythematous papules or pustules that progress to vesicles or bullae, which rupture, leaving moist, honey-colored, crusty lesions on mildly erythematous, eroded skin; less than 2 cm in size; little pain but rapid spread
- Bullous impetigo—large, flaccid, thin-wall, superficial, annular, or oval pustular blisters or bullae that rupture, leaving thin varnishlike coating or scale

TABLE 36-2   Diagnosis and Treatment of Common Bacterial Infections

Infection	Causative Organism	Presentation	Area of Involvement	Treatment	Prevention
Impetigo	*S. aureus* or *Streptococcus*	Honey-colored crust on erythematous base, or blisters that rupture, leaving varnishlike coat	Superficial layers of skin (epidermis)	Topical antibiotic if minor, oral antibiotics if more significant infection	Moisturize skin; thorough cleansing of any break in skin
Cellulitis	Most commonly group A *Streptococcus* (GAS) or *S. aureus*	Erythema, swelling, tenderness; irregular borders with significant induration resembling an orange peel is associated with GAS	Dermis and subcutaneous tissue	Oral antibiotic depending on likely organism; often cephalexin (first-line) amoxicillin/clavulanate or dicloxacillin	Same as above
Folliculitis	*S. aureus*	Pruritus, erythematous papule or pustule at hair follicle	Hair follicle	Warm compresses, topical keratolytics, topical antibiotics, or antistaphylococcal antibiotic if severe	Same as above; good hygiene and antibacterial soap

- *S. aureus* lesions—usually on the face, trunk, extremities; superficial blisters that rupture, leaving the skin with a scalded appearance; commonly appear as tender shallow erosions surrounded by the remnant of the blister roof
- *S. pyogenes* lesions—on traumatized skin, lower extremities; punched-out ulcers with crusts
- Lesions most common on face, hands, neck, extremities, or perineum; satellite lesions near the primary site, although they can be found anywhere on the body
- Lymphadenopathy in up to 90% (Darmstadt & Sidbury, 2004)

Laboratory Studies. Gram stain and culture are ordered if identification of the organism is needed in recalcitrant or severe cases.

Differential Diagnosis
Herpes simplex, varicella, nummular eczema, contact dermatitis, tinea, kerion, and scabies are included in the differential diagnosis.

Management
Management involves the following:
- Topical antibiotics may be used if the impetigo is superficial, nonbullous, or localized to one or two small lesions. Topical treatment alone provides clinical improvement, but may prolong the carrier state (Weston et al, 2007). Mupirocin ointment, polymyxin B, gentamicin, erythromycin, or bacitracin (Cohen, 2005; Paller & Mancini, 2006) is used three times a day for 7 to 10 days. If there is no improvement in 3 days, oral antibiotics should be started.
- Oral antibiotics. Treatment for *S. aureus* and *S. pyogenes* is usually recommended because coexistence is common.
  - Cephalexin 40 mg/kg/day for 10 days.
  - Dicloxacillin 15 to 50 mg/kg/day for 10 days.
  - Cloxacillin 50 to 100 mg/kg/day for 10 days.
  - Erythromycin 40 mg/kg/day for 10 days; note that there is increasing resistance in some communities (Weston et al, 2007).
  - If streptococcus is cultured, treat with penicillin V 125 to 250 mg twice a day for 10 days.
- For widespread infection with constitutional symptoms and deeper skin involvement, use an oral antibiotic active against ß-lactamase-producing strains of *S. aureus*, such as dicloxacillin, cloxacillin, or cephalexin.
- If an infant has bullous impetigo, use parenteral ß-lactamase-resistant antistaphylococcal penicillin, such as methicillin, oxacillin, or nafcillin.
- If there is failure to respond in 7 days, swab beneath the crust and do Gram stain, culture, and sensitivities. Community-acquired methicillin-resistant *S. aureus* (MRSA) should be considered. This organism is more susceptible to clindamycin and trimethoprim-sulfamethoxazole (TMP-SMZ) (Paller & Mancini, 2006).
- If there is recurrence, evaluate with nasal culture and treat with topical mupirocin to the nares twice a day for 1 to 5 days to eradicate staphylococcus carriage (Paller & Mancini, 2006).
- Local care of lesions before applying ointment may be helpful. Soak with wet dressings or Burow's solution compresses to remove crusts and cleanse with soap.
- Educate regarding cleanliness, hand washing, and spread of disease.
- Exclude from day care or school until treated for 24 hours.
- Schedule a follow-up appointment in 48 to 72 hours if not improved and in 10 to 14 days.

Complications
- Cellulitis may occur in up to 10% of cases with nonbullous form (Darmstadt & Sidbury, 2004), ecthyma (infection involving entire epidermis), or erysipelas (spreading cellulitis with induration).
- Lymphangitis, suppurative lymphadenitis, guttate psoriasis, erythema multiforme (EM), scarlet fever, or glomerulonephritis may occur following infection with some strains of streptococcus. Acute rheumatic fever does not follow streptococcal skin infections in the U.S.
- *Staphylococcal scalded skin syndrome (SSSS)*, a blistering skin disease, results from circulating epidermolytic toxin-producing *S. aureus*. The unusual occurrence is in children older than 5 years, but does occur in young infants and neonates. SSSS manifests abruptly with fever, malaise, and tender erythematous skin, especially in the neck folds and axillae, rapidly becoming crusty around the eyes, nose, and mouth. The Nikolsky sign (peeling of skin with a light rub to reveal a moist red surface) is a key finding. Treat with oral dicloxacillin, a penicillinase-resistant penicillin, first-or-second generation cephalosporin, or clindamycin. Avoidance of steroids, minimal handling, and use of ointments as the skin heals result in quicker healing without scarring over 10 to 14 days (Paller & Mancini, 2006; Weston et al, 2007). Severe cases are dealt with as burn victims.

Patient Education and Prevention
- Thorough cleansing of any breaks in the skin helps prevent impetigo.
- Postinflammatory pigment changes can last weeks to months.
- Should not return to school or day care until 24 hours of antibiotic treatment is completed.

CELLULITIS
Description
Cellulitis is a localized bacterial infection often involving the dermis and subcutaneous layers of the skin. It is commonly seen following a disruption of the skin surface from an insect or animal bite, trauma, or a penetrating wound. Periorbital cellulitis is discussed in Chapter 28.

Epidemiology
In children, cellulitis is often facial (one cheek), perivaginal, or perianal or involves a joint or an extremity. Most cases of cellulitis are caused by group A streptococci, although *Haemophilus influenzae* (especially in children under 2 years old, but less common with immunization with the conjugate HIB vaccine), *S. pyrogenes*, and *S. aureus* (increasing incidence

of community-acquired MRSA) are also found. *S. aureus* commonly lives on or colonizes in the skin of children and is commonly found in the nose. It can be spread easily as children often pick their nose. Seventy percent of cases of perianal cellulitis are found in males 6 months to 10 years old. Cellulitis of the cheek is most common in 3-month-olds to 3-year-olds (Weston et al, 2007). Periorbital and orbital cellulitis are now generally caused by streptococcal species (*S. pneumoniae* and group A β-hemolytic streptococcus [GABHS]) and *S. aureus*.

Clinical Findings

History
- A previous skin disruption at the site
- Fever, malaise, irritability, anorexia, vomiting, and chills can be reported
- Recent sore throat or upper respiratory infection
- Anal pruritus, blood-streaked stools, and stool retention (perianal cellulitis)

Physical Examination.   The following can be seen:
- Erythematous, indurated, tender, swollen, warm areas of skin with irregular borders
- Blue to purple tinge to the skin, often produced when the causative organism is *H. influenzae* (in 3-month-olds to 3-year-olds)
- Lymphadenitis proximal to the site
- Bright erythema 2 to 3 cm around anus, superficial, well marginated, not indurated "ring around the anus" (perianal cellulitis)
- Erysipelas—a superficial variant of cellulitis—present with rapidly advancing lesions that are tender, bright red, have sharp margins and an "orange peel" look and feel

Laboratory Studies.   CBC and blood culture are done if the child appears ill or toxic or is under 1 year old. Gram stain and culture of the area can also be done if unusual organisms are suspected, pus is present, which is more typical of MRSA, or the child looks toxic; aspirate the leading edge of the cellulitis. Blood culture should be done if *H. influenzae* or *S. pyogenes* is suspected (Jenson & Baltimore, 2006; Weston et al, 2007).

Differential Diagnosis
Early erythema nodosum, subcutaneous fat necrosis, giant urticaria, contact dermatitis, and panniculitis are included in the differential diagnosis. Blood culture should be done if *H. influenzae* or MRSA is suspected.

Management
Immediate antibiotic therapy is needed.
- Significant infection: An initial intramuscular (IM) dose of antibiotic chosen according to suspected organism (systemic penicillin, such as benzathine penicillin 600,000 to 1,200,000 units if *Streptococcus* is suspected) or a third-generation cephalosporin, such as ceftriaxone 50 to 75 mg/kg IM every 12 hours. Hospitalization may be required if the child is very young, febrile, and acutely ill or has facial, hand, feet, perineum, orbital, or periorbital cellulitis.

- If community-associated MRSA cellulitis, folliculitis and/or pustular lesions, furuncle or carbuncle, or abscess "insect bite" is suspected, incision and drainage of any abscess is needed and a specimen sent for culture.
- Oral antibiotics:
  - Cephalexin 50 to 75 mg/kg/day for 10 days.
  - Dicloxacillin 50 to 100 mg/kg/day for 10 days if *Staphylococcus* is suspected.
  - Penicillin 30 to 60 mg/kg/day for 10 days if *Streptococcus* is suspected (usually perianal).
  - Amoxicillin clavulanate 50 to 80 mg/kg/day for 10 days if *H. influenzae* is suspected; methicillin or a third-generation cephalosporin.
  - TMP-SMZ, clindamycin, or doxycycline (if older than 8 years) are currently the drugs of choice for soft tissue infections caused by community-associated MRSA.
- Follow up in 24 hours to assess response and observe toxicity. Continue daily visits until child is recovering.
- Suspect MRSA if the skin infection is not responding to usual treatment or is more virulent than expected. Also counsel parents if the infection is not improving or getting worse, to call the provider immediately or return for an urgent visit.

Complications
Recurrent perianal streptococcal infection, septicemia, necrotizing fasciitis, and toxic shock syndrome (TSS) are possible complications.
- *Necrotizing fasciitis*, commonly called *flesh-eating strep*, is an acute, rapidly progressing necrotic invasion of group A streptococcus through the skin and subcutaneous tissue to the fascial compartments. It is found when local resistance is decreased, general debilitation is present, or perforating trauma has occurred. Necrotizing fasciitis occurs most commonly in children with decreased local resistance from a skin injury, surgery, or varicella and in children who are malnourished or chronically ill. Children with diabetes who are in ketoacidosis and immunosuppressed children are most susceptible (Weston et al, 2007). Necrotizing fasciitis begins as cellulitis (usually on the leg or on the abdomen in infants) with severe pain, edema, fever, and bullae on an erythematous surface. It quickly progresses to ulcer, eschar, and gangrene within 2 days. Prompt treatment (surgical débridement, fluid management, and prolonged antibiotic treatment) may be lifesaving because the overall mortality rate is high.
- *Toxic shock syndrome* is an acute febrile illness with rapid onset that causes significant fever, vomiting and diarrhea, engorged mucous membranes, hypotension, a diffuse macular or sunburnlike rash, conjunctival injection, and multiple organ system involvement. *S. aureus* or *S. pyogenes* (Group A streptococci) are the causative agents associated with TSS, and incubation can be as little as 14 hours. Initially recognized in menstruating adolescents, TSS is also found in males and younger children. *S. aureus* is usually the causative agent in menstruating females. Nasal packing, surgical procedures, and postpartum are some factors linked to nonmenstrual TSS. Both organisms can be associated with invasive infection

(e.g., pneumonia, osteomyelitis, bacteremia, or endocarditis) or focal tissue invasion that is rapidly progressive (American Academy of Pediatrics [AAP], 2006). Treatment is intensive, requires hospitalization, and consists of fluid management, antibiotics, and other supportive measures. Mortality rates of up to 10% have been reported (Paller & Mancini, 2006). It is a reportable disease in most states. See Chapter 23 for a more in-depth discussion and management recommendations for TSS.

Prevention
- Thorough cleansing of any break in the skin helps prevent cellulitis.
- Keep bites, scrapes, and rashes clean and bandaged until healed to prevent them from being infected by staph bacteria.
- Frequent hand washing is essential, even more so now with MRSA.
- Perianal spread can occur through shared bath water.
- See Chapter 23 regarding treatment of family members to prevent colonization with staph when a family member is diagnosed with an MRSA infection.

FOLLICULITIS AND FURUNCLE
Description
A superficial bacterial inflammation of the hair follicle is called *folliculitis*; a deeper infection with involvement of the base of the follicle and deep dermis is called a *furuncle* (boil). See Color Plate that illustrates staphylococcal superficial folliculitis.

Etiology
Obstruction of the follicular orifice is the most important factor contributing to the development of folliculitis, but a moist environment, maceration, poor hygiene, occlusive emollients, and prolonged submersion in contaminated water are also factors. *S. aureus* is the most common causative organism, except for *Pseudomonas aeruginosa*, which causes hot-tub folliculitis. *Escherichia coli* is also implicated. These infections are more common in males than in females.

Clinical Findings
History. The following can be reported:
- Pruritus with folliculitis; tenderness with furuncle
- Hot-tub exposure
- Irritating surface agent
- Occasional fever, malaise, or lymphadenopathy

Physical Examination. The child often is asymptomatic, but the following can be seen:
- Discrete, erythematous 1- to 2-mm papules or pustules on an inflamed base centered around a hair follicle
- Involvement of face, scalp, extremities (typically thighs and upper arms), buttocks, and back
- Nodules with larger areas of erythema and tenderness (furuncle)
- Pruritic papules, pustules, or nodules deep red to purple in color, most dense in areas covered by swimsuit 8 to 48 hours after exposure (hot-tub folliculitis)

Diagnostic Studies. Gram stain and culture are occasionally ordered (e.g., in the case of persistent or difficult to treat folliculitis consider the possibility of MRSA).

Differential Diagnosis
Candida infection, tinea, acne pustules, and chemical folliculitis constitute the differential diagnosis.

Management
The following steps are taken:
- Warm compresses after washing with soap and water several times a day
- Topical keratolytics, such as benzoyl peroxide 5% to 10% (twice a day for 5 days), especially if chronic or recurrent
- Superficial folliculitis: apply topical antibiotic, such as erythromycin or clindamycin, in cream, gel, solution, or ointment (twice a day for 10 to 14 days)
- Antistaphylococcal ß-lactamase-resistant antibiotics, such as dicloxacillin 15 to 50 mg/kg/day for 7 to 10 days or cephalexin 40 to 50 mg/kg/day for 7 to 10 days in severe or widespread cases
- Review of good personal hygiene habits
- Follow-up treatment in 1 week for folliculitis, in 1 day for furuncle or abscess, which may need incision and drainage
- Identify and eliminate predisposing factors
- If recurrent, look for nasal or skin carrier state

Complications
Deep abscess formation or carbuncles can occur. Sycosis barbae occurs on the chin, upper lip, and jaw, especially in adolescent black males.

Patient Education and Prevention
Good personal hygiene and an antibacterial soap minimize spread to other household members. Hot-tub folliculitis resolves in 5 to 14 days, but can recur up to 3 months after exposure.

▬ FUNGAL INFECTIONS OF THE SKIN
Diagnosis and treatment of common fungal infections are listed in Table 36-3.

CANDIDIASIS (MONILIASIS)
Description
Candidiasis is a fungal infection of the skin or mucous membranes commonly called a *yeast infection* or *thrush*. See Chapters 33 and 35 for discussion of oral and vaginal candidiasis.

Etiology
Candida albicans, a yeastlike fungus, is commonly found on skin and oral, vaginal, and intestinal mucosal tissue. Although *Candida* is part of the normal flora, overgrowth, and penetration of inflamed skin can occur on the skin or mucous membranes when there is a localized or systemic alteration in host

TABLE 36-3   Diagnosis and Treatment of Common Fungal Infections

Infection	Causative Organism	Clinical Findings	Management	Complications
Candidiasis	*C. albicans*	Moist, bright-red diaper rash with sharp borders, satellite lesions; may have associated white spots in mouth, mucous membranes, or corner of mouth	Topical or oral antifungal, generally nystatin; diaper area hygiene	Paronychia or onychomycosis
Tinea corporis	*T. tonsurans, T. rubrum, T. verrucosum, T. mentagrophytes, M. canis, E. floccosum*	Pruritic, slightly erythematous circular lesion with a slightly raised border and central clearing; well demarcated	Topical antifungals; identify and treat source; exclude from day care until treated; use oral medications for resistant cases	Tinea incognita from steroid treatment
Tinea cruris	*E. floccosum, T. rubrum, T. mentagrophytes*	Raised-border, scaly lesion on upper thighs and groin; penis and scrotum spared; symmetric	Same as for tinea corporis; loose clothes, absorbent medicated powder	Possible secondary infection
Tinea pedis	*T. rubrum, T. mentagrophytes* with *E. floccosum* and *T. tonsurans* less often	Vesicles and erosions on instep; fissure between toes with scaling and erythema; diffuse scaling on weight-bearing surfaces with exaggerated scaling in creases; pruritus	Same as for tinea corporis; absorbent medicated powder; cotton socks; open-toed shoes; moisturize	Reinfection common
Tinea versicolor	*M. furfur (P. orbiculare* and *P. ovale)*	Multiple scaly, discrete oval macules on neck, shoulders, upper back, and chest; hypopigmented to hyperpigmented areas; fail to tan in summer	Selenium shampoo; ketoconazole shampoo; topical imidazoles	50% recurrence rate

defenses. Candidiasis is more common in infants, obese children, adolescents, and chronically ill or immunocompromised children. It also is often seen as a secondary infection in persistent diaper rashes or with antibiotic, oral steroid, or oral contraceptive use. Systemic infection with candidiasis is not discussed in this textbook.

Clinical Findings

History. The history often includes antibiotic or steroid use over the previous weeks and occurrence of a rash in a moist, warm area.

Physical Examination. The following can be seen:
- Mouth—white plaques on an erythematous base that adhere to mucous membranes tightly and bleed when scraped; outer lips cracked (cheilitis)
- Corners of mouth—fissured and inflamed (perlèche or angular cheilitis)
- Intertriginous areas (neck, axillae, or groin)—bright erythema in flexural folds
- Diaper area—moist, beefy-red macules and papules with sharply marked borders and satellite lesions; erosions may also be present

- Vulvovaginal area—thick, cheesy, yellow discharge; erythema; edema; and itching
- Nail plates—transverse ridging of the nail plate, loss of cuticle, and mild proximal lateral periungual erythema (chronic paronychia)

Diagnostic Studies. If treatment failure or questionable diagnosis occurs, KOH-treated scrapings of satellite lesions or mucosa reveal yeast cells and pseudohyphae (see Fig. 36-2).

Differential Diagnosis

The differential diagnosis includes erythema toxicum, miliaria, staphylococcal pustulosis, transient neonatal pustulosis, neonatal herpes simplex, and congenital syphilis.

Management

The following steps are taken:
- Skin infection: Topical antifungals (Table 36-4), such as nystatin, miconazole, clotrimazole, ketoconazole, ciclopirox, or econazole applied to skin result in improvement within 3 to 5 days. These may be used at every diaper change for 2 to 3 days until improvement begins.

TABLE 36-4   Antifungal Medications

Drug (Trade Name)	Strength and Formulation	Application	Mode of Action, Indications, Side Effects, and Comments
Topical Medications			
Imidazoles			
Clotrimazole (Lotrimin)	1% C, L, S, P	bid	Fungistatic; erythema, stinging, blistering, peeling, edema, pruritus, hives, burning
Econazole nitrate (Spectazole)	1% C	daily/bid	Fungistatic; burning, pruritus, stinging, erythema; may have antibacterial effects
Ketoconazole (Nizoral)	2% C, Sh	daily/bid	Fungistatic, irritation, dry skin, pruritus, stinging
Miconazole nitrate (Micatin, Monistat)	2% C, P, S, L	daily/bid	Fungistatic, irritation, maceration, urticaria, allergic contact dermatitis, pruritus; economical
Oxiconazole nitrate (Oxistat)	1% C, L	daily/bid	Fungistatic; pruritus, burning, irritation, erythema, folliculitis
Sulconazole nitrate (Exelderm)	1% C, S	daily/bid	Fungistatic; pruritus, burning, stinging
Allylamines			
Butenafine HCl (Mentax)	C	daily	Fungicidal; irritation
Naftifine HCl (Naftin)	1% C, G	daily/bid	Fungicidal; burning, stinging, erythema, pruritus, irritation
Terbinafine HCl (Lamisil)	1% C, S	daily/bid	Fungicidal; pruritus, irritation, burning
Ethanolamine			
Ciclopirox olamine (Loprox)	1% C, L, G (Penlac Nail Lacquer 8% solution)	bid. Penlac applied daily preferably at bedtime	Fungicidal; irritation, erythema, burning
Others			
Calcium undecylenate (Caldesene, Cruex)	10%-20% P, C, O, L	bid	Irritation
Gentian violet	1%-2% S	bid	Topical antiseptic/germicide; staining, vesicle formation
Nystatin (Mycolog-II,* Mycostatin, Nilstat, Mytrex*)	100,000 units/g C, P, O, Su	bid/tid	Fungistatic; rare adverse reactions; effective against yeast only
Selenium sulfide (Excel; Head & Shoulders Intensive Treatment Dandruff Shampoo; Selsun Blue)	1% Sh, 2.5% L, Sh	daily	Thought to block the enzymes involved in growth of epithelial tissues; discoloration of hair, alopecia; used for tinea capitis (reduces transmission), tinea versicolor, and seborrheic dermatitis (shampoo may be used as lotion)
Sodium thiosulfate; salicylic acid (Tinver)	25% L	daily/bid	For tinea versicolor
Tolnaftate (Desenex, Tinactin)	1% C, P, S, G	bid	Fungistatic; rare adverse reactions
Oral Medications			
Clotrimazole	10 mg troche	1 troche 5 times a day dissolved slowly in mouth	Treatment of oral candidiasis; gastrointestinal symptoms; hepatotoxicity
Fluconazole	10-40 mg/mL; 50-, 100-, 150-, 200-mg capsules	3-6 mg/kg/day in single dose for 2 wk for oropharyngeal candidiasis; day one dosage is 6 mg/kg (pediatric patients) and 200 mg/dose (adults) followed by daily therapy of 3 mg/kg/dose (pediatric) and 100 mg/dose (adults)	Approved for pediatric use for oropharyngeal, esophageal, or disseminated candidiasis; possible drug interactions; elevated AST, ALT, or alkaline phosphatase, hepatitis

Continued

| TABLE 36-4 | Antifungal Medications—Cont'd |

Drug (Trade Name)	Strength and Formulation	Application	Mode of Action, Indications, Side Effects, and Comments
Griseofulvin	Ultramicrosized	>2 yr: 5-10 mg/kg in single or divided dose; max dose 750 mg/day	Fungistatic; mainstay of therapy; excellent safety profile and extensive use; monitor CBC
	Microsized	10-20 mg/kg/day given daily or bid; max dose 1000 mg/kg	LFTs, renal function at 4-6 wk and every 4-6 wk while on treatment; possible drug interactions
			Duration of treatment: tinea corporis: 2-4 wk; tinea capitis: 4-6 wk or longer; tinea pedis: 4-8 wk; unguium: 3-6 mo or longer
Itraconazole	Liquid Su not recommended;	5-10 mg/kg/day as single dose or	Not approved for pediatric use; used in treatment failures or for onychomycosis by some; monitor CBC, LFTs; pulse doses often used at 4-6 wk and every 4-6 wk while on treatment; broadest spectrum; possible drug interactions
	100- or 200-mg capsules	given in 2 doses; 3- to 16-yr-olds treated with 100 mg/day or 3-5 mg/kg/day	
Ketoconazole	100 mg/tsp Su 200-mg tab	3.3-6.6 mg/kg/day in single dose	Less effective than griseofulvin and higher risk of hepatotoxicity
Nystatin	100,000 units/mL	Infants: 2 mL qid after meals: Children/adolescents 400,000-600,000 units qid—swished about mouth	Treatment of oral candidiasis
Terbinafine	250-mg tab	<20 kg, ¼ tab; 20-40 kg, ½ tab; >40 kg, 1 tab	Not approved for pediatric use; few studies in children; costly; possible drug interactions
			Duration of the treatment: tinea capitus 4 wk, tinea corporis 2 wk, tinea pedis 2 wk, finger onychomycosis 6 wk, toenail onychomycosis 12 wk

*Nystatin; triamcinolone acetonide.
Data from Taketomo DK, Hodding JH, Kraus DM: *Pediatric dosage handbook*, ed 13, Hudson, OH, 2006, Lexi-Comp. Paller AS, Mancini AJ: *Hurwitz clinical dermatology: a textbook of skin disorders of childhood and adolescence*, ed 3, Philadelphia, 2006, Elsevier Saunders, p 457.
bid, Twice a day; *C*, cream; *CBC*, complete blood count; *G*, gel; *L*, lotion; *LFTs*, liver function tests; *O*, ointment; *P*, powder; *qid*, 4 times daily; *S*, solution; *Sh*, shampoo; *Su*, suspension; *tid*, 3 times daily; *wk*, weeks.

- If inflammation is present, alternate nystatin cream and 1% hydrocortisone for 1 or 2 days. Secondary bacterial infections can occur; in such cases, add an oral antibiotic (Paller & Mancini, 2006).
- Cold milk compresses (if child is not allergic to milk): Mix equal parts skim milk and water with ice cubes in a bowl; saturate cloth and apply repeatedly until warm for 5 to 10 minutes three times a day in conjunction with hydrocortisone and antifungal creams (Weinberg, 1998).
- Keep area dry and cool. Minimize skin irritation:
  - Frequent diaper changes.
  - Leave diaper area open to air.
  - Blow-dry with warm air for 3 to 5 minutes at diaper change (especially helpful in intertriginous areas in infants and obese children).
  - Avoid rubber pants.
  - Use mild soap and water; rinse well; avoid diaper wipes.
  - Avoid other powders and medications, especially antibiotics and steroids.
  - Discontinue oral antibiotics and steroids when possible.
  - Discard or sterilize pacifiers.

- Oral infection: Administer nystatin oral solution four times a day swabbed onto mucous membranes for 5 to 14 days, gentian violet 1% to 2% aqueous solution applied twice a day, or clotrimazole troches 10-mg tablet dissolved slowly in the mouth five times a day for 14 days in children older than 3 years old. If breastfeeding, the mother should put the solution on her nipples to eliminate reinfection. A second course is sometimes needed to clear the infection.
- Perlèche (fissures in the corners of the mouth): Topical corticosteroid (low-dose) two to three times daily; add a topical antifungal if severe or persistent.
  - Educate about avoiding underlying predisposing factor (e.g., lip licking).
  - Add topical or oral antibiotic if secondary infection is suspected.
- If severe or recalcitrant infection, oral fluconazole or itraconazole 5 mg/kg/day for 21 days may be recommended if older than 6 months.
- Nail involvement (chronic paronychia) can be treated with topical application of antifungal cream twice daily, but it will take several months for the nail plate to grow out normally; oral fluconazole may be needed for severe or resistant involvement.

Complications

Chronic mucocutaneous candidiasis resulting from immunologic deficit can occur and is heralded by widespread involvement (oral, skin, nails). Paronychia may occur with thumb sucking.

Patient Education

Emphasize good hand washing. Treatment failure is usually due to lack of compliance.

TINEA CAPITIS

See later section on alopecia.

TINEA CORPORIS

Description

Tinea corporis, commonly called *ringworm*, is a superficial fungal skin infection found on the face or body. It is also identified by the part of the body affected (e.g., tinea manuum [hand], tinea barbae [beard], tinea faciei [face]) (see Color Plate).

Epidemiology

Tinea corporis is caused by the dermatophytes *Microsporum canis*, *M. audouinii*, *Trichophyton mentagrophytes*, *T. rubrum*, *T. verrucosum*, *T. tonsurans*, and *Epidermophyton floccosum*. Transmission comes as the stratum corneum is invaded following direct contact with infected humans, animals, or fomites. The exact mechanism is unknown, but is probably due to a toxin causing an inflammatory response. Infection is common, and it increases with age, hot and humid climates, and crowded living conditions. Autoinoculation can account for spreading lesions (Paller & Mancini, 2006; Weston et al, 2007).

Clinical Findings

History. Contact with a person or animal with ringworm is sometimes reported.

Physical Examination

- Classical appearance of lesions: annular, oval, or circinate with one or more flat, scaling, mildly erythematous circular patches or plaques with raised borders
- Spread peripherally and clear centrally or may be inflammatory throughout with superficial pustules
- Often prominent over hair follicles
- Multiple secondary lesions may merge into a large area several centimeters in diameter

Diagnostic Studies. If treatment failure or questionable diagnosis occurs:

- KOH-treated scrapings of border of lesion reveal hyphae and spores (see Fig. 36-2).
- Fungal culture.
- Wood's lamp is helpful, but does not fluoresce all tinea infections.

Differential Diagnosis

PR herald patch, nummular eczema, psoriasis, seborrhea, contact dermatitis, tinea versicolor, granuloma annulare, and Lyme disease are in the differential diagnosis.

Management

Management involves the following:

- For superficial or localized tinea corporis, topical antifungals (see Table 36-4), such as miconazole or clotrimazole, are generally effective. Apply two to three times a day. Improvement in lesions and pruritus is generally seen within the first week of therapy, but treatment must continue for 2 to 3 weeks to ensure tinea is resolved, usually a minimum of 4 weeks (Paller & Mancini, 2006). Prescriptive antifungals (e.g., econazole, ciclopirox) penetrate the skin more effectively, but are more expensive.
- Extensive infection, or tinea unresponsive to topical treatment, may be treated orally with griseofulvin (see Table 36-4) for 4 to 8 weeks; it must be taken with fatty foods and can cause headache, nausea, diarrhea, or crampy abdominal pain. Monitor CBC, liver function tests (LFTs), and possibly renal function tests if treatment duration is longer than 3 months; obtain initial laboratory panel at 4 to 6 weeks, and repeat every 4 to 6 weeks during treatment. Tinea corporis gladiatorum seen with wrestling may require systemic therapy and is extensive or endemic among the wrestling team members.
- Identify and treat contacts.
- Educate about communicability of lesions and length of treatment.
- Exclude from day care or school until treatment has begun.
- Follow up in 2 weeks or sooner if lesions are not responding. If unresponsive, diagnosis is incorrect or resistance is possible. Culture to confirm diagnosis and change class of antifungal used.

Complications

Tinea incognito occurs when tinea has been treated with hydrocortisone; signs and symptoms of infection are minimized, but the infection persists.

Patient Education

Find the source of infection and treat or eliminate it to prevent recurrence. Treat skin and 1 cm area beyond the border. Keep skin dry following application of antifungal

TINEA CRURIS

Description

Tinea cruris, commonly called *jock itch*, is a superficial fungal skin infection found on the groin, upper thighs, and intertriginous folds.

Epidemiology

Caused by the dermatophyte *E. floccosum* or, occasionally, *T. rubrum* or *T. mentagrophytes*, tinea cruris rarely occurs before adolescence and is more common in males, obese individuals, or those with hyperhidrosis or experiencing chafing from tight clothes or moisture. It is extremely common and often occurs with tinea pedis (Paller & Mancini, 2006).

Clinical Findings
History
- Hot, humid weather, tight clothing, vigorous physical activity and chafing, or contact sport, such as wrestling
- Often associated with tinea pedis
Physical Examination
- Erythematous to slightly brown, sharply marginated plaques with a raised border of scaling, pustules or vesicles; central clearing may be present
- Usually bilateral and symmetric, but not always
- Occurs on inner thighs and inguinal creases; penis, scrotum, and labia majora generally spared
- Occasionally occurs in perianal region or on the buttocks and/or abdomen

Diagnostic Studies. If treatment failure or questionable diagnosis occurs:
- KOH scraping reveals hyphae and spores
- Fungal culture

Differential Diagnosis

Psoriasis, candidiasis, contact dermatitis, seborrhea, intertrigo, and erythrasma are in the differential diagnosis.

Management

Management is the same as for tinea corporis. Duration of topical treatment is usually 4 to 6 weeks. If griseofulvin is required, a treatment course of 2 to 6 weeks is usually indicated (see Table 36-4). If tinea pedis is present, it must be treated. Additionally:
- Advise the patient to wear cotton underwear and loose clothing and to use absorbent antifungal powder.

- Maintain good hygiene following a wrestling event (e.g., bathing as soon as possible, sole use of towel; dry thoroughly).
- Do not use steroids because of risk of atrophy and striae.

TINEA PEDIS

Description

Tinea pedis is a superficial fungal skin infection found on the feet, commonly called *athlete's foot*. There are three clinical forms: (1) vesicles and erosions on the instep of one or both feet; (2) an occasional fissure between the toes with surrounding scale and erythema; and (3) rare diffuse scaling on the weight-bearing surface of the foot with exaggerated scaling in creases (moccasin foot) often extending to lateral foot margins.

Epidemiology

Caused by the dermatophytes *T. rubrum* and *E. floccosum* or *T. mentagrophytes*, tinea pedis rarely occurs before adolescence and is more common in males (Jenson & Baltimore, 2006). It is acquired through direct contact with contaminated surfaces (e.g., warm moist environment of showers and locker room floors) and often occurs with tinea cruris.

Clinical Findings
History. The following are sometimes reported:
- Sweaty feet
- Use of nylon socks or nonbreathable shoes
- Exposure in family or at school
- Itching, intense burning, stinging, foul odor
- Microtrauma to feet—cracks, abrasions, nicks, cuts
- Contact with damp areas (e.g., swimming pools, locker room, showers)
Physical Examination. Findings include the following:
- Red, scaly, cracked rash on soles or interdigital spaces and instep, especially between the third, fourth, and fifth toes
- Infection initially white, peeling lesions becoming erythematous, vesicular, macerated, or fissured, and scaly
- Dorsum of foot remains clear
- Chronic infection manifested by a moccasin pattern with diffuse scaling (plantar hyperkeratosis) and mild erythema

Diagnostic Studies. Laboratory studies are the same as those for tinea corporis.

Differential Diagnosis

Contact dermatitis, atopic dermatitis, dyshidrotic eczema, psoriasis, and juvenile plantar dermatosis (red, dry fissures of weight-bearing surface) are in the differential diagnosis.

Management

Management is the same as that for tinea corporis. Antifungal medication should be applied 1 cm beyond the borders of the rash twice daily until 7 days after clearing. Usual treatment is 3 to 6 weeks. If griseofulvin is required, treatment for 6 to 8 weeks is usually recommended. Additionally:

- Advise patient to keep feet dry, use absorbent antifungal powder or sprays, wear cotton socks, avoid scratching, and wear shoes that allow the feet to breathe or go barefoot when home. Thoroughly dry feet and between toes after using a commercial showering facility.
- Rinse feet with plain water or water and vinegar; dry carefully, especially between the toes. Moisturize and protect feet to prevent splitting and cracking.
- Aluminum chloride (Drysol, Certain Dri, Xerac AC, Arrid Extra Dry antiperspirant spray) may be used for hyperhidrosis.
- Acute vesicular lesions may need to be treated with wet compresses two to four times daily for 10 to 15 minutes in addition to application of topical antifungals.
- Moccasin-type tinea pedis may need the addition of a keratolytic agent (lactic acid or urea) with the application of antifungals.
- Tennis shoes may be washed in the machine with soap and bleach.
- Physical education or sports may be continued.
- Follow up in 2 to 3 weeks or sooner if lesions are not responding.

Complications

A secondary bacterial infection, indicated by foul odor, can occur. An allergic reaction to fungus, called an *id response*, is manifested by a vesicular eruption on the palms and sides of fingers and occasionally on the trunk and extremities.

TINEA VERSICOLOR

Description

Tinea versicolor is a superficial fungal infection, also called *pityriasis versicolor*, that tends to be persistent and occurs predominantly on the trunk. The lesions do not tan in the summer and become relatively darker in winter months.

Epidemiology

This infection is caused by a yeastlike organism, *Malassezia furfur* (referred to as *P. orbiculare* and *P. ovale*) and occurs more commonly in adolescents than in younger children, in chronically ill and immunocompromised children, and in warmer seasons and humid climates. Breastfeeding infants can acquire the organism from their mother and exhibit facial lesions. Genetic factors also predispose to this problem, and it tends to be a chronic, recurrent disorder (Cohen, 2005).

Clinical Findings

History. The infection is associated with warm, humid weather. Occasional mild itching may occur.

Physical Examination. Multiple, annular, scaling, discrete macules or patches, ranging from hypopigmented in dark-skinned individuals to hyperpigmented (salmon-colored to brown) in light-pigmented individuals, are seen on the neck, shoulders, upper back and arms, chest midline, and face (especially in children). They tend to have a guttate or raindrop pattern.

Diagnostic Studies. KOH scrapings, though not necessary, reveal short curved hyphae and circular spores ("spaghetti and meatballs"). Scrapings fluoresce yellow-orange under Wood's lamp if not cleansed recently.

Differential Diagnosis

Pityriasis alba, PR, vitiligo, postinflammatory hypopigmentation or hyperpigmentation, seborrhea, and secondary syphilis are included in the differential diagnosis.

Management

The following steps are taken:

- Selenium sulfide 2.5% shampoo and ketoconazole 2% shampoo should be applied in a thin layer for 10 minutes followed by rinsing; continue treatment for 1 to 2 weeks. It can be applied every other week or monthly for maintenance treatment. Terbinafine 1% spray can also be used with directions to apply once to twice daily for 1 to 2 weeks (Paller & Mancini, 2006).
- Topical imidazoles (clotrimazole, miconazole, ciclopirox, or terbinafine solution) or topical azoles (ketoconazole or oxiconazole) applied twice daily for 2 to 4 weeks can be used instead of selenium (see Table 36-4). This therapy may be impractical if the lesions cover a wide area of skin.
- Resistant or severe cases or tropical climates are sometimes an indication for oral antifungal treatment, such as with ketoconazole or fluconazole or itraconazole. Dosing recommendations include multiple administration as continuous, intermittent, and single-dose approaches. A single dose of ketoconazole (400 mg), followed by physical activity to promote the secretion of the drug into the skin via sweating and no bathing for 10 to 12 hours, with a repeat dose in 1 week has demonstrated good results. At present there is no "gold" standard for systemic dosing (Paller & Mancini, 2006).
- Follow up in 1 month.

Patient Education

- Fifty percent have recurrences within 1 to 10 years.
- Sun exposure makes lesions appear hypopigmented as the surrounding skin tans.
- Repigmentation takes several months.
- If the patient is taking oral antifungal medication, encourage exercise to induce sweating because this may enhance concentration of medication in the skin.
- Skin irritation occurs with overnight application.
- Absence of flaking when skin is scraped is a sign of effective treatment.

■ VIRAL INFECTIONS OF THE SKIN
HERPES SIMPLEX

Description

In the active state, herpes simplex virus (HSV) causes contagious infections of the skin and mucous membranes ranging from mild to life threatening. Primary infection with HSV type 1 (HSV-1) usually affects the oral mucosa, pharynx, lips, and occasionally the eyes. Acute gingivostomatitis is an example of primary disease (see Chapter 33). The virus then becomes dormant in certain nerve cells until reactivated by triggering factors, such as stress, menses, illness, sunburn windburn, and fatigue. HSV-1 causes recurrent herpes labialis infection, commonly called *cold sores* or *fever blisters* (see Color Plate). HSV-2 infection commonly occurs as a neonatal infection (see Chapter 38) or herpetic vulvovaginitis (see Chapter 35) or progenitalis. Type 1 can also be found in the genital area; type 2 is found on the lips and mouth. Herpetic keratoconjunctivitis is discussed in Chapter 28; other information may be found in Chapter 23.

Epidemiology

HSV infection can be either primary or recurrent. Primary infection occurs in individuals without circulating antibodies after direct contact with secretions or mucocutaneous lesions of an infected individual. Incubation takes days to weeks and then manifests itself anywhere from subclinical to severe infection. Recurrent infection occurs in individuals previously infected who had either clinical or subclinical manifestations of infection. HSV-1 is transmitted by close contact with skin, mucous membranes, and body fluids, often through a break in the skin or by autoinoculation. Lesions occur in children of all ages, are contagious as long as they are present, and have an incubation period of 2 to 12 days. Primary lesions usually occur before 5 years old, are more painful and extensive, and last longer. HSV-1 is responsible for gingivostomatitis, herpes labialis, and hand and finger infections. HSV-2 infection occurs most commonly in adolescents as a sexually transmitted disease and in infants from transmittal during delivery; in children, the possibility of sexual abuse must be considered.

Clinical Findings

History. In primary herpes, fever, malaise, sore throat, and decreased fluid intake can occur. Primary genital HSV presents with painful vesicles in genital areas. In recurrent HSV infection, there is often a painful prodrome of burning, tingling, paresthesia, and itching at the involved site. Recent acute febrile illness or sun exposure may also be reported.

Physical Examination. The following are seen on physical examination:

- HSV-1
  - Gingivostomatitis—pharyngitis with grouped erythematous-based vesicles (grouped vesicles on an erythematous base) that ulcerate and form white plaques on mucosa, gingiva, tongue, palate, lips, chin, and nasolabial folds; lymphadenopathy and halitosis are present
  - Herpes labialis—cluster of small, clear, tense vesicles with an erythematous base that become weepy and ulcerated, progressing to crustiness, usually only on one side of the mouth and on the vermillion border—classic cold sore
  - Hand or fingers—deep-appearing vesicles
  - Common sites of involvement: lips, hand, fingers, nose, cheek, forehead, and eyes; can also occur in the genital area

- HSV-2
  - Grouped vesicopustules and ulceration with edema
  - Primary lesions on vaginal mucosa, labia, or perineum in females and on the penile shaft or perineum in males; females may have cervical involvement; oral lesions are possible
  - Recurrent lesions on labia, vulva, clitoris, or cervix in females and on the prepuce, glans, or sulcus in males; generally less severe cutaneous lesions
  - Regional lymphadenopathy

Laboratory Studies. A Tzanck smear can be done on fluid from the lesions to identify epidermal giant cells; however, it does not distinguish HSV-1 from HSV-2. Viral cultures are the gold standard for definitive diagnosis. Direct fluorescent antibody (DFA) tests, enzyme-linked immunosorbent assay (ELISA) serology, and polymerase chain reaction (PCR) tests can be done, but are usually only used with severe forms of HSV infection.

Differential Diagnosis

The differential diagnosis includes aphthous stomatitis, hand-foot-and-mouth disease, varicella, impetigo, folliculitis, and erythema multiforme (EM).

Management

Management can be guided by considering the host (e.g., age, area and extent of involvement, and immune status), the organism (is it definitely HSV?), and the drug needed (Table 36-5).

1. Burow's solution compresses three times a day to alleviate discomfort
2. Acyclovir 20 to 40 mg/kg/day orally five times a day for 5 days or 200 mg every 4 hours five times a day for 7 to 10 days may be indicated to help shorten the course and alleviate symptoms for children older than 2 years with the following conditions:
   - Any underlying skin disorder (e.g., eczema)
   - A severe case
   - An immunocompromised disease
   - Systemic symptoms with primary genital infection
   - Occasionally for initial severe gingivostomatitis

   Acyclovir is most effective if started within 3 days of disease onset. Famciclovir or valacyclovir are additional antiviral agents approved for use in adults.
3. Topical acyclovir ointment may help for initial genital herpes infections, but often not beneficial for recurrent infections.
4. Antibiotics for secondary bacterial (usually staphylococcal) infection:
   - Mupirocin topically three times a day for 5 days
   - Erythromycin 40 mg/kg/day for 10 days
   - Dicloxacillin 12.5 to 50 mg/kg/day for 10 days
5. Oral anesthetics for comfort; use with caution in children (children should be able to rinse and spit).
   - Viscous lidocaine (Xylocaine) 2% topical
   - Liquid diphenhydramine alone or combined with Maalox (aluminum hydroxide; magnesium hydroxide) as a 1:1 rinse (maximum of 5 mg/kg/day diphenhydramine in

TABLE 36-5 **Diagnosis and Treatment of Herpes Simplex (HS) and Herpes Zoster (HZ)**

	Presentation	Clinical Findings	Treatment	Education
HS	Gingivostomatitis as primary infection; herpes labialis or herpes facialis as recurrent infection	Pharyngitis with erythematous vesicles on and/or in mouth; small, clear vesicles on erythematous base progressing to crusting	Burow's solution; acyclovir in primary case or underlying disorder; antibiotics if secondary infection; oral anesthetics; supportive care	Degree and duration of contagion; triggers to infection
HZ	Reactivation of latent varicella virus, especially after mild cases or in infants <1 year old or immunocompromised host	Two to three clustered groups of vesicles on erythematous base, especially over thoracic or lumbosacral dermatomes; pain, itch, tingle is minimal in children	Burow's solution; antihistamine; drying lotions; possible acyclovir; silver sulfadiazine (Silvadene cream); antibiotics if secondary infection	New vesicles occur for up to 1 week; take 2-3 weeks to resolve; contagious for varicella; varicella vaccine to prevent

case it is swallowed); it can also be applied with Q-Tips to the lesions

6. Newborn infant, immunosuppressed child, child with infected atopic dermatitis, or child with a lesion in the eye or on the eyelid margin: consult with or refer to an appropriate provider.
7. Offer supportive care, such as antipyretics, analgesics, hydration, and good oral hygiene.
8. Exclude from day care only during the initial course (gingivostomatitis) and if the child cannot control secretions.
9. Recurrent, frequent, and severe HSV infection may be treated with acyclovir prophylaxis for 6 months.

Complications
Herpetic whitlow, occurring on a finger or thumb, is a swollen, painful lesion with an erythematous base and ulceration resembling a paronychia. It occurs on fingers of thumb-sucking children with gingivostomatitis or adolescents with genital HSV infection. Therapy with oral acyclovir 200 mg five times a day for 5 to 10 days may speed healing. *Eczema herpeticum* or *Kaposi's varicelliform eruption* is discussed in Chapter 23. HSV has also been implicated as a possible cause of EM and Stevens-Johnson syndrome (SJS).

Patient Education, Prognosis, and Prevention
Recurrence of infection, possible triggering factors, and avoidance measures should be discussed. Triggers can include physical and psychological stress, trauma, fever, exposure to UV light, illness, menses, and extreme weather. Contagiousness of lesions and oral secretions must be understood. Explanation of the course of primary disease, with fever lasting up to 4 days and lesions taking at least 2 weeks to heal, is important. Famciclovir and penciclovir are in clinical trials for use in children. Vaccines are under development to decrease transmission and minimize recurrence.

HERPES ZOSTER
Description
Herpes zoster (HZ) is a recurrent varicella infection commonly called *shingles* (see Color Plate).

Epidemiology
Caused by reactivation of the latent varicella zoster infection from the sensory root ganglia, HZ occurs in 10% to 20% of all persons, is rare in childhood, and occurs more frequently with increasing age (three times more common in adolescents than preschoolers). HZ is more common following mild cases of varicella, following varicella before 1 year old (threefold to twentyfold increased risk), and in immunocompromised children. Reoccurrence of HZ is about 4% (Myers et al, 2004).

Clinical Findings
History. Burning, stinging, pain, tenderness to light touch, hyperanesthesia, or tingling precedes eruption by about 1 week, though this is less common in children. The lesions can be extremely itchy and painful.

Physical Examination. Findings include the following (Paller & Mancini, 2006):
- Two or three clustered groups of macules and papules progress to vesicles on an erythematous base. These vesicles become pustular, rupture, ulcerate, and crust.
- Lesions develop over 3 to 5 days and last 7 to 10 days. Lesions may develop for up to 1 week followed by crusting and healing during the next 2 weeks. In children delayed chronic pain, known as postherpetic neuralgia, is rare.
- Lesions commonly follow the dermatomes of the second cervical to lumbar nerves and the fifth to seventh cranial nerves with scattered lesions outside these areas.
- Lesions do not cross midline (key to diagnosis); sharp demarcation at the midline with occasional contralateral involvement.
- Lymphadenopathy may occur.

HZ may be less common after varicella immunization than after natural varicella infection (Habif, 2004).

Diagnostic Studies.   The diagnosis is a clinical one. However, if needed, Tzanck smear or viral culture can be done to distinguish from HSV infection. Bacterial culture or Gram stain can be used to distinguish from impetigo. A DFA stain of vesicle base scrapings is beneficial in the difficult to diagnosis case and results are timely.

Differential Diagnosis
Local cutaneous HSV infection and impetigo are in the differential diagnosis.

Management
Management steps include the following:
1. Apply Burow's solution compresses three times a day to alleviate discomfort.
2. Administer antihistamines for itching, analgesics for discomfort.
3. Lotions, such as calamine, help dry lesions and decrease itching.
4. Antiviral medications:
   - Acyclovir 800 mg orally every 4 hours five times a day for 7 to 10 days helps shorten the course and alleviate symptoms in immunocompromised or significantly ill children. Acyclovir has not been fully studied in children under 2 years old.
   - Famciclovir 500 mg every 8 hours for 7 days at the earliest sign of HZ or within 48 to 72 hours of onset or valacyclovir 1 g orally three times a day for 7 days at the earliest sign of HZ or within 48 hours of onset has been approved for adults but not for children with HZ (Paller & Mancini, 2006).
5. Antibiotics for secondary bacterial (usually staphylococcal) infection:
   - Mupirocin topically twice a day
   - Dicloxacillin 12.5 to 25 mg/kg/day for 7 to 10 days
6. Refer for immediate ophthalmologic examination if eyes, forehead, or nose is involved.

Complications
Complications are rare except in immunocompromised children. Occasionally, HZ is the initial finding in acquired immunodeficiency syndrome (AIDS), especially if more than one dermatome is involved.

Patient Education, Prevention, and Prognosis
- New vesicles appear for up to 1 week and take 2 to 3 weeks to resolve. Illness is usually mild.
- The child is contagious for varicella until lesions are crusted and should be excluded from day care or school until this occurs (AAP, 2006).

MOLLUSCUM CONTAGIOSUM
Description
A benign, common childhood viral skin infection with little health risk, molluscum contagiosum often disappears on its own in a few weeks to months and is not easily treated (See Color Plate).

Epidemiology
This highly contagious poxvirus replicates in host epithelial cells. It attacks skin and mucous membranes and is spread by direct contact, by fomites, or by autoinoculation (typically scratching). It is commonly found in children and adolescents (Cohen, 2005). Three types are identified. Lesions found on the extremities, neck, and head are usually type 1; genital lesions are usually type 2 or 3. The incubation period is about 2 months; the child is contagious as long as lesions are present.

Clinical Findings
History
- Itching at the site
- Possible exposure to molluscum contagiosum

Physical Examination.   Findings include the following:
- Very small, firm, pink to flesh-colored discrete papules 1 to 6 mm in size (occasionally up to 15 mm).
- Papules progressing to become umbilicated (may not be evident) with a cheesy core; keratinous contents may extrude from the umbilication.
- Surrounding dermatitis is common.
- Face, axillae, antecubital area, trunk, popliteal fossae, crural area, and extremities are the most commonly involved areas; palms, soles, and scalp are spared.
- Single papule to numerous papules; most often numerous clustered papules and linear configurations.
- Sexually active or abused children can have genitally grouped lesions.
- Children with eczema or immunosuppression can have severe cases; those with HIV infection or AIDS can have hundreds of lesions.

Differential Diagnosis
Warts, closed comedones, small epidermal cysts, blisters, folliculitis, and condyloma acuminatum are included in the differential diagnosis.

Management
- Untreated lesions take 1 to 5 years to resolve. Mechanical removal of the central core is often done to prevent spread and autoinoculation. Using eutectic mixture of local anesthetics (EMLA) cream (lidocaine; prilocaine) 30 to 45 minutes before the procedure reduces discomfort. Consult manufacturer recommendations regarding the maximum dose and application area by age and body weight.
- Curettage is done with a sharp blade to remove the papule. Piercing the papule and expressing the plug can also be done, but this procedure is painful.
- Nightly application of surgical tape (Scotch or adhesive tape can be used) for 1 month followed by removal of lesions.
- Topical medications may prove beneficial. Recheck the patient in 1 to 2 weeks to determine need for retreatment.
  - Liquid nitrogen may be applied for 2 to 3 seconds (easiest but also painful).

○ Trichloroacetic acid 25% to 50% applied by dropper to the center of the lesion, followed by alcohol (use with caution). Surround the lesion first with Vaseline.

○ Cantharidin 0.7% in collodion applied by dropper to the center of the lesion, followed by alcohol. Salicylic or lactic acid or potassium hydroxide or podophyllin.

○ Podofilox (Condylox) 0.5% topical solution or gel, or imiquimod 5% (Aldara) applied daily with a toothpick or Q-Tip.

○ Tretinoin or Tazarotene cream or gel applied to lesion nightly.

○ Silver nitrate, iodine 7% to 9%, or phenol 1% applied for 2 to 3 seconds.

○ Cimetidine 30 to 40 mg/kg/day in two divided doses orally.

• Sexual abuse of children with genitally grouped lesions should be suspected and evaluated.

• Evaluate for HIV infection if hundreds of lesions are found.

• Wait and see approach—spontaneous clearing occurs over years.

Complications

Molluscum dermatitis, a scaly, erythematous, hypersensitive reaction, can occur and will respond to moisturizer; avoid hydrocortisone because it will cause molluscum to flare. Inflammation of the eyes or conjunctiva and scarring can occur.

Patient Education and Prevention

Patients are contagious, but there is no need to exclude them from day care or school. Children with impaired immunity, atopic dermatitis, or traumatized skin are at greater risk for broader spread. Severe inflammation is possible several hours after application of cantharidin. Scarring is unusual.

WARTS

Description

Warts are a common childhood skin infection characterized by a proliferation of the epidermis; they can also cause mucosal infection. Cutaneous warts are rarely a serious health concern, but present cosmetic problems for children and their families.

Epidemiology

Warts are viral-induced epithelial tumors caused by DNA-containing human papillomavirus (HPV). There are basically two groups of HPV genotypes: cutaneous and mucosal. Cutaneous warts occur in approximately 10% of children (Paller & Mancini, 2006). They are among the most common skin disorders in children. The transmission of warts from person to person is dependent on viral and host factors, such as quantity of virus, location of warts, preexisting skin injury, and cell-mediated immunity. Transmission is from fomites or skin-to-skin contact, and autoinoculation is frequent. Incubation is from 1 to 6 months.

Although a large percentage of all warts resolve spontaneously within 2 years, there is a high recurrence rate. Certain types of HPV are associated with cutaneous and genital oncogenesis. There are four basic types of warts: verruca vulgaris, verruca plana, verruca plantaris, and condyloma acuminatum. Most warts are on the hands, fingers, elbows, and plantar surfaces of the feet.

Clinical Findings

History. The history can include exposure to someone with warts. Trauma to cutaneous warts promotes inoculation of the virus (Koebner phenomenon); therefore, warts are commonly seen on the extremities. With koebnerization, a line of warts develops in a linear constellation of lesions where the skin was excoriated. Warts can occur anywhere on the body, including the face, scalp, and genitalia.

Physical Examination

• *Common* warts (verruca vulgaris) are usually elevated, flesh-colored single papules with scaly, irregular surfaces and occasionally black pinpoints, which are thrombosed blood vessels. They are usually asymptomatic and multiple in number and are found anywhere on the body, although most commonly on the hands, nails, and feet. They may be dome shaped, filiform, or exophytic (Fig. 36-4). *Filiform* warts project from the skin on a narrow stalk and are usually seen on the face, lips, nose, eyelids, or neck. Periungual warts are common warts occurring around the cuticles of the fingers or toes.

• *Plantar* warts (mosaic) are common warts found on weight-bearing surfaces of the feet. Found alone or grouped, plantar warts (verrucae plantaris) grow inward and disrupt skin markings.

• *Flat* warts (verruca plana or juvenile warts) are seen most commonly on the face, neck, and extremities. They are small, slightly elevated papules and number from few to several hundred.

• *Condylomata acuminata* on genital mucosa and adjacent skin are multiple, confluent warts with irregular surfaces, light in color, and cauliflower-like in appearance. See Chapter 35 for more detail.

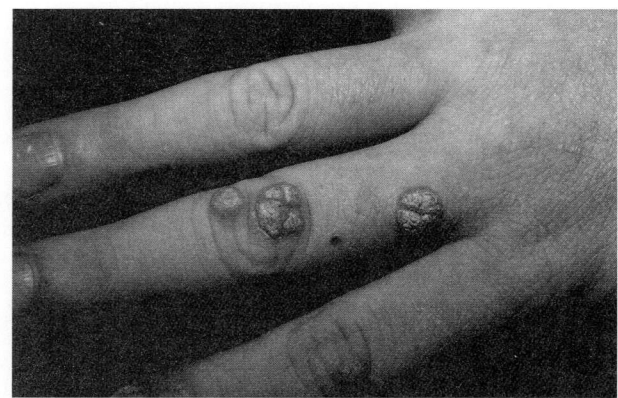

FIG. 36-4 Multiple common warts (verruca vulgaris). (From Weston WL, Lane AT, Morelli JG: *Color textbook of pediatric dermatology*, ed 4, St Louis, 2007, Mosby, p 139.)

Differential Diagnosis

The differential diagnosis includes calluses, corns, foreign bodies, moles, and comedones.

Management

There is no single effective treatment for warts, and watchful waiting is an option. The recurrence rate for warts is high, and it is unlikely that the wart will resolve with a single treatment. No treatment is necessary if the warts are asymptomatic. The decision to treat should be based on location, number and size of lesions, discomfort, and whether the warts are cosmetically objectionable. Treatment should not be harmful, and scarring should be avoided. Genital warts found in young children or in adolescents who are not sexually active should create suspicion of sexual abuse. Specific treatment options are outlined in Box 36-6. Follow up in 2 to 3 weeks to evaluate response.

Complications

Scarring from removal can occur. A ring of satellite warts may develop at the edge of the blister following cantharidin. Immunocompromised hosts can have extensive involvement.

Patient Education

A blister, sometimes hemorrhagic, may form 1 to 2 days after freezing. Redness and itching may herald regression of a wart. Parents and patients must be warned that multiple or prolonged treatment is often necessary.

■ INFESTATIONS OF THE SKIN

Diagnosis and treatment of pediculosis and scabies are listed in Table 36-6.

BOX 36-6 **Treatment Options for Warts**

Keratolytics eliminate the wart by causing topical peeling and an inflammatory response. They are often available over the counter, cause little pain, and are low in cost and risk, but are slow to work.

- Salicylic acid paints with a concentration of greater than 20% are applied with a toothpick once or twice a day for 4-6 weeks. On thick skin, a combination of 16.7% salicylic acid and 16.7% collodion is more effective. This method is useful for common or periungual warts, but it is not effective with warts larger than 5 mm in diameter.
- Salicylic acid plasters with 40% concentration (e.g., Occlusal, Duofilm, Mediplast) are cut to size and taped in place for 3-5 days. After the plaster is taken off, the area should be soaked for 45 minutes and the dead epidermis removed. A new plaster is then applied. Treatment can last 3-6 weeks. This method is useful for plantar warts.
- Retinotic acid gel 0.025% to 0.05% applied once or twice daily brings resolution in 4-6 weeks. This method is useful for flat warts, but it does not work for common, plantar, or periungual warts.
- Occlusion with duct tape for 6 ½ days, off for ½ day, followed by soaking and scraping of epidermis is easy, painless, and inexpensive.

Destructive agents eliminate the wart by causing necrosis and blister formation. Most techniques are painful and require patient cooperation.

- Cryotherapy. Liquid nitrogen is applied for 2-10 seconds after an area 1-3 mm beyond the wart turns white or patient complains of pain; goal is to induce blister formation above the dermal-epidermal junction. Care must be taken not to freeze the wart too vigorously. Caution should be used when freezing warts over joints and the lateral aspects of digits. This method is uncomfortable and often not tolerated by children. Retreatment is often necessary.
- Cantharidin 0.7% is applied directly to the wart with a toothpick and covered with tape for 24 hours. This is a potent blistering agent that creates a blister in 2-3 days that is sloughed after 7-14 days. This method is useful for periungual and some plantar warts. Do not use on other body surfaces.
- Podophyllum 25% solution in compound benzoin tincture is applied to the wart with a toothpick; it should be washed off in 4 hours; may be repeated in 1 week. Podofilox, available over the counter for home use, is applied twice a day for 3 days. After a 4-day rest period, the 3-day cycle may be repeated as necessary. This technique is useful for common or genital warts.
- Surgical excision of warts can lead to scarring that can be more painful than the wart itself, but can be highly effective for large individual warts. Surgery by snipping with scissors, not scalpel, is useful for filiform warts.
- Laser treatments are often as effective as cryosurgery, but can be painful and require several treatments for complete resolution.

Immunotherapy modalities stimulate an immune response to HPV. These newer treatment modalities do not have controlled studies evaluating their effectiveness.

- Oral cimetidine, a histamine$_2$ receptor blocking agent, may improve immunity to HPV. It is used in conjunction with other modalities at a dose of 20-30 mg/kg divided twice a day for 3-4 months.
- Imiquimod cream applied daily creates cell-mediated immunity in surrounding areas and is often effective as a home treatment. It is applied for 1-2 months.
- Contact sensitization and interferon injection are methods used by dermatologists, usually in adult patients.

HPV, Human papillomavirus.

TABLE 36-6 **Diagnosis and Treatment of Pediculosis and Scabies**

	Clinical Findings	Treatment
Pediculosis (head lice)	History of infestation; itchy scalp, scratches; postoccipital nodes; occasional visualization of mites or nits (small white oval cases), commonly on back of head, nape of neck, behind ears, possibly eyelashes	*Key* to treatment is proper technique! *First step* is pediculicide (permethrin or pyrethrin + piperonyl butoxide) *Second step* is removal of nits by combing hair with fine-toothed comb in 1-inch sections with special attention to nape of neck and behind ears *Third step* is to cleanse the environment: check family, friends, day care/school contacts; clean sheets, towels, clothing, headgear; store other items in plastic for 2 weeks; vacuum; soak brushes and combs; follow up in 2 weeks with daily recheck at home by parent; child may return to school after treatment
Scabies	*Key finding*: itching, worse at night, and complaints more significant than findings; fitful sleep, crankiness; curving burrows, especially in webs of fingers, sides of hands, folds of wrist, armpits, forearms, elbows, belt line, buttocks, proximal half of foot and heel; may be <10 lesions total; secondary excoriation; infants may have lesions on palms, soles, scalp, face, posterior auricle and axilla, folds, red-brown in color, dozens in number; lesions may occur in the form of firm nodules in infants	Pharmacologic treatment with permethrin 5%, repeated in 1 week; antihistamine, hydrocortisone, nonsteroidal antiinflammatory drugs for itching; simultaneously treat family members (even if asymptomatic), friends, school/day care contacts; cleanse environment: linens and clothing, vacuum, store anything else in plastic bags for 1 week; rash and itch persist for up to 3 weeks after treatment; return to school 24 hours after treatment

PEDICULOSIS

Description

Pediculosis (lice infestation) affects the head, body, or pubic area. Pediculosis capitis (head) is most common, pediculosis corporis (body) is uncommon, and pediculosis pubis (pubic area) is considered a sexually transmitted disease. Infestation is defined by some as presence of either nits (eggs) or lice and by others as presence of lice alone. The gold standard for diagnosis of pediculosis is finding live lice on the head (Paller & Mancini, 2006).

Epidemiology

Lice infestation is caused by three subspecies, *Pediculus humanus corporis* and *capitis* (head and body) or by *Phthirus pubis* (pubic). The adult female louse, which survives by sucking human blood, deposits six to ten eggs per day at the base of the hair shaft within a waterproof, gluelike substance. The eggs mature in about 1 week and begin laying eggs in another 1 to 2 weeks (Paller & Mancini, 2006). Head lice live approximately 30 days on a host and lay up to 100 nits. Transmission of pediculosis occurs by direct or indirect contact, often by sharing hairbrushes, caps, clothing, or linen or through close living quarters, poor hygiene, or sexual activity (pubic lice).

Pediculosis capitis is considered an epidemic in the U.S., with estimates ranging from 6 to 12 million cases per year (Lembo, 2006). However, head lice are not considered a health hazard because they do not spread disease. All socioeconomic groups are affected, but lice are most common in school-age white females, with the peak season occurring from August to November. Nits incubate for about 1 week and grow into adult lice over 1 to 2 weeks and are transmitted by close contacts and fomites. Lice are uncommon in African Americans (Lembo, 2006). Pediculosis corporis is uncommon in childhood. The nits of the body louse attach to clothing fibers. The louse is rarely seen on the body, rather it attaches to clothing and intermittently pierces the skin. It is the only louse that can carry human disease (e.g., epidemic typhus and trench fever). If pediculosis pubis is found in a child, sexual abuse must be considered. Pubic lice may involve the scalp, eyebrows, or eyelashes, but primarily stay in the pubic area. Clothing and bed linens are a source of residence.

Lice appear to have a growing resistance to available pharmacologic treatment options mainly in children who have been treated multiple times. This has led to the trial of many alternative treatment options.

Clinical Findings

History. The following may be elicited:

- A history of infestation in a family, friend, or day care contact
- Dandrufflike substance in the hair
- Itching of the scalp, scratching, and irritability if infestation has been present for a few weeks
- Reports of a crawling sensation in the scalp

Physical Examination. Findings include the following:

- Head lice:
  - Mites can be visualized; the nits or eggs can be seen as small, white oval cases attached tightly to a hair shaft (Fig. 36-5). Nits are usually laid within 1 to 2 mm of the scalp.
  - Care must be taken to differentiate hair casts, epithelial cells, and other debris from nits.
  - Common sites are the back of the head, nape of the neck, and behind the ears; eyelashes can be involved.
  - Scalp excoriations and occipital or cervical adenopathy can be present.
- Body lice:
  - Excoriated macules or papules may be present (secondary bacterial infection of the skin may develop).
  - Belt line, collar, and underwear areas are common sites.

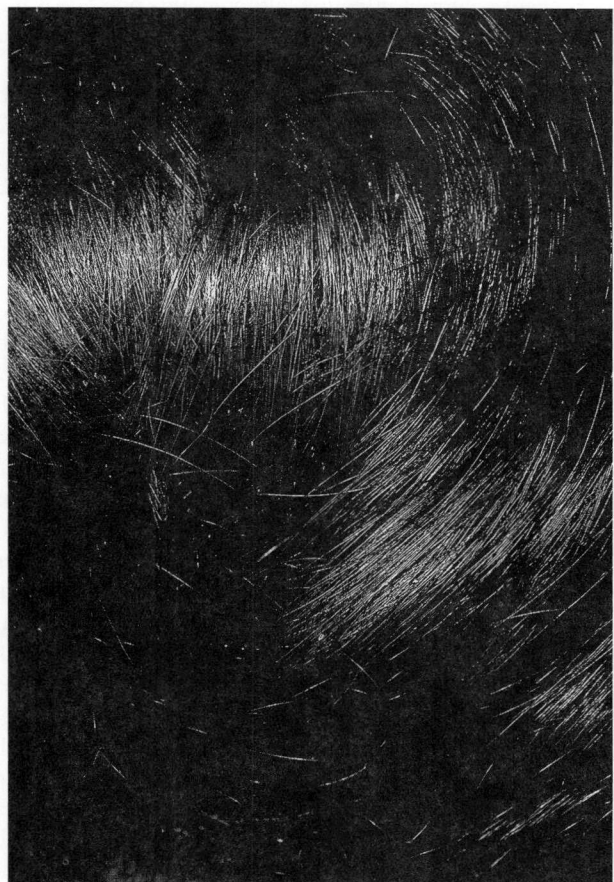

FIG. 36-5 Nits. These eggs are seen as tiny, gray-white specks attached to the hair shafts. (From Paller AS, Mancini AJ: *Hurwitz clinical pediatric dermatology: a textbook of skin disorders of childhood and adolescence,* ed 3, Philadelphia, 2006, WB Saunders, p 489.)

- A hemorrhagic pinpoint macule is seen where the louse extracted blood.
- Axillary, inguinal, or regional lymphadenopathy can be present.
- Pubic lice:
  - Excoriation and small bluish macules and papules may be present.
  - Eyelashes can be involved; spread to other short-haired areas (thighs, trunk, axillae, beard) may occur.

Diagnostic Studies. The following can be helpful:

- Nits fluoresce under a Wood's lamp.
- Microscopic examination of a hair shaft can more clearly identify nits.
- Test for other sexually transmitted diseases, especially gonorrhea and syphilis, with pubic lice.

Differential Diagnosis

Scabies (see Table 36-6), dermatitis herpetiformis, and necrotic excoriations are in the differential diagnosis. Rule out sexual abuse if pubic lice found.

Management

Treatment options are varied and controversial, ranging from standard over-the-counter pharmaceutical products, to prescriptive drugs, to many alternatives, to actually dangerous substances. Correct diagnosis is imperative in determining accurate management. Because nonviable nits can persist on the hair shaft for several months, Paller & Mancini (2006) recommended that a pediculicidal agent be used only when viable nits or live lice are observed. The American Academy of Pediatrics recommends against a "no-nits" policy for schools because such policies have not been effective in controlling head lice transmission and result in excessive lost school and workdays.

Pediculicides are toxic substances and should be used only as directed and with care. If a child is younger than 2 years old, do not use pediculicides, only manual removal. The National Pediculosis Association (NPA) also advises caution in children with chronic illness, undergoing chemotherapy, using medications, or already overexposed to pediculicides and pregnant or nursing mothers who apply the pediculicide (NPA, 2002a). Treatment failure is common, whether as a result of poor technique or actual medication resistance (AAP, 2006). The FDA mandated a change in labeling of over-the-counter lice products in hopes of improving treatment success while minimizing potential harm. Current recommendations are to follow local resistance patterns when determining treatment.

1. The *first step* is application of a pediculicide. Proper technique is key to success. If the hair is to be shampooed, do not use a shampoo containing conditioner or cream rinse. Shampoo the child's hair over a sink, not in the tub or shower. Keep the pediculicide out of the eyes. If applying solution to damp hair, make sure it is damp, not wet (dilutes the pediculicide). Do not rewash the hair for 1 or 2 days following treatment. Retreatment is recommended in 7 to 10 days.
   - Permethrin 1% cream rinse (Nix), also called pyrethrum, is the current treatment of choice for head lice because of its safety, efficacy, and 10-day residual. Hair should be

shampooed and towel dried, permethrin applied and left on for 10 minutes, and then rinsed. Hair should not be rewashed for at least 24 to 48 hours. Many advise retreatment in 7 to 10 days.

- Lindane is an organochloride that kills mites, nits, and ova effectively, but safety is a concern because of potential central nervous system effects on the child and potential environmental effects through ineffective removal from wastewater. It is contraindicated for pregnant women and infants. The AAP (2003) recommends that it be used only in patients who have failed to respond to adequate doses of other approved agents. The NPA, the Cancer Prevention Coalition, and the Public Citizen Health Research Group have all issued statements calling for a ban on Lindane (NPA, 2002b). Eighteen countries outside of the U.S. and California have banned its use, and the FDA issued a warning on the safety of lindane (AAP, 2006). The CDC (2002) has stated that it "is probably safe when used as directed, but overuse, misuse, or accidentally swallowing can be toxic to the brain and nervous system." For head lice, a 1% lindane shampoo is used leaving it on for 4 minutes, then rinsed; for body lice, cream or lotion may be applied for 8 to 12 hours (overnight) and then rinsed off; for pubic lice, a 1% shampoo is used for 10 minutes, then rinsed off and repeated in 1 week (Paller & Mancini, 2006; Weston et al, 2007).
- Pyrethrin is a natural extract from the chrysanthemum plant. It is effective as a pediculicide but not as an ovicide. Commonly found as RID, A-200, Pronto, or Triplex, it is usually a 10-minute shampoo applied to dry hair, with repeat application in 7 to 10 days. It is contraindicated in children with allergy to ragweed. Because these agents are not combination pediculicidal and ovicidal products, treatment failures are more common than is the case with permethrin (that has both functions).
- Malathion lotion 0.5% is an organophosphate with a pine needle oil base. It is a potent lice killer that binds to the hair shaft for 4 weeks. It has been repeatedly withdrawn from the U.S. market, but is once again available by prescription. It is an endocrine disruptor and probable carcinogen (AAP, 2003). The drug is flammable, and if ingested causes severe respiratory distress. Thus, it is not recommended.
- Ivermectin in topical 0.8% solution (not approved by the FDA) or orally as a 200 mcg/kg single-dose tablet is sometimes used to treat apparently resistant lice. It is not for use in children weighing less than 15 kg (AAP, 2006; Paller & Mancini, 2006).

2. The *second step* is ensuring removal of nits, although this is not an absolutely necessary step. Again, proper technique is the key to success. Covering hair with a warm, damp towel for 30 minutes before nit removal may help loosen nits. Hair should be wet when combed. A good light, a magnifying glass, and tweezers are useful. A wide-toothed comb may be used initially to straighten the hair.

- A proper comb has fine teeth. Most pediculicides include a nit-removal comb. The LiceMeister comb from the NPA (see Resource Box at the end of the chapter) has been developed to efficiently remove nits. The correct technique in combing the hair is also essential. A minimum of 20 to 30 minutes should be spent combing damp hair. Working from the top of the scalp down, 1-inch sections should be divided out and combed. Special attention should be paid to the nape of the neck and behind the ears.
- Some products claim to dissolve the substance (cement) that attaches the nit to the hair to facilitate removal. A 1:1 vinegar-to-water solution applied to the scalp for 30 minutes, covered with a warm, moist towel, may also help.
- If eyelashes are involved, coat with petroleum jelly (Vaseline) two to three times a day for 8 to 14 days with manual removal of nits.
- Comb outs and inspection should be repeated every night for 2 to 3 weeks to ensure cure.

3. The *third step* is thorough cleansing of the environment.

- Examination of family members, friends, school, and day care contacts is essential. Treatment of family members, even if nothing is found, is sometimes recommended to prevent recurrent infection, although this practice is now being discouraged because of the emergence of resistant lice and toxicity of pediculicides.
- Cleansing of sheets, towels, clothing, and headgear by hot-water washing and machine drying on hot cycle for 20 minutes, ironing, or dry cleaning is essential.
- Any item that cannot be washed or dry cleaned should be stored in a plastic bag for 2 weeks.
- Hot ironing or vacuuming of play areas, floors, rugs, and furniture is an important step in cleansing.
- Brushes, combs, and hair accessories should be soaked in pediculicide, alcohol, or Lysol for 1 hour, followed by hot-water rinse.
- Spraying or fumigating the house is not recommended.
- Permethrin 0.5% spray (RID) can be used to spray on inanimate objects, such as bedding and furniture. It has dubious efficacy and increases the chemical exposure of the family (AAP, 2006). DO NOT USE ON SKIN.

4. *Alternative treatments* include the use of herbal or essential oils, such as olive oil, pine oil, tea-tree oil, margarine, mayonnaise, dog shampoo, styling gels, and petroleum jelly, all of which are said to suffocate and thereby kill the lice. Further studies are needed regarding these practices. Certain recommendations are definitely to be avoided, including wrapping the hair in plastic and putting the child under a hair dryer or washing the hair with gasoline or kerosene. The *LouseBuster* is a nonchemical treatment for head lice that has demonstrated effectiveness in initial studies (Goates et al, 2006). The *LouseBuster* blows hot air at high volume and has a comblike device at the end of a hose. Because it is expensive, cost is an issue for individual use. Institutional purchase may be an option. Topical application of Cetaphil cleanser also works.

5. *Treatment failure* is not unusual. However, with proper use of a pediculicide, reinfection from contact with an untreated individual is more common (AAP, 2006). Common mistakes include the following:
   - Misdiagnosis
   - Improper use of pediculicide
   - Dilution of pediculicide by applying to wet hair, not damp hair
   - Use of a shampoo with conditioner or cream rinse (decreases adherence of the pediculicide to the hair shaft)
   - Inadequate combing techniques
   - Not cleansing personal care items
   - Not screening and treating family members and close contacts

6. Recommendations for dealing with potential *resistance* are varied. Neither formal recommendations nor FDA approval regarding any of these methods has yet been made. Some methods for treating resistant lice that are currently being discussed include the following:
   - Use Nix creme rinse for 4 to 8 hours instead of 10 minutes.
   - Use Nix creme rinse under a shower cap overnight.
   - Use Elimite cream (five times stronger than Nix) overnight.
   - Use crotamiton 10% (Eurax) lotion applied to the scalp and left for 24 hours before rinsing. (One study showed no difference in resistance [Pollack et al, 2000]).
   - Use TMP-SMZ to kill symbiotic bacteria on which lice survive.
   - Use oral ivermectin 200 mcg/kg as a single dose, repeated in 10 days if the child weighs more than 15 kg. This is an off-label use, and its effectiveness is unclear. (Paller, 2006).

7. Nix creme rinse received FDA approval for *prophylaxis* for institutional use when 20% of the population is infested or for use in immediate household members.

8. Body lice may be treated with improved hygiene and cleaning clothes. Infested clothing should be washed and dried at hot temperatures. The use of 5% permethrin cream or lindane 1% lotion may also be beneficial (Paller & Mancini, 2006).

9. Pubic lice are treated as pediculosis capitis.

Patient Education and Prevention
Items for discussion include the following:
- Follow-up visits in 10 to 14 days are helpful in individual cases to ensure complete resolution of infestation. However, daily to weekly checks for lice or nits should be carried out at home.
- Educate family members about the expected course and that lice infestation is not a social disease.
- Educate family members about the need to avoid excessive or unnecessary retreatment because of the toxic hazard of medications. Do not use extra amounts; do not treat more than three times with the same medication without being seen by a care provider; do not mix pediculocides.
- The child can return to school following initial treatment. The "no nits" policy is controversial and has no documented effectiveness in controlling pediculosis outbreaks

(AAP, 2006). However, close contacts in the neighborhood or at school, camp, or child care should be informed and checked regularly for infestation.

See Resource Box at the end of the chapter for education materials and information.

Complications
Secondary bacterial infection can occur, and school absenteeism can result from the strict enforcement of the "no nit" policy.

SCABIES
Description
Scabies is caused by the itch mite, *Sarcoptes scabiei*, an obligate human parasite that burrows into the epidermis and causes intense itching. There are many different forms of presentation (see Color Plate).

Epidemiology
Scabies is a highly contagious infestation spread through close contact and shared clothing or linen. The female mite burrows into the skin, laying up to three eggs a day as she travels. The eggs hatch in about 3 to 4 days and mature into adult mites in 10 to 14 days; the new mites then repeat the process. The female mite has a life span of 15 to 30 days. Sensitization, which causes intense itching, occurs approximately 3 weeks after infestation. Scabies occurs in all socio-economic groups and in all age groups. However, infestation of African Americans is rare.

Clinical Findings
History.   The following can be reported:
- *Key finding*: Itching, worse at night, initially mild but progressively more intense
- Fitful sleep, crankiness, or rubbing of hands and feet (infants)

Physical Examination.   Findings include the following:
- Complaints are significantly greater than examination findings.
- Characteristic lesions include curving S-shaped burrows, especially on webs of fingers and sides of hands, folds of wrists and armpits, forearms, elbows, belt line, buttocks, genitalia, or proximal half of foot and heel.
- Secondary lesions include itchy papules that can be excoriated, urticarial papules with excoriation, red-brown nodules from inflammatory response, and crusting and excoriation (signs of secondary infection).
- Vesiculopustular lesions tend to be found in infants and young children. They classically have vesicular lesions on palms, soles, scalp, face, posterior auriculae, and axillae, concentrated in the folds; head and neck lesions typically are red-brown vesiculopustules or nodules. However, any child younger than 2 years old can have an unusual manifestation.
- Infants classically have dozens of lesions; older children may have fewer than ten.

Diagnostic Studies.   The following are done as indicated:
- Microscopic examination of scrapings from an unscratched burrow in saline or mineral oil can reveal an eight-legged

mite, eggs, or feces. Do not use KOH because it dissolves the mites, eggs, and feces. Burrows and fresh papules are best for specimen collection.
- Burrow ink test: Apply a drop of ink or rub a washable felt-tipped pen across suspected burrow. Wipe off excess ink and examine with magnifying glass for an ink-stained burrow.

Differential Diagnosis

Papular urticaria, atopic, seborrheic or contact dermatitis, insect bites, folliculitis, lichen planus, and dermatitis herpetiformis are included in the differential diagnosis.

Management

Management involves the following:
1. Pharmacologic treatment begins with applying a thin layer of scabicide to the entire body, excluding the eyes. Areas of special importance are under the fingernails, the scalp, behind the ears, all folds and creases, and the feet and hands. In general, the scabicide should be reapplied in 7 days on all symptomatic patients.
   - Permethrin 5% cream (Elimite) is the drug of choice for treating scabies because of its safety and efficacy. It can be used on infants as young as 2 months old. Apply as a thin, even coat and rub in well from the neck down. Leave on for 8 to 14 hours, then thoroughly rinse off. Retreat in 1 week. In infants, special application is needed to head, postauricular area, and hands and feet; however, be sure to avoid the areas around the eyes and mouth.
   - Crotamiton 10% cream (Eurax) applied to the whole body has been used in infants, but it is not as effective as permethrin and has a high failure rate. Apply from neck down for two consecutive nights, rinsing after 48 hours of last application. It may require up to five daily applications (Paller & Mancini, 2006).
   - Sulfur 6% ointment in petrolatum is an old treatment that is not highly effective, is smelly, and stains. However, it may be used in pregnant or lactating women, infants, and young children; it is applied nightly for three nights and washed off 24 hours after the final application.
   - Ivermectin 200 mcg/kg/dose orally for two doses is effective for crusted (Norwegian) scabies or severe infection. Ivermectin is not FDA approved for this, nor is it recommended under 5 years old or less than 15 kg weight (AAP, 2006; Paller & Mancini, 2006).
2. Antihistamines (hydroxyzine or diphenhydramine) or topical 1% hydrocortisone can be helpful for itching, which can last for several weeks after successful treatment.
3. Simultaneous treatment of family members, friends, and school and day care contacts, even if asymptomatic, is essential.
4. At time of treatment, linens and any clothing worn over the last 48 hours should be washed with hot water, put in a hot dryer for 20 minutes, or dry cleaned. The house should be vacuumed.
5. Nonwashable items should be stored in sealed plastic bags for 1 week.

6. A follow-up visit in 2 weeks can be scheduled to determine success of treatment.
7. Reasons for treatment failure include wrong diagnosis, medication not applied to the whole body, not treating all members of the household, or use of crotamiton. In addition, the child may develop postscabetic eczema that is not indicative of treatment failure. Evaluate and treat with topical corticosteroids.
8. Although resistance has been reported, it is not common and is usually due to treatment failure rather than resistance.

Complications

A secondary bacterial infection is possible and should be treated. Postscabetic syndrome is common, with visible lesions and pruritus persisting for days to weeks following treatment and nodular lesions persisting for weeks to months. Norwegian scabies is a nonpruritic, crusted, scaling infestation with thousands to millions of mites occurring in immunosuppressed or institutionalized patients.

Patient Education, Prognosis, and Prevention
- Educate the family about the course of disease. Rash and itching persist for up to 3 weeks following treatment. Avoid overbathing and further irritation of the skin.
- The child should not be infectious 24 hours after treatment and may return to school or day care.

▄▄▄ ALLERGIC AND INFLAMMATORY REACTIONS OF THE SKIN

ACNE VULGARIS

Description

Acne is an inflammatory disorder of the pilosebaceous unit in which excess sebum, keratinous debris, and bacteria accumulate, producing microcomedones. The microcomedones may be noninflamed or inflamed lesions. Although rarely a serious medical disorder, acne may cause permanent scarring, decreased self-esteem, and occasionally heralds underlying disease. It is often of significant concern to the adolescent, having a serious effect on social development (see Color Plate).

Epidemiology

Acne is the most common skin disorder and affects approximately 80% to 85% of individuals between 11 to 30 years old in the U.S. (Paller & Mancini, 2006). Four mechanisms contribute to the sebaceous follicle disorder: (1) sebaceous follicular plugging with keratinous material; (2) bacterial colonization with overgrowth of anaerobic organisms deep in the follicle, primarily *P. acnes,* but coagulase-negative staphylococci, and *Malassezia furfur* can be involved; (3) sebum overproduction and increased androgen production result in an expansion of the follicle; and (4) inflammation and pustule formation caused by trapping of *P. acnes,* and sometimes coagulase-negative staphylococci and *Malassezia furfur*, and sebum (Lembo, 2006). The bacteria release chemotactic factors that attract neutrophils to ingest the bacteria with resultant release of hydrolytic enzymes and a subsequent inflammatory response. Acne tends to improve in the summer and worsen with menses and stress. (Paller & Mancini, 2006; Weston et al, 2007).

Acne usually begins at the onset of puberty, occurring earlier in girls (12 to 13 years old) than boys (14 to 15 years old) (Paller & Mancini, 2006). The pathogenesis of acne is multifactorial; gender, age, genetic factors, and environment are significant factors. Although not a serious physical disorder, acne has been associated with psychosocial morbidity and decreased emotional well-being. "Patients with even mild to moderate acne have demonstrated high scores on the Carrol Rating Scale for Depression" (Paller & Mancini, 2006, p. 185).

Neonatal acne occurs in about 20% of normal newborns; infants are occasionally affected by acne. Neonatal acne is thought to be related to either stimulation of sebaceous glands by maternal androgens or transient adrenal and gonadal androgen production. Infantile acne may occasionally be associated with hyperandrogenism.

Clinical Findings

History.   Information to obtain includes the following:
- Family history of acne
- Stage of pubertal development and menstrual history
- Facial products used, especially occlusive products or pomades
- Oral and topical prescription medication, especially oral contraceptives, antibiotics, or steroids
- Any current or previous acne treatment and results
- Sports participation, especially if wearing football pads, helmets, headbands, or other protective devices
- Jobs, such as cooking at a fast-food grill or working at a gas station
- Other medical conditions

Physical Examination.   Lesions most commonly are found on the face, back, and chest.
- Noninflammatory lesions:
  - Microcomedone—a follicular plug as a result of obstruction of the pilosebaceous unit (hair follicle and sebaceous gland) typically localized on the face and trunk. They enlarge into comedones with increased sebum production.
  - Open comedo (blackhead)—a noninflammatory lesion or papule, firm in consistency, caused by blockage at the mouth of the follicle and occurring on the face, upper back, shoulders, and chest. The black color is thought to come from oxidized keratinous material at the follicular opening. This is the main lesion in early adolescence.
  - Closed comedo (whitehead)—a noninflammatory lesion, semisoft in consistency, caused by blockage at the neck of the follicle. This is a precursor to inflammatory acne.
- Inflammatory lesions occur secondary to rupture of noninflamed lesions into the dermis.
  - Papule—a "bump" in the follicle caused by bacterial overgrowth and rupture of the follicle wall
  - Pustule—raised, superficial, exudate-filled lesion
  - Excoriation and crusting of lesions—caused by manipulation

- Nodule—firm, erythematous, warm, tender and deeper in location, caused by rupture of a plug
- Cyst—raised, large lesion, soft in consistency without erythema, formed from multiple ruptures and reencapsulations
- Scar—red or purple hue initially, depressed or close to the skin
- Sinus tracts—confluent nodules likely to cause scarring

The severity of acne is determined by the quantity, type, and spread of lesions (Table 36-7). It is helpful to use a diagram of the face or a grading graph to identify the number and type of lesions present. This allows more precise follow-up of the patient. If only open and closed comedones are found, the disorder is called *comedonal acne.* Most adolescents have a combination of comedones, red papules, and pustules called *papulopustular acne,* which can be mild or severe. *Nodulocystic acne* is the most severe form and requires more intensive intervention. Specific types of acne include *frictional,* occurring from rubbing of bras, tight clothes, or headbands; *pomadal,* along the temple and forehead, as a result of pomades or oil-based cosmetics; *athletic,* on forehead, chin, or shoulders, caused by helmets and pads; and *hormonal,* with a beard distribution.

Differential Diagnosis

Cosmetic, mechanical, environmental, or drug-induced acne; rosacea; flat wart; milia; perioral dermatitis; and folliculitis are included in the differential diagnosis.

Management

The goals of acne management are (1) to counteract the excess production of sebum, (2) to counteract the abnormal desquamation of epithelial cells, (3) to decrease the proliferation of *P. acnes,* and (4) to decrease scarring. Choice of treatment depends on the extent, severity, and duration of disease; type of lesions; and psychological effects the adolescent is experiencing (Table 36-8 and Box 36-7).

TABLE 36-7	Grading Scale for Acne Severity
Scale	**Definition**
0	None: skin is clear
1	Few comedones
2	Mild comedones, few papules, minimal erythema
3	Comedones, papules, pustules, erythema
4	Moderate comedones, greater number of papules, pustules extending over wider area of face, chest, shoulders, back, increasing erythema
5	Comedones, increasing number of papules, pustules, nodules with erythema
6	Comedones, papules, pustules, nodules, cysts; scarring may or may not be present with hyperpigmentation

TABLE 36-8 Treatment of Acne

Type of Acne	Lesions	Initial Treatment	If Not Improving
Comedonal	Open or closed comedones	Benzoyl peroxide 5% gel daily (if mild) or Tretinoin (Retin A) 0.025% cream daily (if moderate) or Adapalene 0.1% gel	Combine benzoyl peroxide with tretinoin or Increase strength to 0.05%
Mild papulopustular	Red papules, few pustules	Option 1: Benzoyl peroxide 5%-10% daily or Adapalene 0.1% gel or Azelaic acid bid (if mild) or any 1 of the 3 above **and** a Topical antibiotic bid Option 2: Erythromycin 3% with 5% benzoyl peroxide daily-bid (if moderate) or Clindamycin 1% with 5% benzoyl peroxide daily-bid	Increase benzoyl peroxide to bid or Combine benzoyl peroxide with tretinoin (for comedones) Substitute topical antibiotic bid (for inflammatory
Moderate to severe papulopustular	Red papules, many pustules	Benzoyl peroxide 5% **and** Tretinoin 0.025% or Adapalene 0.1% gel or Azelaic acid (if comedonal) or Topical antibiotic bid (if no comedones) **and** oral antibiotic bid	Increase strength of treatment or Refer to dermatologist
Nodulocystic, scarring, or unresponsive	Red papules, pustules, cysts, and nodules	Oral antibiotics bid **and** tretinoin 0.05% daily or Adapalene 0.1% gel and benzoyl peroxide 10% gel bid (if comedonal) or topical antibiotic	Refer to dermatologist for oral isotretinoin

bid, Twice a day.

BOX 36-7 Medications Commonly Used in Treating Acne

Topical Keratolytic or Comedolytic Agents
Retinoids
  Tretinoin (Retin A, Avita) 0.01% to 0.025% gel; 0.025% to 0.1% cream; 0.1% microgel;
  Tretinoin/Clindamycin (combination topical)
  Tazarotene (Tazorac) 0.05%-0.1% cream, 0.05%-0.1% gel
  Adapalene (Differin) 0.1% gel or cream
Benzoyl peroxide 2.5%-20% gel, 5% and 10% cream, 5%-20% lotion or wash
Azelaic acid (Azelex) 20% cream (Finevin)

Topical Antibiotics
Clindamycin 1% solution, lotion, gel, pledget, foam
Erythromycin 1%-2% solution, 3% gel or swabs
Erythromycin 3% with benzoyl peroxide 5% gel (Benzamycin)
Clindamycin 1% with 5% benzoyl peroxide (BenzaClin or Duac)

Oral Antibiotics (Paller, 2006; Sidbury, 2006)
Tetracycline 250-500 mg per dose twice a day
Erythromycin 250-500 mg per dose twice a day
Minocycline 50-100 mg per dose twice a day (associated with more side effects)
Doxycycline 50-100 mg per dose twice a day
Trimethoprim with sulfamethoxazole, amoxicillin, and azithromycin may benefit acne, but are generally not first-line drugs

1. *Education* is the first priority. The adolescent must have realistic expectations and an understanding of the pathophysiology and the process of treatment, including the fact that the acne often worsens before improving. Providing adolescents with reading materials about acne and its treatment may support them in their self-management efforts with this problem.
   - Wash face twice a day with a mild soap, such as Dove, Neutrogena, or Aveeno Cleansing bar. Scrubbing, rubbing, picking, and squeezing should be avoided. Medication should be applied lightly; do not rub in.
   - Use of a comedo extractor can cause scarring and should be discouraged. Hot soaks applied to pustules may help their resolution.
   - If makeup is used, a nonacnegenic makeup is best.
   - Identify aggravating substances, such as oil-based cosmetics, pomades, hair spray, mousse, and face creams.
   - Identify possible aggravating factors, such as menses; stress; hot, humid weather; and jobs involving frying oil or grease.
   - Reassure the patient that no scientific evidence indicates that any particular foods adversely affect acne; however, a well-balanced diet is important to maintaining healthy skin.
   - Discuss psychosocial concerns and provide support.
   - Remind the patient that results take months and that adherence to treatment is essential to improvement.
   - Sun exposure helps clear acne for some adolescents, but may worsen it for others. Use of sunscreen is recommended, and caution about sun exposure should be given if using medication that increases photosensitivity.

2. *Topical keratolytic* or *comedolytic agents* are used to minimize follicular obstruction and break up microcomedones. They are the first line of treatment. (A minimum of 4 to 6 weeks of treatment is required before improvement). Many strengths and forms are available, the strongest being the gels, if tolerated; creams are the least drying agents A general rule is to start low (in strength) and slowly (in frequency) and advance as tolerated or needed. A useful technique to decrease the incidence of irritation is to start therapy only for three nights weekly and slowly increase to a nightly application over a few weeks (Paller & Mancini, 2006).

   There are three classes of retinoids (tretinoin, adapalene, and tazarotene) and agents that possess both antibacterial and keratolytic propetics (benzoyl peroxide and azelaic acid). Each works by a different mechanism; therefore, they can be used together and interchangeably. Dryness, erythema, irritation, and scaling can occur with these products, and the strength and frequency of use must be adjusted for this.
   - Tretinoin (Retin-A, Retin-A Micro, Avita) is a keratolytic that causes sun sensitivity. A pea-sized application should be made 20 minutes after washing the face. Initially, it is used every other night, advancing to every night. If the skin is very sensitive, applications of 15 to 30 minutes just before bedtime may be used, with the duration gradually advanced.
   - Adapalene (Differin) is a newer formulation with less irritation, more activity, and less photosensitivity.
   - Tazarotene (Tazorac) is a keratolytic to be used once daily.
   - Azelaic acid (Azelex) is antibacterial and keratolytic. Used twice a day, it is useful in individuals with sensitive or dark skin.
   - Benzoyl peroxide (BPO) is the most frequently used topical preparation for acne. It is used once or twice a day, depending on the severity of acne and dryness of skin; it is a powerful antimicrobial and also has comedolytic and antiinflammatory effect.

3. *Topical antibiotics* are used to control the inflammatory process, usually most helpful in moderate inflammatory acne. Additionally, they are used as maintenance to control acne after initial treatment with oral antibiotics. Topical antibiotics are applied to the entire skin surface, not just to problem areas. The solution should not be applied until 30 minutes after shaving. Erythromycin can have up to a 50% resistance rate (Paller & Mancini, 2006).
   - Topical clindamycin is used twice a day.
   - Topical erythromycin is used twice a day (Akne-Mycin is a topical erythromycin product that is used with patients with extremely dry skin).
   - Topical sulfacetamide is used twice a day.
   - Topical erythromycin with benzoyl peroxide (Benzamycin gel) and clindamycin with benzoyl peroxide (BenzaClin or Duac) are combination products that are more effective than either drug alone and have less resistance from *P. acnes*. This combination is especially effective in mild to moderate inflammatory acne or as an adjunct to oral therapy (Paller & Mancini, 2006).

4. *Oral antibiotics* are used in addition to topical keratolytics and topical antibiotics to decrease the concentration of *P. acnes* and to decrease the degree of inflammation if there is no response to topical agents. Antibiotics are taken for 1 to 6 months and often require 3 to 4 weeks to see improvement. Once improvement is noted, the dose should be tapered to a daily dose and then discontinued. Tetracycline and erythromycin are the antibiotics most commonly used, but minocycline, doxycycline, and TMP-SMZ are also used.
   - Tetracycline should be taken 1 hour before or 2 hours after eating with 8 oz of water. Tetracycline should not be used by pregnant or breastfeeding adolescents or in children under 9 years old. Photosensitivity reactions can occur, but it has been used for more than 40 years and is a favorite of many clinicians. Usual dose: 250 to 500 mg twice daily.
   - Erythromycin can be taken with food, but GI upset is common, and vulvovaginal candidiasis can be problematic. Usual dose: 250 to 500 mg twice daily.
   - Minocycline can be taken with food (dairy products decrease absorption) and achieves a higher concentration in the follicles. However, side effects include blue-black discoloration in scars and photosensitivity and hypersensitivity reactions. Usual dose: 50 to 100 mg twice daily.

- Doxycycline also can be taken with food (dairy products decrease absorption), but has the highest rate of photosensitivity reactions. Usual dose: 50 to 100 mg twice daily.
- TMP-SMZ has not been approved for this use, but is sometimes tried before isotretinoin.

5. *Oral retinoids* are used for severe, resistant nodulocystic acne. Isotretinoin (Accutane, Amnesteem, Claravis, Sotret) is contraindicated in pregnancy (pregnancy category X drug known for its teratogenic effect) and usually requires evaluation by a dermatologist before use. Its potential association with depression and suicide remains controversial. The usual course is 20 weeks; there are many side effects, and CBC, LFTs, hCG and urinalysis for pregnancy must be monitored every month while the patient is on the medication. The establishment of the *IPledge* program creates a registry for all patients being treated with isotretinoin. The FDA requires health care providers, patients, and pharmacists to access the *IPledge* website monthly after office visits and before filling their prescription for documentation regarding pregnancy, blood donation, and contraceptive counseling.

6. *Oral contraceptives* (Ortho Tri-Cyclen is the only one approved by the FDA for treatment for acne), antiandrogens (spironolactone), and intralesional steroid therapy are sometimes used in unresponsive cases. Erythromycin-zinc combination is used in Europe and Russia with success, but has not been approved in the U.S.

7. Noncomedogenic moisturizers (Moisturel, Purpose lotion, Neutrogena Moisture, Cetaphil) can be used for dryness, which is common with treatment. Noncomedogenic makeup is also available and helpful in treating these patients.

8. Follow-up visits should occur at least every 4 to 6 weeks until control is established. Control is indicated by clearing of lesions or the appearance of only a few new lesions every 2 weeks. Referral to a dermatologist should be made for nonresponsive or severe cases.

Mild cases of neonatal or infantile acne are best treated with a plan of watchful waiting and gentle daily cleansing with soap and water. In mild comedone acne, sparing use of topical tretinoin is recommended. Use 2.5% BPO or topical antibiotics for mild inflammatory acne. Have the parents apply these agents on an every other night basis. Severe acne may need an oral antibiotic.

Complications

Failure can be due to lack of patient motivation, lack of education, inappropriate treatments, initial treatment that was too strong, or expectations of a quick fix. Psychological effects include decreased self-esteem and poor body image, problems with interpersonal relationships, self-consciousness, embarrassment, depression, and decreased athletic participation, especially in gymnastics, swimming, and wrestling. Resistance of *P. acnes* to tetracycline, erythromycin, and minocycline is increasing.

ATOPIC DERMATITIS

See Chapter 24.

CONTACT DERMATITIS

Description

Contact dermatitis is an acute or chronic inflammation resulting from a hypersensitivity reaction to a substance. The causative agents are either irritants or allergens. Common types of contact dermatitis are the following:

- *Dry skin dermatitis* caused by extremely low humidity (less than 30%) or use of excess soaping or cleansing creams
- *Nickel dermatitis* from contact with jewelry, belts, snaps, or eyeglasses
- *Lip-licker dermatitis* caused by constant lip licking, most often in dry, cold weather
- *Phytophotodermatitis* occurs with sun exposure following contact with plants or juices, such as limes, lemons, carrots, celery, figs, parsnips, or dill; manifests as a blistered lesion on an erythematous base and may be confused with a burn
- *Plant oleoresins*, such as poison ivy, oak, or sumac; contact can be direct or indirect (exposure to burning plant material)
- *Juvenile plantar dermatosis*, manifested as dryness, cracking, and erythema of weight-bearing surfaces of the feet, initially the big toes. It mimics tinea pedis, often found in children with atopic dermatitis (see Chapter 24)
- *Latex dermatitis,* associated with the use of products containing latex, such as protective gloves.

Epidemiology

Irritant dermatitis, the most common form, occurs when a chemical or substance has a toxic effect on the skin. The severity of the rash depends on the length of exposure and the concentration of the irritant. Substances, such as saliva, urine, and feces; baby wipes; bubble bath; overbathing; and adhesives, often cause irritation as do substances that dry the skin. Diaper dermatitis is the most common form (see following section). Allergic reactions occur as an immunologic response to an antigen penetrating the skin. There are two phases: sensitization and elicitation. Allergic dermatitis is seen only after sensitization to an allergen has occurred and a subsequent type IV delayed hypersensitivity response has activated an immune cascade (Ghali, 2006). Common causes are contact with shoes (components, such as rubber and potassium dichromate), nickel, clothes with woolen or rough textures, topical medications (e.g., neomycin and lanolin), perfumed soaps or cosmetics (including lanolin), preservatives, or poison ivy, oak, or sumac. Sometimes the cause is obvious; often no specific cause can be identified. Occurring at any age, contact dermatitis (mostly irritant) is extremely common in children.

Clinical Findings

History. The following information should be sought:

- Contact with any new or unusual substances
- Repeated exposure to any substance or item
- Diarrhea or infrequently changed diapers
- Rash localized to specific area(s)

Physical Examination. The area of involvement offers clues to the causative agent. Often the rash is localized to one area and has sharp borders. Common examples include a linear-type rash secondary to wearing a necklace or bracelet, circular areas from snaps on clothing, or inflammation of the earlobes from jewelry or a reaction pattern on the toes and dorsum of the foot from shoes. The duration and concentration of exposure also affect the intensity of the rash. Minimal contact may produce only mild erythema, whereas prolonged or concentrated contact may produce significant erythema, edema, and blistering with possible crusting and secondary infection. Irritant reactions tend to be immediate, whereas allergic ones are delayed.

- A chafed appearance with shiny, mild to severely erythematous, peeling, or dry, fissured skin or red patches and plaques with secondary scales may be seen if the reaction is due to an irritant. For example, the dorsum of the hand may exhibit the above characteristic appearance with frequent washing of hands with irritating soaps.
- In the diaper area around the anus, the rash is often due to diarrhea; if the skin is affected but the folds are spared, urine is often responsible.
- Erythema, vesicles, and weeping may be present in the acute stage of allergic contact dermatitis. The lesions are pruritic.
- Hyperpigmentation and lichenification are seen in chronic conditions.

Differential Diagnosis
The differential diagnosis includes atopic dermatitis, impetigo, herpes simplex, psoriasis, and seborrhea.

Management
Appropriate skin care, recognizing and eliminating offending agents, and treatment of inflammation are the keys to managing contact dermatitis successfully.

- Identify and avoid the substance (irritant or allergen) causing the dermatitis.
  - Urushiol, the allergen in poison ivy, can remain on contaminated sources, such as clothing, animal hair, toys, and sports equipment resulting in sequential outbreaks with reexposures (Ghali, 2006).
  - A generalized *id* (idiosyncratic) reaction can develop to an allergen. An *id* reaction occurs as a secondary or "sympathy" rash distant from the primary site of exposure.
- For irritant dermatitis in the diaper area, change diapers frequently, keep the area dry and cool (use air-drying as much as possible), and avoid rubber pants. Hydrocortisone 1% may be used cautiously for a period of no more than 5 days. Secondary infection with *Candida* is often present and must be treated with an antifungal agent, such as nystatin. Satellite lesions, small red discrete papules, develop and spread with *Candida* infections.
- Burow's solution soaks or oatmeal baths and cool compresses (1 tsp salt/pint water) applied for 20 minutes every 4 to 6 hours soothe vesicular rashes.
- Apply water and either petrolatum-based or lanolin-and-petrolatum-based emollients to the skin to restore moisture to areas of dryness and chafing.

- Petrolatum-based emollients include dimethicone (Moisturel), white petrolatum, and Vaseline Dermatology Formula.
  - Lanolin-and-petrolatum-based emollients include Aquaphor, Eucerin, Lubriderm, and Alpha Keri. Do not use if there is inflammation.
- Topical corticosteroids used two to three times daily give relief in 2 or 3 days, although it may take 2 or 3 weeks for complete healing. Occasionally, oral corticosteroids are used for short periods of time (10 to 14 days, tapered the last 7 days) if the area of allergic involvement exceeds 10% of the skin surface.
- Oral antihistamines are helpful if itching and scratching are problems.
- Resolution may take 2 to 3 weeks. Referral to a dermatologist or an allergist for patch testing may be indicated if the dermatitis worsens, fails to respond, or recurs.
- Chronic allergic contact dermatitis should be treated with medium potency topical corticosteroids twice daily until resolved (Ghali, 2006).

DIAPER DERMATITIS
Description
Diaper dermatitis is the most frequent contact irritant dermatitis seen in children. It is most commonly an inflammatory disorder of the skin as a result of irritation causing breakdown of the skin's natural barrier (Table 36-9).

Epidemiology
Diaper dermatitis is one of the most common skin disorders of infancy. Factors contributing to diaper dermatitis include the following:
- Improper hygiene and cleansing methods
- Chemical irritation caused by prolonged contact with skin products, urine, feces, or breakdown products
- Mechanical irritation from diapers, rubber pants, or skin folds
- Other skin dermatoses aggravated by wearing diapers (e.g., seborrhea, atopic dermatitis, or psoriasis)

Diaper rash is most commonly due to irritation from the wetness of urine, combined with friction and occlusion from diapers, and the byproducts of feces (the major irritating factor). The initial rash is termed *irritant contact diaper dermatitis*. A variation of this is called *tidewater* or *tidemark dermatitis* and is found at the diaper edges from either chafing or irritation from talcum powder. *Jacquet's dermatitis*, a severe form manifested by punched-out lesions or erosions primarily on the labia and buttocks, is especially prone to secondary infection.

Clinical Findings
History. The following should be assessed:
- Type of diapers and diaper covering used; any recent change in brand
- Frequency of diaper changes and methods of cleansing used
- Any new baby care products used
- Frequency of wet diapers and stools

TABLE 36-9 **Diagnosis and Treatment of Diaper Dermatitis**

Type	Cause	Presentation and Location	Other Characteristics	Treatment
Irritant contact dermatitis	Related to wearing diapers; contact with urine and feces	Chapped, shiny, erythematous, parchment-like skin with possible erosions on convex surfaces; creases spared	Peak at 9-12 months old; may progress to involve creases; skin may be dry	Frequent diaper changes, gentle cleansing; greasy lubricant; sitz bath, air-dry; hydrocortisone for inflammation
Candidiasis	Related to wearing diapers; a superinfection with *Candida*	Shallow pustules, fiery-red scaly plaques on convex surfaces, inguinal folds, labia, and scrotum	Satellite lesions, oral thrush; recent antibiotic or diarrhea; occurs at any age	Antifungal cream plus same measures as for contact dermatitis
Miliaria or intertrigo	Related to wearing diapers; a result of heat and occlusion	Discrete vesicles or papules (miliaria); erythematous, scaly, maceration in folds of skin	Sweat retention or friction associated	Self-limited (miliaria); avoid precipitating factors; care as for contact dermatitis
Seborrhea	Exaggerated by wearing diapers; overgrowth of *Malassezia* yeast in areas of sebaceous gland activity	Greasy, erythematous scales, well circumscribed in creases of skin, groin; spared convex surfaces	Onset at 3-4 weeks old; also occurs on face or body; often superinfected with *Candida*	Ketoconazole is treatment of choice, or hydrocortisone
Atopic dermatitis (AD)	Exaggerated by wearing diapers; exact cause unknown	Increased number of lines in skin; areas of excoriation in folds and convex surfaces and buttocks; less widespread	AD in other areas; usually begins in first year of life; scratches skin with diaper change; hyperlinear skin folds with diffuse borders	Skin care as for contact dermatitis and as indicated for AD (see Chapter 24); antibiotics for bacterial infection
Psoriasis	Exaggerated by wearing diapers; psoriasis evolves as response to chronic trauma	Erythematous, well-defined sharp, scaly plaques on convex surfaces and inguinal folds; less widespread	Psoriasis affects other places; rare occurrence, if found, usually at 6-18 months old	Treatment often required for weeks or until toilet trained; steroids; ketoconazole if *Candida* present
Bacterial dermatitis	Usually caused by staphylococcal or streptococcal infection	Red, denuded areas or fragile blisters; crusting and pustules in suprapubic area and periumbilicus	Usually in newborn, can occur anywhere	Econazole or ketoconazole cream if yeast present as well; mupirocin if minimal; cephalexin, amoxicillin, or erythromycin if extensive

- Medication taken (particularly antibiotics) or used on rash
- Present or recent use of antibiotics

Physical Examination. Erythema, edema, and vesiculation are typically the first characteristic changes observed. Chronic changes include scale, lichenification, and increased or decreased pigmentation. Other findings associated with specific causative factors can include the following:
- Chemical causes
  - Shiny, peeling, erythematous macular or papular rash confluent in the diaper area, sparing folds
  - Head of penis erythematous and dry
  - Erythema primarily on buttocks and around anus (fecal irritation)
- Mechanical causes
  - Erythematous, macerated (acute) or dry (chronic), hyperpigmented area prominent along edges of diaper or plastic pants
  - Erythematous, macerated folds caused by overlapping skin
- Hygiene problems
  - Any finding listed previously
  - Poor hygiene in general

Differential Diagnosis

Differential diagnosis includes contact dermatitis; bacterial, viral, or monilial infection; atopic dermatitis; psoriasis; seborrhea; scabies; and congenital syphilis.

Management

The best treatment is prevention!
1. Keep diaper area dry, clean, and aerated:
   - Frequent diaper changes are essential; every 1 to 2 hours is recommended with one change at night and a minimum of eight changes in a 24-hour period. Cleanse the area well with water at every diaper change and use mild soap, rinsing well following a stool. Avoid vigorous cleansing because this can worsen matters. Avoid using wipes.
   - Use a greasy lubricant if skin is dry.
   - Use a protective barrier ointment or cream, such as Desitin (cod liver oil with zinc oxide), A & D ointment, Aquaphor, petrolatum, or zinc oxide at first sign of irritation.
2. Proper use of diapers:
   - Frequent changes are essential.
   - Use thick or absorbent diapers to pull wetness away from skin.
   - Avoid use of rubber or plastic pants.
   - Cloth diapers should be soaked, prerinsed, washed in a mild soap, double rinsed with ¼ cup of vinegar, and dried in the sun if possible.
   - Disposable diapers must be large enough not to bind and should never be worn with rubber pants.
3. Treatment of diaper rash:
   - Sitz baths in warm water for 10 to 15 minutes four times a day.
   - Expose diaper area to air by leaving diaper off or by blow drying with low heat three or four times a day.
   - Burow's solution soaks or compresses four times a day if skin is weepy.
   - Undecylenic acid (Desenex) or calcium undecylenate (Caldescene) powder to decrease the friction and moisture in tidewater dermatitis.
   - Hydrocortisone 0.5% or 1% applied as a thin layer three times a day for no more than 5 days, especially if skin is dry, for moderate to severe diaper dermatitis. Do not use fluorinated steroids.
   - Increase intake of fluids to dilute urine. In older infants, 2 to 3 oz of cranberry juice acidifies the urine.
   - If the rash has been present for more than 3 days or if there is no response to the aforementioned measures, add a topical antifungal cream, such as clotrimazole or miconazole. If there is still no response, a trial of oral antifungal is indicated (see section on monilial dermatitis).
   - Any recalcitrant rash should be referred to a dermatologist.
   - Follow up by phone in 1 to 2 days. If not improved, reassess within 1 week.

Complications

Secondary infection with bacteria, viruses, or fungi can occur (see previous sections). *Red flags*: severe erosions or ulcers; bullae or pustules; large papules or nodules, purpura, or petechiae; and redness or scaliness over entire body.

SEBORRHEA DERMATITIS

Description

Seborrhea is a chronic inflammatory dermatitis commonly called *cradle cap* in infants or *dandruff* in adolescents.

Epidemiology

The condition is thought to be related to overproduction of sebum, because it commonly occurs in areas with large numbers of sebaceous glands. It may be an overgrowth of *M. ovalis (formerly P. ovale)*, a saprophytic yeast, which is present on everyone's body. Seborrhea occurs most often in early infancy and adolescence, is associated with blepharitis, and is more common in spring and summer.

Clinical Findings

History.   Note age of onset (infancy or adolescence).

Physical Examination.   In infants, erythematous, flaky to thick crusts of yellow, greasy (waxy appearance) scales occur predominantly on the scalp, but also on the face, behind the ears, on the neck and trunk, and in the diaper area. In adolescents, there are mild flakes with some erythema and yellow, greasy scales on the scalp, forehead, nasal bridge, and eyebrows; behind the ears; on the face and flexural surfaces; and in intertriginous areas. The dermatitis is not pruritic and has no pustules.

Differential Diagnosis

Atopic dermatitis, psoriasis, *Candida* infection, contact dermatitis, tinea, scabies, and PR are included in the differential diagnosis.

Management

Seborrhea in infants may be self-limited, typically resolving in the first year of life. However, in adolescents, it is usually chronic and recurring. The following measures are helpful in either age group:
- Shampoo or wash areas daily with a mild soap. In more resistant cases, use antiseborrheic shampoos [e.g., Nizoral, Sebulex, selenium sulfide 1% to 2.5%, Head & Shoulders, salicylic acid (TSal)] to treat scalp scales every other day for infants or daily for adolescents. Tar shampoos can be used by adolescents if needed. Shampoo should be left on the scalp for 5 to 10 minutes before scrubbing crusts and then rinsing.
- Mineral oil, P & S liquid in infants, baby oil, or petroleum jelly placed on thick crusts 10 to 15 minutes before washing softens them, followed by gentle brushing during shampooing to remove crusts. After infancy, P & S liquid or Derma-Smoothe FS can be left on overnight.
- If inflammation is marked, low-potency steroid creams (hydrocortisone 1% to 2.5%) can be applied twice a day to the face or three times a day to other body areas for several days and then weaned. A low- to moderate-strength steroid solution can be applied to the scalp if inflammation is

present. Ketoconazole 2% cream or sulfur-based products are also effective (Dasher & Morrell, 2006).

- Oral biotin can sometimes improve the condition.
- Resistant cases may need 5 to 7 days of medium-potency corticosteroids, and secondary bacterial or fungal infection should be considered.
- Educate parents about the etiology, control measures, and the need to continue treatment for a few days after resolution.
- Follow up in 1 to 2 weeks.

Complications

Secondary infection with bacteria or *Candida* can occur. Severe, generalized seborrhea is commonly found in persons infected with HIV.

SUNBURN

Description

Sunburn is an injury to the skin occurring from overexposure of the skin to the UV rays of the sun. The incidence of skin cancer is increasing as a result of overexposure to the sun and the use of tanning beds.

Epidemiology

Excessive sun exposure causes a change in the skin's blood flow, cell kinetics, and pigment products. Damage to the skin by sun (primarily ultraviolet B [UVB]) includes erythema, pigmentary or texture changes, and potential carcinogenesis. Injury to the skin begins as quickly as 30 minutes after exposure, peaks at 24 hours, and may last for 72 hours. Other factors that contribute to sun sensitivity are medications (especially griseofulvin, NSAIDs, oral contraceptives, tetracycline, topical diphenhydramine, and tretinoin) and some illnesses.

Children are at increased risk for sunburn because of the greater amount of time they spend outdoors. They are also particularly susceptible to UV radiation during their first two decades of life because of age-related structural and immunologic skin differences. Most people receive two thirds of their lifetime exposure to sun by the time they are 18 years old (Benjamin et al, 2006). Blistering sunburns before 20 years old more than double the chance of skin cancer. Factors contributing to the degree of burn include the coloring of skin and hair (Box 36-8) and amount of previous sun exposure. Burns are less common in children with darker hair and skin because of their increased amount of melanin. Timing of sun exposure, latitude, and altitude affect skin sensitivity because UV rays are strongest between 10 AM and 2 PM, at higher altitudes, and nearer the equator. Sunburn can occur on cloudy days, and reflection from sand, water, snow, and concrete increases the risk.

Clinical Findings

History

- Length and time of sun exposure and tanning bed use
- Previous sunburns, especially blistering ones
- Any medications currently taken
- Chills, headache, and fatigue with moderate to severe burn
- Family history of melanoma or other skin cancer

> **BOX 36-8** **Skin Types (I–VI) and Photosensitivity**
>
> Type I: Very sensitive—always burns easily and severely, never tans; has fair skin, blond hair, blue or brown eyes and freckles
> Type II: Very sensitive—usually burns easily, minimally tans; has fair skin, red, blond, or brown hair, and blue, hazel, or brown eyes
> Type III: Moderately sensitive—sometimes burns, gradually and uniformly tans; average white individual
> Type IV: Moderately sensitive—minimally burns, always tans easily; has dark brown hair, dark eyes, and white or light brown skin
> Type V: Minimally sensitive—rarely burns, profusely tans; brown-skinned (middle Eastern and Hispanic)
> Type VI: Heavily pigmented—rarely burns, tans deeply; blacks and other heavy pigmented individuals

Adapted from Paller AS, Mancini AJ, Hurwitz: *Clinical pediatric dermatology: a textbook of skin disorders of children and adolescence,* ed 3, Philadelphia, 2006, Elsevier Inc, p 504.

Physical Examination. Findings include the following:
- Mild or first-degree burns are evidenced by erythema, tenderness, and mild pain.
- Moderate or second-degree burns involve a greater degree of erythema, increased pain, edema, and blisters.
- Severe or third-degree burns involve greater areas of skin and include systemic symptoms of headache, fever, and fatigue.
- Erythema and tenderness are evident from 30 minutes to 4 hours after exposure; 2 to 7 days later, affected layers of the epidermis are shed.

Differential Diagnosis

The differential diagnosis includes photosensitization from medication, xeroderma pigmentosum, lupus erythematosus, viral exanthem, dermatomyositis, and porphyrias.

Management

The degree of burn helps determine which of the following strategies is most appropriate. Prevention is the best intervention (see Patient Education and Prevention).

- Use cool water, saline compresses, or ice packs at least four times a day to ease pain and reduce swelling. Baking soda or cornstarch baths help cool skin. White vinegar or milk compresses help initiate healing.
- Administer prostaglandin inhibitors, such as ibuprofen 5 to 10 mg/kg/dose given as soon as possible and every 6 to 8 hours for the next 2 to 3 days or acetaminophen for fever and pain relief.
- Low-dose cortisone creams 0.5% or 1% two to three times a day, used with caution because of the increased absorption through damaged skin, help reduce inflammation and pain.
- Local anesthetic sprays or first-aid creams with benzocaine are contraindicated because of the risk of sensitization.

- Skin emollients, such as aloe vera gel or moisturizer, are helpful if skin is dry. Jojoba oil and vitamin E creams are sometimes helpful. Avoid petrolatum, butter, or any occlusive ointment because their occlusive properties intensify the burn.
- Extra fluid intake prevents dehydration and restores natural moisture balance.
- If blisters break, dead skin needs to be trimmed and an antibiotic ointment, such as polymyxin B sulfate and bacitracin zinc (Polysporin), applied.

Complications

In addition to skin cancer, photoaging, including telangiectasia and actinic keratosis, cataracts, retinal damage, heat stroke, and a triggering or aggravation of disorders, such as acne rosacea, EM, and herpes labialis, to name a few, are possible complications of sunburn (Cohen, 2005).

The incidence of skin cancer (basal cell carcinoma, squamous cell carcinoma, and malignant melanoma) is increasing rapidly, with 1% to 3% of malignant melanomas occurring in those under 20 years old (Paller & Mancini, 2006). Risk factors for skin cancer include fair skin, history of multiple blistering sunburns, presence of multiple atypical moles, development of new nevi, and family history of melanoma. Basal and squamous cell carcinomas are slow-spreading cancers, directly linked with chronic exposure to UV light. Basal cell carcinomas occur in varied forms, as nodular, pearly, pigmented lesions often on the hand, neck, or head. Squamous cell carcinomas are quickly growing, firm, indurated nodules with or without ulceration on sun-exposed areas, especially the rim of the ear, face, lips, and mouth.

Malignant melanoma is now the most rapidly increasing type of cancer; today a newborn has an estimated 1 in 71 risk of developing melanoma (Benjamin et al, 2006). Melanomas manifest as new pigmented lesions or as changes in existing moles. In preadolescents, melanoma often is nodular, grows rapidly, and itches or bleeds. In adolescents, melanoma manifests as enlarging or changing lesions with irregular color or borders (Chamlin, 2002). There is a link to multiple severe, blistering sunburns, but family history is a more important factor. Any change in a mole, especially with rapid asymmetric growth, crusting, ulceration, or color variation, needs immediate evaluation. Treatment consists of surgical removal and histologic evaluation. All school-age children and adolescents should be taught to do a monthly skin examination (Box 36-9).

Patient Education and Prevention

- Remember that a tan is not a sign of good health, but of skin injury. There is no such thing as a healthy tan. Never seek a tan; seek the shade. Avoid tanning devices or parlors.
- Know your skin type and protection needs (see Box 36-8 and Box 36-10).
- Avoid the sun between 10 AM and 2 PM. Learn the "shadow rule"—seek shade if your shadow is shorter than you are tall. Most newspapers print in the weather section the predicted index of UV exposure (1 to 10) as prepared by the National Weather Service.

BOX 36-9 | **Monthly Skin Examination**

The **ABCDE**s of skin examination:
Asymmetry
Border irregularity or notching
Color variation, especially if multicolored
Diameter greater than 6 mm
Elevation, especially if asymmetric (also **E**volution)
Note any new growths, itchy patches, nonhealing sores, changes in size, irritability, or different sensation in any moles.

Process of Skin Examination
Use a full-length mirror, a hand mirror, and a brightly lit room.
Examine the following areas:
Front and back, right and left sides with arms raised
With elbows bent, forearms, back of arms and palms
Back of legs and feet, toes and soles
Back of neck and scalp
Back and buttocks

From Starr NB: Skin smarts: the essentials of skin protection, *J Pediatr Health Care* 13(3):136-138, 1998.

- Cover up with hats, sunglasses, and clothing.
  - Hats with a wide (3-inch) brim are recommended.
  - Sunglasses should be worn beginning in infancy. Large-framed, wraparound lenses provide the best protection. UV protection is provided by a chemical added to the lenses and is indicated by one of the following labels: UV absorption to 400 nm, special purpose, meets American National Standards Institute (ANSI) UV requirements.
  - Tight-weave, long-sleeved, long-pants clothing with sunscreen applied to the skin underneath provides maximal protection. Color, weight, stretch, wetness, and quality of material all affect the amount of protection offered. *Solumbra* and *SunSkins* offer clothes that provide an SPF of 30 and block 97% of UV rays. *Shades* offers clothes that provide 81% UV protection. *Stingray* offers swimwear that blocks 99% of the sun's rays (see Resource Box at the end of the chapter).
- Use a sunscreen that is broad spectrum and provides protection from both UVB and UVA light (Box 36-10).
- Teach sun protection early on by example and words. "Play Smart When It Comes to the Sun" is an educational program sponsored by the American Academy of Dermatology and the Major League Baseball Players Association. The program's goal is to educate the public to reduce sun exposure and increase protective behaviors. See AAD in Resource Box at the end of the chapter.
- "Choose Your Cover" is a CDC program to increase awareness and change social norms related to skin protection and tanned skin.
- Guidelines for school programs to prevent skin cancer were released by the CDC in 2002 (Glanz et al, 2002).
- Do monthly skin checks (see Box 36-9).

BOX 36-10 **Sunscreen, Clothing, Sunglasses, and Outdoor Activity Time Recommendations**

Sunscreens block the rays of the sun to help prevent sunburn. Sun protection factor (SPF) is the length of time an individual can be exposed to sun without burning if sunscreen is used appropriately. The substantivity of a sunscreen describes its adherence. Sweat resistant (effective for up to 30 minutes of heavy, continuous perspiration), water resistant (effective for up to 40 minutes of swimming), and waterproof (effective for up to 80 minutes of immersion) are different types of substantivity. Specific recommendations include the following:

Use SPF 15 or greater, nonalcohol base, without lanolin, paraben, or fragrance. Use a waterproof product when in water, but reapply every 80 minutes with continuous water exposure.

Apply at least 30 minutes before exposure to sun; reapply at least every 2 hours while in the sun, and after swimming, toweling, or heavy perspiration.

Apply liberally (1 oz for an adult) and, for better coverage, use cream instead of lotion.

Pay special attention to eyelids, nose, cheeks, ears, neck, scalp, shoulders, hands, and feet. Use a lip balm with SPF 15 or greater.

Do not use sunscreen on infants younger than 6 months old, but keep baby out of the sun completely, using shade, brimmed hat, and protective clothing.

Use sunscreen daily in summer or in warm climates. Use even on overcast or cloudy days.

Extra protection is needed with increasing altitude, closer location to the equator, and sand, snow, concrete, or water reflection.

Set an example by using sunscreen.

Sunscreens are available in various chemical combinations (e.g., para-aminobenzoic acid [PABA], PABA esters, cinnamates, benzophenes, salicylates, octocrylene, dibenzoylmethane) and vehicles (e.g., emollient for dry skin, gel or lotion for oily skin, noncomedogenic for acne-prone skin). If a child is sensitive to one, try a sunscreen with different ingredients. A PABA-free sunscreen is recommended for children. Dibenzoylmethane provides the most protection from ultraviolet A.

Sunblocks scatter and reflect light. Zinc oxide, titanium oxide, or a combination product, such as Sportz Bloc, is useful for especially sensitive areas, such as the nose or previously burned areas.

Clothing can help increase protection against the suns rays. Caps and hats with visors or wide brims help to protect the face. Wear clothing made of cotton rather than that made of synthetic fibers—long-sleeved shirts and pants. Children at particular risk for skin cancer may benefit from clothing treated with protection (Solumbra). Cotton T-shirts can be laundered with Rit Sunguard, which provides additional protection from the sun's rays.

Children should wear well-fitted UV protective s*unglasses* when outdoors.

Avoid lengthy outdoor activities during peak sun times from 10:00 AM to 3:00 PM on sunny days; beware that reflective surfaces (water, sand, snow, cement) can reflect up to 85% of sunlight.

From Starr NB: Skin smarts: the essentials of skin protection, *J Pediatr Health Care* 13(3):136-138, 1998; Benjamin LT et al: Sun protection in the pediatric patient. In Burg FD et al, editors: *Current pediatric therapy*, ed 18, Philadelphia, 2006, WB Saunders Elsevier, pp 1091-1093.

DRUG ERUPTIONS

Description

Drugs taken systemically can result in a variety of skin reactions or rashes. The two most common types of drug-related eruptions found in children are (1) morbilliform (measles-like) rash (also called an exanthematous reaction manifested by erythematous macules and/or papules) and (2) urticaria typified by erythematous wheals (Table 36-10). Morbilliform rash is discussed first with urticaria discussed later in this chapter in the section on vascular reactions. Although not described in this chapter, other drug-related reactions manifested by significant dermatologic eruptions include acute generalized exanthematous pustulosis, drug hypersensitivity syndrome, serum sickness-like reaction, vasculitis, fixed drug eruption, acneiform eruptions, and SJS (Paller & Mancini, 2006).

Epidemiology

The morbilliform rash, also called an exanthematous rash, is the most common allergic skin reaction to a drug. The rash may be an immunologic or nonimmunologic reaction to the drug. The most common drugs causing reactions are the penicillins; sulfonamides; cephalosporins, especially cefaclor; erythromycin; NSAIDs; anticonvulsants, barbiturates;

isoniazid; carbamazepine; phenytoin; and fluconazole, ketoconazole, and itraconazole (Weston et al, 2007). The risk of this type of eruption is increased if the patient also has a viral infection (e.g., the rash that appears after penicillin is given to a patient with Epstein-Barr virus). Exanthematous rashes typically have their onset within 1 to 2 weeks of starting a new medication and can occur after the medication has been stopped. If there is a rechallenge of that medication, the reaction can occur within a few days (Paller & Mancini, 2006). Repeated exposure can progress to anaphylaxis.

Clinical Findings

History. The following can be reported:
- Medication taken within the last 3 weeks
- Varying degrees of itching—can be intense
- Rash worsens even after medicine is discontinued for up to 5 days
- Possible systemic symptoms—low-grade fever, arthralgia, arthritis, lymphadenopathy, edema

Physical Examination. Findings include the following (see Color Plate):
- Often begins as a fairly symmetric, macular erythematous rash that becomes papular and confluent.

TABLE 36-10 **Differentiating Drug Eruptions, Urticaria, and Erythema Multiforme**

	Etiology	Clinical Findings	Treatment
Drug eruption	Reaction to medication, especially penicillin, cephalexin, erythromycin, sulfa drugs, NSAIDs, barbiturates, isoniazid, carbamazepine, phenytoin	Symmetric, macular, erythematous to papular, confluent morbilliform rash; intense itching; patches of normal skin throughout; begins on trunk, extends distally, including palms and soles; face with confluent erythema	Stop drug and label as allergen to the child; antihistamine, antipruritics, lubricate skin; prednisone if severe; rash can last 7-14 days; medical alert bracelet
Urticaria	Hypersensitive reaction; immunologic antigen-antibody response to release of histamines; often unknown cause; possible reaction to food, drug, insect bite or sting, pollen; possible reaction to infection, especially streptococcal, sinus, mononucleosis, hepatitis	Family history of hives; rapid onset; possible atopy; intense itching; mild erythema, annular, raised wheals with pale centers; lesions scattered or coalesced; *key finding*: appear suddenly, fade from 20 minutes to 24 hours; blanch with pressure; associated edema of eyelids, lips, tongue, hands, feet	Quick resolution; identify and remove or treat offending agent if possible; stop antibiotic; give oral antihistamines; topical antipruritics; epinephrine or prednisone if anaphylactic, angioedema, or refractory; refer if >6 weeks duration
Erythema multiforme	Immune-mediated hypersensitivity reaction often to infection, especially HSV, also to many other agents	History of infection, especially herpes labialis; variety of lesions on skin and mucous membranes—macules, papules, vesicles, early lesions, such as urticaria; *key finding*: target or iris lesions; *key finding*: lesions fixed, symmetric, typical distribution on hands, feet, elbows, knees, also face, neck, trunk; possible oral mucous membrane involvement	Identify, treat, discontinue trigger if possible; treat infection; supportive measures for hydration, prevention of secondary infection, relief of pain; oral antihistamines, cool compresses; oral lesions—mouthwash, topical anesthetics; lesions last 5-7 days, recur in batches over 2-4 weeks, resolve without scarring or sequelae

- Patches of normal skin scattered throughout areas of involvement.
- Rash begins on the trunk, where it is brighter red, more confluent, and extends distally to the extremities, including the palms and soles.
- Rash may turn brownish-red and desquamate in 7 to 14 days
- The face often has confluent areas of erythema.
- Mucous membranes are typically spared.

   Diagnostic Studies. The following are ordered if necessary for differential diagnosis:
- CBC, monospot test, CRP, antinuclear antibodies, antistreptolysin O (ASO), cold agglutinins
- Chest radiograph

Differential Diagnosis

Viral exanthem; measles; toxic erythema, such as in scarlet fever, staphylococcal scarlatina, or Kawasaki disease; morbilliform rash (if the patient has mononucleosis and is taking amoxicillin); TSS; roseola; and erythema infectiosum are included in the differential diagnosis.

Management

Decisions about whether a drug is to be implicated depend on the patient's previous history of taking the drug, the experience of the general population with the drug, the morphology and timing of the rash, and other possible explanations for the rash (e.g., viral illness). The following steps are taken:

1. Discontinue the suspected drug.
2. Label the patient's medical record with the potential allergen.
3. Prescribe antihistamines if itching is present; recommend a lubricant and antipruritics as adjuncts.
4. Prescribe prednisone 1 to 2 mg/kg/day for 5 to 7 days if significant reaction.
5. Schedule follow-up visit as determined by severity of reaction and other illness.
6. Refer to allergist for skin testing to confirm allergy if there are limited or no alternative medications, for desensitization, to clarify drug allergy, for severe parental anxiety, or if symptoms are severe and life threatening.

Complications

Body heat and water loss can occur if the rash is severe. Progression of the rash if medicine is continued can lead to toxic epidermal necrolysis or SJS (see section on EM) or allergic interstitial nephritis.

Patient Education and Prevention

- The rash can last 7 to 14 days with itching present and worsening before getting better.
- There is potential risk from further exposure to that drug or related ones; alternative therapies should be explained.
- Identification and communication of the child's allergy are imperative. In life-threatening allergies, wearing a medical alert bracelet or necklace is essential.

■ VASCULAR REACTIONS OF THE SKIN
URTICARIA AND ANGIOEDEMA

Description

Urticaria and angioedema are hypersensitivity reactions (usually a type I reaction—IgE mediated) commonly called *hives* (see Color Plate). Transient or acute urticaria lasts less than 6 weeks; chronic, recurrent, or persistent urticaria lasts more than 6 weeks. Papular urticaria occurs in reaction to mosquito or dog and cat flea bites or mites. Contact urticaria can occur from skin exposure to antigens, such as chemicals, latex, or exposure to fish or caterpillars. Physical causes of urticaria include dermatographism, cholinergic reactions (e.g., response to heat, exercise, hot baths), pressure, water, and cold.

Angioedema involves the deeper dermis and subcutaneous tissue; in contrast, urticaria involves the superficial dermis. Patients who get both angioedema and urticaria tend to have more severe reactions (Dalal, 2006).

Epidemiology

Urticaria and angioedema are caused by a complex interplay of immunologically mediated antigen-antibody responses to the release of histamine from mast cells and other vasoactive mediators, such as leukotrienes and prostaglandins. Vasodilation and increased vascular permeability cause erythema and the characteristic wheal of urticaria. Onset is usually rapid, and resolution occurs within a few days of onset. The cause often remains a mystery (idiopathic). Possible causative factors include the following:

- Reactions to foods (e.g., nuts, eggs, shellfish, strawberries, tomatoes), drugs (salicylates and penicillins are the two most common), animal stings (e.g., bees, wasps, scorpion, spider, jellyfish), or pollen
- Response to bacterial, viral, or fungal infections, especially streptococcal or sinus infection, mononucleosis, hepatitis, adenoviruses and enteroviruses, or parasites
- Response to physical stimuli (e.g., heat or cold, sun or water [aquagenic urticaria], tight clothing, vibrations) or stress
- Genetic origin
- Concurrent with inflammatory systemic diseases (e.g., collagen-vascular or inflammatory bowel disease)

Urticaria occurs sometime in the lives of about 15% of the population. Portals of entry include infection (most common), ingestion, injection, inhalation, immunologic (rare), and idiopathic. Drugs are responsible for about 10% of the episodes of urticaria, which are generally acute in nature (Paller & Mancini, 2006). Chronic urticaria is rare in children (Dalal, 2006).

Urticaria and angioedema are more common in children, and about 50% of patients with urticaria have angioedema too. Angioedema is an extension of the reaction into the subcutaneous tissue and tends to involve the face (especially the eyes), the hands, and feet (Dalal, 2006). It is gradual in onset and often involves reactions to medication. There is a hereditary angioedema, which is rare. It is an autosomal dominant disorder that results from either a deficiency or dysfunction of the first component of complement (C-esterase inhibitor). It is life threatening and usually manifests before 10 years old typically with exacerbations in adolescence, often following trauma (e.g., dental work, surgery, accident). It is manifested by repeated episodes of swelling of the extremities, face, and throat (30%), accompanied by abdominal pain that becomes progressively more severe (Paller & Manicini, 2006). Severe airway edema, if untreated, is often the cause of death.

Clinical Findings

History. The following should be assessed:

- Family or previous history of hives, angioedema, connective tissue disease, juvenile arthritis
- Possibility of atopy
- Intense itching and scratching
- Ingestion (within 4 hours) of nuts, shellfish, chocolate, berries, spices, egg white, milk, fish, sesame
- Ingestion or injection of medicines (penicillin, sulfa drugs, sedatives, diuretics, analgesics, acetylsalicylic acid), additives, or preservatives
- Injection of diagnostic agents, vaccine, insect venom, blood, medicine
- Infection with upper respiratory infectious agent, virus, streptococcus, mononucleosis; hepatitis; parasites
- Inhalation of animal danders, pollen, dust, smoke, or aerosols

- Flea or mite bites
- Cold, heat, exercise, sun, water, pressure, or vibration

Physical Examination. Location of lesions may help determine the cause (e.g., a lesion around the mouth or tongue is likely due to an ingested agent). Findings can include the following:

- Urticaria is seen as mildly erythematous, annular, raised wheals or welts with pale centers from 2 mm to 20 cm in diameter; however, they can be of various shapes. Such lesions typically:
  - Are scattered or coalesced but generalized
  - Appear suddenly as individual lesions and fade in anywhere from 20 minutes to less than 24 hours, reappearing in other areas later; if fixed more than 48 hours, it is not urticaria
  - Blanch with pressure
  - Seem to be intensified with heat
  - Appear as wheals after rubbing or stroking the skin (dermatographism)
  - Occur most commonly as papulovesicular lesions with central punctate lesion and wheals in toddlers (papular urticaria)
  - Can appear as large, blotchy, erythematous lesions with 1- to 3-mm central wheals (cholinergic urticaria)
- Angioedema is seen as asymmetric, localized, nondependent and transient edema.
- Typically less pruritic than urticaria
- May involve the upper airway and progress to life-threatening obstruction
- Can cause associated edema of eyelids, lips, tongue, hands, feet, and genitalia

Diagnostic Studies. If urticaria with possible anaphylaxis from an insect bite is suspected, referral to an allergist for testing and hyposensitization is needed. If fever is present, evaluation for underlying disease can be useful.

Differential Diagnosis

Contact dermatitis, atopic dermatitis, scabies, EM (lesions are fixed with dusky centers and appear within 72 hours—see Color Plate), mastocytosis, reactive erythemas, vasculitis, psoriasis, and juvenile arthritis are also included in the differential diagnosis (see Table 36-10).

Management

The following steps are taken:

1. Identify and remove the offending substance if possible. Stop all antibiotics. Avoid any possible food or environmental trigger.
2. Test for dermatographism by stroking the skin, for cholinergic urticaria by applying heat or observing immediately after exercising, for cold urticaria by applying cold packs, for pressure urticaria by applying weighted bands for several minutes, and for water urticaria by applying wet compresses.
3. Administer medications as indicated:
   - Oral antihistamines, such as diphenhydramine 5 mg/kg/day (maximum 50 mg/dose and 300 mg/day) or hydroxyzine 2 to 5 mg/kg/day (400 mg/day maximum) every 4 to 6 hours until itching and urticaria are resolved (Dalal,

2006). Nonsedating antihistamines are less effective, but if needed astemizole, cetirizine, or loratadine is best. Urticaria is less likely to recur if the antihistamine is continued for 1 to 2 weeks after resolution.
   - Topical antipruritics may be helpful.
   - Aqueous epinephrine 1:1000 (subcutaneously 0.01 mL/kg up to 0.3 mL) may be needed if anaphylaxis or significant angioedema with swelling of the face, mucous membranes, and airway is present.
   - Prednisone 1 to 2 mg/kg/day for 1 week with rapid taper only if refractory to other measures or if angioedema is present with swelling of lips and face.
4. Follow-up visit if not improved within 48 hours.
5. Chronic urticaria persisting longer than 6 weeks needs evaluation for infection or systemic causes or referral for further evaluation.
6. An emergency epinephrine kit (EpiPen Jr, 0.15 mg or adult, 0.3 mg) should be prescribed for children after the first episode or with recurrent episodes of life-threatening urticaria or angioedema.

Complications

Angioedema or anaphylaxis occurs by the same mechanism as urticaria.

- Anaphylactic symptoms require emergency intervention.
- Serum sickness begins with hives, but has other systemic symptoms (e.g., fever, arthralgias, malaise, lymphadenopathy, proteinuria).
- If urticaria is from a drug reaction, rechallenge with the drug is more likely to cause anaphylaxis.

Patient Education and Prevention

The following are needed:

- Explanation of causes, course, and treatment. The cause often cannot be found, and control of symptoms is the main goal of treatment. The entire episode usually resolves in 24 to 48 hours, rarely extending beyond 3 to 4 weeks. Further evaluation is needed only if urticaria lasts longer than 8 weeks.
- Papular urticaria hypersensitivity often declines within 6 to 12 months.
- Physical urticarias last 2 to 4 years in most cases, but occasionally persist into adulthood.
- Occasionally, macular blue-brown lesions are found on resolution of urticaria.
- Avoid allergen if known; wear a medical alert bracelet in case severe reaction occurs; refer for hyposensitization if life-threatening symptoms occur.
- Carry an anaphylactic kit if indicated.

ERYTHEMA MULTIFORME (EM), STEVENS–JOHNSON SYNDROME (SJS), TOXIC EPIDERMAL NECROLYSIS (TEN)

Description

Erythema multiforme (EM) is an acute, usually benign, self-limiting eruption of targetoid papules with varying bullae formation. In the past, EM, SJS, and TEN were thought to be related disorders. The current thinking is that EM is a distinct disorder that does not progress to TEN or SJS. EM is rarely associated with complications and has a benign course characterized by the development of target lesions and minor mucosal involvement. SJS and TEN are now considered to represent a distinct syndrome that occurs with variable expression along a continuum. SJS and TEN are associated with significant risk of morbidity and mortality (Cohen 2005; Stein, 2006).

Epidemiology

EM usually follows an infection with approximately 80% of cases of classic EM attributed to HSV. Herpes labialis or progenitalis lesion(s) may or may not be found with the onset of EM. The herpetic lesion may have healed or had a subclinical presentation. EM tends to be recurrent as do herpes lesions. The herpes infection is believed to a precipitating mechanism causing an immune response. Drugs appear to be a rare cause of EM. In contrast, SJS and TEN are commonly triggered by medications, such as sulfasalazine, TMP-SMZ, and aminopenicillins. SJS is less commonly linked to an infectious agent; TEN is a severe drug reaction (Stein, 2006).

Clinical Findings

History. The following are sometimes reported (Cohen, 2005; Stein, 2006):
- With EM
  - Recent or current infection with herpes virus (herpes labialis or progenitalis)
  - Exposure to UV light or trauma to area
  - Low-grade fever, malaise, and myalgia
- With SJS or TEN
  - Use of a triggering medication (SJS and TEN)
  - History of an infection (occurs rarely with SJS)
  - TEN begins with a fever, sore throat, malaise, and generalized sunburnlike erythema
  - SJS can have a prodrome of high fever, cough, sore throat, vomiting, diarrhea, chest pain, and arthralgia that last usually 1 to 3 days (but can be from 1 to 14 days) followed by the onset of lesions.

Physical Examination. It is important to differentiate the clinical findings of EM from SJS and TEN.
- EM:
  - Lesions vary from patient to patient, within a single episode, and with recurrence.
  - Lesions initially appear dusky, as red macules or edematous papules that evolve into target lesions with multiple, concentric rings of color change (Cohen, 2005).
  - Lesions are fixed (another diagnostic clue), tend to be symmetric, and have a typical distribution predominantly on the face, extensor surface of the arms and legs, dorsum of the hands and feet, and the palms and soles.
  - Mucous membranes may be involved with erythema and erosions noted (Stein, 2006).
- SJS or TEN:
  - SJS skin lesions typically are erythematous macules on the head and neck and can spread to the trunk and extremities with blister formation (within hours) that is often

hemorrhagic, extensive, and confluent; mucosal involvement of eyes, nose, and mouth is widespread (Cohen, 2005).
  - The TEN rash has rapidly coalescing target lesions and widespread bullae that become full-thickness epidermal peeling or sloughing within 24 hours; a Nikolsky's sign (peeling of skin with a light rub reveals a moist red surface) is present.
  - Conjunctivae, urethra, rectum, oral and nasal mucosa, larynx, and tracheobronchial mucosa may be or may not be involved with TEN.

Diagnostic Studies. Studies are ordered as indicated by the clinical condition of the child.

Differential Diagnosis

Urticaria can be differentiated by lack of itching, lability of lesions, and shorter-lasting hives that are pale centrally, not target or iris lesions. Viral exanthems are more centrally located, confluent, and less erythematous. Purpura is present in vasculitis. In SSSS, the skin peels superficially (not full thickness) and is significantly red. Also included in the differential diagnosis are Kawasaki disease and lupus erythematosus (see Table 36-10).

Management

Care for EM is generally supportive because the condition is self-limited.
- Symptomatic and supportive care: maintain hydration, prevent secondary infection, and relieve pain.
  - Mild analgesics, cool compresses, and oral antihistamines, such as diphenhydramine.
  - Soothing mouthwashes or topical anesthetics, such as Kaopectate or Maalox, mixed in equal parts with diphenhydramine.
  - Topical intraoral anesthetics, such as dyclonine liquid or viscous lidocaine, are sometimes used with caution in older children and adolescents.
  - Débridement of oral lesions with half-strength hydrogen peroxide
  - Wound care.
  - Intravenous fluids if oral hydration is not adequate.
  - Systemic antihistamines, analgesics, and antimicrobials as needed.
- Prevention of herpes simplex: avoid sun exposure and use sunscreen and protective clothing
- Prophylaxis for recurrent EM treatment:
  - Oral acyclovir, less than 40 kg, 20 mg/kg/day divided twice daily or greater than 40 kg, 400 mg/day divided twice daily, for a 6- to 12-month trial with periodic stopping to reassess.
  - Acyclovir during an acute episode of EM does not alter its course.

SJS and TEN are potentially life-threatening diseases. Children are typically admitted to the PICU or burn unit for wound care, management or hydration and electrolyte issues, nutritional support, and pain control. The use of IVIG interrupts the severe blistering reactions, and administration of corticosteroids has been noted to lead to a longer response time for healing (Stein, 2006).

Complications

EM is typically a self-limiting condition. SJS and TEN are associated with significant morbidity including pneumonitis, sepsis, gastrointestinal bleeding, renal disease, keratitis, and other ophthalmologic disorders.

Patient Education and Prevention

EM lesions can erupt in crops that last 1 to 3 weeks, but resolve without scarring or sequelae, except for transient desquamation, scaling, or hyperpigmentation. Recurrence of EM is common.

■ PAPULOSQUAMOUS ERUPTIONS OF THE SKIN

PITYRIASIS ROSEA

Description

Pityriasis rosea (PR), meaning rose-colored flaking, is a common, mild, self-limited papulosquamous disease (see Color Plate).

Epidemiology

The etiology of PR has not been established. There is debate as to whether PR is caused by human herpesvirus (HHV), 6 or 7 (HHV-6 or HHV-7) or from several other causative agents including enteroviruses and *Mycoplasma pneumoniae* (Cohen, 2005; Paller & Mancini, 2006; Habif, 2004). It is minimally contagious and occurs most commonly in the fall, early winter, and spring months in temperate climates. Fifty percent of all cases occur before 20 years old, most commonly in adolescence with males and females equally affected. Approximately 98% of cases result in lifelong immunity (Paller & Mancini, 2006).

Clinical Findings

History. Although most are otherwise well, a small percentage (5%) of patients experience a prodrome of mild symptoms including malaise, pharyngitis, lymphadenopathy, and headache before onset of rash. Those that have prodromal symptoms tend to have a more florid rash.

Physical Examination. Findings include the following:
- Herald spot or patch (70% of presentations)—a 2- to 5-cm solitary, ovoid, slightly erythematous lesion with a finely scaled, slightly elevated border that enlarges quickly with central clearing); typical locations for the herald patch include the trunk, upper arm, neck, or thigh
- Secondary generalized lesions appear that are symmetric, small macular to papular, and thin, round to oval in shape. The lesions have thin scales centrally with thicker scales peripherally ("collarette" scales surrounds the lesions). They are also pale pink in color; more common on trunk and proximal extremities from neck to knees; typically sparing the face, scalp, and distal extremities; and usually occurring 2 to 21 days after the appearance of the herald patch (*key finding*).
- Christmas tree pattern—rash, especially on back, follows skin lines with oval lesions running parallel and wraps around the trunk horizontally.

- Itching occurs in about 25% of cases particularly with secondary lesions.
- Oral lesions have punctate hemorrhages, erosions or ulcerations, erythematous macules, or annular plaques; such lesions occur in about 16% of patients.
- The face and neck are frequent areas of involvement in young children especially if African American.
- Atypical disease occurs as inverse PR with involvement of usually spared areas (lesions on the face, axilla, groin) most typically occurring in young children (Paller & Mancini, 2006).

Diagnostic Studies. If needed, a KOH preparation of a skin scraping is done to rule out tinea; a Venereal Disease Research Laboratories (VDRL) test is done to rule out secondary syphilis.

Differential Diagnosis

Psoriasis, guttate psoriasis, nummular eczema, scabies, tinea (especially the herald patch), secondary syphilis, drug eruptions, or viral exanthems should be ruled out in the differential diagnosis.

Management

The following steps are taken:
- Application of calamine lotion (or other lotions containing menthol and/or camphor or pramoxine), tepid baths with Aveeno, antihistamines, emollients, or mild topical steroids is done as needed for itching.
- Minimal sun exposure can help lesions resolve more quickly. Prevent sunburn.
- For oral lesions, triamcinolone acetonide (Kenalog in Orabase) in dental paste may be applied or in patients older than 8 years, mouthwash with tetracycline and diphenhydramine.
- Early administration of oral erythromycin has been demonstrated as beneficial in shortening the course of PR (Paller & Mancini, 2006).

Patient Education and Prevention

PR is a benign, self-limited, and noncontagious disease that has three cycles (emerging, persisting, and fading) with spontaneous resolution in 6 to 12 weeks. Transient pigmentary changes can occur, especially in blacks (Cohen, 2005).

PSORIASIS

Description

Psoriasis, a chronic papulosquamous skin disorder with spontaneous remissions and exacerbations, is characterized by thick silvery scales, its distribution pattern, and an isomorphic (Koebner phenomenon) response (see Color Plate). Types of psoriasis include guttate psoriasis (following a streptococcal infection), psoriasis vulgaris, napkin psoriasis (occurring in the diaper area), inverse psoriasis (limited to areas that are normally spared), localized pustular psoriasis, generalized pustular or psoriatic erythroderma, and psoriatic arthritis.

Epidemiology

Psoriasis is an immune-mediated disorder associated with genetic predisposition and environmental risk factors. Though the exact cause is unknown, chromosome 6p21.3 is linked to the development of psoriasis, and the contributing gene is termed PSORS1. An accelerated epidermal proliferation of keratinocytes and dermal vascular abnormalities contribute to the characteristic look of the lesions. Trigger factors including infection, local trauma, stress (physical and psychological), and certain drugs (corticosteroids, lithium, beta blockers, NSAIDs) play a role in psoriasis.

Psoriasis occurs in 2% to 3% of the population, with 31% to 45% of cases appearing before 20 years old. It accounts for 4% of all dermatoses seen in children under 16 years old. Guttate psoriasis is often the first sign of psoriasis in children (Habif, 2004; Paller & Mancini, 2006; Weston et al, 2007).

Clinical Findings

History. The following may be reported:
- Family history in approximately 70% of pediatric patients (Paller & Mancini, 2006)
- Streptococcal infection of the oropharynx or perianal area before onset (guttate)
- Trauma before onset
- Itching (variable)

Physical Examination. Findings include the following:
- The scalp (encircling the hairline and external ears), elbows, knees, and buttocks (especially the diaper area in infants) are the most common sites of involvement. In children, the face may also be involved. Lesions are often found around areas of trauma (e.g., genitalia, palms, soles).
  - *Plaque psoriasis.* Discrete, initially erythematous, symmetric, well-marginated rash becoming papular with silver scales that may be trivial to widespread.
  - *Guttate (teardrop) psoriasis.* Widespread, symmetric, round, or oval 0.5- to 2-cm lesions occurring primarily on the trunk and proximal extremities, occasionally on the face, scalp and ears and rarely on the palms or soles. There is less scaling than in psoriasis vulgaris.
  - *Psoriasis vulgaris.* Well-circumscribed, erythematous plaques with thick, silvery-white scales concentrated on elbows, knees, scalp, and hairline, but also seen on eyebrows, around ears, and in intergluteal fold and genital area.
  - *Koebner phenomenon (isomorphic response).* The occurrence of psoriasis several days after trauma (e.g., bites, scratch, abrasion, sunburn, pressure) is characteristic of psoriasis (Weston et al, 2007).
  - *Auspitz sign.* Bleeding occurs when a scale is removed.
  - *Nail signs.* Nails have "ice pick" pits and ridges, are thick and discolored (yellowing), and can have splinter hemorrhages or subungual hyperkeratosis, and be separated from the nail bed (Cohen, 2005).
  - *Napkin or diaper area psoriasis.* Appears eczematous with sharply defined plaques, bright red coloration, shiny with large drier scales, affecting inguinal and gluteal folds.

Diagnostic Studies. The following are to be considered:
- ASO if guttate pattern
- KOH and culture to rule out fungal infection
- VDRL to rule out secondary syphilis

Differential Diagnosis

PR, seborrhea, *Candida* infection, contact or irritant dermatitis, atopic dermatitis, tinea, dyshidrosis, secondary syphilis, and other nail-pitting conditions are included in the differential diagnosis.

Management

In children, treatment should be as conservative as possible. Medications and treatments should be rotated for best effectiveness. The following are options for management:
- Sun exposure in moderate amounts alleviates lesions. Prevent sunburn.
- Emollient cream, such as petrolatum, Eucerin, Aquaphor, or Cetaphil for dry skin can minimize trauma and subsequent psoriasis and may improve psoriasis.
- Apply topical steroids, moderate or strong and sometimes fluorinated, two to three times a day for 2 to 3 weeks. They should be used intermittently, but not discontinued spontaneously because worsening can occur. Monitoring of the patient during use is important. Small localized lesions can be treated with topical, fluorinated steroids. A moderate-potency steroid can be used on thick plaques and larger areas. Severe plaques on the elbows and knees may need a higher-potency steroid (see Table 36-1). Systemic steroids are not indicated and may worsen the condition, causing pustular flare. Consultation with a dermatologist is often indicated.
- Tar or keratolytic shampoos (ketoconazole [Nizoral], anthralin, salicylic acid [Salex] [P & S]) can be used on the scalp. Tar preparations can also be used on the skin alone or in combination with UV light treatment.
- Mineral or olive oil and warm towels to soak and remove thick plaques.
- Keratolytic agents, such as sulfur 3% or salicylic acid 3% to 6%, to reduce thick, unresponsive plaques. Salicylic acid blocks UVB and should not be used in combination with phototherapy.
- Anthralin ointment for plaques that are resistant to steroids and tar. In high strengths (1% and higher), apply ointment for 10 to 30 minutes once a day and then wash off. In lower strengths, leave ointment on for 8 hours. Strength used is determined by tolerance. Anthralin stains skin and clothing and can irritate skin.
- Calcipotriol, a vitamin D analogue, is effective for mild to moderate plaque psoriasis in adults and children. Available in cream, ointment, and lotion, it is safe, effective and well-tolerated for short- and long-term treatment. Hypercalcemia is reported with application of excessive quantities over large areas; however, calcium metabolism does not change with less than 100 g/week (Habif, 2004; Schachner, 2003).
- Tazarotene (Tazorac) is a retinoid that may be effective in management of plaque psoriasis, but is often too irritating for use in childhood psoriasis (Paller & Mancini, 2006).
- Tacrolimus ointment, a calcineurin inhibitor, has demonstrated benefit when used for facial and intertriginous psoriasis in children (Paller & Mancini, 2006).
- Balneo phototherapy combines magnesium-rich Dead Sea salt baths with UV light treatments for 4 to 6 weeks or 15 to

25 treatments. This natural treatment may bring 80% to 85% clearance of skin lesions or remission (Mikula, 2003).

- Cyclosporine and methotrexate are systemic therapies used for recalcitrant and severe disease.
- Follow up every 2 weeks until psoriasis is controlled and during exacerbations and then as needed.
- Refer to a dermatologist if psoriasis is not responsive. Other treatment options include UV light treatment, psoralens, intralesional steroids, retinoids, cyclosporine, biologic therapy, and immunotherapy.

Complications

The following complications are possible:

- *Candida infection.* As a secondary infection in the diaper area.
- *Erythrodermic* and p*ustular psoriasis.* Unusual in childhood; characterized by generalized or local multiple 1- to 2-mm pustules with erythema and scaling also involving palms and soles; accompanied by malaise, fever, electrolyte and fluid imbalances, and temperature instability and leukocytosis; can be fatal; and should be referred to a dermatologist.
- *Exfoliative erythroderma.* Rare manifestation, including desquamation and loss of hair and nails with previous history of psoriasis. Should be referred to a dermatologist.
- *Psoriatic arthritis.* An inflammatory arthritis that is rare (1%) but increasing in frequency, most common in females 9 to 12 years old (Paller, 1999; Weston et al, 2007). Rheumatoid factor is negative, cutaneous symptoms mild or absent. Prognosis is good.

Patient Education and Prevention

Emotional support and education are the most important aspects in dealing with psoriasis. Areas for discussion include the following:

- Psoriasis is chronic and involves spontaneous remissions and exacerbations. Control and relief are sought, but cure is not available at this time. Treatment may require up to 1 month to determine effectiveness.
- Guttate psoriasis often resolves with antibiotic treatment for streptococcal infection. Psoriasis vulgaris may persist for months to years.
- Lifestyle changes help prevent recurrence. These include avoidance of cutaneous injury, streptococcal infection, sunburn, stress, itching, bites, tight clothes and shoes, some medications (e.g., oral steroids, NSAIDs), and occlusive dressings. Good skin care, including regular use of emollients and avoidance of irritating underarm deodorants and harsh soaps, may improve psoriasis and minimize recurrences. With nail involvement, avoid long fingernails or toenails and use of nail polish. Do not vigorously brush or comb hair if scalp area affected.
- Psoriasis tends to improve during summer and with pregnancy.
- Psoriasis is considered stable if there are either no new plaques or if existing plaques are not enlarging.
- Refer patients to the National Psoriasis Foundation.

LICHEN STRIATUS

Description

Lichen striatus (LS) is peculiar to childhood, characterized by unilateral shiny papules along embryonic lines, or lines of Blaschko.

Epidemiology

Although the etiology is unknown, it is thought to be related to a cutaneous defect from an embryologic mutation of somatic cells. It is most common in school-age children, commonly females. LS is typically located on the extremities, upper back, or neck, but can be found on the palms, soles, nails, genitals or face (Cohen, 2005). Lesions spontaneously disappear after 3 months to 12 months, but may last up to 3 years. Short relapses have occurred on occasion.

Clinical Findings

History. Lesions appear spontaneously without prodrome.
Physical Examination. Findings include the following:

- Linear, shiny hypopigmented or flesh-colored, flat-topped papules with adherent scale
- Limited to one extremity, initially lesions coalesce in a linear distribution down an extremity
- Lesions involving a nail bed will result in nail deformity
- Rarely are lesions noted on the face
- May be asymptomatic or may be intensely pruritic
- May resolve with hypopigmentation that lasts several months

Diagnostic Studies. A skin biopsy is diagnostic when in doubt.

Differential Diagnosis

The unilateral linear lesions are characteristic. However, differential diagnosis includes lichen planus, lichen nitidus, psoriasis, epidermal birthmarks, and linear Darier's disease.

Management

Lesions are resistant to treatment, and treatment is unnecessary for asymptomatic cases. However, pruritus may be relieved with the use of group I or group II topical steroids or topical tacrolimus ointment; however, most cases require no therapy (Cohen, 2005; Paller & Mancini, 2006).

Patient Education and Prevention

LS is a benign, self-limited, noncontagious disorder that results in complete resolution.

KERATOSIS PILARIS

Description

Keratosis pilaris is a common finding on the extensor aspects of the extremities, buttocks, and occasionally the cheeks. The skin has a typical appearance of "chicken skin" with small bumps at the hair follicle.

Epidemiology

The etiology is unknown. It is not present at birth, but is common in early childhood onward. Some believe it to be a disorder of abnormal keratinization; others believe it to be a response to drying of the skin surface. Keratosis pilaris is more common in children with atopic disorders; in those living in cold, dry climates; and in winter months.

Clinical Findings

History. Keratosis pilaris appears spontaneously, without prodrome. It is usually asymptomatic, although most patients are bothered by the appearance and seek treatment.

Physical Examination. Findings include the following:
- Rough dry skin on the posterior upper arms, anterior thighs, buttocks, and cheeks
- Small papules with follicular plugs of stratum corneum
- Occasional diffuse eruption with small sterile pustules

Diagnostic Studies. Skin biopsy reveals inflammation outside the hair follicle; however, this is typically not needed because the diagnosis is easy to determine.

Differential Diagnosis

Microcomedones of acne, molluscum contagiosum, warts, milia, and folliculitis are often confused with keratosis pilaris.

Management

It is important to recognize keratosis pilaris as a benign disorder to avoid detrimental treatment. Management includes the following:
- In mild cases, the use of lubricants and emollients to moisturize skin is sufficient for improvement.
- Topical keratolytics combined with lactic acid 12%, salicylic acid, urea creams, retinoids, and lubricants are applied several times daily.
- Antibiotics active against *S. aureus* are useful for folliculitis.

Treatment takes weeks to months for improvement, and recurrence is common when treatment is stopped.

Patient Education and Prevention

The chronic but benign nature of keratosis pilaris should be stressed. Treatment takes weeks to months, and recurrence is common.

■ CONGENITAL LESIONS OF THE SKIN
VASCULAR AND PIGMENTED NEVI

Description

Nevi are a common finding in children. The two most common types are vascular nevi (vascular malformations and hemangiomas) and pigmented nevi (mongolian spots, café au lait spots, acquired melanocytic nevi, AN, and lentigines).

Epidemiology

Vascular nevi are caused by a structural abnormality (malformations) or by an overgrowth of blood vessels (hemangiomas) and are flat, raised, or cavernous. Flat lesions or vascular malformations include salmon patches (also called macular stains), an innocent malformation that is a light-red macule appearing on the nape of the neck, upper eyelids, and glabella. Approximately 40% of newborns have a salmon patch on the back of the neck. Port-wine stains occur in 3 per 1000 newborns (Cohen, 2005; Weston et al, 2007). At 1 year old, 10% to 12% of white infants will have a hemangioma, with female infants three times more likely than male infants to have a hemangioma. There is also an increased incidence in premature neonates. Vascular lesions are always present at birth and do not resolve spontaneously. Hemangiomas are present at birth 40% of the time. They undergo rapid growth (proliferative stage), stability (plateau phase), and regression (involution phase), with 90% completely resolved by 10 years old (Habif, 2004; Paller & Mancini, 2006).

Pigmented nevi are caused by an overgrowth of pigment cells. Pigmented nevi most commonly seen are mongolian spots (up to 90% in blacks, 81% in Asians, 70% in Hispanics, and in East Indians; less than 10% in whites), café au lait spots (found in 25% to 35% of normal children and in 50% of patients with McCune-Albright syndrome), and acquired melanocytic nevi, the most common tumor of childhood, 2% of which are atypical (Paller & Mancini, 2006; Weston et al, 2007).

Clinical Findings

History. The following should be noted:
- Presence from birth, or age first noted
- Progression of lesion
- Familial tendencies for similar nevi, especially for history of melanoma

Physical Examination. Findings include the following (Box 36-11):
- Vascular malformations or flat vascular nevi are present at birth and grow commensurate with the child's growth.
- Hemangiomas are classified as superficial, deep (cavernous), or mixed. They may or may not be present at birth, but usually emerge by 1 month old. They may manifest as a pale macule, a telangiectatic lesion, or a bright-red nodular papule. Involution occurs slowly (10% per year) but spontaneously: (30% by 3 years old, 50% by 5 years old, 70% by 7 years old, and 90% by 9 to 10 years old). Average involution is between 12 and 24 months old, heralded by gray areas in the lesion followed by flattening from the center outward (Paller & Mancini, 2006). Most are flat by 5 to 7 years old, the remainder by puberty. Most hemangiomas appear as normal skin after involution, but others may have residual changes, such as telangiectasias, atrophy, fibrofatty residue, and scarring (Paller & Mancini, 2006). During the proliferative phase, hemangiomas grow rapidly and form nodular compressible masses, ranging in size from a few millimeters to several centimeters. Occasionally, they may cover an entire limb, resulting in asymmetric limb growth. Rapidly growing lesions may ulcerate.
- Pigmented nevi may be present at birth or may be acquired during childhood.
- Atypical nevi are larger than acquired nevi; have irregular, poorly defined borders; and have variable pigmentation.

BOX 36-11   Common Vascular and Pigmented Lesions

I. Vascular malformations or flat vascular nevi
- A. Salmon p atch or nevus flammeus
  1. Light-pink macule of varying size and configuration
  2. Commonly seen on the glabella, back of neck, forehead, or upper eyelids
- B. Port-wine stain or nevus flammeus
  1. Purple-red macules that occur unilaterally, tend to be large
  2. Usually occur on face, occiput, or neck, although they may be on extremities

II. Hemangiomas
- A. Superficial (strawberry) hemangiomas are found in the upper dermis of the skin and account for the majority of hemangiomas
- B. Deep cavernous hemangiomas are found in the subcutaneous and hypodermal layers of the skin; although similar to superficial hemangiomas, there is a blue tinge to their appearance
  1. With pressure, there is blanching and a feeling of a soft, compressible tumor
  2. Variable in size, they can occur in places other than skin
- C. Mixed hemangiomas have attributes of both superficial and deep hemangiomas

III. Pigmented nevi
- A. Mongolian spots
  1. Blue or slate-gray, irregular, variably sized macules
  2. Common in the presacral or lumbosacral area of dark-skinned infants; also on the upper back, shoulders, and extremities
  3. The majority of the pigment fades as the child gets older and the skin darkens
  4. Solitary or multiple, often covering a large area
- B. Café-au-lait spots
  1. Tan to light-brown macules found anywhere on the skin; oval or irregular in shape; increase in number with age
- C. Acquired melanocytic nevi are benign, light brown, to dark brown, to black, flat, or slightly raised, occurring anywhere on the body, especially on sun-exposed areas, above the waist
  1. *Junctional nevi* represent the initial stage, with tiny, hairless, light brown to black macules
  2. *Compound nevi*—a few junctional nevi progress to these more elevated, warty, or smooth lesions with hair
  3. *Dermal nevi* are the adult form, dome shaped with coarse hair
  4. *Atypical nevi* usually appear at puberty, have irregular borders, variegated pigmentation, are larger than normal nevi (6-15 mm); usually found on trunk, feet, scalp, and buttocks
  5. *Halo nevi* appear in late childhood with an area of depigmentation around a pigmented nevus, usually on trunk (see Color Plate)
- D. *Acanthosis nigricans* is velvety brown rows of hyperpigmentation in irregular folds of skin, usually the neck and axilla; tags may also be present
- E. Lentigines are small brown to black macules 1-2 mm in size appearing anywhere on the body in school-age children
- F. Freckles: 1-5 mm light brown pigmented macules in sun-exposed areas

Differential Diagnosis

Hematomas or ecchymoses of child abuse are occasionally confused with some nevi. Non–insulin-dependent diabetes mellitus (NIDDM) often causes AN.

Management

1. Flat vascular nevi:
   - Salmon patches.
     ◦ Fade with time, usually by 5 or 6 years old.
   - Port-wine stains.
     ◦ A permanent defect that grows with the child, so cosmetic covering is often used.
     ◦ Refer to a dermatologist for possible laser treatment or corrective cosmesis.
     ◦ If forehead and eyelids are involved, there is potential for multiple syndromes, including Sturge-Weber, Klippel-Trenaunay-Weber, and Parkes Weber. Neurodevelopmental and ophthalmologic follow-up is needed.
     ◦ Angiomatous papules and underlying soft tissue hypertrophy develop over years.

2. Hemangiomas:
   - Reassure and educate the family about the nature and course of this nevus. A word that there is no relationship to anything the mother did during pregnancy is often appreciated.
   - Frequent follow-up, especially during the growing phase. Sequential photographs are helpful.
   - If the lesions are strategically placed (eye, lip, oral cavity, ear, airway, diaper area), ulcerating, multiple, very large, or grow very quickly, prompt referral to a dermatologist is indicated because early treatment is most effective.
   - If treatment is required during the proliferative stage, steroids (intralesional and oral) are prescribed until growth is stabilized, then gradually tapered. Indications for steroid treatment are interference with physiologic functions (e.g., breathing, hearing, eating, vision), recurrent bleeding or ulceration, high-output congestive heart failure, Kasabach-Merritt syndrome, rapid growth that distorts facial features, or presence in the diaper area. Interferon-α may also be used.

- Treatment by surgery, cryotherapy, radiation, or injecting sclerosing agents often leads to scarring.
- Danger of cardiovascular complications, disseminated intravascular coagulation, or compression of internal organs with large, deep lesions.
- Regression (without treatment) occurs at a rate of 10% per year. Scarring may be present if ulceration has occurred; fibrofatty masses, atrophy, and telangiectasis can be residual findings following involution (Paller & Mancini, 2006). Laser therapy is effective management for residual telangiectasias (Paller & Mancini, 2006).

3. Pigmented nevi. Educate family about the nature of these lesions:
    - *Mongolian spots*: Document to distinguish from bruise; fade with time, usually no traces by adulthood.
    - *Blue nevus*: Heavily pigmented melanocytes in papule or nodule that can develop melanoma.
    - *Café au lait spots*: If six or more lesions larger than 0.5 cm in diameter are present in children younger than 15 years old and over 1.5 cm in diameter for older individuals or if axillary freckling or tumors are also present, refer child to rule out neurofibromatosis, McCune-Albright syndrome, or other genetic disorder (Cohen, 2005).

4. Other disorders of hyperpigmentation that can appear in early childhood:
    - *Acquired melanocytic nevi*: Giant nevi (e.g., bathing trunk nevus) are at increased risk of developing melanoma and need referral to a dermatologist. If more than fifteen acquired nevi are present, monitor for atypical nevi (Chamlin, 2002).
    - *Atypical nevi* appear most commonly in adolescents and require regular follow-up because of increased risk for melanoma. However, melanoma often manifests with new lesions rather than from transformation of current ones (see section on sunburn complications).
    - *Halo nevus*: A depigmented ring around a pigmented nevi.
    - *Spitz nevus*: A smooth, pink to brown, dome-shaped papule often occurring on head and neck.
    - *Fried-egg mole*: A compound nevi with flat border and raised darker center.
    - *Nevus spilus* is a light-brown speckled lentiginous nevi with darker papules within it; it can be congenital or acquired and has potential to develop melanoma.

5. Guidelines for when a child with a nevus or nevi should be referred to a dermatalogist are listed in Box 36-12.

Complications

Ulceration, infection, platelet trapping, airway or visual obstruction, or cardiac decompensation can occur with large vascular nevi. Kasabach-Merritt syndrome occurs when thrombocytopenic hemorrhage occurs in a large, deep hemangioma. Melanoma in congenital nevi (see discussion in complications of sunburn) is possible, and monitoring of these lesions is important. Changes of particular concern are development of an off-center nodule or papule, color change, bleeding, persistent irritation, erosion, ulceration, and rapid growth.

An autosomal dominant, familial, atypical mole and melanoma syndrome has been identified genetically. Children with

---

| BOX 36-12 | **When to Refer to a Dermatologist** |

- Suspicious appearing nevus (as identified by ABCDE signs [see Box 36-9])
- Rapidly growing or changing nevus
- Greater than 50 nevi
- One or more atypical nevi
- History of one or more first-degree relatives with melanoma
- Presence of a giant or large congenital nevus
- Signs of excessive sun exposure (increased nevi and freckles in exposed areas)
- History of immunosuppression and multiple nevi on examination

---

multiple atypical nevi and family members with melanoma are at risk for childhood melanoma (Chamlin, 2002).

Patient Education and Prevention

Monitoring those nevi that are at risk for developing melanoma is important. Teaching the family to watch nevi for any changes is also important. See sunburn complications section for more information.

■ CUTANEOUS MANIFESTATIONS OF UNDERLYING DISEASE

ACANTHOSIS NIGRICANS

Description and Epidemiology

Acanthosis nigricans (AN) is not a skin disease per se; rather, it is typically a sign of an underlying problem. It may be related to factors of heredity (rare and not associated with endocrinopathies or congenital abnormalities); endocrine disorders (e.g., insulin resistance, hypothyroidism, hyperandrogenic states, Cushing syndrome; obesity [more commonly seen in darker pigmented individuals]); drug administration (e.g., oral contraceptives, stilbestrol use in young males, high levels of nicotinic acid); and malignancy (e.g., adenocarcinoma, Wilms tumor, and less commonly lymphoma). These factors (except for the malignant form of AN) are believed to stimulate epidermal keratinocyte and dermal fibroblast proliferation that results in papillary hypertrophy, hyperkeratosis, and an increase in the number of melanocytes (Habib, 2004). Insulin or an insulin-like growth factor may activate the epidermal cell propagation. In children, insulin resistance and obesity are most commonly associated with the benign form of AN. When it occurs in the hereditary form (autosomal dominant trait with no associated obesity), it may appear at birth or during childhood with proliferation during adolescence. There is no sex predominance. It occurs in Native Americans (40%), blacks (13%), Hispanics (6%), and whites (less than 1%) (Baron & Levine, 2006; Habib, 2004).

Clinical Findings

AN is characterized by symmetric, brown thickening of the skin; as time progresses the skin develops a velvety, leathery, warty, or papillomatous surface. The axillary areas (most commonly), neck, groin, belt line, dorsal surfaces of the fingers, in the mouth, around the areola of the breast, and umbilicus can be affected. In areas of maceration, odor or discomfort may be reported.

Differential Diagnosis

Terra firma-forme dermatosis is often confused with AN and can lead to an extensive and expensive work-up for an endocrine or metabolic disorder. It resembles the appearance of AN, but differs in that the dirt can be rubbed off with isopropyl alcohol; it can occur anywhere on the body. AN lesions involve skin changes and remain despite washing as opposed to dirt on skin (Browning, 2006).

Management

Treatment consists of addressing the underlying causes of AN. This most commonly includes management of overweight (diet changes and weight loss) and correction of metabolic abnormality (hyperinsulinemia). In nonoverweight individuals, an underlying malignancy must be considered. The skin lesions themselves are benign, usually asymptomatic, and do not require intervention. Thicker lesions may cause discomfort and respond to topical retinoic acid cream or gel once daily. Oral agents include etretinate, isotretinoin, metformin, and dietary fish oils. Dermabrasion and long-pulsed alexandrite laser therapy have also been used. Lac-Hydrin (12% lactic acid cream) can help soften lesions.

Patient Education

It is important for patients to understand that AN may be a marker for an underlying disorder (e.g., cutaneous marker for hyperinsulinemia in overweight individuals and present in one third of patients with a malignancy and precedes clinical symptoms of some cancers) (Habib, 2004). AN may completely resolve with adequate treatment of the underlying disorder.

LENTIGINES

Lentigines are small, tan, dark brown, or black, flat, oval or circular, sharply circumscribed lesions that appear in childhood and may increase in number until adulthood. They may also be seen on mucous membranes and may fade or disappear with time. They are also associated with various syndromes, such as Peutz-Jeghers, which is associated with an increased risk of gastrointestinal and genitourinary carcinomas (Paller & Mancini, 2006).

■ OTHER COMMON DERMATOLOGIC ISSUES IN PEDIATRICS

VITILIGO AND HYPOPIGMENTATION DISORDERS

Description

Lack of pigment in the skin causing white or light-colored areas can be either hypopigmentation or vitiligo. The loss of pigment can be congenital or acquired in a diffuse or localized pattern. Vitiligo is a form of patterned loss of pigmentation with location, size, and shapes of individual lesions varying greatly. Postinflammatory hypopigmentation is common in pediatrics. Other less common disorders are incontinentia pigmenti achromians and piebaldism. Albinism and progressive vitiligo are examples of generalized pigmentary disturbances (Cohen, 2005).

Epidemiology

Vitiligo is presumed to be an immune disorder that has a genetic component. It occurs in about 1% of the U.S. population, with 50% of cases beginning before 20 years old. It appears more commonly in children with various systemic or immune disorders (Paller & Mancini, 2006; Weston et al, 2007). Hypopigmentation follows inflammation or injury to the melanocytes in the skin resulting from diseases, such as atopic dermatitis, psoriasis, or PR, or from abrasions, burns, injury from liquid nitrogen, or severe sunburn.

Clinical Findings

History.   The following should be elicited:
- Family history of vitiligo, halo nevi, traumatic depigmentation of skin, or markedly premature graying of the hair (30% of cases) (Paller & Mancini, 2006)
- Onset of depigmentation (birth or more recent)
- Presence of any systemic or skin diseases
- Any recent trauma to the skin; Koebner phenomenon is noted in about 15% of children with vitiligo

Physical Examination.   Findings include the following:
- Vitiligo
  - Flat, milk-white macules or papules with scalloped, distinct borders of varied size
  - Symmetric or asymmetric, possibly following a nerve segment
  - Few to multiple, seen most commonly on face and trunk
- Hypopigmentation
  - Macules and patches with irregular mottling and borders
  - Linear or patterned
  - Possibly associated hyperpigmented areas

Diagnostic Studies.   For vitiligo, a skin biopsy and CBC, fasting glucose, thyroid function and antithyroid antibodies, early-morning serum cortisol, and VDRL are sometimes indicated. The use of a Wood's light may be helpful in fair-skinned individuals to differentiate an area of normal skin from an area of vitiligo (i.e., helps to delineate a contrast between the normal and depigmented skin).

Differential Diagnosis

PR, pityriasis alba, tinea versicolor, and albinism (eye color affected and onset at birth) are included in the differential diagnosis.

Management

The following steps are taken:
- Vitiligo:
  - Broad-spectrum sunscreens are used to decrease the tanning of normal skin.
  - Cover-up agents, such as skin dyes and walnut oil, may be used.
  - Mild to moderate steroids may show success in some patients. Topical calcineurin inhibitors (tacrolimus ointment, pimecrolimus cream) eliminate atrophy, with 40% to 90% of pediatric patients showing a response to these treatments (Paller & Mancini, 2006)
  - Refer for treatment with psoralens. May be used in combination with UVA radiation (best used in children under 9 years old). UVB may also be used.

- ○ Family should be encouraged to be in a support group because this is a highly disfiguring condition, especially for those with dark complexion.
- Hypopigmentation:
  - ○ Reassure family that repigmentation will occur. Post-inflammatory hypopigmentation is self-limited and lasts only a few months.

Complications

Vitiligo may be associated with other immune disorders or their symptoms, such as thyroid disease, diabetes mellitus, pernicious anemia, Addison disease, uveitis, alopecia areata, and severe sunburn.

■ HAIR AND NAIL DISORDERS

Alopecia, hair loss from areas of skin normally producing hair, can be limited to one area or scattered over the scalp, and can be complete or leave residual hairs of differing lengths.

The three main causes of hair loss are tinea capitis, traumatic alopecia, and alopecia areata (Table 36-11).

TINEA CAPITIS

Description

Ringworm of the scalp and hair may be seen in four different manifestations: (1) diffuse fine scaling without obvious hair breaks and with subtle to significant hair loss; (2) discrete areas of hair loss with stubs of broken hairs (black-dot ringworm) (see Color Plate); (3) "classic" patchy hair loss and scaly lesions with raised borders; and (4) scaly, pustular lesions, or kerions. Tinea capitis occurs in a noninflammatory stage for 2 to 8 weeks, then becomes inflammatory.

Epidemiology

The fungus invades the scalp and hair shaft, causing an inflammatory response and fragile hair shaft. *T. tonsurans* is the causative organism 90% to 95% of the time, and the infection is near

---

TABLE 36-11 **Diagnosis and Treatment of Alopecia**

	Etiology	Clinical Findings	Treatment
Tinea capitis	*Trichophyton tonsurans* 90%-95% *Microsporum canis*; others	Fine diffuse scaling without obvious hair breaks and subtle to significant hair loss; hair loss discrete with stubs of broken hair; patchy hair loss with scaling and raised borders to lesions; scaly, pustular lesions or kerions	Griseofulvin taken with fatty food until 2 weeks after negative culture; monitor CBC, LFTs, renal function at 4 weeks and every 4-8 weeks; prednisone if kerion present; culture family members; sporicidal shampoo; keep from school 1 week; follow-up in 2 weeks; launder sheets, clothes, vacuum house
Traumatic alopecia	Chemical, thermal, traction (hairstyling), friction (trichotillomania)	*Traumatic*: incomplete hair loss with varying lengths *Traction*: erythema and pustules, thins and breaks in certain areas, especially linear *Trichotillomania*: circumscribed hair loss with irregular borders and broken hair of varied lengths, no erythema or scarring, especially frontal, parietal, or temporal	*Traction*: avoid hairstyles that precipitate; mild shampoo, gentle brushing; short course of antibiotics if pustules *Trichotillomania*: discussion with parents, oil at night, counseling if entrenched, other interventions if significant
Alopecia areata	Autoimmune mechanism	Family history; single or multiple round or oval patches of complete or near-complete hair loss; no erythema or scaling, scalp smooth with fine new hair growth, usually frontal or parietal; "exclamation hairs" present; nail ridging or pitting; occasional loss of body or pubic hair	Discussion and support; often self-limited course; if extensive, refer to dermatologist for alternative treatments; supportive care—prescription for wig, refer to National Alopecia Foundation

CBC, Complete blood count; *LFTs*, liver function tests.

epidemic in the U.S., but *Microsporum canis* or other species can be responsible (Jenson & Baltimore, 2006). Tinea capitis is transmitted by fomites when humans share hats, combs, and brushes, or by cats, dogs, or rodents. Tinea capitis is the most common dermatophyte infection of children, 3 to 7 years old, in the U.S. (Connelly & Friedlander, 2006; Paller & Mancini, 2006). It is more common in boys than in girls and in black children.

Clinical Findings

History.   Hair loss, itching, and contact with another person or pet with ringworm are sometimes reported.

Physical Examination.   Findings include the following:
- Scaling, erythema, or crusting usually occurs.
- Bald patches or areas of broken hairs are noted.
- Occipital or posterior cervical adenopathy may be significant.
  - *Microsporum* species leaves the hair broken and lusterless with a fine gray scale on the scalp.
  - *T. tonsurans* manifests as black-dot tinea, with tiny black dots that are the remainder of hair that has broken off at the shaft; no scalp scale is present (most common).
- A boggy, inflamed mass filled with pustules (kerion) is a delayed allergy reaction; cervical lymphadenopathy, fever, and leukocytosis may be present.
- The inflammatory stage is noted by widespread pustules, suppuration, and kerion formation.

Diagnostic Studies.   Examine hair scrapings as follows:
- Wood's light fluoresces yellow-green (positive with *M. canis*, negative with *T. tonsurans*).
- KOH examination of scraped hair: Wait 20 to 40 minutes after application of KOH to examine. If Wood's light was positive, under microscopy the KOH-prepared outer surface of hair is coated with tiny mats of spores; if Wood's light was negative, hyphae and spores are present in hair shaft.
- Fungal culture of a completely plucked hair with its root (use a Kelly clamp) is most reliable. The color change in DTM-plated fungal culture plates may begin within 24 to 48 hours if the dermatophytes are fast growing. Evaluate for color generally in 3 to 7 days, the usual time frame for a positive culture; do not evaluate for a color change after 10 days because contaminant fungal growth is then an issue and causes a false-positive result.

Differential Diagnosis

Traumatic alopecia, alopecia areata, hypothyroid and hyperthyroid hair loss, seborrhea, atopic dermatitis, psoriasis, impetigo, and folliculitis are included in the differential diagnosis.

Management

The following steps are taken:
- Griseofulvin ultramicrosize at 10 to 15 mg/kg/day or griseofulvin microsize at 20 to 25 mg/kg/day for 6 to 8 weeks; taken with fatty food, such as ice cream, to enhance absorption. Treatment should be continued until clinical and mycologic cure; however, if more than 8 weeks of therapy are needed, laboratory monitoring is required. Griseofulvin continues to be the "gold standard" (Connelly & Friedlander, 2006; Paller & Mancini, 2006). Topical antifungals are ineffective.

- In addition to griseofulvin therapy, concomitant shampooing with selenium sulfide 2.5% or econazole or ketoconazole 2% (two to three times per week for 4 weeks) decreases spore viability and keeps other household members from being infected.
- Terbinafine (Lamisil) is not approved by the FDA for this indication. However, some studies have been done in children showing it to be effective for resistant cases. See Table 36-4 for dosing.
- If a long-standing kerion with severe inflammation is present, prednisone 1 to 2 mg/kg/day for 5 to 14 days. Antibiotic treatment is not indicated.
- Family members and pets should be checked for infection by fungal culture and treated if positive. More than 50% are positive (Weston et al, 2007), so do not rely on lack of symptoms. Asymptomatic carriers are common.
- Child should be kept out of school for 1 week.
- A follow-up visit should be scheduled after 2 weeks to evaluate response to treatment. Medication should be continued until 2 weeks after culture is negative. Follow-up should be continued every 2 to 4 weeks until new hair growth is evident.
- Monitoring of CBC, LFTs, and possibly renal function tests is recommended at 8 weeks and every 4 to 8 weeks thereafter if griseofulvin is to be continued.
- If resistance to griseofulvin is encountered, oral itraconazole, terbinafine, fluconazole, and ketoconazole have been used, but are not all approved for use in children under 18 years old.

Complications

An "id" reaction is a hypersensitivity reaction to the fungus, not to the medication with which it is being treated. It manifests either as a red, superficial edema or as scaly, red plaques and papules on the scalp and is treated with 1 to 2 weeks of topical or systemic steroids. Permanent hair loss and scarring can occur with an untreated kerion.

Patient Education and Prevention

- Sites and modes of transmission are identified (*M. canis*, animal source; *T. tonsurans*, human source) and treated.
- Side effects of medication should be explained and monitored; griseofulvin typically may result in gastrointestinal disturbances, photosensitivity, skin eruptions, and headache.
- Hair regrowth is slow (3 to 12 months), and, if a kerion was present, hair loss can be permanent.
- Laundering sheets and clothes in a hot-water wash or hot dryer cycle and vacuuming may decrease spread in the family.
- Grooming practices (e.g., hair traction, greasy pomades, infrequent shampooing) may be predisposing factors.
- There is a high rate of asymptomatic carriers; culture is the only definitive means of identification.

TRAUMATIC ALOPECIA

Description

Traumatic hair loss can be due to chemical or thermal traction or friction. The most common forms are traction alopecia and trichotillomania. Trichotillomania is considered a behavior disorder.

Epidemiology

Traction alopecia, commonly seen in black females, is due to hair styling. Common causes are cornrows, ponytails, or braids; tight curlers; or excessive brushing.

Trichotillomania (TTM) is a common disorder seen in children of all ages after infancy. The pattern of hair loss is varied and is caused by repeated pulling and/or excessive twisting of hair with fracturing of the longer hair shafts. Current research indicates etiology is multifactorial, looking at genetic predisposition along with environmental and behavioral variables working together to result in TTM. In preschoolers, it is associated with habitual behaviors and situational stress. It is often seen in children with other obsessive-compulsive habits, such as thumb sucking or nail biting. TTM is classified as an impulse control disorder in the *Diagnostic and Statistical Manual of Mental Disorders*, Fourth Edition (DSM-IV) (Whitaker et al, 2003).

Clinical Findings

History. The history can include the following:
- Various methods of hair styling with tight pull on hair
- Habits, such as nail biting, finger sucking, or hair twirling
- Any recent life changes or stressors
- Medications (anticonvulsants, antithyroids, beta blockers, isotretinoin, lithium, oral contraceptives, vitamin A supplements, warfarin)
- Excess time spent lying in supine position

Physical Examination. The following findings are present:
- Traumatic alopecia
  - Incomplete hair loss with hair of varying lengths
- Traction alopecia
  - Possible erythema and pustules
  - Thinning and breaking in certain areas, tending to occur in a linear pattern related to hairstyle
- TTM
  - Circumscribed hair loss with irregular borders and broken hairs of varied length
  - No erythema or scaling of the scalp
  - Commonly found on frontal eyelashes, parietal, and temporal areas with peripheral sparing, but also eyebrows

Differential Diagnosis

The differential diagnosis includes tinea capitis, alopecia areata, neonatal occipital alopecia, and child abuse (make sure no one but the child is pulling out the hair).

Management

The following steps are taken:
1. Traction alopecia:
   - Avoid any hairstyle or device that causes traction on the hair, including cornrows, ponytails, braids, and curlers.
   - Use only mild shampoo, shampoo infrequently, use wide-toothed combs with rounded ends, and brush gently.
   - A short course of antibiotics is prescribed if pustules are present.

2. TTM:
   - A straightforward discussion and ongoing support of the child and parents are essential. In very young children, TTM is usually benign and resolves spontaneously. Older children and adolescents, however, may require individual and family therapy. Attempt to find means to relieve stress and cope with any traumatic events. The following strategies may be helpful (Thomson, 2002):
     - Helping hands—using the hands "together to solve the problem you used to have"; as one hand lifts, the other gives it a pat for not pulling.
     - Mirroring—the child imagines seeing himself or herself as he or she would like to, noting feelings of pride at the image, enforcing determination to control habit.
   - Applying oil to the hair at night makes it slippery and harder to pull.
   - Medication, behavior therapy, habit reversal, relaxation, and hypnosis are modalities sometimes used.

Complications

Trichobezoars (hairballs) in the child with TTM can cause gastrointestinal symptoms. Some children with TTM have extensive psychopathologic conditions.

Patient Education and Prevention

The cause of the hair loss must be discussed and support offered to resolve issues. New hair growth can take 3 to 6 months.

ALOPECIA AREATA

Description

Alopecia areata is an asymptomatic, complete hair loss occurring primarily in frontal or parietal areas (Fig. 36-6).

Epidemiology

The cause of alopecia areata is unknown, but is thought to be an autoimmune mechanism. It is unusual under 2 years old, but can be seen anytime throughout childhood, with 24% to 50% experiencing their first episode before 16 years old. There is a 10% to 42% (8% to 52%) familial occurrence (Paller & Mancini, 2006; Weston et al, 2007).

Clinical Findings

History. The history can include other family members with alopecia areata.

Physical Examination Findings include the following:
- Single or multiple (up to three) round or oval patches of complete or nearly complete hair loss without erythema or scaling. Scalp is smooth with fine new hair growth.
- The frontal and parietal areas are involved 90% of the time.
- "Exclamation hairs" are narrower at the base, short, and broken off.
- Nail ridging or pitting (a helpful distinguishing factor).
- Occasional loss of body or pubic hair, or eyelashes or eyebrows.
- Possible atopic dermatitis or vitiligo.

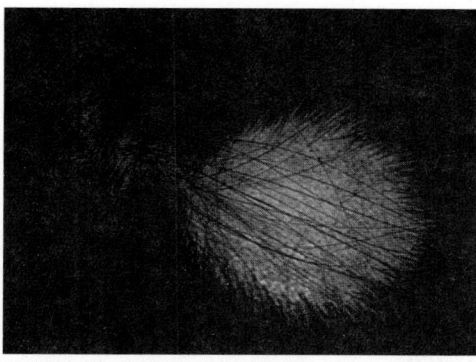

FIG. 36-6 Alopecia areata with sharply defined oval patches of hair loss. (From Hurwitz S: *Clinical pediatric dermatology,* ed 2, Philadelphia, 1993, WB Saunders, p 486.)

Diagnostic Studies. The following are sometimes performed:

- KOH examination or fungal culture to rule out tinea
- Skin biopsy
- Thyroid screening because it can be associated with auto-immune thyroiditis

Differential Diagnosis

Tinea capitis versus traumatic alopecia is the differential diagnosis.

Management

No pharmacologic intervention for this condition has proved helpful. The following steps should be taken:

The most commonly used therapy consists of topical corticosteroids alone or under occlusion (i.e., wig). Intermittent pulse therapy should be used to prevent atrophy and systemic absorption (Paller & Mancini, 2006). Other therapies include topical minoxidil solution, short contact anthralin, and topical immunotherapy (Habif, 2004).

- Open discussion and support of the child and parents. If only one or two patches are present, reassure that regrowth will occur.
- If extensive involvement, refer to a dermatologist for potential treatment options. These include potent topical steroids, intralesional steroids, minoxidil, anthralin, or contact sensitization.
- Recommend wearing a wig, depending on the severity of involvement; prescribing the wig as a medical treatment helps defray the cost (Habif, 2004). Locks of Love is an organization that provides hairpieces to financially disadvantaged children under 16 years old, and the National Alopecia Areata Foundation is a national support group for affected children and families (See Resource Box at the end of the chapter).

Complications

Self-esteem issues are common. *Ophiasis* is a form of alopecia areata that begins in the frontal or occipital hairline and spreads along the hair margins. *Alopecia totalis* is a loss of all the hair on the scalp. *Alopecia universalis* is a loss of all the hair on the body.

Patient Education, Prognosis, and Prevention

All families should be put in touch with the National Alopecia Areata Foundation (see Resource Box at the end of the chapter). The condition is self-limited in most school-age children and adolescents (Weston et al, 2007). Full recovery, often within 1 year, is more likely if three or fewer areas are involved and if onset is in late childhood. However, the greater the hair loss, the longer it takes for regrowth. Prognosis is guarded in infants and toddlers. Approximately one third of patients will have a recurrence within months to years, with a worsening prognosis with each episode.

ONYCHOMYCOSIS

Description

Onychomycosis is a fungal infection of the nail(s) typically with *T. rubrum* or *Candida* (Color Plate). When the nail infection is due to a dermatophyte, is it often called tinea unguium. One or two nails are often involved. The infection may be superficial, hypertrophic (onychauxic), or cause separation of the nail plate from the tissue (onycholytic).

Epidemiology

The infecting organism invades the nail, proliferates, and destroys the nail integrity, causing separation of the nail plate from the nail bed. The infection originates at the distal edge of the nail. It is uncommon during the first two decades of life, limited most commonly to adolescents and adults. When it occurs in children, there is often a concurrent tinea pedis or tinea manuum. There may be a relationship to the use of occlusive shoes. The causative organisms include *T. rubrum, T. mentagrophytes, E. floccosum,* and *C. albicans*. However, 50% of the time another condition is responsible for dystrophic nail.

Clinical Findings

History. The patient may report a thickened, discolored nail.

Physical Examination

- Opaque white or silvery nail that becomes thick, yellow, with subungual debris
- Toenails are involved more often than fingernails with tinea
- Fingernails are involved more often than toenails with *Candida*
- Seldom symmetric; it may be one to three nails on one extremity

Diagnostic Studies. KOH preparations and fungal cultures of the material under the nail are helpful in confirming the diagnosis.

Differential Diagnosis

Psoriasis (involves all nails and includes pitting), hereditary nail defects, dystrophy secondary to eczema or chronic paronychia, lichen planus, and trauma are the differential diagnoses.

Management

1. Successful treatment is difficult and requires oral medication. Griseofulvin can be used, but side effects, length of treatment, low cure rates, and high recurrence rates following treatment make successful management uncommon (Paller & Mancini, 2006).
2. Oral terbinafine, fluconazole, and itraconazole have a better short-term success rate than griseofulvin and a lower relapse rate.

3. Treatment recommendations for onychomycosis are based on the site of infection. Select one of the following options (Connelly & Friedlander, 2006):
   - Toenails
     ◦ Itraconazole 5 mg/kg/day for 12 weeks; see pulse dosing listed as #4.
     ◦ Terbinafine 4 to 6 mg/kg/day for 12 weeks.
     ◦ Griseofulvin 15 to 20 mg/kg/day (decrease dose if using ultramicronized form) for 6 to 18 months.
     ◦ Fluconazole 6 mg/kg/wk for 8 months.
   - Fingernails
     ◦ Itraconazole 5 mg/kg/day for 6 weeks; pulse dose listed as #4.
     ◦ Terbinafine 4 to 6 mg/kg/day for 6 weeks.
     ◦ Fluconazole 6 mg/kg/wk for 4 months.
4. Itraconazole pulse therapy—5 mg/kg/day orally for 1 week each month for 2 months for fingernails and the same dosage but for 3 months for toenails (Connelly & Friedlander, 2006).
5. Ciclopirox in nail lacquer (Penlac) used daily is a new agent that has high cure rates in adults, but has not been studied in children. It has been used as monotherapy and adjunctive therapy (Paller & Mancini, 2006).
6. If triazoles are used, a careful review of current medications must be taken because there are many interactions. Monitoring of CBC and hepatic function is recommended at onset of therapy and every 4 to 6 weeks.
7. *Candida* infection is treated with topical application of ketoconazole (Nizoral) under occlusion (plastic glove covered by a cotton sock at bedtime) for 3 to 4 weeks.
8. Follow-up visits at 1-month intervals to monitor laboratory values are recommended; long-term follow-up every 6 months is suggested.

Patient Education, Prognosis, and Prevention

The unfortunate truth to communicate is that cure is difficult to obtain, and relapse is common.

PARONYCHIA

Description

Chronic or acute inflammation and infection around a fingernail or toenail is called *paronychia*.

Epidemiology

Paronychia is a common disorder seen in childhood and adolescence and is caused by an infection of a nail with bacteria (often *S. aureus*, occasionally *Streptococcus* or *Pseudomonas*), *Candida* (in infants with thrush or thumb sucking or when hands are frequently immersed in water), or herpes. It is more common with tight shoes or when nails are malaligned, cut with rounded edges, or too short.

Clinical Findings

History. Tenderness and drainage are reported and discomfort, especially with walking.

Physical Examination. Findings include the following:
- Proximal nail fold erythematous, swollen, and tender; if chronic, may not be tender

- Purulent exudate expressed
- Cuticle broken or absent
- Nontender erythema and edema with thickened, disrupted nail (*Candida* infection, often with secondary bacterial infection)

Diagnostic Studies. A culture of the exudate is occasionally done.

Differential Diagnosis

Herpetic whitlow (grouped vesicles on an erythematous base) and eczematous inflammation should be ruled out.

Management

Management includes the following:
- Systemic oral antibiotic if acute infection; coverage for staphylococcal infection may be required.
- If *Candida* is suspected, nystatin cream under occlusion (a plastic glove covered by a cotton stocking) every night for 3 to 4 weeks.
- If purulent area is full, loosen cuticle from nail with a no. 11 blade to allow exudate to escape.
- Frequent warm soaks, after which cotton pledgets are inserted beneath the nail to lift it up.
- Instruction on proper trimming of nails and care of toenails:
  ◦ Wear wide-toed shoes.
  ◦ Trim nails straight across and not too short.
  ◦ If condition is recurrent, refer for surgical removal of lateral portion of nail.
- Follow-up visit in 1 month.

Complications

Recurrent infection is possible.

▬ BODY ART

TATTOOS AND BODY PIERCING

Description

A tattoo is an indelible mark fixed on the body by insertion of pigment under the skin. Body piercing is the creation of a hole anywhere in the body (typically the ear, eyebrow, lip, naris, tongue, navel, nipple, or genitalia) to insert jewelry. Both tattoos and piercing are considered forms of *body art*, or embellishment of one's appearance, that have been practiced throughout the ages in many cultures as rites of passage, as means of showing status or membership in a particular group, or as proof of virility.

Epidemiology

A tattoo is accomplished by injection of an insoluble ink via a uniform series of punctures into the dermal layer of the skin. Piercing is accomplished by inserting a sharp implement through the skin. Most tattoos or piercings are done in unregulated, unlicensed tattoo parlors, although some adolescents may tattoo or pierce themselves or their peers. Some states have legislation preventing tattooing of minors in tattoo parlors or requiring parental consent.

Adolescents obtain tattoos for any number of reasons including making a personal statement, seeing it as a form of art or a fashion statement, or wishing to be daring. Piercing is considered less permanent than a tattoo. Adults and parents may see piercing or tattooing as a deviant behavior, a strange new trend, a fetish, a fad, or a fashion.

Both tattooing and piercing have an increased incidence in the U.S., especially in the adolescent population. (Carroll et al, 2002). A study by Carroll and colleagues (2002) surveying 484 teenagers found that 10% to 13% of adolescents 12 to 18 years old have tattoos. Teens who participate in piercing, tattooing, and branding were also more likely to engage in other risk-taking behaviors, such as eating disorders, drug use, increased sexual activity, and suicide. Of note, as the number of body piercings increased, the use of drugs increased.

Clinical Findings

History. Questions to discuss include the following:
- When and where was the body art obtained?
- Where is it located, and what care is being given?
- Were there any complications?

Physical Examination. Any symptoms of infection—erythema, crusting, or scabs?

Differential Diagnosis

Branding, the burning of the skin aimed at creating a permanent scar in a desired design via blowtorch or wire coat hanger in hot oil, is one differential diagnosis. *Self-mutilation*, a self-directed violence that ranges from altering physical appearance (e.g., ear piercing) to extreme forms (e.g., amputation), is another consideration. Some forms are considered normal, but deviant forms are physically damaging, done in response to crisis, and demonstrate disconnectedness and alienation from others.

Management

1. Aftercare for tattoos:
   - Perform basic wound care, including not touching for 24 hours.
   - A moderate amount of oozing and local swelling is normal for 48 hours.
   - Scab should be left alone except for the application of ointment.
   - Protect from rough surfaces that can traumatize; protect from sunburn.
   - Review signs and symptoms of infection.
2. Aftercare for body piercings (Table 36-12):
   - Wash hands before touching; wash area with soap twice daily.
   - A moderate amount of oozing and swelling is normal; if crusts appear, remove with wet swab.
   - Tongue:
     ◦ Use ice to minimize swelling.
     ◦ Rinse mouth ten to twelve times a day with half-strength Listerine, twice a day with carbamide peroxide (Gly-Oxide).
     ◦ No deep kissing for 48 hours; once healed, use dental dams for dental work and avoid smoking.
   - Navel:
     ◦ Slowest to heal, most likely area to reject jewelry.

TABLE 36-12 Healing Time for Body Piercings

Type of Piercing	Time to Heal
Cheek	2-4 months
Clitoris	4-10 weeks
Ear cartilage	2 months-1 years
Ear lobe	6-8 weeks
Eyebrow	6-8 weeks
Frenum (underneath tongue)	2-6 months
Inner labia	4-8 weeks
Lip	2-3 months
Male genitalia	4 weeks-6 months
Nasal septum	6-8 months
Nasal bridge	8-10 weeks
Navel	2 months-1 year
Nipple	2-6 months
Nostril	2 months-1 year
Outer labia	2-4 months
Tongue	4-6 weeks

Data from Martel S, Anderson JE: Decorating the "human canvas": body art and your patient, *Contemp Pediatr* 19(8):86-102, 2002; Schnare SM: Tattooing, branding, and body piercing, *Womens Health Care* 1(4), 2002.

  ◦ Cleanse twice a day with antibacterial soap.
  ◦ Avoid handling; avoid clothing that rubs for up to 1 year.
   - Nipples and genitalia:
     ◦ Cleanse twice a day with antibacterial soap twice a day.
     ◦ Avoid manipulation and tight garments; cotton clothes are ideal.
     ◦ Latex barriers must be used with sexual activity.
3. Healing times are variable and should be considered. A tattoo may take 2 to 3 weeks to heal. Body piercing, depending on the site, can take from 4 to 8 weeks for ears to 6 to 12 months for navel and genital piercings.
4. Infection can be treated with dicloxacillin 500 mg four times a day for 10 days. Whether or not to remove jewelry should be decided by whether it will provide a source of chronic drainage, become an obstacle to healing, or be an ongoing source of infection.
5. Screen for high-risk behaviors.
6. Discuss the need to remove dangling ornaments during contact sports.

Complications

The most common complications of tattooing or body piercing include infections, allergic reactions to the dyes or jewelry, and the transmission of blood-borne diseases, primarily hepatitis B and C, and, potentially, HIV. Other reported complications of tattoos include skin neoplasms, syphilis, leprosy, cutaneous tuberculosis, tetanus, hyperplasia, and granuloma annulare. Complications of piercings also include excessive bleeding, nerve damage, keloids, dental fracture, soft tissue damage, and speech impediments.

Patient Education, Prognosis, and Prevention

Providing information and encouraging teenagers to thoroughly research and consider the idea of getting a tattoo or body piercing is an important area of education. Removal of tattoos is expensive, not necessarily completely successful, and fraught with complication (scarring, rashes). Box 36-13 is a helpful handout that covers much of the important information to be discussed. Maintaining an open, nonjudgmental attitude in discussing the options and in caring for adolescents who have body art is also essential. Alternatives to discuss include temporary stick-on tattoos and use of henna or other body paints (Montgomery & Parks, 2001).

BOX 36-13   So You're Thinking About Getting a Tattoo or Body Piercing

Know the Facts: Make an Informed Decision

Unsterile tattooing and piercing equipment and needles can spread serious infections, hepatitis, or possibly even HIV.

The law in many states prohibits the tattooing of minors.

Asking a friend to apply a tattoo may ruin a friendship if the tattoo does not look like you thought it would.

Tattoos and permanent makeup are not easily removed and in some cases may cause permanent discoloration. Think carefully before getting a tattoo.

Tattoo removal is very expensive. A tattoo that costs $50 to apply may cost more than $1000 to remove.

Blood donations cannot be made for 1 year after getting a tattoo, body piercing, or permanent makeup.

Before You Get a Tattoo or Body Piercing

First: Talk to your friends or others who have been tattooed or pierced.

   Ask them about their experience, the cost, pain, healing time, and so on.

   Ask them what they would do if they had a chance to do it over again.

   Read "Can I get HIV from getting a tattoo or through body piercing" from the CDC (access at www.cdc.gov/hiv/resources/qa/qa27.htm).

Second: Understand that you do not have to tattoo or pierce your body to belong.

   Remember that you are directly involved in decisions that affect your health and body.

   You can always change your mind or wait if you are not sure.

Third: Because of potential complications, if you decide to get a tattoo or body piercing, never tattoo or pierce your own body or let a friend do it.

Health Risks to Consider Before You Act

Both tattooing and piercing involve puncturing the skin to introduce a foreign material, jewelry, or ink, and the procedures carry similar risks. The primary health concern is introducing blood-borne germs or viruses into your body.

Blood-borne illnesses, such as hepatitis B and C, tetanus, tuberculosis, and HIV infection, can lead to serious health problems or death.

Make sure you have had the three series hepatitis B vaccination and a tetanus booster within 10 years.

Localized infections, such as *Staphylococcus* or *Pseudomonas* infection, can lead to illness, deformity, and scarring.

Tattoo troubles: Tattoos are open wounds that may become infected. The new tattoo must be kept clean. It must also be kept moist with an ointment to prevent a scab from forming. If you are allergic to the inks in the tattoo, the site will not heal properly and scarring may occur.

Piercing problems: Complications depend on where the body has been pierced. Navel infections are the most common; it takes approximately 1 year for navel piercings to heal. Ear cartilage heals slowly. Tongue piercings may lead to tooth and enamel damage from biting on the jewelry and jewelry knocking against a tooth, partial paralysis if the jewelry pierces a nerve, and extreme inflammation during the first few days.

Selecting a Tattoo Artist or Piercer

Visit several piercers or tattooists. The work area should be kept clean and have good lighting. If they refuse to discuss cleanliness and infection control with you, go somewhere else.

Consent forms (which the customer must fill out) should be handled before tattooing. Reputable piercing and tattoo studios will not serve a minor without signed consent from parents. Check the laws in your state about tattooing of minors if you are under 18 years old.

The tattooist or piercer should have an *autoclave*—a heat sterilization machine used to sterilize equipment between customers.

Packaged, sterilized needles should be used only once and then disposed of in a biohazard container.

Immediately before tattooing or piercing, the tattooist or piercer should wash and dry his or her hands and wear latex gloves. These gloves should be worn at all times during the tattoo or piercing procedure. If the tattoo artist or piercer leaves the procedure or touches other objects, such as the telephone, new gloves should be put on before the procedure continues.

A piercing gun should not be used because it cannot be sterilized properly. Only jewelry made of a noncorrosive metal, such as surgical stainless steel, niobium, or solid 14-karat gold, is safe for a new piercing.

Leftover tattoo ink should be disposed of after each procedure. Ink should never be poured back into the bottle and reused.

CDC, Centers for disease control and prevention.
From Barbara Freyenberger in Armstrong ML, Murphy KP: Adolescent tattooing, *Prev Researcher* 5(3):1-4, 1998.

RESOURCE BOX

Dermatoogic Conditions

American Academy of Dermatology
www.aad.org

Coppertone
www.coppertone.com
Better Summer 101
An excellent resource for parents about sun protection for the child.

Association of Professional Piercers
www.safepiercing.com

Dermatology Image Atlas
www.dermatlas.org
An interactive clinical and histologic dermatology atlas that has physical findings. Edited by Drs. Bernard Cohen and Christoph Lehmann, Johns Hopkins University School of Medicine

Dermatology Online Journal
http://dermatology.cdlib.org/
Printed journal format with editorials, articles, case reports, and original articles

Electronic Textbook of Dermatology
www.telemedicine.org/stamford.htm

FIRST: Foundation for Ichthyosis and Related Skin Types
www.scalyskin.org
Newsletter, informational materials (including Spanish), networking, referrals to local resources, advocacy, funds research, maintains research registry

Locks of Love
www.locksoflove.org
An organization that provides hairpieces to financially disadvantaged children under 16 years old

Loyola University Dermatology
Medical Education Website
Extensive online image database of dermatologic lesions and diagnoses.
www.meddean.luc.edu/lumen/meded/medicine/dermatology/melton/atlas.htm

National Alopecia Areata Foundation
www.alopeciaareata.com
Newsletter, informational materials (including Spanish), networking, local chapters, advocacy, funds research

National Organization for Albinism and Hypopigmentation (NOAH)
www.albinism.org
Newsletter, informational materials, chapters, advocacy, research

National Pediculosis Association (NPA)
www.headlice.org

National Psoriasis Foundation
www.psoriasis.org
Newsletter, informational materials, networking, referrals to local resources, advocacy, funds research, maintains research registry

National Vitiligo Foundation, Inc.
www.nvfi.org

Nevus Network
www.nevusnetwork.org
Newsletter, informational materials (including Spanish, French), networking, funds research, maintains research registry

OC (Obsessive-Compulsive) Foundation
www.ocfoundation.org
Newsletter, informational materials, networking, referrals to local resources, advocacy, local chapters, funds research

Prevent Cancer Foundation
www.preventcancer.org

Skin Cancer Foundation
www.skincancer.org

Trichotillomania Learning Center, Inc.
www.trich.org

Trichotillomania: A Guide
www.miminc.org/guide_trich01.html

☑ DISCUSSION FORUM

1. What factors do you need to consider when prescribing topicals for skin disorder?
2. What techniques may be helpful in counseling families about caring for a child who has dermatologic problems?
3. There is an outbreak of lice in the community. What role can you play in helping to solve the problem?
4. A 13-year-old male comes for a well visit. He is doing well in school and is a star basketball player. Mom is very concerned about his acne and spends 5 minutes of the visit telling you how she had severe acne growing up. She does not want her son to get severe acne. On exam there are several small whiteheads on his forehead and a few blackheads on his nose. There are no pustules, nodules, or cysts. How severe is his acne? What would be your treatment? What else do you need to discuss with this family?
5. A 5-year-old with impetigo was placed on Keflex 2 days ago. The family reports compliance with the medication, but the impetigo is spreading. What is likely pathogen? How would you manage it?

REFERENCES

American Academy of Pediatrics (AAP): *2006 Red book: report of the Committee on Infectious Diseases*, ed 27, Elk Grove Village, IL, 2006, American Academy of Pediatrics.

American Academy of Pediatrics (AAP), Committee on Environmental Health: *Pediatric environmental health*, ed 2, Elk Grove Village, IL, 2003, American Academy of Pediatrics.

Armstrong ML, Murphy KP: Adolescent tattooing, *Prev Researcher* 5(3):1-4, 1998.

Baron J, Levine N: *Acanthosis nigricans*, updated Oct, 2006. Available at *www.emedicine.com* (accessed Dec 22, 2006).

Benjamin LT et al: Sun protection in the pediatric patient, In Burg FD et al, editors: *Current pediatric therapy*, ed 18, Philadelphia, 2006, Saunders Elsevier.

Browning J: Terra firma-forme dermatosis, *Clin Adv* 9(9):96, 2006.

Carroll ST et al: Tattoos and body piercings as indicators of adolescent risk-taking behaviors, *Pediatrics* 109(6):1021-1027, 2002.

Centers for Disease Control and Prevention (CDC): *Treating head lice*, 2002. Available at *www.dpd.cdc.gov/dpdx/html/headlice.htm* (accessed Nov 6, 2002).

Chamlin SL: Shedding light on moles, melanoma, and the sun, *Contemp Pediatr* 19(6):102-114, 2002.

Cohen BA: *Pediatric dermatology*, ed 3, Philadelphia, 2005, Elsevier Mosby.

Connelly EA, Friedlander SF: Fungal infections of the skin, hair, and nails. In Burg FD et al, editors: *Current pediatric therapy*, ed 18, Philadelphia, 2006, WB Saunders Elsevier.

Dalal I: Urticaria and angioedema. In Burg FD et al, editors: *Current pediatric therapy*, ed 18, Philadelphia, 2006, WB Saunders Elsevier.

Darmstadt GL, Sidbury R: The skin. In Behrman RE, Kliegman RM, Jenson HB, editors: *Nelson textbook of pediatrics*, ed 17, Philadelphia, 2004, WB Saunders.

Dasher DA, Morrell DS: Psoriasis and other papulosquamous disorders. In Burg FD et al, editors: *Current pediatric therapy*, ed 18, Philadelphia, 2006, WB Saunders Elsevier.

Ghali FE: Allergic contact dermatitis. In Burg FD et al, editors: *Current pediatric therapy*, ed 18, Philadelphia, 2006, WB Saunders Elsevier.

Glanz K, Saraiya M, Wechsler H: Guidelines for school programs to prevent skin cancer, *MMWR Morb Mortal Wkly Rep* 51(RR04):1-16, 2002.

Goates BM et al: An effective nonchemical treatment for head lice: a lot of hot air, *Pediatrics* 118(5):1962-1970, 2006.

Habif T: *Clinical dermatology*, ed 4, Philadelphia, 2004, Mosby.

Jenson HB, Baltimore RS: Infectious diseases. In Kliegman RM et al, editors: *Nelson essentials of pediatrics*, ed 5, Philadelphia, 2006, WB Saunders Elsevier.

Lembo R: Dermatology. In Kliegman RM et al, editors: *Nelson essentials of pediatrics*, ed 5, Philadelphia, 2006, WB Saunders Elsevier.

Mikula C: Balneo phototherapy for psoriasis: modern application of an age-old treatment, *Adv Nurse Pract* 11(1):53-56, 2003.

Montgomery DF, Parks D: Tattoos: counseling the adolescent, *J Pediatr Health Care* 15(1):14-19, 2001.

Myers MG, Stanberry LR, Seward JF: Varicella-zoster virus. In Behrman RG, Kliegman RM, Jenson HB, editors: *Nelson textbook of pediatrics*, ed 17, Philadelphia, 2004, WB Saunders.

The National Pediculosis Association: *AAP issues guidelines allowing children in school with lice and nits*, 2002a. Available at *www.headlice.org/news/aapresponse.htm* (accessed Oct 30, 2002).

The National Pediculosis Association: *Lindane educations research network*, 2002b. Available at *www.headlice.org/lindane/index.htm* (accessed Oct 30, 2002).

Paller AS, Mancini AJ: *Hurwitz clinical pediatric dermatology: a textbook of skin disorders of children and adolescence*, ed 3, Philadelphia, 2006, Elsevier.

Paller A: Dermatologic problems. In Dershewitz RA, editor: *Ambulatory pediatric care*, ed 3, Philadelphia, 1999, Lippincott Raven.

Pollack RJ, Kiszewski A, Spielman A: Overdiagnosis and consequent mismanagement of head louse infestations in North America, *Pediatr Infect Dis J* 19:689-693, 2000.

Schachner L, Hansen R: *Pediatric dermatology*, ed 3, Philadelphia, 2003, Mosby.

Sidbury R: Acne vulgaris. In Burg FD et al, editors: *Current pediatric therapy*, ed 18, Philadelphia, 2006, WB Saunders Elsevier.

Spray A, Siegfried E: Dermatologic toxicology in children, *Pediatr Ann* 30(4):197-202, 2001.

Stein SL: Erythema multiforme. In Burg FD et al, editors: *Current pediatric therapy*, ed 18, Philadelphia, 2006, WB Saunders Elsevier.

Thomson L: Hypnosis for habit disorders, *Adv Nurse Pract* 10(7):59-62, 2002.

Weinberg S: Secondary infection often occurs with diaper dermatitis, *Infect Dis J* 11:42-43, 1998.

Weston WL, Lane AT, Morelli JG: *Color textbook of pediatric dermatology*, ed 4, St Louis, 2007, Mosby.

Whitaker H, Wolf KA, Keuthen N: Chronic hair pulling: recognizing trichotillomania, *Clin Rev* 13(3):37-44, 2003.

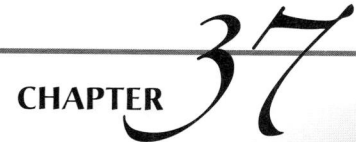

Musculoskeletal Disorders

Jan Bazner-Chandler and Margaret A. Brady

Orthopedic conditions in children are disruptions to the major structural system of the body. A variety of conditions can cause orthopedic findings, including child abuse, trauma, rheumatoid, genetic, hematologic, and bone or muscle conditions. Iatrogenic deformities that result from cultural practices, such as using a cradleboard or from in utero packing problems, can also cause deformities. Disorders of the musculoskeletal system present unique problems because growth and development of this system contribute to the evolution of pathologic conditions over time. For example, untreated developmental dysplasia of the hip (DDH) results in derangement of the hip socket with limping and eventual wearing away of the femoral head. Limited mobility, pain, and deformity interfere with the lifestyle of the child. Children with functional disabilities may not be able to fully participate in all activities with peers and family or have access to various occupations. They may also face challenges related to self-esteem. Primary care providers must be vigilant and seek to help children and their families prevent these problems.

Primary care providers play a significant role in the management of children with orthopedic problems, although, in many cases, specialists manage specific conditions. The primary provider assesses development of the musculoskeletal system, identifies problems for early intervention, focuses on lifestyle and injury prevention, and monitors the long-term outcomes of orthopedic care. When necessary, primary care providers help families to integrate orthopedic care within the daily living activities at home and school. Assisting families to cope with the issues of disability, deformity, and long-term care is another important role that must be addressed in the care of these children.

ANATOMY AND PHYSIOLOGY

Development of the skeletal system begins around the fourth week of gestation, with ossification of the fetal skeleton beginning during the fifth month of gestation. The clavicles and skull bones are the first to ossify, followed by the long bones and spine. The epiphyses of the newborn's long bones are composed of hyaline cartilage. Soon after birth, the cartilage along the epiphyseal plate begins secondary ossification. The shape of the spine also changes from a C shape at birth to a double S curve by late adolescence. As the child starts to walk, the lumbar curve develops. The sacrum starts out as five separate bones at birth only to become fused as one large bone by 18 to 20 years old (Duderstadt & Schapiro, 2006).

Bone age, measured by radiographs of the left hand and wrist, can be used to quantitatively determine somatic maturation and serves as a mirror that reflects the tempo of growth. In adolescents, the skeletal growth spurt begins at about Tanner stage 2 in girls and Tanner stage 3 in boys. It is at its peak around stage 4 and then ends with stage 5. The growth spurt lasts longer in boys than in girls. The pelvis widens early in pubescent girls. In both sexes, the legs usually lengthen before the thighs broaden. Next, the shoulders widen, and the trunk completes its linear growth. Bone growth ends when the epiphyses close.

Long bones have a growth plate, or physis, at each end, which separates the epiphysis from the diaphysis or shaft. Openings through this plate allow blood vessels to penetrate from the epiphysis. In the growth plate, chondrocytes produce cartilage cells, dead cells are absorbed, and the calcified cartilage matrix is converted into bone. The entire growth plate area is weaker than the remaining bone because it is less calcified. Because the blood supply to the growth plate comes primarily through the epiphysis, damage to epiphyseal circulation can jeopardize the survival of the chondrocytes. If chondrocytes stop producing, growth of the bone in that area stops (Fig. 37-1).

There are two ways that children's bones grow. Longitudinal growth occurs in the ossification centers, whereas changes in bone width and strength take place via intramembranous ossification. The length of long bones comes from growth at the epiphyseal plates. The diameter of long bones increases as a result of deposition of new bone on the periosteal surface and resorption on the surface of the medullary cavity. Growth of the small bones, hip, and spine comes from one or more primary ossification centers in each bone. Apophyses are the sites for connection of tendons to bone. In children, these sites, similar to epiphyses, allow for growth and are weaker than bone. These sites can become inflamed with stress.

The development of bones and muscles is influenced by use. Thus, in infants and toddlers, the legs straighten and lengthen with the stimulus of weight bearing and independent walking. The infant is born with the full complement of muscle fibers. Growth in muscle length results from lengthening of the fibers, and growth in bulk comes from hypertrophy. Length of muscles is related to growth in length of the underlying bone. If a limb is not used, it grows minimally. Furthermore, if muscles and bones are not used in their intended normal manner, such as occurs with spastic diplegia, the forces for development tend to stimulate growth in abnormal patterns.

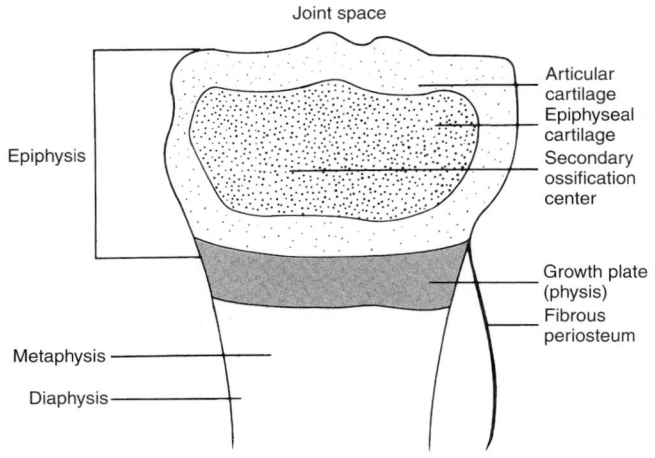

Joint space

Articular cartilage
Epiphyseal cartilage
Secondary ossification center

Epiphysis

Growth plate (physis)
Fibrous periosteum

Metaphysis

Diaphysis

FIG. 37-1 Anatomy of long bones. (Modified from Shapiro F: Epiphyseal disorders, *N Engl J Med* 317:1702-1710, 1987.)

Thus scoliosis can develop or bowlegs may increase in severity. Muscle contractures occur if muscles are not used regularly and put through their full range of motion. The growth of fibrous tissue, tendons, and ligaments is also dependent on mechanical demands.

Nutritional, mechanical, and hormonal factors during the growth process influence the thickness of bones and the health of the marrow. Adequate protein, calcium, and vitamin D in the diet are key nutritional elements that impact the growth and development of a child's musculoskeletal system.

The muscle structures originate from the embryonic mesoderm and include tendons, ligaments, cartilage, and joints. Muscle fibers are developed by the fourth or fifth month of gestation and grow in tangent with their respective bones. The rate of muscle growth (muscle mass and cell sizes) speeds up dramatically around 2 years old with girls exhibiting a greater rate of growth than boys until this gender trend is reversed at puberty (Duderstadt & Schapiro, 2006).

■ PATHOPHYSIOLOGY AND DEFENSE MECHANISMS
PATHOPHYSIOLOGY

Muscles and bones can be affected by localized or systemic problems. Thus the initial orthopedic problem can be symptomatic of a larger problem.

Systemic Problems

Systemic problems can include chronic conditions, such as hemophilia, sickle cell disease, and arthritic diseases; neurologic problems, such as cerebral palsy; and various cancers, including osteosarcomas and leukemias. Children with metabolic problems, such as vitamin D-resistant rickets, have bony deformities. Acute systemic problems can also affect the musculoskeletal system. For example, viruses and bacteria can infect joints and bones. In developing countries, tubercular infections of bones are common and devastating. Thus the pediatric provider must assess patients from a broad perspective,

asking questions about other body systems and ordering appropriate laboratory studies that might identify systemic problems.

Genetic Problems

Many genetic problems have an orthopedic component. For example, osteogenesis imperfecta is a genetically based orthopedic condition known for multiple fractures. Children with Down syndrome are more likely to have hip problems. Children with Marfan syndrome have defective connective tissue, have disproportionately long limbs, and may develop scoliosis or dislocate a patella. Severe scoliosis may develop in children with neurofibromatosis. Mucopolysaccharidosis disorders and other syndromes, such as Turner and Noonan, can result in affected children having short stature.

Many orthopedic problems have a multifactorial inheritance pattern. Thus, if one child in a family has a dislocated hip or scoliosis, the risks increase for other children. The pediatric provider needs to understand the genetic disorder to monitor related orthopedic problems, consider the genetic implications, and provide families with appropriate genetic information or refer them for genetic counseling (see Chapter 40).

Uterine Packing Deformations

The developing fetus moves its body parts frequently, and this movement influences musculoskeletal development. When the baby fills the uterine space, movements are restricted and body parts begin to assume the shape in which they are fixed. With in utero positioning, joints and muscle contractions can develop and are considered generally physiologic in nature. Torsional and angular alignment issues can affect the long bones, most commonly those of the lower extremities. Because much of the bony structure is cartilaginous, molding occurs with relative ease. Thus, in normal newborns, the tibias are normally bowed, and the hips have a 20- to 30-degree flexion (Thompson, 2006). Occasionally, a foot is turned awkwardly, the legs might be fixed straight up with the feet near the ears, or the neck may be tipped to one side. Such positioning issues are outside the range of normal. The outcomes are deformities in various degrees. The longer the position is maintained, the more severe the problems are. In general, there is a tendency for bowing and late deformations to straighten; however, the effects related to in utero positioning may not fully abate until the child is 3 to 4 years old. More severe deformities (i.e., those significantly outside the range of normal) need to be referred to orthopedists for treatment as soon as they are found because a softer skeleton is easier to realign in a positive direction.

Injuries

Ligamentous injuries can produce joint instability. Unstable joints should always be referred to an orthopedist. The most common injuries to muscles produce bleeding in the muscle, at the muscle-tendon junctions, or at tendon insertion points.

Muscle hematomas generally heal in 3 weeks, but significant muscle bleeding can lead to scarring. Injuries sufficient to produce significant soft tissue damage also can damage the underlying bone.

Trauma to the bone can cause a fracture, dislocation of the epiphysis (an orthopedic emergency), or damage to the periosteum covering the bone, with bleeding in the space between the two tissues. The effects of fractures through the growth plates of long bones are discussed later in this chapter. Fractures that are misaligned generally have related soft tissue damage. Damage to the nerves and vascular supply must be carefully assessed. Management of traumatic injuries is discussed in Chapter 39.

The possibility of child abuse should always be considered when orthopedic injuries, especially fractures, are present. The rule of thumb is that the injury history should match the appearance of the problem and be consistent with the child's developmental capabilities. Certain injuries, such as spiral fractures of the long bones, are especially suspect because few independent activities of the child can produce these injuries. They occur with wrenching motions, such as when a child's arm or leg has been jerked. Multiple fractures in various stages of healing must be considered evidence of child abuse until proved otherwise. In contrast to intentionally inflicted injuries associated with fracturing, toddler fractures are typically accidental spiral fractures of the distal one third of the tibia and are often the result of a simple fall associated with running or playing or stepping on an object on the floor. This type of accidental injury occurs in the 2- to 4-year-old child, occasionally up to 6 years old (Thompson, 2004a).

DEFENSE MECHANISMS

Fracture Healing

The lower ash content and greater porosity of young bones allows children's bones to tolerate more energy before deformation and fractures occur than adult bones can tolerate. When fractures occur, they heal by the creation of a callus at the fracture site (Thompson, 2006). The healing process is the same in children as in adults. However, children produce callus more quickly and in greater amounts than adults do. Likewise, young children heal faster because of their growth potential and thicker, more metabolically active periosteum. When the fracture occurs, there is damage to the blood vessels, destruction of bone matrix, and death of bone cells adjoining the fracture site. The body reabsorbs the clot and dead cells, and the periosteum responds by producing new fibroblasts that invade the fracture site. Immature bone is formed with irregular trabeculae, creating the callus. Normal stresses then cause the bone to remodel into the optimal shape, and the callus bone is gradually replaced by lamellar bone.

Growth Plate Fractures. Fractures of the long bones can produce permanent deformities in children if the fracture occurs through the growth plate. The outcomes depend on the fracture location and type, the age of the child, the status of the blood supply to the physis, and the treatment. The Salter-Harris classification is used to describe epiphyseal fractures, which are divided into five types (Fig. 37-2). The number is a guide to the frequency of that type of fracture and an indicator of the prognosis for further epiphyseal growth and indicates the type of treatment needed. Thus type I is the most frequent type of epiphyseal injury and has a good prognosis; type V is the rarest type of epiphyseal fracture and has the worst prognosis because it results in premature closure of the growth plate. There has been some movement to add a type VI to the Salter-Harris classification system. Type VI would describe a perichondral ring injury that is commonly associated with peripheral bony bridge and rapid formation of angular deformities (Thompson, 2006). The radiologist should determine and report the fracture type.

In type I, the epiphysis separates from the metaphysis. The germinal cells remain with the epiphysis, usually uninjured. Type II is similar to type I except that a small piece of metaphysis breaks free to remain with the epiphysis. Type II fractures occur when there is a shearing force applied that fractures a portion of the physis with extension through the metaphysis. For both types, part of the perichondrium is preserved, and the blood supply to the growth plate is maintained. With no disruption to the growth plate, healing is rapid and growth is usually normal. Fracture types I and II do

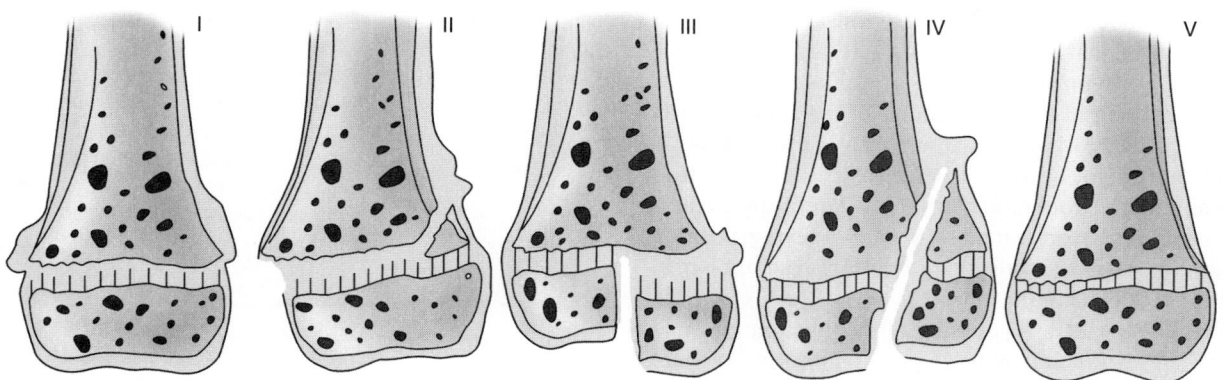

FIG. 37-2 The types of growth plate injury as classified by Salter and Harris. (From Salter RB, Harris WR: Injuries involving the epiphyseal plate, *J Bone Joint Surg Am* 45:587, 1963.)

not require perfect anatomic alignment to heal with a good functional prognosis. Closed reduction is generally the treatment for type I and II fractures. A type II fracture of the distal femur, however, requires anatomic alignment by either open or closed reduction.

Type III involves fracture through a portion of the physis with extension to the epiphysis and into the joint. Type IV fractures involve the metaphysis, physis, and epiphysis. Types III and IV are more serious fractures that must be promptly anatomically realigned, usually with open reduction, to prevent growth arrest. The prognosis for types III and IV is fair and depends on the severity of the injury and the accuracy in achieving anatomic alignment through open reduction. Growth arrest and progressive deformities can result from these fractures.

Type V fractures are rare, but have serious effects when they occur. This fracture results from a crush injury to the physis, often from a fall from a height, and the growth plate cells are crushed. No further growth occurs at that growth plate unless the epiphyseal blood supply was preserved. Sometimes this fracture is missed on radiographic study because no fracture line can be discerned (Thompson, 2004a).

Shaft Fractures. There is a tendency for the long bones to remold into the most normal position possible when they are fractured in places along the shaft. Young children may not fracture bones all the way across, and an incomplete fracture results. This is the typical greenstick fracture, with bone failure on the tension side and a bend deformity on the opposite side. As with adults, young children can experience complete fractures or stress fractures. Complete fractures are common in children and occur when both sides of the bones are fractured. Their classification depends on the direction of the line of fracturing with a spiral, transverse, oblique, or comminuted pattern of fracture (Thompson, 2004a).

▓ ASSESSMENT OF THE ORTHOPEDIC SYSTEM

See Table 37-1 for orthopedic terminology.

HISTORY

- History of present illness
  - *Onset*: appearance of first symptoms; insidious or sudden; association with injury or strain; accompanied by any constitutional symptoms or signs (e.g., fever, malaise, swelling, ecchymosis)
  - *Pain*: location and character, course of radiation, severity, extent of disability produced, effect of various activities including weight bearing, relief measures, changes from day to night or from day to day, child's refusing to move the painful part or assuming a pain-relieving position, effects of previous treatment, presence of pain or discomfort in other parts of the body
  - *Deformity*: character (swelling, inflammation, contracture, joint stiffness, unusual positioning, appearance); first appearance and who noted it; association with injury or disease; rate of change; extent of disability; a cosmetic problem or a cause of embarrassment

TABLE 37-1 Orthopedic Terminology

Term	Definition
Descriptive Terms for Positions	
Abduction	Movement away from midline
Adduction	Movement toward midline
Dorsiflexion	Movement of toes/foot or fingers/hand toward dorsal surface (up)
Eversion	Same as pronation: palmar surface turned away from midline
External rotation	Turning anterior surface of limb outward or away from midline
Internal rotation	Turning anterior surface of limb inward or toward midline
Inversion	Same as supination: palmar surface turned toward midline
Luxation	Dislocation
Plantar flexion	Movement of toes/foot or fingers/hand toward plantar surface (down or toes pointed)
Pronation	Palmar surface turned downward or toward posterior surface of body
Subluxation	Partial dislocation
Supination	Palmar surface turned upward or toward anterior surface of body
Valgus	Deviation away from midline, a >< shape of the two legs, for instance
Varus	Deviation toward midline, a < > shape of the two legs, for instance
Descriptive Positions for Parts of Long Bone	
Apophysis	Insertion point of tendon on long bone
Diaphysis	Shaft or middle part of long bone
Epiphysis	Distal side of growth plate, a secondary ossification center separated from parent bone
Metaphysis	Proximal side of growth plate, on edge of parent bone
Perichondrium	Membrane of fibrous connective tissue surrounding cartilage
Physis	Growth plate
Descriptive Terms for Feet	
Calcaneus	Heel bone articulates with talus (ankle) and cuboid bones
Malleolus	Medial or lateral bony prominence of ankle
Pes cavus	Foot with a high arch
Pes planus	Flatfoot
Pronation	Foot where center of weight lies over medial side of foot rather than being centered—foot sags toward center; often associated with flatfoot
Talipes equinovarus	Clubfoot

- *Injury*: how, when (time and date), why, and where; mechanism or manner in which injury was produced; involvement in organized or competitive sports
- *Altered function*: weakness, limp, decreased range of motion
- *Altered gait patterns*: toe walking, in toeing or out toeing
- *Other factors or constraints*: type of shoe worn (e.g., platform shoes); use of backpack and amount of weight in backpack, amount of time spent at repetitive tasks or at computer station; sitting in TV squat or "W" position
- *Medication use*: steroids
- Family history
  - Any family members with musculoskeletal problems; many orthopedic problems have a genetic component
- Medical history
  - *Pregnancy history and birth history*: breech delivery, shoulder presentation, multiple births, oligohydramnios, asphyxia at birth; maternal alcohol or substance abuse
  - *Development history*: milestones met at appropriate age, such as first walking and sitting; delays in achieving gross or fine motor developmental milestones
  - *Illnesses, accidents or surgeries*: trauma, meningitis, juvenile arthritis
- Review of systems
  - Any infections, constitutional diseases, or congenital problems that might have an orthopedic component

PHYSICAL EXAMINATION

Special orthopedic examination techniques are described in the following paragraphs.

Range-of-Motion Examination

It is necessary to find the bony limits of movement. An excessive range of motion can indicate an unstable joint. Note pain, stiffness, limitations or deviations, and rigidity. The normal values of joint motion are age related, which must be kept in mind (e.g., external hip rotation is greatest in early infancy). Passive range of motion, in which the examiner moves the joint, provides information about joint mobility and stability. It can also provide information about the limits of tendons and muscles that are contracted. To assess such problems as DDH, passive range of motion must be used. Active range of motion, in which the child moves the joint, provides information about both muscle and bony structures working together for functional movement.

Gait Examination

Observe the child walking without shoes and with only minimal covering. Inspect from the front, side, and back as the child walks normally, on his or her toes, and then on heels. The gait should be smooth, rhythmic, and efficient. The gait cycle includes the heel-strike, foot-flat, toe-off, and swing phases. Ankle, knee, and hip movements should be symmetric and full with little side-to-side movement of the trunk.

The smaller child has a faster gait than the larger child, but less distance is covered with each stride. This is related to the smaller child's poorer balance. With a short, quick stride, each leg is off the ground for less time. The feet are spread wider and, in the toddler, the arms may be held up to increase balance. The mature pattern develops by about 3 to 7 years old.

Limping is a disturbance in gait that can be either painless or painful. Painful or antalgic gaits serve to reduce stress or pain at the affected area. The trunk shifts to the opposite side to keep balance and reduce stress; the stance phase and stride length are shortened as compensatory mechanisms. For example, the toe-off phase is restricted if the toe is sore. Causes of a painful gait include infection, trauma, or acquired disorders. A Trendelenburg gait in which the trunk tips over the affected hip indicates hip disease and might or might not be painful because it also involves muscle weakness around the hip joint.

Posture

To assess posture adequately, the child should be examined undressed to his or her underwear. The examiner needs to look at the child from the front, side, and back.
- Pelvis and hips should be level. Place hands on the iliac crest to test for a pelvic tilt caused by limb length discrepancy.
- Legs should be symmetric in shape and size. The patellae should be straight ahead.
- The feet should point straight ahead, with an imaginary line from the center of the heel through the second toe. There should be an arch (except in babies, in whom a fat pad obscures the arch) and straight heel cords.
- The spine should be straight, and the back should look symmetric, with shoulder and scapula heights and waist angles equal. There should be slight lordotic curves at the cervical and lumbar areas.

■ SPECIAL EXAMINATIONS
HIP EXAMINATIONS
Galeazzi Maneuver

The Galeazzi maneuver includes flexing the hips and knees while the infant or child lies supine, placing the soles of the feet on the table near the buttocks, and then looking at the knee heights for equality (Fig. 37-3 *A*). The Galeazzi sign is positive if the knee heights are unequal. However, it is not reliable in children with dislocatable but not dislocated hips or in children with bilateral dislocation.

Barlow Maneuver

The Barlow maneuver dislocates an unstable or dislocatable hip posteriorly (Fig. 37-4, *A*). The infant is placed in the supine position with knees flexed. The hip is flexed, and the thigh is brought into an adducted position applying downward pressure. From that position, the femoral head drops out of the acetabulum or can be gently pushed out of the socket; this is termed a positive Barlow. The dislocation should be palpable as it occurs. The maneuver needs to be done gently in a noncrying neonate to keep from damaging the femoral head. The hips should be examined one at a time. The hip generally spontaneously relocates after release of the posterior force.

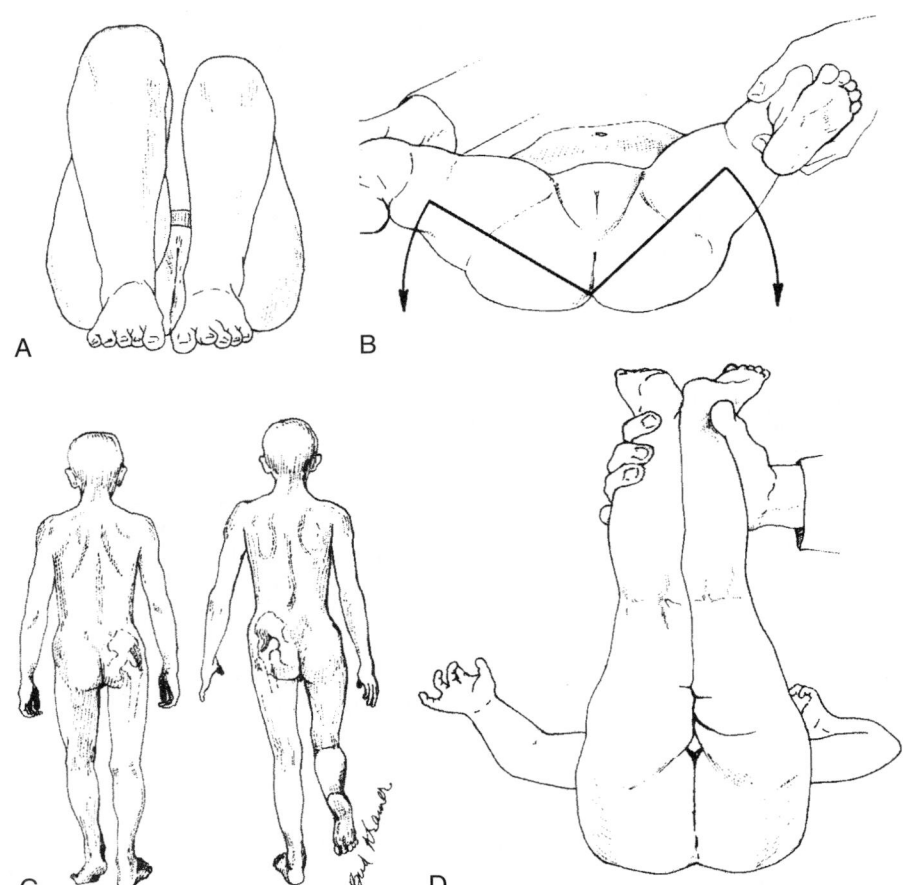

FIG. 37-3 Physical findings in congenital hip dislocation. **A,** Leg length inequality is a sign of unilateral hip dislocation (Galeazzi sign). It is not reliable in children with dislocatable but not dislocated hips or in children with bilateral dislocation. **B,** Limitation of hip abduction is often present in older infants with hip dislocation. Abduction of greater than 60 degrees is usually possible in infants. Restriction or asymmetry indicates the need for careful radiologic examination. **C,** Trendelenburg sign. In single-leg stance, the abductor muscles of the normal hip support the pelvis. Dislocation of the hip functionally shortens and weakens these muscles. When the child attempts to stand on the dislocated hip, the opposite side of the pelvis drops. When bilateral dislocation is present, a wide-based Trendelenburg limp results. **D,** Thigh-fold asymmetry is often present in infants with unilateral hip dislocation. An extra fold can be seen on the abnormal side. The finding is not diagnostic, however. It may be found in normal infants and may be absent in children with hip dislocation or dislocatability. (From Scoles P: *Pediatric orthopedics in clinical practice,* ed 2, St. Louis, 1988, Mosby.)

Ortolani Maneuver

The Ortolani maneuver can be done after the Barlow maneuver or separately (see Fig. 37-4, *B*). The Ortolani maneuver reduces a posteriorly dislocated hip. It is done to reduce a recently dislocated hip and is not done forcefully. The infant is in the supine position with both knees flexed and supported by the thumb and forefinger of the examiner. The thumb is placed near the lesser trochanter, and the pad of the second finger is positioned on the bony prominence of the greater trochanter. The leg is flexed at the hip and then abducted while pushing up with the fingers located over the trochanter posteriorly. The femoral head is lifted anteriorly into the acetabulum. A clunk and a palpable jerk are obtained as the femoral head is relocated. A mild clicking sound is not a positive Ortolani sign. These are common and normal sounds radiating from the knee or ankle that are fine, of short duration, and high pitched (Duderstadt & Schapiro, 2006). Of note, the hip may be dislocated easily only during the first month or two of life. The Ortolani maneuver is most likely to be positive in infants 1 to 2 months old.

The examiner should not still be charting "no hip click" on examinations at 6 months old. Dislocation can occur late in infancy. However, if this occurs, the provider will note limited abduction on the side of the dislocation (Fig. 37-5).

Trendelenburg Sign

The Trendelenburg sign is elicited by having the child stand and then raise one leg off the ground. If the pelvis (iliac crest) drops on the raised leg side, the sign is positive and indicates weak hip abductor muscles on the side that is bearing the weight. Normally, the muscles around a stable hip are strong enough to maintain a level pelvis if one leg is raised (see Fig. 37-3, *D*). With bilaterally dislocated hips, a wide-based Trendelenburg limp is noted.

Medial (Internal) and Lateral (External) Rotations

The child is placed prone, and the knees are flexed 90 degrees. Medial rotation is measured as the legs are allowed to fall apart as far as possible, using gravity alone or with light

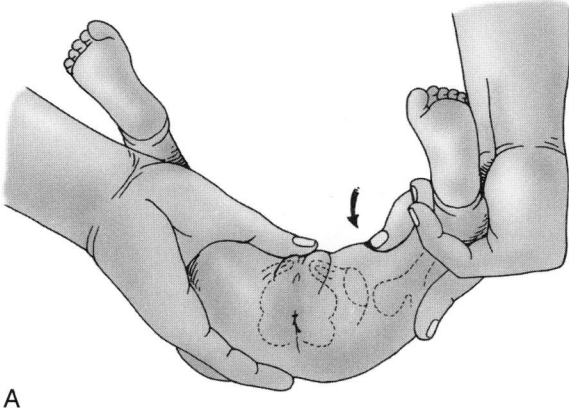

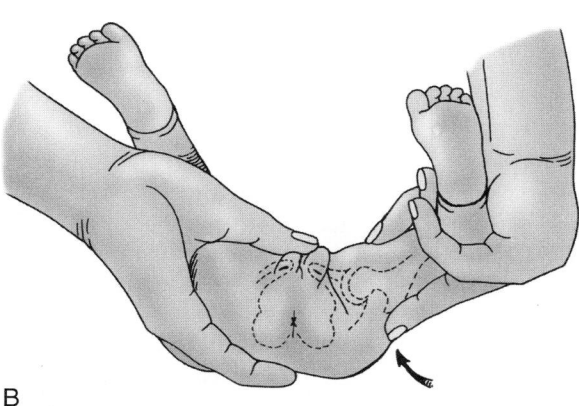

FIG. 37-4 **A,** Barlow (dislocation) test. The "stabilizing hand" is positioned with the thumb on the symphysis and the fingers on the sacrum. The thumb of the abducting hand is placed on the inner aspect of the thigh and gives lateral pressure to the adductor region while the hand (wrapped around the knee with the index finger on the lateral side of the thigh) provides gentle downward pressure. If there is hip instability, dislocation is palpable as the femoral head slips out of the acetabulum. Diagnosis is confirmed with the Ortolani test. **B,** Ortolani (reduction) test. With the infant relaxed on a firm surface, the hips and knees are flexed to 90 degrees. The hips are examined one at a time. Grasp the infant's thigh with the middle finger over the greater trochanter and lift the thigh to bring the femoral head from its dislocated posterior position to opposite the acetabulum. Simultaneously the thigh is gently abducted, reducing the femoral head in the acetabulum. In a positive finding, the examiner senses reduction by a palpable, nearly audible "clunk." Test one hip at a time for both of these tests. (From Kliegman RM et al, editors: *Nelson essentials of pediatrics,* ed 5, Philadelphia, 2006, WB Saunders.)

pressure. The angle between vertical (0 degree) and the leg position is the medial rotation. It is measured for each leg (Fig. 37-6, *A*). Asymmetric hip rotation is abnormal. Lateral rotation is measured by allowing the legs to cross while the child is still prone. The angle between vertical and the leg position is measured for each leg (see Fig. 37-6, *B*). Again, asymmetric hip rotation is abnormal. By 1 year old, a normal child has approximately 45 degrees of internal and external hip rotation (Thompson, 2004b).

Abduction test

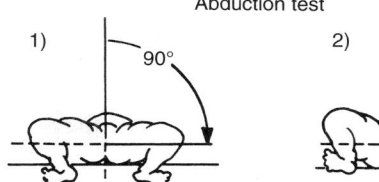
Normal at birth to 1 month of age

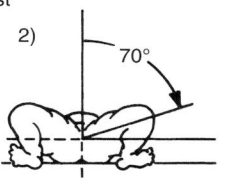
Often normal, 1 to 9 months of age

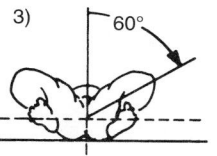
Suspected significant limitation

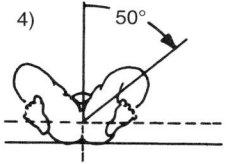
Definite limitation

FIG. 37-5 Hip abduction test. The child is placed supine, and the hips are flexed 90 degrees and fully abducted. Although the normal abduction range is quite broad, one can suspect hip disease in any patient who lacks more than 35 to 45 degrees of abduction. (From Chung SMK: *Hip disorders in infants and children,* Philadelphia, 1981, Lea & Febiger.)

BACK EXAMINATION

Adam's Test or the Adam's Forward Bend Position

Adam's test looks for asymmetry of the posterior chest wall on forward bending. This position allows for evaluation of structural scoliosis. The child bends at the waist to a position of 90 degrees back flexion with straight legs, ankles together, and arms hanging freely or with palms together (in a diving position) but not touching the toes or floor (Fig. 37-7). The back is inspected for asymmetry of the height of the curves on the two sides or rib hump; the provider inspects the child's back by looking at it from the rear and side position. The examiner should be seated in front of the child to best visually scan each level of the spine. If a rib hump is present, a scoliometer, if available, can be used to measure the angular tilt of the trunk. A spinal rotation greater than 5 degrees measured by placing the scoliometer at the peak of the curvature indicates the need for further evaluation (Duderstadt & Schapiro, 2006). Other characteristics of scoliosis to look for include unequal scapula heights, unequal waist angles, unequal iliac crests or shoulders, asymmetry of the elbow to flank distance, and some deviation of the spine from a straight head-to-toe line. Looking primarily at the straightness of the spine, however, can be misleading because scoliosis involves both rotation and misalignment of the vertebrae. The Adam's forward bending position accentuates the rotational deformity of scoliosis.

▇▇ DIAGNOSTIC STUDIES

Radiographs are an important diagnostic tool for the musculoskeletal system. Anteroposterior and lateral views of the affected area, bone, or joint are typically ordered to analyze the anatomic structures. Views of both extremities may be ordered so that comparisons can be made. Computed tomography (CT) scans augment radiographs to detail specific areas of the body, especially in identification of soft tissue lesions.

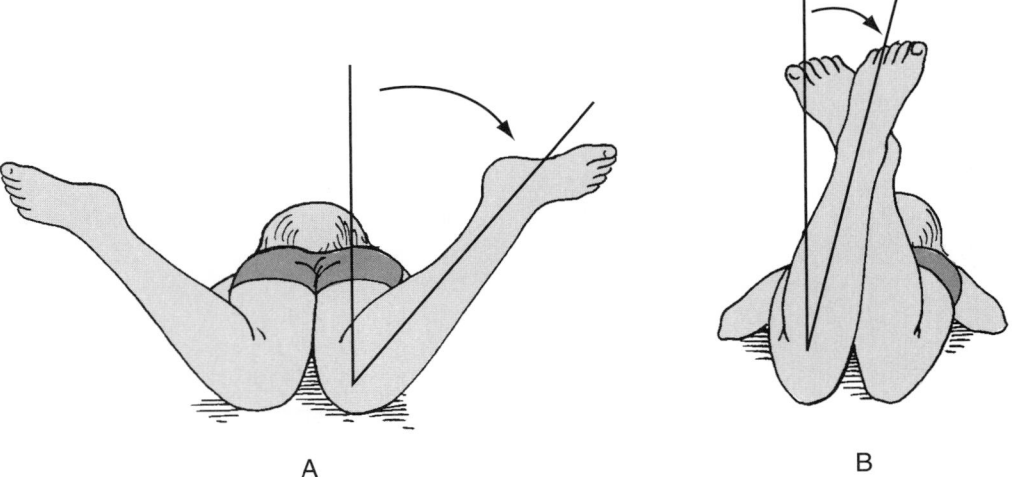

A   B

FIG. 37-6 Hip rotation in extension. This is measured with the child in prone position and the knee flexed 90 degrees. The lower leg is vertically oriented. This is considered the neutral position. On outward rotation (**A**), the leg produces internal hip rotation, and on inward rotation (**B**), the leg produces external hip rotation. (From Thompson GH: Gait disturbances. In Kliegman RM (ed): *Practical strategies in pediatric diagnosis and therapy*, Philadelphia, WB Saunders, 1996.)

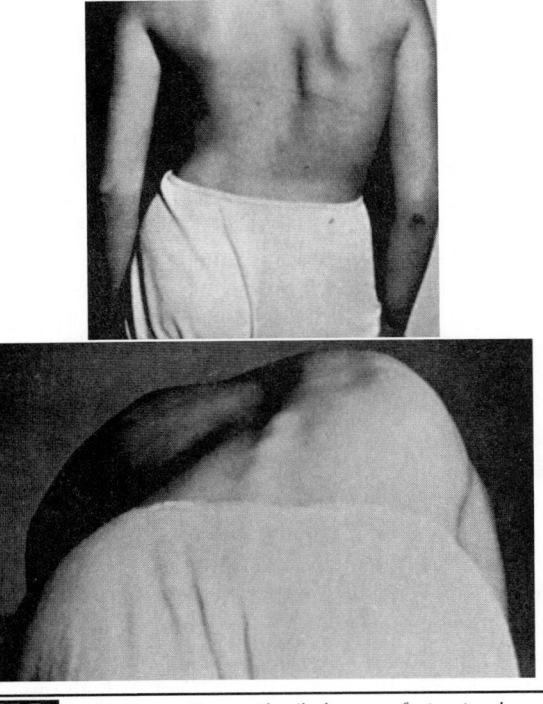

FIG. 37-7 Adam's position with rib hump of structural scoliosis. Lateral curvature of thoracic and lumbar segments of the spine, usually with some rotation of involved vertebral bodies. Functional scoliosis is flexible; it is apparent with standing and disappears with forward bending. It may be compensatory for other abnormalities, such as leg length discrepancy. Structural scoliosis is fixed; the curvature is visible both on standing and on bending forward. *Note rib hump with forward flexions.* At greatest risk are females 10 year old through adolescence. (From Delp MH, Manning RT: *Major's physical diagnosis: an introduction to the clinical process*, ed 9, Philadelphia, 1981, WB Saunders.)

CT is useful in detailing the relationship of bones to their contiguous structures. Magnetic resonance imaging (MRI) can provide additional information, such as the degree of bone demineralization before the tissue loss is radiographically apparent (30% to 50% of bone density must be reduced to show a change on conventional radiography). MRI is particularly useful in assessment of soft tissue lesions and allows distinction among different muscles or muscle groups and among different cartilage structures. It also can distinguish among various physiologic changes that occur in bone marrow related to age and disease process. Ultrasonography also provides information about cartilaginous areas or tissues not visible on radiograph. Bone scans (scintigraphy) are more sensitive than radiographs, demonstrate abnormal uptake earlier than conventional radiographs, and are useful in detecting causes of obscure skeletal pain (Thompson, 2004b).

It is important to remember that false-negative imaging studies results can occur in early stages of disease (e.g., osteomyelitis) or conditions (e.g., developmental hip dysplasia of the newborn). Also, in those circumstances in which a child will most likely be referred to a specialist, it may be more prudent to defer to the specialist to order imaging studies rather than expose the child to unnecessary radiation and potentially increase the cost of health care.

Various laboratory studies can indicate systemic disease, infection, or inflammation. Erythrocyte sedimentation rate, C-reactive protein determination, complete blood count, blood cultures for infectious disorders, rheumatoid factor, and antinuclear antibodies are examples of hematologic tests that can assist in the diagnosis and management of bone disorders. Other laboratory tests also can provide an understanding of muscle metabolism (e.g., lactic acid, pyruvates, carnitine). Some bony lesions may need to be biopsied, and muscle tissue frequently needs to be sampled to determine specific disease pathologic conditions.

■ MANAGEMENT STRATEGIES
COUNSELING

Counseling for orthopedic problems involves several components. The family should understand and have time to ask questions about all of the following issues:
- The pathologic condition, including possible etiologies
- The treatment plan
- The prognosis with and without treatment
- Any genetic implications of the diagnosis
- Long-term care issues

Counseling helps families cope with a poor or challenging diagnosis and its short-term and long-term implications. Congenital problems are often identified prenatally, at birth or shortly thereafter. Families need to be given the diagnosis truthfully, humanely, and as soon as possible. Issues of etiology need to be discussed to address parents' feelings of guilt for causing the problem and to discuss genetic implications, if any. A plan of care that is mutually agreed on by the family and the health care provider must be developed before the infant is discharged from the hospital or clinic.

EXERCISE

All children need exercise to promote their growth and development and prevent overweight or other negative sequelae. Even children with disabling conditions can exercise in some way. Exercise for children should be fun and perceived as play, not work. Often, physical therapists or the child's orthopedist can provide ideas for safe, therapeutic play or sports activities. At school, children with orthopedic problems should engage in physical activities that are as much a part of the regular physical education class as possible.

ANTICIPATORY GUIDANCE: MUSCULOSKELETAL DEVELOPMENT

Families are sometimes concerned about problems that health care providers believe are within normal limits and do not require an orthopedic referral. The pediatric health professional should provide the child's family with a description of the child's predicted musculoskeletal development. Timelines and markers that parents can use to monitor their child's development are particularly helpful in allowing families to understand their child's pattern of growth. Misperceptions about the implications of minor variations need to be clarified, and the family should always be given the opportunity to return for further assessment or discussion if concerns remain. Examples of common concerns are flat feet in infants and toddlers, "bowing" of legs in toddlers, and "knock-knees" in preschool children.

SHOES

The use of therapeutic shoes to correct orthopedic problems is controversial. Studies confirm that therapeutic shoes do little to correct deformities. Shoes for the average child should keep the feet warm and protected from injury. Shoes should be selected to fit properly and comfortably with room for growth. High-top shoes for toddlers may have the advantage of staying on pudgy little feet better, but they do not provide additional support. Toddler feet do not need extra support. Staheli (2003b) identifies five features (the "five Fs") of a good shoe:
- Flexible—to allow as much free motion as possible; for young children, test to see if the shoe can be flexed in the parent's hand
- Flat—do not allow high heels
- Foot shaped—avoid pointed toes or other shapes that are not the normal configuration of the foot
- Fitted generously—better to be too large than too small
- Friction similar to skin—the soles should have the same friction as skin so that they are not slippery

Shoe modifications may be needed in certain conditions. Shoe lifts are needed if limb length differences exceed 2.5 cm. Orthotics also can be used in certain orthopedic situations to more evenly distribute pressure on the sole of the foot and facilitate function.

CARE OF CHILDREN IN CASTS

Children in casts need special attention, and their parents need instructions for care and monitoring for problems. If a plaster cast is used, the major concern is wetness—urine, feces, or environmental substances. The cast absorbs it all. Therefore attention needs to be given to protecting the cast (including a fiberglass cast) from moisture at all times. If the cast becomes wet, a hair dryer can be used for drying small areas; for larger casts, drying may affect only the surface. Pediatric nursing texts can provide ideas for caring for infants in spica casts—the most difficult to manage. For all casts, openings should be inspected and smelled to help identify pressure sores inside the casted areas. The heel is particularly vulnerable to pressure sores.

The child's cast should be kept cool, clean, and dry. Cover the cast with plastic wrap or a plastic bag when the child bathes or is in a situation in which the cast may get wet.

A child in a cast needs to have developmental stimulation, physical contact, changes in environment, and opportunities to make choices and control his or her care within limits, just as any other child does. Parents need to be instructed to use extra care when picking up a child with a cast—the weight can cause trauma if not supported. Depending on cast material used and how quickly they dry, special care must be taken until the cast is completely dry to prevent compression of the cast material.

SPLINTS AND BRACES

Splints and braces need to be monitored for good fit and correct use. Splints are useful to provide temporary immobilization.

GENETICS COUNSELING

See Chapter 40.

PHYSICAL THERAPY

Physical therapists can help restore or maintain function or teach new motor skills. The physical therapist should be accustomed to dealing with children. Physical therapy is especially important to prevent deformities, teach new motor skills, and rehabilitate injuries.

ORTHOPEDIC PROBLEMS SPECIFIC TO CHILDREN
ARM PROBLEMS—BRACHIAL PLEXUS INJURIES
Description

Brachial plexus injuries are typically classified using Narakas criteria as types I through IV (Table 37-2). Narakas type I involves C5 and C6, affecting the shoulder and bicep muscles. Narakas type II involves shoulder, biceps, and forearm extensors with C5 through C7 nerve root injuries. Recovery is usually complete for types I and II. Narakas type III has variable recovery with complete paralysis of the limb caused by C5 through T1 nerve root injury. Narakas type IV also involves C5 through T1 with complete paralysis of the limb and Horner syndrome. Recovery of function in the shoulder and biceps is fair to poor with hand recovery variable in types III and IV. Brachial plexus injuries can also be classified as type I (Erb-Duchenne paralysis) with C5 through C6 involvement that includes the shoulder and upper arm, type II (Erb-Duchenne-Klumpke paralysis) involves the entire brachial plexus (i.e., C5 through T1 involvement) affecting the shoulder, arm, and hand, or type III (Klumpke paralysis) caused by injury to C8 through T1 with involvement of the lower arm and hand. (Drendel et al, 2002; Hansen & Bateman, 2002).

Epidemiology

Brachial plexus injuries are traumatic stretch or traction injuries that occur when excessive lateral traction is applied to the neck and shoulder during birth. The brachiaplexus is damaged, and innervation to the arm is disrupted, resulting in weakness or paralysis of the muscles innervated by spinal nerves C5 through C8 and T1. Shoulder dystocia, fetal macrosomia, prolonged and difficult labor and delivery, the use of forceps or vacuum, and vaginal breech and other abnormal fetal presentation deliveries are linked with this type of birth injury. However, there may be no predisposing risk factor in 40% of children, and there is some evidence that the injury may also occur in utero (Roth, 2006). The incidence ranges from 0.4 to 4.6 per 1000 live births (Stoll & Kliegman, 2004).

Clinical Findings.

History. There may be a history of a traumatic delivery, often of a large baby.

Physical Examination. Findings depend on the type (I through IV) and include the following (Drendel et al, 2002; Hansen & Bateman, 2002):

- Neonate cannot abduct the arm from the shoulder or rotate the arm externally and cannot supinate the forearm; infant keeps the shoulder in adduction and internal rotation (the "waiter's tip"); extension of the elbow; and flexion of the wrist and fingers (Erb's palsy)
- Absent bicep reflex with absent Moro reflex on the affected side
- Limp wrist and hand with absent grasp reflex (lower plexus involvement)
- Horner syndrome (ipsilateral ptosis, miosis, enophthalmos, anhidrosis) if the sympathetic fibers of the T1 nerve root are involved
- Occasionally, hand paralysis with normal shoulder movement, which is a rare occurrence of an isolated C8 through T1 injury

  Traumatic delivery causing brachial plexus injury also can cause the following associated injuries:
- Rupture of intraabdominal structures, especially liver and spleen
- Fracture of the skull, clavicle, or humerus
- Damage to the sternocleidomastoid muscle with resulting limitation of neck movement (a "sternocleidomastoid tumor" indicates the injury, which results in torticollis if prompt and vigorous physical therapy is not initiated)
- Impaired respiratory effort as a result of diaphragmatic paralysis and flaccidity

Diagnostic Studies.

Chest radiograph is needed to rule out fractures of the clavicle or humerus or humeral-epiphyseal separation. Electromyographic studies and radiographs of the clavicle and cervical spine are ordered as indicated.

Differential Diagnosis

Consider dislocation, fracture of the arm or clavicle, cerebral lesions, and cervical column lesions.

Management

The following steps are taken:

- Refer to an orthopedist for immobilization for the first 2 weeks to prevent exacerbation of hemorrhage or edema, followed by physical therapy and splints to prevent contractures.
- Physical therapy may be necessary to maintain a full range of motion.
- Recovery of nerve function needs to be monitored using a standardized tool, such as the Modified British Council

TABLE 37-2   **Brachial Plexus Injury Using Narakas Classification**

Name	Nerve and Muscle Involved	Prognosis
Narakas type I	C5 and C6; shoulder and biceps	Recovery usually complete
Narakas type II	C5-C7; shoulder, biceps, and forearm extensors	Recovery usually complete
Narakas type III	C5-T1	Variable with complete paralysis of limb; shoulder and biceps recovery is fair to poor with hand recovery variable
Narakas type IV	C5-T1	Complete paralysis of the limb and Horner syndrome; shoulder and biceps recovery is fair to poor with hand recovery variable

Scale for muscle strength. Scale (Information on this scale can be found at http://brachialplexus.wustl.edu/medical0.html.) If there is little to no recovery of biceps function by 4 months old, surgical exploration of the brachial plexus with possible nerve grafting or transfer may be necessary.

• Counsel the family, including explanation of the injury, its prognosis, and its management. The child should be held and cared for as any other baby.

Complications

Paralysis can be permanent. Contractures can occur if regular physical therapy is not started and continued for as long as the paralysis lasts. Physical findings are important to rule out concurrent injuries from traumatic delivery. Brachial plexus injury may be associated with phrenic nerve palsy.

Prognosis

Recovery may or may not be complete and requires time, up to 18 months in mild cases. Improvement generally begins within 2 to 4 weeks, with 90% resolving spontaneously during the first year of life. If there has been no improvement by 2 to 3 months old, the infant needs evaluation for nerve root avulsion and, depending on the results, possible surgery. The prognosis for complete recovery of upper brachial plexus injury is excellent, with a more guarded prognosis for lower brachial plexus injury (types III and IV), especially if associated with Horner syndrome or diaphragmatic paralysis (Roth, 2006).

SHOULDER PROBLEMS—CLAVICLE FRACTURE

Epidemiology

In neonates, this fracture occurs often during the birth process. Most clavicle fractures occur during normal labor and delivery. However, risk factors include shoulder dystocia, a large neonate, and increased gestational age. Because the clavicle is the first bone to ossify, it is the bone most frequently fractured at birth, with the right fractured more often than the left. It is often missed as a diagnosis at birth. It may be a complete or greenstick fracture and typically involves the middle third of the clavicle. The incidence of neonatal clavicle fractures is 4.7 per 1000 live births (Hansen & Bateman, 2002). Childhood fractures of the clavicle are related to trauma. A common mechanism of injury is a fall on an outstretched hand, fall onto the shoulder, or direct trauma to the clavicle.

Clinical Findings.

History. In the neonate, assess the following:
• History of difficult delivery—large baby and shoulder dystocia—or a normal labor and delivery
• Irritability when infant is moved or lifted
• In the older child, assess the following:
  ○ History of fall or trauma

Physical Examination. In all children, look for the following:
• Pain occurring with shoulder movement
• Decreased arm movement on affected side (asymmetric spontaneous arm movements) or absent Moro reflex
• Palpable swelling, bony abnormality, discoloration and/or crepitus elicited over fracture site

• Callus felt over fracture site within a few days
• Spasm of sternocleidomastoid muscle on affected side
• An associated Erb's palsy

Diagnostic Studies. In the neonate, radiographs should be used to confirm the diagnosis. Clavicle shaft fractures can be difficult to see radiographically in children, but are clinically identifiable. Radiographs can be helpful in identifying a fracture near the shoulder joint.

Differential Diagnosis. Brachial palsy, shoulder dislocation, or other bony problem should be considered.

Management. Management involves the following:
• Neonate:
  ○ Incomplete fractures that do not cause pain need no treatment.
  ○ Immobilization of the shoulder is an option when movement results in a painful arm (usually with a complete fracture). Pin the sleeve of the infant's arm to the front of the shirt for 1 to 2 weeks.
  ○ Generally, the neonate is just moved gently without undue stress to the arm and shoulder until a callus forms.
• Older child:
  ○ Sling immobilization for comfort to support the affected extremity is often sufficient. Generally, sling immobilization can be discontinued at 3 to 4 weeks (Vidal et al, 2007).
  ○ A figure-eight clavicle brace can be used if displacement results in a decreased shaft length. However, it is uncomfortable to wear, and its effectiveness is questionable.
  ○ Protection for 4 to 5 weeks is generally sufficient because union requires about 4 weeks of healing.
  ○ An older child may need analgesics or a nonsteroidal anti-inflammatory drug (NSAID) for pain.
  ○ The rare open fractures or those with severe tenting may need to be surgically corrected.

Prognosis. The prognosis is excellent. Often the injury in neonates is identified only at later primary care visits, when the callus lump is palpated, though the child may be irritable until the fracture is stable. The infant is usually asymptomatic within 7 to 10 days. Parents need information and emotional support. In older children with fractures, healing is almost always universal with reduction seldom necessary. Bone remodeling is generally complete. A large callus often appears at the healing site; however, the callus typically resolves in 6 to 12 months, making cosmetic surgery unnecessary (Thompson, 2004a).

RIB PROBLEMS—COSTOCHONDRITIS AND STERNOCHONDRITIS

Description. Costochondral disease (costochondritis) is a benign disorder marked by pain that is localized at the junctions of the costal cartilage and rib; sternochondritis is marked by pain at the junction where the costal cartilage and sternum connect (Anderson, 2002). They involve musculoskeletal discomfort and are a common complaint.

Epidemiology. Trauma to the area and unaccustomed physical effort (lifting heavy objects or coughing) are factors known to cause costochondritis. Inflammation is the underlying problem.

Clinical Findings.

History. Pain localized to the costosternal or costochondral junction is the major symptom. It often presents with tenderness over more than one rib as a result of referred pain. The primary rib that is inflamed and usually responsible for the symptoms is most often the one that exhibits the greatest sensitivity to palpation. Characteristics of the pain include the following (Anderson, 2002):

- Acute or gradual onset
- Sharp, darting, or dull quality
- Short duration of hours or lasting days
- Occasional complaints of a feeling of tightness caused by muscle spasm
- No exacerbation of pain with respiratory or mild movements

Physical Examination. The major clinical finding on examination is localized or focal tenderness of one or more costochondral joints with palpation of the costal cartilage. The presence of pain, swelling (a unique bulbous enlargement of the joint) with or without redness, and tenderness at the costal cartilage is referred to as Tietze syndrome.

Diagnostic Studies. No diagnostic studies are needed because history and physical findings are the key to the diagnosis.

Differential Diagnosis.

Rib fractures are the key differential diagnosis if pain is associated with an injury. Childhood rheumatic diseases also can have complaints similar to costochondritis but generally have other characteristic physical findings. Costochondritis is one of the differential diagnoses of pediatric chest pain (see Chapter 30).

Management.

Treatment consists of the use of mild analgesia and NSAIDs to relieve discomfort and avoidance of strenuous activity. Parents and children need to be reassured that this is a benign, self-limited condition and is not related to cardiac disease.

BACK PROBLEMS

Back Pain

Description. Children do not commonly complain of severe back pain. Most episodes of back pain in pediatric patients are brief with nonspecific findings and history (Doyle, 2006). The older the child is the more likely the etiology of back pain is musculoskeletal in origin. Younger children who have such complaints should be carefully evaluated for occult pathologic conditions, and the provider's index of suspicion about underlying pathologic conditions should be raised. Complaints of back pain in adolescents deserve attention, but the index of suspicion for occult pathologic conditions is relatively low. Typically, more than 50% of adolescents report having back pain, but they tend not to seek attention for this symptom. The young athlete is especially susceptible to back injury, with a 10% to 15% incidence. Intense training can cause repetitive microtrauma (Kronberg & Small, 2005). Back pain can result from sprains of the ligaments or muscles (or both) of the back caused by injury.

Clinical Findings. The following findings should alert the pediatric provider to possible pathologic conditions:

- Night pain
- Pain that prohibits play or activities
- Pain that persists or worsens
- History of trauma (vertebral fracture)
- Positive neurologic or musculoskeletal signs on examination

In school-age children and adolescents, back pain can be associated with a history of the following:

- Muscle strain as a result of "overuse syndrome" from excessive muscular exertion, usually related to sports, commonly in sedentary children who recently increased their activity level
- Wearing high heels or platform shoes (females)

Questions about the onset, duration, location, frequency, and intensity of the pain are key questions to ask to form an initial impression (Richards, 2003). Back pain is a commonly reported symptom in somatizing children. Athletes with a history of *low back pain* lasting more than 1 month deserve careful evaluation. A low-back stress fracture or spondylolysis may be the causative factor in 25% of athletes with this history (Small, 2006).

Diagnostic Studies. A complete blood count with differential, erythrocyte sedimentation rate, and C-reactive protein are useful screening tests, particularly in young children with constitutional symptoms or those complaining of night pain (Richards, 2003). Imaging studies may be needed.

Differential Diagnosis. Occult pathologic conditions should be ruled out. Diskitis, vertebral osteomyelitis, vertebral fracture, or tumor can cause significant back pain in toddlers. Older children can experience these same problems, in addition to intervertebral disk herniation or vertebral endplate fractures.

Management. Treatment is determined by the findings on history and physical examination and can include referral for radiographs (anteroposterior and lateral views) and imaging studies or referral to a subspecialist physician or pediatrician. If the back pain is due to injury, pain management and physical therapy may be part of the treatment plan.

Scoliosis

Description. Scoliosis is a structural lateral curvature of the spine greater than 10 degrees in the coronal plane of the spine noted on a standing posterior-anterior (PA) spine radiograph. It also involves significant transverse and sagittal plane rotations (Stewart & Skaggs, 2006). There are seven principle classifications for scoliosis:

- *Idiopathic:* thought to be caused by equilibrium dysfunction, familial or genetic tendency or asymmetric growth; within this classification there are three types divided by age at manifestation:
  - Infantile (0 to 3 years old)
  - Juvenile (3 to 10 years old)
  - Adolescent (puberty to maturity)

Idiopathic scoliosis can progress slowly or rapidly, as great as 1 degree per month until skeletal maturity is reached.

- *Paralytic:* secondary to muscle imbalance in the growing spine caused by primary neuromuscular problems (e.g., cerebral palsy or muscular dystrophy) can worsen rapidly
- *Congenital:* a structural anomaly present at birth (e.g., hemivertebrae), often associated with other congenital abnormalities, such as renal and cardiac anomalies; can worsen slowly, rapidly, or stay the same

- *Mesenchymal:* associated with connective tissue problems (e.g., Marfan syndrome)
- *Posttraumatic:* following injury, thoracoplasty, or irradiation
- *Tumors:* secondary to bone tumors or other lesions constricting the spine
- *Other causes, miscellaneous:* examples include metabolic disturbances or dystrophies

Structural scoliosis is the general term used to indicate a true deformity of the vertebrae rather than a postural problem (*secondary* or *functional scoliosis*). Approximately 10% of the population has mild truncal asymmetry. However, curves greater than 10 degrees in children are abnormal and can progress to significant curves in the growing child (Bennett, 2002a; Reamy & Slakey, 2001).

Epidemiology.   Secondary or functional scoliosis, when there is the appearance of a lateral curvature but no structural change in the vertebral column, is due to such problems as leg length inequality, poor posture, or muscle spasm. Congenital scoliosis is due to bony deformities caused by failure in formation or segmentation of vertebrae during fetal development (e.g., neural tube disorders). Paralytic or neuromuscular scoliosis is caused by myopathies and upper or lower neuron diseases (e.g., muscular dystrophy, cerebral palsy, and polio). Mesenchymal or constitutional scoliosis is associated with genetic syndromes (e.g., Marfan syndrome or diastrophic dwarfism). Miscellaneous scoliosis has numerous etiologies that do not fit one of the other classifications. Idiopathic is the most common type of scoliosis. Its etiology is unknown, but often has a familial or genetic pattern. Approximately 20% have a positive family history, and they typically have an associated right thoracic curve (Thompson, 2006). Hormonal changes play a role in the disease process, and a rapid growth period is believed to be a significant factor in the progress of curvature associated with idiopathic scoliosis. Females with this type of scoliosis are more likely than males to have lateral curvatures that progress (Stewart & Skaggs, 2006). The most common type of idiopathic scoliosis is found in adolescents and is the major focus of the remaining discussion.

Small to moderate scoliotic curves do not increase significantly after skeletal growth is complete. Double "S" curves and more severe curves are more likely to progress during the growth years. For a given child, however, the ability to predict progression is difficult because even small curves can progress to severe deformity. Thus regular monitoring of the curve is important (Table 37-3).

Idiopathic scoliosis is found in children around the world. The overall incidence of idiopathic scoliosis is approximately 2% to 3%, and only 0.3% of those with idiopathic scoliosis have significant curves (greater than 20 degrees of curvature noted on radiographics). The female-to-male ratio increases with increasing curve magnitude. For curves less than 20 degrees, the risk for progression of the curve is low. These curves generally just need to be observed. However, for curves between 20 and 45 degrees, the risk for progression is high during growth, and early intervention is of paramount importance. Thus, young, premenarchal females with large curves are a vulnerable group because their spines are skeletally immature with growth remaining. The majority of adolescents with idiopathic scoliosis have a right thoracic curve. Juvenile manifestation is uncommon, and infantile scoliosis is rare in the U.S. (Doyle, 2006; Stewart & Skaggs, 2006).

Clinical Findings

History.   Scoliosis is generally painless, and insidious onset is typical. Generally, there is no significant history. The provider should assess the following:

- Family history of scoliosis
- Age of menarche
- Etiologic factors related to the various causes of structural scoliosis

The presence of pain with a lateral curvature of the spine suggests an inflammatory or neoplastic lesion as the cause of the scoliosis. Some children with idiopathic scoliosis complain of mild pain that is activity related. Severe, constant, or night pain and point tenderness indicate some other pathologic condition (Stewart & Skaggs, 2006).

Physical Examination.   The predominant features in the child with scoliosis who is standing with weight equally on both feet, legs straight, and arms hanging loosely at the sides include the following, although the location of the curve affects the findings:

- Painless lateral curvature of the spine with greater than 10 degrees of rotation on radiographs.
- The curve can have one turn ("C curve") or may include two compensating curves ("S curve").
- With a large, major double curve, the spine may look balanced when standing erect, but a rib hump becomes noticeable with the Adam's forward bending test.
- Lateral deviation and rotation of each vertebra is accentuated by looking at the ribs and the spinal column itself.
- Unequal shoulder heights.
- Unequal scapula prominences and heights. Note that the muscle masses may be somewhat unequal, especially if the child uses one shoulder more than the other as in carrying books. Look for bony, not muscular, prominence.
- Unequal waist angles—the hip touches one arm, and the contralateral arm hangs free.
- Unequal rib prominences and chest asymmetry.
- Unequal rib heights when the child stands in the Adam's forward bend position (see Fig. 37-7).

The presence of a left-sided curve in a child older than 3 years should be viewed with caution and is suggestive of neurologic abnormality.

Congenital scoliosis may be visible in the infant lying prone; it is sometimes more prominent if the infant is suspended prone. Inspect for skin abnormalities, sacral dimple, and hairy patches.

The physical examination should also include the following:

- Observation for equal leg lengths
- Examination of the skin for hairy patches, nevi, café au lait spots, lipomas, dimples
- Neurologic examination checking for weakness or sensory disturbance
- Cardiac examination for Marfan syndrome

Diagnostic Studies.   The clinical diagnosis is always confirmed by radiograph, although some newer techniques of

TABLE 37-3	Scoliosis, Kyphosis, and Lordosis					
	Curve	**Etiology**	**Clinical Findings**	**Radiographs**	**Management**	**Prognosis**
Scoliosis	Lateral	Classifications: idiopathic (most common); neuromuscular; constitutional; secondary; congenital; miscellaneous; functional (leg length discrepancy—not scoliosis)	Hx: positive family hx; related to etiologies (classifications); painless curvature; typically have right thoracic curve	PA and lateral standing views to identify degree of curve; >10 degrees abnormal; may have 1 curve (C) or 2 curves (S); vertebrae show lateral deviation and rotation	Referral to orthopedic surgeon; brace or surgery; need to monitor progression of curve	Most curves do not increase after growth complete; females with idiopathic scoliosis more likely to have curve progress
Kyphosis	AP curve of thoracic spine	Familial (Scheuermann disease); secondary to tumor, trauma, etc., congenital; postural, not true kyphosis	Postural roundback	Narrow disk space and loss of normal anterior height of vertebrae	Postural: PT, dancing, and swimming can be helpful; if structural: refer to an orthopedic surgeon for observation, bracing, or surgery	
Lordosis	AP curve of lumbar spine	As a result of hip contractures; physiologic; family and racial groups, before puberty	Abdomen and buttock protuberant; if result of hip contractures, lordosis disappears when sitting	Standing lateral views	Lumbar spine flattens, and lordosis disappears when child bends forward, it is physiologic and no treatment; if fixed, refer to an orthopedist	

AP, Anteroposterior; *Hx*, history; *PA*, posteroanterior; *PT*, physical therapy.

curve measurement are being studied. If a scoliometer is used to measure the tilt of the rib hump, readings of greater than 5 degrees indicate the need for radiographs. The anteroposterior (AP) and lateral standing views on trifold, full-length films with shielding are recommended. Standing radiographs are preferred because they demonstrate larger curves than do supine films. The radiograph identifies the degrees of curvature by using the Cobb method to measure the angle of curvature and is the only way to assess the status of the back accurately. This measurement should be determined by the radiologist. A finding of an iliac crest that is significantly higher on one side than the other is suggestive of leg length discrepancy (Stewart & Skaggs, 2006). In infants, the rib vertebral angle difference is an important measurement for orthopedists.

An AP spine radiograph is an important baseline study, in that the rate of change of the curve determines the severity of the problem and appropriate treatment. The curves of idiopathic adolescent scoliosis are classified radiographically as thoracic, double major, thoracolumbar, double thoracic, and lumbar. The Risser sign (grade 0 represents no ossification, and 5 is full ossification with fusion of the apophysis to the ilium) is an iliac apophysis maturation index of bone growth and is useful in determining the likelihood of curvature progression. If the child has a 15-degree curve and a Risser grade of 1, the likelihood of the further curvature progression is high. MRI should be ordered if intraspinal anomalies or neurologic problems are suspected; bone scans are useful if osteoid osteoma is a differential diagnosis (Stewart & Skaggs, 2006).

Differential Diagnosis.   Structural scoliosis must be differentiated from functional scoliosis. The latter disappears when the child is placed in Adam's forward bending position, whereas the former is enhanced in this position. Persistent functional scoliosis to one side in a child with a neuromotor problem can eventually become structural and must be managed with physical therapy or other means to prevent progression.

Consider systemic problems, such as neurofibromatosis, cerebral palsy, multiple sclerosis, Rett syndrome, rickets, tuberculosis, and tumor.

Management.   The goal of treatment is not to fully correct the deformity but to prevent increasing deformity and maximize the child's physical growth and function (Bennett, 2002a; Reamy & Slakey, 2001; Stewart & Skaggs, 2006; Sussman & Turker, 2002). Refer to an orthopedic surgeon. Because most treatment relies on growth to assist in correcting the problem, referrals need to be made as early as possible. Most curves require only observation; however, bracing and surgical correction of large curves may be necessary. Bracing is only effective to control progression of a curve and not to decrease its magnitude. The degree of skeletal maturity is a key factor in whether bracing will be effective. It is effective with skeletally immature spines and is considered when curvatures reach 20 to 25 degrees.

Idiopathic Scoliosis

- Treatment varies depending on age at manifestation. Infantile scoliosis often involves a left thoracic curvature in males and resolves spontaneously in 90% of children. Nonresolving and progressive infantile curves are treated with bracing. Juvenile scoliosis occurs more often in females, is generally progressive, and commonly is a right thoracic curvature that requires treatment with bracing. Adolescent scoliosis has a 3:2 female-to-male ratio and can resolve, remain static, or increase. Mild curves need observation and reassurance only; curves greater than 25 degrees and less than 45 degrees need brace management and observation. Curves greater than 45 degrees or curves expected to progress to that range in children who are not candidates for bracing need surgical intervention (instrumentation and fusion). Bracing and casting after surgery may be necessary.
- Monitoring or treatment (or both) is necessary until growth is complete.
- Physical therapy, electrical stimulation, and chiropractic manipulation have not been shown to alter the progression of curvature.
- Support must be given to the child and family through the diagnostic and treatment phases, considering school and peer factors. Assist the child with psychologic adjustment issues that arise if casting, bracing, or surgery is recommended and instituted. Some specific concerns of the child can include self-esteem problems, managing hostility and anger, learning about the disease and its care, wondering about the long-term prognosis, and concerns about clothing and participation in sports and other activities. Parents often worry about the long-term prognosis and finances to cover care, experience guilt for possibly causing the problem (if it

is thought to be genetic) or not identifying the problem earlier, and feel concern about the possible pain and treatment that the child will experience.

Other Classifications of Scoliosis.   For congenital, constitutional, paralytic, tumor, mesenchymal, posttraumatic, or miscellaneous causes of scoliosis, treatment depends on the etiology and severity of the curve and the rate of its progression. Bracing may be tried, is controversial, and is generally not effective. Bracing may help reduce compensatory curves in congenital scoliosis. Rapidly increasing curves need early operative treatment (e.g., spinal fusion and instrumentation). Supervision needs to be maintained until growth is complete. Exercises are not helpful. Paralytic scoliosis with neuromuscular-related curves greater than 20 degrees is treated with surgery.

Complications.   Progressive scoliosis can result in a severe deformity of the spinal column. Severe deformities can result in impairment of respiratory and cardiovascular function and limitation of physical activities and decreased comfort. The psychological consequences of an untreated scoliosis deformity can be severe.

Prevention.   Prevention is not possible; however, early identification of children with scoliosis can help them avoid more expensive, invasive care and prevent the long-term consequences of the disorder. School screening clinics are recommended by the American Academy of Orthopedic Surgeons and the Scoliosis Research Society. Screening is effective, however, only if identified children are referred for care. Their parents must be notified, a referral arranged, and follow-up ensured.

Kyphosis

Description.   The thoracic spine normally has between 20 to 45 degrees of posterior curvature, which is considered physiologic. Kyphosis is the term used to describe the condition when the normal posterior curvature of the thoracic spine becomes excessive or exaggerated and is outside the physiologic range of normal. With kyphosis there is an AP forward curve of the thoracic spine with the apex posterior (i.e., the back is prominent). The most common clinical type of kyphosis is postural (postural roundback). The curvature of the spinal column points backward, and when viewed from the side, gives the appearance of being humpbacked. In postural kyphosis, the Adam's forward bending test demonstrates normalization of the lateral spine profile when viewed from the side (see Table 37-3), and the child can reverse the roundback appearance with active extension (Doyle, 2006). Kyphosis in children can also be secondary to congenital deformity, tumor, trauma, infection, or such problems as achondroplasia. A radiograph can be useful to identify these nonpostural causes. The radiograph shows narrowed disk space, loss of normal anterior height of the involved vertebrae, and other findings.

Scheuermann disease is a common pathologic form of kyphosis that is most often seen in late childhood and adolescence. It causes back pain at the apex of the curve, is progressive, and has an unknown etiology, though it may have hereditary factors. In Scheuermann kyphosis, radiographs demonstrate wedging of three adjacent thoracic vertebrae and the presence of end-plate intrusions, known as Schmorl's nodes. The curve remains when the child stands or is prone in the hyperextended position. The Adam's forward bending test demonstrates more or less acute angulation of the back when observed from the side (Thompson, 2006).

Management. Postural kyphosis needs to be managed by referral to a physical therapist. Activities, such as dancing or swimming, which require a full range of motion of the shoulders, back, and arms, can be helpful. If the problem is structural and not functional, a referral to an orthopedic surgeon is warranted. If pain is a problem, immobilization of the back in a brace is an option. For mild curves, observation and bracing are the usual options for skeletally immature spines. This is the usual therapy for Scheuermann kyphosis. For severe and congenital kyphosis (greater than 65 degree curves), anterior and posterior spinal surgery with instrumentation and fusion is the appropriate management strategy.

Lumbar Lordosis

Description. Lumbar lordosis, or hyperlordosis, is an AP curve of the lumbar area of the spine (i.e., the child stands with the abdomen and buttocks protuberant). It sometimes occurs with kyphosis. Lordosis can be a secondary result of a hip problem in which full extension is limited by hip flexion contractures or from lumbosacral deformities. Physiologic lordosis is commonly seen in families, certain racial groups, and just before onset of puberty. Physiologic lordosis is not a fixed deformity. In lordosis the curvature points forward; the apex of the curve is anterior (Neyt & Weinstein, 2003).

Management. If the pediatric provider suspects lumbar lordosis, have the child bend forward. If the lumbar spine flattens and the lordosis disappears in the forward bending position, it indicates that the spine is flexible and the lordosis is only physiologic. This child should be seen for follow-up in 6 to 12 months. If the lordosis persists in the forward bending position, this indicates a fixed structural deformity and needs referral to an orthopedist. Lordosis resulting from hip flexion contractures is absent while sitting and commonly seen in children with cerebral palsy, spina bifida, and DDH (see Table 37-3).

HIP PROBLEMS

Developmental Dysplasia of the Hip

Description. Developmental dysplasia of the hip (DDH), formerly congenital dislocated hip, is the term used to describe a variety of disorders resulting in abnormal development of the hip joint. These disorders include dysplasia, subluxation, or complete dislocation of the femoral head out of the pelvic acetabulum. Dysplasia is characterized by a shallow more vertical acetabular socket with an immature hip/acetabulum. In subluxation, the hip is unstable, and the head of the femur can slide in and out of the acetabulum. DDH occurs congenitally or develops in infancy or childhood. Dysplasia may be diagnosed many years after the newborn period.

Epidemiology. The etiology of DDH is multifactorial, with mechanical, environmental, and physiologic factors and a genetic predisposition for the condition. Physiologic factors include the hormonal effect of maternal estrogen and relaxin on joint laxity that can contribute to DDH in the neonatal period. Mechanical factors include uterine packing stresses (e.g., breech position), especially during the last trimester if the fetal pelvis becomes locked in the maternal pelvis. Sometimes the condition is found at birth, but frequently the actual dislocation occurs postnatally, even after some months. In cultures that swaddle infants in an extended position or place them on cradleboards, the incidence of DDH is greater than normal because of such neonatal positioning.

The mechanism for dislocation is considered to be related to distention of the joint capsule, which allows the femoral head to disengage from the acetabulum. If the head is relocated soon after birth, the soft tissues tighten around the joint within a few weeks. All newborns have normal laxity of their joints. However, if the hip is persistently dislocated, soft tissue and bony parts become deformed. The left hip is most often involved because this hip typically is the one in a forced adduction position against the mother's sacrum.

The hip can dislocate noncongenitally or in utero in children with certain muscular or neurologic disorders that affect the use of the lower extremities, such as cerebral palsy, arthrogryposis, or myelomeningocele. Dislocation results from the abnormal use of the extremity over time.

The incidence of DDH is estimated to be 10 per 1000 live births in the U.S. It is found more commonly with breech births and is four times more common in girls than boys. A positive family history (genetic risk factors) increases the risk for having a child with this problem. Other risk factors seen in infants that are associated with DDH include oligohydramnios, torticollis, and lower limb deformities, such as clubfoot, metatarsus adductus (MA), and dislocated knee (Shah & Stankovits, 2006). It is uncommon in African-American infants. Bilateral dislocation occurs in approximately 25% of cases (Cady, 2006).

Clinical Findings.

History. The history may include a positive family history; associated neck, knee, and foot deformities noted at or shortly after birth; and breech delivery.

Physical Examination. A hip examination should be performed on children as part of their well-child supervision until they are 2 years old. Findings of DDH include the following (Bennett, 2002b):

- The early phase, or loose phase, can extend for the first 6 months and is characterized by positive Ortolani or Barlow sign (or both). These signs are seen in infants typically for the first 2 to 3 months of life. Around 2 months old, soft tissue contractures develop, which prevent manual reduction of the dislocated hip.
- The late phase occurs by 6 months old and is characterized by the following:
  - Limited abduction of the affected hip and shortening of the thigh, which becomes well established and must be relied on as the primary sign in the older infant (see Fig. 37-5).

○ Normal abduction with comfort is 70 to 80 degrees bilaterally. Limited abduction includes those cases with less than 60 degrees of abduction or unequal abduction from one side to the other (see Fig. 37-5).

○ Unequal knee heights (positive Galeazzi sign [see Fig. 37-3*A*]).

• Other findings include asymmetry of inguinal or gluteal folds (thigh-fold asymmetry is not related to the disorder [see Fig. 37-3]) and unequal leg lengths, shorter on the affected side.

In the ambulatory child who was not diagnosed earlier or was not corrected, the following might also be noted:

• Short leg with toe walking on the affected side
• Positive Trendelenburg sign (see Fig. 37-3*D*)
• Marked lordosis or toe walking
• Painless limping or waddling gait with child leaning to the affected side

If the hips are dislocated bilaterally, asymmetries are not observed. Limited abduction is the primary indicator in this situation (see Fig. 37-5). Also, in the subluxed hip (not frankly dislocated), limited abduction again is the primary indicator.

Diagnostic Studies. Radiologic evaluation of the newborn to detect DDH is unreliable because so much of the hip joint is cartilaginous in young infants. Also, the dislocation may be so recent that pathologic changes in addition to the loose capsule may not yet have developed. Ultrasound study provides useful information in newborns and infants (less than 3 months old), especially in neonates with suspicious findings or when hip risk factors are present. If an infant's hip is unstable by examination, the diagnosis is made. By around 3 months old, radiography is reliable. AP and Lauenstein (frog-leg) position lateral radiographs of the pelvis are adequate. CT and MRI are reserved for difficult cases (Thompson, 2006).

Differential Diagnosis. The condition is relatively unique.

Management. The goal of management is to restore the articulation of the femur within the acetabulum.

• Refer to an orthopedist promptly while the infant is still in the newborn nursery, if possible. Any child with subluxed, dislocatable, and dislocated hips needs to be referred. The earlier treatment is begun, the better the prognosis is for functional development of the acetabulum. The treatment of choice for subluxation and reducible dislocations identified in the early phase is a Pavlik harness. If the hip is irreducible in the early phase, a Pavlik harness may be tried. However, if it is not successful, a closed reduction followed by Pavlik harness or spica cast is the preferred treatment. The harness is fitted to gently hold the hip in flexion and abduction, which guides the femoral head into the acetabulum until stable, permitting flexion motion. If Pavlik harness treatment fails, a closed reduction of the hip is the next step. If the diagnosis is delayed past about 6 months old, traction with closed reduction is often first tried. However, traction with open reduction is often necessary to bring the femoral head into place. A femoral and pelvic osteotomy is the treatment of choice in children 18 months or older. Surgery is done to bring the acetabulum down over the femoral head when the possibility of further positive development of the joint ceases.

• Triple diapering is *not* helpful because the musculoskeletal forces far outweigh the force that can be exerted by the diaper material.

• Continue long-term monitoring of hip development if neonatal hip instability was noted at birth. A small percentage of infants are noted to have hip instability at birth, versus the 1% of infants with classic DDH. The majority of neonatal hip instability resolves spontaneously. Close observation of these children is recommended.

• The child with a Pavlik harness should be seen weekly to ensure that it fits properly and the femur is properly seated in the socket. It is worn 24 hours a day except for bathing until a normal pelvic radiograph is obtained.

• The earlier treatment is started with the Pavlik harness, the better the prognosis for a successful outcome. Generally the harness is worn full time for 2 months and then worn during waking hours for decreasing periods of time.

• Support the child and family through the treatment phases. Explain management goals clearly. Caring for a child in a Pavlik harness or spica cast requires special knowledge. Cast care, skin care, and car safety when the child cannot easily be placed in a car seat are all issues to be addressed. Also see Chapter 10 for reference to safety restraints for children with special conditions or in a hip spica cast. Furthermore, the child needs special attention to maintain developmental stimulation while immobilized.

• Immediately refer an infant seen in a primary care setting who is in a Pavlik harness and exhibits excessive hip flexion (beyond 100 degrees) or abduction (beyond 60 degrees) to the orthopedist. These degrees of flexion or abduction can be harmful (Shah & Stankovits, 2006).

Complications. The long-term outcomes depend on the age at diagnosis, the severity of the joint deformity, and the effectiveness of therapy. Untreated cases may result in a permanent dislocation of the femoral head so that it lies just under the iliac crest posteriorly. Clinically, the child has limited mobility of this artificial joint and related short leg. Forceful reduction can result in avascular necrosis of the femoral head with permanent hip deformity. Redislocation or persistent dysplasia can occur. Adult degenerative arthritis is associated with acetabular dysplasia.

Prevention. The condition cannot be prevented, but early identification resulting in early treatment significantly reduces the long-term consequences of the problem. Screening of all neonates and infants should include full hip abduction, examination for unequal folds and unequal leg lengths, and Barlow, Ortolani, and Galeazzi maneuvers at every examination. The hip can dislocate at any point in early development, even up to the point of first ambulation. In older children, limited abduction, gait, and standing position, including the Trendelenburg position, add important information. Charting should always include notation about hip findings because these can change at subsequent visits.

Legg-Calvé-Perthes Disease

Description. Legg-Calvé-Perthes disease (LCPD) is idiopathic, juvenile avascular necrosis of the femoral head.

Epidemiology.   There is an initial ischemic episode of unknown etiology that interrupts vascular circulation to the capital femoral epiphysis. The articular cartilage hypertrophies, and the epiphyseal marrow becomes necrotic. The area revascularizes, and the necrotic bone is replaced by new bone. This process can take 18 to 24 months. There is a critical point in these dual processes when the subchondral area becomes weak enough that fracture of the epiphysis occurs. At this time, the child becomes symptomatic. With fracturing, further reabsorption and replacement by fibrous bone occurs, and the shape of the femoral head is altered. Articulation of the head in the hip joint is interrupted. The bone reossifies with or without treatment, but without treatment the femoral head flattens and enlarges, causing joint deformity.

The disorder is five times more common in boys and most commonly occurs between 4 and 8 years old. It occurs bilaterally in approximately 10% of cases (Shah & Stankovits, 2006). Children with bilateral LCPD typically are treated at a younger age and have more associated anomalies. Genetics do not appear to be a major predisposing factor. Approximately 10% of children with LCPD have a history of breech delivery, low birth weight, or abnormal birth presentations; 17% have a history of preceding trauma. LCPD in girls tends to be a more serious problem with a poor prognosis (Warren, 2002b).

Clinical Findings.

History.   There can be an acute or chronic onset with or without a history of trauma to the hip, such as jumping from a high place.

- Acute onset (Warren, 2002b)
  ○ Sudden onset of pain in the groin or knee often occurring at night with pain on weight bearing or stiffness
  ○ Some children may have little restriction in motion of the hip
- Chronic
  ○ Recurring pain (mild or aching) at the hip or referred to the knee, anterior medial thigh, or groin for days to weeks and limp
  ○ Insidious limping generally in the morning and after activities; a "painless" limp is a classic presentation
  ○ Stiffness in the morning or after rest

Physical Examination.   Findings may include the following:
- Antalgic gait (usually the first sign) with a component of shortening and positive Trendelenburg sign
- Muscle spasm
- Thigh atrophy
- Decreased abduction, internal rotation, and extension of the hip
- Pain on rolling the leg internally
- Short stature (mild) if bone age is delayed

Diagnostic Studies.   Routine AP pelvis and frog-leg lateral views are used to confirm the diagnosis and follow disease progression and response to treatment. Alterations seen can include smaller epiphysis, increased epiphyseal density, subchondral fracture line, lateralization of the femoral head, and other features. Changes in the epiphysis margin are discerned by the orthopedist and radiologist (Fig. 37-8). However, there may be no radiographic findings early in LCDP. Bone scans and MRI are helpful in recognizing early disease, but are of limited value in assessing the extent of involvement or following disease progression. Radiographic changes are helpful in predicting poorer outcomes and the need for aggressive management (Thompson, 2006).

Differential Diagnosis.   Acute and chronic infections, sickle cell disease, toxic synovitis, Gaucher disease, slipped capital femoral epiphysis (SCFE), and other hip dysplasia problems may occur with similar features. Generally, SCFE occurs in obese preadolescent and adolescent boys.

Management.   The following steps are taken (Shah & Stankovits, 2006; Thompson, 2006):
- Refer to an orthopedist immediately and ensure access to care for the child and family. Most cases of LCPD are mild and need no treatment because they are self-limited. However, all children with LCPD require frequent follow-up and monitoring by the orthopedist. Initial bed rest and possibly femoral abduction traction (to relieve muscle spasms) may be used to eliminate or reduce hip irritability (1 to 2 weeks). Physical therapy may then be needed to reduce residual stiffness. The orthopedist works to prevent extrusion and collapse of the femoral head and attain or

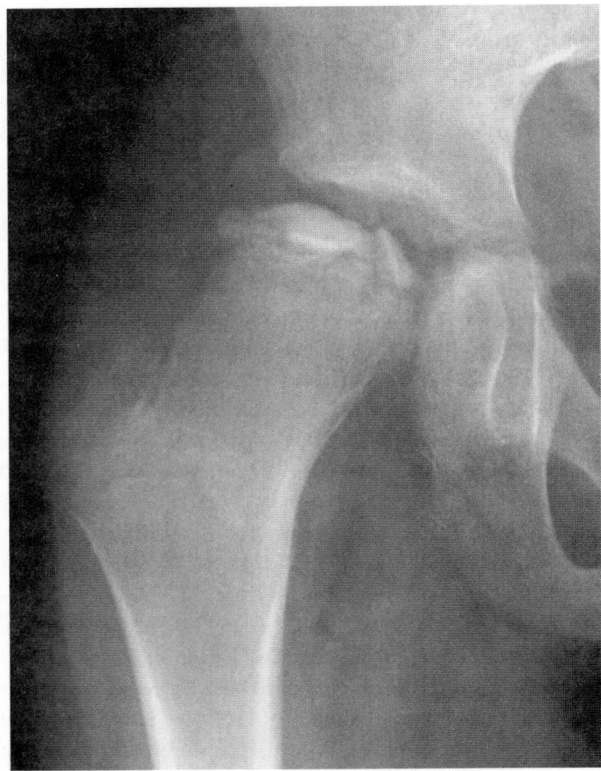

FIG. 37-8   AP radiograph of the right hip of an 8-year-old boy with LCPD. There is a collapsed yet dense capital femoral epiphysis with early fragmentation. The small medial triangle of the capital femoral epiphysis is uninvolved in the disease process. (From Behrman RE, Kliegman RM, Jenson HB, editors: *Nelson textbook of pediatrics*, ed 17, Philadelphia, 2004, WB Saunders.)

maintain a round shape using nonoperative or operative procedures, or both. Containment of the femoral head within the acetabulum is important. For moderate to severe cases, bracing and surgical intervention are the treatment options. Bracing is continued 24 hours a day for 6 to 18 months. Operative treatment is generally used in older children, for those who are not satisfactory candidates for bracing, or for those with extensive necrosis of the femoral head.

- Educate the family regarding the condition and its management and the risk for development of the condition on the other side.
- Support and monitor the child throughout treatment and recovery, including during interruption of school or other activities. The management of LCPD often involves several years of treatment and monitoring.

Complications.   Osteoarthritis related to femoral head deformity and decreased use of the hip joint may occur, depending on the femoral head remodeling status. Older children have a poorer prognosis owing to the decreased opportunity for femoral head remodeling in the remaining growth period. Females with LCPD also have a poor prognosis.

Prevention.   The condition is not preventable, but early identification and treatment reduce the long-term complications of the disorder, such as premature degenerative arthritis in early adult life.

Slipped Capital Femoral Epiphysis

Description.   Slipped capital femoral epiphysis (SCFE) is a condition in which the upper femoral epiphysis slips from its functional position in the hip joint, and the femoral neck assumes a more varus angle. During the process, the physis of the femur (the growth plate area) becomes less competent, resulting in a weakening of the perichondrial ring. This weakening allows the epiphysis to slip posteriorly and medially, while the femoral neck moves anteriorly and proximally. Because the blood supply to the epiphysis crosses the weakened area, the epiphysis is at risk for avascular necrosis. The slippage is generally gradual, and the condition is generally classified as stable or unstable based on the continuity of the capital femoral epiphysis and the femoral neck. SCFE resolves when the growth plate closes with whatever position the epiphysis has taken in relation to the femoral shaft (Shah & Stankovits, 2006).

Epidemiology.   SCFE is the most common hip disorder in adolescents and is associated with genetic, racial, and geographic risk factors. The exact etiology is unknown in most cases and thought to be multifactorial. Other possible causes include mechanical susceptibility or vulnerability of the hip, endocrinopathies or systemic disease (e.g., hypothyroidism, hypopituitarism, hypogonadism, and chronic renal failure), trauma resulting from repetitive shear stress, and inflammatory changes. Obesity increases the shear forces across the femoral head and growth plate. Obese children develop SCFE; the mechanism is thought to be related to low levels of sex hormones. An overabundance of growth hormone is thought to be a factor with tall children who develop SCFE (Thompson, 2006).

SCFE is associated with chronic shear forces on the physis before its closure. The problem occurs two to three times more often in males than females, especially those who are skeletally immature and obese. Affected males are generally between 10 and 16 years old, and females are between 9 and 15 years old (before menarche) (Shah & Stankovits, 2006). African-American males and females have a higher incidence, and about 5% have a positive family history. Polynesian populations are also at risk. Bilateral involvement occurs in 20% to 25% of cases. The majority of children are above the 90th percentile for weight (Warren, 2002c).

Clinical Findings.   The findings are similar to those of younger children with LCPD and depend on the degree of slippage and stability of the capital femoral epiphysis.

History.   The following may be reported (Katz, 2006):
- Acute (symptoms within 3 weeks) or chronic (more than 3 weeks).
- Acute-on-chronic slip can also be reported (acute episode of further slippage in a child with previous slippage).
- Hip pain is a common complaint, but some have no hip-related complaints; instead they complain of referred thigh or knee pain or no pain at all.
- Some have complaints of limping, out toeing, or unspecified gait problem.
- Infrequently, a history of mild trauma to the hip area with excruciating pain afterwards.

Physical Examination.   Findings include the following:
- Pain in the groin or diffusely over the knee or anterior thigh
- Pain and decreased internal rotation
- Antalgic limp with short leg component (50% are up to 1 inch shorter on affected side)
- External rotation of the leg when walking
- External rotation of the thigh when the hip is flexed; lack of internal rotation of the hip with range of motion
- Thigh atrophy
- Limited abduction and extension

Diagnostic Studies.   AP pelvis, frog-leg lateral, and true lateral views of the pelvis are obtained. Radiographic findings include flattening of the epiphyseal prominence, widening or irregularity of the growth plate, and narrowing of the area if the epiphysis has slipped posteriorly. The varus angle between the femoral head and the shaft is also assessed (Fig. 37-9). CT is used for preoperative planning because it provides measurements of the percentage of epiphysial slip and the head-shaft and head-neck angles. SCFE is classified by grade and severity of the slip.

Differential Diagnosis.   LCPD, sepsis of the hip joint, and osteoarthritis should be considered.

Management.   The following steps are taken:
- Refer immediately to an orthopedic surgeon because there is risk of an acute and more devastating slip, which can occur at any time. Assist the family to attain prompt intervention. Immediate hospitalization is needed once the diagnosis is made.

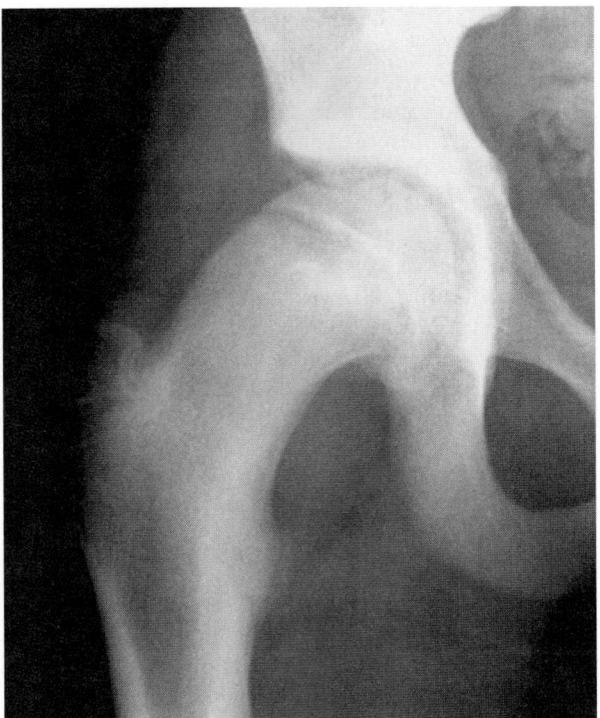

FIG. 37-9 AP radiograph of the right hip of a 13-year-old boy with a moderately severe chronic slipped femoral epiphysis. Notice the physeal widening and the distorted relationship between the capital femoral epiphysis and femoral neck. (From Behrman RE, Kliegman RM, Jenson HB, editors: *Nelson textbook of pediatrics*, ed 17, Philadelphia, 2004, WB Saunders.)

- Place the patient on non–weight-bearing crutches until admitted to the hospital. Wheelchair sitting is not advised because acute flexion can cause further slippage. Adequate instruction should be given so that the child will not fall on the crutches, another risk factor for an acute slip.
- For mild to moderate slips, in situ fixation of the epiphysis to the femur with a metallic screw or pins is the accepted treatment of choice. The screw or pins are removed after the growth plate closes. For very severe slippage, an osteotomy is sometimes required. Spica cast immobilization is sometimes used for acute slips, but has disadvantages. Traction can be used to gently reduce an acute-on-chronic slip.
- Inform the family about the condition and its management and the risk for slippage on the other side if only one side is treated.
- Support and monitor the child throughout the treatment phase, which includes interruption of school and activities during the recovery period. Contact sports are usually restricted by the orthopedist until growth is complete.

Complications. Avascular necrosis of the femoral head or, more commonly, chondrolysis of the cartilage lining the hip joint with narrowing of the hip joint is possible. A bilateral slip may have occurred at the time of diagnosis or can occur at a later time (Thompson, 2006).

Prevention. SCFE is not a preventable condition. However, identification of the condition during the preslip period, when complaints of hip or referred knee pain, loss of motion, or weakness in the hip are present, allows early intervention that can prevent deformity and long-term sequelae, such as premature degenerative arthritis in early adult life. If the child is overweight, advise about the need for weight reduction (Kocher et al, 2004).

Femoral Anteversion

Description. Everyone has some degree of femoral anteversion. By 10 to 12 years old, the normal angle of anteversion is 10 to 15 degrees. Younger children have a somewhat wider angle. Increased femoral anteversion (more than 2 SD [standard deviations] from the mean) is called femoral torsion and can be either medial or lateral. Medial femoral torsion or medial antetorsion generally occurs around 2 to 3 years old and lasts until about 5 years old. It is a condition in which the head and neck of the femur are rotated at an increased angle anteriorly in relation to the femoral shaft. Femoral anteversion is also called *internal femoral torsion*.

Epidemiology. A family history is often identified, and it occurs more commonly in girls. "W" sitting can increase the deformity. Physiologically, the condition produces an in-toeing gait because the anteriorly directed femoral neck internally rotates to a more neutral position and the head of the femur fits neatly into the acetabulum. This results in internal rotation of the lower femur and leg with the feet in-toeing. Increased femoral anteversion generally is more severe between 4 and 6 years old, but resolves as the child grows and the tibia rotates laterally.

Clinical Findings.

History. The following may be reported:
- In-toeing gait, perhaps more severe with fatigue
- Runs awkwardly (looks like an "eggbeater"); may actually trip as a result of crossing the feet while walking or running.
- Possible family history
- Usually a history of "W" sitting (TV squat)

Physical Examination. Findings include the following:
- In-toeing gait with patellae medial
- Internal (medial) rotation normally less than 70 degrees (mild deformity—70 to 80 degrees; moderate—between 80 and 90 degrees; severe—greater than 90 degrees [Sass & Hassan, 2003; Staheli, 2003a] [see Fig. 37-6])
- External (lateral) rotation decreased (limited to 0 to 10 degrees)
- Knees medially rotated ("kissing patella") when standing

Diagnostic Studies. Radiographs are not merited unless surgery is contemplated.

Differential Diagnosis. Consider other rotational deformities, such as internal tibial torsion or MA. Cerebral palsy with a "scissoring gait" might be mistaken for severe femoral anteversion.

Management. Management includes observation of the child and referral to an orthopedist if medial rotations are significant (no external rotation of the hip in extension) or the child or family has significant concerns. Nonoperative management strategies, such as shoe modifications, twister cables, and night splints, have all been found to be ineffective. Operative correction is successful, but carries the risk of complications. Osteotomy is rarely performed and is done only in the child older than 8 years with significant cosmetic and functional deformity. The natural history of the condition is for the medial, or internal, rotation to decrease, giving some improvement (Sass & Hassan, 2003; Staheli, 2003a; Thompson, 2006).

Complications.   Studies have shown that the condition does not cause flatfoot, bunions, knee problems, back difficulties, difficulties in running, or degenerative arthritis of the hip in adults (Staheli, 2003a). It is primarily a cosmetic problem unless severe enough to interfere with activities. Self-esteem can be affected.

Prevention.   The condition cannot be prevented, but its aggravation can be minimized by discouraging "W" sitting, which places the weight of the upper body directly on the femoral neck, thus increasing the molding in the abnormal direction. Ballet lessons or activities, such as skating, bicycle riding, or skiing, can help mildly affected children learn to point their feet straight ahead, but such activities do not modify the bony structures (Sawyer & Drendel, 2006).

KNEE PROBLEMS
Genu Varum
Description.   Genu varum, or bowing of the legs, can be a physiologic or developmental variation of normal or a pathologic condition, which involves a rotational deformity. The term *bowlegs* is used to describe physiologic variations of the normal knee angle resulting in bowing of the legs that is typically seen in children up to 2 years old, but can be considered normal until 3 years old. The typical pattern of normal bowing seen in children is a symmetric lateral bowing of both tibias in the first year followed by bowlegs in the second year. Most bowing resolves spontaneously, but can progress to persistent or pathologic varus. The angle between the tibia and femur is in pronounced varus (up to 15 degrees) in normal children before 1 year old. This is considered a uterine packing effect. The angle approaches neutral by 18 months old and then proceeds to a valgus angle, with an average angle of 12 degrees from 2 to 3 years old. The angle then gradually decreases to 8 degrees in females and 7 degrees in males by adulthood. If the varus angle is greater than 15 degrees in infants, does not begin to decrease in the second year, is asymmetric, is associated with short stature, or is rapidly progressing, the condition is considered pathologic. Knee angle variations that fall 2 SD beyond the mean are outside the normal range of varus and are considered pathologic.

If the varus persists after 30 months old or increases, it may represent Blount disease, rickets, tumor, neurologic problems, infection, or other conditions. A Salter fracture through the tibial growth plate can result in later genu varum as growth across the plate progresses unevenly.

With Blount disease (idiopathic tibia vara that affects the proximal tibia), there is an abnormal growth of the medial aspect of the proximal tibial epiphysis that results in progressive varus angulation of the tibia. Blount disease is rare, but can occur in infancy (18 months to 3 years old), school years (4 to 10 years old), and during adolescence (11 years and older). It is seen more frequently in the African-American, Hispanic, and Scandinavian populations, is associated with obesity and early walkers, and commonly has a positive family history and affects the proximal tibia. Onset in infancy presents the highest risk for greatest deformity (Thompson, 2004b; Sass & Hassan, 2003; Thompson, 2006).

Clinical Findings.
History.   When considering a diagnosis of pathologic genu varum, the primary care provider should assess the following:
- Progression since birth; increasing deformation is problematic
- Risk factors, such as metabolic disease
- Older children may complain of pain (Thompson, 2004b)

Physical Examination.   Findings include the following:
- Tibial-femoral angle greater than 15 degrees
- Associated internal tibial torsion is common
- Intercondylar (knees) distance with the ankles together—measurement greater than 4 to 5 inches is suggestive of the need for additional evaluation
- Joint laxity of the lateral collateral ligaments in older children

Diagnostic Studies.   Radiographs are not necessary for physiologic bowlegs. Irregularity in the proximal medial tibia metaphysis with medial slipping of the physis and lateralization of the tibia are characteristic radiographic findings seen in infantile Blount disease. The radiographic findings in adolescent Blount disease differ in that the typical finding is narrowing of the medial physis only, with epiphysis not affected (Warren, 2002a).

Differential Diagnosis.   Physiologic, persistent, and pathologic genu varum must be differentiated. Metabolic (rickets) or neurologic problems, Blount disease, infections, tumor, osteochondrodysplasias, and internal tibial torsion should be ruled out.

Management.
- In physiologic genu varum (no increasing deformity):
  - No active treatment and resolves spontaneously. Denis Browne sleeping splints, corrective shoes, and passive exercises have not proved useful.
  - Reassure parents; provide information about the natural progression of the problem.
  - Observe the child's condition over time (in 3 to 6 months) to be sure the problem is resolving, especially during the second year of life. Photographs of the legs for the chart can be helpful.
- In pathologic genu varum (increasing deformity):
  - Refer to an orthopedist. Blount disease may be treated with a Blount brace in the early stages of the disease because the bowing is reversible. In later stages of the disease, in older children, or if the disease is progressing, osteotomy is the treatment of choice. Other conditions need to be treated according to the etiology.

○ Monitor to be sure braces are used consistently with good fit.

○ Observe to be sure the problem is not worsening.

Complications. Knee degeneration and deformity result if pathologic genu varum is not treated.

Prevention. Early identification and referral reduce the complexity and expense of treatment and the residual deformities.

Genu Valgum

Description. Genu valgum is commonly referred to as *knock-knees*. Females tend to have a somewhat higher degree of valgus knee posture than males, leveling off by 7 years old at 5 to 9 degrees compared with 4 to 7 degrees for boys. Physiologic genu valgum tends to peak at around 24 to 36 months old and lasts until about 7 to 8 years old.

Epidemiology. The condition can be considered developmental or physiologic in children starting anywhere from 2 to 4 years old. It can be pathologic in the following situations: found in child older than 6 to 7 years; tibial-femoral angle greater than 15 degrees valgus; increasing in severity; and found in the presence of asymmetry, short stature, or obesity (Warren, 2002a). Causes of pathologic genu valgum include osteochondrodysplasias, physeal injury, tumor, myelodysplasia, and cerebral palsy.

Clinical Findings.

History. The pediatric provider should assess the following:
- Progression of the deformity
- Risk factors as listed under epidemiology
- Joint pains or stiff gait caused by adduction of the thighs and abrasions

Physical Examination. Findings include the following (Warren, 2002a):
- Bilateral tibial-femoral angle less than 15 degrees of valgus in the child up to 7 years old is considered normal and can be safely ignored; a valgus angle greater than 15 degrees is outside the range of normal.
- Unilateral deformity.
- Awkwardness of gait.
- Subluxing patella.
- Intermalleolar (ankles) distance with the knees together—measurement greater than 4 to 5 inches suggests the need for additional evaluation (Sass & Hassan, 2003).
- Genu valgum associated with short stature should be referred.

Diagnostic Studies. No radiographic studies are needed unless a pathologic condition is suspected.

Differential Diagnosis. Rule out pathologic conditions of genu valgum.

Management. Management is the same as for physiologic and pathologic genu varum. However, for pathologic genu valgum, the types of braces prescribed are different, as are the surgical procedures. Bracing, usually at night, is used with deformities greater than 15 to 20 degrees, especially if there is a family history. Epiphyseal stapling or osteotomy may be needed if the deformity persists after 10 years old or if ligamentous or patellofemoral instability is present (Warren, 2002a). For most children with genu valgum before 6 years old, the condition resolves spontaneously.

Prevention. Preventive measures are the same as those for genu varum.

Osgood-Schlatter Disease

Description. Osgood-Schlatter disease (OSD) is caused by inflammation of the tibial tubercle, an apophysis site.

Epidemiology. OSD is caused by repetitive microtrauma to the growing tibial tubercle apophysis, which results in inflammation, microfractures, and new bone formation at the site. It is a traction apophysitis with overuse of the muscles that attach to the apophysis as an associated factor. Tight muscles resulting from the slow rate of muscle growth relative to bone growth also are believed to be a factor. With the end of growth, the apophysis fuses to the shaft of the tibia and pain diminishes. Thus the incidence declines in older adolescents and in adults (Grudziak & Musahl, 2007).

OSD is the most common cause of knee pain in adolescents who engage in active sports that typically entail sprinting and jumping. However, it can also occur in children who are inactive. It is most often unilateral, and pain can last up to 2 years (Grudziak & Musahl, 2007).

Clinical Findings.

History. The following may be reported:
- Recent physical activity, such as playing track, soccer, or football; surfboarding commonly produces the condition.
- Pain increases during and immediately after the activity and decreases when the activity is stopped for awhile.

Physical Examination. Characteristic findings include the following:
- Point tenderness, pain, prominence over the tibial tubercle (pathognomonic for OSD)
- Pain at the tibial tubercle with knee extension against passive resistance or with full passive knee flexion
- Possibly reduced knee range of motion
- Bilateral findings (frequent)

The diagnosis is based on history and physical examination. Radiographs are not needed unless another pathologic condition is suspected.

Differential Diagnosis. Other knee derangements, tumors (osteosarcoma), and hip problems with referred pain should be considered. The referred pain of hip problems is diffuse across the distal femur without point tenderness at the tibial tubercle.

Management. OSD is a self-limiting condition with symptom management the key consideration. The following steps are taken:
- Avoid or modify activities that cause pain until the inflammation subsides; symptoms can last up to 2 years.
- Applying ice to the site after activity may help.
- Try hamstring, calf, and quadriceps muscle stretching exercises before sports.
- Use of NSAIDs is recommended by some, but thought ineffective by others. Because this condition may last up to 2 years, chronic use of NSAIDs may be problematic.

- A neoprene sleeve over the knee may help stabilize the patella.
- Apply a knee immobilizer if pain is severe and persistent.
- Cylinder casting for 2 to 3 weeks may be suggested for the noncompliant adolescent.

Complications. In the postpubertal child, a residual ossicle in the tendon next to the bone may cause persistent pain. Surgical removal is indicated and will relieve the pain.

Prevention. The condition cannot be prevented, but earlier management may decrease the length of disability and the discomfort associated with it. Avoid overuse and encourage balanced training and adequate warm-up before exercise or sports participation. The use of kneepads may help protect the tibial tuberosity from direct injury for adolescents who engage in sports that result in knee contact (e.g., volleyball) (Grudziak & Musahl, 2007).

Tibial Torsion

Description. Tibial torsion is a common problem in children that involves the twisting of the long bone along its long axis. *Tibial version* is the term used to describe the normal variation in tibial rotation. At birth, the tibias have a mean lateral rotation of 2.2 degrees and rotate laterally over time, with an adult mean lateral tibial rotation of about 23 degrees. Tibial torsion describes those rotations that are outside the range of normal. Medial tibial torsion (MTT), also known as internal tibial torsion, consists of abnormal medial rotation or twisting, resulting in in toeing of the feet; lateral tibial torsion (LTT) consists of abnormal lateral rotation resulting in out toeing (Dise, 2002; Sawyer & Drendel, 2006).

Epidemiology. Tibial torsion may be congenital, developmental, or acquired. MTT is the most common cause of in toeing during the second year of life and is often noted around 6 to 12 months of life. In most cases, it is a physiologic condition that is the result of in utero positioning. In 90% of cases, internal tibial torsion gradually resolves on its own by the time the child reaches 8 years old (Sass & Hassan, 2003). LTT is a cause of out toeing in late childhood and is usually an acquired deformity. Contracture of the iliotibial band is the underlying problem.

Clinical Findings.

Physical Examination. Observe the child's gait for in toeing. The thigh-foot angle (TFA) is used to assess tibial rotation. With the child prone and the knees flexed 90 degrees, the foot and thigh are viewed from directly above (looking downward at the angle of the thigh and foot). The foot should be relaxed. MTT exists if the TFA is negative by more than 10 to 20 degrees (−10 to −20 degrees), bearing in mind the child's age. In toeing is expressed in negative values (Fig. 37-10). The normal range at 13 years old is −5 to +30 degrees. Abnormal lateral torsion is associated with forward-pointing patellae and outward-pointing feet. A TFA measurement of greater than +30 degrees indicates abnormal LTT (Dise, 2002).

Diagnostic Studies. Radiographs are usually not necessary.

Differential Diagnosis. Genu varum in which the problem originates at the knee with a tibial-femoral angle, femoral torsion (femoral anteversion), adducted great toe, and MA also produce in-toeing gaits. Adducted great toe (the searching toe) is a benign condition that resolves spontaneously. Lateral femoral torsion also causes an out-toeing gait.

Management.

- Treatment of tibial version (the normal variation in tibial rotation) is observation and monitoring of the child.
- MTT should be referred to an orthopedist if the problem is significant (TFA greater than −20 by 3 years old). Stretching exercises or external rotational splints may be recommended. Surgical intervention may be needed for severe cases that persist into late childhood and cause significant functional problems.

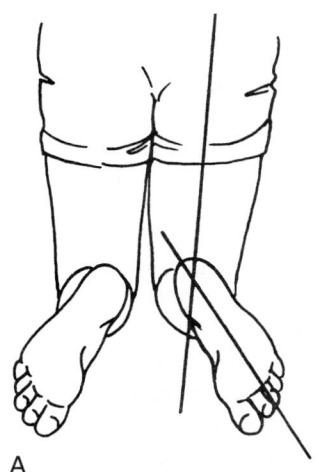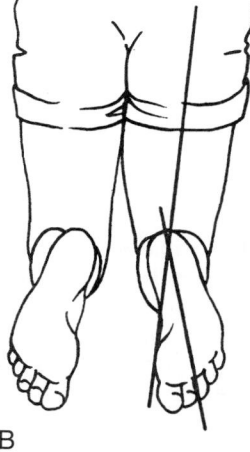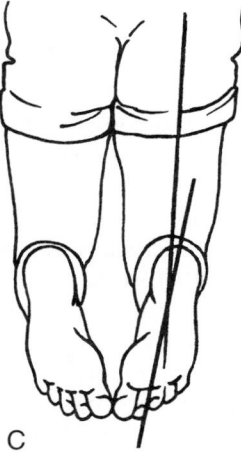

A   B   C

FIG. 37-10 Thigh-foot angle. With the child in the prone position and the knees flexed and approximated, the long axis of the foot can be compared with the long axis of the thigh. The long axis of the foot bisects the heel and the second toe or lies between the second and third toes. External tibial torsion, **A,** produces excessive outward rotation. Normal alignment, **B,** is characterized by slight external rotation. Internal tibial torsion produces inward rotation of the foot and is a negative angle, **C.** (From Thompson GH: Gait disturbances. In Kliegman RM, Nieder ML, Super DM, editors: *Practical strategies in pediatric diagnosis and therapy*, Philadelphia, 1996, WB Saunders.)

- Shoes have been shown to be ineffective for the treatment of MTT. The avoidance of certain postures (e.g., sleeping in the knee-chest position and sitting with the feet tucked under the buttocks) thought to exacerbate MTT is controversial.
- LTT with TFA greater than +30 degrees should be referred to an orthopedist. It usually worsens with growth and does not correct spontaneously. Medial femoral torsion with pain also should be referred (Dise, 2002).

Complications. There are no complications with normal tibial version and no interference with activities. Tibial torsion (the TFA is outside the acceptable range of normal) can lead to significant functional problems in severe cases.

Popliteal Cysts

Description. Popliteal cysts, or Baker cysts, are synovial lesions that result from herniation of the synovium of the knee joint into the popliteal space. In children, they are benign cysts and are not associated with intraarticular defects.

Clinical Findings. The major findings are swelling behind the knee with or without mild discomfort.

Diagnostic Studies. Ultrasonography, transillumination of cyst, and diagnostic aspiration of synovial fluid are the usual diagnostic studies.

Management. Observation is the treatment of choice because the majority of these cysts resolve on their own, although it may take several years (Thompson, 2006). The rare, large, painful, and persistent cyst should be referred to an orthopedic surgeon.

■■■ KNEE INJURIES AND FOOT PROBLEMS
KNEE INJURIES

Chapters 14 and 39 discuss issues related to the musculoskeletal examination and common sports injuries. Table 37-4 outlines the etiology, assessment, management, and differential diagnosis of common knee injuries that are seen in children and young adults.

FOOT PROBLEMS
Pes Planus

Description. Physiologic or flexible pes planus (flatfoot) is commonly seen in neonates and toddlers and is due to a fat pad in the arch that makes the appearance of the arch seem flat. This generally resolves by 2 to 3 years old, but in a small percentage of cases, can persist into adulthood. Flexible flatfoot is often familial, common, and benign. The arch is seen when the foot is suspended, but flattens with weight bearing. Rigid flatfoot is pathologic.

Epidemiology. Flatfoot is the result of soft tissue laxity, muscular weakness, or a tight Achilles tendon. There is often a familial tendency toward the problem. Flatfoot also is associated with certain syndromes (Marfan and Down syndromes), myelodysplasia, cerebral palsy, and obesity. Flatfoot may be secondary to muscle imbalance or weakness, a bony abnormality, or shortened heel cords (Sass & Hassan, 2003).

Clinical Findings.

History. Onset is noticed with weight bearing. The flexible flatfoot is painless and asymptomatic.

Physical Examination. The pediatric health care provider should assess the following:
- Is there an arch in the suspended foot or when the child toe stands?
- Can an arch be molded with pressure by the examiner's fingers?
- Is the Achilles tendon tight?
- Is there abnormal shoe wear on the inner side?

Differential Diagnosis. Congenital vertical talus should be considered if the foot is rigid and no arch can be molded or if the foot has a rocker-bottom appearance. Calcaneovalgus foot might be considered also.

Management. Management involves the following:
- Only symptomatic feet and rigid flatfoot should be treated; refer to an orthopedist.
- For painful, flexible flatfoot, a removable, longitudinal arch support may be recommended by the orthopedist.
- If the Achilles tendon is tight, passive stretching may be helpful.
- Routine radiographs are not indicated unless pathologic flatfoot is suspected.

Complications. Flatfoot should be considered a variation of normal unless there is pain or rigidity. Congenital vertical talus is difficult to treat and should not be missed. Some cases of flatfoot are symptomatic in adulthood, and in severe cases, the bones of the feet adapt to abnormal position with pronation and possible development of bunions.

Patient Education. Parents need to understand that special shoes do not cure the problem, and arch supports do not help the foot to "grow" an arch. The so-called Thomas heel is considered ineffective as a treatment.

Metatarsus Adductus

Description. Metatarsus adductus (MA) is a condition in which the hindfoot is straight but the forefoot is adducted, giving the foot a curved, in-toeing shape. It is often bilateral.

Epidemiology. When the foot is flexible, the condition is usually considered a result of intrauterine packing, with some tightness of the soft tissues in the area of the arch. A nonflexible foot, especially with heel valgus, or persistence may indicate a more serious problem.

Flexible MA is common (1 in 1000 births) and is seen equally in girls and boys. In 10% of cases, it is associated with DDH (Sawyer & Drendel, 2006; Thompson, 2006).

Clinical Findings.

History. There can be a family history.

Physical Examination. Findings include the following:
- The lateral border of the foot has a convex shape with the base of the fifth metatarsal appearing prominent. Normally, this border should look straight. Sometimes spreading of the toes is noted with a wider space between the first and second toes.
- The foot should normally be straight. If one draws a line from the middle of the heel, it should pass through the

TABLE 37-4   **Characteristics of Various Types of Knee Injuries and Conditions**

Condition	History, Mechanism of Injury	Clinical Findings	Management	Differential Diagnosis, Prognosis, Comments
Quadriceps contusion	Typically a sports injury that results in bruising/contusion of the quadriceps muscle. Injury can sometime result from minor trauma or indirectly from tensile overload	Acute pain, swelling, and restriction of active and passive range of motion of hip and knee; tenderness over quadriceps	Rest not to exceed 48 hr, ice, compression wrap, and elevation (RICE) Progressive leg and gravity-assisted ROM after rest Flexion of the knee is the last function to return to normal, so is a good indicator for return to sport NSAID for pain relief	In teens, rule out rhabdomyosarcoma of the quadriceps, Ewing sarcoma, and osteosarcoma if there is swelling and pain in thigh without clear history of trauma
Meniscal tear (torn cartilage)	Associated with a significant injury in a youth; results from axial loading with rotation Tear of a normal meniscus is rarely seen in children <12 yr Congenital abnormal cartilage (discoid) can tear at any age	Pain, swelling and limping Joint line tenderness and positive McMurray sign May report a sensation of a clicking or catching in the knee or a locking of the knee Can be isolated or occur in combination with ACL or MCL injuries	RICE initially MRI if suspected tear; arthrography with MRI to rule out nerve injury with a prior tear Pain management Surgical intervention: meniscectomy generally relieves symptoms	75% of patients develop degenerative articular changes on x-ray by 30 yr A small percentage of youths develop degenerative changes 3 to 5 yr after injury Chondral fractures or injuries to articular cartilage have similar history and physical findings
Sprain of the anterior cruciate ligament (ACL)	Acute injury; typically there is a twisting or hyperextension while the foot is planted and knee extended Report of a "popping" feeling and knee shifting or pulling apart	Swelling/effusion and pain Instability with lateral movement Positive Lachman test	Following the injury, a knee brace or immobilizer is used until swelling and pain subside ACL reconstruction Pain management Neuromuscular training to prevent injury	Associated with MCL and meniscal tears
Sprains of the medial collateral ligament (MCL)	Most commonly injured ligament of the knee Valgus stress to an extended knee Reports tearing sensation with medial pain, swelling, stiffness	Instability with lateral movement and medial knee pain Tenderness over the MCL If tenderness extends along the distal femoral physis, suspect physeal fracture	Ice, elevation, compression, splint or hinged knee brace to protect against valgus stress Pain management Plain radiographs to look for physeal and epiphyseal fractures in skeletally immature children Surgical repair on an isolated collateral ligament is not beneficial; nonoperative treatment is the standard of care	Combined ACL and MCL injuries are common Physeal fractures are more common than MCL sprains in youths
Osteochon-dritis dissecans	Juvenile and adolescent types Common 10-15 yr; boys more common than girls	Activity-related pain and swelling Tenderness of the femoral condyle	Plain radiographs or MRI; 4-6 wk on immobilization and non–weight-bearing if <12 yr Youths >12 yr, arthroscopic surgery	Mimics symptoms of a torn meniscus Articular cartilage transplantation for selected patients

Continued

TABLE 37-4	Characteristics of Various Types of Knee Injuries and Conditions—Cont'd			
Condition	History, Mechanism of Injury	Clinical Findings	Management	Differential Diagnosis, Prognosis, Comments
	Isolation and sometimes sequestration of an osteochondral fragment without significant trauma May be caused by microtrauma, trauma, or may involve metabolic or genetic factors Pain increased with activity and diminished with rest plus intermittent effusions Locking and catching are unusual findings but may be present if bone fragments are detached		Eliminate high-impact activities—non–weight-bearing for several wk until symptoms abate About 50% heal spontaneously with rest and protected weight bearing Surgical intervention if still symptomatic despite 6-12 mo of conservative treatment, symptomatic loose body, or nonunion	
Dislocation of the patella	Associated with patellar malalignment Most cases involve lateral dislocation Pain and swelling Most occur in youths <20 yr Family history in 20%-30% More frequently in girls than boys	Massive and tense effusion Tenderness at the medial border of the patella and medial retinaculum Guarding with gentle pressure on the medial patella with lateral displacement	Nonoperative management: 2-3 wk of joint rest with splint or knee immobilizer, then intensive rehabilitation Isometric exercises, especially of quadriceps 80%-85% of cases are successfully managed with nonoperative treatment Surgical correction for recurrent dislocations or chronic instability	Outcomes with nonoperative therapy vs. acute surgery are similar Patellar dislocation tends to recur (recurrence is more frequent in younger child) but decreases over time Degenerative arthritis is common with or without surgery with recurrent dislocations

hr, Hours; *mo*, months; *MRI*, magnetic resonance imaging; *ROM*, range of motion; *wk*, weeks; *yr*, years.
Data from Anderson SJ: Lower extremity injuries in youth sports, *Pediatr Clin North Am* 49:627-641, 2002; McMahon P, editor: *Current diagnosis and treatment: sports medicine*, New York, 2007, Lange Medical Books/McGraw-Hill; Staheli LT, editor: *Pediatric orthopedic secrets*, ed 2, Philadelphia, 2003, Hanley & Blefus; Drendel AL, Esterhai JL, Sawyer JR: Orthopedic problems of the extremities. In Burg FD et al, editors: *Gellis and Kagan's current pediatric therapy*, ed 17, Philadelphia, 2002, WB Saunders.

second toe or between the second and third toes. In MA, the forefoot has an increased angle (greater than 15 degrees) or resists stretching (Fig. 37-11).

- To determine whether the foot is flexible or rigid, the heel is grasped with one hand while the forefoot is abducted with the other hand. In flexible MA, the forefoot can be abducted past midline.

Diagnostic Studies. Radiographic studies need to be ordered if the foot is not flexible or MA persists beyond 6 months old.

Differential Diagnosis. Consider congenital vertical talus, which will be rigid, or clubfoot, in which the foot is inverted and in the pointed-toe position.

Management. Management involves the following:

- For the flexible foot that can be brought past midline, the soft tissues can be stretched by the parents with each diaper change. Stretching is done as described under physical examination when the examiner determines whether the foot is flexible. Instruct the parents to hold the hindfoot in one hand and stretch the midfoot to overcorrect the deformity

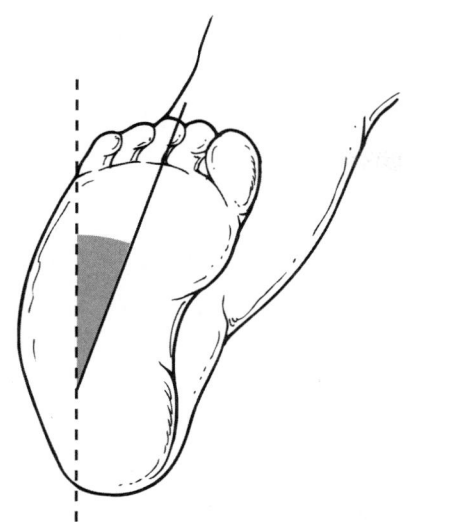

FIG. 37-11 MA angle. An angle (created by the intersecting lines) that is greater than 15 degrees indicates MA.

to the count of five and repeat five times. The soft tissues should blanch with each stretch. Be sure that the parent is not just pushing on the great toe. If no improvement is evident by 6 months old, a short course of serial stretching and casting is appropriate. However, most cases resolve spontaneously (Sawyer & Drendel, 2006).
- For the nonflexible foot:
  ○ Refer to an orthopedist when the problem is identified.
  ○ Educate the family that the treatment for infants may include serial short-leg casts or braces to stretch the foot (two or three casts for 2 weeks per cast) or other management if the bones of the foot are more severely affected. If the child is older than 2 to 3 years old, surgery may be needed to correct the problem.
- Corrective shoes, having the child wear shoes on the opposite foot, or night splints are not helpful for flexible MA.
  Complications. Early intervention can prevent more intensive therapeutic measures to correct the deformity.

Talipes Equinovarus
Description. Talipes equinovarus (clubfoot) has three elements: the ankle is in equinus (the foot is in a pointed-toe position), the sole of the foot is inverted as a result of hindfoot varus or inversion deformity of the heel, and the forefoot has the convex shape of MA (forefoot adduction). The foot cannot be manually corrected to a neutral position with the heel down.
Epidemiology. The etiology of clubfoot may be idiopathic (which tends to be hereditary), neurogenic as seen with myelomeningocele, or associated with certain syndromes, such as arthrogryposis and Larsen syndrome. It varies in severity, with uterine positioning a factor in mild clubfoot. The incidence is 1:1000 live births, with approximately 50% of cases being bilateral. The problem is congenital and can be identified in neonates. It is more common in boys. The risk increases to 3% for subsequent siblings and is 20% to 30% for offspring of involved parents (Thompson, 2006).

Clinical Findings.
History. Clubfoot is present at birth.
Physical Examination. The foot appears as described previously.
Diagnostic Studies. AP and lateral standing or simulated weight bearing radiographs with maximal dorsiflexion lateral views of the foot are done.
Management. The following steps are taken:
- Refer to an orthopedist as early as possible, ideally in the newborn nursery, because the joints are most flexible in the first hours and days of life. The foot can become rigid in a matter of days. The orthopedist may begin with serial manipulation and casting for 6 weeks. The Ponseti method of manipulation and casting technique has shown excellent long-term results and is now the gold standard of treatment. Serial casting is followed by a percutaneous Achilles tenotomy performed under local anesthesia. A foot-abduction brace is used to prevent relapse (Morcuende, 2006). Surgical correction may be required for severe cases that do not respond to serial casting and is usually performed between 9 and 12 months old.
- Monitor throughout childhood because the condition can recur. Postcorrection night splinting may be needed. Older children with rigid bony deformities often require osteotomy, tendon transfers, and fusions.
Complications. With growth, the abnormality can become increasingly distorted, making correction more difficult. Calf hypoplasia and a shorter than normal foot can occur even with correction.

Overriding Toes
Overriding toes are generally identified at birth. Efforts to tape them into a correct position or otherwise modify their position are usually futile. Overriding of the second, third, and fourth toes generally resolves with time. Occasionally, if severe, they can be surgically improved. Shoe fit can be a problem.

In-Toeing and Out-Toeing Rotational Problems
When a child has an in-toeing or out-toeing gait, the degree of rotation and source of the rotational deformity must be assessed. These include internal femoral torsion (femoral anteversion), internal tibial torsion, and MA. The causes of in toeing usually are physiologic, are related to age, and resolve as the child grows (Table 37-5). In addition, in toeing in children can vary with activities and from step to step.
Clinical Findings.
History. The primary care provider assesses the following:
- Onset of problem
- Increasing or decreasing deformity
- Treatments used to date
- Degree of interference with activities
- Effects on self-image for older children
- Neurologic history
Physical Examination. The physical examination involves the following:

TABLE 37-5 **Typical Cause of In-Toeing and Out-Toeing Rotational Problems**

	Cause	Typical Finding	Age at Manifestation
In toeing	Equinovarus	Plantar foot flexion, forefoot adduction, and hindfoot varus	At birth
	Metatarsal adductus	Curved foot—refer if not flexible	Birth-6 months
	Abducted great toe	Searching toe—resolves spontaneously	Toddler period
	Medial tibial torsion	Refer if thigh-foot angle (TFA) >−10 to −20 degrees	12-18 months
	Internal femoral torsion	Refer if >70 degrees medial and <10 degrees lateral hip rotation	2-5 years
Out toeing	Physiologic infantile out toeing	Feet may turn out when infant is positioned upright—resolves spontaneously	Early infancy
	Lateral tibial torsion	Refer if TFA >+30 degrees	Late childhood
	Lateral femoral torsion	Refer if >2 SD of the mean	Late childhood

SD, Standard deviation; >, greater than; <, less than.

- Observe the gait. Note that the slightly older child may consciously or unconsciously improve or worsen the gait for the examiner. Asking the child to run may also be helpful.
- Lay the child prone on the examining table.
- Examine for femoral anteversion (medial and lateral rotations).
- Examine for internal or external tibial torsion (TFA).
- Examine for MA or other deformity.

The child may have a combination of any or all of the aforementioned problems.

Management. See the individual diagnoses for management strategies.

OTHER COMMON MUSCULOSKELETAL SYSTEM FINDINGS NEEDING ATTENTION

TOE WALKING

Description
Most young children walk on their toes until they establish the heel-toe pattern, usually within the first 6 months of walking. Consistent toe walking is frequently associated with neurologic problems, such as cerebral palsy. Autistic children or those with early muscular dystrophy may toe walk. Children with tight heel cords may toe walk. Unilateral toe walking can be associated with a short leg, as found with a dislocated hip. Toe walking also can be a habit, especially in children who used walkers. In these children, toe walking generally resolves before 3 years old and is not associated with any musculoskeletal deformity. It is important to differentiate between the idiopathic toe walker and the child who toe walks because of a neuromusculoskeletal condition associated with tight heel cords and contractures.

Clinical Findings.
History. The pediatric provider should assess:
- Onset
- Severity
- Neurologic history
- Use of walker

Physical Examination. The pediatric provider should:
- Look at shoe wear to assess extent of toe walking. For example, is the heel worn?
- Assess for tight heel cords. The foot should be brought beyond a 90-degree angle.
- Conduct a neurologic assessment.
- Measure leg lengths and examine hips.

Management
Management depends on the etiology. Orthopedic management is needed for tight heel cords, unequal leg lengths, and hip problems.

GANGLIONS OF THE HANDS

Description
Ganglions are the most common benign lesions of soft tissue in children (see discussion of popliteal cysts). A ganglionic cyst is an acquired, mucinous, fluid-filled, painless lesion that originates from the synovial-lined space.

Physical Examination
Ganglions of the hand are hard, fixed masses commonly found on the wrist (commonly dorsal) and flexor aspects of the finger. Transillumination of the cyst with an otoscope or examination by ultrasonography plus findings on physical examination are keys to the diagnosis.

Management
Ganglionic cysts in children are rarely symptomatic and usually regress spontaneously. The likelihood of recurrence with any form of treatment is higher in children than the recurrence rate in adults with ganglionic lesions (Ezake & Hollier, 2003). Conservative care with rest and splinting can be tried. If conservative care fails to result in partial or complete resolution, refer for needle aspiration or surgical excision (the most reliable method to eliminate a ganglion because the tract that extends into the joint is removed). Steroid injections are not advised.

LEG ACHES OF CHILDHOOD

Description

Transient aches are common complaints during childhood that have been reported to occur in 13% of boys and 18% of girls, usually involving the lower extremities. The term *growing pains* has been used to describe this discomfort, but not without controversy because musculoskeletal growth has never been proved to be the cause of these aches or pains. *Leg aches* is the term now most commonly used. Their cause is unknown or idiopathic; a common theory is that thigh and calf muscle fatigue is responsible. Differentiating benign leg aches of childhood from more serious pathologic conditions is important. Onset is common at about 4 years old, and they can affect children up to 12 years old (McCarthy, 2003).

Clinical Findings

History. Pain or leg aches are typically described as:
- Occurring characteristically in the evening or late in the day; may wake child up from sleep
- Pain gone in the morning with no limitation of activity
- Poorly localized and bilateral
- Occurring commonly in the front of the thighs, in the calves, and behind the knees
- Transient and occurring over a period of time as long as several years
- Not associated with a limp or disability (McCarthy, 2003)

Clinical Findings. Normal physical examination with no tenderness, guarding, or reduced range of joint motion. Have the child stand on tiptoes and heels. Measurement of leg lengths should be taken if leg length inequality is suspected.

Diagnostic Studies. Radiographs and blood work are not necessary if a classic history is given and there are no physical findings.

Differential Diagnosis

Neoplastic lesions, leukemia, sickle cell anemia, and subacute osteomyelitis must be ruled out.

Management

Reassure the parents that these are common complaints that are benign and generally resolve spontaneously. Symptomatic treatment with heat and analgesic may be of benefit. Stress the need for parents to bring the child in for reevaluation if there is a change in symptoms or other signs emerge. Refer a child if the pain is localized to one region, is associated with swelling or other constitutional symptoms, is increasing in severity, or alters gait.

LIMPS

Description

Children limp for reasons including pain, deformity, or weakness. Limps must always be carefully assessed and managed. Limps may be of several types.
- *Antalgic.* This is a gait caused by pain that increases with the normal stresses of walking. The child tries to get weight off the affected side quickly; thus the normal walking cadence is off, with a shortened stance phase. Examples of antalgic gaits: The child with a sore knee walks with a fixed knee, whereas the child with a sore toe tries not to roll off the toe at the toe-off phase of the stride. A child with appendicitis may also have an antalgic gait, with a slight slumping posture and a shortened stride on the right resulting from psoas muscle irritation.
- *Trendelenburg gait* or *abductor lurch*. This gait is caused by a hip problem, such as hip dysplasia. The child tilts over the affected hip with each stride to decrease the mechanical stresses while the opposite side is off the ground during the swing-through phase of the gait.
- *Equinus* or *toe-to-heel gait*. This is caused by lack of neurologic coordination, creating an unsteady, wide-based gait. For example, children with cerebral palsy often exhibit this characteristic toe-to-heel sequence during the stance phase of their gait because of heel-cord contractures.
- *Circumduction*. This gait allows a functionally longer leg to progress forward using a circular swing motion. Children with leg length inequality and painful foot or ankle conditions use this gait.

Clinical Findings

History. A careful history is needed, including:
- Onset
- Location of pain, if any
- Changes in limp or pain during the day or since onset
- Interference with activities
- Past medical history, including injury or illness
- Review of systems

Physical Examination. The pediatric provider should do the following:
- Identify the type of limp from the gait.
- Examine the hips, legs, feet, and back for range of motion, asymmetry, changes in tissues, and signs of infection.
- Complete a neurologic examination, including strength, reflexes, balance, and coordination.
- Assess Trendelenburg sign for hip stability.

Diagnostic Studies. Studies are ordered appropriate to the findings and history. Knee pain and limp may be referred from the hip.

Differential Diagnosis

Age is an important factor in diagnosing the many causes of limping. Fracture, DDH, LCPD, SCFE, tumor, infection, juvenile arthritis, and others should be considered (Table 37-6).

Management

Refer the patient to an orthopedist immediately unless the etiology is a mild strain or a local lesion that can be managed conservatively by the primary care provider.

OVERUSE SYNDROMES OF CHILDHOOD AND ADOLESCENCE

Description

Overuse syndrome is caused by repetitive movement injury that causes microtrauma. OSD, discussed earlier, is a classic example

TABLE 37-6 **Differential Diagnosis of Limping**

Condition	Age	Pain ±	Historical Findings	Clinical Findings	Causative Factors	Management
Developmental dysplasia of the hip	I, T, C, A	−	Breech delivery; metatarsus adductus; torticollis; poor treatment outcomes if not diagnosed at birth or shortly	Limited abduction; Trendelenburg; radiography at 2-3 mo; shortening of leg; acetabular dysplasia	Familial; joint laxity, positioning, maternal hormones	Newborn: no triple diapers; Pavlik harness to hold hips in flexion—see weekly; after 6 mo, traction or open reduction; after 18 mo old, osteotomy
Leg length inequality	T, C, A	−	None	Circumduction gait; joint contracture; >1 cm discrepancy in leg lengths	Congenital; neurogenic; vascular; tumor; trauma; infection	Shoe lifts; epiphysiodesis (fusion of growth plate to arrest growth of the opposite side), if discrepancy 2-6 cm
Neuromuscular (NM) disease	T, C, A	−	Depends on cause	Depends on cause; equinus or abductor gait	Cerebral palsy, muscular dystrophy, and other NM diseases	Referral to appropriate specialists
Diskitis	T, C, A	+	Varied: fever, malaise, unwilling to walk, backache	Stiff back, ↑ ESR; positive x-ray 2-3 wk; early bone scan will have typical findings	Bacterial infection in disk space (*Staphylococcus aureus*) or inflammatory response	Immobilization and antistaphylococcal antibiotic therapy
Septic arthritis	T, C, A	++	Moderate to high fever, malaise, arthralgias; irritability; progressive course	Redness, warmth and swelling of joint— knee or hip; limited hip motion; ESR >25 mm/hr	*S. aureus* likely organism	Appropriate antibiotic coverage (7 days, IV; 3-4 wk total)
Acute hematogenous osteomyelitis	T, C, A	+	Varied: malaise, low-grade to high fever; may have severe constitutional symptoms; toxicity	Refusal to walk or move limb; point tenderness; limp; 7-10 days to see radiographic bony changes; 25% ↑ WBCs; ↑ CRP	*S. aureus* likely organism	Appropriate antibiotic coverage (generally 7 days, IV; 4-6 wk total or until ESR normal)
Neoplasm	T, C, A	+	Depends on type of neoplasm	Varied	Neoplasm—benign or malignant	Referral to oncologist
Trauma	T, C, A	+	Depends on type (fractures, strains, sprains)	Varied	Varied	Rule out physical abuse if discrepancy related to developmental capabilities, injury history, and type of injury

TABLE 37-6 **Differential Diagnosis of Limping—Cont'd**

Occult trauma: toddler fracture	T	+	Well child	Commonly radiograph shows spiral fracture of tibia; refusal to walk, mild soft tissue swelling	Trauma	See trauma above
Transient synovitis	3-8 yr	+	Mild to moderate fever, mild irritability; resolves within 1 wk	Limited hip motion; ESR <25 mm/hr	Inflammatory reaction; unknown etiology; often URI (50%) prior	Rest
Juvenile arthritis (JA)	Childhood until 16 yr	+	Fever, rashes, ↑ WBC count; some iritis; joint stiffness and swelling; S & S >3 mo	Mono/polyarticular arthropathy; + ANA (25%-88%); ↑ ESR in moderate/severe JA	Unknown; genetic (HLA) or environmental	Treat with nonsteroidal antiinflammatory agents initially; may need sulfasalazine, methotrexate; corticosteroids; joint replacements when older
Slipped capital femoral epiphysis	9-15 yr	+	>90th percentile weight; African American; male	Limited abduction and extension; external rotation of thigh if hip flexed	Multifactorial: mechanical; endocrine; trauma; familial	Needs immediate surgery; non–weight-bearing crutches until admitted (sitting not advised); bilateral involvement does occur
Legg-Calvé-Perthes disease	4-8 yr	+	Acute or chronic onset; pain in hip, groin, knee; stiffness; male	+ Trendelenburg, shortening; ↓ abduction, internal rotation, hip extension; + radiographs but not early	Familial; breech birth; prior trauma (17%)	In female tends to be more serious problem; bed rest, traction, then PT; bracing and surgery may be needed; bilateral involvement does occur

A, Adolescent (≥11 yr); *ANA*, antinuclear antibody; *C*, child (4-10 yr); *CRP*, C-reactive protein; *ESR*, erythrocyte sedimentation rate; *HLA*, human leukocyte antigen; *I*, infant (newborn to 12 mo); *mo*, months; *PT*, physical therapy; *S & S*, signs and symptoms; *T*, toddler (1-3 yr); *URI*, upper respiratory infection; *WBC*, white blood cell; *wk*, weeks; *yr*, years.

of an overuse injury commonly seen in children 10 to 14 years old. Other typical overuse injuries of childhood are varus overload of the elbow ("Little League elbow"), proximal humeral epiphysiolysis ("Little League shoulder"), patellofemoral pain syndrome, shin splints, and stress fractures (Table 37-7).

Management

Treatment often involves resting and icing the extremity or joint, doing retraining and strengthening exercises, gradually reintroducing activities, and using analgesics. NSAIDs help reduce the inflammatory component of the trauma. Patient and parent education is important to prevent further injury and disability and to allow the child to return to safe sport participation.

MUSCLE DISEASES

Description

Muscle diseases in children are rare. However, there are many types of problems that can affect muscle metabolism or function. It can be difficult to discern whether the lack of good muscular function is due to problems of enervation or an inability of the muscle to contract efficiently.

TABLE 37-7   Overuse Injuries of Childhood: Characteristic Features and Their Treatment

Condition	Clinical Findings	Treatment	Comments
Osgood-Schlatter disease	Swelling and tenderness/ pain over tibial tubercle	NSAIDs, kneepad, knee immobilizer if severe pain for 1-2 weeks	Most resolve with time (12-18 months), x-ray only if pain persists (shows soft tissue swelling and possible residual ossicle); if pain persists, consider surgical incision of ossicle
Patellofemoral pain syndrome	Anterior knee pain	Rest, NSAIDs, retraining, and strengthening of quadriceps muscles	Arthroscopic surgery only if recurring problems
Proximal humeral epiphysiolysis ("Little League shoulder")	Shoulder pain—gradual onset; pain ↑ with throwing, especially curve ball	Modify activity; gradual restart, but limit intensity and frequency of throwing with retraining and muscle strengthening	Seen in skeletally immature children; radiographs show widening proximal humeral physis
Shin splints	Pain along medial border of tibia; child has a history of prolonged running	NSAIDs; ice after running; retraining and muscle strengthening after inflammation ↓; gradual return to running	Associated with poor running technique, hard running surface, muscle weakness; inadequate running shoes; sudden increase in running; is an inflammatory response; may need to consider exertional compartment syndrome (see Chapter 39)
Stress fractures	Tenderness and swelling at site	Reduce or eliminate activity that caused injury for 10-14 days; may need to cast	Caused by microtrauma; most commonly seen in active teens, but can occur during childhood; proximal tibia most common site
Varus overload of the elbow ("Little League elbow")	Elbow pain with activity; locking and ↓ extension of elbow; medial humeral epicondyle tenderness	Rest; NSAIDs; ice; when pain free, gradual return to activity with retraining; surgery if elbow instability	Leads to osteochondral lesions and stress fractures if severe; radiographs reveal widening proximal physis; also seen in gymnasts

Clinical Findings

History.   The following may be reported:

- Failure to achieve motor milestones
- Loss of motor skills, such as the ability to climb stairs easily
- Easy fatigue with physical activity
- A history of good days and bad days with relation to ability to accomplish physical activities
- Increasing difficulties with motor activities

Physical Examination.   Findings include the following:

- Fibrotic or "doughy" feel to the muscles
- Muscle hypertrophy, especially of the calf muscles
- Muscle wasting
- Fibrillations or fasciculations
- Muscle contractures
- Weakness
- Positive Gowers' sign

Gowers' sign is obtained by asking the child to get up off the floor without help. The sign is positive if the child uses his or her arms to push off from the legs, gradually standing in a segmented fashion.

Management

Referral is necessary. These conditions may need to be handled by an interdisciplinary team with orthopedic, metabolic, and physical therapy, social service, and nursing care. Genetics counseling may be necessary, depending on the diagnosis. The muscular dystrophies, for instance, are autosomal dominant and can appear in several children in a family.

Patient and family support is needed. Muscle diseases are chronic, debilitating, and sometimes fatal conditions. Helping the child to lead as normal a life as possible while coping with his or her condition is a major task. The family may need help maintaining caregiving and coping with the implications of the diagnosis.

RESOURCE BOX

National Organizations for Musculoskeletal Disorders

ORTHOPEDIC CONDITIONS
United Brachial Plexus Network, Inc. —Erb's Palsy Support and Information Network
www.ubpn.org

STEPS – national charity in the United Kingdom for those affected by a lower limb condition
www.steps-charity.org.uk

SCOLIOSIS AND KYPHOSIS
Scoliosis Research Society
www.srs.org
A pamphlet with information and advice for parents; order from Scoliosis Research Society

The Spinal Connection
www.scoliosis.org/resources/spinalconnection.php
A newsletter published by the National Scoliosis Foundation, Inc.

MUSCLE DISEASES
Muscular Dystrophy Association
www.mdausa.org

OTHER PROFESSIONAL ORGANIZATIONS
American Academy of Family Practice
www.aafp.org
Use the search option for specific orthopedic conditions of interest. Access is free to several excellent clinical articles including topics, such as the evaluation of the limping child and pediatric septic arthritis.

American Academy of Orthopaedic Surgeons
www.aaos.org
Excellent patient education brochures and videos on common pediatric orthopedic conditions and their treatment available for sale

Connecticut Children's Medical Center
www.ccmckids.org
Excellent patient education materials about common pediatric orthopedic conditions. Go to the website toolbar and click on Services/Programs. Go to the "services" option and select orthopedics from the choices listed. A listing of all available orthopedic materials will be displayed.

☑ DISCUSSION FORUM

1. Compare and contrast the musculoskeletal assessment of a 2-month-old, a 4-year-old, and a 10-year-old. Include developmental variances and physiologic differences.
2. A brachial plexus injury is noted during the newborn exam of a postterm, large-for-gestational-age infant. The right shoulder, biceps, and forearm do not move; but the baby can flex the wrist. Create a plan of care for this child that includes diagnostic testing and management of the infant and family's physical, education, and developmental needs.
3. A 11-year-old girl had a scoliosis screening done at school today. The school nurse told the mother that the child had a nine-degree lumbar curvature on the scoliometer. How do you respond to the mother? What treatment, diagnostic evaluation, and follow-up do you suggest?
4. What would be the differential for a 7-year-old male with a new-onset limp and complaint of anterior thigh pain? What physical examination, medical history, and diagnostic testing findings would you expect for your top three diagnoses? How would your answers change if the boy were 13 years old?
5. A 12-month-old has marked in toeing with a thigh-foot angle of −16 degrees. Other exam findings are normal including the child's gait. What diagnostic testing and management do you prescribe?
6. A mother notes that her 18-month-old's foot is "curved," and the curving has worsened during the last 6 months since the toddler began walking. Physical exam reveals a normal right foot and a convex left foot. The defect can be straightened by applying lateral pressure to the anterior foot. Grandma told the mother that placing the child's shoes on the wrong foot would fix the problem. How do you respond? What management do you initiate?

REFERENCES

Anderson SJ: Lower extremity injuries in youth sports, *Pediatr Clin North Am* 49:627-641, 2002.

Bennett J: Scoliosis and kyphosis. In Finberg L, editor: *Saunders manual of pediatric practice*, ed 2, Philadelphia, 2002a, WB Saunders.

Bennett J: Dysplasia of the hip. In Finberg L, Kleinman RE, editors: *Saunders manual of pediatric practice*, ed 2, Philadelphia, 2002b, WB Saunders.

Cady RB: Developmental dysplasia of the hip: definition, recognition, and prevention of late sequelae, *Pediatric Annals* 25:92-101, 2006.

Dise TL: Flatfleet and tibial torsion. In Finberg L, Kleinman RE, editors: *Saunders manual of pediatric practice*, ed 2, Philadelphia, 2002, WB Saunders.

Doyle JS: Disorders of the spine and shoulder girdle. In Burg FD et al, editors: *Current pediatric therapy*, ed 18, Philadelphia, 2006, WB Saunders Elsevier.

Drendel A, Esterhai JL, Sawyer JR: Orthopedic problems of the extremities. In Burg FD et al, editors: *Gellis and Kagan's current pediatric therapy*, ed 17, Philadelphia, 2002, WB Saunders.

Duderstadt KG, Schapiro NA: Musculoskeletal system. In Duderstadt KG, editor: *Pediatric physical examination: an illustrated handbook*, Philadelphia, 2006, Mosby Elsevier.

Ezake M, Hollier LH: Acquired hand problems. In Staheli LT, editor: *Pediatric orthopedic secrets*, ed 2, Philadelphia, 2003, Hanley & Belfus.

Grudziak JS, Musahl V: The youth athlete. In McMahon PJ, editor, *Current diagnosis & treatment: sports medicine*, New York, 2007, Lange Medical Books/McGraw-Hill.

Hansen CA, Bateman DA: Birth injuries. In Burg FD et al, editors: *Gellis and Kagan's current pediatric therapy*, ed 17, Philadelphia, 2002, WB Saunders.

Katz DA: Slipped capital femoral epiphysis: the importance of early diagnosis, *Pediatric Annals* 35:102-127, 2006.

Kocher MS et al: Delay in diagnosis of slipped capital femoral epiphysis, *Pediatrics* 133(4):e322-e325, 2004.

Kronberg J, Small E: Tackling back pain in a young athlete, *Contemp Pediatr*, 2005. Available at *http://contemporarypediatrics.com/contpeds/content/pringContentPopup.jsp?id=197* (accessed Nov 28, 2006).

McCarthy RE: Leg aches. In Staheli LT, editor: *Pediatric orthopedic secrets*, ed 2, Philadelphia, 2003, Hanley & Belfus.

Morcuende JA: Congenital idiopathic clubfoot: prevention of late deformity and disability by conservative treatment with the Ponseti Technique, *Pediatric Annals* 35:128-136, 2006.

Neyt JG, Weinstein SL: Kyphosis and lordosis. In Staheli LT, editor: *Pediatric orthopedic secrets*, ed 2, Philadelphia, 2003, Hanley & Belfus.

Reamy BV, Slakey JB: Adolescent idiopathic scoliosis: review and current concepts, *Am Fam Physician* 11(1):111-116, 2001.

Richards BS: Back pain. In Staheli LT, editor: *Pediatric orthopedic secrets*, ed 2, Philadelphia, 2003, Hanley & Belfus.

Roth P: Birth injuries. In Burg FD et al, editors: *Current pediatric therapy*, ed 18, Philadelphia, 2006, Saunders Elsevier.

Sass P, Hassan G: Lower extremity abnormalities in children, *Am Fam Physician* 68(3):461-467, 2003.

Sawyer JR, Drendel AL: Rotational orthopedic problems of the extremities. In Burg FD et al, editors: *Current pediatric therapy*, ed 18, Philadelphia, 2006, WB Saunders Elsevier.

Shah SA, Stankovits LM: The hip. In Burg FD et al, editors: *Current pediatric therapy*, ed 18, Philadelphia, 2006, Saunders Elsevier.

Small E: The sports physical. In Burg FD et al, editors: *Current pediatric therapy*, ed 18, Philadelphia, 2006, WB Saunders Elsevier.

Staheli LT: In-toeing and out-toeing. In Staheli LT, editor: *Pediatric orthopedic secrets*, ed 2, Philadelphia, 2003a, Hanley & Belfus.

Staheli LT: Shoes for children. In Staheli LT, editor: *Pediatric orthopedic secrets*, ed 2, Philadelphia, 2003b, Hanley & Belfus.

Stewart DG, Skaggs DL: Adolescent idiopathic scoliosis, *Pediatr Rev* 27:299-305, 2006.

Stoll BJ, Kliegman RM: Nervous system disorders. In Behrman RE, Kliegman RM, Jenson HB, editors: *Nelson textbook of pediatrics*, ed 17, Philadelphia, 2004, WB Saunders Elsevier.

Sussman M, Turker RJ: Disorders of the shoulder girdle and spine. In Burg FD et al, editors: *Gellis and Kagan's current pediatric therapy*, ed 17, Philadelphia, 2002, WB Saunders.

Thompson GH: Common fractures. In Behrman RE, Kliegman RM, Jenson HB, editors: *Nelson textbook of pediatrics*, ed 17, Philadelphia, 2004a, WB Saunders Elsevier.

Thompson, GH: Torsional and angular deformities. In Behrman RE, Kliegman RM, Jenson HB, editors: *Nelson textbook of pediatrics*, ed 17, Philadelphia, 2004b, WB Saunders Elsevier.

Thompson GH: Orthopedics. In Kliegman RM et al, editors: *Nelson essentials of pediatric practice*, ed 5, Philadelphia, 2006, Elsevier WB Saunders.

Vidal LS, Vidal AF, McMahon PJ: Shoulder injuries. In McMahon PJ, editor: *Current diagnosis & treatment*, New York, 2007, Lange Medical Books/McGraw-Hill.

Warren FH: Genu varum and genu valgum. In Finberg L, Kleinman RE, editors: *Saunders manual of pediatric practice*, ed 2, Philadelphia, 2002a, WB Saunders.

Warren FH: Legg-Calvé-Perthes disease. In Finberg L, Kleinman RE, editors: *Saunders manual of pediatric practice*, ed 2, Philadelphia, 2002b, WB Saunders.

Warren FH: Slipped capital femoral epiphysis. In Finberg L, Kleinman RE, editors: *Saunders manual of pediatric practice*, ed 2, Philadelphia 2002c, WB Saunders.

CHAPTER 38

Perinatal Conditions

Nan M. Gaylord and Robert J. Yetman

The neonatal period is remarkable for the vast array of physiologic changes that occur as the infant transitions from the intrauterine to extrauterine life. This period is a highly vulnerable time for the infant. In the U.S., about two-thirds of all deaths in the first year of life occur among infants less than 28 days old with the highest risk being in the first 24 hours of life (Stoll & Kliegman, 2004). Because serious health problems can arise for the infant in the hours after the initial transition to extrauterine life, the primary care provider must be prepared to manage these problems while providing psychosocial support and education for the families. An understanding of the physiology of fetal development, risk factors for potential problems, and pertinent physical findings is necessary to effectively assist the newborn's transition to extrauterine life.

STANDARDS OF CARE

The *Healthy People 2010* objectives (U.S. Department of Health and Human Services, 2003) related to maternal, infant, and child care are available online. The overall goal of these objectives is to improve maternal health and pregnancy outcomes and reduce rates of disability in infants, thereby improving the health and well-being of women, infants, children, and families in the U.S. *Healthy People 2010* suggests that the health of a population is reflected in the health of its most vulnerable members. A major focus of many public health efforts, therefore, is improving the health of pregnant women and their infants, including reductions in the rate of birth defects, risk factors for infant death, and death of infants and their mothers. Included among these goals are improvements in the rates of breastfeeding, ensuring that all newborns are screened for state-mandated diseases, and increasing the proportion of newborns screened for hearing loss in the first month of life.

The *Guide to Clinical Preventive Services* (U.S. Preventive Services Task Force, 2002) recommends the following preventive services for neonates:

- Prenatal screening for Rh (D) incompatibility; HIV; hepatitis B; syphilis; chlamydia and gonorrhea; neural tube defects (including provision of appropriate folic acid prophylaxis).
- Promotion of breastfeeding.
- Neonatal screening for sickle hemoglobinopathies to identify infants who may benefit from antibiotic prophylaxis to prevent sepsis. All screening efforts must be accompanied by comprehensive counseling and treatment services.

- Screening for congenital hypothyroidism with thyroid function tests on dried blood spot specimens for all newborns during the first week of life.
- Screening for phenylketonuria (PKU) with a phenylalanine level on a dried blood spot for all newborns before discharge from the nursery. Infants who are tested before 24 hours old should receive a repeat screening test by 2 weeks old.
- Ocular antibiotic prophylaxis of all newborn infants to prevent gonococcal ophthalmia neonatorum.
- Routine newborn hearing screening is less clear. The group concluded that newborn hearing screening led to earlier identification of hearing loss, but few data supported long-term benefit.

Put Prevention into Practice: The Clinician's Handbook of Preventive Services (U.S. Public Health Services, 2006) outlines recommendations from major organizations, such as the American Academy of Pediatrics (AAP), the American Academy of Family Physicians, and the Canadian Task Force on the Periodic Health Examination. These authorities recommend that newborn screening be performed according to each state's regulations. Specific recommendations regarding screening for hypothyroidism, PKU, galactosemia, and hemoglobinopathies are detailed in this handbook.

Bright Futures: Guidelines for Health Supervision of Infants, Children, and Adolescents (Green & Palfrey, 2002) and the AAP's Committee on Practice and Ambulatory Medicine (AAP, 2000) have detailed anticipatory guidelines for the newborn, first-week, and 1-month health supervision visits. *Guidelines for Perinatal Care* from the AAP and the American College of Obstetricians and Gynecologists (Gilstrap & Oh, 2002) is another thorough compendium of standards of caring for the newborn.

ANATOMY AND PHYSIOLOGY
INTRAUTERINE-TO-EXTRAUTERINE TRANSITION

The infant's intrauterine-to-extrauterine transition requires an extraordinary number of biochemical and physiologic changes. In utero, the placenta provides metabolic functions for the fetus. Oxygenated blood from the placenta arrives to the fetus through the umbilical vein. Because of high pulmonary vascular pressure, this blood is shunted from the right to the left side of the fetus' heart through the foramen ovale or to the systemic circulation through the ductus arteriosus. At birth, the umbilical cord is severed. Simultaneously, the infant begins to breathe and the high pulmonary vascular pressure drops, allowing blood flow to the lungs for oxygenation. The foramen ovale and ductus arteriosus are no longer necessary and close after birth. The newborn becomes dependent on gastrointestinal tract function to absorb nutrients, renal function to excrete wastes and maintain chemical balance, liver function to metabolize and excrete toxins, and the functions of the immunologic system to protect against infection. Many newborn problems are related to poor transition to extrauterine life as a result of asphyxia, premature birth, congenital anomalies, or adverse effects of delivery.

A predictable series of changes or reactivities in vital signs and clinical appearance take place after the delivery of most normal infants (Fig. 38-1). The first period of reactivity includes sympathetic system changes, such as tachycardia, rapid respirations, transient rales, grunting, flaring and retractions, a falling body temperature, hypertonus, and alerting exploratory behavior. Parasympathetic system changes during the first period of reactivity include the initiation of bowel sounds and the production of oral mucus. After an interval of sleep, the infant enters the second period of reactivity. During this time, the oral mucus production again becomes evident, the heart rate becomes labile, the infant becomes more responsive to endogenous and exogenous stimuli, and meconium is often passed.

■ PATHOPHYSIOLOGY
HIGH-RISK PREGNANCY

High-risk pregnancies are defined as those in which factors exist that increase the chances of abortion, fetal death, premature delivery, intrauterine growth retardation, fetal or neonatal

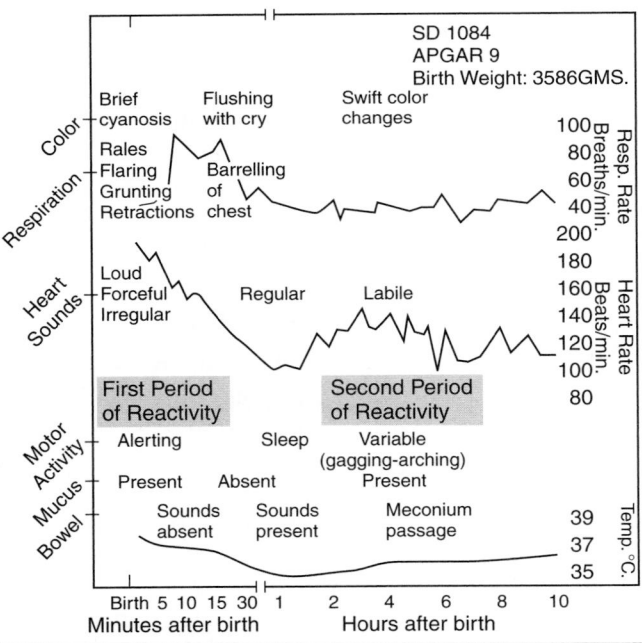

FIG. 38-1 Summary of normal transition. (From Desmond MM, Rudolph AJ, Phitaksphraiwan P: The transitional care nursery, *Pediatr Clin North Am* 13:651-668, 1966.)

disease, congenital malformations, mental retardation, and other handicaps. Identification of a high-risk pregnancy is the first step toward prevention of neonatal problems (Box 38-1). Comprehensive and frequent prenatal visits for women with high-risk pregnancies are aimed at preventing complications in the newborn.

ACQUIRED HEALTH PROBLEMS

In utero exposure to poor nutrition, alcohol, drugs, viruses or bacteria, and maternal conditions, such as hypertension and diabetes, can result in prematurity and abnormalities at birth. The risk of neonatal problems increases with maternal age younger than 20 years and older than 35 years (See Box 38-1).

GENETIC PROBLEMS

The presence of chromosomal abnormalities, congenital anomalies, inborn errors of metabolism, mental retardation, and familial diseases increases the risk of the same condition in the infant. Because many conditions are not easily identifiable on physical examination, exploring family histories to identify newborns at risk for any inheritable diseases is important. Anticipation of various inherited conditions leads to their early identification and management of potential problems.

PERINATAL COMPLICATIONS AND INJURIES

Perinatal complications occur immediately before or during birth. Prolonged or dysfunctional labor increases the risk of fetal distress. Prolonged rupture of the membranes and chorioamnionitis increase the risk of infant infection, and ruptured placenta previa increases the risk of infant blood loss. Cesarean deliveries, the use of forceps or vacuum extraction, and the type of maternal anesthesia used also pose risks. The term *birth injury* includes mechanical and anoxic trauma incurred by an infant during labor and delivery. Predisposing risk factors for birth injury include macrosomia, prematurity, cephalopelvic disproportion, dystocia, prolonged labor, and breech presentation. Birth injuries include caput succedaneum, cephalhematoma, subcutaneous fat necrosis of the face or scalp, fractures of the skull, subconjunctival and retinal hemorrhages, intracranial hemorrhage, peripheral nerve palsies (brachial, phrenic, facial), fractured clavicle or humerus, ruptured liver or spleen, and hypoxic-ischemic insults. Proper steps to monitor and treat an infant with perinatal complications and injuries must be undertaken immediately after birth. The provider must be familiar with perinatal conditions that subject the newborn to a higher risk and be prepared to intervene quickly based on the available perinatal information.

■ ASSESSMENT OF THE NEONATE
HISTORY

The history includes the following:
- Past maternal health history
- Past obstetric history

BOX 38-1 Factors Associated With High-Risk Pregnancies

Demographic Social Factors
Maternal age less than 20 years or greater than 35 years
Developmentally delayed mother or low educational status
Illicit drug, alcohol, cigarette use
Poverty, homelessness
Unmarried or lack of support
Emotional or physical stress including depression and other mental health problems
Poor access to prenatal care, underinsured or uninsured

Medical History
Diabetes mellitus
Hypertension or maternal hypercoagulable state or sickle cell disease
Asymptomatic bacteriuria
Autoimmune disease including rheumatologic illness (SLE)
Chronic medication
Sexually transmitted infections (colonization: herpes simplex, GBS, syphilis, HIV)

Prior Pregnancy
Intrauterine fetal demise or neonatal death
Previous infertility
Prematurity or low-birth-weight infant
Intrauterine growth retardation
Congenital malformation
Incompetent cervix
Blood group sensitization, neonatal jaundice
Neonatal thrombocytopenia
Hydrops
Inborn errors of metabolism

Present Pregnancy
Uterine bleeding (abruptio placentae, placenta previa)
Inception by reproductive technology
Poor weight gain or abnormal fetal growth
Multiple gestation, parity more than 5
Preeclampsia or eclampsia
Premature rupture of membranes
Short interpregnancy time
Polyhydramnios or oligohydramnios

Labor and Delivery
Premature labor (<37 weeks) or prolonged labor
Postdates (>42 weeks) or prolonged gestation
Fetal distress
Immature L/S ratio: absent phosphatidylglycerol
Breech presentation
Meconium-stained fluid
Nuchal cord
Cesarean delivery
Forceps delivery
Apgar score less than 4 at 1 minute

Neonate
Birth weight less than 2500 g or greater than 4000 g
Birth before 37 or after 42 weeks of gestation
Small or large for gestational age
Hypoglycemia
Tachypnea, cyanosis
Congenital malformation
Pallor, plethora, petechiae

GBS, Group B streptococcus; *HIV*, human immunodeficiency virus; *L/S*, lecithin-sphingomyelin ratio; *SLE*, systemic lupus erythematosus,
Adapted from Stoll BJ & Kliegman RM: High risk pregnancies. In Behrman RE, Kliegman RM, Jenson HM, editors: *Nelson textbook of pediatrics*, ed 17, Philadelphia, 2004, WB Saunders, p 532.

○ Number of previous pregnancies; number of infants born alive or stillborn
○ Number of elective or spontaneous abortions; number of preterm and term deliveries
○ Cesarean deliveries and indications for them
○ Health status of living children; if deceased, age and cause of death
• Family history
○ Genetically acquired conditions, birth defects, mental retardation, or other diseases
○ Hypertension, hyperlipidemias, heart disease, or familial cancers
○ Age and health status of living relatives
○ Causes of death of family members
• Current obstetric history
○ Present health and medical history including depression or other mental health conditions
○ Age of mother
○ Prenatal care—duration of
○ Medications used during pregnancy including prescription, over-the-counter, and natural health products

○ Use of pregnancy-enhancing drugs or technology
○ Infections (including group B streptococcus [GBS] status and results of other screening tests) and illnesses during pregnancy
○ Alcohol, cigarettes, or other drugs used during pregnancy
○ Hypertension or glucose intolerance
○ Duration of labor, duration of ruptured membranes, analgesia, anesthesia, presentation and route of delivery, use of forceps
○ Polyhydramnios (excessive fluid) or oligohydramnios (little to no fluid)
○ Infant meconium stained or amniotic fluid foul smelling
○ Fever
• Social history
○ Emotional stressors during pregnancy including homelessness
○ Unplanned or unwanted pregnancy
○ Financial and emotional support
○ Dietary considerations (e.g., strict vegan diet)
○ Educational background of parents
○ Father's anticipated involvement in raising infant
○ Age of other children in the home

PHYSICAL EXAMINATION

Immediately After Birth

Apgar Score. Immediate evaluation of the newborn infant at 1 and 5 minutes old can be a valuable routine procedure. An Apgar score is assigned to the baby based on the criteria in Table 38-1.

- Apgar score 8 to 10
  - Vigorous, pink, and crying
  - Requires only warming, drying, gentle stimulation
  - Occasionally requires oxygen for a short period of time
- Apgar score 5 to 7
  - Cyanotic
  - Slow, irregular respirations
  - Good muscle tone and reflexes
  - Responds to bag-and-mask ventilation
- *Apgar score 4 or less
  - Limp, pale, or blue
  - Apneic, slow heart rate
  - Maximal resuscitative efforts with bag and mask, chest compressions, intravenous volume expansion, and drug therapy

The 5-minute Apgar score is an indication of how well the resuscitation efforts have succeeded. Caution must be exercised when using the Apgar score to predict long-term outcomes of mortality and developmental delay. Only when combined with other factors, such as fetal status, umbilical cord or scalp blood pH, evidence of organ injury, or seizures, can the Apgar score be useful in determining long-term outcome (AAP, 2006a). In actual practice, the decision to resuscitate an infant typically is based on a quick assessment of the heart rate, color, and respiratory rate rather than the full 1-minute Apgar score (Fig. 38-2).

Gestational Age. Maturational assessment of an infant's gestational age is based on the physical examination (Fig. 38-3). The assessment is:

- Done promptly after birth to confirm maternal estimated dates
- Interpreted with information on the mother's menstrual history, obstetric milestones achieved during pregnancy, and prenatal ultrasonograms

An infant's length, weight, and frontooccipital head circumference are measured and plotted on growth curves based on gestational age (Fig. 38-4). Infants whose weights fall above the 90th percentile for age are classified as large for gestational age (LGA); those whose measurements fall below the 10th percentile for age are classified as small for gestational age (SGA). Those whose measurements fall between the 10th and 90th percentiles are classified as appropriate for gestational age (AGA).

Temperature. Body surface area of the newborn infant relative to its weight is approximately three times that of the adult. Estimated rate of heat loss in the newborn is four times that of an adult (Stoll & Kliegman, 2004). Body temperature falls precipitously in a cool environment unless adequate precautions are taken.

- Towel dry infant after birth to prevent evaporative heat loss.
- Use radiant warmer.
- Wrap infant in warm blankets and cover head to reduce heat loss when baby is to be held by parents.

Lungs. During a vaginal delivery, the squeezing action on an infant's chest as it passes through the pelvis and vagina assists in expulsion of amniotic fluid from the lungs. Further expulsion of amniotic fluid from the lungs and reversal of high pulmonary vascular resistance ensue with an infant's first large breaths. Careful bulb suctioning assists in clearing the amniotic fluid from the oropharynx. An infant born by cesarean delivery does not experience the squeezing action of a vaginal birth and is dependent on respiratory efforts and appropriate bulb suctioning to adequately clear the amniotic fluid. Auscultation of the newborn's lungs reveals bronchovesicular or bronchial breath sounds. Fine crackles can be present during the first few hours of life and is a variant of normal.

Umbilical Cord. The normal umbilical cord contains two thick-walled arteries and a single thin-walled vein. Vessel numbers other than this are abnormal and can be associated with congenital anomalies. The umbilical cord is clamped using sterile technique to prevent infection and bleeding.

After Stabilization

After a quick initial assessment in the delivery room to evaluate for obvious problems, a more complete physical examination

---

TABLE 38-1 Apgar Scores

	Score		
Sign	**0**	**1**	**2**
Heart rate (BPM)	Absent	Slow (<100)	>100
Respiratory effort	Absent	Weak cry; hypoventilation	Good; strong cry
Muscle tone	Limp	Some flexion of extremities	Well flexed
Reflex irritability (response of skin stimulation to feet)	No response	Some motion	Cry
Color	Blue; pale	Body pink; extremities blue	Completely pink

From Apgar V et al: Evaluation of the newborn infant. Second report, *JAMA* 168:1985.

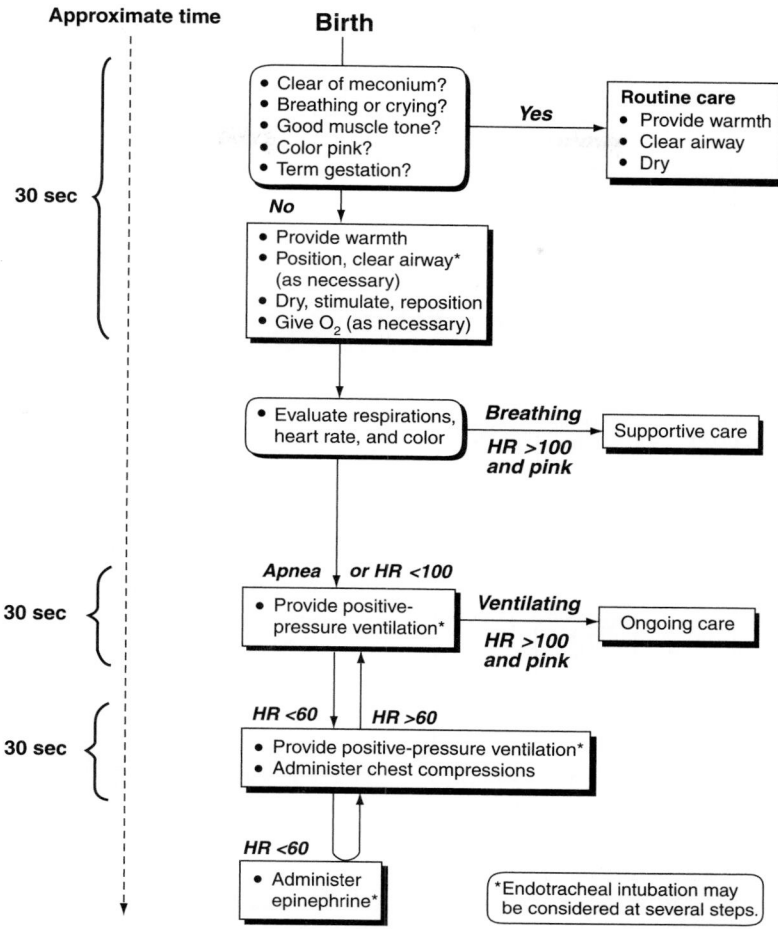

Approximate time

Birth

30 sec
- Clear of meconium?
- Breathing or crying?
- Good muscle tone?
- Color pink?
- Term gestation?

Yes →

Routine care
- Provide warmth
- Clear airway
- Dry

No ↓

- Provide warmth
- Position, clear airway* (as necessary)
- Dry, stimulate, reposition
- Give O₂ (as necessary)

↓

- Evaluate respirations, heart rate, and color

Breathing
HR >100 and pink → Supportive care

Apnea   or HR <100 ↓

30 sec
- Provide positive-pressure ventilation*

Ventilating
HR >100 and pink → Ongoing care

HR <60   *HR >60* ↓

30 sec
- Provide positive-pressure ventilation*
- Administer chest compressions

HR <60 ↓

- Administer epinephrine*

*Endotracheal intubation may be considered at several steps.

FIG. 38-2   Resuscitation in the delivery room. (From Niermeyer S, Kattwinkel J, Van Reempts P: International guidelines for neonatal resuscitation: an excerpt from the Guidelines 2000 for Cardiopulmonary Resuscitation and Emergency Cardiovascular Care: International Consensus on Science, *Pediatrics* 106(3):29, 2000.)

is done (Table 38-2). When performing the physical examination, the infant's gestational age, age in hours, and stage of transition must be considered.

DIAGNOSTIC STUDIES
Newborn Screening
All states require screening of infants for a variety of congenital abnormalities, although the screening tests performed vary from state to state. Screening panels may include PKU, congenital hypothyroidism, galactosemia, hemoglobin type, homocystinuria, tyrosinemia, maple syrup urine disease, sickle cell trait, cystic fibrosis, and congenital adrenal hyperplasia. Testing for the organic acidemias is less widely performed. The ideal timing of these tests is usually after the infant is older than 24 hours to ensure the baby is feeding and has had adequate time for production of metabolites. Early discharge often necessitates repeating some tests. Two screenings approximately 2 weeks apart are required in some states and increase the chances of picking up one of the metabolic disorders. Box 38-2 details specifics related to newborn testing. The National Newborn Screening and Genetics Resource

Center (see Resource Box) maintains an updated report on all 50 states delineating the testing status for core conditions and metabolic disorders.

Special Screening
Although most infants require no special screening tests, some are at risk for predictable complications in the newborn period. Infants born to mothers with poorly controlled diabetes and LGA or SGA infants are at higher risk for hypoglycemia and requiring serum glucose levels screening. Similarly, infants demonstrating Coombs test positivity because of maternal-child blood incompatibility are screened for evidence of hemolysis. Some nurseries screen both mothers and infants for syphilis; mothers should be screened for HIV and hepatitis B unless done prenatally. Universal hearing screening is recommended by many experts (Joint Committee on Infant Hearing et al, 2000), and special attention is paid to any newborn at higher risk for hearing loss as a result of low birth weight, rubella or other infection, malformation, trauma, asphyxia, prematurity, intensive care unit stay, or antibiotic use.

MATURATIONAL ASSESSMENT OF GESTATIONAL AGE (New Ballard Score)

NAME _____   SEX _____

HOSPITAL NO. _____   BIRTH WEIGHT _____

RACE _____   LENGTH _____

DATE/TIME OF BIRTH _____   HEAD CIRC. _____

DATE/TIME OF EXAM _____   EXAMINER _____

AGE WHEN EXAMINED _____

APGAR SCORE: 1 MINUTE _____ 5 MINUTES _____ 10 MINUTES _____

NEUROMUSCULAR MATURITY

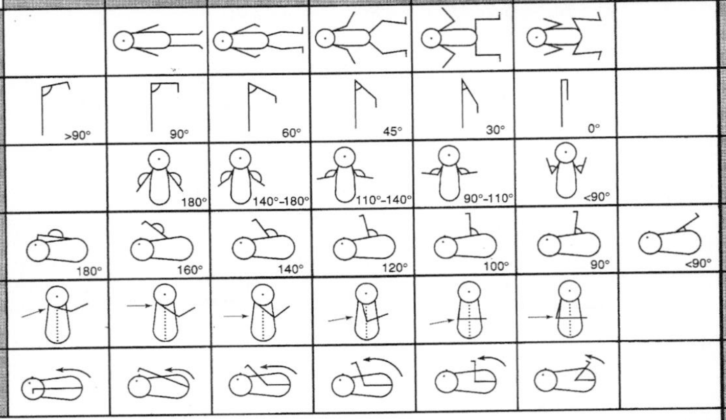

NEUROMUSCULAR MATURITY SIGN	SCORE							RECORD SCORE HERE
	-1	0	1	2	3	4	5	
POSTURE								
SQUARE WINDOW (Wrist)	>90°	90°	60°	45°	30°	0°		
ARM RECOIL		180°	140°-180°	110°-140°	90°-110°	<90°		
POPLITEAL ANGLE	180°	160°	140°	120°	100°	90°	<90°	
SCARF SIGN								
HEEL TO EAR								

TOTAL NEUROMUSCULAR MATURITY SCORE

SCORE

Neuromuscular _____

Physical _____

Total _____

MATURITY RATING

score	weeks
-10	20
-5	22
0	24
5	26
10	28
15	30
20	32
25	34
30	36
35	38
40	40
45	42
50	44

PHYSICAL MATURITY

PHYSICAL MATURITY SIGN	SCORE							RECORD SCORE HERE
	-1	0	1	2	3	4	5	
SKIN	sticky friable transparent	gelatinous red translucent	smooth pink visible veins	superficial peeling &/or rash, few veins	cracking pale areas rare veins	parchment deep cracking no vessels	leathery cracked wrinkled	
LANUGO	none	sparse	abundant	thinning	bald areas	mostly bald		
PLANTAR SURFACE	heel-toe 40-50 mm:-1 <40 mm:-2	>50 mm no crease	faint red marks	anterior transverse crease only	creases ant. 2/3	creases over entire sole		
BREAST	imperceptible	barely perceptible	flat areola no bud	stippled areola 1-2 mm bud	raised areola 3-4 mm bud	full areola 5-10 mm bud		
EYE/EAR	lids fused loosely: -1 tightly: -2	lids open pinna flat stays folded	sl. curved pinna; soft; slow recoil	well-curved pinna; soft but ready recoil	formed & firm instant recoil	thick cartilage ear stiff		
GENITALS (Male)	scrotum flat, smooth	scrotum empty faint rugae	testes in upper canal rare rugae	testes descending few rugae	testes down good rugae	testes pendulous deep rugae		
GENITALS (Female)	clitoris prominent & labia flat	prominent clitoris & small labia minora	prominent clitoris & enlarging minora	majora & minora equally prominent	majora large minora small	majora cover clitoris & minora		

TOTAL PHYSICAL MATURITY SCORE

GESTATIONAL AGE (weeks)

By dates _____

By ultrasound _____

By exam _____

Reference
Ballard JL, Khoury JC, Wedig K, et al: New Ballard Score, expanded to include extremely premature infants. *J Pediatr* 1991; 119:417-423. Reprinted by permission of Dr Ballard and Mosby-Year Book, Inc.

FIG. 38-3 Classification of newborns by intrauterine growth and gestational age. (From Ballard JL et al: New Ballard score, expanded to include extremely premature infants, *J Pediatr* 119:417–423, 1991.)

■ MANAGEMENT STRATEGIES

INITIAL CARE

Following birth, newborns require special care and observation as they master the transition to the extrauterine environment. Additional components of care at this period include prophylaxis for eye infection with antibiotic ointment and vitamin K injection for hemorrhagic disease.

ESTABLISHING FEEDING

Regardless of the route of feeding the family has chosen, the provider must ensure that the infant and parents have well-established feeding patterns before discharge. Follow-up care is scheduled in 2 or 3 days to ensure adequate nutrition is ongoing. See Chapters 11 and 12 for more detailed information on breastfeeding and formulas.

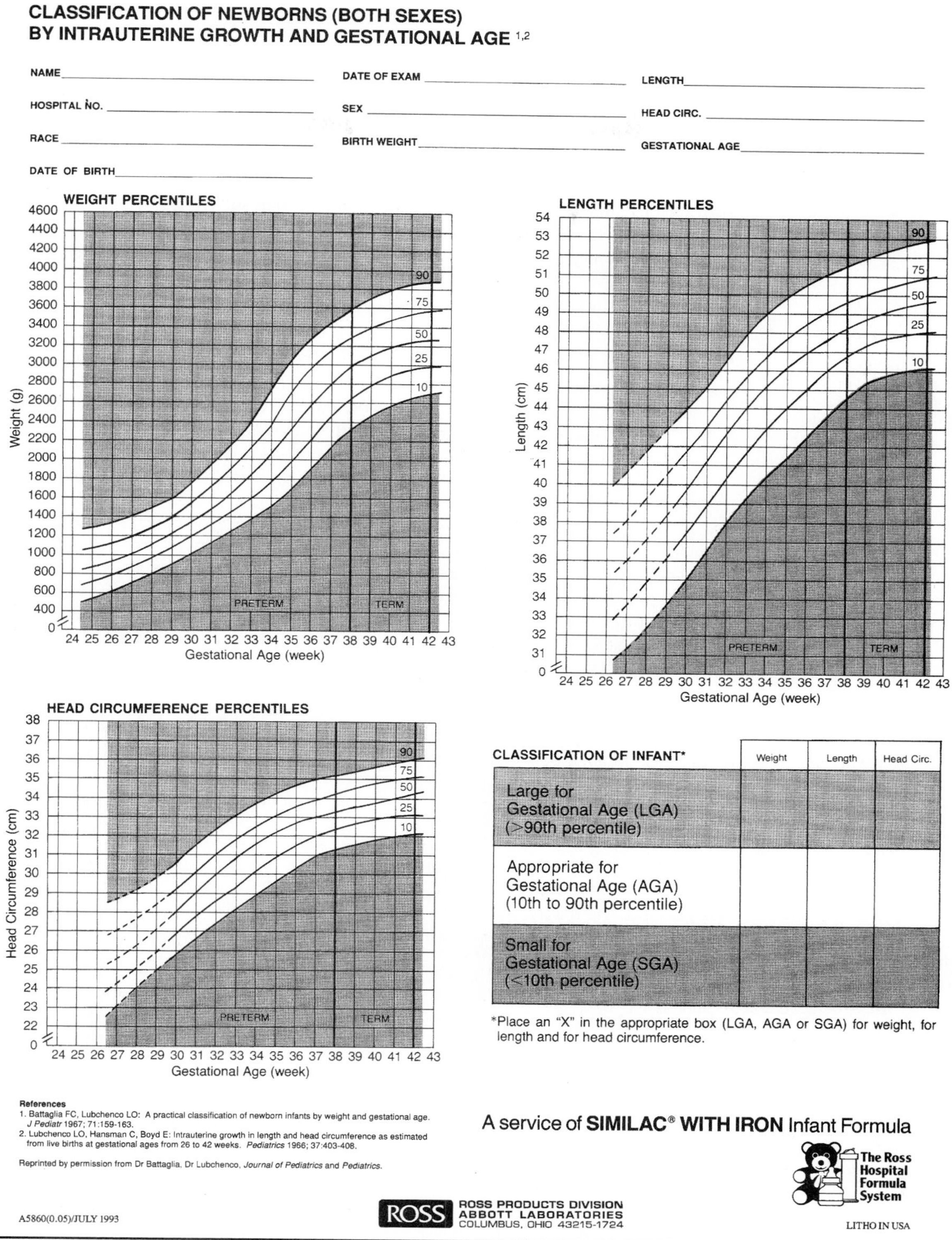

CLASSIFICATION OF NEWBORNS (BOTH SEXES)
BY INTRAUTERINE GROWTH AND GESTATIONAL AGE [1,2]

NAME _____   DATE OF EXAM _____   LENGTH _____

HOSPITAL NO. _____   SEX _____   HEAD CIRC. _____

RACE _____   BIRTH WEIGHT _____   GESTATIONAL AGE _____

DATE OF BIRTH _____

WEIGHT PERCENTILES

LENGTH PERCENTILES

HEAD CIRCUMFERENCE PERCENTILES

CLASSIFICATION OF INFANT*	Weight	Length	Head Circ.
Large for Gestational Age (LGA) (>90th percentile)			
Appropriate for Gestational Age (AGA) (10th to 90th percentile)			
Small for Gestational Age (SGA) (<10th percentile)			

*Place an "X" in the appropriate box (LGA, AGA or SGA) for weight, for length and for head circumference.

References
1. Battaglia FC, Lubchenco LO: A practical classification of newborn infants by weight and gestational age. *J Pediatr* 1967; 71:159-163.
2. Lubchenco LO, Hansman C, Boyd E: Intrauterine growth in length and head circumference as estimated from live births at gestational ages from 26 to 42 weeks. *Pediatrics* 1966; 37:403-408.

Reprinted by permission from Dr Battaglia, Dr Lubchenco, *Journal of Pediatrics* and *Pediatrics*.

A5860(0.05)/JULY 1993

A service of **SIMILAC® WITH IRON** Infant Formula

The Ross Hospital Formula System

ROSS PRODUCTS DIVISION
ABBOTT LABORATORIES
COLUMBUS, OHIO 43215-1724

LITHO IN USA

FIG. 38-4   Newborn maturity rating and classification. (From Ross Hospital Formula System, Ross Products Division, Abbott Laboratories, Columbus, OH; adapted from Battaglia FC, Lubchenco LO: A practical classification of newborn infants by weight and gestational age, *J Pediatr* 71:159-163, 1967; Lubchenco LO, Hansman C, Boyd E: Intrauterine growth in length and head circumference as estimated from live births at gestational ages from 26 to 42 weeks, *Pediatrics* 37:403-408, 1966.)

ANTICIPATORY GUIDANCE BEFORE DISCHARGE
Physical Care
Umbilical Cord.   Applying alcohol to the base of the cord traditionally has been recommended to aid in cord sepa-ration, although the utility of this practice has been questioned; air-drying by tucking the diaper below the cord may be pref-erable (Lin et al, 2005). After cord separation, which usually occurs at 10 to 14 days of life, a slight bloody discharge can

Text continued on p.1047

TABLE 38-2   Physical Examination Findings

System	Findings
Vital signs and measurements	Check vital signs frequently in the first hours after birth, then every 6-8 hr when stable. Evaluate ability to maintain temperature (36.5° C to 37.4° C [97.7° F to 99.3° F]) in open crib after transition to extrauterine environment. *Failure to maintain temperature* requires evaluation for other problems, particularly sepsis. Respirations should remain between 30 and 60 breaths/min. Heart rate should remain between 100 and 160 bpm. Significant molding of the head requires repeated measurements to verify size. Daily weight losses of up to 10% or so in the first 2-3 days of life are not abnormal because normal infants excrete a large amount of water in the first days of life. *Weight loss of greater than 10%* is unexpected and is often due to poor intake or excessive losses
Skin	Lanugo and vernix. Lanugo is fine dark hair, prominent over the trunk and shoulders. It is seen in infants born prematurely, becoming less prominent as the gestation approaches term. Thick, greasy, white vernix is more common on prematurely born infants' skin. Dry and cracked skin. This is normal over the first several days of life. If associated with thin subcutaneous fat (parchmentlike), it is suggestive of a postmature infant, fetal growth retardation, or both. *Cyanosis.* Acrocyanosis, bluish changes in the color of the hands and feet, and generalized mottling of the skin are frequently noted in the first several days of life when an infant loses body heat. *Central cyanosis* beyond the first few moments of life is abnormal and can represent a significant problem with oxygenation. *Pallor.* Many perinatal events can result in pallor, indicating a significant disruption of the infant's circulatory system. Specific causes include anemia, sepsis, cold stress, hypoglycemia, and seizures. Plethora. An excessively reddish discoloration to the skin can be caused by polycythemia or hyperthermia. Infants born to diabetic mothers can be plethoric. *Meconium staining.* Antenatal stress can cause the first stool to pass in utero. If this greenish-black meconium remains in the amniotic fluid for a prolonged period, staining of the infant's skin and fingernails results. *Jaundice.* See the discussion of jaundice in the text under Hematologic Conditions.
Head	Sutures and molding. Vaginally delivered infants demonstrate some degree of molding, usually elongation of the anteroposterior diameter of the skull; if delivered by cesarean method, there are minimal alterations to the shape of the head. Fontanelles. The anterior fontanelle is usually about 2-3 cm in diameter; the posterior fontanelle is about 1 cm in diameter. Both are usually slightly depressed (see Fig. 38-5).
Face	Symmetric structures of the face should be apparent, although unilateral facial edema as a result of delivery conditions can occur normally. Overall view of the face may reveal maxillary or mandibular hypoplasia, distortion, or hemifacial hypoplasia.
Eyes	Size, shape, and position of eyes. Too small or large, too widely spaced, or abnormal upward or downward slanting of palpebral fissures should alert the practitioner to potential congenital problems. Uncoordinated eye movements. Intermittent uncoordinated eye movements (disconjugate gaze) during the first weeks after birth are common, improving by 2-4 months old and resolving by 6 months old. *Fixed disconjugate gaze* is abnormal, even in the neonate. Conjunctivae. Reddening in the first 24-48 hours of life caused by chemical irritation of the eyes from silver nitrate drops or erythromycin ointment is normal. *Purulent discharge* in the first days or weeks of life can be associated with gonococcus, chlamydia, or herpes. Conjunctival hemorrhages secondary to delivery resolve spontaneously over the first weeks of life. Sclerae. Yellowing is associated with hyperbilirubinemia. Small hemorrhages secondary to delivery resolve spontaneously over the first weeks of life.

TABLE 38-2	Physical Examination Findings—Cont'd
System	**Findings**
	Thinning of the sclera, common in blacks, is manifested by dark blue or black patches. Blue sclerae are associated with osteogenesis imperfecta. Red reflex. Shining an ophthalmoscope white light through the pupil reveals the "red reflex," a disc ranging from pearly gray to orange in color. *Absence of a red reflex* may indicate the presence of lens opacities secondary to cataracts, congenital infection (rubella), or calcium metabolism abnormality. A *white reflex* can indicate retinoblastoma. Absence of the expected red reflex indicates the need for an immediate ophthalmologic evaluation.
Ears	Identify normalcy in the size, rotation, shape, position, and patency of the external auditory canal. Presence of low-set ears should prompt careful examination for other dysmorphic features. Abnormalities in shape require thorough physical examination, especially of the genitourinary system. Assessment of hearing is done by noting a startle response to a loud noise, avoiding any tactile sensations, such as a wind current on the face as a result of clapping near the ear. Auditory brain response testing should be ordered for any infant in whom a question of hearing exists. Screening for universal detection of infants with hearing loss is recommended and is especially important for high-risk infants (e.g., family history, in utero infection, craniofacial anomalies). Preauricular skin tags or significant pits should be noted (can be a genetic red flag). See text section on skin dimpling.
Nose	Patency of the nasal passages can be tested by closing the mouth and one nostril at a time or by passing a small catheter into the nasopharynx to see if the passage is clear. Nasal flaring is a sign of respiratory distress that can be caused by any number of abnormalities, including mechanical obstruction, parenchymal lung disease, or acidosis.
Mouth	Size and symmetry of the lips: • Thin lips with a smooth philtrum (the area between lips and nose) are associated with fetal alcohol syndrome. • *Asymmetric movements* while crying can be due to nerve palsies or absence of perioral muscles. Cleft lip and palate can be associated with midline CNS abnormalities. Incomplete cleft palates are recognized by digital examination of the mouth for bony defects of the hard palate in the presence of normal palatal mucosa. Excessive salivation can be related to reflux of gastric contents or esophageal atresia. Epstein pearls are small, white epithelial inclusion cysts on the palate and gums. An excessively large tongue can be associated with genetic or metabolic abnormalities, such as hypothyroidism or Down syndrome. Natal teeth are sometimes seen at birth (approximately 1 in 3000 live births). If they are extremely loose, aspiration is a concern. Consultation with a pediatric dentist is indicated. Webbing. Redundant skin is seen in trisomy 21, Turner syndrome, and Noonan syndrome.
Neck	Short neck indicates the possibility of Klippel-Feil syndrome or other vertebral problems. Masses: • Thyroglossal duct cysts (midline) or branchial cleft cyst (along the edge of the sternocleidomastoid muscles) can be found. • Other masses that can be seen include a hematoma in the sternocleidomastoid muscle, cystic hygromas, and, rarely, goiters. • Torticollis. Asymmetric shortening of the sternocleidomastoid muscle results in preferential turning of the head to one side, not to be confused with irritability on neck movement associated with meningitis or subarachnoid hemorrhage. Hematoma of the sternocleidomastoid muscle can result in the development of torticollis and requires early management.
Thorax	Shape, symmetry. Rounded appearance measuring about 2 cm less than the frontooccipital head circumference (approximately 33 cm):

Continued

| TABLE 38-2 | Physical Examination Findings—Cont'd |

System	Findings
Thorax—cont'd	• *Minimization of rounding* occurs with RDS, atelectasis, and other diseases of decreased expansion of the chest. • Accentuation is seen in meconium aspiration. Wide-spaced nipples and a shieldlike appearance are characteristic of Turner syndrome. Chest movement on inspiration should be symmetric and unlabored. Movement of the abdomen with respirations is normal. *Asymmetric movement* occurs with unilateral pneumothorax. *Intercostal, subcostal, or supracostal retractions* indicate respiratory distress. Clavicles. Vaginally delivered LGA babies are especially prone to fractures of the clavicle (see perinatal injury section in text). Breast bones. Pectus excavatum (concave chest) and pectus carinatum (pigeon chest) are occasionally seen. If severe both can lead to restrictive lung disease later in life. Nipples: • Fullness and sometimes secretion of a white milky substance are normal and are secondary to maternal hormonal stimulation. • Redness surrounding the nipple, especially with purulent drainage, occurs in neonatal mastitis.
Lungs	General. Coughing, retractions, and an intermittently increased respiratory rate occur immediately after birth, resolving by about 12 hours of life to smooth and unlabored respirations at a rate of 30 to 60 breaths/min. Respiratory distress. *Tachypnea, apnea* (pauses in respiration > about 15 seconds), *grunting* (an infant's attempt to increase functional residual capacity, thereby improving gas exchange), *interclavicular, subclavicular, or supraclavicular retractions, nasal flaring*, and *central cyanosis* all indicate distress. Auscultation: • Rales or crackles are commonly heard immediately after birth as lung fluid is resorbed. Beyond the immediate postpartum period, *rales* can indicate pneumonia, delayed resorption of lung fluid, meconium aspiration, or pulmonary edema. • *Unilateral absence of breath sounds* occurs in pneumothorax, atelectasis, and pleural effusion. • *Bowel sounds over the chest*, especially with a scaphoid abdomen and significant respiratory distress, indicate a diaphragmatic hernia with displacement of abdominal contents into the chest.
Heart	Inspection. Observe neonate for adequacy of perfusion. Respiratory distress is common with cardiac abnormalities. Edema as a result of cardiac failure is rarely seen in the newborn. Palpation: • *Point of maximal impulse is displaced* from the fourth left intercostal space with pneumothorax, situs inversus, or dextrocardia. • *Thrills or heaves* are associated with murmurs and cardiac abnormalities. Auscultation. Heart rate is normally 100 to 160 bpm. Detection of skipped beats warrants electrocardiogram. *Heart sounds may be muffled or displaced* in the infant with a pneumothorax. Murmurs. Common in the newborn period, many murmurs disappear after a few hours or a few days. Significant murmurs need to be investigated. Pulses. Brachial or radial pulses are compared with femoral or dorsalis pedis pulses for symmetry of impulse and strength in pulse. Delay or relative weakness of lower extremity pulses occurs in coarctation of the aorta. Blood pressure. By Doppler device using a 2.5-4 cm wide and 5-9 cm long cuff, compare with normals for age and gestation. Systolic blood pressures greater than 96 mm Hg are considered significant hypertension in the newborn, and systolic blood pressures exceeding 106 mm Hg are considered severe hypertension (National High Blood Pressure Education Program Working Group, 1996).
Abdomen	General: • Normal abdomen is slightly protuberant, is soft, moves smoothly with respirations, and has fine bowel sounds scattered throughout. *Absent bowel sounds* can indicate ileus.

TABLE 38-2 **Physical Examination Findings—Cont'd**

System	Findings
	• The liver is usually palpated 1-2 cm below the right costal margin; the spleen tip is sometimes felt at the left costal margin; kidneys, deep within lateral aspects of the abdomen measuring 3-4 cm in size, may be palpated.
	• Pain is indicated by crying, grimacing, or forceful resistance with palpation.
	Umbilical hernias. Midline outpouching from the sternum to the umbilicus is seen with weak abdominal musculature (diastasis recti); a large and protuberant umbilicus occurs with an umbilical hernia.
	Umbilical vessels. The normal cord contains two arteries and a single vein.
	Absence of the second artery can be associated with congenital abnormalities.
	Vomiting and abdominal distention. Regurgitation of large volumes of feeding is not expected. *Bilious vomiting* is always abnormal and usually a sign of obstruction. *Abdominal distention* with enlargement of any of the organs of the abdomen or failure to pass stool is abnormal. Meconium ileus with failure to pass stool in the first 24-48 hours of life is associated with cystic fibrosis.
Genitalia	Male:
	• The penis should have the urethral opening at the tip of the phallus with completely developed foreskin. Chordee means that the distal end of the penis is bent.
	• Testes not located in the scrotal sac or inguinal canal but retrievable to the scrotum are normal. Testes not located in or relocated in the scrotal sac from the canal are considered to be undescended.
	• Hydrocele is identified by transilluminating fluid collection around the testis and is regarded as normal unless it is associated with inguinal hernia or it lasts more than 12 months.
	• Inguinal hernia with displacement of intestines into the scrotal sac is frequently nontransilluminating and is associated with bowel sounds. Inguinal hernias are sometimes apparent and reduced at other times. A surgical consultation is indicated.
	Female:
	• Labia majora are large and completely surround the labia minora.
	• Labia and vagina should be open, often with a white discharge.
	• Blood-tinged fluid in small amounts by day 2-3 is normal.
	Ambiguous genitalia are genitalia that do not appear to be completely masculinized or feminized. An endocrine referral is essential.
	Anus and rectum. Patency of the rectum and placement of the anus should be noted. A small amount of blood streaking in the diaper, especially with a small anal fissure, is common.
Extremities, back, hips	Molding. Intrauterine constraint and resultant molding cause mild curvatures of the forefeet (metatarsus adductus vs. varus [in toeing or out toeing]) or the tibia (genu varum [bowleg], genu valgum [knock-knee]), or both. See Chapter 37 for more information.
	Contractures of the joints and molding of the bones occur if amniotic fluid was decreased and is abnormal.
	Fractures:
	• Skull fractures can occur as a result of extensive molding of a large head.
	• Femora and humeri can fracture with difficult deliveries and use of instrumentation.
	• *Multiple fractures* can indicate osteogenesis imperfecta.
	Spine. Dimples, hemangiomas, tufts of hair, or other lesions along the spine may be associated with spinal abnormalities, such as spina bifida occulta.
	Hips. See Chapter 37 for information about eliciting Ortolani and Barlow signs. Both are indicators of dislocated or dislocatable hips.
Neurologic examination	Muscle tone. Observe tone, movement, and symmetry of the extremities while the infant is awake.
	Reflexes. Elicit the following:
	• Rooting
	• Sucking
	• Palmar grasp

Continued

TABLE 38-2	Physical Examination Findings—Cont'd

System	Findings
Neurologic examination—Cont'd	• Moro reflex • Ankle clonus (3-4 beats of clonus at ankle is normal) • Stepping and placing response • Galant reflex • Asymmetric tonic neck reflex Cranial nerves. Cranial nerve I (olfactory) is rarely tested. Vision (cranial nerve II) is tested by an infant's response to a bright light. Cranial nerves III, IV, and VI are tested by noting an infant's ability to gaze in all directions, although intermittent disconjugate gaze is normal through 6 months old. Adequate sucking and swallowing confirm presence of cranial nerves V, IX, X, and XII. Symmetric movement of the face with crying confirms presence of cranial nerve VII. Hearing (cranial nerve VIII) is assessed by startle to loud noise.

Italicized findings indicate "red flags."
bpm, Beats per minute; *cm*, centimeters; *CNS*, central nervous system; *LGA*, large for gestational age; *min*, minute; *RDS*, respiratory distress syndrome.

BOX 38-2	Newborn Screening

- All infants should be screened before discharge.
- All infants initially screened before 24 hours old should be rescreened before 14 days old.
- All infants should be tested before the seventh day of life.
  1. For some diseases, such as PKU, the infant needs to be fed so that the intake or production of amino acids exceeds the infant's capacity to metabolize or excrete them.
  2. Rescreening is now recommended in many states. Providers need to be aware of the need for retesting, especially when infants are discharged early.
  3. Cord blood is not acceptable for newborn screening because most metabolites accumulate after birth.
  4. Filter papers should be used, preferably with 1 drop of blood filling the entire circle. Blood should not be added from the other side of the paper. If a capillary tube is used, it should not touch the paper. For sick infants, venous blood may be used, but care must be taken that no heparin or hyperalimentation components are included. To prevent hemolysis, the needle should not touch the paper.
  5. The filter paper must not be contaminated in any way. The specimen should be dried while lying flat and not exposed to heat or sunlight. Remember that mailboxes may be hot in the summer!
  6. Demographic data must be clearly written to ensure follow-up of abnormal results.
  7. Specimens should be mailed within 24 hours of collection via first-class mail to prevent delays in reaching the laboratory.
  8. Premature or sick infants should be screened by the seventh day of life.
  9. Transfusions may temporarily affect results, so specimens should be collected before plasma or blood products are administered.

be seen for 1 to 2 days. Bellybands or coins to cover the navel are avoided because these increase the chance of infection. If a foul-smelling discharge or erythema appears around the umbilicus, the infant should be evaluated immediately for sepsis. If a granuloma appears after the cord falls off, an application of silver nitrate helps to heal it.

Circumcision. Circumcision, the removal of the foreskin that normally covers the glans penis, is a controversial procedure. The decision to circumcise is the parents' responsibility, although the provider can provide factual information on the risks and potential benefits of the procedure.

Proponents of circumcision claim that it keeps the glans cleaner; the chance for developing urinary tract infections is reduced (although the chance of urinary tract infections in uncircumcised males is only 1%); it reduces the incidence of penile cancer, phimosis, balanitis, adhesions, and occlusion of the urethral meatus; and the boy may look more like his peers. The opponents of circumcision claim that it does not prevent sexually transmitted disease; that good hygiene prevents penile cancer; that circumcision leaves the glans open to the chance of cautery burns and meatal stenosis; and that because fewer boys are being circumcised, these boys will not be different from many of their peers.

Contraindications to circumcision include epispadias or hypospadias, ambiguous genitalia, exstrophy of the bladder, familial bleeding disorders, and illness. Complications of circumcisions include infections, bleeding, gangrene, scarring, meatal stenosis, cautery burns, urethral fistula, amputation or trauma to the glans, and pain. For infants who undergo circumcision, procedural anesthesia is recommended. A variety of anesthesia techniques are available, including application of topical anesthetics (EMLA cream), dorsal penile nerve block, and subcutaneous ring block. Postoperative pain relief measures in the form of sucrose

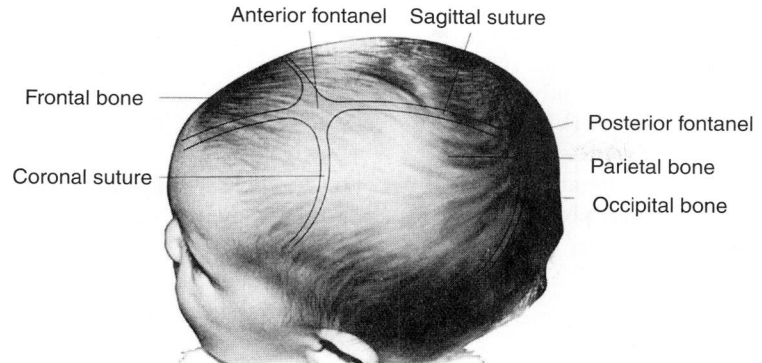

FIG. 38-5   Fontanelles and sutures. (From Betz CL, Hunsberger M, Wright S: *Family-centered nursing care of children*, ed 2, Philadelphia, 1994, WB Saunders, p. 124.)

on a pacifier, acetaminophen, soft music, and physiologic positioning of the infant in a padded environment are helpful (Brady-Fryer et al, 2004).

Care of the uncircumcised baby includes gentle cleaning around the genital area. The skin normally adheres to the penis and is not retractable at birth, but loosens as the baby grows. The parents are counseled not to force the foreskin back. If the baby is circumcised, the penis should be cleansed daily with cotton balls dipped in tap water followed by the application of a small amount of petroleum jelly to the tip of the penis with each diaper change to prevent discharge from the penis sticking to the diaper. The petroleum jelly is needed only for the first 2 to 3 days after the circumcision.

Bathing, Oils, and Powders.   Counsel parents to test the temperature of the water before bathing the infant. Tradition favors that the infant not be immersed in a tub of water, but rather should be sponge bathed until the umbilical cord separates and the navel appears healed. Mild cleansing agents, such as Dove, Caress, Neutrogena, and Basis, are gentle enough for infants' skin. Encourage parents to hold the baby to make him or her feel secure in the water and to never leave the baby alone in the tub.

Oils and powders are not recommended for infants' skin. Oils and greasy substances tend to clog the skin's pores and can cause acne or rashes. Powders should be avoided because inhaling the talc could lead to respiratory problems. For dry skin, a lotion such as Keri, Eucerin, Aveeno, or Cetaphil is recommended.

Diapers.   There is much controversy about whether disposable or cloth diapers are the better choice for infants. The need for frequent changing and proper cleansing is the important message to deliver.

Sleep Position

By 1992, the preponderance of available evidence suggested that the prone sleeping position was associated with an increased incidence of sudden infant death syndrome (SIDS). Current recommendations for *healthy* infants include: placing infant in a nonprone position (flat on the back preferred);

avoiding soft surfaces and gas-trapping objects in an infant's sleeping environment; advising that co-sleeping can be hazardous, but sleeping in the same room as the caregiver for the first 6 months of life may be beneficial; avoiding overheating; offering pacifiers may be helpful; "tummy time" during the awake period is recommended for developmental reasons and to help prevent flat spots on the occiput (AAP, 2005). Encourage parents to ensure that their child care center and other caregivers (e.g., grandparents) are following these guidelines. SIDS is discussed later in this chapter.

Injury Prevention

Counsel parents on the appropriate use and installation of a crash-tested safety seat when driving with their infant. The best child safety seat is the one that fits the child properly, is easy to use, and fits in the parent's vehicle correctly. The National Highway Traffic Safety Administration rated 135 backward facing infant child restraint systems for ease of parental use (see Resource Box at the end of the chapter). Correct installation of the infant safety seat can be checked at a child safety seat inspection station (often located in fire stations) or by a certified child passenger safety technician. Most hospitals have a certified person on-site who can assist parents when the infant leaves the hospital, or one can be located by searching the internet. At the first visit it is ideal to have a trained staff member check for appropriate positioning and belt use. It is disconcerting that 80% of car seats are used inappropriately (AAP, 2002).

The house should be childproofed before the infant is taken home. Falls and burns are the most common injuries to neonates. Parents should be counseled to avoid shaking their baby for any reason. Refer to Chapter 10 and 39 for more information.

Parenting

The parenting role is stressful, even if all goes well. Fatigue and maternal depression resulting from hormonal shifts are common. Encourage parents to identify and make use of supportive people, arrange time for rest and time alone, and keep their expectations reasonable. When a mother seems to be having significant difficulty in adjusting to her new infant, it is imperative that the provider also keep in mind the possibility of severe postpartum depression and be ready to intervene on the behalf of the infant, the mother, and the family. The 10-question Edinburgh Postnatal Depression Scale (EPDS) is an easy-to-administer tool that has been demonstrated to be a valuable and efficient way of identifying mothers at risk for "perinatal" depression (Fig. 38-6). Women with postpartum depression need not feel alone; intervention, with possible referral for mothers whose score indicates a depressive illness, should be individualized.

EARLY DISCHARGE AND FOLLOW-UP

Newborns are often discharged after a relatively short period of hospital observation. Although "early discharge" is a common practice, infants can experience difficulty with breastfeeding, poor weight gain, jaundice, and dehydration (Madden et al, 2004). Guidelines for early discharge of normal, healthy newborns are listed in Box 38-3. Plans for follow-up care within 48 to 72 hours and plans for ongoing health maintenance should be confirmed before discharge (Box 38-4). Even some newborns who are hospitalized longer may need follow-up care within the first few days of life. All parents leaving the hospital with a newborn should have a confirmed time and place for follow-up, in addition to contacts in case of an emergency or questions.

PREMATURE INFANTS AND NEWBORNS WITH SPECIAL NEEDS

Premature infants have special needs that must be addressed before discharge (Box 38-5). Newborns with special needs (e.g., anomalies, disease states, social situations) require early assessment, intervention, and referral before discharge to ensure that support, education, and follow-up are in place.

■ COMMON NEONATAL CONDITIONS
SKIN CONDITIONS
Milia

Description and Epidemiology. Milia are multiple, firm, pearly, opalescent, white papules scattered over the forehead, nose, and cheeks. Their intraoral counterparts are called Epsteins pearls. Histologically, milia represent superficial epidermal inclusion cysts filled with keratinous material associated with the developing pilosebaceous follicle.

Management. No treatment is necessary because milia exfoliate spontaneously in most infants over the first few weeks of life.

Sebaceous Hyperplasia

Description and Epidemiology. Sebaceous hyperplasia is characterized by prominent yellow-white papules at the opening of each pilosebaceous follicle, predominantly over the nose, forehead, upper lip, and cheeks. The overgrowth of sebaceous glands in response to the same androgenic stimulation that occurs in adolescence causes sebaceous hyperplasia.

Management. No treatment is required. These tiny papules diminish in size and disappear entirely within the first few weeks of life.

Erythema Toxicum

Description and Epidemiology. Firm, yellow-white 1- to 2-mm papules or pustules with a surrounding erythematous flare characterize erythema toxicum. Lesions are clustered in several sites. These lesions usually develop at 24 to 48 hours old. The cause is unknown, although examination of a Wrights-stained smear of the lesion reveals numerous eosinophils. Up to 50% of infants develop erythema toxicum, with the incidence higher in term than in premature infants.

Differential Diagnosis. Pyoderma, candidiasis, herpes simplex, transient neonatal pustular melanosis, and miliaria should be considered (Table 38-3).

Management. No treatment is required because the course is brief and transient.

Transient Neonatal Pustular Melanosis

Description and Epidemiology. Transient neonatal pustular melanosis is characterized by superficial vesiculopustules that rupture easily and leave a halo of white scales around a central pinhead-sized macule of hyperpigmentation. Pustular melanosis is caused by increased melanization of the epidermal cells, with sites of predilection being the trunk, limbs, palms, and soles. It is more common in black than in white infants.

Differential Diagnosis. Pyoderma and erythema toxicum are the differential diagnoses.

Management. No treatment is required. The pustular phase rarely lasts more than 2 to 3 days; hyperpigmented macules can persist for as long as 3 months.

Sucking Blisters

Description and Epidemiology. Sucking blisters are solitary or scattered superficial bullae on the upper limbs and lips of infants at birth, commonly found on the radial aspect of the forearm, the thumb, and the index finger. These blisters result from vigorous sucking on the affected part in utero.

Management. No treatment is required. These bullae resolve rapidly without sequelae.

Cutis Marmorata

Description and Epidemiology. Cutis marmorata is a lacy, reticulated, red or blue cutaneous vascular pattern appearing over most of the body surface. The vascular change is a response to exposure to low environmental temperatures. It represents an accentuated physiologic vasomotor response that disappears with increasing age. Persistent and pronounced cutis marmorata occurs in Down and trisomy 18 syndromes.

Management. Cutis marmorata usually resolves with warming of the infant.

Edinburgh Postnatal Depression Scale (EPDS)

Name: _____   Address: _____

Your date of birth: _____

Baby's date of birth: _____   Phone: _____

As you are pregnant or have recently had a baby, we would like to know how you are feeling. Please check the answer that comes closest to how you have felt IN THE PAST 7 DAYS, not just how you feel today.

Here is an example, already completed.

I have felt happy:
- ○ Yes, all the time
- X Yes, most of the time
- ○ No, not very often
- ○ No, not at all

This would mean: "I have felt happy most of the time" during the past week.

Please complete the other questions in the same way.

In the past 7 days:

1. I have been able to laugh and see the funny side of things
   - ○ As much as I always could
   - ○ Not quite so much now
   - ○ Definitely not so much now
   - ○ Not at all

2. I have looked forward with enjoyment to things
   - ○ As much as I ever did
   - ○ Rather less than I used to
   - ○ Definitely less than I used to
   - ○ Hardly at all

*3. I have blamed myself unnecessarily when things went wrong
   - ○ Yes, most of the time
   - ○ Yes, some of the time
   - ○ Not very often
   - ○ No, never

4. I have been anxious or worried for no good reason
   - ○ No, not at all
   - ○ Hardly ever
   - ○ Yes, sometimes
   - ○ Yes, very often

*5. I have felt scared or panicky for no very good reason
   - ○ Yes, quite a lot
   - ○ Yes, sometimes
   - ○ No, not much
   - ○ No, not at all

*6. Things have been getting on top of me
   - ○ Yes, most of the time I haven't been able to cope at all
   - ○ Yes, sometimes I haven't been coping as well as usual
   - ○ No, most of the time I have coped quite well
   - ○ No, I have been coping as well as ever

*7. I have been so unhappy that I have had difficulty sleeping
   - ○ Yes, most of the time
   - ○ Yes, sometimes
   - ○ Not very often
   - ○ No, not at all

*8. I have felt sad or miserable
   - ○ Yes, most of the time
   - ○ Yes, quite often
   - ○ Only occasionally
   - ○ No, never

*9. I have been so unhappy that I have been crying
   - ○ Yes, most of the time
   - ○ Yes, quite often
   - ○ Only occasionally
   - ○ No, never

*10. The thought of harming myself has occurred to me
   - ○ Yes, quite often
   - ○ Sometimes
   - ○ Hardly ever
   - ○ Never

Administered/reviewed by _____   Date _____

SCORING
QUESTIONS 1, 2, and 4 (without an *) are scored 0, 1, 2 or 3 with top box scored as 0
QUESTIONS 3, 5, 6, 7, 8, 9, and 10 (marked with an *) are reverse scored, with the top box scored as a 3
   Maximum score: 30
   Possible depression: 10 or greater
   Always look at item 10 (suicidal thoughts)

Instructions for using the Edinburgh Postnatal Depression Scale:
1. The mother is asked to check the response that comes closest to how she has been feeling in the previous 7 days.
2. All the items must be completed.
3. Care should be taken to avoid the possibility of the mother discussing her answers with others. (Answers come from the mother or pregnant woman.)
4. The mother should complete the scale herself, unless she has limited English or has difficulty with reading.

Users may reproduce the scale without further permission providing they respect copyright by quoting the names of the authors, the title and the source of the paper in all reproduced copies.

FIG. 38-6   Edinburgh Postnatal Depression Scale (EPDS). (From Cox JL, Holden JM, Sagovsky R: Detection of postnatal depression: development of the 10-item Edinburgh Postnatal Depression Scale, *Br J Psychiatry* 150:782-786, 1987 and from Wisner KL, Parry BL, Piontek CM: Postpartum depression, *N Engl J Med* 347(3):194–199, July 18, 2002.)

BOX 38-3 Guidelines for Early Discharge of Normal, Healthy Newborns

Antepartum, intrapartum, and postpartum course for baby and mother must be normal

Vaginal delivery

Single, appropriate for gestational age, term (38 to 42 weeks) baby

Stable vital signs for at least 12 hours before discharge:

Axillary temperature of 36.5° C to 37.4° C [97.7° F to 99.3° F] in open crib

Heart rate 100 to 160 bpm

Respiratory rate less than 60 breaths/minute

Passage of urine and stool

Two successful feedings have been accomplished

Normal physical examination

No excessive bleeding at circumcision site for at least 2 hours

The clinical significance of jaundice has been determined and appropriate follow-up plans made

Infant laboratory data, including maternal syphilis, hepatitis B, and HIV, and infant blood type and Coombs testing (as indicated) completed

Appropriately timed neonatal screening completed

Mother knowledgeable in the care of the infant, including the following:

- Feeding
- Normal stool and urine frequency
- Skin, genital, and cord care
- Ability to identify illness (especially jaundice)
- Proper safety (car seat, sleeping position)
- Smoke alarms in the home

Social support and continuing health care identified

Social situation adequate: screen for drug abuse, previous child abuse, mental illness, lack of social support, lack of permanent home, history of domestic violence, teenage mother, inadequate transportation or communication abilities

Appropriate early follow-up care within 48 hours of discharge identified

bpm, Beats per minute.
Data from American Academy of Pediatrics (AAP): Hospital stay for healthy term newborns, *Pediatrics* 113:1434-1436, 2004.

Harlequin Color Change

Description and Epidemiology. Harlequin color change is a division of the body skin coloring from forehead to pubis into red and pale halves. The cause is unknown.

Management. No treatment is indicated with this transient and benign condition.

Mongolian Spots, Café au Lait Spots, Salmon Patch (Nevus Simplex), and Port-Wine Stain (Nevus Flammeus, Port-Wine Nevus)

See Chapter 36 for a discussion of these skin conditions.

Nevus Sebaceous

Description and Epidemiology. Nevus sebaceous is a yellowish, hairless, sharply demarcated smooth plaque usually on the head and neck. Histologically, these nevi

BOX 38-4 Guidelines for 48- to 72-Hour Follow-up Visit of the Normal, Healthy Newborn

1. Review delivery and discharge summary for any identified follow-up needs (e.g., hearing screening, specialty referrals, etc.)
2. Assess the infant's general health, weight, hydration, and jaundice; identify any new problems; review feeding, stooling, and urination
3. Assess quality of bonding
4. Reinforce maternal and family education
5. Review outstanding laboratory data
6. Perform neonatal screen if indicated
7. Develop plan for health care maintenance, including emergency care, preventive care, and periodic screenings
8. Refer to WIC eligibility screening as appropriate.

contain an abundance of sebaceous glands. With maturity, usually during adolescence, the lesions become verrucous with large rubbery nodules. During adulthood, the lesions are complicated by secondary malignancies, most commonly basal cell carcinoma.

Management. Total excision before the onset of adolescence is recommended. Referral to a pediatric dermatologist is warranted.

Skin Dimpling

Description and Epidemiology. Deep skin dimples, in addition to pits and creases, can occur over bony prominences and in the sacral area. They occur in normal infants and in those with dysmorphologic syndromes, such as congenital rubella, deletion of the long arm of chromosome 18, and cerebrohepatorenal syndromes.

Management. No treatment is indicated if isolated and not associated with other findings.

Preauricular Sinus Tracts and Pits

Description and Epidemiology. Sinus tracts and pits occur anterior to the pinna and can be unilateral or bilateral. They result from imperfect fusion of the tubercles of the first and second branchial arches during gestational development; are familial, more common in females and blacks, and occasionally are associated with other anomalies of the ears and face.

Management. Excision rarely is required and only if tracts and pits are chronically infected and draining.

Amniotic Constriction Bands

Description and Epidemiology. In utero fibrous strands that encircle fetal parts can cause permanent depression of the underlying tissue, producing defects in the extremities and digits. Found in otherwise normal infants, these bands are thought to result from intrauterine rupture of the amnion with formation of fibrous strands. Sometimes there are associated abnormalities, including craniofacial anomalies and thoracic or abdominal wall defects.

BOX 38-5   Guidelines for Discharge and Follow-up of the High-Risk Neonate

Discharge Planning

Demonstrate adequate weight gain, temperature control in open crib, adequate feeding without cardiorespiratory compromise, and mature and stable cardiorespiratory function

Identify all active medical or social problems through a review of the medical record and physical examination of infant

Ensure adequacy of immunizations based on infant's chronologic age and appropriate metabolic screenings

Screen for anemia, and begin iron or vitamins if necessary

Review with family member medications, feeding schedules, well child care, signs of illness, safety instruction, and appropriate response and follow-up for infants with active medical conditions

Identify family and community resources if infant is to be discharged on home oxygen therapy

Ensure adequate training of appropriate family members in cardiopulmonary resuscitation and, if applicable, home apnea monitor use

Counsel family in car seat adaptations for the premature infant

Consider need for visiting nurse, social service, respite care, support groups, early intervention services, or referral to the Women, Infants, and Children (WIC) Program

Ensure appropriate hearing screen has been completed

Ensure that follow-up care within 48 hours of discharge is scheduled

Follow-up Planning

Schedule follow-up hearing screen (if necessary) for infants with:
- Craniofacial abnormalities
- In utero infections
- Birth weight less than 1500 g
- Meningitis
- Exchange transfusion for hyperbilirubinemia
- Use of ototoxic medications
- Apgar score of 0 to 4 at 1 minutes or 0 to 6 at 5 minutes
- Mechanical ventilation for 5 days or longer
- Stigmata of syndrome associated with hearing loss
- Family history of deafness

At 4 to 6 weeks of chronologic age, schedule a dilated binocular indirect ophthalmoscopic examination for neonates with a birth weight of 1500 g or less or with a gestational age of <32 weeks and for infants between 1500 and 2000 g or gestational age of more than 32 weeks with an unstable clinical course including cardiorespiratory support thought to be at high risk for retinopathy of prematurity by their attending physician (Section on Ophthalmology American Academy of Pediatrics; American Academy of Ophthalmology, American Association for Pediatric Ophthalmology and Strabismus, American Academy of Ophthalmology, 2006)

Follow-up visits every 1 to 2 weeks, especially if infant is on oxygen therapy

Growth and development should be of prime interest at each routine outpatient visit with referral for formal developmental assessment if any concerns are identified

---

TABLE 38-3   Comparison of Erythema Toxicum and Herpes Simplex Virus

Erythema Toxicum	Herpes Simplex Virus
Benign, self-limited	Pathologic, progressive
No specific maternal history	Frequently a history of maternal disease
Usually seen only in term infants	Can occur in infants of any gestational age
Begins on the second or third day of life, lasting as long as 1 week	Often begins late in the first week of life or early in the second week of life
Rash is evanescent, often involving the face, trunk, and extremities	Can be superficial and localized only to the presenting part (vertex or buttocks) or widespread and disseminated without cutaneous involvement
1-2 mm white papules or pustules on an erythematous base that occasionally may become somewhat vesicular	May manifest similar to sepsis without cutaneous findings or as grouped vesicles on an erythematous base on the presenting part about days 9-11 of life
Wright or Giemsa stain of lesion scraping demonstrates large numbers of eosinophils and no organisms; cultures are sterile	DFA staining or ELISA detection of HSV antigens of vesicle scrapings or growth of the organism from vesicle fluid is diagnostic
No specific therapy necessary	Acyclovir and other antiviral agents

Management. Treatment depends on the severity of deformities produced. Constriction bands on the limbs are often managed in consultation with plastic surgery.

Supernumerary Nipples

Description and Epidemiology. Solitary or multiple accessory nipples and sometimes areolae occur in unilateral or bilateral distribution along a line from the midaxilla to the inguinal area. The cause is unknown. Urinary tract anomalies do occur, but are rare.

Management. Usually no treatment is necessary.

Branchial Cleft and Thyroglossal Cysts and Sinuses

Description and Epidemiology. Cysts and sinuses in the neck can be unilateral or bilateral and can open onto the cutaneous surface or drain into the pharynx. Thyroglossal cysts and fistulas are similar defects located in or near the midline of the neck, extending to the base of the tongue. Thyroglossal cysts occasionally contain aberrant thyroid tissue and mucinous material. Cysts and sinuses in the neck can be formed along the course of the first and second branchial clefts as a result of improper closure during embryonic life. These anomalies can be inherited as autosomal dominant traits.

Management. Antibiotic therapy is indicated for infections of the cysts or sinuses, which are rare in the neonatal period. Surgical excision is recommended for thyroglossal cysts.

HEAD, FACE, AND EYE CONDITIONS

Caput Succedaneum

Description and Epidemiology. Caput succedaneum is a diffuse swelling of the soft tissue of the scalp with possible underlying bruising; the swelling usually crosses the suture lines (Fig. 38-7). Caput succedaneum originates from trauma as the baby descends through the birth canal.

Clinical Findings.

History. Primigravida and traumatic delivery may be part of the history.

Physical Examination. Findings include the following:
- Obvious swelling and bruising in the parietal regions of the scalp
- Swelling that crosses suture lines
- Frequently associated with molding

Differential Diagnosis. Cephalhematoma is the differential diagnosis.

Management. No treatment is necessary because swelling resolves spontaneously over a few days. If the lesion is large, observe the baby for the development of jaundice as the blood from bruising is reabsorbed.

Cephalhematoma

Description and Epidemiology. Cephalhematoma is a collection of blood in the subperiosteal area of the scalp that does not cross the suture lines. Frequently, no noticeable bruising of the area is seen (Fig. 38-8). Cephalhematoma

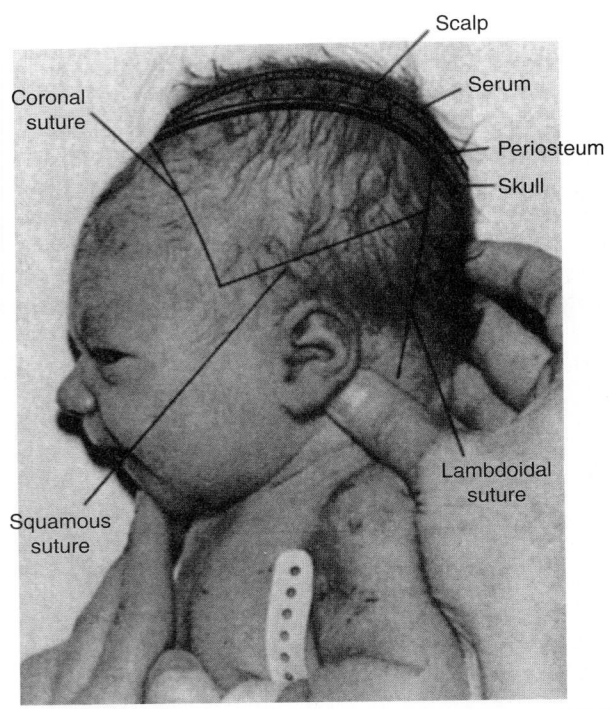

FIG. 38-7 Caput succedaneum. (From Betz CL, Hunsberger M, Wright S: *Family-centered nursing care of children*, ed 2, Philadelphia, 1994, WB Saunders, p 124.)

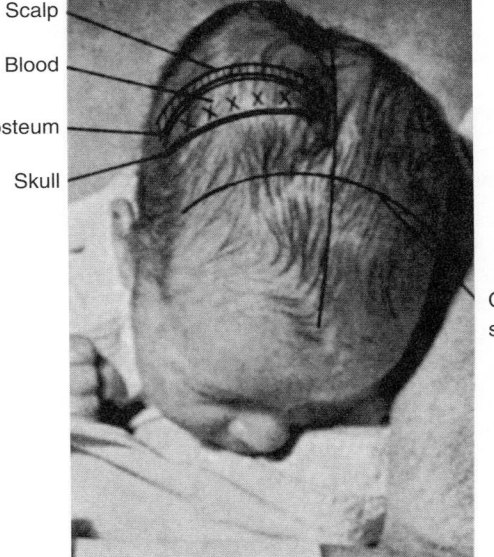

FIG. 38-8 Cephalhematoma. (From Betz CL, Hunsberger M, Wright S: *Family-centered nursing care of children*, ed 2, Philadelphia, 1994, WB Saunders, p 124.)

results from trauma occurring during a difficult delivery. The swelling appears hours to days after delivery.

Clinical Findings.

History.   Primigravida and traumatic delivery may be part of the history.

Physical Examination.   Findings include the following:

• Swelling in the parietal area that does not cross suture lines
• Rarely associated with a skull fracture, coagulopathy, or intracranial hemorrhage

Differential Diagnosis.   Caput succedaneum and cranial meningocele should be considered.

Management.   No treatment is indicated because the condition resolves in a few weeks to months. Calcification of the hematoma can occur, which will be felt as bony prominences on the cranium. Observe for hyperbilirubinemia.

Craniotabes

Description and Epidemiology.   Craniotabes is thinning of the bone of the scalp. This is a normal variation of the parietal bone, usually near the sagittal suture line.

Clinical Findings.

History.   Prematurity can be part of the history.

Physical Examination.   Findings include a "ping-pong ball" effect when pressing on the parietal bone.

Management.   No treatment is necessary because craniotabes resolves spontaneously. If persistent, pathologic causes, such as rickets, should be investigated.

Cleft Lip and Palate

Description and Epidemiology.   Cleft lip results from failure of embryonic structures surrounding the oral cavity to join. Cleft palate appears when the palatal shelves fail to fuse. There are various degrees of clefts. Genetic factors influence the development of cleft lip more than cleft palate; however, both occur sporadically. A combination of cleft lip and cleft palate is more common than one without the other. Cleft lip with or without cleft palate occurs in about 1 in 1000 births. Cleft palate alone occurs in 1 in 2500 births (Tinanoff, 2004). Clefts are more common in males than in females. In most cases, a genetics consultation is warranted.

Clinical Findings.

Physical Examination.   Findings include the following:

• A varying degree of cleft, from a small notch to a complete separation
• Unilateral or bilateral cleft
• Involvement of the soft palate, hard palate, or both
• A bifid uvula, which may indicate a submucosal cleft palate

Management and Complications.   Surgical repair is indicated, and the timing is individualized. Special nipples and feeding techniques are used until surgery can be performed. Breastfeeding and bottle feeding may be successful depending on the severity of the cleft. Speech evaluation and perhaps therapy are necessary in later years. Dental restoration is often needed. Team management is beneficial. Middle ear, nasopharyngeal, sinus infections, and associated hearing loss can occur.

Congenital Cataracts, Glaucoma, and Retinopathy of Prematurity

See Chapter 28.

CARDIAC CONDITIONS

See Chapter 30.

RESPIRATORY CONDITIONS

Respiratory Distress Syndrome

Description and Epidemiology.   Respiratory distress syndrome (RDS), formerly called hyaline membrane disease, occurs secondary to atelectasis of the lungs. This is the most common pulmonary disease in the newborn (Table 38-4). Surfactant deficiency is the underlying cause of the disease, resulting in alveolar atelectasis and decreased lung compliance. The incidence is 1% of all live births, but only 0.5% of term births. The incidence rises rapidly below 33 to 34 weeks of gestational age. An estimated 50% of all neonatal deaths result from RDS or its complications (Stoll & Kliegman, 2004). The incidence increases with decreasing gestational age and/or weight.

Clinical Findings.

History.   The history can include the following:

• Diabetic mother (incidence increased at older gestational ages in infants of diabetic mothers)
• Preterm delivery
• Multiple prior pregnancies
• Cesarean delivery
• Precipitous delivery
• Asphyxia
• Cold stress
• Previously affected siblings

Physical Examination.   Findings include the following:

• Tachypnea
• Grunting
• Intercostal retractions
• Nasal flaring
• Duskiness, cyanosis
• Breath sounds may be normal, but often are diminished with harsh tubular quality
• Fine rales on deep inspiration

Diagnostic Studies.   A radiograph of the chest shows a fine reticular granularity of the parenchyma and air bronchograms. Blood gas results indicate hypoxemia, hypercarbia, and metabolic acidosis.

Management, Prognosis, and Prevention.   Supportive care and mechanical ventilation are used as indicated. The immediate use of exogenous surfactant has been found to reduce mortality rates and improve short-term respiratory status in preterm infants. The prognosis depends on the severity of the disease and the birth weight of the infant. The only fully effective preventive measure is elimination of prematurity. Administration of synthetic corticosteroids to selected women 48 to 72 hours before delivery is also used to reduce the severity of the problem (Soll & Pfister, 2006).

TABLE 38-4   **Clinical Comparison of Transient Tachypnea of the Newborn and Respiratory Distress Syndrome**

Transient Tachypnea of the Newborn	Respiratory Distress Syndrome
Seen only in infants delivered at or near term, often in infants born by cesarean section	Found only in premature infants, with the greatest incidence in infants weighing <1500 g
Increased respiratory rate is invariably present; grunting and intercostal retractions are not always present	Usually, respiratory rate is increased, infants grunt at expiration, nasal flaring is noted, and sternal and intercostal retractions are commonly seen
Cyanosis is not a prominent feature	Cyanosis in room air is a prominent feature
Air exchange is good; rales and rhonchi are usually absent	Auscultation reveals diminished air entry
Begins at birth, usually resolving in the first 24-48 hours of life	Progressive respiratory distress in the first hours of life
Chest radiograph shows central perihilar streaking with slightly enlarged heart	Chest radiograph demonstrates reticulogranular, ground-glass appearance and air bronchograms
Typical course involves gradual decrease in respiratory rate with resolution in the first 5 days of life	Course variable depending on infant's gestational weight and age; classically, RDS begins to improve after about 72 hours of symptoms
No specific therapy other than maintaining oxygenation is usually necessary	Artificial surfactant and administration of steroids to the mother can reduce the severity of this disease; mechanical ventilation is commonly needed

Transient Tachypnea of the Newborn

Description and Epidemiology.   Transient tachypnea of the newborn (TTN) is a respiratory condition that results from incomplete evacuation of fetal lung fluid in full-term infants. TTN results from decreased pulmonary compliance and tidal volume and increased dead space secondary to slow absorption of fetal lung fluid. It is more common in cesarean deliveries.

Clinical Findings.

History.   TTN usually disappears within 24 to 48 hours.

Physical Examination.   Findings include the following:

- Tachypnea
- Expiratory grunting
- Auscultation without findings
- Intercostal retractions
- Occasionally, cyanosis can be seen, but it responds to minimal oxygen

Diagnostic Studies.   A chest radiograph shows prominent pulmonary vascular markings, fluid lines along fissures, over-aeration, flat diaphragms, and occasionally pleural fluid.

Differential Diagnosis.   The differential diagnosis is RDS (see Table 38-4).

Management and Prognosis.   If the infant is not in significant respiratory distress, close observation and transcutaneous oxygen saturation monitoring can be sufficient until the tachypnea resolves. The need for supplemental oxygen therapy provided in a hood should be based on close oxygen monitoring. The use of mechanical ventilation in TTN is rare. Infants usually recover rapidly within 24 to 48 hours with no intervention.

Meconium Aspiration Syndrome

Description and Epidemiology.   Meconium aspiration syndrome occurs in term or postterm infants. This syndrome is a serious pulmonary disorder characterized by small airway obstruction, chemical pneumonitis, and secondary respiratory distress. In utero fetal distress and anoxia increase intestinal peristalsis and relax the anal sphincter resulting in release of meconium into the amniotic fluid. Thick meconium is aspirated either in utero or with the first breath. Approximately 10% to 15% of all newborns are meconium stained, but only 5% of these infants develop respiratory problems (Stoll & Kliegman, 2004).

Clinical Findings.

History.   The history includes meconium in the amniotic fluid and below the vocal cords on resuscitation.

Physical Examination.   Findings include the following:

- Tachypnea
- Intercostal retractions
- Grunting
- Cyanosis within hours of delivery

Diagnostic Studies.   A chest radiograph shows patchy infiltrates, coarse streaking of both lung fields, and flattening of the diaphragm.

Management, Prognosis, and Prevention.   An infant born with meconium present in the amniotic fluid but who is vigorous (strong respiratory effort, good muscle tone, and a heart rate of higher than 100 beats per minute [BPM]) does not need intubation and suctioning. Meconium-stained depressed infants do benefit from intubation and suctioning before the initiation of positive pressure ventilation (Vain et al, 2004). Ongoing treatment includes supportive care and standard management of respiratory distress. Severe meconium aspiration cases are managed by extracorporeal membrane oxygenation (ECMO). The mortality rate of meconium-stained infants is higher than that of nonstained infants. Meconium aspiration accounts for a significant proportion of neonatal deaths. Residual lung problems are possible. Ultimate prognosis depends on the extent of central nervous system (CNS) injury from asphyxia. DeLee suctioning after the infant's head is delivered was previously felt by some to reduce the risk of meconium aspiration, especially if the baby had not yet breathed deeply. However, it is no longer recommended.

GASTROINTESTINAL AND ABDOMINAL CONDITIONS

Esophageal Atresia and Tracheoesophageal Fistula

Description and Epidemiology. In esophageal atresia, a blind pouch occurs in the esophagus with or without an associated fistula. Most infants (90%) have a proximal pouch, with the associated fistula connecting the distal esophagus and the trachea (Fig. 38-9). This defect occurs in 1 in 3500 births. Approximately one third of affected infants are born prematurely (Orenstein et al, 2004).

Clinical Findings.

History. The history includes maternal polyhydramnios and inability to pass a nasogastric tube during resuscitation at birth or afterward in the nursery, especially in the child with vomiting.

Physical Examination. Findings include the following:
- Excessive oral secretions that require frequent suctioning
- Choking, coughing, and cyanosis, particularly during feedings
- Spitting or vomiting

Diagnostic Studies. Chest and abdominal radiographs show the nasogastric tube coiled in the thoracic region. Carefully performed water-soluble x-ray evaluation of the upper esophagus demonstrates the exact location of the atresia and rules out tracheoesophageal fistula.

Differential Diagnosis. RDS, meconium aspiration, and congenital heart disease should be considered.

Management, Complications, and Prognosis. This is a surgical emergency requiring immediate intervention. A nasogastric tube can be inserted into the blind pouch to prevent aspiration until surgical repair can be accomplished. Preoperatively the infant should be placed in a prone position

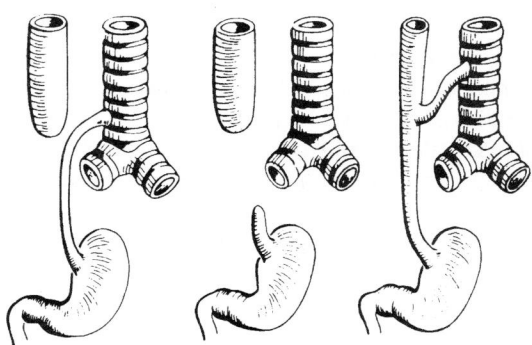

FIG. 38-9 The three most common types of esophageal atresia and tracheoesophageal fistula (TEF). (From Ein SH: Congenital malformations of the esophagus. In Wyllie R, Hyams JS, editors: *Pediatric gastrointestinal disease*, Philadelphia, 2006, WB Saunders.)

and suctioned frequently. Pneumonia, atelectasis, aspiration, strictures, and repeated surgery are possible complications. The survival rate postoperatively is almost 100% unless other congenital anomalies are present. Approximately 50% to 70% of affected infants have other congenital anomalies (Ulshen, 2006; Orenstein et al, 2004).

Duodenal Atresia

Description and Epidemiology. Duodenal atresia is a complete obstruction of the duodenum, ending blindly just distal to the ampulla of Vater. Duodenal atresia occurs in 1 in 10,000 to 30,000 births. It is associated with prematurity in 50% of cases, Down syndrome in 40% of cases, and other anomalies in up to 20% of cases (Ulshen, 2006; Wyllie, 2004).

Clinical Findings.

History. The history may include the following:
- Maternal polyhydramnios
- Down syndrome
- Premature birth

Physical Examination. Findings include the following:
- Bile-stained vomitus
- Abdominal distention
- Jaundice

Diagnostic Studies. Abdominal radiographs show a "double-bubble" pattern in the upright position secondary to air in the stomach and a distended duodenum.

Differential Diagnosis. Malrotation, duodenal obstruction, and annular pancreas should be considered.

Management, Complications, and Prognosis. Surgical intervention is indicated. Feedings should be discontinued and gastric suctioning applied. The prognosis depends on early identification and treatment and other associated anomalies. Aspiration of gastric contents can occur as a complication of this condition.

Volvulus

Description. Volvulus is the twisting of a loop of bowel, causing intermittent or acute pain and obstruction, occurring in 1 in 6000 live births (Ulshen, 2006).

Clinical Findings.

Physical Examination. Findings include abdominal distention and bilious vomiting.

Diagnostic Studies. Intestinal obstruction is demonstrated on abdominal radiograph.

Differential Diagnosis. Duodenal obstruction or atresia and annular pancreas are in the differential diagnosis.

Management, Complications, and Prognosis. Surgical repair and fluid replacement are indicated. The prognosis depends on identification and the urgency of surgery. Perforation, necrosis of the bowel, sepsis, and peritonitis are possible complications.

Pyloric Stenosis

Description and Epidemiology. Pyloric stenosis is characterized by hypertrophied pyloric muscle, causing a narrowing of the pyloric sphincter. Pyloric stenosis occurs in 3 per 1000 live births, with a fourfold increase in males as compared with females (Wyllie, 2004). It tends to be familial and is seen more commonly in white first-born males.

Clinical Findings.

History. The history may include the following:
- Regurgitation and nonprojectile vomiting during the first few weeks of life
- Projectile vomiting beginning at 2 to 3 weeks old
- Insatiable appetite with weight loss, dehydration, and constipation

An association of pyloric stenosis with the early administration of erythromycin has been demonstrated (Mahon et al, 2001).

Physical Examination. Findings include the following:
- Weight loss
- Vomitus that is nonbilious and can contain blood
- A distinct "olive" mass that is often palpated in the epigastrium to the right of midline
- Reverse peristalsis visualized across the abdomen

Diagnostic Studies. An upper gastrointestinal series demonstrates a "string sign," indicating a fine, elongated pyloric canal. Ultrasound, with measurement of the pyloric muscle thickness, is used in many centers.

Management and Prognosis.
Surgical intervention (pyloromyotomy) is indicated after correction of fluid and electrolyte imbalance. Vomiting can continue for a few days after surgery, although it is not as significant as it was preoperatively; feedings should be introduced gradually. The prognosis is excellent.

Hirschsprung Disease (Congenital Aganglionic Megacolon)

Description and Epidemiology. Hirschsprung disease is an absence of ganglion cells in the bowel wall, most often in the rectosigmoid region, resulting in a portion of the colon having no motility. This disorder occurs in 1 in 5000 births and is more common in boys. It is the most common cause of neonatal obstruction of the colon and accounts for approximately 33% of all neonatal obstructions. The disease is familial, affects males four times more commonly than females, and is common in children with trisomy 21. Additional anomalies are sometimes present (Middlesworth & Kodenhe-Chiweshe, 2006; Wyllie, 2004).

Clinical Findings.

History. The history may include the following:
- Failure to pass meconium within the first 48 hours of life
- Failure to thrive
- Poor feeding
- Chronic constipation
- Down syndrome

Physical Examination. Findings include the following:
- Vomiting
- Abdominal obstruction
- Failure to pass stools
- Diarrhea, explosive bowel movements, or flatus

Diagnostic Studies. Radiographs indicate dilated loops of bowel (Fig. 38-10). A biopsy determines the absence of ganglion cells.

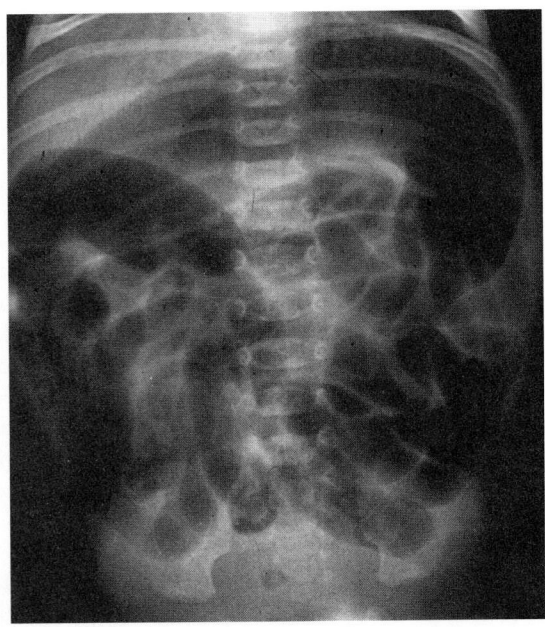

FIG. 38-10 Dramatic dilation of bowel consistent with Hirschsprung disease. (Photo courtesy Lawrence H. Robinson, Professor of Radiology and Pediatrics, University of Texas Medical School, Houston, TX.)

Differential Diagnosis. The differential diagnosis includes acquired functional megacolon, colonic inertia, chronic idiopathic constipation, obstipation, small left colon syndrome, meconium plug syndrome, and ileal atresia with microcolon.

Management. Surgical resection of the affected bowel is indicated, with or without a colostomy.

Imperforate Anus

Description and Epidemiology. Imperforate anus is the lack of a rectal opening. This condition occurs in about 1 in 4000 births, about half associated with another anomaly (often the VACTERL syndrome consisting of vertebral dysgenesis, anal atresia [imperforate anus], cardiac anomalies, tracheoesophageal fistula, renal anomalies, and limb anomalies (Pena, 2004).

Clinical Findings.

History. The history includes no passage of meconium.

Physical Examination. Findings include no obvious opening in the rectal area.

Diagnostic Studies. Endoscopic examination and ultrasound indicate the degree of malformation.

Associated Conditions. Congenital heart disease, esophageal atresia, intestinal atresia, annular pancreas, intestinal malrotation or duplication, bicornuate absence of the musculus rectus abdominis, trisomy 21, finger and hand anomalies, omphalocele, bladder exstrophy, and exstrophy of the ileocecal area are associated conditions (Pena, 2004).

Management. Immediate surgical repair with or without performing a colostomy is indicated. Long-term management related to bowel functioning may be needed because some children will have trouble with bowel emptying or incontinence.

Omphalocele and Gastroschisis

Description and Epidemiology. An omphalocele is a protrusion of the sac of intestines into the base of the umbilical cord. The intestines are covered by the peritoneum without overlying skin. Occurrence is 1 in 5000 to 10,000 births (Stoll & Kliegman, 2004). Gastroschisis is similar in appearance with intestinal contents protruding through the abdomen with no protective peritoneal covering. Gastroschisis occurs in about 1 in 10,000 to 20,000 live births when there is failure to close the lateral ventral folds of the developing abdominal wall.

Clinical Findings.

Physical Examination. Examination reveals a saclike protrusion covered by the peritoneum without overlying skin at the midabdomen.

Associated Conditions. With omphalocele, serious associated conditions occur in 50% of newborns including chromosomal abnormalities (trisomy 13 & 18), congenital diaphragmatic hernia, and a variety of cardiac problems. Concomitant hypoglycemia and macroglossia suggest Beckwith syndrome (Stoll & Kliegman, 2004). Associated congenital anomalies are rare with gastroschisis.

Management and Complications. Maintain body temperature. Apply protective gauze and wrap abdomen with cellophane to prevent heat and fluid loss. When the infant is stable, surgical repair is indicated. Ileus is a common complication.

Necrotizing Enterocolitis

Description and Epidemiology. Necrotizing enterocolitis (NEC) is characterized by varying degrees of mucosal or transmural necrosis of the intestine. The usual onset is in the first 2 weeks of life, but can be later in very-low-birth-weight infants. The cause is unknown, but it is much less common in infants that are breastfed and have minimal feeds before bolus feeds. High-risk infants are found to have immature colons that become necrosed from trauma or injury. NEC occurs in 3% to 5% of neonates in the NICU, with the vast majority (90% to 93%) of these cases occurring in premature infants, especially those between 500 and 750 g (Brown & Neu, 2006; Semeao, 2005; Stoll & Kliegman, 2004).

Clinical Findings.

History. The history can include the following:
- Prematurity, SGA
- Maternal hemorrhage, preeclampsia
- Cocaine exposure in utero
- Exchange transfusions, umbilical catheters
- Asphyxia
- Polycythemia

Physical Examination. Findings include the following:
- Abdominal distention
- Vomiting
- Bloody stools (25%)
- Lethargy
- Apnea
- Disseminated intravascular coagulation
- Rapid progression of shock

Diagnostic Studies
- Sepsis work-up should be done.
- An abdominal radiograph shows pneumatosis intestinalis, a specific air pattern.

Differential Diagnosis. The differential diagnosis includes sepsis, intestinal obstruction, volvulus, Hirschsprung disease, anal fissures, and neonatal appendicitis.

Management, Complications, and Prognosis. Take the following steps:

1. Prescribe systemic antibiotics following sepsis work-up.
2. Stop feedings, initiate gastric suctioning, maintain electrolyte balance, give oxygen as needed, and initiate surgical consultation.
3. Obtain serial abdominal radiographs to follow course of disease.
4. Delay oral feedings in very-low-birth-weight infants for at least 1 week after definitive diagnosis; when feedings are begun, they should be continuous slow drip before advancing to bolus.

The mortality rate is 10% to 50%, causing 1000 deaths per year. Ileus and perforation are early complications. Sequelae to NEC include feeding intolerance, stricture formation, and short-bowel syndrome, especially after intestinal resection (Brown & Neu, 2006; Semeao, 2005; Stoll & Kliegman, 2004).

Meconium Ileus

Description and Epidemiology. Meconium ileus is an impaction of the bowel with meconium, causing intestinal obstruction. Meconium ileus is associated with cystic fibrosis and maternal polyhydramnios. About 80% to 90% of patients with meconium ileus have cystic fibrosis; about 10% to 20% of patients with cystic fibrosis have meconium ileus (Stoll & Kliegman, 2004).

Clinical Findings.

History. There is a failure to pass meconium within 48 hours of life.

Physical Examination. Findings include abdominal distention and persistent vomiting.

Diagnostic Studies. A radiograph shows bowel loops of varying width. There is a grainy appearance at points of heaviest meconium concentration.

Associated Conditions. Infants with complicated meconium ileus may have associated intestinal disorders, including atresia, stenosis, volvulus, or perforations, and symptoms suggestive of cystic fibrosis (Wyllie, 2004).

Management and Prognosis. Treatment is individualized; high enemas (with water-soluble contrast material) or laparotomy can be used. The survival rate is good. Identification of any underlying disorders should be undertaken, and referral to a gastrointestinal specialist may be considered.

Diaphragmatic Hernia

Description and Epidemiology. In diaphragmatic hernia, abdominal contents herniate into the thoracic cavity. A diaphragmatic hernia is caused by failure of the pleuroperitoneal canal to close completely during embryologic development. It occurs on the left side 80% to 90% of the time with a frequency of about 1 in 2000 to 5000 live births and is more common in males (Lovrekovic, 2005).

Clinical Findings.
History. After birth, immediate respiratory failure occurs secondary to pulmonary hypertension or pulmonary hypoplasia.

Physical Examination. Findings include the following:
- Respiratory distress with tachypnea
- Cyanosis
- Scaphoid abdomen
- Rarely, bowel sounds heard in the chest
- Absence of breath sounds
- Heart tones best heard in the contralateral chest

The amount of respiratory distress depends on the amount of functional lung capacity. Any newborn with respiratory distress should be evaluated for diaphragmatic hernia.

Diagnostic Studies. A chest radiograph shows fluid and air-filled loops of intestine in the chest. The mediastinum is displaced toward the unaffected side, usually to the right.

Management. Treatment involves the following:
- As soon as the diagnosis is suspected, the infant should be positioned with the head and chest higher than the abdomen.
- Intensive respiratory support, which often includes ECMO
- Surgery
- After surgery, intensive respiratory and metabolic support

Prognosis. The mortality rate is 55% to 65%, depending on the degree of hypoplastic lung (Lovrekovic, 2005).

Hydrocele and Inguinal Hernia
See Chapter 34.

Umbilical Hernia
Definition. Umbilical hernia is a weakness or imperfect closure of the umbilical ring.

Clinical Findings.
Physical Examination. Findings include a soft swelling in the umbilical area that can be reduced, often associated with diastasis recti.

Management, Prognosis, and Education. Surgery is not required unless the hernia persists beyond 5 years old, strangulates, is nonreducible, or dramatically enlarges. Most umbilical hernias resolve spontaneously by 1 year old, but can take up to 4 to 5 years; those with fascial defects greater than 1.5 cm in diameter have a lower rate of spontaneous closure. Incarceration is extremely rare. Counsel parents to avoid taping coins or placing bellybands over the umbilicus because these efforts do not help and can contribute to infection.

RENAL CONDITIONS
Acute Renal Failure
Description and Epidemiology. The newborn normally produces 1 to 3 mL/kg/hour of urine and urinates within the first 48 hours of life. A stressed neonate may develop decreased renal function. Urine output less than 0.5 mL/kg/hour can indicate acute renal failure and puts the infant at risk for disrupted body fluid homeostasis. Multiple causes of renal failure can be identified, including stress during the prenatal period, dehydration, sepsis, anoxia, shock, administration of nephrotoxic drugs, renal dysgenesis, obstructive uropathy, congenital heart disease, hemorrhage, and renal vein thrombosis.

Clinical Findings.
History. Maternal oligohydramnios may be noted.
Physical Examination. Findings include the following:
- Decreased or no urinary output
- Abdominal mass
- Pallor, edema, lethargy, vomiting, seizures, coma
- High blood pressure
- Pulmonary edema, congestive heart failure, or arrhythmias
- Meningomyelocele
- Prune-belly syndrome

Diagnostic Studies. Order the following, as indicated:
- Bladder tap or catheterization to confirm inadequate urinary output
- Urinalysis to identify hematuria or pyuria
- Urine osmolarity, sodium, and potassium values to indicate kidney filtration ability
- Serum blood urea nitrogen, creatinine, sodium, and potassium values to indicate poor filtration
- Complete blood count including differential and platelets for evidence of thrombocytopenia, sepsis, or renal vein thrombosis

Management and Prognosis.
- Replace fluid loss (approximately 30 mL/kg/24 hours), then restrict fluid and diet.
- Maintain strict intake, output, and fluid and electrolyte balance.
- Monitor blood pressure.
- Peritoneal dialysis is sometimes indicated.

The prognosis depends on the cause and the degree of renal failure.

Hydronephrosis
Description and Epidemiology. Hydronephrosis is a dilation of one or both kidneys frequently caused by an obstruction of the ureteropelvic junction, posterior urethral valves, ectopic ureterocele, prune-belly syndrome, or ureteral or ureterovesical obstructions. Obstructive uropathy is slightly more common in males.

Clinical Findings.
History. The history can include the following:
- Decreased urinary output
- Occasionally found on prenatal ultrasonogram
- Asymptomatic in early stages

Physical Examination. Findings include an abdominal mass.

Management and Prognosis. Surgical repair may be necessary depending on the cause of the hydronephrosis and if spontaneous resolution does not occur by 6 to 12 months old. The longer the obstruction lasts, the less likely renal function will return to normal.

Cystic Kidney Disease

Description and Epidemiology. The presence of multiple cysts of various sizes and shapes in the kidney can be either an autosomal dominant or autosomal recessive disease. The autosomal dominant form usually appears in the fourth or fifth decade of life and can be associated with hepatic cysts or cerebral aneurysms. In the autosomal recessive form, which also usually has hepatic cysts, the infant has abdominal masses at birth. The adult form (autosomal dominant) occurs in 1 per 1000 to 2000 persons; the juvenile form (autosomal recessive) occurs in 1 per 10,000 to 40,000 live births (Leonard, 2005).

Clinical Findings.

History. Maternal oligohydramnios may be noted in the juvenile form.

Physical Examination. Findings include the following:
- Abdominal lobular mass
- Hematuria
- Hypertension

Diagnostic Studies. A renal scan is done to document the disorder.

Differential Diagnosis. Multicystic dysplastic kidney, hydronephrosis, Wilms tumor, and renal vein thrombosis are included in the differential diagnosis.

Management and Prognosis. Monitor kidney function and check for enlargement of cysts (with a renal ultrasound) or infection. Nephrectomy may be necessary if no regression is seen or a complication occurs. Dialysis or transplantation is sometimes considered. With severe involvement, the neonate dies from pulmonary or renal insufficiency. Hypertension may be difficult to control.

Renal Artery or Vein Thrombosis

Description. Decreased blood flow to the kidney because of thrombus formation is seen.

Clinical Findings.

History. In the newborn, this condition is often associated with asphyxia, dehydration, shock, and sepsis. Maternal diabetes is a rare cause. Sudden onset of gross hematuria may be noted.

Physical Examination. Findings include a firm flank mass.

Diagnostic Studies. Ultrasonography shows marked enlargement of the kidney. The hematocrit is low. The urine contains protein and often blood.

Differential Diagnosis. Other causes of hematuria, such as hydronephrosis, cystic disease, Wilms tumor, hemolytic-uremic syndrome, and renal abscess, are included in the differential diagnosis.

Management.
- Maintain fluid and electrolyte balance.
- Monitor blood pressure.
- Prophylactic anticoagulation therapy is occasionally given to prevent thrombosis in the other kidney.
- Nephrectomy is not necessary unless chronic infection or uncontrollable hypertension occurs.

Neuroblastoma

Description and Epidemiology. A neuroblastoma is a solid tumor that originates from neural crest tissue along the craniospinal axis. The majority of neuroblastomas develop in the abdomen, usually in the adrenal gland. The cause is unknown. It occurs in 1 in 7000 births and is slightly more common in males (Stern, 2005).

Clinical Findings.

History. An unexplained fever, mass, and symptoms related to the site of the tumor are part of the history.

Physical Examination. Findings include the following:
- Firm, irregular, nontender mass in abdomen
- Pallor
- Hypotension
- Ascites
- Irritability
- Possible external tumors in newborn

Diagnostic Studies. The following help assess and stage the disease:
- CBC, basic chemistry panel
- Renal radiographs to detect calcifications
- Ultrasound, computed tomography (CT) or magnetic resonance imaging (MRI) of abdomen
- Radiograph or CT scan of chest
- Skeletal survey or bone scan
- Urine catecholamines, homovanillic acid (HMA) and vanillylmandelic acid (VMA)
- Bone marrow aspirate and biopsy

Differential Diagnosis. Wilms tumor, hydronephrosis, renal vein thrombosis, and lymphoma are included in the differential diagnosis.

Management and Prognosis. Although some neuroblastomas regress without therapy, usually only those in children under 1 year old, treatment generally involves surgical removal followed by radiation therapy or chemotherapy. The prognosis depends on the age of the patient and the stage of the tumor. The prognosis is better if complete resection of the tumor is performed or if the patient is younger than 1 year old.

Renal Agenesis

Description and Epidemiology. Renal agenesis is failure of the kidney to form normally. Bilateral agenesis is incompatible with life. Bilateral renal agenesis occurs in 1 in 3000 births (Elder, 2004).

Clinical Findings.

History. Maternal oligohydramnios is noted in bilateral agenesis. Unilateral renal agenesis usually is detected when the child is evaluated for other congenital anomalies or for urinary tract infection.

Physical Examination. Findings include the following:
- Single umbilical artery associated with unilateral agenesis
- Associated anomalies involving the gastrointestinal or urinary tract and skeleton, especially with Potter syndrome (bilateral agenesis)
- Low-set ears, senile appearance, broad nose, and receding chin consistent with Potter syndrome

Management and Prognosis. Monitor for proteinuria and hypertension. Patients with bilateral disease die within a few months of life.

ENDOCRINE CONDITIONS

Congenital Hypothyroidism, Congenital Adrenal Hyperplasia
See Chapter 25.

METABOLIC CONDITIONS

Hypoglycemia
Description and Epidemiology. In the term infant, serum glucose levels rarely fall below 35 mg/dL in the first 3 hours of life, below 40 mg/dL between 3 and 24 hours of life, or below 40 mg/dL thereafter. Infants at higher risk of developing hypoglycemia include SGA infants and those with diabetic mothers, asphyxia at birth, sepsis, erythroblastosis fetalis, glycogen storage disease, or galactosemia (Table 38-5).

Clinical Findings.
History. The history can include the following:
- Risk factors for sepsis or asphyxia
- Infant of a diabetic mother
- SGA

Physical Examination. Findings include the following:
- Lethargy
- Poor feeding and regurgitation

TABLE 38-5 **Identification and Management of Hypoglycemia, Infant of Diabetic Mother, and Polycythemia in the Newborn**

Condition	Clinical Findings	Work-up	Management
Hypoglycemia	Blood glucose <30 mg/dL Infant with history of SGA; poorly controlled diabetic mother (IDDM); at risk for sepsis; asphyxia; erythroblastosis fetalis Lethargy Poor feeding and regurgitation Apnea Jitteriness Pallor, sweating, cool extremities Seizures	Serum glucose—measure within 1 hr of birth, every 2 hr until 6-8 hr of life, then every 4-6 hr until 24 hr of life	Give normoglycemic high-risk infants oral or gavage feedings with breast milk or formula at 1-3 hr of life and continue every 2-3 hr for 24-48 hr; intravenous glucose at 8 mg/kg/min if serum glucose less than 30-35 mg/dL and oral feedings poorly tolerated (Robertson & Shilkofski, 2005).
Infant of diabetic mother (IDM)	IDDM: large, plump infant with large viscera; puffy facies; plethora; hyperactivity first 3 days; ± hypotonicity, lethargy, poor suck; ± cardiomegaly and murmurs	Intensive observation and care Serum glucose—measure within 1 hr of birth, then every 1 hr for the next 6-8 hr	If clinically well and normoglycemic, initially give oral or gavage feedings with infant formula or breast milk started within 2-3 hr old and continued at 3-hr intervals If infant is unable to tolerate oral feeding, discontinue feeding and give 10% glucose by peripheral intravenous infusion at a rate of 4-8 mg/kg/hr (Robertson & Shilkofski, 2005). Treat hypoglycemia, even in asymptomatic infants, with intravenous infusions of glucose
Polycythemia	Cyanosis, tachypnea, respiratory distress Hyperbilirubinemia Infant with history of diabetic mother, IUGR, postmaturity; SGA exposed to chronic hypoxia; recipient of twin-twin transfusion; delayed clamping of umbilical cord Plethora Feeding disturbance	Hematocrit ≥65%	Phlebotomy and replacement with saline or albumin or partial exchange transfusion to reduce hematocrit to 50% (Robertson & Shilkofski, 2005).

hr, Hours; *IDDM,* insulin-dependent diabetes mellitus; *IUGR,* intrauterine growth retardation; *SGA,* small for gestational age.

- Apnea
- Jitteriness
- Pallor, sweating, cool extremities
- Seizures

Management and Prognosis. See Management in Table 38-5. Infants with symptomatic hypoglycemia, particularly low-birth-weight infants and infants of diabetic mothers, are less likely to have normal intellectual development than are asymptomatic infants. Prognosis for normal intellectual function is guarded in infants with prolonged and severe hypoglycemia.

Infant of a Diabetic Mother (IDM)

Description and Epidemiology. An infant born to a mother whose pregnancy is complicated by poorly controlled gestational or insulin-dependent diabetes mellitus is referred to as an infant of a diabetic mother (IDM). Maternal hyperglycemia causes fetal hyperglycemia and hyperinsulinemia, leading to increased hepatic glucose uptake and glycogen synthesis, accelerated lipogenesis, and augmented protein synthesis (Hendricks-Munoz, 2006). See Table 38-5.

Clinical Findings.

History. The history includes a mother with diabetes, especially those who are poorly controlled.

Physical Examination. Findings include the following:
- Large and plump neonate with large viscera
- Puffy facies
- Plethora
- Hyperexcitability during the first 3 days of life, although hypotonia, lethargy, and poor sucking also occur

Management, Complications, and Prevention. See Table 38-5. Cardiomegaly is common (30%), and heart failure occurs in 5% to 10% of infants. Congenital anomalies are increased threefold; cardiac malformations (15 times greater) and lumbosacral agenesis are most common (Hendricks-Munoz, 2006). There is a predisposition to obesity in childhood that can extend into adult life. Symptomatic hypoglycemia increases the risk of impaired intellectual development.

Strict management of blood glucose levels in mothers with diabetes decreases the risk of severe problems in the infant.

ORTHOPEDIC CONDITIONS

Fractured Clavicle and Brachial Palsy
See Chapter 37.

Polydactyly and Syndactyly

Description and Epidemiology. Polydactyly is a condition that varies from a skin tag to a formed finger with a nail that extends from the postaxial side. Polydactyly occurs in 2 per 1000 births, more commonly in the black population (Thompson, 2004). In contrast, syndactyly can be identified by finding fingers or toes fused by skin and sometimes bone. Syndactyly can be seen as part of a variety of syndromes.

Clinical Findings.

History. Positive family history in 30% (Thompson, 2004).

Physical Examination. In polydactyly, a floppy digit is seen on the foot or hand. It varies in degree of formation.

Syndactyly is webbing of two digits, partially or to the tip of the digit.

Management. For polydactyly surgical removal of the floppy extra digit is indicated. If the digit is stabilized by bone, surgical removal is deferred until the patient is older, when function can be assessed. For patients with syndactyly, treatment is not indicated in the neonate. Surgical separation is recommended at 2 to 3 years old.

CENTRAL NERVOUS SYSTEM CONDITIONS

Congenital Hydrocephalus

Description and Epidemiology. Congenital hydrocephalus is an accumulation of cerebrospinal fluid (CSF) in the brain's ventricles at birth occurring in 1 of 1000 live births (Feldstein & Anderson, 2006). Malformations, infections, intraventricular hemorrhage, and disorders in brain development can lead to congenital hydrocephalus. The incidence varies depending on which of these conditions is causative.

Clinical Findings.

History. The history can include projectile vomiting, lethargy, irritability, and poor feeding.

Physical Examination. Findings include the following:
- Enlarged head circumference or rapidly increasing in size
- Cranial sutures separated by large, tense fontanelles

Diagnostic Studies. Cranial ultrasonography shows dilated ventricles. Often an MRI is obtained to further define anatomy.

Management. Medications that decrease CSF production (e.g., acetazolamide), a ventriculoperitoneal shunt, or both are used. Referral should be prompt.

Intraventricular Hemorrhage

Description and Epidemiology. Intraventricular hemorrhage (IVH) occurs within the ventricles of the brain, usually within the first 72 hours of life. Risk factors include prematurity, RDS, hypoxic-ischemic or hypotensive injury, increased or decreased cerebral blood flow, hypertension, hypervolemia, and reduced vascular integrity. The incidence of IVH decreases with increasing gestational age. Infants weighing under 1000 g are especially prone to severe IVH (Stoll & Kliegman, 2004).

Clinical Findings.

History. Risk factors for IVH include SGA, prematurity, and others mentioned previously.

Physical Examination. Findings include the following:
- Diminished or absent Moro reflex
- Poor muscle tone, lethargy, somnolence
- Apnea
- Periods of pallor or cyanosis
- Failure to suck well
- High-pitched, shrill cry, seizures

Diagnostic Studies. Ultrasonography is used to classify IVH into grades I to IV based on the presence and quantity of blood in the ventricles or brain tissue. Screening cranial ultrasounds should be performed on all infants between 1250 to 1500 g at 3 to 5 days and before discharge; on infants between 1000 to 1250 g at 3 to 5 days, at 28 days, and before discharge; and on infants under 1000 g at 3 to 5 days, at 10 to 14 days, at 28 days, and before discharge (Perlman, 2006).

Management and Prognosis. Treatment may include the following:

- Glucocorticoid given antenatally to reduce severe IVH
- Supportive management and minimal stimulation
- Indomethacin to reduce the severity of IVH
- Acetazolamide to decrease CSF production
- Repeated lumbar punctures
- Ventriculoperitoneal shunt or external ventriculostomy

Outcome is related to associated white matter involvement, with grade IV being associated with the most adverse outcome (Perlman, 2006).

Hypoxic-Ischemic Insults

Description and Epidemiology. Hypoxic-ischemic insult in the newborn is divided into three levels of injury (grades I, II, and III, or mild, moderate, and severe). See Table 38-6. Brain damage results from fetal hypoxia or ischemia over an extended period of time. The initial hypoxic or ischemic insult is followed by metabolic and respiratory acidosis. Compensatory mechanisms, such as shunting blood through the ductus to maintain perfusion of the brain, heart, adrenals, kidneys, liver, and intestines, ultimately fail if the insult is severe enough. Depending on the organ most damaged, a variety of signs and symptoms can be seen. Fifteen percent to 20% of infants with hypoxic-ischemic encephalopathy die in the neonatal period; up to 30% develop permanent neurodevelopmental disabilities. Causes of the initial hypoxic or ischemic insult include abruptio placentae, hemorrhage, cord compression, mechanical injury, severe maternal hypertension or diabetes, and inadequate resuscitation of the infant (Stoll & Kliegman, 2004).

Clinical Findings.
Physical Examination. Findings include the following:
- Seizure activity
- Pallor

- Cyanosis, apnea
- Bradycardia and unresponsiveness to stimulation

Management and Prognosis. The prognosis depends on the effectiveness of managing the underlying symptoms. Severe complications (hypoxia, hypoglycemia, shock) and encephalopathy characterized by flaccid coma, apnea, and seizures are associated with a poor prognosis (Stoll & Kliegman, 2004). An infant who remains neurologically abnormal after the initial recovery phase (2 weeks) likely has suffered permanent neurologic impairment. A low Apgar score at 20 minutes, absence of spontaneous respirations, and persistence of abnormal neurologic signs at 2 weeks old predict death or severe cognitive and motor deficits; Apgar scores done at 1 and 5 minutes are far less predictive of outcome (AAP, 2006a).

Myelomeningocele

Description and Epidemiology. A myelomeningocele is the result of failure to close the posterior neural tube and the vertebral column. This is the most severe form of neural tube defect occurring in 1 per 4000 live births (Johnston & Kinsman, 2004). Genetic and environmental factors are both believed to play a causative role. See Chapter 27 for more information.

Clinical Findings.
History. Poor intake of folic acid and exposure to hyperthermia or valproic acid are risk factors.
Physical Examination. Findings include the following:
- Saclike cyst containing meninges and spinal fluid covered by thin layer of partially epithelialized skin; 75% found in the lumbosacral area
- Flaccid paralysis of lower extremities
- Absence of deep tendon reflexes
- Lack of response to touch and pain
- Constant urinary dribbling

Management, Prognosis, and Prevention. Surgical repair and multidisciplinary supportive management are indi-

---

TABLE 38-6 Hypoxic-Ischemic Encephalopathy in Term Infants

Signs	Stage 1	Stage 2	Stage 3
Level of consciousness	Hyperalert	Lethargic	Stuporous, coma
Muscle tone	Normal	Hypotonic	Flaccid
Posture	Normal	Flexion	Decerebrate
Tendon reflexes/clonus	Hyperactive	Hyperactive	Absent
Myoclonus	Present	Present	Absent
Moro reflex	Strong	Weak	Absent
Pupils	Mydriasis	Miosis	Unequal, poor light reflex
Seizures	None	Common	Decerebration
Electroencephalograph	Normal	Low-voltage changing to seizure activity	Burst suppression to isoelectric
Duration	<24 hours if progresses, otherwise may remain normal	24 hours to 24 days	Days to weeks
Outcome	Good	Variable	Death, severe deficits

Adapted from Sarnat H, Sarnat M: Neonatal encephalopathy following fetal distress: a clinical and electroencephalopathic study, *Arch Neurol* 33:696, 1976.

cated. The mortality rate is 10% to 15% in aggressively treated children with most deaths occurring before 4 years old. At least 70% have normal intelligence, but seizure disorders, hydrocephalus, learning disabilities, and neurogenic bowel and bladder are more common than in the general population (Johnston & Kinsman, 2004). Folic acid supplementation (400 mcg/day) with a daily multivitamin is helpful in preventing neural tube defects and should be taken by all females of childbearing age. Prenatal vitamins have at least 400 mcg/vitamin; however, additional folic acid supplementation (4000 mcg) is recommended for those women who have had a previous child with any neural tube defect (March of Dimes, 2006).

HEMATOLOGIC CONDITIONS

Polycythemia

Description and Epidemiology. Polycythemia is characterized by a central hematocrit of 65% or higher. Polycythemia can occur in a variety of conditions, including IDM, cyanotic congenital heart disease, and infants with growth retardation who were exposed to chronic fetal hypoxia that stimulated erythropoietin production and increased red blood cell production. Polycythemia occurs in 1% to 2% of term AGA births, depending on the etiology. See Table 38-5.

Clinical Findings.

History. The history includes the following:
- Diabetic mother
- Recipient of a twin-twin transfusion
- Delayed clamping of umbilical cord
- Postmature infant
- SGA

Physical Examination. Infants with polycythemia may be asymptomatic, or findings may include the following:
- Plethora
- Feeding disturbances
- Hypoglycemia
- Cyanosis (persistent fetal circulation), tachypnea, respiratory distress
- Hyperbilirubinemia

Management and Prognosis. See Table 38-5. Long-term problems may include speech deficits, abnormal fine motor control, reduced IQ, and other neurologic abnormalities as a result of the decreased brain tissue perfusion both with and without intervention.

Hemorrhagic Disease in the Newborn

Description and Epidemiology. Severe transient deficiencies of vitamin K–dependent clotting factors lead to bleeding. Hemorrhagic disease is caused by a lack of free vitamin K in the mother and absence of bacterial intestinal flora normally responsible for synthesis of vitamin K in the infant. Vitamin K–dependent clotting factors (factors II, VII, IX, X) are normal at birth, but decrease within 2 to 3 days. Breast milk is a poor source of vitamin K; late-onset bleeding (occurring 1 to 3 months after birth) is rare, but may be seen in exclusively breastfed infants. A particularly severe form of

deficiency of vitamin K–dependent coagulation factors occurring in the first day of life has been reported in women receiving the anticonvulsants phenytoin and/or phenobarbital.

Clinical Findings.

History. The history may include the following:
- Anticonvulsant (phenytoin or phenobarbital) use by the mother
- Prematurity
- Exclusive breastfeeding without vitamin K supplementation
- Failure to administer parenteral vitamin K at birth
- Neonatal hepatitis or biliary atresia

Physical Examination. Findings include gastrointestinal, nasal, subgaleal, or intracranial bleeding or bleeding at the site of an injection or circumcision.

Diagnostic Studies. Prothrombin time, blood coagulation time, and partial thromboplastin time are prolonged.

Differential Diagnosis. This disorder may be the result of disseminated intravascular coagulation or congenital bleeding disorders unrelated to vitamin K.

Management, Prevention, and Prognosis
- Intravenous infusion of 1 to 5 mg of vitamin K is needed. Improvement of coagulation defects and cessation of bleeding should occur within a few hours.
- If a newborn is delivered at home, confirm vitamin K was given.
- Prevention of both early- and late-onset bleeding is achieved by routinely giving 1 mg of natural oil-soluble vitamin K intramuscularly within 1 hour of birth. Prognosis depends on the site and extent of bleeding.

Anemia

Description and Epidemiology. Anemia is characterized by less than the normal range of hemoglobin for birth weight and postnatal age. Anemia occurs secondary to acute blood loss before or during delivery. Acute blood loss after delivery can be external (gastrointestinal, circumcision site, umbilical stump), internal (fracture site, cephalhematoma, pulmonary hemorrhage, injured internal organ), or secondary to hemolysis or congenital aplastic or hypoplastic anemia.

Clinical Findings.

History. The history can include the following:
- Twin-twin transfusion
- Unexpected tearing or delayed clamping of umbilical cord resulting in neonate blood loss
- Internal hemorrhage (caused by fracture, cephalhematoma, or internal organ trauma)
- Umbilical stump or circumcision bleeding

Physical Examination. Pallor, congestive heart failure, and shock are possible findings.

Management and Prognosis. Treatment depends on the cause. An asymptomatic full-term infant with a hemoglobin level of 10 g/dL can be observed, whereas a symptomatic neonate born after abruptio placentae or with severe hemolytic disease of the newborn warrants transfusion. Treatment with blood should be balanced by concern about transfusion-acquired infection with cytomegalovirus (CMV), human immunodeficiency virus (HIV), and hepatitis B and C viruses. Prognosis depends on the cause and severity of the anemia.

Blood in Vomitus or Stool

Description and Epidemiology.   Bright-red or dark-red blood in the vomitus or stool can be seen without clinical evidence of blood loss. This problem often is caused by ingestion of maternal blood during delivery.

Clinical Findings.

Physical Examination.   Bright-red or dark-red blood is seen in vomitus or stool.

Diagnostic Studies.   Blood of maternal origin can be differentiated from infant blood by testing for fetal hemoglobin using the Apt test.

Differential Diagnosis.   The differential diagnosis includes infant gastrointestinal bleeding caused by trauma, duplication of bowel, intussusception, volvulus, hemangioma or telangiectasia of bowel, rectal prolapse, vitamin K deficiency, or anal fissure.

Management.   No treatment is necessary if blood is of maternal origin.

Jaundice

Description and Epidemiology.   Jaundice, a clinically apparent accumulation of bilirubin in the skin, causes a yellowish orange or sometimes green hue to the skin. Jaundice becomes apparent when serum bilirubin levels exceed 5 to 7 mg/dL and usually advances in a pattern from the infant's head to the toes (Table 38-7). Physiologic jaundice is the most common type of jaundice in the newborn period with the infant showing no signs of illness. Classic physiologic jaundice is characterized by a rise in bilirubin from 1.5 mg/dL in cord blood to 5 to 6 mg/dL on the third day of life, declining to a normal adult level (less than 1.3 to 1.5 mg/dL) by 10 to 12 days in white and black infants. Asian infants reach 8 to 12 mg/dL on day 4 to 5 and decline more slowly. Two percent of Asian newborns and 1% of whites and blacks have serum bilirubin higher than 20 mg/dL in the first week of life. Breast milk jaundice can be divided into early-onset and late-onset types. Early-onset breast milk jaundice develops within 2 to 4 days of birth and is believed to occur as a result of infrequent breastfeeding and insufficient intake leading to decreased intestinal motility. Late-onset breast milk jaundice develops 4 to 7 days after birth, peaks at 10 to 15 days of life, and frequently persists. See Chapter 12 on breastfeeding for more information. Nonphysiologic (pathologic) jaundice appears at less than 24 hours old and may last longer than 8 days. The rate of increase in total bilirubin is rapid at greater than 0.5 mg/dL/hour. Total bilirubin levels are frequently greater than 12.5 mg/dL before 48 hours old, or the direct bilirubin exceeds 1.5 to 2 mg/dL. Kernicterus or bilirubin encephalopathy involves toxicity of the nervous system resulting from very high levels of bilirubin. The current estimated minimal level of risk for kernicterus and thus considering exchange transfusion is probably at 25 to 30 mg/dL in HEALTHY term infants (AAP, 2004).

Jaundice is observed during the first week of life in approximately 60% of term infants (Stoll & Kliegman, 2004). Causes include:

- Increased rate of hemolysis: ABO incompatibility, Rh incompatibility, abnormal red blood cell shapes (spherocytosis, elliptocytosis, pyknocytosis, and stomatocytosis), red blood cell enzyme abnormalities (glucose-6-phosphate dehydrogenase deficiency, pyruvate kinase deficiency)
- Decreased rate of conjugation: immaturity of bilirubin conjugation (physiologic jaundice), congenital familial nonhemolytic jaundice (inborn errors of metabolism affecting glucuronyl transferase system and bilirubin transport), breast milk jaundice
- Abnormalities of excretion or absorption: sepsis, hepatitis (viral, parasitic, bacterial, toxic), metabolic abnormalities (galactosemia, glycogen storage disease, IDM, cystic fibrosis), biliary atresia, choledochal cyst, obstruction of ampulla of Vater (annular pancreas), drugs

Clinical Findings.

Family History.   The family history may include the following risk factors for the development of hyperbilirubinemia:

- Significant hemolytic disease, anemia
- Inborn errors of metabolism
- Early or severe jaundice
- Ethnic or geographic origin associated with hemolytic anemia
- Hepatobiliary disease
- Previous sibling received phototherapy

History.

- ABO or Rh incompatibilities in previous pregnancies
- Sepsis risk for the infant, such as prolonged rupture of maternal membranes
- Macrosomic infant of a diabetic mother

Physical Examination.   Findings include the following:

- Jaundice at birth or at any time during the neonatal period, depending on the underlying condition, with face affected first, followed by the shoulders, chest, and abdomen. Jaundice from deposition of indirect bilirubin in the skin tends to appear bright yellow or orange; jaundice of the obstructive type (direct bilirubin) appears greenish or muddy yellow, with the difference apparent only in severe jaundice. There is no dependable relationship between the intensity of jaundice and the degree of hyperbilirubinemia.
- A crude estimate of the level of jaundice can be based on the dermal zone in which the jaundice is noticed. This estimate should not be used to determine bilirubin levels or management, but it can help determine whether acquiring a total serum bilirubin (TSB) or a transcutaneous bilirubin (TcB) is warranted.
  - Head and neck—a mean bilirubin of 6 mg/dL
  - Trunk and umbilicus—a mean bilirubin of 9 mg/dL
  - Groin including the upper thighs—a mean bilirubin of 12 mg/dL
  - Knees and elbows (including the ankles and wrists) or to the feet and hands (including the palms and soles)—a mean bilirubin of 15 mg/dL
- Petechiae, bruising, hepatosplenomegaly, or signs of infection.

TABLE 38-7　Diagnostic Features of the Various Types of Neonatal Jaundice

Diagnosis	Nature of Van Den Bergh Reaction	Jaundice Appears	Jaundice Disappears	Peak Bilirubin Concentration mg/dL	Peak Bilirubin Concentration Age (days)	Bilirubin Rate of Accumulation (mg/dL/day)	Remarks
Physiologic jaundice							Usually relates to degree of maturity; infant shows no signs of illness
Full-term	Indirect	2-3 days	4-5 days	10-12	2-3	<5	
Premature	Indirect	3-4 days	7-9 days	15	6-8	<5	Metabolic factors: hypoxia, respiratory distress, lack of carbohydrate
Hyperbilirubinemia caused by metabolic factors							Hormonal influences: cretinism
Full-term	Indirect	2-3 days	Variable	>12	First week	<5	Genetic factors:
Premature	Indirect	3-4 days	Variable	>15	First week	<5	Crigler-Najjar syndrome, transient familial hyperbilirubinemia
							Drugs: vitamin K, novobiocin
Hemolytic states and hematoma	Indirect	May appear in first 24 hours	Variable	Unlimited	Variable	Usually >5	Erythroblastosis: Rh, ABO
							Congenital hemolytic states: spherocytic, nonspherocytic
							Infantile pyknocytosis
							Drugs: vitamin K; enclosed hemorrhage—hematoma
Mixed hemolytic and hepatotoxic factors	Indirect and direct	May appear in first 24 hours	Variable	Unlimited	Variable	Usually >5	Infection: bacterial sepsis, pyelonephritis, hepatitis, toxoplasmosis, cytomegalic inclusion disease, rubella
							Drugs: vitamin K
Hepatocellular damage	Indirect and direct	Usually 2-3 days	Variable	Unlimited	Variable	Variable; can be >5	Biliary atresia; galactosemia; hepatitis; infection

From Brown AK: Diagnostic features of the various types of neonatal jaundice, *Pediatr Clin North Am* 9:589, 1962.

- Lethargy, hypotonia, poor feeding, and loss of the Moro reflex are common initial signs of bilirubin toxicity to the brain (kernicterus). These symptoms are subtle and indistinguishable from those of sepsis, asphyxia, hypoglycemia, intracranial hemorrhage, and other acute illnesses in the neonate.
- Diminished tendon reflexes, respiratory distress, failure to suck, opisthotonos, bulging fontanelle, twitching of face or limbs, seizures, and a shrill, high-pitched cry are later signs of kernicterus.

   Diagnostic Studies. The following labs may be ordered:

- TcB
- TSB level (indirect and direct) for infants who have a TcB more than 15, for darker skinned infants, or for infants under phototherapy
- If the provider suspects that the total bilirubin is significantly elevated for the age of the infant, extra blood can be drawn and held for further testing, eliminating a return visit, stick, and/or unnecessary expense if all of the tests are not later indicated. Tests that may be indicated include:
  - ABO, Rh, blood type, isoimmune antibodies on mother (should be available at prenatal and delivering hospital)
  - ABO, Rh, blood type, Coombs test on infant (many times this is done at delivery and held in the hospital's laboratory)
  - Hemoglobin, hematocrit, reticulocyte count

   Elevated indirect (unconjugated) serum bilirubin with a normal reticulocyte count and negative Coombs test indicates conditions such as physiologic jaundice, breast milk jaundice, or congenital familial nonhemolytic jaundice.

   Elevated indirect serum bilirubin with an increased reticulocyte count indicates increased hemolysis secondary to conditions such as isoimmunization (positive Coombs test, such as caused by ABO or Rh incompatibility), abnormal red blood cell shape, or red blood cell enzyme abnormalities.

   Elevated indirect and direct serum bilirubin with a negative Coombs test and a normal reticulocyte count indicates hepatitis, metabolic abnormalities, biliary atresia, choledochal cyst (in the bile duct), gastrointestinal or pancreatic obstruction, sepsis, or drugs.

   Pathologic jaundice requires a more in-depth work-up for the cause. Risk factors include:

- Appearance of jaundice in first 24 hours of life
- Rise of bilirubin greater than 0.5 mg/dL/hour
- Conjugated bilirubin greater than 2 mg/dL

   Management and Prevention.

Prevention of severe hyperbilirubinemia and bilirubin encephalopathy in infants requires the promotion and support of successful breastfeeding, systematic assessment of the newborn for the risk of hyperbilirubinemia, early and focused follow-up based on the risk assessment and treatment when indicated.

- Promote breastfeeding by advising mothers to put the baby to the breast 8 to 12 times per day for the first several days and discourage the use of routine supplementation of water or dextrose water.
- In the healthy full-term (greater than 35 weeks) infant, physical findings, bilirubin level according to age and designation of risk are helpful in determining the course of treatment (Figs. 38-11, 38-12, and 38-13).
- Phototherapy is used to treat elevated indirect hyperbilirubinemia. Home phototherapy can be used for those infants without risk factors and with TSB levels 2 to 3 mg/dL below those shown in the Fig. 38-12. Phototherapy is contraindicated with elevated direct bilirubin. The infant should be dressed only in a diaper and should have eye shields on. Three types of phototherapy are used:
  - Phototherapy via banks of overhead lights placed close to the infant requires eye patches removed at regular intervals, taking care to prevent corneal abrasions; monitoring of temperature; increased fluid intake in response to evaporative water losses; and avoidance of oral drugs because of decreased absorption.

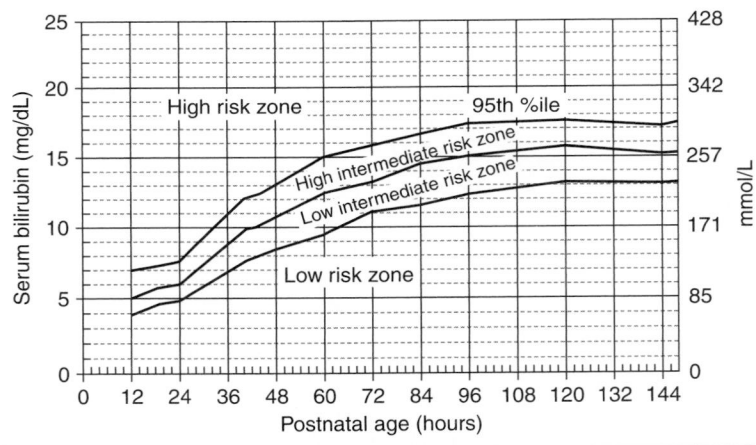

FIG. 38-11 Nomogram for designation of risk in 2840 well newborns at 36 or more weeks gestational age with birth weight of 2000 g or more or 35 or more weeks gestational age and birth weight of 2500 g or more based on the hour-specific serum bilirubin values. (From the Academy of Pediatrics Subcommittee on Hyperbilirubinemia: Clinical practice guideline: management of hyperbilirubinemia in the newborn infant 35 or more weeks of gestation, *Pediatrics* 114:297-316, 2004.)

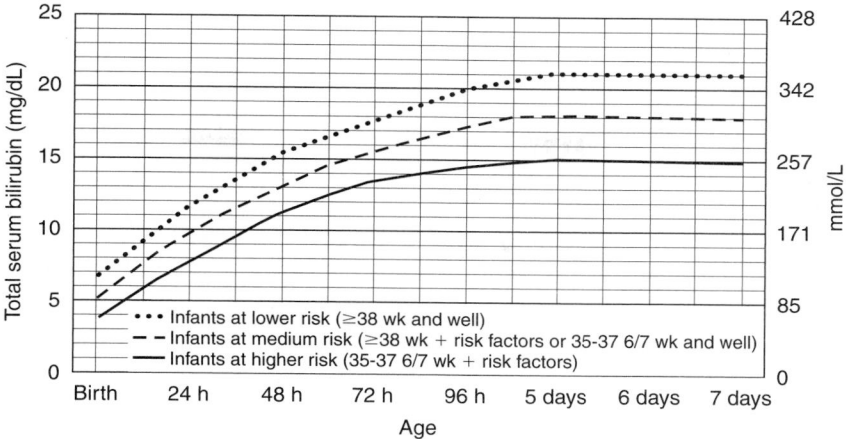

- Use total bilirubin. Do not subtract direct-reacting or conjugated bilirubin.
- Risk factors = isoimmune hemolytic disease, G6PD deficiency, asphyxia, significant lethargy, temperature instability, sepsis, acidosis, or albumin <3 g/dL (if measured)
- For well infants 35-37 6/7 weeks can adjust TSB levels for intervention around the medium risk line. It is an option to intervene at lower TSB levels for infants closer to 35 wks and at higher TSB levels for those closer to 37 6/7 weeks.
- It is an option to provide conventional phototherapy in hospital or at home at TSB levels 2-3 mg/dL (35-50 mmol/L) below those shown but home phototherapy should not be used in any infant with risk factors.

FIG. 38-12 Guidelines for phototherapy in hospitalized infants of 35 or more weeks gestation. (From the Academy of Pediatrics Subcommittee on Hyperbilirubinemia: Clinical practice guideline: management of hyperbilirubinemia in the newborn infant 35 or more weeks of gestation, *Pediatrics* 114:297-316, 2004.)

- ○ Phototherapy via Biliblanket (fiberoptic pad) allows ongoing interaction between mother and infant.
- ○ Phototherapy via Bilibed.
- If the breastfeeding infant requires phototherapy, breastfeeding should be continued. It is also an option to temporarily interrupt breastfeeding (have the mother pump to maintain her supply) and substitute formula for 24 hours. In breastfed infants receiving phototherapy, supplementation with expressed breast milk or milk-based formula is appropriate if the infant's intake is inadequate, weight loss excessive (greater than 10% of birth weight), or the infant seems dehydrated (AAP, 2004).
- Rebound bilirubin testing (measurement of bilirubin after phototherapy is discontinued) is not required in full-term newborns with physiologic jaundice (AAP, 2004).
- Guidelines for exchange transfusion levels are available in the AAP practice parameter on the management of hyperbilirubinemia.

INFECTIONS OF THE NEWBORN

Three mechanisms for acquiring neonatal infections exist:
- Transplacental, when the mother acquires an organism that invades her bloodstream and passes through the placenta
- Vertical, when organisms in the vagina invade the amniotic fluid within the uterus
- Horizontal, when the newborn is exposed to environmental agents after birth

Syphilis is transplacentally acquired; herpes, gonorrhea, GBS, *Listeria, Escherichia coli,* and *Chlamydia trachomatis* are typically vertically acquired (Fanaroff & Martin, 2006; Remington et al, 2005). Staphylococcal infection is the most common horizontal infection. The most common means for horizontal transmission are the unwashed hands of health care providers.

Risk factors for sepsis (systemic infection) in the newborn include early rupture of amniotic membranes followed by preterm labor, prolonged rupture of membranes, maternal fever, maternal diagnosis of chorioamnionitis, maternal tachycardia, fetal tachycardia, and malodorous amniotic fluid. The neonate with sepsis can be asymptomatic or have nonspecific symptoms (Fanaroff & Martin, 2006; Remington et al, 2005). This is in part caused by a delayed immune response to local infection, allowing the neonate to bypass the typical signs and symptoms of infection (e.g., fever). Organisms quickly invade the systemic circulation, and significant deterioration occurs before it can be clinically recognized. Because of the serious nature of neonatal sepsis, significant risk factors or a clinically unstable neonate without perinatal risk factors warrants investigation and initiation of appropriate antibiotics. See Box 38-6 for an overview of neonatal sepsis.

Toxoplasmosis
Description and Epidemiology. Toxoplasmosis is an infection caused by *Toxoplasma gondii,* an obligate intracellular protozoan. *T. gondii* infects most species of warm-blooded animals, particularly cats. Cats excrete oocysts in their stools; intermediate hosts include cattle, pigs, and sheep. Humans become infected by consumption of poorly cooked meat or by accidental

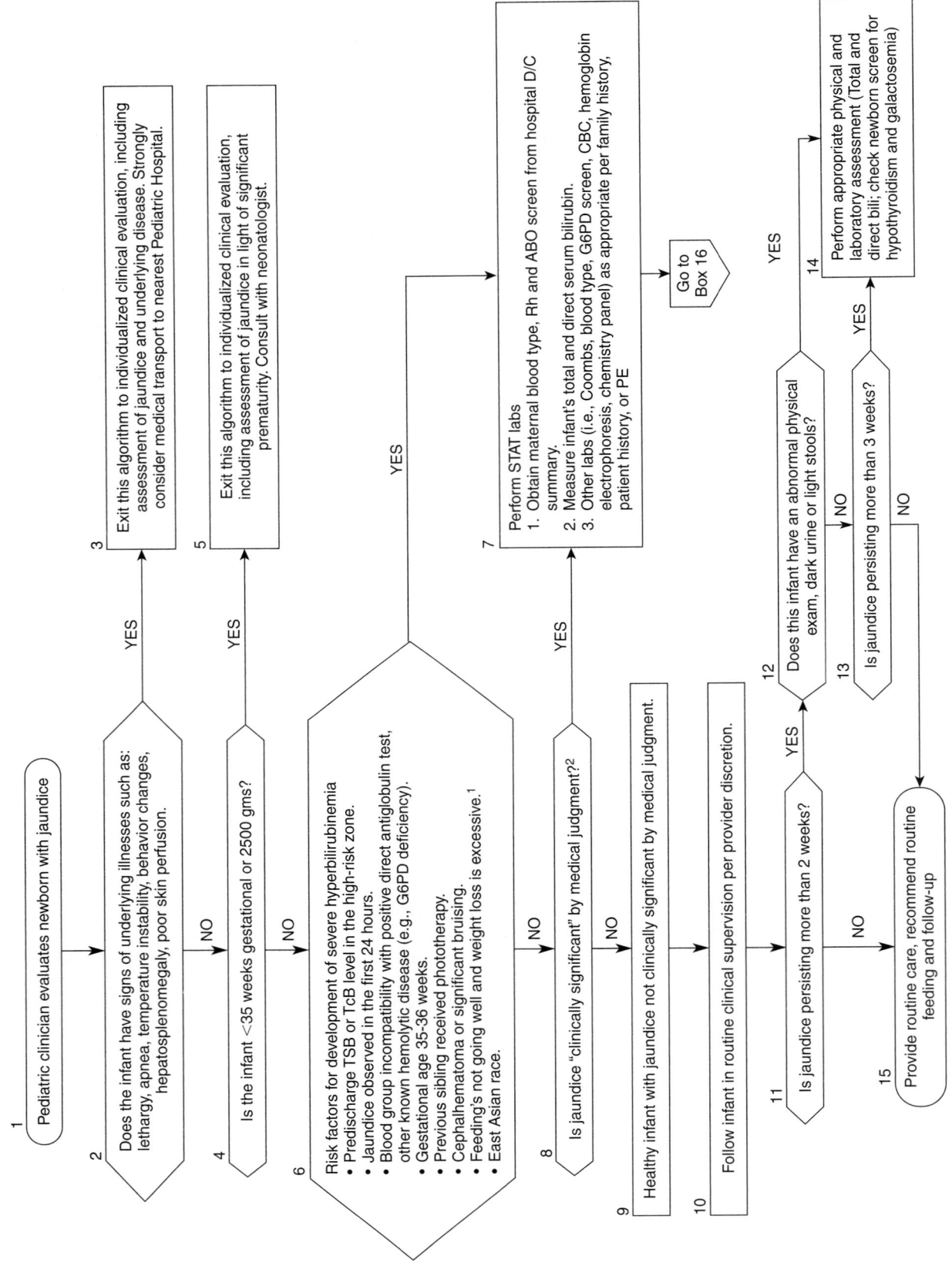

1 Pediatric clinician evaluates newborn with jaundice

2 Does the infant have signs of underlying illnesses such as: lethargy, apnea, temperature instability, behavior changes, hepatosplenomegaly, poor skin perfusion.

YES → 3 Exit this algorithm to individualized clinical evaluation, including assessment of jaundice and underlying disease. Strongly consider medical transport to nearest Pediatric Hospital.

NO

4 Is the infant <35 weeks gestational or 2500 gms?

YES → 5 Exit this algorithm to individualized clinical evaluation, including assessment of jaundice in light of significant prematurity. Consult with neonatologist.

NO

6 Risk factors for development of severe hyperbilirubinemia
• Predischarge TSB or TcB level in the high-risk zone.
• Jaundice observed in the first 24 hours.
• Blood group incompatibility with positive direct antiglobulin test, other known hemolytic disease (e.g., G6PD deficiency).
• Gestational age 35-36 weeks.
• Previous sibling received phototherapy.
• Cephalhematoma or significant bruising.
• Feeding's not going well and weight loss is excessive.[1]
• East Asian race.

YES → 7 Perform STAT labs
1. Obtain maternal blood type, Rh and ABO screen from hospital D/C summary.
2. Measure infant's total and direct serum bilirubin.
3. Other labs (i.e., Coombs, blood type, G6PD screen, CBC, hemoglobin electrophoresis, chemistry panel) as appropriate per family history, patient history, or PE

→ Go to Box 16

NO

8 Is jaundice "clinically significant" by medical judgment?[2]

YES → 7

NO

9 Healthy infant with jaundice not clinically significant by medical judgment.

10 Follow infant in routine clinical supervision per provider discretion.

11 Is jaundice persisting more than 2 weeks?

YES → 12 Does this infant have an abnormal physical exam, dark urine or light stools?

YES → 14 Perform appropriate physical and laboratory assessment (Total and direct bili; check newborn screen for hypothyroidism and galactosemia)

NO → 13 Is jaundice persisting more than 3 weeks?

YES → 14

NO → 15 Provide routine care, recommend routine feeding and follow-up

NO → 15

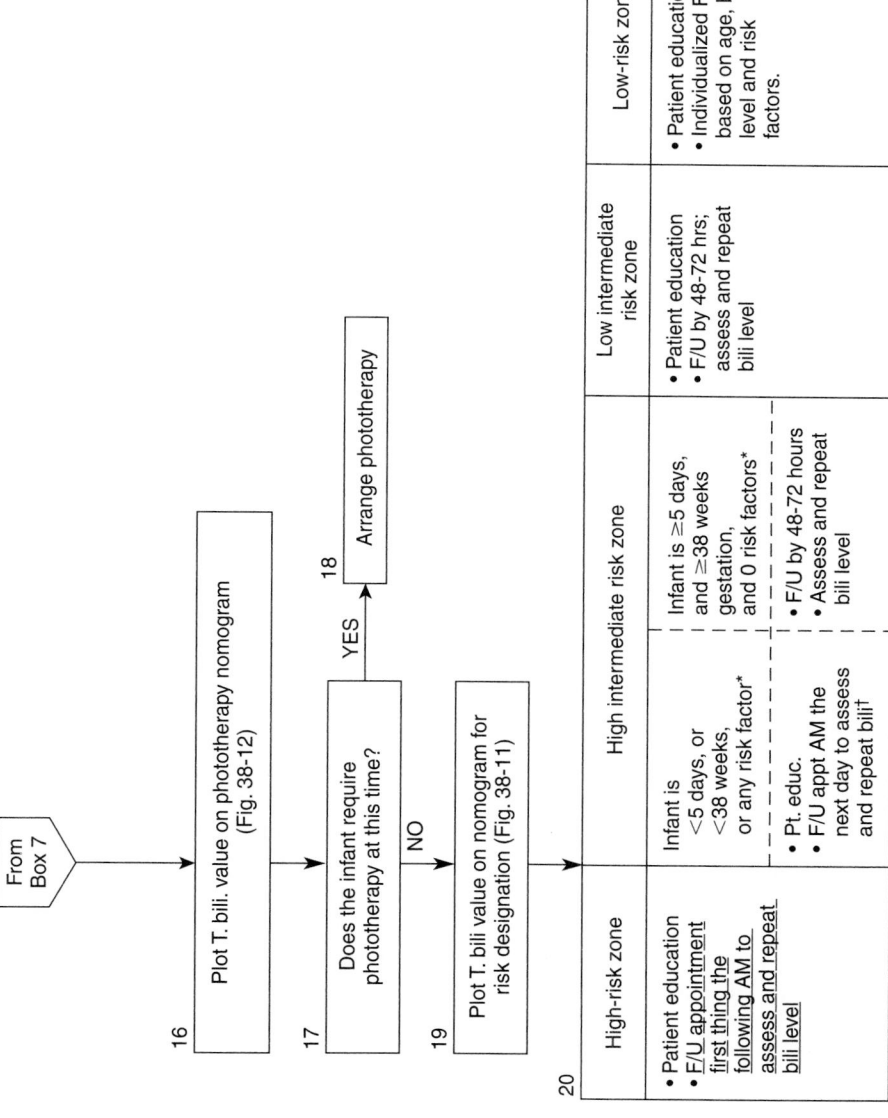

16 Plot T. bili. value on phototherapy nomogram (Fig. 38-12)

17 Does the infant require phototherapy at this time?

YES → **18** Arrange phototherapy

NO

19 Plot T. bili value on nomogram for risk designation (Fig. 38-11)

20

High-risk zone	High intermediate risk zone		Low intermediate risk zone	Low-risk zone
• Patient education • F/U appointment first thing the following AM to assess and repeat bili level	Infant is <5 days, or <38 weeks, or any risk factor* • Pt. educ. • F/U appt AM the next day to assess and repeat bili†	Infant is ≥5 days, and ≥38 weeks gestation, and 0 risk factors* • F/U by 48-72 hours • Assess and repeat bili level	• Patient education • F/U by 48-72 hrs; assess and repeat bili level	• Patient education • Individualized F/U based on age, bili level and risk factors.

* Risk factors as defined in Box #6

† If infant's bilirubin levels have stabilized at the high intermediate risk zone or below, follow up can be slightly later than the above recommendations

¹ Weight loss of >10% of birth weight is excessive at 72-96 hrs, or >12% after 96 hrs. Breastfed babies usually reach their maximum weight loss on day three. To additionally assess adequacy of intake in breastfed infants consider normal 4-6 wet diapers/24 hours; 3-4 stools/day by day four. Change from meconium to yellow soft breast stool by day four.

² Severely jaundiced infants should be referred immediately to the ED for assessment in order to expedite medical intervention.

ABO, Blood types; *AM,* morning; *bili,* bilirubin; *CBC,* complete blood count; *ED,* emergency department; *F/U,* follow-up; *G6PD* glucose-6-phosphate dehydrogenase; *hr,* hour; *PE,* physical exam; *Rh,* rhesus; *T.bili,* total bilirubin; *TcB,* transcutaneus bilirubin; *TSB,* total serum bilirubin; *wk,* week.

FIG. 38-13 Algorithm for the management of neonatal hyperbilirubinemia in the outpatient setting. (Modified and used with permission of the Multnomah County Health Department, Primary Care Division, Portland, OR.)

From Box 7

BOX 38-6 Neonatal Sepsis

History
"Not doing well"
Temperature instability (often hypothermia)
Jitteriness
Poor feeding, vomiting
Irritability or lethargy
Apnea
Respiratory distress
Seizures

Physical Examination
Jaundice
Pallor
Petechiae or purpura
Rash
Hepatosplenomegaly
Poor tone and perfusion
Tachycardia or bradycardia
Tachypnea
Cyanosis, grunting, flaring, retractions

Laboratory Evaluation
Blood for CBC with differential, platelet count, and culture—anemia; increase or decrease in WBC count with left shift; thrombocytopenia, serum ammonia for urea cycle defects
Urine—urine culture usually not done in the first 72 hours of life because of low yield
CSF often obtained for protein, glucose, cell count, and culture—elevated protein and WBC count; depressed glucose

Management
Combination broad-spectrum antibiotic coverage for gram-positive cocci, gram-negative bacilli, and *Listeria* is recommended. Consider adding coverage for *herpes* infection when suspected. *Listeria* is treated with ampicillin; *GBS* can be treated with the penicillins and the cephalosporins; gram-negative organisms are well covered by aminoglycosides and some cephalosporins.

CBC, Complete blood count; *CSF*, cerebrospinal fluid; *GBS*, group B streptococcus; *WBC*, white blood cell.

---

ingestion of oocysts from soil or in contaminated food. Depending on the timing of the infection, 17% to 65% of untreated women who acquire toxoplasmosis during gestation transmit the parasite to their fetuses (McLeod & Remington, 2004).

Clinical Findings.

History. Prematurity and low Apgar scores are included in the history.

Physical Examination. Infants with congenital infection are asymptomatic at birth in 70% to 90% of the cases (AAP, 2006b). Findings include the following:

- Jaundice
- Anemia
- Hepatosplenomegaly
- Chorioretinitis
- Microcephaly

Diagnostic Studies. CT of the brain shows calcifications or hydrocephalus. The CSF shows high protein, low glucose, and evidence of *T. gondii*. Serum immunoglobulin IgG, IgM, IgA, and IgE antibodies against toxoplasmosis are seen. The organism can be isolated by inoculation into mice or tissue culture of blood from the placenta, the umbilical cord, or the infant.

Differential Diagnosis. Sepsis, syphilis, and hemolytic disease are considered in the differential diagnosis.

Management, Prognosis, and Prevention. Pyrimethamine plus sulfadiazine (with folic acid supplementation) for up to 1 year is often recommended. Treatment usually eliminates the manifestations of toxoplasmosis, such as active chorioretinitis, meningitis, encephalitis, hepatitis, splenomegaly, and thrombocytopenia. Infants with extensive involvement at birth have mild to severe impairment of vision, hearing, cognitive function, and other neurologic functions. No protective vaccine is available. Pregnant women should be informed not to handle raw meat or contaminated cat litter, to wash fruits and vegetables before consumption, to cook meat and eggs well, and to drink pasteurized milk.

Congenital Rubella

Description and Epidemiology. Rubella is an RNA virus. Rubella is transmitted by person-to-person contact; the virus infects the placenta and is transmitted to the fetus. It occurs more frequently in the winter and spring.

Clinical Findings.

History. The history can include the following:
- Maternal infection before 16 weeks of gestation
- Negative rubella titers in mother

As many as 50% of infected women are asymptomatic (AAP, 2006b).

Physical Examination. Many infected infants may be asymptomatic in the newborn period. Findings include the following:
- Hearing loss
- Congenital heart disease
- Mental retardation
- Cataract or glaucoma and microphthalmia
- "Blueberry muffin" skin lesions

Diagnostic Studies. The rubella virus can be isolated from nasopharyngeal secretions, conjunctiva, urine, stool, and CSF.

Management and Prevention. No specific drug therapy is available. Monitoring and intervention for developmental, auditory, visual, and medical needs improve the quality of life for these children. Congenital rubella is now a rare occurrence because of widespread administration of an effective vaccine (AAP, 2006b). All women of childbearing age should have rubella serology titers, and vaccine should be given to IgG-seronegative women who are not pregnant.

Cytomegalovirus

Description and Epidemiology. Cytomegalovirus (CMV), a member of the herpesvirus family, is transmitted via intimate and household contact with virus-containing secretions and blood products. When CMV is introduced into a household, it is likely that all members will acquire the infection. CMV is transmitted to the infant via the placenta. Infections are distributed worldwide, and most humans have become infected by the time they reach adulthood. CMV causes congenital infection in 1% to 2% of all live births in the U.S. When pregnant women acquire the virus, there is a 30% to 40% transmission rate to the fetus (AAP, 2006b; Fanaroff & Martin, 2006; Remington et al, 2005).

Clinical Findings.

History.   Maternal infection (though many women are asymptomatic) and intrauterine growth retardation can be part of the history.

Physical Examination.   As many as 90% of infected newborns are asymptomatic. Findings include the following:

- SGA
- Hepatosplenomegaly
- Jaundice
- Petechial rash
- Chorioretinitis
- Cerebral calcifications
- Microcephaly

Diagnostic Studies.   CMV is isolated in cell cultures from urine, saliva, or other body fluids. Techniques for detection of viral DNA by polymerase chain reaction (PCR) are available from selected reference laboratories. Proof of congenital infection requires obtaining specimens within 3 weeks of birth. Viral isolation or a strongly positive test for serum IgM anti-CMV antibody is considered diagnostic.

Management, Prognosis, and Prevention.

No specific treatment is routinely recommended for infected neonates, although some data suggest that ganciclovir may be helpful in decreasing progression of hearing impairment; consultation with an expert is recommended (AAP, 2006b). Monitor urine for CMV for 18 to 24 months. The outcome of symptomatic congenital CMV infection is poor; there is a 20% to 30% mortality rate and a 90% to 95% morbidity rate, characterized by psychomotor retardation, microcephaly, hearing loss, seizures, chorioretinitis, optic atrophy, mental retardation, and learning disabilities. At greatest risk are susceptible pregnant women exposed to the urine and saliva of CMV-infected children who attend day care centers (AAP, 2006b). Hand washing and simple hygienic measures should be reinforced in this population.

Group B Streptococcus

Description and Epidemiology.   Group B streptococcus (GBS) is a gram-positive diplococcus that is the leading cause of sepsis in infants from birth to 3 months old resulting in significant perinatal morbidity and mortality rates. Early-onset disease usually occurs at birth or within the first 24 hours of life; late-onset disease occurs during the second week of life.

The organism forms colonies in the maternal genitourinary and gastrointestinal tracts. Pregnant women are usually asymptomatic, but can manifest chorioamnionitis, endometritis, or urinary tract infection. Infants born of women who are highly colonized are more likely to become colonized. GBS is acquired by newborns following vertical transmission (e.g., ascending infection through ruptured amniotic membranes or contamination following passage through the colonized birth canal). As many as 50% of infants with early-onset disease are symptomatic at birth, indicating an intrauterine infection. The highest attack rate of early-onset GBS is in high-risk deliveries, premature SGA infants, very-low-birth-weight infants, or those with prolonged ruptured membranes; full-term infants account for 50% of cases. Colonization of pregnant women and newborns ranges from 15% to 40%. Incidence of early-onset GBS disease has been reduced from about 1 to 4 cases per 1000 live births to about 0.3 cases per 1000 live births owing to widespread chemoprophylaxis (AAP, 2006b).

Clinical Findings.

History.   Risk factors include the following:

- Infants who are less than 37 weeks of gestation
- Rupture of membranes (ROM) of 18 hours or greater
- Maternal fever during labor of greater than 100.4° F oral
- Previous delivery of a sibling with invasive GBS disease
- Maternal chorioamnionitis to include ROM and maternal fever with at least two of the following:
  - Maternal tachycardia (heart rate greater than 90 BPM)
  - Fetal tachycardia (heart rate greater than 170 BPM)
  - Maternal leukocytosis (white blood cell count greater than 15,000)
  - Uterine tenderness
  - Foul-smelling amniotic fluid

Physical Examination.   Findings include the following:

- Poor feeding
- Temperature instability
- Cyanosis, apnea, tachypnea, grunting, flaring, and retracting
- Seizures, lethargy, bulging fontanelle
- Rapid onset and deterioration

Diagnostic Studies.   Cultures of blood, CSF, or both are definitive; antigen identification tests are available, but have poor specificity.

Differential Diagnosis.

RDS, amniotic fluid aspiration syndrome, persistent fetal circulation, meningitis, osteomyelitis, septic arthritis, sepsis from other infections, and metabolic problems are included in the differential diagnosis.

Management, Prognosis, and Prevention.

Initiate antibiotic therapy with a penicillin (usually ampicillin) and an aminoglycoside, often gentamicin, until GBS has been differentiated from *E. coli* or *Listeria* sepsis or meningitis (AAP, 2006b).

- Ampicillin intravenous:
  - Infant less than 7 days old, give 200 to 300 mg/kg/day in three divided doses
  - Infant older than 7 days old, give 300 mg/kg/day in four to six divided doses
- Gentamicin doses are found in Table 38-8.

TABLE 38-8 **Gentamicin Doses**

Gestational Age (weeks)	Age (days)	Dose
≤29 or asphyxia, decreased renal function	0-7	5 mg/kg every 48 hours
	8-28	4 mg/kg every 36 hours
	>28	4 mg/kg every 24 hours
30-33	0-7	4.5 mg/kg every 36 hours
	>7	4 mg/kg every 24 hours
≥34	0-7	4 mg/kg every 24 hours
	>7	4 mg/kg every 12-18 hours

- Penicillin G given intravenously is the treatment of choice for documented GBS infection.
- Infant less than 7 days old, give 250,000 to 400,000 units/kg/day in three divided doses
- Infant older than 7 days old, give 450,000 to 500,000 units/kg/day in four to six divided doses
- Duration of therapy is 10 days (bacteremia without tows) to 14 days (uncomplicated meningitis)
- Consultation with pediatric infectious disease specialists is recommended.

Screening of all pregnant women for GBS at 35 to 37 weeks of gestation is recommended. Antepartum treatment of asymptomatic mothers carrying GBS is not recommended. The mortality rate of early-onset disease ranges from 10% to 40%; mortality rate is highest in very-low-birth-weight infants and in those with low neutrophil count (less than 1500), low Apgar scores, hypotension, apnea, and a delay in starting antimicrobial therapy. Chemoprophylaxis of high-risk, colonized, pregnant women is an effective method of preventing early-onset GBS infection. Consensus guidelines developed by the Centers for Disease Control and Prevention (CDC) outline steps for a screening-based and risk-factor strategy to prevent GBS (AAP, 2006b; CDC, 2002). Treatment consists of intravenous penicillin or ampicillin given to high-risk women at the onset of labor, repeated every 4 hours until the infant is born.

Listeriosis

Description and Epidemiology. *Listeria monocytogenes* is a small, gram-positive rod isolated from soil, streams, sewage, certain foods, silage, dust, and slaughterhouses. The food-borne transmission of disease is related to Mexican (soft ripened) cheese, whole and 2% milk, uncooked hot dogs, undercooked chicken, raw vegetables, and shellfish. The newborn infant acquires the organism transplacentally or by aspiration or ingestion at the time of delivery.

Clinical Findings.

History. Brown-stained amniotic fluid is seen.

Physical Examination. Findings include the following:
- Generalized symptoms of sepsis
- Whitish posterior pharyngeal and cutaneous granulomas
- Disseminated erythematous papules on skin

Diagnostic Studies. Cultures of the blood, CSF, meconium, and urine are done. The CSF shows elevated protein, depressed glucose, and a high leukocyte count. Cultures of the placenta and amniotic fluid also may be helpful.

Management and Prognosis.

- Administer intravenous ampicillin and an aminoglycoside (gentamicin) as initial therapy for severe infections.
- After clinical response occurs or for less severe infections in normal hosts, administer ampicillin alone.
- The duration of therapy is 10 to 14 days for infections without meningitis and 14 to 21 days for infections with meningitis (AAP, 2006b).

Transplacentally acquired listeriosis often results in spontaneous abortion. The death rate of premature infants with *Listeria* pneumonia noted within 12 hours of birth approaches 100%. Mortality rate varies from 20% to 50% if disease develops between 5 and 30 days of birth, and is especially high in premature infants. Mental retardation, paralysis, and hydrocephalus have been noted in survivors of *Listeria* meningitis (Fanaroff & Martin, 2006; Remington et al, 2005).

Congenital Varicella

Description and Epidemiology. Varicella-zoster virus (VZV) is a herpesvirus. Humans are the only source of infection for this highly contagious virus. The infectivity rate for congenital varicella syndrome in infants born to mothers with chickenpox during the first trimester is 0.4%; it is 2% when infection occurs between 12 and 20 weeks of gestation (Watson, 2005).

Clinical Findings

History. There is a history of maternal chickenpox infection.

Physical Examination. Findings may include the following:
- Limb atrophy
- Scarring of the skin
- Eye manifestations

Diagnostic Studies. Diagnosis of VZV is made by immunofluorescent staining of vesicular scrapings.

Management, Prognosis, and Prevention. Some experts recommend acyclovir for pregnant women with varicella, especially in the second or third trimester (AAP, 2006b). Varicella-zoster immune globulin (VZIG) is recommended for the term newborn infant whose mother had an onset of chickenpox within 5 days before delivery or within 48 hours after delivery. All exposed premature infants less than 28 weeks gestation or less than 1000 g birth weight should receive VZIG; exposed premature infants more than 28 weeks gestation whose mothers lack serologic evidence of disease or a reliable history of disease also require VZIG (AAP, 2006b). VZIG is not indicated if the mother has varicella zoster (shingles) only. Airborne and contact precautions are recommended for neonates born to mothers with varicella. If still hospitalized, such precautions are continued until 21 days old or 28 days if they received VZIG.

Prevention efforts are targeted to potential mothers. Varicella vaccination is recommended for nonpregnant women of childbearing age who have no history of varicella infection (AAP, 2006b; CDC, 2005).

SEXUALLY TRANSMITTED DISEASES

Gonorrhea

Description and Epidemiology. *Neisseria gonorrhoeae* is a gram-negative diplococcus infection that occurs only in humans. The organism lives in exudate and secretions of infected mucous membranes. The organism is transmitted primarily through sexual contact and parturition. Gonococcal infections in the newborn are acquired primarily during delivery.

Clinical Findings.

History. There is a history of maternal gonococcal infection.

Physical Examination. Findings include conjunctivitis.

Diagnostic Studies. Culture of eye exudate is positive for *N. gonorrhoeae.*

Management and Prevention. Administer a single dose of intramuscular ceftriaxone 25 to 50 mg/kg (not to exceed 125 mg) for prophylaxis of infants born to mothers with active gonorrhea. Because gonorrheal conjunctivitis can rapidly lead to blindness, all infants are given eye prophylaxis at birth with either 1% silver nitrate, 1% tetracycline ophthalmic ointment, or erythromycin 0.5% ophthalmic ointment (AAP, 2006b; CDC, 2006).

Chlamydia

Description and Epidemiology. Chlamydial infection is caused by an obligate intracellular parasite. *C. trachomatis* infection is the most common sexually transmitted disease in the U.S. Acquisition occurs in approximately 50% of infants born vaginally to infected mothers and in some infants delivered by cesarean section with intact membranes. Of infants acquiring *C. trachomatis* infection, the risk of developing conjunctivitis is 25% to 50% and of pneumonia is 5% to 20% (AAP, 2006b).

Clinical Findings.

History. There is a history of maternal chlamydial infection.

Physical Examination. Assess for the following:

- Conjunctivitis a few days to several weeks after birth
- Infant commonly afebrile with normal activity level
- Pneumonia 2 to 19 weeks after birth

Diagnostic Studies.

- Tests for detection of *C. trachomatis* without cell culture include DNA probe, direct fluorescent antibody (DFA) staining, enzyme immunoassay (EIA), and nucleic acid amplification (PCR, ligase chain reaction [LCR]).
- Routine bacterial cultures are not helpful.
- Gram stain and culture of discharge from the eye (must include epithelial cells from the palpebral conjunctival sac because chlamydia is an obligate parasite) are necessary for diagnosis.

Management and Prevention. Oral erythromycin suspension (50 mg/kg/day in four divided doses for 10 to 14 days) is given for both conjunctivitis and pneumonia (CDC, 2006). Appropriate treatment of the pregnant woman before delivery prevents disease in the newborn. Prophylaxis with oral erythromycin of the asymptomatic infant born to an untreated but chlamydia-positive woman is contraindicated

because of the increased risk of developing hypertrophic pyloric stenosis in the infant exposed to erythromycin.

Syphilis

Description and Epidemiology. Syphilis is caused by the spirochete *Treponema pallidum* which crosses the placenta in an infected mother. Routine maternal serologic testing is legally required during prenatal care in all states.

Clinical Findings.

History. A history of maternal infection and positive serologic testing in the mother is found.

Physical Examination. The majority of neonates are asymptomatic at birth. Findings include the following:

- Hepatosplenomegaly
- Persistent rhinorrhea
- Maculopapular or bullous dermal lesions
- Failure to thrive, restlessness, fever

Diagnostic Studies. Evaluation needs to be individualized depending on the adequacy of maternal treatment and follow-up for syphilis. Consultation with infectious disease may be indicated. CSF evaluation shows high protein, low glucose, high white blood cell count, and positivity on Venereal Disease Research Laboratories (VDRL) test; serum liver enzymes are elevated with liver involvement, and serum rapid plasma reagin (RPR) test is positive.

Management and Prognosis. For proven or highly probable congenital syphilis, the CDC (2006) recommends 10 consecutive days of crystalline penicillin G 100,000 to 150,000 units/kg/day, given as 50,000 units/kg intravenously every 12 hours during the first 7 days of life and every 8 hours thereafter. Procaine penicillin G 50,000 units/kg intramuscularly daily in a single dose is the **only** acceptable treatment regimen for congenital syphilis and for all infants born to seropositive mothers without a documented history of adequate treatment. If more than 1 day is missed, the entire course must be restarted. For infants with less certain evidence of syphilis, alternative regimens are available; referral to the latest CDC guidelines is recommended (CDC, 2006). Untreated congenital syphilis can lead to severe multiorgan involvement. Infants who are appropriately treated have a good prognosis.

Herpes Simplex Virus

Description and Epidemiology. Three clinically distinguishable categories of herpes simplex virus (HSV) infection exist: (1) disseminated disease, (2) CNS disease, and (3) disease restricted to the skin, eyes, and mouth (AAP, 2006b) (see Table 38-3). HSV is transmitted by direct contact with infected maternal genitalia during the birth process. Transplacental transmission occurs, but has been reported in only a few cases. The risk of neonatal infection is highest with primary genital infection (see Chapter 23 for further discussion).

Clinical Findings.

History. The mother may have active lesions and deliver vaginally.

Physical Examination. Vesicles in the skin, eye, and mouth are found. Signs or symptoms of encephalitis, pneumonia, or sepsis can also be present.

Diagnostic Studies. The virus is isolated in tissue cultures obtained from vesicles, nasopharyngeal or conjunctival swabs, urine, stool, and tracheal secretions; alternatively, vesicle scrapings can be evaluated for antigens with rapid diagnostic tests.

Management, Prognosis, and Prevention. Acyclovir 60 mg/kg/day intravenously every 8 hours is given for 14 days (skin, eyes, and mouth infection) or 21 days (disseminated or involving the CNS) (AAP, 2006b; CDC, 2006). Additionally, treatment with ophthalmic drugs (1% trifluridine, 0.1% iododeoxyuridine, or 3% vidarabine) is used for infants with ocular involvement (AAP, 2006b). Despite effective antiviral therapy, disseminated neonatal HSV infections and localized encephalitis are associated with considerable morbidity and mortality. The risk of acquiring this serious infection is lowered by performing cesarean delivery before rupture of membranes in any pregnancy in which signs or symptoms of HSV infection occur.

Human Immunodeficiency Virus

Description and Epidemiology. Human immunodeficiency virus (HIV), a retrovirus, is transmitted to the newborn via the placenta or at birth secondary to exposure to maternal blood. It is estimated that an infant born to an untreated mother who is HIV positive has a 13% to 39% chance of becoming HIV positive. About 15% to 20% of untreated infants die in the first 4 years of life (median age 11 months). The remainder are relatively well during infancy, but gradually become chronically ill during childhood. Perinatally acquired HIV infections are increasing rapidly in the U.S. Most cases of preadolescent HIV infection occur as a result of mother-to-child transmission (Abrams, 2005). See Chapter 23 for further discussion.

Clinical Findings.

History. The history includes an HIV-positive mother. It can also include the following:
- Maternal intravenous drug abuse
- Maternal intercourse with a high-risk male
- Maternal receipt of blood products before April 1985

Physical Examination. Most infants are asymptomatic. Findings *may* include the following:
- Low birth weight
- Microcephaly
- Failure to thrive

Diagnostic Studies. HIV DNA PCR is the preferred virologic method for diagnosing HIV infection during infancy. Because of concerns regarding potential contamination with maternal blood, blood samples from the umbilical cord should not be used for diagnostic evaluations. HIV infection can be reasonably excluded among nonbreastfed children with two negative HIV DNA or RNA PCR virologic tests (one performed at 1 month or older and one at 4 months or older); it can definitely be excluded in these same children at 12 to 18 months old with a negative HIV antibody test. See Chapter 23 for the screening schedule for the HIV-exposed infant.

Management, Prognosis, and Prevention. The principal antiretroviral agents undergo frequent change as new research is published. The latest recommendations are available at *www.aidsinfo.nih.gov*. Once a definitive diagnosis of HIV is established, combination therapy (often three antiretroviral drugs) is provided, two of which are nucleoside analogue reverse transcriptase inhibitors in combination with either a protease inhibitor or a nonnucleoside reverse transcriptase inhibitor. In all cases, the goal of therapy is to reduce viral concentrations to undetectable levels. Additionally, some recommend intravenous immune globulin (IVIG) in children with hypogammaglobulinemia who also experience serious bacterial infections lasting over a 1-year period.

Ideally, the above antiretroviral therapy regimen should be initiated in all HIV-infected infants less than 12 months old. Until the diagnosis of HIV disease is excluded, trimethoprim-sulfamethoxazole prophylaxis is recommended for the first year of life and is continued in HIV-positive infants beyond this period depending on CD4 cell counts. See Chapter 23 for more detail. Breastfeeding is contraindicated in HIV-positive mothers (the exception may be in third world countries where no other feeding source is available) because of documented transmission via breast milk (CDC, 2006).

Improving the outcomes for HIV-infected infants depends on identifying infants at risk early so that prompt prophylactic strategies and therapeutic interventions can be initiated. Early identification of maternal HIV infection during the antenatal period enables the mother to be treated with antiretroviral chemoprophylaxis during pregnancy and labor. The newborn begins treatment immediately after birth to reduce the risk of HIV transmission from mother to infant. The use of prenatal antiviral agents, such as zidovudine or nevirapine, and elective cesarean section at 38 weeks can reduce the perinatal transmission to as little as 2% (AAP, 2006b; CDC, 2006). Although research is continuing, vaccines are not yet available. Prevention efforts are targeted at potential mothers, including the reduction of risk factors through behavioral changes.

DRUG-EXPOSED INFANTS

Cocaine (Crack) Exposure

Description. Cocaine is a local anesthetic and CNS stimulant that is believed to be a teratogen that crosses the placenta.

Clinical Findings.

History. Maternal exposure to cocaine or crack and positive maternal and/or infant urine drug screen for cocaine are found. Premature labor, abruptio placentae, and fetal asphyxia are possible.

Physical Examination. Many infants will show no adverse affects from maternal use of cocaine. Findings may include the following:
- Low birth weight, IUGR or prematurity
- Fetal distress and meconium staining
- Microcephaly
- Anomalies of the urinary or gastrointestinal tract
- Feeding difficulties, including voracious appetite, poorly coordinated sucking and swallowing, and vomiting

- CNS symptoms of transient irritability, abnormal sleeping patterns, tremors, hypertonia, and lability of mood

There is no clinically documented neonatal withdrawal syndrome for cocaine (Stoll & Kliegman, 2004).

Management, Complications, and Prevention. Take the following steps:

- Offer quiet and pacification techniques, such as swaddling and decreased environmental stimuli.
- If symptoms suggest that further treatment is indicated, see following section (Heroin and Methadone Exposure).
- Because cocaine is detectable in breast milk, mothers who use cocaine should not breastfed.
- Involvement of the Department of Child and Family Services is essential.

In one study, authors found that mothers who stated they had used cocaine or had a positive drug screen had a significantly higher risk of infections, including syphilis, gonorrhea, hepatitis, and HIV; psychiatric, nervous, and emotional disorders; and abruptio placentae. The prevalence of serious and life-threatening medical outcomes is low in drug-abusing pregnant women; however, the disadvantaged social and environmental conditions that are often characteristic of the lifestyle of these women may compound the risk for infection and poor neurodevelopmental outcome (Bauer et al, 2002). Prenatal cocaine exposure has been associated in some studies with long-term changes in behavior, including neurobehavioral dysfunction, hyperactivity, aggression, and short attention span; further research is underway (Campbell, 2003). Elimination of in utero exposure to cocaine can occur only if there is identification of a potential problem in a high-risk mother and referral to a substance abuse prevention program.

Heroin and Methadone Exposure

Description. Heroin and methadone are narcotics that cross the placenta.

Clinical Findings.

History.

- Maternal exposure to heroin or methadone
- Urine drug screen positive for opiates in mother and/or infant
- Increased incidence of stillbirths and SGA infants, but probably not congenital anomalies

Physical Examination. Findings include the following:

- Tremors and hyperirritability often more coarse than those with hypoglycemia
- Limbs rigid and hyperreflexic
- Skin abrasions secondary to hyperactivity
- Tachypnea
- Poor feeding
- Diarrhea
- Vomiting
- High-pitched cry
- Fist sucking
- Low birth weight or SGA in 50% (Stoll & Kliegman, 2004)

Symptoms of heroin withdrawal occur in up to 75% of infants, usually beginning in the first 48 hours of life, depending on the daily maternal dose, duration of addiction, and time of last maternal dose. Symptoms of methadone withdrawal occur in up to 90% of infants. A higher incidence of symptomatology is seen if the last dose was taken within 24 hours of birth. Overall the withdrawal syndrome is more severe and more prolonged with methadone than with heroin (Stoll & Kliegman, 2004).

Differential Diagnosis. The differential diagnosis includes hypoglycemia and hypocalcemia.

Management and Prevention. Supportive management, such as swaddling, frequent feedings, and protection from external stimuli, is needed. Education regarding SIDS is imperative because these infants are at increased risk. The Department of Child and Family Services must be involved before discharge. Medications, such as phenobarbital and methadone, can be used if symptoms, such as severe irritability, vomiting and diarrhea, seizures, temperature instability, or severe tachypnea, are noted. Pregnant women who are addicted to heroin should be encouraged to enter a treatment program.

Fetal Alcohol Syndrome

See Chapter 40.

■ SUDDEN INFANT DEATH SYNDROME AND APPARENT LIFE-THREATENING EVENTS

DESCRIPTION AND EPIDEMIOLOGY

The accepted definition of *sudden infant death syndrome* (SIDS) is the sudden death of an infant under 1 year old that remains unexplained after a complete case investigation, including performance of a complete autopsy, examination of the death scene, and review of the clinical history (Hunt & Hauck, 2004). SIDS rarely occurs in the first month of life, with 90% of deaths occurring between 1 and 6 months old, peaking at 12 weeks old (85% occur between 2 and 4 months old). SIDS is the most common cause of death in infants between 1 and 6 months old, accounting for 5000 deaths per year. Black infants are at twice the risk; there is a higher frequency of SIDS in male infants and in the winter months, although the seasonal difference in rates is decreasing (AAP, 2005; Christian & Cox, 2005; Hunt & Hauck, 2004).

An *apparent life-threatening event* (ALTE) is defined as an episode that is frightening to the observer and that is characterized by some combination of apnea (central or occasionally obstructive), color change, marked change in muscle tone, choking, or gagging. In some cases, the observer fears that the infant has died.

The diagnosis is one of exclusion because the specific cause of SIDS remains unknown. It cannot be predicted nor prevented, although placing the infant in a supine position has been shown to decrease the incidence of SIDS and is now the recommended sleep position for infants. The National Institutes of Health has monitored sleep position since 1992, and prone sleeping has decreased from 70% to about 13%. At the same time, the SIDS death rate has fallen by about 53% in the U.S. (AAP, 2005).

Three main pathophysiologic mechanisms are considered to contribute to SIDS: decreased arousal, asphyxia and rebreathing, and thermal stress. Experts have considered as possible causes respiratory obstruction, restrictive clothing, and hyperthermia. Factors associated with SIDS include ALTE, poverty, lack of prenatal care, low birth weight, SGA, preterm birth, young maternal age, high parity, maternal smoking and drug use, and co-sleeping.

CLINICAL FINDINGS

History

The following risk factors may be identified:
- Maternal: cigarette smoking, drug or alcohol use; no or poor prenatal care; bottle feeding; poor education; unmarried; multiparity; maternal age less than 20 years; short intervals between pregnancies; anemia
- Infant: prematurity (less than 37 weeks); low birth weight (less than 2500 g) or SGA; twins or other multiple births; Apgar score less than 6 at 5 minutes; apnea; poor weight gain; anemia; intensive care unit stay; neonatal respiratory abnormality, bronchopulmonary dysplasia, previous ALTE; previously healthy infant with or without recent URI symptoms
- Socioeconomic, other: low-income family; crowded living conditions; poor housing conditions; prior SIDS in family; prone sleeping position, soft bedding, overheating; co-sleeping, especially with smoke, alcohol or mind-altering drug use; race, ethnicity, culture (higher rates in black and American Indian and Alaska Native children).

Physical Examination

Findings include the following:
- No sign of injury (nonaccidental trauma must be ruled out)
- Frothy blood-tinged secretions in mouth and nares
- Intrathoracic petechiae on autopsy
- Retention of periadrenal brown fat on autopsy

Diagnostic Studies

Autopsy and death scene evaluation must be done. A skeletal bone survey may be done if there is concern about abuse.

DIFFERENTIAL DIAGNOSIS

Aspiration; suffocation; infant botulism or poisoning; cardiac or respiratory disease; hypoxemia; infection; metabolic disorders; child abuse, Munchausen syndrome, or shaken baby syndrome; and CNS abnormalities should be ruled out. Bed sharing, especially if the parent is large, appears to be associated with an increased likelihood of some SIDS-like deaths (AAP, 2005).

MANAGEMENT AND PREVENTION

Management is aimed at assisting the family to cope with the loss of the child. The first response of the family is disbelief and shock.

1. Obtain a thorough history from the caretaker within a short period of time after the death. Do not accuse the family of any wrongdoing. Focus the questioning on the cause of death to better understand the circumstances.
2. Reassure caretaker and family that it was not their fault and could not have been prevented.
3. Offer support and counsel to families as soon as possible after death.
4. Supply names of different support groups to help the family overcome grief. Agencies to contact are listed in the Resource Box at the end of the chapter.
5. Provide follow-up for 1 year.
6. Assist surviving siblings. Observe their reaction to the death and refer for counseling if necessary. Help them to understand that it was not their fault and alleviate their feelings of guilt. Allow children to verbalize their feelings. Assist parents to deal with the other children; suggest that parents give extra love, attention, and reassurance to their other children.
7. Evaluate need for home monitoring. Because the rate of SIDS in succeeding children is low (less than 2%) and because monitoring a child cannot prevent a SIDS episode from occurring, the controversy remains about whether to monitor succeeding children (AAP, 2005). Monitors are recommended by some in the following instances: when more than one child in a family has died from SIDS; in infants with ALTE; in infants with tracheostomy or other airway problems; in infants with neurologic problems affecting respiratory control; in infants with chronic lung disease.

Box 38-7 lists measures that aid in the prevention of SIDS.

BOX 38-7 **Measures That Aid in the Prevention of Sudden Infant Death Syndrome**

- Place infants on their backs to sleep until at least 6 months old. The National Institutes of Health has a "Back to Sleep" program with parent information, stickers, and video (see Resource Box).
- Use a firm mattress. Do not use soft bedding or have stuffed animals in bed. Infants should not sleep on a sofa or chair or in a waterbed or in bed with adult.
- Avoid overheating and overbundling; room temperature should be 68° F to 72° F (20° C to 22.2° C).
- Avoid alcohol and drugs (including smoking) while pregnant and breastfeeding, and while in bed.
- Avoid bed sharing and co-sleeping.
- Do not allow cigarette smoking within the house or car.
- Separate but proximate caregiver sleeping environments are recommended.
- Consider pacifier use at nap time and bedtime (but not in breastfed infants until after the first month of life when feedings are established)
- A variety of products to maintain an infant's sleep position are commercially available; their efficacy and safety have not been thoroughly investigated and cannot be recommended.
- For at-risk infants, educate parents and caregivers regarding pros and cons of apnea monitor use. Cardiopulmonary resuscitation instruction is recommended.

✓ DISCUSSION FORUM

1. Create a discharge plan for a healthy, term newborn. Make sure you include the newborn's and the family's needs. Create a similar discharge plan for an infant with one of the high-risk conditions listed in Box 38-1. How do the plans differ? How are they the same?

2. You do a prenatal visit with the parents of a baby diagnosed with cleft lip and cleft palate during the second trimester ultrasound. The mother's due date is in 4 weeks, and the parents voice concern about the child's immediate and long-term care needs. What do you tell the parents? What management will the baby need after birth?

3. Compare and contrast the risk factors and physical exam findings for newborn RDS and TTN.

4. You are called to the newborn nursery to evaluate a term, newborn with Apgar of 9/9 born via vaginal delivery to a 34-year-old primigravida. Pregnancy history was normal except for oligohydramnios. The nursery nurses inform you the infant has had 1 wet diaper in the last 8 hours and is now lethargic. Physical examination reveals a palpable abdominal mass. What diagnostic testing do you order, and what do you expect to find? What management do you prescribe?

5. Develop a plan of care for a 10-week-old with an acute life-threatening event. Be sure to list parameters for evaluation, referral, consultation and follow-up.

6. You see a 36-week gestation newborn at 3 days old for follow-up following a discharge bilirubin of 9.4 mg/dL (obtained yesterday afternoon). The parents report an intake of 16 oz iron-fortified cow's milk formula over the last 24 hours. The newborn had 3 wet diapers and 1 bowel movement in the last 16 hours. Physical examination reveals marked jaundice of the face, trunk, and upper thighs with scleral yellowing. Prenatal history was negative, and the Coombs test was negative at birth. Total bilirubin today is 15.2. What management do you prescribe?

ℛESOURCE BOX

National Perinatal Resources

Birth Defect Research for Children, Inc.
www.birthdefects.org
Provides parents and expectant parents with information about birth defects and support services for their children

Association for SIDS and Infant Mortality Programs
www.asip1.org

SIDS: Back to Sleep Campaign (National Institute of Child Health and Human Development)
www.nichd.nih.gov/sids

Centers for Disease Control and Prevention: Infectious Disease Information
www.cdc.gov/ncidod/diseases
Guidelines for disease management, such as GBS, varicella, sexually transmitted diseases

Cleft Palate Foundation
www.cleftline.org
Informational materials (including Spanish), networking, referrals to local resources, advocacy, funds research

Compassionate Friends
www.compassionatefriends.org
Assists families with grief following the death of a child of any age

Family Empowerment Network: Families Affected by Fetal Alcohol Syndrome/Fetal Alcohol Effects
Informational materials (including Spanish), networking, referrals to local resources
www.fammed.wisc.edu/fen/

Group B Strep Association
www.groupbstrep.org
Newsletter, informational materials, networking, referrals to local resources, advocacy, funds research, maintains research registry

March of Dimes (local chapters found online)
www.marchofdimes.com

National Highway Traffic Safety Administration
www.nhtsa.gov/cps/cpsfitting

Child Safety Seat Inspection Station Locator
www.seatcheck.org
Information on safety seat checks.

National Newborn Screening and Genetics Resource Center
http://genes-r-us.uthscsa.edu

National Perinatal Association
www.nationalperinatal.org

National SIDS Resource Center
www.sidscenter.org

POSTPARTUM DEPRESSION RESOURCES

National Women's Health Information Center
www.4women.gov

Postpartum Support International
www.chss.iup.edu/postpartum

Depression after Delivery
www.depressionafterdelivery.com

First Candle (formerly the National SIDS Foundation)
www.sidsalliance.org

TEF/VATER International Support Network
www.tefvater.org
Support group for parents with infants with tracheal or esophageal fistulas.

REFERENCES

Abrams EJ: Human immunodeficiency virus infection. In Schwartz MN, editor: *The 5-minute pediatric consult*, ed 4, Philadelphia, 2005, Lippincott.

American Academy of Pediatrics (AAP): The Apgar score, *Pediatrics* 117:1444-1447, 2006a.

American Academy of Pediatrics (AAP): *2006 Red book: report of the committee on infectious diseases*, ed 27, Elk Grove Village, IL, 2006b, American Academy of Pediatrics.

American Academy of Pediatrics (AAP): The changing concept of sudden infant death syndrome: diagnostic coding shifts, controversies regarding the sleeping environment, and new variables to consider in reducing risk, *Pediatrics* 116:1245-1255, 2005.

American Academy of Pediatrics (AAP): Clinical practice guideline: management of hyperbilirubinemia in the newborn infant 35 or more weeks of gestation, *Pediatrics* 114:297-316, 2004.

American Academy of Pediatrics (AAP): Recommendations for preventive pediatric health care, *Pediatrics* 105:645-646, 2000.

American Academy of Pediatrics (AAP): Selecting and using the most appropriate car safety seats for growing children: guidelines for counseling parents, *Pediatrics* 109:550-553, 2002.

Apgar V et al: Evaluation of the newborn infant. Second report, *JAMA* 168:1985, 1958.

Bauer CR, et al: The maternal lifestyle study: drug exposure during pregnancy and short-term maternal outcomes, *Am J Obstet Gynecol* 186: 487-495, 2002.

Brady-Fryer B, Wiebe N, Lander JA: Pain relief for neonatal circumcision, *Cochrane Database Syst Rev* 18:CD004217, 2004.

Brown RE, Neu J: Necrotizing enterocolitis. In Burg FD et al, editors: *Current pediatric therapy*, ed 18, Philadelphia, 2006, WB Saunders.

Campbell S: Prenatal cocaine exposure and neonatal/infant outcomes, *Neonatal Network* 22:19-21, 2003.

Centers for Disease Control and Prevention (CDC): Prevention of perinatal group B streptococcal disease: revised guidelines from CDC, *MMWR Morb Mortal Wkly Rep* 51(RR-11):1-22, 2002.

Centers for Disease Control and Prevention (CDC): Recommended adult immunization schedule — United States, October 2005–September 2006, *MMWR Morb Mortal Wkly Rep* 54(RR-40):Q1-Q4, 2005.

Centers for Disease Control and Prevention (CDC): Sexually transmitted diseases guidelines, 2006, *MMWR Morb Mortal Wkly Rep* 55(R-11):1-94, 2006.

Christian CW, Cox MJ: Sudden infant death syndrome. In Schwartz MN, editor: *The 5-minute pediatric consult*, ed 4, Philadelphia, 2005, Lippincott.

Elder JS: Urologic disorders in infants and children. In Behrman RE, Kliegman RM, Jenson HB, editors: Nelson textbook of pediatrics, ed 17, Philadelphia, 2004, WB Saunders, p.1783-1826.

Fanaroff AA, Martin RJ: *Fanaroff & Martin's neonatal-perinatal medicine: diseases of the fetus and infant*, ed 8, Philadelphia, 2006, Mosby Yearbook.

Feldstein NA, Anderson RCE: Diagnosis & management of hydrocephalus. In Burg FD et al, editors: *Current pediatric therapy*, ed 18, Philadelphia, 2006, WB Saunders.

Gilstrap LC, Oh W, editors: *Guidelines for perinatal care*, ed 5, Elk Grove Village, IL, 2002, American Academy of Pediatrics and American College of Obstetricians and Gynecologists.

Green M & Palfrey JS editors: *Bright futures: guidelines for health supervision of infants, children, and adolescents*, rev ed 2, Arlington, VA, 2002, National Center for Education in Maternal and Child Health.

Hendricks-Munoz: Infants of diabetic mothers. In Burg FD et al, editors: *Current pediatric therapy*, ed 18, Philadelphia, 2006, WB Saunders.

Hunt CE, Hauck FR: Sudden infant death syndrome. In Behrman RE, Kliegman RM, Jenson HB, editors: *Nelson textbook of pediatrics*, ed 17, Philadelphia, 2004, WB Saunders.

Johnston MV, Kinsman S: Congenital anomalies of the central nervous system. In Behrman RE, Kliegman RM, Jenson HB, editors: *Nelson textbook of pediatrics*, ed 17, Philadelphia, 2004, WB Saunders.

Joint Committee on Infant Hearing; American Academy of Audiology; American Academy of Pediatrics (AAP); American Speech-Language-Hearing Association; Directors of Speech and Hearing Programs in State

Health and Welfare Agencies: Year 2000 position statement: principles and guidelines for early hearing detection and intervention programs. Joint Committee on Infant Hearing, American Academy of Audiology, American Academy of Pediatrics, American Speech-Language-Hearing Association, and Directors of Speech and Hearing Programs in State Health and Welfare Agencies, *Pediatrics* 106:798-817, 2000.

Leonard MB: Polycystic kidney disease. In Schwartz MN, editor: *The 5-minute pediatric consult*, ed 4, Philadelphia, 2005, Lippincott.

Lin RL, Tinkle LL, Janniger CK: Skin care of the healthy newborn, *Cutis* 75:25-30, 2005.

Lovrekovic G: Diaphragmatic hernia (congenital). In Schwartz MN, editor: *The 5-minute pediatric consult*, ed 4, Philadelphia, 2005, Lippincott.

Madden JM et al: Length-of-stay policies and ascertainment of postdischarge problems in newborns, *Pediatrics* 113:442-9, 2004.

Mahon BE, Rosenman MB, Kleiman MB: Maternal and infant use of erythromycin and other macrolide antibiotics as risk factors for infantile hypertrophic pyloric stenosis, *J Pediatr* 139:380-384, 2001.

March of Dimes: US Government Recommendations on Folid Acid. Available from www.marchofdimes.com/professionals/690_4089. asp (accessed December 28, 2007).

McLeod R, Remington JS: Toxoplasmosis. In Behrman RE, Kliegman RM, Jenson HB, editors: *Nelson textbook of pediatrics*, ed 17, Philadelphia, 2004, WB Saunders. pp.1144-1153.

Middlesworth W, Kadenhe-Chiweshe A: Neonatal intestinal obstruction. In Burg FD et al, editors: *Current pediatric therapy*, ed 18, Philadelphia, 2006, WB Saunders.

Orenstein S et al: Embryology, anatomy & function of the esophagus. In Behrman RE, Kliegman RM, Jenson HB, editors: *Nelson textbook of pediatrics*, ed 17, Philadelphia, 2004, WB Saunders.

Pena A: Surgical conditions of the anus, rectum, and colon. In Behrman RE, Kliegman RM, Jenson HB, editors: *Nelson textbook of pediatrics*, ed 17, Philadelphia, 2004, WB Saunders.

Perlman JM: Intracranial hemorrhage in the newborn. In Burg FD et al, editors: *Current pediatric therapy*, ed 18, Philadelphia, 2006, WB Saunders.

Remington JS, Klein J: *Infectious diseases of the fetus and newborn infant*, ed 6, Philadelphia, 2005, Elsevier.

Robertson J, Shilkofski N: *The Harriet Lane handbook*, ed 17, St Louis, 2005, Mosby.

Section on Ophthalmology American Academy of Pediatrics (AAP); American Academy of Ophthalmology; American Association for Pediatric Ophthalmology and Strabismus: Screening examination of premature infants for retinopathy of prematurity, *Pediatrics* 117:572-576, 2006.

Semeao E: Necrotizing enterocolitis. In Schwartz MN, editor: *The 5-minute pediatric consult*, ed 4, Philadelphia, 2005, Lippincott.

Soll RF, Pfister RH: Respiratory distress syndrome. In Burg FD et al, editors: *Current pediatric therapy*, ed 18, Philadelphia, 2006, WB Saunders.

Stern JW: Neuroblastoma. In Schwartz MN, editor: *The 5-minute pediatric consult*, ed 4, Philadelphia, 2005, Lippincott.

Stoll BJ, Kliegman RM: The fetus and the neonatal infant. In Behrman RE, Kliegman RM, Jenson HB, editors: *Nelson textbook of pediatrics*, ed 17, Philadelphia, 2004, WB Saunders.

Tinanoff N: The oral cavity. In Behrman RE, Kliegman RM, Jenson HB, editors: *Nelson textbook of pediatrics,* ed 17, Philadelphia, 2004, WB Saunders.

Thompson GH: The foot & toes. In Behrman RE, Kliegman RM, Jenson HB, editors: *Nelson textbook of pediatrics*, ed 17, Philadelphia, 2004, WB Saunders.

Ulshen MH: Intestinal malformations. In Burg FD et al, editors: *Current pediatric therapy*, ed 18, Philadelphia, 2006, WB Saunders.

US Department of Health and Human Services: *Healthy People 2010 objectives*, Washington, DC, 2003. Available from *www.healthypeople. gov* (accessed Aug 2006).

US Preventive Services Task Force: *Guide to clinical preventive services*, 2002. Available from *www.ahrq.gov/clinic/uspstfix.htm* (accessed Aug 2006).

US Public Health Services: *Put prevention into practice: clinician's handbook of preventive services*, ed 2, 1998. Available from *www.ahcpr.gov/clinic/ppiphand.htm* (accessed Aug 2006).

Vain NE et al: Oropharyngeal and nasopharyngeal suctioning of meconium-stained neonates before delivery of their shoulders: multicentre, randomised controlled trial, *Lancet* 364:597-602, 2004.

Watson B: Chickenpox. In Schwartz MN, editor: *The 5-minute pediatric consult*, ed 4, Philadelphia, 2005, Lippincott.

Wisner KL, Parry BL, Piontek CM: Postpartum depression, *N Engl J Med* 347(3):194-199, 2002.

Wyllie R: Stomach & intestines. In Behrman RE, Kliegman RM, Jenson HB, editors: *Nelson textbook of pediatrics*, ed 17, Philadelphia, 2004, WB Saunders.

CHAPTER 39

Common Injuries

Constance B. Brehm

Injuries are major pediatric health problems that are best managed with both treatment and prevention strategies. A child with an injury might respond best to (1) a simple home treatment by the parent, caregiver, or supervising adult; (2) intervention by the provider in the primary care setting; (3) referral to a medical specialist or inpatient facility; or (4) a combination of these. Health care professionals have a responsibility to assist families to prevent injuries from occurring. Chapter 10 discusses strategies for treatment of common injuries and prevention as part of ongoing health maintenance.

The term *accident prevention* has been replaced by *injury control*, to avoid the connotation that "accidents will happen," implying that nothing can be done to prevent them. Most injuries occur under fairly predictable circumstances to high-risk children and families (Rivara & Grossman, 2004). Beyond the first few months of life, injuries are the most common cause of death during childhood and are likewise an important cause of preventable pediatric morbidity and mortality in other age groups. Unintentional injuries cause more than 36% of the deaths among children 1 to 14 years old and more than 45% of deaths in youths 15 to 24 years old (National Center for Health Statistics, 2006).

This chapter focuses on the identification and management of common unintentional pediatric injuries frequently seen in primary care settings. Prevention of nonintentional injuries involves anticipatory guidance to help parents provide a safe environment for their children. Strategies to prevent injuries in children now focus on understanding and modifying risk factors, developing communitywide program approaches, and promoting health policy legislative agendas that focus on injury prevention.

◼ PRINCIPLES OF INJURY CONTROL

In the past, there was an underlying assumption that children were simply "accident prone" because of their highly active and impulsive nature. Earlier prevention efforts often focused on these childhood characteristics. Emphasizing accident proneness is now considered a counterproductive strategy. Injury control plans now focus on education or persuasion of parents and caregivers, changes in product design, and modification of the environment. This is an epidemiologic approach that looks at the interdependent host-agent issues, including the child, parent, and the environment within the social context. These agents may cause, prevent, or modify the injury process (Bass, 2006).

Another approach to preventing injury was suggested by Dr. William Haddon in 1997, who developed a matrix framework. Haddon advocated a triphasic temporal approach for intervention strategies looking at pre-event, event, and post-event issues and identifying appropriate educational and technological strategies, along with government action during each of these three time frames. The goals for the various stages would be: pre-event strategies—prevent the injury from occurring; event—reduce the severity of the injury; and post-event—improve the treatment of the injury (Bass, 2006).

Those involved in parent safety education agree that it is more advantageous to speak with parents specifically about using child car seat restraints and bike helmets than giving advice that is too general, such as recommendations to closely supervise children and "childproofing" the home. Anticipatory guidance provided by health providers at well-child visits should be geared to the developmental stage of the child. Written materials, audiovisual presentations, peer counseling, and one-to-one interaction with a health professional are all effective teaching and learning strategies. However, safety information should be provided in moderate doses, with reinforcement or repetition at subsequent visits.

Passive injury prevention has been an effective intervention and includes modification of everyday items in the child's environment. Examples include household products, such as the use of child-resistant caps on medicines and cleaning products, and caution in the design of toys so that they do not contain small parts, which are a choking hazard. Other effective strategies for environmental modification include use of smoke and carbon monoxide detectors, safe roadway design, reduction in traffic volume and speed in residential neighborhoods, and elimination of guns from the child's environment. Providers can advocate for local and national prevention strategies and support such programs as the *SafeKids USA* campaign (see Resource Box at the end of the chapter). They can also play a key role by supporting injury prevention legislation or initiatives. Public and consumer awareness is crucial for successful prevention programs.

Although most children with serious injuries are seen first in emergency departments (EDs), primary care providers have a professional obligation to remain current in basic life support techniques. Competence in performing emergency cardiopulmonary resuscitation and emergency intervention for choking (whether it be for infants, children, or adults) should be a requirement of all licensed health professionals employed in clinical practice settings. Likewise, all parents and caregivers should be encouraged to enroll in a basic pediatric life support program, especially parents and caregivers of infants and children at risk for cardiopulmonary arrest.

COMMON PEDIATRIC INJURIES
APPROACH TO TRAUMA

Any child sustaining more than trivial injury must be considered at risk of dying, and the pediatric provider needs to make an immediate assessment about the severity of the trauma. The approach includes primary assessment, evaluation of vital signs, and a quick review of essential functions for all organ systems. Resuscitation must be initiated if indicated. This takes place in the first 5 to 10 minutes of the assessment process. Secondary assessment follows and includes additional physical examination, radiographs, and laboratory tests, if indicated. Physical examination should be repeated serially and compared throughout treatment. Definitive care includes stabilization of the specific local injuries and possible preparation of the patient for transport to an ED if the injury is moderate to severe (Table 39-1).

TRAUMA TO THE SKIN AND SOFT TISSUE
Abrasions

Description.   A simple abrasion represents the loss of mucous membrane or the superficial layer (epidermis) of the skin without loss of dermal integrity. Abrasions are the equivalent of second-degree burns.

Epidemiology.   Abrasions often result from falls or friction accidents. Mechanical means, such as dermabrasion, can remove the superficial layer of the skin.

Clinical Findings.

History.   Seek information about the cause and type of injury and the presence of a foreign object or dirt at the accident scene.

Physical Examination.   The extent of the abrasion and the presence of dirt, grime, or other foreign body (e.g., tar) should be determined. Findings include an area of skin that appears scraped off with oozing of serum and blood. Be sure to note redness, heat, and swelling of the area, which may indicate presence of infection. Also assess any punctured body part (most commonly the foot) for circulation, sensation, and function.

Differential Diagnosis.   The history of an injury and physical findings are the key to diagnosis. Any other skin condition that can cause loss of epidermis, such as a burn, is included in the differential diagnosis.

Management.   Appropriate first aid care is important to prevent infection. Most abrasions can be managed at home unless the abrasion is deep, involves a large area, is associated with severe pain, or has significant dirt, grime, tar, or a foreign body in the wound. The immunocompromised patient may need to be seen. Corneal abrasions are discussed in Chapter 28.

Management of an abrasion includes the following points:
- Thoroughly cleanse the wound. The area can be scrubbed with an antibacterial cleanser using a wet gauze or soft surgical nail brush. Harsh agents such as Betadine, alcohol, or peroxide should not be used on open wounds. If dirt or dark-colored matter is not adequately removed, new skin may grow over the particles, resulting in a permanent tattoo. Gentle irrigation with copious amounts of normal saline or water (300 to 1000 ml) is the preferred method to thoroughly cleanse a wound and prevent infection.
- Débride pieces of loose skin with a sterile scissors and remove foreign particles with a tweezers. If tar particles are present, the area can be rubbed with petrolatum and then irrigated again.
- Leave small abrasions open to the air or apply a sterile bandage if desired.
- Cover larger abrasions with a sterile nonadherent dressing. Antibiotic ointment such as Bacitracin may be applied to abrasions of the elbows or knees to prevent cracking or reopening of the wound because of constant movement and stretching of the joints.
- Protect abrasions of the hands, feet, or areas overlying joints from friction and dirt until a protective dry scab is formed.
- Instruct the parent to wash the area at least every 24 hours and reapply the dressing and antibiotic ointments until a protective dry scab is formed. Instructions regarding the signs and symptoms of infection should also be provided.
- Antitetanus prophylaxis should be administered if the wound is significant. The use of Tdap is now the preferred vaccination (see Chapter 23).

TABLE 39-1   Classification and Disposition of Trauma by Severity

| | | | | Physical Examination | |
| | | | | Laboratory/Radiographic Studies | Probable Disposition |
Category	History	Vital Signs	Local Findings		
Mild	Minimal force	Normal	Superficial only	Few	Discharge
Moderate	Significant force	Normal	Suspicious for internal injury	Intermediate	Evaluate
Severe	Critical force	Abnormal	Indicative of internal injury	Many	Immediate therapy; admit

From Ruddy RM, Fleischer GR: Trauma—an approach to the injured child. In Fleischer GR, Ludwig S, Silverman B, editors: *Synopsis of pediatric emergency medicine,* Philadelphia, 2002, Williams & Wilkins, p 462.

Puncture Wounds

Description. Puncture wounds result from penetration of varying levels of the skin and its underlying tissue or structures. These wounds are typically classified as superficial or deep. Because of the potential for serious infection, puncture wounds must be carefully evaluated and treated if indicated. The location and depth of the wound, plus retention of a foreign object, are key risk factors for the subsequent development of infection. For example, deep penetrating wounds and injuries to the forefoot, especially if they involve the plantar fascia, have a higher risk of infection than wounds to the arch or heel area. The forefoot has less overlying soft tissue than other plantar surfaces and is the major weight-bearing area of the foot; therefore cartilage and bone can be involved. In contrast, puncture wounds to muscle, if clean, can be quite deep and still have a relatively low risk of infection.

Epidemiology. Puncture wounds are common pediatric injuries, generally first seen in children about 2 years old. A nail, often rusty, is the classic cause of an injury that requires health care intervention. Glass, wood splinters and toothpicks, needles, metal and wire, staples, and thumbtacks are other common sources of injury. Bites also produce puncture wounds and are especially infection-prone.

Although the majority of puncture wounds heal without problems, a sizable minority of these injuries are complicated by infections that may lead to cellulitis or soft tissue abscesses. The most common causative organisms are *Pseudomonas aeruginosa* and *Staphylococcus aureus*. *Pseudomonas* osteomyelitis can occur if the puncture wound has penetrated a bone or joint. A classic history is puncture to the foot through a sneaker, as *P. aeruginosa* colonizes on the foam-rubber sole of the sneaker and enters the wound when a nail or other object (toothpick or pins) punctures the foot. The end result can be a subacute focal osteomyelitis (Krogstad, 2006; Lampe, 2004).

Clinical Findings. In assessing a child with a minor wound, the provider should first exclude more serious, sometimes occult injuries that take precedence in management. Always consider nonaccidental trauma (child abuse), especially when the details of the accident, as told during the history-taking, fail to explain adequately the child's injury (Jenkins & Braen, 2005). Sometimes parents and children will seek care only after symptoms of secondary infection develop.

History. Important information to elicit after a report or suspicion of a puncture wound includes the following:
- Date of injury and wound care provided at the time of initial injury.
- Identification of the agent of injury. If it is not known what object penetrated the skin, the likelihood of an imbedded foreign body is high.
- Condition of the penetrating object. Was the object clean or rusty, jagged or smooth?
- Whether all or part of the foreign object was removed.
- Whether the child was barefoot or what type and condition of footwear was being worn (pertinent to injuries to the foot).
- Immunization status for tetanus coverage (see Chapter 23).
- Presence of any medical condition that increases the risk for infectious complications.

Physical Examination. Physical examination of the wound must include an assessment of the length and depth of the injury, circulatory status, motor and sensory function, the presence of foreign bodies and contaminants, and the involvement of underlying structures (nerves, tendons, muscles, ligaments, vessels, bones, joints, and ducts) (Jenkins & Braen, 2005). To examine the foot area (the most likely site of puncture wounds), have the patient lie prone and backward on an examination table, so that the head of the table or bed flexes the knee and brings the sole of the foot into clear view. Clean the surrounding skin (irrigate with saline), provide good lighting, and take time to carefully inspect the wound. Local anesthetic may be required.

The following examination findings indicate cellulitis:
- Localized pain or tenderness, swelling, and erythema at the puncture site, but may be more obvious on the dorsum of the foot
- Possible fever
- Pain with flexion or extension of the extremity involved
- Decreased ability to bear weight
- Pain along the plantar aspect of the foot during extension or flexion of the toes (may indicate deep tissue injury)

Findings indicative of osteomyelitis-osteochondritis are similar to those for cellulitis, with extension of pain and swelling around the puncture wound and to adjacent bony structures. There can be exquisite point tenderness over the bone, erythema, and decreased use of the affected extremity as well. In pyarthrosis (septic arthritis), there are findings of pain, swelling, warmth, and erythema over the affected joint and decreased range of motion and decreased weight-bearing ability of the affected joint. In the foot, the metatarsophalangeal joint of the great toe is most frequently involved.

Diagnostic Studies. The following are ordered as indicated (Jenson & Baltimore, 2006):
- Plain film radiograph should be ordered if a retained foreign body is suspected; if the object is still embedded; if there was penetration of a joint space, the bone or growth cartilage, or the plantar fascia of the foot; or if the puncture site is due to a nail injury and has signs of infection.
- If the radiograph is negative but a retained foreign object is still suspected, computed tomography (CT), ultrasound, and magnetic resonance imaging (MRI) are useful tools.
- Bone scan can be positive within 24 hours of the first appearance of symptoms of osteomyelitis.
- Complete blood count (CBC) may be needed. Assess for elevated WBC.
- Erythrocyte sedimentation rate (ESR) and C-reactive protein (CRP) may be mild to moderately elevated in osteomyelitis. ESR and CRP are sensitive tests for inflammatory response but are nonspecific. They are helpful in evaluating the effectiveness of treatment.
- Some recommend a baseline culture of the wound if it is infected.

Differential Diagnosis. A history of penetrating injury and the child's symptoms are the keys to whether the injury represents a superficial wound that will heal uneventfully or develop infectious complications.

Management. Buttaravoli & Stair (2000) outline a practical and straightforward approach to management of puncture wounds:

- If the puncture was created by a slender object, such as a needle or thumbtack, that was positively removed intact, no treatment other than gentle débridement and irrigation (with large amounts of normal saline) is necessary. For débridement, the puncture wound can be gently shaved using a No. 10 scalpel blade to remove the cornified epithelium and debris. If debris is found in the wound, gently slide the plastic sheath of an over-the-needle catheter (such as from an angiocatheter) down the wound track and slowly irrigate with physiologic saline solution, moving the catheter sheath in and out until debris no longer flows from the wound. At times, a small amount of local anesthetic will be necessary to accomplish this.
- If there is any question that a portion of a foreign body may have broken off in the tissues, obtain radiographs. Glass and metal may be visualized on plain films; plastic, aluminum, and wood are more radiolucent and may require ultrasound, CT scan, or MRI for visualization. If radiographs demonstrate that an embedded object has invaded bone, growth cartilage, or a joint space, refer the child immediately to an orthopedic surgeon. Retained foreign bodies increase the potential for infection and should be suspected in patients who have infection or are not responding to treatment of infection. Deep, highly contaminated wounds should also be referred, because débridement in the operating room may be necessary to prevent the catastrophic complications of osteomyelitis (Buttaravoli & Stair, 2000).
- If signs of infection or cellulitis are present, the wound should be cultured. Cultures can also be obtained by needle aspiration if necessary. Incision and drainage is recommended and methicillin-resistant *Staphylococcus aureus* (MRSA) resistant antibiotics started if MRSA is suspected (pus and/or signs of systemic infection).
- All wound management requires tetanus prophylaxis, if it has been more than 5 years since the last tetanus booster or if the date of the last booster is not known. Consider passive immunization with tetanus immune globulin (TIG) and initiation of primary tetanus series (DTap or Tdap as appropriate) in all children who may never have been immunized. This is sometimes the case among immigrant children or those whose parents have refused immunizations for reasons of personal belief (see Chapter 23).
- Once the wound has been adequately cleansed and débrided, coverage with a Band-Aid or gauze dressing is sufficient. For deep wounds, a small sterile wick of iodoform gauze may be placed inside the wound to keep the edges open. This gauze can be removed after 2 to 3 days, and the subsequent granulation tissue will aid healing. If signs of infection (minor redness or swelling) have appeared, or if the wound was particularly deep and contained debris, prescribe antibiotic coverage with Augmentin, cephalexin, or clindamycin and ciprofloxin (best choice if allergic to penicillin) for 10 to 14 days. If pus is present or MRSA is suspected, provide antibiotic coverage to treat MRSA. Change

antibiotic coverage if warranted after culture results are known. Schedule a return visit to recheck within 48 hours. If pain, erythema, and swelling do not improve within 48 hours of beginning oral antibiotics, consider intravenous antibiotics and possible hospitalization (Jenkins & Braen, 2005). Simple, uncomplicated clean wounds do not need antibiotic coverage in healthy older children.
- Ceftazidime or piperacillin-tazobactam and an aminoglycoside are used for the treatment of subacute focal osteomyelitis (Jenson & Baltimore, 2006).

Patient and Parent Education. Instruct parents to allow no weight bearing for 3 to 4 days for a foot injury. Patient education should include observation for signs and symptoms of infection, with the importance of prompt medical attention if there is persistent aching or discomfort.

Ingrown Toenails and Nail Hematoma

Description. Two problems commonly seen in pediatrics are ingrown toenails and nail hematomas from trauma to the nail. Ingrown toenails are a common disorder caused by any of the following: anatomic predisposition, improper nail trimming, trauma, or compression from constrictive shoes or stockings. The lateral edges of the nail curve inward and penetrate the underlying tissue, which results in erythema, pain, and swelling. With chronic ingrown toe nails, granulation tissue is often seen. Infants often exhibit pseudo-ingrown toenails that correct on their own by approximately 12 months (Paller & Mancini, 2006). Nail hematomas are due to injury and the formation of a subungual hematoma. Nail injuries that involve lacerations or fracture of the distal phalanx should be referred to an orthopedist; uncomplicated nail hematomas can be drained (nail trephination) by primary care providers, typically without local anesthetic.

Management. The treatment for these problems is as follows:

- For ingrown toenail:
  - Pack cotton under the nail edge to elevate the nail from inflamed nailbed.
  - Recommend elevation and soaking of the foot. Cleaning and promotion of drainage may be needed for more severe inflammation.
  - Instruct about wearing properly fitting shoes and correctly trimming the nails (i.e., straight across). Toenails should be trimmed so that a concave end is left to extend the nail edge beyond the skin.
  - Systemic antibiotics may be required with acute infection
- For nail hematoma:
  - Determine whether a digital or regional nerve block is needed (proper training is required).
  - Attempt to lift the nail to examine for the presence of significant nailbed injuries.
  - Irrigate nail surface with saline solution.
  - Make one or more holes in the area of the nail hematoma with either a portable heat cautery device or the end of an untwisted heated paperclip (heated to ensure sterility). A No. 11 scalpel blade is an alternative instrument. Create

a small hole or holes in the nail by applying downward pressure with a rotary motion of the scalpel.

- One or more holes will need to be made to permit continued drainage.
- Antibiotics generally are not needed.

Lacerations

Description. Lacerations are cuts through the skin; after contusions, they are the most common type of soft tissue injury seen in EDs. The face, scalp, and hands are the most common sites of injury in children. Lacerations often require more complicated treatment than other minor wounds because they can be associated with occult injuries to the deeper tissues and therefore require careful exploration. Prevention of infection is another major consideration. There are three main classes of lacerations: shear, tension, and compression injuries (Lipton, 2002).

Shear injuries are caused by sharp objects and usually cause little damage to surrounding tissues but can cause nerve, tendon, and vascular damage. They usually heal the fastest and have the lowest incidence of wound infection. The biggest danger of shear injuries is the potential damage to nerve, tendon, and vascular structures. Such injuries require repair of these delicate structures, which should only be attempted in EDs or in the operating room by a skilled surgeon.

Tension lacerations occur when stresses cause the skin to tear. These are accompanied by damage to surrounding tissues. A classic example is when a child falls and bumps his or her head on a dull edge of a piece of furniture, causing the skin to break open in the appearance of a laceration. These lacerations are irregularly shaped.

Compression lacerations occur during a crush injury and have irregular, often stellate wound edges. They can happen from a direct blow by a large blunt object. Because of their association with significant injury to the adjacent skin, they have the highest incidence of wound infection compared with other types of lacerations.

Epidemiology. Lacerations are caused by various forms of trauma. They are common reasons for pediatric health care visits.

Clinical Findings.

History. Important questions to ask include the following:

- How did the injury happen? Determining the mechanism of injury is essential in identifying the presence of contaminants or possible presence of a foreign body, such as dirt, debris, glass, and splinters.
- How long ago (number of hours) did the injury occur? Length of time since injury is a critical factor to consider.
- Does the child have allergies to antibiotics or anesthetics?
- What is the child's tetanus immunization status? Is there a need for further immunization?

Physical Examination. Important points in the examination of the injury are as follows:

- Cleanse the wound (see Management) and cover with saline-soaked gauze until a thorough examination can be made.

- Perform a neurovascular examination of pulses, motor function, and sensation distal to the laceration, and then search for foreign bodies and nerve or tendon injury. Evaluation of range of motion is especially important with wounds involving the distal forearm, wrist, and hand.
- Prepare the wound for exploration and repair (see Management).

Differential Diagnosis.
The history and physical examination provide the diagnosis.

Management. Depending on their preparation and experience in the treatment of minor wounds that require closure, providers may suture wounds or use medical grade cyanoacrylate glue when appropriate, and provide follow-up care. Significant wounds to the face, hands, or genital areas should be referred to a specialist, such as an orthopedic surgeon, who specializes in hand repair, or a plastic surgeon for plastic and reconstructive surgery (particularly for the face). Minor lacerations to the scalp or the arms and legs are commonly managed by care providers who have been trained in these techniques.

The steps in wound management are summarized as follows (Selbst & Attia, 2002):

1. *Decision to close the wound.* Compared with adults, children are less likely to get wound infections. In children, the infection rate is about 2% for all sutured wounds. Thus most wounds may be closed *primarily* (i.e., bringing the edges of the skin together, known as "approximation") as soon after the injury as possible to speed healing, prevent infection, and improve the cosmetic result. Delayed closure increases the risk of infection. Some researchers suggest a "golden period" for wound closure of 6 hours. However, wounds considered low risk for infection, such as a clean knife wound to an extremity, can be closed even 12 to 24 hours after the injury. Other guidelines to consider in wound closure include the following:
   - Most wounds to the face are best closed primarily even up to 24 hours after the injury to achieve an optimal cosmetic effect. If the wound is extensive or has high potential for infection (such as a dog bite), the operating room may be the best place for closure.
   - The risk of a laceration becoming infected is greater in areas with lower blood flow. For example, a hand or foot laceration is far more likely to become infected than a scalp laceration because the extremities of the body have lower blood perfusion than the head and scalp. Contaminated or crush wounds and those involving immunocompromised individuals should be closed promptly, within 6 hours of injury, because they are at high risk of infection.
   - Some contaminated wounds (animal or human bites or those occurring in a barnyard or in an immunocompromised individual) should be left open for healing by *secondary intention*, a process of healing by granulation and reepithelialization, although the scar formation may be more unsatisfactory with this method.
   - If a wound is not closed initially, *delayed primary closure (tertiary closure)* should be considered after the risk of infection decreases (about 3 to 5 days later). This is

recommended for selected heavily contaminated wounds and those associated with extensive damage, such as high-velocity missile injuries, crush injuries, and explosion injuries. The wound should be cleaned and débrided and covered at the time of initial treatment and then reassessed in a few days for infection and reconsidered for closure (Selbst & Attia, 2002).

2. *Anesthesia.* Appropriate use of conscious sedation and local anesthetics is essential for successful repair of lacerations in children. Proper wound care includes wound exploration and careful cleansing, which, when added to fear and anxiety, may be extremely painful. Infiltration of the wound with local anesthetic (such as lidocaine) can also help control bleeding. Discussion of anesthetic administration and the details of wound closure techniques are beyond the scope of this text. However, published texts are available that address procedures in primary/ambulatory care that include excellent information on local anesthetic and wound closure. Attendance at workshops that focus on wound management is also helpful.

3. *Hair.* Hair near the wound usually creates minimal difficulty during repair and generally does not need to be removed. In any case, hair should not be shaved because to do so can damage hair follicles and increase the risk of infection. Instead, the hair should be clipped with scissors when necessary. Alternatively, petroleum jelly can be used to keep unwanted scalp hair away from the wound while suturing. Eyebrow hair should not be removed because this may lead to abnormal or slow regrowth.

4. *Wound cleansing.* Use of chlorhexidine or povidone-iodine surgical scrub preparations, hydrogen peroxide, or alcohol in the wound itself is *not* recommended. These agents may be irritating to tissues and may increase infection by damaging white blood cells. The preferred method of wound cleansing is *irrigation* to reduce bacterial contamination and prevent subsequent infection. Normal saline remains the safest and most cost-effective choice for irrigation. The wound should be irrigated with at least 100 to 200 mL for the average 2 cm laceration. More solution may be needed if the wound is unusually large or contaminated. A large irrigating syringe (20 to 50 mL) with an attached splash guard can be used to reduce splatter during irrigation. *Scrubbing* the wound should be reserved for particularly "dirty" wounds in which contaminants are not effectively removed with irrigation alone. It may be necessary to extract some foreign material with fine forceps if it remains adherent after copious irrigation. This will prevent tattooing of the skin and reduce the risk of infection.

5. *Exploration of the wound.* The wound must be explored for presence of foreign bodies, deep tissue layer damage, injury to nerve or blood vessel, or joint involvement. It is imperative that the depth of the wound be determined. Wound probing is done with a Q-Tip, a hemostat, or a needle holder. Deep lacerations should be referred to an ED for layered closure. If tendon injury is suspected or if bone is exposed, referral to an orthopedist is the standard of care.

6. *Wound débridement.* Gentle removal of unattached loose tissues may be done with sterile instruments. Débridement is advantageous because it creates well-defined wound edges that can be more easily opposed. Although it is helpful to excise necrotic skin, excessive trimming of irregular lacerations should not be attempted. Existing wound irregularity (such as a zigzag wound) is actually helpful in approximation of the edges and allows for a more natural appearance in the scar. Excessive removal of tissue can create a defect that is difficult to close or that may increase tension at the wound margin, making scarring more likely.

7. *Wound closure.* There are several methods available for wound closure. Topical skin adhesive is one of the newest innovations in skin closure. The adhesive is applied on top of the skin while the edges of the wound are held together. Adhesive in the wound or between wound margins should be avoided. The adhesive takes less time to apply than stitches and forms a strong, flexible bond over the top of the wound and does not require a bandage. The topical skin adhesive sloughs off the wound as it heals, usually in 5 to 10 days, and does not require a return visit to the physician for suture removal.

Traditional stitches (or sutures) are often used to close cuts. This involves "sewing" the skin together with a needle and surgical thread. This procedure usually requires an injection of anesthetic and a bandage applied to the wound afterward.

Simple, uncomplicated lacerations to the scalp, trunk, arms, or legs may be closed with sutures (called *primary closure*). An absorbable suture material is used for closure of structures deeper than the epidermis and nonabsorbable sutures used to close the outermost layer of a laceration. Deep sutures relieve skin tension, decrease dead space, and probably improve cosmetic outcome.

Staples are gaining in popularity for wound closure, particularly in EDs. Staples can be applied rapidly and are associated with a lower infection rate, but can be more painful to remove. Surgical tape (Steri-Strips) are rarely used for primary closure because of inadequate strength in areas subject to tension. Table 39-2 compares wound closure techniques.

8. *Dressing.* Dress the wound using a nonadherent gauze for the first layer followed by a second layer of plain gauze if needed. Elasticized gauze (tubular net bandage) can be used to secure dressings.

9. *Immunization.* Give tetanus booster or tetanus immunoglobulin as indicated (see Chapter 23).

10. *Antibiotic controversy.* Antibiotic prophylaxis of clean wounds is not indicated. Its use in contaminated wounds may be helpful, but careful wound cleaning with extensive irrigation followed by prompt wound closure (when indicated) are the most effective safeguards in preventing infection.

11. *Suture and staple removal.* Remove sutures or staples depending on their location. See Table 39-3 for a useful guide.

12. *Bandage.* A nonocclusive bandage can be used to cover the sutured wound.

TABLE 39-2 **Advantages and Disadvantages of Common Wound Closure Techniques**

Technique	Advantages	Disadvantages
Suture	Time honored Meticulous closure Greatest tensile strength Lowest dehiscence rate	Requires removal Requires anesthetic Greatest tissue reactivity Highest cost Slowest application Highest risk of needle stick
Staples	Rapid application Low tissue reactivity Low cost Low risk of needle stick	Less meticulous closure May interfere with imaging techniques
Tissue adhesive	Rapid application Patient comfort Resistant to bacterial growth No need for removal Low cost Low or no risk of needle stick	Lower tensile strength than sutures Dehiscence over high-tension areas Not useful on hands Cannot bathe or swim
Surgical tape	Least reactive Lowest infection rate Rapid application Patient comfort Low cost No risk of needle stick	Frequently falls off Lower tensile strength than sutures Highest rate of dehiscence Requires use of toxic adjuncts Cannot be used in areas with hair Cannot get wet

From Lipton JD: Soft tissue injury and wound repair. In Strange GR et al, editors: *Pediatric emergency medicine: a comprehensive study guide*, ed 2, New York, 2002, McGraw-Hill.

TABLE 39-3 **Suture and Staple Removal Guide**

Location of Sutures	Length of Time Before Removal
Facial	3-5 days
Upper extremity	7-10 days
Trunk	10 days
Lower extremity	14 days
Over a joint	10-14 days

Patient and Parent Education. Instructions for wound care at home are best given in writing and should include the following information:

- The patient can briefly shower 48 hours after sutures are in place without worrying about the risk of possible infection. However, dry the area well and keep it dry at all other times.
- Note signs and symptoms of infection that warrant an early recheck (redness, swelling, discharge, increasing pain).
- Give instructions about cleansing and bandaging the wound.
- List any restrictions on activities.
- Identify a date for a return appointment.

Burns

Description. A burn injury to one or more layers of the skin and underlying tissues can cause varying degrees of damage. Burns are classified by depth of injury, percent of body surface area involved, location of the burn, and association with other injuries. The traditional classification of the depth of burns as first, second, third, or fourth degree is being replaced by the designations of superficial, partial thickness (superficial or deep partial thickness), and full thickness (Jenkins & Braen, 2005; Marcdante, 2006).

- Superficial burns (formerly first degree) involve only the epidermis. The skin is erythematous, but there are no blisters. Sensation is preserved. A common example is sunburn. Superficial burns usually heal within 1 week with little risk of scarring and infection and require only symptomatic treatment.
- Partial-thickness burns (formerly second degree) involve the epidermis and the dermis to a variable degree. The dermal appendages are always preserved and provide a source for regeneration.
  - Superficial partial thickness burns are red, painful, mottled, and blistered and heal in 10 to 21 days with no or little scarring.
  - Deep dermal partial-thickness burned areas appear pale and yellow, are weepy, and are painfully hypersensitive. They take longer to heal (3 weeks) and may result in scarring. The most common causes are exposure to hot liquids (immersion) and flames.
- Full-thickness burns (formerly third degree) are major thermal injuries. The dermis and dermal appendages/elements are destroyed. The skin appears whitish (a waxy white appearance) or leathery. The surface is dry and nontender

TABLE 39-4 Estimation of Surface Area Burned Based on Age*

Area	Birth to 1	1-4	5-9	10-14	15	Adult
Head	19	17	13	11	9	7
Neck	2	2	2	2	2	2
Anterior trunk	13	13	13	13	13	13
Posterior trunk	13	13	13	13	13	13
Right buttock	2.5	2.5	2.5	2.5	2.5	2.5
Left buttock	2.5	2.5	2.5	2.5	2.5	2.5
Genitalia	1	1	1	1	1	1
Right upper arm	4	4	4	4	4	4
Left upper arm	4	4	4	4	4	4
Right lower arm	3	3	3	3	3	3
Left lower arm	3	3	3	3	3	3
Right hand	2.5	2.5	2.5	2.5	2.5	2.5
Left hand	2.5	2.5	2.5	2.5	2.5	2.5
Right thigh	5.5	6.5	8	8.5	9	9.5
Left thigh	5.5	6.5	8	8.5	9	9.5
Right leg	5	5	5.5	6	6.5	7
Left leg	5	5	5.5	6	6.5	7
Right foot	3.5	3.5	3.5	3.5	3.5	3.5
Left foot	3.5	3.5	3.5	3.5	3.5	3.5

Age (years) spans the columns Birth to 1, 1-4, 5-9, 10-14, 15, Adult.

*This modification by O'Neill of the Brooke Army Burn Center Diagram shows the change in surface area of the head from 19% in an infant to 7% in an adult. Proper use of this chart provides an accurate basis for subsequent management of the burned child.
From Joffee M: Burns. In Fleisher GR, Ludwig S, Silverman B, editors: *Synopsis of pediatric emergency medicine*, Philadelphia, 2002, Lippincott Williams & Wilkins, p 529.

to palpation. These burn areas are characterized by coagulation and are avascular. Full-thickness burns result from prolonged exposure to fire or hot liquids and are associated with permanent scarring.

- Full-thickness burns with extension into deep tissues (formerly fourth degree), such as muscle, fascia, nerves, tendons, vessels, and bone, involve extensive injury. They typically require surgical intervention.

Burns involving large surfaces of the body generally vary as to their degree of depth. Burn wounds are dynamic, and the effect of dermal ischemia (affected by infection, exposure, and dehydration) may not be readily apparent at first. Their depth can also change from day to day. The percentage of body surface area (BSA) and the part(s) of the body affected are also key factors to determine treatment, disposition, and prognosis (Table 39-4). Multiple methods have been devised to estimate the BSA affected. For example, the area covered by a child's hand is considered to represent 1% of total BSA. This may be helpful for estimating the extent of small or patchy burns (Lukish, 2006).

Children with burn injuries who meet the following criteria are considered to have major burns and should be admitted to a children's hospital or burn center (Lukish, 2006).

- Partial-thickness burns involving 10% or more of BSA (considered serious)
- Burns involving the hands, face, feet, genitalia, perineum, or major joints; burns in certain body locations are high

risk for disability. These include greater than 1% burns to the face, perineum, hands, or feet; circumferential burns; or burns overlying joints; they are also high risk for disability.

- Full-thickness burns
- Chemical burns, electrical burns (including lightning injury), inhalation injury
- Burns associated with another injury (e.g., motor vehicle accident) or in a child with a preexisting medical disorder

Children with inhalation injury or associated trauma may also require hospital admission. Airway complications should be suspected if there is loss of consciousness, presence of facial burns, burns over nasal passages or oral cavity, hoarseness, change in voice, or presence of cough or wheezing (Jenkins & Braen, 2005).

Epidemiology. Burn statistics in children reveal that nearly 1% of all children sustain burn injuries each year. Approximately 25,000 children require hospitalizations for these injuries, and more than 800 children 1 to 14 years old die each year (Marcdante, 2006). In 2001, approximately 99,000 children less than 14 years old were treated in emergency departments for burn-related injuries. Thermal injuries are the fifth most common cause of unintentional death in children in the U.S. (Lukish, 2006). Modern technology has increased the exposure of children to potentially injurious thermal energy in their environment. Common modes of injury include scalding, flash injuries from ignition of volatile substances, and contact of clothing with a flame, resulting in ignition of fabrics. However, the house fire is by far the most lethal cause of burns in children and typically results in thermal and concomitant inhalation injury. Much has been done to reduce these injuries through the use of smoke detectors and fire safety instruction programs, yet house fires continue to take the lives of far too many children every year. Grease-related scald burns often have devastating results because they typically involve the face and hands (Lukish, 2006).

Boys younger than 5 years old have the highest rate of burn-related injury, with African-American, Native American, and Hispanic children at greater risk for such injuries than white children (Marcdante, 2006). Because younger children's skin is thinner than adults, their skin burns at lower temperatures with resultant deeper injuries than adults (Lukish, 2006).

The intentional inflicting of burns to a child is, unfortunately, a common form of abuse. Every burn injury in a child should be evaluated for a potential etiology of abuse or neglect. Intentionally inflicted burn injuries often leave a characteristic pattern (see Chapter 18).

Clinical Findings.

History. The following information should be obtained:

- Description of how the burn occurred, including agent of injury and length of time agent was in contact with the skin, circumstances surrounding the injury, when it occurred, and likelihood of other injuries, such as trauma or smoke inhalation
- Initial and subsequent treatment of the burn
- Previous history of burn injuries
- Other current medical problems, medications, allergies, and tetanus status
- Suspect child abuse if the accident occurred when the child was reportedly alone, is attributed to a sibling, the history varies from one interview to another, there is a previous history of accidental trauma, the history is incompatible with the observed injury, or there was delay in seeking medical attention (Ciorciari & Chou, 2003).

Physical Examination. The physical examination should begin by conducting a primary assessment of the airways. The most common cause of death during the first hour after a burn injury is respiratory impairment. Inhalation injury produces upper airway edema that can proceed with alarming speed to complete airway obstruction. Inhalation injury should be suspected if there is hoarseness, wheezing, rales, singed nasal hairs, carbonized sputum, cyanosis, or altered mental status. Inhalation injury may also be associated with facial or neck burns. In such cases, immediate emergency intervention (paramedics and immediate transport to the ED) is warranted. Once the patient is stable, a thorough physical examination requires the following determinations:

- Percentage of BSA affected (see Table 39-4)
- Type of burn and associated injuries
- Distribution and pattern of the burn with particular concern for circumferential burns to the thorax that may cause poor chest expansion and declining oxygen saturation

- Depth of the burn, classified as superficial, partial thickness, or full thickness
- Assessment of the vascular status of extremities
- Presence of any complicating medical condition

Diagnostic Studies.

- A CBC is indicated to establish baseline levels. The hematocrit will often be elevated secondary to fluid loss. White cell count may also be elevated as an acute phase reaction, but later may be an indicator of infection.
- Serum electrolytes may reveal elevated potassium due to cell breakdown.
- Renal function tests (blood urea nitrogen and creatinine) are used to assess renal and tissue perfusion. A urinalysis, particularly the specific gravity, helps determine hydration status, and presence of myoglobin may suggest acute tubular necrosis.
- Baseline clotting studies and typing and crossmatching may be indicated if there is associated trauma or if surgical intervention, such as grafting, is considered.
- Pulse oximetry, arterial blood gases, carboxyhemoglobin (for inhalation or suspected inhalation injury), and chest radiograph are indicated if there is airway involvement or vascular instability.
- Culturing of critical burn wounds may need to be done weekly or more frequently if infection develops.

Differential Diagnosis. Chapter 18 discusses intentional burn injuries resulting from child abuse. Scalded skin syndrome caused by staphylococcal infection can cause skin exfoliation, but the clinical presentation clearly differentiates it from an accidental burn injury. Management is similar to that used for burn management.

Management. Most children with major or serious burns require treatment in the hospital setting and management by a burn surgeon. Electric and chemical burns also require hospitalization for observation. Children with a burn injury associated with inhalation injury, fractures, suspicion of abuse, uncertainty of follow-up by the parent, or severe pain should also be admitted. The outpatient treatment of minor burns is an option only for superficial burns (first degree) or superficial partial-thickness burns (second degree) to less than 10% of BSA or a burn of less than 1% of BSA to the hands, feet, face, ears, and genitalia. Box 39-1 outlines the primary care management of superficial and partial-thickness burns. Deep partial-thickness burns covering greater than 10% of BSA or full-thickness burns covering more than 2% of BSA should be referred for hospital management by burn specialists.

Patient and Parent Education. The following points are important components of patient and parent education:

- Emphasize use of sunscreen protection to prevent sunburn (see Chapter 36). This is also very important for skin that is recovering from a burn because the skin will be prone to hyperpigmentation from sunlight for up to a year following the burn injury. Thus all skin that has been burned should be protected from sun for at least 12 months. Healed burns remain sensitive to the sun and sunburn more severely than nonburned skin. Encourage parents to avoid sun exposure

BOX 39-1   Management of Superficial and Partial-Thickness Burns in the Primary Care Setting

1. Maintain proper nutrition and hydration to enhance healing.
2. Management of superficial burns such as sunburn (Paller & Mancini, 2006):
   - Apply cool compresses (do not apply ice) or cool tub baths with colloidal oatmeal, baking soda, or cornstarch.
   - Apply moisturizers to the skin (emollient creams).
   - Administer analgesics, such as acetaminophen or ibuprofen topical formulations with pramoxine or menthol.
   - Apply topical preparations such as formulations containing pramoxine or menthol and a mild topical corticosteroid.
3. Management of superficial partial-thickness burns (Marcdante, 2006):
   - Cleanse the wound by generous irrigation with normal saline solution.
   - Monitor the burn daily for the first few days to ensure proper healing and assess for infection.
   - Treat very small areas, especially facial wounds, with polymyxin B/bacitracin/neomycin (Neosporin) ointment only and leave area open to air.
   - If bullae or blisters are present, do not open or "pop" them. They act as a natural bandage to keep bacteria out. Most will open eventually on their own, but while left intact they protect the underlying skin from infection and allow time for internal healing.
   - Gently débride open blisters to remove devitalized tissue and residue from prior dressing changes.
   - If the burn is less than or equal to 3% of the body surface area, Vaseline gauze (or fine gauze with Bacitracin ointment) in strips may be applied to the clean débrided area, followed by a dry gauze outer dressing.
   - For burn wounds greater than 3% of the total body surface area, apply silver sulfadiazine 1% (SSD or Silvadene) after the wound is cleansed unless the child has a known sulfa allergy. SSD is an antimicrobial and a soothing agent.
   - Apply strips of fine-mesh gauze over the wound. Do not wrap the wound with gauze because wrapped gauze can impair circulation if swelling occurs. Apply additional SSD to gauze strips.
   - Apply a dry outer gauze dressing that can be held in place by a tubular net bandage.
   - Administer adequate analgesic medication. Acetaminophen with codeine may be needed before the wound care is performed and during the day. Switch to over-the-counter acetaminophen or ibuprofen as the pain subsides. See Chapter 22 for pain management discussion.
   - Use mittens for young children to prevent scratching if itching occurs as the burn heals; if needed, administer an antihistamine such as diphenhydramine.
   - If a partial-thickness burn involves an extremity, keep it elevated to reduce edema and compromise of blood flow to the burned area. Persons with circumferential burns of an extremity may need to be admitted to the hospital for observation so that compartment syndrome does not develop.

---

as much as possible and to use a sunscreen with a sun protection factor (SPF) of 30 (or higher) if sun exposure is unavoidable.

- Discuss home and environmental safety issues related to burn prevention at health maintenance visits.
- Reinforce safety issues after a burn injury has occurred (e.g., scald prevention, use of smoke detectors, safekeeping of matches and cigarette lighters, safe use of electric cords and outlets).
- Teach first aid measures for burns (e.g., submerge minor burned area in cold water; rinse chemical burns in cold water, flushing skin thoroughly for at least 20 minutes).
- Inform parents of serious or long-term consequences of burns (e.g., frequent and significant sunburns during early childhood can predispose an individual to skin cancers in later life; electric burns cause thermal injury to skin [contact burn]; if an arc is created and there is passage of electrical current through the body, there is a potential for cardiac dysrhythmias and neurologic impairment following the burn episode).
- Inform parents that the extent of scarring is difficult to predict with certainty; that scarring depends on depth of the burn, length of time needed for healing, whether grafting was done, and the child's age and skin color; and that scars remain immature for the first 12 to 18 months and go through color and texture changes as the child grows. Most scald injuries from hot liquids heal quickly with little or no scarring.

Contusions and Hematomas

Description.   A contusion, or bruise, is an injury in which the skin is not broken but trauma has caused effusion into muscle and subcutaneous tissue with injury to the vessels and possibly the nerves. In children, contusions are most often seen on the extremities but can also be found on the face or head.

Epidemiology.   Contusions are common in children and are caused by blunt trauma, most often as a result of falling or bumping into objects during play. Participation in contact sports puts children at increased risk for contusions. Bruises to the trunk, face, or head should raise a red flag for possible child abuse. A careful history must be taken to determine whether the explanation of the injury is consistent with the child's condition and his or her independent report of what happened.

Hematomas are localized collections of extravasated blood that are relatively or completely confined within a space or potential space. In essence, a hematoma is a raised, palpable ecchymosis or bruise. Hematomas can be associated with most types of minor and major wounds; they must be observed closely for signs of infection and, in some instances, drained.

Clinical Findings.

History. The following should be assessed:

- Cause of bruise
- Treatment given
- History of easy bleeding or bruising, slow healing

Physical Examination. The following should be determined:

- Circulatory status and discoloration
- Motor and sensory function: reduced mobility or range of motion
- Involvement of underlying structures
- Presence of swelling
- Pain or point tenderness
- Limited mobility
- If there is any evidence of circulatory compromise, such as lack of pulse, it is important to seek care in the ED immediately.

Differential Diagnosis. Hemophilia, von Willebrand disease, and purpura should be considered. Myositis ossificans, a complication of contusions rarely seen in children, can be confused with osteogenic sarcoma.

Management. With contusions involving extremities:

1. Acute phase, first 24 hours (Grudziak & Musahl, 2007)
   - Prescribe rest, ice, compression, and elevation (RICE):
      - Rest and immobilize the affected part (this is best achieved with a splint in extremity injuries).
      - Ice (or cold compress with an ice bag wrapped in a towel) applied to the injury for 10 to 20 minutes per hour for the first 24 hours.
      - Compression: application of a pressure bandage to help prevent swelling.
      - Elevation of the affected part (ideally, above the level of the heart) to prevent swelling.
   - Provide appropriate analgesia. A nonsteroidal antiinflammatory medication, such as ibuprofen, is a good choice.
2. Twenty-four to 48 hours after the acute phase of tenderness and swelling:
   - Apply warm compresses or soaks.
   - Stretch.
   - Do range-of-motion and strengthening exercises.
3. For 5 to 7 days, avoid exercise that involves the contused area.
4. Reserve radiographs for suspected foreign bodies or bone fractures.
5. Refer severe injuries for orthopedic management.

Complications. Most contusions heal quickly without sequelae, but severe trauma to the quadriceps muscle can lead to myositis ossificans if not treated properly or, with large hemorrhage, to compartment syndrome.

Patient and Parent Education. Explain to parents the expected color changes of ecchymosis from the purple discoloration to greenish and that the ecchymosis may also migrate to other surrounding tissues. Arrange for follow-up if there is continuing or increasing discomfort. Encourage parents to provide their children with a physical environment that minimizes risk of injury. Return to activities is determined by the degree of injury and resolution of subjective symptoms. A program of rehabilitation may be needed (Grudziak & Musahl, 2007).

Sprains and Strains

Description. Ligaments act to help stabilize a joint. A sprain is a tear of a ligament joining bone to bone around the joint and is caused most commonly by outside forces, especially contact sports. Strains are tears of the muscle or of fascia joining muscle to bone, often resulting from a dynamic injury and usually not a contact sport.

Sprains and strains may occur concurrently, and both can be graded by severity as a first-degree, second-degree, or third-degree injury. A grade I sprain involves minimal stretching of a ligament with no major change in the affected joint. However, small hemorrhagic areas are noted on histologic examination. A grade II sprain results in more tearing and hemorrhaging of the ligament than seen with a grade I sprain. There is mild-to-moderate functional loss and bleeding but the ligament is still holding. A grade III sprain is a complete disruption of the ligament with ligamentous instability and often requires casting (Eustace et al, 2007).

Ankle injuries are common in children and account for 25% to 38% of all physeal injuries with the vast majority of injuries occurring during sports participation. Injuries causing ankle sprains are due to ankle inversion, eversion, or a combination of the two. In pediatrics, 5.5% of ankle injuries are fractures; the others are strains and sprains. Approximately 85% of ankle sprains are due to inversion injuries, 5% are due to eversion injuries, and 10% are combinations of the two (Hergenroeder & Chorley, 2004).

Epidemiology. Sprains are a common athletic injury in children. They most commonly affect the ankle, knee, shoulder, elbow, or wrist and are caused by falls or contact in which the extremity is immobile or moving on one plane and a countervailing force is applied to the joint. In general, the degree of disability immediately after the injury correlates with the severity. For example, if an athlete is injured during a game and cannot walk off the playing field, he or she is more likely to have a serious injury than one who is able to continue playing. Ankle sprains in the child or preadolescent are less common than fractures because the ligaments in this age group are much stronger than the growth plates or even bone. If a ligamentous injury occurs in a child with an open growth plate, an associated avulsion fracture is almost always present. Once skeletal maturity is reached, however, ankle sprains become the most common sports injuries (Anderson, 2002; Hyman & Moore, 2006).

Muscle strain is a common injury and can indicate delayed muscle soreness (muscle pain 24 to 72 hours after intense physical activity) and a partial or complete muscle tear. This injury is commonly seen in fatigued muscles that are not able to lengthen in a controlled fashion (Eustace et al, 2007).

Clinical Findings.

History. The following are assessed (McMahon, 2007):

- Detailed history of the mechanism of injury (e.g., fall, collision, twisting of joint).
- Description of symptoms (e.g., onset, location, duration, characteristics, aggravating and relieving factors).
- Type of first aid treatment given.
- Sprain complaints depend on the site of ligamentous injury:

○ Calf—some children may describe an immediate sharp pain, hear or feel a "pop" or "snap," and are unable to raise their lower leg, or complain of calf pain when raising their leg.

○ Ankle—inversion injury. In younger children, tears of the lateral ankle ligament often disrupt the open growth plate of the distal fibular. In contrast, with skeletal maturity, classic lateral ankle sprain is more common in an adolescent than a Salter-Harris I fracture of the distal fibula.

○ Wrist—swelling and pain along the dorsum of the wrist; positive Watson sign (pain and an audible click heard when dorsal pressure is placed over the distal scaphoid while performing ulnar and radial deviation)

○ Lumbar—midline tenderness as these sprains are often due to injury to the interspinous process ligament; low back pain and paraspinal muscle spasm are common; neurologic symptoms are absent

• Strain complaints depend on the site of muscular injury (McMahon, 2007):

○ Calf— may describe an immediate sharp pain, hear or feel a "pop" or "snap," and are unable to raise the lower leg or complain of pain when raising the lower leg

○ Cervical—limited range of motion and tenderness over the involved neck muscles

○ Lumbar—either acute or chronic back pain; pain is limited to the back or paraspinal muscles and there is no radiating pain to the lower extremities; may have a painful trigger point with palpation

Note: An orthopedic injury should be suspected if there is a history of significant trauma (fall from height, motor vehicle accident, etc.) or if the patient complains of pain after an injury. However, the cause may have been unwitnessed or not noticed, so that an injury is not suspected until significant swelling becomes apparent. Toddlers and young children may present with crying after an unwitnessed fall. In addition, children can self splint injuries, particularly buckle fractures of the distal forearm, so that the discomfort may appear minimal (Mann, 2003).

Physical Examination. The approach to the physical examination depends on the joint involved, the severity of the injury, and the child's ability to cooperate. If the injury is acute, it can be difficult to distinguish the extent of damage. The child may require additional visits for a more careful examination as the swelling and pain subside. Always examine the joints and structures located above and below the injury for possible involvement, check function of the injured part, and check circulation and sensation. Any circulatory compromise or notable reduction in sensation (numbness or paralysis) suggests a more serious injury and should be referred to the ED or an orthopedist. During the examination, use the corresponding joint and muscle mass in the other extremity as a control for comparison. Inspect for degree of swelling and ecchymosis over the affected side of the ankle. In differentiating ankle fractures versus ankle sprains, findings on physical examination can be helpful. Ankle strains are marked by swelling and tenderness directly over the talofibular ligament; distal fibular physis fractures are associated with tenderness over the lateral malleolus growth plate (Hyman & Moore, 2006).

Diagnostic Studies. Radiographs are indicated if a fracture or dislocation is suspected. Suspicious findings that suggest the need for radiographs include gross deformity, serious impairment in mobility of the injured area, point tenderness examination, and moderate-to-severe swelling. Simple radiographs of extremities or other major joint systems are relatively inexpensive and can be useful in distinguishing a sprain or strain from a fracture. Table 39-5 identifies a grading system for ankle injuries. With ankle injuries, carefully assess the ankle area for proximal fibula tenderness and, if present, include tibial-fibula radiographs to check for a high fibula fracture (Hyman & Moore, 2006). To rule out fractures and dislocations of the cervical spine, two orthogonal radiographic views from the occiput to the T1 junction are needed. MRI is necessary if there is cervical instability or neurologic compromise.

Stiell and colleagues (1995) developed the Ottawa Ankle Rules to guide clinical decision-making regarding when radiographs are indicated for certain foot and ankle injuries. Fig. 39-1 depicts the Ottawa Ankle Rules (OAR). These rules have been applied successfully in adult populations and are shown

TABLE 39-5	Grading of Ankle Injuries	
Severity	**Signs and Symptoms**	**Disability**
Grade I (mild)	Minimal swelling (clear definition of Achilles tendon), small area of tenderness, little or no hemorrhage, minimal decreased range of motion	Little or no limp with walking; minimal difficulty hopping
Grade II (moderate)	Moderate swelling (margin of Achilles tendon less defined), more generalized tenderness, some hemorrhage, decreased range of motion	Obvious limping with walking; unable to run, unable to hop, unable to do toe raise
Grade III (severe)	Diffuse swelling (no clear margins of Achilles tendon), widespread tenderness, hemorrhage evident, pronounced decreased range of motion	Unable to bear weight; involuntary guarding with examination

Adapted from Hergenroeder A, Chorley JN: Sports medicine. In Behrman RE, Kliegman RM, Jenson HB, editors: *Nelson textbook of pediatrics*, ed 17, Philadelphia, 2004, WB Saunders, pp 2302-2320.

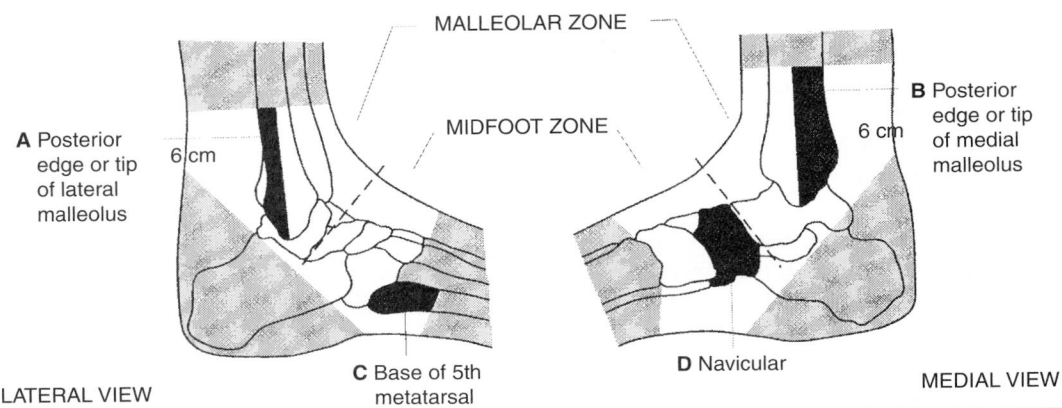

FIG. 39-1 The use of radiography in acute ankle injuries: Ottawa Ankle Rules. (From Stiell IG et al: A study to develop clinical decision rules for the use of radiography in acute ankle injuries, *Ann Emerg Med* 21:384-390, 1992, with permission from the American Academy of Emergency Physicians.)

An ankle x-ray series is required only if there is any pain in the malleolar zone and any of these findings:

- Bone tenderness at **A**
- Bone tenderness at **B**
- Inability to bear weight both immediately and in emergency department

A foot x-ray series is required only if there is any foot pain in midfoot zone and any of these findings:

- Bone tenderness at **C**
- Bone tenderness at **D**
- Inability to bear weight both immediately and in emergency department

to save time and money in the health care system without compromising quality of care. Because their appropriateness in pediatric populations is still not confirmed, it is recommended that their use be limited to older children (postpubertal).

The study by Stiell and colleagues (1995) demonstrated that "use of these rules led to a decrease in ankle radiography, waiting time, and costs without an increased rate of missed fractures." The rules state that an ankle radiograph series is required only if there is any pain in the malleolar zone. A foot radiograph is required only if there is any pain in the midfoot zone (see Fig. 39-1). Several studies have supported the use of the Ottawa Ankle Rules to help avoid unnecessary radiographs for ankle injuries. However, Clark & Tanner (2003) conducted a prospective research study involving 195 pediatric patients. They concluded that the OAR is not as sensitive in predicting ankle fractures in children as in adults. These researchers identified three additional variables useful in predicting possible fracture (and indication for radiograph) with these being: (1) inability to walk immediately after the injury event; (2) inability to bear weight for four steps in the ED, and (3) tender deltoid ligament. The OAR should be used in conjunction with the additional variables in decision-making regarding use of radiograph to determine the presence of fracture after ankle injury (Clark & Tanner, 2003).

The Ottawa Knee Rules (OKR) are also available to use as guides for when to order radiographs in cases of acute knee injury in patients over 18 years old. Studies have demonstrated that relying on the OKR in pediatric populations does not always identify all patients with knee fractures (Khine et al, 2001). However, a multicenter study investigated the use of OKR in 750 children between 2 to 14 years old who came to the ED with a knee injury (Bulloch et al, 2003). The findings of Bulloch and colleagues indicated that OKR identified fractures in children with a high degree of accuracy. The four OKR criteria used in this study as indicators for the presence of a fracture were: tenderness at the head of the fibula (it must

be the only area of bone tenderness), isolated tenderness of the patella, inability to flex 90 degrees, and inability to bear weight (4 steps) immediately and in the ED. However, until greater certainty is established about the use of OKR in children, liberal referral for radiograph in cases of knee injury in children is still recommended.

Differential Diagnosis. If there is excessive swelling or discoloration around the joint, suspect a fracture or dislocation, especially of the epiphysis. The degree of pain or pain behavior (i.e., dramatic) does not distinguish a sprain or strain from a fracture. Preverbal children, in particular, may have difficulty localizing pain, may complain of generalized pain, or may experience referred pain in one area caused by injury in an adjacent area. Although trauma is the most common cause of joint pain in children, infectious, rheumatologic, inflammatory, neoplastic, and hematologic abnormalities also should be considered, especially with fever, joint effusion, swelling, or erythema.

Management. Care of sprains and strains differs depending on the grade of injury. Children with severe sprains or strains (third-degree injury) should always be referred to an orthopedist. Management for lesser injuries is as follows:

1. Acute management for grade I or II sprains and strains:
   - RICE (rest, ice, compression, and elevation of the injured part, as discussed previously). Apply ice immediately for 15 to 20 minutes, and then, depending on the severity of the injury, every 2 to 6 hours for the first 24 to 48 hours. Ice may be applied using massage (a paper cup filled with water and frozen is ideal), ice packs, or immersion of the injured part in an ice water bath. A pressure bandage, preferably an adhesive tape athletic wrapping, may then be applied with gentle, steady pressure. An ace wrap is less effective. Take care not to allow impairment of circulation. Elevate the limb. There should be non-weight bearing until pain diminishes.

- Give nonsteroidal antiinflammatory medication with food. Initially, NSAIDs can be used for 7 to 10 days without affecting muscle healing, but longer use may interfere with muscle healing at a later stage.
- Heat may be used after 48 hours for mild sprains to facilitate healing.
2. Nonacute/chronic management:
   - May be weight bearing as tolerated.
   - Apply stabilizer or brace for unstable joint; may be needed for 3 to 6 weeks.
   - Recommend rehabilitation exercises, including range of motion, stretching, and strengthening. Rehabilitation should be gradual, beginning with isometric exercises of muscles and progressing to fuller range of motion and strengthening exercises. There should be no pain or swelling as exercise progresses. A general rule of thumb for return to sport activities for ankle sprains is 1 month for grade I, 2 months for grade II, and up to 3 months for grade III sprains. Ultrasound therapy may be beneficial.
   - Apply ice after exercise.
   - Athletes should not return to competition after a sprain until they are pain free and can perform all sports-specific activities.
3. Severe sprains may need casting or surgery (Latterman et al, 2007).

Patient and Parent Education.   Prevention of injury is key. Teach children and parents the importance of using protective gear (e.g., wrist guards for skaters). Children should also be encouraged to maintain a continuous level of physical activity to maximize muscle strength. See Chapter 14 for a discussion of children's participation in athletic activities.

Prevention of strains can be achieved with consistent stretching, warm-up exercises, and maintenance of muscle strength through regular activity. Strength training may reduce the incidence and severity of overuse injuries. For children who wish to participate in sports activities, advise them to structure a period of conditioning into their schedules.

Fractures and Dislocations

Description.   A fracture involves a disruption in the continuity of bone tissue, with bowing or a break, with or without separation. Pediatric patients have unique patterns of fractures due to the immaturity of bone and the dynamic nature of skeletal growth. Fractures are more common than ligamentous injuries or sprains in children due to the relative weakness of the physis or growth plate (Dobiesz & Greenfield, 2002; Hyman & Moore, 2006). Fractures that occur in the physis, epiphysis, metaphysis, or diaphysis may be complete, greenstick, buckle, comminuted, avulsed, transverse, oblique, or spiral. Various types of epiphyseal fractures based on the Salter-Harris classification system are discussed in Chapter 37. Stress fractures are discussed later in this chapter.

Dislocations are characterized by displacement of bone ends from their normal position in a joint. There can be wide variation in degree of displacement.

Epidemiology.   Fractures are relatively common in children, accounting for 10% to 15% of all childhood injuries (Thompson, 2006), with Salter II being seen most often (75%). Each year approximately 3.5 million children are seen in emergency departments for orthopedic injuries (Hyman & Moore, 2006). The majority of these injuries occur in children older than 10 years old. Clavicular fractures may be due to birth trauma and are discussed in Chapter 37. Accidents in which the child tries to break a fall using outstretched arms can result in fractures of the wrist, ulna, radius, or humerus. Direct trauma to bones or joints (e.g., resulting from contact sports, auto accidents, falls) can cause fractures or dislocations.

Clinical Findings.

History.   A description of the acute trauma, and the signs and symptoms occurring at the time of trauma, provides useful data. An accurate history of the time of the event, mechanism of injury, and direction of forces is important and helps define the type of injury. Often such orthopedic injuries are not witnessed. A child may be too frightened, in too much pain, or too immature to articulate what happened to give a reliable history. However, children rarely complain about persistent pain unless there is an abnormality. Be sure to ask about any history of previous injury and aggravating disease processes, such as preexisting bleeding abnormality, rickets, renal failure, liver disease, or malignancy. A delay in seeking medical care or a history that is vague or inconsistent with injuries is suggestive of child abuse (see Chapter 18).

Physical Examination.   Carefully inspect the injured part and the adjacent body parts, keeping in mind that pain and tenderness may be referred from injury in another area. Meticulously check for the following three functions:
1. Motor function, including range of motion, both passive and active. Note any limitations, particularly problems with tendon functioning. This is especially important with hand or finger injuries.
2. Sensory function, especially for any loss of sensation or numbness. Use a body chart to map the location. The existence of point tenderness, produced by palpating over a particular area, is suggestive of possible fracture.
3. Vascular function, especially for evidence of any vascular compromise.

These three functions are easily remembered by using the initials M/S/V. The provider should carefully document findings before and after any manipulation that is done. Significant findings include the following:
- Deformity
- Swelling
- Ecchymosis
- Misalignment of bone or joint
- Loss of function or mobility (especially with dislocation); limping or inability to bear weight
- Muscle spasm
- Discoloration (pallor or cyanosis)
- Decrease in vascular function, such as capillary refill, diminished or absent pulses

Lacerations with open fractures must be treated promptly in the ED. Dislocations are rare, and when they do occur, they most commonly involve the radial head or patella. Fractures often accompany dislocations because the ligamentous structures are more resistant to trauma (Table 39-6).

TABLE 39-6	Assessment and Management of Fractures		
Injury	**Clinical Findings**	**Diagnostic Studies**	**Management**
Fracture/ dislocation	Point tenderness over site, generalized pain, deformity, misalignment of bone or joint, loss of function or mobility (especially in dislocation), muscle spasm, discoloration, swelling, lacerations (if open fracture) *Clinical pearl:* tenderness below the lateral malleolus is typically ankle sprain, not fracture; if excessive swelling or discoloration along the joint, suspect fracture or dislocation, especially of epiphysis	Lateral and anteroposterior radiographs; may need to repeat in 10-14 days because early and Salter I fractures may not appear on first films	Referral for casting or other orthopedic interventions
Stress fracture (repeated microtrauma)	Gradual onset of pain with activity that decreases with rest, point tenderness, local swelling; distal atrophy may be noted	Radiograph; if normal, do a bone scan/ ultrasonography	Rest and eliminate activity that caused microtrauma for 10-14 days; casting if complete fracture; retraining

Diagnostic Studies. Because of pain, anxiety, and the possibility of an unreliable or incomplete history, the health provider must maintain a high index of suspicion for possible fracture. Radiography must be considered for findings of deformity, marked swelling, pain, ecchymosis, point tenderness, numbness, and loss of function. See Fig. 39-1 for the use of radiography in acute ankle injuries using the Ottawa Ankle Rules. Diagnostic findings suggestive of a patient having a positive extremity radiograph are found in Table 39-7.

Lateral and anteroposterior radiographic views should be obtained along with radiographs of the joint above and below an injury. Because of the growth plates, comparison views may be obtained on a selective basis. Always request contralateral radiographs if a suspected fracture is in a region where ossification is not complete (Hyman & Moore, 2006). This is especially helpful for elbow fractures in children. Early fractures and Salter I fractures do not always appear on radiographs at the time of injury. However, follow-up radiographic studies 7 to 10 days after the trauma may reveal a fracture line. Guidelines for ordering radiography after ankle injuries are discussed earlier in this chapter.

A CT scan may be necessary to delineate articular fractures or for complex physeal fractures (e.g., in the area of the distal tibia). Toddler's fracture (an oblique fracture of the distal one third of the tibia without a fibula fracture) may not be seen radiographically. An oblique view may help to visualize the fracture.

Differential Diagnosis. The cause of a fracture should be determined because fractures can also be due to pathologic conditions, such as osteogenesis imperfecta, sarcoma, hyperparathyroidism, and nutritional deficit (rickets, copper deficiency). Chronic use of the drug phenytoin can produce a rickets-like picture (Mann, 2003). Children who are physically abused may have multiple fractures at different

TABLE 39-7	Diagnostic Findings Suggestive of a Patient Having a Positive Extremity Radiograph	
Upper Extremity		**Lower Extremity**
Gross deformity		Gross deformity
Activity restricted		Activity restricted
Bone point tenderness		Bone point tenderness
Pain on motion		Pain on motion
Swelling moderate or severe		Knee injury
Time since injury >6 hours		Foot injury

From Mayeda DV: Orthopedic injuries: management principles. In Barkin RM, Rosen P, editors: *Emergency pediatrics: a guide to ambulatory care,* ed 5, St Louis, 1999, Mosby, p 518.

stages of healing or have a history of repeated fractures. The fractures typically seen in cases of child abuse involve the skull, ribs, or vertebrae, or spiral, oblique, or transverse fractures in the long bones (especially in children before the age of walking). Chapter 18 discusses findings of child abuse in more detail.

Management. All suspected fractures should be splinted promptly. This stabilizes the fracture to prevent damage to the surrounding soft tissues and reduces pain by reducing movement. If the injury is to an extremity, immediate intervention requires application of ice and elevation of the body part to prevent swelling. Uncontrolled swelling can cause neurovascular compromise if confined to a compartment.

Simple fractures can usually be reduced and immobilized easily. They typically heal quickly with no disruption in the child's growth. The potential for impairment to growth plates, joints, tendons, or neurovascular structures following trauma is of serious concern. All children with fractures, other than simple fractures or dislocations need immediate referral to an orthopedic specialist for management. Open reduction is often necessary with severe fractures. Pediatric elbow fractures are often difficult to diagnose and are prone to complications. Referral of these fractures to a pediatric orthopedist is usually needed.

Because dislocations often involve fractures in addition to the stretching and deforming of the ligaments, it is best to have an orthopedist involved for the dislocation reduction procedure. Analgesia is usually required before the reduction, and radiographic studies should be obtained before and after the reduction. Open dislocations or those associated with neurovascular compromise are true emergencies and must be referred immediately for emergency care. Patients recovering from fractures and dislocations should be provided with appropriate and adequate analgesia because both fractures and dislocations are painful injuries.

Indications for orthopedic consultation include (Mann, 2003):
- Compound, complete, or pathologic fracture
- Displaced fracture requiring reduction
- Growth plate (Salter) injury
- Grade II or III sprain
- Suspected neurovascular compromise
- Specific fractures: supracondylar, pelvic, hip, femoral
- Specific dislocations: shoulder, patellar, tarsometatarsal

Patient and Parent Education.   Patients and parents should be provided with information concerning cast care or application of compression bandages, use of ice to minimize swelling, and keeping the injured part immobilized and elevated as much as possible. They should also be cautioned to carefully observe the injury for signs of worsening pain, circulatory compromise, or delayed healing and should promptly notify their health care provider if any such signs occur. As with strains and sprains, prevention of injury through use of protective devices, proper conditioning, and attention to the child's physical environment is essential.

Stress Fractures

Description.   Stress fractures are classified as overuse injuries and are becoming more common in children. They are caused by repeated muscular action on a bony insertion site or repetitive direct trauma. Bone remodeling cannot keep up with the repeated microtrauma, which leads to bone reabsorption and fracture. Stress fractures in athletes are typically associated with too much training and minimal recovery time.

Epidemiology.   Stress fractures occur in typical locations and are associated with activities and sports. Common sites and causes include the following:
- Metatarsal shaft—running, marching, and ballet
- Tarsal navicular—running, high-impact aerobics
- Distal fibula and proximal tibia—running
- Ribs—coughing and golf
- Neck and shaft of the femur—running, ballet, and gymnastics

Clinical Findings.   Characteristic history includes:
- Gradual onset of pain (insidious) with activity that decreases with rest

- Point tenderness over the fracture site, and local swelling
- Distal atrophy may be noted

The typical history is that of excessive exercising or beginning an aggressive exercise program without preconditioning (see Table 39-6).

Diagnostic Studies.   Most stress fractures typically show normal radiographic findings or a zone of radiolucency. Only 10% of stress fractures are initially positive on radiograph. Bone scan (the more sensitive test) may be needed to identify the fracture if radiographs are normal. It identifies a "hot spot" at the fracture site and helps to identify other bones that are at risk (Latterman et al, 2007).

Management.   Management includes rest and eliminating the repetitive activity that is the source of the microtrauma for 10 to 14 weeks. Noncompliant patients may need to be casted for immobilization, usually for 6 to 8 weeks. For fractures of the forefoot (metatarsal fracture), a hard soled shoe (e.g., cast shoe) or removable boot with a rocking sole can be used. A tarsal fracture can be treated by being protected or with non-weight bearing for 6 to 8 weeks. Complete fractures need to be referred to an orthopedic surgeon and most likely will be casted. Retraining is necessary to eliminate the source of the problem, with a gradual return to activity. If symptoms reappear, more rest is needed (Drendel et al, 2002; Hergenroeder & Chorley, 2004; Latterman et al, 2007).

Subluxation of the Radial Head

Description.   Subluxation of the radial head, also known as "nursemaid's elbow" or "pulled elbow," occurs frequently in infants and children from 2 to 5 years old. Recurrence is an issue in 5% to 39% of cases but generally is no longer a problem after 5 years old (Hyman & Moore, 2006). The injury occurs when abrupt longitudinal (axial) traction is applied to the wrist or hand of the extended, pronated forearm of the young child. This action causes the annular ligament to become partially detached from the head of the radius. It then slips into the radiohumeral joint, where it becomes entrapped (Bachman & Santora, 2002).

Epidemiology.   Often subluxation results from an unintentional injury when a child's arm is suddenly tugged when stepping off of a curb or when the child is swung by the forearm. It can be a recurrent problem (not related to child maltreatment). It can also occur if the arm of an infant is trapped beneath the child's trunk as the child is rolled over. The injury is occasionally reported as the result of a fall. However, pulling of the child's arm, especially if this is a recurrent problem, may be the result of inappropriate disciplining, ignorance, or child maltreatment.

Clinical Findings.

History.   Often the history is nonspecific as to a report of an injury, and the parent may not have been aware of when the injury occurred. The classic presentation is that of a child who cries with pain and refuses to use an arm after being pulled or lifted by that same arm (Bachman & Santora, 2002). The toddler with nursemaid's elbow may be comfortable, but refuses to actively flex the elbow. There is no swelling and minimal tenderness around the elbow or wrist unless passive flexion of the elbow is attempted (Hyman & Moore, 2006; Mann, 2003).

Physical Examination. Common findings in children include the following:

- The child uniformly holds the arm in pronation with the elbow slightly flexed. The degree of distress may appear minimal, but range of motion of the elbow elicits pain.
- Mild tenderness may be noted with palpation of the radial head and pain is localized to the lateral aspect of the elbow.

Diagnostic Studies. Radiographs are not routinely recommended when the history and clinical presentation are classic. However, if obtained, radiography of the elbow is normal.

Differential Diagnosis. Subluxation has a classic history and presentation. If the child does not improve after the reduction procedure (see next section), a fracture of the elbow or clavicle should be considered. The clinical presentation of a fracture may be similar to that of a subluxation injury. Consider maltreatment if recurrent dislocations or other symptoms or signs are present.

Management. Reduction of a subluxed radial head is one of the most gratifying procedures for a primary care provider and parents alike. Two techniques can be used to reduce the radial head: supination and flexion or pronation and flexion. The steps to correct the subluxation involve the following:

- Approach the child in a slow, nonthreatening way and distract the child by talking or other diversionary tactics.
- Use either the supination and flexion technique as illustrated in Fig. 39-2 or the pronation and flexion technique. With the pronation and flexion technique, the examiner hyperpronates the child's forearm by a slight counterclockwise motion and flexes the elbow while applying gentle longitudinal traction (Shah, 2002).
- A palpable or audible "pop or click" usually signals successful reduction. Typically the patient again reaches for objects with the affected arm within 15 minutes of reduction. No further treatment is necessary.

Several attempts (up to three at reduction may be necessary) before the patient resumes normal use of the arm. If normal use does not follow reduction attempts, alternative diagnoses should be considered. In these cases, immobilization with prompt orthopedic follow-up is indicated.

Patient and Parent Education. Key points to cover include the following:

- Instruct parents not to lift or pull the child by the hand or elbow.
- The condition tends to recur until the child is approximately 5 years old in up to 30% of cases.

Compartment Syndrome

Description. Compartment syndrome is a complication of soft tissue injuries (e.g., fractures, crush injuries, and strenuous running). It generally affects the leg and forearm; however, any muscle that is contained by fascia can develop compartment syndrome. This complication tends to occur after supracondylar fractures at the distal humerus and tibial shaft fractures. Compartment syndrome develops when there

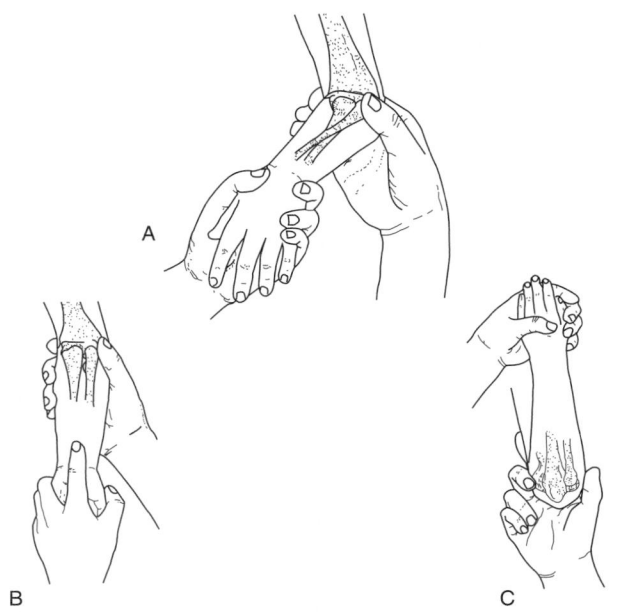

FIG. 39-2 Reduction of radial head subluxation by supination and flexion technique. **A,** Grasp the palm of the child's hand as if to shake it. Axial traction is applied to the forearm with the wrist adducted to the ulnar side. Pressure is also applied directly over the radial head at the elbow. **B,** The forearm is supinated while axial traction and pressure are maintained over the forearm and radial head, flex the elbow to the shoulder while supination and pressure are maintained over the radial head (**C**). (From Shah B: Reduction of radial head subluxation. In Finberg L, Kleinman RE, editors: *Saunders manual of pediatric practice,* ed 2, Philadelphia, 2002, WB Saunders, p. 1162.)

is bleeding or soft tissue swelling within a closed fascial space (compartment), producing progressive swelling and an increase in intracompartmental pressure. As the pressure increases, venous blood flow is impaired, followed by ischemia, which, if prolonged, results in cell death of the surrounding muscle and nerves. A cast that is too tight can be an iatrogenic cause of compartment syndrome (i.e., cast-induced compartment syndrome) (Thompson, 2006).

Clinical Findings. Compartment syndrome is characterized by the "six *P*s": pain, pallor, paresthesia, pulselessness, pressure, and paralysis, with pain being the earliest sign. Pain with passive stretch of toes or fingers is a characteristic finding. A child with a splinted fracture should be comfortable with mild analgesia. Acute pain in such a child raises the possibility of compartment syndrome (Doyle JR et al, 2005; Smith, 2002; Thompson, 2006).

Chronic compartment syndrome can be seen in runners and is called exertional compartment syndrome. It is associated with a history of a local dull ache or pain confined to the muscle (not the bone) with exercise, relief with rest. The affected compartment may be tender and feel significantly swollen. The pain can be reproduced after a period of time following onset of the activity or intensity of the exercise. Runners will complain of pain with passive stretch, numbness, weakness, and the area may feel significantly swollen. The tibial muscle compartment (usually anterolateral) is typically involved in runners, and was previously called "classic shin splints." (Latterman et al, 2007).

Management.   Prompt recognition of acute compartment syndrome and referral to an orthopedic surgeon are important. The diagnosis is made by direct measurement of compartment pressures. If the syndrome is confirmed, it is treated by immediate fasciotomy. Without treatment, irreversible damage to the compartment structures occurs within 6 to 8 hours after onset of symptoms and leads to muscle necrosis, fibrosis, and ischemic contracture. With exertional or chronic compartment syndrome caused by running, pain prevents resumption of exercise and limits the risk of muscle and nerve damage.

BITES

Animal and Child Bites

Description.   Children can be bitten by pets, stray animals, or humans, especially other children. Most bites are to the hand, although pet ferrets may attack a child's face. Human bites, cat bites, and bites to the hand carry the greatest risk of infection (Sonnett et al, 2006).

Epidemiology.   An estimated 1% of ED visits annually in the U.S. are due to mammalian bites. About 80% are dog bites (both provoked and unprovoked). Boys are attacked more often than girls. Dog bites are often caused by animals known to the child; in contrast, cat bites are more commonly caused by strays. The risk of infection from a dog bite is between 5% and 16%. By contrast, the risk of infection from a cat bite (despite early medical attention) is at least 50%. Cat bites cause puncture wounds and tend to be deeper than dog bites (Sonnett et al, 2006). Dog bites can cause abrasions, puncture wounds, and lacerations, with or without an associated avulsion of tissue. Limited data define the incidence of human bite injuries, but it is suspected that human bites are the leading cause of injury in child care centers in the U.S. All human bite wounds, regardless of mechanism of injury, should be considered at high risk for infection. Other animal bites, such as rat bites, are not reportable, so there is a paucity of information about their epidemiology (Ginsburg, 2004). Clenched-fist bites are the most serious of human bites and typically are the result of fighting. In this type of injury, the closed fist hits the teeth of another with laceration(s) of the skin typically over the third and fourth metacarpals. These human bite injuries are high risk for infection and joint compromise (Sonnett et al, 2006).

Clinical Findings.

History.   Ask about the circumstances surrounding the bite, including the type of animal, domestic or sylvatic, provoked or unprovoked, and location of the attack. History of drug allergies and immunization status of the child also should be ascertained.

Physical Examination.   During physical examination, the wound should be assessed for the type, size, and depth of injury. Explore for the presence of foreign material and the status of underlying structures. If the bite is on an extremity, assess its range of motion and sensory intactness. Likewise, assess functioning of the facial nerve with deep facial bite injuries. A diagram of the injury should be recorded in the child's chart (Ginsburg, 2004). The provider may be wise to consider photographing the injury for documentation.

Secondary infection is the most common complication of mammalian bites and can lead to cellulitis and lymphangitis, requiring hospitalization. *Streptococcus* and *Staphylococcus* are common organisms associated with infected animal and human bites; anaerobic infection is also possible. Species of gram-negative bacteria, such as *Pasteurella, Moraxella,* and *Enterococcus* from dog and cat bites, and *Eikenella corrodens* and *Corynebacterium* from human bites can also cause infections (Ciorciari & Touger, 2003). The potential for rabies exposure must also be considered.

Diagnostic Studies.   Obtain wound cultures if indicated to look for aerobic and anaerobic microorganisms. A roentgenogram of the affected part should be obtained if it is likely that a bone or joint could have been penetrated or fractured or if retained foreign material is present.

Differential Diagnosis.   The differential diagnosis includes lacerations or puncture wounds from other causes.

Management.   Management involves both physical and psychologic care of the child and includes the following (Baldwin & Mannheimer, 2002; Sonnett et al, 2006):

- Administer tetanus booster and rabies prophylaxis if indicated (consult with local animal control or public health department).
- Swab the wound with a moistened gauze to remove gross debris and culture the wound if indicated.
- Superficial wounds not extending further than the epidermis need cleansing with normal saline or standard agents.
- Anesthetize, clean, and vigorously irrigate the wound that extends through the epidermis with copious amounts of normal saline under pressure. Puncture wounds should be thoroughly cleaned and gently irrigated with a 16- to 18-gauge angiocatheter, a blunt-tipped needle, or a splash-guard device. Use a 20- to 50-mL syringe filled with normal saline and flush directly into the wound. Typically, 300 to 500 mL will sufficiently clean most wounds, unless heavily contaminated or extensive.
- If rabies is a possibility, cleansing with soap and water after initial irrigation is recommended.
- Débride avulsed or devitalized tissue.
- Superficial wounds that do not involve high-risk structures, such as the fingers, cartilaginous tissue, tendons, bones, and joints, generally do not need to be treated with prophylactic antibiotics.
- Prescribe prophylactic antibiotics for all human and cat bites, and the following types of bite or wound characteristics: hand, puncture, overlying bone fracture, substantial crushing tissue injuries or if required débridement, or those involving tendons, muscles, or joint spaces. In addition, antibiotic coverage is needed for wounds in children who are immunosuppressed. For outpatients, prescribe a broad-spectrum antibiotic such as amoxicillin clavulanate (first choice). Alternate choices are trimethoprim-sulfamethoxazole, azithromycin, or cefuroxime. Prescribe a 3 to 5 day course of prophylactic antibiotics. Clindamycin needs to be added to the regimen if symptoms of infection are present (Sonnett et al, 2006). Some sources recommend prophylactic antibiotics for facial wounds only because of the potential for scarring from infection.

- Rabies exposure prophylaxis should also be considered if there is any question about possible exposure. Refer to *Human Rabies Prevention - U.S. Recommendations of the Immunization Practices Advisory Committee (ACIP)* available though the U.S. Centers for Disease Control: *www.cdc.gov/vaccines/vpd-vac/rabies/*
- Some controversy exists over whether bite wounds should be closed primarily with delayed closure (3 to 5 days after injury) or should be allowed to heal by secondary intention (leaving the wound open). Factors to consider are the type, size, and depth of the wound, the anatomic location, presence of infection, the time interval since the injury, and the potential for cosmetic disfigurement. Surgical consultation should be obtained for all deep or extensive wounds and those involving the bones, joints, or hands. Because of the excellent blood supply to the face, facial lacerations are at less risk for infection. Many plastic surgeons advocate primary closure of facial bite wounds that have been brought to medical attention within 5 hours and have been thoroughly irrigated and débrided. Because of concern about scarring, the provider may refer facial wounds for plastic surgery repair.
  - There is consensus that bites involving the hand or foot should not be sutured but allowed to drain. Hand and foot bites less than 1.5 cm are best left to heal by secondary intention; bites greater than 1.5 cm should have delayed primary closure.
  - Bite wounds greater than 8 to 12 hours old should not be sutured except for facial wounds that can be sutured up to 24 hours but no longer than that.
  - A single layer of nonabsorbable sutures is best (avoid multiple closure layers).
- Refer children with severe bites. Obtain a surgical consult if evidence of or concern about nerve, tendon, and/or ligament injury or if a joint space was involved (Sonnett et al, 2006). Hospitalization, reconstructive surgery, and long-term follow-up can also be indicated.
- Discuss the child's fears and management of any behavioral problems that may result.
- Report dog and wild animal bites to animal control.

Patient and Parent Education. Preventive education and actions should include the following:

- Teach children to avoid stray animals, be cautious around domesticated animals, and not tease or provoke any animal.
- Emphasize the importance of parental supervision of children as they play with pets. Young children, especially, are often unaware of the risks that animals present, and their interactions must be carefully monitored.
- Do not keep typically wild animals as pets in families with very young children.
- Do not allow pets to roam freely.
- Never leave infants or young children alone with dogs or cats; animals with histories of aggression are inappropriate in households with children.
- Report stray animals promptly to animal control officials.

Hymenoptera

Description. Bees, hornets, yellow jackets, fire and harvester ants, and wasps belong to the *Hymenoptera* order of insects and have common antigens in their venom. Bees and wasps ordinarily do not sting unless frightened, bothered, or hurt. Yellow jackets are aggressive. Fire ants may cause multiple, painful stings. Reactions to stings by these insects are caused by the *Hymenoptera* venom and can vary from mild, local responses to life-threatening anaphylaxis with wheezing and urticaria. Most children experience only a local reaction, but some children suffer severe systemic reactions, which can progress to medical emergencies unless prompt intervention is initiated.

Epidemiology. Immunoglobulin E-dependent hypersensitivity is the underlying cause of reactions. Histamines, leukotrienes, prostaglandins, and other inflammatory factors are released, causing local or systemic symptoms. The venom of bees, wasps, and yellow jackets is similar and can cause cross-reactivity (Sorrentino & Monroe, 2002).

Clinical Findings.

History. The child usually reports being bitten or stung. There may be a past history of a local or systemic reaction following an insect bite.

Physical Examination. Findings include the following:

- Mild reaction consists of local redness, pruritus, pain, edema, and possibly generalized urticaria.
- Severe reactions, including anaphylaxis, are characterized by local signs plus any of the following:
  - Difficulty in breathing, wheezing
  - Difficulty swallowing
  - Hoarseness, thickened speech
  - Gastrointestinal disturbances, abdominal pain
  - Dizziness, weakness, confusion
  - Collapse, unconsciousness, even death
  - Fire ant bites are characterized by vesicles that develop into sterile pustules.

Diagnostic Studies. Skin testing is not necessary and can be dangerous if there is a history of an allergic response to *Hymenoptera* sting.

Differential Diagnosis. Other insect bites or dermatologic eruptions that produce similar symptoms are included in the differential diagnosis.

Management. The following steps are taken:

1. For mild local reactions:
   - If the stinger is visible, flick it off with the edge of a sharp object (e.g., knife blade or credit card), taking care to not squeeze the attached venom sac.
   - Apply cool compresses locally or cool baths.
   - Administer an antihistamine, such as diphenhydramine (Benadryl) at 5 mg/kg per day or hydroxyzine 2 mg/kg/day, in divided doses every 8 hours daily (hydroxyzine has a 50 mg maximum dosage) for treatment of pruritus (Ciorciari & Touger, 2003).
   - Calamine lotion or one part meat tenderizer mixed with four parts water may help relieve discomfort (Paller & Mancini, 2006).
2. For moderate to severe allergic reaction:
   - Moderate reactions may need to be treated with oral antihistamines, corticosteroids, and inhaled bronchodilators (if wheezing).

- Institute emergency measures for treatment of anaphylactic reactions and transport to the ED as quickly as possible (Erickson et al, 2002; McGintee et al, 2006):
  - Epinephrine (0.01 mL/kg of 1:1000 aqueous epinephrine per dose subcutaneously or intramuscularly, repeated at 5 minute intervals up to three times, not to exceed 0.5 mL total). IM administration of epinephrine into the thigh results in more rapid absorption and higher peak plasma levels than does administration in the arm.
  - Antihistamines should be given immediately following epinephrine, but not as a substitute for epinephrine; give both H_1 and H_2 histamine blockers parentally every 6 hours. The H2 class of antihistamines may be helpful in reducing histamine-induced cardiac arrhythmias in selected cases. Give famotidine 1 to 2 mg/kg (50 mg maximum) slowly IV (Leickly, 2003).
  - Glucocorticoids are not helpful for treating acute reaction, but may help in the late-phase inflammatory response and prevention of serum sickness. Give IV hydrocortisone (5 mg/kg every 6 hours) or methylprednisolone (1 to 2 mg/kg every 6 hours to a maximum of 60 mg) or oral prednisolone (2 mg/kg with 60 mg maximum) (Leickly, 2003).
  - Bronchodilators are also given if bronchospasm occurs, typically albuterol 0.5% in nebulizer at 0.03 mL/kg (1 mL maximum) per dose in 2 mL of saline.
  - Persistent hypotension is treated with vasopressors (e.g., dopamine); glucagon is preferred in the treatment of persistent hypotension in individuals taking ß-blocking agents.
  - IV fluids should be administered if the child is hypotensive as a result of anaphylactic shock.
  - Administer oxygen.
  - Tracheostomy if laryngeal edema is life threatening.
  - Hospitalize for anaphylactic shock.
3. Referral to an allergist is indicated for any child who has life-threatening respiratory symptoms (e.g., stridor or wheezing) or hypotension. Venom immunotherapy desensitization is highly effective (98% protective) in preventing further systemic reactions (McGintee et al, 2006). Children less than 16 years old who have only urticaria or angioedema do not require venom immunotherapy because only 10% of these children will have systemic reactions with subsequent stings (Erickson et al, 2002).

Patient and Parent Education.   Key issues to discuss include the following:
- Importance of wearing a medical alert tag or bracelet
- Proper use of an insect sting kit that includes self-injectable epinephrine pen (Epi-Pen) and need to have kit always readily available for emergency use
- Prevention of stings by avoiding areas likely to be infested with these insects, not wearing bright-colored clothing, and not using perfumed products

Mosquitoes, Fleas, and Chiggers (Red Bug Mites)

Description.   Mosquitoes are the vectors of many important diseases in humans (see Chapter 23) and also cause irritating local skin reactions when they bite. Similarly, flea and chigger bites produce local skin eruptions. The chigger is also known as red bug mite or harvest mite.

Epidemiology.   Mosquito bites are the most common insect bites of infants and children. Fleas that commonly attack humans in the U.S. include the human flea, cat flea, and dog flea. The six-legged larvae of harvest mites are responsible for the skin eruption characteristic of chigger bites. Harvest mites live on grain stems, shrubs, grass, and vines. As humans or animals pass by, the larvae attach themselves to the skin and inject an irritating secretion. The harvest mites then drop to the ground or are scratched off within 1 to 2 days. A seasonal pattern is characteristic of mosquito, flea, and chigger bites (Paller & Mancini, 2006).

Clinical Findings.

History.   The following may be reported:
- Mosquito or flea bites
  - Known mosquito or flea bite or seasonal time
  - Presence of cat or dog in child's environment
  - Complaints of a brief stinging sensation followed by itching after mosquito bite
- Chigger bites
  - Complaints of itching followed by dermatitis after chigger bite
  - History of playing or walking in grassy areas, parks, or other harvest mite habitat near woods and water

Physical Examination.   Mosquito bites are characterized by the following:
- Local irritation in unsensitized children
- Urticarial wheals that itch and last several hours to days in sensitized children or firm papules or nodules that last a long period of time
- Central punctum (sometimes noted)
- Secondary impetigo from scratching of skin lesions
  Flea bites are characterized by the following:
- Urticarial wheal or papule surrounded by redness in a sensitized person
- Often, central hemorrhagic punctum
- Progression of wheals into bullae in highly sensitized individuals, especially young children
- Grouping of multiple lesions, commonly found on arms, ankles, legs, feet, thighs, waist, buttocks, and lower abdomen
- Bites are commonly in a classic linear configuration, which is referred to as the "breakfast, lunch, and dinner" sign
  Chigger bites are characterized by the following:
- Discrete, bright-red papules 1 to 2 mm in diameter that often have hemorrhagic puncta
- Lesions mainly seen on legs (sock area) and belt line but can be widespread
- Wheals, papules, or papulovesicles in sensitized individuals
- Blisters if a secondary hypersensitivity reaction; purpuric lesions or bullae
- Intense pruritus reaching a peak on the second day and decreasing over the next 5 to 6 days, but can persist for months
- Possible secondary impetigo from scratching lesions
- May see the embedded chiggers

Diagnostic Studies. The presence of fleas or harvest mites is diagnostic; otherwise, no studies are done.

Differential Diagnosis. The diagnosis is often obvious, but the differential diagnosis can include insect bites that produce similar papular, vesicular lesions, or other skin conditions.

Management. Management consists of controlling pruritus and can include such measures as the following:

- Cool compresses
- Topical corticosteroids (e.g., 1% hydrocortisone cream)
- Topical antipruritic agents such as calamine lotion; avoid topical diphenhydramine
- Oral antihistamines (e.g., diphenhydramine) if topical corticosteroids do not provide relief
- Removal of embedded chiggers (can be withdrawn by covering the insect with alcohol, mineral oil, nail polish, or ointment)
- Treatment of secondary skin lesions as indicated
- Elimination of fleas by treating animals and cleaning carpets, bedding, upholstered furniture; avoid areas that are potentially infested with mosquitoes, fleas, or chiggers
- Insecticides should be used with caution

Patient and Parent Education. Prevention of insect bites is a key component in education. Bites can be prevented by eliminating mosquitoes, fleas, and chiggers from the environment or by preventing their contact with the skin.

- Use insect repellents (generally effective against mosquitoes and harvest mites).
- Wear protective clothing to cover body and tuck pants into shoes or socks.
- Wear neutral-colored clothes (white, green, tan, and khaki do not attract mosquitoes).
- Avoid scented hair sprays, powders, soaps, lotions, creams, and perfumes because these products can attract all forms of stinging insects.
- Mosquitos are attracted to bright clothing and sweaty skin and are drawn to humans by scent.
- Treat suspected animal carrier for fleas, and spray carpets and other infested areas; spray yards and grassy places for fleas in those environments that the child frequents.
- Vacuum carpets daily if fleas are seen on household pets.
- Avoid playing in areas of harvest mite habitat.

Ticks

Description. Ticks are blood-sucking arachnids and are classified into three families: *Ixodidae* (hard ticks), *Argasidae* (soft ticks), and *Nuttalliellidae* (soft ticks). They are vectors of significant diseases such as rickettsial infection (e.g., Rocky Mountain spotted fever and Q fever), Colorado tick fever, tularemia, and Lyme disease. (See discussion of Lyme disease in Chapter 23).

Epidemiology. Ticks are found in grass, shrubs, vines, and brush and attach themselves to various animals and humans. The female tick sucks blood from the skin and can inject a toxin while sucking blood. Transmission of Lyme disease in the U.S. is primarily by the *Ixodes scapularis* (deer) tick. However, *Ixodes ricinus* is the vector of Lyme disease in northern California and Oregon. Transmission of Lyme disease requires at least a 24-hour tick attachment. Tick bites are most common from early spring to early fall and are associated with both acute and chronic dermatoses.

Clinical Findings.

History. The practitioner assesses a report of known tick bite and exposure to a tick habitat.

Physical Examination. Findings include the following:

- The initial bite is painless and innocuous; thus the tick is frequently undetected or detected only after several days of attachment.
- Acute reactions can include papules, nodules, bullae, ulceration, and necrosis.
- An infiltrated lesion with a distinct surrounding erythematous halo develops and can last for 1 to 2 weeks.
- A small pruritic nodule, lasting for months or years, can result if the tick's mouth parts are left in the skin.
- Tick bite pyrexia or tick paralysis, occurring about 6 days after attachment, can result; both disorders are reversible, and symptoms quickly resolve if the tick is removed (Hodge & Tecklenburg, 2002; Paller & Mancini, 2006).
- Other signs depend on the tick-related illness that can develop; erythema chronicum migrans can develop around the bite in 2 to 3 weeks and progress to a disseminated rash and Lyme disease.

Diagnostic Studies. Identification of the tick is diagnostic. Diagnostic studies are ordered depending on the disease for which the tick is the vector.

Differential Diagnosis. The differential diagnosis of local reactions to simple tick bites includes other insect bites. Many different diseases result from tick bites and their sequelae. The presentation of tick-related diseases is variable and depends on the illness for which the tick is the vector.

Management. Although intervention varies with the specific disease, illnesses resulting from tick bites are best managed with prompt introduction of antibiotics, such as amoxicillin or doxycycline. Antibiotic prophylaxis for asymptomatic deer tick bites is generally not recommended especially if the tick had been attached for less than 24 hours (Paller & Mancini, 2006).

Complete removal of the tick is essential. If fragments of mouth parts or proboscis are left in the skin, local symptoms can continue. To remove ticks, wear gloves and firmly grasp the tick with forceps, tweezers, or gloved fingers as close to the skin as possible (try to grasp its head and not crush the tick). Gently pull straight upward with steady, even pressure. Wash the area with soap and water and save the tick for identification. If any part remains, a skin punch biopsy will remove the rest. Symptoms of tick bite paralysis can resolve within 24 hours after the tick is removed.

Patient and Parent Education. The following key points should be made:

- Avoid areas known to be infested with ticks.
- Wear protective clothing—preferably light colored to see ticks better (e.g., long-sleeved shirts tucked into pants and pants tucked into socks).

- Use of insect repellents sprayed onto clothes and hats or directly on the skin can help prevent tick bites, but do not apply to face or nonintact skin. Also inform parents that repellents occasionally cause allergic or toxic effects. Skedaddle™ 7.25% and OFF®10% are effective agents and have a good safety profile (Cohen, 2005). Use a higher sun protection factor (SPF) of sunscreen if applying insect repellents because the SPF may be decreased.
- Inspect for ticks after exposure or walking in areas likely to be infested; check for ticks every 2 to 3 hours during a hike; carefully check the scalp, hairline, neck, behind the ears, armpits, legs, back of knees, and groin because these areas are favorite hiding places of ticks.
- Take a brisk shower after a hike to help remove ticks that are not firmly attached. Wash off tick repellents with soap.

Spiders and Scorpions

Description. Most spider bites are innocuous, causing no reaction or a minor, localized response that can be mistaken for a flea, bedbug, or some other insect bite. There are three spiders common in the North American continent whose bite can cause serious complications: the black widow (*Latrodectus mactans),* the brown recluse (*Loxosceles reclusa),* and the hobo (*Tegenaria agrestis)* spiders. The black widow spider has a globular body about 1 cm across that is coal black in color with a red or orange hourglass marking on its underside. It is found throughout the U.S. The brown recluse spider, one of the most dangerous spiders in the U.S., has an oval light fawn to dark chocolate-brown body; it is approximately 1 cm in length (adults range from 1 to 5 cm in total length), with a dark-brown violin-shaped band extending from its eyes partially down its back. It bites humans only in self-defense. The brown recluse is found in southern and Midwestern states. The hobo spider, common to the Pacific Northwest and also found in Montana, Utah, and northern California, measures 1 to 1.5 inches across, including its legs, is brown with gray markings, and has parallel marks on its head and herringbone marks on its rear section. It is often mistaken for the brown recluse.

Scorpions have a stinging apparatus in their tail. They are found in the southwestern and southern U.S. and live in cool, dark places during the day.

Epidemiology. The black widow spider prefers to live in cool, dark, dry places in building and little-used structures, such as woodpiles, garages, basements, and tool sheds (less frequented outbuildings). It often spins its web on outdoor furniture, which explains why many black widow spider bites are received around the genital and buttock areas. The brown recluse spider typically lives in dark, dry places (attics, basements, boxes) and storage closets among clothes; when living outdoors, it resides in grasses, rocky bluffs, and barns. The brown recluse prefers dark recesses and bites only in self-defense. The hobo spider is found in crawl spaces, wood piles, and other dark areas. Like the brown recluse, the hobo spider bites in self-defense. The venom of the brown recluse can be hemolytic and necrotizing with extension caused by a spreading factor. Scorpions come

out at night and hide by day; they are nonaggressive unless disturbed (Paller & Mancini, 2006).

Clinical Findings.

History. Assess the known history of a spider bite or activities in, or travel to, an environment that is frequented by these spiders. The characteristic appearance of the spider helps in its identification. Children are more vulnerable to spider and scorpion bites.

Physical Examination. The characteristic features are identified for each type of spider bite (Paller & Mancini, 2006):
- Black widow spider bites:
  - Slight erythema and mild pain. A prick sensation is followed by regional lymph node tenderness (30 to 120 minutes later) and two red punctuate marks, burning or stinging, and local swelling at the bite site.
  - Severe, muscle cramping pain starts from 10 minutes to 1 hour after the bite and increases to maximum intensity within 3 hours.
  - Sweating, irritability, and agitation noted in children
  - Central nervous system symptoms include nausea, vomiting, headache, anxiety, salivation, lacrimation, sweating, hypertension, and tachycardia.
  - Most children recover in 2 to 3 days; some experience milder symptoms and some die.
- Brown recluse spider bites:
  - Localized reaction is characterized by mild itching or stinging at the time of bite (bite can be painless) with mild to severe pain in about 2 to 8 hours. This is followed by swelling, itching, tenderness, a hemorrhagic vesicle (a red ring followed by blue-purple discoloration) 12 to 24 hours later, and finally a gangrenous eschar. Lymphangitis is common if a bite is on an extremity. The lesion frequently takes weeks to months to resolve.
  - Systemic reaction may include nausea, vomiting, chills, fever, malaise, muscle aches and pains, thrombocytopenia, and hemolysis (Paller & Mancini, 2006).
- Hobo spider bites:
  - Similar to brown recluse spider bites.
- Scorpion bites:
  - Severe, local, and painful burning sensation with redness, discoloration, edema, and severe necrosis.
  - Systemic reactions include uncontrolled jerking, muscle fasciculation, facial twitching, hypersalivation, diaphoresis, and respiratory paralysis.

Differential Diagnosis. Other spider bites and conditions that result in similar cutaneous manifestations or systemic findings, or both, are included in the differential diagnosis.

Management. In cases in which venomous spider bites are suspected or confirmed, the patient should be referred to the appropriate medical specialist. Treatment for black widow spider bites includes administration of specific antivenin (in selected cases), intravenous calcium gluconate, muscle relaxants, pain medications, tetanus prophylaxis, and antibiotics if secondary infection develops. Most brown recluse bites tend to heal without incident. Bites with necrotic centers generally require tetanus prophylaxis, pain medication, application of ice or cold compresses, and elevation of the extremity. Children are at greatest risk of developing severe scorpion envenomation. Scorpion stings may be managed immediately with application of a restrictive bandage above the sting area and application of ice or cold water. Children experiencing severe reactions may require the use of antivenin therapy; however, this therapy is controversial (Paller & Mancini, 2006).

Patient and Parent Education. The focus of patient and parent education is prevention. Careful monitoring of environments in which these spiders tend to live and prompt treatment, if bitten, are important points to cover.

Snakebites

Description. Most snakes in the U.S. are not venomous. However, approximately 2500 children per year receive poisonous snakebites causing approximately 5 to 15 deaths. Poisonous snakes include indigenous pit vipers (*Crotalidae*), such as rattlesnakes, cottonmouths, water moccasins, and copperheads and the *Elapidae* (coral snake). The *Crotalidae* cause 99% of venomous snakebites occurring in the wild and *Elapidae* are responsible for the other 1%. Victims are occasionally bitten by exotic snakes that are kept as pets (Ciorciari & Touger, 2003).

Epidemiology. The snake injects venom that contains a variety of toxins into the soft tissue, and the venom can be carried throughout the body via the blood and lymph systems. Snake venom reactions can be divided into three presentations: cytotoxic, hemotoxic, and neurotoxic. Cytotoxicity presents with localized pain, swelling, and ecchymoses; compartment syndrome may develop in severe cases. Hematologic toxicity can include ecchymoses, coagulopathy, and thrombocytopenia. Neurologic toxicity can include taste abnormalities, local paresthesia, and in severe cases, bulbar and respiratory muscle weakness (Ciorciari & Touger, 2003).

Clinical Findings.

History. Assess for a report of a snakebite. It is helpful to determine the type of snake. Snakes with large triangular head and vertically oriented elliptical pupils are likely venomous viper. Copperheads and rattlesnakes have diamond-shaped patterns of varying colors. Coral snakes are brightly banded with red, yellow, and black rings.

Physical Examination. Characteristic features indicating the presence of venom include the following:

- Severe local reaction soon after the bite, with pain, discoloration, edema, and hemorrhagic effects
- Proximal extension of ecchymosis and swelling during the first few hours after the bite with later fluid-filled or hemorrhagic bullae and necrosis
- Peripheral and central neurologic symptoms (numbness or tingling around the face and/or limbs)
- Increased salivation and sweating; nausea and vomiting
- Evidence of hematologic coagulopathy, such as hematemesis, melena, hemoptysis
- Respiratory distress and shock that can lead to death

Diagnostic Studies. Coagulation studies and other laboratory tests are ordered as indicated by the child's condition.

Management. For nonvenomous bites, simply clean the wound, give tetanus prophylaxis if necessary, and appropriate pain medication. Give oral antibiotic therapy for 5 days with Augmentin. If there is any uncertainty about the identity of the snake, contact poison control and observe for venomous symptoms for at least 3 to 4 hours.

If a venomous snakebite is suspected, the effects (including possible death) will depend on the size of the child, site of the bite, type of snake, and degree of envenomation, plus the effectiveness of treatment. Up to 20% of venomous snake bites are "dry" bites and are therefore asymptomatic. In the case of a venomous bite by a rattlesnake there is a period of 6 to 8 hours between the bite and death in which effective treatment can be instituted to reverse the effects of rattlesnake venom. Treatment includes rapid transportation to a medical center, referral to appropriate medical specialists, antivenin therapy, and treatment for shock and respiratory difficulties.

Patient and Parent Education. Prevention of snakebite is important. Parents and patients who live or vacation in areas where pit vipers are found should be familiar with emergency first aid treatment of snakebites. First aid measures include the following (Ciorciari & Touger, 2003):

- Splint the affected extremity and minimize the patient's movements.
- Remove any jewelry that could cause a tourniquet effect.
- Do not elevate the affected extremity; lay or sit the person down with the bite below the level of the heart.
- Do not give the person alcohol as a pain killer nor give the individual a caffeinated beverage to drink.
- Cover the bite with a clean, dry dressing.
- Do not use a tourniquet or ice packs.
- Do not cut the bite area and attempt to suction the venom out.
- Transport immediately to a medical facility.

HEAD INJURIES

Description

The skull of an infant or child is anatomically different from the skull of an adult, a factor that influences how effectively it protects the brain from injury. The brain can better withstand trauma after myelination is complete, the anterior fontanel is closed, and the cranial sutures are fused. Before these events occur, children are particularly vulnerable to cerebral trauma, and this trauma has more severe effects.

In head injuries, irreparable cell damage occurs at the time of the initial trauma, followed by secondary events that can lead to further tissue death. These secondary events are potentially reversible. The mechanisms of head injury are direct contact and acceleration-deceleration forces. The acceleration-deceleration can result in cerebral concussion, diffuse axonal injury, and subdural hematoma. Cerebral concussion is characterized by an alteration in mental state, with confusion and amnesia, with or without loss of consciousness, occurring immediately after a brain injury. See Chapter 27 for an in-depth discussion of the brain and its functions and Chapter 14 for a discussion on the evaluation, management, and return-to-play policies for athletes.

The discussion of head injury in this chapter is limited to minor closed head injuries and is based on a joint American Academy of Pediatrics and American Academy of Family Physicians practice parameter titled "The Management of Minor Closed Head Injury in Children," and other current documents. In addition, indications of impending central nervous system compromise are presented. Head injuries can also be classified as mild, moderate, and severe. Table 39-8 identifies key characteristics that are used in this classification system.

Epidemiology

Traumatic brain injury (TBI) is a common cause of trauma in pediatrics, resulting in 2,685 deaths, 37,000 hospitalizations, and 435,000 emergency department visits annually in the U.S. for children 0 to 14 years old (*www.cdc.gov/Ncipe/ tbi/TBI.htm*). Approximately 2 to 5 million children sustain head traumas of varying intensities each year in the U.S. when all ages during childhood and adolescence are considered. Approximately 30,000 suffer permanent disability, including seizures, cognitive impairment, learning and motor disorders, and behavioral and emotional problems (Rosman, 2006). Boys experience head injury twice as frequently as girls. Many children die each year from head trauma, and children who survive their injuries have significant long-term disability. Children can also experience subtle symptoms of TBI that may not appear until days or weeks after the injury. Various types of head injuries can result in pathologic conditions: skull fracture, concussion, posttraumatic seizure, cerebral contusion, epidural hematoma, subdural hematoma, cerebral edema, and penetrating injury. A brief description of each is presented in Table 39-9.

TABLE 39-8   **Classification of Head Injuries Based on Key Characteristics**

Classification	Glasgow Coma Scale*	Neurologic Focal Deficit†	Loss of Consciousness	Other Neurologic Findings
Mild	13-15	No	No or brief loss (<30 minutes)	May have linear skull fractures
Moderate	9-12	Focal signs	Variable loss	May have depressed skull fracture or intracranial hematoma
Severe	≤8	Focal signs	Prolonged loss	Often have depressed skull fractures and intracranial hematoma

*Either initial or subsequent scores.
†Neurologic focal deficit (e.g., hemiparesis, reflex asymmetry, Babinski sign, abnormal cranial nerve findings).

TABLE 39-9   **Common Types of Head Injuries in Children**

Type of Injury	Characteristics
Skull fracture	Linear, compound, basilar, depressed, and diastatic. Less common in children owing to more elastic skull. Linear is most common type.
Concussion	Transient loss of consciousness with amnesia. Computed tomography scan is normal. Child's level of consciousness may be depressed, child may vomit, but neurologic examination becomes normal within hours of treatment.
Posttraumatic seizure	Convulsion resulting from injury that occurs immediately, early (within the first 24 hours), or late (>1 week after injury). A seizure is the result of a focal injury to the brain.
Cerebral contusion	Bruising of the brain. Injury results from acceleration/deceleration forces. Common features include depressed level of consciousness, headache, and vomiting.
Epidural hematoma	Collection of blood between skull and dura. An overlying fracture is a common association. Classic clinical picture is an initial loss of consciousness, then a lucid interval with subsequent neurologic deterioration.
Subdural hematoma	Collection of blood between dura and brain parenchyma. More common than epidural hematoma. Associated with cerebral contusion following skull fracture or direct trauma or with child abuse. Unconsciousness common with acute subdural hematoma; with chronic subdural hematoma, note increasing head size in infants or gradual progressive symptoms in older child.
Cerebral edema	Caused by vasogenic, cytotoxic, hydrostatic, or osmotic forces. Significant cause of increased intracranial pressure following injury.
Penetrating injury	Trauma caused by an object such as a bullet entering the brain. In the case of a bullet, the kinetic energy released during its passage through the brain can cause major damage.

Clinical Findings

History. The following information should be obtained:

- History of how injury occurred; if injury involved a fall, determine height from which the child fell
- Loss of or alteration in consciousness or memory, confusion, irritability, inappropriate behavior, repetitive questioning
- Presence of vomiting and frequency
- Presence of headache, description of the headache pain
- Presence of blurred vision, diplopia, or other vision problem
- Numbness or loss of sensation, loss of balance, or difficulty walking

A child who is being maltreated may be seen in the ED with head trauma. Reece & Sege (2000) reviewed the histories of a sample of 287 children, 1 week to 6 years old, who were admitted to a pediatric hospital with head injuries. Eighteen percent of these cases involved suspected child abuse. Based on the findings of this study and others, child abuse should be strongly suspected when a head injury is present in a child without a history of fall or with a history of fall from a relatively low height of less than 4 feet. It is also recommended that a skeletal survey be obtained in children younger than 3 years when inflicted head injuries are suspected because younger children are at higher risk for skeletal trauma as well (Christian & Blum, 2006). (See Chapter 18 for further discussion of child abuse.)

Physical Examination. Check vital signs (temperature, blood pressure, pulse, and respiration) and compare findings with normal parameters expected for children of varying ages. Changes in vital signs can indicate shock or intracranial hypertension. Perform a thorough physical examination (including a careful oral examination) and a careful neurologic examination. The neurologic examination should include level of consciousness, mental status, motor function (both gross and fine motor), sensory function, cranial nerve functioning, and reflexes. The examiner should be alert to any signs of central nervous system involvement. Evaluation of mental status can be based on the Glasgow Coma Scale (Table 39-10). Always remember to examine the entire child for other signs of trauma such as neck injury internal abdominal injuries, or bone fractures. Periorbital hemorrhage ("raccoon-eyes"), ecchymosis behind the ear (Battle sign), blood behind the eardrum, and bleeding from the ears or nose indicate a basilar skull fracture.

Diagnostic Studies. The severity of the head trauma dictates the need for investigative studies. All children with moderate (GCS 9 to 12) and severe (GCS 3 to 8) acute trauma should have a cranial computed tomography (CT) scan. In addition, the need for skull radiographs and other views is determined by the severity of the head trauma. Rosman (2006) recommends including plain radiographs (cervical spine and a series of skull views) with significant loss of consciousness, focal neurologic signs (GCS score of 3 to 8), and further neurologic study. Indications for obtaining a CT scan include any of the following (Rosman, 2006):

- History of loss of consciousness (exceeding 1 minute)
- Amnesia about the injury
- Depressed level of consciousness (lethargy)

TABLE 39-10 Glasgow Coma Scale

Category	Best Response	Score*
Eye opening (E)	Spontaneous	4
	To speech (command)	3
	To pain	2
	None	1
Motor (M)	Obeys (command)	6
	Localizes	5
	Withdraws	4
	Abnormal flexion	3
	Extensor response	2
	None	1
Verbal (V)	Oriented	5
	Confused conversation	4
	Inappropriate words	3
	Incomprehensible sounds	2
	None	1

*Total score (E + M + V): maximum 15; minimum 3.
From Coulter DL: Head trauma. In Finberg LL, editor: *Saunders manual of pediatric practice*, Philadelphia, 1998, WB Saunders, pp 883-885.

- Focal neurologic signs or deficit
- Depressed skull fracture or signs of basilar injury
- Seizures
- Persistent vomiting

CT is the preferred imaging technique because it can be obtained rapidly, and the child can be monitored easily during the study. Skull fractures are better visualized on skull radiographs. Acute hemorrhage is detected more easily by CT (order without contrast) than by MRI. However, MRI is the preferred imaging modality for examination of the brain during the recovery period following head trauma and for imagery of the posterior fossa, or to detect hemorrhage when CT is normal but bleeding is suspected (Rosman, 2006). If CT is ordered after several days (3 or more days past injury), it should be done both with contrast (to pick up extravasated blood) and without. CT can demonstrate brain edema, midline displacements, hydrocephalus, loss of brain tissue, and most skull fractures. Although CT itself is a safe procedure, some healthy children require sedation or anesthetic (with some risk), so the benefits gained from CT should be carefully weighed against the possible harm of sedating or anesthetizing a child. In addition, CT scans obtained for asymptomatic children may show incidental findings that lead to subsequent unnecessary medical or surgical interventions.

CT scans, MRI, or skull radiographs are generally not indicated for mild or minor closed head trauma without focal neurologic signs or loss of consciousness (AAP, 1999; Rosman, 2006).

Differential Diagnosis

History of a head injury is the key to diagnosis. Differentiating minor head trauma that will resolve on its own from more extensive brain injury is problematic at times. Head trauma may cause injuries of the scalp, skull, and intracranial contents. Remember that these injuries may occur alone or in combination

(Schutzman, 2002). Children with intracranial lesions after minor closed head injury are not easily distinguishable clinically from the large majority with no intracranial injury. Children with mild nonspecific signs such as headache, vomiting, or lethargy after minor closed head injury may be more likely to have intracranial lesions than children without such signs. However, these clinical signs are of limited predictive value, and most children with headache, lethargy, or vomiting after minor closed head injury do not have demonstrable intracranial injury. In addition, some children with intracranial injury do not have any such signs or symptoms, showing a normal neurologic assessment (AAP, 1999). Because of these findings, some experts recommend a liberal policy on the ordering of cranial CT scans following any head trauma; however, there are drawbacks to routine CT scanning (see discussion in prior section).

Management

Management issues related to only mild and moderate head injuries are discussed in this chapter. The level of consciousness is a key determinant of the child's prognosis. Prompt identification of a deteriorating level of consciousness and quick medical and/or surgical intervention are essential components of the management plan.

Management of the Child with Minor Closed Head Injury and No Loss of Consciousness.   Observation in the clinic, office, ED, or home, under the care of a competent caregiver, is recommended for children with minor closed head injury and no loss of consciousness. Observation implies regular monitoring by a competent adult who would be able to recognize abnormalities and seek appropriate assistance.

Management of the Child with Minor Closed Head Injury and Brief Loss of Consciousness.   For children with minor closed head injury and brief loss of consciousness (several minutes) and no other neurologic or physical deficits reported or detected on examination, observation in the office, clinic, ED, hospital, or home, when under the care of a competent caregiver (see definition in preceding paragraph), may be used to evaluate such a child. The use of CT scan, skull radiographs, or MRI in the initial management of children with minor closed head injury and loss of consciousness is not routinely recommended. However, CT scanning along with observation is also accepted. If the provider is not assured that the child will be closely and reliably monitored at home, hospitalization is indicated (Rosman, 2006).

Management of the Child with Moderate Head Injury or Worrisome Symptoms.   Children with moderate head injuries (GCS score of 9 to 12) may require admission or prolonged observation in the ED until their mental status stabilizes; children with severe head injuries (GCS score of less than 8 or coma and physical findings) need immediate hospital admission. Children with any of the following should be hospitalized (Rosman, 2006):

- Changing vital signs
- Seizures
- Altered mental status

- Prolonged unconsciousness
- Persisting memory deficit or focal neurologic signs
- Depressed or basilar skull fractures
- Persistent headache (particularly with stiff neck)
- Recurrent vomiting or unexplained fever
- Unexplained injury (suspected child abuse)
- CT scan or MRI findings that are worrisome

A child with a skull fracture or transient neurologic findings whose level of consciousness is normal may be admitted for overnight observation.

Complications

Complications of head injury can include concussion, posttraumatic seizures, cerebral contusion, epidural hematoma, subdural hematoma, intracerebral hematoma, subarachnoid hemorrhage, acute brain swelling, and penetrating injuries. Second impact syndrome is described in Chapter 14. Intracranial lesions, particularly epidural hematomas, are life threatening and have significant complications. Features indicative of serious injury include loss of consciousness (longer than 1 minute), persistent vomiting, depressed level of consciousness, seizures, unequal pupil size, severe headache, and GCS score of less than 15.

Patient and Parent Education

Give all parents or caregivers a "head injury sheet," and make every effort to ensure that they understand the instructions and will comply with them. Salient points to cover in a pediatric head injury information sheet include instructions about when to contact the health care provider or take the child to an ED. Indications are the following:

- Increased drowsiness, sleepiness, inability to wake up, unconsciousness
- Vomiting more than one or two times
- Neck pain
- Watery or bloody drainage from ear or nose
- Convulsion, "fit," or fainting
- Unusual irritability, personality change, confusion, or any unusual behavior
- Headache that gets worse or lasts more than a day
- Unequal pupils
- Trouble with vision (blurred), hearing, or speech
- Trouble with walking (e.g., clumsiness or stumbling) or weakness of any muscle of arms, legs, or face

In addition, parents or caregivers should be given the following specific instructions:

- Wake up child every 2 to 4 hours for the first 24 hours after injury; child should wake easily and be able to stay awake for a few minutes.
- Make sure child is moving his or her arms and legs normally.
- Give only acetaminophen, if needed for headache or relief of pain of bumps and bruises.

Parents should also be informed that sometimes symptoms from head trauma occur days, weeks, or months after the initial trauma.

Neurologic sequelae following mild head injury in children often improve or resolve within 9 to 12 months. These sequelae include the following:

- Headache
- Vertigo or dizziness
- Difficulty concentrating or loss of memory
- Depression, fatigue
- Poor school performance and neurobehavioral problems

Postconcussive Syndrome and Return to Contact Sports

Typical postconcussive syndrome in adolescents is manifested by headache, dizziness, irritability, and impaired ability to concentrate. In younger children, it is manifested as aggression, disobedience, behavioral regression, inattention, and anxiety.

The American Academy of Neurology has established guidelines related to concussions (grade I, II, or III) and when or if a child can return to a contact sport. Caution needs to be exercised in allowing a child to return to a contact sport as repeated concussion can cause cumulative neuropsychological damage. Chapter 14 discusses second-impact syndrome, a second (even minor) blow to a brain that is still symptomatic from a recent mild head injury. It can result in death or other catastrophic sequelae (Rosman, 2006). See the Resource Box at the end of the chapter for free information about concussions that can be shared with coaches.

HEAT AND COLD INJURIES

Frostbite

Description. Frostbite occurs when ice crystals form within the soft tissues as a consequence of exposure to cold. The freezing of tissue impairs circulation to the affected area and results in constriction and vasoocclusion. This causes microvascular changes leading to cellular destruction and the release of inflammatory mediators that also cause damage (Paller & Mancini, 2006). Frostbite most commonly involves distal, relatively poorly perfused regions of the body, such as fingertips, toes, earlobes, and the nose. In children, areas that have poor heat-generating ability and insulation, including the cheeks and chin, are also at high risk for frostbite. However, any area of skin that is exposed to prolonged cold can be affected (Ciorciari & Chou, 2003).

Epidemiology. Exposure to temperatures ranging from $-2°$ C to $-10°$ C ($28.4°$ F to $14°$ F) can cause frostbite. Factors such as duration of exposure, increased wind velocity, dependency of the extremity (limb in a dependent not elevated position), application of emollients, fatigue, injury, high altitude, immobility, and general health can potentiate the effects of cold. Exposure to very cold chemicals (e.g., liquid oxygen) also produces instant frostbite.

Clinical Findings

History. The provider should assess the following:
- Exposure to cold temperatures
- Sensory changes (initially painful, then numbness if deeply frostbitten)
- Complaints of throbbing pain after thawing

Physical Examination. Typical initial findings include the following:
- Frozen area is cold.
- Skin is red at first, then appears pale or waxy white or slightly yellow or may have a bluish tint if deeply frostbitten.
- In early stages, tissue blanches; in later stages, it feels doughy or rock hard.

On rewarming, the extent of tissue damage becomes apparent. Deep frostbite occurs when tissues are icy hard and without deep tissue resilience. With deep frostbite the following signs and symptoms appear with rewarming:
- Cyanosis or mottling
- Erythema and swelling
- Numbness that evolves into complaints of burning pain
- Vesicles and bullae that appear within 24 to 48 hours
- Gangrene in severe frostbite

See Table 39-11 for a description of the four-levels of frostbite.

Differential Diagnosis. The differential diagnosis includes other conditions that produce similar cutaneous manifestations and injury; a history of exposure to extreme temperatures is the key to the diagnosis.

Management. Severe frostbite should be managed by medical specialists. Treatment includes rapid rewarming procedures, pain management, medical and surgical management of tissue necrosis, prevention of infection, and amputation if needed. Damaged skin should never be massaged or rubbed with snow or ice. Early treatment of mild frostbite includes the following:

TABLE 39-11 **The Four Categories of Frostbite**

Category by Degree	Description	Complication
First (frostnip)	Redness, edema, transient discomfort; reversible within a few hours	Normal skin appearance within a few hours; may have mild desquamation
Second	Notable redness and swelling; numbness becomes burning pain in 12-24 hours; bullae and vesicles form	Sensory neuropathy and cold sensitivity are residuals after healing
Third	Hemorrhagic bullae or waxy, mummified skin	Extensive tissue loss
Fourth	Involvement of full-thickness skin, muscle, tendon, bone	Amputation is likely

- Cover affected area with other body surfaces and warm clothing.
- Avoid pressure or any contact on the affected area
- *Do not use local dry heat*; this practice is dangerous and can cause tissue damage.

Patient and Parent Education. Education of children and parents about the prevention and initial management of frostbite is important. Essential points include advice about the following:

- Use of appropriate clothing when exposed to extreme cold temperatures
- Survival skills for travelers, hikers, or winter sports participants who are exposed to cold temperatures or who could become lost
- Immediate rewarming of skin that is white by covering with warm clothing or another body surface
- Danger of rubbing affected area with snow or ice or massaging; these practices are contraindicated because they lead to mechanical trauma.

Hypothermia

Description. Hypothermia is the condition in which body core temperature falls below 35° C (95° F). At less than 35° C (95° F), the human body loses its ability to generate sufficient heat to maintain bodily functions. Predisposing factors include malnutrition, hypoglycemia, major trauma, hypothyroidism, Addison disease, and drug use or abuse. Although most cases of accidental exposure are seen in winter, hypothermia can occur in other seasons during wet, windy weather. It can also come on quickly in the case of cold water emersion (Ciorciari & Chou, 2003).

Epidemiology. Hypothermia can be the result of environmental exposure. Body heat is lost by radiation of heat to nearby objects, evaporation of moisture from the skin and respiratory system, convection of heat from the skin's surface into cooler air, or conduction of heat to objects in direct contact with the body. The effect of cool ambient temperatures is exacerbated by wind, moisture, and lack of appropriate clothing or shelter.

Children are at increased risk of hypothermia because of their relatively larger body surface area, proportionately larger head, smaller body fluid volume, less developed temperature-regulating mechanisms, and less protective body fat. Children are also less able to escape on their own from a cold environment and are more likely to wander off from adult supervision. Newborns, particularly low-birth-weight or premature infants, very young children, and children who are ill, fatigued, poorly nourished, or have experienced trauma are at high risk.

Hypothermia results in cutaneous vasoconstriction and increased heat production by shivering and thyroxine releases. Hypothermia, not associated with environmental exposure, may be a sign of other life-threatening illnesses or injuries (e.g., near-drowning in cold water). This secondary hypothermia is not discussed here.

Clinical Findings

History. The following are assessed:

- Exposure to low ambient temperatures
- Risk factors (e.g., age, physical condition)

Physical Examination. Signs of hypothermia progress from early to late stages and include the following:

- Decreasing body temperature
- Shivering that disappears in late hypothermia
- Pallor or blue lips and skin
- Disorientation, listlessness, sleepiness
- Decreased pulse and respiration
- Coma and death

Diagnostic Studies. No studies are done if hypothermia is mild and responds to basic treatment measures.

Differential Diagnosis. Shock is the differential diagnosis.

Management. For mild hypothermia (greater than 32° C [89.6° F] body temperature), in early stages of cooling, remove the child from the cold environment, replace wet clothing, and provide warm liquids. Placing the child in a warm water bath can be effective. As the body cools further, it can no longer generate adequate heat itself, so external sources of heat must be provided. Again, remove the child from the cold environment, replace wet clothing, and provide heat with warm blankets, heat lamps, hot water bottles, or, if none of these is available, use the classic technique of placing the child skin-to-skin with a warm person of normal temperature in a sleeping bag or blanket.

Active rewarming by external or core rewarming techniques (e.g., warmed, humidified oxygen and warmed intravenous fluids) is necessary for children with severe hypothermia (less than 32° C [89.6° F] body temperature) who are in danger of cardiovascular instability (Kilbaugh et al, 2006).

Patient and Parent Education. Instruct parents on the risks of hypothermia in young children. Emphasize the need to monitor children's activities in cold weather and to provide adequate supervision and protection from exposure. The higher metabolic rate of normal, healthy children keeps them warm, and they may not feel the effects of short-term exposure to the cold. Thus they may not want a jacket, sweater, hat, or mittens when their parents believe they need them. Having a survival kit along with families or teens on camping trips or traveling in uninhabited areas may save a life (see Resource Box at the end of the chapter).

Hyperthermia: Common Heat-Related Illness

Description. Hyperthermia is a life-threatening increase in body core temperature. Heat cramps, heat exhaustion, and heat stroke are types of hyperthermia. Heat cramps are painful muscle cramps that are probably caused by electrolyte depletion associated with insufficient blood supply to an exercising muscle. Heat exhaustion is caused by excessive sweating associated with inadequate intake of water and salt in a hot environment. Heat stroke is a life-threatening condition and is associated with core temperatures of over 40° C (104° F) (Ciorciari & Chou, 2003). Heat cramps and heat exhaustion are discussed in more detail in Chapter 14 because they often occur during sports activities. They are reversible changes; in contrast, heat stroke is a life-threatening condition. This section more specifically discusses heat stroke.

Etiology. Heat-related illness results from an ineffective response of the body's thermoregulatory mechanisms to environmental conditions. Hyperthermia causes cutaneous vasodilation, sweating, and decreased heat production by inhibition of shivering. Children with some genetic myopathies have malignant hyperthermia, a reaction to anesthetic. All children are at risk for hyperthermia or heat stroke when exposed to high air temperature, especially if the heat is combined with high humidity and if steps are not taken to keep the child cool. Evaporation through sweating is the body's primary cooling mechanism with activity. If air temperature is higher than body temperature, if humidity is high, or if the body is dehydrated, the body's cooling mechanisms and the process of evaporation are compromised. Internal body temperature then increases. Age, exertion, illness, obesity, and poor nutrition also exacerbate the risk of hyperthermia. Compared with adults, children sweat less, begin to sweat at a higher internal temperature (or set-point), have a higher metabolic rate (thus producing more body heat) and lower cardiac output, and are more susceptible to dehydration (because of proportionately larger body surface area).

Clinical Findings

History. The provider assesses the following:
- Exposure
- Excessive exercise
- Wearing inappropriate clothing
- Inadequate fluid intake or the use of water or other low-sodium fluids during prolonged and strenuous exercise
- Previous episode of heat stroke
- Heat cramps: complaints of intermittent muscle cramping (no rigidity)
- Heat exhaustion: complaints of thirst, headache, fatigue, dizziness, malaise, myalgias and muscle cramps, nausea, and vomiting; core temperature is normal or slightly elevated and the patient still sweats
- Heat stroke: delirium, stupor, or coma—central nervous system dysfunction

Physical Examination. Signs of heat exhaustion include the following:
- Appears anxious and diaphoretic
- Tachycardia with temperature less than 40° C (104° F)
- Orthostatic hypotension

Signs of heat stroke, include all the symptoms of heat exhaustion listed above, are progressive, and also include the following:
- Body temperature greater than 104° F (40° C)
- Hot, dry, red skin
- May or may not sweat
- Initially has a rapid, strong pulse that becomes progressively weaker
- Initially constricted pupils, progressively dilated
- Initially has a deep, rapid "snorelike" breathing that becomes progressively weaker
- Tremors, increasing dizziness, and weakness
- Confusion, irritability, anxiety (central nervous system dysfunction)
- Headache
- Loss of appetite, nausea, vomiting
- Decreasing blood pressure, tachyarrhythmia
- Seizures, collapse
- Renal insufficiency, coma, and death

Diagnostic Studies. CBC and urinalysis, along with electrolyte monitoring may be necessary for significant heat cramps and heat exhaustion. Heat stroke requires extensive laboratory studies and monitoring of physiologic parameters.

Differential Diagnosis. Fever differs from hyperthermia in that it is an alteration of the body's hypothalamic set point in response to a pathologic illness or condition.

Management. The management of heat-related illness includes the following:
1. Heat cramps
   - Cooling measures
   - Oral sodium replacement with electrolyte fluids or liberally salted foods (occasionally IV saline may be needed)
2. Heat exhaustion
   - Cool environment
   - Intravenous replacement of electrolytes (initial bolus of 10 to 20 mL/kg of normal saline)
3. Heat stroke
   - All individuals with heat stroke die without treatment. Heat stroke patients should be transported to a medical facility as quickly as possible. The goal of treatment is to reduce the temperature to less than 100° F (37.8° C) or about 5.4° F (3° C) over a 30- to 60-minute period. First aid management includes the following steps:
     - Remove the child from the source of heat.
     - Apply cold packs, wet sheets, or towels, or spray the body with lukewarm water. The body responds quickly to cooling of the neck, head, abdomen, and inner thighs.
     - Use a fan to cool and circulate air over the child and to facilitate evaporation.
     - Be alert for vomiting; prevent aspiration.
     - Administer IV lorazepam to prevent shivering, which generates heat
   - When the body temperature is lowered to the desired level, stop cold packs, monitor, and be prepared to reapply cold packs if temperature increases.
   - Alcohol baths are contraindicated due to the potential for alcohol poisoning. Acetaminophen and ibuprofen have no role in the treatment of heat stroke.
   - Other therapies are instituted based on the child's condition—IV hydration and therapy for myoglobinuria (Ciorciari & Chou, 2003; Kilbaugh et al, 2006).

Patient and Parent Education. Instruct parents on the risks of hyperthermia (e.g., never leave an infant or a child in a closed car or continuously exposed to direct sunlight). Inform parents that children who suffer heat stroke are at a higher risk for subsequent heat-related illnesses. Teach ways to prevent hyperthermia, including the following:
- Keep children well hydrated. Offer water often during active play and athletic events or practices. Water is an adequate replacement fluid, although children can also use electrolyte-based sports drinks.
- Make sure children are well rested and have good nutritional intake.
- Provide appropriate clothing (e.g., sunshades, hats, and light-reflective shirts that allow ventilation).
- Regulate children's activity levels to the conditions (e.g., limit active play if it is very hot or humid).
- Acclimatize child gradually to changes in environment.

RESOURCE BOX

National Injury Resources

American Academy of Neurology
www.aan.com/professionals/practice/guidelines/pda/Concussion sports.pdf
Download a copy of the Practice Parameter: *The Management of Concussion in Sports* (Summary Statement).

American Burn Association
www.ameriburn.org
This organization is dedicated to improving the lives of those affected by burn injury through education, research, patient care, and advocacy.

Equipped to Survive
www.equipped.com
Information on survival equipment and supplies, outdoors and camping gear, and survival tips.

Kids Don't Leave Home Without It Equipment
www.equipped.com/kidequip.htm
Lists information on survival equipment and skills for children.

Local Poison Control Center
The number is listed among emergency numbers in the local telephone book. A call can be made to the local hospital emergency room and advice given according to the local poison control center. One can also call 911 and be transferred to the poison control center; however, not every state or city has a poison control center. The website for the Poison Control and Prevention Center Directory is www.aapcc.org/findyourcenter.htm

SafeKids USA
www.safekids.org
Safe Kids Worldwide is a global network of groups dedicated to the prevention of accidental childhood injury. Safe Kids creates programs and educational resources aimed at the reduction of childhood injuries.

U.S. Department of Health & Human Services (Center for Disease Control and Prevention)
www.cdc.gov
Has several fact sheets to educate the public about prevention of injuries (i.e., How to Prevent or Respond to a Snake Bite, Dog Bite, and other animals. Go to www.cdc.gov and search for the injury topic of interest.
Send away for "Heads Up: Concussion in High School Sports"— free information for coaches.

✓ DISCUSSION QUESTIONS

1. There are several guidelines for the management of concussions in the pediatric population. What would you do for an 11-year-old with a history of being tackled during a football game who 1 month later has a persistent headache? Do the guidelines agree with each other?
2. You are seeing a patient with a fractured wrist for the first time in an ED? What are key history points that may be helpful in trying to determine whether there is a pattern of injuries that may be suspicious of abuse?
3. Given the paucity of time in an office-based visit, what interventions can you use to prevent childhood injuries? What community-based interventions can be used to prevent injuries in children?
4. A family is planning a 1-week camping excursion. They ask you what they should bring on their trip in case of injuries. Can you develop a list for use in your practice based on recommendations from reliable resources (see Resource Box)?
5. A 15-year-old comes in following a fight at school. He has multiple abrasions and a few puncture wounds on the right knuckle. How do you treat these abrasions? The mother tells you that she put peroxide on them at home. What are key teaching points in this patient? What else about the presentation concerns you and why?
6. A 6-year-old who was playing basketball when his foot overturned has point tenderness on the right lateral malleolus. What is on your differential diagnosis? What are the physiologic differences between the skeleton of a 6-year-old versus the skeleton of a 15-year-old?

REFERENCES

American Academy of Pediatrics (AAP): The management of minor closed head injury in children, *Pediatrics* 104:1407-1415, 1999.

Anderson AC: Injury-ankle. In Fleisher GR, Ludwig S, Silverman BK, editors: *Synopsis of pediatric emergency medicine*, ed 4, Philadelphia, 2002, Lippincott Williams & Wilkins.

Bachman D, Santora S: Orthopedic trauma. In Fleisher GR, Ludwig S, Silverman BK, editors: *Synopsis of pediatric emergency medicine*, ed 4, Philadelphia, 2002, Lippincott Williams & Wilkins.

Baldwin S, Mannheimer A: Animal and human bites and bite-related infections. In Burg FD et al, editors: *Gellis and Kagan's current pediatric therapy*, ed 17, Philadelphia, 2002, WB Saunders.

Bass JL: Preventing childhood injuries. In Burg FD et al, editors: *Current pediatric therapy*, ed 18, Philadelphia, 2006, WB Saunders.

Bulloch B et al: Pediatric Emergency Researchers of Canada. Validation of the Ottawa Knee Rule in children: a multicenter study, *Ann Emerg Med* 42:48-55, 2003.

Buttaravoli P, Stair T: *Minor emergencies: splinters to fractures*, St Louis, 2000, Mosby.

Christian CW, Blum NJ: Psychosocial issues. In Kliegman RM et al, editors: *Nelson essentials of pediatrics*, ed 5, Philadelphia, 2006, Elsevier Saunders.

Ciorciari AJ, Chou KJ: Environmental injuries. In Crain EF, Gershel JC, editors: *Clinical manual of emergency pediatrics*, ed 4, New York, 2003, McGraw-Hill.

Ciorciari A, Touger M: Wound care. In Crain EF, Gershel JC, editors: *Clinical manual of emergency pediatrics*, ed 4, New York, 2003, McGraw-Hill.

Clark KD, Tanner S: Evaluation of the Ottawa Ankle Rules in children, *Pediatr Emerg Care*, 19 (2):73-8, 2003.

Cohen BA. *Pediatric dermatology*, ed 3, Philadelphia, 2005, Elsevier Mosby.

Coulter DL: Head trauma. In Finberg LL, editor: *Saunders manual of pediatric practice*, Philadelphia, 1998, WB Saunders.

Dobiesz VA, Greenfield RH: Orthopedic injuries. In Strange GR et al, editors: *Pediatric emergency medicine: a comprehensive study guide*, ed 2, New York, 2002, McGraw-Hill.

Drendel AL, Esterhal JL, Sawyer JR: Orthopedic problems of the extremities. In Burg FD et al, editors: *Gellis and Kagen's current pediatric therapy*, ed 17, Philadelphia, 2002, WB Saunders.

Doyle JR, Tornelta P, Ernhorn TA. Hand and Wrist, Philadelphia, 2005, Lippencott Williams & Wilkins.

Erickson T, Herman BE, Bowman MJ: Spider and arthropod bites. In Strange GR et al, editors: *Pediatric emergency medicine: a comprehensive study guide*, ed 2, New York, 2002, McGraw-Hill.

Eustace S, et al: *Sports injuries: examination, imaging and management*, Edinburgh, 2007, Churchill Livingstone, Elsevier.

Ginsburg CM: Animal and human bites. In Behrman RE, Kliegman RM, Jenson HB, editors: *Nelson textbook of pediatrics*, ed 17, Philadelphia, 2004, WB Saunders.

Grudziak JS, Musahl V: The youth athlete. In McMahon PJ, editor: *Current diagnosis & treatment in sports medicine*, New York, 2007, McGraw-Hill.

Hergenroeder A, Chorley JN: Sports medicine. In Behrman RE, Kliegman RM, Jenson HB, editors: *Nelson textbook of pediatrics*, ed 17, Philadelphia, 2004, WB Saunders.

Hodge D, Tecklenburg FW: Bites and stings. In Fleisher GR, Ludwig S, Silverman BK, editors: *Synopsis of pediatric emergency medicine*, ed 4, Philadelphia, 2002, Lippincott Williams & Wilkins.

Hyman, JE, Moore DW: Orthopedic trauma. In Burg FD et al, editors: *Current pediatric therapy*, ed 18, Philadephia, 2006, WB Saunders Elsevier.

Jenkins JL, Braen GR: *Manual of emergency medicine*, ed 5, Philadelphia, 2005, Lippincott, Williams & Wilkins.

Jenson HB, Baltimore RS: Infectious diseases. In Kliegman RM et al, editors: *Nelson essentials of pediatrics*, ed 5, Philadelphia, 2006, WB Saunders, Elsevier.

Joffee M: Burns. In Fleisher GR, Ludwig S, Silverman BK, editors: *Synopsis of pediatric emergency medicine*, ed 4, Philadelphia, 2002, Lippincott Williams & Wilkins.

Kilbaugh TJ, Huh JW, Helfaer MA: Disorders of temperature control. In Burg FD et al, editors. *Current pediatric therapy*, ed 18, Philadelphia, 2006, Saunders Elsevier.

Khine H, Dorfman DH, Avner JR: Applicability of Ottawa Knee Rule for knee injury in children, *Pediatr Emerg Care* 17(6):401-404, 2001.

Krogstad P: Osteomyelitis. In Burg FD et al, editors: *Current pediatric therapy*, ed 18, Philadelphia, 2006, WB Saunders Elsevier.

Lampe RM: Osteomyelitis and suppurative arthritis. In Behrman RE, Kliegman RM, Jenson HB, editors: *Nelson textbook of pediatrics*, ed 17, Philadelphia, 2004, WB Saunders.

Latterman C, Armfield D, Wukich DK: Lower leg, ankle, & foot injuries. In McMahon PJ, editor, *Current diagnosis & treatment sports medicine*, New York, 2007, McGraw-Hill.

Leickly F: Allergic emergencies. In Crain EF, Gershel JC, editors: *Clinical manual of emergency pediatrics*, ed 4, New York, 2003, McGraw-Hill.

Lipton JD: Soft tissue injury and wound repair. In Strange GR et al, editors: *Pediatric emergency medicine: a comprehensive study guide*, ed 2, New York, 2002, McGraw-Hill.

Lukish J: Burns. In Burg FD et al, editors. *Current pediatric therapy*, ed 18, Philadelphia, 2006, WB Saunders Elsevier.

Mann RL: Orthopedic emergencies. In Crain EF, Gershel JC, editors: *Clinical manual of emergency pediatrics*, ed 4, New York, 2003, McGraw-Hill.

Marcdante KJ: The acutely ill or injured child. In Kliegman RM et al, editors. *Nelson essentials of pediatrics*, ed 5, Philadelphia, 2006, WB Saunders, Elsevier.

Mayeda DV: Orthopedic injuries: management principles. In Barkin RM, Rosen P, editors: *Emergency pediatrics: a guide to ambulatory care*, ed 5, St Louis, 1999, Mosby.

McGintee EE, Beno S, Brown-Whitehorn T: Anaphylaxis. In Burg FD et al, editors. *Current pediatric therapy*, ed 18, Philadelphia, 2006, WB Saunders, Elsevier.

McMahon PJ: *Current diagnosis & treatment sports medicine*, New York, 2007, McGraw-Hill.

National Center for Health Statistics: Health, United States, 2006 with chartbook on trends in the health of Americans. Hyattsville, MD, U.S. Department of Health and Human Services, Centers for Disease Control and Prevention, National Center for Health Statistics, 2006.

National Center for Injury Prevention and Control: How many people have traumatic brain injury? Available at www.cdc.gov/Ncipc/tbi/TBI.htm (accessed Dec. 16, 2007).

Paller AS, Mancini AJ: *Hurwitz clinical pediatric dermatology: a textbook of skin disorders of childhood and adolescence*, ed 3, Philadelphia, 2006, WB Saunders, Elsevier.

Reece RM, Sege R: Childhood head injuries. Accidental or inflicted? *Arch Pediatr Adolesc Med* 154:11-15, 2000.

Rivara FP, Grossman D: Injury control. In Behrman RE, Kliegman RM, Jenson HB, editors: *Nelson textbook of pediatrics*, ed 17, Philadelphia, 2004, WB Saunders.

Rosman NP: Head injury. In Burg FD et al, editors: *Current pediatric therapy*, ed 18, Philadelphia, 2006, WB Saunders Elsevier.

Schutzman SA: Injury-head. In Fleisher GR, Ludwig S, Silverman BK, editors: *Synopsis of pediatric emergency medicine*, ed 4, Philadelphia, 2002, Lippincott Williams & Wilkins.

Selbst SM, Attia M: Minor trauma—lacerations. In Fleisher GR, Ludwig S, Silverman BK, editors: *Synopsis of pediatric emergency medicine*, ed 4, Philadelphia, 2002, Lippincott Williams & Wilkins.

Shah B: Reduction of radial head subluxation. In Finberg L, Kleinman RE, editors: *Saunders manual of pediatric practice*, ed 2, Philadelphia, 2002, WB Saunders.

Smith JT: Orthopedic problems in children. In Rudolph AM, Kamei RK, Overby KJ, editors: *Rudolph's fundamentals of pediatrics*, ed 3, New York, 2002, McGraw-Hill.

Sonnett FM, Green RA, Dayan PS: Mammalian bites and bite-related infections. In Burg FD et al, editors: *Current pediatric therapy*, ed 18, Philadelphia, 2006, WB Saunders Elsevier.

Sorrentino A, Monroe K: Insect stings. In Burg FD et al, editors: *Gellis and Kagan's current pediatric therapy*, ed 17, Philadelphia, 2002, WB Saunders.

Stiell IG et al: Multicentre trial to introduce the Ottawa Rules for use of radiography in acute ankle injuries, *BMJ* 311:594-597, 1995.

Thompson GH: Orthopedics. In Kliegman RM et al, editors. *Nelson essentials of pediatrics*, ed 5, Philadelphia, 2006, WB Saunders Elsevier.

40

Genetic Disorders

Janet K. Williams and Catherine E. Burns

Genetic factors are linked to many disorders found in children. Some of these disorders are considered to be classic genetic diseases. Examples include cystic fibrosis, Down syndrome, and Duchenne muscular dystrophy. However, many of the most prevalent disorders of childhood have some genetic components. The chance that a child has or will develop a single gene, chromosomal, or malformation condition during his/her life is between 3.15% to 7.3% (Jorde et al, 2006).

The manifestations of genetic diseases can appear immediately after birth or after many years, such as in patients with Huntington chorea. The manifestations can be evidenced in biochemical, reproductive, growth, developmental, or behavioral ways. Therefore, the primary health care provider must be constantly vigilant for the possibility of genetic disease. Furthermore, once a genetic condition is suspected, referral to a medical geneticist will not always be required or possible. Primary care providers need to be knowledgeable, yet know their own limitations and set personal criteria for referral to specialists.

Caring for children with significant, long-term problems confers enormous responsibilities on the provider, family, community, and society. Primary care providers assume a variety of roles related to the care of children with genetic disorders. These roles include promoting health of persons with genetic conditions and assisting children and families to reduce risk for medical problems by helping families make decisions about childbearing, screening for early detection to prevent disability, assisting parents to use specialized services, teaching health principles, monitoring and evaluating clients with genetic diseases, and working with families under the stress of caregiving. Ethical decision-making has a particularly important role in the area of genetics and genetic counseling.

▨ CELLULAR AND MOLECULAR GENETICS

Humans have forty-six chromosomes arranged in twenty-three pairs. Twenty-two pairs are autosomes (the same in males and females) and are homologous because their deoxyribonucleic acid, commonly referred to as DNA, is very similar. The remaining pair is the sex chromosomes, with two X chromosomes

for females and one X and one Y chromosome for males. They are not homologous. Each chromosome has a long arm (q) and a short arm (p) and is numbered according to its distinct appearance from the largest to the smallest. The gametes (egg and sperm) have half the chromosome complement from the parents (twenty-three). During meiosis (formation of the haploid with twenty-three chromosomes from the egg or sperm), the original paired chromosomes from paternal and maternal sides cross over and exchange genetic material, resulting in genetic diversity. The resultant interindividual variation is much greater than intergroup variation. Fusion at fertilization restores the forty-six-chromosome (twenty-three pair) complement, with one of each chromosome pair from each gamete. As a result of genetic variation, a gene may differ from one individual to another in its DNA sequence. These differences in sequencing are called *alleles*. If the two alleles at any given location of a pair of homologous chromosomes are identical, the locus is *homozygous*. If the two alleles are different, the locus is *heterozygous*.

Genes, which carry the information about inherited characteristics from parent to child, are arranged linearly on the chromosomes, each with a specific locus. Thousands of genes are located on each chromosome. Not all genes are active at once; certain mechanisms activate them at various developmental points. In homozygous loci, the genes from a pair of chromosomes carry similar instructions regarding the trait of interest; in heterozygous loci, the instructions are different for each gene. In the latter case, one gene may be dominant, with its instructions manifested in the phenotype, as in Huntington disease, or the genes can be co-dominant, as in the case of individuals with blood type AB.

The human genome contains approximately 30,000 genes. Genes are composed of deoxyribonucleic acid. Each DNA molecule includes pairs of nitrogenous bases—adenine, cytosine, guanine, and thymine (labeled A, C, G, T)—wound around a histone protein core in a double helix. There are more than 3 billion base pairs in the human genome for an individual. From the four nitrogenous bases, 64 triple-base combination sequences (codons) of A, C, G, and U (uracil is substituted for thymine in the messenger ribonucleic acid [RNA] at this point) such as GUA, UUG, and CGG are possible (Jorde et al, 2006). Three codons signal the end of a gene (stop codons) and 61 define the 20 amino acids. Thus, each amino acid may be specified by more than one codon. The sequence of the amino acids directs the synthesis of proteins in the cell cytoplasm (Nussbaum et al, 2001) (Fig. 40-1).

The authors would like to acknowledge Pamela J. Hellings for her contributions that remain unchanged from the previous edition of this textbook.

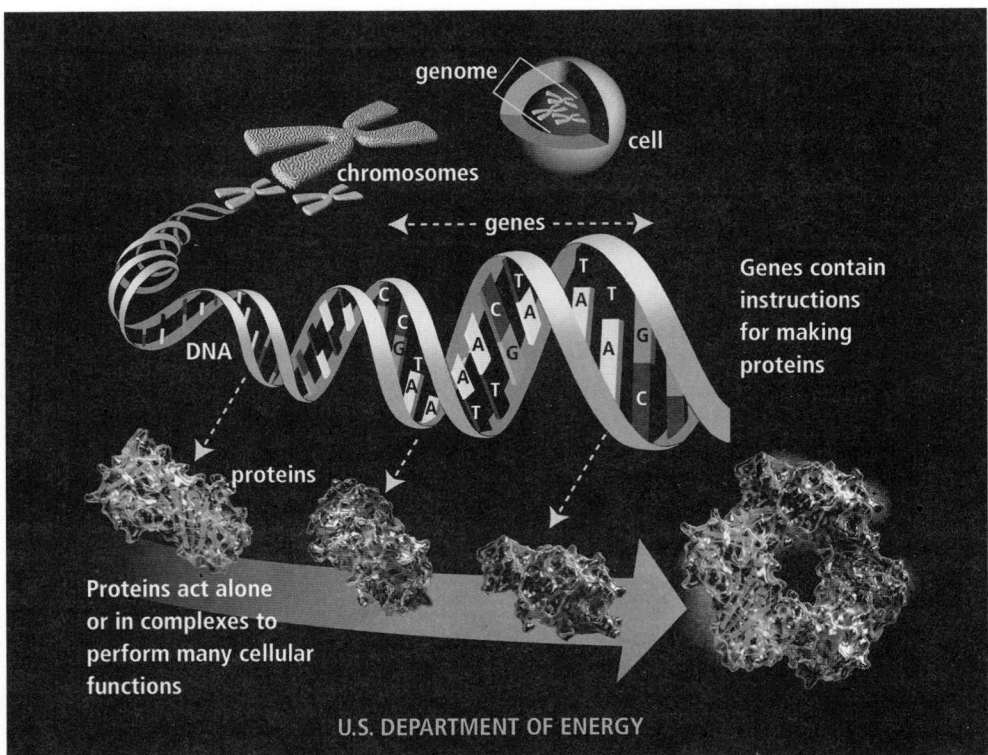

genome

cell

chromosomes

genes

DNA

Genes contain instructions for making proteins

proteins

Proteins act alone or in complexes to perform many cellular functions

U.S. DEPARTMENT OF ENERGY

FIG. 40-1 Genetic diagram. From the U.S. Department of Energy, Washington, D.C.

CAUSES OF GENETIC VARIATION AND GENETIC DISORDERS

Mutations occur when genetic material is permanently changed through alteration, deletion, duplication, or misplacement. Sometimes mutations arise spontaneously, but once the change occurs in the germ cells, it is transmitted to future generations. Mutations are defined as characteristics being present in less than 1% of the population. A change in greater than 1% is called a *polymorphism*. Mutations and polymorphisms may be benign, beneficial, or detrimental.

Genetic disorders are classified as *chromosomal disorders*, in which the entire chromosome or large segments of it are duplicated or missing; *single-gene disorders*, in which single genes are altered; and *multifactorial problems*, in which multiple genetic and environmental factors interact. Although the majority of genetic conditions fit in these categories, other patterns of inheritance, such as mitochondrial inheritance may lead to genetic disorders. Conditions that result from mutation in mitochondrial DNA are inherited through the maternal line.

CHROMOSOMAL DISORDERS

Chromosomal disorders are present in 0.6% to 0.9% of the general population (Jorde et al, 2006). There is also a high frequency of chromosomal disorders in spontaneous abortions and stillbirths. Such disorders are commonly linked to alterations in cognitive development; linear growth, usually short stature; and congenital anomalies. The chromosomal disorders include problems of chromosome number (increase or decrease in the number of chromosomes), structure, or both.

The prevalence of chromosomal disorders due to nondisjunction (failure of homologous pairs to separate properly during meiosis) increases with advancing maternal age. Testing to diagnose a chromosome disorder is done through cell culture and chromosome analysis. In addition to the more traditional method of karyotype analysis, in which the total number of each chromosome is identified, staining techniques to identify chromosomal banding assist in the identification of deletions and duplications of chromosomal material. Techniques such as fluorescence in situ hybridization (FISH) provide the ability to identify missing, additional, or rearranged chromosomal material for some of the more common abnormalities but must be ordered for the specific location of interest (Jorde et al, 2006).

SINGLE-GENE DISORDERS

Mendelian theory describes four patterns of inheritance: autosomal dominant, autosomal recessive, X-linked dominant, and X-linked recessive. Dominant inheritance disorders occur in heterozygotes, where one gene dominates its counterpart from the other parent. Recessive inheritance disorders occur only when a person is homozygous, when the gene with a disease-causing mutation appears on both of the chromosomes of the pair. However, genetic mutations for some conditions have reduced *penetrance*, in which a person may have the affected gene (genotype) without expressing the observable characteristics (phenotype), and variable *expressivity*, in which the severity of the disease condition varies greatly. The result is that some children have clinically severe disease whereas others, with mutations in the same gene, are more mildly affected.

MULTIFACTORIAL OR MULTIPLE GENE DISORDERS

Multifactorial problems result from the complex interaction of multiple genes in various sites and/or interaction of genes with the environment. Several terms are used for this group of conditions (e.g., *multifactorial, multiple gene*, and *polygenic*). Cleft lip and palate, spina bifida, hypertension, schizophrenia, pyloric stenosis, diabetes, hypercholesterolemia, Hirschsprung disease, and asthma all fall into this category (Johnson & Robin, 2000).

Multifactorial problems are more likely to cluster in families. The exact recurrence risk is more difficult to predict because the precise genetic and environmental risks are usually not known. However, in general, the risk for the condition increases if more family members are affected, and if the disease has a more severe expression (Jorde et al, 2006).

NONTRADITIONAL INHERITANCE

Three additional patterns of transmission of genetic material from generation to generation have been identified—germline mosaicism, uniparental disomy, and mitochondrial inheritance.

Germline Mosaicism

In this pattern, a mutation occurs in a cell of the developing organism sometime after fertilization. Thus, as cells are multiplying, some will begin to reproduce with the mutation while others will not contain the gene mutation. The outcome is a person with "mosaicism"—some normal and some abnormal cells. Whether the gametes are affected will dictate inheritance to the next generation. Thus, the term *germline mosaicism* is used to indicate inheritability of the trait. With germline mosaicism, parents appear normal but have some gametes with the gene mutation. The challenge, clinically, is to identify the condition as inheritable. If normal-appearing parents have a first child with a condition such as achondroplasia, which is normally autosomal dominant, the clinician would deduce that the achondroplasia was not inherited in an autosomal dominant manner (in which case one parent would have had the disorder), so a new mutation, and the possibility of germline mosaicism, must be considered. If germline mutation is present, the risk of recurrence in a second offspring is increased. It is because of such situations that genetic counseling for parents is important to help determine the risk to subsequent children.

Uniparental Disomy

Generally, children receive one chromosome from each parental pair at the time of fertilization. If, by some chance, the child receives two copies of one chromosome of a pair from one parent and none from the other parent, uniparental disomy has occurred. The result is that the child will be homozygous for every gene located on that chromosome, which increases the possibilities of an autosomal recessive disorder in the child. The process has been described in some patients with cystic fibrosis. The same process also may result in either Prader-Willi or Angelman syndrome, which involve the same gene loci but the disease differs depending on whether the copies are from the mother or the father (Jorde et al, 2006).

Mitochondrial DNA Inheritance

Mitochondria in cells also have DNA (mtDNA). Unlike chromosomal DNA, mtDNA is circular. All inherited mtDNA comes from the ovum—thus it has a maternal transmission pattern. Because each cell has more than one mitochondrion, there are more opportunities for mutations and also for variable expressivity; if many normal mitochondria are present, the effects from the aberrant mtDNA may be minimal. Several biopsies of different tissues will be subjected to both enzymatic and DNA analyses for diagnosis of mtDNA-related diseases. Although rare, mitochondrial diseases do play a role in some more common conditions such as deafness and non-insulin-dependent diabetes (Jorde et al, 2006).

TERATOGENS

Although not strictly genetic in origin, teratogens are often discussed with genetic disorders because the differential diagnosis includes factors that affect the embryo after fertilization and those that affect the DNA of the germ cells or their joining with fertilization. Fetal alcohol syndrome is an example of a condition in this category. Viral diseases, such as rubella, certain drugs, and environmental toxins—such as mercury—are also considered teratogens. The Pregnancy Exposure InfoLine contains current information on potential teratogenic effects of specific environmental substances (see Resource Box at the end of the chapter).

■ HUMAN GENOME PROJECT

The Human Genome Project (HGP) is an international effort begun in 1990 with the following goals:
- Sequence the entire genome by 2003 (the sequence is now publicly available)
- Identify genes and their function
- Expand database and data analysis capabilities
- Study the ethical, legal, and social implications of current and anticipated information and technology outcomes of the HGP

Final sequencing of the genome is completed; however, the remaining challenges include further understanding of structure and function of genes, genetic aspects of risk for disease and responses to treatments; and social consequences of new genetic technologies and information. Knowledge about genetics for delivery of primary care clinical services is increasingly important. Primary care providers must have a firm grasp on genetic principles and, at a minimum, meet the core competencies for all health care professionals developed by a coalition of member organizations representing nursing, medicine, psychology, genetic counseling, and others (National Coalition for Health Professional Education in Genetics [NCHPEG], 2005). The three basic competencies are as follows:
- Appreciate the limitations of one's own genetic expertise
- Understand the social and psychologic implications of genetic services
- Know how and when to make a referral to a genetics professional

In addition, there are detailed recommendations for knowledge, skills, and attitudes that all health professionals need to have to apply genetics to their health care practices. Finally, the resultant ethical and legal issues will continue to provide formidable challenges for society. Primary care providers must continue to be a part of the societal debate and resolution.

More specific nursing practice guidelines were developed in 2005 by a consensus panel of expert nurses as a resource for educators, practitioners, and credentialing organizations (Essential Nursing Competencies and Curricula Guidelines for Genetics and Genomics, 2005).

ETHICAL ISSUES

Since 1990, largely due to the work of the HGP, the ability to diagnose a hereditary condition for those who are currently symptomatic or who are presymptomatic, the ability to identify those who are carriers of a genetic condition, and the ability to determine susceptibility to a genetic condition have increased dramatically. However, the availability of this technology raises significant ethical issues. The HGP was concerned about these issues from the beginning and has a branch specifically devoted to oversight of these concerns (the Ethical, Legal, and Social Initiative [ELSI]).

Maintenance of confidentiality is a challenge. The presence of genetic information in the medical record, health insurance diagnostic database, or in DNA databases such as newborn screening specimens mandates policies to maintain the integrity of these records. The Health Insurance Portability and Accountability Act (HIPAA) of 1996 specifies the duty for clinicians not to disclose medical information without the signed consent of the patient or the child's parents (U.S. Department of Health and Human Services, 2006).

During the collection of genetics information and tests, it is also possible to discover unanticipated information, for instance, regarding the parentage of the child being tested. Situations such as misattribution of paternity and children being raised by nonbiologic parents may be discovered. There is not agreement about whether these findings should be routinely disclosed. Prior agreement in the consent process can assist in the decision about whether to disclose this information or not.

The availability of presymptomatic testing for conditions that may not become apparent until adulthood, such as Huntington disease and breast cancer, has raised another set of questions. Should children and adolescents be tested for such conditions? Generally, it is recommended that genetic testing for late-onset conditions be deferred until adulthood when individuals, rather than their parents, can make the decision, unless there is evidence that early diagnosis can result in treatment strategies that will alter the progression of the disease (AAP Committee on Bioethics, 2001). However, providers should explore parents' reasons for requesting genetic testing of their child or children (Ross, 2004).

The ability to screen for a large number of genetic disorders via the newborn screening process has increased the number and types of conditions that can be included. Because these programs are organized by and paid for through state governments, there is some variability in required tests between states (National Newborn Screening & Genetics Resource

Center, 2006). Three principles have been suggested by the Institute of Medicine (IOM) to be used in making decisions about the introduction or continuation of tests:

- Identification of the genetic condition must provide a clear benefit to the child.
- A system must be in place to confirm the diagnosis.
- Treatment and follow-up must be available for affected infants (IOM, 1994).

Congenital hypothyroidism, sickle cell disease, sickle-C, sickle-beta thalassemia, classical galactosemia, and phenylketonuria are mandated in newborn screening programs in all U.S. states. An additional sixty-one conditions are included in individual state newborn screening programs.

These are only a few of the ethical issues under current discussion. Primary care providers must be part of the ongoing debate and be aware of the issues, policies, and laws as they work with families who are trying to make decisions.

ASSESSMENT

Primary care providers identify possible genetic disorders by using the same skills as those used for other pediatric health problems: knowledge of risk factors, collection of a good history, and a complete physical examination augmented with appropriate laboratory or other studies. After the assessment, providers determine the operative genetic mechanism and develop and implement a plan of care for the patient and family with consideration of individual, family, and cultural factors. Box 40-1 identifies some common features of children or family members with genetic disorders that should lead providers to explore issues of possible genetic problems in the child and family.

RISK FACTORS

Risk factors that may be identified in the child or family members include the following:
- Family history of known genetic disorder or recurrent pathologic condition
- Malformations (see Box 40-3)

BOX 40-1 Features Suggesting a Genetic Disorder

Mental retardation/developmental delays
Seizures with mental retardation
Severe hypotonia in infancy
Loss of developmental milestones
Short stature
Failure to thrive/growth retardation
Microcephaly
Dysmorphic features
Two or more physical malformations
Ambiguous genitalia
Pigmentary skin lesions
Ocular findings such as colobomas or blindness
Deafness

- Mental retardation
- Metabolic disorders
- Delayed development of secondary sex characteristics
- Sensory deficits
- Progressive disorders
- Neuromuscular disorders
- Affective disorders (e.g., schizophrenia)
- Presence of birth defects
- Developmental delays or learning problems
- Repeated spontaneous abortions or stillbirths
- Maternal factors, including alcohol or drug exposure, medication exposure, age older than 35 years, environmental or occupational toxin exposure
- Family ethnic background (Table 40-1)

HISTORY

The history of genetic diseases usually includes the following main areas: family history of the disease using a pedigree format, environmental and occupational history, reproductive history, dietary history, medical history of the child, and developmental data (see Figs. 40-2 and 40-3 for an example of the pedigree notation format). The pedigree provides a visual map of the occurrence of specific traits and helps identify other family members who might be at risk. Screening questions for genetic disorders that should be asked of all patients are included in Table 40-2. Families can be encouraged to record their own family history information by using programs, such as the U.S. Surgeon General's Family History Initiative (2005). Parents and children should be encouraged to learn about the health of members of their family, which may, in turn, provide clues as to specific health risks for themselves (Siegel & Milunsky, 2004).

When a genetic disorder is suspected, the history must become more specific, as outlined in Table 40-3. Questions need to address the following:

- A family history is needed to identify family members with conditions that may be genetically transmitted. A pedigree helps providers display the potential pattern of inheritance and visualize the relationships among affected family members. Past and current health of each person in the pedigree, birth histories of other family members, and mental retardation or learning problems of family members are all

TABLE 40-1   Genetic Risks Associated With Ethnic Background

Ethnic Background	Genetic Disorder at Higher Risk
Northern European	Cystic fibrosis, phenylketonuria
Jewish (Ashkenazi descent)	Tay-Sachs, Canavan, Gaucher
West African	Sickle cell, sickle cell–hemoglobin C
Mediterranean	β-thalassemia, sickle cell
French-Canadian	Tay-Sachs, branched-chain ketoaciduria

important areas to explore. Consanguinity should be noted; persons who have a common ancestor may each be carriers of a gene mutation present in that family.

- The environmental and occupational history may provide information about specific teratogenic factors, which might be involved.
- The mother's reproductive history may give information about malformations, genetic conditions, or infectious diseases transmitted to other offspring. Her pregnancy and delivery of the child in question may give other information to determine whether the condition was the result of genetic factors or whether the condition was a result of trauma, infection, or some other factor occurring during the pregnancy or delivery.

PHYSICAL EXAMINATION

When a genetic disease is being considered, the physical examination focuses on growth, major and minor anomalies, and comparisons with family members. Any major anomaly can have a genetic cause. A known genetic cause is identified in approximately 30% of newborn infants with a congenital malformation (Nelson & Holmes, 1989). Three minor anomalies should raise the suspicion of a major anomaly and a genetic disorder.

First, general appearance and familial similarities are assessed. Note if a parent with similar physical features has specific health problems. Body size and proportions, measurements and percentiles, and a careful assessment of all systems constitute the remainder of the examination.

Common minor anomalies are identified in Box 40-2. Box 40-3 lists various anomalies by body parts. *Smith's Recognizable Patterns of Human Malformations* includes tables on the size, length, and shape of various body parts that can be used to validate observations presumed to represent pathology (Jones, 2006). About 3% of infants are born with any one of 45 birth defects (CDC, 2006).

Dysmorphic features may be recognized and can result from the following:

- *Deformation* - abnormal shape or position of body part caused by external mechanical forces (e.g., clubfoot)
- *Disruption* - defect of organ or large body part caused by external disruption of originally normal process (e.g., amniotic bands)
- *Dysplasia* - abnormal organization of cells into tissues (e.g., polycystic kidneys)
- *Malformation* - abnormal development of an organ or large body part from an intrinsically abnormal process (e.g., cleft palate)

Visual recognition, combined with family history evaluation, are major factors in diagnosing genetic diseases. The provider can hone skills by reviewing pictures of patients with various disorders and consulting with experts.

DEVELOPMENTAL ASSESSMENT

Many genetic disorders cause some degree of mental retardation and central nervous system effects. Developmental assessment is a key component in planning a comprehensive approach to the evaluation of a child with developmental delay (Roberts

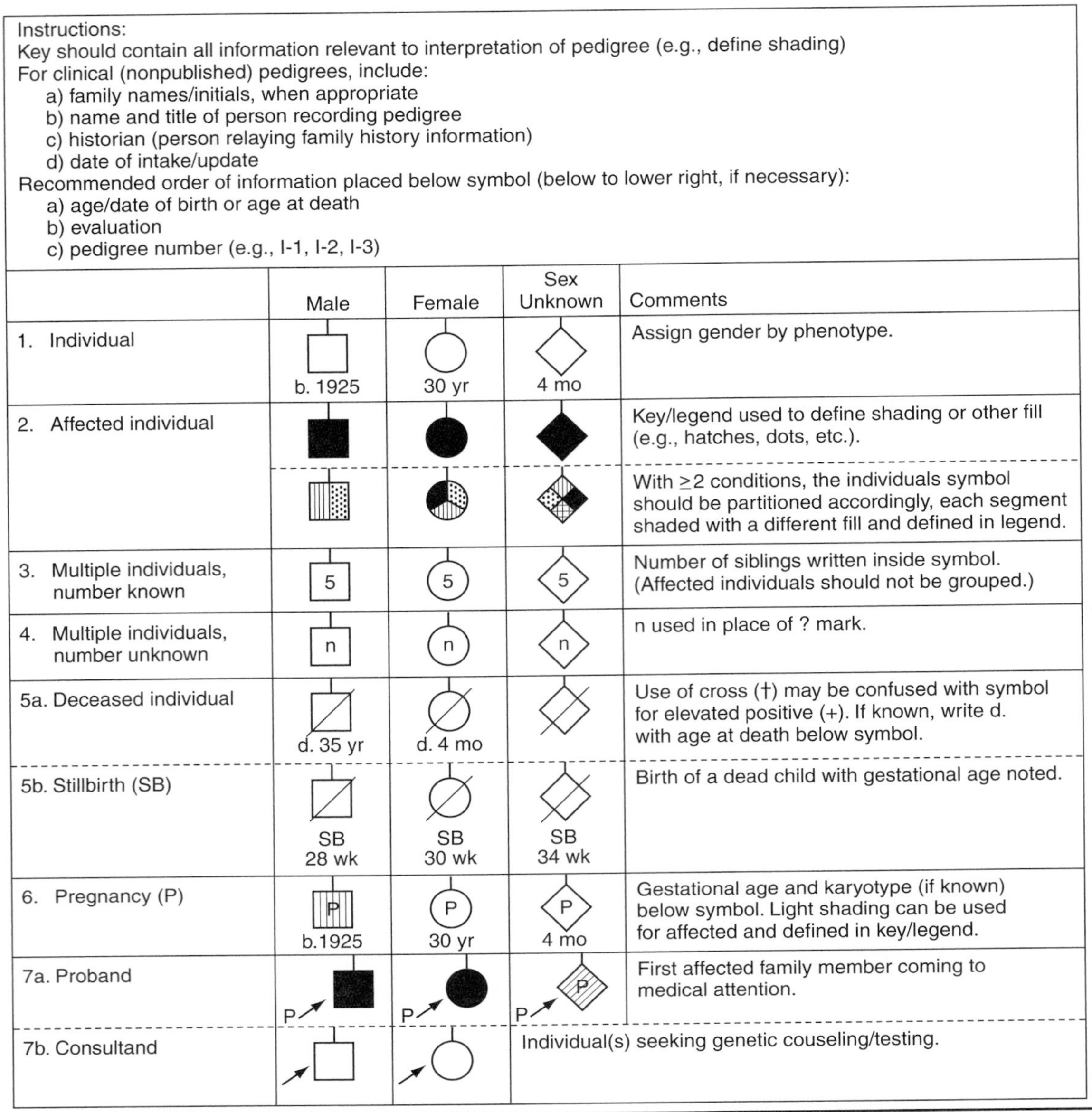

Instructions:
Key should contain all information relevant to interpretation of pedigree (e.g., define shading)
For clinical (nonpublished) pedigrees, include:
   a) family names/initials, when appropriate
   b) name and title of person recording pedigree
   c) historian (person relaying family history information)
   d) date of intake/update
Recommended order of information placed below symbol (below to lower right, if necessary):
   a) age/date of birth or age at death
   b) evaluation
   c) pedigree number (e.g., I-1, I-2, I-3)

	Male	Female	Sex Unknown	Comments
1. Individual	b. 1925	30 yr	4 mo	Assign gender by phenotype.
2. Affected individual	(filled)	(filled)	(filled)	Key/legend used to define shading or other fill (e.g., hatches, dots, etc.).
	(hatched)	(part filled)	(part filled)	With ≥2 conditions, the individuals symbol should be partitioned accordingly, each segment shaded with a different fill and defined in legend.
3. Multiple individuals, number known	5	5	5	Number of siblings written inside symbol. (Affected individuals should not be grouped.)
4. Multiple individuals, number unknown	n	n	n	n used in place of ? mark.
5a. Deceased individual	d. 35 yr	d. 4 mo		Use of cross (†) may be confused with symbol for elevated positive (+). If known, write d. with age at death below symbol.
5b. Stillbirth (SB)	SB 28 wk	SB 30 wk	SB 34 wk	Birth of a dead child with gestational age noted.
6. Pregnancy (P)	P b.1925	P 30 yr	P 4 mo	Gestational age and karyotype (if known) below symbol. Light shading can be used for affected and defined in key/legend.
7a. Proband	P (filled)	P (filled)	P (filled)	First affected family member coming to medical attention.
7b. Consultand	(open)	(open)		Individual(s) seeking genetic couseling/testing.

FIG. 40-2 Pedigree model. Common pedigree symbols, definitions, and abbreviations. *mo*, Month; *wk*, week; *yr*, year. (Adapted from Bennett R et al: Recommendations for standardized human pedigree nomenclature, *Am J Hum Genet* 56:745–752, 1995.)

et al, 2004). Based on findings from the family history, physical examination, and developmental assessment, specific laboratory studies may be useful in determining if a specific diagnosis can be identified. The genetic evaluation of a child with mental retardation is diagrammed in Figure 40-4.

DIAGNOSTIC STUDIES

Biochemical Studies

Many screening tests are available to check for inborn errors of metabolism. Such tests include those for phenylketonuria (PKU), galactosemia, and others. See Chapter 38 for further discussion.

Molecular Analyses (DNA Studies)

Blood tests are commonly used to screen for sickle cell disease, the thalassemias, and Tay-Sachs disease. Molecular genetic methods are increasingly being used for many dis-

orders, such as cystic fibrosis. Generally, the tests must be ordered with some specificity. Linkage analysis, direct mutation analysis, and molecular cytogenetic analyses are all types of DNA studies. Each has its own advantages and disadvantages (Roberts et al, 2004; AAP Committee on Genetics, 2000).

Cytogenetics: Chromosome Studies

Chromosome tests may be needed to identify specific genetic diseases. Fluorescent in situ hybridization (FISH) combines elements of standard cytogenetic technique with molecular technology; probes for specific, extremely small chromosome abnormalities are used. For instance, FISH analysis might identify the deletion of chromosome site 15q11-q13 associated with Prader-Willi. Subtelomeric screening examines gene-rich regions of chromosomes where specific translocations may be

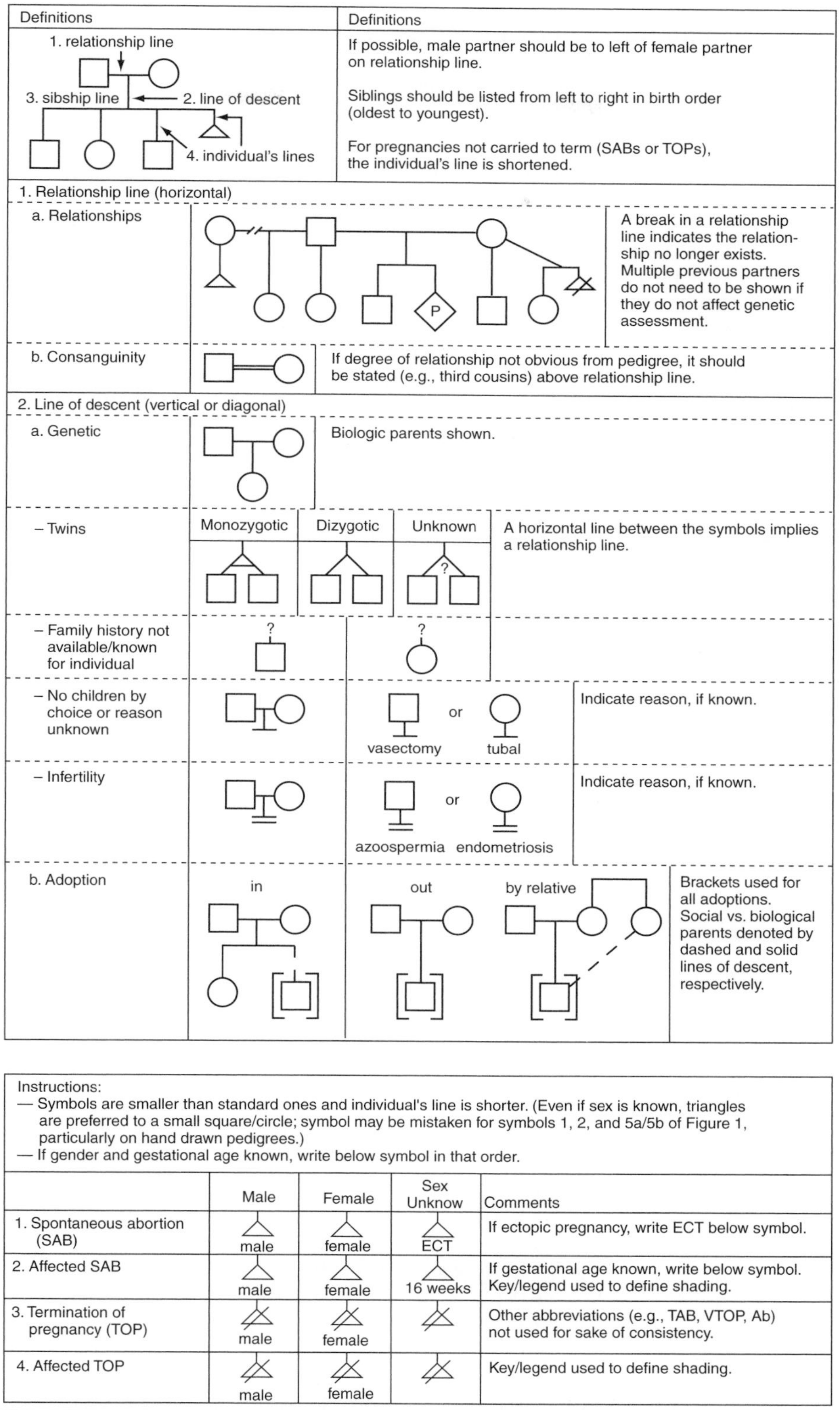

Definitions	Definitions
1. relationship line 3. sibship line · 2. line of descent 4. individual's lines	If possible, male partner should be to left of female partner on relationship line. Siblings should be listed from left to right in birth order (oldest to youngest). For pregnancies not carried to term (SABs or TOPs), the individual's line is shortened.

1. Relationship line (horizontal)

a. Relationships		A break in a relationship line indicates the relationship no longer exists. Multiple previous partners do not need to be shown if they do not affect genetic assessment.
b. Consanguinity		If degree of relationship not obvious from pedigree, it should be stated (e.g., third cousins) above relationship line.

2. Line of descent (vertical or diagonal)

a. Genetic		Biologic parents shown.
– Twins	Monozygotic Dizygotic Unknown	A horizontal line between the symbols implies a relationship line.
– Family history not available/known for individual		
– No children by choice or reason unknown	vasectomy or tubal	Indicate reason, if known.
– Infertility	azoospermia endometriosis or	Indicate reason, if known.
b. Adoption	in out by relative	Brackets used for all adoptions. Social vs. biological parents denoted by dashed and solid lines of descent, respectively.

Instructions:
— Symbols are smaller than standard ones and individual's line is shorter. (Even if sex is known, triangles are preferred to a small square/circle; symbol may be mistaken for symbols 1, 2, and 5a/5b of Figure 1, particularly on hand drawn pedigrees.)
— If gender and gestational age known, write below symbol in that order.

	Male	Female	Sex Unknow	Comments
1. Spontaneous abortion (SAB)	male	female	ECT	If ectopic pregnancy, write ECT below symbol.
2. Affected SAB	male	female	16 weeks	If gestational age known, write below symbol. Key/legend used to define shading.
3. Termination of pregnancy (TOP)	male	female		Other abbreviations (e.g., TAB, VTOP, Ab) not used for sake of consistency.
4. Affected TOP	male	female		Key/legend used to define shading.

FIG. 40-3   Pedigree line definitions. (Adapted from Bennett R et al: Recommendations for standardized human pedigree nomenclature, *Am J Hum Genet* 56:745–752, 1995.)

TABLE 40-2   General Screening for Genetic Conditions: The History

Question	Rationale/Comments
Has anyone in the family had a birth defect?	To identify conditions that affect others in the family. If answer is yes, try to get more information about the nature of the defect.
Is there anyone in the family with a stillborn baby or baby who died early in life?	To identify unrecognized genetic disorders. Babies who died very early may have inheritable metabolic disorders. Distinguish from sudden infant death syndrome.
Is there any chance that you and your partner are blood related? Is this pregnancy a product of incest?	Consanguinity of partners closer than first cousins is a risk factor for autosomal recessive disorders. If yes, recommend genetics consultation.
Are there any diseases or traits that run in your family?	Significant if early onset, two or more close relatives affected. Genetic heart disease and genetic cancer risks are important. If yes, recommend genetic consultation and monitoring.
Have you or any of your parents or siblings had three or more miscarriages?	May indicate a chromosome translocation. If yes, order a karyotype of the mother or father (or both).
Does anyone in the family have mental retardation?	Look for multiple members affected and associated with dysmorphic features. If yes, recommend genetic consultation.
What is your ethnic background? Your partner's?	Consider ethnic risk factors and screen if at risk.

TABLE 40-3   Specific Genetic History Questions

Topic	Specific Items of History
Family history: Helps identify family members with conditions that may be genetically transmitted	• The pedigree should focus on at least three generations and look for people with similar characteristics. • Consanguinity of partners (closer than first cousins) is very important. • Note the past and current health of each person listed on the pedigree. • Note the age of onset for family members' illnesses. • Note multiple miscarriages, stillbirths, and anomalies within family. • Family members with learning disabilities or mental retardation are important to document.
Environmental and occupational history	Exposure to environmental toxins, alcohol, cigarette smoke, drugs, or radiation that might affect offspring
Reproductive history: Helps identify malformations, genetic conditions, or infectious diseases transmitted from mother to child: 1. Maternal medical history 2. Prenatal history 3. Pregnancy and delivery history	Maternal medical history: • Uterine anomalies • Maternal illnesses and diseases (e.g., phenylketonuria, diabetes) • Immunization status Prenatal history. The reproductive history should list every pregnancy, stillbirth, and abortion. Fetuses with significant chromosomal disorders are often aborted, and 5%-7% of stillbirths and perinatal deaths are related to genetic problems: • Recurrent miscarriages • Parity • Advanced maternal or paternal age • Complications of pregnancy • Polyhydramnios or oligohydramnios • Fetal movements • Fetal growth assessments • Prenatal screening results Pregnancy and delivery history: • Breech position • Birth measurements • Gestational age • Results of newborn screening tests • Presence of three or more minor anomalies in neonate • Failure of neonate to adapt to extrauterine life • Complications of delivery

TABLE 40-3   **Specific Genetic History Questions—Cont'd**

Topic	Specific Items of History
Dietary history: Helps identify infants with single-gene-related metabolic disorders	• Infant feeding behavior • Formula or food intolerance • Temporal relation of symptoms to meals • Relation of signs and symptoms to types of food
Medical history of affected child	Use routine past medical history questions—history and current status of illnesses, hospitalizations, surgeries, allergies, injuries, immunizations. List all health care providers involved with the child's care.
Developmental history	• Achievements of milestones • Speech and language development • School performance • Developmental evaluations • Growth

located. This test may be useful in identifying abnormalities in a child with serious mental retardation and abnormal physical examination (Roberts et al, 2004).

Imaging Studies

Radiographs and other imaging studies are used to identify skeletal, central nervous system, cardiac, and other anomalies.

Photography

Photographs provide a visual record of facial and other anatomic variations. They may also be useful in identifying other family members with similar characteristics.

BOX 40-2   **Minor Malformations and Variations of Normal**

Large fontanel
Epicanthal folds
Hair whorls
Widow's peak
Low posterior hairline
Preauricular tags or pits
Minor ear anomalies
Protruding ears
Rotated ears
Low-set ears
Darwinian tubercle (blunt point protruding from upper edge of helix)
Digital anomalies
Clinodactyly (curved finger)
Camptodactyly (bent finger)
Syndactyly (webbed finger)
Transverse palmar crease
Shawl scrotum
Redundant umbilicus
Widespread nipples
Supernumerary nipples

MANAGEMENT STRATEGIES

Primary care management of children with genetic disorders includes a variety of strategies, depending on what diagnosis has been made.

PRENATAL SCREENING AND DIAGNOSIS

Prenatal evaluations can be done for many diseases if the family history indicates the possibility of a specific disease appearing in offspring. Prenatal carrier tests of parents may be conducted if these parents are at risk to be carriers of gene mutations for sickle cell disease, Tay-Sachs disease, the thalassemias, cystic fibrosis, or other conditions based on the couple's family history. Childbearing women should be referred to obstetric or genetic clinics for prenatal genetic counseling, testing, and diagnosis. Chorionic villus biopsy sampling for diagnosis of some conditions may be performed at 8 to 12 weeks of gestation at some specialized centers, and amniocentesis may be performed in the second trimester. By the fourteenth to sixteenth week of gestation, many imaging studies can also be performed to look for structural anomalies. A combination of tests including maternal serum α-fetoprotein, ultrasound, and maternal serum markers may be offered during the end of the first trimester and early weeks of the second trimester. Efficacy of prenatal testing options continues to be evaluated, and prenatal diagnostic centers may vary regarding screening procedures. These tests can identify fetuses likely to have chromosome abnormalities, neural tube defects and other prenatally identifiable disorders. Prenatal diagnosis gives the family information to make decisions regarding reproductive alternatives, such as possible termination of pregnancies with affected fetuses, artificial insemination, egg donor, deferral of childbearing, or special preparations at childbirth.

NEWBORN GENETIC SCREENING

Newborn genetic screening for a variety of metabolic diseases is done routinely. As mentioned above, different states include different groups of diseases in their panels. The provider should be sure that the routine newborn statewide screening

BOX 40-3 Malformations of the Body

Central nervous system (not mental deficiency)
- Hypotonic
- Hypertonic
- Ataxia
- Seizures
- Deafness

Brain: major anomalies
- Anencephaly
- Encephalocele
- Hydrocephalus
- Microcephaly
- Macrocephaly
- Meningomyelocele

Cranium
- Craniosynostosis
- Occiput shapes, flat or prominent
- Delayed fontanel closures
- Frontal bossing

Scalp and facial hair patterning
- Multiple hair whorls
- Anterior upsweep
- Posterior midline scalp defects

Facies
- Flat
- Round
- Broad
- Triangular
- Masklike
- Coarse

Ocular region
- Hypotelorism
- Hypertelorism
- Short palpebral fissures
- Inner canthus placement
- Inner epicanthal folds
- Slanted palpebral fissures
- Depth of orbital ridges
- Eye prominence
- Periorbital fullness
- Eyebrow shape and extension
- Ptosis
- Nystagmus
- Strabismus

Eye
- Blue sclera
- Myopia
- Microphthalmos
- Colobomas of iris
- Patterning or color of iris
- Glaucoma
- Keratoconus
- Microcornea
- Corneal opacity

- Lens discolorations/opacities
- Retinal pigmentation

Nose
- Nasal bridge shape
- Short with or without anteverted nostrils
- Hypoplasia of nares
- Prominent nose
- Choanal atresia

Maxilla and mandible
- Malar hypoplasia
- Maxillary hypoplasia often with narrow or high arched palate
- Micrognathia
- Prognathism

Oral region and mouth
- Cleft lip with or without cleft palate
- Abnormal philtrum
- Full lips
- Downturning mouth corners
- Microstomia
- Macrostomia
- Cleft palate or bifid uvula with cleft in lip
- Macroglossia/microglossia
- Hypertrophied alveolar ridges

Teeth
- Adontia
- Hypodontia (including conical teeth)
- Enamel hypoplasia
- Caries
- Early loss
- Irregular placement
- Late eruption
- Other tooth anomalies

External ears
- Low set
- Malformed auricles
- Preauricular tags or pits

Neck, thorax, and vertebrae
- Web neck
- Short neck
- Nipple anomaly
- Clavicle anomalies
- Pectus excavatum or carinatum
- Small thoracic cage
- Rib defects
- Scoliosis
- Other vertebral defects

Limbs
- Arachnodactyly
- Short limbs
- Limb reductions
- Small hands or feet
- Clinodactyly of fifth fingers

BOX 40-3   Malformations of the Body—Cont'd

- Thumb hypoplasia
- Radius hypoplasia
- Metacarpal hypoplasia
- Polydactyly
- Broad thumb or toe (or both)
- Syndactyly
- Elbow dysplasia
- Patellar dysplasia

Limbs: nails, creases, dermatoglyphics
- Nail hypoplasia or dysplasia
- Single crease (simian)
- Dermal ridge pattern abnormalities

Limbs: joints
- Joint limitations/contractures
- Clubfoot
- Clenched hand
- Joint hypermobility or lax ligaments (or both)
- Joint dislocations

Skin and hair
- Loose/redundant skin
- Pigmentation alterations
- Ichthyotic changes
- Hemangiomas and telangiectasias
- Dimples
- Alopecia
- Hirsutism
- Assorted abnormalities of hair (amount, quality, distribution, color)

Cardiac anomalies
Abdominal
- Hernias

- Hepatosplenomegaly
- Pyloric stenosis
- Incomplete rotation of colon
- Single umbilical artery

Renal
- Kidney malformations
- Renal insufficiency

Genital
- Hypospadias or ambiguous external genitalia
- Micropenis
- Cryptorchidism
- Hypoplasia of labia majora
- Anal defects

Endocrine and metabolic
- Hypothyroidism
- Hypogonadism
- Other endocrine abnormalities
  Hypocalcemia/hypercalcemia
  Hyperlipidemia
  Immunoglobulin
  Immunoglobulin deficiency

Hematology-oncology
- Anemia
- Thrombocytopenia
- Lymphoreticular malignancy
- Other malignancies

Unusual growth patterns
- Obesity
- Early macrosomia
- Asymmetry

Adapted from Jones K: *Smith's recognizable patterns of human malformations*, ed 6, Philadelphia, 2006, WB Saunders.

panel blood test is completed correctly, and that infants who have a presumptive positive result on their screening test are promptly referred for further evaluation. The provider can help parents understand that a positive result from a screening test indicates that further testing is needed to determine if their child has the condition in question.

GENETIC DISORDER DIAGNOSIS

Careful history taking and physical examinations of children will help providers identify children with genetic diseases. Newborn infants with malformations or dysmorphic features should be evaluated. Children with two major, one major and two minor, or three minor anomalies with other indicators as noted in Box 40-4 should be referred for further genetic evaluation.

In the case of a stillbirth or neonatal death, the infant's features should be documented—preferably photographed. A karyotype on blood and establishment of a fibroblast culture are also important. Head and renal ultrasound should be done if no autopsy is performed.

Children and their families should be referred for diagnosis if a genetic disease is suspected. Establishing the correct diagnosis is important for the family and the provider. The recurrence risk, prognosis given the natural history of the condition, guide to appropriate laboratory testing, plan of treatment and management, and facilitation of family coping all require knowledge of the nature of the disorder.

Telling new parents that their child may have a genetic disorder needs to happen as soon as possible—even if a diagnosis cannot be confirmed. It should be done in a quiet, comfortable place when both parents are present, by someone with credibility. When the diagnosis is made in a newborn infant, the baby should be present and referred to by name if possible. The discussion should include some positive points and the problems to be faced. A follow-up phone call should be planned and additional sources of information identified, including credible information resources, support organizations, clinical resources, and/or contact with other parents, if that is desired. The parents should have some uninterrupted time with their baby.

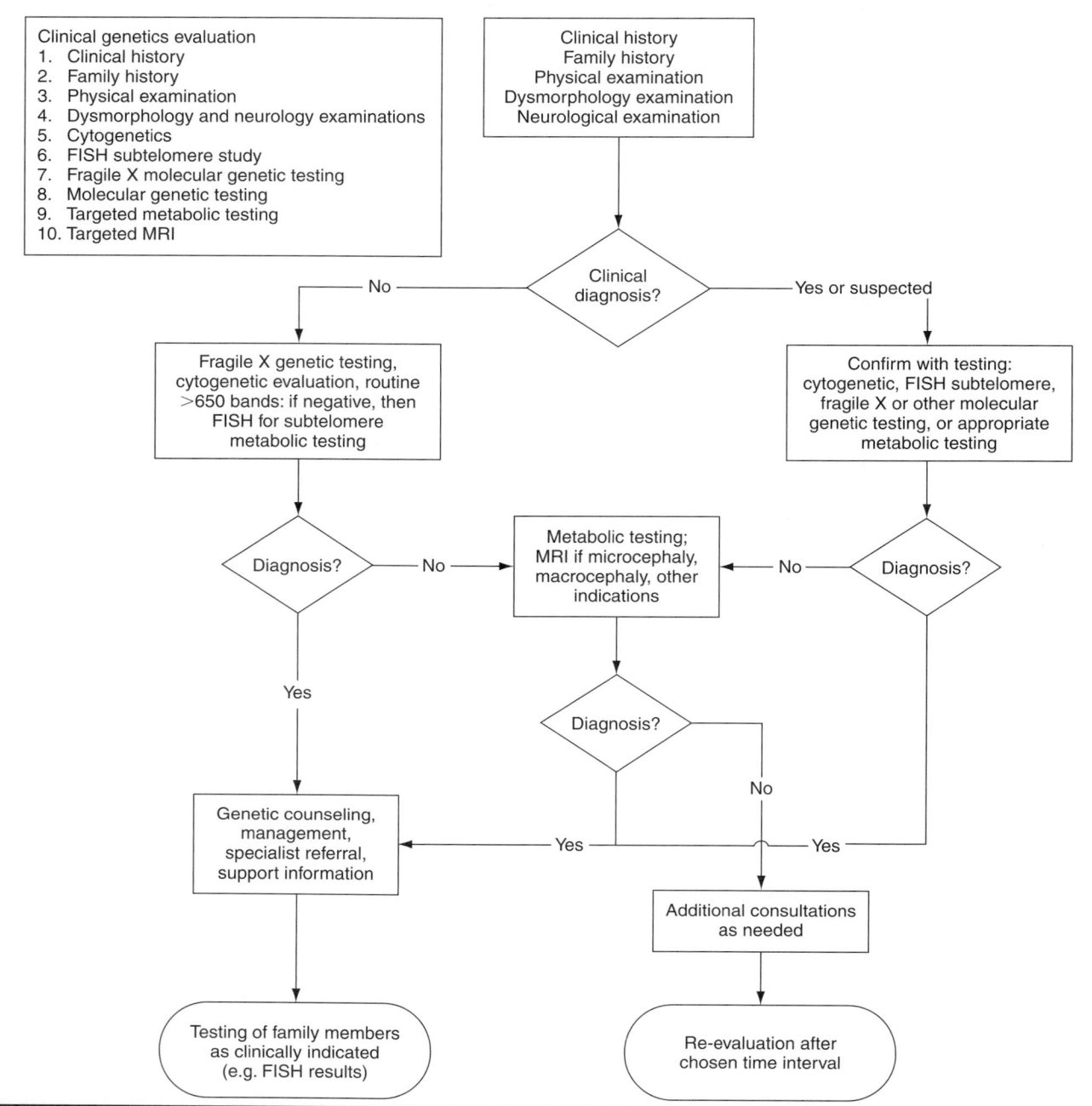

FIG. 40-4 Clinical genetic evaluation of the child with mental retardation or developmental delays. (From Moeschler JB, Shevell M, and Committee on Genetics, AAP: Clinical genetic evaluation of the child with mental retardation or developmental delays, *Pediatrics* 117:2304–2316, p. 2307, 2006.)

GENETIC COUNSELING

Genetic counseling involves open communication with families who are at risk for, or who have a genetic disease. A nondirective approach is used to allow families to determine what decisions, especially regarding reproductive plans, are best for them. However, when management or ongoing surveillance is discussed for some conditions, (e.g., for familial cancers), the family may expect health care providers to be more directive regarding recommended screening or treatment options. Genetic counseling goals include helping the family to do the following:

• Understand the diagnosis, its course, and its management

• Appreciate the way heredity influences the disorder and the risks of recurrence and carrier status to specific family members
• Understand the alternatives available to reduce the risk of recurrence
• Choose the course of action that is appropriate in view of the risks, family ethics and values, and family goals
• Adjust as well as possible to the disorder, its prognosis, and the risks of recurrence

The process takes time and may require many visits (Skirton & Patch, 2002; Johnson & Brensinger, 2000). Generally, genetic counseling is provided by specialists. Ethical genetic counsel-

BOX 40-4   Indications for Karyotype Analysis

Suspected chromosomal problem
Two major malformations
One major and two minor malformations
Ambiguous genitalia
Congenital heart disease
Hypotonia
Malformed stillborns and normal stillborns when demise is of
   undetermined etiology
Mental retardation or developmental delay
Growth retardation or short stature
Couple with two or more miscarriages or infertility

Adapted from Pacific Northwest Regional Genetics Group: Practical
genetics for primary care, Portland, OR, 1996, Oregon Health Science
Center, Pacific Northwest Regional Genetics Group.

ing takes into consideration the principles of beneficence (helping the patient and family) and nonmaleficence (do no harm).

The primary care provider's role in genetic counseling is to
perform the following:

• Identify individuals at risk for genetic disorders
• Teach children and families about the genetic counseling
  process
• Initiate referrals with screening pedigrees, medical records,
  and appropriate histories and physical examinations

• Evaluate the family's understanding of genetic counseling
  and provide support as the family makes decisions based on
  genetic testing information
• Provide health care as indicated

All families with genetic diseases should receive genetic
counseling. The extent of counseling needed, and the ongoing needs of the child and family determine when the primary
care provider can manage the child and family and when
referral to a genetic or specialty clinic would be necessary.

PRIMARY HEALTH CARE OF CHILDREN WITH GENETIC DISORDERS

Primary care and chronic disease management of children
with genetic disorders need to be integrated. Health supervision,
screening for complications, and management of the health of
the child given the genetic condition at hand are all important.
The American Academy of Pediatrics (AAP) has developed
an example of health supervision guidelines for children with
Down syndrome (AAP Committee on Genetics, 2001a). It
incorporates developmental, psychological, educational, and
medical components. Monitoring for high-risk conditions,
including congenital heart disease, thyroid disorders, hearing loss, atlantoaxial subluxation, ophthalmic abnormalities,
and growth and development, needs to be integrated into the
plan for primary health care. There are similar guidelines
for the care of children with neurofibromatosis type 1 (AAP
Committee on Genetics, 1995), Turner syndrome (Frias et al,

BOX 40-5   Primary Care Monitoring of Children with Common Genetic Disorders

This box highlights some of the specific monitoring that can be done by primary care providers. It does not serve as a comprehensive
   guide and assumes the following:
• General health supervision guidelines for all children will be followed as much as possible.
• Genetic counseling will be provided to all families.
• Family support and counseling services will be provided.
• Support groups that might be helpful will be identified for the family.
• Long-term planning will occur.
• Sexual and reproductive issues will be addressed when the child approaches adolescence, including information/referrals for both
   the child directly and the parents.
• School placement and ongoing educational evaluations will occur.
• Care will be coordinated with a clinic specializing in services for children with the specific condition.
• Developmental and behavioral issues will be addressed, with referrals as needed.

Down Syndrome
Cardiac echocardiography: at diagnosis and follow-up as needed if defects identified*
Screen for mitral valve prolapse at adolescence[†]
Hearing: at 9 months (or sooner if concerns) and follow-up as needed* (50%-70% will have hearing loss)
Ophthalmologic: at 4 months (sooner if concerns), 12 months, 24 months, then every 2 years and follow-up as needed*
Thyroid: newborn screen and every 6 months to 2 years old, yearly to 5 years old, then as indicated*
Cervical spine for atlantoaxial instability: at 3 years, 12 years, and 18 years*
Down clinic assessment at 4 months, 12 months, then annually to 6 years, then biannually[‡]
Early intervention services[‡] for developmental delays
Supplemental Security Income referral[‡]
Use Down syndrome growth charts to evaluate shorter stature and increased weight[†] and manage obesity
Screen for hip dislocation through 10 years old[†]

Continued

| BOX 40-5 | **Primary Care Monitoring of Children with Common Genetic Disorders—Cont'd** |

Neurofibromatosis

To be done at initial evaluation with follow-up as indicated:

Head and spine MRI at diagnosis*

Hearing*[§]

Blood pressure*[§] (renal artery stenosis, aortic stenosis, pheochromocytomas, adrenal tumors, vascular hypertrophic lesions)

Imaging studies of identified affected areas as indicated*[§]

Vision screening[§]

Skin evaluations for new neurofibromas and progression of lesions[§]

Skeletal evaluations for scoliosis, limb abnormalities, localized hypertrophy[§]

Monitor for developmental, academic, behavioral difficulties.

Turner Syndrome

To be done at initial evaluation with follow-up as indicated:[‡‡]

Cardiac,* echocardiography, or MRI for aortic abnormalities[¶]

Renal sonogram*[¶]

Blood pressure because hypertension is common, even without cardiac or renal abnormalities[¶]

Hearing*[¶]

Karyotype*[¶]

Developmental assessment at 3 years (or sooner if indicated) for mild learning disabilities*

Prepubertal pelvic ultrasonography at time of referral to endocrinology*

Possible referral for growth hormone therapy in mid to late childhood*

Thyroid function at diagnosis and every 1–2 years because 10%–30% have primary hypothyroidism[¶]

Vision screening because strabismus, amblyopia, and ptosis are common[¶]

Orthopedic evaluation of developmental dislocated hip and scoliosis[¶]

Obesity monitoring and management[¶]

Lymphedema monitoring and management[¶]

Short stature management, including growth hormone therapy if the girl drops below the fifth percentile for the normal female growth curve, estrogen therapy for induction of puberty and feminization[¶]

Fertility counseling and family planning because some women with Turner syndrome can achieve pregnancy using a donor egg[¶]

Achondroplasia[‡‡]

MRI of foramen magnum at diagnosis; if small, repeat at 3–6 months and similarly thereafter; if normal, repeat at 1 year*

Ultrasonography/CT or MRI of brain at diagnosis; repeat if head growth exceeds achondroplasia growth curves or if symptoms of increased intracranial pressure are present*

Physical therapy to focus on development of gross and fine motor skills*

Monitoring of upper airway restriction, obstructive sleep apnea, and potential for cor pulmonale*

Orthopedic evaluation if bowing of lower extremities progresses because of fibular overgrowth*

Hemophilia and von Willebrand Disease

Developmental screen as follow-up to head trauma[‖]

Adequate protein and calcium intake for bone formation[‖]

Safety: protective helmets and knee pads as needed[‖]

ID bracelet with diagnosis, treatment product, blood type; remember to update annually[‖]

Noncontact sports participation[‖]

Regular dental hygiene care; may need clotting replacement products for dental extractions[‖]

Annual hematocrit[‖]

Annual screen for microscopic hematuria[‖]

Hemophilia management through a regional hemophilia treatment center with copy of active bleed plan shared with primary care provider and family.

*Toomey K: Medical genetics for the practitioner, *Pediatr Rev* 17:163-174, 1996.

[†]Vessey J: Down syndrome. In Jackson P, Vessey J, editors: *Primary care of the child with a chronic condition*, ed 2, St Louis, 1996, Mosby, pp 371-379.

[‡]American Academy of Pediatrics (AAP), Committee on Genetics: Health supervision for children with Down syndrome, *Pediatrics* 107:442-449, 2001.

[§]American Academy of Pediatrics (AAP), Committee on Genetics: Health supervision for children with neurofibromatosis, *Pediatrics* 96:368-372, 1995.

[¶]Rosenfeld R et al: Recommendations for diagnosis, treatment, and management of individuals with Turner syndrome, *Endocrinologist* 4:351-358, 1994.

[‖]Dragone M, Karp S: Bleeding disorders. In Jackson P, Vessey J, editors: *Primary care of the child with a chronic condition*, ed 2, St Louis, 1996, Mosby, pp 145-170.

[††]Frias JL, Davenport ML, and the Committee on Genetics and the Section on Endocrinology: Health supervision for children with Turner syndrome, *Pediatrics* 111:692, 2003.

[‡‡]Trotter TL, Hall, JG, and the Committee on Genetics: Health supervision for children with achondroplasia, *Pediatrics* 116:771, 2005.

CT, Computed tomography; *MRI*, magnetic resonance imaging.

2003), achondroplasia (Trotter et al, 2005), sickle cell disease (AAP Committee on Genetics, 2002), Marfan syndrome (AAP, 1996b), Williams syndrome (AAP, 2001b), and fragile X syndrome (AAP Committee on Genetics, 1996a). Key features for several genetic disorders are listed in Box 40-5. They illustrate the integration of monitoring for the physiologic, developmental, and psychological consequences that may occur.

Families with a child with a genetic condition or chronic disease face many challenges and stresses. Stresses can be emotional, social, and financial and demand that families deal with bureaucracies in the health care delivery, education, and health insurance systems. The family's adjustment is a long-term process that requires monitoring and support with new information and resources as the child grows and changes. Some areas to include in planning care are as follows:

- Health education:
  - Educate the family about the condition and its management, including family responsibilities.
  - Answer questions about health care services, and respect the confidentiality of the patient and parents so that information is not shared with insurance companies, employers, or other family members without the client's consent.
- Assist the child and family to evaluate information they obtain from Internet, print, and other sources.
  - Provide children who have genetic conditions, within developmental limits, with health education and support to understand and manage their own care.
- Health care services:
  - Provide primary care for health promotion and disease prevention services.
  - Monitor the child for growth, development, emergence of new disease manifestations, and complications.
  - Assess the child's developmental age, and recommend appropriate interventions.
  - Work with the family regarding long-term planning for the child's care, including attention to psychologic, developmental, social, and sexual factors.
  - For conditions unresponsive to known medical therapies, offer on-going, help families with support for ongoing management, decision-making related to experimental treatments that may be offered, and assistance in deciding when residential care or withdrawal of supportive care might be considered.
  - Be an advocate for the family with schools, insurance companies, and others.
  - Support and monitor the care of children with inborn errors of metabolism who need treatment to decrease the offending substrate, increase a deficient substance, provide an enzymatic cofactor, or a combination of these.
- Resources:
  - Know community resources for specific problems that the family may face.
  - Direct the family to financial resources or social services to be sure that necessary care is provided.
  - Direct the family to support groups and local resources.
  - Provide the family with written materials from disease-related organizations.

- Refer to early intervention and other special educational programs as needed.
- Direct the family to respite care services as needed.
- Family coping:
  - Evaluate all family members, including siblings and grandparents, for their responses to the child with the diagnosed condition.
  - Support the family through the grief process.
  - Evaluate the parents' coping skills, family dynamics, and psychosocial responses.
  - Assess the adjustment of siblings.

Care needs to be especially vigilant during times of transition. Parents need a support person who will listen to their concerns, joys, and sorrows over time. The primary care provider can be that person.

▆▆▆ GENETIC DISORDERS

Various genetic disorders are described in this section. Information is summarized in Tables 40-4 and 40-5.

CHROMOSOMAL DISORDERS

As described earlier, chromosomal disorders are problems of chromosome number or structure. Thus, with thousands of genes involved for a given chromosome, chromosomal disorders usually result in major, multisystem problems. Only the most common of the many chromosomal disorders are described here.

Changes in Chromosome Number

The trisomies are the most common chromosomal disorders involving a change in chromosome number.

Trisomy 21. *Trisomy 21* (also called Down syndrome) occurs in 1 in 660 live births (Jones, 2006). A person with trisomy 21 may not have all of the features that are found in this condition. Common characteristics include brachycephaly; hypotonia; hyperlaxity; oblique palpebral fissures; protruding tongue; flat nasal bridge; small ears; Brushfield spots on the iris; short, wide hands with palmar simian creases; epicanthal folds; wide gap between the first and second toes; and mental retardation. Complications may include cardiac anomalies (40% to 50%), ocular abnormalities (20%), myopia (70%), serous otitis media (60% to 80%), hearing loss (66% to 75%), thyroid disease (15%), gastrointestinal tract anomalies (12%), and leukemia (close to 1%) among others (Jones, 2006; Van Cleve & Cohen, 2006). Screening tests to indicate the likelihood that a fetus has Down syndrome include ultrasonography and maternal serum screening (Cunnif & Committee on Genetics, 2004). Prenatal diagnosis from chorionic villus sampling or amniocentesis confirms the condition.

Health care guidelines have been developed and revised by the AAP and are summarized in Box 40-5. Early intervention begins in infancy and continues throughout childhood. Education in integrated classrooms in a neighborhood school has been shown to be successful (OMIM Online Mendelian Inheritance in Man, 2006). Many people with Down syndrome

| TABLE 40-4 | **Inheritance Patterns With Examples** |

Inheritance Pattern	Characteristics	Examples
Chromosomal Abnormalities		
Changes in number of chromosomes	Generally major anomalies and multisystem problems with the trisomies	Trisomies 21, 18, 13
	Sex chromosome disorders cause sterility and changes in growth patterns. Other changes may be more subtle	XXY (Klinefelter) XO (Turner)
Changes in structure of chromosomes	Changes may include deletions, duplications	Cri du chat (46, XY, deletion [5p]) Cornelia de Lange (duplicated 3q segment), fragile X
Single-Gene Defects		
Autosomal dominant	Person with condition has parent with condition	Neurofibromatosis, osteogenesis imperfecta, achondroplasia, Huntington chorea, familial hypercholesterolemia
	Sexes equally affected. Normal offspring will have normal children	
Autosomal recessive	Both parents heterozygous for trait. Sexes equally affected. Newborn screening may pick up these disorders. Family history usually negative except that siblings may be affected	Cystic fibrosis, sickle cell, Tay-Sachs, phenylketonuria
X-linked recessive	Males have condition. Female carriers usually do not have condition unless they are homozygous for the abnormal gene	Hemophilia, Duchenne muscular dystrophy, glucose-6-phosphate dehydrogenase deficiency
Multifactorial	Familial clustering. Sex difference in frequency No clear biochemical or molecular defect Considerable variation in expression Both genetic and environmental components are important	Cardiac defects, cleft lip/palate, clubfoot, scoliosis, dislocated hip
Germline mosaicism	Two or more cell lines with differing genotypes in an individual. Consider if parents seem normal but offspring has an autosomal dominant condition	Achondroplastic siblings from normal-appearing parents
Uniparental disomy	Proband has two copies of a chromosome from one parent and none from the other	Prader-Willi, Angelman
Mitochondrial DNA disorder	Circular, double-stranded mitochondrial DNA defect, not in nuclear DNA Variable expression depends on how many mitochondria carry defect	Leber hereditary optic neuropathy, myoclonic epilepsy Kearns-Sayre syndrome

will enter the workforce after high school and may live in group homes as adults. Immunizations are important because these children are more susceptible to infections. Cardiac care, hearing screening, growth monitoring, and prevention of overweight are important roles for providers. Thyroid screening; gastrointestinal care for disorders such as pyloric stenosis, duodenal atresia, Hirschsprung disease, or imperforate anus; atlantoaxial instability screening for those involved in sports; and awareness that leukemia may emerge as a problem are further issues that the provider should monitor (AAP Committee on Genetics, 2001a; Van Cleve & Cohen, 2001).

Trisomy 18. *Trisomy 18*, or a third chromosome 18, occurs in 1 in 6000 live births (Jorde, 2006). It is the second most common autosomal chromosomal disorder. Features of trisomy 18 include mental retardation, failure to thrive,

rocker-bottom feet, prominent occiput, small features, short sternum, low-set malformed ears, hypoplasia of the nails, horseshoe kidneys, hernias, flexed and overlapping fingers, micrognathia, and other deformities. More than 50% have cardiac defects, and only about 5% survive the first year of life. The potential for scoliosis, deafness, and central apnea need to be monitored.

Trisomy 13. Children with *trisomy 13* have problems so severe that 50% die in the first month of life and 95% die by 1 year old. Characteristics include mental retardation, failure to thrive, capillary hemangiomas, persistent fetal hemoglobin, microcephaly, cleft lip or cleft palate (or both), microphthalmia, colobomas, apparent deafness, cardiac septal defects, polycystic kidneys, polydactyly, and other features. The incidence is about 1 in 10,000 live births (Jorde, 2006).

TABLE 40-5   **Characteristics of Common Chromosomal Disorders**

Chromosomal Disorder	Principal Clinical Findings of the Diagnosis*
Down syndrome (trisomy 21)	Short stature, brachycephaly, small midface with upturned nose, hypoplastic frontal sinuses, speckled iris, epicanthal folds with palpebral fissures that slant down to midline, small mandible with resulting appearance of large tongue, myopia, small ears, lax joints (including atlantoaxial articulation), short broad hands and feet and digits, single palmar crease, clinodactyly, exaggerated space between great and second toes, developmental delays, hypotonia as infant, congenital heart disease
	At risk for leukemia, Alzheimer disease, hypothyroidism
Turner syndrome (XO)	Fetal edema—neonatal carpal or pedal edema (or both), short stature, sexual infantilism, low hairline, webbed neck, increased carrying angle of arms (cubitus valgus), wide-spaced nipples, horseshoe kidney
	At risk for bicuspid aortic valve, coarctation of aorta, problems with spatial relationships and visual problem-solving, hypertension
	Difficulties with arithmetic
	Social development often impaired secondary to not understanding nonverbal communications
Klinefelter syndrome (XXY)	Mild mental retardation, long limbs, gynecomastia; postpubertal males—infertility, hypogonadism
Neurofibromatosis	More than five café au lait spots greater than 5 mm, axillary freckles, Lisch nodules, neurofibromas, optic glioma, megalencephaly
	At risk for pheochromocytoma, skeletal dysplasia, renovascular hypertension, mental retardation, scoliosis, compromised organs, and neurologic system from neurofibroma invasion
Fragile X syndrome	Large ears, macro-orchidism, long narrow face, mental retardation, autistic behavior
Fetal alcohol syndrome	Growth deficiencies, decreased adipose tissue, mental retardation, infant irritability/child hyperactivity, poor coordination/hypotonia, microcephaly, short palpebral fissures, ptosis, retrognathia in infancy, maxillary hypoplasia, hypoplastic long or smooth philtrum, thin vermilion border of upper lip, short upturned nose, micrognathia in adolescence
	At risk for heart defects, myopia, small teeth with poor enamel, hypospadias, hydronephrosis, hernias

*Not all children will exhibit all findings.

Other Trisomies.   Generally, other trisomies are not compatible with life.

Sex Chromosome Disorders

Sex chromosome disorders involve changes in the number or structure of X or Y chromosomes. Turner syndrome and Klinefelter syndrome are examples of changes in number, and fragile X syndrome (discussed later in greater detail) involves change in a gene on the X chromosome leading to an apparent fragility of a portion of the chromosome.

Turner Syndrome.   Turner syndrome (XO) is a disorder of girls in which one X chromosome is present instead of two. The incidence is 1 in 2500 girls. However, about 25% of chromosomally abnormal spontaneous abortions are XO. The girls have short stature and absence of ovarian function. Other features that may be present in a girl with Turner syndrome include a broad chest, webbed neck, lymphedema of the hands and feet as newborns, cubitus valgus, congenital heart disease (10% to 30%), urinary tract anomalies (greater than 60%), and a low hairline. They will be infertile, but some may be able to successfully complete a pregnancy through assisted reproductive technology using a donor egg. Girls with Turner syndrome are at higher risk for learning disabilities but generally have normal intelligence. Hormone therapy is important to help with both growth and development of female characteristics. Five percent to 10% of women with Turner syndrome have some Y genetic material and are at increased risk for gonadoblastomas (Jorde et al, 2006).

Klinefelter Syndrome.   Klinefelter syndrome (XXY) occurs in 1 in 500 boys. Boys with the problem are often not identified until adolescence, when testes fail to enlarge. In addition to hypogonadism, they can have gynecomastia and decreased body hair. They are usually tall and lanky. They are not feminine in behavior or sexual orientation and usually have normal sexual function. However, they are always sterile. Boys with Klinefelter syndrome may have learning disabilities.

Other changes in the number of sex chromosomes such as XYY may or may not have clinical implications.

Structural Chromosome Defects

Structural chromosome defects can be of several types. First, *deletions* can occur in which a part of a chromosome is lost. Cri du chat syndrome involves loss of the 5p segment. Some deletions are called *microdeletions* because they can only be identified with high-quality studies. Prader-Willi syndrome is a condition in which a small segment of chromosome 15q inherited from the father is missing. Children with Prader-Willi syndrome have mental retardation and obesity, with small hands and feet, among other characteristics. If the problem stems from the chromosome 15 inherited from the mother, Angelman syndrome occurs. Characteristics of this disorder include mental retardation and recurrent bouts of laughter that are very different from those of Prader-Willi syndrome (Jorde, 2006). Prader-Willi and Angelman syndromes may also be caused by uniparental disomy as described previously.

Duchenne' muscular dystrophy, Williams syndrome, and DiGeorge syndrome have all been found to include some microdeletions.

Duplications of sections of chromosomes can occur, such as a duplication of the 3q segment resulting in a Cornelia de Lange-like syndrome. Unbalanced inversions, or the wrong order of genes, are not usually compatible with life. However, children with *translocations* where genetic material is exchanged between nonhomologous pairs may survive. Some children with Down syndrome (3.3%) have a translocation rather than a duplication of chromosome 21.

SINGLE-GENE DISORDERS

Single-gene disorders follow Mendelian rules of inheritance. The online catalogue, *Online Mendelian Inheritance in Man (OMIM)*, describes more than 17,000 entries (OMIM Online Mendelian Inheritance in Man, 2006). Inherited biochemical (metabolic) disorders are generally single-gene defects. The reported incidence of inborn errors of metabolism is thought to be 1% to 2% of live births, but this may be underreported because not all are apparent at birth (Lea, 2000).

Autosomal Dominant Disorders

Chromosome pairs 1 to 22 are the autosomes, and pair 23 consists of the sex chromosomes. In autosomal dominant disorders, a mutation in only one gene of a pair is needed for the problem to appear. The risk for recurrence is 50% if one parent has the gene mutation. Offspring who inherit the normal gene from the parent who has the gene mutation will not have the condition, nor would they be able to pass the mutated gene on to their children; males and females are equally likely to inherit the gene mutation. A Punnett square is used to diagram the inheritance risk for the genotype for each pregnancy and is shown in Fig. 40-5, *A*, for autosomal dominant disorders. Often vertical transmission of the disease phenotype through several generations is identified by a family history, although wide variability in expression can occur. It is also possible that nonpenetrance can be observed in a family where there are several people with an autosomal dominant condition. This is illustrated when a grandparent and a grandchild have the same autosomal dominant disorder, yet the condition is not apparent in the parent who has inherited the gene mutation and has passed it on to his or her child. Although it can appear that the gene mutation has "skipped a generation," this can be explained by the principle of nonpenetrance. If DNA testing is available for the condition, a DNA test would confirm that the parent has the gene mutation, even though there are no signs of the disease.

This parent could pass the gene mutation on to other offspring. When there is no evidence of an autosomal dominant condition in either parent, the cause may be a new mutation in the child. Increased paternal age can be associated with the likelihood of a new mutation (Jorde, 2006). Neurofibromatosis (1 in 3000), tuberous sclerosis (1 in 10,000), achondroplasia (1 in 6000), Huntington disease (1 in 20,000), osteogenesis imperfecta (1 in 10,000), and familial hypercholesterolemia (1 in 500) are examples of autosomal dominant disorders (Jorde, 2006).

Neurofibromatosis is one of the most common genetic disorders seen in children. About two thirds of affected individuals have only mild disease manifestations (café au lait spots and cutaneous neurofibromas). Neurofibromatosis I is diagnosed if an individual has at least one of the following seven:

- Five or more café au lait spots greater than 5 mm in diameter in prepubertal individuals or greater than 15 mm in postpubertal individuals (100% of cases)
- Axillary or inguinal freckling (20% to 50% of cases)
- Two or more Lisch nodules on the iris
- Two or more neurofibromas usually appearing in late childhood or with puberty
- A distinctive osseous lesion, such as sphenoid dysplasia or scoliosis
- Optic gliomas along the pathway (15% of cases)
- A first-degree relative diagnosed with neurofibromatosis or who meets the previously listed characteristics for diagnosis.

Children may have learning disabilities (50%) or ADHD. Speech abnormalities may occur and need to be screened for periodically. Malignancies occur in less than 10% (see Box 40-5). Psychologic problems can occur because of the uncertainty of the disease, which is progressive in nature. Care should be multidimensional with attention to neurologic, ophthalmologic, orthopedic, educational, and behavioral issues (Jorde, 2006).

Autosomal Recessive Disorders

These disorders occur when two carriers mate and the offspring inherits the gene mutation for the condition from each parent. Each pregnancy has a 25% chance that the offspring will inherit two gene mutations for the condition and a 50% chance that the offspring will be a carrier. Carriers will be heterozygous, but an individual with the condition will be homozygous; that is, both chromosomes of a pair must have the same defect present for expression. The Punnett square for autosomal recessive disorders is shown in Fig. 40-5, *B*. Males and females are affected in equal numbers. The family history is usually negative, although siblings from the same parents may have the condition. Consanguinity increases the risk for autosomal recessive disorders, and fresh gene mutations are rare. The age of onset of the disease is usually in infancy and often involves an enzyme deficiency or defect; these diseases may be severe. Prenatal diagnosis and carrier detection are often available. Ethnicity risk factors are most significant for autosomal recessive disorders (see Table 40-1). Uniparental disomy may also result in an autosomal recessive condition (see discussion earlier in this chapter).

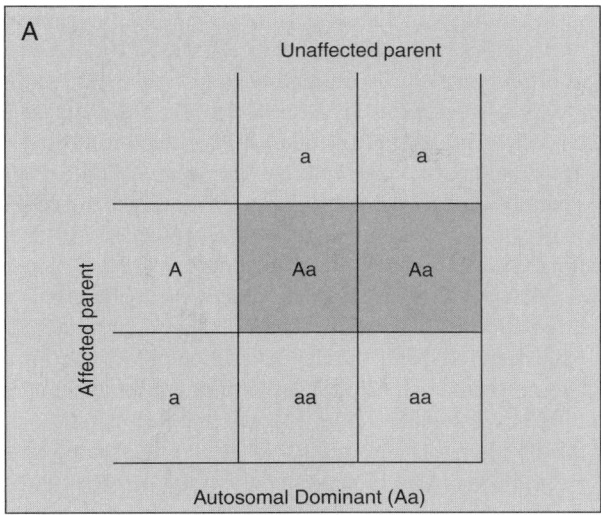

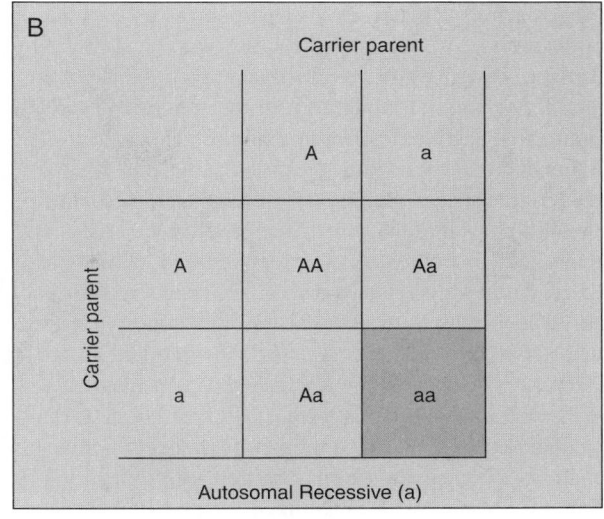

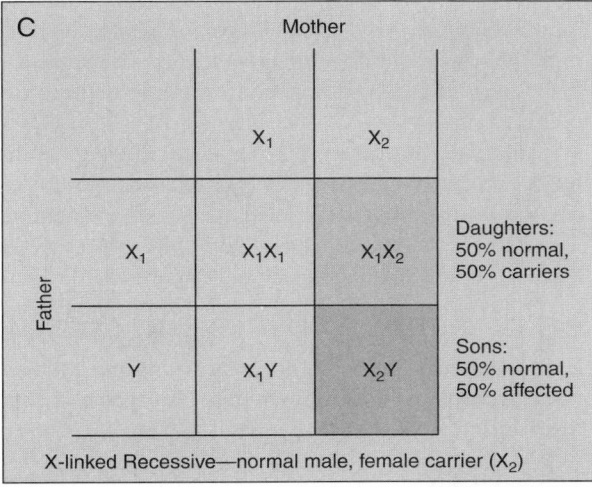

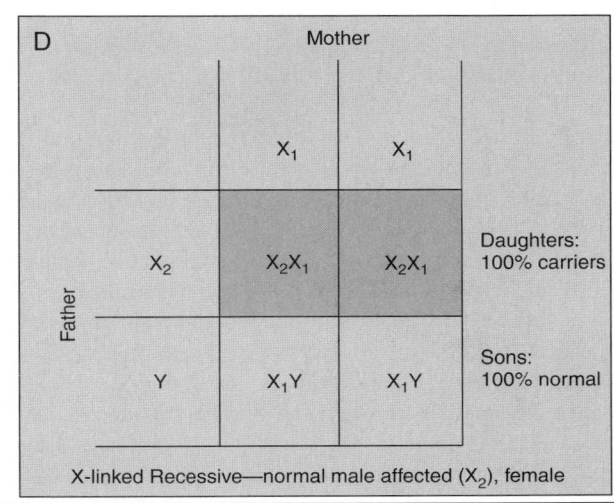

FIG. 40-5   Punnett squares. (Adapted from Jorde L et al: *Medical genetics*, ed 3, St Louis, 2006, Mosby, pp. 63, 65, 94.)

Examples of these disorders include cystic fibrosis (1 in 2000 U.S. Caucasians), Tay-Sachs disease (1 in 3900 Ashkenazi Jews), and sickle cell disease (1 in 400 African Americans). Congenital adrenal hyperplasia which may produce ambiguous genitalia in females and adrenal crises in males and females is also autosomal recessive.

Newborn blood screening tests are used to identify children with some of these disorders. A metabolic disorder may need to be included in the differential diagnosis in any child with developmental delay or regression, seizures or other neurologic abnormalities, psychosis, failure to thrive, hypoglycemia, unusual odor, abnormal eating patterns, liver disease, or metabolic acidosis.

X-Linked Disorders

In all X-linked disorders, the gene with the mutation lies on the X chromosome. Both X-linked dominant and recessive disorders occur. Because men have only one X chromosome, disorders here always yield effects. The Lyon principle explains that one X chromosome in each cell of females is inactivated

randomly in early female embryonic development. If a high number of normal chromosomes are inactivated by chance, the female can exhibit pathology from the gene with the mutation on the active X chromosomes, which then predominate. In other words, females who are carriers of an X-linked disorder may or may not exhibit signs of that condition. Prenatal diagnosis is available for many of the X-linked diseases, and the carrier state of the mother can often be determined.

In X-linked dominant disorders, males with the condition transmit the disorder to their daughters, all of whom will be affected, but to none of their sons. There is no carrier state. Fifty percent of the offspring of the daughters have a chance of receiving the gene with the mutation. X inactivation lessens the clinical effect in females, and families with the gene often have an excess of female offspring. These disorders are very rare but are characterized by vertical transmission, twice as many affected females as males, and no male-to-male transmission. This pattern of inheritance is observed in Rett syndrome, a neurodevelopmental disorder present in 1:10,000 to 1:15,000 females and in a smaller proportion of males.

Vitamin D-resistant rickets is another example of an X-linked dominant disorder.

X-linked recessive disorders require two copies of the mutant gene in females or, a mutated X chromosome in males. There is a 50% chance that each male offspring of a female carrier will inherit the gene mutation and have the disorder. All daughters of affected males are carriers, and no sons of affected males inherit the gene mutation. The Punnett squares for X-linked recessive disorders in which one parent is a carrier and in which one parent has the disorder are shown in Fig. 40-5C, and Fig. 40-5D, respectively. Generally, females who are homozygous for the gene mutation will have the disorder, those in whom the majority of X chromosomes with the normal gene are inactivated may have milder signs of the condition. X-linked recessive disorders are characterized by much greater prevalence in males, lack of male-to-male transmission, and transmission through carrier females. Some of the X-linked recessive disorders include hemophilia A (1 in 5000 to 10,000 males), Duchenne muscular dystrophy (1 in 3500 males), and glucose-6-phosphate dehydrogenase deficiency (1 in 10 African-American males).

Fragile X Syndrome. An X-linked disorder due to an *expansion repeat* is fragile X syndrome. Fragile X syndrome is the most common inherited cause of mental retardation and is responsible for about 40% of cases of X-linked mental retardation (Jorde, 2006) (Fig. 40-6). Fragile X occurs in both boys (1 in 4000) and girls (1 in 8000), but is more common in males. It is named for the fragile site on the long arm at Xq27.3. The DNA of a normal person contains 10 to 60 copies of the CGG trinucleotide repeat in the region of the FMR-1 gene. A small increase in the number of repeats to between 61 and 200 increases the instability of the area and is called a *premutation*. A man who carries the premutation is a phenotypically normal male and has normal intelligence, but passes the premutation to all of his daughters. If these daughters have sons, there is a likelihood of further increases

in the number of repeats of the CGG/CGG sequence. When the number of repeats exceeds 200, a full mutation (called *symptomatic*) causes moderate to severe mental retardation (ACOG Committee on Genetics, 2006). The increase in number of CGG repeats is called *repeat expansion* and may be associated with *anticipation,* a progressively earlier and more severe expression of a disease in more recent generations. It may take several generations of expansion in females to finally reach the symptomatic point.

Males with the syndrome are likely to have a long face, large ears, prominent forehead and jaw, high-arched palate, macrocephaly, and single palmar crease. Macro-orchidism is significant in postpubescent males. Mental retardation is found in essentially all people with the full mutation, although the problem may be milder in females. Behavioral features are important and include hyperactivity, short attention span, perseveration of speech, hand flapping, hand biting, poor eye contact, excessive chewing on clothes, tactile defensiveness, mood instability, shyness, and social anxiety. Seizures occur in approximately 20% of individuals (Hagerman, 1997). Females with the syndrome show varying degrees of mental retardation.

Children with fragile X syndrome and their families need follow-up for connective tissue dysplasias, multidisciplinary team assessment of developmental issues, treatment of behavioral problems and attention-deficit/hyperactivity disorder (ADHD), and genetic counseling (Hagerman, 1997).

OTHER CONDITIONS WITH REPEAT EXPANSION

Expansions can occur at other sites on autosomes as well, causing problems such as myotonic dystrophy and Huntington disease.

TERATOGENS

A variety of drugs and diseases, as well as irradiation, can have significant effects on the developing fetus. Congenital

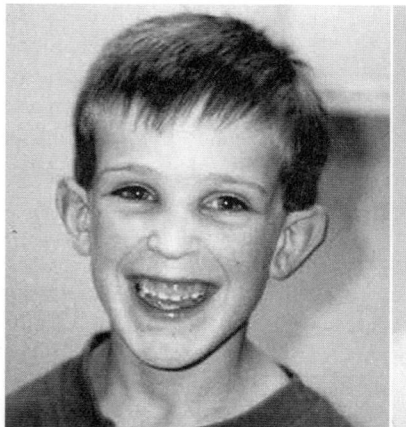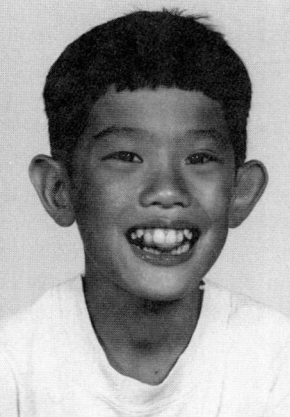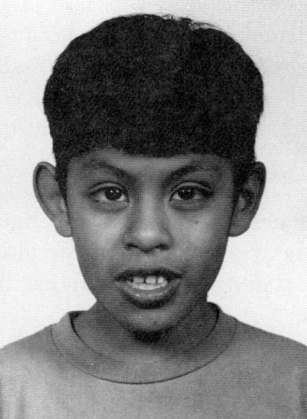

FIG. 40-6 Children with fragile X syndrome. (From Jorde L et al. *Medical genetics,* ed 3, St. Louis, 2006, Mosby/Elsevier p.99.)

infections include syphilis, rubella, and many others. Maternal PKU and diabetes can also affect fetuses. Fetal alcohol, fetal hydantoin, and fetal warfarin (Coumadin) effects are all described. Alcohol is the most common human teratogen.

Fetal Alcohol Syndrome

Fetal alcohol syndrome (FAS) is severe and occurs in approximately 1 to 2 per 1000 children. Fetal alcohol effects (FAE) occurs more frequently. Characteristics of FAS include growth retardation; facial dysmorphology with an underdeveloped philtrum, thin upper lip, flat midface, short or upturned nose, low nasal bridge, ear anomalies, short palpebral fissures, ptosis, micrognathia, and epicanthal folds; and central nervous system involvement, including microcephaly, structural brain abnormalities, and other neurologic signs such as developmental delays, retardation, poor motor control, attention deficits, hyperactivity, and muscle weakness (Fig. 40-7). The average IQ is 65 with a range of 20 to 120 (Jones, 2006). Many other anomalies have also been described, including scoliosis, clubfoot, renal and hepatic defects, cardiac defects, cleft lip and palate, ophthalmic abnormalities, hearing loss, and limb reduction.

Other terms used to describe alcohol-related effects not meeting the criteria for FAS include alcohol-related birth defects (ARBDs) and alcohol-related neurodevelopmental disorder (ARND) (Thackray & Tifft, 2001; AAP Committee on Substance Abuse, 2000).

Differential diagnoses include Williams syndrome, Noonan syndrome, Dubowitz syndrome, Bloom syndrome, fetal hydantoin syndrome, and maternal phenylketonuria fetal

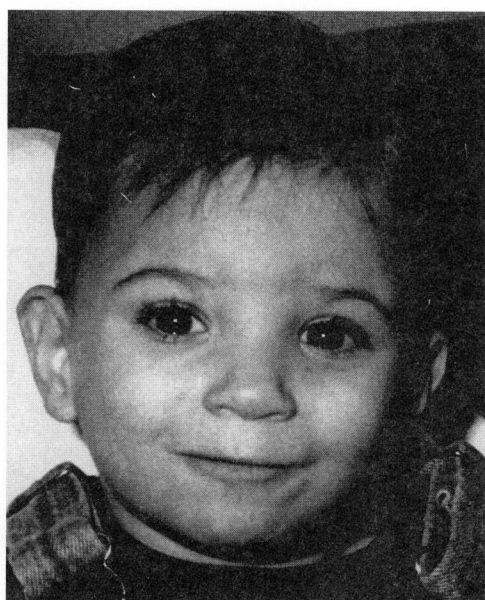

FIG. 40-7   Children with fetal alcohol syndrome. (From Jorde L et al, *Medical Genetics*, ed 3, St. Louis, 2006, Mosby/Elsevier, p. 321.)

effects. Fragile X syndrome, Turner syndrome, and others may also have some similar physical, central nervous system, or behavioral features.

Management includes evaluation of growth and nutrition, management of medical problems related to the birth defects, and identification of other medical issues. Educational evaluation and support with community resources will help the child reach his or her potential. Maternal and family help may be useful when children live in homes with continued alcohol use. Other siblings may also be diagnosed with one of the alcohol-related conditions. Abstinence from alcohol during pregnancy is the best prevention for the problem.

GENETICS AND CANCER

Gene mutations occur in cells of the human body throughout one's lifespan. Cells have the ability to recognize alterations in DNA and, in most instances, cells correct the change before it is passed on to subsequent cells through cell division. Cells' capacities to repair damage from gene mutations may diminish over time, leading to an accumulation of genetic changes, some of which can lead to disease (ACOG Committee on Genetics, 2006). Cancer is a genetic disease because alterations in the genetic material of somatic and/or germ cells can result in the aberrant cellular growth. Cancer genes are classified into three categories: (1) tumor suppressors–inhibit cellular proliferation; (2) oncogenes–activate cellular proliferation; and (3) defects in DNA repair–increase in number of somatic mutations. Errors in any of these areas will result in abnormal cell growth. Chromosomal instability associated with specific conditions also puts the child at risk for certain cancers; for example, Down syndrome is associated with a risk of acute leukemia. Rhabdomyosarcoma, Ewing sarcoma, lymphoma, neuroblastoma, and other cancers are under study. In some cases, the risk for cancer can be associated with cancer susceptibility mutations, which are passed from parent to child. A thorough family history is a component of recognizing families in which several family members have a cancer diagnosis and in which children may also be at risk for a familial form of cancer. Familial adenomatous polyposis is an example of an autosomal dominant subtype of colon cancer in which people who have the gene mutation for this condition are recommended to begin colonoscopy in the second decade of life to identify the presence of polyps (Jorde, 2006).

In summary, the field of genetics is expanding with greater understanding of how the human genome is constructed and functions. The applications of genetic concepts to clinical practice will expand at an ever-increasing rate of speed over the coming decades. Primary care providers will need to remain knowledgeable about the new information and be ready to after their practices, using the latest information for more astute assessments and effective and ethical practice with children and their families.

*R*ESOURCE BOX

National Resources for Genetic Disorders

GENERAL INFORMATION
Birth Defect Research for Children, Inc.
www.birthdefects.org

Genetic Alliance
www.geneticalliance.org
Referrals to genetic support groups and genetic services via online and toll-free help lines

Genetic Conditions/Rare Conditions: University of Kansas Medical Center
www.kumc.edu/gec/support
Provides information on various genetic conditions and support groups

Information About the Human Genome Project
www.ornl.gov/hgmis
Human Genome Project Information

March of Dimes Foundation
www.marchofdimes.com/professionals/professionals.asp
Resource for health care providers with contact information for genetic clinics and teratology information for all states

National Coalition for Health Professional Education in Genetics
www.nchpeg.org
For health professionals of all types; includes an information center with a collection of links to high-quality genetic education-related websites

National Organization for Rare Disorders (NORD), Inc.
www.rarediseases.org
Federation of more than 140 nonprofit volunteer organizations offering information and family support referrals for rare disorders

National Office of Public Health Genomics (Centers for Disease Control and Prevention)
www.cdc.gov/genetics

Office of Rare Diseases (National Institutes of Health)
www.rarediseases.info.nih.gov
Excellent list of links to genetic resources

Online Mendelian Inheritance in Man (OMIM)
www.ncbi.nlm.nih.gov/entrez/query.fcgi?db=OMIM
Database created by V. McKusick, MD; provides a searchable catalogue of virtually all hereditary disorders.

Pregnancy Exposure InfoLine
www.thegenesisfund.org/InfoLine.php
Confidential telephone information service for pregnant women, their partners, and health care providers

DOWN SYNDROME
National Down Syndrome Congress
www.ndsccenter.org

National Down Syndrome Society
www.ndss.org

FETAL ALCOHOL SYNDROME
Family Empowerment Network
www.fammed.wisc.edu/fen
A national resource, referral, support, and research program serving families affected by fetal alcohol syndrome (FAS) and fetal alcohol effects (FAE) and the providers who work with them; includes information on family retreats, family assessment tools, educational and training programs, resource materials and technical assistance, and a newsletter, the FEN Pen.

National Organization for Fetal Alcohol Syndrome (NOFAS)
www.nofas.org

FRAGILE X SYNDROME
National Fragile X Foundation
www.fragilex.org
Newsletter, informational materials, networking, local chapters, advocacy, funds research

NEUROFIBROMATOSIS
National Neurofibromatosis Foundation and Children's Tumor Foundation
www.neurofibromatosis.org

SHORT STATURE/DWARFISM
Little People of America
www.lpaonline.org
Newsletter, informational materials (including Spanish), networking, local chapters for people of short stature and their families.

TRISOMIES 13, 18
Support Organization for Trisomy 18, 13, and Related Disorders (SOFT)
www.trisomy.org
Offers support for parents who have had or are expecting a child with a chromosome disorder and education to families and professionals interested in the care of these children.

TURNER SYNDROME
Turner Syndrome Society of the United States
www.turner-syndrome-us.org
Creates awareness, promotes research and provides support for all persons touched by Turner Syndrome.

Turner Syndrome Support Society
www.tss.org.uk

✓ DISCUSSION FORUM

1. Conduct a family history on a child with asthma. Create a family pedigree paying special attention to atopic diseases (i.e., asthma, allergies, and eczema). Look at the inheritance pattern. Does asthma appear to be a multifactorial problem or a single gene disorder? Why?

2. The mother of a child with an autosomal recessive disorder wants to know the likelihood of her next child contracting the disease? What would you tell her? How would your answer be different if the disease were x-linked recessive?

3. How would you explain to the parent the role of spontaneous mutations in childhood genetic disease?

4. A 3-year-old child with fetal alcohol syndrome comes to your office for the first time. Create a care plan for this child that includes interventions for this child's physical, psychosocial, and emotional needs. Include interventions for the family's needs. Make sure you include referrals to agencies in your area.

REFERENCES

American Academy of Pediatrics (AAP), Committee on Bioethics: Ethical issues with genetic testing in pediatrics (RE9924), *Pediatrics* 107:1451-1455, 2001.

American Academy of Pediatrics (AAP), Committee on Genetics: Health supervision for children with neurofibromatosis, *Pediatrics* 96:368-372, 1995.

American Academy of Pediatrics (AAP), Committee on Genetics: Health supervision for children with fragile X syndrome (RE9626), *Pediatrics* 98:297-300, 1996a.

American Academy of Pediatrics (AAP), Committee on Genetics: Health supervision of children with Marfan syndrome (RE9639), *Pediatrics* 98:978-982, 1996b.

American Academy of Pediatrics (AAP), Committee on Genetics: Molecular testing in pediatric practice: a subject review (RE0023), *Pediatrics* 106:1494-1497, 2000.

American Academy of Pediatrics (AAP), Committee on Genetics: Health supervision for children with Down syndrome (RE0016), *Pediatrics* 107:442-449, 2001a.

American Academy of Pediatrics (AAP), Committee on Genetics: Health care supervision for children with William syndrome (RE0034), *Pediatrics* 107:1192-1204, 2001b.

American Academy of Pediatrics (AAP), Committee on Genetics: Health supervision for children with sickle cell disease, *Pediatrics* 109:526-535, 2002.

American Academy of Pediatrics (AAP), Committee on Substance Abuse and Committee on Children with Disabilities: Fetal alcohol syndrome and alcohol-related neurodevelopmental disorders (RE 9948), *Pediatrics* 106:358-361, 2000.

American College of Obstetrics and Gynecology, Committee on Genetics: Screening for fragile X syndrome, *Obstet Gynecol* 107:1483, 2006.

Centers for Disease Control and Prevention (CDC) (2006). Improved national prevalence estimates for 18 selected major birth defects—United States, 1999-2001. *MMWR morbid mortal wkly Rep* 54(51):1301-1305.

Cunniff C, Committee on Genetics: Prenatal screening and diagnosis for pediatricians, *Pediatrics* 114:889, 2004.

Essential Nursing Competencies and Curricula Guidelines for Genetics and Genomics (2005). Available at *www.nursingworld.org/ethics/genetics/* (accessed Aug 28, 2006).

Frias JL, Davenport ML, and the Committee on Genetics and the Section on Endocrinology: Health supervision for children with Turner syndrome, *Pediatrics* 111:692, 2003.

Hagerman R: Fragile X syndrome: meeting the challenges of diagnosis and care, *Contemp Pediatr* 14:31-59, 1997.

Institute of Medicine (IOM): *Assessing genetic risks: implications for health and social policy*, Washington, DC, 1994, National Academy Press.

Johnson K, Brensinger J: Genetic counseling and testing, *Nurs Clin North Am* 35:615-626, 2000.

Johnson M, Robin N: Pediatrics and the human genome project, *Contemp Pediatr* 17:100-112, 2000.

Jones KL: *Smith's recognizable patterns of human malformation*, ed 6, Philadelphia, 2006, WB Saunders.

Jorde LB et al: *Medical genetics,* St Louis, 2006, Mosby.

Lea D: A clinician's primer to human genetics: what nurses need to know, *Nurs Clin North Am* 35:583-614, 2000.

National Newborn Screening & Genetics Resource Center (2006). Available at *http://genes-r-us.uthscsa.edu/* (accessed Aug 28, 2006).

National Coalition for Health Professionals Education in Genetics (NCHPEG) *Core Competencies for Health Professionals* (2005). Available at *www.nchpeg.org/content.asp?dbsection=basic&dbid=1* (accessed Aug 29, 2006).

Nelson K, Holmes LB. Malformations due to spontaneous mutations in newborn infants, *N Engl J Med* 320:19, 1989.

Nussbaum R, McInness R, Willard H: *Thompson and Thompson genetics in medicine*, ed 6, Philadelphia, 2001, WB Saunders.

OMIM online mendelian inheritance in man (2006). Available at *www.ncbi.nlm.nih.gov/entrez/query.fcgi?db=OMIM* (accessed Sept 2, 2006).

Roberts G, Palfrey J, Bridgemohan C: A rational approach to the medical evaluation of a child with developmental delay, *Contemp Pediatr* 21:76, 2004.

Ross LF: Should children and adolescents undergo genetic testing? *Pediatr Ann* 33:763, 2004.

Siegel B, Milunsky J: When should the possibility of a genetic disorder cross your radar screen? *Contemp Pediatr* 21:30, 2004.

Skirton H, Patch C: *Genetics for healthcare professionals*, Oxford, 2002, BIOS Scientific Publishers.

Thackray H, Tifft C: Fetal alcohol syndrome, *Pediatr Rev* 22:47-55, 2001.

Trotter TL, Hall, JG, Committee on Genetics: Health supervision for children with achondroplasia, *Pediatrics* 116:771, 2005.

United States Department of Health & Human Services. Office for Civil Rights-HIPAA. *Medical privacy: National standards to protect the privacy of personal health information.* Available at *www.hhs.gov/ocr/hipaa/finalreg.html* (accessed Aug 28, 2006).

United States Surgeon General's Family History Initiative (2005). Available at *www.hhs.gov/familyhistory* (accessed Aug 28, 2006).

Van Cleve SN, Cohen WI: Part I: Clinical practice guidelines with Down syndrome from birth to 12 years, *J Pediatr Health Care* 20:47, 2006.

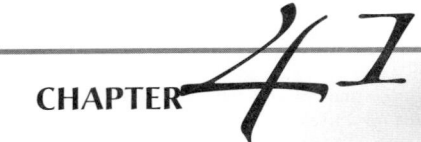

CHAPTER 41

Environmental Health Issues

Catherine E. Burns and Ardys M. Dunn

The environment is a basic determinant of human health and illness. It is estimated that 25% to 33% of the global burden of disease can be attributed to environmental risk factors, with children less than 5 years old bearing the greatest burden (Smith et al, 1999). Environmental factors contribute to 100% of lead poisoning, 30% of asthma, 5% of cancers, and about 10% of neurobehavioral disorders; based on these estimates, the *annual* cost of environment-related illness in children in the U.S. has been calculated to be $54.9 billion dollars (Landrigan et al, 2002).

Chemicals, both natural and synthetic, constitute a large part of the environmental risk to health. Five major industrial chemicals (lead, methyl mercury, polychlorinated biphenyls, solvents, and pesticides) are recognized causes of neurodevelopmental disorders, and an additional 200 chemicals are known to have neurologic effects in adults. Approximately 80,000 chemicals are registered for use in the U.S., however, fewer than half of these have any laboratory testing at all. Almost 3000 of these chemicals are produced in quantities of 120 tons or more annually and 80% of these have no information available about developmental or pediatric toxicity. Further, the information available almost never considers interactions among chemicals or genetic susceptibility (Grandjean & Landrigan, 2006).

Many European nations have adopted the *Precautionary Principle*, which stipulates that chemicals should not be introduced into the environment until they have been proven to be safe. The U.S. government, in contrast, resists using this principle, arguing for a "cost-benefit" approach in which the cost of testing and regulating chemicals to ensure they are safe is balanced against the health problems those chemicals might cause. Because it can be difficult to prove an immediate, direct connection between a chemical and illness, because a limited number of people are exposed, or because the long-term cost of illness is impossible to assess, U.S. industry has been able to assert it would be "too costly" to control pollution and restrict exposure for many chemicals. As a result, many people are unnecessarily exposed. Health care providers across the U.S. must advocate for use of the precautionary principle to control exposure to environmental toxins nationally and internationally.

Significant research is being done to assess the exposure of Americans to chemical toxins. In July 2005, the U.S. Department of Health and Human Services (USDHHS) and the Centers for Disease Control and Prevention (CDC) released the Third National Report on Human Exposures to Environmental Chemicals (USDHHS & CDC, 2005). Although it does not examine the relationship between health and exposure, this study provides information on 148 environmental chemicals found in the blood and urine of humans. It also includes information from the first and second reports. The CDC plans to publish reports every 2 years and, as more data is collected, evaluate trends in exposure to and contamination with environmental toxins. The report can be accessed at *www.cdc.gov/exposurereport/report.htm*.

In 2000, the U.S. Congress authorized the National Children's Study to specifically investigate the root causes of many childhood and adult diseases. It was proposed that 100,000 children would be in the study group. Their mothers would be studied before and during pregnancy, and the children would be followed until they reached 21 years old. Environmental influences on health would be examined, including the effects of diet, ambient air, and home and school environments as well as interactions with various genetic traits. Unfortunately, President Bush did not include funding for the study in his 2007 budget and "instructed the study to cease activities as of Sept. 30, 2006". Congress, however, appropriated $69 million for this project in 2007, and further work is contingent on federal funding. Providers should lobby for continued support of this important study (National Children's Study, 2007).

Health care providers need to be able to give their clients accurate information about environmental health issues. In many cases, parents or providers may suspect that an illness is associated with environmental conditions, but a direct cause-and-effect relationship is unclear. The provider who is knowledgeable about the potential hazards of environmental exposure will be able to explain the possible connections, collect clear assessment data, and work closely with families to make appropriate treatment choices, including referral and consultation with public health authorities. If not personally knowledgeable, the provider should know where to get information. A core competency for all nurse practitioners (NPs) states that the NP "recognizes environmental health problems affecting patients and provides health protection interventions that promote healthy environments for individuals, families, and communities (USDHHS, 2002)."

In addition to direct patient care and education, primary health care providers can collaborate with other health care providers, conduct research to identify environmental problems, and advocate in the public arena (e.g., industry, policy, funding, and regulation) for more responsible management of environmental agents that affect health.

RELATIONSHIP BETWEEN ENVIRONMENTAL FACTORS AND HUMAN HEALTH

CHILDREN'S INCREASED RISK FOR ENVIRONMENT-RELATED ILLNESS

Children, because of their developmental immaturity, rapid growth, size, and behavior, are particularly susceptible to environmental threats (Table 41-1). Exposure to toxins or other harmful substances can affect growth and damage organs or body systems during critical developmental periods or *windows of vulnerability*,

both prenatally and during childhood. It is known, for instance, that a 50 mg dose of thalidomide, administered during the 26th day of gestation will likely result in major malformations to an embryo but that same dose taken at the 10th week of gestation will have no effects (Brent, 2004). Toxicants that cross the placenta (e.g., drugs, carbon monoxide, mercury, lead, and cotinine from environmental tobacco smoke) can contribute to low birth weight, spontaneous abortion, intrauterine growth retardation, increased risk of cancer, poor cognitive and behavioral development, and birth defects. Approximately 3% of all babies born in

---

TABLE 41-1   **Environmental Risk Factors for Children at Different Stages of Development**

Developmental Stage	Developmental Characteristics	Exposure Pathways (Physical Environment)	Biologic Vulnerabilities	Appropriate Responses in the Social Environment
Preconception	Maternal and paternal health status	Maternal/paternal reproductive organs may be compromised Maternal stores of toxicants in bones and fatty tissue can be mobilized during pregnancy	Problems with fertilization, implantation of ovum Damage to ovum or sperm	Need for research and education regarding long-term effects of environmental contaminants on reproductive system and subsequent offspring
Prenatal	Fetal development dependent on maternal health status and environmental exposure	Maternal blood supply via placenta Radiation Noise Heat	Tissue differentiation Rapid cell division and growth Organ development Metabolic pathways incomplete	Need for prenatal programs and regulations regarding: Alcohol Cigarettes Drugs Metals
Newborn (0-2 months)	Nonambulatory Restricted environment High calorie, water intake High air intake Highly permeable skin Alkaline gastric secretions (low gastric acidity)	Food: Breast milk, infant formula Dyes in clothing Soaps and shampoos Indoor air Tap/well water in home	Brain: Cell migration Neuron myelination Creation of neuron synapses Lungs: Developing alveoli Rapid air exchange Narrow airways Bones: Rapid growth and hardening Other organs: Rapid growth Poor enzyme detoxification	Need for newborn-sensitive programs and regulations regarding: Polychlorinated biphenyls (PCBs) Lead in drinking water Environmental tobacco smoke Need to educate parents and policy makers concerning environmental hazards
Infant/toddler (2 months-2 years)	Beginning to walk Oral exploration (mouthing) Restricted environment and near floors Increased time away from parents Minimal variation in diet High intake of fruits, vegetables, and milk products per body weight	Food: Baby food, food additives, milk and milk products Air indoor layer effects: air near floor contains more toxicants Tap/well water in home and day care Surfaces: Rugs, floors. lawns	Brain: Creation of synapses Lungs: Developing alveoli Rapid air exchange Narrow airways	Need for child-sensitive programs and regulations regarding: Radon in the home Residential pesticide use Lead abatement Environmental tobacco smoke Need to educate parents and policy makers concerning environmental hazards

Continued

TABLE 41-1   **Environmental Risk Factors for Children at Different Stages of Development—Cont'd**

Developmental Stage	Developmental Characteristics	Exposure Pathways (Physical Environment)	Biologic Vulnerabilities	Appropriate Responses in the Social Environment
School-age child (6-12 years)	Beginning school Playground activities Increased involvement in group activities	Food at home and school Air: School Outdoor Water: School water fountains Tap/well water Swimming areas Playgrounds: Wood preservatives, pesticides, and fertilizers Other: Arts and crafts supplies	Brain: Specific synapse formation, dendritic trimming Lung: Volume expansion Metabolic enzymes more active than in younger child	Need for child-sensitive programs and regulations regarding: Asbestos abatement Lead in school drinking water Hazards in arts and crafts materials Environmental tobacco smoke Need to educate parents and policy makers concerning environmental hazards
Adolescent (12-18 years)	Development of abstract thinking Puberty Growth spurt Increased adherence to peer norms	Food Air Water Other occupation Self-determination: smoking, inhalations	Brain: Continued synapse formation Lung: Volume expansion Gonad maturation Ova and sperm maturation Breast development Bone growth and calcification Muscle growth	Need for adolescent-sensitive programs and regulations regarding: Child labor and other issues, especially environmental tobacco smoke Need to educate parents and policy makers concerning environmental hazards

Adapted from Gitterman BA, Bearer CF: A developmental approach to pediatric environmental health, *Pediatr Clin N Am* 48(5):1071-1083, 2001.

the U.S. are born with a severe birth defect, and the rate of some birth defects is increasing (Brent, 2004; Martin et al, 2006).

Children's rapidly growing tissues more readily absorb environmental toxins; the lungs, skin, and gastrointestinal (GI) tract of newborns are highly permeable and gastric pH is high, facilitating absorption. At the same time, newborns' immature organ systems more slowly metabolize drugs, making it more difficult for infants to detoxify and excrete harmful substances. Children consume more fresh fruit, water, milk, and juice per pound of body weight than adults; many of these products are treated with pesticides or other chemicals. Children engage in more outdoor activities than adults, breathe more pollutants per pound of body weight, and are physically closer to many potentially harmful substances. Crawling on floors, chewing on objects, and running and rolling in grass are behaviors that expose children to environmental toxins and can result in respiratory problems, lead poisoning, and pesticide poisoning. Asthma and other respiratory conditions in children have been linked to air pollution in a variety of studies (American Academy of Pediatrics, 2004). Adolescents are particularly susceptible to environmental tobacco smoke and occupational hazards.

Children living in poorer communities are at higher risk than others. Poor housing and nutrition, high levels of lead,

toxic waste deposits, and limited access to health screening and treatment all contribute to increased risk (Powell & Stewart, 2001; Perera et al, 2005). The Perera study found decreased head circumference, birth weight and length, and cognitive functioning (7 points) in infants whose mothers had higher levels of exposure to environmental tobacco smoke, benzo[a]pyrene (B[a]P), polycyclic aromatic hydrocarbons, and residential pesticides while pregnant.

In addition to the immediate risk during childhood, children have a longer time span for exposure to environmental toxins, and, with some conditions, children are more likely to suffer health problems than adults exposed to the same substance.

UNDERSTANDING ENVIRONMENTAL HEALTH HAZARDS

Although many environmental health hazards have been identified, data still do not exist on any large scale for many contaminants of land, air, and water. Even when data are available, it is not always possible to determine direct cause and effect. Several difficulties have been noted in making this determination: (1) the extent of exposure may be unclear; (2) there can be a long latency period between exposure and appearance of illness; (3) an individual may have exposure to multiple confounding agents; (4) exposure may need to occur during a "window of vulnerability" (e.g., during the period when a particular body system is forming prenatally) for the agent to have an effect; (5) some individuals may have a genetic susceptibility to an exposure, whereas others do not; and (6) much research in environmental health has been short term, or conducted on animals so results may not translate to human development. Using principles of epidemiologic relationships and toxicology, however, providers can better understand and explain to their patients the relationship between environment and health.

EPIDEMIOLOGIC MODEL: RISK ASSESSMENT

A first step in an epidemiologic approach (Fig. 41-1) identifies the interactive factors in the environment, including *receptors* (i.e., hosts or living things that are susceptible or exposed to environmental agents); *toxins*, or harmful substances that might cause damage (i.e., the agent); and the environmental *medium*, or route by which exposure could occur (e.g., air, water, or food).

A second step of risk assessment using an epidemiologic model is to determine the possibility that harm could occur. A number of questions are asked when making this determination:

- How *susceptible* is the receptor to the agent (e.g., age, sex, genetics, diet, and general health)?

- At what quantity (i.e., dose) will the agent present a problem or cause a response in this receptor? This amount is called the *applied action* or dose-response level.
- What is the concentration of the toxic agent? How much is there? How strong is it? How long will it stay around? What is the extent of contact of the toxic agent with the receptor?

A final step in this process compares the actual environmental condition with the applied action level, asking the following question: With the amount of exposure present, is the individual at risk for health problems?

TOXICOLOGIC PRINCIPLES

Toxicologic principles are the same as those the primary care provider has learned related to pharmacologic therapy: exposure, absorption, distribution, metabolism, tissue sensitivity, and effects—therapeutic or toxic. In fact, Paracelsus (1493–1541), considered the "father of toxicology," is reputed to have said, "All substances are poisons; there is none that is not a poison. The right dose differentiates a poison from a remedy."

Exposure

Contact of a biologic, chemical, or physical agent with the outer boundary of an organism (e.g., skin, lungs, GI tract)

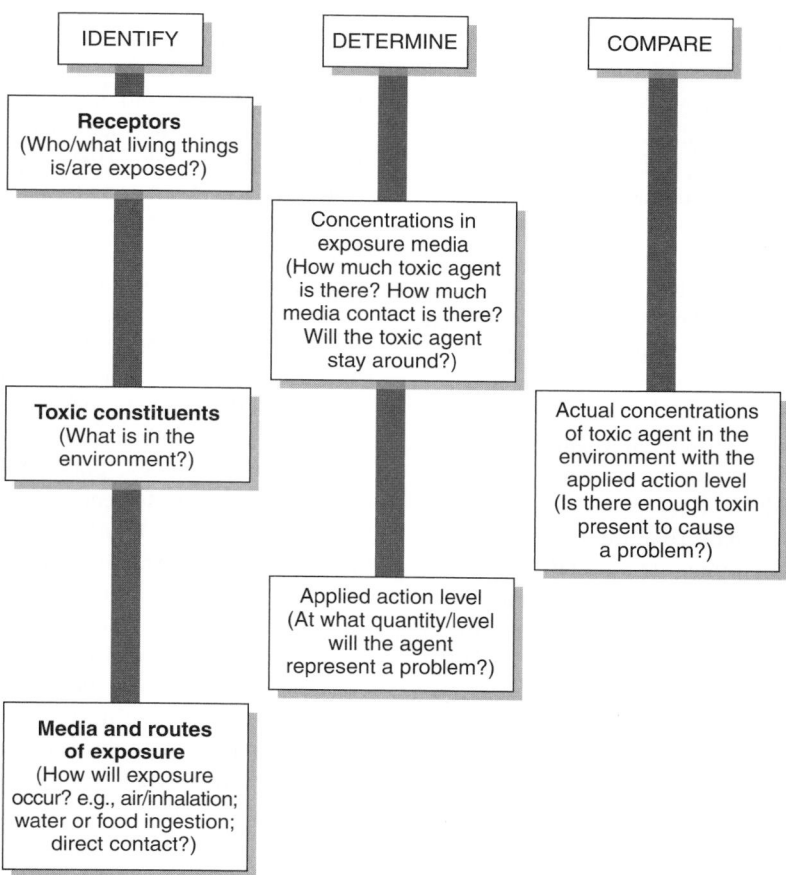

FIG. 41-1   Risk assessment of environmental hazards. (Adapted from Oregon Poison Center and Health Division, Oregon Department of Human Resources: *Environmental hazards in perspective: seminar syllabus and environmental health resource notebook,* Portland, OR, 1994, Oregon Department of Human Resources.)

constitutes exposure. The extent to which exposure creates a problem is an epidemiologic issue (see previous discussion) and depends on factors such as frequency and duration of exposure, concentration of the agent at the point of contact, and the susceptibility of the organism (e.g., an infant's skin burns much more easily than an adult's).

Absorption

Absorption is the process by which an agent is taken into the organism. It occurs in the skin, mucous membranes, lungs, or GI tract (e.g., carbon tetrachloride is absorbed via the skin). Absorption involves active or passive transport (e.g., lipid-soluble chemicals such as polychlorinated biphenyls [PCBs] are passively absorbed through the gut and stored in fat; lead is taken up through active transport in the GI tract and stored in bone or other tissues).

Distribution

Toxic agents are distributed throughout the organism via the blood or lymph systems. The ability of an agent to cross the blood-brain barrier, the amount of blood flow to an organ, and the affinity of tissues to take up a particular agent (e.g., lipid-soluble chemicals are found in fatty tissues) all influence the degree to which a toxicant will be distributed throughout the body.

Metabolism

Metabolic enzymes in the body interact with toxic agents in several ways: (1) oxidation, reduction, and hydrolysis of the agent—the agent can be detoxified, but chemicals can also be activated and made more toxic; and (2) conjugation and breakdown to enhance elimination, usually through the kidney. Metabolism is influenced by the individual's age, sex, nutritional status, genetic makeup, presence of other drugs, and disease or illness.

Tissue Sensitivity

Susceptibility and reaction of tissue to a particular agent can vary. The example of thalidomide (above) illustrates increased tissue susceptibility during a critical point of gestation.

Toxic Effects

Toxic effects vary by agent, dose, and organ or system affected. They include a wide range of pathologic conditions. Prenatal exposures can result in sterility, infertility, miscarriage, stillbirth, congenital malformations, fetal growth retardation, prematurity, and chronic illnesses (Brent, 2004). Paradoxically, for some environmental toxins, such as endocrine disruptors, small doses may have deleterious effects whereas large doses do not; the larger doses simply kill the exposed cells rather than being used by the cells in an abnormal fashion.

ASSESSMENT

Assessment of environmental health hazards should be integrated into regular health appraisals, as well as examinations of ill children. Tables 41-2, 41-3, and 41-4 list essential questions to ask for an environmental history, including questions related to asthma.

Physical Examination

The physical examination should cover all body systems thoroughly. Evaluate agent-specific findings (e.g., burns caused by chemicals and neurotoxicity caused by mercury), but also look for subtle, nonspecific signs and symptoms (e.g., skin rashes and headaches). The effects of toxicants on the body can be subclinical in many cases, and effects can occur long after exposure.

Diagnositc Studies

Laboratory studies can be performed on patients as indicated, based on signs and symptoms. Agent-specific laboratory studies, if available and reliable, can be helpful in determining treatment plans. However, few tests are appropriate for use in primary care settings because of the following limitations:

- For most toxins, valid and reliable tests have not been developed.
- For those toxins that do have tests, not all laboratories are capable of performing them. The provider should consult with individual laboratories regarding their capabilities.
- Many tests show a wide range of reference levels at which "toxicity" appears.
- There may be little correlation between exposure and levels present in the body at the time the test is done. Levels may have returned to normal, despite damage done to the body; or a one-time sample can reflect recent active exposure, but not measure the total body burden of the contaminant.
  Some available tests include the following:
- Plasma lead levels
- Gas-liquid chromatography (for PCBs)
- Atomic absorption spectrometry (for mercury)
- Carboxyhemoglobin (for CO poisoning)
- Twenty-four-hour urine (for heavy metals)
- Urinary cotinine assays (for tobacco metabolites)
- Plasma cholinesterase (ChE) levels (for pesticide metabolites, organophosphates)

MANAGEMENT OF ENVIRONMENTAL CONDITIONS

Management of illness related to environmental factors uses a public health model of primary, secondary, and tertiary prevention. A multidisciplinary approach that includes epidemiology, pediatrics, toxicology, public health, and health economics is necessary to treat specific conditions, as well as to prevent exposure to toxins. In addition to caring for acute exposures, providers can serve to inform patients and families about health risks and the nature of environmental contaminants, advocate for healthy environments in the creation of public policy, and work with other professionals to report, monitor, and control exposures. The regional Pediatric Environmental Health Specialty Units (PEHSUs) and many online sources provide information and support for clinical, toxicologic, educational, and policy work (see Resource Box at the end of the chapter).

Primary Prevention

The goal of primary prevention is to keep a condition from occurring and to maintain a level of wellness. Potential environmental hazards can be identified before a health problem

TABLE 41-2	**Pediatric Environmental History (0–18 Years of Age): The Screening Environmental History**

For all of the questions below, most are often asked about the child's primary residence. Although some questions may specify certain locations, one should always consider all places where the child spends time, such as daycare centers, schools, and relative's houses.

Where does your child live and spend most of his/her time?	_____
What are the age, condition, and location of your home?	_____
Does anyone in the family smoke?	❑ Yes ❑ No ❑ Not sure
Do you have a carbon monoxide detector?	❑ Yes ❑ No ❑ Not sure
Do you have any indoor furry pets?	❑ Yes ❑ No ❑ Not sure
What type of heating/air system does your home have? ❑ Radiator ❑ Forced air ❑ Gas stove ❑ Wood stove ❑ Other_____	
What is the source of your drinking water? ❑ Well water ❑ City water ❑ Bottled water	
Is your child protected from excessive sun exposure?	❑ Yes ❑ No ❑ Not sure
Is your child exposed to any toxic chemicals of which you are aware?	❑ Yes ❑ No ❑ Not sure
What are the occupations of all adults in the household?	_____
Have you tested your home for radon?	❑ Yes ❑ No ❑ Not sure
Do you have any other questions or concerns about your child's home environment or symptoms that may be a result of his or her environment?	_____

Follow up/ Notes

_____

_____

_____

_____

This screening environmental history is designed to capture most of the common environmental exposures to children. The screening history can be administered regularly during well-child exams as well as to assess whether an environmental exposure plays a role in a child's symptoms. If a positive response is given to one or more of the screening questions, the primary care provider can consider asking further questions on the topic provided in the Additional Categories and Questions to Supplement the Screening Environmental History.

The Screening Environmental History is taken in part from the following sources:

■ Etzel RA, Balk SJ, ed: *Pediatric Environmental Health*, 2nd ed. Chapter 4: How to take an Environmental History. Elk Grove Village, IL, 2003, American Academy of Pediatrics.

■ Balk SJ. The environmental history: asking the right questions. *Contemp Pediatr.* 13:19-36, 1996.

■ Frank A et al. Case Studies in Environmental Medicine. Taking an Exposure History. Atlanta GA, 2000, Agency for Toxic Substances and Disease Registry.

Used with permission of the National Environmental Education Foundation, Washington, DC.

has occurred. Health promotion and health education of the individual or public are forms of primary prevention. Providers can find a wealth of information about specific toxins, patient support groups, advocate activities, and safety practices and regulations by accessing sources identified in the Resource Box at the end of the chapter. Primary prevention also includes assessment of communities and populations. Safety inspections in industry and public areas (e.g., school playgrounds); monitoring of lead or radon in buildings; and scientific research to determine connections between environmental agents and disease are all examples of early assessment. It is important to conduct research on children, adapt research methodologies to the unique characteristics of children, and develop biologic markers to better assess the impact of environmental hazards on children (Schwenk et al, 2003; Patton, 2005).

TABLE 41-3 **Pediatric Environmental History (0–18 Years of Age): Additional Categories and Questions to Supplement** *The Screening Environmental History*

For all of the questions below, most are often asked about the child's primary residence. Although some questions may specify certain locations, one should always consider all places where the child spends time, such as daycare centers, schools, and relative's houses.

General Housing Characteristics (For lead poisoning, see Fig. 41-2, Management recommendations for lead poisoning)

Do you own or rent your home?	_____
What year was your home built? (Or: Was your home built before 1978? 1950?)	_____
Has your child been tested for lead?	❑ Yes ❑ No ❑ Not sure
Is there a family member or playmate with an elevated blood lead level?	❑ Yes ❑ No ❑ Not sure
Does your child spend significant time at another location? (e.g., baby sitters, school, daycare?)	_____

Indoor home environment (For asthma, refer to *Environmental History Form for Pediatric Asthma Patient*)

If a family member smokes, does this person want to quit smoking?	❑ Yes ❑ No ❑ Not sure
Is your child exposed to smoke at the baby sitters, school, or daycare center?	❑ Yes ❑ No ❑ Not sure
Do regular visitors to your home smoke?	❑ Yes ❑ No ❑ Not sure
Have there been renovations or new carpet or furniture in the home during the past year?	❑ Yes ❑ No ❑ Not sure
Does your home have carpet?	❑ Yes ❑ No ❑ Not sure
Is the room where your child sleeps carpeted?	❑ Yes ❑ No ❑ Not sure
Do you use a wood stove or fire place?	❑ Yes ❑ No ❑ Not sure
Have you had water damage, leaks, or a flood in your home?	❑ Yes ❑ No ❑ Not sure
Do you see cockroaches in your home daily or weekly?	❑ Yes ❑ No ❑ Not sure
Do you see rats and/or mice in your home weekly?	❑ Yes ❑ No ❑ Not sure
Do you have smoke detectors in your home?	❑ Yes ❑ No ❑ Not sure

Air Pollution/Outdoor Environment (For asthma, refer to *Environmental History Form for Pediatric Asthma Patient*)

Is your home near an industrial site, hazardous waste site, or landfill?	❑ Yes ❑ No ❑ Not sure
Is your home near major highways or other high traffic roads?	❑ Yes ❑ No ❑ Not sure
Are you aware of Air Quality Alerts in your community?	❑ Yes ❑ No ❑ Not sure
Do you change your child's activity when an Air Quality Alert is issued?	❑ Yes ❑ No ❑ Not sure
Do you live on or near a farm where pesticides are used frequently?	❑ Yes ❑ No ❑ Not sure

Food and Water Contamination

If you use well water for drinking, when was the last time the water was tested?
   Coliform bacteria_____ Other microbials_____ Nitrites/nitrates_____ Arsenic_____ Pesticides_____

For all types of water sources:

Have you tested your water for lead?	❑ Yes ❑ No ❑ Not sure
Do you mix infant formula with tap water?	❑ Yes ❑ No ❑ Not sure
Which types of seafood do you normally eat?	_____
How many times per month do you eat that particular fish or shellfish?	_____

How many times a week do you eat any of the following types of fish?
   Shark_____ Swordfish_____ Tile fish_____ King mackerel_____ Albacore tuna_____ Other_____

How often do you wash fruits and vegetables before giving them to your child? _____

What type of produce do you buy? ❑ Organic ❑ Local ❑ Grocery store ❑ Other

Continued

TABLE 41-3 **Pediatric Environmental History (0–18 Years of Age): Additional Categories and Questions to Supplement *The Screening Environmental History*—Cont'd**

Toxic Chemical Exposures

Consider this set of questions for patients with seizures, frequent headaches, or other unusual or chronic symptoms

How often are pesticides applied inside your home?	_____
How often are pesticides applied outside your home?	_____
Where do you store chemicals/pesticides?	_____
Do you often use solvents or other cleaning or disinfectant chemicals?	_____
Do you have a deck or play structure made from pressure treated wood?	❑ Yes ❑ No ❑ Not sure
Have you applied a sealant to the wood in the past year?	❑ Yes ❑ No ❑ Not sure
What do you use to prevent mosquito bites to your children?	_____
How often do you apply that product?	_____

Occupations and Hobbies

What type of work does your child/teenager do?	_____
Do any adults work around toxic chemicals?	❑ Yes ❑ No ❑ Not sure
If so, do they shower and change clothes before returning home from work?	❑ Yes ❑ No ❑ Not sure
Does the child or any family member have arts, crafts, ceramics, stained glass work or similar hobbies?	❑ Yes ❑ No ❑ Not sure

Health Related Questions

Have you ever relocated due to concerns about an environmental exposure?	❑ Yes ❑ No ❑ Not sure
Do symptoms seem to occur at the same time of day?	❑ Yes ❑ No ❑ Not sure
Do symptoms seem to occur after being at the same place every day?	❑ Yes ❑ No ❑ Not sure
Do symptoms seem to occur during a certain season?	❑ Yes ❑ No ❑ Not sure
Are family members/neighbors/co-workers experiencing similar symptoms?	❑ Yes ❑ No ❑ Not sure
Are there environmental concerns in your neighborhood, child's school, or day care?	❑ Yes ❑ No ❑ Not sure

Has any family member had a diagnosis of any of the following?
❑ Asthma ❑ Autism ❑ Cancer ❑ Learning disability

Does your child suffer from any of the following recurrent symptoms?
❑ Cough ❑ Headaches ❑ Fatigue ❑ Unexplained pain_____

Used with permission of the National Environmental Education Foundation, Washington, DC.

Primary prevention also takes place at the public policy level. Regulations or legal restrictions can prevent health problems (e.g., through implementation of air and water quality standards, restaurant and food handling regulations, or bans on the use of hydrofluorocarbons). Various U.S. federal agencies function to regulate development and use of hazardous materials (e.g., the Environmental Protection Agency [EPA], the U.S. Consumer Product Safety Commission, and the Occupational Safety and Health Administration [OSHA]). In 1997, the U.S. joined seven other countries (the G-8) in creating the 1997 Declaration of the Environment Leaders of the Eight on Children's Environmental Health, raising the issue of protection of children from environmental threats to an international level (EPA, 1997).

Secondary Prevention

Secondary prevention involves early detection, treatment, and referral for identified diseases. Testing for serum lead levels is one form of early detection. Reporting exposures to county and state public health officials helps prevent further contact with the contaminant and can lead to the implementation of abatement procedures. Poisoning due to environmental contaminants is reportable in most states.

Tertiary Prevention

Tertiary prevention seeks to rehabilitate and restore the environment to a healthful state (e.g., asbestos and lead abatement, "Superfund" and "brownfields" cleanup, restoration of wetlands). Individually, patients can take steps to end exposure

TABLE 41-4   Environmental History Form for Pediatric Asthma Patient

Specify that questions related to the child's home also apply to other indoor environments where the child spends time, including school, daycare, car, school bus, work, and recreational facilities.

				Follow up/ Notes
Is your child's asthma worse at night?	❑ Yes	❑ No	❑ Not sure	
Is your child's asthma worse at specific locations? If so, where? _____	❑ Yes	❑ No	❑ Not sure	
Is your child's asthma worse during a particular season? If so, which one? _____	❑ Yes	❑ No	❑ Not sure	
Is your child's asthma worse with a particular change in climate? If so, which?_____	❑ Yes	❑ No	❑ Not sure	
Can you identify any specific trigger(s) that makes your child's asthma worse? If so, what? _____	❑ Yes	❑ No	❑ Not sure	
Have you noticed whether dust exposure makes your child's asthma worse?	❑ Yes	❑ No	❑ Not sure	
Does your child sleep with stuffed animals?	❑ Yes	❑ No	❑ Not sure	
Is there wall-to-wall carpet in your child's bedroom?	❑ Yes	❑ No	❑ Not sure	
Have you used any means for dust mite control? If so, which ones? _____	❑ Yes	❑ No	❑ Not sure	
Do you have any furry pets?	❑ Yes	❑ No	❑ Not sure	
Do you see evidence of rats or mice in your home weekly?	❑ Yes	❑ No	❑ Not sure	
Do you see cockroaches in your home daily?	❑ Yes	❑ No	❑ Not sure	
Do any family members, caregivers or friends smoke?	❑ Yes	❑ No	❑ Not sure	
Does this person(s) have an interest or desire to quit?	❑ Yes	❑ No	❑ Not sure	
Does your child/teenager smoke?	❑ Yes	❑ No	❑ Not sure	
Do you see or smell mold/mildew in your home?	❑ Yes	❑ No	❑ Not sure	
Is there evidence of water damage in your home?	❑ Yes	❑ No	❑ Not sure	
Do you use a humidifier or swamp cooler?	❑ Yes	❑ No	❑ Not sure	
Have you had new carpets, paint, floor refinishing, or other changes at your house in the past year?	❑ Yes	❑ No	❑ Not sure	
Does your child or another family member have a hobby that uses materials that are toxic or give off fumes?	❑ Yes	❑ No	❑ Not sure	
Has outdoor air pollution ever made your child's asthma worse?	❑ Yes	❑ No	❑ Not sure	
Does your child limit outdoor activities during a Code Orange or Code Red air quality alert for ozone or particle pollution?	❑ Yes	❑ No	❑ Not sure	
Do you use a wood burning fireplace or stove?	❑ Yes	❑ No	❑ Not sure	
Do you use unvented appliances such as a gas stove for heating your home?	❑ Yes	❑ No	❑ Not sure	
Does your child have contact with other irritants (e.g., perfumes, cleaning agents, or sprays)?	❑ Yes	❑ No	❑ Not sure	

What other concerns do you have regarding your child's asthma that have not yet been discussed?

Used with permission of the National Environmental Education Foundation, Washington, DC.

to a contaminant (e.g., stop using pesticides in the home and follow directions on pesticide usage exactly) or change other behaviors that exacerbate adverse effects (e.g., radon in combination with tobacco smoke is more harmful). Follow-up is essential because effects of environmental agents may not appear for months or years.

PREVENTION AND PATIENT EDUCATION

Many health problems are related to environmental factors, but the relationship is not always clear. This uncertainty can be frustrating. Providers may have to tell patients they do not know if there is a connection between a particular environmental factor and illness. It is important to listen to and validate patient concerns; this gives the message that the provider is also concerned and will work with patients to minimize problems. Blanket reassurances are inappropriate, but providers can provide perspective to patients by explaining the process of environmental effects on health and encouraging patients to actively control their environment. All providers are encouraged to serve as liaisons and advocates between the family and environmental, community, and specialty health care resources.

■ COMMON ENVIRONMENTAL AGENTS AND ADVERSE EFFECTS

This section presents a brief discussion of general pediatric poisoning and some common environmental agents that are particularly hazardous to children.

GENERAL PEDIATRIC POISONING

Description

Poisoning is the process in which a substance that interferes with the body's normal function is taken in by ingestion, inhalation, absorption, or injection. Medications, plants, and chemicals are common causes of poisoning in children.

Epidemiology

Poisoning is a major cause of pediatric injury. The mouthing behavior of infants and normal curiosity of toddlers and preschoolers puts them at high risk for accidental ingestion of toxic materials, and cultural factors and views of medications and vitamins may influence storage practices (Agran et al, 2003). More than 2 million poisonings occur each year in the U.S. and more than 50% are among children 5 years old or less (Rodgers & Matyunas, 2004).

Assessment

History. The following are assessed:
- Type and amount of substance taken in
- Exact time of intake or exposure
- Route or method of intake
- Reaction or signs and symptoms and their progression over time
- Emergency care given
- Child's health status before poisoning (e.g., any significant chronic illness? Is child taking prescription medication?)
- Contact information including phone and address if the assessment is via phone

Physical Examination. Findings vary greatly depending on the type and amount of poisonous substance, time since exposure, and susceptibility of the child. Consulting with a poison control center can provide the provider with the information needed to proceed with the physical examination. Reactions can be local or systemic. Questions to consider while conducting the physical examination include the following:
- When did exposure occur?
- Which body system or systems does the poison affect?
- What are specific signs of the poison's effect?
- How quickly does the poison have an effect?
- How susceptible is the child?
- What is the child's age and weight?

Diagnostic Studies. Analysis of specimens (e.g., emesis) can be helpful in determining the type of poison, if unknown. Serum levels of the poison can be assessed for some toxicants to determine appropriate treatment of the hospitalized child. In general, however, toxicology screens are not necessary, and diagnosis is made on the basis of history and in consultation with a poison control or pediatric environmental health center.

Differential Diagnosis

A history of exposure distinguishes poisoning or potential poisoning from acute-onset illness. Because there is not always an obvious episode of exposure, the provider should be suspicious of poisoning in otherwise well children who experience sudden seizures, GI distress, or cardiorespiratory collapse.

Management

Management approaches for ingested poisons vary with the type of poison, amount of exposure, time lapse since exposure, and susceptibility of the child. Initial management focuses on airway, breathing, and circulation (the ABCs). No matter what poison was taken in, vital body functions must be maintained.

If the patient is to be treated at home initially, the provider needs to talk with the parent or caregiver approximately one-half, 1, and 4 hours after the ingestion. Changes in the child's condition will dictate changes in the plan of care. If the child requires hospital care, an ambulance may be necessary and the emergency department personnel informed so that they can be prepared appropriately (Rodgers & Matyunas, 2004).

Subsequent management involves counteracting or neutralizing the effects of the poison (administration of antidotes), decreasing the amount of poison in the system (gastric decontamination), and providing life-support measures while the body detoxifies itself. For some poisons (e.g., warfarin), observation alone may be sufficient.

Basic decontamination guidelines for contact contaminants are listed in Box 41-1. Most liquid products are absorbed completely within 30 minutes of ingestion and solids within 1 to 2 hours. Thus, timing is critical, and since decontamination procedures also contain risks, one must consider whether the technique chosen is likely to be of sufficient value to merit its

BOX 41-1	**Basic Decontamination Protocol**

Determine the need for decontamination by calling the poison control center in your area.

If clothing has been contaminated, strip the patient and double bag clothing, then flush the entire body with plain water for 2 to 5 minutes. If contaminated with dust, keep clothing dry; remove carefully to minimize dust becoming airborne; if possible, apply dust mask or respirator to patient before removing clothing (brush dust from face first).

Chemical contamination:

Scrub or irrigate open wounds for 5 to 10 minutes or longer using lukewarm water.

Irrigate eyes with sterile saline, balanced salt solution, or Ringer's lactate for at least 15 to 30 minutes.

Irrigate face, nose, and ear canals with normal saline using frequent suction.

Wash appendages (if that is only body part contaminated) without wetting the whole body, if possible.

Clean under nails with scrub brush and nail cleaner.

Oily or greasy contamination:

Cleanse with soap or shampoo, followed by water flushing.

---

use. Activated charcoal, an adsorbent agent, has been demonstrated to have good efficacy for many, but not all, toxins. The toxins adhere to its surface, rather than being absorbed from the gastrointestinal mucosa. The use of gastric lavage is coming into question more and more, because it only removes a small portion of gastric contents. Syrup of ipecac is no longer recommended for use in poisoning (AAP, 2003b). Cathartics are often used with activated charcoal but without good evidence to support use. Whole-bowel irrigation with a polyethylene glycol electrolyte into the stomach to cleanse the entire GI tract has been shown to be somewhat successful for substances which are absorbed slowly, such as iron or sustained release medications (Rodgers & Matyunas, 2004).

Prevention and Patient Education

Prevention is the best management for poisonings. Teach parents how to "poison-proof" their home, pointing out connections between the developmental stages of children and sources of poisoning. If a child is exposed to a toxic or potentially toxic substance, instruct parents to call the poison control center *before* instituting treatment.

HEAVY METALS

Several heavy metals can cause severe toxic effects in children. These include lead, mercury, and arsenic among others. Intoxications have diverse multiorgan effects through widespread disruption of cellular functioning. Lead and mercury are particularly well known for their neurodevelopmental effects.

Lead

Description. Lead poisoning is the presence of serum lead levels that cause toxic effects on multiple organ systems. The major pathway of exposure is via ingestion. Once

ingested, lead circulates through the body attached to erythrocytes. It affects heme production, competes with calcium for calcium binding sites on proteins and may affect any calcium-mediated process. It affects certain enzyme functions (e.g., ferrochelatase in bone marrow) and damages the nervous system, both through direct nerve cell damage and interference with nerve conduction. It also affects brain development as it inhibits the normal pruning process that eliminates multiple intercellular connections (Markowitz, 2004). Environmental lead exposure has been linked with an increasing number of conditions and diseases, including reading problems, school failure, delinquent behavior, tooth decay, spontaneous abortions, renal disease, and cardiovascular disease (Lanphear et al, 2005). A review of research connects prenatal lead exposure with schizophrenia (Opler & Susser, 2005).

Children and adults differ in the lead exposure sources, metabolism, and specific ways in which toxicities are expressed. Children are more likely to be exposed via hand-to-mouth behaviors, the fraction of lead absorbed from the gut is higher in infants and children, and the amount absorbed increases in children when nutritional deficiencies, such as iron and calcium, are present. Temporary peripheral neuropathies from lead toxicities predominate in adults while permanent central nervous system effects predominate in children. There is no window of vulnerability for lead exposure in children (Bellinger, 2004).

Over the past 30 years, the definition of the blood lead level considered to be toxic has been revised downward. The current toxic level for clinical assessment in the U.S. is 10mcg/dL or more, but even at lower levels, impairment of cognitive function occurs. Studies show clear, persistent intellectual impairments at levels of less than 7.5mcg/dL (Lanphear et al, 2005). Some experts are now calling for a level of 2mcg/dL, recognizing that no level is totally safe (Gilbert & Weiss, 2006).

Epidemiology. Although environmental lead sources have decreased in the U.S., lead poisoning continues to be a serious environmental health problem for young children. It is estimated that more than 500,000 children 1 to 5 years old in the U.S. have lead levels above 10mcg/dL (Markowitz, 2004).

The major source of lead poisoning in children is dust and chips from deteriorating paint on interior surfaces (AAP, 2005). Before 1950, much white house paint was 50% lead and 50% linseed oil. Limits on the lead content of paint began in 1955 and were augmented in 1971 and 1977. Homes built before 1960 have been found to have five to eight times the prevalence of lead hazards of homes built between 1960 and 1977 and 14 to 23 times the hazard of homes built between 1978 and 1998 (Jacobs et al, 2002). Children are at greatest risk in houses where paint is peeling or those where renovation with paint removal is occurring. Lead dust is more readily absorbed than chips. Soil near deteriorating homes, mines, lead-using industries, and smelters can have high lead levels. Acidic water with low mineral content can leach lead from lead pipes or solder. Hot water may be of more concern than cold. Brass fixtures also contain lead. Food can be a source of lead.

For example, lead from soil can contaminate root vegetables. Some other sources of lead are listed in Table 41-3. Lead crosses the placenta so that the fetal blood level will be close to that of the mother's, but little lead is transferred in breast milk.

Clinical Findings.

Screening. Providers should use state and local recommendations or policies to guide their practice. Routine screening of all children for lead is not recommended unless children have any sign of lead toxicity or are at risk. The American Academy of Pediatrics (2005) notes that most children are at sufficient risk to have their blood lead level measured at least once. All Medicaid-eligible children should be screened, since children living in poverty have significantly higher levels (Zabel & Castellano, 2006). Children who have recently emigrated from other countries should be screened upon arrival to the U.S. Screening for lead poisoning involves two processes: (1) assessing the risk of high-dose exposure through history-taking, and (2) testing blood lead levels.

In addition to questions found in the environmental assessment screening tools (Table 41-2 and Table 41-3), assessment for lead risk should include questions such as:

- How does the family control dust or dirt particles that might be contaminated with lead?
- Does the child live near a lead smelter, battery recycling plant, or other industry likely to release lead?
- Does the parent or guardian have a job or hobby that uses lead?
- Does the family use ceramic pottery for cooking or storing food?
- Does the family use traditional or folk healing remedies?
- Does the child demonstrate pica behavior?
- Does the child have a retained lead bullet?

In 2006, the Food and Drug Administration approved wider use of a rapid screening test that gives results in as little as 3 minutes. If this preliminary screening test is positive, a follow-up test is required, but the second sample can be drawn immediately, rather than having the patient return (FDA, 2006). If the screening blood lead level is 10 mcg/dL or greater, additional assessment and management is required (Fig. 41-2).

Physical Examination. Most lead retained by the body is stored in the bones and is not measured by blood lead levels. Although lead affects almost all organ systems, the nervous system, kidneys, and blood are particularly susceptible. Toxicity is a function of both dose and duration of exposure, but clinical signs of toxicity may not accurately reflect the amount of lead in the body. A child can have high blood lead levels (e.g., 45 mcg/dL) with no obvious clinical signs. Another child may complain of severe gastrointestinal (GI) problems with a lower lead level (e.g., 15 to 20 mcg/dL). Low level chronic exposure is very difficult to identify.

Subclinical Effects. In most cases, changes caused by lead toxicity are subtle enough not to be identified as a clinical problem (Table 41-5). Findings from early studies related to decreased cognitive function and increased behavior problems continue to be confirmed, and IQ can decrease as much as

seven points for each 10 mcg/dL (AAP, 2005; Lanphear et al, 2005).

Clinical Effects. Many children do not demonstrate signs of acute toxicity until late in the disease. At higher levels, lead affects vitamin D metabolism, nerve conduction velocities, and hemoglobin synthesis. See Table 41-5 for clinical signs and symptoms.

Diagnostic Studies. Blood lead testing should be done using venous blood rather than a capillary sample to confirm the diagnosis. Assessment of free erythrocyte protoporphyrin (FEP) and zinc protoporphyrin (ZPP) is helpful because these are elevated due to the biochemical effects of lead. Evaluate iron deficiency, including serum ferritin or low ratio of serum iron to iron-binding capacity.

Differential Diagnosis.
GI infections, other causes of anemia, growth retardation, behavior disorders, attention-deficit/hyperactivity disorder (ADHD), and central nervous system (CNS) infections are all included in the differential diagnosis.

Management.
Management involves preventing the child's exposure to lead in the environment, treating the child for toxicity, monitoring lead levels, correcting dietary deficiencies (if any), and removing lead from the environment (see Table 41-5 and Fig. 41-2). Other children in the same household or environment where exposure could have occurred also should be tested and treated as appropriate. There is no evidence that chelation will reverse cognitive impairments, so prevention is critical (AAP, 2005). It is also critical that providers do follow-up testing for children with positive lead screens. Lack of follow-up is an error of omission, which is common and which can lead to permanent damage in the child (Kemper et al, 2005).

Prevention and Patient Education.
Table 41-5 outlines prevention strategies. Parents need to know that lead abatement is essential; treatments such as chelation therapy and dietary changes are ineffective unless the child is returned to a clean house. Until lead abatement can be implemented, however, parents can work to control lead dust and paint chips in older homes. Conventional vacuums can be used to help control lead dust and high-efficiency particulate air (HEPA) filtering vacuum cleaners can temporarily reduce lead loads, but levels soon rise if the source of lead remains (Yiin et al, 2002). Other strategies parents can use include the following:

- Block access to areas of the room where large peeling paint areas are found.
- Cover smaller peeling areas with sticky-backed paper.
- Damp-mop and damp-dust with household cleaners or lead-specific cleaning products (e.g., Ledizolv) twice weekly to decrease lead dust in the air; do not dry mop or sweep.
- Pick up and dispose of paint chips with a disposable rag or paper towel soaked in phosphate cleaner.

Inform parents that chelation therapy leads to a rapid fall in blood lead levels, but that most children have a rebound increase within days or weeks of treatment and repeated treatment may be necessary until the lead level is in a safe range.

Text continued on p. 1151

Child has risk factor from screening criteria		
Yes: Draw venous blood sample and complete laboratory assessment		**No:** Routine screening not recommended; provide caregiver dietary and environmental education

Screening sample: blood lead levels (BLLs)	Actions to be taken*	Follow-up BLL monitoring
<10 mcg/dL	Not considered lead poisoning: • Provide caregiver dietary and environmental education • Refer to social services if necessary	If high risk, retest in 6 months If low risk, no further testing needed
10-14 mcg/dL	Borderline: Confirmatory venous blood testing within 3 months	Early follow-up within 3 months If follow-up level is 15-19 mcg/dL or higher in two tests taken 3 months apart, retest every 1-2 months until results <15 mcg/dL for at least 6 months, then retest every 6-9 months
15-19 mcg/dL	Confirmatory venous blood testing within 3 months Proceed according to actions for 20-44 mcg/dL if: • A follow-up BLL is in this range at least 3 months after initial venous testing or • BLLs increase	Early follow-up within 2 months If levels continue >15 mcg/dL, retest every 1-2 months until results <15 mcg/dL for at least 6 months, then retest every 3 months until child is 36 months old
20-44 mcg/dL	Confirmatory venous blood testing shortly (within 1 week to 1 month; the higher levels in the shorter time) Complete history and physical exam Neurodevelopmental monitoring Lab work: Hgb or Hct and iron status (FEP or ZPP) Abdominal x-ray (if particulate lead ingestion is suspected) with bowel decontamination if indicated	Early follow-up in 1-3 months for BLLs 20-24 mcg/dL; in 2 weeks-1 month for BLLs 24-44 mcg/dL Retest every 1-2 months until results <15 mcg/dL for at least 6 months, then retest every 3 months until child is 36 months old
45-69 mcg/dL	Diagnostic venous blood testing within 24-48 hours Complete history and physical examination Complete neurologic exam Lab work: Hgb or Hct and iron status (FEP or ZPP) Abdominal x-ray with bowel decontamination if indicated Chelation therapy	Early follow-up as soon as possible Retest every month until results <15 mcg/dL for at least 6 months, then retest every 3 months until child is 36 months old
>70 mcg/dL	Medical emergency: Retest immediately as an emergency lab test with venous blood sample Hospitalize for intravenous chelation Proceed according to action for 45-69 mcg/dL	Early follow-up as soon as possible Retest every month until results <15 mcg/dL for at least 6 months, then retest every 3 months until child is 36 months old

*In all cases of lead toxicity:
• Provide caregiver dietary and environmental education
• Remove child from source of lead if known
• Report to Public Health Department
• Initiate environmental investigation
• Initiate lead hazard control/abatement
• Refer to social services
Adapted from CDC, 1997, pp. 92, 104; CDC, 2002a, pp. 41, 51.
Hgb, Hemoglobin; *Hct*, hematocrit; *FEP*, free erythrocytes protoporphyrin, *ZPP*, zinc protoporphyrin.

FIG. 41-2 Management recommendations for lead poisoning. (Adapted from Centers for Disease Control and Prevention (CDC): *Screening young children for lead poisoning: guidance for state and local public health officials,* Atlanta, 1997, Centers for Disease Control and Prevention; Centers for Disease Control and Prevention (CDC): *Managing elevated blood lead levels among young children: recommendations from the Advisory Committee on Childhood Lead Poisoning Prevention,* Atlanta, 2002, Centers for Disease Control and Prevention.)

TABLE 41-5   **Common Pediatric Toxicants and Relationship to Disease**

| Substance | Source | Health Effects | | Prevention Strategies |
		Systems Affected	Signs and Symptoms	
Lead	Ingestion of particles or inhalation of fumes and particles from: Lead-based paint, caulk Dust, soil, water (lead pipes) Cosmetics Solder, ammunition Bearings, fishing weights Folk medicine remedies (e.g., greta, azarcon, pay-loo-ah) Pottery, lead crystal Some dyes used in paper, magazines, plastic wrappers Lead-based insecticides Industries that use/process lead (e.g., smelters, battery manufacturers) Hobbies, stained glass, jewelry	Central nervous system (CNS) Cardiac Gastrointestinal (GI) Renal Some enzymes Thyroid	Anemia Constipation Abdominal pain Anorexia, vomiting Learning disabilities; lower IQ scores Impaired hearing Delayed growth and development Hyperactivity or other behavior problems Agitation or clumsiness Myocardial excitability (with high levels) Headache, increased intracranial pressure Seizures, coma (usually above 70-100 mcg/dL), and death	Test blood for lead levels Test soil, water, dust for lead Begin lead abatement as required, using professional experts Repair/replace deteriorating paint Keep children away from remodeling/demolition projects where lead dust could be released Clean surfaces with cleaning solution; do not dry dust Teach handwashing Keep children from chewing on painted surfaces, eating dirt Use fresh, cold water from taps; when faucet has not been used for 2 hours or more, flush 30-60 seconds until water is noticeably colder Make sure diet has adequate iron, calcium, zinc, and ascorbate because deficiencies in these enhance lead absorption, retention, and toxicity Use lead-free paints, gasoline, materials for hobbies Do not store or cook food in lead crystal, old or imported pottery Be sure folk remedies are lead free Change work clothes before returning home if job is lead related
Mercury	Food chain; accumulated and concentrated in animals (especially fish), grains, and flour Fungicides Antiseptics Medications Latex paints (added to paints until 1991; older paints still contain Hg)	CNS; GI Respiratory Renal	Five manifestations (see text): Acrodynia: Erythema of palms and soles Pruritis Chronic inorganic mercury intoxication: Tremors Irritability Memory loss Metallic taste in the mouth	Do not eat fish or other food sources suspected of being contaminated with mercury; limit intake of fresh water fish caught by family or friends: 6 oz cooked fish per week for pregnant women, women of childbearing years, and nursing mothers; 2 oz for young children (EPA, 2004) Pregnant women should avoid eating swordfish, shark, king mackerel, and tile fish; can eat up to 12 oz of other fish per week; should not eat >6 oz albacore tuna per week (EPA, 2004)

Continued

| TABLE 41-5 | **Common Pediatric Toxicants and Relationship to Disease—Cont'd** | | | |

| | | Health Effects | | |
Substance	Source	Systems Affected	Signs and Symptoms	Prevention Strategies

	Thermometers and thermostats
	Fluorescent lights
	Button/disk batteries
	Folk medicine remedies or religious practices (e.g., *azogue*)
	
	Burning fossil fuels
	Mining
	Smelting
	Incineration (especially of medical wastes)
	Industrial discharge
	Natural seepage from rocks
			Gingivostomatitis
			Renal dysfunction
			Methyl mercury intoxication:
			  Impaired vision or hearing
			  Numbness or pain in extremities
			  Birth defects
			  Hypotonia
			  Ataxia
			Acute inhalation of elemental mercury:
			  Necrotizing bronchitis
			  Pneumonia Fever
			Acute ingestion of inorganic mercury salts:
			  Nausea and vomiting
			  Intestinal pain
			  Bloody diarrhea
			  Renal necrosis and failure
			  Seizures, coma, and death
				Do not allow children to play with glass thermometers, electrical wires, paints, or other materials with mercury
				Replace mercury thermometers and thermostats
				Never vacuum up mercury spills (this vaporizes and spreads the mercury)
				Call hazardous materials officials for advice on mercury spills
				Safely store and dispose of products containing mercury
				Be sure folk remedies are mercury free.
				Advise families from cultures that use elemental mercury in religious ceremonies of the danger, especially to children.

Environmental tobacco smoke (ETS)	Side stream smoke from tobacco products being used by others (child is inhaling unfiltered smoke)	Respiratory Cardiac Growth Neurologic	Bronchitis Pneumonia Asthma Otitis media Middle ear effusion Premature coronary artery disease Low birth weight Sudden infant death syndrome Cognitive delays	Adults and siblings in child's environment stop smoking Enroll child in day care that is smoke free Prevent child from starting smoking Recommend smoking cessation programs Health care provider recommendation of and support for decision to stop smoking

Radon	Air
	Water
	Is concentrated in basements and low areas
		Respiratory	Lung cancer
			May be some other health effects
				Test air in basements and first floor of home for radon levels (see text)
				Avoid having children play in basements of homes with radon
				Reduce amount of radon in basements:
				  Seal cracks in foundation of house
				  Cover dirt crawl spaces with impermeable plastic
				  Seal drains
				  Pour concrete floors
				  Provide good ventilation
				  Stop smoking (tobacco smoke acts as a vehicle for radon to enter the body)

TABLE 41-5   **Common Pediatric Toxicants and Relationship to Disease—Cont'd**

Substance	Source	Health Effects		Prevention Strategies
		Systems Affected	Signs and Symptoms	
Particulate matter	Outdoor: Industrial pollution Gasoline and diesel exhaust Pollens Natural phenomena Forest fires Volcanic activity Indoor: Wood-burning stoves Dust mites Animal dander Cockroach particles Molds Tobacco smoke	Respiratory Cardiovascular	Bronchitis Pneumonia Wheezing Chronic cough Decreased lung function Asthma Cardiovascular conditions Lung cancer	When outdoor air pollution is high, keep children indoors, decrease outdoor playtime Air-condition the home (HEPA systems are most effective) Check heating system to ensure it is clean Cover mattresses, wash bedding frequently Launder or discard stuffed animals
Molds	Damp areas in the home or school (leaking roofs or plumbing, flooding in basements, backed-up sewers) Humidifiers Steam from shower, bath, or cooking Wet clothes House plants Dry leaves	Respiratory Skin CNS	Allergic reactions: Cough Wheezing or shortness of breath Sinus congestion Watery, itchy, light- sensitive eyes Sore throat Skin rash Headaches, memory loss, mood changes Aches and pains Fever	Maintain dry, clean environment: Clean with hot water and detergent Clean surfaces where mold grows with solution 1 part bleach: 4 parts water If unable to thoroughly clean, discard moldy materials to prevent spores from being released when materials dry
Asbestos	Construction materials: Insulation Ceiling and floor tiles Shingles	Respiratory	Lung irritation Lung disease later in life with repeated exposure	Prevent exposure to asbestos products: If buildings that contain asbestos are in good repair, it may be best to leave asbestos in place; if there is a question, contact a certified asbestos professional to check it Use asbestos abatement measures as appropriate when renovating If parents' workplace is a source of asbestos exposure, remove clothing and bathe before coming in contact with children
Pesticides	Food Water Direct contact with plants, grass, and other areas treated with pesticides, insecticides, herbicides, or fungicides Direct contact with pesticide through dust, mists, sprays	CNS Immune Endocrine Skin GI	Skin rash Increased risk of cancer Developmental delay Neurotoxicity: Impaired sensation Dizziness Restlessness, confusion, irritability Impaired coordination	Use few or no pesticides in the home; use nonchemical treatments Use only amount recommended for purpose stated Protect skin from exposure when using; was thoroughly after use Do not inhale or use on windy day

Continued

TABLE 41-5 **Common Pediatric Toxicants and Relationship to Disease—Cont'd**

| Substance | Source | Health Effects | | Prevention Strategies |
		Systems Affected	Signs and Symptoms	
			May disrupt endocrine function	Keep children and pets from treated areas
			May contribute to immune dysfunction	Clean up any spills
			Nausea/vomiting	Keep pesticides from food/dishes
			Seizures	Store pesticides safely out of childre n's reach, in original container
			Death by poisoning	Do not mix pesticides
				Dispose of pesticides at a registered disposal site
				Keep a copy of the label handy
				Decrease exposure in foods: Vary kinds of fruits and vegetables children eat Grow your own
				Buy organically grown foods; check USDA labels: "100% organic," "organic" (at least 95% organic content), "made with organic" (70% organic content for up to 3 ingredients), and "organic components" (products with less than 70% organic content)
				Wash and peel fruits and vegetables (many pesticides are in the product itself; washing and peeling will not remove them)
				Try to use in-season fruits and vegetables to avoid those sprayed for transport and preservation
Polychlorinated biphenyls (PCBs)	Foods and cooking oil Fish; concentrated in fatty tissues of animals Prenatal exposure via maternal ingestion of contaminated food Breastfeeding Older and deteriorating electrical equipment or wiring; transformers Hydraulic fluids, plasticizers, caulking compounds, paints, adhesives, and flame retardants Pesticides Inks and carbonless paper	CNS Respiratory Hepatic Skin	Low birth weight Growth delay Developmental delay Decreased IQ scores Neurologic and intellectual impairment Increased respiratory infections Increased behavior problems Smaller male genitalia Chloracne, including cysts (1-10mm diameter), comedones, papules, hyperpigmentation, conjunctiva, gingiva, and nail changes	Avoid PCB-contaminated foods, especially prenatally Avoid environmental exposure from electrical leakage Use professional abatement procedures to dispose of or clean up contaminated materials

TABLE 41-5	Common Pediatric Toxicants and Relationship to Disease—Cont'd			
		Health Effects		
Substance	**Source**	**Systems Affected**	**Signs and Symptoms**	**Prevention Strategies**
			Childhood exposure leads to: Developmental delays Premature pubertal changes in both boys and girls Acute dermatologic and neurologic problems Chronic liver disease Tooth enamel defects (Jan & Vrbic, 2000)	

HEPA, High-efficiency particulate air; *USDA*, U.S. Department of Agriculture.
Data from American Academy of Pediatrics, Committee on Environmental Health: *Handbook of pediatric environmental health*, ed. 2, Elk Grove Village, IL, 2003a, American Academy of Pediatrics; Landrigan PJ: Pesticides and PCBs: does the evidence show that they threaten children's health? *Contemp Pediatr* 18:110-126, 2001; Reigert JR, Roberts JR: Pesticides in children, *Pediatr Clin North Am* 48:1185-1198, 2001; Reigert JR, Roberts JR: *Recognition and management of pesticide poisonings*, ed. 5, Washington, DC, 1999, U.S. Environmental Protection Agency.

Mercury

Description. Mercury, like lead, is a heavy metal, and is the second most common cause of heavy metal poisoning. A blood mercury level of 5.8 mcg/L is considered within the safe limit. Mercury exists in elemental forms (liquid or vapor), inorganic mercury salts, and organic forms. Organic mercury compounds, such as methyl mercury, are the most toxic and are found in the food chain. CNS tissue is the main target organ for mercury in humans. Once absorbed into the brain, mercury metabolizes to its inorganic form and cannot cross the blood-brain barrier to exit the brain; significant neurologic symptoms can result. The fetus and child are more susceptible to mercury toxicity than are others. Permanent damage to the developing fetal brain can occur. Reductions to IQ due to methyl mercury exposure have been estimated to affect between 300,000 and 600,000 children each year with economic costs due to loss of productivity amounting to an estimated $8.7 billion annually (Trasande et al, 2005). Offspring of pregnant women who ingested methyl mercury have been affected by a severe, irreversible central and peripheral neurologic condition (referred to as Minamata disease). The kidney is another major target organ, especially for inorganic mercury poisoning. Mercury may be corrosive to the GI system.

Epidemiology. Each year 7.8% to 15% of the annual birth cohort are born with cord blood methyl mercury levels above 5.8 mcg/L (Trasande et al, 2005). Blood levels are higher in women from Asian, Pacific Islander, Native American, and multiracial populations—groups that include more fish in their diets. Approximately 16.6% of women in these ethnic groups who were sampled through the National Health and Nutrition Examination Survey (NHANES) study for 1999-2002 had

levels above 5.8 mcg/L. This is of concern since cord blood levels of fetuses will be 70% higher than maternal concentrations (Hightower et al, 2006).

Mercury is pervasive in the environment. Common sources are listed in Table 41-5; exposure and contamination varies for each type of mercury. Coal-fired electric utilities are the only remaining unregulated commercial source of mercury emissions in the U.S. (Charnley, 2006).

Children can be exposed to *elemental mercury* through accidents, magico-religious rituals, and vapors from amalgam burning in gold mining operations (more often seen internationally). This is the form of mercury found in thermometers and used in dental amalgams. It is poorly absorbed in the GI tract, so dental fillings are not considered a health risk (DeRouen et al, 2006), but it can vaporize (e.g., vacuuming up spills can spread the mercury through airborne particles; heating during industrial processing releases vapors), be inhaled, and is readily absorbed through the lungs. In the body, it is oxidized to the inorganic form that is toxic to the kidneys and nervous system. Elemental mercury is being removed from the manufacturing of instruments and switches so that it does not enter the environmental waste stream.

Inorganic mercury, found in some fungicides, antiseptics, and medications, is poorly absorbed by the gut or through the skin, and does not readily cross the blood-brain barrier. It can be absorbed through inhalation and will cross the placenta. It is excreted in breast milk and urine and affects the kidneys.

Organic mercury (e.g., methyl mercury, ethyl mercury) accumulates in the biologic organism, is concentrated in food products (especially fish) and is readily absorbed from the GI

TABLE 41-6 **Levels of Mercury in Fish and Shellfish**

Fish and Shellfish Source	Average Hg concentration (microgram/g)
Shark	1.3
Swordfish	0.95
Walleye	0.52
Bass, freshwater	0.38
Northern pike	0.31
Halibut	0.25
Snapper	0.25
Lobster	0.23
Tuna, albacore and skipjack	0.21
Catfish, channel and flathead	0.16
Trout	0.15
Sea bass	0.13
Cod	0.12
Crab	0.12
Perch	0.11
Sardines	0.10
Carp, common	0.09
Other catfish	0.08
Shrimp	0.04
Scallops	0.04
Salmon	0.03
Clams	0.02
Oysters	0.02
Herring	0.01

Adapted from Mahaffey KR, Clickner RP, Bodurow CC: Blood organic mercury and dietary mercury intake: National Health and Nutrition Examination Survey, 1999 and 2000, *Environ Health Perspect* 112: 562-570, 2004.

tract (90%) and through the skin. Methyl mercury easily enters the brain, crosses the placenta, and has been found in breast milk. It bioaccumulates up the food chain, is a neurotoxin and teratogen, and is the most widespread source of mercury toxicity. Ethyl mercury is less toxic. It is not thought to be actively transported across the blood-brain barrier, has a larger molecular size, and decomposes at a faster rate than methyl mercury. It is found in thimerosal, a vaccine preservative, now out of use in the U.S. except in influenza vaccine. Multiple international studies have shown that there is "no substantial evidence that EtHg in the amounts contained in vaccines is associated with neurodevelopmental disorders, including autism spectrum disorder" (Counter & Buchanan, 2004).

Clinical Findings.

History. A thorough history is essential to identify the source of exposure because the signs and symptoms can be very confusing. Questions focus on potential exposure, workplace environment, diet, and whether others in the family are experiencing similar symptoms.

Physical Examination. Five manifestations of mercury poisoning are found clinically (Goto, 2004):

1. Acrodynia ("pink disease"), most often seen in children:

- Hypersensitivity reaction with generalized pain, paresthesias
- Pink, papular, pruritic rash that may involve face, hands, and feet
- May have morbilliform, vesicular, or hemorrhagic rash
- Anorexia
- Weakness, hypotonia, especially of pelvic area
- Good prognosis when mercury source is removed

2. Chronic inorganic mercury intoxication (signs and symptoms may also be seen with chronic exposure to elemental and organic mercury):

- Classic triad: tremor, neuropsychiatric disturbance, gingivostomatitis
- May have sensorimotor neuropathy and visual disturbances
- Renal dysfunction, nephrotic syndrome

3. Methyl mercury intoxication (Minamata disease):

- Delayed neurotoxicity, ataxia, paresthesias, tremors, sensory impairment, dementia, death
- Fetal involvement most severe: low birth weight, profound developmental delays, cerebral palsy, deafness, blindness, seizures

4. Acute inhalation of elemental mercury vapor:

- Cough, dyspnea, chest pain, fever, headache, GI disturbance
- Can be self-limited
- Can progress to necrotizing bronchiolitis; may be fatal

5. Acute ingestion of inorganic mercury salts:

- Corrosive gastroenteritis within hours, severe GI pain, hematemesis, cardiovascular collapse, renal failure
- Can be fatal

Diagnostic Studies. Blood mercury levels can be used to determine acute mercury exposure, but the blood half-life is short, and levels may not reflect toxicity. A blood level of less than 2 mcg/L is considered normal. A 24-hour urine sample in an acid-washed container gives the optimal sample of mercury contamination (less than 10 mcg/L is considered normal), but a first morning void may give good information. Hair or nail analysis provides a measure of long-term exposure (Nuttall, 2006).

Differential Diagnosis. The differential diagnosis includes other poisonings, infections of the CNS, and CNS conditions.

Management. Patients should be referred to a center for clinical management of acute poisoning. Chelation is the treatment of choice and needs to be conducted at a center where supportive therapy can stabilize the patient during the procedure. Decontamination through gastric lavage may be appropriate to remove ingested inorganic mercury, depending on how recently exposure occurred. Because of the corrosive effects of inorganic mercury salts, emesis is not recommended.

Prevention and Patient Education. For all forms of mercury, stopping exposure is essential.

Methyl mercury. Women of childbearing age, pregnant women, nursing mothers, infants, and young children should not eat shark, swordfish, king mackerel, or tilefish. They should limit their intake of albacore tuna to no more than 4 to

6oz per week, and other fish to no more than 12oz per week (USDHHS, 2004). A list of fish and seafood with levels of mercury is found in Table 41-6.

Elemental mercury. Children have been known to innocently play with mercury. Parents need to be reminded of the deadly effect of mercury and encouraged to keep all materials that contain mercury out of children's reach. Mercury spills should be handled by a professional abatement team or cleaned with wet, occlusive materials. Any mercury switches, mercury thermometers, sphygmomanometers, switches containing mercury, or fluorescent light bulbs should be recycled at recycling centers.

Arsenic

Description. Arsenic is a highly poisonous chemical element, a heavy metal that occurs naturally in the environment in organic and inorganic forms. Arsenic is found in many different compound forms and salts, such as arsenic acid, arsenic trioxide, and arsenate; some compounds (e.g., arsine) are gaseous, colorless, nonirritating substances with an odor of garlic. Arsenic acts as an enzyme poison in the body and can affect all systems. Long-term, low-level exposure can lead to chronic poisoning and cancer. Acute poisoning is usually paralytic or gastrointestinal in nature. Stillbirths are higher in mothers exposed to arsenic in drinking water (von Ehrenstein et al, 2006).

Epidemiology. In addition to its natural occurrence, arsenic is used commercially in pesticides, herbicides, rodenticides, and wood preservatives. Arsenic trioxide is also used in glassmaking and some pigments. Exposure to arsenic occurs primarily through drinking water and contaminated foods. Children can also be exposed through contact with wood used to construct playgrounds that has been treated with chromated copper arsenate (CCA) to prevent decay. Leaching of arsenate into soil and sand of playground areas from treated wood presents a further danger to children. Burning treated wood releases arsenic into the air where it can be inhaled.

Clinical Findings. An exposure history is essential in determining whether arsenic poisoning has occurred. Physical signs and symptoms depend on the type of exposure and include the following:

Acute exposure to high levels such as with arsine gas results in massive hemolysis after a latent period of 2 to 24 hours along with malaise, headache, weakness, abdominal pain, nausea, vomiting, diarrhea, hepatomegaly, pallor, jaundice, hemoglobinuria, and renal failure (Goto, 2004). Other signs of acute toxicity include cardiovascular effects with decreased circulation to extremities, arrhythmias, liver damage, delirium, and coma (Calderon et al, 2004).

Chronic exposure to low levels such as from well water results in some of the effects listed: cancer, often in the skin; other dermatologic lesions; encephalopathy; peripheral neuropathy; hepatomegaly; splenomegaly; noncirrhotic portal fibrosis; and portal hypertension (Goto, 2004).

Diagnostic Studies. Twenty-four-hour urine sample is the preferred specimen, but serum levels can also be measured.

Management. Prevent exposure by keeping children away from arsenic-containing pesticides. Parents and providers can work with schools and communities to assess for and clean up arsenic contamination of playground areas (Tran et al, 2003). If there is a possibility of arsenic in the water supply, testing is recommended. Bottled water, distilled water, or home treatment units that remove arsenic should be used if drinking water is contaminated. Providers should also support standards for use and production of arsenic products, such as a 2001 EPA action that lowers the allowable arsenic in drinking water from 50 to 10 parts per billion, and the voluntary agreement by the pressure-treated wood industry to phase out use of CCA in wood produced for residential use by December 2003. Chelation may help with acute toxicity.

AMBIENT AIR POLLUTION: INDOOR AND OUTDOOR

Air quality is an important environmental factor in childhood illness, especially respiratory conditions. Since the 1970s, outdoor air quality has improved in many areas as a result of local, state, and federal regulations, but outdoor air pollution continues to contribute significantly to adverse health effects. Both children and adults are affected by carbon monoxide, sulfur oxides, hydrocarbons, ozone, particulate matter including ultrafine particles that are especially toxic because they penetrate cells, and nitrogen oxides. Diesel engines are potent polluters of the environment. The exhaust contains ultrafine, fine, and course particles plus a mixture of toxic chemicals and respiratory irritants which chemically promotes expression of the T-helper cell type 2 associated with developing asthma (Pandya et al, 2002).

Indoor air quality has declined in the same time period, largely due to an increase in the use of carpets, wood stove heating, and synthetic and chemically formulated building materials (e.g., pressed wood made with formaldehyde) coupled with more "energy-conserving" construction that makes new homes more "airtight" and reduces ventilation. Because up to 90% of an individual's time is spent indoors, exposure to airborne toxicants has increased markedly.

As discussed earlier, children are especially susceptible to air quality problems because they are experiencing rapid lung development; have smaller, narrower airways; breathe more rapidly; are more physically active than adults; and spend more time on the floor. Very young children spend notably more time indoors. This section discusses several of the more common indoor and outdoor airborne toxicants that influence children's health status: environmental tobacco smoke, carbon monoxide, radon, particulate matter, asbestos, and molds.

Environmental Tobacco Smoke

Description. Environmental tobacco smoke (ETS), the presence of tobacco smoke in the air smokers and nonsmokers breathe, has been associated with a wide range of health problems during pregnancy and among infants and children. Spontaneous abortion is higher among women who smoke. Prenatal ETS exposure affects the respiratory health of children after birth. Neonates born to smoking mothers are more likely to have low birth weight and cleft lip and palate. Children who live with ETS have more problems with chronic and acute respiratory disease, recurrent otitis media, middle ear effusions, bronchitis, pneumonia, sudden infant death syndrome (SIDS), asthma, and invasive meningococcal disease. ETS also affects physical growth and is associated with cognitive and behavioral problems in children (Kum-Nji et al, 2006; Yolton et al, 2005). ETS may also be related to gastrointestinal problems (colic and acid reflux) (Shenassa & Brown, 2004). Pubertal children with a history of long-term exposure to passive cigarette smoke, especially white males, are at increased risk of premature coronary artery disease (Moskowitz et al, 1999) In some conditions, tobacco may be a complicating rather than causal factor and other variables such as socioeconomic status and diet must also be considered (Denson, 2001). ETS is perhaps the most hazardous of children's environmental exposures, causing an estimated 6000 excess deaths among American children less than 5 years old annually, and there are no levels at which exposure to ETS can be considered safe (DiFranza et al, 2004).

Epidemiology. ETS contains more than 4000 chemicals, which cause a variety of illnesses. Nicotine, carbon monoxide, formaldehyde, hydrogen cyanide, sulfur dioxide, nitrogen dioxide, ammonia, polycyclic aromatic hydrocarbons, and nitrosamines are the most common (Kum-Nji et al, 2006). ETS is also absorbed into clothing, so even if smokers abstain in the house or around children, their clothes may present a hazard (Noble, 2000).

At least 4 different reasons for increased infections among children exposed to ETS have been proposed:

- Nicotine suppresses or inhibits phagocytic activity of neutrophils or macrocytes in alveolar pulmonary cells and the oral mucosa.
- Nicotine suppresses Th1 cells responsible for Ig production and stimulates Th2 cell function to produce cytokines and interleukins responsible for clinical symptoms of atopic diseases, including asthma, eczema, allergic rhinitis, and others.
- Nicotine allows pathogenic bacteria to adhere more easily to mucociliary epithelial tissue.
- ETS exposure causes prolonged inflammation and congestion of airways and decreased ciliary action (Kum-Nji et al, 2006).

Nicotine, carbon monoxide, oxidant gases, and polycyclic aromatic hydrocarbons of ETS contribute to cardiovascular disease. Combined, they accelerate atherogenesis and are implicated in sudden cardiac death. Thrombosis, endothelial dysfunction, inflammation, lipid abnormalities, and platelet activation are all involved (Benuck, 2006).

Children, especially very young children, are exposed to tobacco smoke primarily through cigarettes, cigars, or pipes used by parents, other family members, or visitors in the home. Day care providers or teachers also may smoke. Although smoking has decreased in the U.S. adult popula-

tion, it is estimated that 35% to 80% of children, depending on the method of measurement used and population studied, are exposed to ETS. About 12% of all pregnant women smoke and 20% of teen mothers smoke (Kum-Nji et al, 2006). The National Youth Tobacco Survey (2001-2002 data) found that in the week before the survey, 88% of middle school children and 91% of high school students were exposed to ETS (Marshall et al, 2006). The Youth Risk Behavior Surveillance (2004-2006 data) revealed that 28.4% of high school students across the U.S. currently use tobacco products, with cigarette use being most common (23% of high school students use cigarettes) (Eaton et al, 2006). Older, white students tend to smoke more than younger students from other ethnic groups; and more girls smoke until their senior year when 29% of boys smoke cigarettes compared with 26% of girls. Boys also tend to be heavier smokers, smoking more than 10 cigarettes a day than girls. Data from these studies indicate that it is easy for children to purchase cigarettes; nearly half of the high school students (48.5%) stated they did so without being asked for proof of age. Interestingly, 70.4% of all ninth graders purchased cigarettes without being asked for proof of age, while only 32.7% of twelfth graders were *not* asked (Eaton et al, 2006).

Assessment. Assessment of the extent to which ETS affects a child's health requires a thorough and accurate history. The physical problems for which children are treated vary, and the pediatric health care provider should suspect tobacco smoke as a factor in children who have recurrent respiratory and ear infections.

History. Collect data about the following:
- The amount of smoke in the child's environment. Three screening questions have proven effective for identifying risks of ETS for children:
  "Does the mother smoke?"
  "Do others smoke?"
  "Do others smoke inside?" (Groner et al, 2005)
- The amount of time the child spends in ETS environments: How long is the child exposed to ETS? Is the child ever in a car with a smoker?
- Any symptoms related to ETS: Has the child experienced health problems that may be associated with ETS (cough, colds, ear infections, etc.)?

Physical Examination and Diagnostic Studies. These will be specific to the physical signs and symptoms of the child (see Table 41-5).

Management. The best treatment for adverse affects of ETS is prevention; every effort should be made to ensure that the child's environment begins and stays smoke free (see Table 41-5). Children should be discouraged from starting to smoke, and those who do smoke should be helped to quit. All children should be informed about the dangers associated with smoking, and nonsmoking youth should be praised for their decision to not smoke. Parents can help prevent their children from becoming smokers by communicating their disapproval (Sargent & Dalton, 2001), and when parents stop smoking, children do not start, or are more likely to also stop (Chassin et al, 2002).

Parents must be discouraged from smoking. An extensive research review of eighteen programs designed to reduce ETS exposure to children showed only four studies that had success. Brief counseling and intensive counseling with parents to stop smoking were the strategies most likely to succeed, although intensive counseling led to somewhat limited changes (Roseby et al, 2003). Winickoff et al (2003) found that engaging parents in smoking cessation interventions while their child was hospitalized for a respiratory illness tended to strengthen the decision for parents to quit.

Smoking cessation is a difficult process for youth, just as it is for adults, and depends on a number of biologic, behavioral, and psychosocial factors. In a recent National Youth Tobacco Survey, more than 62% of high school students who smoked reported a desire to stop and 53% had made at least one attempt to stop (Marshall et al, 2006). Over half (54.6%) of the students surveyed in the Youth Risk Surveillance study had tried to quit in the year before the study (Eaton et al, 2006). Earlier studies indicate the desire to quit, attempts to quit, and actually quitting may not match, as only about 15% of youth were able to say they had quit (defined as "not smoking for the past 30 days") (Zhu et al, 1999).

Predictors for success in quitting include (1) being an "occasional" smoker; (2) never having quit or having quit for 14 or more days previously; (3) making a self-prediction that he or she would not be smoking in 1 year; (4) having lower depression scores; and (5) having a mother who does not smoke.

In the general population, many providers ask their patients about smoking and urge them to stop, but do not provide support and follow-up intervention. Pediatric providers can use the U.S. Agency for Health Care Policy and Research (USAHCPR) guidelines, *Treating Tobacco Use and Dependence: A Clinical Practice Guideline*, to structure their smoking cessation counseling (USAHCPR, 2000). These include the "five *As*":

- *Ask about us*: Systematically identify tobacco users and document their status.
- *Advise to quit*: Strongly urge all smokers to quit.
- *Assess willingness to quit*: Identify smokers willing to make an attempt to quit.
- *Assist in quit attempt*: Aid the patient in quitting by offering a plan, providing education and support with nicotine replacement therapy as needed, or referring to a smoking cessation program in the community.
- *Arrange follow-up*: Schedule follow-up contact.

Since it is difficult to stop smoking, however, the environment in which there is a smoker must be altered to protect the child. If parents continue to smoke, smoking outside the home, not smoking in cars, and using adequate ventilation are essential. Alternative day care arrangements should be explored if there is smoking at the child's care center.

Carbon Monoxide

Description. Carbon monoxide (CO) is a poisonous gas. It is formed by incomplete combustion of any fossil fuel.

Improperly vented gas water heaters, kerosene space heaters, charcoal grills, hibachis and Sterno stoves all emit CO, as do wood stoves, gas stoves, pool heaters, and gas-powered engines (e.g., car exhaust fumes). Methylene chloride, a paint stripping agent, is metabolized in the liver to CO. Cigarette smokers also have measurable CO blood levels of 3% to 10% (Qureshi & Mahajan, 2005).

Epidemiology. Carbon monoxide is not easily detected because it is tasteless and colorless and not irritating. In the body, it binds to hemoglobin 200 to 250 times more easily than oxygen does, thus diminishing oxygen-carrying capacities. It may also affect the body through some other more complex mechanisms. It crosses the placenta and has a particular affinity for fetal hemoglobin so that the fetus of a pregnant woman exposed to CO will be affected more than the mother is. In all cases, the net result is tissue hypoxia.

Clinical Findings. Children often have nonspecific neurologic and gastrointestinal symptoms, including headache, drowsiness, loss of consciousness, seizure, confusion, nausea, vomiting, blurred or double vision, shortness of breath, chest pain, and palpitations. Because the symptoms are vague, a key indicator will be similar symptoms in more than one person in a specific setting. Some long term, low-level exposure symptoms that have been reported include chronic headaches, learning difficulties, and behavioral problems. Autism, blindness, seizures, urinary and fecal incontinence, psychosis, paralysis, and a Parkinson-like syndrome have been reported. Cardiac symptoms may appear as the cardiovascular system tries to supply adequate oxygen to the body. Multiorgan failure can occur with acute, severe poisoning (Qureshi & Mahajan, 2005; Rodgers & Matyunas, 2004).

Management. Acute carbon monoxide poisoning is treated with high concentrations of oxygen, even with hyperbaric oxygen therapy.

Prevention. Carbon monoxide detectors are available for installation in homes and are the best assurance against carbon monoxide exposure. Family and community education should include warnings against using space heaters, barbeques, or gas stoves in unventilated areas.

Radon

Description. Radon is a colorless, odorless, radioactive gas that enters homes through soil or water (e.g., basement floors, cracks in concrete foundations, sumps, or drains) (see Table 41-5). As radon decays, some of its products change to an isotope of polonium, which, when inhaled, can cause lung damage leading to cancer. In the atmosphere, radon is diluted and has no health effect. When concentrated in an enclosed area, it represents a risk. Tobacco smoke provides a vehicle for radon to enter the lungs, adding to the risk of radon-induced cancer for smokers and individuals exposed to ETS. Water that has been filtered through the soil can contain radon (e.g., well water), and about 2% to 5% of radon in homes is found in the water supply. Radon in water has been associated with a slightly increased incidence of gastric cancer and leukemia, and occupational exposure leads to changes in chromosomal structure.

Epidemiology. Radon is the second leading cause of lung cancer in Americans (EPA, 1994). Radon is more prevalent in certain geographic areas. Local health departments can be consulted to determine if radon is a local health risk.

Assessment. In 1988, the Surgeon General recommended that all homes, except residences above the second floor in multilevel buildings, be tested for radon. Radon detector kits can be purchased in hardware, home improvement, or department stores and are available from the National Safety Council (see Resource Box at the end of the chapter). Short-term (2 to 7 days) or long-term (3 to 12 months) testing can be done. The long-term testing gives a more accurate measure of the average radon exposure, because levels fluctuate over time and with changes in seasons; however, the EPA recommends using the short-term test.

Management. Radon remediation involves decreasing the amount of radon entering the home and removing radon that is present (see Table 41-5). Although the EPA does not yet have standards for safe radon levels in water, it recommends that homes with a radon level of 4 picoCuries per liter (pCi/L) or higher in indoor air be repaired. Higher levels require immediate action. Children and families should not spend significant amounts of time in high-risk areas of the home (e.g., basements). Parents will need education to understand the risks, since radon is not a widely known contaminant. Only 21% of parents in a recent study correctly understood their risk status from radon exposure, despite the fact that 32% of the homes in the area had radon levels above 40 pCi/L (Hill et al, 2006).

Particulate Matter

Description. Particulate matter (PM) is one of a cluster of indoor and outdoor air pollutants that have an adverse effect on respiratory and cardiovascular function. Other outdoor air pollutants include ozone, sulfur dioxide (SO_2), nitrogen oxides (NO and NO_2), and carbon monoxide (CO). The diameter of PM is measured in microns, and standards have been set for concentrations of PM_{10} and $PM_{2.5}$. Fine PM (2.5 micrometers in diameter or smaller) is of growing concern because it can be inhaled and carried deep into lung tissue. Coarse PM (2.5 to 10 micrometers in diameter) can be filtered by the nasal mucosa or trachea and removed by coughing or sneezing. Ultrafine particles represent a growing health problem. These particles are so small (less than 100 nanometers) that they can penetrate into cells, carrying toxic compounds into a person's DNA and other critical areas. To date, they are not regulated. They cause allergic inflammation of the lung (Alessandrini et al, 2006) and are prevalent near major roadways; children who live within 80 yards of the road are 50% more likely to have had asthma symptoms in the previous year (McConnell et al, 2006).

Epidemiology. Eighty percent of alveoli are developed after birth, so the infant and young child's developing lungs are highly susceptible to environmental toxins with demonstrated effects on both lung function and lung growth. Exposure to PM creates an inflammatory response in the body and, in combination with other pollutants, is associated with increased hospitalization rates for respiratory or cardiovascular problems. The anatomic structure of the lung may contribute to differential distribution of PM in the pulmonary tree, with subsequent cancer in particular sites (Balashazy et al, 2003). Recent studies have also shown relationships between ambient air pollution and/or carbon monoxide and infant mortality, low birth weight, and preterm birth (AAP, 2004).

PM is a pervasive by-product of industrial production, gasoline and diesel engines, wood-burning stoves, and natural phenomena (e.g., volcanic activity, grass and forest fires, and blowing dust). Residents of urban and industrial areas are exposed to high levels of PM, and concentrations increase in summer months and when there is more combustion present (e.g., rush-hour traffic). The amount of indoor PM, including dust, mites, cockroach particles, and animal dander, varies among households, but many low-income urban residences have high levels of dust, mouse, and cockroach residue.

Assessment. Parents can keep a record of their child's illness episodes to determine if increased air pollution, dust, insects, or pets in the home are associated with illness.

Management. The goal of management is to decrease the amount of PM in the environment and limit the child's contact with PM (see Table 41-5). Minimizing exposure to diesel exhaust is one measure that families and schools can take.

Molds

Description. Molds are microscopic organisms in the class of bioaerosols, living organisms that can affect health through immune or nonimmune mechanisms. The cell walls of mold and the enzymes and metabolites produced during fungal growth cause allergic reactions (immune mechanism) and elicit irritant and toxic responses (Mazur & Kim, 2006). Molds thrive in damp spaces, but spores can be found in dust, dry leaves, and storage areas. *Aspergillus* (black mold), *Alternaria, Penicillium, Streptomyces, Epicoccum,* and *Cladosporium* are the most common household molds.

Epidemiology. Children have an increased risk of cough and wheezing when exposed to damp and mold in the home or school. Allergic rhinitis, conjunctivitis, and asthma are common responses to mold. Pneumonitis, sinusitis, and bronchopulmonary aspergillosis are also seen with mold exposure (Mazur & Kim, 2006). Mycotoxins produced by mold spores can also cause GI, skin, neurologic, or renal problems. Infants are especially susceptible to effects of mycotoxins (Knapp et al, 1999). Common sources of mold exposure for children are listed in Table 41-5.

Assessment. Assessment questions clarify the nature of symptoms, usually a spectrum of allergic reactions (see Table 41-5), and identify the cause of the symptoms:

- Is there a pattern to the symptoms?
- Are they aggravated by any particular environment?
- Are they relieved when the child changes environments?
- What has the family done to remediate the environment?

Laboratory tests to measure antigens, antibodies, or to conduct immunoassays do not reliably indicate exposure or establish causal relationships between mold and illness.

Differential Diagnosis. The differential diagnosis includes other causes of allergic reactions and upper respiratory infections. Reaction to molds can be confused with pesticide poisoning.

Management. Treatment involves control of allergic symptoms (e.g., antihistamines to control itching or sneezing; see Chapters 24 and 36 for discussion of allergies and their management) and removal of the cause of the problem. Ultimately, the source of moisture must be removed because maintaining a dry, clean environment minimizes the growth of molds (see Table 41-5). Ozone air cleaners are not effective against molds and may cause respiratory problems by creating ozone.

Provide information regarding the connection between exposure to molds, allergic reactions, and respiratory and other health problems. Parents may need support during cleanup because it may be difficult or nearly impossible to do a thorough job (e.g., mold may have permeated the walls in a rental unit and the family is not able to have them replaced or to move to a more suitable apartment) (Regional Asthma Management & Prevention, 2006).

Asbestos

Description. Asbestos is the name given to a group of incombustible fibrous magnesium silicate minerals used most often in construction materials. Chrysolite is the only asbestos product still on the market; other forms are found in older buildings. Contamination by asbestos is measured in fibers per cubic centimeter of air. The OSHA workplace standard is 0.1 fibers per cubic centimeter averaged over an 8-hour shift (OSHA, 1994). Levels in schools may range from 0.05 to 0.2 fibers per cubic centimeter, placing schoolchildren at relatively low risk.

Epidemiology. Asbestosis is considered an occupational problem of adults, and smokers are at higher risk of asbestos-induced lung disease than nonsmokers. Any exposure to asbestos fibers is a risk, but repeated inhalation of the fibers is associated with significant lung disease later in life. There may be a latency period of 10 to 40 years or more before conditions such as pleural effusion, lung fibrosis, lung cancer, and mesothelioma in the pleura or peritoneum appear. Childhood exposure to asbestos may contribute to serious illness as an adult. Children can be exposed through direct contact with air in a contaminated building or with material or clothing parents bring home from their work site. Parents who work with asbestos should shower and change clothes before returning to the home. Although asbestos is found in many buildings (e.g., tiles, pipes, and insulation), it is considered a hazard only if the material is disrupted through deterioration or renovation and fibers become airborne.

Clinical Findings. Assessment of disease is based on a history of exposure and signs and symptoms of respiratory distress. Exposure to asbestos does not typically produce acute symptoms, although high concentrations of asbestos dust can cause lung irritation, including cough, dyspnea, fatigue, and chest pain in both children and adults.

Management. Preventing unnecessary exposure to asbestos fibers reduces the risk of inhalation and subsequent disease (see Table 41-5). If asbestos is present in the workplace, OSHA standards (not always enforced) require employers to provide workers with full body suits and shoe covers that are left at the work site; parents should be encouraged to work with their employers to minimize the possibility of bringing fibers into the home. The Asbestos Hazard Emergency Response Act of 1986 (AHERA) sets standards for schools to inspect and manage asbestos contamination (EPA, 2006b). The EPA has also adopted OSHA standards and extended protection to school employees (EPA, 2000). Parents should be informed of the adverse effects of asbestos exposure and reassured that their children are at low risk unless they spend significant amounts of time in older buildings that are in poor repair or undergoing renovation.

PESTICIDES

Description
Pesticides are chemicals used to kill or control unwanted pests, including plants; among these products are herbicides, fungicides, and insecticides. Pesticides are classified as "general-use" or "restricted-use" pesticides, depending on their toxicity to humans or the environment. Restricted-use pesticides require special handling by certified applicators. Labeling of pesticides varies by toxicity, with a skull and crossbones and the statement "DANGER-POISON" on the most toxic; "WARNING" on less toxic; and "CAUTION" on the labels of the least toxic pesticides. All pesticides are hazardous and, although they have improved lives, they also carry significant health risks. The Environmental Protection Agency is responsible for regulating pesticides.

Epidemiology
Approximately 5 billion pounds of pesticides are used in the U.S. annually; chlorine and hypochlorites are the major category in use (52% of all pesticides) (EPA, 2006a). They are used in agriculture; in forests to control insects; on boat hulls to control fungi; in and around houses, schools, and commercial and office buildings to control insects and rodents; in landscaping and recreational areas to control weeds and insects; and in aquatic areas to control mosquitoes. Wood products may be impregnated with chemicals to retard decay. Humans and animals may be treated with insecticides.

Herbicides are the most widely used pesticide, and contaminated food products are a major source of exposure. Because of children's small size and large fruit and vegetable intake per unit of body weight, they ingest pesticides in foods at a disproportionate rate. Farm workers and children who live on or near farms are exposed to agricultural pesticides. Garden and lawn use increases risks to children playing outdoors in these areas. Pesticide routes of exposure are oral, inhalation, and dermal. Incidental exposure via residues is most common among children.

Pesticides are increasingly implicated in fetal development and childhood illness (Perera et al, 2005). Although they are now being phased out, chlorpyrifos and diazinon, which are organophosphate insecticides, have been heavily used in inner cities. They are transferred to the fetus if the mother is exposed, and both have been linked to decreased birth weight and birth length. If both pesticides are present, a synergistic effect has been found (Perera et al, 2005). A study of clinical exposures to agricultural pesticides and birth defects in South Africa found that babies born to women exposed to chemicals used in gardens and fields were seven times more likely to have birth defects than babies of women who reported no exposures. Pregnant women who participated in dipping livestock for ticks were twice as likely to have infants with birth defects (Heeren et al, 2003). A study of children's developmental capacity has demonstrated significant developmental differences in native Yaqui children from Mexico exposed to pesticides versus a cohort not exposed (Guillette, 2000). Indoor pesticides are associated with an increased risk of leukemia (Ma et al, 2002).

Clinical Findings

Adverse effects of pesticide exposure can be acute or chronic, and all body systems can be affected, depending on the nature of the toxin and the extent of exposure. Assessment must be comprehensive (see Table 41-5). In acute exposure, assessment is the same as with general poisoning. Chronic exposure presents a more complicated picture, since much data about pesticide poisoning are based only on studies in adults. There is concern that the effect of pesticides on children differs, and the risk children face for long-term health problems is seriously underestimated.

Management

Specifics of management depend on the type and amount of pesticide taken in and the route of absorption. Information on treatment is available on product labels. When treating an individual who may have been exposed to pesticides, health care providers, by law, are entitled to access information about the implicated pesticides (see National Pesticide Information Center in the Resource Box at the end of the chapter). The EPA's Worker Protection Standard (WPS) also ensures that providers will be able to access information on general- and restricted-use pesticides. Under the WPS, this information can be obtained from employers or manufacturers. Patients may be able to provide the pesticide label. Treatment focuses on supporting life functions:

- ABCs
  - Maintain gas exchange; may need to intubate
  - Prevent aspiration of vomitus
- Consult with a poison control center for direction in management (refer to a center or provider with expertise in this area as soon as possible; see previous discussion for management of general poisonings)
- Seizure control
- Report pesticide exposure to the state health department
- Work with parents, schools, and community agencies to prevent pesticide exposure

Prevention and Patient Education

The risks pesticides present to children are immense. Pesticide exposure occurs in a number of ways and is additive. Regulating the amount of pesticide children take in from any one source is good, but the pattern of multiple contamination must be recognized and a plan to regulate overall exposure developed. Education of parents is the key to preventing pesticide poisoning

in children (see Table 41-7). Steps can be taken to reduce pesticide use, which in turn reduces exposure. Integrated pest management combines physical, cultural, biologic, and other means of pest control with minimal use of pesticides. For example, farms might encourage cats to catch mice rather than using rodenticides, or school cafeterias might use bait traps for cockroaches rather than chemical spray. Herbicides on athletic fields could be applied as spot treatments rather than broadcast widely.

To reduce pesticide ingestion by children, fruits and vegetables should be washed with water to remove surface residues. But pesticides used in growing the products may be incorporated throughout the plant, so families should choose foods that are local, in season, and organically raised as much as possible. A list of hazardous and safer fruits and vegetables is found in Table 41-7. Organic diets significantly lower children's dietary exposure to organophosphorus pesticides (Chensheng et al, 2006).

ENDOCRINE DISRUPTORS

Description

Endocrine disruptors are chemicals that may have the most serious effects upon living organisms on our planet. The book. *Our Stolen Future*, by Colborn and colleagues (1996) brought their existence to the forefront. Endocrine disruptors are found extensively in the environment including in food, water, soil, air, plastics, cosmetics, and drugs. They work by altering the function of endocrine hormones through a variety of mechanisms. Their actions include binding to hormone receptors to mimic

TABLE 41-7	**Pesticide Content of Common Fruits and Vegetables**
Highest in pesticides	Apples
	Bell peppers
	Celery
	Cherries
	Grapes
	Nectarines
	Peaches
	Pears
	Potatoes
	Red raspberries
	Spinach
	Strawberries
Lowest in pesticides	Asparagus
	Avocados
	Bananas
	Broccoli
	Cauliflower
	Corn
	Kiwi
	Mangos
	Onions
	Papaya
	Peas
	Pineapple

Adapted from *FoodNews* Environmental Working Group: From *Shopper's Guide*. Available at *www.foodnews.org* (accessed Dec 17, 2007).

natural hormones, blocking hormone receptors, or altering the production or metabolism of endogenous hormones. It is hypothesized that a "U"-shape impact occurs: extremely low doses and extremely high doses have significant effects, thus traditional toxicological concepts such as "dose-response" may not apply.

Epidemiology

Many conditions and illnesses that are affected by endocrine function have increased in the last few decades. Between 1973 and 1999, rates of prostate cancer rose about 80% in Americans. The rate of hypospadias and related disorders, such as cryptorchidism and testicular cancer, now collectively referred to as testicular dysgenesis syndrome, have also risen significantly. Male fertility has declined over the past 50 years with sperm counts 50% less than they were 50 years ago in some agricultural states. Breast cancer has also increased, rising from 1:22 in the 1940s to 1:8 in 2006. Neurologic problems such as ADHD and autism have increased significantly in the past several decades. Colborn and colleagues (1996) also pointed out that birds, reptiles, fish, and other animals have the same endocrine hormones as humans do—thyroid, testosterone, and estrogen, for instance, and endocrine-related disorders have occurred over the past several decades in many animal species. Male fish filled with eggs, and fish contaminated with polychlorinated biphenyls in the Great Lakes with reproductive disorders and enlarged thyroid glands have been found.

The relationship between endocrine disruptors and disease in humans becomes clearer as more studies are done (Bay et al, 2006). Cancer caused by diethylstilbestrol is a classic example of disease following prenatal exposure to an endocrine disruptor. Phthalates have been linked to asthma symptoms in children in at least one study (Bornehag et al, 2004), with reduced anogenital distance in male infants (Marsee et al, 2006), and with altered semen quality in subfertile men (Hauser et al, 2006). A list of the cognitive and behavioral characteristics of humans that are regulated by endocrine hormones is found in Box 41-2. Some common endocrine disruptors, their sources, effects, and alternatives for use are found in Table 41-8.

BOX 41-2   **Hormonal Determinants of Behavior in Humans**

- Sexual differentiation of the brain
- Sexual behavior
- Courtship, mating, motivation
- Maternal behavior
- Aggressive and attack behaviors
- Sensory-motor function
- Stress responses
- Cognitive function
- Learning and performance
- Play behavior

POLYCHLORINATED BIPHENYLS

Description

Polychlorinated biphenyls (PCBs), a family of up to 209 chemicals, are one type of extremely stable organochlorines. Many organochlorines are endocrine disruptors. PCBs used commercially are always mixtures of the various types and are frequently contaminated with furans and dioxins. PCBs are structurally similar to thyroid hormones. They probably work through changes in hormonal function, altering concentrations of hormones or affecting receptor numbers or affinity. PCBs have been shown to affect levels of circulating THs, especially T-4. Effects have also been found on the human immune system.

Epidemiology

Although banned from production since 1977, PCBs are so stable that they are still commonly found in the environment, even in Arctic mammals (Colborn et al, 1996). Low levels are found throughout the world, evaporating and returning to earth by rainfall and settling in dust particles. PCBs are not very water soluble, and as a result are not found in high concentrations in drinking water. They dissolve readily in oils, accumulating in the fatty tissues of fish, birds, and mammals. Human exposure comes primarily through ingestion of contaminated foods. Channel catfish, large lake trout, and carp may have high levels. Yellow perch, lake whitefish, smelt, sunfish, and wild ocean salmon have low levels. For children, fetal and neonatal exposures are common, usually via maternal ingestion of contaminated food. Schoolchildren can be exposed through deteriorating building materials. The workplace is a major source of exposure to PCBs in the U.S. A recently identified source of PCBs is in caulking material for windows in older buildings (Herrick et al, 2004).

Clinical Findings
History.
- History of maternal ingestion of contaminated food
- Skin disorders, including hyperpigmentation, nail changes, and chloracne
- Hepatic dysfunction
- Low birth weight and developmental delays
- Behavioral symptoms
- Frequent respiratory infections

Physical Examination. Clinical effects are listed in Table 41-5.

Diagnostic Studies. Increased liver enzymes with severe exposure, although these findings are nonspecific.

Differential Diagnosis

The differential diagnosis includes acne vulgaris, other causes of developmental delay, lead poisoning, and hypothyroidism.

Management

Avoid contact with PCB-contaminated food and environmental sources, especially prenatally. Breastfeeding should not be stopped.

TABLE 41-8 **Endocrine Disruptors**

Type	Agent	Chemical Group	Products Containing the Chemical	Known Toxic Effects	Alternatives
Industrial chemicals		Bisphenol A (BPA)	Plastics: polycarbonates and polystyrene used in flame retardants and plastic food containers, bottles, dental sealants, linings for metal cans, most baby bottles may leach BPA	Rodent studies: mammary tissue, reduced sperm production, increased prostate weight, accelerated growth, early puberty in females	High density polyethylene (HDPE) (opaque or translucent plastics such as milk bottles). Avoid use of products with BPA or wash with mild detergent, rinse well. Use glass or ceramic containers for storage and reheating of food.
		Polychlorinated biphenyls (PCBs), dioxins, furans	Electrical capacitors, transformers, carbonless copy paper, produced with some manufacturing of paper and plastic, some chemicals. Recently found in caulking for old windows.	PCBs: decreased birth weight, increases weight in adolescent females. No effect on pubertal development. Changes thyroid utilization; neurodevelopmental delays and learning problems; increased breast cancer risk. Dioxins: cancer, birth defects, learning disabilities, infertility, endometriosis, immune suppression	No longer manufactured in U.S. but may be found in fish which have lived in contaminated waters. Limit fish consumption of fish at risk. Bioaccumulates.
		Phthalates	Plastics: polyvinyl chloride and other plastic products, nail polish, hair spray, inks, adhesives	Premature thelarche, endometriosis, shorter gestation; lower serum testosterone levels in infants exposed to high phthalates from breast milk. Animal studies: testicular dysgenesis in males, suppression of endogenous testosterone, suspected carcinogen	Do not use polyethylene terephthalate (PETE or PET) found in clear containers such as soda bottles, bottled water; do not use PVC cling wraps. Do not reheat foods in Styrofoam. Low-density polyethylene (LDPE) used in many food storage bags is OK. Polypropylene (PP) found in storage containers such as Rubbermaid, Ziploc, Gladware, Tupperware is considered safe.
		Polybrominated phenyls (PBB, PBDEs)	Fire retardants	Early onset of menstruation following in utero exposure	Avoid using these materials
		Persistent aromatic hydrocarbons (PAEs)	Industrial pollution, tobacco tar, charred foods	Carcinogen	
Pesticides		DDT/DDE, dieldrin, alachlor, atrazine, malathion, pentachlorophenol, benomyl, aldrin	Insecticides, fungicides, herbicides, wood preservatives	DDT/DDE: possible links to breast cancer; Alachlor: probable carcinogen; Alachlor and atrazine: antiestrogenic activity with decreased semen quality	Vary food intake of produce to limit exposure; wash produce before eating, choose organic and local, in-season produce if possible. Use traps for insects rather than spraying. Avoid pesticide-sprayed areas for a few days. For pest prevention indoors, clean up food and spills, don't leave pet food out overnight, keep lids on trash, clean dirty dishes right away, eat at the table only, get rid of stacks of paper.

Adapted from DiDiego ML et al: Unmasking the truth behind endocrine disruptors, *Nurse Pract* 30:54-59, 2005.

PHTHALATES

Description

Phthalates are industrial compounds used in the production of soft plastics; they subsequently leach from the plastic into the environment. Di-(2-ethylhexyl) phthalate (DEHP) is the most commonly used compound. Phthalates are endocrine disruptors. In utero phthalate exposure has been associated with preterm birth. It is believed that phthalates interfere with the way the mother uses essential fatty acids that are critical to fetal development (Latini et al, 2006). They also interfere with thyroid homeostasis. Phthalates are associated with testicular dysgenesis (decreased sperm counts, testicular cancer, cryptorchidism, and hypospadias) in male offspring (Shakkebaek, 2002), and have been linked to decreased semen quality and endometriosis.

Humans are exposed through dermal, ingestion, and inhalation routes. Many hospitals are removing all DEHP-containing products from patient care, especially from neonatal units. This includes IV tubing, IV bags, umbilical catheters, and other soft plastic materials (see Resource Box at the end of the chapter for information on the Health Care Without Harm's PVC/DEHP Audit Tool for hospitals). Phthalates are also found in PVC toys, vinyl shower curtains, car seats, wallpaper, floor coverings, and many other products (Hall, 2006).

NOISE

Description

Noise is defined as any sound, but is usually considered loud, harsh, unpleasant, or unwanted. Noise pollution is the presence of irritating, distracting, or physically dangerous noise. Sound has qualities of frequency or pitch (measured in cycles per minute and stated in Hertz [Hz]), intensity or loudness (measured in decibels [dB]), periodicity, and duration (either continuous, short-term, or episodic). The human voice is approximately 50 dB sound pressure levels (AAP, 2003a). The National Institute for Occupational Safety and Health (NIOSH) defines hazardous noise as 85 decibels for an average of 8 hours sound exposure (Chepesiuk, 2005). Table 41-9 lists the decibels of common environmental noises.

Epidemiology

The impact of noise on human health is varied. Noise-induced hearing loss (NIHL) and tinnitus are the most obvious effects. Hearing loss is a growing problem in the pediatric population, especially among adolescents. Approximately 9.9 per 100,000 individuals suffer NIHL in the total population. Although this number is small, the ratio is significantly higher for children and young adults than other age groups, with 28 per 100,000 in 6- to 25-year-olds, and 107 per 100,000 in 19-year-old boys (Plontke et al, 2002). As many as 12.5% of 6- to 19-year-olds have evidence of a noise-induced hearing threshold loss (Niskar et al, 2001).

Humans are subject to NIHL from exposure to continuous noise or to sudden acoustic trauma that causes damage to the hair cells of the cochlea due to excessive vibration; extreme noise can rupture the tympanic membrane. Noise of more than 85 dB but less than 140 dB leads to temporary hearing loss, most often in the 4000 Hz range. Permanent hearing loss can result from one exposure to a sudden, extreme noise (greater than 140 dB) of

TABLE 41-9 Noise in the Environment	
Noise Source	**Decibels**
Quiet room	28–33
Computer	37–45
Refrigerator	40–43
Normal conversation	40
Forced-air heating system	42–52
Dishwasher	54–85
Microwave oven	55–59
Alarm clock	60–80
Vacuum cleaner	62–85
Telephone	66–75
Inside car, windows closed, 30 mph	68–73
Electric shaver	75
Gas-powered lawn mower	87–92
Average motorcycle	90
Leaf blower	95–105
Max output of stereo	100–120
Average snowmobile	120
Average rock concert	140

Data from Chepesiuk R: Decibel hell: the effects of living in a noisy world, *Environ Health Perspect* 113(1):A34-A47, 2005.

short duration, or from ongoing lower levels of noise. Permanent loss is often in the 3000 to 6000 Hz range. Music listened to on headphones and at concerts, firecrackers, electrical tools, airport noise, and even everyday noise of traffic can cause problems (Lercher et al, 2002). The American Academy of Pediatrics Committee on Environmental Health published a policy statement concluding that excessive noise exposure results in high-frequency hearing loss in newborns and that excessive noise in intensive care units may disrupt the natural growth and development of premature infants (Etzel et al, 1997).

Noise can also cause tinnitus, a problem for more than 12 million Americans (Chepesiuk, 2005). Chronic, everyday noise causes sleep disturbance, distraction, decreased concentration, and an increased stress response (e.g., increased heart rate, blood pressure, adrenalin, and cortisol production); these in turn result in personality changes, irritability, poor coping, and lower achievement in children. A recent cross-national study found that aircraft noise was directly associated with impaired reading comprehension and could impair cognitive function (Clark et al, 2006).

Assessment

History.   A careful history looks at the following:
- Type of noise in child's environment
- Exposure to chronic noise
- Episodic acoustic trauma
- History of ear disease

Physical Examination.   Many states require assessment of newborns for congenital or birth-related hearing loss. This testing establishes a baseline; thereafter children should be assessed for hearing using a pure-tone audiometer at well-child examinations at 4, 5, 10, 12, and 18 years old. Tympanography and visual examination of the tympanic membrane help rule out otitis media and middle ear effusion.

Management

Noise-induced hearing loss is virtually 100% preventable. The goals of management are to:

- Increase awareness of the health hazard noise represents. Parents and children need to understand the relationship between noise and the auditory system. Every well-child visit should include questions related to the child's noise environment, and both children and parents should be given information on the dangers of excessive noise and how to avoid them. Primary care providers can work with parents and schools to offer a hearing loss management curriculum.
- Decrease noise in the environment. Parents and children should be encouraged to minimize noise in their environment, including efforts to:
  - Reduce volume on television and radios; turn off "background" TVs and radios.
  - Use headphones cautiously, keeping the volume low enough to hear normal conversation.
  - Avoid loud music, firecrackers, popguns, and other sources of episodic, extreme noise.
  - Avoid loud noises; for example, do not vacuum or use appliances (e.g., blender) with infants nearby.
  - Create a "quiet" place in the home.
- Mitigate exposure to noise. Wear earplugs and earmuffs to protect against "unavoidable" noise. Commercial-quality ear protectors are available for use in the home (e.g., when electrical saws or other loud tools are used). Earplugs can be purchased at any drugstore.
- Implement standards to regulate noise. The Federal Noise Control Act of 1972 provides the mechanism to set standards, rules, and regulations for occupational, industrial, and residential noise (e.g., automobiles and construction). States and municipalities have also established standards for noise control. Pediatric providers can be a resource to policy makers by providing information about the health effects of excessive and chronic noise.

SUMMARY

In summary, environmental hazards and toxins are pervasive and have significant impact upon the health of children everywhere beginning with fetal life and persisting into adulthood. Although many of the health outcomes are unknown, and most are difficult to manage, prevention is possible by reducing hazards in the environment and reducing children's exposures to existing hazards. This is an area of health care where the provider must take a public health perspective, recognizing that the patient at hand is likely not the only person in the family or community who has been exposed to a given hazard and is affected by it. Generally, the local clinician will want to enlist the help of experts in the field—the local or state health department, the Environmental Protection Agency, a regional Pediatric Environmental Health Specialty Unit, or other sources. Through advocacy and policy development, the worst of the hazards can be eliminated from our air, water, food, and soil, creating a healthier environment for future generations than exists today.

"All things are connected. Whatever befalls the earth befalls the children of the earth."
Chief Seattle
From The Soul of an Indian

NURSING DIAGNOSES

Nursing Diagnoses Related to Environmental Health

- Contamination
  - Risk for contamination
- Risk for poisoning

From NANDA International: *NANDA-I nursing diagnoses: definitions & classification 2007-2008*, Philadelphia, 2007. From Jorde L et al, Medical Genetics, ed 3, St. Louis, 2006, Mosby/Elsevier, p. 321.

RESOURCE BOX

Environmental Health Issues

Agency for Toxic Substances and Disease Registry (ATSDR)
www.atsdr.cdc.gov

Alliance to End Childhood Lead Poisoning
www.aeclp.org

American Academy of Clinical Toxicology
clintox.org
Position statements on treatment of poisonings

Association of Occupational and Environmental Clinics (AOEC)
www.aoec.org

Center for Children's Health and the Environment
www.childenvironment.org
Academic and research policy center on environmental health of children

RESOURCE BOX

Environmental Health Issues—Cont'd

Centers for Disease Control and Prevention (CDC)
National Center for Environmental Health
www.cdc.gov/nceh

Children's Environmental Health Network
www.cehn.org

Consumer Product Safety Commission Office
of Information
www.cpsc.gov

Environmental Health Perspectives
http://ehp.niehs.nih.gov/children
Link to Pediatric Environmental Health Specialty Units (PEHSUs)

Environmental Working Group (EWG)
www.ewg.org
Public advocacy and information

EnviRN (University of Maryland Environmental Health
Site for Nurses)
www.enviRN.umaryland.edu
Environmental news and information for nurses and others

Health Care Without Harm
www.noharm.org
Publication: Going Green: A Resource Kit for Pollution
Tool Kit: PVC/DEHP audit tool for hospitals to remove phthalates
www.noharm.org/pvcDehp/reducingPVC

Project KISS: Keeping Infants Safe from Smoke
www2.dfci.harvard.edu/ccbr/projects_events/past/project
   kiss.html
Program to help smokers lower their children's exposure to
tobacco smoke

Material Safety Data Sheets
www.ilpi.com/msds
Information on effects of substances on body

National Environmental Education and Training
Foundation (NEETF)
www.neefusa.org
Developing initiative to educate health care providers on
management of pesticide poisoning (National Pesticide
Competency Guidelines) and tools for environmental history-
taking

National Environmental Health Association
www.neha.org

National Institute of Environmental Health Sciences
www.niehs.nih.gov
Links to Children's Environmental Health Centers

National Institute for Occupational Safety and Health
www.cdc.gov/niosh/topics/pesticides
Lists state-based pesticide poisoning surveillance programs

National Pesticide Information Center (NPIC)
www.npic.orst.edu

National Safety Council
www.nsc.org
form to obtain radon testing kits at www.nsc.org/ehc/radon/
coupon.htm

Rocky Mountain Drug Consultation Center
www.rmpdc.org
Pharmaceutical and over-the-counter medication and drug
information and consultation services for health care providers;
information on poisoning

Scorecard: The pollution information site
www.scorecard.org
Provides information about major pollutants for all zip codes
in the U.S.

U.S. Environmental Protection Agency (EPA)
www.epa.gov
The EPA has information on a wide range of environmental
toxins. For example:
Molds: *www.epa.gov/iaq/molds*
Superfunds: *www.epa.gov/superfund*
Brownfields: *www.epa.gov/brownfields*
Worker Protection Standard: *www.epa.gov/oppfead1/safety/workers/
amendment.htm*
Radon and indoor air: *www.epa.gov/iaq/whereyoulive.html*

INFORMATION ABOUT TOXICANTS
Collaborative on Health and the Environment: CHE
Toxicants and Disease Database
http://database.healthandenvironment.org
Scientifically based, web-interactive database summarizing the
evidence of links between exposure to chemical contaminants
and more than 180 associated human diseases or conditions

TOXNET: Hazardous substances Data Bank
www.toxnet.nlm.nih.gov/cgi-bin/sis/htmlgen?HSDB
Peer reviewed data on more than 4800 chemicals

TOXMAP
www.toxmap.nlm.nih.gov/toxmap/main/index.jsp
Displays toxic release inventory data on interactive maps and
provides additional information on chemicals

✓ DISCUSSION FORUM

1. How can you integrate the use of the Pediatric Environmental Health History into your well child care visits? How can the use of survey tools like these improve your practice?

2. What are the principal environmental hazards in your local community? What community resources are there to assist families to clean up hazards?

3. What environmental hazards are more common in rural and urban settings? What do you need to think about in terms of environmental hazards in caring for children who travel or have extended families in other parts of the world?

4. What steps would you take if a parent brought a child in to you reporting that he had been playing with a jar of elemental mercury that he found? What information would you need to collect initially? What agencies would you call for help?

5. What steps would you take if your patient was the child of a migrant farm worker and the parent reported that pesticide spraying had drifted across the farm worker housing area several times in the past few weeks?

REFERENCES

Agran PF et al: Rates of pediatric injuries by 3-month intervals for children 0 to 3 years of age, *Pediatrics* 111(6):e683-e692, 2003.

Alessandrini F et al: Effects of ultrafine carbon particle inhalation on allergic inflammation of the lung, *J Allergy Clin Immunol* 117(4):824-830, 2006.

American Academy of Pediatrics (AAP) Committee on Environmental Health: Lead exposure in children: prevention, detection, and management, *Pediatrics* 116(4):1036-1046, 2005.

American Academy of Pediatrics (AAP) Committee on Environmental Health: Policy statement: ambient air pollution: health hazards to children, *Pediatrics* 114(6):1699-1707, 2004.

American Academy of Pediatrics (AAP) Committee on Environmental Health: *Handbook of pediatric environmental health*, ed 2, Elk Grove Village, IL, 2003a, American Academy of Pediatrics.

American Academy of Pediatrics (AAP) Committee on Injury, Violence, and Poison Prevention: Policy statement: poison treatment in the home, *Pediatrics* 112:1182-1185, 2003b.

Balashazy I, Hofmann W, Heistracher T: Local particle deposition patterns may play a key role in the development of lung cancer, *J Appl Physiol* 94:1719-1725, 2003.

Bay K et al: Testicular dysgenesis syndrome: possible role of endocrine disrupters, *Best Pract Res Clin Endocrinol Metab* 20(1):77-90, 2006.

Bellinger DC: Lead, *Pediatrics* 113:1016-1022, 2004.

Benuck I: Tobacco, heart disease, and practical counseling, *Pediatr Ann* 35(11):802-807, 2006.

Bornehag CG et al: The association between asthma and allergic symptoms in children and phthalates in house dust: a nested case-control study, *Environ Health Perspect* 112(14):1393-1397, 2004.

Brent RL: Environmental causes of human congenital malformations: the pediatrician's role in dealing with these complex clinical problems caused by a multiplicity of environmental and genetic factors, *Pediatrics* 113(4):957-968, 2004.

Calderon RL, Abernathy CO, Thomas DJ: Consequences of acute and chronic exposure to arsenic in children, *Pediatr Ann* 33(7):461-466, 2004.

Charnley G: Assessing and managing methylmercury risks associated with power plant mercury emissions in the United States, *Medscape General Medicine* 8(1):64, 2006. Available at *www.medscape.com/viewarticle/522270* (accessed Jan 7, 2007).

Chassin L et al: Parental smoking cessation and adolescent smoking, *J Pediatr Psychol* 27:485-496, 2002.

Chensheng L et al: Organic diets significantly lower children's dietary exposure to organophosphorus pesticides, *Environ Health Perspect* 114(2):260-263, 2006.

Chepesiuk R: Decibel hell: the effects of living in a noisy world, *Environ Health Perspect* 113(1):A34-A41, 2005.

Clark C et al: Exposure-effect relations between aircraft and road traffic noise exposure at school and reading comprehension: the RANCH project, *Am J Epidemiol* 163(1):27-37, 2006.

Colborn T, Dumanoski D, Myers JP: *Our stolen future: are we threatening our fertility, intelligence, and survival? A scientific detective story,* New York, 1996, Penguin Group.

Counter SA, Buchanan LH: Mercury exposure in children: a review, *Toxicol Appl Pharmacol* 198(2):209-230, 2004.

Denson KW: Passive smoking in infants, children and adolescents: the effects of diet and socioeconomic factors, *Int Arch Occup Environ Health* 74:525-532, 2001.

DeRouen TA et al, 2006: Neurobehavioral effects of dental amalgam in children: a randomized clinical trial, *JAMA* 295(15):1784-92, 2006.

DiFranza JR, Aligne CA, Weitzman M: Prenatal and postnatal environmental tobacco smoke exposure and children's health, *Pediatrics* 113(4 supp): 1007-1015, 2004.

Eaton DK et al: *Youth risk behavior surveillance—United States, 2005, MMWR Surveill Summ* 55(SS-5), Atlanta, GA, 2006, Centers for Disease Control and Prevention.

Environmental Protection Agency (EPA): *About pesticides: 2000-2001 pesticide market estimates,* 2006a. Available at *www.epa.gov/oppbead1/pestsales/01pestsales/usage2001.html%233_3* (accessed Jan 9, 2007).

Environmental Protection Agency (EPA): *Asbestos in schools.* 2006b. Available at *www.epa.gov/asbestos/pubs/asbestos_in_schools.html* (accessed Jan 9, 2007).

Environmental Protection Agency (EPA): Asbestos worker protection: final rule, *Federal Register* 65(221): 69210-69217, 2000.

Environmental Protection Agency (EPA): *FDA and EPA announce the revised consumer advisory on methylmercury in fish.* Available at *www.fda.gov/bbs/topics/news/2004/NEW01038.html* (accessed Jan 7, 2007).

Environmental Protection Agency (EPA): *Indoor air: mold,* 2006c. Available at *www.epa.gov/iaq/molds* (accessed Jan 9, 2007).

Environmental Protection Agency (EPA): *Radon-induced lung cancer,* Washington, DC, 1994, Environmental Protection Agency.

Environmental Protection Agency (EPA) Office of Children's Health Protection: *1997 declaration of the environment leaders of the eight on children's environmental health.* Available at *http://yosemite.epa.gov/ochp/ochpweb.nsf/content/declara.htm* (accessed Jan 5, 2007).

Etzel RA et al: Noise: A hazard for the fetus and newborn, *Pediatrics* 100(4):724-727, 1997.

Food and Drug Administration: *FDA broadens access to lead screening test that gives immediate results: waiver allows community-based testing.* Available at *www.fda.gov/bbs/topics/NEWS/2006/NEW01456.html* (accessed Jan 7, 2007).

Gilbert SG, Weiss B: A rationale for lowering the blood action level from 10 to 2 microg/dL, *Neurotoxicology* 27(5):693-701, 2006.

Goto C: Heavy metal intoxication. In Behrman R, Kliegman R, Jenson H, editors: *Nelson textbook of pediatrics,* ed 17, Philadelphia, 2004, WB Saunders.

Grandjean P, Landrigan PJ: Developmental neurotoxicity of industrial chemicals, *Lancet* 368(9553):2167-2178, 2006.

Groner J et al: Screening for children's exposure to environmental tobacco smoke in a pediatric primary care setting, *Arch Pediatr Adolesc Med* 159(5):450-455, 2005.

Guillette EA: A broad-based evaluation of pesticide-exposed children, *Cent Eur J Public Health* 8(suppl):58-59, 2000.

Hall AG: Nurses: taking precautionary action on a pediatric environmental exposure: DEHP, *Pediatr Nurs* 32(1):91-94, 2006.

Hauser R et al: Altered semen quality in relation to urinary concentrations of phthalate monoester and oxidative metabolites, *Epidemiology* 17(6): 682-691, 2006.

Heeren GA, Tyler J, Mandeya A: Agricultural chemical exposures and birth defects in the Eastern Cape Province, South Africa: a case-control study, *Environ Health* 2(1):11, 2003.

Herrick R et al: An unrecognized source of PCB contamination in schools and other buildings, *Environ Health Perspect* 12(10):1051-1053, 2004.

Hightower JM, O'Hare A, Hernandez GT: Blood mercury reporting in NHANES: identifying Asian, Pacific Islander, Native American and multiracial groups, *Environ Health Perspect* 114(2):173-175, 2006.

Hill WG, Butterfield P, Larsson LS: Rural parents' perceptions of risks associated with their children's exposure to radon, *Public Health Nurs* 23(5):392-399, 2006.

Jacobs DE et al: The prevalence of lead-based paint hazards in US housing, *Environ Health Perspect* 110:A599-A606, 2002.

Jan J, Vrbic V: Polychlorinated biphenyls cause developmental enamel defects in children, *Caries Res* 34:469-473, 2000.

Kemper AR et al: Follow-up testing among children with elevated screening blood lead tests, *JAMA*, 293(18):2232-2237, 2005.

Knapp JF et al: Case records of the Childrens' Mercy Hospital, case 02-1999: a 1-month-old infant with respiratory distress and shock, *Pediatr Emerg Care* 15:288-293, 1999.

Kum-Nji P, Meloy L, Herrod H: Environmental tobacco smoke exposure prevalence and mechanisms of causation of infections in children, *Pediatrics* 117(5):1745-1754, 2006.

Landrigan PJ: Pesticides and PCBs: does the evidence show that they threaten children's health? *Contemp Pediatr* 18:110-126, 2001.

Landrigan et al: Environmental pollutants and disease in American children: estimates of morbidity, mortality, and costs of lead poisoning, asthma, cancer, and developmental disabilities, *Environ Health Perspect* 110: 721-728, 2002.

Lanphear B et al: Low-level environmental lead exposure and children's intellectual function: an international pooled analysis, *Environ Health Perspect* 113(7):894-899, 2005.

Latini G et al: In utero exposure to phthalates and fetal development, *Curr Med Chem* 13(21):2527-2534, 2006.

Lercher P et al: Ambient neighbourhood noise and children's mental health, *Occup Environ Med* 59:380-386, 2002.

Ma X et al: Critical windows of exposure to household pesticides and risk of childhood leukemia, *Environ Health Perspect* 110:955-960, 2002.

Markowitz M: Lead poisoning. In Behrman RE, Kliegman RM, Jenson HB, editors: *Nelson textbook of pediatrics,* ed 17, Philadelphia, 2004, WB Saunders.

Marsee K et al: Estimated daily phthalate exposures in a population of mothers of male infants exhibiting reduced anogenital distance, *Environ Health Perspect* 114(6):805-809, 2006.

Marshall L et al: Youth tobacco surveillance—United States, 2001-2002, *MMWR Surveill Summ* 55(3):1-56, 2006.

Martin JA et al: Births: final data for 2004, *Natl Vital Stat Rep* 55(1):1-101, 2006.

Mazur LJ, Kim J, Committee on Environmental Health: Technical report: spectrum of noninfectious health effects from molds, *Pediatrics* 118(6): e1909-e1926, 2006.

McConnell R et al: Traffic, susceptibility, and childhood asthma, *Environ Health Perspect* 114(5):766-772, 2006.

Moskowitz WB, Schwartz PF, Schieken RM: Childhood passive smoking, race, and coronary artery disease risk: the MCV Twin Study, *Arch Pediatr Adolesc Med* 153:446-453, 1999.

National Children's Study, October 2007 update. Available at *www. nationalchildrensstudy.gov* (accessed Dec 17, 2007).

Niskar AS et al: Estimated prevalence of noise-induced hearing threshold shifts among children 6 to 19 years of age: the Third National Health and Nutrition Examination Survey, 1988-1994, United States, *Pediatrics* 108:40-43, 2001.

Noble RE: Environmental tobacco smoke uptake by clothing fabrics, *Sci Total Environ* 262:1-3, 2000.

Nuttall KL: Interpreting hair mercury levels in individual patients, *Ann Clin Lab Sci* 36(3):248-261, 2006.

Occupational Safety and Health Administration (OSHA): *Occupational exposure to asbestos,* Washington, DC, 1994, US Department of Labor. Available at *www.osha.gov/pls/oshaweb/owadisp.show_document?p_ table=FEDERAL_REGISTER&p_id=13404* (accessed Jan 9, 2007).

Opler MG, Susser ES: Fetal environment and schizophrenia, *Environ Health Perspect* 113(9):1239-1242, 2005.

Pandya RJ: Diesel exhaust and asthma: hypotheses and molecular mechanisms of action, *Environ Health Perspect* 110(Suppl 1):103-112, 2002.

Patton S: Biomonitoring: measuring toxins in our bodies as a tool in protecting children's health, *Zero to Three* 26(2):33-37, 2005.

Perera FP et al: A summary of recent findings on birth outcomes and developmental effects of prenatal ETS, PAH, and pesticide exposures, *Neurotoxicity* 26:573-587, 2005.

Plontke SK et al: The incidence of acoustic trauma due to New Year's firecrackers, *Eur Arch Otorhinolaryngol* 259:247-252, 2002.

Powell DL, Stewart V: Children: the unwitting target of environmental injustices, *Pediatr Clin North Am* 48:1291-1305, 2001.

Qureshi ST, Mahajan P: Carbon monoxide poisoning: clues to unmasking the great masquerader, *Consultant Pediatricians* 4(10):477-479, 482, 2005.

Regional Asthma Management & Prevention: *Companion to CTS's people with asthma: appropriate rental housing accommodations, 2006,* California Thoracic Society. Available at *www.rampasthma.org/CTS% 20Housing%20Guidelines.htm* (accessed Jan 9, 2007).

Reigart JR, Roberts JR: Pesticides in children, *Pediatr Clin North Am* 48:1185-1198, 2001.

Reigart JR, Roberts JR: *Recognition and management of pesticide poisonings,* ed 5, Washington, DC, 1999, US Environmental Protection Agency.

Rodgers GA, Matyunas N: Poisonings: drugs, chemicals, and plants, In Behrman RE, Kliegman RM, Jenson HB, editors, *Nelson textbook of pediatrics,* ed 17, Philadelphia, 2004, WB Saunders.

Roseby R et al: Family and career smoking control programmes for reducing children's exposure to environmental tobacco smoke, *Cochrane Database of Systematic Reviews* 3:CD001746, 2003.

Sargent JD, Dalton M: Does parental disapproval of smoking prevent adolescents from becoming established smokers? *Pediatrics* 108:1256-1262, 2001.

Schwenk M et al: Children as a sensitive subgroup and their role in regulatory toxicology: DGPT workshop report, *Arch Toxicol* 77:2-6, 2003.

Shakkebaek NE: Endocrine disrupters and testicular dysgenesis syndrome, *Horm Res* 57(Suppl 2):43, 2002.

Shenassa ED, Brown M-J: Maternal smoking and infantile gastrointestinal dysregulation: the case of colic, *Pediatrics* 114:e497-e505, 2004.

Smith KR, Corvalan CF, Kjellstrom T: How much global ill health is attributable to environmental factors? *Epidemiology* 10 573-584, 1999.

Tran B et al: *Arsenic lurks in Canadian playgrounds: is your child safe?* Toronto, 2003, Environmental Defence Canada.

Trasande L, Landrigan PJ, Schechter C: Public health and economic consequences of methylmercury toxicity to the developing brain, *Environ Health Perspect* 113(5):590-596, 2005.

US Agency for Health Care Policy and Research (USAHCPR): *Treating tobacco use and dependence: a clinical practice guideline 2000.* Available at *www.ncbi.nlm.nih.gov/books/bv.fcgi?rid=hstat2.chapter.7644* (accessed Dec 17, 2007).

US Department of Health and Human Services (USDHHS): *Nurse practitioner primary care competencies in specialty areas: adult, family, gerontological, pediatric, and women's health,* Rockville, MD, 2002, USDHHS.

US Department of Health and Human Services (USDHHS), Environmental Protection Agency (EPA): *FDA and EPA announce the revised consumer advisory on methylmercury in fish.* Available at *www.fda.gov/bbs/topics/ news/2004/NEW01038.html* (accessed Jan 7, 2007).

US Department of Health and Human Services (USDHHS), Centers for Disease Control and Prevention (CDC): *Third National Report on Human Exposure to Environmental Chemicals,* Atlanta, GA, 2005, National Center for Environmental Health.

von Ehrenstein OS et al: Pregnancy outcomes, infant mortality, and arsenic in drinking water in West Bengal, India, *Am J Epidemiol* 163(7):662-669, 2006.

Winickoff JP et al: A smoking cessation intervention for parents of children who are hospitalized for respiratory illness: the Stop Tobacco Outreach Program, *Pediatrics* 111(1):140-145, 2004.

Yiin LM et al: Comparison of techniques to reduce residential lead dust on carpet and upholstery: the New Jersey assessment of cleaning techniques trial, *Environ Health Perspect* 110:1233-1237, 2002.

Yolton K et al: Exposure to environmental tobacco smoke and cognitive abilities among U.S. children and adolescents, *Environ Health Perspect* 113(1):98-103, 2005.

Zabel EW, Castellano S: Lead poisoning in Minnesota Medicaid children, *Minnesota Med* 89(5):45-49, 2006.

Zhu SH et al: Predictors of smoking cessation in US adolescents, *Am J Prev Med* 16:202-207, 1999

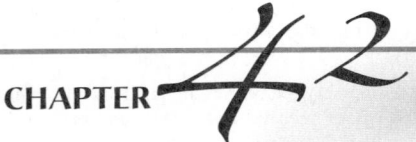

CHAPTER 42

Complementary Medicine

Catherine G. Blosser

■ USE OF COMPLEMENTARY THERAPIES

Since this chapter was originally published in 2000, a transition has been occurring in the clinical, academic, and philosophical foundations that drive conventional Western medicine. There is a growing institutionalization of what was once regarded to be unconventional therapy into the more mainstream education and practices of nursing and medicine. The academic realization that change was needed is best summed up by Dr. Ralph Synderman, of the Bravewell Collaborative: "We as a healthcare system have had our way over the last two decades and have become so enamored with [sic] technology and specialization that we lost sight of the individual—a very complex entity. We need to return to the patient as the center of our focus" (Bravewell, 2006a). What follows will bring the reader a better understanding of how the health care system model may be changing as a "gathering" of human wisdom endeavors to join rather than continue to divide up a patient into small pieces. The journey is an interesting one.

It is estimated that 65% to 80% of the world's population relies on some form of non-Western medicine practice for primary health care (McNeil, 2002). A 1993 landmark study in the U.S. brought the use of complementary therapies into the national spotlight. In this study, patients reported more office visits to practitioners who offered alternative approaches to health and illness than to conventional primary care providers (Eisenberg et al, 1993). Depending on the region, up to 68% of American adults may have used some type of complementary or alternative medicine (CAM) therapy in their lifetime, and 50% continue to do so (Kessler et al, 2001). In a 2002 federal National Health Interview Survey, 36% of adults reported using some form of CAM therapy. This number increased to 62% when megavitamin therapy and prayer were included in the CAM definition (Centers for Disease Control and Prevention [CDC], 2004). Rates of CAM use among patients with chronic, recurrent, or incurable conditions tend to be higher (Kemper, 2001). For example, use of specific psychotropic herbal preparations has been reported as high as 67% (Ting et al, 2002), and another study revealed that 80% of adolescents reported using CAM therapies for asthma (Reznik et al, 2002).

Vitamin or other nutritional supplementation, elimination diets, herbal preparations, aromatherapy, homeopathy, and chiropractics lead the list of the most frequently used CAM therapies in children (Kemper, 2001; Ottolini et al, 2001; Simpson & Roman, 2001). Dietary supplement (multivitamins, minerals, iron, ergogenic agents) use among young children exceeds 50%. More than 30% of adolescents have reported the use of such supplements (Gardiner et al, 2004).

Tu and Hargraves, using the data from the 2002 CDC National Health Interview Survey, reported on the socioeconomic parameters of the respondents. They found that 6 million adults in the U.S. turned to CAM because they found conventional medical care too expensive. These same respondents were four times more likely to be uninsured and twice as likely to have incomes 200 percent below the federal poverty level. Most of these patients had specific medical issues they needed addressed, such as depression and/or chronic pain. They were more likely to use herbal products for their depression, such as St. John's wort or Kava (Tu & Hargraves, 2004).

Until the late 1990s, the prevalence of use of CAM therapies in the pediatric population was unknown. Two studies in 1999 provided data that revealed that approximately 20% to 30% of general pediatric patients had used CAM therapies. Adolescent use was higher, ranging from 50% to 75% (Kemper, 2001).

More recent studies reveal the following usage rates: 20% for the treatment of attention-deficit/hyperactivity disorder (ADHD) or depression; 41% for the treatment of inflammatory bowel disease; 89% by inner-city parents for treating asthma in their children; 12.8% herbal products taken presurgery; and approximately 80% sought information about herbal or dietary supplements in an inpatient, holistic, pediatric oncology consult service. Forty-one percent of adolescents reported use of CAM products (Cala, 2003; Heuschkel et al 2002; Kemper & Wornham, 2001; Wilson & Klein, 2002; Braganza, 2003; Lin et al, 2004). It is notable that one of these studies showed that caregivers were combining both herbal preparations and prescription drugs 13% of the time without informing the pharmacist or care provider (Cala, 2003). Generally, there is an increase in use among patients with chronic, recurrent, or incurable diseases (30% to 70%) (Kemper, 2001).

Reasons cited by parents for choosing an array of CAM therapies for their children include the following (Spiegelblatt, 1997; Turow, 1997; Gardiner et al, 2004):

- Maintenance of health and prevention of diseases
- Limited access to or dissatisfaction with traditional care; ready access to CAM practitioners
- Failure of traditional medicine to have an impact on chronic conditions, such as degenerative diseases, allergies, asthma, otitis media, musculoskeletal ailments, cancer, rheumatoid arthritis, and cystic fibrosis

- Awareness of complications and side effects produced by pharmaceuticals
- Inadequacy of invasive procedures or diagnostics
- Desire for a more holistic, individualistic form of health care
- Ethnic and cultural beliefs
- Belief that alternative practices are more natural, less harmful, and more effective
- Parents are CAM users
- Belief that by combining conventional and nonconventional treatment a more effective approach to health care is achieved than either practice alone affords
- Awareness of the mind-body connection to affect the immune system response
- Desire for more parental, active participation in their child's treatment

In 1990, approximately 40% of patients told their conventional providers about using nonconventional treatments (Eisenberg et al, 1993). Surveys from the late 1990s to 2002 show that this number had increased by only about 10% to 14% (Eisenberg et al, 1998; Landmark Healthcare, 1998; Winslow & Shapiro, 2002; Tu & Hargraves, 2004).

In a study by Ottolini and colleagues (2001), less than half of the families who voiced a desire to discuss the use of CAM options with their physicians had done so. Konefal (2002) observed that physicians were reluctant to respond to patients about CAM modalities because of their traditionally poor communication with CAM practitioners, doubts about CAM practitioner competence, inability to sort out efficacious complementary procedures, and reluctance to participate in offering false hope of obtaining cures.

■ INTEGRATION OF WESTERN AND COMPLEMENTARY THERAPY MODELS

Various phrases have been used to describe health practices that are not fully embraced by conventional Western medicine practices. These terms include *alternative, complementary, contemporary, holistic, integrative, folk, irregular, mind-body medicine, natural, New Age, new medicine, nonconventional, nontraditional, quackery,* and *vernacular medicine*. Dr. Jonas, the first Director of the Office of Alternative Medicine at the National Institutes of Health (NIH), observed that these terms represented "practices that aren't part of the politically dominant medical system of a country" (Wysocki, 1997, p. 4). To be acknowledged as a component of the dominant medical system, a particular medical practice must be taught in medical schools, be available in hospitals or conventional health clinics, and be reimbursable by third-party payers (Wysocki, 1997). As the reader will see, medical education and health care clinics are rapidly integrating and advocating that such practices become part of mainstream medicine. Complementary therapies are being regarded as one of many "tools" that are available to the practice of medicine.

Representatives of both the dominant and nondominant medical practices have more routinely used the terms *complementary* and *integrative* instead of *alternative*. The current mainstream view is to "transform medicine and healthcare through rigorous scientific studies, new models of clinical care, and innovative educational programs that integrate biomedicine, the complexity of human beings, the intrinsic nature of healing, and the rich diversity of therapeutic systems" (Bravewell Collaborative, 2006b). This new movement is being referred to as the "integrative medicine" model. The updated "role" of the physician who uses the integrative medicine model focuses on the patient as a unique individual, similar to the focus of practitioners of complementary therapies discussed in the next paragraph. Advocates of both practices point out that patients benefit when nonconventional and conventional health practices are used collaboratively and when one practice is not an "alternative" to the other. Patients seem to demonstrate this preference because the 2002 National Health Interview Survey (NHIS) reported that CAM users were more likely to also use conventional medical services (Barnes et al, 2004).

Practitioners of complementary therapies view each individual as having unique inner resources for healing, maintaining health, or both. Patients are seen as the primary agents influencing the status of their own health; the practitioner helps mobilize these inherent resources rather than simply administering a "magic bullet." One practitioner describes the effort as one of augmenting host resistance (enhancing the overall immune response or constitutional state) rather than one of attacking (treating, controlling, and suppressing symptoms) the disease (Schoch, 1999). Western medicine–oriented physicians propose incorporation of the best of science and technologic tools (including complementary practices with proven scientific efficacy) with a focus on health prevention and the "therapeutic relationship and healing power of nature" (Snyderman & Weil, 2006).

Table 42-1 lists many of the complementary therapies in use. Specific applications to pediatric or adolescent diagnoses are discussed at the end of the chapter in Table 42-4. Primary care providers need to become familiar with complementary therapies, routinely inquire into their use, be cognizant of allopathic drug and herbal product interactions, and foster open discussion with clients who may be combining conventional and nonconventional treatments. In fact, the most effective treatment may involve using therapeutic applications from several different approaches. Successful primary health care providers benefit from moving between paradigms without prejudice, gleaning what is of value, and knowing when referral to a complementary medical practitioner is appropriate. As Dr. Jonas so aptly stated, "Alternative medicine is here to stay. It is no longer an option to ignore it or treat it as something outside the normal process of science and medicine" (Jonas, 1998).

■ HISTORY OF COMPLEMENTARY MEDICAL PRACTICES

Before 1910, many different medical and apprenticeship schools allowed graduates to be licensed and referred to as "doctors." With acceptance of the 1910 Flexner report, all medical training, licensure, and regulation in the U.S. became standardized; since then "approved" medical education has been

TABLE 42-1   Complementary Therapies and Their Applications

Nonconventional Therapy	Theory Behind Use	Treatment Applications*
Acupressure	Similar principle as acupuncture but uses fingertips instead of needles to apply pressure (see Acupuncture); also incorporates breathing techniques to aid healing by balancing mind-body-spirit; shiatsu, reflexology, jin shin use similar techniques.	Muscle tension, targeting a specific organ or glandular systems Usually more acceptable to children than acupuncture
Acupuncture	Hair-thin needles inserted at specific anatomic points alter blockages in energy flow patterns along "meridians" and stimulate body to produce pain-relieving and mood-lifting chemicals or antiinflammatory substances (sterile, disposable needles should always be used) (University of California, Berkeley, 1998).	Morning sickness of pregnancy Postoperative dental pain Chronic pain (including headaches) Allergies Asthma Nausea and vomiting (including morning sickness, chemotherapy-induced, and postsurgical) Menstrual cramps Migraine headaches Low back pain Addictions (e.g., smoking) Musculoskeletal pain (e.g., arthritis, fibromyalgia, carpal tunnel syndrome, tendinitis)
Aromatherapy	Uses pure, essential, volatile oils containing oxygenated molecules to transport nutrients to cells of the body; believed to promote immunity and create a cellular environment in which disease-causing bacteria, fungi, and viruses cannot live; aromas of essential oils are either inhaled or absorbed through the skin. When inhaled, believed to activate the brain's amygdala (associated with memory and emotions). Taught in medical schools in France; Japanese use in factories to increase productivity (Krebs, 2006).	Stress, anxiety, depression, agitation Fatigue Immune disorders Acute and chronic pain Insomnia Intrapartum: strengthens contractions
Ayurvedic medicine	The traditional form of medicine practiced in Indian cultures; treats imbalances or "dosnas" within body that cause illness by using diet changes, herbal remedies, breath work, physical exercise, hatha yoga, meditation, and rejuvenation or detoxification programs; focuses on preventing disease by enhancing the mind-body connection.	For primary health care disorders involving GI systems, GYN, respiratory tract, bones and muscles, circulation (including cardiovascular), emotional, and psychological, addictions, ENT
Balneotherapy	Therapy focuses on the beneficial effects of medicinal waters and involves bathing in water of various types (e.g., in reduced-sulfurous mineral water).	Low back pain, muscle spasm, stress, promotion of healing (Balogh et al, 2005)
Biofeedback	Empowers the mind to take control of conscious and autonomic processes (Frishberg, 1998); relaxation is focused on one muscle or function rather than on the whole body.	Chronic pain, HTN, Insomnia, circulation Tension and migraine headaches Incontinence (urine and fecal) Stroke rehabilitation PTSD and depression Chronic tinnitus Chronic facial nerve palsy Torticollis In children: chronic pain (e.g., sickle cell crises), JRA, RAP, functional voice disorders, improve sphincter control associated with urinary and fecal incontinence, postural training for scoliosis, ADHD (Allen, 2004)

TABLE 42-1   Complementary Therapies and Their Applications—Cont'd

Nonconventional Therapy	Theory Behind Use	Treatment Applications*
Chelation	Involves IV injections of binding (chelating) agents that attach to toxic metals and wastes in the body that are then excreted in the urine.	Lead poisoning Arteriosclerosis Autism (experimental)
Chiropractic (contraindications: malignancies, bone or joint infections, acute fractures, arthropathies)	Regards the spinal column as the center of body's well-being; uses manipulation and massage of spinal vertebrae to restore proper flow of nerve impulses necessary for health.	Musculoskeletal pain, including chronic low back pain (Abrams, 1997)[†] and headaches Torticollis Whiplash following MVA
Chromotherapy (color or light therapy	Uses human sensitivity to color to identify energy pattern imbalances. Each of the 7 colors used is regarded as having healing energies (e.g., blue is sedating).	Stress, depression Fatigue
Craniosacral mobilization	Manipulates craniosacral mechanisms to free the flow of cerebrospinal fluid pathways that surround brain and spinal cord; flow can be inhibited by injury to the brain, spinal cord, skull, sacrum, and related membranes.	TMJ Headaches Skull injuries with resultant chronic pain Poorly fitting dentures Colic, vomiting, hypertonicity, tremor, irritability in infancy Obstetrically complicated delivery for infant ADHD
Deep breathing	Helps quiet the mind; involves taking slow, deep inhalations through the nose while counting to 10, then slowly and completely exhaling for another count of 10. This is repeated 5-10 times, a few times a day.	Stress and/or tension, anxiety Insomnia HTN, headaches
Diet (vegetarian, macrobiotic, Atkins, Ornish, Pritikin Zone)	Desired effects achieved by eliminating calories, increasing fiber, decreasing fat, and/or restricting fluids. Zone diet has goal of altering body's metabolism by manipulating production of key hormones.	Weight loss Prevention of heart disease and arteriosclerosis, HTN, diabetes, to enhance athletic performance
Folk medicine (e.g., Curanderismo, Native American healing, Shamanism)	Form of healing embedded in many cultures; administered by folk healers often believed to have a gift passed down through generations. Practices may involve prayer, healing touch, charms, herbal teas, tinctures, and magic rituals.	Maladies treated run the gamut of those seen in primary health care; many symptoms culturally-based or have culturally-based interpretation of disease
Guided imagery	Involves relaxation followed by visualization of calming images; technique practiced 20-30 min, several times a week.	Chronic conditions including headaches, stress, HTN, anxiety; adjunct to cancer treatment
Herbalism (many phytomedicinals are not recommended for use in children; see Table 42-2)	Natural herbs are used over pharmaceutical derivatives, practitioners believe them to be as efficacious, gentler, and less toxic; used extensively by naturopathic, homeopathic, and holistic practitioners; appropriate preparation (tea, capsule, topical) of the herb important; the dried or extract form of the plant may be used.	Used in place of many pharmaceuticals to treat a myriad of primary health care entities, including PMS, cardiovascular, insomnia, stress, menopause, GI, respiratory, immunity, energy, and memory
Hippotherapy	Uses the unique movements of a horse to achieve therapeutic benefits.	Balance, fear, anxiety, lack of confidence, motor (may also improve energy expenditure during walking in those who have CP) and social delays in children Mental illness

Continued

TABLE 42-1	Complementary Therapies and Their Applications—Cont'd	

Nonconventional Therapy	Theory Behind Use	Treatment Applications*
Homeopathy	Stimulates a healing response by introducing a substance that is either the same as or similar to the patient's disease; infinitesimal doses of plants, minerals, and animal matter are used; medicinal products are prescribed on the basis of the "law of similars"—the medicine used is "homeopathic" to the symptoms presented.	Used by many for wide range of primary care illnesses (e.g., respiratory ailments, headaches, diarrhea, teething, toothaches, arthritis, dermatology problems, GI ailments, depression, and anxiety)
Hypnosis	Employs an altered state of consciousness to access various levels of the mind to effect changes. Can be self-learned; usually practiced by a hypnotist or hypnotherapist.	Weight loss, drug addictions, smoking cessation, insomnia, pain and stress reduction, phobias
Magnets, electromagnetic therapy (contraindications: pacemakers, defibrillators, acute injuries to bone and muscles, first-trimester pregnancy). Not to be confused with *static magnetic therapy* (sold as pads, shoe inserts, jewelry).	The use of magnetic field or biofields purport to produce vascular responses by releasing chemicals in response to injury and inflammation. The resulting vasodilation increases blood flow and directs it more quickly to stressed or injured areas, aiding the healing process; may interfere with electric impulses triggering pain or stimulate release of natural body painkillers (endorphins). Mechanism not clear (Miller, 2004).	Musculoskeletal pain Headaches Nausea Osteoarthritis of knee and cervical spine Neck pain Chronic pelvic pain Fracture therapy, soft tissue injury Parkinson disease (experimental)
Massage therapy (contraindications: clotting tendencies or communicable skin condition)	Hands-on bodywork techniques that knead and manipulate muscles, soft tissues, and connective tissues of the body; used to promote healing and relaxation, relieve sore and injured muscles, and improve one's overall sense of well-being and health.	Premature infants, low birth weight Cocaine- and HIV-exposed infants Colic in infants Infants with disturbed sleep patterns Autistic children Diabetic children to help normalize glucose levels Asthma Arthritis HIV patients Chronic fatigue syndrome Stress-induced maladies Acute and chronic pain Digestive disorders Circulatory problems, lymphedema Musculoskeletal injuries Headaches
Meditation	A deep relaxation technique that can take many forms, from repeating a mantra to Sufi dancing.	Stress-induced maladies Chronic illnesses
Megavitamin or high-dose vitamins	Use of vitamins beyond the RDA; can produce adverse and/or toxic effects.	Prevention and treatment of such illnesses as cancer, heart disease, schizophrenia, viral infections
Music therapy	Music used to provide rhythmic cues to stimulate brain's motor systems to help build and strengthen connections among nerve cells in the cerebral cortex; boosts immune function in children.	Physical rehabilitation of stroke, cerebral palsy, Alzheimer (O'Brien, 1998), Parkinson, ADHD, learning disabilities, Down syndrome, depression and anxiety, hypertension Pain relief (surgical, during labor) Premature infants (speeds the discharge rate from hospitals [Gideonse, 1998])

TABLE 42-1 **Complementary Therapies and Their Applications—Cont'd**

Nonconventional Therapy	Theory Behind Use	Treatment Applications*
Naturopathy	Use natural remedies to help restore health and balance in the body, such as diet, herbal medicine, hydrotherapy, acupuncture, homeopathy, and therapeutic massage; practitioners often use similar diagnostic and testing procedures as Western medicine practitioners.	Used by many for most primary health care issues
Nutrition	Stresses wisdom of following healthy, balanced diet to affect diet-related health issues; advocate the food pyramid guidelines.	Weight loss Food allergies Vitamin and mineral deficiencies Nonpathologic GI conditions (e.g., constipation) Chronic diseases
Osteopathy	Remobilization of joints and tissues to restore them to normal, structural positions and mobility, thus releasing tension in muscles and ligaments.	Musculoskeletal pain, including chronic back pain and headaches Torticollis Whiplash following MVA
Pet therapy	Therapy uses dogs, cats, and birds to help those with psychological issues.	Anxiety, social isolation, poor sense of well-being, antipathy
Pilates	Works on mind-body connection with exercise techniques; relies on exercising with firm support and stretching without straining to improve overall body flexibility and fitness.	Restricted body flexibility
Prayer	Works on mind-body connection by employing the strongly held belief of the connection between the self and a higher power. The most commonly relied upon healing practice by people of all cultures and religious beliefs.	All forms of health, illness, disease, and disability
Progressive relaxation	Successive tensing and relaxing each of the 15 major muscle groups, starting from the head; often used with deep breathing.	Stress, tension, insomnia, anxiety, pain, HTN
Qi gong	Ancient Chinese practice combining gentle physical movements, mental focus, and deep breathing. Believed to integrate mind, body, spirit, and stimulate movement of vital life energy (qi). A learned series of movements—often organ specific—done 2+ times a week for 30 minutes.	Asthma, arthritis, stress, lower back pain, allergies, diabetes, headaches, CVD, HTN, chronic pain
Reflexology (use with caution in patients with: deep vein thrombosis, leg ulcers, phlebitis in lower extremities, pregnancy, pacemakers; avoid renal reflexes in patients with suspected renal calculi; avoid kidney and gallbladder reflexes in patients with gallstones)	Massage technique based on the principle that proprioceptive nerve receptors in hands and feet correspond to all parts of the body, including organs and glands; use thumb and fingers to massage reflex areas to detect diseases and to rebalance vital energy; practitioners believe that more than 100 medical conditions can be helped.	Stress and anxiety Promote circulation Colic, irritability and reflux in infants Headaches Low back pain Some allergic responses Some dermatology conditions GI tract disorders Menstrual problems Arthritis and sciatica
Reiki (aka energy healing therapy)	A bodywork technique to stimulate healing energy within body.	Musculoskeletal maladies Low blood hemoglobin levels Pain control (including from cancer, fractured bones) Stress and grief

Continued

TABLE 42-1	Complementary Therapies and Their Applications—Cont'd	
Nonconventional Therapy	**Theory Behind Use**	**Treatment Applications***
Tai chi	Stimulates and balances flow of *chi* or vital energy along acupuncture meridians.	Restricted body flexibility, fitness, stamina and energy, stress
Traditional Oriental (Chinese) medicine	Combines practices and beliefs of acupuncture, acupressure, herbal remedies, massage, dietary changes, and bodywork, such as tai chi, breathing, and meditation, to stimulate vital body energy to rebalance life force.	Used by one fourth of world's population for primary health care disorders involving GI systems, GYN, respiratory tract, bones and muscles, circulation (including cardiovascular), emotional and psychological, addictions, ENT
Touch, therapeutic or healing	Based on autonomic nervous system effects using the subtle energy fields, vibration field, nonlinear electromagnetic energy, spirit or vital force to produce relaxation, reduce anxiety, pain and enhance sense of well-being. Similar to Qi gong, Reiki.	In children: reduces anxiety, worry; insomnia, asthma, fatigue, isolation, pain (abdominal, arthritis, backache, burn, bruises, cancer, fibromyalgia, headache, postoperative [Kemper & Kelly, 2004])
Yoga	Works on breathing, body alignment, and posture to improve health; preventive.	Chronic musculoskeletal ailments Stress-related maladies Improving overall body flexibility, fitness, stamina, mental health Asthma Hypertension

*These applications may or may not be supported by scientific research; the listing of these therapies does not imply endorsement of proven efficacy.
†Guidelines for the advocacy of spinal manipulation for acute lower back pain were endorsed in 1994 by the Agency for Health Care Policy and Research of the U.S. Department of Health and Human Services.
Some data from Barnes P, Powel-Griner E, McFann K et al: Complementary and alternative medicine use among adults: U.S. 2002, *CDC Advance Data Rep 343*, May 27, 2004. Available at *www.cdc.gov* (accessed Aug 26, 2006); Gasalberti D: Alternative therapies for children and youth with special health care needs, *JPed Health Care* 20(2): 133-136, 2006.
ADHD, Attention-deficit hyperactivity disorder; *CP*, cerebral palsy; *CVD*, cardiovascular disease; *ENT*, Ears, nose, and throat; *GI*, gastrointestinal; *GYN*, gynecology; *HIV*, human immunodeficiency virus; *HTN*, hypertension; *IV*, intravenous; *JRA*, juvenile rheumatoid arthritis; *MVA*, motor vehicle accident; *PMS*, premenstrual syndrome; *PTSS*, posttraumatic stress syndrome; *RAP*, recurrent abdominal pain; *RDA*, Recommended Daily Allowances established by the National Academy of Science; *TMJ*, temporomandibular joint.

based on science and research. Only training schools that could meet the rigorous Flexner standards were accredited and their graduates recognized as legitimate medical doctors. Although these standards effectively put many charlatans and snake oil medical practitioners out of work, many other nonconventional medical practitioners were also disqualified or their practices severely limited. The philosophies and practices of chiropractic, naturopathy, osteopathy, homeopathy, herbal treatments, and others fell into the unaccredited category. By excluding these disciplines, the medical community failed to consider the efficacy, benefits, and applications of the healing and treatment theories that these other practices had to offer. Rapid advances in immunology, pathology, and the seduction of technology solidly secured the dominance of the rational-empirical approach, which became known as Western, allopathic, conventional, biomedical, scientific, rational, regular, orthodox, or mainstream medicine. All ailments were expected to fit within a scientific conceptual framework (Janiger & Goldberg, 1993). However, this caused medical physicians to become separated from their roots as healers, working with patients to incorporate instrinsic healing powers with conventional and nonconventional practices.

The 1960s brought civil unrest and the questioning of authority in the U.S. At the same time, a number of doctors and patients began to express disillusionment with the strict limitations of accepted medical practices. The "holistic" health care movement of the 1970s evolved as patients and disaffected medical providers began to refocus health care toward healing, prevention, and the spiritual and environmental factors that affect health. From these contexts, the current trend toward combining the best of Western and nontraditional medicine grew.

Certain basic principles are common to all nonconventional treatment modalities (Micozzi, 1997). These principles include the following:

- A focus on wellness—which in turn prevents illness
- Self-healing—focusing external manipulations that stimulate the body's internal healing processes
- Bioenergy—ensuring that the body's energy forces are balanced
- Nutrition, plants, and other natural products—obtaining nutrients from natural food sources to maintain or return to health
- Individuality—recognition and use of the individual's unique constitution, inner resources, and so forth to achieve health

SCIENTIFIC OBSERVATION AND COMPLEMENTARY MEDICINE

Many CAM therapies are effective and are increasingly being subjected to the rigorous scientific study that would meet Western criteria. Many mainstream medical providers still refute claims about the efficacy of CAM treatments and label them quackery or "not scientifically validated". The Office of Technology Assessment points out, in response to this argument, that only about 20% of routine allopathic biomedical therapies have been subjected to the same rigorous, scientific testing standards demanded of complementary medicine treatments (Micozzi, 1997). One only needs to reflect on the recent studies regarding the once-accepted-yet recently disproved benefit of hormone replacement therapy for cardiovascular health in women (Clinical Evidence Concise editorial staff, 2003). Also, only 20% of all drugs marketed in the U.S. have been approved by the Food and Drug Administration (FDA) for use in children or have limited approval for use in children because of the lack of rigorous, scientific clinical trials regarding efficacy of the drugs (Bell, 2002).

Micozzi writes that "one way of studying and understanding alternative medicine is to view it in light of contemporary physics and biology-ecology, and to focus not just on the subtle manipulations of the alternative practitioners but on the physiologic response of the body" (Micozzi, 1996, p 5). Medical researchers of both disciplines are challenged to apply both Western treatments and successful complementary treatments until advances in physics and biology can explain the mechanisms of their effectiveness.

The NIH created the Office of Alternative Medicine in 1992 to provide evidence-based research that would move complementary treatments into mainstream medicine, thus enabling greater access and further advancements in the therapies themselves. The name was changed to the National Center for Complementary and Alternative Medicine (NCCAM), and there are now 27 NCCAM-funded centers that are identifying and studying promising CAM practices using scientific methods to determine effectiveness. The current NCCAM-sponsored portfolio is heavily weighted toward mind-body medical practices; biologically based practices (defining composition, mechanisms of action, properties, safety and efficacy of botanicals, diets, CAM products); manipulative and body-based practices; energy medicine; whole medical systems using an array of CAM modalities; international research; health services (how CAM is integrated into the health care systems); ethical, legal, and social implications of CAM research and integrated medicine; expansion of outreach to medical professionals; and the training of investigators. More than 1000 research projects are underway, which represents a tenfold increase over the last 4 years (NCCAM, 2006).

The goals behind the NCCAM-sponsored research efforts include the following:

- Conduct and support basic and applied research in complementary and alternative medical treatments
- Identify, investigate, and validate the role that complementary medical treatments play in diagnosis and prevention
- Provide training for CAM research within the complementary medicine community
- Encourage the establishment of multidisciplinary research approaches and networking between both conventional and complementary communities
- Base results on rigorous scientifically supported research
- Disseminate data to the public and professionals regarding what CAM therapies may be beneficial, ineffective, or unsafe

Other studies focus on CAM approaches to arthritis, flu, asthma and allergy, cardiovascular diseases, menopause and "andropause," digestive diseases, immunology, infectious diseases, manual therapies, mental health, mind-body medicine, neurologic diseases, and pain.

Clinical evidence-based medicine research projects involving children have studied the use of echinacea, probiotics, and fish oil. The first Pediatric Integrative Medicine Conference in the U.S. was held in 2000, is now held annually each fall, and lectures are delivered by nationally recognized experts in their field. The conference focuses on ways to integrate CAM practices into clinical pediatric practice, how to evaluate current CAM research, and hands-on workshops.

Proven research discoveries about CAM therapies in children will help improve the quality of mainstream health care in pediatrics. Examples of some current NCCAM CAM-related research projects applicable to pediatrics involve melatonin and sleep; probiotics and otitis media; herbal treatments for Crohn disease, dermatitis, and epilepsy; nutritionals for psoriasis; biophysics of acupuncture; food additives and ADHD; and an evaluation of East Asian herbal medicines. Three dietary supplements were recently studied in children, echinacea, lactobacillus, and fish oil. The results of these studies are incorporated into Table 42-4 on pp. 1180-1181.

The general trend in the U.S. for CAM academic centers is to investigate integrative medicine across the age and disease spectrum. The Center for Holistic Pediatric Education and Research, located at Children's Hospital in Boston (now called the Osher Institute with a broader scope), was initially established in 1998 as the first academic center devoted to pediatric complementary therapies. The initial director is the same pediatric researcher and educator that is now chairing the new Provisional Section of the American Academy of Pediatrics (AAP) on complementary and integrative medicine for children. The Osher Institute at Harvard University has previously been involved in clinical trials in acupuncture and botanical supplements for cancer treatment in children. Other research centers have had clinical studies with potential applicability to children's illnesses (e.g., arthritis, asthma, immunology).

A great body of research into complementary therapies has been generated outside the U.S. However, these may not meet U.S. standards of double-blinded, placebo-controlled research models. European and Indian studies are most closely aligned with our own research designs; the Chinese do not regard double-blind, placebo-controlled human studies as ethical. Many of the large, randomized, controlled studies have been done in Germany, where herbal extracts are regulated and used much the same way as pharmaceutical drugs to treat diseases.

COMPLEMENTARY PRACTICES BY HEALTH CARE PROVIDERS IN THE U.S.

Eighty-one percent of surveyed health care providers incorporate vitamins, minerals, or other nonherbal dietary supplements in their personal health regimens (Gardiner et al, 2006). A 2001 survey of pediatricians in the U.S. showed that 87% of them had at least one inquiry about a complementary medicine therapy from patients or families; however, few proactively asked their patients if they were using any type of CAM therapy. When faced with a hypothetical patient that had a recurrent upper respiratory illness, it was rare for them to recommend an adjunctive therapy (other than chicken soup or a vaporizer with or without eucalyptus oil). Yet, 72.8% of the pediatricians felt that they should be providing more information about all forms of treatment modalities to their patients. They estimated that about 70% of their patients were probably using CAM therapies (AAP, 2006).

In 2005, the AAP established the Provisional Section on Complementary, Holistic and Integrative Medicine (PSOCHIM) with the intent to educate clinicians, collaborate with other diverse health professionals working with children, and integrate evidence-based, safe, and effective CAM therapies into pediatric practice. There are no current practice guidelines for the use of CAM therapies in children with chronic or disabling conditions. A 2001 AAP policy statement and other providers offer guidance for clinicians counseling families about CAM to minimize legal risks of malpractice and/or professional discipline (AAP, 2001; Cohen & Kemper, 2005). Their advice consists of the following:

- Determine whether or not the parents intend to abandon known effective, allopathic treatments if the child's illness is life threatening or serious
- Seek information about complementary practices, being prepared to discuss them with patients, and providing information about different approaches to treatment
- Evaluate the scientific evidence for CAM therapies, including their safety and efficacy
- Identify risks or possible deleterious effects, including diverting the child from an imminently necessary allopathic treatment
- Educate families about evaluating information regarding CAM treatments
- Avoid communication of a negative bias or defensiveness about CAM therapies
- Offer to assist in monitoring and evaluating CAM therapies, if chosen by the family
- Evaluate the risk-benefit ratio of the CAM therapy as if you were another equally qualified clinician considering the same therapy; base your judgment upon support from medical literature

Nurse Practitioners (NPs) recommend CAM therapies at a higher rate. One study reported that nine out of every ten NPs did so (Sohn & Loveland Cook, 2002). This interest in such therapies was also mirrored in another survey conducted of faculty and students employed or enrolled at the University of Minnesota schools of medicine, nursing, and pharmacology. Ninety percent of the combined groups believed that a model that integrated both CAM and allopathic medicine would be most efficacious for clinical care. Eighty-eight percent of the faculty members thought that CAM should be included in their school's curriculum; the nursing faculty reported the highest interest in practicing such therapies (Kreitzer et al, 2002).

INTEGRATING COMPLEMENTARY AND ALTERNATIVE MEDICINE INTO TRADITIONAL MEDICIAL AND NURSING EDUCATION

Eighty-two medical schools in the U.S. offered CAM courses in 2002 (Gordon, 2004). Thirty academic health centers or medical schools in the U.S. and Canada now belong to the Consortium of Academic Health Centers for Integrative Medicine (CAHCIM). They all offer clinical programs for medical students, residents, and other allied health professionals in integrative health care, clinical services, research, and/or education (CAHCIM, 2006).

A search of the nursing literature by this author documents numerous articles that discuss and/or encourage the incorporation of holistic nursing practices and complementary and alternative modalities into schools of nursing curricula at both the baccalaureate and graduate levels. Richardson (2003) showed that 77% of the 105 baccalaureate nursing programs surveyed offered some content and/or experiential learning on CAM therapies. Fenton and Morris (2003) documented that, of the 125 schools of nursing sampled, 60% incorporated such educational framework. In every case, the researchers and academicians noted that this integration was largely in response to consumer demand and that it was imperative that "nursing education find room for CAM in its curriculum to meet the needs of 21st century patients, so that nurses can effectively practice CAM with skills useful for participation in CAM research and safe clinical practice" (Wyatt & Post-White, 2005, p. 2).

The NCCAM, American Medical Association, American Academy of Family Practice, American Nurses Association, American Nurse's Holistic Association, and other institutions (including hospitals) are providing patient and professional education (including hospital staff) in nonconventional treatment options.

Rigorous scientific clinical research into complementary therapies is burgeoning, and studies are readily available in the literature and from well-regarded Internet reference sites (Pubmed, NCCAM, National Library of Medicine to name of few). Many courses about CAM and herbal products are now online, and certifications of completion are offered (see Resource box at the end of the chapter).

THE ATTRACTION OF COMPLEMENTARY MEDICAL PRACTICES

The CAM therapy literature from 1990 to the present indicates a shift toward a cultural norm of acceptance of complementary therapies rather than a rejection of allopathic medicine. The 2002 NHIS survey revealed that use varied by race, gender, and geographic areas. Those who used complementary forms of care were more likely to be women, to have achieved higher educational levels, to have been hospitalized in the past year, and to have been former smokers (NCCAM, 2004). Blacks reported using CAM more than white, Latino, or Asian responders. Mind-body therapy (including prayer) or biologically based therapies were more commonly used; nonlicensed CAM practitioners were more likely to be employed; and there was more CAM sought by those living in urban areas. Treatment was more likely sought for anxiety, back or neck problems, headaches, colds, muscle sprains or strains, GI, sleeping issues, or for chronic or recurring pain. Prayer for one's own health or the health of others was used most often; herbal and vitamin regimens and body therapy (yoga, massage, meditation) were used to a lesser extent (Barnes et al, 2004).

Why did the respondents in the NHIS survey choose CAM therapies? Most said they believed that they worked in combination with conventional medical care, that Western medicine was not helping them, or that they were curious to try it. The researchers proposed further rationale for the surge in popularity of CAM. These included the increase in CAM marketing forces, Internet access for information, a desire to be more fully involved in one's medical decision-making, and dissatisfaction with conventional medicine. Literature reviews by this author over the past 8 years also note that CAM users regard CAM practices as more reflective of their own values and beliefs about the nature of life and spirituality.

THE ROLE OF PRIMARY HEALTH CARE PROVIDERS

Primary health care providers are increasingly challenged to offer a more comprehensive management partnership with patients and to form more collaborative and integrative relationships with CAM practitioners. Although care providers may not personally embrace the integration of these therapies in their own practices, they need to have sufficient knowledge, sensitivity, and willingness to support and help patients make informed decisions about their use.

Sixty-three percent of adults believed that their own medical care would improve if communication between their medical doctor and their alternative care provider increased (Landmark Healthcare, 1998). This expectation is one that primary care providers could readily fulfill. By being broad-minded about the use of alternative therapies, the provider can prevent perceptions similar to the one voiced by one patient: "Why would I bother sharing any kind of

information that I might know about how this seemed to help me—they don't want to hear it and I don't want to get yelled at by them" (Elder et al, 1997, p. 183). This feeling, however, seems to be held by a small minority of patients (del Mundo et al, 2002).

The increasing use of complementary therapies suggests that patients' needs are not being adequately met by allopathic methods. The conventional care provider can help identify a better medical approach to illness and prevention for each patient by being more cognizant of that individual's core values, beliefs, and approach to life (Adams et al, 2002). Medicine needs to return to an "art of healing," or as Rakel so aptly stated, "dependence on the 'quick fix' has made us less self-reliant regarding matters of health. The focus in medicine should be on creating an environment in which the body needs as few of these fixes as possible, and people become less dependent on the medical system, not more" (Rakel, 2003, p. 8).

An estimated $36 to $47 billion was remitted in the U.S. in 1997 to CAM practitioners; of which $12.2 to $19.6 billion was paid out of pocket. This was one half of the amount spent out-of-pocket for physician services that same year (Barnes et al, 2004). Insurance companies are continuing to study the issue of offering premium coverage for "alternative medical treatments" in response to pressure from policy holders, including employers. One survey of forty-three insurance plans in three large eastern states showed that all offered chiropractic services; others covered or discounted fees for massage, acupressure, acupuncture, or other CAM treatments (Cleary-Guida et al, 2001). White and Ernsts' study interestingly showed that there was a reduction in referrals and treatment costs when primary care providers included an array of CAM therapies in their treatment recommendations (White & Ernst, 2000).

TALKING WITH PATIENTS

Patients' perceptions of the acceptance they feel from Western health care providers provide an opportunity for open discussion regarding the possible risks and benefits of CAM therapies. Care providers are better able to monitor patients when they know the complementary practitioners in their area and establish communication with them, even to the point of sharing the management of patients.

In particular, the patient's health history should be expanded to include the following:

- Alternative products that the patient may be taking, including herbs, "natural products," and homeopathic and nutritional supplements from a health food store
- Other practitioners whom the patient may be seeing
- Other kinds of activities engaged in to address a particular problem
- The perception of any benefit gained from the complementary treatment
- The philosophy and self-care approaches to wellness and illness

The topic must be broached nonjudgmentally to help the family clarify the safety issues and explore how these products or services might fit into their child's management plan. Dr. Jonas states that "the practitioner-patient relationship and the trust that's been developed by looking at mutual goals form the foundation" for ongoing dialogue (Wysocki, 1997). Furthermore, an open, sensitive attitude implies a commitment "to patients' welfare rather than to the particular system of medicine in which they trained" (Gordon, 1996, p. 2209).

THE ROLE OF ALLERGIES AS VIEWED BY COMPLEMENTARY MEDICINE PRACTITIONERS

Complementary practitioners are more likely to identify allergies as being the etiology for many common childhood conditions. Childhood afflictions such as otitis media, upper respiratory infections and other immunologic conditions, atopic dermatitis, asthma, headaches, and hyperactivity/attention-deficit hyperactivity disorder (Box 42-1) are mentioned as being caused by allergies to foods and food additives.

BOX 42-1 **Elimination and Challenge Diet Regimen***

Elimination Phase

The initial step of the elimination diet is to completely stop one suspected food, a few suspected foods, or many foods at once, depending upon the clinician's initial evaluation. The help of a dietician or nutritionist may be needed in the case of many foods being eliminated to ensure adequate nutrition and calories. This elimination step should be followed for at least 10 days (some suggest 2-4 weeks), but for no more than for 4 weeks.

Symptoms caused by food allergens will usually disappear by the fifth or sixth day of the diet, when the body has thoroughly cleansed itself of the allergen-antibody complexes, and the intestines have completely eliminated the allergen-containing food. Should symptoms not disappear, it is recommended that the diet become further restricted. Generally, the fewer known allergens included in the diet, the easier it is to establish a cause (see Box 42-2). If used for ADHD,* behavioral changes may be evidenced. *Eat only these foods before reintroduction of other foods*: lamb, chicken, rice, potatoes, bananas, apples, and vegetables in the cabbage family (cabbage, Brussels sprouts, broccoli, cauliflower, mustard, radish, turnip, watercress). Do not eat foods that contain artificial colors or preservatives (see Box 42-2).

Reintroduction Phase

This phase adds foods back one at a time; a diary or log needs to be kept to track symptoms. One food is reintroduced every 3 days. The challenged food should be introduced in sequential incremental doses, starting in the morning with a small bite and increasing the amount during the challenge day. The food should be in its most identifiable state (e.g., eating a scrambled egg rather than incorporating it in pancakes). Symptoms may be seen within hours, or a delayed response may take up to 3 days. No other foods should be reintroduced during this 3-day period. After a food is reintroduced, it should again be eliminated until all of the eliminated foods have been reintroduced per directions.

If there is a positive response, more pronounced or acute symptoms will recur upon reintroduction of the eliminated food.

Upon reintroduction, the most common foods that produce symptoms are often found to be eggs, wheat, chocolate, nuts, cow's milk, citrus, and cheese. Corn, soy, beef, food colorings and additives, refined sugar, and caffeine have also been implicated. Avoidance means both eliminating the food and identifying it in hidden foods (e.g., breads prepared with eggs).

A diary should be kept and wrist pulse recorded because the pulse may change when an allergen is eaten (Murray & Pizzorno, 1998). Children with atopy are more likely to respond to this diet (Boris & Mandel, 1994).

Final Phase

This can be done in one of two ways. A final diet can be planned that totally eliminates all of the foods that produced symptoms, or the foods can be eliminated for 3 to 6 months and then reintroduced on a rotational basis. This rotation diet adds the suspected food on an infrequent but consistent basis from every 4 days to once a month. This is believed to allow the levels of non-IgE antibodies to fall since the body is exposed to reduced antigen. The IgE levels are not likely to rise with this approach (Johnson, 2003).

General Guidelines

Is it important to be diligent about avoiding any exposure to the eliminated foods. Failing to do so may result in unclear symptoms during the reintroduction phase. Closely reading ingredient labels is imperative. If the elimination phase fails to reduce symptoms, one of three things may be occurring. Either food hypersensitivity or intolerance is not the cause of the symptoms, the foods may still being eaten, or something else—in addition to food—may be causative. The elimination diet is only a tool, not a treatment. If possible ensure that the patient understands that this is not a "diet" in the traditional sense. Foods should not be permanently eliminated if they did not cause symptoms (Johnson, 2003).

---

*The role that diet plays as a causative factor of some ADHD symptoms is controversial. However, some more recent studies have demonstrated that children with ADHD have shown significant improvement in symptoms with the elimination of certain foods or additives or with diet modifications (Bateman B, Warner JO, Hutchinson E et al: The effects of a double blind, placebo controlled artificial food colouring and benzoate preservative challenge on hyperactivity in a general population sample of preschool children, *Arch Dis Child* 89[6]: 506–511, 2004; Schnoll R, Burshteyn D, Cea-Aravena J: Nutrition in the treatment of attention deficit hyperactivity disorder: a neglected but important aspect, *Appl Psychophysio Bio Feedback* 28[1]: 63–75, 2003).

These health conditions are believed to result from reactions of the "inner being" to external environmental stimuli, notably foods (Micozzi, 1996). Naturopathic physicians cite genetics, the early introduction of solids, early weaning, genetic reengineering of food components, limited consumption of a variety of foods, hidden foods, additives and colorings, and impaired digestion as possible reasons for an increase in food sensitivities (Pizzorno, 2002).

ALLERGY TESTING

Nonallopathic practitioners may advocate laboratory testing for food allergies. Blood testing (ELISA, IgE, and ALCAT) remains unproven and controversial in conventional medical settings, less so with nutritionally-oriented practitioners, such as naturopaths. It is also of note that a positive skin prick test reaction to egg in infancy was higher in infants with atopic disease (Schoetzau et al, 2002).

▉ SAFETY AND REGULATORY ISSUES

The clinician may find the following risk-benefit issues helpful when recommending or advising against CAM therapies (Adams et al, 2002). These include considering the:

- Severity and acuteness of the illness
- Curability of the illness by conventional, allopathic treatment
- Degree of invasiveness of the CAM therapy
- Associated toxicities of the CAM therapy
- Availability and quality of evidence for the CAM therapy
- Patient's knowledge of and willingness to accept the risk and benefits of therapy
- Level of patient's intent to use the CAM therapy
- Concurrent use of any prescribed medications

It is particularly important to ascertain the safety of certain treatment modalities by learning about any alternative product that the patient may be using, including its side effects, possible interactions with other medications, and mechanism of action. Mind-body techniques (e.g., prayer, guided imagery, spiritual healing, relaxation) and acupuncture are unlikely to interact with conventional medications. Providers should be aware of the possible harmful effect of products that are taken at high doses, such as herbal or phytomedicinal products, megadose combination nutritional supplements, colonics, or products taken in unconventional ways. Any treatment must be viewed as hazardous if its use delays the provision of proven conventional care for a serious medical condition.

BOX 42-2   Foods, Factors, and Labels Implicated in Hypersensitivity or Intolerance

Foods Accounting for Hypersensitivity Reactions*
  Eggs
  Wheat
  Citrus
  Peanuts, walnuts, pecans, almonds
  Shellfish and fish
  Milk and dairy products
  Other gluten-containing grains (oats, rye, barley)
  Soy

***Substances Implicated in Food Intolerance** (these occur naturally in food, are additives, or implicated in food intolerance)
  Lactose
  Biogenic amines (histamine, tyramine)
  Other disaccharides
  Preservatives (benzoates, BHA [butylated hydroxyanisole], BHT [butylated hydroxytoluene], sulfites)
  Artificial colors, especially tartrazine
  Salicylates
  Monosodium glutamate and other artificial flavors
  Nitrates

***Other Factors Implicated With Hypersensitivity** (increase the likelihood of hypersensitivities in those genetically predisposed)
  Family history of allergic reactions
  Frequency of exposure

Other allergic reactions (e.g., inhalant allergies)
Increased intestinal permeability to allergens ("leaky gut")
Vigorous exercise
Concurrent consumption of alcohol
Hormone levels
Stress

Food Label Ingredients That May Signal Hyperallergenic Foods

Dairy
  Casein, caseinate
  Lactalbumin
  Milk solids
  Whey

Wheat
  Semolina
  Durum
  Modified food starch
  Malt, malt syrup

Soy
  Hydrolyzed vegetable protein
  Textured vegetable protein
  Miso
  Lecithin

*For a more complete list see Chapter 11, Table 11-14, Common Foods Containing Allergens.
Adapted from Johnson K: The elimination diet and diagnosing food hypersensitivities. In Rakel D: *Integrative medicine,* Philadelphia, 2003, WB Saunders.

Contamination and potency are other concerns when patients use herbal or folk remedies. Some traditional folk remedies or herbal preparations manufactured in third world countries contain heavy metals, such as lead, zinc, mercury, arsenic, aluminum, and tin. Approximately 32% of Asian patent medicines (compounded herbal pills) have been found to be spiked with steroids and antibiotics to enhance their effectiveness. Other problems with herbal products were noted, such as improper labeling of contents and failure to provide adequate amounts of the substance noted on the label (Gardiner & Kemper, 2000; Mortimore & Fischer, 2001). Prior, nonproblematic use of a product by an individual may not be a predictor of a future drug reaction because:

- Consistency of potency between batches of herbal preparations varies
- Herbal products can lack standardization regarding which parts of a plant are used
- Plant ripeness, storage, and regional growth conditions vary
- The influence of fertilizers, pesticides, and herbicides used for cultivating the herbal product is unknown

Contamination of plant materials, substitutions, adulterations, incorrect preparations or dosages, and inappropriate labeling and advertising have also contributed to adverse patient reactions. However, few reports of adverse reactions to herbal preparations have been documented, which may be a reflection of either the relatively low risk of these products or underreporting. England and Australia have provided the most complete data to date on documented adverse reactions to herbal preparations. A 2001 survey in the United Kingdom showed a rate of 0.38%; in 2000, Australia reported a 1.16% adverse reaction rate (Ramsay, 2002). The American Association of Poison Control Centers (AAPCC) has consistently reported more deaths and adverse reactions caused by drugs rather than vitamins, nutritionals, or herbal preparations. Their 2004 report revealed that 133 nonsuicidal deaths were caused by prescription drugs and over-the-counter preparations (analgesics, antidepressants, stimulants, and heart drugs in order of prevalence) versus ten deaths from dietary supplements, herbals, or homeopathics. Seven of the ten deaths were due to ma huang as an ingredient. Their surveillance report of children under 6 years old showed no deaths were reported from plants or essential oils, although there were adverse reactions under the plant category (AAPPC, 2004). Ingestion of toxic ornamental plants rather than herbs accounted for most reports of plant poisonings.

In children, the most dangerous elements are the pyrrolizidine alkaloids, which can cause liver complications or death. These compounds occur in comfrey, borage, coltsfoot, and species of *Crotalaria* and *Senecio*. These plants are often found in herbal teas, particularly from Jamaica, Africa, and South and Central America. Chaparral, germander, and a Chinese medicine called jin bu huan can also cause liver toxicity. See Box 42-3 for a summary list of these herbs.

BOX 42-3 **Herbals, Botanicals, and Diet Supplements: Precautions About Use in Children**

DO NOT USE
- Aristolochic acid-containing products:
- "Liqiang Xiao Ke Ling Thirst Quenching Efficacious" (aka: birthwort, snakeroot, snakeweed, sangree root, sangrel, serpentary, wild ginger)
- Glyburide-containing supplements:
- "Liquiang 4"
- Tiratricol-containing supplements (often marketed for weight loss)
- Fenfluramine-containing products (often marketed for weight loss)
- "Better than Formula Ultra Infant Immune Booster 17"
- Flu or avian flu preventive or treatment-promoting dietary supplements
- Body-building supplements:
- Gamma hydroxybutyrate (GHB)
- Gamma butyrolactone (GBL)
- 1,4 butanediol (BD)
- Dieter's teas containing senna, aloe, cascara, castor oil, rhubarb root, buckthorn, or other plant-derived stimulant laxative

- Ephedra (ma huang)
- Comfrey (symphytum)
- Borage *(Borago officinalis)*
- Coltsfoot *(Tussilago farfara)* and species of *Crotalaria* and *Sececio* in herbal teas
- Chaparral *(Larrea divaricata)*
- Germander *(Teucrium chamaedrys)*
- Jin bu huan
- Monkshood/wolfbane/aconite
- Heliotropes
- Rattlebox *(Leguminosae)*
- Sassafras
- Kava kava
- Pennyroyal oil
- Lobelia
- Organ or glandular extracts

USE WITH RESTRICTIONS
- Goldenseal/roots—not for use in infants under 1 month old
- Tea tree oil—do not prescribe for internal use
- Echinacea—do not use in children under 2 years old
- Pennyroyal—do not prescribe for internal use

Data from Eisenberg (1997); Fugh-Berman (1997); Gardiner & Kemper (2000); Mack (1998); Food and Drug Administration: Medical Product Safety Information. Available at *www.fda.gov/medwatch/safety.htm* (accessed Aug. 29, 2007); Clinical Advisor, editorial staff: Warn patients away from these supplements, *Clin Advisor* 7(5):12, 2004.

Even though 25% of pharmaceutical drugs are made from herbs, Western medical providers often regard herbal, natural health products (NHPs) as dangerous or ineffective. Since 1993, the FDA has had a voluntary system in place, called MedWatch, for reporting adverse reactions to nutritionals and botanicals. Access to MedWatch is available from the FDA's Internet website (see Resource Box at the end of the chapter). Complaints reported to the FDA have principally involved drugs rather than NHPs (forty-seven drug and therapeutic biological products alerts issued versus five alerts for NHPs in the first 8 months of 2006) (Food and Drug Administration, 2007).

With 250,000 flowering plant species, the burden of knowing what is safe to use or not use becomes cumbersome. There are, however, some useful guidelines that clinicians can use when either advocating or advising about herbal and dietary supplements for their patients (Sego, 2006; Gardiner et al, 2004; The Oregonian, 2006). These include:
- Use only single-herb supplements instead of combinations to prevent any side-effect confusion
- Stop herbals at least 1 week before any scheduled surgical procedure to prevent coagulation time influenced by the herb or an interaction with anesthesia
- Research the herb or NHP as thoroughly as possible:
  ○ USP Dietary Supplement Verified seal means the product has met certain manufacturing standards
  ○ If possible determine that the manufacturer complies with Good Manufacturing Practices that set standards for cleanliness, maintenance, and documented quality checks. Other quality standards are set by the National Nutritional Food Association TruLabel program, National Sanitation Foundation International certification program, and the U.S. Pharmacopeia (USP) Dietary Supplement Verification Program (USP noted on the product label). Refer to the Resource box at the end of the chapter for contact information
  ○ Check the American Herbal Products Association safety rating system (discussed below)
  ○ Herbal and NHPs manufactured and imported from Europe are generally regarded as safe because they have had to comply with standards set forth by Commission E (Europe's equivalent of the U.S. FDA). For example, a label noting "original German formula" would be a good choice
  ○ Should the patient be on a drug involving the hepatic cytochrome P-450 enzyme system (e.g., warfarin), avoid the use of herbs starting with the letter "G"-gingko, ginseng, garlic, ginger, green tea because these can either potentiate or inhibit that system

Use websites, such as the American Botanical Council HerbClip Database, to determine if the product has been tested or reviewed (3000 articles available). Also, Natural Medicines Comprehensive Database (subscription fee) discusses clinically tested products and their interactions with pharmacologic drugs.

Although many herbs are harmless even in large amounts, others should be prescribed only by a knowledgeable herbalist or botanic professional. *Standardized extracts* are more likely to ensure that a specific amount of an active compound is present, thus avoiding the discrepancies found when different parts of a plant are used or when seasonal or climatic variations occur during cultivation for any given plant or plant part. Western herbalists often use *simples* (the compound is made from one herb), whereas Chinese and Indian (Ayurvedic) medicines often blend together more than one herb. A general rule is that all herbs need to be respected; they are neither completely safe nor poisonous. Herbs can interact with other herbs or with pharmaceutical drugs. See Table 42-2 for a list of drug categories and herbal product interactions and Table 42-3 for herbs contraindicated in pregnancy and lactation.

The appropriate herb in the appropriate quantity—like pharmaceutical medicines—is necessary to obtain the intended benefits. The medicinal effect of any one herb is thought to be the result of dozens of pharmacologically distinct actions. The herb may be causing physiologic changes in numerous subtle ways, none of which alone would produce the desired response. This mechanism contrasts with conventional medicines, which generally act by one of a few mechanisms of action and use "physiologically more significant pharmacologic" dosing (Clinical Advisor, editorial staff, 1998).

The Dietary Supplement Health and Education Act of 1994 required cautionary labeling for all dietary supplements containing herbs. The American Herbal Products Association has evaluated herbal safety for all botanical ingredients sold in North America (see Resource Box at the end of the chapter). Each herb has been placed in one of the following classes:

Class 1: herb can be safely consumed when used appropriately
Class 2: the following use restrictions apply:
    Class 2a: for external use only
    Class 2b: not to be used during pregnancy
    Class 2c: not to be used while nursing
    Class 2d: other specific use restrictions as noted
Class 3: data exist to recommend the following labeling: "To be used only under the supervision of an expert qualified in the appropriate use of this substance."
Class 4: insufficient date available for classification

Herbal supplements that carry the USP designation indicate that the manufacturers have voluntarily met USP standards for purity, potency, disintegration, and dissolution. Information on USP-verified dietary supplements by manufacturer are available.

Before expanding their practice, NPs are advised to check the advanced nurse practice act of their state, the policies of their employer, and the relevant standards of practice. NPs may have to pursue a broader interpretation and additional training or certification to ensure compliance with the terms of the nurse practice act.

For providers who are incorporating CAM therapies into their practices, it is recommended that informed consent be obtained and reference made to any conventional treatments that may be foregone. A good patient intake form can be

TABLE 42-2 **Drug–Herb Interactions for Some Pharmaceuticals Used in Children**

Drug Category	Herbs	Effect of Herb on the Drug's Action
Acetaminophen	Ginkgo	May cause intracranial bleeding
Anesthetics	Kava, valerian	Prolonged sedation—an additive effect
Antibiotics (ampicillin, ciprofloxacin)	Dandelion, fennel, khat	Decrease drug availability
Anticonvulsants, general	Cis-gamma-linolenic acid–rich herbs (evening primrose oil) Thujone-containing herbs (cedar, tansy, sage)	Decreased therapeutic effect—may decrease seizure threshold, per case reports; mechanism of action unknown
	Salicylate-rich herbs (e.g., cramp bark, willow, wintergreen)	Increased therapeutic effect with transient effects, per case reports; mechanism of action unknown
Anticonvulsants (Zarontin, Cerebyx, Dilantin)	Shankapulshpi (an ayurvedic product with many herbs)	Decreases effectiveness of phenytoin; decreased drug levels in case reports
Antidepressants—general		
Bupropion (Wellbutrin)	Evening primrose oil, ginkgo, kava ginseng	May interfere with seizure control
	Cis-gamma-linolenic acid–rich herbs (evening primrose oil)	May cause mania Lowers seizure threshold and may cause epileptic seizures
Tricyclics	Ma huang, St. John's wort, ginkgo, yohimbe	May enhance drug effects, causing restlessness May cause high blood pressure
SSRIs	St. John's wort, ma huang	May enhance drug effects, causing restlessness
Barbiturates	Valerian, St. John's wort, kava	Potentiate side effects of drug, causing sleepiness, lethargy
Benzodiazepines	St. John's wort	Decreased drug effect; may increase side effects and sedation; herb binds to GABA receptor sites, per animal and pharmacology studies
	Kava, valerian	Enhance drug effects of sleepiness, lethargy
Mood stabilizers	Psyllium, ginseng	Psyllium, decreases drug concentration; ginseng, may cause mania
Monoamine oxidase inhibitors (MAOIs)	St. John's wort	May decrease effect of MAOIs
	Yohimbe	Increases toxic effect of MAOIs
	Ma huang	Potentiates action of MAOIs, possibly causing life-threatening high blood pressure, high fever, coma
	Panax ginseng, bioactive amines, licorice	Increased side effects that may lead to toxicity; licorice is reported to be a very strong MAOI, per case reports
Corticosteroids	Laxative herbs (e.g., aloe, cascara, senna, yellow dock), diuretic herbs (e.g., celery seed, corn silk, horsetail, juniper)	Increases side effects; increased potassium loss, per theoretical evidence
	Licorice	Increased plasma levels as a result of increase in bioavailability, per case reports and some pharmacologic evidence
	Panax ginseng	CNS stimulation and insomnia, per case reports
Diabetes medications, Type II diabetes	Fenugreek, ginseng, karela or bitter melon	May decrease blood sugar
	Echinacea	Can alter metabolic control
General medications	High-fiber herbs (e.g., flax, psyllium, acacia, slippery elm, marshmallow)	Decreased absorption of drugs, per pharmacologic studies
	"Hot" remedies (e.g., ginger, garlic, black pepper, red pepper)	Increased absorption by causing vasodilation of intestinal wall, per traditional use
Iron	Tannin-rich herbs (e.g., caffeine-containing herbs, cat's claw, tea, uva ursi)	Decreased drug effect because tannin binds with iron to decrease absorption, per theoretic and pharmacologic evidence
Laxative, stimulant (e.g., Dulcolax)	Aloe, cascara sagrada, senna, yellow dock	May increase laxative effect
Minerals	Fiber-containing herbs (flax, psyllium, acacia, slippery elm, marshmallow)	Decreased bioavailability, especially of Ca, Mg, Cu, Zn with psyllium, per case reports

TABLE 42-2   Herb–Drug Interactions for Some Drugs Used in Children—Cont'd

Drug Category	Herbs	Effect of Herb on the Drug's Action
NSAIDs	Gastric irritant herbs (e.g., caffeine, rue, uva ursi)	Increased side effects and may increase gastric erosion and bleeding, per theoretical evidence
	Nettles	Increased therapeutic effect—increases effect of antiinflammatory activity, per controlled trials
Oral contraceptives (Alesse, Levlen, Levlite, Brevicon, Genora, Jenest, Ortho 7/7/7)	Licorice, St. John's wort	Both may increase blood pressure; St. John's wort may also cause breakthrough bleeding
Salicylates (e.g., aspirin)	Herbs that alkalinize urine (e.g., uva ursi)	Decreased plasma levels caused by increased urine secretion, per pharmacology studies
	Tamarind	Increases blood level of aspirin
	Ginkgo, garlic	May cause prolonged bleeding by decreasing platelet aggregation; eye hemorrhage
Theophylline	St. John's wort	May inhibit drug's effectiveness
Thyroid hormone	Horseradish	Decreased therapeutic effect by decreasing thyroid function
	Kelp	Increased therapeutic effect because kelp contains iodine, which may lead to hyperthyroidism, per theoretical evidence

Ca, Calcium; *CNS,* central nervous system; *Cu,* copper; *GABA,* gamma-aminobutyric acid; *Mg,* magnesium; *SSRI,* selective serotonin reuptake inhibitor; *MAOI,* monoamine oxidase inhibitors; *NSAIDS,* nonsteroidal antiinflammatory drugs; *Zn,* zinc.
Data from Hardy M: Herb-drug interactions: an evidence-based table, *Int Med Alert* Jan 29, 2001, pp 1-8; Graedon J, Graedon T: *The people's pharmacy: guide to home and herbal remedies,* New York, 1999, Graedon Enterprises; Golub C: Herb-medication interactions: what you don't know can hurt you, *Environ Nutr* 24(10):1-5, 2001; Simkins A, Thurston D, Colyar M et al: Nature's wrath?: a closer look at complication with five popular herbs, *Adv Nurs Pract* 13(6):55-58, 2005.

downloaded from *www.integrativemedicine.arizona.edu/clinic/ptintakeform118C3.* One should not refer patients to a CAM practitioner without first having done a complete diagnostic evaluation that should also include (Kemper & Cohen, 2004):

- Discussing treatment options, including the use of CAM treatment
- Studying the literature about the safety and efficacy of the chosen CAM treatment for the particular malady
- Being aware of the licensure status of the recommended CAM practitioner
- Applying common sense regarding the risks and benefits of the CAM therapy
- Monitoring the patient's response to the CAM treatment

After the diagnostic evaluation of the patient's complaint, the following steps should be taken by a clinician to assist a patient who wishes to try a CAM therapy:

- Assist the patient in identifying a suitable licensed practitioner.
- Provide the patient with questions to ask the alternative provider during the first consultative visit, including issues of safety, efficacy of any treatment, reasonable expectations of measurable improvement.
- Monitor the patient to review the recommended treatment plan; encourage the patient to keep a symptom diary.
- Monitor the patient's response to treatment at monthly intervals.
- Document all interactions with the patient.

Many states have licensing boards and professional organizations that set standards for nonconventional practitioners, including a requirement to carry malpractice insurance. The Federation of State Medical Boards (see Resource Box at the end of the chapter) has established policy and model guidelines for the use of CAM therapies both when practicing the therapy or when co-managing the patient with a CAM provider. Licensing requirements are subject to change, and patients should be encouraged to review the credentials of any practitioner whom they are considering using. Doctorates in acupuncture or Oriental medicine (OMD degree) are not recognized in the U.S.

■ SPECIFIC COMPLEMENTARY TREATMENTS FOR CHILDREN AND ADOLESCENTS

Table 42-4 lists some of the complementary treatments that parents of pediatric-age children may be considering

TABLE 42-3 Herbs in Pregnancy and Lactation

Avoid in Pregnancy	Avoid During Lactation	May Be Used in Small, Limited Quantities During Lactation
Aloe	Aloe	Commercial Herbal Teas (available from Celestial Seasonings) such as orange, cinnamon, lemon lift, raspberry, rose hips
Autumn crocus	Black cohosh	Fennel (NOT in oil form)
Black cohosh root	Bladderwrack	Blessed thistle
Buckthorn bark and berry	Borage	Echinacea
Cascara sagrada bark	Buckthorn bark	
Chaste tree fruit	Buckthorn berry	
Cinchona bark	Bugleweed	
Cinnamon bark	Caraway oil	
Coltsfoot leaf	Cascara sagrada bark	
Comfrey herb, leaf, and root	Chaste tree	
Dong quai	Comfrey	
Echinacea purpurea herb, injectable form	Coltsfoot leaf	
Ephedra	Elecampane	
Fennel oil and seed	Ephedra	
Ginger root	Fenugreek (causes notable maple syrup smell in mother and infant).	
Ginkgo biloba	*Note: This is used widely in some communities.*	
Indian snakeroot	Garlic	
Juniper root	Ginkgo biloba	
Kava kava	Ginseng	
Licorice root (above 100 mg glycyrrhizin)	Indian snakeroot	
Mayapple root and resin	Joe Pye	
Parsley herb and root	Kava kava	
Pennyroyal	Licorice	
Petasites root	Male fern	
Red raspberry leaf	Peppermint oil	
Rhubarb root	Petasites root	
Rosemary	Rhubarb root	
Thuga	Senna leaf	
Sage leaf	Stillinga	
Senna leaf	St. John's wort	
St. John's wort	Uva ursi	
Uva ursi leaf	Valerian	
	Wormwood	

Herbal Combinations

Angelica root with gentian root and fennel seed
Anise oil with fennel oil and caraway oil
Anise oil with fennel oil, licorice root, and thyme
Anise oil with fennel seed and caraway seed
Anise seed with ivy leaf, fennel seed, and licorice root
Anise seed with marshmallow root, eucalyptus oil, and licorice root >100 mg glycyrrhizin
Caraway oil and fennel oil
Caraway oil, fennel oil, chamomile flower
Caraway seed and fennel seed
Caraway seed, fennel seed, chamomile flower

TABLE 42-3	Herbs in Pregnancy and Lactation—Cont'd

Avoid in Pregnancy	Avoid During Lactation	May Be Used in Small, Limited Quantities During Lactation
Ivy leaf, licorice root (>100 mg glycyrrhizin), and thyme		
Licorice root, peppermint leaf, German chamomile flower		
Licorice root, primrose root, marshmallow root, and anise seed		
Marshmallow root, fennel seed, Iceland moss, and thyme		
Marshmallow root, primrose root, licorice root (>100 mg glycyrrhizin), and thyme oil		
Peppermint leaf and fennel seed		
Peppermint leaf, caraway seed, and fennel seed		
Peppermint oil and fennel oil		
Peppermint oil, caraway oil, fennel oil		
Peppermint oil, caraway oil, fennel oil, chamomile flower		
Peppermint oil, fennel oil, chamomile flower		
Senna leaf, peppermint oil, caraway oil		

Note: Botanical product elixirs and liquid preparations may be mixed with alcohol; such preparations should be avoided.
Adapted from Mattison D: *Herbal supplements: their safety, a concern for health care providers. www.hpakids.org/holistic-health/articles/115/1/Safety-of-Herbal-Supplements-with-Breastfeedingmarchofdimes.com* (accessed Dec 28, 2007). Additional data from Lawrence RA: Herbs and breastfeeding. Available at *www.breastfeeding.com/reading_room/herbs.html* (accessed on Sept 4, 2006); McGuffin M, Goldberg A, editors: *American Herbal Products Association's botanical safety handbook*, New York, 1998, CRC Press, p 188; Conover E, Buehler BA: Use of herbal agents by breastfeeding women may affect infants, *Pediatr Annals* 33(4):235-240, 2004.

or are actually using. Health care providers may personally want to begin incorporating some complementary approaches into their own practices according to their own comfort level. The families' desires for more integrative health care are more likely to be met when conventional providers act as advocates, active participants, listeners, and facilitators.

The complementary therapeutics in Table 42-4 were chosen by the specific referenced authors on the basis of evidence-based research, as being clinically reasonable, or holding clues to promising areas needing further research. Physician authors from both Western medicine and naturopathic professions have been used to compile this table. This information is included for the reader's reference. *Inclusion of a complementary treatment in Table 42-4 does not imply endorsement by this textbook's authors.* Herbal remedies are too numerous to list; it is suggested that the clinician take one of the myriad of classes now being offered and use a good reference source that cites research and safety precautions. The Resource Box at the end of this chapter provides several suggestions.

■ GLOSSARY OF TERMS USED IN THE PREPARATION OF HERBAL TREATMENTS

Knowledge of the following terms will be useful for using Table 42-4 for reference.

Standardized: An herbal product that contains a *specified concentration of one ingredient* of the plant; it may contain other nonstandardized ingredients from the same plant.

Essential oils: Also known as volatile or aromatic oils and found in many plants. These oils are highly concentrated and potent and are not to be taken internally.

Infusion: Preparation similar to tea. The dried herb is steeped in boiling water for 5 to 10 minutes and strained; the preparation can be sweetened to make it more palatable; drink warm or cold.

Tincture: A concentrated extract of an herb made with a mixture of cold water and alcohol (typically 25%, 40%, 60%, or 90% alcohol). The tincture usually is diluted four to five times with water or juice for children; tinctures should not be given internally to children younger than 2 years old.

TABLE 42-4   **Complementary Treatments* for Some Common Conditions in Children and Adolescents**

Diagnosis	Treatment Approach	Dosage	Benefit	Possible Side Effects[†]	Research/Citations
Acne					
	Herbal *Goldenseal*	Adolescents: use as infusion (wash face)	Antibacterial properties	Nontoxic at recommended dose *Class 2b*	Murray & Pizzorno (1998)
	Tea tree oil	Adolescents: 5% topically, diluted with water twice daily (use 15% concentration for severe acne)	Effective against *Propionibacterium acnes*—antiseptic and antifungal properties	Contact dermatitis	Studies show 5% tea tree oil as effective as 5% benzoyl peroxide (Gardiner et al, 2001; Pizzorno, 2002)
	Salicyclic acid	Adolescents: topically twice daily (start with 0.5% until tolerated and increase to 2% concentration)	Breaks apart sebum plugs	Redness and irritation	Kemper (2002a)
	Azelaic acid (20%)	Apply bid for 1-6mo	Antibiotic against *P. acnes*	Redness and irritation	Pizzorno (2002)
	Diet	Omit refined and/or concentrated CHO, milk, and foods with trans fats, iodine	High concentrated CHOs decrease immunosuppression; milk contains hormones; in acne-prone skin, glucose tolerance is impaired	None	Pizzorno (2002)
	Nutritional *Vitamin A*	100,000 international units daily × 3mo	For premenstrual aggravation of acne		Kemper (2002a) cites uncertain benefit; Pizzorno (2002)
	Vitamin E	400 international units daily			
	Vitamin C	1000mg daily			
	Selenium	200mcg daily			
	Zinc	50mg daily (picolinate or monomethionine)			
	Brewers yeast	1 tbsp bid			Pizzorno (2002).
	Acupuncture		Hormonal influence	None	Kemper (2002a)—costly; needs more study
	Calendula soap	Twice daily	For cleansing	None	Pizzorno (2002)
	Homeopathy	*Antimonium crudum, carbo animalis, Hepar sulfur, Kali bromatum, sulfur*		None	Kemper (2002a) (need more studies)
Abdominal pain, recurrent	Mind-body therapies (biofeedback, touch, hypnosis, deep breathing)	Depends upon practitioner		None	Kemper & Kelly (2004); Allen, (2004)—several studies cited

Anxiety	Herbal *Peppermint oil, enteric-coated*	1 capsule for children (that can swallow capsule)	Decreases pain	None	Ditchek & Greenfield (2002); Scharff & Kemper (2003)—**do not use any other form of oil**
	Yoga		Decreases need for medication, improved self-esteem and ability to cope	Limit some postures in pregnancy, after recent surgery, HTN, glaucoma, acute sciatica, herniated disk, or joint replacement	Ott (2002) (cites studies)
	Aromatherapy *Chamomile*	Infants/children: put in vaporizer using 2-3 drops of the essential oil	Decreases irritability from illnesses (GI upset, varicella, fevers)	Rare allergic reactions in those hypersensitive to ragweed, aster, chrysanthemums (daisy family of plants) consisting of dermatitis, asthma, dyspnea, anaphylaxis *Class 2b*	Kemper (2002a)
	Lavender, rosemary	Can be inhaled from vaporizer or added to massage oil	Studies showed increase in beta waves with lavender; a decrease in alpha and beta waves with rosemary (Krebs, 2006)	None	Krebs (2006); Kemper (2002a)
	Belly breathing	Place child's hand over his or her belly button and picture it as a balloon. Have child breathe in through nose slowly, counting to 3-4, meanwhile blowing up "belly balloon"; breathe out through mouth slowly to a count of 6-8, deflating "balloon." Do for 1-2min, working up to 10-20min	Reduces stress, anxiety, pain, panic; slows heart rate	None	Ditchek & Greenfield (2002)

Continued

TABLE 42-4 **Complementary Treatments* for Some Common Conditions in Children and Adolescents—Cont'd**

Diagnosis	Treatment Approach	Dosage	Benefit	Possible Side Effects†	Research/Citations
	Music therapy		Listening to music directly influences pulse, BP, electrical activity of muscles; may help nerve cell connections within the cerebral cortex	None	Gideonese (1998); Kemper & Jennings (2005)
	Massage		Improved behavior, reduced cortisol levels, BP	Rare reactions to too much pressure; allergic reaction to oil	Field et al (1998); Reilly (2005)
	Meditation Therapeutic touch		Increases relaxation, diminishes pain and anxiety	None	Kemper & Kelly (2004)
Aphthous stomatitis	Herbal				
	Aloe vera	Apply topically several times daily	Accelerates healing; under investigation as antiviral and immunomodulator	Rare allergic reactions if taken internally; rare skin eruptions with topical use *Class 1*	Marcolina (2001)—cites studies
	Tea tree oil	Apply topically twice daily	Antifungal, antibacterial	Rare allergic reaction DO NOT INGEST	LaValle et al (2000)
	Lactobacillus acidophilus	<12yr: 2 tabs daily up to 3 times daily >12yr: 4 tabs up to 3 times daily	Antifungal, antibacterial	None	Graedon & Graedon (1999)
	Nutritional Vitamins B, B₂, B₆, Zinc gluconate	Multivitamin with minerals for age	Nutritional deficiencies in B vitamins occur more frequently in those with canker sores	None	Rini & Bloom (2002); Graedon & Graedon (1999)
	Black tea bag	Hold a tepid tea bag over ulcerated area for 3-5min	Tannins relieve pain and coat the sore to speed healing	None	Graedon & Graedon (2006d)
	Sauerkraut juice	1 tbsp swished in mouth, then swallowed			Graedon & Graedon (2006d)

Continued

Asthma

Nutritional			
Diet exclusions	Eliminate milk, chocolate, wheat, citrus, food colorings (tartrazine, sunset yellow, amaranth), food additives (sodium benzoate, 4-hydroxybenzoate esters, sulfites) and tryptophan (amino acid in milk, cheese, turkey, bananas). Ensure adequate vitamin C, magnesium, extra onions and garlic, fatty fish in diet.	In severe asthma, combined treatment with pharmaceuticals is recommended— nutritionals reduce allergic threshold and can help prevent acute attacks	Requires diet compliance	Many studies cited in Pizzorno (2002) for nutritional recommendation Kemper (2002a)
Vegan diet	Vegan diet with exception of cold-water fish for their omega-3 fatty acids—try for 4 mo; use onions and garlic liberally PLUS Omega-3 fatty acids (supplement with fish oil)	Alters prostaglandin metabolism, increases intake of antioxidant nutrients and magnesium, eliminates food allergens; onions and garlic inhibit release of inflammatory chemicals; omega-3 fatty acids improve airway responsiveness to allergens; asthmatics that regularly eat fresh, fatty fish have significantly better lung function and decrease risk of asthma		Description of diet in Pizzorno (2002, p 53) Kemper (2002a) (flaxseed oil or fresh fish several times a wk rather than fish oil supplements
Green tea extract OR	Give as watered-down tea, prn	Inhibits histamine release from mast cells by increasing absorption of flavonoids		Pizzorno (2002)

TABLE 42-4 Complementary Treatments* for Some Common Conditions in Children and Adolescents—Cont'd

Diagnosis	Treatment Approach	Dosage	Benefit	Possible Side Effects†	Research/Citations
	Ginkgo biloba extract	<50lb: 25mg tid 50-100lb: 40mg tid >100lb: 80mg tid	Improves respiratory function and reduces bronchial reactivity	Rare side effects (headaches, GI upset) Class 2d—may potentiate effect of MAO inhibitors	McGuffin et al (1997); Pizzorno (2002)
	Astralgalus	2-6yr: 2g in tea 6-12yr: 5g in tea	May boost the immune system	Can interfere with anesthesia and Coumadin	Ditchek & Greenfield (2002); Graedon & Graedon (1999)
	Vitamin B6 (effects seen after 1mo)	<50lb: 8-15mg/day 50-100lb: 12-25mg/day >100lb: 25-50mg/day	Reduces side effects in asthmatics being treated with theophylline and reduces number and severity of attacks and other medication use		Pizzorno (2002); Kemper (2002a)
	Magnesium	<50lb: 60-125mg/day 50-100lb: 100-200mg/day >100lb: 200-400mg/day	Adequate levels necessary for lung function; affects asthma severity		Pizzorno (2002); Kemper (2002a); Patel et al (2006)
	Vitamin B12	<50lb: 300mcg/day 50-100lb: 500mcg/day >100lb: 1000mcg/day	Possibly reduces reactions to sulfites		Pizzorno (2002)
	Vitamin C	10-30mg/kg/day in divided doses	A major antioxidant in lung lining; asthmatics have higher need for vitamin C; inhibits histamine release		Pizzorno (2002); Kemper (2002a); Patel et al (2006): study demonstrated lower levels of vit C and magnesium in adults with asthma—symptoms may be modifiable with increase in eating fruits with vit C)
	Vitamin E	>100#: 200-400 international units daily			Pizzorno (2002)
	Quercetin	>100# 400mg 20min before meals			Pizzorno (2002)
	Acupuncture		Study results mixed; some show modest, temporary effect; ineffective for long-term control		Fugh-Berman (1997); Micozzi (1996) (evidence is mixed). Can be used as an adjunct (Kemper, 2002a)
	Chiropractic				Kemper (2002a) (no evidence of efficacy)

Condition	Therapy	Dosage/Application	Effects	Cautions	References
	Homeopathy	Immunotherapy using whatever substance patient is allergic to	Possibly some positive effect in allergic asthma	Possible initial exacerbation of symptoms	Fugh-Berman (1997) (one study cited); Kemper (2002a) (no published studies using homeopathic treatments for children, but showed promise in adults; if child has both allergies and asthma, may be tried as adjunct therapy)
	Hypnosis	Requires subjects highly susceptible to hypnosis	Reduced symptoms and medication use		Kemper (2002a) (controlled studies cited)
	Biofeedback	Age-appropriate	Improved breathing, fewer and less severe asthma attacks		Kemper (2002a) (studies cited)
	Massage		Improves peak air flow, decreases asthma attacks, relieves anxiety, depression.	None reported	Kemper (2002a) (studies cited)
	Yoga		May be helpful in reducing symptoms and reducing medication use; ↑ lung capacity	None	Kemper (2002a); Ott (2002) (cites studies)
Breastfeeding (mothers)	Fish oil *(salmon oil is better rather than cod liver oil)*	750mg, 2-3 times daily	Important for hormone, nervous tissue, cellular membrane production	Use with caution in those with diabetes, hypoglycemia, if taking aspirin, NSAIDs, anticoagulants **Do NOT use in those with bleeding disorders Stop before surgery or dental procedures**	LaValle et al (2000)
Burns—first or second degree	Herbal *Aloe vera*	Prepared gel (70% aloe vera) or gel directly from leaves: apply topically several times daily	Antiinflammatory, antibacterial, promotes wound healing	Contact dermatitis *Class 1*	Kemper (2002a) (recommends using fresh leaves)

Continued

TABLE 42-4 Complementary Treatments* for Some Common Conditions in Children and Adolescents—Cont'd

Diagnosis	Treatment Approach	Dosage	Benefit	Possible Side Effects[†]	Research/Citations
	Calendula (no other homeopathic remedies recommended)	Popular skin soother, available in skin creams	Some antiinflammatory properties	Rare rash *Class 1*	Kemper (2002a). Warns against using gotu kola, arnica, geranium oil, Eupolin ointment (*Chromolaena odoratum* or *Eupatorium odoratum*), marshmallow root, plantain, comfrey, mullein leaves, tea tree oil, topical garlic because of skin reactions, unproven efficacy, or contamination
	Nutritional *Vitamin A*	10,000 international units daily			
	Vitamin C	60-250 mg 3-4 times daily	Vit C aids in skin healing; vit E seems to improve resistance to infection	Diarrhea with vit C; decrease dose if occurs.	Kemper (2002a) (Vit E is experimental)
	Vitamin E	<100 lbs: 100-200 international units daily >100 lbs 200-400 international units daily PO or as a salve			
	Hypnosis		Decreases pain, improves sleep and appetite, reduces anxiety with dressing changes	None	Kemper (2002a) (cites studies)
	Therapeutic touch		Increased healing	None reported	Kemper (2002a) (cites double-blind study showing statistically significant results)
	Massage (of nonburned areas during healing; of burned areas after healing)		For comfort, relaxation, decreases pain, lowers stress hormones; decreases itching, tightness, pain, improves circulation and promotes flexibility.	None	Kemper (2002a).

Colic

Therapy	Instructions	Effect	Side Effects	References
Nutritional *12% sucrose solution*	Infants: 5½ tsp sugar in 8oz water: give 2ml over 30-60sec for 1-2 days during inconsolable crying	Sucrose analgesia—works by stimulating secretion of endogenous endorphins	None	Markestad (1997) (small double-blind crossover study)
Herbal *Tea with chamomile, mint, fennel, licorice, vervain. Other herbs used by different cultures: anise, catnip, peppermint leaf, fennel, caraway seed, ginger root, dill.*	Infants: Give in weak tea form (mix ½ to 1 tsp of herb in boiling water; steep 5min): give ½-4oz tid-qid. Give no more than 4-6oz per day.	Calming, sedating effects (antispasmodic on smooth muscles of digestive tract)	Rare allergic reaction (dermatitis, asthma, dyspnea, anaphylaxis) in people with hypersensitivity to daisy family (see Anxiety section, chamomile) Class 2b	Kemper (2002a) (cites study. Discourages using any pharmacologic drugs, including simethicone, sedatives, antihistamines, dicyclomine, motion sickness medications. Do not use alcohol).
Chiropractic	Average of 3 treatments	Colic relieved	None reported	Kemper (2002a); (noncontrolled study showed 94% resolution, but subjects were 6wk old at which time spontaneous resolution may have occurred)
Nutritional *Eliminate certain foods in mother's diet if breastfed*	Mother should eliminate the following for 1wk: cow's milk, chocolate, coffee, tea, cola, soy, corn, wheat, eggs, cabbage, broccoli, onion, peppers, beans, garlic.	Colic symptoms improved	None—counsel mother on other appropriate foods of equal nutritional value	Kemper (2002a) (studies equivocal—elimination diet helps in some infants; 25% colicky babies sensitive to cow's milk protein)
Therapeutic touch		Calming	None reported	Kemper (2002a) (no studies cited)
Massage	Can be taught to parents; used prn: massage tummy lightly with baby on side, head somewhat down and bottom elevated; give 20-30min after a meal; can extend massage to include entire body. Use lavender oil as massage vehicle.	Calming, relaxes	None if done gently	Kemper (2002a); Ditchek & Greenfield (2002)

Continued

TABLE 42-4 Complementary Treatments* for Some Common Conditions in Children and Adolescents—Cont'd

Diagnosis	Treatment Approach	Dosage	Benefit	Possible Side Effects†	Research/Citations
	Motion	Gentle rocking or rolling in rhythmic and relaxed manner; wear in a front or backpack.	Calming, relaxes	None	Ditchek & Greenfield (2002)
	Music therapy	When colicky baby is quiet, calm, not crying, play a recording of some music baby likes; pay extra attention at this time to infant. When infant starts crying, turn off the music and withdraw attention. Follow procedure throughout the day; within days colic and crying should decrease significantly. Also, white noise in background may sooth (e.g., turn on the dryer).	Conditioning response	None; requires fair amount of discipline and dedication for parents to comply.	Kemper (2002a) (cites study showing significant results)
	Aromatherapy *Lavender*	Place lavender oil in a vaporizer/diffuser in infant's room.			
Common cold/flu	Herbal		Stimulates immune system by boosting macrophages' ability to destroy germs, increases T-cell production, and may have interferon-like effects	None	Note: Echinacea is commonly used for the common cold. However, new studies show no evidence that it prevents, reduces, speeds recovery of colds, nor stimulates immune system (University of California, Berkeley, 2005).
	Astralgus root	2-6 yr: 4-8 gtts liquid standardized extract or tincture every 12 hr. 6-12 yr: 8-15 gtts every 12 hr (capsules: 250-500 mg every 12 hr)		*Do NOT use in patients with progressive infections (e.g., TB, HIV) or autoimmune diseases;* can interfere with immunosuppressive therapy	Kemper (2002a); Ditchek & Greenfield (2002). Astralgus root may be used as a daily tonic to prevent URIs.

Maitake mushroom liquid extract or tincture (can also use shiitake or reishi)	1-5yr: 5gtts in chocolate syrup, 1-3 times daily 6+ yr: 10gtts	May boost immunity	None	Ditchek & Greenfield (2002)
Tea made from ginger, cinnamon, cloves, allspice, cardamom	Put ⅛ tsp of each into 2 cups of water to make a tea. Sip slowly. Or cut up 1-2 inches of ginger root, boil pieces in a quart of water for 10-20min; strain, let cool; sweeten if desired.	Helps fight chills and fatigue. Ginger combats one of the common cold viruses.	None	Kemper (2002a) (cites study)
Elderberry extract	Sambucol preparations	Antiviral properties, especially against influenza and herpes simplex; increases inflammatory cytokine production and activates immune system	None reported	Barak et al (2001); Zakay-Rones et al (2004) (cite studies showing decrease in length of flu symptoms; studies done in 18+-yr-olds)
Nutritionals Vitamin C	Children: 250mg qid or 4-5 glasses of orange juice daily at onset of cold. Increase other citrus fruit, kiwi, berries, melon, bell pepper, broccoli.	Reduces symptoms and length of illness by activating neutrophils to oxidize inflammatory mediators and increase extracellular vitamin C	Regarded as safe; diarrhea in high doses	Kemper (2002a); Ditchek & Greenfield (2002)
Chicken soup: peppers (inc. cayenne), mustard, horseradish, salsa, other spicy foods	Sip soup slowly throughout the day.	Thins nasal secretions, increases nasal and sinus mucous mobility	None reported but use cautiously in children with diarrhea-associated illnesses because of chance of causing hypernatremic dehydration	Kemper (2002a) (proven efficacy incomplete in children but worthwhile to try)
Garlic	Raw clove minced in mashed potatoes (1 medium clove = 100,000 units penicillin); do not exceed 2 cloves in 1 day. Kyolic liquid garlic: 1-5yr: ½ tsp; 6+ yr: 1tsp in grape juice twice daily.	Kills cold viruses; supports immune function	Safe, occasional GI upset *Class 2c*	Kemper (2002a); Ditcheck & Greenfield (2002)

Continued

TABLE 42-4   Complementary Treatments* for Some Common Conditions in Children and Adolescents—Cont'd

Diagnosis	Treatment Approach	Dosage	Benefit	Possible Side Effects†	Research/Citations
	Zinc lozenges	Children: 15-25mg sucked every 2hr for 7 days only	May reduce severity and length of illness by binding rhinoviral docking sites with somatic cells, inhibiting infectivity	Mouth irritation, nausea, vomiting, diarrhea, abdominal pain; can suppress immune system if taken longer than 7 days	Kemper (2002a); has not been tested or proven effective in children
	Biochemical *Saline nose drops or spray*	Recipe: ½ tsp salt in 1 cup warm water; instill as drops nasally prn	Helps thin nasal secretions	None reported at recommended dilution	Kemper (2002a)
	Aromatherapy *Oils of camphor, eucalyptus, menthol, pine, rosemary, wintergreen, tea tree*	Inhaled by vaporizer or steam	Helps relieve congestion; heats nasal passages to a degree that inhibits viral replication	*Class 1*	Kemper (2002a)
	Massage *Oils of menthol (Vicks VapoRub), Tiger Balm*	Infant older than 1mo: massage face, head, back, lymph glands, chest in gentle downward motion. Vicks VapoRub on soles of feet can decrease coughing.	May cool the nose causing perception of decreased nasal congestion	Safe *Class 1*	Kemper (2002a); Graedon & Graedon (2006c)
	Acupuncture		Aids blocked sinuses	Included in 1979 WHO list of recognized therapies influenced by acupuncture	Micozzi (1996); Kemper (2002a) cites inadequate study in adults; does not recommend for children
Crohn's disease/ IBD	Nutritional *Coconut*	Eat 2 coconut macaroon cookies daily (Archway®) or add flaked coconut to cereal (1-2tsp) or as much as needed for control.	Possible antibacterial effect from lauric acid in coconut fat that decreases inflammation	None	Graedon & Graedon (1999) (anecdotal information of efficacy)
	Reduce undigested or unabsorbed carbohydrates	Diet available in Gottschall E: *Breaking the vicious cycle: intestinal health through diet*, Baltimore, 1994 Kirkton Press.)	Avoids carbohydrate overload and excessive fermentation in the intestines	Diet very restrictive	Ditchek & Greenfield (2002) (patients have been able to avoid immunosuppressive therapy when on the diet)

Condition	Remedy	Dose	Benefits	Side Effects/Cautions	Reference
Dental caries	Xylitol	6-10 g daily. 1 piece of gum chewed for 5 min qid (or 2 mints sucked). See Appendix A.	Encourages remineralization and inhibits plaque formation; bacteria cannot colonize	None; diarrhea if recommended dose exceeded	Ly et al (2006) (cites well-documented, scientific studies)
Diabetes, type II	Nutritional *Whey protein supplementation for those eating high glycemic index meals*		Whey proteins have insulinotropic effects and reduce postprandial glycemia in healthy people; stimulates insulin release	None	Frid et al (2005) (study cited)
	Herbal Cinnamon	½ tsp daily	Lowers blood-sugar levels; also lowers HDL cholesterol	None	Pratt & Matthews (2004) (cites study by USDA)
Diarrhea	Herbal *Berberine-containing plants (goldenseal, barberry, or Chinese remedy "huanglian coptis chinonsis")*	***Goldenseal:*** toddlers and older children ¼-½ tsp tincture or ⅛ tsp fluid extract tid-qid—can be mixed with water or juice ***Giardia:*** children, 5mg/ kg/day for 6 days	Demonstrated benefits for antimicrobial activity against bacteria (includes *E. coli, Shigella, Salmonella, Klebsiella, F. aerogenes*), fungi, protozoa, including *Giardia*. When used with any indicated antibiotics, decreased length of illness.	Hypotension or hypertension, nausea, vomiting, diarrhea; **NOT recommended for infants younger than 1 mo old** *Class 2b* More effective than Flagyl in treating symptoms but not as effective in clearing from GI tract; best approach to use with standard antibiotic therapy	Kemper (2002a) (also, stop vit C); Pizzorno (2002) (cite studies). Only use Chinese herbal preparations if prepared by a licensed herbalist because of contamination. Avoid herbal diarrhea remedies that contain agrimony or cocklebur, alder, and leaves and tops of betony because they contain high levels of cancer-causing tannins.
	Lactobacillus acidophilus or *Bifidobacterium bifidum*	5-7 billion organisms/ day (check bottle ingredients). If using yogurt, make sure it contains these bacteria.	Can also be used to decrease incidence of rotavirus diarrhea in infants 5-24mo old; reinforces mucosal wall barrier	Flatulence, constipation ***Do NOT use in those with impaired immune systems***	Kemper (2002a) (study cited); Pettit (2002)

Continued

TABLE 42-4 Complementary Treatments* for Some Common Conditions in Children and Adolescents—Cont'd

Diagnosis	Treatment Approach	Dosage	Benefit	Possible Side Effects†	Research/Citations
	5% carob pod powder	Infants to 1yr: 1.5g/kg/day in formula or in Oral Rehydration Solution (ORS) Children > 1yr: 1-15g/kg/day in ORS or milk; stop 24hr after appearance of formed stools	Acute diarrhea in infants and children; tannins inhibit growth of bacteria and bind bacterial toxins; controlled studies of hospitalized infants showed efficacy of treatment	None Used for centuries in Mediterranean regions *Class 1*	Kemper (2002a) (recommends not relying solely on this remedy until more studies prove its efficacy).
	Garlic *Best formulations are enteric coated tabs/capsules/dried or powdered garlic, standardized for allilin content*	All ages: 1 clove (or 4g) chewed, chopped, bruised, or crushed; do not use more than 2 cloves of raw garlic daily	Treats *Entamoeba histolytica*, athlete's foot, vaginal candidiasis; is antimicrobial; organosulfur compounds are believed to interfere with microbial structures and functions	Garlic breath (try chewing fennel, parsley, fenugreek to counter garlic breath); has anticlotting effect; GI upset, rash, burning mouth, sweating, lightheadedness; raw garlic is toxic in high doses	Castleman (1995); Therapeutic Research Center (1997)
	Oral rehydration solution 4 cups water ½ tsp salt 1-1½ cups rice cereal for babies (2tbsp sugar can also be added); ½ tsp instant Jell-O powder for flavor	Offer 1 tbsp to 1oz every 15-30min; increase as tolerated.			WHO (2003); Kemper (2002a).
	Homeopathy	Arsenic trioxide, calcium carbonate, German chamomile, May apple, flowers of sulfur are choices depending upon clinical presentation	Decrease number of stools and duration of symptoms	None	Kemper & Jacobs (2003) (2 studies cited that showed efficacy of homeopathy)
Eczema/atopic dermatitis	Herbal				
	Evening primrose oil (EPO, Efamol), borage oil, black currant oil	3g PO daily Requires 4-12wk for benefit	Decreased scaling, itching, and general severity; contains high amounts of a fatty acid (gamma linolenic acid) that children with eczema are thought to have a defect in metabolizing	Very safe; rare, mild GI effects, headache *Class 1*	Kemper (2002a); Gardiner et al, (2001) (studies cited)

Echinacea	Apply topically	Promotes healing by stimulating formation of new tissue	Contact dermatitis; use with caution in patients allergic to ragweed and daisy family of plants *Class I*	Kemper (2002a) (remains untested)
Oolong tea	3 cups daily	Improvement in skin symptoms	None	Kemper (2002a) (cites study showing 63% of patients reported moderate or marked improvement; more than 50% continued to benefit for up to 6mo) Pizzorno (2002); Kemper (2002a)
Licorice (Glycyrrhiza glabra)	Apply topically as pure glycyrrhetinic acid (commercial product: Simicort from Enzymatic Therapy). Can be used as a compress, using licorice tea.	Exerts effect similar to hydrocortisone cream	None *Class 2b*	
Chamomile extracts, witch hazel, calendula, aloe vera, St. John's wort oil	Apply topically (commercial product: CamoCare)	May help reduce itching and inflammation; promotes healing	Contact dermatitis; use with caution in patients with allergy to ragweed or daisy family of plants	Kemper (2002a); Gardiner & Kemper (2000)
Nutritional and naturopathic Rotation diet	4-day rotation diet, eliminating all major allergens (milk, eggs, peanuts); as patient improves, slowly reintroduce allergens and reduce stringency of rotation diet; limit animal products (see Box 42-1)	Improvement in symptoms	Ensure adequate calcium, nutrients	Pizzorno (2002). Kemper (2002a) (does not rec. elimination diet unless eczema affects >20% of body)
Breast milk Vitamin C (after diet exclusion and rechallenge)	Infants/children: one 8-oz glass of orange juice daily		None at recommended doses	Refer to Colic, nutritional Kemper (2002a) (cites double-blind, controlled crossover trial of vit C with significant improvement of eczema. Do not give added vit A, vit E, or zinc to eczema prone children.)

Continued

TABLE 42-4 **Complementary Treatments* for Some Common Conditions in Children and Adolescents—Cont'd**

Diagnosis	Treatment Approach	Dosage	Benefit	Possible Side Effects†	Research/Citations
	Yogurt	Daily	Helps keep the immune system balanced		Kemper (2002a) (mothers who consume yogurt or probiotics 2 wk before delivery and 6 mo after delivery had infants who developed eczema at ½ the rate of control group)
	Fatty fish(wild salmon, herring, mackerel, tuna)	Once weekly	An omega-3 series of fatty acids; see evening primrose oil discussed earlier		
	Mind-body techniques Biofeedback, visualization, progressive relaxation, meditation, deep breathing		Affects oversensitive immune system by decreasing stress		Kemper (2002a)
	Massage	Add 1-2 drop of chamomile or yarrow oil to 1 tsp vegetable oil	Enhances healing, decreased stress		Kemper (2002a)
Elevated lead level	Herbal				
	Garlic	Add liberally to foods; see under Common Cold/Flu for dosing information	Helps eliminate lead and heavy metals	Use with caution in patients with clotting disorders	Castleman (1995) (based on some European studies)
	Teas from red clover, lemon grass, milk thistle	Tea drinks	Herbalists believe these help detoxify heavy metals	Do not give red clover to children under 2yr old (Castleman, 1995)	Kemper (1996) (no scientific studies done to date)
	Nutritional	Ensure adequate intake of calcium and iron	May speed elimination of lead	None	Ditchek & Greenfield (2002)
Enuresis	Biofeedback	Children > 4 yr: program—child voids in front of a uroflow device while being coached; pelvic floor relaxation techniques in front of electromyogram	80%-100% resolution; decreases postresidual void and improves voiding curves	None	Schulman et al (2001) (cites study)
	Acupuncture	Several weeks of acupuncture treatments		None	Kemper (2002a) (cites study showing comparable results with use of DDAVP)

Headaches

	Dosage	Action	Side Effects	References
Herbal				
Feverfew (Tanacetum parthenium)	Children > 2yr: 0.25-0.5mg parthenolide bid (start with lower dose and increase as necessary) OR Chew 1-3 leaves daily Change brands if no results seen after a few wk; try for several months	Prevention of migraines: inhibits release of blood vessel–dilating substances from platelets to decrease production of inflammatory substances and reestablish proper blood vessel tone; benefits are similar to aspirin and NSAIDs, but if NSAIDs do not work, feverfew will [work] because properties are similar	Mouth sores, abdominal pain, allergic reactions usually within first wk of use; not to be used during pregnancy or in patients with clotting disorders; sudden cessation may result in rebound headaches *Class 2b*	Pizzorno (2002) (double-blind studies cited that showed reduction in number and severity of migraines—not for acute attacks); Holroyd & Mauskop (2003) (study showed reduction number of attacks but not duration; reduced nausea and vomiting); Kemper (2002a)
Ginger	Fresh: 6mm slice daily Dried: 500mg qid	Antiinflammatory	None	Pizzorno (2002) (needs further study; best results from fresh ginger or ginger oil)
Thermal biofeedback	6yr and up: as needed to master techniques (4-12 sessions over 6-10wk); daily home practice results in greater improvement in pain	For tension and migraine headaches: patients learn to dilate blood vessels in body to affect blood flow to the head and relax muscles; reduces frequency and intensity of pain	None. Technique very popular with children familiar with computer age technology.	Fugh-Berman (1997; cites studies showing success rates of 44%-65% for muscle-contraction headaches and 38% for migraines); Kemper (2002a) (50% decrease in headaches); Pizzorno (2002); Grazzi et al (2001); Allen, (2004); (technique best at preventing recurrent pain rather than helping once pain has started)
Massage	Head, neck, shoulder massage techniques using 1-2 drops peppermint or eucalyptus oil to 1 tsp vegetable oil as massage lotion. Foot massage is an alternative, using reflexology points	Muscle relaxation; oil may help decrease pain sensitivity	None reported	Kemper (2002a) (cites studies showing proven effectiveness)

Continued

TABLE 42-4 Complementary Treatments* for Some Common Conditions in Children and Adolescents—Cont'd

Diagnosis	Treatment Approach	Dosage	Benefit	Possible Side Effects†	Research/Citations
	Hypnosis				Kemper (2002a); Holroyd & Mausckop (2003)
	Therapeutic touch				
	Progressive relaxation				
	Acupuncture	Age when tolerant to needles; nonneedle techniques or Japanese-style acupuncture also available	Use in conjunction with massage and relaxation	None reported	Kemper (2002a) (cites many studies showing effectiveness for migraine prevention and tension headaches); Holroyd & Mauskop (2003)
	Chiropractic	Chiropractors "adjust" all ages: manipulation of cervical and thoracic vertebrae	Pain reduction, acute and chronic	Few complications with cervical manipulation, less with other areas; issues with chiropractics occur when only manipulation is used and more appropriate medical diagnosis and treatment was delayed (e.g., encopresis, ear infections, diabetes, anemia, HTN, tumors)	Fugh-Berman (1997); Nickerson & Silberman (1992); Kemper (2002a) (cites studies showing no better relief of headaches than with massage alone).
	Naturopathy and nutritional				
	Elimination diet	Avoid nitrates, nitrites, aspartame, MSG, chocolate, aged cheeses, caffeine, wheat, oranges, eggs, milk, beef, corn, sugar, yeast, shellfish Avoid vit A and D, zinc Limit caffeine intake; ↑ water	Benefits children with other allergy symptoms and frequent headaches; vit A excess increases intracranial pressure, vit D and zinc can cause headaches	None reported	Kemper (2002a); Pizzorno (2002) (cites nonrandomized study showing 85% reduction in headaches)
	Riboflavin (B₂)	400 mg daily for 3 mo	Increases mitochondrial energy efficiency	None reported	Scharff & Kemper (2003)
				None	Pizzorno (2002) (more research needed; 50%-68% patients improved in studies)

Condition	Therapy	Application/Dosage	Effect	Precautions/Side Effects	References
		Increase magnesium-rich foods (nuts, legumes, dark, leafy green vegetables, whole grain cereals and breads, seafood) and include ginger and hot peppers, garlic, onion, vegetable oils, fish oils	Adolescents: magnesium 250-400mg tid plus vitamin B_6 25mg tid Ginger: daily ¼ slice fresh or 500mg qid dried or 100-200mg tid extract (20% gingerol and shogaol) (for prevention) and 200mg every 2hr acute migraine	Low magnesium levels often found in patients with all types of headaches; magnesium maintains blood vessel tone and prevents overexcitability of nerve cells; vit B_6 increases intracellular Mg; ginger (contains aspirin-like compounds) exerts antiinflammatory effects and decreases platelet aggregation	Diarrhea, gastric irritation	Kemper (2002a); Pizzorno (2002); Holroyd & Mauskop (2003) (double-blind study in children showed significantly decreased frequency and severity of headaches)
	Homeopathy	Individualized homeopathic remedies (belladonna, *Bryonia, Gelsemium, Nux vomica*	Reduction in intensity and frequency of attacks	Not recommended for children (Kemper, 2002b)	Fugh-Berman (1997) (cites a double-blind, placebo-controlled study)
	Aromatherapy	Peppermint oil in diffuser or vaporizer	Analgesic effect for tension headaches	None	Holroyd & Mauskop (2003)
Head lice	Bug Buster kit (contains 4 combs for use on wet conditioned hair)	Sequential combing regimen	Elimination of lice	None—more advantageous than using pediculicides	Hill (2005): (significantly more elimination of lice over those using permethrin and malathion treatments; results may not be applicable outside UK, as a result of resistance patterns in different countries)
	Margarine; mayonnaise; Vaseline; Dr. Weil's mixture‡	Apply heavy coating to hair and scalp; cover with shower cap overnight; wash out; comb repeatedly with nit comb		None; messy	Ditchek & Greenfield (2002)
Herpes simplex labialis	Herbal *1% lemon balm extract*	Apply topically: 1% dried lemon balm extract cream qid with onset of symptoms or within 72hr of symptoms for best result	Antiviral compounds; complete healing by eighth day	Use with caution if taking thyroid medication; increases effects of barbiturates	Gardiner et al (2001)

Continued

TABLE 42-4   **Complementary Treatments* for Some Common Conditions in Children and Adolescents—Cont'd**

Diagnosis	Treatment Approach	Dosage	Benefit	Possible Side Effects†	Research/Citations
	Aloe vera	0.5% aloe vera extract cream applied topically several times daily at onset of symptoms	Speeds healing; antiinflammatory	Contact dermatitis *Class 1*	Same as above
Hyperactivity/ ADHD	Music therapy	Have children listen to calm, low-pitched, slow-tempo music	Improved work performance, decrease tension and activity, calming effect on autonomic nervous system	High-pitched music creates tension; low pitch stimulates relaxation; slow tempo is soothing; fast or stimulating music increases anxiety and activity	Kemper (1996, 2002a) (cited one study done in Israel showing hyperactive boys doing as well as normal boys when listening to calming music vs no music vs fast-paced music); Klein & Winkelstein (1996); Thaut (1998)
	Biofeedback *(Two types: electromyogram and electroencephalogram)*	Takes 6-8 wk (35-50 sessions) to learn techniques, age dependent	More relaxed behavior, improved attention, improved language skills; technique focuses on reducing muscle tension in the forehead and ways to exercise different neurologic pathways to control impulses; ↑ attention, and process information better		Kemper (2002a) (cites studies showing behavioral improvement equal to Ritalin; technique works best if also used with structured scheduling and behavioral rewards)
	Homeopathy Herbal treatments commonly tried: *Stramonium, Cina, Hyoscyamus niger, Veratrum album, Tarentula hispanica*			None	Chan (2002) Chan et al (2000); Kemper (2002a) (does not routinely recommend, but safe)
	Evening primrose oil (EPO)	Children: 500-1000 g/ daily standardized to contain 8% gamma linolenic acid (GLA)	Improvement on parent and teacher behavioral scales	Safe to try; nausea, diarrhea, headache with high dose or chronic use; flatus, halitosis; increases bleeding time	Chan et al (2000) (2 studies cited); Ditcheck & Greenfield (2002)

	Dose	Benefit	Side effects/cautions	Reference
Nutritional/ naturopathic				
Elimination diet	See Box 42-1 Also recommended: elimination of refined sugars and supplementation with a multivitamin that includes thiamin, niacin, vitamin B_6, magnesium, manganese, potassium, and zinc	Decrease in irritability, insomnia, fidgetiness; improvement seen in up to 73% (Boris & Mandel, 1994) Vitamin deficiencies can result in impaired brain and nervous system function. Refined sugars thought to promote reactive hypoglycemia causing increased adrenalin secretion and hyperactivity (Pizzorno, 2002).	Elimination diet can put strain on family; dietary management less likely to produce results with discordant marital relationships present (Carter et al, 1993); may need consultation with nutritionist	Studies showed some behavioral changes in hyperactive children (not all studies used subjects meeting DSM III criteria) when challenged by specific food allergens (Carter et al, 1993; Egger et al, 1992; Rowe & Rowe, 1994; Boris & Mandel, 1994); Pizzorno (2002); Kemper (2002a) (try elimination diet only after other measures have failed to help; does not recommend Feingold diet)
Nutritional				
Magnesium	<12yr: 400mg daily >12yr: 400-600mg daily. These doses are greater than RDA.	Regulates muscles and nerve function, helps with restlessness, irritability, anxiety	Diarrhea, drowsiness, weakness, lethargy if overdose	Starobrat-Hermelin & Kozielec (1997) (cite study)
Fish oil (omega-3, EPA, DHA)	500-1000mg/daily or more	Improves visual processing and motor coordination in children with dyslexia and dyspraxia—may help with ADHD	Safe to try	Chan et al (2000); (no studies on ADHD); Ditcheck & Greenfield (2002)
Caffeine	Low doses	May boost benefit of Ritalin without increasing side effects	Effects of caffeine (jittery, nervous, anxious, tired with withdrawal)	Kemper (2002a)
Yoga, Tai Chi, Gi gong Meditation Guided therapy		Enhances relaxation	None reported	Kemper (2002a)
Exercise *Martial arts*	Any sport that involves close interaction between child and coach		None	Kemper (2002a) Kemper (2002a)
Massage				Kemper (2002a) (cites limited study showing efficacy)

Continued

TABLE 42-4 **Complementary Treatments* for Some Common Conditions in Children and Adolescents—Cont'd**

Diagnosis	Treatment Approach	Dosage	Benefit	Possible Side Effects†	Research/Citations
Jaundice	Therapeutic touch			None reported	Kemper (2002a) (studies done in adults only)
	Prayer therapy		Prayer healing has been shown to prevent RBCs from breaking down in test tubes; increase in hemoglobin in adults		Kemper (1996) (studies done in adults only)
Jock itch (fungal infection)	Herbal			*DO NOT USE*	Kemper (2002a)
	Listerine mouthwash	Apply to groin area	Antifungal activity from the herbal oils contained in the product (eucalyptol, menthol, methyl salicylate and thymol)	Stings if placed in more delicate areas	Graedon & Graedon (2006a)
Nausea and vomiting	Herbal				
	Combination tea with chamomile, lemon balm, peppermint	Small, frequent sips	Soothing to stomach upsets	Safe unless existing allergy to ragweed or daisy family of plants *Class 1*	Kemper (2002a)
	Goldenseal or barberry	Tincture: 2-3 drops in 4 oz water; sipped slowly over 1 hr	Especially helpful if child has vomiting and diarrhea	None reported at therapeutic levels; excessive levels can cause GI upset, CNS stimulation *Class 2b*	Kemper (2002a)
	Basil tea	Make with ½ oz dry basil and 1 cup boiling water, steeped 5 min and strained		Not recommended for infants or toddlers *Class 2b*	Kemper (2002a); McGuffin et al (1997)
	Ginger root	<3 yr: 25 mg qid 3-6 yr: 50-75 mg qid 6-12 yr: 125 mg. qid >13 yr: 250 mg qid OR Ginger tea: 1 cup water to 2 slices ginger root (simmer 5 min) OR ¼ tsp fresh grated ginger in juice, applesauce, or cereal OR Ginger soda (with real ginger)	Helps to reduce nausea by promoting elimination of intestinal gas and reducing GI spasms	Not for long-term use; use only in recommended doses. Large doses can depress CNS, cause cardiac arrhythmias, compromise platelet aggregation *Do NOT use in pregnancy* *Class 2b*	Kemper (2002a); Therapeutic Research Center (1997)

Therapy	Application/Dosage	Indication	Side Effects	Reference
Poultice	Soak cotton flannel cloth in castor oil, lay cloth over abdomen, and cover with towel; have child rest 1hr, then remove cloth and rinse abdomen with baking soda/water solution	Old folk remedy for nausea		Kemper (2002a)
Nutritional *Vitamin B$_6$*	Motion sickness and nausea of radiation therapy: 10mg 1hr before traveling; Pregnancy: 10-25mg every 8hr; Age dependent	May help minimize nausea	None reported	Kemper (2002a)
Hypnosis		Helpful in reducing recurrent vomiting and nausea associated with chemotherapy or motion sickness	None reported	Kemper (2002a)
Therapeutic Touch/Reiki				Kemper (2002a) (has found it useful in her practice)
Acupressure	Apply pressure 1 inch above wrist crease, between the two tendons leading to the palm; repeat every 2 hr as needed to control nausea	Controls nausea symptoms	None reported	Kemper (2002a) (few studies to date involving children but safe to try)
Acupuncture	At P6 point (can use Sea-Bands)	Useful before and after surgery, for morning sickness, motion sickness, chemotherapy	None	Kemper (2002a)
Onychomycosis Herbal *Tea tree oil Vicks VapoRub*	Apply topically to affected nails twice daily for 3mo	Antifungal, antibacterial	Allergic dermatitis in sensitive patients	Gardiner et al (2001); Graedon & Graedon (1999)
Vinegar	Soak affected nails in 50:50 solution white vinegar and water for 30min daily for several mo			

Continued

TABLE 42-4 Complementary Treatments* for Some Common Conditions in Children and Adolescents—Cont'd

Diagnosis	Treatment Approach	Dosage	Benefit	Possible Side Effects†	Research/Citations
	Vitamin E	Puncture one vitamin E capsule; apply oil to affected nail at bedtime (cover with cotton sock) until new nail begins to grow out			
	Cornmeal soaks	Place 1 inch of cornmeal in dishpan; add hot water and stir to dissolve cornmeal; when just cooled enough to tolerate, soak feet for 1 hr. Repeat regularly.			Graedon & Graedon (2006b)
Otitis media	Nutritional *Elimination diet*	Eliminate milk and dairy products, eggs, wheat, corn, oranges, peanut butter, concentrated simple carbohydrates (sugar, honey, dried fruit, concentrated fruit juices, etc.)	Boosts immune system by eliminating allergens known to impede it; decreases congestion of nasal mucous membranes that affect drainage of the eustachian tubes or insults to the integrity of the middle ear	None reported	After elimination diet 86% of food-sensitive patients (71% of subjects) showed significant improvement in serous otitis media recurrence; most subjects allergic to 2-4 foods, most to milk, wheat, egg, peanuts, soy, and corn (Nsouli et al, 1994); tympanostomy tubes deemed inappropriate or of equivocal use in 58% of children (Kleinman et al, 1994)
	Breast milk Xylitol chewing gum, syrup, mints (see Appendix A)	All infants 2-3 mg qid (< 30 g daily)	Bacteriostatic effect against *S. pneumoniae*; interferes with bacterial adhesion to mucous membranes		Kemper (2002b) (studies cited that showed 30%-40% decrease in infections)
Pain • **Acute**	Combination of acupuncture and hypnosis	10-15 min tid	Significant decrease in pain, per studies	None	Zeltzer et al (2002) (cites study)

Category	Therapy	Dose/Form	Effect/Mechanism	Side Effects	References
Postsurgical or procedural	Music therapy; Deep breathing; Imagery; Distraction; Relaxation		Reduce anxiety and pain		Cites studies showing efficacy: Kankkunen et al (2003); He et al (2006); Voss et al (2004); Good et al (2001)
	Infants: Breastfeeding or breast milk supplementation		Significant decrease in pain scores vs when infants swaddled or held for painful procedures		Shah et al (2006); Walach et al (2003)
Chronic	Mind-body techniques				
	Music therapy		See Hyperactivity/ADHD section		Voss et al (2004); Good et al (2001)
	Yoga		Delays muscle soreness		Boyle et al (2004)(cites study; consider for preseason training)
	Acupuncture		Acute and chronic pain analgesia	None reported	Kemper (2000; 2002a)
	Therapeutic Touch			None reported	Kemper (2002a)
	Relaxation			None reported	Kemper (2002a)
	Deep breathing			None reported	Koh et al (2005); He et al (2006)
	Distraction			None reported	Kemper (2002a)
	Massage				
	Magnet therapy	Electromagnetic, not static	Mechanism not understood; suspected neuronal effect.		Miller (2004) (cites studies showing improvement of various pain syndromes, including soft tissue, bone, musculoskeletal pain, OA) Shah et al (2006); Walach et al (2003)
	Nutritional				
	Infants: Breastfeeding or breast milk supplementation		Significant decrease in pain scores vs when infants swaddled or held for painful procedures		
	Omega-3 fatty acids	Fish oil omega-3 fatty acids (3 g/daily) plus 9.6cc of olive oil daily	Inhibits proinflammatory eicosanoid and cytokine production by peripheral tissues and glial cells; blocks voltage-gated sodium channels	Mild GI distress	Berbert et al (2005) (adult study showed significant improvement in joint mobility, fatigue, pain over 12wk; better than when just taking omega-3 fatty acids alone)
	Glucosamine, Chondroitin, SAM-e	Adult doses: Glucosamine: 1600-2000mg daily	Reduces cartilage destruction, enhances chondrocyte anabolism, decreases inflammation by inhibiting PGs	Do not take if diabetic or have seafood allergies	Soeken (2004) (adult studies show these help with mild knee pain caused by OA)

Continued

TABLE 42-4   Complementary Treatments* for Some Common Conditions in Children and Adolescents—Cont'd

Diagnosis	Treatment Approach	Dosage	Benefit	Possible Side Effects†	Research/Citations
	Natural proteases	Chondroitin: 400-500mg bid-tid		None	Miller et al (2004) (study of men running downhill showed superior recovery of contractile function and decreased soreness)
		SAM-e: 200-1600mg daily		None; very expensive	
		Adults: 2 tabs qid (containing 325mg pancreatic enzymes, 75mg trypsin, 50mg papain, 50mg bromelain, 10mg amylase, 10mg lipase, 10mg lysozyme, 2mg chymotrypsin)	Promotes production of cartilage proteoglycans	None	
	Herbal				
	Boswellia	>120 lbs: 500mg bid	Attenuates soft tissue injury after intense exercise	None to mild GI upset	Kimmatkar et al (2003) (adult studies show significant decrease in knee pain, swelling, mobility with OA and RA)
	Bromelain	Individually tailored program	Antiinflammatory, antiarthritic, analgesic properties	Rare, including allergic reactions	Walker et al (2002) (adult studies show effective for ankle sprain, muscular trauma, OA and RA, mild knee pain)
	Willow bark		Antiinflammatory, analgesic properties		Under study
	Rosa canina		Antiinflammatory, analgesic properties		Under study
Premature infants	Massage		Facilitates growth and development and decreases medical complications	None reported; less duration of massage seems to produce less positive results	Fugh-Berman (1997) (cites several studies supporting massage or stroking)
	Music therapy	Used in preemie nurseries Slow, soothing music	Reduces stress	None	Kemper & Martin (2004)
Presurgery Precautions	STOP THE FOLLOWING: *Vitamin E* *Ginkgo biloba* *Ginseng* *Garlic* *Ginger* *Green tea* *Flax* *NSAIDs, ASA* *Fish oil*		Interfere with platelet function, causing prolonged bleeding		Graedon & Graedon (1999); Sego (2006)

PMS

Herbal	Dosage	Action	Cautions	References
Herbal Black currant seed oil OR Flaxseed oil OR Evening primrose oil	As directed on label tid *or* 1000 mg tid	Important fatty acids help relieve PMS symptoms and aid glandular function	None Flax needs to be taken with at least 6 oz of water; contraindicated with bowel obstruction	Balch & Balch (1997) (other helpful suggestions offered in this reference); McGuffin et al (1997); Gardiner & Kemper (2000) *Class 1*
Angelica or Dong Quai (*Angelica sinensis*)	Powered root or tea: 1-2 g tid Tincture (1:5): 4 mL tid Fluid extract: 1 mL tid	Roots contain phytoestrogens, which nourish and tone female glandular and organ system	**Do NOT use if patient is pregnant, is nursing, or has a history of cancer, cardiac disease, or photosensitivity; occasional light laxative effect** *Class 2b*	Pizzorno (2002) (other helpful preparations offered in this reference); Gardiner & Kemper (2000)
Licorice root (*Glycyrrhiza glabra*)	Powered root or tea: 1-2 g tid Fluid extract (1:1): 4 mL tid Dry powdered extract (1:4): 250-500 mg tid	Reduces water retention of PMS; believed to lower estrogen levels and increase progesterone levels	**Do NOT use if patient is pregnant, is breastfeeding or has glaucoma, diabetes, HTN, or cardiac disease** *Class 2b*	McGuffin et al (1997); Therapeutic Research Center (1998)
Black cohosh (*Cimicifuga racemosa*)	1 tab once or twice daily	Useful for relieving cramps; may help with depression, anxiety, tension, mood swings	Use only with nonpregnant, nonnursing patients; not to be used in patients with cardiac disease or estrogen-dependent cancers. Overdose symptoms: nausea, diarrhea, abdominal pain, vomiting, dizziness, headache, tremors, arthralgias *Class 2b*	Gardiner & Kemper (2000); McGuffin et al (1997); Pizzorno (2002)
Chasteberry (*Vitex agnus-castus*)	Powdered extract tabs (0.5% agnuside content) 175-225 mg/day Liquid extract: 20-40 mg/day	Useful with breast tenderness symptoms of PMS; appears to alter GnRH and FSH-RH to normalize secretion of prolactin and estrogen/progesterone ratio; dopaminergic effect	**Do NOT** use in pregnant, lactating patients; occasional minor skin irritations *Class 2b*	McGuffin et al (1997); Pizzorno (2002); Mancho & Edwards (2005) (cites study showing 50% symptom relief)

Continued

TABLE 42-4   Complementary Treatments* for Some Common Conditions in Children and Adolescents—Cont'd

Diagnosis	Treatment Approach	Dosage	Benefit	Possible Side Effects[†]	Research/Citations
	Nutritional and naturopathic				
	Calcium	1000 mg/day	Relieves cramping, backache, nervousness		Pizzorno (2002)
	Magnesium Vitamin B complex plus extra vitamin B$_6$	12 mg/kg/day 100 mg tid 50-100 mg/day	Helps with headaches B vitamins complement each other. Decreases water and increases circulation to female organs; helps restore estrogen levels.		Balch & Balch (1997); Pizzorno (2002)
	Vitamin E	400 international units/day	Helps with breast tenderness, depression, irritability; improves oxygen profusion to body		
	Zinc	15-20 mg/day	Promotes hormone balance; controls prolactin secretion		Micozzi (1996)
	Diet	Eat plenty of fresh fruits, vegetables, whole-grain cereals and breads, beans, peas, lentil, nuts and seeds, broiled fowl, fish, high-protein foods as snacks, and soy products; avoid salt, red meats, processed foods, junk and fast foods, caffeine, refined sugar, and dairy products 1 wk before menses; increase water intake to 1 quart distilled water/day 1 wk before menses and continue 1 wk after onset	Red meats and dairy products believed to contribute to hormonal fluctuations; other recommended foods aid in metabolism, glucose, and absorption of nutrients, and decrease free estrogen in blood; excluding salt decreases bloating and water retention; dairy products and refined sugars also believed to increase excretion of magnesium with resulting impaired estrogen metabolism and moodiness		
	Isolated soya protein (ISP) containing soy isoflavones (IF)	ISP containing 68 mg (aglycone equivalents) of IF daily	Influence endogenous estrogen effects on specific tissues	None reported	Bryant et al (2005) (study showed some improvement in headaches and breast tenderness; significant improvement in swelling and cramps)

Continued

	Treatment	Dosage/Application	Action/Use	Cautions	References
	Chiropractic		For cramps: possibly alters prostaglandin levels		Fugh-Berman (1997) (cites studies)
	Acupuncture		For cramps		Fugh-Berman (1997) (cites studies); NIH (1998)
Skin irritation/ diaper rashes	Yoga				
	Herbal				
	Aloe vera	All ages: pure gel form, applied topically several times daily	Antibacterial effects; accelerates healing	Contact dermatitis *Class 1*	Kemper (2002a); Murray & Pizzorno (1998); Gardiner et al (2001)
	Chamomile	Add essential oil to bath or make as tea and rub affected area	Soothes diaper rash, varicella, contact dermatitis	Contact dermatitis; use in caution in patients with allergy to ragweed or daisy family of plants *Class 1*	Kemper (2002a)
	Nutritional				
	Zinc	Formula-fed infants: 10mg/day for formula-fed infants with history of yeast diaper rashes	May help prevent yeast diaper rashes in formula-fed infants (does not apply to breastfed infants)	None noted	Kemper (2002a) (cites study showing that infants with frequent diaper rashes have lower levels of zinc in their bodies)
	Live Lactobacillus acidophilus bacteria OR *Bifidobacterium bifidum*	Infants ≥ 6 mo: give as yogurt; ½-1 cup daily PO / < 6 mo: apply directly to diaper area	Thought to help replace the yeast on the skin	None noted	Kemper (2002a)
Sleep/Sedation	Music therapy (before sleep deprived EEG)	1-5yr: soothing music of voice, guitar, and/or soft percussion; culturally appropriate	Produces sleep for procedure	None	Loewy et al (2005) (study compared music therapy vs. chloral hydrate for successful completion of EEG; 97% of music therapy vs. 50% drug subjects were successful)
Teething	Herbal				
	Tea tree oil	Dilute with water and apply topically to gums with Q-Tip *NOT FOR INGESTION*	Antifungal, antibacterial; mouthwash for oral health	Allergic dermatitis in sensitive patients	LaValle et al (2000)
	Clove oil	Apply topically; do not use > 48hr	Antiseptic: good for toothaches, teething; analgesic on mucous membranes; antibacterial and antiviral		

TABLE 42-4 **Complementary Treatments* for Some Common Conditions in Children and Adolescents—Cont'd**

Diagnosis	Treatment Approach	Dosage	Benefit	Possible Side Effects†	Research/Citations
Toothache, temporary relief	Acupressure	Rub ice cube in the V-shaped area where bones of your thumb and forefinger meet ("anatomical saltbox," "Hoku" point) for 5-7 min.	Dulls pain	None	Shedletsky et al (1984) (repeated in later studies; 60%-90% effective)
UTI prevention	Herbal *Cranberry juice, juice extract capsules, or pure cranberry liquid extract mixed with orange juice to decrease tangy taste*	150-600mL/day children and adolescents; 1-2 capsules once or twice daily for adolescents	Reduces adhesion of gram-negative and gram-positive bacteria to bladder wall cells	Safe: can increase urinary oxalate levels; those with sugar sensitivity should use with caution	Pettit (2002); Gardiner et al (2000) (cites studies)
Warts (*Verruca Vulgaris*)	Duct tape occlusive therapy	Cover wart(s) with piece of duct tape for 6 days (if falls off, replace); remove tape: soak wart in warm water and file with emery board; replace tape the next day and repeat regimen for 2mo or until wart disappears (most resolve in 1mo)		Allergic reaction to tape	Focht et al (2002)

*Inclusion of a complementary treatment in this table does not imply endorsement by this textbook's authors; for reference only.
†Food supplements and herbal labeling classifications. *Class 1*, Herb can be safely consumed when used appropriately; *Class 2*, the following use restrictions apply: *2a*, for external use only; *2b*, not to be used during pregnancy; *2c*, not to be used while nursing; *2d*, other specific use restrictions as noted; *3*, requires label stating to be used only under supervision of an expert; *4*, insufficient data for classification.
‡Dr. Andrew Weil's mixture for head lice. Mix together:

2 oz olive or coconut oil

20gtts Tea-tree oil

10gtts either rosemary, lavender, or lemon essential oil

Rub into scalp and hair; cover with towel or shower cap for 1hr only; wash thoroughly and comb repeatedly with nit comb (Ditcheck & Greenfield, 2002, p. 350-351).

ADHD, Attention-deficit hyperactivity disorder; *bid*, twice daily; *BP*, blood pressure; *cap*, capsule; *CHO*, carbohydrate; *CNS*, central nervous system; *DHA*, docosahexaenoic acid; *DSM III*, *Diagnostic and Statistical Manual of Disorders*, third edition; *EPA*, eicosahexaenoic acid; *FDA*, Food and Drug Administration; *FSH-RH*, follicle-stimulating hormone; *GI*, gastrointestinal; *GnRH*, gonadotropin-releasing hormone; *HIV*, human immunodeficiency virus; *hr*, hour(s); *HTN*, hypertension; *IBD*, irritable bowel disease; *MAO*, monoamine oxidase; *min*, minutes; *mo*, month(s); *MSG*, monosodium glutamate; *NIH*, National Institutes of Health; *NSAID*, nonsteroidal antiinflammatory drug; *OA*, osteoarthritis; *ORS*, oral rehydration solution; *PMS*, premenstrual syndrome; *PO*, by mouth; *prn*, as needed; *qid*, 4 times daily; *RA*, rheumatoid arthritis; *RBC*, red blood cell; *RDA*, recommended dietary allowance; *sec*, seconds; *tabs*, tablets; *TB*, tuberculosis; *tbsp*, tablespoon; *tid*, 3 times daily; *tsp*, teaspoon; *USDA*, U.S. Department of Agriculture; *UTI*, urinary tract infection; *wk*, week(s); *yr*, year(s); *#*, pounds.

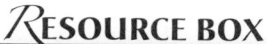
RESOURCE BOX

Complementary Therapies

RESEARCH STUDIES

Harvard Medical School Osher Institute: Division for Research and Education in Complementary and Integrative Medicine
www.osher.hms.harvard.edu

National Center for Complementary and Alternative Medicine (NCCAM), National Institutes of Health
www.nccam.nih.gov

Wake Forest University Baptist Medical Center: Program for Holistic and Integrative Medicine
www1.wfubmc.edu/phim

REGULATORY

Federation of State Medical Boards
www.fsmb.org

INTEGRATIVE EDUCATIONAL MODELS

Consortium of Academic Health Centers for Integrative Medicine (CAHCIM)
www.imconsortium.org

OTHER INFORMATION SOURCES

American Academy of Pediatrics Provisional Section on Complimentary, Holistic, and Integrative Medicine
www.aap.org/sections/chim/p&r.htm

Center for Studying Health System Change (HSC)
www.hschange.com
Designs and conducts studies about the U.S. health care system to understand forces driving change

Cochrane Electronic Library
www.theCochraneLibrary.com or www3.interscience.wiley.com/cgi-bin/mrwhome/106568753/Home?CRETRY=18.5Retry=O

HERBALS, DIETARY SUPPLEMENTS, OR NATURAL HEALTH PRODUCTS

American Herbal Products Association
www.ahpa.org
Evaluates safety of botanical ingredients

Consumer Laboratory
www.consumerlabs.com

Herb Gram
www.herbalgram.org
Journal of the American Botanical Council

Longwood Herbal Task Force
www.longwoodherbal.org
Monographs on common pediatric herbs

MedWatch (U.S. FDA)
www.fda.gov/medwatch

Natural Medicines Comprehensive Database
www.naturaldatabase.com
Subscription service; 1000 monographs of natural medicines available including evidence-based information, daily updates, drug interactions, safety ratings

NSF (National Sanitation Foundation) International
www.nsf.org

ONLINE COURSES IN COMPLEMENTARY, ALTERNATIVE, OR INTEGRATIVE MEDICINE

American College for Advancement in Medicine (ACAM)
www.acam.org

National Center for Complementary and Alternative Medicine (NCCAM)
www.nccam.nih.gov/videolectures

National Training Center and Clearinghouse
www.nnlm.gov/ntcc/ch

University of Arizona Program in Integrative Medicine
www.integrativemedicine.arizona.edu
Further Reading
Kemper K: *The holistic pediatrician*, New York, 2002, HarperCollins.

Wake Forest University Baptist Medical Center
www.wfubmc.edu
Class on herbs and dietary supplements

☑ DISCUSSION FORUM

1. Are there medicolegal implications for the use of complementary and alternative therapy?
2. What principles govern the use of CAM therapies?
3. Does your malpractice cover you for using CAM? Discuss areas of your clinical practice you feel lend themselves to incorporating CAM practices.
4. You are asked about dosage of an herbal preparation. How do you answer? Where do you get your information? Are there risks in giving information about herbal preparations? Where do you get current information about CAM?
5. Discuss how you would go about compiling a list of reliable complementary providers in your practice community. How would you go about setting up a collegial working relationship with them?

REFERENCES

Abrams G: Chiropractic treatment holds promise for low back pain, *Complement Med Physician* 2(9):66, 1997.

Adams KE, Cohen MH, Eisenberg D, et al: Ethical considerations of complementary and alternative medical therapies in conventional medical settings, *Ann Intern Med* 137(8):660-664, 2002.

Allen K: Using biofeedback to make childhood headaches less of a pain, *Ped Annals* 33(4):241-245, 2004.

American Academy of Pediatrics (AAP): Policy statement: counseling families who choose complementary and alternative medicine for their child with chronic illness or disability (RE0049), *Pediatrics* 107(3):598-601, 2001.

American Academy of Pediatrics (AAP): *Periodic survey #49: Complementary and alternative medicine (CAM) therapies in pediatric practices.* Available at *www.aap.org/research/periodicsurvey/ps496exs.htm* (accessed Aug 29, 2006).

American Association of Poison Control Centers: *2004 Annual report of the American Association of Poison Control Centers Toxic Exposure Surveillance System.* Available at *www.aapcc.org/2004.htm* (accessed on Aug 29, 2006).

Balch J, Balch P: *Prescription for nutritional healing,* ed 2, Garden City, NY, 1997, Avery.

Balogh Z, Ordögh J, Gász A, et al: Effectiveness of balneotherapy in chronic low back pain-a randomized single-blind controlled follow-up study, *Forsch Complementarmed Klass Naturheilkd* (Research in Complementary Natural Medicine) 12(4):196-201, 2005.

Barak V, Halperin T, Kalickman I: The effect of Sambucol, a black elderberry-based, natural product, on the production of human cytokines: I. inflammatory cytokines, *Eur Cytokine Netw* 12(2):290-296, 2001.

Barnes P, Powell-Griner E, McFann K, et al: Complementary and alternative medicine use among adults: United States, 2002, *CDC Advance Data Rep #343,* May 27, 2004. Available at *http://www.mbcrc.med.ucla.edu/PDFs/camsurvey2.pdf* (accessed Aug 26, 2006).

Bell E: Implications of using drugs "off-label," *Infect Dis Child* 15(11): 10-11, 2002.

Berbert AA, Kondo CR, Almendra CL, et al: Supplementatin of fish oil and olive oil in patients with rheumatoid arthritis, *Nutrition* 21(2):131-136, 2005.

Boris M, Mandel F: Foods and additives are common causes of the attention deficit hyperactive disorder in children, *Ann Allergy* 72:462-468, 1994.

Boyle CA, Sayers SP, Jensen BE, et al: The effects of yoga training and a single bout of yoga on delayed onset muscle soreness in the lower extremity, *J Strength Cond Res* 18(4):723-729, 2004.

Braganza S: The use of complementary therapies in inner-city asthmatic children, *J Asthma* 40(7):823-827, 2003.

Bravewell Collaborative, Philosophical Foundation for Integrative Medicine: Statement by Ralph Snyderman, MD. Available at *www.bravewell.org/integrative_medicine/philosophical_foundation* (accessed Aug 27, 2006a).

Bravewell Collaborative, Philosophical Foundation for Integrative Medicine: Mission statement. Available at *www.bravewell.org/transforming_healthcare/* (accessed Aug 27, 2006b).

Bryant M, Cassidy A, Hill C, et al: Effect of consumption of soy isoflavones on behavioral, somatic and affective symptoms in women with premenstrual syndrome, *Br J Nutr* 93(5):731-739, 2005.

Cala S: A survey of herbal use in children with attention-deficit-hyperactivity disorder or depression, *Pharmacotherapy* 23(2):222-230, 2003.

Carter CM et al: Effects of a few food diet in attention deficit disorder, *Arch Dis Child* 69:564-568, 1993.

Castleman M: *The healing herbs: the ultimate guide to the curative power of nature's medicines,* New York, 1995, Bantam.

Centers for Disease Control and Prevention (CDC), National Center for Health Statistics: *Complementary and alternative medicine use among adults: United States, 2002,* prepared by Barnes PA et al, No. 343, May 27, 2004. Available at *www.cdc.gov/nchs/pressroom/04news/adultsmedicine.htm* (accessed on Aug 26, 2006).

Chan E: The role of complementary and alternative medicine in attention-deficit hyperactivity disorder, *J Dev Behav Pediatr* 23(1S):S37-S44, 2002.

Chan E, Gardiner P, Kemper K: "At least it's natural …": herbs and dietary supplements in ADHD, *Contemp Pediatr* 17(9):116-130, 2000.

Cleary-Guida MB, Okvat HA, Oz MC, et al: A regional study of health insurance coverage for complementary and alternative medicine: current status and future ramifications, *J Alt Compl Med* 7(3):269-73, 2001.

Clinical Advisor editorial staff: Herbal medicine taken as a whole, *Clin Advisor* 1(11/12):51, 1998.

Clinical Evidence Concise, editorial staff: Secondary prevention of ischaemic cardiac events, *Clinical Evidence Concise,* Issue 9, London, 2003, BMJ Publishing Group.

Cohen MH, Kemper KJ: Complementary therapies in pediatrics: a legal perspective, *Pediatrics* 115(3):774-780, 2005.

Consortium of Academic Health Centers for Integrative Medicine (CAHCIM): Role. Available at *http://www.ahc.umn.edu/cahcim/about/home.html* (accessed on Aug 29, 2006).

del Mundo W, Shepherd W, Marose R: Use of alternative medicine by patients in a rural family practice clinic, *Fam Med* 34:206-212, 2002.

Ditchek SH, Greenfield RH: *Healthy child, whole child: integrating the best of conventional and alternative medicine to keep your kids healthy,* New York, Quill, 2002.

Egger J, Stolla A, McEwen L: Controlled trial of hyposensitisation in children with food-induced hyperkinetic syndrome, *Lancet* 339:1150-1153, 1992.

Eisenberg DM: Advising patients who seek alternative therapies, *Ann Intern Med* 127:61-69, 1997.

Eisenberg DM, Davis RB, Ettner SL, et al: Trends in alternative medicine use in the United States, 1990-1997: results of a follow-up national survey, *JAMA* 280:1569-1575, 1998.

Eisenberg DM, Kessler RC, Foster C, et al: Unconventional medicine in the United States: prevalence, costs and patterns of use, *N Engl J Med* 328:246-252, 1993.

Elder NC, Gillcrist A, Minz R: Use of alternative health care by family practice patients, *Arch Fam Med* 6:181-184, 1997.

Fenton MV, Morris DL: The integration of holistic nursing practices and complementary and alternative modalities into curricula of schools of nursing, *Altern Ther Health Med* 9(4):62-67, 2003.

Field T, Henteleff T, Hernandez-Reif M, et al: Children with asthma have improved pulmonary functions with massage therapy, *J Pediatr* 132:854-858, 1998.

Focht D, Spicer C, Fairchok M: The efficacy of duct tape vs cryotherapy in the treatment of *verruca vulgaris* (the common wart), *Arch Pediatr Adolesc Med* 156(10):971-977, 2002.

Food and Drug Administration: Medical Product Safety Information. Available at *www.fda.gov/medwatch/safety.htm* (accessed Aug 29, 2007).

Frid AH, Nilsson M, Holst JJ, et al: Effect of whey on blood glucose and insulin responses to composite breakfast and lunch meals in type 2 diabetic subjects, *Am J Clin Nutr* 82(1):69-75, 2005.

Frishberg M: Alternative medicine gaining wider acceptance, *Common Ground Reflections* 8-24, Jan 1998.

Fugh-Berman A: *Alternative medicine: what works,* Baltimore, 1997, Williams & Wilkins.

Gardiner P, Conboy L, Kemper K: Herbs and adolescent girls: avoiding the hazards of self-treatment, *Contemp Pediatr* 17(3):133-154, 2000.

Gardiner P, Kemper K: Herbs in pediatric and adolescent medicine, *Pediatr Rev* 21(2):44-57, 2000.

Gardiner P, Coles D, Kemper K: The skinny on herbal remedies for dermatologic disorders, *Contemp Pediatr* 18(7):103-113, 2001.

Gardiner P, Dvorkin L, Kemper KJ: Supplement use growing among children and adolescents, *Ped Ann* 33(4):227-232, 2004.

Gardiner P, Wood C, Kemper KJ: Dietary supplement use among healthcare professionals enrolled in an online curriculum on herbs and dietary supplements, *Complement Altern Med* 6: 21, 2006.

Gasalberti D: Alternative therapies for children and youth with special health care needs, *J Ped Health Care* 20(2):133-136, 2006.

Gideonse T: Music is good medicine, *Newsweek,* Sept 1998, p 103.

Good M, Stanton-Hicks M, Grass JA, et al: Relaxation and music to reduce postsurgical pain, *J Adv Nurs* 33(2):208-215, 2001.

Gordon J: Alternative medicine and the family physician, *Am Fam Physician* 54:2205-2212, 1996.

Gordon R: Close-up on complementary care: Is that all there is? Why more patients are seeking alternative therapies, *Adv Nurs Pract* 12(5):45-48, 2004.

Graedon J, Graedon T: *The people's pharmacy: guide to home and herbal remedies,* New York, 1999, Graedon Enterprises.

Graedon J, Graedon T: *Mouthwash may relieve pesky case of "jock itch."* Available at *www.peoplespharmacy.com/archives/herb_home_remedy_qa/listerine_works_against_jock_itch_and_dandruff.asp* (accessed Sept 15, 2006a).

Graedon J, Graedon T: *Cornmeal fights fungus on rose and toes.* Available at *www.peoplespharmacy.com/archives/herb_home_remedy_qa/cornmeal_fights_Fungus_on_roses_and_toes.asp* (accessed Sept 10, 2006b).

Graedon J, Graedon T: *Calming a cough calls for creativity.* Available at *wwww.peoplespharmacy.com/archives/editorial/calming_a_cough_calls_for_creativity.php* (accessed Sept 10, 2006c).

Graedon J, Graedon T: *Home remedy may ease misery of canker sores.* Available at *www. peoplespharmacy.com/archives/herb_home_remedy_qa/home_remedy_may_ease_misery_of_canker_sores.asp* (accessed Sept 10, 2006d).

Grazzi L, Andrasik F, D'Amico D, et al: Electromyographic biofeedback-assisted relaxation training in juvenile episodic tension-type headache: clinical outcome at three-year follow-up, *Cephalalgia* 21(8):798-803, 2001.

He HG, Pölkki T, Pietilä AM, et al: Chinese parent's use of nonpharmacological methods in children's postoperative pain relief, *Scand J Caring Sci* 20(1):2-9, 2006.

Heuschkel R, Afzal N, Wuerth A, et al: Complementary medicine use in children and young adults with inflammatory bowel disease, *Am J Gastroenterol* 97(2):382-388, 2002.

Hill N, Moor G, Cameron MM, et al: Single blind, randomized, comparative study of the Bug Buster kit and over the counter pediculicide treatments against head lice in the United Kingdom, *BMJ* 331(7513):326-3, 2005.

Holroyd KA, Mauskop A: Complementary and alternative treatments, *Neurology* 60(7):S58, 2003.

Janiger O, Goldberg P: *A different kind of healing,* New York, 1993, Putnam.

Johnson K: The elimination diet and diagnosing food hypersensitivities. In Rakel O: *Integrative medicine,* Philadelphia, 2003, WB Saunders.

Jonas W: Alternative medicine-learning from the past, examining the present, advancing to the future, *JAMA* 280:1616-1617, 1998.

Kankkunen P, Vehviläinen-Julkunen K, Pietilä AM, et al: Parents' use of nonpharmacological methods to alleviate children's postoperative pain at home, *J Adv Nurs* 41(4):367-375, 2003.

Kemper KJ: *The holistic pediatrician,* New York, HarperCollins, 1996.

Kemper KJ, Sarah R, Silver-Highfield E, et al: On pins and needles? Pediatric pain patients' experience with acupuncture, *Pediatrics* 105(4 pt 2):941-947, 2000.

Kemper KJ: Complementary and alternative medicine for children: does it work? *West J Med* 174:272-276, 2001.

Kemper KJ, Wornham W: Consultations for holistic pediatric services for inpatients and outpatient oncology patients at a children's hospital, *Arch Pediatr Adolesc Med* 155(4):449-454, 2001.

Kemper KJ: *The holistic pediatrician,* ed 2, New York, 2002a, HarperCollins.

Kemper KJ: Otitis media: when parents don't want antibiotics or tubes, *Cont Pediatr* 4:47, 2002b.

Kemper KJ, Jacobs J: Homeopathy in pediatrics-no harm likely, but how much good? *Contemp Pediatr* 20(5):97, 2003.

Kemper KJ, Cohen M: Ethics meet complementary and alternative medicine: new light on old principles, *Contemp Pediatr* 21:61, 2004.

Kemper KJ, Kelly EA: Treating children with therapeutic and healing touch, *Ped Ann* 33(4):249-252, 2004.

Kemper KJ et al: Attitudes and expectations about music therapy for premature infants among staff in a neonatal intensive care unit, *Altern Ther Health Med* 10(2):50-54, 2004.

Kemper KJ, Jennings D: Consider the benefits of music therapy for your patients, *Contemp Pediatr* 22(2):59, 2005.

Kessler RC, Davis RB, Foster DF, et al: Long-term trends in the use of complementary and alternative medical therapies in the United States, *Ann Intern Med* 135(4):262-268, 2001.

Kimmatkar J, Thawani V, Hingorani L, et al: Efficacy and tolerability of *Boswellia serrata* extract in treatment of osteoarthritis of the knee-a randomizeddouble blind placebo controlled trial, *Phytomedicine* 10(1):3-7, 2003.

Klein S, Winkelstein M: Enhancing pediatric health care with music, *J Pediatr Health Care* 10:74-81, 1996.

Kleinman L, Kosecoff J, Dubois RW, et al: The medical appropriateness of tympanostomy tubes proposed for children younger than 16 years in the United States, *JAMA* 271:1250-1255, 1994.

Koh JL, Harrison D, Palermo TM, et al: Assessment of acute and chronic pain symptoms in children with cystic fibrosis, *Pediatr Pulmonol* 40(4):330-335, 2005.

Konefal J: The challenge of educating physicians about complementary and alternative medicine, *Acad Med* 77(9):847-850, 2002.

Krebs M: The sweet smell of healing: promote wellness with aromatherapy, *Adv Nurs Practi* 14 (5):41-44, 2006.

Kreitzer MJ, Mitten D, Harris I, et al: Attitudes toward CAM among medical, nursing, and pharmacy faculty and students: a comparative analysis, *Altern Ther Health Med* 8(6):50-53, 2002.

Landmark Healthcare: *Landmark report on public perceptions of alternative care,* Sacramento, 1998, Landmark Healthcare.

LaValle J, Krinsky DL, Hawkins EB, et al: *Natural therapeutics pocket guide 2000-2001,* Hudson, OH, 2000, Lexi-Comp.

Lin YC, Bioteau AB, Ferrari LR, et al: The use of herbs and complementary and alternative medicine in pediatric preoperative patients, *J Clin Anesth* 16(1):4-6, 2004.

Loewy J, Hallan C, Friedman E, et al: Sleep-sedation in children undergoing EEG testing: a comparison of chloral hydrate and music therapy, *J Perianaest Nurs* 20(5):323-332, 2005.

Ly KA, Milgrom P, Rothen M: Xylitol, sweeteners, and dental caries, *Pediatr Dent* 28(2):154-163, 2006.

Mack R: "Something wicked this way comes"—herbs even witches should avoid, *Contemp Pediatr* 15(6):49-64, 1998.

Mancho P, Edwards QT: Chaste tree for premenstrual syndrome, *Adv Nurs Practi* 13(5):43-46, 2005.

Marcolina S: Topical aloe vera for skin and oral wounds, *Altern Med Alert* 1:8-11, 2001.

Markestad T: Use of sucrose as a treatment for infant colic, *Arch Dis Child* 76:356-358, 1997.

McGuffin M, Goldberg A, editors: *American Herbal Products Association's botanical Safety handbook,* New York, 1998, CRC Press.

McNeil D: Health agency embarks on survey of alternative medicine, *Oregonian: International,* Friday, May 17, 2002, p A10.

Micozzi M: *Fundamentals of complementary and alternative medicine,* New York, 1996, Churchill Livingstone.

Micozzi M: The common principles of complementary health care systems: enduring concepts with current clinical relevance, *Complement Med Physician* 2(8):1, 1997.

Miller PC, Bailey SP, Barnes ME, et al: The effects of protease supplementation on skeletal muscle function and DOMS following downhill running, *J Sports Sci* 22(4):365-372, 2004.

Miller SK: Magnet therapy for pain control, *Adv Nurs Practi* 12(5):49-52, 2004.

Mortimore J, Fischer S: Are we ready to give herbal remedies to children? Health Care Agency, County of Orange, California, *Nutrition Times* 3(1):1-3, 2001.

Murray M, Pizzorno J: *Encyclopedia of natural medicine,* ed 2, Rocklin, 1998, Prima Health.

National Center for Complementary and Alternative Medicine (NCCAM): National Institutes for Health, National Center for Health Statistics *National Health Interview Survey—2002,* published 2004. Available at *www.NCCAM.nih.gov/ccamonpubmed* (accessed Aug 26, 2006).

National Center for Complementary and Alternative Medicine (NCCAM): Strategic Plan 2005-2009. Available at *www.nccam.nih.gov/research* (accessed Aug 26, 2006).

National Institutes of Health: Consensus conference: acupuncture, *JAMA* 280:1518-1524, 1998.

Nickerson J, Silberman T: Chiropractic manipulation in children, *J Pediatr* 12:172, 1992.

Nsouli TM, Nsouli SM, Linde RE, et al: Role of food allergy in serous otitis media, *Ann Allergy* 73:215-219, 1994.

O'Brien M: Integrated geriatrics: optimizing and gentling health care for the elderly, *Complement Med Physician* 3(5):1, 1998.

Ott M: Yoga as a clinical intervention: pain control and stress reduction may be just a breath away, *Adv Nurse Pract* 10(1):81-90, 2002.

Ottolini MC, Hamburger EK, Loprieato JO, et al: Complementary and alternative medicine use among children in the Washington, DC area, *Ambul Pediatr* 1(2):122-125, 2001.

Patel BD, Welch AA, Bingham SA, et al: Dietary antioxidants and asthma in adults, *Thorax* 61(5):388-393, 2006.

Pettit J: Alternative medicine: cranberry, *Clin Rev* 12(1):43-44, 2002.

Pizzorno J: *The clinician's handbook of natural medicine,* ed 1, Philadelphia, Churchill Livingstone, 2002.

Pratt SG, Matthews K: *SuperFoods Rx: fourteen foods that will change your life,* New York, 2004, HarperCollins.

Rakel D: *Rakel's integrative medicine,* Philadelphia, WB Saunders, 2003.

Ramsay C: *Overkill: The regulation of natural health products in Canada.* Fraser Forum, Feb 2002. The Fraser Institute Web page. Available at *www.Fraserinstitute.org/commerce.web/publication_details.aspx?pubID=2630* (accessed Jan 11, 2003).

Reilly AM: Massage therapy: integration with traditional medicine, *Adv Nurs Practi* 13(5):37-42, 2005.

Reznik M, Ozuah PO, Franco K, et al: Use of complementary therapy by adolescents with asthma, *Arch Pediatr Adolesc Med* 156(10):1042-1044, 2002.

Richardson SF: Complementary health and healing in nursing education, *J Holistic Nurs* 21 (1):20-23, 2003.

Rini A, Bloom K: Down in the mouth: update on treatment of oral aphthous ulcers, *Clin Advisor* 5(2):67-72, 2002.

Rowe K, Rowe K: Synthetic food coloring and behavior: a dose response effect in a double-blind placebo-controlled, repeated-measure study, *J Pediatr* 125:691-697, 1994.

Scharff C, Kemper KJ: For chronic pain, complementary and alternative medical approaches, *Contemp Pediatr* 20:117, 2003.

Schoch R: A conversation with Dana Ullman, *Calif Monthly*, Feb 1999, pp 27-30.

Schoetzau A, Filipiak-Pittroff B, Franke K, et al: Effect of exclusive breast-feeding and early solid food avoidance on the incidence of atopic dermatitis in high-risk infants at 1 year of age, *Pediatr Allergy Immunol* 13(4):234-242, 2002.

Schulman SL, Von Zuben FC, Plachter, N et al: Biofeedback methodology: does it matter how we teach children how to relax the pelvic floor during voiding? *J Urol* 166(6):2423-2426, 2001.

Sego S: What clinicians should know about herbals, *Clin Adv* 10(1):46-51, 2006.

Shah PS, Aliwalas LI Shah V: Breastfeeding or breast milk for procedural pain in neonates, *Cochrane Database Syst Rev* 19 (CD004950): 3, 2006.

Shedletsky P, Gale EN, Levine MS: The effects of ice massage applied over the "Koku" acupuncture point I reducing spontaneous pain of endodontic origin, *J Can Dent Assoc* 50(8):635-638, 1984.

Simpson N, Roman K: Complementary medicine use in children: extent and reasons. A population-based study, *Br J Gen Pract* 51(472):914-916, 2001.

Snyderman R, Weil W: *Abstract: Integrative medicine: bringing medicine back to its roots.* Available at *www.bravewell.org/content/pdf/14_Synderman_Weil_Article.pdf* (accessed on Aug 27, 2006).

Soeken KL: Selected CAM therapies for arthritis-related pain: the evidence from systematic reviews, *Clin J Pain* 20(1):13-18, 2004.

Sohn PM, Loveland Cook CA: Nurse practitioner knowledge of complementary alternative healthcare, *J Adv Nurs* 39(1):9-16, 2002.

Spiegelblatt L: Alternative medicine: a pediatric conundrum, *Contemp Pediatr* 14(8):51-64, 1997.

Starobrat-Hermelin B, Kozielec T: The effects of magnesium physiological supplementation on hyperactivity in children with ADHD. Positive response to magnesium oral loading test, *Magnes Res* 10(2):149-156, 1997.

Thaut M: Music therapy: the unsung modality, *Complement Med Physician* 3(6):1, 1998.

The Oregonian: Want to know if natural remedies work? April 5, 2006, pF3.

Therapeutic Research Center: Therapeutic uses of herbs. Continuing Education #97-005, *Prescriber's Letter,* Fall 1997.

Therapeutic Research Center: Therapeutic uses of herbs. Continuing Education Booklet, *Prescriber's Letter*, Spring 1998.

Ting W, Gross M, Oz M: The Internet as a research tool in complementary and alternative medicine: a pilot study, *Altern Ther Health Med* 8(3): 84-86, 2002.

Tu HT, Hargraves JL: High cost of medical care prompts consumers to seek alternatives. Center for Studying Health System Change, *Data Bulletin No. 28,* 2004. Available at *www.hschange.com/content/722/?words.* (accessed on Aug 31, 2006).

Turow V: Chiropractic for children, *Arch Pediatr Adolesc Med* 151:527-528, 1997.

University of California, Berkeley: *Wellness Letter: the newsletter of nutrition, fitness, and self-care* 22(1):1, 2005.

University of California Berkeley: *Acupuncture scores points, University of California wellness Letter* 14(8):2, 1998.

Voss JA, Good M, Yates B et al: Sedative music reduces anxiety and pain during chair rest after open-heart surgery, *Pain* 112(1-2):197-203, 2004.

Walach J, Guthlin C, Konig M: Efficacy of massage therapy in chronic pain: a pragmatic randomized trial, *J Altern Complement Med* 9(6):837-846, 2003.

Walker AF, Bundy R, Hicks SM, et al: Bromelain reduces mild acute knee pain and improves well-being in a dose-dependent fashion in an open study of otherwise healthy adults, *Phytomedicine* 9(8):681-686, 2002.

Wilson KM, Klein JD: Adolescents' use of complementary medicine, *Ambul Pediatr* 2(2):104-110, 2002.

Winslow C, Shapiro H: Physicians want education about complementary and alternative medicine to enhance communication with their patients, *Arch Intern Med* 162(10):1176-1181, 2002.

White AR, Ernst E: Economic analysis of complementary medicine: a systemic review, *Complement Ther Med* 8 (2):111-118, 2000.

World Health Organization: Oral Rehydration Salts (ORS): A new reduced osmolarity formulation. Available at *www.who.int/child-adolescant-health/New_Publications/News/Statement.htm* (accessed Feb 23, 2003).

Wyatt G, Post-White J: Future direction of complementary and alternative medicine (CAM) education and research, *Semin Oncol Nurs* 21(3): 2005.

Wysocki S: Unconventional and conventional medicine: searching for common ground, *Contemp Nurse Pract,* Winter 1997, pp 3-15.

Zakay-Rones A, Thom E, Wollan T, et al: Randomized study of the efficacy and safety of oral elderberry extract in the treatment of influenza A and B virus infections, *J Int Med Res* 32(2):132-40, 2004.

Zeltzer LK, Tsao JC, Stelling C, et al: A phase I study on the feasibility and acceptability of an acupuncture/hypnosis intervention for chronic pediatric pain, *J Pain Symptom Manage* 24(4):437-446, 2002.

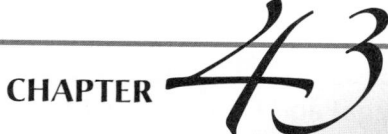

Practice Management Strategies for a Health Care Practice

Denise A. Hall

A successful health care practice requires the provision of excellent clinical care, a commitment to good customer service, sound business planning, efficient day-to-day operations, and ongoing attention to administrative and risk management operations. If the practice has excellent clinical providers but does not pay attention to or does not devote equal resources to its business operation, its future ability to operate will be compromised. This chapter is a primer for setting up and managing a health care practice and provides brief overviews of key administrative and clinical management strategies necessary for successful practice operations.

Paying attention to business operations in a medical practice can seem like a daunting task at times. Staying current with state and federal regulations, employment laws, and risk management issues requires constant vigilance and attention. Compliance with these legal requirements is only the beginning of ensuring good business operations. Strategic planning; financial management; staff recruiting, training, and retention; efficient administrative and clinical operations; ongoing practice benchmarking; risk management awareness; marketing; customer service and patient education are all areas that can make a practice either mediocre or outstanding and are basic and necessary elements of successful medical practice management.

The development of a business plan and an operations plan are two practice management strategies that can provide the structure for many of the administrative and clinical recommendations that make the practice successful.

THE BUSINESS PLAN

Developing a business plan is a requisite first step in the development of a new practice and is also recommended for established practices when considering a new project or change in business operations (e.g., adding a new provider, opening a new office, or offering new services). The business plan clearly declares the philosophy and goals of the practice on which an overall strategic plan will be based and how these goals will be reached. Even a simple one- or two-page plan can help provide a formal structure for present and future planning. A *vision statement, market analysis, strategic plan,* and *organizational chart* make up a simple business plan for the practice and provide the necessary framework for clinical and administrative operations. If the practice is seeking

funds from a financial institution or granting organization, a business plan will most certainly be requested as part of the application process.

VISION STATEMENT

This vision statement is the foundation for all clinical and administrative operations of the practice. It may be one or two simple sentences or one or two paragraphs, but it should summarize the practice's reason for being and the philosophy of the organization. It is a good idea to revisit the vision statement annually to ensure that it continues to reflect the mission and values of the practice.

MARKET ANALYSIS

A market analysis is a primary and critical key task that should be done to better understand the specific demographic makeup of the targeted patient population. This analysis looks at the current and future demand or need for (pediatric) health care services in a particular area and the current capacity or options for providing these services. Factors, such as population data, growth projections, primary care competition, and the current economic and business climate, are important areas to review. Gathering this information requires time and effort, but is important for good decision-making for new business operations and for short- and long-range planning.

STRATEGIC PLAN

The vision statement and market analysis are used together to formulate the strategic plan for the practice. A strategic plan is useful for starting a new practice, planning practice growth, or simply developing new projects. It provides both framework and direction for the task at hand and sets the business plan in motion. The strategic plan normally includes the following:

- Goals and objectives identified by the practice
- Budget or financial plan
- Physical and human resource requirements of the project
- Operations plan for development and implementation, including a timeline

ORGANIZATIONAL CHART

An organizational chart is a helpful administrative resource for the strategic plan and ongoing practice operations. The organizational chart normally shows names, titles, and reporting responsibilities of the people involved in implementing the business and operations plans of the practice. It not only provides a visual snapshot of the management structure of the practice, but also connects its business plan with the practice's personnel resources. An organizational chart can be valuable in assisting the practice in clarifying roles and responsibilities for ownership, management, and staff.

■ THE OPERATIONS PLAN

Successfully moving the business plan from paper to reality requires additional planning and implementation. The operations plan provides structure during this process and helps ensure that key elements for successful practice management are not overlooked. It uses the formal business plan for its initial direction, but has a different purpose. Its goal is to take more of a micromanagement view of the business and strategic plan and make them fully functional. The development of an annual operations plan and corresponding budget is a valuable process and tool for ensuring that the practice's clinical, administrative, and financial goals and operations are integrated. Although every practice is individual and distinct, and business plans differ by design and need, the operating plan establishes systems and processes by which to:

- Identify key practice management areas and practice resources.
- Develop policies and procedures to ensure administrative and clinical quality assurance.
- Monitor, report, and benchmark clinical and administrative results.
- Emphasize quality improvement and customer service.

Operational checklists are included in this chapter for the areas of legal and governance operations, financial, human resources, and clinical operations. The checklists include a basic list of elements and issues that are important in practice operations, regardless of size or strategy.

LEGAL AND GOVERNANCE OPERATIONS

Legal counsel and a certified public accountant (CPA) are valuable resources to consult when establishing the practice's legal and governance operations. Developing a strong business relationship with an attorney and accountant with experience in health care operations is valuable, not only for the start-up phase of a health care practice, but also for ongoing consultation. Box 43-1 includes a checklist of major items included in this category that need to be taken into consideration, especially for a new practice.

Organizational Structure and Tax Status

Choosing an organizational structure (normally a partnership or corporation) and a tax status are two initial decisions required when starting a practice or in subsequent years if the practice undergoes ownership changes or it is beneficial to take advantage of new tax laws relating to business structures. Because of the numerous legal and financial implications involved when choosing an organizational structure, it is imperative to have good legal advice during this process. Trusted financial and legal advice is also essential when drafting the practice's

---

BOX 43-1	**Legal and Governance Checklist**

- Legal counsel
- Accountant
- Organizational structure
  - ○ Partnership, corporation
  - ○ Tax status
  - ○ Governance documents
- Federal tax employer identification number (EIN)
- National practice identification number (NPI)
- State and local tax identification numbers
- Business licenses
- Provider clinical license and DEA
- National provider identification number (NPI)
- Insurance requirements
  - ○ General liability
  - ○ Professional liability
  - ○ Workers' compensation
- Government regulations
  - ○ Occupational Safety and Health Administration (OSHA)
  - ○ Health Insurance Portability and Accountability Act (HIPAA)
  - ○ Clinical Laboratory and Improvement Amendments of 1988 (CLIA)
- Legal guidelines
  - ○ Record retention

---

governance documents, such as bylaws, articles of incorporation, employment agreements, and buy-sell agreements, and when reviewing lease documents and contracts.

Federal Tax Identification, National Provider Identification and Required Licenses

In addition to appropriate legal documents, the practice will require a federal tax identification number, also called an employer identification number (EIN), and a national provider identification number (NPI). A state tax identification number is required for state tax reporting, and most cities require a local business license.

There are also identification and licensing requirements for health care providers. All providers should have an NPI. Most states require a state license and a Drug Enforcement Administration (DEA) number as minimum requirements.

Insurance Requirements

Basic insurance requirements for the practice include general liability, professional liability, and workers' compensation insurance. *General liability insurance* protects the assets of the business from casualty damage, employee dishonesty, theft, business interruption, and personal injury. *Professional liability insurance* provides coverage for both individual providers and the practice in the event of a claim of medical malpractice. Professional liability insurance is written on either a claims-made or an occurrence basis. Because claims-made policies normally require the purchase of a "tail" or extended coverage in the event that the policy is terminated, it is important to understand the differences and which type of coverage is offered under the policy. When purchasing professional liability insurance, it is wise to insure the practice and the individual providers. Insuring the practice provides an added layer of protection in the event of a medical malpractice claim and also includes coverage for clinical and administrative support staff. Limits of $1.5 million to $2 million for each occurrence with an aggregate limit of $3 million to $4 million are currently considered minimal standards of protection. The practice will need to review the pros and cons of individual policies for providers versus obtaining coverage on a group basis. This decision may vary based on practice preference, organizational structure, or legal or insurance company recommendations.

Workers' compensation insurance protects the practice and its employees against accidents or injuries on the job. Examples of accidents that most often happen in a health care practice are needle-stick injuries; injuries caused by lifting or moving patients, equipment, or files; and repetitive motion types of injuries suffered by administrative staff. The practice's annual claims experience will impact its premiums for workers' compensation coverage; consequently an ongoing training program regarding safety in the workplace is important for good risk management and managing practice expenses.

Government Regulations

There are numerous and important regulations for health care practices. Special attention must be given to these regulations to ensure awareness, training, and compliance.

Health Insurance Portability and Accountability Act. The newest regulation affecting health care providers is the Health Insurance Portability and Accountability Act (HIPAA). Although the section of this regulation dealing with the portability of health insurance (Consolidated Omnibus Budget Reconciliation Act [COBRA]) has been in effect since 1996, two new sections on privacy and security have important relevance for health care providers. The primary purpose of the privacy section of HIPAA is to protect the rights of patients. HIPAA regulations define how providers must treat protected health information (PHI). HIPAA regulations now require health care providers to provide all patients with a "Notice of Privacy Practices." This notice informs patients of their rights under HIPAA and how the practice will use and disclose their PHI for treatment, payment, or health care operations purposes. Other parts of this regulation include requirements for the electronic transfer of PHI and for the development of business associate contracts with organizations with which the practice may share confidential information (outside billing or collection agencies, medical records couriers, transcription companies, answering services, etc.). Other sections of HIPAA contain regulations that require specific security precautions for the safety and confidentiality of electronic health information. Being HIPAA compliant requires the practice to develop policies and procedures that ensure confidentiality of patient information within the practice and to orient and train staff in these areas.

Occupational Safety and Health Administration. The Occupational Safety and Health Administration (OSHA), a division of the Department of Labor, regulates health and safety in the workplace. Medical offices are required to meet safety standards regarding universal precautions, blood-borne pathogens, and tuberculosis and are required to have written policies that enforce these standards. Practices must also provide education and annual training to staff and keep accurate records regarding any injuries and exposures that may have occurred. OSHA standards focus on infection control and contain guidelines for personal protective equipment, frequent hand washing, decontamination, and waste disposal.

Clinical Laboratory and Improvement Amendments of 1988. The Clinical Laboratory and Improvement Amendments of 1988 (CLIA) set performance standards and licensing requirements for hospital and physician-office laboratories based on the complexity of the tests being performed. CLIA standards focus on personnel qualifications of laboratory staff, quality control, quality assurance, and proficiency testing. A procedure manual that details how to perform every test conducted in the laboratory must be kept up to date. Based on the complexity of tests performed, the laboratory will have a CLIA designation of waived, physician-performed microscopy (PPM), moderate complexity, or high complexity. When determining what types of laboratory tests or services will be performed in the office, it is important to ensure that the practice has the necessary CLIA designation before providing those services. For example, a rapid strep test could be categorized as waived, PPM, or moderate based on the particular brand of the test. A cost-benefit analysis should be undertaken as part of any decision regarding laboratory services. The cost of CLIA compliance, proficiency testing, equipment, and staffing of the laboratory are costs that should be included along with the price of the individual tests when analyzing clinical needs, potential reimbursement, and customer service.

Retention of Records

There are specific guidelines for the retention of all records and business documents in the health care practice. Requirements vary depending on the type of records (medical records, financial records, claims and billing records, staff and employment records). Table 43-1 contains general recommendations for records retention. As the practice gets larger, the retention of records can become an expensive storage problem. New technologies, such as optical scanners and electronic file cabinets, can help practices meet these requirements in an efficient manner.

▆ FINANCIAL OPERATIONS

Managing the revenues and expenses of a practice requires the establishment of good financial and accounting systems. This includes the development and implementation of financial policies and processes to ensure necessary cash flow for the financial health of the practice and regular monitoring, review, and reporting of its revenues and expenses (Box 43-2). The following steps are recommended when establishing the financial operations of the practice.

- Establish a professional relationship with a bank or other financial institution for the purposes of opening a checking account, a payroll checking account, a savings account, and a line of credit.

TABLE 43-1 **Guidelines for Record Retention**

Document/Records	Months to Keep
Agenda or schedules	24
Bank statements	60
Budgets	60
Cancelled checks	60
Committee meeting minutes	60
Contracts	60 (after expiration)
Employment applications	36
Financial reports	60
Financial statements	Life of organization
Insurance documents	36
Insurance policies	72 (after expiration)
Invoices	72
Policies	Life of organization
Accounts receivable	84
Account reconciliations	24
Reports	60
Tax returns	72
Medical records	Pediatric records should be kept a minimum of 7 year past age of majority

Developed from Recommendations of the American Society of Association Executives and the U.S. Code of Federal Regulations.

BOX 43-2 **Financial Operations Checklist**

- Accountant
- Bank accounts
- Accounting software
- Chart of accounts
- Budgets
  - Operations
  - Personnel
  - Capital expense
- Payroll
- Financial reports
- Revenue cycle

- Work closely with an accountant to develop the bookkeeping and accounting systems to meet the needs of the practice. Depending on the size and sophistication of the practice this may mean that the accountant actively reviews financial operations on a monthly basis and prepares the financial reports or is used more as a business consultant. In either case, the accountant will probably be responsible for preparing annual tax returns.
- Choose computerized accounting software. A packaged accounting software, such as Quick Books or Quicken, usually meets the needs of a small- to medium-sized practice, whereas larger organizations with multiple locations and many cost centers may require a more powerful and sophisticated system. The accountant should be able to suggest a system that will best meet the needs of the practice. The

system should not only be able to manage accounts payables and write checks, but should also be able to develop budgets, automate payroll, and provide a standard set of financial reports. The practice's accountant can also help decide whether to operate the accounting system on a cash basis, an accrual basis, or a modified cash basis. Most medical practices use a cash or modified cash basis of accounting.

- Establish a chart of accounts. The chart of accounts plays a key role in budgeting and financial reporting. Although any chart of accounts that can break out and report on revenue sources and track expenses by similar types will suffice, the practice may wish to adopt a chart of accounts similar to the one recommended by the Medical Group Management Association (MGMA). Setting up the chart of accounts so that financial reports are comparable with those of other similar medical groups can be helpful not only for the management of revenue and expenses in the practice, but also for comparison or benchmarking purposes.
- Establish internal controls. Safeguarding the assets of the practice is an important part of good financial operations. Policies and procedures for the handling and depositing of cash and checks, reconciling bank statements, check signing, and petty cash management are several issues that need attention in this area.
- Prepare an operations budget. The development of an operations budget is important as a tool for (1) synchronizing the clinical and administrative operations of the practice with the anticipated revenues and expenses, (2) monitoring the revenues and expenses throughout the year, and (3) reporting the status of actual financial operations compared with the budgeted plan.

OPERATIONS BUDGET

An annual operations budget should be developed in conjunction with the practice's operations plan and usually starts with a detailed look at the anticipated revenues of the practice (revenues from third-party payers or insurance payers, patient payments, and ancillary services). The fee schedule, insurance reimbursement data, average collection rates, and patient visit data are all important elements used to forecast practice revenues. Revenue projections should not only look back at historical data and current contracts, but should also take into account any anticipated changes that will affect the practice. Potential new sources of revenues, anticipated growth, and changes in contracts can all affect practice revenue and should be included in the budget process.

Practice Expenses

Salaries and Benefits. In most instances, the biggest expense for a health care practice is personnel. Personnel and supporting expenses are listed in the budget as salaries and benefits. Development of this part of the budget will also require projections based on past and projected patient visit data. The anticipated patient visit data will be helpful in determining the number of providers and support staff required. A separate *personnel budget* developed using spreadsheet software, such as Excel, can help with planning this part of the expense budget. The personnel budget should identify titles, departments, full-time equivalent (FTE) status, hourly rate or salary, and projected annual compensation, including estimated salary increases and overtime. The chart of accounts normally specifies separate line items for budgeted salaries for physicians, nurse practitioners, physician assistants, management, and support staff. After the total salary expense is determined, the amount to budget for payroll taxes can be calculated (usually a percentage of the total salary expense). Benefit costs, such as health or dental insurance, can also be projected using a spreadsheet and then transferred to the operating budget. If practice policies or employment agreements provide additional benefits, such as continuing medical education or professional dues, these totals should also be added as a specific line item in the benefits budget category.

Other Expenses.   Other operating expenses in the budget will fall under the categories of *physical resources, general and administrative expenses,* or *purchased services,* and these should be included as separate sections in the budget and in financial reports. Examples of expenses budgeted as physical resources are occupancy costs (rent or mortgage payments), janitorial expense, medical supplies (including vaccines), printing of clinical forms, or any expense directly used for the provision of medical services. General and administrative expenses are those that pay for the administrative operations of the practice. Office supplies, administrative printing, telephone (including pagers), insurance, and depreciation expenses are examples of expenses that belong in this category. Expenses that fall under the classification of purchased services are fees paid to others for specific services provided. Accounting and legal services, answering service, telephone support, computer support, and marketing services are examples of purchased services.

Fixed Asset Expenses.   If the practice is planning to purchase any furniture or equipment or make significant improvements to the facility that are considered "major" in nature (usually over $500), a capital expense budget and corresponding depreciation schedules should also be developed.

After the budget is finalized, the revenue and expense line items should be spread over a 12-month period so that they can be tracked, monitored, and reported by month. These expenses can either be spread equally over the 12 months of the year, or they can be adjusted based on known revenue or expense patterns.

FINANCIAL REPORTS

At a minimum, a basic set of monthly financial reports should include a profit and loss (income/expense), a year-to-date profit and loss compared with budget, and a balance sheet. The practice's accounting software system should be able to produce these basic reports and other financial reports that can be beneficial in tracking the financial performance of the practice. The practice may want to review additional reports on a quarterly or annual basis.

PAYROLL

In a small practice, the accounting software can usually be used to prepare the payroll, calculate withholding taxes, and help ensure that tax deposits are made in a timely manner. Practices with more than 20 employees, or even small practices without the staff or the desire to manage this function, may want to explore using a payroll service for convenience and cost efficiencies. In any case, a method for hourly employees to record and report hours worked will be necessary. There are a variety of ways for employees to track and report time—from manual time sheets to electronic systems that integrate with the payroll or accounting system. If the practice has both exempt (salaried) and nonexempt (hourly) staff, it is usually advisable to have two separate payroll schedules. For example, hourly staff can be paid on a biweekly basis (every 2 weeks) and salaried staff on a semimonthly or monthly basis. This schedule assists with cash flow and balancing time management for payroll preparation.

REVENUE CYCLE

The revenue cycle of the practice is a critical concept to understand and manage. It is the all-inclusive system that starts with the development of a fee schedule and ends with reimbursement for services performed. Good policies and procedures and knowledgeable staff are important to ensure optimal revenue and cash flow for the practice. Included in the revenue cycle are the following elements:

• Contracts with commercial insurance, Medicare, and Medicaid—Contracts may be for individual providers or for the practice with individual providers listed under the group contract. Providers will need to be "credentialed" with the insurance company before being added to a contract or receiving an individual contract. A standard universal credentialing is often used (e.g., CAQH) for the initial and renewal credentialing process. Besides the reimbursement rate or fee schedule, important things to review in a contract include timely filing guidelines, methods for appeals, prompt payment guidelines, product lines, length of contract, specific requirements for patient access, and claims filing requirements.

• Fee schedule—The practice will need a fee schedule that lists its prices for the services it provides. A highly recommended process for development of the fee schedule is to use the Medicare RBRVS (Resource Based Relative Value Scale). The RBRVS schedule is based on a formula of work values and practice and professional liability expenses and is adjusted by geographic region. The Medicare RBRVS table is adjusted annually and is the amount used for Medicare reimbursement. Many commercial payers also use the RBRVS formula in determining reimbursement rates. Similarly, the practice can use the RBRVS formula to develop its own fee schedule. It is important to coordinate the fee schedule with practice contracts (e.g., if the practice's highest reimbursement contract is negotiated at 130% of RBRVS, the practice's fee schedule will normally be set at a minimum of 135% to 140% of RBRVS). This ensures that the practice receives full reimbursement under its contracts and maintains a buffer for new contracts, contract changes, and those contracts that may not be based on RBRVS. At the same time, it is important to not set the RBRVS percentage of the fee schedule too high. A fee schedule that is too high will (1) falsely inflate the practice's accounts receivables and (2) place a higher burden on uninsured patients or patients with deductibles. See the Resource Box at the end of the chapter for more information on RBRVS.

- Charge ticket—The charge ticket or "superbill" is the document the provider uses to communicate the services provided and the diagnosis for the visit. It should be as comprehensive as possible and easy for the provider to use to ensure that all services provided are identified and billed. It is also important to have a system that accounts for all charge tickets so that if one comes up missing it can be identified and recreated by the provider using the documentation in the medical record. Plan on reviewing and revising the charge ticket at least once a year to make annual CPT and ICD revisions.
- Patient registration form—The patient registration form provides several important functions. Primarily, it is a record of the patient's current demographic and insurance information. It can also function as a consent-to-treat form, and it can often be a valuable resource for additional data if needed for collection purposes (employment, social security, additional family members, etc.). Patient demographic and insurance information should be reviewed at each visit to ensure the practice has accurate information on file and in the chart for both clinical and administrative operations.
- Verification of insurance eligibility—Verification of a patient's insurance eligibility should be done as early as possible in the revenue cycle. Ideally, it should be done before the visit, but in any case, it should be done before submitting a claim. Verifying insurance before the claim is submitted may add a day or two longer to the billing process, but is a proactive step that can prevent denials and save time and money for the practice.
- Accurate CPT and ICD-9 coding—Choosing the correct CPT code for services provided can be challenging for even the most experienced provider, and modifiers and special situations can add more uncertainty to the process. Continuing education and coding assistance for providers and billing staff are important not only for ensuring that the practice is getting adequate reimbursement, but also to guard against fraud and overcoding.
- Charge entry (manual or electronic)—Entering the charges from the charge tickets into the practice management system should be done accurately and in a timely fashion. In most cases, setting a guideline of having charges posted by three to five days after the date of service should give the billing staff adequate time to ensure the correct insurance data and perform any necessary coding reviews. Having some type of audit process for charge tickets is recommended to ensure that all charge tickets are accounted for and all services have been captured and correctly coded before being submitted.
- Electronic claims submission—Most insurance companies require electronic claims submission for the majority of their claims. Exceptions will be the few claims that require attachments or special handling. Sending claims electronically also allows better tracking and faster processing of the claims.
- Payment posting (manual or electronic)—Payment posting can be done several ways depending on the functions and sophistication of the practice management system. Insurance companies can still mail a check with a corresponding explanation of benefits (EOB), although more are requesting that offices be able to accept an electronic deposit with corresponding online EOB or even an automatic electronic posting to the practice management system. In any case, it is important for the billing or payment staff to ensure that the correct reimbursement was received and that adjustments are posted correctly, that denials and adjustments reviewed and appealed if necessary, and that there is a good system in place for quickly identifying claims that are overdue for payment.
- Patient statements—Patients should receive statements whenever there is activity on their account and most importantly should receive a statement as soon as there is a patient balance on the account. Statements should be patient friendly by being easy to read and understand.
- Accounts receivable management—The business office or billing staff should have processes in place to identify as early as possible any claims that have been billed but not paid. Most states have guidelines that require insurance companies to process and pay claims within 30 days. Accounts receivable reports in the practice management system should be used to help this process. A process for monitoring, analyzing and appealing denials is important to have in place. Accounts receivable management also includes development of collection policies and procedures, including collection letters and use of a collection agency. This is often a good time for the practice to discuss what kind of charity care or discounts for payment at time of service they are prepared to offer.
- Practice management reports—In addition to financial reports, monthly practice management reports are important business tools. Individual and practice production reports, CPT distributions, average charge, average collection, and days in AR are all basic and important measurements for the practice to collect and monitor.

FINANCIAL POLICIES

The development of policies and procedures for financial operations should include guidelines for internal cash controls, making bank deposits, collection of co-payments at time of service, insurance verification, methods of payment accepted (check, cash, credit card), timeliness of entry of charges into the practice management system, regular attention to accounts receivable, and collection policies, including potential discharge of patients from the practice. If the practice has decided to outsource any of its accounting, financial, or billing functions, similar policies should be developed and made part of any service contract.

■ HUMAN RESOURCE OPERATIONS

The employees of a practice are instrumental in making a practice successful. They are either an asset to the practice or detrimental to its operations. The staff is not only the largest expense in the practice budget, but also functions as the day-to-day marketing and customer service team. Whether by providing clinical or administrative services, the staff represents the practice to current and potential patients every day. Managing staff and the human resource function of a practice is complex and requires a sound knowledge of employment law. Job descriptions are recommended for all employees and can be a valuable tool for use in the hiring, training, and evaluation of practice staff. A basic human resources operations checklist is provided in Box 43-3.

LEGAL ISSUES FOR HUMAN RESOURCES

Knowledge of a state's wage and hour laws is necessary. These wage and hour laws help in the development of human resource policies and procedures for the practice. State wage and hour laws will help in the development of the following standards:

- Identification of a "work week" for the practice (e.g., 12:01 AM Sunday to 12 PM Saturday). This standard is necessary for calculating overtime.
- Compliance with minimum hourly wage laws (federal and state).
- Identification of staff as "nonexempt" or "exempt" from overtime. Nonexempt staff members are normally paid hourly, whereas exempt staff members are paid by salary. The correct classification of staff is critical; misclassification and the failure to pay overtime when required can result in legal recourse and back pay and fines.
- Development of policies for employee rest breaks during the workday.
- Payment of wages on involuntary or voluntary termination.
- Requirements of the practice for employee's civic obligations, such as jury duty or military leave.

   The practice, depending on its size and its contracts, must be in compliance with the following federal employment laws:

BOX 43-3   **Human Resources Checklist**

- State wage and hour laws
- Federal employment laws
  - Americans with Disabilities Act (ADA)
  - Fair Labor Standards Act (FLSA)
  - Family and Medical Leave Act (FMLA)
  - Equal Employment Opportunity Commission (EEOC)
  - Consolidated Omnibus Budget Reconciliation Act (COBRA)
- Staffing
  - Exempt and nonexempt
  - Employment agreements
  - Personnel forms
- Salaries and benefits
- Employee handbook
- Job descriptions
- Performance evaluation process
- Orientation and training
- Important policies
  - Confidentiality
  - Harassment
  - Nonviolence

- Americans with Disabilities Act (ADA)
- Family and Medical Leave Act (FMLA)
- Equal Employment Opportunity Commission (EEOC)
- Fair Labor Standards Act (FLSA)
- Consolidated Omnibus Budget Reconciliation Act (COBRA)

   Other legal requirements that affect the human resource function include the completion by employees of I-9 (immigration) and W-4 (payroll withholding) forms. These two forms should be completed before the beginning of employment. It is generally recommended that the I-9 form be kept separately from the employee's personnel file for confidentiality purposes in the event of an audit. A separate medical file should be created if an employee has documents relating to medical treatments, such as workers' compensation or FMLA medical reports.

COMPENSATION AND BENEFITS

Compensation and the use of salary structures or salary ranges are an essential part of human resource management. The marketplace normally plays a large role in establishing these ranges by cities, states, or other specific regions of the country. In addition, the development of job descriptions and a method to evaluate employees' performance are elements that affect salary structure and consequently the personnel costs of the practice. Many human resource consultants suggest directly linking the performance evaluation to the job description. Various professional organizations and websites provide salary statistics that may be helpful in the development of salary ranges or structures and at the very least can be used as a method of comparison with the local market.

   By offering good benefits, the practice can increase its competitiveness in the marketplace and also provide security for employees. A basic benefit package usually includes health and dental insurance, life insurance, vision insurance, vacation, sick leave, or more widely recommended, a combination of vacation and sick leave in a paid time off (PTO) account. More extensive benefits can include 401K retirement plan, tuition allowance, uniform allowance, continuing education, bus passes, parking allowances, long- or short-term disability insurance, or employee assistance programs. A standard benefit package combined with required payroll taxes can add an additional 10% to 20% to the personnel costs of the practice.

EMPLOYEE HANDBOOK

An employee handbook is an excellent way to communicate personnel policies to staff members. An employee handbook should include the practice's mission statement, confidentiality requirements and agreements, and policies on benefits, vacation, sick leave, time off for bereavement or jury duty, calling in when ill, and leaves of absence. The handbook also communicates the practice's compliance with state and federal regulations. In addition, the practice should develop and include policies on a professional code of conduct, harassment, and nonviolence for inclusion in the handbook. Although extremely valuable, an employee handbook is a legal document and should always be reviewed by an attorney or a professional human resources organization to ensure that it does not contain or imply any language that could be construed as a contract of employment.

EMPLOYMENT AGREEMENTS

Health care practices often incorporate employment agreements or a contract of employment for their professional and senior management staff. An employment agreement is a legal contract that specifies the employees' and employers' duties to each other in detail. Counsel from the practice's attorney should be sought when deciding if employment agreements are right for the practice. In any event, an employment agreement should never be construed as a guarantee of employment and should always include a method for termination of the employment by either the employee or the employer during the contract term.

■ PRACTICE OPERATIONS

An efficient and well-run health care practice often gives the impression that operating or managing a practice is an easy task. Nothing could be further from the truth! A health care practice is a complex business requiring multiple clinical and administrative systems that work well together. Successful day-to-day operations require that both systems operate in conjunction with good customer service. A basic practice operations checklist is provided in Box 43-4.

APPOINTMENT SCHEDULING

The practice's scheduling system provides the structure for the clinician's day and either helps to create an office that runs smoothly or contributes to one that is in constant chaos. Important issues in pediatric scheduling require decisions on how to handle well-child visits, sick-child visits, and newborns—how they should be arranged in the schedule and how much time should be allotted for each type of visit.

| BOX 43-4 | **Practice Operations Checklist** |

- Appointment scheduling and phones
  - Patient flow
  - Phone system
  - Phone messages
  - Telephone triage
  - Answering service
- Medical records
  - Electronic medical record
  - Charting and documentation
  - Quality assurance
  - Medical record forms
- Practice management information system
- Standardized procedures
- Emergency procedures
- Quality Assurance
- Risk Management

In a multiprovider practice, a single scheduling philosophy and consistent scheduling rules for the entire practice is highly recommended.

Most pediatric practices keep a substantial portion of the daily schedule open for same-day visits. Additionally, the practice may want to consider keeping the first half hour of the morning open for patients who have been instructed to come in to the office during that time by the provider or after-hours service taking night call. Patients like the fact that they can be assured of being seen first thing in the morning without having to wait until the office opens to phone for an appointment. Many offices have reported good success with open access types of schedules where even well-care appointments are available on a same-day basis.

Other scheduling concerns that should be addressed in office policy statements and standard protocols include how the practice will confirm appointments and how it will deal with late patients, no-show patients, walk-in patients, and urgent or emergency patients.

Practices serving pediatric patients also have found it beneficial to have seasonal schedules. For example, during the winter months, it is a good idea to think about reducing the number of well-child appointment slots on Mondays and increasing the number of sick-child slots. Likewise, practices can implement a schedule in the summer months that contains more slots for well-child visits or physical examinations to help meet the demand for school and camp physicals.

PATIENT PHONE CALLS

Patient phone calls are a significant factor in the day-to-day operations of any health care practice. Whether calling to schedule an appointment, for a prescription refill, for test results, to request a referral, or to ask for advice on home care suggestions during an illness, patients want their concerns handled efficiently and in a timely manner. The practice should have policies and procedures on how these and other types of phone inquiries will be handled and by which staff members. Many of these responsibilities can be handled by clinical support staff, such as registered nurses and medical assistants, or administrative staff. Registered nurses can take patient phone calls, assess the patient, and depending on the situation and following specific triage protocols, either give medical advice or recommend that an appointment be made. Medical assistants can take messages off a prescription refill line and call in refills. Medical assistants or administrative support staff can assist the patient in obtaining a referral or an appointment to instigate a referral. Care should be given that staff members functioning in these capacities are neither expected nor allowed to act outside of their clinical competency or scope of practice as designated by state laws.

The phone system itself plays a critical role in the scheduling process, practice operations, and good customer service. Does the practice want to have an automated greeting or a live person answer the phone? Both require backup systems to make them work successfully. If the practice uses an automated system, the greeting and subsequent choices for obtaining service should be simple, with only a few choices. If the practice opts for live operators, it should make sure that there are sufficient lines and staff members to handle anticipated volume at various times of the day and week.

MEDICAL RECORDS

Developing an effective medical records system to meet the needs of the practice has traditionally revolved around determining how to organize the paper medical chart, what type of filing system to use, and development of the policies and procedures required for the medical record functions. With numerous electronic systems available, a new practice should also seriously consider an electronic medical records (EMR) system as a way to not only record the clinical and demographic information on each patient, but also as a way to improve coordination of care. Established practices should also consider an EMR system for all of the aforementioned benefits, realizing, however, that additional planning for incorporating current paper records with the electronic system will be required. Large practices and practices with multiple locations often find that the benefits of the EMR system outweigh the difficulties involved in moving to the electronic system, even if it is a time- and labor-intensive process. There are many types of EMR and electronic medical chart (EMC) systems. Adequately researching how a system works and knowledge of practice styles and outcomes are necessary when deciding on an EMR system. The federal government through the Certification Commission for Healthcare Information Technology (CCHIT) has developed standards for EMR systems and publishes these standards and lists the companies that have successfully met the CCHIT standards.

PRACTICE MANAGEMENT INFORMATION SYSTEM

A practice management computer system or practice management information system is essential to a modern health care office. The basic system should integrate patient demographic information, the scheduling process, and billing functions. If the practice is interested in adopting an EMR or EMC system immediately or in the future, the software should have an EMR component or be compatible with the desired EMR or EMC system. Many good systems have basic or entry-level systems for small offices that can be upgraded as the practice size and demands of the practice increase. When considering the purchase of a new system, it is a good idea to arrange to visit another practice of similar size that is using the system to see the functions demonstrated in a real-time environment. Scheduling functions, reporting capabilities, and billing functions—including the ability to send claims electronically—are key areas to research in a system. In addition, technical support, initial and ongoing training, and system upgrades are important aspects about which to become knowledgeable.

STANDARDIZATION IN THE PRACTICE

A medical practice can realize some important benefits by standardizing its practices and procedures. In addition to a standardized appointment schedule, policies and procedures for chart organization and documentation, immunization and well-child schedules, and nursing procedures are areas that lend themselves to conformity. For example, if there are uniform policies and procedures for preparing patients before the clinician's entry into the examination room (vital signs, weighing, measuring, appropriate charting and graphing), support staff can more easily cover for each other and the provider can be confident that all necessary tasks are accomplished.

EMERGENCY PROCEDURES

Practices should develop and implement policies and procedures for handling emergencies in the practice. Some topics to consider when developing these policies and procedures include:
- Identification of an emergency
- Calling 911
- Definition of levels of emergency to be handled in the practice
- Leadership and communication during the emergency
- Provider and support staff responsibilities
- Stocking and monitoring of an "emergency cart" for true emergencies
- Initial and ongoing staff training in cardiopulmonary resuscitation/basic life support (CPR or BLS) or advanced life support (ALS) as appropriate
- Documentation and charting of emergencies
- Staff training for emergency situations
- Assessment or critique of emergencies or training sessions

QUALITY ASSURANCE

Developing clinical quality standards for the practice should be a major focus of any clinical checklist for risk management, in addition to improving clinical care. Organizations, such as the National Committee for Quality Assurance (NCQA), the American Health Information Management Association (AHIMA), and the Joint Commission on Accreditation of Healthcare Organizations (JCAHO), can provide valuable information and guidance for the development of clinical quality standards. NCQA is a national organization with a primary function of accrediting managed care health plans. Accreditation by NCQA requires health plans to meet standards ranging from access and customer service to preventive medical care; the plans are rated based on their compliance in these areas. Accordingly, NCQA standards are used by health plans when setting quality assurance guidelines for providers in their networks. Many professional liability insurers also use NCQA standards when developing risk management guidelines for their policyholders.

RISK MANAGEMENT

Risk management is an extremely important aspect of practice operations. Keeping up to date on legal requirements and developing and implementing policies and processes that encourage sound clinical and administrative practices can prevent many problems. Some areas that require special attention include medical record documentation, confidentiality and adolescent issues, informed consent, release of records, and clinical practices, such as communicating test results, and follow-up of recommended tests and treatment.

The Medical Record

A review of the medical chart is a primary focus of accreditation and impromptu site visits by insurance companies. This is because the record serves as legal documentation of all clinical activity. Consequently, the organization, content, and completeness of the medical record can be valuable to ensure quality assurance. Guidelines suggested by AHIMA and JCAHO are included in Box 43-5.

Clinical Tracking Systems

Systems that focus on the tracking of necessary medical follow-up appointments, high-risk referrals, and clinical tests ordered are other risk management tools that benefit coordination of care and customer service. A newborn requiring a repeat bilirubin test is an example of a critical appointment that requires tracking to ensure that the patient complies with the provider's instruction for the repeat testing.

Appointment Tracking

An appointment tracking system helps ensure that patients return to the office as instructed (e.g., ADHD medication evaluations, annual well-care exams, etc).

Referral Tracking

If the provider refers the patient to a specialist for a high-risk problem, a tracking system will ensure that the visit was completed and the report from the specialist has been received and reviewed.

Tests Ordered

A tracking and follow-up system should be implemented to ensure that diagnostic test results are completed and the results are received and reviewed in a timely manner. The system should also include verification that the patient was notified of the test results.

BOX 43-5　Medical Records Guidelines

- Only authorized individuals may make entries in the medical record, and individuals should be trained in documentation practices and documentation standards.
- Every page in the medical record must identify the patient by name and an identifying number.
- Entries made into the medical record should be made as soon as possible after the visit or communication with the patient.
- Every entry in the medical record must be signed or initialed and include a complete date (month, day, year) and time. Entries must be dated at the date and time they are made.
- A signature legend should be maintained by the practice that identifies all signatures and initials appearing in the medical record.
- The medical record should always use factual information. Documentation should clearly identify speculation versus factual information.
- A standard set of abbreviations to be used in the medical record should be developed by the practice.
- All entries in the medical record should be legible.
- If using forms or checklists, all fields should have some entry. If a field is not applicable, an entry, such as "N/A," should be made.
- Informed consent should be documented whenever applicable.
- All pertinent communication (and attempts at communication) with the patient or the patient's family should be documented. Messages left on answering machines or voice mail are not considered a valid form of notification.
- When an incident occurs, document the facts of the occurrence in the progress note. Do not chart that an incident report has been completed or refer to the report in charting.
- All entries in the medical record are considered permanent.
- All entries in the medical record should be in blue or black ink. Pencils should never be used.
- If an error is made in an entry, it should be corrected by (1) drawing a thin line through the incorrect entry, ensuring that the inaccurate information is still legible; (2) signing and dating the entry; (3) stating the reason for the error in the margin or above the note; and (4) documenting the correct information.
- If a late entry, addendum, or clarification is added to the medical record, identify it as such and enter the current date and time. The reason for the late entry should also be noted.
- The medical record should not be removed from the practice site. If it is necessary to transport the medical record, a tracking system and safeguards should be in place to protect confidentiality and protect against loss.
- Policies and procedures should be developed for the destruction of medical records.

Other components of the medical record that ensure both good clinical processes and risk management include:

- A *problem list* that identifies the patient's chronic and significant illnesses. The problem list should appear in a prominent location in the medical record (usually at the front of the medical record).
- *Allergy flags* that indicate known allergies or no known allergies. Allergy flags should be documented on the outside of the medical record and on the problem list. Patients should be questioned about allergies at each visit.
- A *medication list* that contains the patient's acute and chronic medications. This list should be maintained in a prominent location in the medical record. The medication prescribed, the dosage, the date prescribed, and the prescriber should be entered on the medication list. The medication list should also include a record of prescription refills.

Being proactive in the area of risk management will benefit the practice by ensuring optimal clinical care and follow-up, but it will also prevent potential care oversights or patient compliance issues.

■ SUMMARY

The topics reviewed in this chapter briefly touch upon the many important components of the successful medical practice with most of the operational examples focused on pediatric or family medicine. In one chapter, it is simply not possible to be completely thorough or to discuss many other interesting and important subjects pertaining to practice management. New technologies are bringing exciting possibilities along with new challenges to medical practices today as patients expect their health care providers to use modern technology for clinical and administrative operations and for communications. Practice websites, online communication between patient and provider, electronic prescribing, and EMRs are just a few examples of ways modern technology is changing medical practices.

It is extremely important for the principals of a medical practice to be business savvy and to take advantage of the knowledge and expertise that is available. The Resource Box at the end of the chapter lists several professional organizations that provide excellent information on the topics covered in the chapter and many subjects that were not covered. There is a wealth of excellent information available through websites, books, journals, educational offerings, and networking that can help answer a specific question, explain a complicated subject, assist with solving a problem, or introduce a new concept. Good practice management is also good business, and regular business books can offer new ideas and perspectives on technology, finance, operations, personnel, etc., that can also benefit the medical practice. Although medical practice management often seems complex and overwhelming, there is an abundance of resources to help manage the challenges and establish the practice as a leader in the community for children's health care.

*R*ESOURCE BOX

Practice Management Strategies for Health Care

ORGANIZATIONS
American Academy of Family Physicians (AAFP)
www.aafp.org

American Academy of Pediatrics (AAP)
www.aap.org

American Health Information Management Association (AHIMA)
www.ahima.org

Medical Group Management Association (MGMA)
www.mgma.com

Society of Human Resource Management (SHRM)
www.shrm.org

BOOKS (AVAILABLE THROUGH MGMA)
Chart of accounts for healthcare organizations, 1999, MGMA.
Floreen N: *Collections manual for healthcare providers,* Englewood, CO, 1999, MGMA.
Kuehn L: *Health information management: medical record processes in group practice,* 1997, MGMA.
Lucash PD: *Medical practice business plan workbook,* 1999, McGraw-Hill.
Medisphere Health Partners: *Managed care contract reference guide,* 1998, MGMA.
Novak A: *Governing policies manual for medical practices,* 1996, MGMA.
Pavlock E: *Financial management for medical groups,* 2000, MGMA.
Physician office safety guide, 1998, MGMA.

Price C, Novak A: *MBA job description manual for medical practices,* 1999, MGMA.
Rowell JC, Green MA: *Understanding health insurance: a guide to professional billing,* 2002, Delmar Thomson Learning.
Schryver D, editor: *An assessment manual for medical groups,* 2002, MGMA.
Woodcock E, Warn B: *Operating policies and procedures manual for medical practices,* ed 3, 2006, MGMA.

BOOKS (AVAILABLE THROUGH AAP)
A guide to starting a medical office, Elk Grove Village, IL, 1997, American Academy of Pediatrics.
Medical liability for pediatricians, ed 6, 2006, American Academy of Pediatrics.
Poole SR: *Developing a telephone triage and advice system for a pediatric office practice,* July 2003, American Academy of Pediatrics.
Schmitt BD: *Pediatric telephone protocols: office version,* ed 11, 2006, American Academy of Pediatrics.
Seidel J, Knapp J: *Childhood emergencies in the office, hospital, and community,* 1992, American Academy of Pediatrics.

ANNUAL BUSINESS GUIDES
Reel SJ: *Developing a business plan: getting down to specifics,* Adv Nurse Pract 11(6):53-54, 90, 2003.
Robnett M: *Planning your private practice: setting realistic expectations,* Adv Nurse Pract 11(6):48-49, 2003.
Rollet J: *Marketing your practice: strategies that work,* Adv Nurse Pract 11(6):59-60, 62, 2003.
Zaumeyer C: *Financing a private practice: investigating the options,* Adv Nurse Pract 11(6):56-57, 2003.

Continued

$\mathcal{R}$ESOURCE BOX

Practice Management Strategies for Health Care—Cont'd

OTHER RESOURCES
Certification Commission for Healthcare Information Technology Standards
www.cchit.org

Pediatric Coding Alert
www.codinginstitute.com
Monthly newsletter for ethically optimizing coding reimbursement and efficiency for pediatric practices

RBRVS
www.cms.hhs.gov/PFSlookup

☑ DISCUSSION FORUM

1. Create your own personal vision statement that reflects your philosophy and role as a primary care provider.
2. Create a simple business plan for a one-provider practice. Be sure to cover organizational structure, insurance requirements, and financial operations.
3. Create an appointment scheduling process for a pediatric primary care provider.

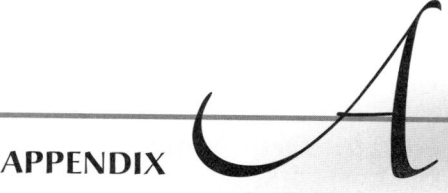

Medications in Pediatric Practice

Catherine G. Blosser

■ MEDICATION ADHERENCE

Historically, whether or not a patient was taking the recommended pharmaceutical or following a recommended treatment regimen was referred to as "compliance" or "non-compliance." The term "adherence" is now a more favorable term and used more often in medical literature. Research into adherence has lead to the following conclusions (Bell, 2005; Daiichi Pharmaceutical Corporation, 2004):

- A provider obtains a better idea of the actual adherence rate if the question is framed in terms of nonadherence, such as "how many doses did you miss" rather than "did you take all of your medicine."
- Adolescents are less likely to be adherent.
- A patient's or his/her parents' perception of the seriousness of an illness and consequences of not taking the medicine increases adherence rates.
- Have the patient and/or parent devise a plan for when they will take or administer the medicine, especially if they link the administration with a specific activity (e.g., toothbrushing, eating breakfast) with stickers as reinforcement, which increases rates of adherence.
- The more complex the treatment regimen, the lower the adherence rate.
- Past experience regarding the ease or difficulty administering a drug will increase or decrease adherence.
- The better the relationship and communication between provider and patient and parent the better the adherence rate.
- Written instructions increase adherence rates.

Table A-1 discusses additional factors that predispose to lower adherence rates and strategies a provider may use to increase those rates.

■ PRESCRIBING MEDICATIONS FOR CHILDREN

Prescribing medications for pediatric patients presents a special challenge. When making treatment decisions, the provider must consider the child's age, the child's developmental level, and any family social and functional issues. Factors that influence compliance, such as taste, dosing regimen, and collaborative decision-making, also need to be considered.

A child's developmental level and age will determine the amount of parental control over the medication administration and assist the provider in determining a successful teaching

The authors would like to acknowledge Teri Moser Woo for her contributions that remain unchanged from the previous edition of this textbook.

strategy. For *infants* it is important to take the following into consideration:

- The parent is in total control of administering the medication.
- The parent should be taught how to properly administer medications.
- Determine whether other caregivers will be administering the medication.
- Determine whether a simplified dosing schedule is necessary for a family with children in day care.

Toddlers and *preschoolers* are beginning to exert their independence, and administering medication to this age can be challenging. The key to success with this age is to:

- Discuss medication administration with the parent.
- Choose a medication regimen with the fewest problems with administration.
- Take into account palatability and doses per day to increase compliance.

School-age children developmentally are industrious and are often the easiest age to which to administer medications. Education should focus on:

- Both the parent *and* the child who will be taking the medication.
- Letting the child choose the formulation, if possible (liquid, chewable, or pills to swallow).
- Avoid dosing during school hours, if possible, to increase compliance.

Adolescent patients often administer their own medication, and compliance rates may vary. The provider needs to closely collaborate with adolescent patients regarding their medication regimen by:

- Allowing them to have input on dosing schedule and what will work best for them.
- Assisting the family with the transition from parent-controlled to teen-controlled administration.

PRESCRIBING DRUGS "OFF-LABEL"

Approximately 75% of drugs approved by the Food and Drug Administration (FDA) in the U.S. have never been tested for use in the pediatric population (Groopman, 2005; Tyre, 2005). Eighty percent are without specific dosing and safety information for this age group (Adcock, 2006). Using drugs "off-label" refers to prescribing the drug outside of the approved indications, dosing recommendations, or age groups according to the official FDA-approved drug's labeling. Using a drug in such a way does not imply unethical use.

Many off-label drugs are used in pediatrics despite lack of pediatric labeling. This has largely resulted from two interrelated

TABLE A-1   Factors That Influence Adherence in Prescribing Pediatric Medications

Factors That Influence Adherence	Interventions That Improve Adherence
Length of treatment. • Poorer adherence for longer length of treatment.	*Shorten length of treatment if possible.* An example would be to use 5 days of therapy for otitis media rather than 10; this can be accomplished with a number of antibiotics (azithromycin and cefpodoxime at all ages, amoxicillin in children > 5 years old).
• Adherence rates vary with chronic illness.	*Creative solutions to encourage adherence:* When a child is on medications for a chronic illness, the provider needs to be creative to encourage adherence because adherence rates vary significantly. Sticker charts or calendars with a small reward for completing a set amount of therapy (e.g., 1 month) is one strategy.
• Doses per day: Adherence research in children indicates that the more doses of a medication that need to be administered per day, the poorer the adherence rate. This is particularly significant with working parents and children in school, who often miss midday doses.	*Simplify dosing regimen.* Prescribing medications that require fewer doses per day will increase adherence. Rates range from 65%-93% for once a day dosing and 54%-84% for twice-daily regimens, compared with 49%-81% for 3 times a day and 31%-71% for a 4-daily dosing regimen (Claxton et al, 2001). When the child needs to take the medication at day care or school, dispense 2 bottles: 1 for school and 1 for home. This will ensure fewer missed doses as a result of forgetting to transport the medication back and forth.
Palatability.	*Choose the best-tasting medication or mask the taste.* If a medication has the same efficacy profile, the best-tasting medication will be easier to administer to young children. There is also the option of using flavoring syrups or crushing tablets, such as prednisone, and mixing with sweet foods, such as chocolate syrup, jam, or pudding (Woo, 2002). Before crushing any tab or mixing a medication with syrup, the provider should check with a pharmacist to determine if the flavoring is compatible with the medication.
Out-of-pocket costs and family finances.	*Choose the medication that has the lowest out-of-pocket expense for the family.* Asking families about insurance coverage and resources and problem-solving with them increases the likelihood that they will fill the prescription.
Family issues: Concerns, such as working parents, lack of social support, fatigue, family disruption, and dysfunction, affect the family's ability to adhere to the prescribed treatment regimen.	*Assess the family for issues that affect successful outcome.* If there is poor or less than expected outcome with a treatment regimen, the provider will need to determine if family issues are a factor in adherence and address interventions to assist the family in identifying strategies that will improve success.

factors: (a) pharmaceutical manufacturers did not test the safety and efficacy of drugs in the pediatric age group, and (b) the preponderance of off-label use in pediatrics has provided little incentive for manufacturers to perform official pediatric clinical trials. All providers caring for pediatric patients are familiar with the statement in pharmaceutical reference materials that state under "Pediatric Use" that "safety and effectiveness in pediatric patients have not been established." Determining the dosage for any pediatric patient using an off-label drug has been a result of proportionately reducing the dose based on weight. However, this does not take into account pediatric metabolism, the drug's pharmacokinetics, adverse effects (e.g., the connection between SSRIs and potential suicide risk), and medication delivery form. Furthermore, the emerging field of ethnopharmacology could eventually add another consideration: dosing based upon ethnicity whereby genetic variations in certain enzymes can influence one's response to certain drugs (Muñoz & Hilgenberg, 2005).

In the U.S., an assessment of adverse events in pediatric children that were reported to the FDA's Adverse Event Reporting System revealed that 17% of 28 identified drugs (50 drugs were reviewed) needed labeling changes as to safety for this age group (Grassia, 2005). Subsequently, the FDA's Pediatric Advisory Committee recommended that labels carry warnings about suicide, neonatal withdrawal and toxicity, and risk of off-label use for some drugs. It is surmised, however, that many postmarket drug adverse effects in this age group go unreported, so the true nature of drug safety is not fully known. All providers are encouraged to report adverse effects to the FDA MedWatch website at *www.fda.gov/medwatch*.

The federal Pediatric Rule of 1994 was passed to correct this deficit in pediatric dosing knowledge. It was revamped in 1996 and 1997 and then reinvigorated in 2003 by the U.S. Congress. The Rule dictates that a drug company that is working on a new drug treatment that affects an illness shared by both adults and children is mandated to perform clinical trials that include the pediatric population. In exchange, they are allowed a 6-month patent extension. Loopholes, however, have resulted in few studies being done. Additionally, generic drugs are not included in the law, and the law "sunsets" in 2007 unless renewed.

■ DRUG LABELING CHANGES

The U.S. Department of Health and Human Services mandated a pharmaceutical labeling change, the first one in 25 years. The goal is to present information about a drug in a more easily accessible and understandable way for providers.

Information regarding the most important prescribing information about the benefits and risk of a drug (in a section called *Highlights*), the date of initial product approval, and phone number and/or Web address to report adverse effects are now placed at the beginning of prescribing information and package inserts. Similar formatting must be included in electronic prescribing tools and other information resources. This change initially affects only newly and recently approved prescription drugs (those approved within the last 5 years) and drugs approved for new uses. Older drugs' labeling will be phased in over time (Brunell, 2006).

■ DISPOSAL OF DRUGS

Over-the-counter and prescription drugs should not be flushed down the drain or toilet. Trace amounts are showing up in rivers, streams, and treated water (University of California,

Berkeley, 2006). It is advisable to instruct parents to inquire if pharmacies will take back unused or expired products, take them to hazardous recycling facilities, or place them in the trash in their original packaging and secure tightly.

■ MEDICATIONS

Table A-2 is an abbreviated listing of medications. It is the responsibility of the reader or prescriber to seek detailed information and thoroughly investigate the drug being prescribed. The textbook's authors take no responsibility for any errors in prescribing. Pharmaceutical references and the FDA often indicate dosages in terms of broad categories of ages, such as "pediatric," "children," and "adult." Wherever possible specific age- or weight-based dosages (or both) are given. The prescriber needs to use professional judgment when dosing "adolescent" patients; adult dosing is included for that reason.

TABLE A-2 Medications

Generic/Trade *Classification*	Indications/Dose	Supplied	Remarks
Acetaminophen (Tylenol, Tempra, and others) *Miscellaneous analgesic and antipyretic*	*Treatment of mild to moderate pain and fever:* Neonates: 10-15 mg/kg/dose every 6-8 hr prn ≤12 yr: 10-15 mg/kg/dose every 4-6 hr PO (max 5 doses/day) >12 yr: 325-650 mg every 4-6 hr PO (max 4 g/day)	80 mg/0.8 mL drops 160 mg/5 mL, 500/15 mL elixir 80 mg chewable 325, 500 mg tabs 500 mg caplet 80, 120, 325, 650 mg suppository	Drug interactions: barbiturates, carbamazepine, hydantoins, rifampin, sulfinpyrazone. Can cause severe hepatic toxicity with overdose.
Acetaminophen with codeine *Analgesic and antipyretic*	Children: 0.5-1 mg codeine/kg/dose every 4-6 hr PO Adults: 15-60 mg every 4-6 hr PO	Tylenol 120 mg and codeine 12 mg/5 mL elixir Various combination tabs with Tylenol and codeine	Can cause respiratory depression. Codeine can cause nausea, vomiting, constipation.
Acyclovir (Zovirax) *Antiviral*	*Genital herpes infection:* Children >12 yr & adults: initial: 200 mg PO every 4 hr (5 capsules/day) for 10 days; recurrent infection: treat for 5 days; chronic HSV infections: 400 mg PO bid or 200 mg PO 3-5 times a day for 12 mo, then reevaluate; intermittent: 200 mg every 4 hr (5 times a day) for 5 days *Herpes zoster (shingles):* ≥2 yr or <40 kg: 20 mg/kg qid (max 80 mg/kg × 5 days) >40 kg: 800 mg qid × 5 days Children ≥12 yr and adult dose: 800 mg PO every 4 hr (5 times a day) for 5-10 days (best if started within 48 hr of onset) *HSV encephalitis or other severe HSV infection:* Neonates: 0-3 mo: 20 mg/kg IV every 8 hr for 14-21 days	200 mg/5 mL suspension 200 mg capsules 400 mg, 800 mg tab 500 mg vial for injection 5% ointment (15, 30 g)	Contraindications: valacyclovir hypersensitivity. Drug interactions: avoid nephrotoxic drugs. Potentiated by probenecid. Therapy should be started at the first sign of infection. Use gloves when applying ointment; apply a thin layer. Adverse effects: renal toxicity (reversible), neurotoxicity, GI disturbances. May have stinging or pain with topical application. Avoid contact with eyes when using ointment. Do not crush/break tabs.

Continued

TABLE A-2   Medications—Cont'd

Generic/Trade Classification	Indications/Dose	Supplied	Remarks
	3 mo-12 yr: 20 mg/kg IV every 8 hr for 14-21 days ≥12 yr: 10-15 mg/kg IV every 8 hr for 14-21 days *HSV infections in immuno-compromised patients, in those with underlying skin disorders:* <12 yr: 10 mg/kg IV every 8 hr for 7-14 days (5 days for genital herpes) Children ≥12 yr and adults: 5 mg/kg IV every 8 hr for 7-14 days (5 days for genital herpes) *Varicella infections:* ≥2 yr or <40 kg: 20 mg/kg/dose PO qid (max 80 mg/kg) for 5 days Children >40 kg and adults: 800 mg/dose PO qid for 5 days *Mucocutaneous HSV infections:* Children and adolescents: cover all lesions with a thin layer of ointment every 3 hr, 3-6 times/day for 7 days		
Adapalene (Differin) *Topical retinoid*	*Treatment of acne vulgaris:* Apply to affected acne areas once daily at bedtime after washing	0.1% cream or gel	Effects seen after 8-12 wk; exacerbation is common early in the course of treatment. Adverse effects: erythema, scaling, dryness, pruritus, burning, acne flares. Drug interactions: avoid use until the effects of sulfur or salicylic acid have subsided. Avoid waxed areas. Precautions: avoid use on irritated, eczematous, or sunburned skin. Avoid contact with eyes, lips, mucous membranes, sun, UV light.
Albuterol sulfate (Proventil, Ventolin, AccuNeb, Volmax, Proventil Repetabs, Vospire ER) *Bronchodilator*	*Treatment of bronchospasm:* **For current asthma guideline, refer to Appendix D** *Exercise-induced bronchospasm:* 2 inhalations 15 min before exercise	2 mg/5 mL syrup 2, 4 mg tab 4, 8 mg sustained-release tab 5 mg/mL (0.5%), 0.083% unit-dosed vials (2.5 mg albuterol per vial); 0.75 mg/3 mL (0.63 mg/3 mL albuterol), 1.5 mg/3 mL (1.25 mg/3 mL albuterol) inhalation solution 90 mcg/metered spray	Common side effects: tachycardia, tremor, palpitations. Do not administer with MAOIs or tricyclic antidepressants. Inhaler use most effective if spacer is used. For nebulization, dilute 0.5 mL of 0.5% solution with 0.9% NaCl to reach a volume of 2.5 mL (equals 2.5 mg); give over 5-10 min.
Amantadine HCl (Symmetrel) *Antiviral*	*Prophylaxis or symptomatic relief of influenza A:* 1-9 yr or <45 kg: 5 mg/kg/day PO divided bid-tid (max 150 mg/day)	50 mg/5 mL syrup 100 mg capsule, tab	Not recommended for children <1 yr. Do not administer with alcohol or stimulants. Reduce dose for renal dysfunction (creatinine clearance

TABLE A-2 Medications—Cont'd

Generic/Trade Classification	Indications/Dose	Supplied	Remarks
	≥9-12 yr 100 mg bid (max 100 mg bid) >13 yr and >45 kg: 100 mg PO bid or 200 mg PO single dose; start within 24-48 hr of symptom onset and continue until symptoms resolve		<50 mL/min) or hepatic dysfunction. Precautions with seizure disorders, psychiatric disorders, and heart failure. Can cause insomnia
Amitriptyline HCL (Elavil, generics) *Tricyclic antidepressant*	*For migraine prophylaxis, tension HA:* ≥12 yr: 10 mg PO at hs; increase every 3 days to 30 mg PO at hs	10, 25, 50, 75, 100, 150 mg tab 10 mg/mL parenteral	Adverse effects: drug mouth, constipation, weight gain, postural hypotension, drowsiness, confusion, HA, visual disturbance, suicidal ideation/behaviors.
Ammonium lactate (LAC-Hydrin 12%) *Miscellaneous emollient*	*Used in the treatment of moderate to severe xerosis and ichthyosis vulgaris* Apply twice daily to affected areas	Lotion (225, 400 g) Cream (280 g, 385 g)	Avoid contact with lips, eyes, mucous membranes. Minimize exposure to sun or UV light. Transient stinging, burning, erythema. Irritation (especially on face), rash, peeling, dryness, hyperpigmentation.
Amoxicillin (Amoxil, Polymox, Trimox, Biomox, DisperMox, Moxilin, Novamoxin, Wymox); generics available. *Penicillin, β-lactam*	*Community-acquired pneumonia, sinusitis, skin, otitis, urinary tract, gonorrhea, streptococcal infections* Children <2 yr: high-dose for OM, 80-90 mg/kg/day divided bid or tid (see below comment) Children ≥2 yr: 40-90 mg/kg/day PO divided bid-tid (do not exceed adult recommended dose) If child has received 3 doses of pneumococcal vaccine, dose at 40-45 mg/kg/day regardless of age or child's care situation (Garbutt et al, 2006) Adults: 250 mg PO bid-tid or 500 mg bid (max 2-3 g/day) *Prophylaxis for otitis media with effusion:* 20 mg/kg/day	50 mg/mL drops (15, 30 mL) 125, 200, 250, 400 mg/5 mL suspension reconstituted 125, 200, 250, 400 mg chewable 250, 500 mg capsule 500, 875 mg tab 200, 400 mg tab for suspension	Can cause a rash if given to a patient with mononucleosis. Usually treat infections for 10 days. Low-risk children >5 yr may treat OM for 5-7 days. Drug interactions: cross allergy with cephalosporins or imipenem. May decrease effectiveness of OCPs. Probenecid may increase amoxicillin blood concentration. Side effects: GI, especially with high-dose (80-90 mg/kg) dosing; penicillin allergy symptoms. One study demonstrated an increase in fluorosis on permanent first molars and maxillary central incisors in those treated in infancy (notably between 3-6 mo old) (Hong et al, 2005).
Amoxicillin and clavulanate (Augmentin) *Penicillin, beta-lactamase inhibitor*	*Community-acquired pneumonia, otitis media, sinusitis, skin (periorbital cellulitis, human/ animal bites):* *Dosing based on amoxicillin component* ≤40 kg: <12 wk, 30 mg/kg day divided bid; >12 wk, 40 mg/kg/day PO tid or 45 mg/kg/day PO bid; do not exceed adult dose *Otitis media specific* ≤2 yr: 80 to 90 mg/kg/day amoxicillin component divided bid or tid	125, 200, 250, 400, 600 mg/5 mL suspension (75, 150 mL) 125, 200, 250, 400 mg chewable 250, 500, 875 mg tab (two 250 mg tabs do not equal one 500 mg tab because of the clavulanate dose component) 1000 mg XR tab	Drug interactions: cross allergy with cephalosporins or imipenem. Fewer side effects at bid dosing with 45 mg/kg/day. GI side effects—give with food. Peanut butter and cherry yogurt have been shown to decrease GI side effects. Reduce dose for renal impairment. Penicillin allergy symptoms.

Continued

TABLE A-2 Medications—Cont'd

Generic/Trade Classification	Indications/Dose	Supplied	Remarks
	If child has received 3 doses of pneumococcal vaccine, dose at 40-45mg/kg/day amoxicillin component regardless of age or child's care situation (Garbutt et al, 2006) Children ≥40kg and adults: 250mg PO tid (max 2g/day) or 875mg bid; for severe infection may use 500mg tid		
Antipyrine and benzocaine (Auralgan, A/B otic, Otocalm and others) *Local anesthetic (otic)*	*Used for temporary relief of pain associated with otitis media:* Fill ear canal with drops; may use every 2-4hr	Otic solution (antipyrine 5.4%, benzocaine 1.4%)	Not for prolonged use. Do not use if TM is perforated.
Aripiprazole (Abilify) *Antipsychotic*	Used for bipolar disorder, schizophrenia, and/or associated agitation *Bipolar disorder:* Adolescents: 30mg/day; decrease to 15mg if symptoms controlled *Schizophrenia:* Adolescent: 10-15mg PO once daily; increase to 30mg daily after at least 2 weeks if needed *Agitation:* Adolescent: 5.25 to 15mg deep IM (9.75mg recommended, may in repeat 2hrs ([max dose 30mg/d]; switch to PO form as soon as possible.)	2, 5, 10, 15, 20, 30mg tab 10, 15, 20, 30mg ODTs 1mg/5mL solution	Safety in younger children not established. Check pharmacologic reference regarding drug interactions before starting. Monitor weight, BP, pulse. Adverse effects: extrapyramidal symptoms, somnolence, impaired judgment/thinking/motor skills, suicidal ideation/behaviors.
Atomoxetine HCl (Strattera) *Norepinephrine reuptake inhibitor*	*ADHD (nonstimulant) for children, adolescents, adults:* ≥6yr and adolescents: ≤70kg: start at 0.5mg/kg/day and ↑ after minimum of 3 days to target dose of 1.2mg/kg/day divided AM and late afternoon (max 1.4mg/kg/day or 100mg whichever is less). >70kg: initial 40mg/day, ↑ after minimum of 3 days to target dose of 80mg in AM or divided between AM and late afternoon (max 1.4mg/kg/day or 100mg/day if needed after trial of 2-4wk at lower dose).	5, 10, 18, 25, 40, 60mg capsule	Close monitoring is imperative, including parental observation, especially at initiation of treatment and when changing dosages. Possible drug interactions (use with caution): Paxil, Prozac, quinidine, albuterol. Adverse reactions: possible suicidal thinking and behavior, agitation, irritability, unusual cha0nges in behavior, abdominal pain, constipation, dyspepsia, nausea/vomiting, decreased weight, anorexia, mood swings, irritability, dry mouth, insomnia. Use with caution in individuals with HTN, tachycardia, cardiovascular disease, asthma.
Azelastine hydrochloride (Astelin) *Antihistamine*	*Seasonal allergic rhinitis:* 5-11yr: 1 spray each nostril bid; >12yr: 2 sprays per nostril bid; not recommended <5yr	137mcg in 100 and 200 metered spray bottles	Drug interactions: cimetidine, CNS depressants, antacids. Caution with concurrent use of other antihistamines. Side effects: bitter taste, fatigue, HA, weight increase, nasal irritation or burning. Children: also conjunctivitis, cough, asthma.

TABLE A-2   Medications—Cont'd

Generic/Trade *Classification*	Indications/Dose	Supplied	Remarks
Azithromycin (Zithromax) *Macrolide antibiotic*	Pharyngitis, pneumonia, uncomplicated skin and soft tissue disorders, otitis media, sinusitis, pneumonia, streptococcal pharyngitis; nontuberculous mycobacterial infections; nongonococcal urethritis and cervicitis caused by *C. trachomatis* (single dose). Atypical, community-acquired pneumonia, pharyngitis/tonsillitis (as second-line therapy) *Otitis media*: ≥ 6 mo: 30 mg/kg single dose, OR 10 mg/kg once daily × 3 days, OR 10 mg/kg on day 1, 5 mg/kg on days 2-5, given once daily *Pharyngitis*: > 2 yr: 12 mg/kg/day, days 1-5 (max 500 mg/dose) *Community-acquired pneumonia*: ≥ 6 mo: 10 mg/kg PO (max 500 mg) day 1, 5 mg/kg (max 250 mg/ dose) on days 2-5. *Nongonococcal urethritis, cervicitis caused by* C. trachomatis, *chancroid*: adults: 1 g as a single dose	250 mg capsule 200, 500, 600 mg tab 100 mg/5 mL, 200 mg/5 mL suspension 1 g single-dose packet	Food decreases bioavailability of capsules. Theophylline effect unknown. Alternative when erythromycin ethylsuccinate not tolerated. Some strains of streptococcus are resistant to azithromycin. Drug interactions: Propulsid, digoxin, theophylline, phenytoin, carbamazepine, triazolam, fluconazole. Side effects: GI upset, abdominal pain. Rare: allergy.
Bacitracin, neomycin, polymyxin B (Neosporin) *Topical antibiotic*	*Used to prevent infection in minor wounds*: Apply 1-3 times daily	Ointment or cream	High incidence of sensitivity reactions, which can include redness, itching, edema. Do not use in large areas, serious burns, puncture wounds, blisters.
Bacitracin, neomycin, polymyxin B pramoxine (Neosporin Plus) *Topical antibiotic and anesthetic*	*Used to prevent infection in minor wounds*: ≥ 2 yr: apply 1-3 times daily	Ointment or cream	High incidence of sensitivity reactions, which can include redness, itching, edema. Not recommended for children <2 yr. Do not use in large areas, serious burns, puncture wounds, blisters.
Bacitracin, neomycin, polymyxin B (Neosporin ophthalmic) *Antibiotic (ophthalmic)*	*Treatment of external ocular infections*: Ointment: apply every 3-4 hr for 7-10 days Solution: 3 or 4 times daily	Ophthalmic ointment, solution	Side effects: sensitization, local irritation.
Bacitracin, neomycin, polymyxin B, and hydrocortisone (Cortisporin otic) *Antibiotic, antiinflammatory*	*Treatment of topical infections of the external auditory canal*: Otic suspension: 2-3 drops 3-4 times daily for 7 days	Otic suspension, solution	Otic suspension should be used if tympanic membrane is not intact.
Beclomethasone dipropionate *Oral inhalation systems* (Beclovent, Vanceril, QVAR)	*Maintenance and prophylactic therapy for asthma*: See Appendix D for NIH asthma management guidelines.	Beclovent (42-80 mcg/ spray); Vanceril (42 mcg/ spray, 84 mcg/spray); QVAR (40 mcg/puff, 80 mcg/puff MDIs)	Contraindicated in patients with status asthmaticus. Use cautiously in patients with tuberculosis and those on oral steroids.

Continued

TABLE A-2 Medications—Cont'd

Generic/Trade Classification	Indications/Dose	Supplied	Remarks
Glucocorticoid, antiinflammatory			Adverse reactions: hypothalamic-pituitary-adrenal axis suppression during and after the switch from systemic steroids to less systemically available inhaled corticosteroids, oral candidiasis, HA (oral or nasal delivery systems), nasal irritation (nasal system only). Monitor for linear growth suppression in children if on long-term high-dose therapy. Rinse mouth well following oral inhalation. When changing from oral to inhaled steroids, allow an overlap of at least 2 wk.
Nasal inhalation system (Beconase, Beconase AQ, Vancenase AQ, Vanceril DS, Vancenase AQ DS) *Glucocorticoid, antiinflammatory*	*Used in the treatment of seasonal allergic rhinitis and nasal polyps:* Nonaqueous (AQ) sprays: 6-12 yr: 1 spray/nostril bid (max 336 mcg/day) ≥12 yr: 1-2 spray/nostril bid (max 336 mcg/day) Aqueous (AQ) sprays: 6-12 yr: initially 1 spray/nostril bid increasing to 2 sprays/nostril bid depending on response ≥12 yr: 1-2 sprays/nostril bid	Beconase (42-84 mcg/spray), Beconase AQ (42 mcg/spray), Vancenase AQ (42 mcg/spray),	Relief may not occur for 2 wk; stop if symptomatic relief has not occurred after 3 wk. If severely congested, instruct patient to use a nasal vasoconstrictor the first 2-3 days before using the nasal inhalation system.
Benzonatate (Tessalon Perles) *Nonnarcotic antitussive*	*Used for cough suppression:* Children ≥10 yr: 100 mg PO tid (max 6 perles/day)	100 mg perles	Side effects: drowsiness, HA, dizziness, confusion, GI upset, pruritus No respiratory depression. Do not chew perles—can cause oropharyngeal anesthesia.
Benzoyl peroxide (5%, 10%) (Benzagel wash, Desquam-E, Desquam-X, Ersa-Gel, Benzashave, NeoBenz, others) *Antibacterial/keratolytic agent*	*Used in mild to moderate acne:* Gel: apply sparingly to clean face 1-3 times daily Wash: wash face before use; apply to affected areas 1-2 times per day; rinse well. Often best to start by using product once a day for the first wk, then ↑ to bid	5%, 10% gel, wash 4%, 8% lotion 3.5%, 5.5% cream	Avoid contact with eyes, lips, mucous membranes. Adverse reactions: burning, swelling, peeling, excessive drying. Areas should be cleaned before applying. Can bleach fabrics.
Bethanechol chloride (Duvoid, Urecholine) *Urinary tract and GI tract stimulant*	*Used to treat nonobstructive urinary retention, abdominal distention, gastroesophageal reflux, familial dysautonomia, and to induce sweating in the diagnosis of cystic fibrosis:* Children: 0.3-0.6 mg/kg/day PO divided 3 or 4 times daily (for gastroesophageal reflux give 30 min-1 hr before meals) Children: Familial dysautonomia: 0.02-0.4 mg/kg SC qid 30 min before meals with an oral	1 mg/mL solution (not available at all pharmacies) 5, 10, 25, 50 mg tab 5 mg/mL injection	Adjunctive therapy for irritable bowel syndrome, colitis, spastic bladder, peptic ulcer disease. Drug usually effective within 5-15 min. Contraindicated in patients with hyperthyroidism, hypotension, coronary artery disease, peptic ulcer disease, asthma. Give on empty stomach to prevent nausea and

TABLE A-2   Medications—Cont'd

Generic/Trade *Classification*	Indications/Dose	Supplied	Remarks
	antacid. After 2wk, stop giving SC and give 1-2mg PO qid.		vomiting. Adverse reactions: cramping, nausea, flushing, dizziness, urgency, bronchospasms, fainting. Use in caution in children <8yr if their urinary retention is due to obstruction.
Bisacodyl (Dulcolax) *Stimulant laxative*	*Used to treat chronic constipation, bowel preparation:* <2yr: 5mg rectally >2-5yr: 10mg rectally ≥6-11yr: 5-10mg PO or PR at hs or breakfast. Children ≥12yr-adults: 10-15mg PO once daily; 10mg rectally; up to 30mg can be used for preparation for bowel procedure	5mg enteric-coated tab 10mg rectal suppository 10mg/30mL enema	Drug interactions: antacids. Do not crush tabs. Administer in the evening or before breakfast to maintain regularity.
Bismuth subsalicylate (Bismatrol, Children's Kaopectate, Kaopectate*)(OTC) *Antidiarrheal*	*Used to treat mild diarrhea:* <3yr: do not use 3-6yr: 1 tsp or ⅓ tab following each loose stool (max 4 tsp/12hr) 6-9yr: 2 tsp or ⅔ tab each dose (max 4 tsp/12hr) >9-12yr: 1 tbsp or 1 tab (max 8 doses/24hr) ≥12yr: 2 tbsp or 2 tab (max 8 doses/24hr)	600mg/15mL Children's kaopectate; 750/15mL regular kaopectate suspensions Chewable tab, tab	*Generic kaopectate may contain kaolin and pectin (old formula), and the dosage is different (check ingredients of product before dosing). Do not administer for longer than 48hr. Drug interactions: tetracycline, theophylline, chloroquine, digoxin. Avoid using in those with aspirin or oil of wintergreen sensitivities or in those with influenza or chicken pox. May cause tongue and stool gray-black discoloration.
Bitolterol mesylate (Tornalate) *Bronchodilator*	*For treatment of acute bronchial asthma, bronchospasms:* **See Appendix D for asthma treatment guidelines**	0.2% inhalation solution	Cardiotoxic effects can be increased if used in conjunction with theophylline. Decreases effects of beta-adrenergic blockers (propranolol). Ipratropium may increase duration of bronchodilation. Increased toxicity with MAOIs.
Brompheniramine maleate (Bromarest, Bromphen, Chlorphed, Cophene-B, Dehist, Dimetane, Nasahist B, Oraminic II, Sinusol-B, Veltane, others) *Antihistamine*	2-6yr: 1mg PO given every 4-6hr 6-12yr: 2mg PO every 4-6hr; max 12-16mg/day ≥12yr: 4mg PO every 4-6hr, or 8mg of sustained-release form every 8-12hr or 12mg of sustained-release form every 12hr (max 24mg/day) IM/SC/IV: <12yr: 0.5mg/kg/day divided every 6-8hr ≥12yr and adults: 10mg (range 5-20mg) every 3-12hr (max 40mg/day); usually bid is sufficient	2mg/5mL (alcohol base) 4, 8, 12mg tab 8, 12mg time-released tab 10mg/mL injection	Adverse effects: drowsiness, sedation, anorexia, dry mouth. Less drowsiness than with other antihistamines. Children <6yr can experience hyperexcitability, hallucinations, convulsions, death. Not for use in children <2yr Drug interactions: alcohol and other CNS depressants.

Continued

TABLE A-2 | Medications—Cont'd

Generic/Trade Classification	Indications/Dose	Supplied	Remarks
Brompheniramine and pseudoephedrine (Dimetapp Elixir, Dimetapp tablets, Dimetapp Liquigel, Dimetapp Extentabs) *Antihistamine, decongestant*	2-6yr: elixir 2.5mL (½ tsp) every 4hr 6-12yr: ½ tab every 4hr; elixir 5mL every 4hr ≥12yr: 1 liquigel PO every 4hr; 1 tab PO every 4hr; 1 extentab PO every 12hr; elixir 10mL every 4hr	2mg/12.5mg (brompheniramine/ pseudoephedrine) elixir 4mg/25mg tab, liquigel 12mg/75mg extentabs	Adverse effects: Drowsiness, excitability; should not be taken by those with HTN, heart disease, diabetes, thyroid disease, hallucinations. Drug interactions: MAOIs, alcohol. Pseudoephedrine requires a prescription in some states; its OTC use is regulated. Should not be used in children <2yr because deaths have been reported.
Budesonide (Pulmicort Rhinocort, Turbuhaler) *Corticosteroid*	*Maintenance and prophylactic therapy for asthma or allergic or perennial rhinitis:* **For current use in asthma treatment, refer to Appendix D**	Turbuhaler (200mcg/ inhalation) Aerosol 50mcg preactivated (32mcg delivered to patient)	Drug interactions: ketoconazole (CYP3A4 inhibitors). Side effects: dry mouth, oral candidiasis, HA, insomnia, GI disturbance. Rinse mouth after use. Rinse face after use if face mask is used with nebulized budesonide.
Calcium (Citracal, Os-Cal, Tums, Caltrate 600, Caltrate Jr, Viactiv, Children's Mylanta) *Antacid, calcium salt*	*Adequate intake in terms of elemental calcium (1997 National Academy of Science Recommendations):* <6mo: 210mg/day PO 6-12mo: 270mg/day PO 1-3yr: 500mg/day PO 4-8yr: 800mg/day PO 9-18yr: 1300mg/day PO *Antacid use:* 2-5yr, 400mg up to tid; 6-11yr, 800mg up to tid as needed Children >11yr and adults: 1000-1500mg of elemental calcium chewed every hr, up to 8g/day	Refer to product listings	Drug interactions: may potentiate digoxin toxicity, may antagonize the effects of calcium channel blockers. Oral calcium administration decreases the absorption of tetracycline, iron, atenolol, quinolone antibiotics, sodium fluoride, and zinc. Adverse reactions: constipation, hypercalcemia.
Carbamazepine (Carbatrol, Epitol, Tegretol, Tegretol XR) *Miscellaneous anticonvulsant*	*Partial, generalized tonic-clonic seizures in children >2yr:* <6yr: initial, 5mg/kg/day PO: can increase every wk by 5mg/kg divided bid-qid (max 20mg/kg/ day) 6-12yr: initially, 10mg/kg/day divided bid-qid; can increase weekly by 100mg/day or 5mg/ kg/day until therapeutic levels (usual dose 800-1200mg/day) >12yr: 200mg PO bid initially; increase by 200mg/day at wkly intervals to therapeutic levels; usual dose: 1.6 to 2.4g/day divided every 6-8hr Maintenance: 10-20mg/kg/day PO divided every 6-12hr	100mg/5mL 100mg chewable 200mg tab 100, 200, 400mg XR	Therapeutic range 4-12mcg/ mL. Take with food. CBC before therapy (baseline), at 6-12wk, then annually during long-term therapy. Suspension has to be given 3-4 times daily, tab 2-4 times daily. XR tab dosed bid and should not be crushed. Drug interactions: increased plasma levels with CYP3A4 inhibitors (cimetidine, propoxyphene, isoniazid, macrolides, calcium channel blockers, loratadine, fluoxetine, ketoconazole, itraconazole, valproate); decreased plasma levels

TABLE A-2 **Medications—Cont'd**

Generic/Trade Classification	Indications/Dose	Supplied	Remarks
			with CYP3A4 inducers (phenobarbital, phenytoin, rifampin, theophylline). May increase levels of clomipramine, phenytoin, primidone. May decrease levels of phenytoin, warfarin, doxycycline, theophylline, haloperidol, acetaminophen, alprazolam, clozapine, oral contraceptives, anticonvulsants, and others metabolized by CYP3A4. Cross-sensitivity with tricyclic antidepressants. Adverse reactions: vertigo, diplopia, hyponatremia, drowsiness, hepatotoxicity, aplastic anemia, bone marrow suppression, rash, Stevens-Johnson syndrome, photosensitivity.
Cefadroxil monohydrate (Duricef, Ultracef) *First-generation cephalosporin*	*Serious skin infections, urinary tract, bone and joint, streptococcal infections:* <1yr: 25mg/kg/day PO bid for 10 days 1-6yr: 250mg PO bid for 10 days >6yr: 500mg PO bid (up to 2g/day) >40kg: 0.5-1g bid *Skin, soft tissue, UTI*: 1g daily for 7-10 days	125, 250, 500mg/5mL (50, 100mL) 500mg capsule, 1g tab	Can dose daily for streptococcal pharyngitis. Use cautiously in patients with serious penicillin hypersensitivity.
Cefdinir (Omnicef) *Cephalosporin antibiotic* *Third-generation cephalosporin*	*Otitis, sinusitis, pharyngitis, skin infections, community-acquired pneumonia, bronchitis:* 6mo-12yr: 7mg/kg PO every12hr or 14mg/kg PO daily (max 600mg/day) ≥13yr: 300mg PO bid or 600mg daily Twice-daily dosing for pneumonia and skin infections; once-daily dosing for other infections	300mg capsule 125mg/5mL suspension	Drug interaction: antagonized by magnesium- or aluminum-containing antacids and iron (separate dose by 2hr). Side effects: GI disturbances, vaginitis.
Cefixime (Suprax) *Third-generation cephalosporin*	*Uncomplicated urinary tract infections, bronchitis, pharyngitis, tonsillitis, skin disorders (poor* Staphylococcus aureus *coverage),* Shigella *gastroenteritis, otitis media:* Children: 8mg/kg/day PO divided daily-bid (max dose 400mg) > 50kg or >12yr: 200mg bid or 400mg daily PO Gonorrhea: 400mg PO once	100mg/5mL (50, 100mL) 200, 400mg tab	Can be given as a single dose. Not indicated for infants <6mo. Treat otitis media with suspension—gives higher therapeutic levels. GI symptoms common, administer with food to decrease GI distress.

Continued

TABLE A-2 **Medications—Cont'd**

Generic/Trade Classification	Indications/Dose	Supplied	Remarks
Cefotaxime sodium (Claforan) *Third-generation cephalosporin*	*Serious infections: skin, septicemia, bone, urinary tract, lower respiratory tract, gynecologic infections, meningitis, and ventriculitis:* 1mo to 12yr: <50kg: 100-150mg/ kg/day divided every 6-8hr IV/IM >50kg or >12yr with moderate to severe infection: 1-2g IV/IM every 6-8hr (max 12g/day) *Life-threatening infection:* 2g IV every 4hr (max dose 12g/day)	0.5, 1.2g vial	GI side effects.
Cefpodoxime proxetil (Vantin) *Third-generation cephalosporin*	2mo-12yr: *Acute otitis media:* 5mg/kg PO every 12hr for 5 days (max 400mg/day) *Pharyngitis/tonsillitis and urinary tract infections:* 5mg/kg PO every 12hr for 5-10 days (max 200mg/day) *Sinusitis:* 5mg/kg PO every 12hr for 10 days (max 400mg/day) ≥13yr: *Pneumonia:* 200mg PO every 12hr for 14 days *Gonorrhea:* 200mg PO once as a single dose *Skin:* 400mg PO every 12hr for 7-14 days *Pharyngitis:* 100mg PO every 12hr for 5-10 days *Sinusitis:* 200mg PO every 12hr for 10 days *Complicated urinary tract:* 100mg every 12hr for 7 days	50, 100mg/5mL 100, 200mg tab	Drug interactions: Antacids, H$_2$antagonists, oral anticholinergics may decrease efficacy. Precautions: Penicillin allergy. Impaired renal function. Not indicated for infants <2mo. Adverse reactions: GI upset.
Cefprozil (Cefzil) *Second-generation cephalosporin*	*Pharyngitis, skin infections, tonsillitis, acute sinusitis, secondary bacterial infection of acute or chronic bronchitis:* urinary tract infection 6mo-12yr: *otitis media, sinusitis, lower respiratory tract*—15mg/ kg PO every 12hr for 10 days—*pharyngitis, urinary tract;* 7.5mg/kg PO every 12hr—*uncomplicated skin infections;*—20mg/kg PO every 24hr for 10 days *Children ≥13yr and adults: pharyngitis, tonsillitis, acute sinusitis, lower respiratory tract infections, urinary tract*—500-1000mg/day divided bid PO (max 1.5g/day); *uncomplicated skin*—250mg every 12hr (or 500mg every 24hr)— *skin structure infections*—500mg every 12hr	125, 250mg/5mL 250, 500mg tab	Adverse reactions: GI upset, elevated liver enzymes. May be taken without regard to meals. Not indicated for infants <6mo. Use with caution in penicillin-sensitive patients.

TABLE A-2 Medications—Cont'd

Generic/Trade Classification	Indications/Dose	Supplied	Remarks
Ceftibuten (Cedax) *Cephalosporin*	Bronchitis, otitis media, pharyngitis, and tonsillitis (limited coverage) >6 mo (≤45 kg): 9 mg/kg PO every 24 hr for 10 days (max 400 mg/day) >45 kg or ≥12 yr: 400 mg PO every 24 hr for 10 days	90 mg/5 mL 180 mg/5 mL 400 mg capsule	Reduce dose in patients with renal impairment. Use with caution in patients with penicillin sensitivity. Active against beta-lactamase-producing strains. Give suspension on empty stomach; capsule may be taken with food.
Ceftriaxone sodium (Rocephin) *Third-generation cephalosporin*	*Skin, bone and joint, urinary tract, gynecologic, respiratory tract, intraabdominal infections, bacteremia:* ≤12 yr: 50-75 mg/kg/day IV/IM divided 1-2 times daily (max 2 g/day) >12 yr: 1-2 g every 12-24 hr IV/IM (max 4 g/day) *Prophylaxis for high-risk contacts of patients with invasive meningococcal disease:* ≤12 yr: 125 mg IM once; >12 yr: 250 mg IM once *OM:* 50 mg/kg IM once (alternative OM therapy: 50 mg/kg/day for 3 days) max 1 g/day *Meningitis:* initially 100 mg/kg/day IV/IM (max 4 g daily), then 100 mg/kg IV/IM once daily or in divided doses every 12 hr (max 4 g) for 7-14 days.	0.25, 0.5, 1, 5, 10 g vial	Precautions: do not give to hyperbilirubinemic neonates (especially if premature). GI side effects. Mix with lidocaine to prevent pain at IM injection site.
Cefuroxime axetil (Ceftin) **Sodium** (Zinacef) *Second-generation cephalosporin*	*Pharyngitis, tonsillitis, skin, otitis media, lower respiratory tract, urinary tract, uncomplicated gonorrhea:* *Otitis media:* <2 yr: 30 mg/kg/day PO divided bid for 10 d 2-12 yr: 250 mg PO bid for 10 d *Secondary bacterial infection of acute bronchitis, uncomplicated skin, skin structure infections:* ≥13 yr: 250-500 mg PO bid *Gonorrhea:* 1 g PO as single dose *Lyme disease:* ≥13 yr: 500 mg PO bid for 20 days ≥13 yr: *Pharyngitis/tonsillitis:* ≥13 yr: 250 mg PO bid for 10 d 3 mos-12 yr: 125 mg PO bid for 10 d or 20 mg/kg/d divided bid for 10 d (max 500 mg/d) *UTI:* ≥13 yr: 125-250 mg PO bid for 7-10 d	125, 250, 500 mg tab 125 mg/5 mL suspension	Cefuroxime film-coated tabs and suspension are not bioequivalent and are not to be substituted on a mg/mg basis. Suspension must be administered with food to decrease GI side effects. Tab may be taken without regard to meals. Swallow tab whole, do not crush or chew because of bitter taste.

Continued

TABLE A-2   Medications—Cont'd

Generic/Trade Classification	Indications/Dose	Supplied	Remarks
Cephalexin monohydrate (Keflex, Keftab) *First-generation cephalosporin*	*Skin, bone and joint, septicemia, respiratory tract, urinary tract, otitis media, pharyngitis* <12 yr: 25-50 mg/kg/day PO divided bid-qid; in severe infections, dose can be doubled (max 4 g/day) ≥12 yr: 250 mg to 1 g PO every 6 hr or 500 mg every 12 hr (max 4 g/d)	100 mg/mL drops 125, 250 mg/5 mL 250, 500 mg Pulvule capsules 500 mg, 1 g tab	Caution: do not use in patients with immediate-type hypersensitivity to penicillins. Administer on empty stomach. Administer with food if GI upset occurs. Adjust dose in those with impaired renal function.
Cetirizine (Zyrtec) *Antihistamine*	*Seasonal or perennial rhinitis, chronic idiopathic urticaria*: <2 yr (limited data): 0.25 mg/kg/day PO as a single dose 2-5 yr: 2.5 mg daily to max of 5 mg PO daily or divided bid 6-12 yr: 5-10 mg PO daily as a single dose or divided bid ≥12 yr: 10 mg/day single dose	5, 10 mg tab 5 mg/5 mL syrup	Drug interaction: potentiates CNS depression with alcohol or other CNS depressants. Large doses of theophylline may decrease cetirizine clearance with potential increased toxicity. Contraindications: hydroxyzine sensitivity Warning: doses >10 mg/day may cause significant drowsiness. Side effects: fatigue, dry mouth, somnolence, HA. Children may also have abdominal pain, nausea, vomiting, bronchospasm.
Chloral hydrate (Aquachloral, Chloral Hydrate generic) *Anxiolytic, sedative, hypnotic*	*Used preoperatively to produce sedation and relieve anxiety:* Neonates: 25 mg/kg/dose PO or PR sedation before procedure Children: 8 mg/kg PO or PR tid (max 500 mg tid) ≥12 yr: 500 mg to 1 g PO or PR 30 min before surgery *Before EEG*: Children: 20-25 mg/ kg/dose PR or PO 30-60 min before EEG, up to 500 mg/single dose. May give divided doses 30 min apart. *Nonpainful procedures requiring sedation*: <12 yr: 50 mg/kg PO 30-60 min before procedure; may repeat in 30 min for a total of 120 mg/kg or 1 g total for children ≥12 yr: 250 mg PO tid for anxiety; 500-1000 mg at hs for insomnia or 30 min before procedure for sedation (max 2 g/day)	500 mg/5 mL 500 mg capsules 324, 500, 648 mg suppository	Drug interactions: warfarin, furosemide. Prolonged use in newborns can cause hyperbilirubinemia. Administer syrup in ½ glass of water, fruit juice, or ginger ale; may be mixed in infant formula. Adverse effects: Rare residual sedation or hangover at hypnotic dosages. Other possible effects include somnambulism, confusion, ataxia, HA, respiratory arrest with overdose.

TABLE A-2   Medications—Cont'd

Generic/Trade *Classification*	Indications/Dose	Supplied	Remarks
Chlorpheniramine maleate (Chlor-Trimeton, generics) *Antihistamine*	*Allergic rhinitis, urticaria:* 2-6yr: 0.35mg/kg/day divided every 4-6hr PO or 1mg every 4-6hr, PO (max 12mg/day) ≥6-12yr: 2mg every 4-6hr PO ≥12yr: 4mg every 4-6hr PO (max 24mg/day) or 8-12mg every 12hr (time-released)	2mg/5mL syrup 4, 8, 12mg tab 8, 12mg time-released tab, capsule	Adverse effects: CNS sedation, anticholinergic effects.
Ciclopirox olamine (Loprox) *Local antiinfective,* *antifungal*	Tinea cruris, tinea corporis, tinea pedis, tinea versicolor; also for cutaneous candidiasis, seborrhea dermatitis, onychomycosis *Tinea cruris, tinea corporis, tinea pedis, tinea versicolor; also for cutaneous candidiasis:* >10yr: topical—massage into affected area bid for at least 2wk; treat tinea pedis for 4wk (safety and efficacy <10yr not established) *Seborrhea:* use gel bid up to 4wk; shampoo: 5mL applied to wet hair and scalp; lather and leave on 3min. Rinse well; use twice wkly for 2-4 weeks with minimum of 3 days between applications. *Onychomycosis:* apply lacquer daily to nail and 5mm around adjoining skin at hs and allow to dry; remove every 7 days and reapply	0.77% base cream, lotion, gel, shampoo, nail lacquer	Side effects: erythema; rare rash, acne with gel. Requires treatment for 36-48 weeks
Cimetidine (Tagamet) *Histamine-receptor* *antagonist*	*Duodenal ulcers, hypersecretory conditions, gastroesophageal reflux:* Infants: 10-20mg/kg/day PO divided every 6-12hr Children: 20-40mg/kg/day PO divided qid Adults: 300mg PO qid before meals and at hs	300mg/5mL liquid 200, 300, 400, 800mg tab	Used cautiously in patients with impaired renal or hepatic function. Adverse reactions: dizziness, confusion, HA. Drug interactions: diazepam, theophylline, propranolol, antacids, phenytoin, tricyclic antidepressants, oral contraceptives, warfarin.

Continued

TABLE A-2 Medications—Cont'd

Generic/Trade Classification	Indications/Dose	Supplied	Remarks
Ciprofloxacin (Cipro, Ciloxan Ophthalmic) *Fluoroquinolone*	Lower respiratory tract, sinus, prostate, stomach, skin, bone and joint, urinary tract, infectious diarrhea, gonorrhea, anthrax, tularemia, bacterial conjunctivitis, corneal ulcers Children (oral preparations usually not recommended for children <18 yr): *complicated UTI or pyelonephritis:* 1-17 yr: 10-20 mg/kg/day PO divided bid (max 1.5 g/day) or 6-10 mg/kg IV every 8 hr for 10-21 days (max dose 400 mg) ≥18 yr: 250-750 mg PO every 12 hr depending upon type of injection (consult drug reference) *Postexposure prophylaxis of inhalational anthrax or treatment of cutaneous anthrax:* Children: 15 mg/kg PO every 12 hr for 60 days (max 1 g/day) Adults: 500 mg PO bid for 60 days *Tularemia:* Children: max dose 1 g/day PO for 14 days *Conjunctivitis:* Ophthalmic solution: ≥1 yr 1-2 drops each eye every 2 hr while awake for 2 days, then every 4 hr while awake for 5 more days Ophthalmic ointment: ≥2 yr 0.5 inch ribbon in conjunctival sac tid for 2 days then bid for 5 days	250, 500 mg/5 mL suspensions 100, 250, 500, 750 mg tab 0.3% ophthalmic solution and ointment	Oral medication not indicated for children <18 yr unless justified by multidrug-resistant gram (−) bacteria or no other drug available; used in children for anthrax. Can be considered for children 9-18 yr with cystic fibrosis or typhoid fever. Increases serum theophylline. Antacids decrease absorption. Causes photosensitivity.
Ciprofloxacin hydrochloride and hydrocortisone (CiproDex, Cipro HC Otic) *Antibiotic and steroid*	*Otitis externa:* Children ≥1 yr and adolescents: 3 drops to affected ear bid for 7 days. Probably OK to use in ≥6 mo. OM with PE tubes: ≥6 mo: 4 drops bid × 7 days. Pump ear to get solution through PE tubes.	0.2% cipro with 1% hydrocortisone; 0.3% cipro with 0.1% dexamethasone 10, 30 mL bottle	Do not use for otitis externa if TM is perforated. Side effects: HA, pruritus, rash.
Citalopram hydrobromide (Celexa) *Antidepressant*	*Treatment of depression:* ≥12 yr: 20 mg/day PO in AM or at hs; titrated by 20 mg/day in a wkly interval to 40 mg/day	10 mg/5 mL solution 10, 20, 40 mg tab	Do not give if patient is on MAOIs. Drug interactions: MAOIs, tricyclic antidepressants, alcohol, cimetidine, lithium, sumatriptan, metoprolol, St. Johns Wort, alcohol. Adverse reactions: suicide ideation or behaviors, nausea, dry mouth, insomnia, sweating, sexual dysfunction, tremor, diarrhea, fatigue. Do not abruptly stop drug. Safety and efficacy not established in pediatric patients. Close monitoring and parental observation is imperative.

TABLE A-2   Medications—Cont'd

Generic/Trade Classification	Indications/Dose	Supplied	Remarks
Clarithromycin (Biaxin, Biaxin XL) *Macrolide antibiotic*	*Pharyngitis, tonsillitis, sinusitis, lower respiratory tract, upper respiratory tract, skin, community-acquired pneumonia:* ≥ 6 mo and to 35 kg: 15 mg/kg/day PO divided every 12 hr for 10 days (max 500 mg bid) >35 kg or ≥12 yr: 250-500 mg PO every 12 hr for 10-14 days (max 1 g/day)	250, 500 mg tab 125, 250 mg/5 mL granules for suspension	Decrease dose in renal impairment. Drug interactions: theophylline (increased serum levels by 20%), carbamazepine (increased serum levels after only 1 dose of clarithromycin), terfenadine, digoxin, astemizole, propulsid, and other drugs metabolized by CYP-450 isoenzyme CYP3A3/4. Rinse mouth following suspension. Do NOT refrigerate suspension because it may gel.
Clemastine fumarate (OTC) (Anti-Hist-1, Dayhist-1, Tavist) *Antihistamine*	*Allergic rhinitis, urticaria, allergies:* <6 yr: 0.335-0.67 mg/day divided bid (max 1.34 mg daily, 1 mg base) 6-12 yr: 0.67-1.34 mg PO bid (max 4.02 mg/day) ≥12 yr: 1.34 PO bid (max 8.04 mg/day of syrup or 2.68 mg/d of tablets) *Urticaria:* 6-12 yr: 1.34 mg bid (max 4.02 mg/day) ≥12 yr of 2.68 mg once-tid (max 8.04 mg/day)	0.67 mg/5 mL (0.5 mg/5 mL base) syrup 1.34 (1 mg base), 2.68 mg (2 mg base) tab	Administer with food. May cause drowsiness.
Clindamycin (Cleocin T, generics) *Topical antibiotic*	*Mild to moderate acne, candidiasis vaginitis, vaginal pruritus:* *Acne:* >2 yr: apply thin film to all acne-affected areas twice daily *Bacterial vaginosis:* Nonpregnant: insert 1 full applicator (100 mg) intravaginally once daily before bedtime for 3 or 7 days, OR 1 suppository intravaginally at bedtime for 3 days	1% topical lotion, gel, solution 2% vaginal cream, 100 mg vaginal suppository 75 mg/5 mL solution Also available in combination with 1.2% clindamycin and 0.025% tretinoin gel (Ziana)	Use if comedones become inflamed; may use alone or with benzoyl peroxide (see below). Solution is flammable—no smoking following application. Discontinue if significant diarrhea occurs. Adverse reactions: dryness, oily skin, irritation; rare: diarrhea, colitis; use with caution in those with atopy. Avoid eyes and mucous membranes. Discontinue if significant diarrhea occurs. Vaginal cream may weaken latex in condoms and contraceptive diaphragms for 5 days after completion of therapy. Wait 30 min after washing face before applying. Can take 6-8 wk to see improvement in acne.

Continued

TABLE A-2   Medications—Cont'd

Generic/Trade *Classification*	Indications/Dose	Supplied	Remarks
Clindamycin and benzoyl peroxide (Benzaclin, Duac) *Topical antibiotic*	*Used in mild to moderate acne; use if comedones become inflamed. Apply thin film to all acne-affected areas twice daily (Benzaclin) or once daily (Duac).*	1% clindamycin-5% benzoyl peroxide	Drug interactions: additive irritation with other topical agents. Avoid erythromycin. Avoid eyes and mucous membranes. Discontinue if significant diarrhea occurs. Wait 30 min after washing before applying. Can take 6-8 wk to see improvement.
Clindamycin hydrochloride (Cleocin HCl) *Miscellaneous antibiotic*	*Serious infections involving skin, respiratory tract, sepsis, pelvic and genital tract, intraabdominal areas, bone (staphylococcal and streptococcal organisms)* >1 mo-12 yr: 8-20 mg/kg/day divided every 6-8 hr (15-40 mg/kg IM or IV daily divided every 6-8 hr) Adolescents: 150-300 mg PO every 6-8 hr (max 1.8 g/day); *more serious infections*, 300-450 mg every 6 hr for 10 days (300-600 mg IM or IV every 6, 8, 12 hrs) Adults: 150-450 mg every 6-8 hr (max 2 g/day) (IM/IV dose same as adolescents)	75 mg/5 mL 75, 150, 300 mg capsule	Can cause severe colitis. Do not refrigerate suspension; take with a full glass of water.
Clonidine (Catapres) *Antihypertensive, ADHD treatment*	Hypertension, improves attention in ADHD, tic disorder (including Tourette syndrome) *Hypertension*: ≥12 yr: 0.1 mg bid PO; may ↑ by 0.1 mg wkly; usual effective dose range 0.05-0.4 mg bid (max 2.4 mg/day) *ADHD*: 0.05 mg PO at hs, gradually increasing number of daily doses by 0.05 mg/day every 3-7 days given in 3-4 divided doses (max 0.3-0.4 mg/day) Maintenance dose usually 0.05-0.4 mg/day	0.1, 0.2, 0.3 mg tab 0.1, 0.2, 0.3 mg patch (lasts up to 7 days) (consult pharmacology reference before using transdermal patch)	Drug interactions: methylphenidate may potentially increase ECG effects (ECG abnormalities and 4 cases of sudden death reported); tricyclic antidepressants, beta-blockers, CNS depressants, and alcohol. Do not abruptly discontinue because rapid increase in blood pressure and sympathetic overactivity may occur (increased heart rate, tremors, agitation, anxiety, insomnia, palpitations, sweating). Taper over at least 1 wk. Decrease methylphenidate dose by 40% if using concurrently with clonidine, consider ECG monitoring.
Clotrimazole (OTC) (Mycelex, Lotrimin, generics) *Local antiinfective, antifungal*	*Oral candidiasis*: Children >3 yr and adults: 10 mg troche PO—dissolve slowly, 5 times daily for 2 wk *Vaginal candidiasis*: 1 applicator at hs for 1-2 wk *Tinea pedis, tinea cruris, tinea corporis, or tinea versicolor*: Topical application of cream bid for 1-8 wk (use for 7 days after rash clears)	10 mg troche 1% cream, solution, lotion	Adverse reactions: nausea, vomiting, abnormal liver function tests.

TABLE A-2   **Medications—Cont'd**

Generic/Trade Classification	Indications/Dose	Supplied	Remarks
Codeine *Opiate agonist, antitussive, analgesic*	Children: Analgesic: 0.5-1 mg/kg every 4-6 hr PO, IM, SC (max 60 mg/dose) Antitussive: 2-12 yr: 1-1.5 mg/kg/day divided every 4-6 hr PO (max 30 mg/day); 7-12 yr: 5-10 mg every 4-6 hr PO (max 60 mg/day) >12 yr and adolescents: Analgesic: 15-60 mg/dose every 4-6 hr (max 120 mg/day) Antitussive: 10-20 mg/dose every 4-6 hr (max 120 mg/day)	15 mg/5 mL solution 15, 30, 60 mg tab 30, 60 mg/mL injection	Respiratory depression, nausea, vomiting, constipation.
Cromolyn sodium (Crolom, Gastrocrom, Intal, Nasalcrom) *Mast cell stabilizer*	*Prophylaxis in treatment of allergic disorders and asthma:* Children >2 yr (oral inhalation): 10 mg (1 mL) via nebulizer tid-qid Children >5 yr and adolescents (oral inhalation): 1-2 inhalations tid-qid by metered-dose inhaler or 20 mg (2 mL), nebulizer tid-qid; 1 spray, intranasally, 3 or 4 times daily *Prevention of exercise-induced bronchospasm:* 2 inhalations 10-60 min before exercise	Aerosol: 800 mcg/metered spray Solution: 10 mg/mL (2 mL) ampule for nebulization Solution, nasal: 40 mg/spray	Not to be used to treat acute asthmatic attacks; may take 3-4 wk for max effectiveness in asthma treatment. Adverse reactions: HA, bronchospasm, urticaria, cough, throat irritation. Do not withdraw drug abruptly.
Cromolyn sodium (Opticrom, Crolom, cromolyn sodium generic) *Mast cell stabilizer*	*Used for allergic conjunctivitis:* >4 yr: 1-2 drops 4-6 times daily	4% ophthalmic solution	Side effect: transient ocular burning/stinging.
Cyclobenzaprine (Flexeril, generic) *Skeletal muscle relaxant*	*Treatment of muscle spasms associated with acute painful musculoskeletal conditions:* >15 yr: 5-10 mg 3 times/day	5, 10 mg tab	Drug interactions: MAOIs. Use only for 2-3 wk.
Cyproheptadine HCl (Periactin, generic) *Antihistamine*	*Allergic rhinitis, urticaria, allergic conjunctivitis:* Children: 0.25 mg/kg/day PO divided bid-tid or 2-6 yr: 2 mg PO bid-tid (max 12 mg/day) 7-14 yr: 4 mg PO bid-tid (max 16 mg/day) >14 yr: 12-16 mg/day divided tid (max 0.5 mg/kg/day) *Migraine HA:* Children: 4 mg bid-tid Adolescents: 4-8 mg 3 times a day	2 mg/5 mL syrup 4 mg tab	Experimentally used to stimulate appetite and increase weight gain in children. Side effect: weight gain; in some patients, sedative effect disappears within 3-4 days.
Desloratadine (Aerius, Clarinex, Claramax, NeoClarityn) *Antihistamine*	*Allergic rhinitis (seasonal or perennial); chronic idiopathic urticaria:* 6-11 mo: 1 mg syrup once daily 1-5 yr: 1.25 mg syrup once daily	2.5, 5 mg tab (regular or disintegrating wafer) 0.5 mg/mL syrup Clarinex-D 24 hr XR product combo with Clarinex 5 mg and pseudoephedrine 240 mg	Adverse effects: dry mouth or throat, somnolence, myalgia, dizziness. Safety not established in children <2 yr with seasonal rhinitis or in those <6 mo with perennial rhinitis or urticaria.

Continued

TABLE A-2   Medications—Cont'd

Generic/Trade Classification	Indications/Dose	Supplied	Remarks
	6-11yr: 2.5mg syrup once daily ≥12yr and adolescents: 5mg PO once daily; renal or hepatic impairment: 5mg every other day		
Desmopressin acetate (DDAVP, Stimate, Minirin) *Posterior pituitary hormone; antidiuretic*	Used in the treatment of diabetes insipidus, temporary polyuria, and some forms of hemophilia *Diabetes insipidus:* 3mo-12yr: 0.05mg tab daily or bid ≥12yr: 0.05mg PO bid; adjust dose to patient response; or 2-4mcg/day SC or IV divided bid *Nocturnal enuresis:* >6yr: 0.2mg PO **tabs only** at hs; adjust up to max 0.6mg. *Hemophilia A and type I von Willebrand disease:* >3mo and adolescents: 0.3mcg/kg slow IV preoperative	Injection: 4mcg/mL 0.1, 0.2mg tab, scored	Upper respiratory infections can decrease the absorption of the drug. High incidence of relapse in the treatment of nocturnal enuresis when drug is stopped. Nasal spray is no longer recommended for treatment of nocturnal enuresis because of hyponatremia-related seizures and death. Tablets may still be used but treatment should be stopped during acute illnesses that may cause fluid and/or electrolyte imbalance (e.g., fever, vomiting, diarrhea) or vigorous exercise or conditions that may increase water consumption. Restrict fluids 1 hour prior to and 8 hours following administration. Report any adverse events related to use of this drug to Medwatch*. Drug interactions: chlorpropamide, lithium, heparin, carbamazepine, epinephrine, fludrocortisone. Observe for signs of water intoxication: HA, drowsiness, listlessness, shortness of breath. Adverse reactions: HA, flushing, ↑BP, nausea, nasal congestion, abdominal cramps. Wake children within 10hr to urinate after taking drug. Give on an empty stomach. When switching to tabs, give first dose 24hr after last nasal dose.
Dexamethasone (Decadron, Decaject, Solurex, generic) *Glucocorticoid, antiinflammatory*	Used in the treatment of chronic inflammatory disorders, cerebral edema, shock, allergies, croup, hematologic disorders, bacterial meningitis *Antiinflammatory:* Children: 0.024-0.34mg/kg/day PO, IV, or IM divided qid *Antiinflammatory, other uses:* Adults: 0.5-9mg/day PO, IV, or IM divided bid-qid *Croup:* 0.6mg/kg once. Use Decadron IV solution and give PO, mixed in acetaminophen elixir per age to improve compliance over the bitter-tasting suspension	0.5mg/5mL elixir 0.5mg/0.5mL solution 0.5, 0.75, 1.5, 2, 4, 6mg tab 4, 8, 10mg/mL IM or IV	Contraindicated in patients with systemic fungal infections. Use cautiously in patients with untreated viral or bacterial infections, renal disease, heart disease, tuberculosis, ulcerative colitis, hypothyroidism, diabetes. Do not give live vaccines to patients on dexamethasone. Can mask signs and symptoms of infection. Drug interactions: oral anticoagulants, oral contraceptives, rifampin, phenytoin, barbiturates, hypoglycemics. Suspension tastes bitter.

*Medwatch 1-800-FDA-1088; fax, 1-800-FDA-0178; on-line, www.fda.gov/medwatch.

TABLE A-2   **Medications—Cont'd**

Generic/Trade Classification	Indications/Dose	Supplied	Remarks
Dexmethylphenidate HCL (Focalin, Focalin XR) *CNS stimulant similar to amphetamine*	*ADHD* Dosage depends upon patient's current drug treatment (if presently on racemic methylphenidate or other stimulant)—Consult a pharmacologic reference for dosing recommendations If initially starting ADHD treatment: ≥6yr: 2.5mg PO bid given at least 4 hrs apart. Increase weekly by 2.5-5mg daily up to max 20mg daily in divided doses XR caps once in the AM (may be sprinkled on applesauce).	2.5, 5, 10mg tab 5,10, 20mg XR capsule	Careful history for cardiovascular (structural abnormalities or other severe cardiac condition) and psychiatric (suicide, bipolar, depression) problems in patient and family. Sudden withdrawal may cause severe depression. Adverse effects: abdominal pain, anorexia, insomnia, tachycardia, anxiety, tension, agitation, psychotic or manic symptoms, growth suppression, seizures, blurred vision. Drug interactions: with racemic methylphenidate; ↓ metabolism of anticonvulsants or SSRIs; possible hypotensive crisis with MAOIs.
Dextroamphetamine saccharate; dextroamphetamine sulfate; amphetamine aspartate; amphetamine sulfate (Adderall, Adderall XR) *Amphetamine, CNS stimulant*	*Used in the treatment of ADHD/ ADD* *Tab:* 3-5yr: 2.5mg daily; increase 2.5mg/day wkly increments until desired response attained ≥6yr: 5mg daily or bid; increase by 5mg/day wkly increments until desired response attained Give first dose on awakening; additional doses (1 or 2) in 4-6hr intervals (max 40mg/day) *XR capsule:* 6yr and older: 5-10mg daily AM; increase by 5-10mg/ day at wkly intervals (max 30mg/day)	5, 7.5, 10, 12.5, 15, 20, 30mg tab; all tabs are double scored 5, 10, 15, 20, 25, 30 XR capsule	Drug interactions: MAOIs, tricyclic antidepressants, antihypertensives, phenobarbital, meperidine, phenytoin. Abuse potential. Side effects: HTN, insomnia, anorexia, dry mouth, GI disturbance. Can exacerbate tics and Tourette syndrome. Monitor growth in children. XR capsule may be opened and sprinkled on a small amount of applesauce (do not chew).
Dextroamphetamine sulfate (Dexedrine, generic) *Amphetamine, CNS stimulant*	Used in the treatment of ADHD and narcolepsy *Narcolepsy:* Children 6-12yr: 5mg PO initially; increase by 5mg at wkly intervals (max 60mg/day) until desired response attained ≥12yr: 10mg PO initially; increase by 10mg at wkly intervals (max 60mg/day); give in divided doses or use long-acting forms	5, 10, 15mg capsule (spansule), sustained release 5, 10mg tab	Contraindicated in patients with hypertension, hyperthyroidism, glaucoma, or cardiovascular disease. Drug interactions: MAOIs, tricyclic antidepressants, phenobarbital, phenytoin; insulin requirements may be altered. Do not give within 6hr of bedtime. Adverse reactions: GI disturbances, insomnia, dry mouth, anorexia, hypertension, tremor, tachycardia. Avoid caffeine.

Continued

TABLE A-2 Medications—Cont'd

Generic/Trade Classification	Indications/Dose	Supplied	Remarks
	Spansules: give once daily; if using tabs, give first dose in the morning after eating; additional doses (1-2) at 4-6 hr intervals *ADHD*: 3-5 yr: 2.5 mg/day PO initially; increase by 2.5 mg/day in wkly intervals; usual dose 0.1-0.5 mg/kg/day, given in the AM (range 5-15 mg bid or 5-10 mg tid; max 40 mg/day) >6 yr: 5 mg/day PO initially given daily or bid; increase by 5 mg/day in wkly intervals; usual dose 0.1-0.5 mg/kg/day, given in the AM (max 40 mg/day); additional doses (1-2) at intervals of 4-6 hr		
Dextromethorphan hydrobromide (Benylin, Delsym, Hold, Robitussin DM, Sucrets Cough, others) *Nonnarcotic antitussive*	*Cough suppression*: 2-5 yr: 2.5-5 mg every 4 hr PO (max 30 mg/day) or 15 mg XR syrup bid > 6 yr-11 yr: 5-10 mg every 4 hr PO (max 60 mg/day) or 30 mg XR syrup bid ≥12 yr: 10-20 mg every 4 hr PO (max 120 mg/day); or 60 mg XR syrup bid	5, 7.5, 10, 15 mg/5 mL syrup 5, 15 mg lozenge 7.5 mg chewable 15 mg capsule 30 mg/5 mL extended-release syrup	"Robo-tripping" has been reported in teenagers abusing dextromethorphan-containing cough medications and has led to these products being stocked behind counters. Should not be used in children <2 yr because deaths have been reported.
Diazepam (Valium, Diastat rectal, generic) *Anxiolytic, benzodiazepine*	Status epilepticus (slow IV push over 2-3 min) Neonate: (Not first-line drug) ≥30 days and <5 yr: 0.05-0.3 mg/kg/dose every 30 min to a max total dose of 5-10 mg. Repeat every 2-4 hr prn >5 yr: 1 mg/dose every 2-5 min up to a max of 10 mg. Repeat every 2-4 hr prn Adults: 5-10 mg; may repeat in 10-15 min intervals to a max of 30 mg. Repeat every 2-4 hr prn *Repetitive seizures* 2-5 yr: 0.5 mg/kg PR rounding up to nearest available dose form. May repeat in 4-12 hrs. 6-11 yr: 0.3 mg/kg PR (rounded to closest available dose form). May repeat in 4-12 hr ≥12 yr: 0.2 mg/kg PR (rounded to nearest available dose form). May repeat in 4-12 hr. *Sedation/relaxation*: >6 mos-11 yr: 0.12-0.8 mg/kg/day PO divided tid-qid ≥12 yr: 2-10 mg PO bid-qid	5 mg/mL injection 5 mg/mL solution 2, 5, 10 mg tab 2.5, 5, 10, 20 mg rectal gel system (pediatric and adult applicator tips)	Controlled substance, schedule IV. Do not use in patients with narrow-angle glaucoma, severe pain. Causes CNS depression. Tab can be crushed. Complete blood count, liver and kidney function tests should be performed regularly with long-term use. IV lorazepam often preferred because it is longer acting than diazepam. Also used in neonates for opiate withdrawal.

TABLE A-2   Medications—Cont'd

Generic/Trade Classification	Indications/Dose	Supplied	Remarks
Dicloxacillin monohydrate (Dycill, Dynapen, Pathocil, generic) *Penicillinase-resistant penicillin*	*Sinusitis, skin, bone and joint, respiratory tract* (infections caused by penicillinase-producing staphylococcus) Children >1mo but <40kg: 25-50mg/kg/day PO divided every 6hr (max 2g/day) Children >40kg and adults: 125-500mg PO every 6hr (max 2g/day)	62.5mg/5mL suspension 250, 500mg capsule	Drug interactions: warfarin, rifampin, aminoglycosides. Decreases effectiveness of oral contraceptives. Food decreases absorption.
Dicyclomine HCl (Bentyl, generic) *Antimuscarinic, antispasmodic*	*Used as adjunctive therapy to treat peptic ulcer disease, functional GI disturbances (acute enterocolitis):* >6mo: 5mg PO tid-qid Children: 10mg/dose PO tid-qid Adults: 20mg PO qid; may increase to 40mg qid if tolerated and adequate response not obtained at lower dose	10mg/5mL syrup 20mg tab 10mg capsule	Contraindicated in patients with glaucoma, obstructive GI or GU conditions, myasthenia gravis. Use cautiously in patients with hyperthyroidism, cardiac disease, hypertension. Adverse reactions: hypotonia, dry mouth, blurred vision, palpitations.
Dimenhydrinate (Dramamine, generic) *Antiemetic*	*Treat and prevent nausea, vertigo, and vomiting associated with motion sickness:* 2-5yr: 12.5-25mg PO every 6-8hr (max 75mg/day) 6-12yr: 25-50mg PO every 6-8hr (max 150mg/day) Children ≥12yr and adults: 50-100mg PO every 4-6hr (max 400mg/day)	12.5mg/5mL liquid 50mg scored tab, chewable tab, capsule	Contraindicated in patients with glaucoma, asthma, seizures. Adverse reactions: drowsiness, dizziness, hypotension, dry mouth, blurred vision.
Diphenhydramine hydrochloride (OTC) (Benadryl, generic) *Antihistamine*	*Allergic rhinitis, urticaria, allergic reaction to blood or plasma, motion sickness, vertigo, cough, insomnia, control of dyskinetic movement:* Children: 5mg/kg/day divided every 6-8hr PO/IM/IV (max 300mg/day) Adults: 10-50mg/dose every 4-6hr PO/IM/IV (max 400mg/day) Topical: apply tid-qid	12.5mg/5mL syrup, elixir 12.5mg chewable 25, 50mg tab, capsule 10, 50mg/mL injection 1% cream, lotion	Can cause respiratory suppression. Topical diphenhydramine should not be used to treat chickenpox, poison oak, or sunburn or over large areas of the body or on blistered or oozing skin. May cause paradoxic excitation in children.
Diphenoxylate HCl and atropine sulfate (Lomotil, Lonox, generic) *Antidiarrheal*	*Used to treat nonspecific diarrhea* <2yr: not recommended 2-5yr: 4mL (2mg diphenoxylate component) tid 5-8yr: 4mL qid 8-12yr: 4mL 5 times daily OR 2-12yr: 0.3-0.4mg/kg/day PO divided qid; dose calculated as the diphenoxylate component >12yr: 5mg PO tid-qid (diphenoxylate component)	Solution: diphenoxylate 2.5mg and atropine 0.025mg/5mL Tab: diphenoxylate 2.5mg and atropine 0.025mg	Use cautiously in pediatric patients and those with liver disease or ulcerative colitis. Use solution in children ≤12yr. Drug interactions: MAOIs. Adverse reactions: dizziness, HA, dry mouth, tachycardia, drowsiness. If no response in 48hr, drug is not likely to be effective.

Continued

TABLE A-2   Medications—Cont'd

Generic/Trade Classification	Indications/Dose	Supplied	Remarks
Docusate sodium (Colace, Correctol, Ducusoft S, DOK, DOS, Liqui-gels, Diocto, Ex-Lax, others, generic) *Laxative*	*Stool softener oral:* 5 mg/kg/day in 1-4 divided doses or dose by age <3 yr: 10-40 mg/day divided in 1 or more doses 3-6 yr: 20-60 mg/day PO 6-12 yr: 40-120 mg/day PO >12 yr: 50-360 mg/day PO divided 1-4 times daily	10 mg/mL solution; 16.7 mg/5 mL syrup; 20 mg/5 mL solution 50, 100, 250 mg capsule 100 mg tab	Drug interactions: mineral oil. Mix liquid with fruit juice or milk to mask taste. Docusate sodium liquid (5-10 mL) instilled into the ear as a ceruminolytic produces ear wax softening within 15 min.
Doxycycline calcium (Doryx, Vibramycin, Vibra-Tabs, Monodox, generic) *Tetracycline*	*Used in treatment of infections caused by* Rickettsia, Chlamydia, Mycoplasma; *syphilis, gonorrhea, traveler's diarrhea, postexposure of inhaled or cutaneous anthrax:* >8 yr and <45 kg: 2.2 mg/kg PO bid (max 200 mg/day) × 5-7 days >8 yr and >45 kg: 100 mg PO bid × 5-7 days *For postexposure prophylaxis of inhalational anthrax or treatment of cutaneous anthrax:* ≤8 yr: 2.2 mg/kg every 12 hr for 60 days >8 yr (>45 kg) and adolescents: 100 mg every 12 hr or 2.2 mg/kg bid for 7-10 days	25 mg/5 mL, 50 mg/5 mL suspension 50, 75, 100 mg tab 50, 75, 100 mg capsule	Syrup not available at many pharmacies. Use of outdated product can cause Fanconi-like syndrome. Can cause photosensitivity. Drug interactions: antacids, iron products, zinc, calcium, magnesium reduce absorption. Note: see *MMWR* vol. 50:1014-1016, 2001 for more information on anthrax dosing.
Econazole nitrate (Spectazole, generic) *Local antiinfective, antifungal*	*For treatment of tinea pedis, tinea cruris, tinea corporis, tinea versicolor:* Children >3 yr and adolescents: apply topically once daily Treat tinea pedis for 4-6 wk, all others for 2 wk *Cutaneous candidiasis:* Apply topically twice daily for 2 wk (morning and evening)	1% cream	Adverse effects: transient burning/stinging, pruritus, erythema. Instruct patients to use for full length of treatment; do not use around eyes or vaginally.
EMLA cream (lidocaine 2.5% and prilocaine 2.5%) *Topical anesthetic*	*Used for topical anesthesia before painful procedures,* including dental work. The following are max doses: 1-3 mo or <5 kg: 1 g with max application area of 10 cm² 4-12 mo or >5 kg: 2 g with max application area of 20 cm² 1-6 yr or >10 kg: 10 g with max application area of 100 cm² 7-12 yr or >20 kg: 20 g with max application area of 200 cm²	Gel/jelly (subgingival), cream, film, kit	Do not use on open wounds. Do not use near eyes. Clean and disinfect area before applying. Apply at least 1 hr before procedure.
Epinephrine HCl (Epinephrine Mist, Primatene Mist, AsthmaHaler, Adrenalin, Ana-Guard, EpiPen, EpiPen Jr; racepinephrine preparations: Breatheasy Inhalant, S-2 Inhalant)	*Bronchodilation; anaphylactic reactions:* Children: *anaphylaxis or asthma:* 0.01 mg/kg (1:1000) SC repeat every 15 min for 2 doses, then every 4 hr prn (max 0.5 mg/dose)	1:1000 (1 mg/mL), 1:2000 (0.5 mg/mL), 1:10,000 (0.1 mg/mL) injection 160, 220 mcg/metered spray, powder	Inhaled beta$_2$-agonist preferred. Rotate injection sites. Adverse effects: ECG changes, restlessness, tremor, nausea, vomiting.

Generic/Trade *Classification*	Indications/Dose	Supplied	Remarks
Bronchodilator, vasopressor, cardiac stimulant	Adults: *anaphylaxis*: 0.1-0.5 mg (1:1000) SC every 5-15 min; *asthma*: 0.3 mg SC every 20 min up to 3 times (max 1 mg/dose) Inhaler: *Asthma*: ≥4 yr: 160-250 mcg/spray; repeat once if necessary after 1 min, then no sooner than every 3 hr Nebulizer: *Asthma*: ≥4 yr: 1-3 deep inhalations of 0.25-0.5 mL of 2.25% diluted in 3 mL NaCl (depending on response; do not repeat more often than every 3 hr) of racepinephrine or epinephrine solutions	1% solution (1:100 epinephrine) or 2.25% racepinephrine	
Ertaczo *Antifungal*	*For tinea pedis* ≥12 yr: apply cream bid to affected areas for 4 wks	2% cream	Contact dermatitis, erythema, dryness, burning, hyperpigmentation
Erythromycin topical (Emgel, Erygel, Akne-Mycin, T-Stat, generic) *Topical antibiotic*	*For mild-to-moderate acne* Apply bid to acne-prone areas	2% solution, gel	Cleanse area first, wait 30 min before applying. Wash hands after applying. Additive irritant effects when used with other topical acne products. Contraindicated in patients with known sensitivity to erythromycin.
Erythromycin and benzoyl peroxide topical (Benzamycin Pak) *Topical antibiotic, keratolytic agent*	*Used in mild to moderate acne:* Apply twice daily	3% gel pak (60 per carton) or gel	Should be refrigerated. Expires every 3 mo. Contraindicated in patients with known sensitivity to erythromycin. Should be applied following cleansing. Wash hands after applying.
Erythromycin base, estolate, stearate, ethylsuccinate (generic) *Antibiotic*	*Upper and lower respiratory tract, otitis media, pharyngitis, syphilis, gonorrhea, skin, gynecologic disorders, and Legionnaires disease:* *Erythromycin base* (ERYC, Ery-Tab, PCE Dispertab, Erythromycin base filmtab) *Erythromycin estolate* (Erythromycin Estolate generic) *Erythromycin stearate* (Erythrocin) *Erythromycin ethylsuccinate* (EES) (E.E.S., EryPed, E.E.E. filmtabs)	*Erythromycin base:* 250, 500 mg tab 250, 333, 500 mg delayed-release tab or capsule *Erythromycin estolate:* 250 mg capsule 125, 250 mg/5 mL suspension *Erythromycin stearate:* 250, 500 mg tab *Erythromycin ethylsuccinate:* 125 mg pellets in capsule 250 tab, 333 mg delayed-release tab 250 mg capsule 100 mg/2.5 mL drops 200, 400 mg/5 mL 200 mg chewable tab; 400 mg tab	Most prescribe tid. GI upset common. Give with food to decrease side effects. Drug interactions: theophylline, carbamazepine, cyclosporine, digoxin, terfenadine, warfarin. Useful in patients allergic to penicillin.

Continued

TABLE A-2 Medications—Cont'd

Generic/Trade Classification	Indications/Dose	Supplied	Remarks
	Preparations dosed as follows: Base: *Children to 12yrs:* 30-50 mg/kg/day PO divided every 6-8 hr (do not exceed 2 g/day of base) Estolate *Children to 12yrs:* 30-50 mg/kg/day divided every 8-12 hr (max 250-500 mg qid) Stearate: *Children to 12yrs:* 20-40 mg/kg/day divided every 6 hr (max 250-500 mg qid) ≥12yr-*adults:* estolate/stearate/base: 250-500 mg every 6 hr or 400-800 mg ethylsuccinate PO every 6 hrs. *Pneumonia due to C. trachomatis:* base/estolate/sterate: Infants: 50 mg/kg/day PO divided qid for 21 days		
EES and sulfisoxazole combination (Pediazole, Eryzole, generic) *Erythromycin and sulfonamide*	Upper and lower respiratory tract disorders, otitis media. Dose according to EES component ≥3 mo: 50 mg/kg/day PO (of EES) divided tid-qid (max 2 g erythromycin, 6 g sulfisoxazole/day)	EES 200 mg and sulfisoxazole 600 mg/5 mL	Can be prescribed bid-qid. Drug interactions as with erythromycin.
Erythromycin ethylsuccinate ophthalmic (Romycin, generic) *Ocular antibiotic*	Treatment of ocular infections; prophylaxis of ophthalmia neonatorum *Prophylaxis of ophthalmia neonatorum:* instill 0.5-1 cm ribbon of ointment in each conjunctival sac within first hr following birth *Chlamydia infections:* 0.25-inch ribbon twice daily for 2 mo *Other eye infections:* instill 0.25-inch ribbon of ointment in each eye 3 or 4 times daily	Ophthalmic ointment 0.5%	Side effects: ocular irritation or redness after application.
Estrogens, conjugated (Premarin cream) *Hormone*	*Treatment of vaginal adhesions:* Apply small amount daily until agglutination resolves	Vaginal cream, 0.625%	Apply small amount of cream to Q-Tip and then gently use Q-Tip to rub cream over labial adhesions. Use for 2 wk, then stop. If excessive amounts used or if prolonged use, estrogen effects may be noted.
Ethosuximide (Zarontin, Ethosuximide Syrup) *Anticonvulsant*	*Controls absence seizures:* 3-6 yr: 10-15 mg/kg/24 hr to start divided bid; ↑ every 4-7 days to therapeutic level. Usual maintenance dose 15-40 mg/kg/day (max 250 mg in 1 dose/day) >6 yr: initially 250 mg bid, increase as needed by 250 mg/day every 4-7 days until seizures controlled; usual maintenance dose 20-40 mg/kg/day (max 1.5 g/day in 2 divided doses). Dose dependent on drug levels	250 mg capsule 250 mg/5 mL syrup	Therapeutic range: 40-100 mcg/mL; toxic: >150 mcg/mL. Drug interactions: phenytoin, valproic acid. Side effects: GI disturbances, blood dyscrasias, fatigue, sedation.

TABLE A-2 **Medications—Cont'd**

Generic/Trade *Classification*	Indications/Dose	Supplied	Remarks
Famotidine (Pepcid, Pepcid AC, generic) *GI histamine H$_2$ agonist*	Duodenal or gastric ulcers, gastroesophageal reflux disease (GERD) *Peptic ulcer:* 1-16 yr: 0.5 mg/kg/day PO daily or divided bid (max 40 mg/day) > 16 yr: 20 mg bid or 40 mg daily *GERD:* 1-16 yr: 1-2 mg/kg/day PO divided bid (max 80 mg/day) > 16 yr: 20 mg bid up to 6 wk	40 mg/5 mL suspension 10 mg chewable tab; 10 mg tab (OTC), 20 mg, 40 mg tab	Drug interactions: may give antacids concomitantly. Adverse reactions: HA, constipation, dizziness, diarrhea, somnolence.
Felbamate (Felbatol) *Anticonvulsant*	*For partial, generalized seizures and Lennox-Gastaut syndrome:* Consult with a neurologist before using 2-14 yr: 15 mg/kg/day PO tid-qid; ↑ by 15 mg/k/day wkly to max of 45 mg/kg/day or 3600 mg, whichever is less. >14 yr: initially, 1.2 g/day divided tid-qid; ↑ by 1.2 g/day wkly (max 3.6 g/day)	600 mg/5 mL suspension 400, 600 mg tab	Adverse reactions: drowsiness, lethargy, nausea, vomiting, aplastic anemia, hepatitis, anorexia, ataxia, behavioral changes. LFTs, CBC with differential, platelets, reticulocyte count need to be monitored monthly; blood drug levels are not monitored.
Ferrous sulfate (OTC) (Feosol, Fer-In-Sol, Fer-Gen-Sol, Mol-Iron, Feratab, many products with varying levels of elemental iron) *Oral iron supplement*	*Prevention and treatment of iron deficiency anemia:* <5 yr: 1-2 mg/kg/day to 15 mg/day *for prophylaxis;* 3-6 mg/kg/day in divided doses bid-tid for 2-3 mo for treatment of iron deficiency 5-12 yr: *prophylaxis:* 15-18 mg/day; treatment for iron deficiency anemia: 60 mg elemental iron/ day for 2-3 mo Menstruating adolescent females 12-18 yr: *prophylaxis:* 60-120 mg/day elemental iron ≥12 yr: *prophylaxis:* 60 mg elemental iron/day; iron deficiency anemia: 50-100 mg elemental iron tid for 2-3 mo	Fer-In-Sol drops: 125 mg (25 mg elemental iron)/mL Elixirs (elemental iron): 44 mg/5 mL; 60 mg/5 mL; 125 mg/mL Tab: 150 mg (50 mg elemental iron); 100 mg (33 mg elemental iron); 200 mg (66 mg elemental iron) Chewable tab (Feostat): 100 mg (33 mg elemental iron)	Concurrent vitamin C (e.g., orange juice) enhances absorption. Best taken 2 hr before or 1 hr after meals for max absorption. Contraindicated in patients with enteritis, ulcers, ulcerative colitis, hemochromatosis, hemolytic anemia, hepatitis. Drug interactions: tetracycline, vitamin C, antacids, chloramphenicol. Adverse reactions: GI symptoms, staining of teeth, dark stools. Overdosage can be fatal, at levels between 30-300 mg/kg elemental iron.
Fexofenadine HCl (Allegra, Allegra-D, generic) *Antihistamine*	*Treatment of seasonal allergic rhinitis* (Allegra-D not recommended for those <12 yr): 2-11 yr: 30 mg PO bid ≥12 yr: 60 mg bid or 180 mg daily; 60 mg daily if decreased renal function *Chronic idiopathic urticaria:* 6 mo-11 yr: 15 mg PO bid ≥12 yr: dose as for seasonal allergic rhinitis	30 mg, 60 mg, 180 mg tab 60 mg capsule Allegra-D (combo with pseudoephedrine): 60/120 mg/12 hr; 180/240/24 hr extended release 30 mg/5 mL Allegra oral suspension	Drug interactions: MAOIs, antihypertensives. Side effects: HA, GI upset, insomnia, dry mouth.
Fluconazole (Diflucan, generic) Antifungal	For oral, esophageal, systemic candidiasis *Oral candidiasis:* Children >2 wk: 6 mg/kg on day 1, then 3 mg/kg/day for 14-21 days	50 mg/5 mL suspension 50, 100, 150, 200 mg tab	Renal and hepatotoxicity have been reported; if abnormal liver or renal function tests occur during therapy, discontinue drug or monitor closely for more severe renal or hepatic injury.

Continued

TABLE A-2	Medications—Cont'd		
Generic/Trade *Classification*	**Indications/Dose**	**Supplied**	**Remarks**
	Adults: 200 mg on day 1, then 100-200 mg/day for 14 days *Vaginal candidiasis:* Severe, nonpregnant adult: two, 150 mg tabs PO given 3 days apart. *Recurrent vaginal candidiasis nonpregnant adult*: 150 mg every third day × 3. *Maintenance*: 150 mg once wkly × 6 mo		Can cause nausea, HA, rash, vomiting, abdominal pain, diarrhea. Decrease dose in renal failure. Drug interactions: warfarin, theophylline, oral hypoglycemics, phenytoin, cyclosporine, rifampin, hydrochlorothiazide, propulsid, astemizole.
Flunisolide (AeroBid, Nasarel, generic) *Glucocorticoid, antiinflammatory*	For treatment of asthma requiring chronic steroid use; nasal solution used to treat seasonal allergic rhinitis *Allergic rhinitis*: Nasal spray: Children 6-14 yr: initially, 1 spray each nostril tid or 2 sprays each nostril bid (max 4 inhalations or sprays daily); titrate dose to lowest effective amount; maintenance, 1 spray each nostril daily Adults: initially, 2 sprays each nostril bid (max 8 inhalations or sprays daily); titrate dose to lowest effective amount; maintenance, 1 spray each nostril daily *Asthma prophylaxis*: Metered inhaler: 6-15 yr: 2 oral inhalations bid >15 yr: 2 oral inhalations bid (max 8 inhalations/day) **For current asthma guidelines see Appendix D**	250 mcg/metered spray for oral inhalation 25 mcg/metered spray for nasal inhalation	Rinse mouth following oral inhalation. Not recommended for use in children <6 yr. Contraindicated in patients with fungal, untreated bacterial, or viral infections. Not to be used to treat acute asthmatic attacks. Adverse reactions: oral candidal infections, nasal irritation, adrenal suppression, HA. Do not stop drug abruptly. Use caution when transferring from systemic steroids to inhaled steroids.
Fluoride (many preparations, generic) *Mineral supplement*	*Used to prevent dental caries and in the treatment of osteoporosis:* Caries prevention depends on content of fluoride in child's source of drinking water: *<0.3 ppm fluoride content of water*: 6 mo-3 yr: 0.25 mg PO daily 3-6 yr: 0.5 mg PO daily 6-16 yr: 1 mg PO daily *0.3-0.6 ppm fluoride content of water*: 6 mo-3 yr: no supplement required 3-6 yr: 0.25 mg PO daily 6-16 yr: 0.5 mg PO daily	Drops calibrated by fluoride ion Luride drops: 0.125 mg/drop Pediaflor drops: 0.5 mg/mL Tri-Vi-Flor drops: 0.25, 0.5 mg/mL Oral solution: 1 mg/mL fluoride ion Chewable tab: 0.25, 0.5, 1 mg fluoride ion Tab: 0.25 mg fluoride ion	Do not give if fluoride content of drinking water is >0.6 ppm. Do not give with milk products. Adverse reactions: GI upset; do not swallow rinse or gel. Dental fluorosis can occur if supplements are given unnecessarily. Infants <6 mo should not receive fluoride supplements. This includes those exclusively breastfed.

TABLE A-2 Medications—Cont'd

Generic/Trade Classification	Indications/Dose	Supplied	Remarks
Fluoxetine (Prozac, Prozac Weekly, Sarafem, generic) *Antidepressant*	*Depression or obsessive-compulsive disorder:* <5 yr: no dosing information available 8-18 yr: initial dose of 5-10 mg/day or 10 mg given 3 times a wk may result in less adverse effects; dose titrated upward wkly (max 20 mg/day) >18 yr: initially 5 mg/day or 20 mg every 2-3 days; increase dose after several wk by 20 mg/day increments, titrate dose every few wk up to max dose of 80 mg/day if needed *Bulimia:* Adults: 60 mg/day administered in the morning; may need to titrate up or down to this dose, depending on response and side effects *Premenstrual dysphoric disorder:* Adults: 20 mg/day titrated as necessary up to 60-80 mg/day; start 14 days before expected start of menses and continue through first full day of menses *Obsessive-compulsive disorder:* 7-17 yr: 10 mg/day, titrating up in those with higher weights to 20-60 mg/day after 2 wk; in lower weight children titrate up after 2 wk to 20-30 mg/day as needed	10, 20, 40 mg tab In combo with olanzapine (Symbyax)—refer to a pharmacologic reference 20 mg/5 mL solution	Drug interactions: do not use within 14 days of MAOIs. May increase phenytoin, carbamazepine levels. Black box precautions with antipsychotics, benzodiazepines, and other CNS drugs. Adverse effects: suicidal ideation/behaviors, nausea, CNS stimulation, somnolence, HA, tremor, fatigue, mania/hypomania, anorexia, weight loss, GI upset. Slow titration up to effective dose decreases adverse effects. Give last dose of the day before 4 PM to prevent insomnia.
Fluticasone propionate (Flonase) *Inhaled steroid*	Treatment of seasonal or perennial allergic rhinitis and as asthma therapy *Allergic rhinitis (nasal inhalation):* Children <4 yr: not recommended Children ≥4 yr: 1 spray per nostril/day to max 2 sprays per nostril/day Adults: 2 sprays each nostril daily **See current asthma guidelines (oral inhalation) in Appendix D**	50 mcg/metered nasal spray 50, 100, 250 mcg powder, Rotadisk oral inhalation 44 mcg, 110 mcg, 220 mcg/inhalation inhalers	Side effects: nasal irritation, HA, candidiasis, pharyngitis. If exposed to varicella, consider prophylactic therapy to prevent varicella (e.g., varicella zoster immune globulin). Rinse mouth following use.

Continued

TABLE A-2 | Medications—Cont'd

Generic/Trade Classification	Indications/Dose	Supplied	Remarks
Fluticasone propionate and salmeterol combination (Advair Diskus 100/50, 250/50, 500/50) *Inhaled steroid + long-acting beta agonist*	*For long-term asthma control only*; prescribe a short-acting inhaled beta-agonist for acute asthma symptoms >12 yr *Not previously on an inhaled steroid:* 1 inhalation of 100/50 every 12 hr; if insufficient response after wk use next higher strength (max 1 inhalation 500/50 every 12 hr) and reevaluate in 1 week *Currently using another inhaled steroid:* initial, every 12 hr dose depends on dosage of inhaled corticosteroid currently in use (guidelines provided in a pharmacology reference book and also see Appendix D)	Fluticasone propionate/ salmeterol diskus 100 mcg/50 mcg, 250 mcg/50 mcg, 500 mcg/50 mcg	Drug interactions: antagonized by beta-blockers. Avoid other sympathomimetics (except short-acting beta-agonists).
Furazolidone (Furoxone) *Antibacterial, antiprotozoal*	*For treatment of bacterial or protozoal diarrhea and enteritis:* <12 yr: 5-9 mg/kg/day, divided every 6 hr (not to exceed 400 mg) for 7 days >12 yr: 100 mg PO qid for 7 days	50 mg/15 mL liquid 100 mg tab	Interactions: alcohol, tricyclic antidepressants, tyramine-containing foods, sympathomimetic drugs. Duration of therapy not to exceed 7 days.
Gabapentin (Neurontin, gabarone, gabapetin, generic) *Anticonvulsant*	*For refractory partial-onset seizures (an adjunct drug only) and neuropathic pain (mechanism unclear):* 3-12 yr: initially 10-15 mg/kg/day PO divided tid; maintenance, 30-50 mg/kg/day PO divided tid >12 yr: 300 mg/day initially with daily increases by 300 mg to 900-3600 mg/day divided tid	250 mg/5 mL solution 100, 300, 400 mg capsule 100, 300, 400, 600, 800 mg tab	Therapeutic blood level: 5-15 mcg/mL. An adjunct drug only with other convulsants. Adverse reactions: somnolence, dizziness, ataxia, HA, tremor, vomiting, nystagmus, fatigue, behavioral problems in developmentally delayed patients. Other laboratory values that may need monitoring depend on other concurrent anticonvulsants used.
Gentamicin sulfate (Gentak, Gentasol, Ocu-Mycin, Gentasol, generic) *Antibiotic, ophthalmic*	*Treatment of ocular infections:* Solution: 1-2 drops every 4 hr for 5-7 days Ointment: use bid-tid for 5-7 days *For severe infection:* 2 drops every hr	0.3% ophthalmic solution, ointment	Transient irritation, burning/ stinging, rarely redness and lacrimation. Discontinue if allergic contact dermatitis results.
Griseofulvin (Grifulvin V, Gris-PEG) *Penicillium griseofulvum derivative*	For treatment of tinea corporis, tinea pedis, tinea capitis, tinea unguium, tinea cruris *Tinea pedis, tinea cruris, tinea unguium:* >2 yr: 7.3 mg/kg/day PO (alternative: 10-15 mg/kg/day PO of ultramicrosize for areas highly resistant) or 10-20 mg/kg/day PO divided bid (microsize); treat tinea pedis for 4-8 wk; treat tinea unguium for 4-6 mo Adults: 660-750 mg/day PO (ultramicrosize) or 1 g/day PO (microsize)	Microsize: 125 mg/5 mL suspension 500 mg tab scored Ultramicrosize: 125, 250 mg tab	Give with fatty foods to increase absorption. Use with caution in penicillin-sensitive patients. Adverse reactions: blood dyscrasias, nausea, vomiting, photosensitivity. Drug interactions: alcohol, barbiturates, warfarin, anticoagulants. Monitor CBC and LFTs after 4-6 wk of treatment and every 4-6 wk of continuing treatment.

TABLE A-2 **Medications—Cont'd**

Generic/Trade Classification	Indications/Dose	Supplied	Remarks
	Tinea capitis, tinea corporis: Children >2yr (ultramicrosize): 5-10mg/kg PO once daily (max 750mg) for 2-4wk for tinea corporis; 4-12wk for tinea capitis Adult: 330-375mg/day PO (ultramicrosize) or 500mg/day PO (microsize)		
Guaifenesin (many products plus in combinations) *Expectorant*	*Controls cough from minor throat, bronchial irritation:* 2-5yr: 50-100mg PO every 4hr (max 600mg/day) or 300mg XR every 12hr (max dose) 6-11yr: 100-200mg PO every 4hr (max 1.2g/day) or 600mg XR every 12hr (max 1.2g/day) ≥12yr: 200-400mg PO every 4hr or 600mg XR every 12hr (max 2.4g/d)	33.3mg/5mL syrup in combo with dyphylline 100, 200mg tab 200, 300mg capsule 200, 250, 300, 600mg extended-release with pseudoephedrine or phenylephrine	Side effects: rarely GI upset. Should not be used to treat the chronic coughs of asthma, smoking, or bronchitis. Not for use in children <2yr.
Guaifenesin and dextromethorphan (Robitussin DM, Tussin DM, many others) *Expectorant and cough suppressant*	Children (dose based on dextromethorphan component): 1-2mg/kg/day PO divided every 6-8hr Adults: DM 60-129mg/day PO divided every 6-8hr	Syrup: many strengths available; Robitussin DM: guaifenesin 100mg and dextromethorphan 10mg/5mL	See dextromethorphan and guaifenesin listings. Not for use in children <2yr because of reported deaths.
Hydrocodone and acetaminophen (Vicodin, Bancap, Ceta-Plus, Lorcet, Lortab elixir, others, generic) *Opiate agonist, analgesic, antipyretic, antitussive*	*Relief of moderate to severe pain; antitussive:* *Antitussive (based on hydrocodone content):* Children: 0.6mg/kg/day PO divided every 4-6hr (<2yr: do not exceed 1.25mg/dose PO) 2-12yr: do not exceed 5mg/dose PO >12yr: do not exceed 10mg/dose PO *Analgesic:* Children: dose has not been established Adults: 1-2 tabs PO every 4-6hr	2.5mg, 5mg, 7.5mg hydrocodone with 500mg acetaminophen; 7.5mg/650mg; 7.5mg/750mg acetaminophen tab 2.5mg hydrocodone and 167mg acetaminophen/ 5mL; 10mg hydrocodone and 400mg, or 500mg, or 650mg, or 660mg, or 750mg acetaminophen per 5mL	Avoid alcohol and other CNS depressants. Elixir is 7% alcohol. If taking other drugs containing acetominophen, can result in overdose.
Hydroxyzine hydrochloride (Atarax, Anx, Vistaril, generic) *Miscellaneous anxiolytics, sedative, hypnotic, antihistamine*	*Antiemetic:* Children: 1.1mg/kg IM Adults: 25-100mg IM *Anxiety:* Children <6yr: 50mg PO divided qid Children ≥6yr: 50-100mg PO divided qid (max 600mg) Adults: 50-100mg PO qid *Preoperative:* Children: 0.6mg/kg PO or 1.1mg/ kg IM; adults: 50-100mg PO or 25-100mg IM	10mg/5mL syrup (Atarax); 25mg/5mL suspension (Vistaril) 10, 25, 50, 100mg tab (Atarax, Anx) 25, 50, 100mg capsule (Vistaril) 25, 50mg/mL injection	Interacts with other CNS depressants. Adverse reactions: drowsiness, dry mouth.

Continued

TABLE A-2	Medications—Cont'd		
Generic/Trade **Classification**	**Indications/Dose**	**Supplied**	**Remarks**
	Pruritus: < 6yr: 50mg/day PO divided every 6-8hr ≥ 6yr: 50-100mg/day PO divided every 6-8hr Adults: 25mg PO every 6-8hr		
Ibuprofen (Advil, Motrin, Nuprin, generic) *Nonsteroidal antiinflammatory, antipyretic*	Management of inflammatory disorders; analgesic for mild/ moderate pain; antipyretic; dysmenorrhea > 6mo: *Antipyretic*: 5-10mg/kg/dose every 6-8hr PO (max 40mg/kg/dose) *Juvenile arthritis*: 30-70mg/kg/day PO divided tid *Analgesic*: 6mo-12yr: 10mg/ kg/dose PO divided every 6-8hr ≥ 12yr: 400-800mg/dose every 4-6hr (max 1.2g/day)	40mg/mL, 100mg/5mL suspension 50mg, 100mg chewable 100, 200mg tab (OTC), 400, 600, 800mg tab (Rx)	Drug interactions: digoxin, methotrexate. Can cause GI upset. Contraindicated in patients with aspirin sensitivities or bleeding disorders.
Imipramine (Tofranil, Tofranil-PM, generic) *Tricyclic antidepressant*	Used in the treatment of childhood enuresis, depression, ADHD *Enuresis*: ≥ 6yr: 10-25mg PO initially 1hr before hs; increase by 10-25mg/ dose increments wkly (max 2.5mg/ kg/day or max of 50mg PO at hs for 6-12yr and 75mg PO ≥12yr) Slowly reduce dosage after desired response for several wk *ADHD*: ≥ 6yr: 2-5mg/kg/day PO divided bid-tid *Depression*: <12yr initial 1.5mg/kg/day PO, increasing as necessary by 1mg/kg every 3-4 days to max of 5mg/kg/day Children >12yr: initial 30-40mg/ day PO (to 100mg/day) Adults: 50-100mg/day PO initially divided tid; increase by 25-50mg to max of 300mg/day	10, 25, 50mg tab (imipramine HCL) 75, 100, 125, 150mg capsule (Tofranil-PM) (imipramine pamoate)	Children should have supine and standing blood pressures, ECG to rule out long QT conduction disorder, and CBC before therapy and before any increase in dosages ≥ 3.5mg/kg/day. Use with caution in patients with cardiac disease, glaucoma, seizure disorders, diabetes. Drug has suicidal ideation/behaviors warning label. Drug interactions: MAOIs (if given within 14 days), warfarin, CNS depressants, antihypertensive agents. Adverse reactions: drowsiness, dry mouth, GI upset, photosensitivity, arrhythmias. Can take 2-4wk to see full effects of therapy.
Ipratropium bromide (Atrovent, Combivent, DuoNeb, generic) *Anticholinergic bronchodilator*	*Used as adjunctive therapy in asthma with short-acting beta-agonist:* 5-12yr (nebulization): 125-250mcg every 4-6hr (dilute ¼-½ dose vial [2.5mL] of 0.02% solution to final volume of 3-5mL with 0.9% sodium chloride inhalation solution)	18mcg/spray inhaler (Atrovent); 18mcg ipratropium with 90mcg albuterol (Combivent); 0.02% (500mcg ipratropium in 2.5mL NS [Atrovent] solution for nebulization); 0.5mg ipratropium with 2.5mg albuterol per 3mL (DuoNeb) solution for nebulization	Side effects: nervousness, GI disturbances, HA. Albuterol may also be mixed with the nebulized Atrovent solution if used within 1hr. Refer also to Appendix D.

TABLE A-2   Medications—Cont'd

Generic/Trade Classification	Indications/Dose	Supplied	Remarks
	>12 yr (nebulization): 250-500 mcg (½-1 unit dose [2.5 mL] vial of 0.02% solution) every 6-8 hr; inhaler: 2 inhalations qid ≥12 yr (oral inhalation): initial 2 inhalations (36 mcg) every 6 hr (max 12/day)		
Isoniazid (INH, Laniazid) *Antituberculosis Agent*	*Active tuberculosis* (adjunct with other drugs): Infants/children up to 15 yr: 10-15 mg/kg/day PO (max 300 mg/day); if compliance in question: 20-30 mg/kg/dose PO biwkly (max 900 mg), preferably after 1 mo of daily isoniazid treatment ≥15 yr: 5-10 mg/kg/day PO daily (usual dose 300 mg/day); 15 mg/kg/dose PO biwkly (max 900 mg) *Latent tuberculosis or preventive treatment:* Children: 10-15 mg/kg/day PO (max 300 mg/day) for 9-12 mo Adolescents: 300 mg/day PO for 9-12 mo	10 mg/5 mL 100, 300 mg tab scored	Tab may be crushed and put into applesauce for children because the solution is very bitter tasting. Take on empty stomach. Avoid food containing tyramine. Avoid alcohol. Drug interactions: phenytoin, diazepam, carbamazepine. Adverse reactions: peripheral neuritis, seizures, ataxia, stupor, tinnitus, diarrhea. Note: INH is usually used in combination with other antituberculosis agents in cases of active disease. Consultation with TB specialist is indicated to prevent development of multidrug-resistant TB.
Isotretinoin (Accutane, Amnesteem, Claravis) *Antiacne agent*	*Management of severe recalcitrant cystic acne:* ≥12 yr: 0.5-1 mg/kg/day PO divided bid with food for 15-20 wk (face); may stop earlier if number of nodular cysts has ↓ by 70%; 0.5-2 mg/kg/day PO divided bid (chest and back); if relapse occurs, therapy can be reinstated after 8 wk break	10, 20, 30, 40 mg capsule	Monitor CBC, platelets, sedimentation rate, triglycerides, lipids. Pregnancy category X. Note: Isotretinoin therapy is reserved for use by dermatologists or primary care providers who have completed special training and are registered to use the product because of its serious adverse effects; program provided by the manufacturer. Patients required to sign iPLEDGE agreement before treatment. Two negative serum pregnancy tests need to be done at least 19 days apart before treatment. Avoid pregnancy during therapy. Two methods of contraception must be used; at least one method needs to be started at least 1 mo before and following cessation of Rx.

Continued

TABLE A-2 Medications—Cont'd

Generic/Trade Classification	Indications/Dose	Supplied	Remarks
			Acne worsens during first few wk of therapy and subsides by 4-6 wk. Relapses more likely to occur at the lower doses. No blood donation for at least 1 mo following discontinuation of drug. Avoid other vitamin A products. Adverse reactions: pruritus, photosensitivity, conjunctivitis, GI upset, lethargy, fatigue, HA, cheilitis, epistaxis, bone pain, onset IBS, skeletal hyperostosis, possible ↓ bone mineral density, corneal opacities. Depression and suicidal ideation have been reported.
Itraconazole (Itraconazole, Sporanox, generic) *Antifungal*	For onychomycosis; oropharyngeal and esophageal candidiasis in the immunocompromised *Onychomycosis*: ≥18 yr: Toenails: 200 mg/day PO for 12 wk or pulsed 400 mg/d PO for 1 wk each mo for 3 mo Fingernails: pulsed 200 mg bid for 1 wk, stop wk 2-4, then resume at 200 mg bid wk 5 If recalcitrant: 100 mg bid for 2-4 wk; may relapse after drug stopped *Oropharyngeal/esophageal candidiasis* (solution): ≥100-200 mg/day swished in mouth for 1-3 wk. Use 10 mL at a time, swishing for several sec; then swallow and continue for 2 wk after symptoms resolve	10 mg/mL solution; 100 mg capsule	Drug interactions: Prolonged effect of benzodiazepines. Adverse reactions: GI, rash, pruritus, urticaria, HA, dizziness, hepatic function abnormalities, hypokalemia, fatigue, fever, myalgia, decreased bone plate activity in animal studies. Drug has been used in children 6 mo-12 yr without unusual adverse effects, but long-term effect of therapy in children is not known. Baseline and monthly CBC and LFTs recommended.
Ketoconazole (Nizoral, generic) *Antifungal*	*Systemic candidiasis, histoplasmosis, blastomycosis, chromomycosis, onychomycosis* >2 yr: 3.3-6.6 mg/kg/day PO >40 kg and adolescents: initially 200 mg PO daily; may increase to 400 mg daily if no response to lower dose	200 mg tab (scored) 2% cream 1%, 2% shampoo	Adverse reactions: hepatotoxicity, nausea, vomiting. Most effective oral antifungal. Drug interactions: phenytoin, cimetidine, ranitidine, rifampin, terfenadine,

TABLE A-2   Medications—Cont'd

Generic/Trade Classification	Indications/Dose	Supplied	Remarks
	Minimum treatment for candidiasis is 1-4 wk; chronic mucocutaneous candidiasis use for 6-12 mo *Tinea capitus, tinea pedis, extensive or recalcitrant tinea corporis, tinea cruris, tinea unguium:* >40 kg and adolescents: 200-400 mg/day PO for 1-2 mo; for tinea unguium treat for 6-12 mo *Topical treatment of tinea corporis, tinea cruris, tinea versicolor, tinea unguium (onychomycosis):* Adults and children: apply cream 1 or 2 times daily for 2 wk (tinea pedis for 6 wk); for onychomycosis apply once at bedtime and cover with cotton socks; treat for 3-4 wk *Tinea versicolor:* Use shampoo—lather and apply to skin for 5 min, then rinse. Use once/day 1-2 wk *Seborrhea dermatitis or dandruff:* Use 2% cream bid up to 4 wk or 1% shampoo every 3-4 days up to 8 wk then prn *Uncomplicated vulvovaginal candidiasis:* in nonpregnant individual: 200-400 mg bid for 5 days; maintenance 100 mg/day up to 6 mo		antacids, HIV protease inhibitors, loratadine and others, quinolones, theophylline. Limited experience with this drug in children—need to outweigh risks with benefits. LFTs and bilirubin should be monitored before treatment and biwkly the first 2 mo, then monthly or bimonthly, especially in prolonged therapy.
Ketorolac tromethamine 0.5% (Acular) *Nonsteroidal antiinflammatory (ophthalmic)*	*Used for treatment of ocular itching as a result of seasonal allergic conjunctivitis:* <3 yr: not recommended ≥3 yr and adolescents: 1 drop qid for up to 7 days	Ophthalmic solution 0.4%, 0.5%	Can have transient stinging and burning following instillation. Refrigeration decreases stinging. Contraindicated in patients with soft contact lenses.
Lactulose (Constilac, Constulose, Evalose, Kristalose, generic) *Laxative*	*Laxative:* Children: 5 g/day after breakfast Adolescents: 10-20 g daily PO (max 40 g/day) or 10-20 g dissolved in 4 oz water	3.33 g/5 mL solution 10, 20 g packets	Contraindicated in patients with fecal impaction or in those with acute abdomen. Use with caution in diabetic patients. Can take up to 24-48 hr for normal bowel function to be restored.

Continued

TABLE A-2 Medications—Cont'd

Generic/Trade Classification	Indications/Dose	Supplied	Remarks
Kunecatechins (Veregen) *Keratolytic*	*For treating genital and perianal warts:* ≥18 yr: apply with fingers 0.5 cm strand of ointment tid to each wart for up to 16 wk	15% ointment	Not for treating urethral, intravaginal, cervical, rectal, intraanal warts. Wash hands thoroughly before and after use; may stain clothing/bedsheets. Adverse effects: local pain, erythema, vesicles, ulceration, induration. Weakens condoms/diaphragms so alternative contraception should be discussed with individual.
Lamotrigine (Lamictal) *Anticonvulsant*	Partial, absence, atonic, juvenile myoclonic seizures; Lennox-Gastaut syndrome (an adjunct drug with valproic acid), bipolar disorder. *Lennox-Gastaut syndrome* (in combination with valproic acid): 2-12 yr: initially, 0.15 mg/kg/day PO divided bid; titrate by 0.15 mg/kg wkly until maintenance dose of 1-5 mg/kg/day is reached (max 200 mg once or divided bid) ≥12 yr: 25 mg every other day for 2 wk, followed by 25 mg once daily for 2 wk; after 4 wk, daily dose may be increased by 25-50 mg every 1-2 wk until effective maintenance dose of 100-400 mg once or twice daily *Partial seizures*: Monotherapy: 2-12 yr: 0.6 mg/kg/day divided 1-2 doses for 2 wk; then 1.2 mg/kg/day divided in 2 doses × 2 wk; then 5-15 mg/kg/day in 2 doses per response (max 400 mg/day). ≥12 yr: 50 mg daily for 2 wk, followed by 100 mg/day divided bid for 2 wk; then increase by 100 mg every 1-2 wk until maintenance dose of 500 mg/day divided bid	2, 5, 25 mg chewable tab 25, 100, 150, 200 mg tab	Adverse reactions: Stevens-Johnson syndrome, drowsiness, HA, blurred vision, vomiting. Blood levels 2-20 mcg/mL. Monitor LFTs, ammonia, prothrombin, partial thromboplastin because of the co-valproic acid therapy.
Levalbuterol HCl (Xopenex, Xopenex HFA) *Bronchodilator for nebulization*	*Prevention and treatment of bronchospasm* (<6 yr: no clinical trials have been done) ≥4 yr: Xopenex HFA (90 mcg): 2 inhalations every 4-6 hr. (1 inhalation is sufficient for some individuals) 6-11 yr: 0.31 mg via nebulization every 6-8 hr, may increase to 0.63-1.25 mg every 6-8 hr >12 yr: 0.63 mg every 6-8 hr; may be increased to 1.25 mg every 6-8 hr	0.31 mg/3 mL; 0.63 mg/3 mL unit dose, 1.25 mg/3 mL inhalation solution 15 g (200 activations) inhalation aerosol	Drug interactions: beta-blockers, diuretics, digoxin, MAOIs, tricyclic antidepressants. Side effects: tachycardia, elevated heart rate, tremor, nervousness, pain, flu syndrome.

TABLE A-2 **Medications—Cont'd**

Generic/Trade Classification	Indications/Dose	Supplied	Remarks
Levetiracetam (Keppra) *Anticonvulsant*	Adjunct treatment for partial and myoclonic seizures *Partial seizures*: 4-16 yr (consult with a neurologist before using in this age group): initially, 10- mg/kg PO bid; increase by 10 mg/kg bid every 2 wk to max of 30 mg/kg bid ≥16 yr: initially, 500 mg PO bid; increase by 500 mg bid every 2 wk to max 3000 mg/day *Myoclonic*: ≥12 yr: same schedule as ≥16 yr above	250, 500, 750 mg tab 100 mg/mL solution	Therapeutic level: 20-60 mcg/mL. Adverse reactions: somnolence, anxiety, fatigue, behavioral changes, coordination difficulties, dizziness.
Lindane (Kwell, Kwildane, Scabene) *Scabicide, pediculicide*	For treating scabies, head and body lice *Scabies*: this is never the drug of first choice, especially in children <2 yr Infants: apply thin layer of lotion from head to toe and wash off after 6 hr >2 yr and adolescents: apply thin layer, massage, moving from neck to toes; shower after 8-12 hr *Lice*: Children >50 kg (use with caution if <50 kg) and adolescents: apply to hairy areas and adjacent areas, wash off in 8-12 hr; for scalp, shampoo well for 4 min only, rinse, and comb hair to remove nits	1% lotion, shampoo	Not for use in preemies; exercise caution using in infants, small children, those <50 kg, and in those with atopic dermatitis or psoriasis. Only used if individual fails treatment with a safer medication. Wear gloves when applying; avoid applying if pregnant. Refer to pharmacologic reference regarding medication interactions before prescribing. Do not use if individual has seizures. Avoid contact with eyes, mucous membranes, face, and urethral meatus. Body should be clean and dry before application. Do not apply to broken or inflamed skin. Itching may continue for 4-6 wk because of the body's reaction to the infestation rather than to the therapy. Adverse effects: neurotoxic (seizures, death with repeated exposure).
Linezolid (Zyvox) *Antiinfective*	For pneumonia, complicated and uncomplicated skin infection, active towards vancomycin-resistant *E. faecium*, MRSA, multidrug-resistant *S. pneumoniae*	100 mg/5 mL suspension 600 mg tab	Use with caution in those with hyperytension and in those taking SSRI because serotonin syndrome can result (agitation, hallucinations, coma, tachycardia, etc.) Can interact with cold medicines.

Continued

TABLE A-2   Medications—Cont'd

Generic/Trade Classification	Indications/Dose	Supplied	Remarks
	Uncomplicated skin/skin structure infection: < 5 yr: 10 mg/kg PO every 8 hr × 10-14 days 5-11 yr: 10 mg/kg every 12 hr × 10-14 days ≥12 yr: 600 mg PO every 12 hr × 10-14 days *Complicated skin/skin structure infection:* Birth-11 yr: 10 mg/kg IV or PO every 8 hr × 10-14 days ≥12 yr: 600 mg IV or PO every 12 hr × 10-14 days		Adverse effects: infrequent diarrhea, HA, pseudo-membranous colitis, visual changes, myelosuppression (CBC should be monitored if drug used >14 days). Instruct patient to consult if onset of any nausea/vomiting. Contains aspartamine; individual should not indulge in high tyramine diet while taking.
Lodoxamide (Alomide) *Mast cell stabilizer (ophthalmic)*	*Used to treat vernal conjunctivitis, vernal keratitis, and vernal keratoconjunctivitis:* ≥2 yr and adolescents: 1-2 drops qid for up to 3 mo	Ophthalmic solution 0.1%	Contraindicated in patients with contact lenses. Adverse reactions: stinging, blurred vision, transient burning, itching, dry eyes.
Loperamide (OTC) (Imodium, Anti-Diarrheal Formula, Kaopectate II, and others; generic) *Antidiarrheal*	*For the treatment of acute and chronic diarrhea:* 2-5 yr (13-20 kg): initially, 1 mg tid PO 6-8 yr (20-30 kg): initially, 2 mg bid PO 8-12 yr (>30 kg): initially, 2 mg tid PO Second and subsequent doses: 0.1 mg/kg/dose on second and subsequent days of unformed stool >12 yr: 2 capsules initially, then 1 capsule following each stool (max 8 capsules/day)	1 mg/5 mL liquid 2 mg capsule, tab	Contraindicated in patients with ulcerative colitis, pseudomembranous colitis, or hepatic disease. Adverse reactions: constipation, abdominal cramping, nausea, vomiting, dizziness. Use cautiously in pediatric patients.
Loracarbef (Lorabid) *Carbacephem*	Upper and lower respiratory tract (non–β-lactamase-producing strains only), otitis, sinusitis, pharyngitis, tonsillitis, uncomplicated cystitis, and pyelonephritis *Otitis media:* > 6 mo-13 yr: 30 mg/kg/day PO divided bid; *sinusitis:* 30 mg/kg/day PO divided bid; *skin, pharyngitis, tonsillitis:* 15 mg/kg/day PO divided bid. Treat all of above for 10 days ≥13 yr: 200-400 mg PO every 12 hr (max 500 mg/day) × 7-10 days (14 days for *pyelonephritis*)	100, 200 mg/5 mL 200, 400 mg pulvules	Food limits bioavailability. Strawberry/bubble gum taste. Treat otitis with suspension—better therapeutic outcome. 10% cross-sensitivity in patients with penicillin and cephalosporin allergies.

TABLE A-2 **Medications—Cont'd**

Generic/Trade Classification	Indications/Dose	Supplied	Remarks
Loratadine (Claritin, Claritin-D 12 Hour, Claritin 24 Hour, generic) *Antihistamine*	*Nasal and nonnasal symptoms of seasonal allergic rhinitis:* 2-5yr: 5mg/day PO (use syrup) ≥6yr: 5mg/day PO bid (do not use Claritin-D combination in children <12yr) OR <30kg: 5mg/day PO; >30kg: 5mg/day PO bid ≥12yr: 10mg/day XR *Chronic urticaria:* 2-5yr: 5mg/day ≥6yr: 10mg/day	10mg tab 10mg redi-tab 5mg loratadine/120mg pseudoephedrine, 10mg/240mg extended-release tab 5mg/5mL syrup tab	Give on empty stomach. Possible increased plasma levels when given concurrently with macrolide antibiotics, ketoconazole, cimetidine, ranitidine, or theophylline, although no adverse effects reported. May alter tuberculin skin test results.
Magnesium citrate (Evac-Q-Mag, generic) *Cathartic, laxative*	2-5yr: 2.7-6.25g PO once or in divided doses 6-11yr: 5.5-12.5g PO once or in divided doses ≥12yr: 11-25g PO daily or in divided doses	77.5-95mg/5mL solution when powder mixed	Contraindicated in patients with renal impairment, acute abdominal pain, bowel obstruction, or appendicitis. Drug interactions: tetracycline, digoxin, indomethacin, ketoconazole, iron salts, ciprofloxacin, benzo-diazepines, and calcium channel blockers. Chilling magnesium citrate will increase palatability.
Magnesium hydroxide (OTC) (Phillips' Milk of Magnesia, Milk of Magnesia, generic) *Laxative*	Used to treat constipation and to induce bowel evacuation *Constipation:* 2-5yr: 5-15mL PO daily 6-11yr: 15-30mL PO daily >12yr: 30-60mL as single dose	400, 800mg/5mL and 1.2g/5mL suspension 300, 600mg tab	Contraindicated in patients with renal failure, intestinal obstruction, fecal impaction. Adverse reactions: abdominal cramps, hypotension, nausea, vomiting. Drug interactions: tetracycline, digoxin, indomethacin, ketoconazole.
Mebendazole (Vermox) *Anthelmintic*	Roundworms, whipworms, hookworms, pinworms *Pinworms:* Children >2yr and adults: 100mg PO as single dose; can repeat in 2wk if infection persists *Roundworm, whipworm, hookworm:* >2yr and older: 100mg PO bid for 3 days; can repeat in 3wk; OR 500mg once	100mg tab (chewable)	Few side effects at low doses. Occasional abdominal pain and diarrhea. Can swallow tab or crush and mix with food. Administer with food.
Medroxyprogesterone acetate (Depo-sub-Q-Provera) *Progestin*	For abnormal uterine bleeding, secondary amenorrhea, or as contraception *Dysfunctional uterine bleeding:* 5-10mg PO for 5-10 days beginning on day 16 or 21 of cycle	2.5, 5, 10mg tab 150mg/mL, 104mg/0.65mL vial or prefilled syringe for injection	Contraindicated in patients with thromboembolic disease, pregnancy, hepatic disease, breast or genital cancer, cardiovascular disease, undiagnosed vaginal bleeding.

Continued

TABLE A-2 Medications—Cont'd

Generic/Trade Classification	Indications/Dose	Supplied	Remarks
	Secondary amenorrhea: 5-10mg PO for 5-10 days *Contraception:* 150mg IM or 104mg SubQ preparation every 3mo, first dose given only during first 5 days of normal menstrual period; may give within 5 days postpartum if not breast-feeding or at 6wk postpartum if breastfeeding		Drug interactions: bromocriptine. Adverse reactions: depression, weight fluctuations, loss of bone mineral density, irregular bleeding, edema, breast tenderness, acne, galactorrhea. Counsel to notify prescriber for visual disturbances or onset of acute HA, chest or leg pain, shortness of breath
Mefenamic acid (Ponstel) *Nonsteroidal antiinflammatory*	*Mild to moderate pain, dysmenorrhea, inflammatory disease:* >14yr: 500mg PO, then 250mg PO every 6hr × 2-3 days—not to exceed 1wk	250mg tab	Adverse reactions: blood dyscrasias. Drug interactions: anticoagulants, phenytoin, sulfonamides, corticosteroids. Take with food.
Metaproterenol sulfate (Alupent) *Bronchodilator*	*For reversible airway obstruction as a result of asthma or chronic obstructive pulmonary disease (COPD):* For current asthma treatment guidelines see Appendix D.	10mg/5mL solution 10, 20mg tab (scored) 0.65mg/metered spray 0.4%, 0.6% nebulization solution	Can cause nervousness, restlessness, or tremor. Drug interactions: MAOIs, propranolol. Do not use concurrently with other sympathomimetic bronchodilators. Best results if second inhalation is given 10min following first.
Metformin HCL (Riomet, Glucophage) *Antidiabetic*	*For treating Type II diabetes:* 10-16yr: 500mg bid (morning and evening) with meals. ↑dose by 500mg prn weekly (max 2000mg/d in divided doses) Use only the conventional (regular-release) tabs or oral solution (safety and efficacy not established with the extended-release preparations) >16yr: 500mg PO bid (morning and evening meals) increase by 500mg weekly prn (max 2500mg/d in divided doses) OR 800mg PO once daily (AM meal) of regular-release tab OR 850mg every other week prn (max 2550mg/d in divided doses). For XR dosing, consult pharmacology reference book.	500mg/5mL 500, 850mg tab 1g tab 500, 750mg, 1gXR tab	Adverse effects: GI (diarrhea, nausea, vomiting), hypoglycemia (rare if drug used as monotherapy), HA, dizziness. Consider serum hemoglobin and vit B_{12} drawn annually. Use with caution in those with decreased renal function.

TABLE A-2 Medications—Cont'd

Generic/Trade Classification	Indications/Dose	Supplied	Remarks
Methylphenidate (Concerta, Ritalin, Ritalin-SR, Ritalin-LA, Methylin, Methyline-ER, Metadate-ER, Metadate-CD, Daytrana patch) *CNS stimulant*	Used for the treatment of narcolepsy and ADHD *ADHD:* >6yr: initially, 5mg PO 1 or 2 times daily with breakfast and lunch; increase by 5-10mg wkly. Usual dose 5-20mg 2 or 3 times daily (max 60mg/day). For weight-based dosing, initial dose 0.25mg/kg/day given 2 or 3 times daily, doubled wkly to optimum dose of 2mg/k/day Adolescents: dose up to 65mg/day divided bid-tid Extended-release or long-acting preparation can be used after adequate control is first achieved with a conventional preparation: Refer to a pharmacology reference for switching to Concerta, Daytrana, or Methylin. *Narcolepsy: consult pharmacology reference*	5, 10, 20mg immediate-release ("conventional") tab (Methylin, Ritalin) 10, 20mg extended-release tab (Metadate-ER, Methylin-ER, Ritalin-SR) 10, 20, 30, 40, 50, 60mg sustained-release ("long-acting") tab (Metadate-CD, Ritalin-LA) 18, 27, 36, 54mg core, extended-release tab (Concerta) 10mg, 15mg, 20mg, 30mg per 9hr transdermal patches (Daytrana) 1mg/mL, 2mg/mL solution (Methylin)	Dosage does not need to be weight-based. Schedule II drug. May change to extended-release (Metadate ER, Methylin ER, Ritalin-SR) or long-acting, sustained release (Metadate-CD, Ritalin-LA, Concerta) after individual is established on conventional therapy. Discontinue if no improvement seen in 1mo. Contraindicated in patients with hyperthyroidism, cardiovascular disease, glaucoma, hypertension. Cautious use in patients with tics or Tourette syndrome. Drug interactions: MAOIs, tricyclic antidepressants, anticonvulsants. Adverse reactions: anorexia, insomnia, nausea, weight loss, tachycardia, abdominal pain, psychosis, hallucinations; may lower seizure threshold in those with a seizure disorder. May sprinkle Metadate CD or Ritalin LA extended-release capsule contents on cold applesauce to administer; do not chew or crush. Residual part of the Concerta tab may be seen in stools. Transdermal patch applied once daily in the morning; takes 2hr before effect seen; remove 9hr later. Place on hip; do not expose to high temperature.
Metronidazole (Flagyl, Protostat; MetroGel/Cream/Lotion, Noritate vaginal, generics) *Antiinfective*	*Trichomoniasis,* amebiasis, giardiasis, *H. pylori, C. difficile,* anaerobic and mixed aerobic-anaerobic bacterial infections *Amebiasis:* Children: 35-50mg/kg/day PO divided tid × 7-10 days; adults 500-750mg every 8hr for 10 days	250, 500mg tab 375mg capsule; 750mg extended-release tab 0.75% cream	Adverse reactions: HA, metallic taste, nausea, diarrhea, dizziness, dry mouth. Avoid alcohol (may cause disulfiram-like reaction). Extended-release given 1hr before or 2hr after eating. Drug interactions: warfarin, phenobarbital, cimetidine. Liquid preparations can be made by a compounding pharmacy.

Continued

TABLE A-2 Medications—Cont'd

Generic/Trade Classification	Indications/Dose	Supplied	Remarks
	Trichomoniasis: <45kg: 15mg/kg/day PO divided tid for 7 days (max 2g); >45kg: 500mg bid for 7 days; or 2g single dose; or 2g divided bid in 1 day *Giardiasis:* Children: 15mg/kg/day PO divided tid for 5-7 days; adults 250mg PO tid for 5-7 days or 2g as single dose for 3 days *H. pylori:* Children: 15-20mg/kg/day divided bid for 4wk Adults: 250-500mg PO tid in combination with at least one other agent effective against *H. pylori* for 14 days *Anaerobic infections should initially be treated per IV:* Children: 30mg/kg/day PO divided every 6hr; adults: 30mg/kg/day PO divided every 6hr *Clostridium difficile* (antibiotic-associated colitis): Children: 30-50mg/kg/day PO divided every 6-8hr (max 2g/day) for 7-10 days; adults: 250mg PO qid or 500mg tid for 10 days *Pelvic inflammatory disease:* Adults: 500mg PO bid for 14 days in combination with other antibiotics *Bacterial vaginosis:* <45kg: 15mg/kg/day divided bid × 7days (max 1g) Adolescent, nonpregnant: 500mg bid × 7 days OR 2g dose once with 750mg extended-release daily × 7 days Adolescent, pregnant: 500mg bid OR 250mg tid for 7 days *Prophylaxis after sexual assault:* Adolescent: 2g dose (in conjunction with single dose of Ceftriaxone plus either doxycycline or azithromycin)		
Miconazole nitrate (Micatin, Desenex, Lotrimin, Ting, Monistat-Derm, Monistat -1, -3, -7; others, generic) *Local antifungal*	*Topical treatment of tinea pedis, tinea cruris, tinea corporis, tinea versicolor:* >2yr and adolescents: apply daily (for tinea versicolor) or bid for 2-4wk (tinea versicolor for 2wk)	1%, 2% cream, lotion, spray, kit, powder for topical use 100, 200, 1200mg vaginal suppository	Adverse effects: irritation, burning; vulvovaginal burning, itching, irritation. Rarely HA, pelvic cramps, hives, skin rashes, contact dermatitis.

TABLE A-2   **Medications—Cont'd**

Generic/Trade Classification	Indications/Dose	Supplied	Remarks
	Vulvovaginal candidiasis: 1 applicator or 100 mg vaginal suppository at hs for 7 days or 200 mg suppository at hs for 3 days or one 1200 mg suppository at bedtime. OR apply topical cream lightly to affected area bid for 7 days.		
Mineral oil (OTC) (Fleet, Kondremul, generic) *Laxative*	6-11 yr: 5-15 mL daily (may be divided bid) ≥12 yr: 15-45 mL/day PO as single dose or divided *Retention enema:* 2-11 yr: 30-60 mL ≥12 yr: 60-150 mL single dose	Sterile liquid Fleet enema— 133 mL	Liquid form contraindicated in children <4 yr because of aspiration potential. Enema form not for use in children <2 yr. Give on empty stomach. Take a multivitamin if on prolonged therapy. Can be mixed with a small amount of ice cream to improve compliance.
Minocycline HCl (Minocin, Dynacin, generic) *Semisynthetic tetracycline derivative*	*Mycoplasma, Chlamydia, Rickettsia, neisserial meningitis carriers (alternative drugs are recommended for prophylaxis when in close contact of individuals with invasive meningococcal disease):* Children >8 yr: 4 mg/kg/day PO once, followed by 2 mg/kg every 12 hr for 5-7 days Adults: 200 mg initially, then 100 mg bid for 5-7 days *Acne resistant to tetracycline or erythromycin:* Adolescents: 50 mg/day divided 1-tid decrease dose after improvement	2.5 mL, 4.75 mL per 5 mL oil suspension 50, 75, 100 mg capsule	Drug interactions: increases digoxin levels. Avoid penicillins and methoxyflurane. Oral contraceptives may be less effective. Adverse effects: photosensitivity. Nausea, dizziness, blood dyscrasias, pseudotumor cerebri (signs/symptoms include HA and blurred vision), hepatotoxicity. HA at higher doses. Outdated products can be toxic.
Mometasone furoate monohydrate (Nasonex) *Corticosteroid*	*Treatment of seasonal and perennial allergic rhinitis:* < 3 yr: not recommended ≥ 3-11 yr: 1 spray each nostril daily >12 yr: 2 sprays per nostril daily	0.05% (50 mcg/spray) nasal suspension	Improvement of symptoms should begin in 2 days. If used for longer than brief periods of time, secondary adrenocortical insufficiency may occur that can result in patient being more susceptible to infection. Therefore if exposed to varicella, consider prophylactic therapy to prevent varicella. Side effects: HA, pharyngitis, epistaxis, cough, URI.
Montelukast sodium (Singulair) *Leukotriene receptor antagonist*	*Prophylaxis and chronic treatment of asthma:*	4, 5 mg chewable tab/ granules	Drug interactions: drugs that induce CYP-450 (phenobarbital, rifampin).

Continued

TABLE A-2   Medications—Cont'd

Generic/Trade Classification	Indications/Dose	Supplied	Remarks
	<6 mo: not recommended for allergic rhinitis 6-23 mo: 4 mg/day at hs oral granules (*allergic rhinitis only*) 12-23 mo: 4 mg/day at hs oral granules (*for asthma only*) 2-5 yr: 4 mg/day chewable tab or 4 mg oral granules at hs 6-14 yr: 5 mg/day chewable tab at hs ≥15 yr: 10 mg/day PO at hs Also see Appendix D	10 mg tab	Side effects: asthenia/fatigue, abdominal pain, HA, cough. Not for primary treatment of asthma. Not for monotherapy. Advise patient to take regularly, even during symptom-free periods. Granules may be mixed ONLY with unheated formula or breast milk or applesauce, rice, carrots or ice cream.
Mupirocin (Bactroban) *Topical antibiotic*	*Useful in the treatment of impetigo caused by Staphylococcus, Streptococcus:* Apply 3 times daily	2% ointment or cream	Rare reactions: burning/stinging, pain, pruritus, rash, erythema, nausea, abdominal pain, HA, dizziness, stomatitis.
Naproxen OTC (Naprosyn, Aleve, Anaprox, Naprelan, generic) *Nonsteroidal Antiinflammatory, analgesic*	*Juvenile arthritis:* children: 10 mg/kg/day PO every 12 hr (use suspension); *analgesic:* 5-7 mg/kg/dose every 8-12 hr *Rheumatoid arthritis:* Adults: 250-500 mg bid; *Analgesia:* 500 mg PO every 12 hr (max 1250 mg/day) *Mild to moderate dysmenorrhea:* initially 500 mg, then 250 mg PO every 6-8 hr (max 1250 mg/day)	125 mg/5 mL suspension 220, 250, 375, 500 mg tab 250, 375, 500 mg delayed release	Use cautiously in patients with impaired renal function or burns. Side effects: constipation, heartburn, abdominal pain, nausea. Take with milk, antacids, or food to minimize GI effects. Drug interactions: warfarin, methotrexate.
Nedocromil sodium (Tilade) *Nonsteroidal antiinflammatory*	*Used as prophylaxis in treatment of asthma:* <6 yr: safety not established ≥6 yr (inhalation): 2 inhalations qid; frequency may be reduced to bid-tid, depending on response	1.75 mg/metered spray oral inhalant	Not to be used for acute asthma attacks. Adverse reactions: bad taste, HA.
Neomycin/polymyxin B/ hydrocortisone combination (Antibiotic Ear Solution, Cortisporin Otic, generic) *Otic antibiotic, antiinflammatory*	*Used for treatment of superficial bacterial infections of the external ear:* Infants and children: 3 drops every 6-8 hr for 7-10 days only Adolescent: 4-5 drops 3-4 times daily	0.35%/10,000 units/1% HCL otic suspension or solution	A wick can be used to instill drops—saturate cotton with drops and leave in ear canal. The wick should be replaced daily.
Nitrofurantoin (Macrodantin, generic) *Urinary antiinfective*	*Prevention and treatment of urinary tract infections; Pseudomonas, Serratia,* and *Proteus* are resistant to this drug	25 mg/5 mL 25, 50, 100 mg capsule	Drug interactions: avoid magnesium-containing antacids.

TABLE A-2   Medications—Cont'd

Generic/Trade Classification	Indications/Dose	Supplied	Remarks
	Children ≥1 mo: 5-7 mg/kg/day PO divided every 6 hr (max 400 mg/day) for at least 7 days; *prophylaxis therapy:* 1-2 mg/kg/day PO as a single daily dose (max 100 mg/day) Adults: 50 mg/dose PO every 6 hr for at least 7 days; *prophylaxis:* 50-100 mg/dose PO at hs		Can cause discoloration of urine. Do not crush tab. Rinse mouth following administration of suspension to prevent staining of teeth.
Nystatin (Nystop, Pedi-Ori, Mycostatin, generic) *Antifungal*	*Oral Monilia* (give all of the below for 14 days, including a span of 48 hr when all symptoms have resolved): Do not feed or eat for 5-10 min after administering. Neonates: 100,000 units (1 mL) qid (50,000 units in each cheek). Infants: 200,000 units (2 mL) qid (100,000 units in each cheek) Children and adults: troche 200,000-400,000 units qid or 400,000-600,000 units qid *Gastrointestinal infections:* Adults: 500,000-1 million units PO as tab qid *Cutaneous and mucocutaneous candidal infections:* Topical: apply 2 or 3 times daily × 7-10 days (up to 14 days) Vaginal: 1 tab at hs for 2 wk	100,000 units/mL suspension 500,000 units tab 100,000 units vaginal tab 100,000 units/g cream, ointment, powder	Not for treating systemic fungal infection. Swab oral suspension in infant's mouth to coat lesions. Vaginal tab can be used orally by immunosuppressed patients to provide prolonged drug contact with oral mucosa.
Ofloxacin otic solution (Floxin Otic, Ocuflox ophthalmic) *Antibiotic, quinolone*	Otitis media with tympanostomy tubes in place, otitis externa, bacterial conjunctivitis, keratitis *Otitis media, otitis externa:* 6 mo-13 yr: 5 drops in affected ear, daily, for 7 days ≥13 yr: 10 drops (or 1 single-use container) in affected ear daily for 7 days; use bid for 14 days in chronic suppurative otitis media. **If PE Tubes in place:** 1-12 yr: 5 drops bid × 10 days or single-dose container bid × 10 days—pump tragus after instillation × 4 *Conjunctivitis:* Children ≥1 yr: 1-2 drops every 2-4 hr while awake for 2 days, then 1-2 drops qid for 5 days (used also for keratitis at increased frequency of instillation—refer to pharmacology reference)	0.3% otic, ophthalmic solution	Side effects: pruritus, dizziness, vertigo, earache, taste perversion, rash, ocular burning or discomfort. Warm bottle in hand 1-2 min before administering otic solution. Position child with affected ear up, instill drops and keep child stationary for 5 min.

Continued

TABLE A-2 **Medications—Cont'd**

Generic/Trade Classification	Indications/Dose	Supplied	Remarks
Oseltamivir phosphate (Tamiflu) *Antiviral*	Prophylaxis and treatment of symptomatic, uncomplicated acute influenza A or B *Treatment:* ≥1 yr: if <15 kg, 30 mg (2.5 mL oral suspension) bid >15 to 23 kg: 45 mg (3.8 mL oral suspension) bid >23 to 40 kg: 60 mg (5 mL) bid >40 kg: 75 mg (6.2 mL) bid *Prophylaxis:* ≥13 yr: 75 mg once daily for at least 7 days	12 mg/mL suspension 75 mg capsule	Before prescribing, check with CDC at beginning of influenza season to see if this drug is efficacious for the circulating virus. Start drug within 24-48 hr of onset of symptoms. Start prophylaxis within 2 days of exposure to an infected person; can be used up to 6 wk for prophylaxis. Efficacy has not been established in those with underlying pulmonary disease; adjust dose in those with impaired creatinine clearance. Drug is not to be a substitution for influenza vaccination. Adverse effects: vomiting, abdominal pain, epistaxis, otic disorder, conjunctivitis.
Oxcarbazepine (Trileptal) *Anticonvulsant*	Partial seizures (monotherapy or as adjunct therapy)* *New onset seizures:* Children 4-16 yr (monotherapy): initially, 8-10 mg/kg/day PO divided bid; ↑ dose by 5 mg/kg every 3rd day to reach maintenance dose, depending upon weight (max 600-1800 mg/day) Children ≥16 yr (monotherapy): 600 mg/day divided bid, titrated by 300 mg daily every 3rd day for desired response (max 1200 mg/day)	300 mg/5 mL suspension 150, 300, 600 mg tab	Therapeutic blood level: 5-50 mcg/mL. Side effects: hyponatremia, dizziness, somnolence, diplopia, fatigue, nausea, ataxia; contraindicated if carbamazepine sensitive. *Doses differ if the individual has been on a prior anticonvulsant or if oxcarbazepine is being used as an adjunct drug for control of partial seizures—consult a pharmacologic reference.
Oxybutynin chloride (Ditropan) *Antispasmodic*	*For bladder spasms associated with neurogenic bladder or urinary urgency, leakage, or dysuria:* >5 yr: 5 mg PO bid (max 15 mg/day) Adults: 5 mg PO 2-3 times daily (max 20 mg/day)	5 mg/5 mL syrup 5 mg tab; 5, 10, 15 mg extended-release tab (best for daytime enuresis)	Contraindicated in patients with GI or GU obstruction, myasthenia gravis, glaucoma, ulcerative colitis, unstable cardiac disorders. Drug interactions: CNS depressants. Adverse reactions: GI disturbances, dry mouth, dizziness, decreased sweating, tachycardia. Do not use in children <5 yr.
Palivizumab (Synagis) *Humanized monoclonal antibody*	*Prevention of RSV in high-risk pediatric patients:*	50 mg/0.5 mL, 100 mg/mL parenteral only	See Chapter 23 for indications for use

TABLE A-2 Medications—Cont'd

Generic/Trade Classification	Indications/Dose	Supplied	Remarks
Penicillin G benzathine (Bicillin LA parenteral, Permapen) *Penicillin*	Pediatric patients: 15 mg/kg per dose given IM once a mo, beginning in the fall before RSV season and continuing monthly through RSV season (November through April in most regions) Children: *Streptococcal pharyngitis:* <27 kg: 600,000 units IM as a single dose; ≥27 kg: 1.2 million units IM as a single dose *Secondary prophylaxis of rheumatic fever:* 1.2 million units/ dose IM every 3-4 wk or once monthly *Syphilis,* >4 wks: 50,000 units/kg IM in 3 weekly doses after 10 day course of IV therapy (if indicated based upon lab results) (max 2.4 million units) Adolescent: *Streptococcal pharyngitis:* 1.2 million units IM for 1 dose *Secondary prophylaxis of rheumatic fever:* 1.2 million units IM every 3-4 wk or 600,000 units bimonthly *Syphilis:* 2.4 million units IM for 1 dose (dose increased depending upon latency of syphilis infection)	300,000, 600,000 units/mL injection	Side effects: GI disturbances, pain and redness at injection site, URI, rash, SGOT increases. Doses >1 mL should be divided. Give deep IM in upper, outer quadrant of buttocks. Give midlateral thigh in infants and small children. Adverse reactions: hypersensitivity, pain at injection site. *Duration of secondary prophylaxis for rheumatic fever depends upon degree of carditis.
Penicillin G benzathine/ penicillin G procaine (Bicillin CR parenteral) *Penicillin*	*Streptococcal pharyngitis:* >1 mo and <14 kg: 600,000 units IM as single dose 14-27 kg: 900,000-1.2 million units IM as a single dose ≥27 kg and adults: 2.4 million units IM as a single dose	150,000/150,000, 300,000/300,000, 900,000/300,000, 600,000/600,000 units/mL injection 1.2 million units isojet	Give deep IM in upper, outer quadrant of buttocks. Give midlateral thigh in infants and small children. Adverse reactions: hypersensitivity, pain at injection site. Preferred over Bicillin LA for treatment of streptococcal pharyngitis because Bicillin CR has earlier peak levels of antibiotic.
Penicillin V potassium (Veetids, generic) *Penicillin*	Skin and soft tissue disorders, streptococcal pharyngitis, prophylaxis pneumococcal infection, anthrax *Streptococcal pharyngitis, erysipelas, scarlet fever:* >1 mo: 15-62.5 mg/kg/day PO divided 3-6 doses ≥12 yr: 125-250 mg PO every 6-8 hr or 500 mg PO every 12 hr for 10 days	125, 250 mg/5 mL solution 250, 500 mg tab	Food interferes with absorption. May be dosed bid for streptococcal pharyngitis. Drug interactions: tetracycline. Suspension has unpleasant taste.

Continued

TABLE A-2   Medications—Cont'd

Generic/Trade Classification	Indications/Dose	Supplied	Remarks
	Streptococcus pneumoniae, skin, or skin structure infections: ≥12 yr: 250-500 mg PO every 6 hr (every 6-8 hr for skin-related infections) *Prophylaxis of pneumococcal infection:* <5 yr: 125 mg PO bid; >5 yr: 250 mg PO bid *Cutaneous anthrax:* ≥2 yr: 25-50 mg/kg/day PO divided bid-qid for 60 days; Adults: 200-500 mg/day PO divided qid (children <2 yr should initially be treated with IV rather than oral therapy) *Prophylaxis aerosolized anthrax spores if anthrax found to be penicillin sensitive:* <9 yr: 50 mg/kg PO divided qid >9 yr and adults: 7.5 mg/kg PO qid for 60 days (duration of treatment will also depend on use of anthrax vaccine postexposure) *Secondary prophylaxis rheumatic fever:* Children and adolescents: 250 mg bid, long term *Necrotizing ulcerative gingivitis:* ≥12 yr: 250-500 mg every 6-8 hr × 10 days		
Permethrin (Elimite, Nix, generic) *Pediculicide*	*Head, pubic lice and their eggs (use 1% cream rinse*):* Adults and children >2 mo: apply cream rinse to hair after shampooing and towel drying, leave on for 10 min, then rinse; can repeat treatment in 7-10 days if lice are observed *Scabies (use 5% cream):* Adults and children >2 mo: apply cream from head to toe; leave on for 8-14 hr before washing off with water; in infants also apply to hairline, neck, scalp, temple, and forehead; may repeat in 1 wk if live mites appear	1% lotion/cream rinse 5% cream	Thorough combing to remove nits from hair is required and cleansing of the equipment. Permethrin 5% cream was shown to be safe and effective when applied to infants <1 mo old for neonatal scabies. Permethrin is a safer alternative than lindane for treating scabies and head lice in young infants. Dispensing 30 g is sufficient to treat an adult. *Some clinicians recommend using 5% cream for both head and pubic lice.

TABLE A-2 **Medications—Cont'd**

Generic/Trade *Classification*	Indications/Dose	Supplied	Remarks
Phenazopyridine HCl (Pyridium, generic) *Urinary analgesic*	*For pain associated with urinary tract infections or irritation:* 6-12 yr: 12 mg/kg/d PO divided every 8 hr for 2 days only >12: 100-200 mg PO every 6-8 hr	100, 200 mg tab	Contraindicated in patients with liver or kidney disease/insufficiency. Adverse reactions: GI disturbances, HA, vertigo, methemoglobinemia, skin pigmentation. Urine discoloration occurs (orange or red) and stains clothing. May stain soft contact lenses.
Phenobarbital (generic) *Barbiturate, anticonvulsant, sedative*	Simple partial, tonic-clonic, febrile seizures; status epilepticus,* hyperbilirubinemia, chronic cholestasis *Loading dose for convulsion:* Children and adolescent: 15-20 mg/kg PO *Maintenance for grand mal, partial seizures:* Neonates: 3-4 mg/kg/day PO once daily or divided every 12 hr Children: 5-6 mg/kg/day PO divided bid Adults: 1-3 mg/kg/d PO at hs (can be divided every 12 hr, but there is no advantage) *Febrile seizures:* 3-4 mg/kg/day PO maintenance *Hyperbilirubinemia:* Children: 3-8 mg/kg/day PO divided bid if desired Adolescent: 90-180 mg/day PO (may be divided every 12 hr) *Sedation:* Children: 2 mg/kg per dose	20 mg/5 mL elixir 15, 16, 30, 32, 60, 65, 100 mg tab 30, 60, 65 mg/mL injection	2-3 wk may be required to achieve full anticonvulsant effect. Therapeutic level 10-45 mcg/mL (>50 mcg/mL is potentially toxic).* Not the drug of choice for status epilepticus—see diazepam. Drug interactions: primidone, valproic acid, warfarin, corticosteroids, oral contraceptives, doxycycline. Do not withdraw drug abruptly. Side effects: sedation, irritability, hyperkinesis, ataxia, slurred speech, nystagmus, Stevens-Johnson syndrome, attention/memory/learning changes.
Phenylephrine HCl (Mydfrin ophthalmic, Neo-Synephrine, Neofrin, Ocu-Phrin, *Vasoconstrictor, mydriatic, decongestant*	Relief of nasal and nasopharyngeal mucosal congestion; ocular congestion, itching *Nasal congestion:* 0.25-0.05% solution ≥6 yr, 2-3 drops or sprays bid for 2-3 days 1% solution: use in adults with *severe congestion*, 1-2 sprays each nostril no more frequently than every 4 hr	0.16%, 0.25%, 0.5%, 1% nasal solution 0.12%, 2.5%, 10% ophthalmic solution	Available in various combinations, usually 5 mg/mL. Side effects: transient burning, stinging, sneezing, increased nasal discharge, nasal dryness; overuse can cause rebound nasal congestion, which subsides 1 wk or more after discontinuance; rare systemic effects as a result of absorption. Do not use in those with HTN. Not for use in children <6 yrs.

Continued

TABLE A-2   Medications—Cont'd

Generic/Trade Classification	Indications/Dose	Supplied	Remarks
Phenytoin (Dilantin, generic) *Hydantoin derivative, anticonvulsant*	Partial, generalized seizures, status epilepticus, migraines, arrhythmias *Seizures:* Neonates: 4-7 mg/kg/day PO divided every 6-8 hr Children: initially, 5 mg/kg/day PO divided every 8-12 hr; maintenance, 4-8 mg/kg/day (max 300 mg/day) Adults: initially, 100 mg PO tid, increasing 100 mg every 2-3 wk to reach desired effect; maintenance, 6-7 mg/kg/day divided tid-qid (300-600 mg/day)	125 mg/5 mL suspension (shake well before administering) 50 mg chewable tab 30, 100, 200, 300 mg capsule	Therapeutic blood level in neonates: 8-15 mcg/mL; children and adults: 10-20 mcg/mL, but clinical response is more meaningful than plasma concentrations. Monitor CBC with differential, and liver enzymes before onset and at regular intervals during first few months of treatment; then blood levels and lab every 6 mo. Phenytoin may alter thyroid hormone demands, requiring monitoring. Plasma levels may be decreased if used with acyclovir. Drug interactions: alcohol, antihistamines, folic acid, rifampin, antacids. Barbiturates, carbamazepine, theophylline, and calcium can all cause decreased plasma levels of hydantoins. Adverse reactions: gingival hyperplasia, blood dyscrasias, rash, hirsutism, anemia, lymphadenopathy, Stevens-Johnson syndrome. Can cause discoloration of urine. Is poorly absorbed in infants and young children.
Polyethylene glycol (Miralax, Glycolax, generic) (OTC) *Osmotic laxative*	*Constipation, encopresis:* Children: 0.5-1 mg/kg/dose PO bid in 4-8 oz water or juice depending on response Adults: 1 heaping tbsp/day PO (17 g) in 4-8 oz water, juice, soda, coffee, tea	255, 527 g packets	Do not use in patients with known or suspected bowel obstruction. In encopresis, goal is a daily soft, easily passed bowel movement; treatment duration is usually about 6 mo for effective normalization of bowel function.
Posaconazole (Noxafil) *Antifungal*	*For oropharyngeal candida refractory to other treatments and to prevent invasive* Aspergillus *and* Candida *infections in the immunocompromised:* ≥13 yr: 200 mg PO tid; duration of treatment depends upon response	40 mg/mL suspension	Take with meals or liquid nutritional supplement. Use with caution in those with decreased renal/hepatic function. Adverse reactions: HA, anxiety, altered taste, blurred vision, abdominal pain, anemia, neutropenia, anorexia, arthalgia, cough, others.

TABLE A-2   Medications—Cont'd

Generic/Trade Classification	Indications/Dose	Supplied	Remarks
Prednisolone sodium phosphate (Prelone, Pediapred, Oraped, generic) *Glucocorticoid, anti-inflammatory*	For treatment of inflammatory disorders of respiratory and GI tracts, allergic disorders, and rheumatic disease Children: *antiinflammatory,* 0.1-2 mg/kg/day PO divided 1-4 times daily; *asthma,* 1-2 mg/kg/day PO divided every 6-12 hr for 3-10 days Adults: 4-60 mg/day PO single dose or divided bid-qid	5, 15 mg/5 mL solution 5, 10 mg tab	Contraindicated in patients with active, untreated infections, including varicella. Can mask symptoms of infections. Do not abruptly stop drug if given >5 days. Adverse reactions: growth suppression, fractures, GI discomfort, vertigo, acne. Oraped better tolerated because of taste.
Prednisone (Meticorten, Sterapred, generic) *Glucocorticoid, antiinflammatory*	*Used in the treatment of inflammatory disorders, allergic disorders, and hematologic diseases:* Children: 0.1-2 mg/kg/day PO in 4 divided doses Adults: 5-60 mg/day PO divided in 2-4 doses	5 mg/mL (concentrated), 5 mg/5 mL solution 1, 2.5, 5, 10, 20, 50 mg tab	See contraindications and adverse reactions for prednisolone.
Primidone (Mysoline, generic) *Anticonvulsant*	*Partial, tonic-clonic, myoclonic seizures:* <8 yr: 50 mg PO at hs for 3 days; 50 mg PO bid for days 4-6; 100 mg tid for days 7-9; maintenance of 125-250 mg tid (10-25 mg/kg/day divided tid) ≥8 yr: 100-125 mg PO at hs for 3 days; 100-125 mg PO bid for days 4-6; 100-125 mg PO tid for days 7-9; maintenance of 250 mg tid	250 mg/5 mL suspension 50, 250 mg tab	Therapeutic level: 5-12 mcg/mL. Side effects: drowsiness, ataxia, vertigo, anorexia, nausea/vomiting, rash, aggression.
Promethazine HCl (Phenergan, Phenadoz, generic) *Antihistamine, antiemetic, antivertigo, sedative*	Used to treat vertigo, nausea, vomiting Children: *Antihistamine:* 0.1 mg/kg PO every 6 hr during the day and 0.5 mg/kg PO at hs prn (max 25 mg/dose) *Antiemetic:* 0.25-0.5 mg/kg every 4-6 hr PO, IM, IV, rectally (max 25 mg/dose) *Motion sickness:* 0.5 mg/kg PO 30-60 min before departure and every 8-12 hr as needed (max 25 mg/dose) *Sedation:* 0.5-1.1 mg/kg/dose every 5 hr as needed PO, IV, IM, rectal Adolescent: *Antihistamine:* 12.5 mg PO or rectally tid and 25 mg PO or rectally at bedtime; 25 mg IV, IM may be given and repeated in 2 hr; switch to oral route as soon as possible	6.25 mg/5 mL syrup 12.5, 25, 50 mg tab 12.5, 25, 50 mg suppository 25, 50 mg/mL injection	Drug interactions: MAOIs, CNS depressants. Adverse reactions: confusion, dry mouth, dizziness, drowsiness, blurred vision. IM administration preferred to IV. IV administration can cause hypotension (rapid administration) or hypertension (slow administration). Avoid SC administration—can cause tissue necrosis.

Continued

TABLE A-2 Medications—Cont'd

Generic/Trade *Classification*	Indications/Dose	Supplied	Remarks
	Antiemetic: 12.5-25 mg every 4-6 hr PO, IM, IV, rectally *Motion sickness:* 25 mg PO 30 min-1 hr before departure, then every 12 hr as needed *Sedation:* 25-50 mg/kg every 6 hr PO, rectal, IM, IV		
Propranolol (Inderal, Innopran, Inderide, generic) *Nonselective β-adrenergic blocking agent*	*Migraine prophylaxis (use conventional tab in children):* ≥7 yr: 1-4 mg/kg/day divided bid-tid and gradually increase dose (max 16 mg/kg/day). To discontinue, slowly decrease dose over 1-2 wk	4, 8 mg/mL solution 80 mg/mL concentrated solution 10, 40,60, 80 mg tab 60, 80, 120, 160 mg sustained-release 1 mg/mL parenteral	Adverse effects: Decreased cardiac contractility, hypotension, bradycardia, hypoglycemia, bronchospasm.
Pseudoephedrine (OTC; some states require a prescription*) (Sudafed, many others, generic) *Decongestant, sympathomimetic*	*Upper respiratory infections:* 2-5 yr: 15 mg PO every 6 hr (max 60 mg/day) 6-12 yr: 30 mg PO every 6 hr (max 120 mg/day) ≥12 yr: 60 mg PO every 6 hr (max 240 mg/day) OR extended-release product: 120 mg PO every 12 hr	Pseudoephedrine hydrochloride: 15, 30 mg/5 mL; 75 mg/0.8 mL oral solutions 30, 60 mg tab 15 mg chewable tab 120 mg, 240 mg extended-release tab	*Pseudoephedrine is one of the crucial ingredients required to make methamphetamines. Drug interactions: additive effects with other sympathomimetics. Hypertensive crisis with MAOIs. Adverse effects: tachycardia, palpitations, arrhythmias, CNS excitement. Not to be used in those <2 yr because of side effects of death.
Pyrantel pamoate (Ascarel, Pin-X, Reese's Pinworm Medicine) *Anthelmintic*	*Roundworms, hookworm, pinworms:* >2 yr and adolescents: 11 mg/kg PO as single dose (max 1 g); for pinworms, repeat in 2 wk	250 mg/5 mL suspension 62.5 mg tab	Suspension can be mixed with milk or juice; can be given with food. Treat all family members. Minimal toxicity. Use with caution in patient who is malnourished, anemic, or has hepatic disease.
Pyrethrins (OTC) (A-200, Licide, Pyrinyl, Pronto, RID, Tisit) *Pediculicide*	*Pediculosis:* Apply to *dry* hair and affected body areas, leave on 10-20 min (time varies by brand), rinse; repeat in 7-10 days regardless if there is evidence of infestation; do not repeat in <24 hr	Available as gel, shampoo, liquid	Avoid contact with eyes, face.
Ramantadine hydrochloride (Flumadine, generic) *Antiviral*	*For prophylaxis or symptomatic treatment of influenza A:* If <40 kg and regardless of age: 5 mg/kg daily in 1-2 divided doses 1-9 yr: 5 mg/kg daily in 1 or 2 divided doses (max 150 mg/day); alternative dosing if ≥20 kg: 100 mg/day in 1 or 2 divided doses ≥10 yr: 100 mg bid; alternative dosing if ≥10 yr and ≥40 kg: 200 mg daily in 1 or 2 divided doses	50 mg/5 mL solution 100 mg coated tab	Before prescribing, check with CDC at beginning of influenza season to see if this drug is efficacious for the circulating virus. Drug should be started within 48 hr of symptom onset; discontinue treatment after 3-5 days or within 24-48 hr after signs and symptoms of illness resolve. For prophylaxis in high-risk individuals, start drug as soon as possible after recognition of the outbreak and continue for at least

TABLE A-2 Medications—Cont'd

Generic/Trade Classification	Indications/Dose	Supplied	Remarks
			2 wk or until about 1 wk after end of outbreak. Children receiving influenza virus vaccine for the first time may require prophylaxis for up to 6 wk following the vaccine or until 2 wk after the second dose of vaccine. For those immunocompromised and unable to take the vaccine, prophylaxis can be used 6-12 wk during the influenza A outbreak. Possible adverse effects: CNS (insomnia, nervousness/jitteriness, dizziness/lightheadedness, impaired concentration) and GI (nausea, anorexia, abdominal pain), rash, tinnitus, dyspnea.
Ranitidine HCl (Zantac, Ranitidine, generic) (OTC) *Antiulcer agent*	For treatment of duodenal or gastric ulcers (acute and long-term prophylaxis), GERD, erosive esophagitis *Gastric/duodenal ulcer:* 1 mo-16 yr: 2-4 mg/kg bid PO (max 300 mg/day); maintenance: 2-4 mg/kg/day PO once daily (max 150 mg/day) × 2-4 wk. Some may require an additional 4 wk of treatment. >16 yr: 150 mg bid or 300 mg at hs; maintenance 150 mg/day at hs *GERD and erosive esophagitis:* 1 mo-16 yr: 5-10 mg/kg/day PO divided bid (GERD max 300 mg/day; erosive esophagitis max 600 mg/day) ≥16 yr: 150 mg bid or 300 mg at hs. If erosive esophagitis, 150 mg PO qid	25 mg/mL injection 75 mg/5 mL solution 75, 150, 300 mg tab 150, 300 mg capsule 25, 150 mg tab for solution	Use with caution if liver and renal impairment. Take with water. Adverse reactions: HA, dizziness, sedation, malaise, mental confusion, nausea, vomiting, constipation, rash, arthralgia, bradycardia, or tachycardia.
Rifampin (Rifadin, Rimactane; Rifamate, Rifater [combinations with isoniazid], generic) *Antituberculosis agent, antibiotic*	*Tuberculosis (should be given in combination with other drugs):* <1 wk: max 10 mg/kg/day PO Children: 10-20 mg/kg/day PO single dose (max 600 mg/day) OR 10-20 mg/kg twice wkly ≥15 yr: 10 mg/kg/day PO once daily up to 600 mg/day OR 10 mg/kg 2-3 times wkly	50 mg/mL 150, 300 mg capsule Combinations: 300/150 isoniazid (ISO) 120/50 ISO/300 pyrazinamide	Prophylaxis is most effective within 24 hr of exposure and no later than 2 wk. Take on empty stomach. Can discolor body fluids.

Continued

TABLE A-2 | **Medications—Cont'd**

Generic/Trade Classification	Indications/Dose	Supplied	Remarks
	H. influenzae prophylaxis: <1 mo: 10 mg/kg/day PO for 4 days; ≥1 mo: 20 mg/kg/day PO for 4 days (max 600 mg) Adults: 600 mg/day PO for 4 days Meningococcal prophylaxis, nasal carriers of N. meningitidis: <1 mo: 5 mg/kg/dose PO every 12 hr for 2 days ≥1 mo: 10 mg/kg PO every 12 hr for 2 days (max 600 mg/day) Adults: 600 mg PO every 12 hr for 2 days		Drug interactions: verapamil, methadone, digoxin, cyclosporine steroids, oral contraceptives (an alternate form of birth control should be used). Adverse reactions: nausea, vomiting, heartburn, epigastric distress, anorexia, abdominal cramps, flatulence, diarrhea, HA, drowsiness, fatigue, ataxia, confusion. Monitor liver function, CBC, bilirubin during therapy for tuberculosis.
Salicylic acid preparations (DuoFilm; Compound W, Fostex, Clearasil Stri-Dex, Oxy, Noxzema, and others) *Keratolytic agent*	For treatment of seborrheic dermatitis, psoriasis, dandruff, warts, and other benign epithelial tumors *Warts*: apply once daily to wart *Seborrhea and dandruff of scalp*: follow package directions *Acne*: use per package directions; usual use is application to all acne-affected areas once or twice daily	Cream, gel, shampoo, bar, lotion, ointment, pledget, solution, plaster	Avoid contact with healthy skin; if used in concentrations >10%, protect surrounding area with application of petrolatum to surrounding normal tissue. Contraindicated in diabetics, those with impaired circulation. Not to be used on moles, birthmarks, unusual skin lesions.
Salmeterol xinafoate (Serevent Diskus, Advair-FHA) *Bronchodilator*	*For long-term control therapy in the treatment of asthma:* >4 yr: use 1 diskus inhalation every 12 hr (equals 50 mcg salmeterol) See Appendix D for asthma treatment guidelines for using Advair-HFA	50 mcg/inhalation discus (Serevent) 21 mcg/inhalation metered-dose inhaler either with 100, 250, 500 mcg fluticasone (Advair-HFA)	Not used as treatment for acute asthma attack. Use cautiously (high incidence of overuse). Patient education is very important. Small increase in risk of life-threatening asthma episodes or asthma-related deaths, especially in African Americans and in those not taking a concomitant inhaled corticosteroid. Drug interactions: MAOIs, tricyclic antidepressants. Also available in combination with fluticasone propionate (Advair).
Selenium sulfide (OTC and Rx) (Selsun, Selsun Gold, Selsun Blue) *Local antiseborrheic, Antifungal*	For treatment of dandruff, seborrhea, dermatitis of scalp, tinea versicolor *Dandruff, seborrhea, dermatitis of scalp* (may use the lotion or shampoo): Children and adolescents: wash with 1-2 tsp, leave on 2-3 min, rinse well; 2 applications/wk for 2 wk, then every 3-4 wk. Maintenance once every 1-4 wk prn for control.	1% selenium sulfide shampoo and lotion (OTC) 2.5% selenium sulfide lotion—Rx	Safety in infants has not been established. Do not use on excoriated or inflamed areas. Avoid getting in eyes.

TABLE A-2   **Medications—Cont'd**

Generic/Trade *Classification*	**Indications/Dose**	**Supplied**	**Remarks**
	Tinea versicolor: Apply 2.5% lotion or shampoo in thin layer on affected area, leave on for 10 min, then rinse; apply once daily for 7 days; may be used prophylactically once a mo *Seborrhea* Apply 1% selenium sulfide shampoo in very small amount to scalp, massage in, and rinse well; apply twice wkly for 2 wk; avoid getting in eyes		
Sertaconazole (Ertaczo) *Antifungal agent*	*For treating tinea pedis, tinea cruris, tenia manuum, tinea versicolor, cutaneous candidiasis:* ≥12 yr: for all of the above apply bid for 4 wk	2% cream	Reevaluate diagnosis if no improvement seen in 2 wk. Dry skin thoroughly before applying cream. Adverse effects: contact dermatitis, dry skin, burning sensation.
Sertraline hydrochloride (Zoloft) *Selective serotonin reuptake inhibitor*	*Treatment of depression and obsessive-compulsive disorder:* 6-12 yr: 25 mg PO daily (max 200 mg/day) ≥13-17 yr: 50 mg PO daily; increase at 1 wk intervals (max 200 mg/day)	25 mg/mL solution 25, 50, 100 mg tab	Drug interactions: cimetidine, diazepam, tricyclic antidepressants, warfarin, tolbutamide. MAOIs may cause hypertensive crisis. Also used in adults for PTSD, panic disorder, premenstrual dysphoric disorder, social phobias. Drug should not be abruptly stopped. Black box warning. Side effects: GI disturbances, sweating, agitation, insomnia, suicidal ideation/behaviors, hyperkinesia, malaise, fever.
Simethicone (OTC) (Gas-X, Mylicon, Phazyme, Mylanta, Maalox, others, generic) *Antiflatulent*	*Used to treat flatulence and functional gastric bloating:* <2 yr: 20 mg PO qid 2-12 yr: 40 mg PO qid >12 yr: 40-125 mg PO after meals and at hs	40 mg/0.6 mL; 50 mg/5 mL suspension 80, 125, 150, 166 mg chewable tab 62.5 mg tab; 125, 166 mg capsule	Administer after meals or at bedtime.
Sodium citrate and citric acid (Bicitra, Cytra-2, Shohl's Solution) *Alkalinizing agent*	*Used in the management of metabolic acidosis and in conditions requiring alkaline urine:* Consult a specialist before using.	Solutions of sodium citrate citric acid or bicarbonate	Contraindicated in patients with renal insufficiency and in those with a sodium restriction. Drug interactions: antihypertensives. Adverse reactions: hypernatremia, metabolic alkalosis, diarrhea.
Sitagliptin phosphate (Januvia) *Antidiabetic*	*For those with Type II diabetes:* (used as monotherapy in conjunction with other diabetic drugs) ≥18 yr: 100 mg once daily (safety and efficacy in those <18 yr not yet studied)	100 mg tab	Adverse effects: Upper respiratory infection, sore throat and/or HA. Use with caution in those with decreased renal function.

Continued

TABLE A-2 Medications—Cont'd

Generic/Trade Classification	Indications/Dose	Supplied	Remarks
Sodium phosphate (Fleet Enema) *Laxative*	>2yr: 1oz/20lb of weight Adolescents and adults: 4oz (max 8oz)	2.25 and 4.5oz squeeze bottle	Enemas are not recommended for children <2yr.
Sulfacetamide sodium (Bleph, Blephamide, AK-Sulf, Sulf, generic) *Sulfonamide ophthalmic*	*For treatment of ocular infections:* >2 mos: Solution: 1-2 drops every 2-3hr and hs for 7-10 days; 0.25-inch ribbon of ointment is used every 3-4hr × 7-10 days	10%, ophthalmic solution 10% ophthalmic ointment Also above found in combination with 0.25% prednisolone or 0.1% fluorometholone	Do not use in children <2mo. Solution will burn with instillation. Eyes should be cleansed before instillation—inactivated by purulent discharge. As an alternative, the solution can be used during the days and ointment for hs dosage.
Sulfasalazine (Azulfidine, Azulfidine EN, generic) *Sulfonamide* *Antibacterial and antiinflammatory*	For management of ulcerative colitis, Crohn disease, polyarticular course juvenile arthritis *Ulcerative colitis:* >2yr: 40-60mg/kg/day PO divided every 4-8hr; maintenance: 20-30mg/kg/day PO divided every 6hr (max 2g/day) >6yr: delayed-release tab: 40-60mg/kg/day divided every 4-8hr (maintenance 30mg/kg/d divided qid) Adults: 1-2g PO every 6-8hr; maintenance: 2g/day (max 4g/day) *Juvenile arthritis:* ≥6yr: delayed-release tab: 30-50mg/kg/day PO divided bid (max 2g/day); increase drug slowly in wkly increments to maintenance	500mg tab; 500mg delayed-release tab	Can cause discoloration of urine and skin. GI intolerance is common during first few days (may start out with ¼ to ⅓ of planned maintenance dose to minimize GI symptoms). Drug interactions: folic acid, phenytoin, methotrexate, anticoagulants, oral hypoglycemics. Adverse effects: Seizures, nausea, vomiting, diarrhea, Stevens-Johnson or other skin eruptions, leukopenia, and others.
Sulfisoxazole (Gantrisin) *Sulfonamide*	*Urinary tract infections:* >2mo: 60-75mg/kg PO initially, then 120-150mg/kg PO divided every 6hr (max 6 g/day) × 10 days *Adults:* 2-4g PO initially, then 4-8g divided every 4-6hr × 10 days *Otitis media* with effusion prophylaxis: 50-75mg once daily	500mg/5mL syrup 500mg tab	Not indicated for infants <2mo. Take on empty stomach. May decrease hormonal contraceptive effectiveness; may cause photosensitivity reactions in sunlight.
Sumatriptan (Imitrex) *Selective agonist of vascular serotonin type 1-like receptors*	Acute treatment of migraine HA (Limited evidence for use in those 6-18yr: but may be considered in those >12yr: 4-6mg/kg/dose SC; may repeat once in 2hr) >18yr: 6mg SC; repeat in 1hr to max 2 doses per 24hr	6mg/0.5mL unit dose syringe/vial; 25, 50, 100mg tab 5, 20mg nasal/0.1mL spray	Consult a pharmacologic reference for using oral doses following an injection dose. Drug interactions: MAOIs, SSRIs. Contraindicated in patients with ischemic heart disease or HTN.

TABLE A-2   Medications—Cont'd

Generic/Trade Classification	Indications/Dose	Supplied	Remarks
	Oral: 25 mg once; if unsatisfactory response repeat dose at 2 hr intervals to max 200 mg/day Nasal spray: 5, 10, 20 mg intranasally; can repeat once after 2 hr; max 40 mg or 4 sprays		Side effects: increased blood pressure, flushing, nausea, drowsiness, sweating; local reactions with spray and injection.
Terbinafine HCl (Lamisil) *Antifungal*	*For treating tinea pedis, tinea corporis, tinea cruris, tinea versicolor* ≥12 yr: apply cream or solution twice daily for 1-2 wk	1% cream, solution	Adverse reactions: erythema, pruritus, burning, blistering, swelling, oozing with topical application.
Terbutaline sulfate (Brethine) *Bronchodilator (short-acting beta-adrenergic agonist)*	*For asthma exacerbations and COPD:* <12 yr: 0.05 mg/kg/dose PO every 6-8 hr (max 0.15 mg/kg/dose tid or 5 mg/day); 0.01 mg/kg/dose SC (max 0.3 mg/dose every 15-20 min for 2 doses only) 12-15 yr: 2.5 mg PO tid (max 7.5 mg/day); SC dose same as above >15 yr: 2.5-5 mg PO tid, titrated up as necessary (max 15 mg/day); SC 0.25 mg, repeated once within 15-30 min if necessary (max 0.5 mg within a 4 hr period of time). See Appendix D for asthma guidelines	2.5, 5 mg tab 1 mg/mL injection	Drug interactions: MAOIs, tricyclic antidepressants, beta-blockers. Can cause tachycardia, tremor, hypertension, HA, palpitations.
Tetracycline (Sumycin, generic) *Tetracycline*	Mycoplasma, *Chlamydia*, rickettsia, acne, exacerbation of bronchitis, *H. pylori* (in combination with other drugs), gonorrhea, tularemia, syphilis (in patients sensitive to penicillin), anthrax. **Inappropriate to use in children with severe infection.** Children >8 yr: 25-50 mg/kg/day PO divided qid, max 2 g/day × 10 days Adults: 250-500 mg PO qid × 10 days *Acne:* initially, 500-1000 mg qid for 1-2 wk, then lower dose to 125-500 mg daily for 1-2 mo and for maintenance	125 mg/5 mL suspension 250, 500 mg capsule/tab	Combination therapy packet (Helidac Therapy) available for treating *H. pylori*. Take on empty stomach. Photosensitivity. Outdated drugs may be toxic. Drug interactions: antacids, milk, zinc, iron, calcium. Pregnancy category D; contraception must be used by sexually active females.

Continued

TABLE A-2 Medications—Cont'd

Generic/Trade Classification	Indications/Dose	Supplied	Remarks
Theophylline (Elixophyllin, Quibron, Theo-24, Uniphyl, Theochron, generic) (aminophylline, dyphylline are other substituted preparations) *Respiratory smooth muscle relaxant*	Used as a bronchodilator in the treatment of asthma, COPD; also used for apnea of prematurity *Apnea of prematurity:* loading dose 6-10mg/kg; maintenance dose: 2-4mg/kg/dose every 12hr 6wk-6mo: 10mg/kg/day PO divided every 6hr 6mo-1yr: 12-18mg/kg/day PO divided every 6hr 1-9yr: 20-24mg/kg/day PO divided every 6hr 9-12yr: 16mg/kg/day PO 12-16yr (nonsmokers): 13mg/kg/day PO Smokers: 15mg/kg/day PO ≥16yr (nonsmoking, healthy): 10mg/kg/day PO	27, 33.3, 80mg/5mL solution 125, 250, 300 tab 100, 125, 200, 300, 400, 600mg extended-release tab (12 and 24hr) 150/90, 300/180 capsule in combination with guaifenesin Injection form (for acute bronchospasm—consult pharmacologic reference for dosing based upon serum theophylline levels)	Therapeutic levels: 10-15mcg/mL (toxic level >20mcg/mL). After therapeutic level obtained, serum levels should be monitored every 6-12mo. Factors that affect serum levels: smoking cigarettes or marijuana, charcoal-broiled beef, phenytoin, phenobarbital, carbamazepine, rifampin, IV isoproterenol, fever, illnesses, propranolol, allopurinol, erythromycin, cimetidine, oral contraceptives, ciprofloxacin, troleandomycin. Use cautiously and decrease dose in patients with hypothyroidism, enzyme inhibitors, hypertension, cardiac disease, or liver disease. Dose may be increased in smokers and enzyme-inducing drugs.
Thiabendazole (Mintezol) *Anthelmintic*	*Pinworms, roundworms, whipworms, trichinosis, threadworm, cutaneous larva migrans (dog and cat hookworm):* Children and adolescents: 22-25mg/kg/day PO divided every 12hr for 2 days (max 3g/day); duration of treatment depends on type of helminthic infection	500mg/5mL suspension 500mg chewable tab	Can inhibit metabolism of aminophylline. Side effects: 50% of patients experience nausea, vomiting, dizziness, anorexia. Administer after meals. Chew well before swallowing.
Tiagabine HCl (Gabitril) *Anticonvulsant*	*Partial, generalized seizures.* Used as adjunct therapy only: <12yr: consult with a neurologist for dosing 12yr-18yr: initially, 4mg daily for 1wk, increasing to 4mg bid on the second wk; thereafter, titrate wkly in 4-8mg increments divided bid-qid until clinical response or maintenance of 32mg/day is reached divided bid-qid >18yr: initially, 4mg/day for 1wk, increasing by 4-8mg/day (divided bid-qid) in wkly increments until maintenance (or clinical response) of 32-56mg/day is reached divided bid-qid	2, 4, 6, 8, 10, 12, 16, 20mg tab	Therapeutic level: not determined, but 5-70mcg/mL has been suggested. Drug interactions: valproic acid possibly. Adverse reactions: drowsiness, concentration problems, increase of spike and wave of EEG, withdrawal seizures. Titrate doses more slowly in those with renal and hepatic impairment.

TABLE A-2   **Medications—Cont'd**

Generic/Trade Classification	Indications/Dose	Supplied	Remarks
Tobramycin sulfate (Tobrex, TobraDex, generic) *Antibiotic (ophthalmic)*	For treating ocular infections of Chlamydia, fungi, viruses, most anaerobic bacteria. Parenteral preparation used to treat meningitis and infections in those with CF *Mild to moderate infections:* Suspension: 1-2 drops every 4 hr; ointment: 0.5-inch ribbon 2-3 times daily; use for 5-7 days *Severe infections:* Suspension: 2 drops every 60 min, decreasing to every 4 hr when improvement occurs; ointment: 0.5-inch ribbon every 3-4 hr until improvement occurs, then every 6-12 hr	0.3% ophthalmic suspension, solution 40 mg/mL solution Also available in combination with steroids (consult pharmacologic reference)	Adverse reactions: increased lacrimation, itching, eyelid edema, erythema, punctate keratitis.
Tolnaftate (OTC) (Aftate, Tinactin, Ting, Breezee Mist, generic) *Antifungal*	*Topical treatment of tinea pedis, tinea manuum, tinea cruris, tinea corporis, tinea versicolor:* Children and adolescents: apply to affected area bid for 2-6 wk Continue treatment for 2 wk after symptoms resolve; 2nd and 3rd courses may be required	1% cream, powder, solution, spray	Rare local skin sensitivity/ irritation, especially if applied to excoriated skin.
Tolterodine (Detrol, Detrol-LA) *Genitourinary tract smooth muscle relaxant*	*Used for urinary dysfunction as a result of detrusor muscle instability* Children 5-10 yr: 1 mg PO bid or 2 mg XR ≥10 yr: 2 mg PO bid or 4 mg XR, decreasing dosage to 1 mg PO bid or 2 mg XR according to response	1, 2 mg tab 2, 4 mg extended-release cap	Has fewer side effects than oxybutynin chloride. Use lower dose for those with decreased renal/kidney function. Adverse effects: dry mouth, constipation, abnormal vision, urinary retention, abdominal pain, HA, dizziness.
Topiramate (Topamax) *Anticonvulsant*	*Partial, generalized seizures, and migraine HA prophylaxis Partial, generalized seizures:* 2-16 yr: initially, 1-3 mg/kg/day PO given nightly the first wk, increasing at 1-2 wk intervals by increments of 1-3 mg/kg/day divided bid to achieve optimal clinical response or 5-9 mg/kg/day divided bid ≥17 yr: initially, 25-50 mg/day PO divided bid, titrating upward by 25-50 mg at wkly intervals to achieve optimal response or maintenance of 400 mg/day divided morning and evening *Prophylaxis migraine headache:*	15, 25 mg sprinkle capsule 25, 50, 100, 200 mg tab	Therapeutic range: 2-25 mcg/mL. Adverse reactions: language and coordination difficulties, difficulty concentrating, nervousness, somnolence, fatigue, abnormal vision, anorexia, weight loss, kidney stones. Reevaluate use of this drug during pregnancy.

Continued

TABLE A-2 | **Medications—Cont'd**

Generic/Trade Classification	Indications/Dose	Supplied	Remarks
	6-15 yr: Start with 25 mg at hs for 1 wk; increase to 25 mg PO bid for 1 wk; increase to 25 mg PO every AM and 50 mg PO every PM for 1 wk; then 50 mg PO bid. Effective prophylaxis 100-200 mg/day.		
Tretinoin (Retin-A, Renova, Resanoid) *Cell stimulant and proliferant*	*Used in the treatment of mild to moderate acne:* Apply a thin layer to acne areas once daily at bedtime; begin with 0.025% cream and increase frequency to bid if needed; patients with sensitive skin may need every other night dosing	0.025%, 0.05%, 0.1% cream 0.01%, 0.025% gel Also available in combination of 0.025% tretinoin gel and 1.2% clindamycin (Ziana)	Do not apply immediately following hydration of skin. Can have exacerbation of acne initially, including hyperpigmentation or hypopigmentation of skin. Avoid contact with abraded skin, eyes, and mucous membranes.
Triamcinolone acetonide (Azmacort, Nasacort AQ, Aristocort, Nasacort-HFA, Kenalog) *Glucocorticoid, antiinflammatory*	Long-term control medication for asthma; seasonal and perennial allergic rhinitis; atopic dermatitis Topical: Children and adults: apply thin film 2-3 times daily *Allergic rhinitis:* 6-11 yr: 1-2 sprays/day each nostril (max 2 sprays/nostril/day) ≥12 yr: 2 sprays/day each nostril (max 4 sprays/nostril/day). Titrate to lowest possible, effective dose *Asthma:* See Appendix D for guidelines (oral inhalation)	0.025%, 0.1%, 0.5% cream, lotion, paste, ointment 55 mcg/nasal spray and suspension 0.2 mg per 2-sec skin spray 100 mcg/metered dose, oral inhalation	See contraindications and side effects for flunisolide. Monitor linear growth in children using high-dose inhaled steroids. Rinse mouth with water after using oral inhaled steroids. Reduce oral inhalations from high doses as soon as effective response is achieved.
Trifluridine (Trifluridine Solution, Viroptic, generic) *Antiviral (ophthalmic)*	*For treating herpes simplex keratitis (HSV-1 and HSV-2) and keratoconjunctivitis* <6 yr: not recommended ≥6 yr: 1 drop every 2 hr during day (max 9 drops/day) until reepithelialization, decreasing dose to 1 drop every 4 hr after reepithelialization for 7 days more (max 5 drops); do not use for longer than 21 days. If reepithelializatoin is not complete after 14 days, consider other treatment agent.	1% ophthalmic solution	Adverse effects: transient stinging or burning. Ocular toxicity can occur if used >21 days.
Trimethobenzamide HCl (Tigan, Tebamide, generic) *Antiemetic*	*Used for the treatment of nausea and vomiting* <13.6 kg: 100 mg rectally tid-qid ≥13.6-45 kg: 100-200 mg PO or rectally tid-qid	100, 200 mg capsule 100, 200 mg suppository 100 mg/mL injection	Use cautiously in infants and children and in patients with acute febrile illness. Not effective in the treatment of motion sickness. Can mimic or mask symptoms of Reye syndrome.

TABLE A-2   **Medications—Cont'd**

Generic/Trade Classification	Indications/Dose	Supplied	Remarks
	Alternative dose for children ≤ 45 kg: 15-20 mg/kg/day divided tid-qid rectally or orally >45 kg: 250 mg PO tid-qid, or 200 mg IM or rectally tid-qid		
Trimethoprim HCl (Proloprim, Tripex) *Antibiotic (folic acid inhibitor)*	For treating acute uncomplicated UTIs; prophylaxis for UTIs and traveler's diarrhea; *P. carinii* pneumonia (conjunctive therapy with Dapsone) *UTI:* < 12 yr: 4-6 mg/kg/day PO divided every 12 hr for 10 days ≥12 yr: 100-200 mg PO every 12 hr or 200 mg once daily for 10 days *P. carinii* (with Dapsone—refer to pharmacologic reference): 15-20 mg/kg/day divided every 6 hr for 21 days	50 mg/5 mL bubblegum-flavored solution 100 mg, 200 mg tab	Adverse effects: rash, diarrhea, rare hematologic effects. May cause folate deficiencies with subsequent bone marrow suppression and blood dyscrasias (avoid large doses or prolonged administration). Use with caution in patients with impaired renal or hepatic function, with known folic acid deficiency, or in children with fragile X chromosome associated with mental retardation.
Trimethoprim (TMP)-sulfamethoxazole (SMX) (Bactrim, Bactrim DS, Septra, Septra DS, Sulfatrim, generic) *Sulfonamide + folic acid inhibitor antibiotic*	Urinary tract infections, bronchitis in adults, otitis media, shigellosis, traveler's diarrhea; *P. carinii* pneumonia (dosage differs—consult pharmacology reference) Children <2 mo: do not use Children ≥2 mo: 8 mg TMP/kg/day PO (40 mg/kg SMX/day) PO divided bid or 1 mL/kg/day divided bid (max 160 mg TMP, 800 mg SMX/day) Adults: 1 DS tab, 2 regular tabs, or 20 mL of suspension PO bid Treat *otitis media and UTI for* 10 days; shigella for 5 days.	TMP 40 mg and SMX 200 mg/5 mL suspension TMP 80 mg and SMX 400 mg/tab TMP 160 mg and SMX 800 mg/DS tab	Adverse reactions: Stevens-Johnson syndrome, drug fever, rash. GI side effects minimal. Not effective against streptococcal infections. Drug interactions: warfarin, methotrexate, phenytoin.
Trimethoprim sulfate, polymyxin B sulfate (Polytrim, generic) *Antibiotic ophthalmic*	For ocular bacterial infections (including *P. aeruginosa)* and other bacteria, otitis externa Children ≥2 mo and adults: 1 drop every 3-4 hr for 7-10 days (max 6 drops/day) × 3-5 days *Otitis externa:* use tid-qid	Ophthalmic solution TMP 0.1%/10,000 units Poly B	Contraindicated in children <2 mo. Less burning than with other preparations.
Valproic acid (Depakene, Depakote) *Carboxylic acid derivative, anticonvulsant*	Generalized seizures, myoclonic, absence seizures; also used for migraine prophylaxis, bipolar and schizophrenia as an adjunct drug to other antipsychotics, and aggressive outbursts in children with ADHD. *Generalized seizures if >10 yr and the other seizures* listed above:	250 mg/5 mL syrup 125 mg sprinkle 125, 250, 500 mg delayed-release 250, 500 mg extended-release tab 250 mg cap	Therapeutic range: 50-120 mcg/mL. Take with food. Do not take with carbonated soda. Do not crush or chew tab. Blood monitoring (baseline, after 1 mo, then every 6-12 mo, and before surgery): LFTs, ammonia, prothrombin, partial thromboplastin, bilirubin. Children <2 yr and those

Continued

TABLE A-2 | Medications—Cont'd

Generic/Trade *Classification*	Indications/Dose	Supplied	Remarks
	Children and adults: initially, 10-15 mg/kg/day PO divided bid-tid; may increase by 5-10 mg/kg/day wkly to max of 100 mg/kg/day divided tid-qid; tab given bid; syrup and sprinkle given tid-qid *Migraine prophylaxis*: 250 mg PO bid (max 1 g/day) or 10-30 mg/kg/day PO bid (max 40 mg/kg/day) (studies have included children 7-17 yr)		on multiple anticonvulsants are at increased risk of developing hepatotoxicity. Concurrent use with acyclovir may decrease plasma levels of valproic acid.
Vancomycin HCl (Vancocin, Luphocin) *Miscellaneous antiinfective*	*Methicillin-resistant staphylococcal enterocolitis, C. difficile-associated diarrhea/colitis, pseudomembranous colitis:* Only oral doses effective for above Infants and children: 40 mg/kg/day PO divided every 6-8 hr for 7-10 days (max 2 g/day) Adults: 500 mg-2 g/day PO divided every 6-8 hr for 7-10 days (max 2 g/day)	125, 250 mg pulvules 1, 10 g solution	Use with caution in neonates and young infants. Unpleasant taste. Adverse effects: rare anaphylaxis, Stevens-Johnson, rashes, nausea.
Varenicline (Chantix) *Nicotinic agonist*	*Adjunct for tobacco cessation:* ≥18 yr: Start 1 wk before set cessation date: 0.5 mg daily days 1-3; 0.5 mg bid days 4-7; 1 mg bid day 8 through 12 wk. If successful, continue 12 wk more to increase long-term abstinence.	0.5 mg tab; 1 mg tab card pack; 0.5 mg and 1 mg tab kit	No contraindications. Adverse effects: nausea, abdominal pain, dyspepsia, constipation, HA. If breastfeeding, woman should stop nursing or wait until infant is weaned.
Xylitol (OTC) (Epic, Omnii "Theragum", Spry, B-FRESH, WellDent, Altoids sugar-free gum, Trident gum with xylitol and others; also in mints) *Natural sweetener*	*Used to inhibit dental decay by encouraging remineralization and inhibits plaque formation:* Children and older (oral): 1 piece of gum chewed for 5 min qid; or 2 mints sucked for 5 min qid	Gum, mints	Caries-causing bacteria cannot colonize in the presence of Xylitol.
Zafirlukast (Accolate) *Leukotriene receptor antagonist*	*Long-term control medication for mild persistent asthma;* not for acute asthma attacks 5-11 yr: 10 mg PO bid taken 1 hr before or 2 hr after meals ≥12 yr: 20 mg PO bid as above See Appendix D for asthma guidelines	10, 20 mg tab	Not recommended for use in children <7 yr. Drug interactions: potentiates warfarin. Plasma levels reduced by erythromycin, theophylline. Plasma levels increased by aspirin. Caution with drugs metabolized by CYP2C9 (tolbutamide, phenytoin, carbamazepine) or CYP3A4 (dihydropyrinine calcium channel blockers, cyclosporine). Cautious use with calcium channel blockers, cyclosporine, astemizole. Side effects: HA, GI disturbances, dizziness. Rarely hepatic dysfunction.

TABLE A-2   **Medications—Cont'd**

Generic/Trade Classification	Indications/Dose	Supplied	Remarks
Zanamivir (Relenza) *Antiviral*	*Treatment of symptomatic, uncomplicated acute influenza A or B;* prophylaxis use remains to be established ≥7 yr: 2 inhalations PO (one 5 mg blister per inhalation) twice daily about every 12 hr for 5 days. Two doses should be taken the first day, as long as 2 hr has passed between doses	5 mg powder for inhalation per Rotadisk foil blister pack used in a Diskhaler	Before prescribing, check with CDC at beginning of influenza season to see if this drug is efficacious for the circulating virus. Drug must be started within 24-48 hr of symptom onset. Consult before using in patients with underlying respiratory disease (asthma, COPD). Patients needing to use an inhaled bronchodilator at the same time as zanamivir should use the bronchodilator first. Adverse effects: possible bronchospasm and decline in pulmonary function tests; diarrhea, nausea, vomiting; nasal symptoms, sinusitis, cough; ENT infections; HA; dizziness; rash. Drug should not be used as a substitute for influenza vaccine.
Zidovudine (AZT) (Retrovir) *Antiviral*	*Human immunodeficiency virus (HIV) in combination with other drugs* (consult CDC for latest treatment recommendations): <2 wk: 2 mg/kg every 6 hr 2-4 wk: 3 mg/kg every 6 hr <6 wk: 2 mg/kg every 6 hr (dosage differs for preemies) 6 wk-12 yr: 160 mg/m² PO every 8 hr (max 200 mg every 8 hr) OR 180-240 mg/m² every 12 hr to increase compliance >12 yr and adolescents: 600 mg/day PO divided bid-tid See Chapter 23 for dosing for prophylaxis of neonatal infection if born to an HIV-positive mother and for postexposure prophylaxis	50 mg/5 mL syrup 300 mg tab 100 mg capsule 10 mg/mL injection Also in combination with Abacavir and Lamivudine	Must be taken frequently—around the clock. Adverse effects: GI symptoms, anemia (<8 g/dL), granulocytopenia, thrombocytopenia. Monitor CBC, platelets every mo × 3 mo, then once every 3 mo for asymptomatic or early symptomatic HIV infection.
Zileuton (Zyflo) *Leukotriene receptor agonist*	*Long-term control medication for mild persistent asthma;* not for acute asthma attacks Children ≥12 yr and adults: 600 mg PO qid (with meals and at bedtime) See Appendix D for asthma guidelines	600 mg tab	Drug interactions: propranolol (doubles serum propranolol concentrations), theophylline (doubles serum theophylline levels), warfarin (decreased warfarin clearance, leading to increased prothrombin time). Monitor drugs metabolized by CYP3A4.

Continued

TABLE A-2 Medications—Cont'd

Generic/Trade Classification	Indications/Dose	Supplied	Remarks
Zonisamide (Zonegran, generic) *Anticonvulsant*	*Partial, generalized seizures:* ≥16 yr: initially, 100 mg PO daily for 2 wk, increasing to 200 mg once daily or divided bid for 2 wk, and then by 100 mg increments every 2 wk thereafter until effective response achieved; usual maintenance, 100-600 mg once daily or divided bid	25, 50, 100 mg capsule	Adverse effects: altered liver function, dyspepsia, HA, myalgia. Monitor liver function every mo for the first 3 mo of administration, every 2-3 mo for the first yr, and periodically thereafter. Therapeutic blood levels: 10-40 mcg/mL. Plasma clearance is increased with concomitant use of phenytoin or carbamazepine; half-life is decreased with concomitant use of phenytoin, phenobarbital, and carbamazepine. Adverse reactions: behavioral problems, kidney stones, drowsiness, anorexia, abdominal pain, taste perversion, HA, dizziness, ataxia, nystagmus, and others.

ADD, Attention-deficit disorder; *ADHD,* attention-deficit hyperactivity disorder; *bid,* twice daily; *CBC,* complete blood count; *CDC,* Centers for Disease Control and Prevention; *CF,* cystic fibrosis; *CNS,* central nervous system; *dL,* deciliter; *ECG,* electrocardiogram; *EEG,* electroencephalogram; *ele,* elemental; *GI,* gastrointestinal; *g,* grams; *GU,* genitourinary; *HA,* headache; *HSV,* herpes simplex virus; *hr,* hour(s); *hs,* bedtime; *HTN,* hypertension; *IBS,* irritable bowel syndrome; *IM,* intramuscular; *IV,* intravenous; *LFTs,* liver function tests; *MAOI,* monoamine oxidase inhibitor; *max,* maximum; *MDI,* metered-dose inhaler; *mcg,* micrograms; *min,* minute(s); *mL,* milliliters; *mo,* month(s); *NIH,* National Institutes of Health; *NS,* normal saline; *ODTs,* orally disintegrating tablets; *OTC,* over the counter; *OM,* otitis media; *PR,* per rectum; *PO,* by mouth; *prn,* as needed; *qid,* 4 times daily; *RSV,* respiratory syncytial virus; *Rx,* prescription; *SC,* subcutaneous; *SGOT,* serum glutamic-oxaloacetic transaminase; *SL,* sublingual; *SSRIs,* selective serotonin reuptake inhibitors; *tab,* tablet(s); *tid,* 3 times daily; *TM,* tympanic membrane; *URI,* upper respiratory infection; *UTI,* urinary tract infection; *UV,* ultraviolet; *wk,* week(s); *wkly,* weekly; *XR,* extended release; *yr,* years; >, greater than; <, less than; ≥, greater than or equal to; ≤, less than or equal to; and; ~, approximately; ×, times.
Data from American Society of Health-System Pharmacists: *American Hospital Formulary Service (AHFS) drug information 2007,* Bethesda, MD, 2007, American Society of Health-System Pharmacists. Behrman RE, Kliegman RM, Jenson HB: *Nelson textbook of pediatrics,* ed 17, Philadelphia, 2004, WB Saunders. *Mosby's drug consult,* ed 16, St Louis, 2006, Mosby/Elsevier; *Nursing 2008 Drug Handbook,* ed 28, Philadelphia, 2008, Lippincott-Williams & Wilkins.

REFERENCES

Adcock KG: Prescribing principles for children: foundations of a rational approach, *Adv Nurse Pract* 14(3):30-35, 2006.

Bell E: Are your patients taking their medication? *Infect Dis Child* 18(9): 12-13, 2005.

Brunell P: FDA announces revisions to prescription drug package inserts, *Inf Dis Child* 19(3):46, 2006.

Claxton AJ, Cramer J, Pierce C: A systematic review of the associations between dose regimens and medication compliance, *Clin Ther* 23 (8): 1296-1310, 2001.

Daiichi Pharmaceutical Corporation: Adherence and dosing, *Sound Advice* 1(12):1-8, 2004.

Garbutt J et al: Empiric first-line antibiotic treatment of acute otitis in the era of the heptavalent pneumococcal conjugate vaccine, *Pediatrics* 117(6): e1087-1094, 2006.

Grassia T: FDA review of pediatric drug adverse events leads to label changes, *Inf Dis Child* 18(12):17-18, 2005.

Groopman J: Annals of medicine: the pediatric gap, *The New Yorker* LXXX(42):32-37, 2005.

Hong L et al: Association of amoxicillin use during early childhood with developmental tooth enamel defects, *Arch Pediatr Adolesc Med* 159(10):943-948, 2005.

Muñoz C, Hilgenberg C: Ethnopharmacology, *AJN* 105(8) 40-48 2005.

Tyre P: Your health in the 21st century. An Rx for kids-with warnings, *Newsweek* 145(26A):74-5, 2005.

University of California, Berkeley: *Wellness letter* 23(2):8, 2006.

Woo T: Pediatric patients. In Wynne A, Woo T, Millard M: *Pharmacotherapeutics for nurse practitioner prescribers,* Philadelphia, 2002, FA Davis.

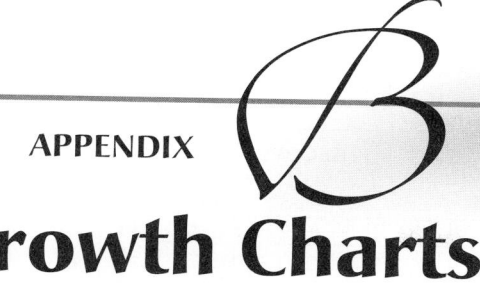

Growth Charts

Catherine E. Burns

Growth in height, weight, and head circumference is an important indicator of health for children. However, the health care provider must remember that growth must be assessed accurately to be valid. Growth is modified by a variety of factors including, but not limited to, nutrition, general health, and genetics. Some of the following points may be helpful:

- Measure height of infants and children less than 2 years old in a recumbent position, holding the head stable against a headboard and using a footboard against both feet.
- Measure height of children greater than 2 years old using a stadiometer or against a wall using a right angle against the head rather than the height measure on a standing scale.
- Measure the head circumference for all infants less than 2 years old and older children who seem to have a small or large head. Measure the largest circumference 3 times and take the largest of the three measures.
- The Body Mass Index (BMI) is now used for assessing the height-weight proportions for all children older than 2 years.

To calculate BMI:
- Weight (cm)/stature (cm) × 10,000 OR
- Weight (lb)/stature (inches)/stature (inches) × 703
- Measure height without shoes and infant weight without diapers.
- Chart the height, weight, and head circumference on grids for all visits, not just well-child visits.
- An estimate of adult height in inches can be calculated as follows:

$$\text{Boys: } \frac{(\text{Mother's height} + 5 \text{ inches}) + (\text{Father's height})}{2}$$

$$\text{Girls: } \frac{(\text{Father's height} - 5 \text{ inches}) + (\text{Mother's height})}{2}$$

When possible use growth charts that are specific for children with certain genetic conditions. Down syndrome, Turner syndrome, Williams syndrome, and others have growth charts (see Resource Box).

RESOURCE BOX

Growth Charts

Down Syndrome Growth Charts
American Academy of Pediatrics: Health supervision guidelines for children with Down syndrome (RE0016), *Pediatrics* 107(2):442–449, 2001. Available online at **aap.org/policy/re0016.html**.

Turner Syndrome Growth Charts
American Academy of Pediatrics: Health supervision guidelines for children with Turner syndrome, *Pediatrics* 111(3):692–702, 2003. Available online at **aap.org/policy/0202.html**

Williams Syndrome Growth Charts
American Academy of Pediatrics: Health supervision guidelines for children with Williams syndrome (RE0034), *Pediatrics* 107 (5):1192–1204, 2001. Available online at **aap.org/policy/re0034. html**

World Health Organization. Child Growth Standards.
International growth charts, birth to 6 years old. Available online at **www.who.int/childgrowth/standards/en/**

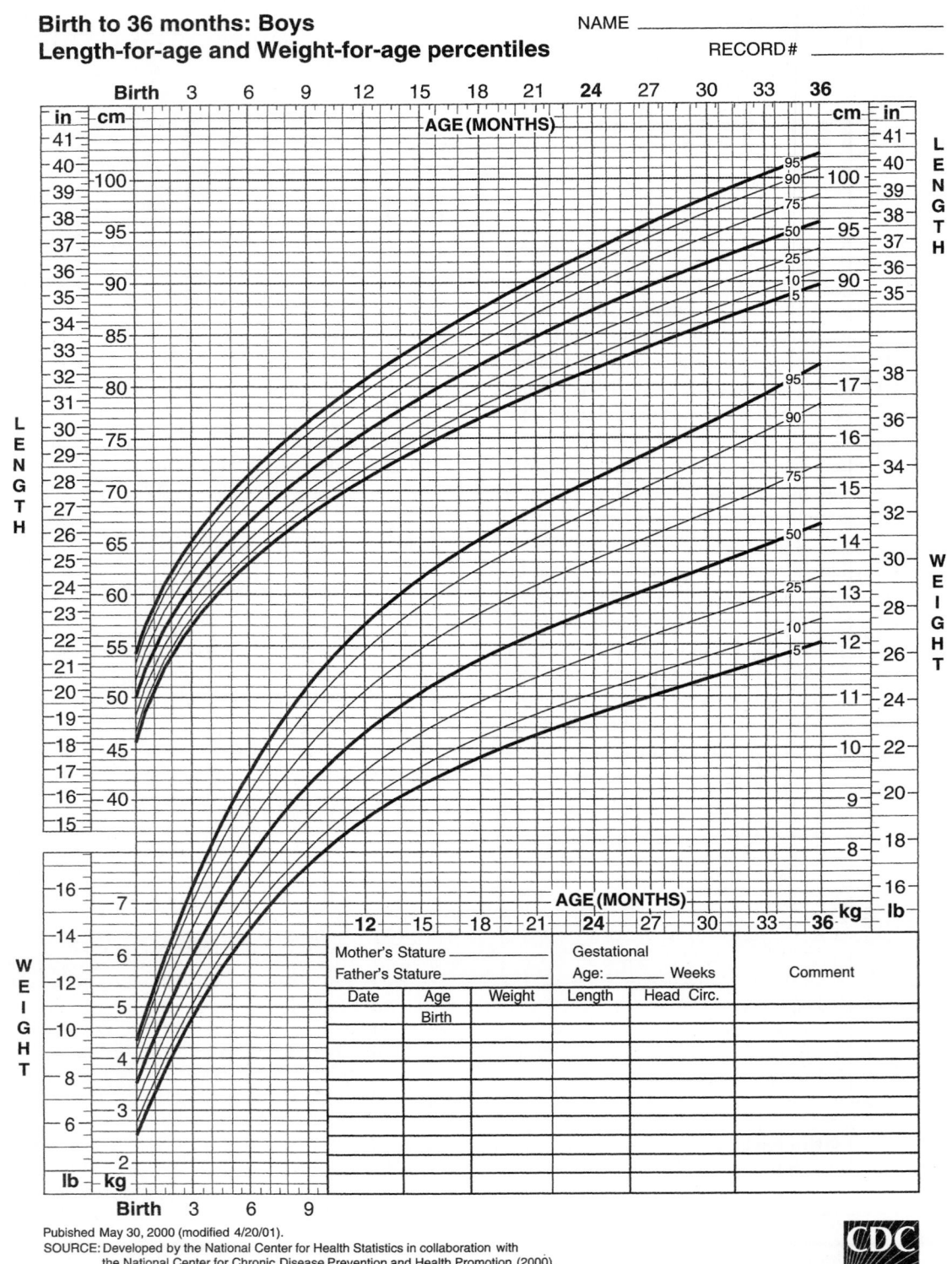

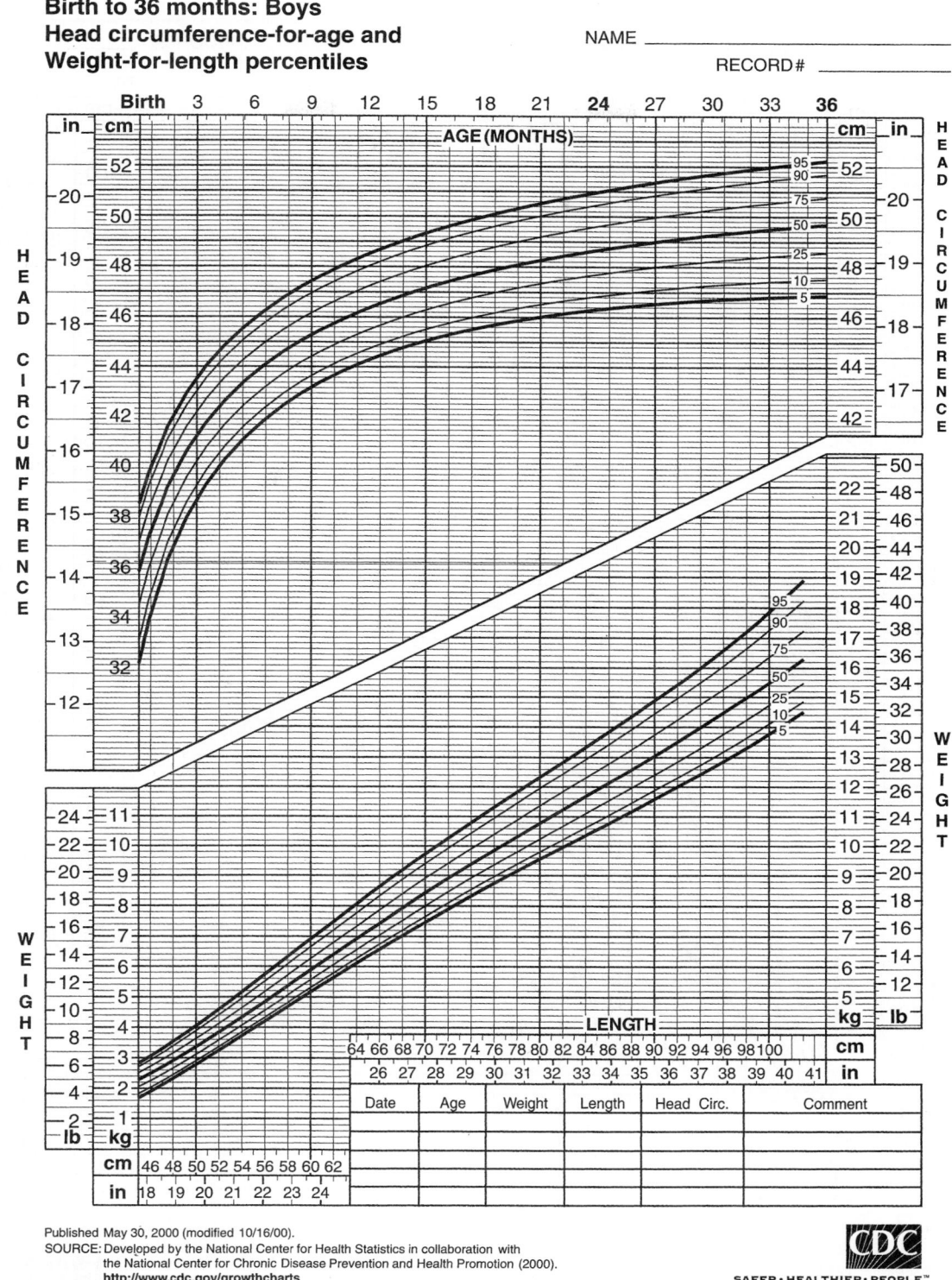

**Birth to 36 months: Boys
Head circumference-for-age and
Weight-for-length percentiles**

NAME _____

RECORD# _____

Published May 30, 2000 (modified 10/16/00).
SOURCE: Developed by the National Center for Health Statistics in collaboration with
the National Center for Chronic Disease Prevention and Health Promotion (2000).
http://www.cdc.gov/growthcharts

FIG. B-2 Birth to 36 months: boys' head circumference-for-age and weight-for-length percentiles. (From the National Center for Health Statistics in collaboration with the National Center for Chronic Disease Prevention and Health Promotion, 2000. Available at *www.cdc.gov/growthcharts*.)

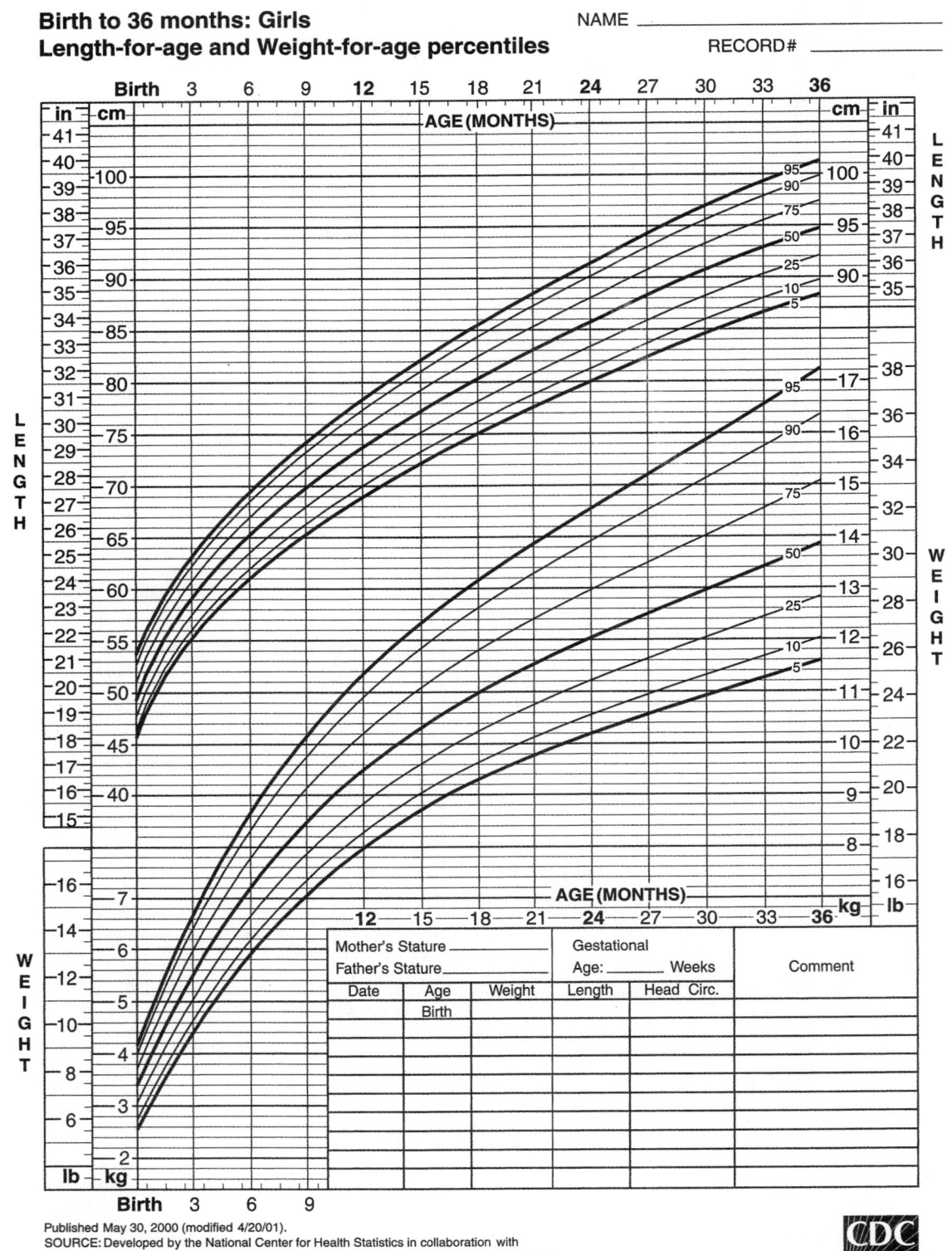

Birth to 36 months: Girls
Length-for-age and Weight-for-age percentiles

NAME _____

RECORD# _____

Published May 30, 2000 (modified 4/20/01).
SOURCE: Developed by the National Center for Health Statistics in collaboration with
the National Center for Chronic Disease Prevention and Health Promotion (2000).
http://www.cdc.gov/growthcharts

FIG. B-3 Birth to 36 months: girls' length-for-age and weight-for-age percentiles. (From the National Center for Health Statistics in collaboration with the National Center for Chronic Disease Prevention and Health Promotion, 2000. Available at *www.cdc.gov/growthcharts*.)

Birth to 36 months: Girls
Head circumference-for-age and
Weight-for-length percentiles

NAME _____

RECORD# _____

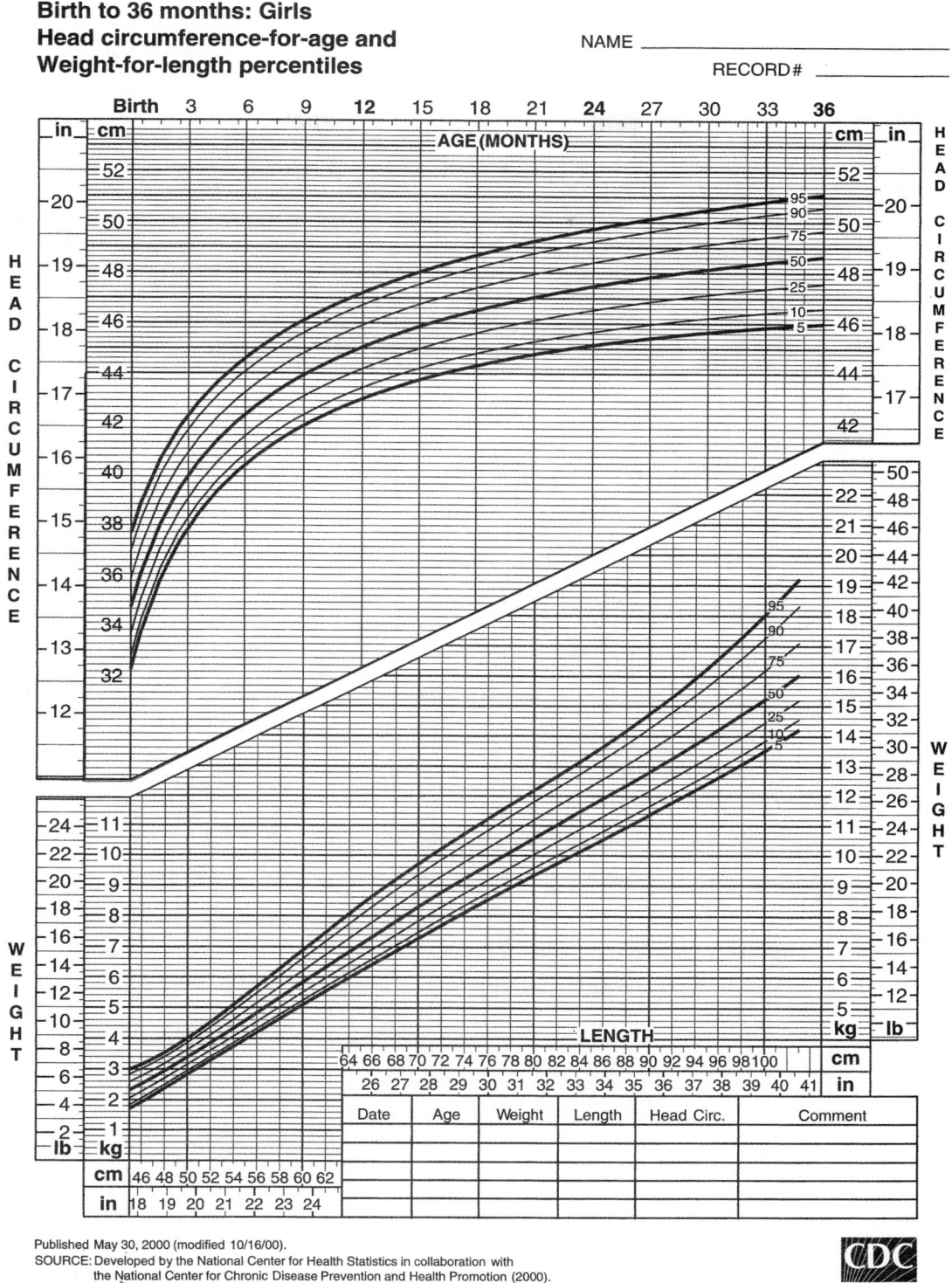

Published May 30, 2000 (modified 10/16/00).
SOURCE: Developed by the National Center for Health Statistics in collaboration with
the National Center for Chronic Disease Prevention and Health Promotion (2000).
http://www.cdc.gov/growthcharts

FIG. B-4 Birth to 36 mo: girls' head circumference-for-age and weight-for-length percentiles. (From the National Center for Health Statistics in collaboration with the National Center for Chronic Disease Prevention and Health Promotion, 2000. Available at *www.cdc.gov/growthcharts*.)

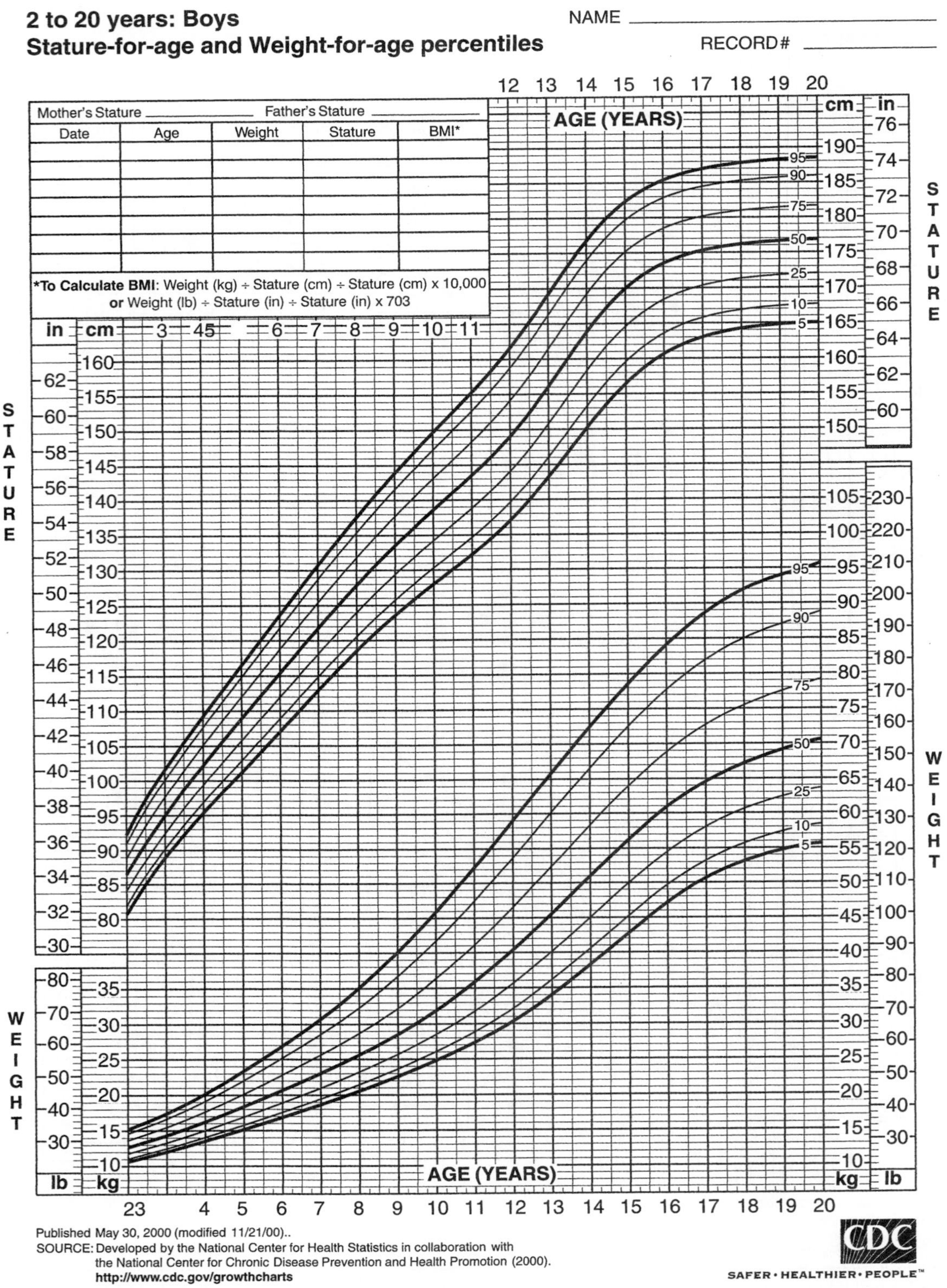

2 to 20 years: Boys
Stature-for-age and Weight-for-age percentiles

NAME _____

RECORD# _____

*To Calculate BMI: Weight (kg) ÷ Stature (cm) ÷ Stature (cm) x 10,000
or Weight (lb) ÷ Stature (in) ÷ Stature (in) x 703

Date	Age	Weight	Stature	BMI*

Mother's Stature _____ Father's Stature _____

AGE (YEARS)

Published May 30, 2000 (modified 11/21/00)..
SOURCE: Developed by the National Center for Health Statistics in collaboration with
the National Center for Chronic Disease Prevention and Health Promotion (2000).
http://www.cdc.gov/growthcharts

CDC
SAFER · HEALTHIER · PEOPLE™

FIG. B-5 2 to 20 years old: boys' weight-for-age and stature-for-age percentiles. (From the National Center for Health Statistics in collaboration with the National Center for Chronic Disease Prevention and Health Promotion, 2000. Available at *www.cdc.gov/growthcharts*.)

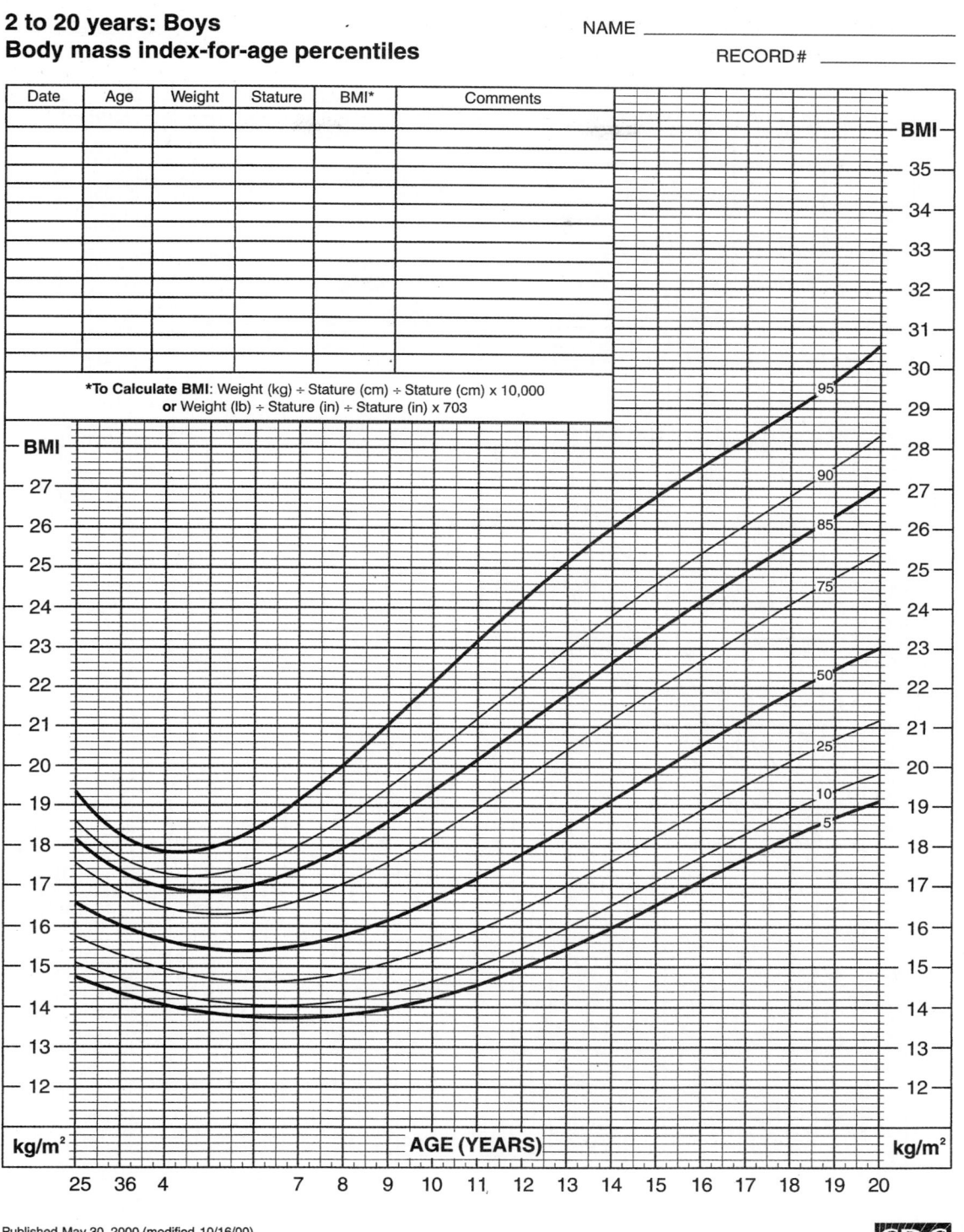

2 to 20 years: Boys
Body mass index-for-age percentiles

NAME _____

RECORD# _____

*To Calculate BMI: Weight (kg) ÷ Stature (cm) ÷ Stature (cm) x 10,000
or Weight (lb) ÷ Stature (in) ÷ Stature (in) x 703

Published May 30, 2000 (modified 10/16/00).
SOURCE: Developed by the National Center for Health Statistics in collaboration with
the National Center for Chronic Disease Prevention and Health Promotion (2000).
http://www.cdc.gov/growthcharts

FIG. B-6 2 to 20 years old: boys' body mass index-for-age percentiles. (From the National Center for Health Statistics in collaboration with the National Center for Chronic Disease Prevention and Health Promotion, 2000. Available at *www.cdc.gov/growthcharts*.)

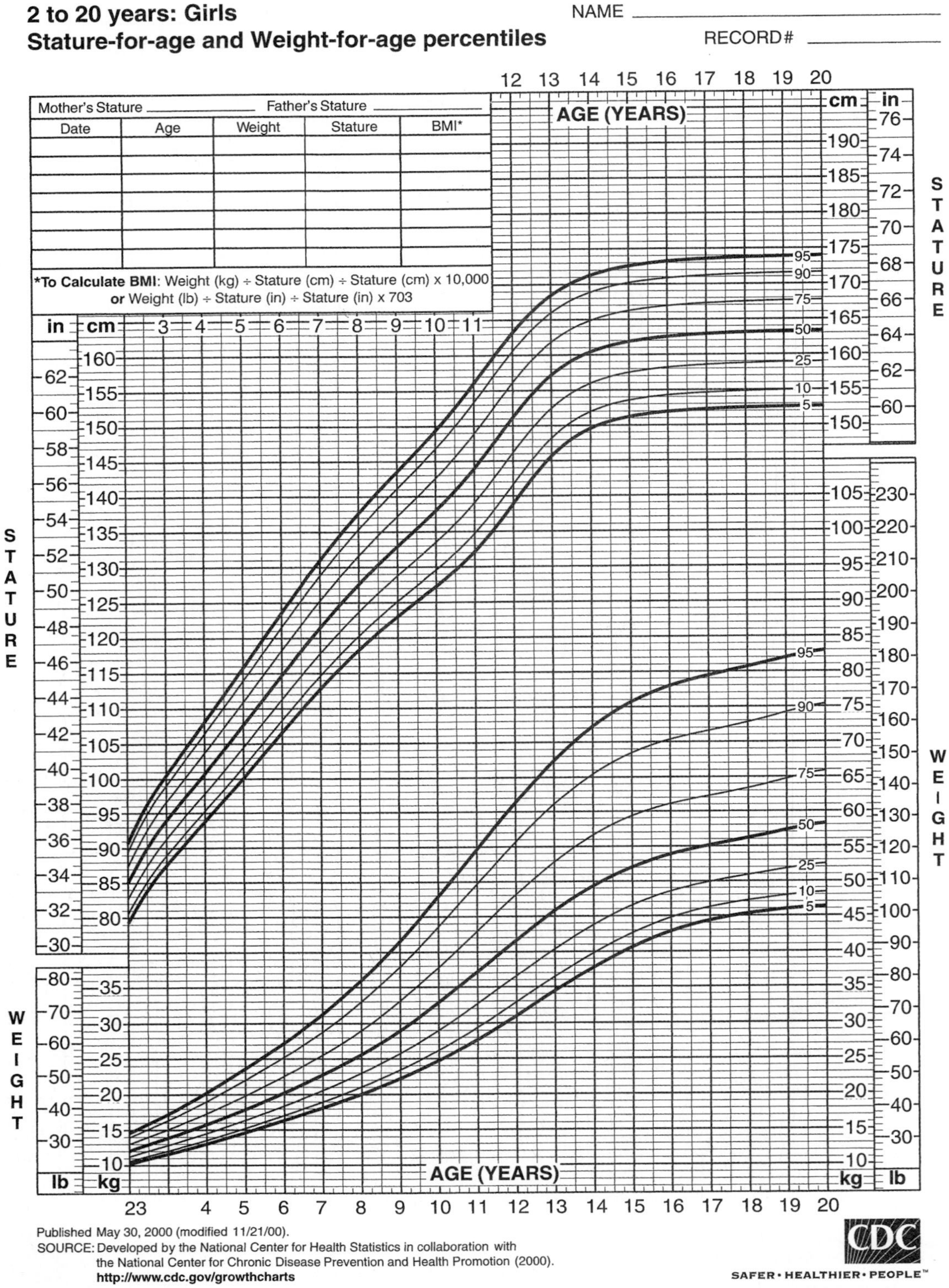

2 to 20 years: Girls
Stature-for-age and Weight-for-age percentiles

NAME _____

RECORD# _____

Mother's Stature _____		Father's Stature _____		
Date	Age	Weight	Stature	BMI*

*To Calculate BMI: Weight (kg) ÷ Stature (cm) ÷ Stature (cm) x 10,000
   or Weight (lb) ÷ Stature (in) ÷ Stature (in) x 703

AGE (YEARS)

STATURE

WEIGHT

12 13 14 15 16 17 18 19 20

Published May 30, 2000 (modified 11/21/00).
SOURCE: Developed by the National Center for Health Statistics in collaboration with
the National Center for Chronic Disease Prevention and Health Promotion (2000).
http://www.cdc.gov/growthcharts

CDC
SAFER · HEALTHIER · PEOPLE™

FIG. B-7   2 to 20 years old: girls' weight-for-age and stature-for-age percentiles. (From the National Center for Health Statistics in collaboration with the National Center for Chronic Disease Prevention and Health Promotion, 2000. Available at *www.cdc.gov/growthcharts*.)

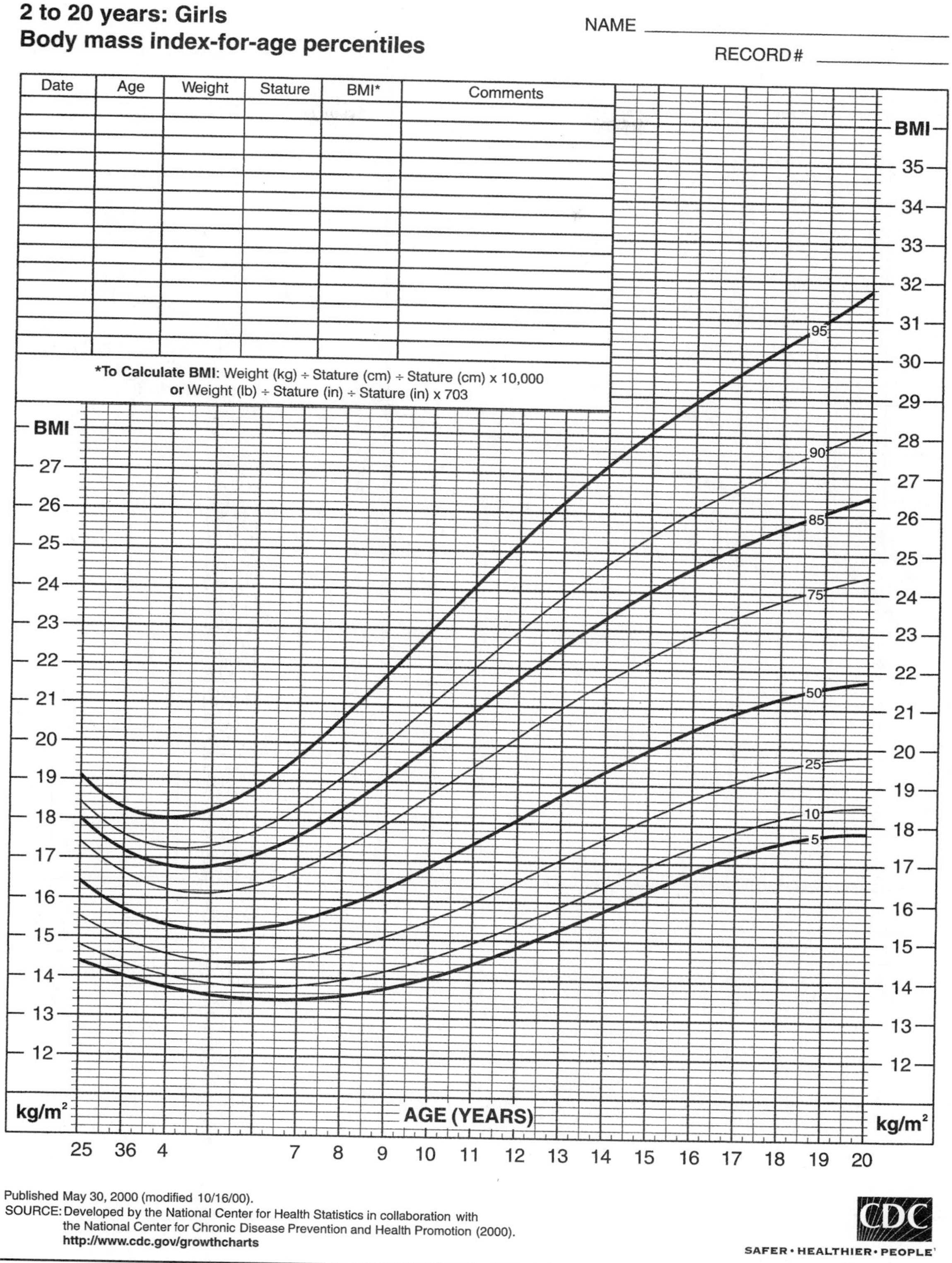

2 to 20 years: Girls
Body mass index-for-age percentiles

NAME _____

RECORD# _____

Date	Age	Weight	Stature	BMI*	Comments

*To Calculate BMI: Weight (kg) ÷ Stature (cm) ÷ Stature (cm) x 10,000
or Weight (lb) ÷ Stature (in) ÷ Stature (in) x 703

AGE (YEARS)

Published May 30, 2000 (modified 10/16/00).
SOURCE: Developed by the National Center for Health Statistics in collaboration with
the National Center for Chronic Disease Prevention and Health Promotion (2000).
http://www.cdc.gov/growthcharts

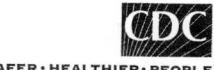

SAFER · HEALTHIER · PEOPLE'

FIG. B-8   2–20 years old: girls' body mass index-for-age percentiles. (From the National Center for Health Statistics in collaboration with the National Center for Chronic Disease Prevention and Health Promotion, 2000. Available at *www.cdc.gov/growthcharts*.)

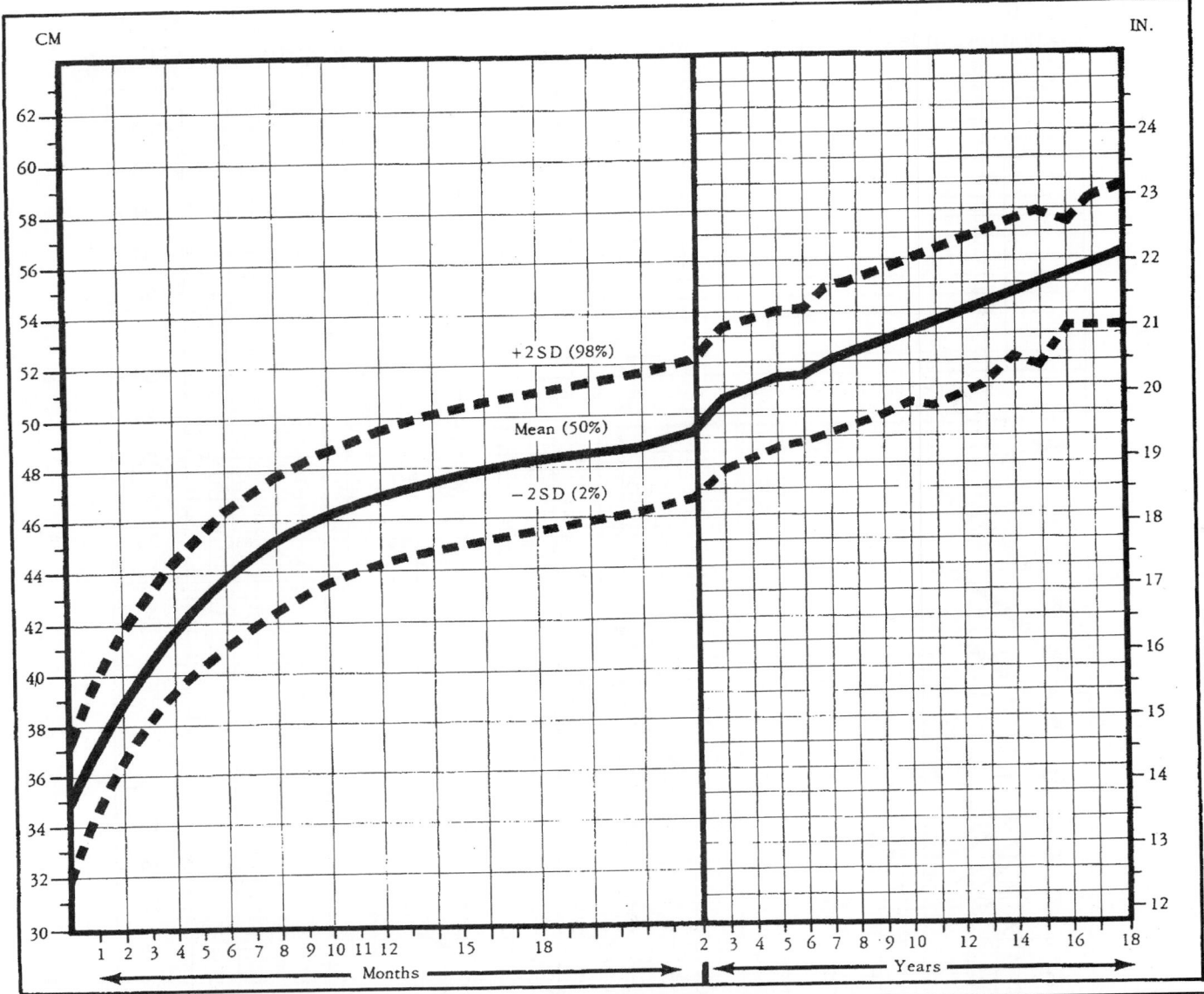

FIG. B-9 Birth to 18 years old: boys' head circumference percentiles. (From Nellhaus G: Head circumference from birth to eighteen years. Practical composite international and interracial graphs, *Pediatrics* 41:106–114, 1968.)

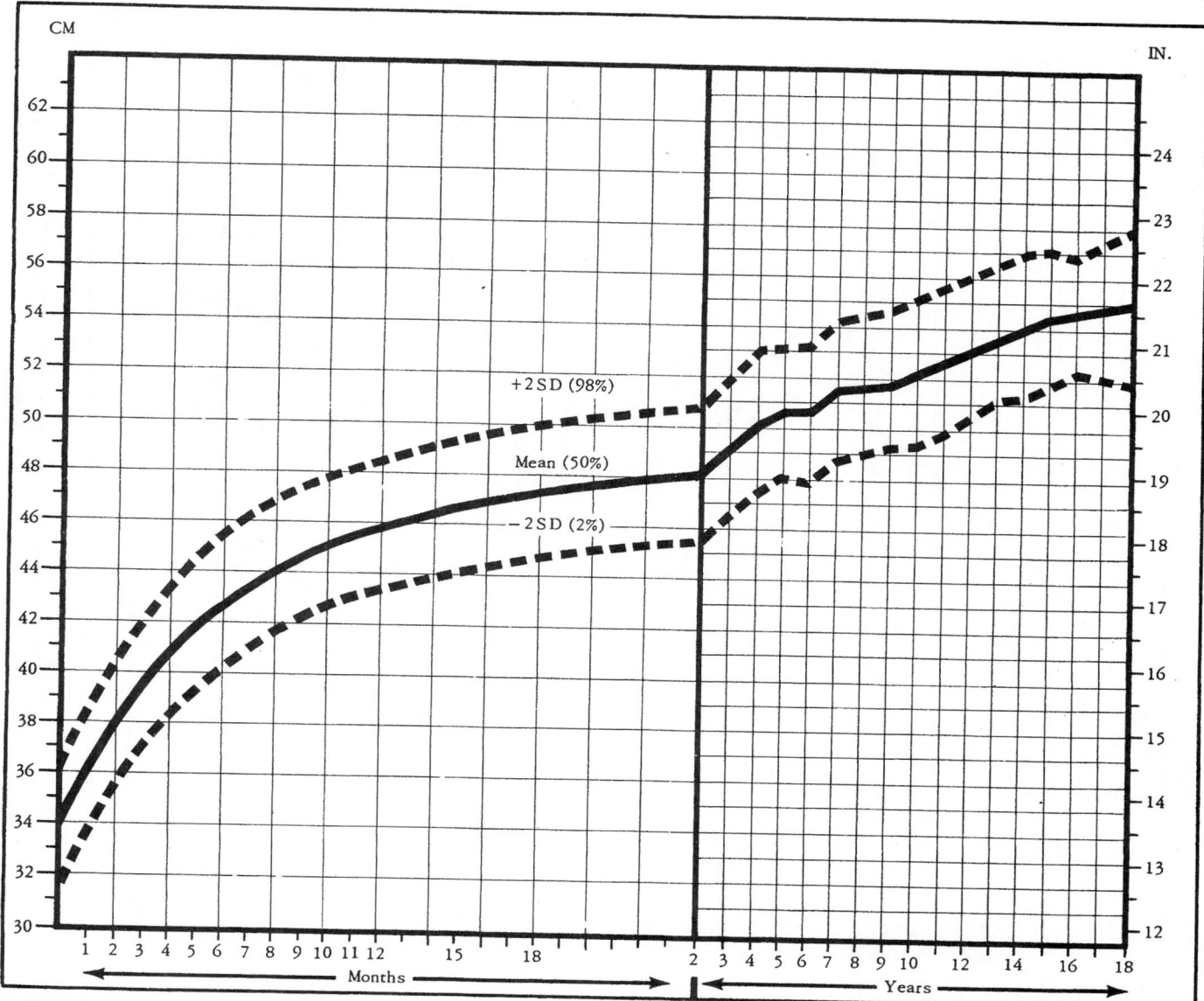

FIG. B-10 Birth to 18 years old: girls' head circumference percentiles. (From Nellhaus G: Head circumference from birth to eighteen years. Practical composite international and interracial graphs, *Pediatrics* 41:106–114, 1968.)

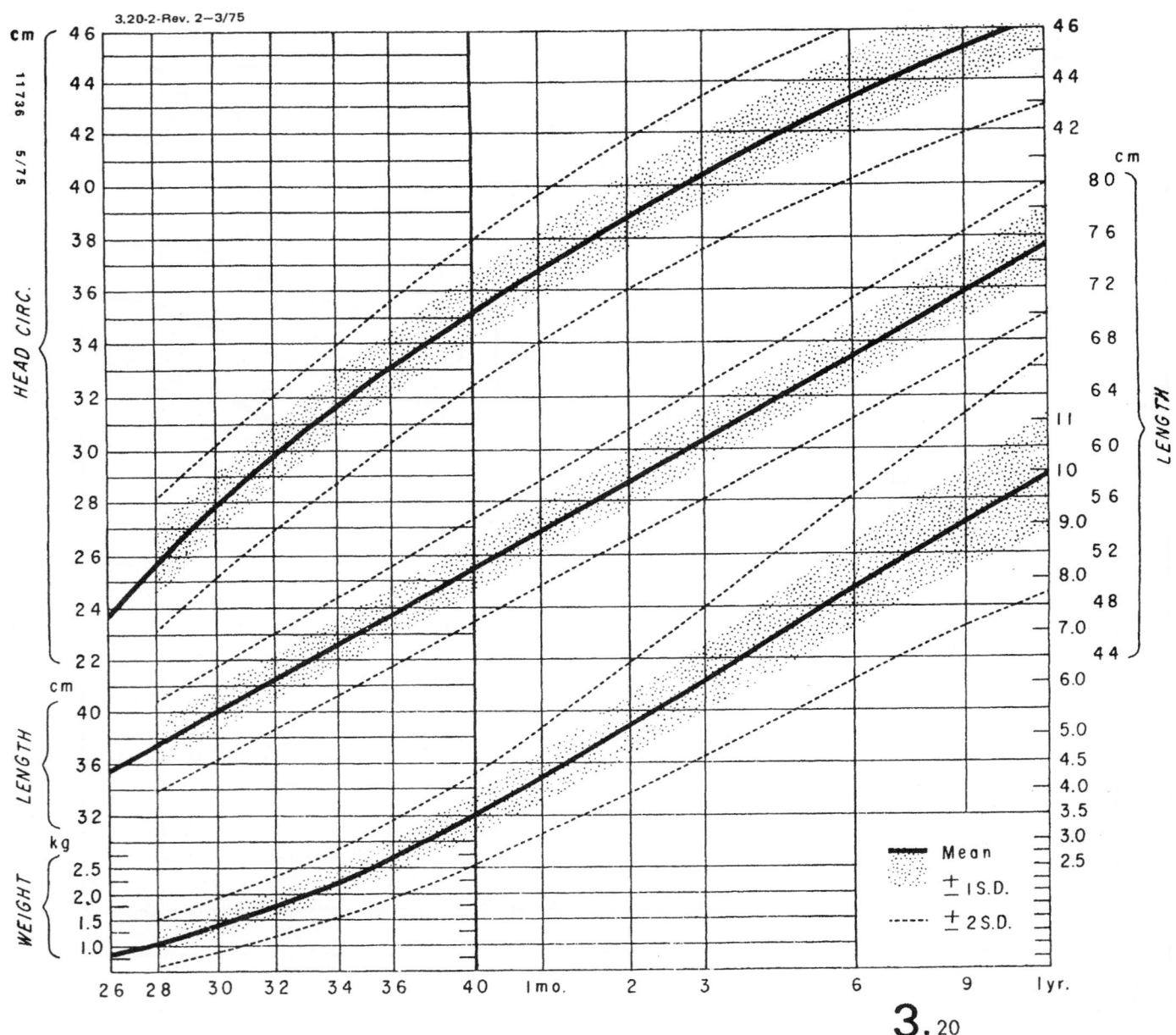

3.20-2-Rev. 2—3/75

FIG. B-11 Growth record for premature infants in relation to gestational age and fetal and infant norms. (From Fenton T: A new growth chart for preterm babies: Babson and Benda's chart updated with recent data and a new format, *BMC Pediatrics* 3:13, 2003. Available at *www.biomedcentral. com/1471-2431/3/13.*)

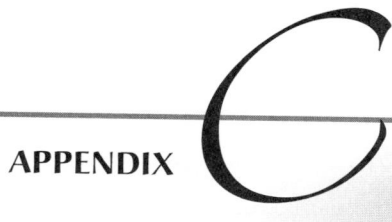

APPENDIX

Normal Laboratory Values

Catherine E. Burns and Steven Goodstein

A limited selection of blood chemistry, urine, and hematologic values is presented as the most common laboratory screening tests requested. The authors recognize that the primary care provider may have a need for more complex tests (e.g., cerebrospinal fluid studies, immunoglobulins, and therapeutic drug levels). The reader is directed to seek the source of these values from the performing laboratory and its respective standards in comparison with control specimens. Some pediatric specimens need to be sent to a special laboratory for appropriate testing.

Laboratories use a variety of analytic methods to determine biochemical and hematologic values. Normal values for laboratory tests vary depending on the procedure used. Normal ranges reflect a combination of the population served, individual biologic differences, specimen collection and handling techniques, and intrinsic laboratory variation. Given this variability, if any questions arise, it is recommended that the reader consult with the reference laboratory for its methods and the established normal range of values for the methods used.

Interpretation of laboratory values can be a complex diagnostic exercise. In Table C-1, the comments in the Interpretation column are intended to offer the reader general ideas about each test and its common use. A skilled clinician uses laboratory data with other clinical data to make decisions, sometimes combining several tests to best understand the physiologic status of the client.

The laboratory values for this appendix have been compiled from tables in Behrman and colleagues (2004), Burtis and Ashwood (1999), Fishbach (2000), and Free (1996).

TABLE C-1 Pediatric Laboratory Values

Test Name	Reference Range		Interpretation
Blood Chemistry (from Serum)			
Alanine aminotransferase (ALT, SGPT) (units/L)	Newborn/infant	13-45	Liver, heart, and skeletal muscle have significant levels. High levels are associated with hepatic cell damage.
	Adult		
	M	10-40	
	F	7-35	
Amylase (units/L)	Newborn	5-65	Marked rise generally indicates acute pancreatitis.
	Adult	27-131	
Aspartate aminotransferase (AST, SGOT) (units/L)	Newborn	25-75	Elevated levels occur with heart, liver, and muscle disease.
	Infant	15-60	
	Adult	8-20	
Bilirubin, total (mg/dL)	Premature		Elevated levels occur with increased destruction of RBCs or impairment of liver excretory function.
	Cord blood	<2	
	0-1 day	<8	
	1-2 days	<12	
	3-5 days	<16	
	Full term		
	Cord blood	<2	
	0-1 day	1.4-8.7	
	1-2 days	3.4-11.5	
	3-5 days	1.5-12	
	Adult	0.3-1.2	

Continued

TABLE C-1	Pediatric Laboratory Values—Cont'd

Test Name	Reference Range		Interpretation
Chloride (mmol/L)	Cord blood	96-104	Values increase in metabolic acidosis and other conditions. Decreased values occur with diuresis, GI losses, and other conditions.
	0-30 days	98-113	
	>30 days	98-107	
Cholesterol (5th-95th percentile, mg/dL)	Cord blood		Elevated levels indicate disorders of blood lipids.
	M	44-103	
	F	50-108	
	0-4 yr		
	M	114-203	
	F	112-200	
	5-9 yr		
	M	121-203	
	F	126-205	
	10-14 yr		
	M	119-202	
	F	124-201	
	15-19 yr		
	M	113-197	
	F	119-200	
	20-24 yr		
	M	124-218	
	F	122-216	
Creatinine (mg/dL)	Cord blood	0.6-1.2	Elevated levels indicate impaired renal function, muscle disease, congestive heart failure, shock, dehydration, and other conditions.
	Newborn	0.3-1	
	Infant	0.2-0.4	
	Child	0.3-0.7	
	Adolescent	0.5-1	
	Adult		
	M	0.7-1.3	
	F	0.6-1.1	
Ferritin (mg/mL)	Newborn	25-200	Ferritin is a more sensitive indicator than iron or TIBC for diagnosing iron deficiency or overload.
	1 mo	200-600	
	2-5 mo	50-200	
	6 mo-15 y	7-140	
	Adult		
	M	20-250	
	F	10-120	
Glucose (fasting) (mg/dL)	Cord blood	45-96	Fasting low levels may indicate a physiologic response or a disorder in glucose metabolism. Increased fasting levels may indicate diabetes mellitus, pancreatic disorders, endocrine diseases, drugs, and other conditions.
	Premature	20-60	
	Neonate	30-60	
	Newborn	40-60	
	1 day	50-80	
	>1 day	60-100	
	Child	74-106	
	Adult		
Iron (mcg/dL)	Newborn	100-250	Decreased levels occur with iron deficiency, blood loss, and other conditions. Elevated levels occur with hemolytic anemias, iron intoxication, hepatitis, and other conditions.
	Infant	40-100	
	Child	50-120	
	Thereafter		
	M	65-175	
	F	50-170	

TABLE C-1 **Pediatric Laboratory Values—Cont'd**

Test Name	Reference Range		Interpretation
Lead (whole blood specimen) (mcg/dL)	Child	<10	Increased levels indicate lead toxicity. Any level indicates some degree of toxicity.
	Adult	<25	
	Toxic	≥100	
Potassium (mmol/L)	Newborn	3.7-5.9	Decreased levels may indicate shifting of potassium into cells, GI loss, biliary loss, renal loss, and reduced uptake. Increased levels occur with shifts to intracellular fluid, decreased excretion, or increased uptake.
	Infant	4.1-5.3	
	Child	3.4-4.7	
	Thereafter	3.5-5.1	
Sodium (mmol/L)	Newborn	133-146	Decreased levels indicate sodium loss or water excess (caused by numerous conditions). Increased levels may occur with an increase in sodium or an excessive loss of water (caused by numerous conditions).
	Infant	139-146	
	Child	138-145	
	Thereafter	136-145	
Thyrotropin (thyroid-stimulating hormone [TSH]) (microunits/L)	Adult	0.4-4.2	Decreased levels are associated with hyperthyroidism. Increased levels are associated with hypothyroidism.
	Birth-4 days	1-39	
	2-20 wk	1.7-9.1	
	21 wk-20 yr	0.7-6.4	
Thyroxine, free (FT_4) (ng/dL)	Newborn	2.6-6.3	Decreased levels are associated with hypothyroidism or overproduction of T_3. Increased levels are associated with Graves disease and thyrotoxicosis from overproduction of T_4.
	Adult	0.8-2.7	
Thyroxine, total (T_4) (mcg/dL)	1-3 days	11.8-22.6	T_4 serves as a good index of thyroid function only if binding globulin (TBG) is normal.
	1-2 wk	9.8-16.6	
	1-4 mo	7.2-14.4	
	4-12 mo	7.8-16.5	
	1-5 yr	7.3-15	
	5-10 yr	6.4-13.3	
	10-15 yr	5.6-11.7	
	Adult	4.6-10.5	
	M	5.5-11	
	F		
Urea nitrogen (BUN) (mg/dL)	Premature (1 wk)	3-25	Measures glomerular function and production/excretion of urea. Decreased with liver failure, malnutrition, and other conditions. Increased with impaired renal function, congestive heart failure, salt/water depletion, shock, and other conditions.
	Newborn	4-12	
	Infant/child	5-18	
	Adult	6-20	

Hematology (Whole Blood Specimens)

Test Name	Reference Range		Interpretation
Erythrocyte count (RBC) (millions of cells/mm³ [microliters])	1-3 days (capillary)	4-6.6	Measures total number of RBCs. Decreased with anemia, cell destruction, and decreased production. Increased with increased RBC production, renal disease, tumors, altitude, pulmonary disease, cardiovascular diseases, and other conditions. A relative increase may occur with dehydration.
		3.9-6.3	
	1 wk	3.6-6.2	
	2 wk	3-5.4	
	1 mo	2.7-4.9	
	2 mo		
	3-6 mo	3.1-4.5	
	0.5-2 yr	3.7-5.3	
	2-6 yr	3.9-5.3	
	6-12 yr	4-5.2	
	12-18 yr		
	M	4.5-5.3	
	F	4.1-5.1	
	18-49 yr		
	M	4.5-5.9	
	F	4-5.2	

Continued

TABLE C-1 **Pediatric Laboratory Values—Cont'd**

Test Name	Reference Range		Interpretation
Erythrocyte sedimentation rate (ESR, sed rate) (mm/hr)			Not diagnostic, but indicates a disease process. Increases occur with collagen diseases, infections, inflammatory conditions, neoplasms, heavy metal poisoning, tissue destruction, and other conditions.
Westergren, modified	Child	0-10	
	Adult		
	M <50 yr	0-15	
	F <50 yr	0-20	
Wintrobe	Child	0-13	
	Adult		
	M	0-9	
	F	0-20	
Hematocrit (HCT, Hct) (% packed erythrocyte volume [erythrocyte volume/whole blood × 100])	1 day	48-69	Low values indicate blood loss or inadequate production or excess destruction of RBCs. High values indicate erythrocytosis, severe dehydration, shock, and other conditions.
	2 days	48-75	
	3 days	44-72	
	2 mo-6 yr	28-42	
	6-12 yr	35-45	
	12-18 yr		
	M	37-49	
	F	36-46	
	18-49 yr		
	M	41-53	
	F	36-46	
Hemoglobin, total (Hb) (g/dL)	1-3 days	14.5-22.5	Decreased levels are found with anemia, hyperthyroidism, cirrhosis, severe hemorrhage, hemolysis, and systemic diseases. Very low values may lead to heart failure and death.
	2 mo-6 yr	9-14	
	6-12 yr	11.5-15.5	
	12-18 yr		
	M	13-16	
	F	12-16	
	18-49 yr		
	M	13.5-17.5	
	F	12-16	
Leukocyte count (white blood cell [WBC] count) (× 1000 cells/mm^3)	Birth	9-30	Indicates total WBC count circulating in the blood. With some infections, WBCs increase as cells are transported. A low count may occur in overwhelming bacterial infection (sepsis) or with the use of immunosuppressive agents. Elevated levels may occur in response to an underlying disease, a primary cellular disorder (leukemia), pregnancy, corticosteroid treatment, strenuous exercise, and other conditions.
	24 hr	9.4-34	
	1 mo	5-19.5	
	1-3 yr	6-17.5	
	4-7 yr	5.5-15.5	
	8-13 yr	4.5-13.5	
	Adult	4.5-11	
Leukocyte differential (%)	Myelocytes	0-0	Describes the proportion of the types of WBCs. Used in conjunction with the total leukocyte count to determine absolute cell counts.
	Neutrophils ("bands")	3-5	
	Neutrophils ("segs")	54-62	Myelocytes: involved in the early maturation of neutrophils, eosinophils, basophils, and monocytes.
	Lymphocytes	25-33	Neutrophils: usually increased during bacterial infections. May be decreased in viral infections. Bands are immature; segmented are more mature forms.
	Monocytes	3-7	Lymphocytes: increased in viral infections. T, B, and natural killer types.
	Eosinophils	1-3	
	Basophils	0-0.75	Monocytes: increased in severe and recovery stages of infections (phagocytosis).
			Eosinophils: increased during allergic responses and parasitic infections.
			Basophils: increased in allergic reactions, hematologic disorders, and other conditions.

TABLE C-1 **Pediatric Laboratory Values—Cont'd**

Test Name	Reference Range		Interpretation
Platelet count (thrombocyte count)	Newborn 1 wk-adult	84-478 × 10³/mm³ 150-400 × 10³/mm³	Decreased platelet counts occur with anemias, some infections, congestive heart failure, bone marrow lesions, and other conditions. Increases occur with malignancies, splenectomy, collagen diseases, some anemias, and other conditions.
Reticulocyte count (%)	1 day 7 days 1-4 wk 5-6 wk 7-8 wk 9-10 wk 11-12 wk Adult	<0.4-6 <0.1-1.3 <0.1-1.2 <0.1-2.4 <0.1-2.9 <0.1-2.6 <0.1-1.3 <0.5-1.5	Provides an estimate of the rate of RBC production. The percentage may be used to calculate the absolute value. An elevated count with normal hemoglobin indicates RBC loss with bone marrow compensation. A normal reticulocyte count with a low hemoglobin level indicates an inadequate response to anemia. Reticulocyte turns to erythrocyte in 24 hr.
Urine			
Urine, macroscopic	All ages		
Bilirubin		Negative	Increased in hepatocellular disease or intrahepatic/extrahepatic biliary obstruction.
Blood, occult		Negative	RBCs increased in acute glomerulonephritis, acute infections, renal calculi, trauma, and other conditions.
Glucose, qualitative		Negative	Increased when blood glucose level exceeds the reabsorption capacity of the renal tubes (pathologic or benign).
Hemoglobin		Negative	Hemoglobinuria may occur in intravascular hemolysis and other conditions.
Ketones		Negative	Increased with adequate carbohydrate intake or a defect in carbohydrate metabolism. Especially significant with diabetes mellitus.
Leukocyte esterase		Negative	Measures WBCs. Increase indicates inflammation or infection (or both). Associated with certain renal diseases and diseases of the urinary tract or vaginitis.
Nitrite		Negative	Positive associated with urinary tract infection.
pH		4.6-8	Indication of acid-base balance.
Protein, qualitative		Negative	Increased in pathologic or physiologic conditions (e.g., fever, stress, strenuous exercises).
Specific gravity		1.001-1.030	Measures the concentrating and diluting ability of the kidney. Associated with tubular damage.
Urobilinogen		0.2-1 mg/dL	Increased in liver disease. Decreased in obstruction of bile ducts and other conditions.
Urine, microscopic			
Casts	Hyaline	0-1/lpf	Hyaline casts: increased in pathologic or physiologic conditions. Implies damage to the glomerular capillary membrane permitting leakage of proteins through the glomerular filtrate.
	Other	None	Other casts: involved in a variety of conditions depending on the type of cast. Involved in tubular epithelial damage (epithelial cell cast), renal infection (WBC cast), vascular disorder (RBC cast), renal disease (granular cast), chronic renal condition (waxy cast), severe renal disease (broad cast), and degenerative tubular disease (fatty cast).
Red blood cells (RBCs)		0-2/hpf	RBCs: denote bleeding into the urinary system.

Continued

TABLE C-1   Pediatric Laboratory Values—Cont'd

Test Name	Reference Range		Interpretation
White blood cells (WBCs)	M	0-3/hpf	WBCs: associated with an inflammatory process.
	F and children	0-5/hpf	
Urine volume (mL/24 hr)	Newborn	50-300	Decreased in dehydration, renal ischemia, renal disease,
	Infant	350-550	obstruction, and other conditions. Increased in diabetes
	Child	500-1000	insipidus, diabetes mellitus, chronic progressive renal failure,
	Adolescent	700-1400	and other conditions.
	Thereafter		
	M	800-1800	
	F	600-1600	

BUN, Blood urea nitrogen; *F,* female; *GI,* gastrointestinal; *hpf,* high-power field; *hr,* hours; *lpf,* low-power field; *M,* male; *mo,* month(s); *T₃,* triiodothyronine; *TBG,* thyroxin-binding globulin; *TIBC,* total iron-binding capacity; *wk,* week(s); *yr,* years.

TABLE C-2   Evaluation of Bleeding Disorders

Test	Mechanism	Normal Values*	Examples of Disorders
Prothrombin time	Extrinsic to common pathway	Neonate: 12-18 sec Postneonate: <12 sec	Defect in vitamin K–dependent factors, hemorrhagic disease of newborn, malabsorption; liver disease, DIC, oral anticoagulants
Activated partial thromboplastin time (APTT, PTT)	Intrinsic and common pathway	Neonate: 70 sec Postneonate: 25-40 sec	Hemophilia, von Willebrand, heparin, DIC, deficient factors
Thrombin time (TT)	Fibrinogen to fibrin	Neonate: 12-17 sec Postneonate: 10-15 sec	Fibrin split products, DIC, low fibrin level, heparin, uremia
Bleeding time (BT)	Hemostasis, capillary and platelet function	Postneonate: 3-7 min	Platelet dysfunctions, low platelet count, von Willebrand, aspirin
Platelet count (see Table C-1)	—	—	—
Peripheral blood smear	Number and shape of blood cells	—	Platelets: peripheral destruction disorder RBCs: suggest microangiopathic process (e.g., HUS, hemangioma, DIC) WBCs: number and differential suggest infections, leukemias, etc.

*Values will vary from laboratory to laboratory based on the technology used. The values here are typical, but should not be considered as absolute normal values. Use the norms recorded on laboratory slips as another guide to decide whether a given value is abnormal or normal. And, of course, use clinical judgment because most disorders are defined by a variety of signs, symptoms, and test values.

DIC, Disseminated intravascular coagulation; *HUS,* hemolytic-uremic syndrome; *min,* minutes; *RBCs,* red blood cells; *sec,* seconds; *WBCs,* white blood cells.

TABLE C-3   Red Blood Cell Indices (May Be Used to Differentiate Anemias)

Index	Definition	Calculation (Usually Done Electronically)
Mean corpuscular volume (MCV)	Average volume of RBC expressed as femtoliters (fL)	Hct (%) × 10/RBC count (×10^{12}/L)
Mean corpuscular hemoglobin (MCH)	Average weight of hemoglobin in an RBC expressed in picograms (pg)	Hb (g/dL) × 10/RBC count (×10^{12}/L)
Mean corpuscular hemoglobin concentration (MCHC)	Average concentration of hemoglobin in the RBC expressed as grams per deciliter (g/dL)	Hb (g/dL) × 100/Hct (%)
Red cell distribution width (RDW)	A measure of anisocytosis; the coefficient of variation of the RBC size determined on automated blood cell counting instruments expressed as a percent	Standard deviation of RBC size/mean corpuscular volume. Normal range: 11.5%-14.5%

NOTE: Normal values will vary depending on the technology used. Generally all of these values are calculated electronically.

Age	MCV (fL)	MCH (pg)	MCHC (g/dL)
0-1 day	95-125	30-42	30-34
2-4 days	98-118	30-42	30-34
5-7 days	100-120	30-42	30-34
8-14 days	95-115	30-42	30-34
15-30 days	93-113	28-40	30-34
1-2 months	83-107	27-37	31-36
3-5 months	83-107	25-35	32-36
6-11 months	78-102	23-31	32-36
1-3 years	76-92	23-31	32-36
4-7 years	78-94	23-31	32-36
8 years-adult	80-94	26-32	32036

Hb, Hemoglobin; *Hct*, hematocrit; *RBC*, red blood cell.
Data from Rodak B: *Hematology clinical principles and applications,* ed 2, Philadelphia, 2002, WB Saunders.

REFERENCES

Behrman R, Kliegman R, Jenson H, editors: *Nelson textbook of pediatrics,* ed 17, Philadelphia, 2004, WB Saunders.

Burtis C, Ashwood E: *Tietz textbook of clinical chemistry,* ed 3, Philadelphia, 1999, WB Saunders.

Fishbach F: *A manual of laboratory and diagnostic tests,* ed 6, Philadelphia, 2000, JB Lippincott.

Free HM, editor: *Modern urine chemistry,* Tarrytown, NY, 1996, Bayer.

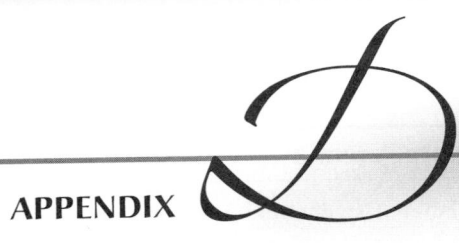
Supplementary Asthma Information: Expert Panel Guidelines for the Diagnosis and Management of Asthma*

Intermittent Asthma	**Persistent Asthma: Daily Medication** Consult with asthma specialist if step 3 care or higher is required. Consider consultation at step 2.

Step 6
Preferred:

High-dose ICS + either LABA or Montelukast

Oral systemic corticosteroids

Step 5
Preferred:

High-dose ICS + either LABA or Montelukast

Step 4
Preferred:

Medium-dose ICS + either LABA or Montelukast

Step 3
Preferred:

Medium-dose ICS

Step 2
Preferred:

Low-dose ICS

Alternative:

Cromolyn or Montelukast

Step 1
Preferred:

SABA PRN

Step up if needed

(first, check adherence, inhaler technique, and environmental control)

Assess control

Step down if possible

(and asthma is well controlled at least 3 months)

Patient Education and Environmental Control at Each Step

Quick-Relief Medication for All Patients

- SABA as needed for symptoms. Intensity of treatment depends on severity of symptoms.
- With viral respiratory infection: SABA q 4-6 hours up to 24 hours (longer with physician consult). Consider short course of oral systemic corticosteroids if exacerbation is severe or patient has history of previous severe exacerbations.
- Caution: Frequent use of SABA may indicate the need to step up treatment. See text for recommendations on initiating daily long-term-control therapy.

Key: **Alphabetical order is used when more than one treatment option is listed within either preferred or alternative therapy.** *ICS*, Inhaled corticosteroid; *LABA*, inhaled long-acting beta2-agonist; *q*, every; *SABA*, inhaled short-acting beta2-agonist.

Notes:
- The stepwise approach is meant to assist, not replace, the clinical decisionmaking required to meet individual patient needs.
- If alternative treatment is used and response is inadequate, discontinue it and use the preferred treatment before stepping up.
- If clear benefit is not observed within 4-6 weeks and patient/family medication technique and adherence are satisfactory, consider adjusting therapy or alternative diagnosis.
- Studies on children 0-4 years of age are limited. Step 2 preferred therapy is based on Evidence A. All other recommendations are based on expert opinion and extrapolation from studies in older children.

FIG. D-1 Stepwise Approach for Managing Asthma in Children 0-4 Years of Age.

*Figures contained in Appendix D are from National Heart, Lung, and Blood Institute, National Asthma Education and Prevention Program: *Expert Panel Report 3: Guidelines for the Diagnosis and Management of Asthma* (Full Report), 2007.

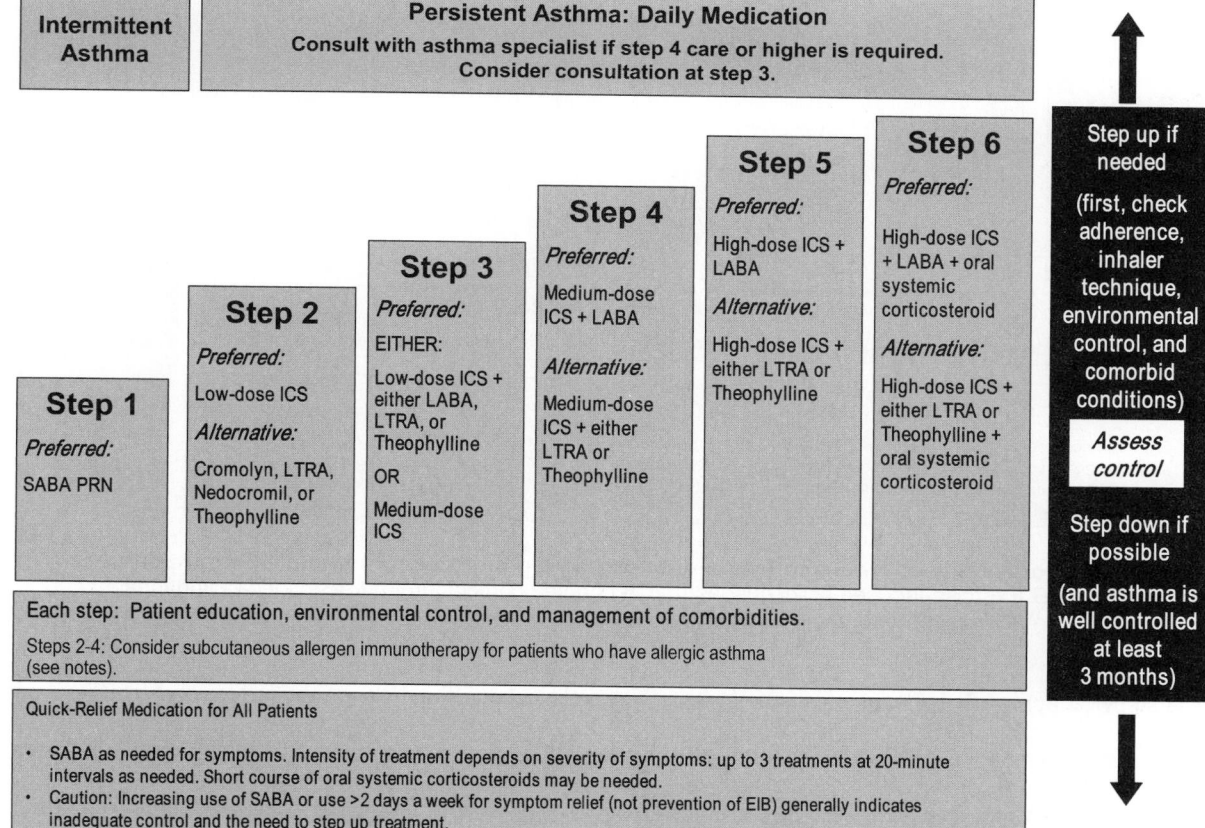

Intermittent Asthma

Persistent Asthma: Daily Medication
Consult with asthma specialist if step 4 care or higher is required.
Consider consultation at step 3.

Step 1
Preferred:
SABA PRN

Step 2
Preferred:
Low-dose ICS
Alternative:
Cromolyn, LTRA, Nedocromil, or Theophylline

Step 3
Preferred:
EITHER:
Low-dose ICS + either LABA, LTRA, or Theophylline
OR
Medium-dose ICS

Step 4
Preferred:
Medium-dose ICS + LABA
Alternative:
Medium-dose ICS + either LTRA or Theophylline

Step 5
Preferred:
High-dose ICS + LABA
Alternative:
High-dose ICS + either LTRA or Theophylline

Step 6
Preferred:
High-dose ICS + LABA + oral systemic corticosteroid
Alternative:
High-dose ICS + either LTRA or Theophylline + oral systemic corticosteroid

Step up if needed
(first, check adherence, inhaler technique, environmental control, and comorbid conditions)

Assess control

Step down if possible
(and asthma is well controlled at least 3 months)

Each step: Patient education, environmental control, and management of comorbidities.

Steps 2-4: Consider subcutaneous allergen immunotherapy for patients who have allergic asthma (see notes).

Quick-Relief Medication for All Patients

· SABA as needed for symptoms. Intensity of treatment depends on severity of symptoms: up to 3 treatments at 20-minute intervals as needed. Short course of oral systemic corticosteroids may be needed.
· Caution: Increasing use of SABA or use >2 days a week for symptom relief (not prevention of EIB) generally indicates inadequate control and the need to step up treatment.

Key: **Alphabetical order is used when more than one treatment option is listed within either preferred or alternative therapy.** *ICS*, Inhaled corticosteroid; *LABA*, inhaled long-acting beta$_2$-agonist, *LTRA*, leukotriene receptor antagonist; *SABA*, inhaled short-acting beta$_2$-agonist.

Notes:

■ The stepwise approach is meant to assist, not replace, the clinical decisionmaking required to meet individual patient needs.

■ If alternative treatment is used and response is inadequate, discontinue it and use the preferred treatment before stepping up.

■ Theophylline is a less desirable alternative due to the need to monitor serum concentration levels.

■ Step 1 and step 2 medications are based on Evidence A. Step 3 ICS + adjunctive therapy and ICS are based on Evidence B for efficacy of each treatment and extrapolation from comparator trials in older children and adults— comparator trials are not available for this age group; steps 4-6 are based on expert opinion and extrapolation from studies in older children and adults.

■ Immunotherapy for steps 2–4 is based on Evidence B for house-dust mites, animal danders, and pollens; evidence is weak or lacking for molds and cockroaches. Evidence is strongest for immunotherapy with single allergens. The role of allergy in asthma is greater in children than in adults. Clinicians who administer immunotherapy should be prepared and equipped to identify and treat anaphylaxis that may occur.

FIG. D-2   Stepwise Approach for Managing Asthma in Children 5–11 Years of Age.

					Step 6	Step up if needed

Intermittent Asthma

Persistent Asthma: Daily Medication
Consult with asthma specialist if step 4 care or higher is required.
Consider consultation at step 3.

Step 6
Preferred:
High-dose ICS + LABA + oral corticosteroid
AND
Consider Omalizumab for patients who have allergies

Step 5
Preferred:
High-dose ICS + LABA
AND
Consider Omalizumab for patients who have allergies

Step 4
Preferred:
Medium-dose ICS + LABA
Alternative:
Medium-dose ICS + either LTRA, Theophylline, or Zileuton

Step 3
Preferred:
Low-dose ICS + LABA
OR
Medium-dose ICS
Alternative:
Low-dose ICS + either LTRA, Theophylline, or Zileuton

Step 2
Preferred:
Low-dose ICS
Alternative:
Cromolyn, LTRA, Nedocromil, or Theophylline

Step 1
Preferred:
SABA PRN

Step up if needed
(first, check adherence, environmental control, and comorbid conditions)

Assess control

Step down if possible
(and asthma is well controlled at least 3 months)

Each step: Patient education, environmental control, and management of comorbidities.

Steps 2-4:   Consider subcutaneous allergen immunotherapy for patients who have allergic asthma (see notes).

Quick-Relief Medication for All Patients

- SABA as needed for symptoms. Intensity of treatment depends on severity of symptoms: up to 3 treatments at 20-minute intervals as needed. Short course of oral systemic corticosteroids may be needed.
- Use of SABA > 2 days a week for symptom relief (not prevention of EIB) generally indicates inadequate control and the need to step up treatment.

Key: **Alphabetical order is used when more than one treatment option is listed within either preferred or alternative therapy.** *EIB,* Exercise-induced bronchospasm; *ICS,* inhaled corticosteroid; *LABA,* long-acting inhaled beta$_2$-agonist; *LTRA,* leukotriene receptor antagonist; *PRN,* as needed; *SABA* inhaled short-acting beta$_2$-agonist.

Notes:

■ The stepwise approach is meant to assist, not replace, the clinical decisionmaking required to meet individual patient needs.

■ If alternative treatment is used and response is inadequate, discontinue it and use the preferred treatment before stepping up.

■ Zileuton is a less desirable alternative due to limited studies as adjunctive therapy and the need to monitor liver function. Theophylline requires monitoring of serum concentration levels.

■ In step 6, before oral systemic corticosteroids are introduced, a trial of high-dose ICS + LABA + either LTRA, theophylline, or zileuton may be considered, although this approach has not been studied in clinical trials.

■ Step 1, 2, and 3 preferred therapies are based on Evidence A; step 3 alternative therapy is based on Evidence A for LTRA, Evidence B for theophylline, and Evidence D for zileuton. Step 4 preferred therapy is based on Evidence B, and alternative therapy is based on Evidence B for LTRA and theophylline and Evidence D for zileuton. Step 5 preferred therapy is based on Evidence B. Step 6 preferred therapy is based on (EPR—2 1997) and Evidence B for omalizumab.

■ Immunotherapy for steps 2-4 is based on Evidence B for house-dust mites, animal danders, and pollens; evidence is weak or lacking for molds and cockroaches. Evidence is strongest for immunotherapy with single allergens. The role of allergy in asthma is greater in children than in adults.

■ Clinicians who administer immunotherapy or omalizumab should be prepared and equipped to identify and treat anaphylaxis that may occur.

FIG. D-3   Stepwise Approach for Managing Asthma in Youths ≥12 Years of Age and Adults.

Assessing severity and initiating therapy in children who are not currently taking long-term control medication

Components of Severity		Classification of Asthma Severity (0-4 years of age)			
		Intermittent	Persistent		
			Mild	Moderate	Severe
Impairment	Symptoms	≤ 2 days/week	> 2 days/week but not daily	Daily	Throughout the day
	Nighttime awakenings	0	1-2x/month	3-4x/month	> 1x/week
	Short-acting beta$_2$-agonist use for symptom control (not prevention of EIB)	≤ 2 days/week	> 2 days/week but not daily	Daily	Several times per day
	Interference with normal activity	None	Minor limitation	Some limitation	Extremely limited
Risk	Exacerbations requiring oral systemic corticosteroids	0-1/year	≥ 2 exacerbations in 6 months requiring oral systemic corticosteroids, or ≥ 4 wheezing episodes/1 year lasting > 1 day AND risk factors for persistent asthma		
		← Consider severity and interval since last exacerbation. Frequency and severity may fluctuate over time. →			
		Exacerbations of any severity may occur in patients in any severity category.			
Recommended Step for Initiating Therapy **(See Fig. D-1 [p. 1312] for treatment steps.)**		Step 1	Step 2	Step 3 and consider short course of oral systemic corticosteroids	
		In 2-6 weeks, depending on severity, evaluate level of asthma control that is achieved. If no clear benefit is observed in 4-6 weeks, consider adjusting therapy or alternative diagnoses.			

Key: *EIB*, Exercise-induced bronchospasm.

Notes

- The stepwise approach is meant to assist, not replace, the clinical decisionmaking required to meet individual patient needs.

- Level of severity is determined by both impairment and risk. Assess impairment domain by patient's/caregiver's recall of previous 2-4 weeks. Symptom assessment for longer periods should reflect a global assessment such as inquiring whether the patient's asthma is better or worse since the last visit. Assign severity to the most severe category in which any feature occurs.

- At present, there are inadequate data to correspond frequencies of exacerbations with different levels of asthma severity. For treatment purposes, patients who had ≥ 2 exacerbations requiring oral systemic corticosteroids in the past 6 months, or ≥ 4 wheezing episodes in the past year, and who have risk factors for persistent asthma may be considered the same as patients who have persistent asthma, even in the absence of impairment levels consistent with persistent asthma.

FIG. D-4   Classifying Asthma Severity and Initiating Treatment in Children 0–4 Years of Age.

Assessing severity and initiating therapy in children who are not currently taking long-term control medication

Components of Severity		Classification of Asthma Severity (5-11 years of age)			
				Persistent	
		Intermittent	Mild	Moderate	Severe
Impairment	Symptoms	≤ 2 days/week	> 2 days/week but not daily	Daily	Throughout the day
	Nighttime awakenings	≤ 2x/month	3-4x/month	> 1x/week but not nightly	Often 7x/week
	Short-acting beta₂-agonist use for symptom control (not prevention of EIB)	≤ 2 days/week	> 2 days/week but not daily	Daily	Several times per day
	Interference with normal activity	None	Minor limitation	Some limitation	Extremely limited
	Lung function	• Normal FEV_1 between exacerbations • FEV_1 > 80% predicted • FEV_1/FVC > 85%	• FEV_1 = > 80% predicted • FEV_1/FVC > 80%	• FEV_1 = 60-80% predicted • FEV_1/FVC = 75-80%	• FEV_1 < 60% predicted • FEV_1/FVC < 75%
Risk	Exacerbations requiring oral systemic corticosteroids	0–1/year (see note)	≥ 2/year (see note) ——————————————————→		
		Consider severity and interval since last exacerbation. ←————→ Frequency and severity may fluctuate over time for patients in any severity category.			
		Relative annual risk of exacerbations may be related to FEV_1.			
Recommended Step for Initiating Therapy (See Fig. D-2 [p. 1313] for treatment steps.)		Step 1	Step 2	Step 3, medium-dose ICS option	Step 3, medium-dose ICS option, or step 4 and consider short course of oral systemic corticosteroids
		In 2-6 weeks, evaluate level of asthma control that is achieved, and adjust therapy accordingly.			

Key: *EIB*, Exercise-induced bronchospasm; *FEV₁*, forced expiratory volume in 1 second; *FVC*, forced vital capacity; *ICS*, inhaled corticosteroids.

Notes

■ The stepwise approach is meant to assist, not replace, the clinical decisionmaking required to meet individual patient needs.

■ Level of severity is determined by both impairment and risk. Assess impairment domain by patient's/caregiver's recall of the previous 2-4 weeks and spirometry. Assign severity to the most severe category in which any feature occurs.

■ At present, there are inadequate data to correspond frequencies of exacerbations with different levels of asthma severity. In general, more frequent and intense exacerbations (e.g., requiring urgent, unscheduled care, hospitalization, or ICU admission) indicate greater underlying disease severity. For treatment purposes, patients who had ≥ 2 exacerbations requiring oral systemic corticosteroids in the past year may be considered the same as patients who have persistent asthma, even in the absence of impairment levels consistent with persistent asthma.

FIG. D-5   Classifying Asthma Severity and Initiating Treatment in Children 5-11 Years of Age.

Assessing severity and initiating treatment for patients who are not currently taking long-term control medications

Components of Severity		Classification of Asthma Severity ≥ 12 years of age			
			Persistent		
		Intermittent	Mild	Moderate	Severe
Impairment Normal FEV₁/FVC: 8-19 yr 85% 20-39 yr 80% 40-59 yr 75% 60-80 yr 70%	Symptoms	≤ 2 days/week	> 2 days/week but not daily	Daily	Throughout the day
	Nighttime awakenings	≤ 2x/month	3-4x/month	> 1x/week but not nightly	Often 7x/week
	Short-acting beta₂-agonist use for symptom control (not prevention of EIB)	≤ 2 days/week	> 2 days/week but not daily, and not more than 1x on any day	Daily	Several times per day
	Interference with normal activity	None	Minor limitation	Some limitation	Extremely limited
	Lung function	• Normal FEV₁ between exacerbations • FEV₁ > 80% predicted • FEV₁/FVC normal	• FEV₁ > 80% predicted • FEV₁/FVC normal	• FEV₁ > 60% but <80 % predicted • FEV₁/FVC reduced 5%	• FEV₁ < 60% predicted • FEV₁/FVC reduced > 5%
Risk	Exacerbations requiring oral systemic corticosteroids	0-1/year (see note)	≥ 2/year (see note) ⟵ Consider severity and interval since last exacerbation. ⟶ Frequency and severity may fluctuate over time for patients in any severity category. Relative annual risk of exacerbations may be related to FEV₁.		
Recommended Step for Initiating Treatment (See Fig. D-3 [p. 1314] for treatment steps.)		Step 1	Step 2	Step 3 and consider short course of oral systemic corticosteroids	Step 4 or 5
		In 2-6 weeks, evaluate level of asthma control that is achieved and adjust therapy accordingly.			

Key: *FEV₁*, Forced expiratory volume in 1 second; *FVC*, forced vital capacity; *ICU*, intensive care unit; *x*, times; *yr*, years.

Notes:

- The stepwise approach is meant to assist, not replace, the clinical decisionmaking required to meet individual patient needs.

- Level of severity is determined by assessment of both impairment and risk. Assess impairment domain by patient's/caregiver's recall of previous 2-4 weeks and spirometry. Assign severity to the most severe category in which any feature occurs.

- At present, there are inadequate data to correspond frequencies of exacerbations with different levels of asthma severity. In general, more frequent and intense exacerbations (e.g., requiring urgent, unscheduled care, hospitalization, or ICU admission) indicate greater underlying disease severity. For treatment purposes, patients who had ≥ 2 exacerbations requiring oral systemic corticosteroids in the past year may be considered the same as patients who have persistent asthma, even in the absence of impairment levels consistent with persistent asthma.

FIG. D-6   Classifying Asthma Severity and Initiating Treatment in youths ≥12 Years of Age and Adults.

Components of Control		Classification of Asthma Control (0-4 years of age)		
		Well Controlled	Not Well Controlled	Very Poorly Controlled
Impairment	Symptoms	≤ 2 days/week	> 2 days/week	Throughout the day
	Nighttime awakenings	≤ 1x/month	> 1x/month	> 1x/week
	Interference with normal activity	None	Some limitation	Extremely limited
	Short-acting beta₂-agonist use for symptom control (not prevention of EIB)	≤ 2 days/week	> 2 days/week	Several times per day
Risk	Exacerbations requiring oral systemic corticosteroids	0-1/year	2-3/year	> 3/year
	Treatment-related adverse effects	Medication side effects can vary in intensity from none to very troublesome and worrisome. The level of intensity does not correlate to specific levels of control but should be considered in the overall assessment of risk.		
Recommended Action for Treatment (See Fig. D-1 [p. 1312] for treatment steps.)		• Maintain current treatment. • Regular followup every 1-6 months. • Consider step down if well controlled for at least 3 months.	• Step up (1 step) and • Reevaluate in 2-6 weeks. • If no clear benefit in 4-6 weeks, consider alternative diagnoses or adjusting therapy. • For side effects, consider alternative treatment options.	• Consider short course of oral systemic corticosteroids, • Step up (1-2 steps), and • Reevaluate in 2 weeks. • If no clear benefit in 4-6 weeks, consider alternative diagnoses or adjusting therapy. • For side effects, consider alternative treatment options.

Key: *EIB*, Exercise-induced bronchospasm.

Notes:

■ The stepwise approach is meant to assist, not replace, the clinical decisionmaking required to meet individual patient needs.

■ The level of control is based on the most severe impairment or risk category. Assess impairment domain by caregiver's recall of previous 2-4 weeks. Symptom assessment for longer periods should reflect a global assessment such as inquiring whether the patient's asthma is better or worse since the last visit.

■ At present, there are inadequate data to correspond frequencies of exacerbations with different levels of asthma control. In general, more frequent and intense exacerbations (e.g., requiring urgent, unscheduled care, hospitalization, or ICU admission) indicate poorer disease control. For treatment purposes, patients who had ≥ 2 exacerbations requiring oral systemic corticosteroids in the past year may be considered the same as patients who have not-well-controlled asthma, even in the absence of impairment levels consistent with not-well-controlled asthma.

■ Before step up in therapy:

— Review adherence to medications, inhaler technique, and environmental control.

— If alternative treatment option was used in a step, discontinue it and use preferred treatment for that step.

FIG. D-7 Assessing Asthma Control and Adjusting Therapy in Children 0-4 Years of Age.

Components of Control		Classification of Asthma Control (5-11 years of age)		
		Well Controlled	Not Well Controlled	Very Poorly Controlled
Impairment	Symptoms	≤ 2 days/week but not more than once on each day	> 2 days/week or multiple times on ≤ 2 days/week	Throughout the day
	Nighttime awakenings	≤ 1x/month	≥ 2x/month	≥ 2x/week
	Interference with normal activity	None	Some limitation	Extremely limited
	Short-acting beta$_2$-agonist use for symptom control (not prevention of EIB)	≤ 2 days/week	> 2 days/week	Several times per day
	Lung function • FEV$_1$ or peak flow • FEV$_1$/FVC	> 80% predicted/ personal best > 80%	60-80% predicted/ personal best 75-80%	< 60% predicted/ personal best < 75%
Risk	Exacerbations requiring oral systemic corticosteroids	0-1/year	≥ 2/year (see note)	
		Consider severity and interval since last exacerbation		
	Reduction in lung growth	Evaluation requires long-term followup.		
	Treatment-related adverse effects	Medication side effects can vary in intensity from none to very troublesome and worrisome. The level of intensity does not correlate to specific levels of control but should be considered in the overall assessment of risk.		
Recommended Action for Treatment (See Fig. D-2 [p. 1313] for treatment steps.)		• Maintain current step. • Regular followup every 1-6 months. • Consider step down if well controlled for at least 3 months.	• Step up at least 1 step and • Reevaluate in 2-6 weeks. • For side effects: consider alternative treatment options.	• Consider short course of oral systemic corticosteroids, • Step up 1-2 steps, and • Reevaluate in 2 weeks. • For side effects, consider alternative treatment options.

Key: *EIB*, Exercise-induced bronchospasm; *FEV$_1$*, forced expiratory volume in 1 second; *FVC*, forced vital capacity.

Notes:

■ The stepwise approach is meant to assist, not replace, the clinical decisionmaking required to meet individual patient needs.

■ The level of control is based on the most severe impairment or risk category. Assess impairment domain by patient's/caregiver's recall of previous 2-4 weeks and by spirometry/or peak flow measures. Symptom assessment for longer periods should reflect a global assessment such as inquiring whether the patient's asthma is better or worse since the last visit.

■ At present, there are inadequate data to correspond frequencies of exacerbations with different levels of asthma control. In general, more frequent and intense exacerbations (e.g., requiring urgent, unscheduled care, hospitalization, or ICU admission) indicate poorer disease control. For treatment purposes, patients who had ≥ 2 exacerbations requiring oral systemic corticosteroids in the past year may be considered the same as patients who have persistent asthma, even in the absence of impairment levels consistent with persistent asthma.

■ Before step up in therapy:

— Review adherence to medications, inhaler technique, environmental control, and comorbid conditions.

— If alternative treatment option was used in a step, discontinue it and use preferred treatment for that step.

FIG. D-8   Assessing Asthma Control and Adjusting Therapy in Children 5-11 Years of Age.

Components of Control		Classification of Asthma Control (≥ 12 years of age)		
		Well Controlled	**Not Well Controlled**	**Very Poorly Controlled**
Impairment	Symptoms	≤ 2 days/week	> 2 days/week	Throughout the day
	Nighttime awakenings	≤ 2x/month	1-3x/week	≥ 4x/week
	Interference with normal activity	None	Some limitation	Extremely limited
	Short-acting beta$_2$-agonist use for symptom control (not prevention of EIB)	≤ 2 days/week	> 2 days/week	Several times per day
	FEV$_1$ or peak flow	> 80% predicted/personal best	60-80% predicted/personal best	< 60% predicted/personal best

	Validated questionnaires
	    ATAQ
	    ACQ
	    ACT
		0
		≤ 0.75*
		≥ 20
			1-2
			≥ 1.5
			16-19
				3-4
				N/A
				≤ 15

Risk	Exacerbations requiring oral systemic corticosteroids	0-1/year	≥ 2/year (see note)	
		Consider severity and interval since last exacerbation		
	Progressive loss of lung function	Evaluation requires long-term followup care		
	Treatment-related adverse effects	Medication side effects can vary in intensity from none to very troublesome and worrisome. The level of intensity does not correlate to specific levels of control but should be considered in the overall assessment of risk.		
Recommended Action for Treatment (See Fig. D-3 [p. 1314] for treatment steps.)		• Maintain current step. • Regular followups every 1-6 months to maintain control. • Consider step down if well controlled for at least 3 months.	• Step up 1 step and • Reevaluate in 2-6 weeks. • For side effects, consider alternative treatment options.	• Consider short course of oral systemic corticosteroids, • Step up 1-2 steps, and • Reevaluate in 2 weeks. • For side effects, consider alternative treatment options.

*ACQ values of 0.76-1.4 are indeterminate regarding well-controlled asthma.
Key: *EIB*, Exercise-induced bronchospasm; *ICU*, intensive care unit.

Notes:

■   The stepwise approach is meant to assist, not replace, the clinical decisionmaking required to meet individual patient needs.

■   The level of control is based on the most severe impairment or risk category. Assess impairment domain by patient's recall of previous 2-4 weeks and by spirometry/or peak flow measures. Symptom assessment for longer periods should reflect a global assessment, such as inquiring whether the patient's asthma is better or worse since the last visit.

■   At present, there are inadequate data to correspond frequencies of exacerbations with different levels of asthma control. In general, more frequent and intense exacerbations (e.g., requiring urgent, unscheduled care, hospitalization, or ICU admission) indicate poorer disease control. For treatment purposes, patients who had ≥ 2 exacerbations requiring oral systemic corticosteroids in the past year may be considered the same as patients who have not-well-controlled asthma, even in the absence of impairment levels consistent with not-well-controlled asthma.

■   Validated Questionnaires for the impairment domain (the questionnaires do not assess lung function or the risk domain)
    ATAQ = Asthma Therapy Assessment Questionnaire (See sample in "Component 1: Measures of Asthma Assessment and Monitoring.")
    ACQ = Asthma Control Questionnaire (user package may be obtained at www.qoltech.co.uk or juniper@qoltech.co.uk)
    ACT = Asthma Control Test (See sample in "Component 1: Measures of Asthma Assessment and Monitoring.")
    Minimal Important Difference: 1.0 for the ATAQ; 0.5 for the ACQ; not determined for the ACT.

■   Before step up in therapy:
    —   Review adherence to medication, inhaler technique, environmental control, and comorbid conditions.
    —   If an alternative treatment option was used in a step, discontinue and use the preferred treatment for that step.

FIG. D-9   Assessing Asthma Control and Adjusting Therapy in Youths ≥ 12 Years of Age and Adults.

Assess Severity

- **Patients at high risk for a fatal attack require immediate medical attention after initial treatment.**

- Symptoms and signs suggestive of a more serious exacerbation such as marked breathlessness, inability to speak more than short phrases, use of accessory muscles, or drowsiness should result in initial treatment while immediately consulting with a clinician.

- Less severe signs and symptoms can be treated initially with assessment of response to therapy and further steps as listed below.

- If available, measure PEF—values of 50-79% predicted or personal best indicate the need for quick-relief mediation. Depending on the response to treatment, contact with a clinician may also be indicated. Values below 50% indicate the need for immediate medical care.

Initial Treatment

- Inhaled SABA: up to two treatments 20 minutes apart of 2-6 puffs by metered-dose inhaler (MDI) or nebulizer treatments.

- Note: Medication delivery is highly variable. Children and individuals who have exacerbations of lesser severity may need fewer puffs than suggested above.

Good Response

No wheezing or dyspnea (assess tachypnea in young children).

PEF ≥ 80% predicted or personal best.

- Contact clinician for followup instructions and further management.

- May continue inhaled SABA every 3-4 hours for 24-48 hours.

- Consider short course of oral systemic corticosteroids.

Incomplete Response

Persistent wheezing and dyspnea (tachypnea).

PEF 50-79% predicted or personal best.

- Add oral systemic corticosteroid.

- Continue inhaled SABA.

- Contact clinician urgently (this day) for further instruction.

Poor Response

Marked wheezing and dyspnea.

PEF < 50% predicted or personal best.

- Add oral systemic corticosteroid.

- Repeat inhaled SABA immediately.

- If distress is severe and nonresponsive to initial treatment:
  —Call your doctor AND
  —**PROCEED TO ED;**
  —Consider calling 911 (ambulance transport).

- To ED.

Key: *ED*, Emergency department; *MDI*, metered-dose inhaler; *PEF*, peak expiratory flow; *SABA*, short-acting beta$_2$-agonist (quick-relief inhaler).

FIG. D-10   Management at Asthma Exacerbations: Home Treatment.

Index

A

Abandonment
  child's fear of, 368-369
Abbreviations
  prescription, 459
"ABCDEs"
  of skin examinations, 979b
Abdomen
  assessment of, 36, 205
  examining
    during physical exams, 116t
    in preparticipation physical exam (PPE), 285t
  of neonates, 1044t-1045t
  pain (See abdominal pain)
Abdominal migraine
  description of, 822-823
  signs and symptoms of, 810t
Abdominal pain
  acute
    characteristics of, 810t-814t, 815-818
    decision tree for, 817f
  alarm symptoms of, 820b
  complementary medicine treatments for, 1184t-1185t
  differential diagnoses for GI, 810t-814t
  functional, 819
  red flags concerning, 820b
  as symptom of Type 1 diabetes, 596
  types of, 815
Abrasions, 1081
Absorption, 1138
Abuse; See also alcohol abuse; child abuse; substance abuse
  as parenting red flag, 64b
  related to developmental characteristics
    from infants to adolescents, 182t-195t
  by siblings, 379, 380
Academics
  and attention-deficit/hyperactivity disorder (ADHD), 334, 335b
  and risky behavior
    in adolescents, 145, 146t-147t, 147-148
Acanthosis nigricans, 990-991
Acceptable macronutrient distribution range (AMDR), 192, 193t
Access
  to health care
    as *Healthy People 2010* indicator, 9b
    helping families gain health care, 177
    removing barriers to, 178
Accidents; See injuries; injury control
Acclimatization, 293-294, 1108
Accommodation
  definition of lens, 674-675
Achondroplasia, 1124b
Acid-base
  regulation by genitourinary system, 866
Acid-peptic disease
  medications for, 808t
Acids
  recommended daily allowance
    according to age, 193t
Acne
  complementary medicine treatments for, 1184t
  in puberty, 134
  vulgaris
    description and treatment of, 970-974
Acoustic reflectometry, 709
Acquired heart disease
  acute rheumatic fever (ARF), 760-762
  chest pain, 753-754
  hypertension, 754-756, 757t, 758

Acquired heart disease (*Continued*)
  infective endocarditis, 762-763
  Kawasaki disease, 758-760
  myocarditis, 763
  pericarditis, 763-764
Acquired melanocytic nevi, 989b
Action
  behavior of change, 156
Active immunity, 485-486
Active immunizations, 482
Active sleep, 305
Activities; See physical activities
Activity patterns
  in Gordon's functional health patterns, 158
Acupressure, 1168t
Acupuncture, 1168t
Acute abdominal pain
  characteristics of, 810t-814t, 815-818
  decision tree for, 817f
Acute asthma, 560, 563t-564t
Acute diarrhea, 833t-834t, 835-837
Acute diseases
  approaches to, 453-454
Acute hematogenous osteomyelitis
  limping due to, 1030t
Acute hemorrhagic conjunctivitis, 503
Acute illnesses
  description and treatment of, 453-454
Acute infections
  blood-borne viral pathogens, 290
  human immunodeficiency virus (HIV), 290
  infectious mononucleosis, 289
  skin infections, 289-290
Acute lymphonodular pharyngitis, 503
Acute otitis media
  antibacterial agents for, 718t
  description and epidemiology of, 716
  diagnosing and managing, 717-719, 718f
  medications to treat, 718t, 720t
  risk factors for, 721b
  types of, 716t
Acute pain
  abdominal, 815
  complementary medicine treatments for, 1206t-1208t
Acute purulent rhinitis, 775-776
Acute purulent rhinorrhea, 774t
Acute renal failure
  in newborns, 1058
Acute rheumatic fever (ARF)
  as autoimmune disease, 579-580
  symptoms and management of, 760-762
Acute spasmodic croup, 781
Acute upper respiratory infections
  and sports participation decisions, 276t
Acyanotic congenital heart disease
  symptoms and management of, 739, 742f
Adam's forward bend position, 1007, 1008f
Adam's test, 1007, 1008f
Adaptability; See also adaptive skills
  in healthy families, 366
Adaptive skills
  for ADHD children
    in classroom, 335b
  for cognitive-perceptual problems, 324-325
  definition of, 61t
  in divorce cases, 371b
  first-grade school readiness skills, 122t
Addiction; See also alcohol abuse; drug abuse; substance abuse
  to violence, 380
Adenoidectomy, 772-773
Adenoviruses, 835
Adherence
  factors influencing medication, 1230t
  treatment, 457t

Adolescence
  definition of, 132
  transition to adulthood, 138
Adolescent parents
  challenges of, 375-376
  defining and assessing, 34
Adolescent pregnancy
  challenges of, 375-376
  description and epidemiology of, 921
  goals for reducing, 906
  monitoring and evaluating, 376
  statistics, 3-4, 375
  testing and managing, 922
Adolescents
  appropriate exercise for, 273t
  assessment tools for, 36b
  with attention-deficit/hyperactivity disorder (ADHD), 327
  autism signs and symptoms in, 342
  bedtime routines for, 310-312
  bowel patterns in, 254
  cardiac assessment of, 732b
  cleft lip or palate, 217t
  cognitive-perceptual patterns, 321
  depression
    and brain chemistry, 138
    link to obesity, 7
  development of
    changes during, 135, 138-140
    mental health, 416
  developmental management of
    anticipatory guidance, 141-145
    assessment, 140-141
    common developmental issues, 145, 146t-147t
    physical development, 132-134, 135f-137f, 138-140, 141
    screening and assessment, 140-141
  elimination patterns in, 254
  environmental risk factors for, 1135t
  estimated energy requirements (EER)
    normal ranges, 192t
  exercise for, 273t
  goals for reducing HIV, STIs and teen pregnancy in, 906
  gynecological exam of, 908
  health supervision visits
    daily living and functional health patterns, 173t-176t
  homicides, 138
  immunization coverage, 4
  immunization schedules for, 488t
  inborn errors of metabolism (IEM) in, 603b
  injury prevention in, 184t-185t
  mental health development in, 416
  and nutrition, 203-204
  obesity, 7, 19
  overuse syndromes in, 1029, 1031, 1032t
  pneumonia forms in, 787t
  practical hints concerning violence, 383b
  pregnancy in, 203-204
  problem-oriented health records
    cognitive and perceptual problems, 23b
    development database, 23b-24b
    functional health elements, 22b
    self-concept and perception, 23b
    sexual and menstrual questions, 23b
  recommended eye exams of, 677t
  risk-taking behaviors among, 4
  and self-esteem, 349-350, 359-360
  sexual development of
    function, concept and roles, 398t
    and sex counseling, 404-406, 406t
    sexuality issues in, 395-408
  sexually transmitted diseases in, 933-937
  sleep patterns of, 307
  smoking among, 4, 157, 179-180

Page reference followed by *b* indicates box, *f* indicates figure, and *t* indicates table